Pathology Review
& Practice Guide

Pathology Review & Practice Guide

THIRD EDITION

Edited by Zu-hua Gao,
MD, PhD, FRCPC, FCAHS
with assistant editor
Thomas Shi,
MD, FRCPC, DABP

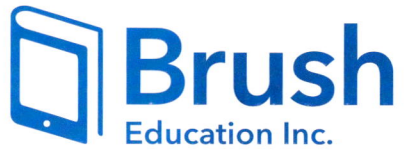

Brush
Education Inc.

Brush Education is located on Treaty 6 territory and is a beneficiary of this treaty. We gratefully acknowledge this land and the many peoples—including the Nêhiyawak, Anishninaabe, Niitsitapi, Saulteaux, Métis, Dene, Nakota Isga, Nakota Sioux, and Inuit—for whom this land continues to be a traditional home, meeting ground, gathering place, and travelling route.

Brush Education Inc.

www.brusheducation.ca

contact@brusheducation.ca

Cover design: Carol Dragich, Dragich Design

Interior design: Carol Dragich, Dragich Design

Index: François Trahan

Library and Archives Canada Cataloguing in Publication

Title: Pathology review and practice guide / edited by Zu-hua Gao, MD, PhD, FRCPC ; with assistant editor Thomas Shi, MD, FRCPC, DABP.
Other titles: Pathology review (Calgary, Alta.)
Names: Gao, Zu-hua, 1962- editor.
Description: Third edition. | Revision of: Pathology review. | Includes bibliographical references and index.
Identifiers: Canadiana (print) 20220468443 | Canadiana (ebook) 20220468478 | ISBN 9781550599169 (hardcover) | ISBN 9781550599183 (EPUB) | ISBN 9781550599176 (PDF)
Subjects: LCSH: Pathology—Examinations, questions, etc.
Classification: LCC RB31 .P38 2023 | DDC 616.07076—dc23

We acknowledge the support of the Government of Canada | Canadä
Nous reconnaissons l'appui du gouvernement du Canada

Acknowledgements

This third edition builds on the excellent work in the first and second editions by the following contributors:

Chapter 1:   Davide Salina, Adrian Box
Chapter 2:   Lisa M. DiFrancesco
Chapter 3:   Arjumand Husain, Travis Ogilvie, Hua Yang
Chapter 4:   Yinong Wang, John P. Veinot
Chapter 5:   Ivan Chebib, Manon Auger
Chapter 6:   Karen Naert, Duane Barber, Thai Yen Li, Sylvia Pasternak, Noreen M. Walsh
Chapter 7:   Moosa Khalil
Chapter 8:   Amy Bromley, Evan Matshes
Chapter 9:   Denise Ng, Vincent Falck, Zu-hua Gao
Chapter 10:   Jennifer Merrimen, Cheng Wang
Chapter 11:   Nicole Bures, Guangming Han, Lawrence Lee
Chapter 12:   Kenneth Berean, Martin Bullock
Chapter 13:   Iwona Auer-Grzesiak, Meer-Taher Shabani-Rad
Chapter 14:   Lik Hang Lee, Daniel Gregson, Yu Shi
Chapter 15:   Davinder Sidhu, Zu-hua Gao
Chapter 16:   Mircea Iftinca, Jeffrey T. Joseph
Chapter 17:   James R. Wright Jr, Weiming Yu, Alfredo Pinto-Rojas
Chapter 18:   Zhaolin Xu, Stefan J. Urbanski
Chapter 19:   Zu-hua Gao

My thanks to all,
Zu-hua Gao

Contents

Preface to the Third Edition

Pathology practice has been changing rapidly, and so is our training model and curriculum. Firstly, since the publication of the second edition, next-generation sequencing of common tumors has become routine practice in most pathology centers. Many tumors are now classified based on their molecular genetic profile and many new molecular markers have become available for targeted therapy. Secondly, whole slide imaging and digital pathology have been adopted across a range of contexts, from education and research, to limited clinical use in frozen section and consultation, to full application in routine sign out of surgical cases. The COVID-19 pandemic has further cascaded the implementation of digital pathology due to its convenience of remote sign out and communication. Completely supervised, partially supervised, and even unsupervised artificial intelligence technology has started to find its way into pathology diagnosis. Thirdly, the Royal College of Physicians and Surgeons of Canada has officially launched the "competency by design" training model, which requires much closer supervision and more frequent feedback to ensure our trainees can truly function as competent pathologists on graduation.

In this third edition, we have:

- Incorporated molecular profiling and new biomarkers of tumors into each chapter.

- Revised the basic science chapter with newly updated molecular information and some basic concepts of artificial intelligence.

- Added a "must know, must see, must do" section to each chapter, in line with the "competency by design" education requirement.

- Invited several national and international leaders to join us as chapter authors, which added significantly to those chapters.

In addition, we have created some resources available on the Brush Education website, including:

- 10 sets of mock exam questions, based on the Canadian exam format. These are meant to familiarize you with the format of the Canadian exam and function as self-evaluation tools. They are not intended to replace attentive study of this book.

- 10 specimen-grossing videos. Specimen handling and grossing is the first critical step for making accurate pathology diagnoses. Understanding the uniqueness of each specimen is key. These videos offer general guidance on appropriate handling and grossing common specimens in a standard manner.

Overall, the third edition is updated and more comprehensive, and offers better training tools that extend beyond the original purpose of exam preparation to cover the entire training of competent pathologists.

This work is a collaborative product of leading Canadian and American pathologists who are passionate about pathology education. I would like to thank all the authors of previous editions and the current edition for their commitment, dedication, and passion for transmitting their knowledge and experiences to our trainees. I would like to thank my wife, Jingjing Xing, for supporting me when I spent my weekends and evenings working on this project.

I hope you enjoy this new edition and I am eager to hear from you with any suggestions that might help to further improve this educational resource.

Zu-hua Gao, MD, PhD, FRCPC

DISCLAIMER

The publisher, authors, contributors, and editors bring substantial expertise to this reference and have made their best efforts to ensure that it is useful, accurate, safe, and reliable.

Nonetheless, practitioners must always rely on their own experience, knowledge and judgment when consulting any of the information contained in this reference or employing it in patient care. When using any of this information, they should remain conscious of their responsibility for their own safety and the safety of others, and for the best interests of those in their care.

To the fullest extent of the law, neither the publishers, the authors, the contributors nor the editors assume any liability for injury or damage to persons or property from any use of information or ideas contained in this reference.

Introduction

Knowledge is the foundation of excellent pathology practice and excellent outcomes on exams. This book helps build that foundation in a comprehensive yet concise format. It is a solid reference for practicing pathologists, and provides excellent preparation for the US and Canadian pathology exams.

The US and Canadian pathology exams differ in format: the US exam is entirely written and multiple choice; the Canadian exam has a written and an oral component, and the written component is entirely short answer.

For this reason, the exam strategies discussed below cover different formats, and the book itself includes multiple choice questions and short answer questions.

Getting Ready for the Exam

A structured study plan

In addition to reading cases, a structured study plan should include a thorough and systematic reading of *Robbins and Cotran Pathologic Basis of Disease* and of a surgical pathology textbook (either *Mills and Sternberg's Diagnostic Surgical Pathology* or *Rosai and Ackerman's Surgical Pathology*). Pay particular attention to definitions, fundamental terms, and concepts. Make lists and tables for comparison and grouping. Focus on subspecialty books during your rotation of that subspecialty. When it is closer to the time of the examination, go over old examination questions and collections of images to help you objectively assess your knowledge and your weaknesses.

Group study

If there are more than 3 people writing the examination, it can be helpful to get together regularly to go over old examination questions, slides, gross images, and so on. As a group, go over a chapter or a topic in *Robbins and Cotran Pathologic Basis of Disease* and brainstorm possible questions on the areas you think are important.

Literature review

Glance over the last 3 years of the *American Journal of Surgical Pathology*. This should be sufficient to keep you up to date on this field. *Advances in Anatomical Pathology* has some very good review articles that can help you quickly update your knowledge on specific topics. You also need to be aware of any new tumor classification systems in the most recent editions of World Health Organization publications.

Trust your program

In the 3 months before the examination, try to systematically gain exposure to all subspecialty experts in your department. Trust yourself and your program. If the resident training committee thinks you are doing well, and you did well on your department exams, you will do fine on the pathology exam.

Taking the exam

The basics

Before you begin taking the exam, make sure you have entered all required personal information. If you forget to enter your name and ID number, your results may not be scored. Do not bring personal electronic devices to the exam. Do not communicate with fellow examinees while the exam is in progress. Do not comment about the wording of questions in your answers.

Strategies for unknown lesions

First, try to categorize the lesion as neoplastic or nonneoplastic.

Nonneoplastic lesions can be classified as congenital, inflammatory, or infectious.

Neoplastic lesions can be classified as benign or malignant. Malignant neoplasms can be primary or secondary. Most neoplasms can be further classified into the following 3 subcategories based on cell lineage or origin: epithelial (carcinomas), stromal (sarcomas), and hematopoietic (lymphomas, leukemias).

Strategies for multiple choice questions (US)

- Anticipate the correct response while you read the question. If you see the response that you anticipated, note it and then check to be sure that none of the other responses is better. If you do not see the response that you expected, use the following strategies to eliminate responses that are probably wrong:

  · Responses that use absolute words, such as "always" or "never," are less likely to be correct than ones that use conditional words such as "usually" or "probably."

  · "Funny" responses are usually wrong.

  · If you can identify more than 1 correct response, "all of the above" is the correct answer. "None of the above" is usually an incorrect response, but be very careful not to be trapped by double negatives.

  · The longest response is often the correct one.

  · A response that repeats key words that are in the body of the question is likely to be correct.

  · If you have no idea of the correct answer, choose response *b* or *c*. Response *a* is least likely to be correct.

- If you cannot answer a question within a minute, skip it and come back to it later.

- Take the time to check your work before you complete the exam. Trust your instincts and try not to change your original answers.

Strategies for short answer questions (Canada)

- There are about 30 questions divided by groups and each question has multiple parts. You have 3 hours to answer them. Pace yourself appropriately.

- Glance through the questions and answer the easy ones first.

- Read the entire question before putting down your answer.

- Use bulleted lists and tables.

- Provide the number of answers that are asked for. If you provide 5 answers when 3 are asked for, only the first 3 will be marked.

- Write down the most important answer first. If a disease has multiple histologic features, write down the most common feature first.

- Do not leave any questions unanswered.

Strategies for examining slides and images

- Both the US and Canadian exams also include images of microscopic slides, gross specimens, forensic specimens, and other visuals.

- Provide 1 answer only to each question unless otherwise specified.

- If you cannot make a satisfactory diagnosis, provide the best answer you can, and move on. Do not leave any questions unanswered.

- Remember "common things are common" and the answer is most likely straightforward. You do not need to rack your brain looking for "rare birds."

- For the Canadian exam, do not write lists of differential diagnoses. Be as specific as you can.

Strategies for oral examinations (Canada)

- Be professional. Dress professionally and act professionally. Look at the examiners with a level of confidence. You have studied hard and prepared yourself well for this day. Accept that you will be a bit nervous, which is expected and appropriate.

- There are 5 to 6 cases to examine in 1 hour. Each case will have 1 or 2 slides with age, gender, and site information. The materials could come from surgical cases, autopsy, or cytology. After reviewing the cases, you will be examined by 2 examiners for 1 hour.

- Make notes while looking at the cases: summarize histologic features, differential diagnoses, and diagnosis; note answers to anticipated questions. Take the notes with you into the examination room. You can also make notes during the oral exam to organize your thoughts.

- The oral examination usually starts with "describe what you see and give a differential diagnosis," followed by "describe how you would work this case up." Do not jump to the diagnosis right away even if you are confident with your diagnosis. Do not be panic when you cannot get a definitive diagnosis. A structured approach with a differential diagnosis is usually what the examiners are looking for.

- Be patient. Wait for the full question to be asked before answering. Think and organize your thoughts before answering. It is fine to ask for clarification or for the question to be repeated if you do not completely understand the question.

- Be honest. When you do not know the answer, say, "I do not know," or "I will look it up," or "I will show it to someone else." Do not guess wildly. Do not ramble wildly. You will be interrupted if you ramble.

- Be independent. Do not expect feedback or comments on how you did during the exam. Do not be misled by inadvertent feedback, or the behavior or attitude of the examiners.

- Take hints from your examiners. If they ask you whether you have anything else on your differential or any other stains you would like to order, it means you are missing something. If they ask whether you are sure, it means you are probably wrong. Do not argue with or question the examiners.

After the exam

- You have done your best. Do not contact your examiner to see how you did.

- In the US, you receive your results through PATH*way* from the American Board of Pathology.

- In Canada, the exam board stratifies candidates into pass, borderline, and fail groups. For all borderline candidates, the exam board reads final in-training evaluations reports (FITER) and considers scores on all components to make the pass/fail decision. Exam results are usually available within 1 week.

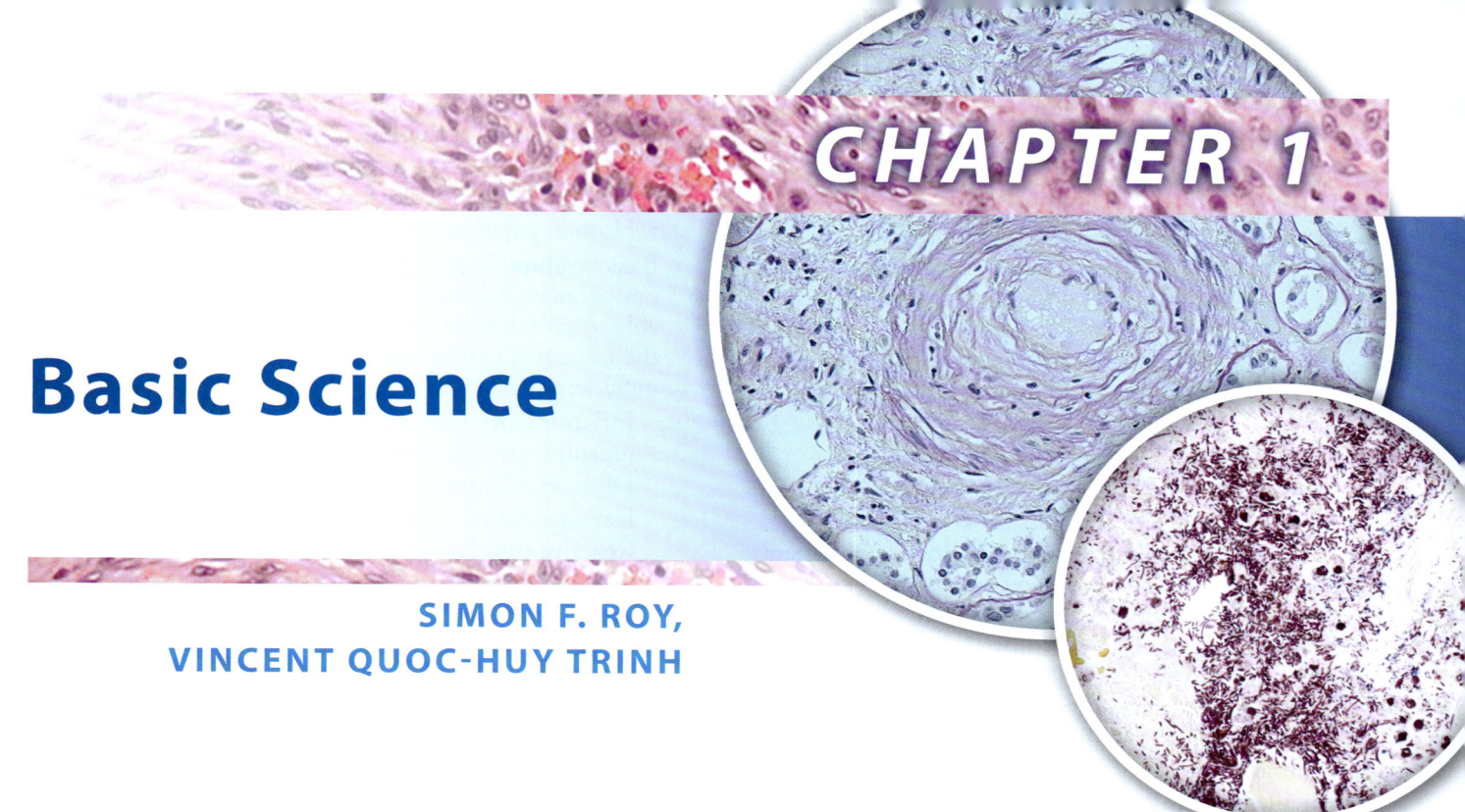

CHAPTER 1

Basic Science

SIMON F. ROY,
VINCENT QUOC-HUY TRINH

Basic Science Exam Essentials

MUST KNOW

Genetics and cell biology

- You should have a solid foundation in genetics and molecular biology, including familiarity with the following basic topics:
  - The organelles of a cell and their function.
  - DNA, RNA, and proteins.
  - The central dogma of molecular biology from transcription, translation, and posttranslational modification to epigenetic mechanisms.
  - Mechanisms of cell death.
  - Autosomal dominant versus recessive modes of transmission.
  - Anticipation, especially in neurodegenerative diseases such as Huntington disease.
  - Various types of DNA mutation, ranging from single nucleotide change to large chromosomal rearrangements.
  - Genomic imprinting and lyonization (also known as the Lyon hypothesis or Lyon law).
- You should be able to give at least 1 or 2 classic examples of large-scale chromosomal changes (e.g., trisomies and monosomies). For each inherited condition discussed in this book, note:
  - The name of the disease, and the gene and protein involved. For frequently encountered genetic diseases, memorize the specific pathogenic mutations or chromosomal changes (e.g., *CFTR* ΔF508 for cystic fibrosis, *HFE* C282Y for hemochromatosis).

  - Its clinical manifestations, including morphological changes, biochemical abnormalities, organ malformations, and predisposition to tumors. Pay special attention to associated malignancies.
  - Any characteristic pathologic finding, the organ it involves, and whether it is benign or malignant (e.g., characteristic polyps in Peutz-Jeghers syndrome).
  - Variants of the syndrome, such as attenuated familial adenomatous polyposis (FAP).

Molecular biology

- You should be able to explain the basic molecular pathway, and how alterations in the pathway, or the gene or protein, lead to diseases. Memorize at least 1 or 2 classic lesions related to the gene or protein. Key topics include:
  - Tumor suppressors, protooncogenes, and oncogenes.
  - The cell cycle and key regulators of the cell cycle.
  - The extrinsic and intrinsic pathways of apoptosis and key regulators.
  - Receptor tyrosine kinases.
  - *JAK-STAT*.
  - PI3K-Akt.
  - G-protein-coupled receptor.
  - Ras-Raf-MEK pathway.

- Dishevelled *APC* β-catenin.
- *p53* and *PTEN*.
- *p16*, *CDK*, *Rb*.
- PD-1 and PD-L1 inhibition.
- Common vitamin deficiencies (vitamins B_1, B_{12}, C, D).

- You should understand each technique of gene sequencing, its advantages and limitations, and common scenarios for its use. Focus on techniques in clinical use more than on experimental techniques. Key topics include:
  - Studies of large-scale chromosomal changes including karyotyping, chromosomal analysis, and fluorescence in situ hybridization (FISH).
  - Studies with higher resolution including polymerase chain reaction (PCR), Sanger sequencing, next-generation sequencing, and CRISPR.
  - Studies to assess RNA or protein expression, such as immunohistochemistry (IHC), in situ hybridization, immunofluorescence, comparative genomic hybridization, tissue microarray, and DNA or RNA microarray.
  - Ancillary techniques including flow cytometry and electron microscopy.
  - Histochemical stains.
- Where applicable, note any special tissue handling requirement or fixative required for special techniques, including:
  - Fresh, frozen, or formalin-fixed tissue.
  - Particular tissue media or fixative requirements.
  - Artifacts and false results.

Histopathology

You should be able to state the pathophysiology, its gross appearance, and its microscopic findings, and give at least 1 or 2 classic examples. For microscopic findings, state the differential diagnosis and any additional stain or ancillary workup. Key topics include:

- Apoptosis versus necrosis.
- Classification of necrosis.
- Types of wound healing and clinical features.
- Angiogenesis in both normal and pathologic conditions.
- Virchow triad, types of emboli, and fates of thrombi.
- Amyloidosis: systemic and local.
- Types of calcification.
- Hyperplasia, hypertrophy, and atrophy.
- Inflammation: signs, types, and cells involved.

Microbiology and immunology

- You should be able to briefly articulate the pathogenesis of infectious diseases caused by different types of pathogens. (See chapter 14, Pathology of Infectious Disease, for details on histopathology.) Key topics include:
  - Oncogenic viruses and bacteria.
  - Common bacteria, fungal, and parasitic organisms. Pay attention to those pertaining to the sinonasal area, lungs, and gastrointestinal (GI) tract.
  - HIV and associated diseases.
  - Human papilloma virus and associated diseases.
- Basic immunology is important for many topics in nonneoplastic diseases. For each topic, you should be able to give at least 1 or 2 classic examples, and state the basic mechanisms of pathogenesis. Key topics include:
  - Inflammatory cells, their function, progenitors, and morphological features.
  - Diseases of immunodeficiency.
  - Key mediators of the inflammatory response.
  - Reactive oxygen species.
  - Types of ANCAs with their associated diseases.
  - The role of the immune system in autoimmune diseases and vasculitides.

Miscellaneous

- You should know common statistical and methodological parameters related to medicine, including:
  - Sensitivity and specificity.
  - Positive predictive value and negative predictive value.
  - Measures of central tendency and error.
  - Positive and negative controls.
  - False positives and false negatives.
  - Factors that affect the internal and external validity of a study.

MUST SEE

- You should seek out clinical images of the following entities and be familiar with the key gross findings:
  - Trisomy 13, 18, and 21.
  - Turner and Klinefelter syndromes.

MUST DO

Create a plan for studying.

- Find study partners.
- Make sure everyone has their own copy of this book so each person can write notes and mark pages of interest. Consider buying additional review books (e.g., *Gross Pathology of Common Diseases*).
- Make a study schedule and stick to the schedule.
- Ask for tips from past residents, departmental staff, and fellows.
- Make a list of high-yield topics in each chapter of this book to study in depth.
- Make a list of knowledge deficiencies, emerging topics, and new guidelines to review.
- Review College of American Pathologists protocols, especially the explanations at the end and special notes throughout the synoptic checklist.

- For inherited conditions and syndromes, make a chart that summarizes the key information (similar to the checklist at the end of this chapter). For ideas on headings, see the Must Know at the beginning of this chapter.
- Gather and share study resources such as notes, books, slide collections, repositories of digital slides, and helpful websites.
- Gather any previous intradepartmental exams and practice questions from previous residents or fellows.

- Consider subscribing to online question banks (note, however, that these question banks target the American qualifying exams only).
- Consider holding informal teaching sessions with junior residents: teaching others a topic is often the best way to learn that topic yourself.
- Revisit topics with your study partners and quiz each other to reinforce key concepts.

MULTIPLE CHOICE QUESTIONS

1. Which of the following syndromes does **not** have an autosomal dominant inheritance pattern?
   a. Huntington disease.
   b. Marfan syndrome.
   c. Familial hypercholesterolemia.
   d. Ehlers-Danlos syndrome.
   e. Achondroplasia.

Answer: d

2. Disseminated intravascular coagulation (DIC) depletes all factors **except**:
   a. Platelet.
   b. Fibrinogen.
   c. Fibrin split products.
   d. Antithrombin 3.
   e. Factor 8.

Answer: c

3. Which inheritable genetic condition exhibits anticipation?
   a. Huntington disease.
   b. Down syndrome.
   c. Gaucher disease.
   d. Klinefelter syndrome.

Answer: a

Anticipation is the phenomenon of earlier and more severe disease onset associated with inheritable trinucleotide repeat diseases, such as Huntington disease.

4. *JAK2* mutations are associated with which condition?
   a. Polycythemia vera.
   b. Crohn disease.
   c. Ulcerative colitis.
   d. Burkitt lymphoma.

Answer: a

Up to 95% of all cases of polycythemia vera are associated with *JAK2* mutations.

5. Which protein is **anti**apoptotic?
   a. *BAX*.
   b. *BAK*.
   c. Caspase 3.
   d. *BCL2*.

Answer: d

BCL2 is antiapoptotic and is upregulated in malignancies as compared to nonmalignant conditions (i.e., follicular lymphoma versus reactive lymph nodes).

6. Pediatric cardiac rhabdomyomas are associated with which condition?
   a. Prader-Willi syndrome.
   b. Tuberous sclerosis.
   c. Niemann-Pick disease.
   d. Down syndrome.

Answer: b

Cardiac rhabdomyomas are detected in > 50% of neonates with tuberous sclerosis.

7. Which is **not** a feature of apoptosis?
   a. Nuclear shrinkage.
   b. DNA laddering.
   c. Associated inflammation.
   d. Membrane blebbing.

Answer: c

Necrosis generally induces a surrounding inflammatory response, unlike apoptosis.

8. Which cellular process is associated with cytochrome c release from the mitochondria?
   a. Intrinsic pathway apoptosis.
   b. Necrosis.
   c. Extrinsic pathway apoptosis.
   d. Autophagy.

Answer: a

The intrinsic pathway of apoptosis is associated with mitochondrial release of cytochrome c into the cytoplasm of the cell.

9. Which disease is associated with HLA-DR3?
   a. Diabetes.
   b. Celiac disease.
   c. Ankylosing spondylitis.
   d. Crohn disease.

Answer: a

10. What is **not** a function of normal p53?
   a. Apoptosis.
   b. Glucose metabolism.
   c. Cell cycle arrest.
   d. Response to DNA damage.

Answer: b

Normal p53 plays a central role in inducing cell cycle arrest and apoptosis due to various stimuli. It also upregulates genes involved in DNA damage from radiation. It has no direct effect on glucose metabolism.

11. Which of the following proteins is a protooncogene?
   a. p53.
   b. p16.
   c. Retinoblastoma.
   d. K-ras.

Answer: d

K-ras is the only protooncogene among the provided list. The other proteins are tumor suppressors.

12. What condition is **not** associated with abnormal genomic imprinting?

a. Down syndrome.
b. Angelman syndrome.
c. Prader-Willi syndrome.
d. Beckwith-Wiede-mann syndrome.

Answer: a

Most cases of Prader-Willi syndrome are associated with 15q11–13 deletion in the paternally derived chromosome. Most cases of Angelman syndrome are associated with a 15q11–13 deletion in the maternally derived chromosome. A subset of Beckwith-Widemann syndrome cases are caused by genomic imprinting abnormalities of 11p15.5.

13. What is the most common type of epidermal growth factor receptor (*EGFR*) gene mutation that occurs in lung adenocarcinoma?

a. Point mutation.
b. Inversion.
c. Deletion.
d. Insertion.

Answer: c

Deletion of *EGFR* exon 19 is the most common mutation occurring in lung adenocarcinoma. Point mutation of L858 is the next most common alteration.

14. Which *EGFR* mutation does **not** confer sensitivity to tyrosine kinase inhibitors?

a. Exon 19 deletion.
b. L858R mutation.
c. T790M mutation.
d. Exon 19 insertion.

Answer: c

Threonine 790 to methionine (T790M) mutation confers resistance to most standard tyrosine kinase inhibitors in adenocarcinomas of the lung. All other mutations listed are sensitive to these therapeutic agents.

15. What is the most common type of mutation that occurs in melanoma?

a. Point mutation.
b. Inversion.
c. Deletion.
d. Insertion.

Answer: a

BRAF point mutations, resulting in the V600E transition, are the most common mutation in melanoma.

16. Calreticulin mutations are associated with which disease?

a. Chronic eosinophilic leukemia (CEL).
b. Primary myelo-fibrosis (PMF).
c. Chronic myelogenous leukemia (CML).
d. Polycythemia rubra vera (PV).

Answer: d

Calreticulin mutations are a newly discovered etiology of primary myelofibrosis. They occur independently of *JAK2* and account for approximately 50–60% of *JAK2* negative cases of PMF.

17. What type of mutation is seen in calreticulin in PMF?

a. Point mutation.
b. Inversion.
c. Deletion.
d. All of the above.

Answer: c

Out of frame deletions of calreticulin exon 9, specifically a 52bp deletion, are the most common mutation seen in PMF. A 5bp insertion can also be seen. These mutations have also been identified in most cases of *JAK2* negative essential thrombocytosis.

SHORT ANSWER QUESTIONS

The Cell

18. Name 3 cell-cell interactions.

- Occluding junctions (tight junctions), which are composed of transmembrane proteins such as claudin and tight junction–associated MARVEL protein.
- Anchoring junctions (adherens junctions and desmosomes), which attach cells to cells of the extracellular matrix.
- Communication junctions (gap junctions), which are formed of connexons (pores) and connexin proteins. Pores allow passage of small molecules.

19. What is the definition of a stem cell? What are the main types?

- Cells that can both self-renew and become differentiated cells.
- Totipotent stems cells are found mostly in embryogenesis and can become any kind of differentiated tissue.
- Adult stem cells can become differentiated cells, but only of the tissue type in which they reside.

20. Name 2 types of cell divisions by which stem cells self-renew their populations.

- Asymmetric division: 1 daughter cell becomes differentiated, while the other keeps self-renewing without differentiation.
- Symmetric division: both daughter cells keep self-renewing (mostly in embryogenesis, for expansion of stem cell populations or after chemotherapy affecting the bone marrow).

21. Briefly explain the main roles associated with each of the following organelles.

ORGANELLE	MAIN ROLES
Cytosol	• Metabolism. • Transport. • Protein translation.
Mitochondria	• Energy output. • Apoptosis.
Rough endoplasmic reticulum Smooth endoplasmic reticulum and Golgi apparatus	• Synthesis of membranous and secreted proteins. • Protein modifications. • Triage. • Catabolism.
Nucleus	• Cellular regulation. • Proliferation. • DNA transcription.
Endosome	• Intracellular and export transportation. • Absorption of extracellular substances.
Lysosome	• Cellular catabolism.
Peroxisome	• Fatty acid metabolism (very long chains).

22. Name the main 5 classes of functional noncoding genetic elements.

- Promoter and enhancer regions.
- Binding sites for functions which organize and maintain higher order chromatin structures.
- Noncoding regulatory RNAs.
- Mobile genetic elements.
- Telomeres and centromeres.

23. Name 2 types of noncoding regulatory RNA and their roles.

- Micro-RNA (miRNA) and long noncoding RNA (lncRNA) (longer than 200 base pairs).
  - miRNA modulates mRNA translation. These short sequences are transcribed in the nucleus, processed by the Dicer protein, and cause translation repression or mRNA cleavage by linking with the RNA-induced silencing complex (RISC).
  - lncRNA modulates gene expression. These longer sequences have a role in gene activation, gene suppression, promoting chromatin modification, and assembly of protein complexes.

24. Name 3 roles associated with growth factors after they bind to a receptor.

- Promotes entry into the cell cycle.
- Relieves blocks on cell cycle progression.
- Prevents apoptosis.
- Enhances synthesis of components required for cell division.

25. Name 5 growth factors and 1 function for each.

GROWTH FACTOR	FUNCTIONS
Epidermal growth factor (EGF)	• Mitogenic. • Stimulates migration. • Promotes formation of granulation tissue.
Transforming growth factor-α (TGF-α)	• Stimulates proliferation of hepatocytes and other cell types.
Hepatocyte growth factor (HGF)	• Enhances proliferation of hepatocytes and other epithelial cells. • Increases cell motility.
Vascular endothelial growth factor (VEGF)	• Stimulates proliferation of endothelial cells. • Increases vascular permeability.
Platelet-derived growth factor (PDGF)	• Chemotactic for neutrophils, macrophages, fibroblasts and smooth muscle. • Activates and stimulates proliferation of fibroblasts, endothelial cells, and other cells. • Stimulates ECM protein synthesis.
Fibroblastic growth factors (FGFs)	• Chemotactic and mitogenic for fibroblasts. • Angiogenesis. • ECM protein synthesis.
Transforming growth factor-β (TGF-β)	• Chemotactic for leukocytes and fibroblasts. • Stimulates ECM protein synthesis. • Suppresses acute inflammation.
Keratinocyte growth factor (KGF)	• Stimulates keratinocyte migration, proliferation, and differentiation.

26. Name the 4 functions of the extracellular matrix (ECM).
- Provides mechanical support for cell anchorage.
- Regulates cell proliferation.
- Provides scaffolding for tissue removal.
- Provides the foundation for establishing tissue microenvironments.

27. Name the 2 forms of extracellular matrix.
- Interstitial matrix.
- Basement membrane.

28. Name 3 components of extracellular matrix.
- Fibrous structural proteins (collagen or elastin).
- Water-hydrated gels (proteoglycans or hyaluronan).
- Adhesive glycoproteins (integrins, fibronectin, or laminin).

29. How is heterochromatin organized?
It is dense and inactive.

30. How is euchromatin organized?
It is dispersed and active.

31. What are the roles of the cytoskeleton?
- Maintains structure.
- Maintains polarity.
- Organizes and moves organelles.

32. What are the 3 main classes of cytoskeletal proteins?
- Actin microfilaments.
- Intermediate filaments.
- Microtubules.

33. Why do most mitochondria come from the maternal side?
The fertilized oocyte contains the vast majority of organelles and thus mitochondria.

34. What is the composition of a plasma cell membrane?
- It is a fluid bilayer of amphipathic phospholipids.
  - Hydrophilic head groups face the aqueous environment;
- Hydrophilic lipid tails interact with each other to form a barrier to passive diffusion or charged molecules.

35. What are 3 important functions of proteins and glycoproteins in the plasma membrane?
- Ion and metabolite transport.
- Fluid-phase and receptor-mediated uptake of macromolecules.
- Cell-ligand, cell-matrix, and cell-cell interaction.

36. What are the classes of signals that most cells respond to?
- Danger (damaged cells) and pathogens.
- Cell-cell contacts, through adhesion molecules and or gap junctions.
- Cell-ECM contacts, through integrins.
- Secreted molecules, such as growth factors and cytokines.

37. It is also possible to classify signals by spatial relationship. What are those classes?
- Paracrine.
- Autocrine.
- Synaptic.
- Endocrine.

38. Name 4 classic types of receptors.
- G-protein coupled receptors.
- Tyrosine kinase receptors.
- Nuclear receptors.
- Others (e.g., notch receptors, frizzled receptors [Wnt pathway]).

39. Name the phases of the cell cycle and their roles.
- G0: quiescence.
- G1: cellular growth through doubling of content, but not DNA.
- S: DNA synthesis.
- G2: premitosis.
- M: mitosis.

40. Name 2 classes of proteins regulating the cell cycle.
- CDK.
- CDK-inhibitors.

41. What are the 2 main checkpoints of the cell cycle?
- G1/S, to verify the integrity of the DNA prior to replication.
- G2/M, to verify the integrity of the DNA after replication and prior to mitosis.

42. What are the 2 main fundamental characteristics of stem cells?
- Self-renewal.
- Asymmetrical division.

43. What are the 2 main types of stem cells?
- Embryonal.
- Tissue specific.

44. Locate tissue-specific niches of stem cells.
- Skin: bulge region of follicles.
- Intestines: crypts.
- Cornea: limbus.
- Brain: subventricular.
- Liver: canal of Hering, at the interface with hepatocytes, and hepatic stellate cells.

Cell Injury, Cell Death, and Adaptations

45. Describe common types of brown pigmentation in tissue.

PIGMENTATION	TISSUE
Bile — green to greenish brown.	• Commonly seen in bile canaliculi. • Intrahepatocellular bile (centrilobular) cannot be distinguished from lipofuscin or iron.
Copper — yellow brown.	• Seen in periportal hepatocytes. • Stain with rhodamine and orcein.
Iron — brown to golden brown.	• Seen in periportal hepatocytes, except in congestive liver. • In Kupffer cells, seen in hemolysis, iron overload, or recent hepatocyte necrosis. • In hepatocytes, seen in hemochromatosis. • Perls' Prussian blue stain shows positive.
Lipofuscin — brown.	• Seen in centrilobular hepatocytes (never periportal). • Can be seen in Kupffer cells in recent hepatocellular necrosis. • Acid fast stain (Fite) shows positive.
Melanin — black/brown.	• Seen in melanoma, nevi, melanocytes. • Not polarizable or refractile.

46. Oxygen toxicity causes what type of damage to cells?
- It causes oxidative damage.
- Excess oxygen (such as reperfusion injury) causes the formation of free radicals and reactive oxygen species, which can lead to direct damage to cell membranes, nuclear DNA, and cellular organelles.

47. Ultraviolet (UV) radiation causes what type of DNA damage?
- UV-A: free radical formation causes indirect DNA damage or breaks.
- UV-B: cross-links between adjacent cytosine and thymidine form pyrimidine dimers (repaired by nucleotide excision repair pathway, enzymes of which are deficient in patients with xeroderma pigmentosum).

48. List 5 types of DNA damage.
- Oxidation of base pairs and DNA strand breaks from reactive oxygen species.
- Alkylation of bases (methylation).
- Hydrolysis, including deamination, depurination, depyrimidination.
- Adduct formation, bulky modification with benzo[a]pyrene (e.g., smokers).
- DNA mismatch, errors in DNA replication.

49. List at least 3 biochemical mechanisms responsible for cell membrane damage.
- Adenosine triphosphate (ATP) depletion, which results in the loss of function of the sodium-potassium pump.
- pH-drop from lactic acid accumulation and anaerobic metabolism, which causes denaturation of cellular enzymes.
- Entry of calcium ions (Ca^{2+}) into cells with activation of proteases, phospholipases, and endonucleases.
- Osmotic changes, which can lead to cell rupture.
- Detachment of ribosomes from endoplasmic reticulum with decreased protein synthesis.

50. Define autophagy and list its steps.
- Autophagy is self-digestion of cellular contents for recycling of these components by the lysosome.
- Steps involve initiation, elongation, maturation of the autophagosome, fusion with the lysosome and degradation (recycling of metabolites).
- It is regulated by autophagy-related genes (*ATGs*).

51. List 4 physiologic processes in which autophagy plays a role.
- Recycling of metabolites of atrophic cells exposed to severe nutrient deprivation.
- Turnover of organelles.
- Recycling of intracellular debris from aging and disease.
- Triggering cell death if cellular stressor.

52. List 4 human diseases in which autophagy plays a role.
- Cancer.
- Neurodegenerative disorders.
- Infectious diseases.
- Inflammatory bowel diseases.

53. By which mechanism are mitochondria degraded?
They are degraded through mitophagy (autophagy of mitochondria) that allows turnover of mitochondria and acts as a quality-control system.

54. Name 5 mechanisms of cell death. Explain each mechanism briefly.
- Necrosis: the morphological changes indicative of cell death caused by progressive enzymatic degradation. It may affect groups of cells, parts of a structure, or an entire organ.
- Apoptosis: the programed cell death pathway, regulated by an intricate enzyme cascade, which ultimately leads to DNA fragmentation, apoptotic bodies, and cytoplasm degradation.
- Necroptosis: a hybrid form of cell death, with shared characteristics of necrosis and apoptosis. It is sometimes called programed necrosis, which is caspase-independent unlike pure apoptosis, but which starts with the same extrinsic pathway as apoptosis. (See Figure 2.16 in *Robbins and Cotran Pathologic Basis of Disease*, 10th edition).
  · Physiologic example: formation of the bone growth plate.
  · Pathologic examples: steatohepatitis, acute pancreatitis, ischemia-reperfusion injury, neurodegenerative diseases (Parkinson disease).
- Pyroptosis: a form of apoptosis that involves the production of the cytokine interleukin-1 (IL-1) and activation of the inflammasome complex, which in turn activates caspase-1 (*pyro* refers to fever).
  · Pathologic example: local inflammation induced by the death of cells infected by microbes.
- Ferroptosis: a recently described form of cell death triggered by excess accumulation of intracellular iron or reactive oxygen species (ROS) that cause membrane lipid peroxidation, ultimately resulting in plasma membrane leakage.
  · Pathologic example: cancer, neurodegenerative diseases, and stroke.

55. Describe the pathogenesis of apoptosis.
- Intrinsic pathway: release of mitochondrial proteins (cytochrome c) activates caspase 9.
  - Proapoptosis: *BAX, BAK*.
  - Anti-apoptosis: *BCL2, BCL-X, MCL1*.
- Extrinsic pathway: plasma membrane receptors containing FADD/death domains can bind their appropriate ligands and activate caspases, resulting in apoptosis (i.e., FAS ligand binding to the FAS receptor).
- The common downstream effect of both pathways is the activation of executioner caspases (3, 6), leading to activation of DNases to cleave DNA. This results in DNA fragmentation into "DNA ladders" of approximately 200 base pairs.

56. List at least 3 morphological differences between apoptosis and cell necrosis.

MORPHOLOGICAL CATEGORY	APOPTOSIS	CELL NECROSIS
Surrounding tissue	• No inflammation.	• Inflammatory reaction frequent.
Histology	• Isolated cells affected in healthy tissue.	• Cells die together cause structure disintegration.
Cytology	• Pyknotic nuclei, condensed chromatin (pyknosis), chromatin fragmentation (karyorrhexis), minor changes in cytoplasmic organelles, and overall cell shrinkage, blebbing of the plasma membrane, and formation of apoptotic bodies that contain nuclear or cytoplasmic material.	• Karyorrhexis, edema, fading of chromatin.
Staining	• Cell membrane not permeable to staining agents.	• Cell membrane permeable to staining agents.
Electron microscopy	• Dense nuclear crescents and apoptotic bodies, intact plasma membrane.	• Swollen mitochondria, vacuoles in the cytoplasm, fragmented organelles, ruptured plasma membrane and nuclear membrane.

57. List 4 physiological situations where apoptosis occurs.
- Programed destruction of cells during embryogenesis.
- Involution of hormone-dependent tissues upon hormone withdrawal, such as endometrial atrophy after menopause.
- Cell loss in proliferating cell populations, such as immature lymphocytes in bone marrow and thymus that fail to express useful antigen receptors.
- Elimination of potentially harmful self-reactive lymphocytes.
- Death of host cells that have served their useful purpose, such as neutrophils in an acute inflammatory response.

58. List 4 pathological situations where apoptosis occurs.
- DNA damage, which can result — directly or indirectly via the production of free radicals — from radiation, cytotoxic anticancer drugs, or hypoxia.
- Accumulation of misfolded proteins, as seen in neurodegenerative disease and α1-antitrypsin deficiency.
- Cell death in certain infections, particularly viral infections such as acute hepatitis.
- Pathologic atrophy in parenchymal organs after duct obstruction, such as occurs in the pancreas, parotid gland, and kidney.

59. What is the key gene involved in regulating apoptosis?
BCL2.

60. Describe some pathological processes involved in cell death.
- Factors external to the cell, such as infections or hypoxia, which lead to irreversible cell injury.
- ATP depletion (ion pump failures), pH changes, osmotic forces, which lead to denaturation of intracellular proteins and loss of plasma membrane integrity.
- Release of enzymes from lysosomes, which leads to degradation.

61. List at least 3 histologic types of cell necrosis and 1 example of each.
- Coagulative necrosis: myocardial infarct, splenic infarct.
- Liquefactive necrosis: abscesses, stroke.
- Gangrenous necrosis: diabetic foot ulcer.
- Caseous necrosis: TB, atypical mycobacterium, histoplasmosis, cryptococcosis, coccidiomycosis.
- Fat necrosis: acute pancreatitis.
- Fibrinoid necrosis: vasculitis (leukocytoclastic vasculitis, Churg-Strauss syndrome, Wegener granulomatosis).

62. Name 2 histologic features of reversible cell damage.
- Cellular swelling.
- Fatty change.

63. Name 3 histologic features of irreversible cell damage.
- Markedly swollen mitochondria containing amorphous densities.
- Disrupted cell membranes.
- Dense pyknotic nuclei.

64. By which mechanisms do cells accumulate injury?
- Mitochondrial injury and depletion of ATP and ROS.
- Calcium entry.
- Membrane injury.
- Abnormal protein folding.

65. By which mechanisms do ischemia and reperfusion cause cellular injury?
- Oxidative stress.
- Intracellular calcium overload.
- Inflammation.
- Complement activation.

66. What happens when necrotic cells and debris are not cleared rapidly?

This leads to calcium salts and other mineral deposition, also known as dystrophic calcifications.

67. List types of calcium crystals.
- Calcium oxalate — polarize as flat rhomboids, refractile pale yellow or clear, positive mammogram. Found in apocrine cysts, giant cell reactions, but not carcinomas. Visible on X-rays but may be invisible on slides.
- Calcium phosphate — purple granular material histologically; fails to polarize; most common source of positive mammogram. Found in chronic inflammation, heart valves, breast cysts, sclerosing adenosis, hyalinized fibroadenomas, ductal carcinoma in situ (DCIS), and invasive breast carcinoma.
- Calcium pyrophosphate — blue to purple rhomboidal crystals found in joints with pseudogout.

68. Describe how to proceed in the case of a suspicious mammogram with calcifications where Ca^{2+} is not found on histology.
- Polarize.
- Cut deeper.
- Perform radiography on the tissue blocks (flat and on edge).
- Check fixation time: calcium can dissolve if left in formalin for over 24 hours.
- Rule out specimen mix-up.

69. Give an example of 1 physiological process and 1 pathological process associated with the following cellular response mechanisms.
- Hypertrophy.
  - Physiological: uterus gravida.
  - Pathological: uncompensated cardiac hypertrophy.
- Hyperplasia.
  - Physiological: breast during pregnancy.
  - Pathological: endometrial hyperplasia.
- Atrophy.
  - Physiological: fetal development.
  - Pathological: muscular atrophy.
- Metaplasia.
  - Physiological: location shift of cervical metaplasia with age.
  - Pathological: Barrett esophagus.

70. What is the mechanism of metaplasia?

Reprograming of progenitor cells.

71. What are the main categories of injurious stimuli to cells?
- Hypoxia.
- Physical agents.
- Chemical agents.
- Drugs.
- Infectious agents.
- Immunological reactions.
- Genetic abnormalities.
- Nutritional imbalance.

72. By which mechanisms can pathological intracellular deposition occur?
- Absence of an enzyme.
- Abnormal metabolism.
- Failure of folding or transport protein formation.
- Ingestion of indigestible material.

73. Name pathological changes due to intracellular accumulation of lipids and their associated diseases.
- Steatosis (fatty change).
  - Liver disease, nonalcoholic steatohepatitis (NASH).
- Atherosclerosis.
  - Spumy macrophages and cholesterol crystals in vessel walls.

(continued on next page)

- Xanthomas.
  - Macrophages full of cholesterol.
  - Acquired or hereditary hyperlipidemia.
- Cholesterolosis.
  - Accumulation of macrophages full of cholesterol in the lamina propria of gallbladders.

- Niemann-Pick C1 disease.
  - Lysosomal storage disease.
  - Cholesterol transport deficiency.

74. What are the 4 main causes of hypercalcemia?
- Hyperparathyroidism (primary or paraneoplastic).
- Accelerated bone resorption secondary to a neoplasm or Paget disease.

- Excess vitamin D (intoxication, sarcoidosis).
- Renal insufficiency.

75. Which organs are prone to metastatic calcifications?
- Stomach mucosa.
- Kidneys.
- Lungs.

- Arteries.
- Pulmonary veins.

76. What are the 4 mechanisms responsible for cellular aging?
- DNA damage.
  - Cells accumulate mutations with age. Werner, Bloom, and ataxia-telangiectasia syndromes are examples of syndromes with DNA repair abnormalities leading to early aging.
- Cellular senescence.
  - This involves telomere shortening, leading to activation of tumor suppressor genes.

- Loss of protein homeostasis.
  - Misfolding of proteins increases with age, possibly due to deficient misfolded protein degradation.
- Abnormal nutrient detection.
  - Caloric restriction has been associated with diminished IGF-1 and activation of sirtuins, leading to lower proliferation, reduced DNA damage, and longevity.

Inflammation and Repair

77. Compare the properties of neutrophils and macrophages.

	NEUTROPHILS	MACROPHAGES
Origin	Bone marrow	Bone marrow and some tissue-resident macrophages
Lifespan in tissues	Days	Circulating macrophages: days or weeks. Tissue resident macrophages: years.
Response timing	Rapid	Slower
Reactive oxygen species	Yes, rapidly induced	No
Nitric oxide	No	Yes
Degranulation	Yes	None
Cytokine production	No	Yes

78. Name the 2 pathways of macrophage activation and their effects.
- Classical activation (M1 macrophages): occurs as a response to microbial products and IFN-γ.
  - Produces ROS, nitric oxide, and lysosomal enzymes to kill bacteria and fungi.
  - Releases IL-1, IL-12, IL-23 and chemokines, which can lead to inflammatory reactions.

- Alternative activation (M2 macrophages): involved in tissue repair and resolution of inflammation.
  - Produces growth factors and TGF-β involved in tissue repair and fibrosis.
  - Produces IL-10 and TGF-β for their antiinflammatory effects.

79. Describe the types of prostaglandins and their function.
- PGI2.
  - Promotes vasodilation.
  - Inhibits platelet aggregation.
- PGE2.
  - Decreases gastric acid.
  - Increases gastric mucous.

- Promotes vasodilatation and gastrointestinal (GI) smooth muscle relaxation.
- PGD2.
  - Promotes vasodilatation.
  - Increases vascular permeability.

80. Name the 3 main pathways of complement activation.
- Classical pathway: this involves binding of C1 to antibodies (IgM or IgG).
- Alternative pathway: this is triggered by microbial surface molecules (e.g., endotoxin, lipopolysaccharide.) without antibodies.
- Lectin pathway: mannose-binding lectin binds to microbe carbohydrates to activate C1.
- Each pathway leads to deposition of cleaved C3b deposited on microbes by activation of the C3 convertase enzyme.

81. Name the 3 main functions of complement activation.
- Inflammation: recruitment and activation of leukocytes to destroy microbes.
- Opsonization/phagocytosis: phagocytes recognizing bound C3b in order to phagocytose microbes.
- Cell lysis: the result of formation of the membrane attack complex (MAC).

82. Name 3 molecules that modulate complement function and a related disease for each.
- C1 inhibitor: blocks the activation of C1.
  · Deficiency in C1 inhibitor is the cause of hereditary angioedema.
- Decay accelerating factor (DAF) and CD59: DAF prevents formation of C3 convertase enzymes; C59 prevents formation of the MAC.
  · Deficiency of these anchoring proteins is involved in paroxysmal nocturnal hemoglobinuria (PNH).
- Complement Factor H (CFH): glycoprotein that inhibits alternative pathway.
  · Deficiency or anti-CFH antibodies are associated with atypical hemolytic uremic syndrome (HUS).
  · CFH single-nucleotide polymorphism variant Y402H is associated with age-related macular degeneration.

83. Define angiogenesis.
- Angiogenesis is the process of developing new blood vessels.
  · Physiological angiogenesis occurs in wound formation; revascularization after trauma, ischemia, or menstruation; and granulation tissue formation.
  · Pathological angiogenesis occurs in tumor growth, diabetic retinopathy, and chronic inflammation.

84. List 5 angiogenic growth factors.
- Vascular endothelial growth factor (VEGF).
- Angiopoietins 1 and 2.
- Platelet derived growth factor (PDGF).
- Transforming growth factor beta (TGF-β).
- Fibroblast growth factor (FGF).

85. How does vascular endothelial growth factor (VEGF) function?
- VEGF is the most important angiogenic factor.
  · It binds to VEGF receptors, which promotes the release of endothelial precursor cells from bone marrow.
  · It stimulates endothelial cells to migrate and proliferate to new vessels from preexisting ones.
  · It is induced by: hypoxia; TGF-β released from fibroblasts (wounds); PDGF released from platelets (wound and injury); and TGF-α (inflammation).

86. Describe the differences between healing by primary intention and by secondary intention.
- Primary intention: occurs in small, clean cuts, where edges can approximate or line up. Heals with minimal scarring.
- Secondary intention: occurs in larger wounds, which heal with larger amounts of granulation tissue, scar, and wound remodeling and contraction. These wounds have broader scar formation; are slow to heal if they get infected; and require wound care.

87. Describe the cells and factors involved in the phases of skin wound healing by primary intention.
- Day 1: blood clot formation and arrival of neutrophils.
  · Cells: platelets, neutrophils.
  · Factors: fibrin, growth factors, chemokines, cytokines, clotting cascade.
- Day 3: replacement of neutrophils by macrophages, formation of prominent granulation tissue; angiogenesis and ECM deposition.
- Day 5: peak of neovascularization; proliferation of fibroblasts, which begin laying down collagen and ECM.
- Day 7: more collagen deposition.
- Day 30: formation of cellular connective tissue scar without inflammatory cells.

88. List 4 local factors and 4 systemic factors that retard wound healing.
- Local factors:
  · Infection.
  · Mechanical factors, such as early motion of wounds.
  · Foreign bodies.
  · Size, location, and type of wound.

(continued on next page)

- Systemic factors:
  - Nutrition, such as protein deficiency and vitamin C deficiency.
  - Metabolic status, such as diabetes mellitus.
  - Circulatory status, such as inadequate blood supply caused by arteriosclerosis.
  - Hormones, such as glucocorticoids.

89. List 2 examples of abnormal wound healing.
- Excess scar formation or keloid.
- Wound dehiscence.

90. List 4 vascular changes in acute inflammation.
- Vasodilation.
- Endothelial permeability.
- Neutrophil recruitment.
- Stasis of blood flow.

91. List 4 endothelial leukocyte adhesion molecules.
- L-selectin (*CD34*).
- VLA-4 (B1) integrins (*VCAM-1*).
- Sialyl-Lewis X–modified proteins (P- and L-selectins).
- B2 integrins (*CD18*), which bind *ICAM*, fibrinogen, and fibronectin.

92. List at least 5 inflammatory mediators.
- Histamine.
- Serotonin.
- Cytokines.
- Tumor necrosis factor (*TNF*).
- Interleukins.
- Chemokines.
- Leukotrienes.
- Complement factors.
- Nitric oxide.
- Reactive oxygen species.

93. Describe the effects of corticosteroids and their mechanisms.
- Effects:
  - Corticosteroids, produced in the adrenal cortex, affect stress response, immune response, carbohydrate metabolism, and lipid and protein metabolism.
- Mechanisms:
  - Inflammation: bind to glucocorticoid receptors and enter nucleus; bind DNA and upregulate genes involved in anti-inflammation (transactivation) and downregulate genes involved with inflammation (transrepression).
  - Metabolism: metabolize glucose via stimulation of gluconeogenesis in liver, mobilization of amino acids from other tissues, inhibition of glucose uptake by adipose tissue, and stimulation of fatty acid release and fat breakdown.
  - Central nervous system (CNS): cross the blood-brain barrier and bind to receptors in the central nervous system to regulate blood pressure, salt excretion, and sympathetic activation (fight or flight).
  - Embryogenesis: promote surfactant synthesis (used in premature deliveries).

94. List the complications of long-term steroid use.
- Immunodeficiency — decreased function and number of neutrophils, lymphocytes, and macrophages. This predisposes patients to infection.
- Adrenal insufficiency crisis — from sudden withdrawal of long-term steroids.
- Cushing syndrome — bilateral adrenal cortical atrophy from exogenous steroids, decreased corticotropin.
- Hyperglycemia, diabetes mellitus, insulin resistance.
- Osteoporosis — reduced bore density.
- Cataracts.
- Hypertension.
- Hypothyroidism.
- Growth failure/pubertal delay.
- Glaucoma — increased intracranial pressure.
- Slow wound healing.

95. Name 5 morphological classes of acute inflammation. Explain their origin and the reason for their morphology.
- Classic inflammation: dilatation of small vessels and accumulation of leukocytes and edema.
- Serous inflammation: exudate of cell-poor fluid.
- Fibrinous inflammation: extraversion of fibrin in the extravascular tissue. An exudate can form with strong procoagulant stimuli and there are significant leaks.
- Purulent inflammation: production of pus by neutrophils, liquified debris, and edema. If severe and prolonged, it can form an abscess with a necrotic center, neutrophils surrounding the center, vascular dilatation, and a fibroblastic reaction.
- Ulcer: excavation of the surface of an organ with sloughing and necrotic tissue. Acutely, a polymorphonuclear infiltrate is associated with vascular dilatation. Chronically, there is a fibroblastic proliferation, scarring, and chronic infiltrate accumulation.

96. What are the outcomes of acute inflammation?
- Complete resolution with limited tissue destruction.
- Scarring or fibrosis in extensive injuries or excessive fibrin deposition.
- Chronic inflammation.

97. Name 3 main classes of chronic inflammation based on etiology.
- Chronic infections.
  · Mycobacteria, viruses, parasites.
  · Delayed hypersensitivity.
  · Granulomatous inflammation.
  · Abscesses.
- Hypersensitivity.
  · Autoimmune diseases.
  · Allergies.
- Chronic exposition to toxic agents.
  · Exogenous.
  · Endogenous.

98. Name 5 systemic responses to inflammation and briefly explain their mechanisms.
- Fever: due to release of pyrogens and prostaglandins.
- Acute-phase proteins: due to inflammatory proteins released by the liver (e.g., CRP, serum amyloid A, fibrinogens), which promote the inflammatory response by opsonization. Hepcidin is also increased, which causes a decrease in iron absorption and "inflammatory anemia."
- Leukocytosis: caused by a left shift hematopoiesis, and direct effects by infectious agents. Generally, bacteria lead to increased neutrophils, viruses lead to increased lymphocytes, and eosinophils arise from parasites.
- Increased cardiac rhythm, shivers, anorexia, somnolence, malaise: due to cytokine activity on the brain.
- Septic shock: may result from bacterial infections leading to production to large quantities of inflammatory cytokines. It can be fatal.

Hemodynamic Disorders

99. What are the 3 components of the Virchow triad?
- The Virchow triad describes the 3 broad categories of factors that are thought to contribute to thrombosis:
  · Hypercoagulability.
    › Inherited — e.g., factor V Leiden.
    › Acquired — e.g., disseminated cancer.
  · Hemodynamic alteration.
    › Stasis — e.g., atrial fibrillation.
    › Turbulence — e.g., atherosclerotic vessel narrowing.
  · Endothelial injury or dysfunction.
    › Hypercholesterolemia.
    › Inflammation.

100. List 2 types of infarcts.
- Red infarct (venous occlusion).
- White infarct (arterial occlusion).

101. List 6 types of emboli.
- Fat emboli.
- Air emboli.
- Amniotic emboli.
- Tumor emboli.
- Bacteria emboli.
- Thrombotic emboli.

102. What are the consequences of a pulmonary embolus?
- No symptoms (i.e., asymptomatic or silent).
- Sudden death.
- Vascular rupture and hemorrhage.
- Pulmonary infarction.
- Pulmonary hypertension.

103. What causes of systemic embolization?
- Postinfarction mural thrombus.
- Aortic aneurysm.
- Atherosclerotic plaques.
- Valvular vegetations.
- Venous thrombosis through paradoxical embolization.

104. What histological findings are present in an amniotic embolus?
Fetal squamous cells, lanugo, fat, and mucin in the vessel.

105. Name 3 causes for each of primary (genetic) and secondary (acquired) hypercoagulable states.
- Primary:
  · Factor V Leiden mutation.
  · Prothrombin mutation.
  · Antithrombin III deficiency.
  · Protein C deficiency.
  · Protein S deficiency.
- Acquired:
  · Prolonged bed rest.
  · Myocardial infarction.
  · Atrial fibrillation.
  · Cancer.
  · Prosthetic cardiac valves.
  · Tissue injury (surgery, fractures).
  · Heparin-induced thrombocytopenia.

106. List normal endothelial factors that inhibit thrombosis.
- Heparin-like molecule and antithrombin III: inactivate thrombin.
- Tissue factor pathway inhibitor: inactivates tissue factor-VIIa complexes.
- Thrombomodulin and thrombin: activate protein C which requires protein S and results in inactivation of factors Va and VIIIa.
- Prostacyclin, nitric oxide, and adenosine diphosphatase: inhibit platelet aggregation.
- Tissue plasminogen activator: activates fibrinolysis.

107. List injured endothelial factors that promote thrombosis.
- Exposure of platelets to subendothelial collagen and platelet adhesion (held together by fibrinogen.
- Von Willebrand factor.
- Exposure of membrane-bound tissue factor, which activates the extrinsic coagulation sequence.

108. List the steps and molecules underlying heparin-induced thrombocytopenia (HIT) syndrome.
- HIT is a complication of administration of unfractionated heparin: it results from antibodies that recognize complexes of heparin and PF4 on the surface of platelets.
- PF4 binds to IgG antibodies forming PF4-IgG immune complexes. This immune complex forms cross-links with the platelet Fc receptors causing platelet aggregation and activation.
- Platelets with bound HIT antibodies are removed by macrophages, leading to thrombocytopenia. Thrombosis is the most serious complication.

109. If a patient survives an initial thrombus, what are the potential fates of the thrombus?
- Propagation.
- Embolization.
- Dissolution.
- Organization.
- Recanalization.

110. Name 3 major types of shock and the mechanisms for each.
- Cardiogenic: myocardial pump failure, resulting from myocardial damage, extrinsic compression, or obstruction to outflow (e.g., myocardial infarction and cardiac tamponade).
- Hypovolemic: inadequate blood or plasma volume (e.g., secondary to fluid loss).
- Shock associated with systemic inflammation: activation of cytokine cascades, peripheral vasodilatation, and pooling of blood (e.g., overwhelming infections and burns).

111. How do you distinguish between antemortem and postmortem thrombi?
- Antemortem: the thrombus adheres to the vascular wall and Zahn lines.
- Postmortem: the thrombus has 2 components, a yellow component that resembles chicken fat and a dark red component.

112. Name 3 high-risk secondary hypercoagulability states and 3 low-risk states.
- High-risk states:
  · Immobilization.
  · Cardiac infarction.
  · Atrial fibrillation.
  · Significant tissue damage (surgery, trauma, burns).
  · Cancer.
  · Mechanical valves.
  · Disseminated intravascular coagulation.
  · HIT.
  · Antiphospholipid syndrome.
- Low-risk states:
  · Cardiomyopathy.
  · Nephrotic syndrome.
  · Hyperestrogenic state.
  · Smoking.

113. What are the 2 main types of infarction by histopathology?
- Red (hemorrhagic): venous occlusions.
- White: arterial occlusions.

114. What is a state of shock?
- Reduction in cardiac output or circulating volume.
- Reduction of tissue perfusion.
- Cellular hypoxia as a result of these reductions.

115. Name 3 clinical consequences of shock
- Immunosuppression.
- Microvascular thrombosis (disseminated intravascular coagulation).
- Multiorgan failure.

116. List 5 pathophysiological factors of septic shock.
- Activation of inflammatory mediators.
- Activation of endothelium and increased permeability.
- Activation of coagulation.
- Metabolic abnormalities such as insulin resistance.
- Organ failure.

117. What are the steps of shock?
- Initial nonprogressive phase, in which the body can still maintain organ perfusion.
- Progressive phase, involving hypoperfusion, vascular collapse, metabolic abnormalities, and lactic acidosis.
- Irreversible phase, involving severe tissue damage leading to death.

Genetic Disorders and Genomic Techniques

118. What is lyonization?
Lyonization (also known as Lyon hypothesis or Lyon law) refers to the random and fixed inactivation (in the form of sex chromatin) of 1 X chromosome in mammalian cells at an early stage of embryogenesis, leading to mosaicism of paternal and maternal X chromosomes in females.

119. List 3 mutations causing familial hypercholesterolemia.
- Mutations in the *LDLR* (low-density lipoprotein receptor) gene.
- Mutations in genes encoding ApoB, found on the surface of LDL receptors.
- Mutations in the *PCSK9* gene, which reduces the number of LDL receptors on the cell.

120. What causes hereditary angioedema?
- Deficiency of the C1 protease inhibitor of the complement cascade.
  - C1 protease inhibitor deficiency causes accumulation of factor XII and bradykinins.
- This leads to episodes of edema of the skin, larynx, and GI tract.

121. What genetic syndrome produces degenerative arthropathy and black urine?
- Alkaptonuria (ochronosis) — an autosomal recessive disorder caused by deficiency in homogentisic oxidase.
  - It is characterized by deposits of phenols (homogentisic acid) into cartilage and connective tissue, with bluish-black pigmentation of joints.
- It looks like solar elastosis in the skin.
- Hardened connective tissue can induce a foreign body–type reaction.
- It can cause excess pigment excretion into ducts (breast, prostate, sweat glands).

122. A person with renal cysts, angiomyolipoma, and cerebral hemangioblastoma has what syndrome?
- Von Hippel-Lindau disease — a rare, autosomal dominant genetic condition.
  - It results from a mutation in the von Hippel-Lindau tumor suppressor gene on chromosome 3p25.3.
- It is associated with several pathologies, including: hemangioblastomas in the cerebellum; spinal cord, kidney, and retina angioma; renal cell carcinoma (clear cell variety); angiomyolipomas and pheochromocytoma; pancreatic cysts, and also renal cysts (75%).

123. A person with renal cysts and berry aneurysm has what syndrome?
- Adult form autosomal dominant polycystic kidney disease or syndrome (ADPKD).
  - ADPKD is 1 of 2 forms of polycystic kidney disease (PKD), a genetic disorder of the kidneys.
  - The other form of PKD is autosomal recessive polycystic kidney disease (ARPKD), which is less common and occurs in childhood.

TYPE OF PKD	INHERITANCE	PATHOLOGIC FEATURES	CLINICAL FEATURES OR COMPLICATIONS	TYPICAL OUTCOME
Adult form polycystic kidney disease (ADPKD)	• Autosomal dominant. • Mutations at chromosome 16p13.3 (*PKD1*) and 4q21 (*PKD2*). • Encodes polycystin-1 and polycystin-2.	• Large multicystic kidneys. • Liver cysts. • Berry aneurysms.	• Hematuria. • Flank pain. • Urinary tract infection. • Renal stones. • Hypertension.	• Chronic renal failure beginning at age 40–60 years.
Childhood form polycystic kidney disease (ARPKD)	• Autosomal recessive. • Mutations of the *PKHD1* gene at chromosome 6p21–p23.	• Enlarged, cystic kidneys at birth.	• Hepatic fibrosis.	• Variable: death in infancy or childhood.

124. Name 3 molecular mechanisms that cause the phenotype of trisomy 21 and explain them briefly.
- Overexpression of genes on chromosome 21.
- Mitochondrial dysfunction due to dysregulation of mitochondria-related genes.
- Increase in the number of noncoding RNAs, which are overrepresented on chromosome 21.

125. Which gene, not subject to X inactivation, is responsible for both tall stature in Klinefelter syndrome and short stature in Turner syndrome?
Short-stature homeobox gene (*SHOX*): copy number gains result in Klinefelter syndrome and copy number deletions result in Turner syndrome.

126. Name 5 triplet repeat diseases, with their corresponding triplet.
- Fragile X syndrome: CGG, transcriptional silencing.
- Fragile X tremor ataxia: CGG, transcriptional dysregulation, and accumulation of toxic mRNA.
- Fragile-X-associated primary ovarian insufficiency: CGG, transcriptional dysregulation, and accumulation of toxic mRNA.
- Friedrich ataxia: GAA, transcriptional silencing.
- Huntington disease: CAG, polyglutamine expansions with misfolding.

127. Define Gaucher disease.
Gaucher disease: a rare hereditary autosome recessive disorder that causes glucocerebroside to build up in the spleen, liver, lungs, bones, and sometimes the brain. Glucocerebrosides also accumulate within phagocytic cells throughout the body.

128. Describe the genetic and clinical variants of Gaucher disease.
- Type 1:
  · Is the most common form.
  · Causes liver and spleen enlargement, bone pain, broken bones, and, sometimes, lung and kidney problems.
  · Has no brain involvement.
  · Can occur at any age.
- Type 2:
  · Causes severe brain damage.
  · Appears in infants — most children who have it die by age 2.
- Type 3:
  · Is intermediate between type 1 and type 2.
  · May involve liver and spleen enlargement.
  · Shows gradual signs of brain involvement.

129. Describe the morphological characteristics of Gaucher disease.
- Gaucher cells (distended phagocytic cells) can be identified in spleen, liver, bone marrow, and lymphoid tissue.
- The phagocytic cells exhibit abundant "tissue paper" cytoplasm.
- Gaucher cells show positive with PAS, and sometimes also with Perls Prussian blue stain (iron).
- Electron microscopy findings: cytoplasm contains numerous elongated and tapering single membrane bound lysosomes.

130. Define Niemann-Pick disease.
Niemann-Pick disease: a hereditary autosome recessive biochemical disorder, caused by intracellular accumulation of sphingomyelin, resulting in progressive hepatosplenomegaly, lymphadenopathy, anemia, and mental and physical deterioration.

131. Describe the clinical variants of Niemann-Pick disease.
- At least 5 forms of Niemann-Pick disease have been distinguished:
  · Classical infantile form (type A).
  · Visceral (organ) form (type B).
  · Subacute or juvenile form (type C).
  · Nova Scotian variant (type D).
  · Adult form (type E).

132. List 3 diseases caused by sex chromosome imbalance.
- XO: Turner syndrome.
- XXY: Klinefelter syndrome.
- XYY: unclear if associated with a genetic syndrome.

133. List 3 diseases caused by autosomal chromosome imbalance.
- Trisomy 21: Down syndrome.
- Trisomy 13: Patau syndrome.
- Trisomy 18: Edward syndrome.

134. List 4 specific HLA subtypes and their associated diseases.
- HLA-DR3: diabetes (type 1), systemic lupus erythematosus, autoimmune hepatitis, Sjögren syndrome, rheumatoid arthritis.
- HLA-B27: ankylosing spondylitis.
- HLA-DQ2/8: celiac disease.
- HLA-DR15: multiple sclerosis.

135. Define phenylketonuria.
- Phenyl ketonuria: an autosomal recessive inheritable mutation in phenylalanine hydroxylase.
  · Patients cannot metabolize phenylalanine, which results in toxic accumulation causing permanent developmental delay, seizures, and retardation.
  · Restriction of phenylalanine in the diet is an effective treatment.

136. Define Down syndrome.
- Down syndrome: a common chromosome disorder due to an extra chromosome number 21 (trisomy 21).
- It causes:
  · Mental deficiency.
  · Characteristic facial features — slight flattening of the face, minimal squaring off of the top of the ear, a low bridge of the nose (lower than the usually flat nasal bridge of the normal newborn), an epicanthic fold (fold of skin over the top of the inner corner of the eye, which can also be seen less frequently in normal babies), a ring of tiny harmless white spots around the iris, and a minor narrowing of the palate.
  · Congenital heart defects — endocardial cushion defect and ventricular septal defects.
  · Other malformations — duodenal atresia; a minor but still significant risk of acute leukemia.

137. Name 3 epigenetic physiological and 3 epigenetic pathological processes.
- Physiological:
  · Gene expression regulation (miRNAs are an example of epigenetics).
  · Lyon's law
  · Transition from stem cell or progenitor cell to differentiated cell states.
- Pathological:
  · Genomic imprinting disorders such as Prader-Willi syndrome.
  · Epigenetic alterations of DNA repair genes or cell cycle control genes in cancer.
  · Epigenetic reprograming of stress-related genes due to abuse and trauma.

138. Describe the genetic abnormality and neoplasms associated with von Hippel-Lindau disease.
- Genetic abnormalities: mutation of the von Hippel-Lindau protein (pVHL) resulting in constitutive hypoxia signaling.
- Associated pathological conditions: renal cell carcinoma, pheochromocytoma, pancreatic neoplasms, retinal and cerebellar hemangiomas, hemangioblastomas, endolymphatic sac tumors, and papillary cystadenoma of the epididymis/broad ligament.

139. Describe the genetic abnormality and findings associated with neurofibromatosis type 1 (NF1).
- Genetic abnormalities: mutation in the *NF1* gene that encodes neurofibromin protein.
- Associated pathological conditions: neurofibromas (plexiform type), café au lait spots, Lisch nodules in the iris, malignant peripheral nerve sheath tumors, scoliosis, somatostatinoma, gangliocytic paraganglioma, gastrointestinal stromal tumor (GIST), pheochromocytoma, juvenile xanthogranuloma, and optic glioma.

140. Name 3 methods to measure cell proliferation, stating advantages and disadvantages of each method.

METHOD	ADVANTAGES	DISADVANTAGES
Ki 67 (MIB-1)	• Easy application in paraffin embed tissue. • Established prognostic marker for some tumors. • Captures all proliferating cells irrespective of the stage in the cell cycle.	• Formalin fixation only. • Not a true measure of mitosis.
Mitotic cell count	• Specific for mitotic cells. • Can identify aberrant mitosis/aneuploidy. • Recognized in H&E sections, no need for special stains.	• Tumor heterogeneity. • Unable to measure proliferating cells outside mitotic phase.
Flow cytometry/FACS analysis	• Can count cells in each phase of cell cycle. • Can determine ploidy status. • Used as an ancillary technique in cytology.	• Equipment cost. • Needs fresh tissue. • Requires technical expertise to perform the test and interpret the result. • 2–3 day turnaround time.

141. Describe the principles of the polymerase chain reaction (PCR) technique.

- PCR is a scientific technique in molecular biology to amplify a single or a few copies of a piece of DNA across several orders of magnitude, generating thousands to millions of copies of a particular DNA sequence.
- It essentially involves amplification of a target sequence of DNA using 3′ and 5′ DNA primers. Each amplification cycle is made up of 3 steps:
  · Step 1: heat denaturation (sequences come apart, dsDNA to ssDNA).
  · Step 2: addition of primers. Cooling to reanneal primers to ssDNA.
  · Step 3: DNA synthesis by DNA polymerase.
- After 25 cycles, 10^7 copies of target DNA sequence are made.

142. List 3 applications of PCR as a diagnostic tool in the laboratory.

- Direct DNA sequencing — forensics, cancer gene/translocations, paternity assays.
- Clonality assays — T cell receptor genes in lymphomas, B cell lymphomas.
- DNA mismatch repair — MSI (microsatellite sequence identification).
- Identification of infectious agents (tuberculosis, *H. pylori*, syphilis, human papillomavirus, hepatitis C, Epstein-Barr virus, toxoplasmosis).

143. Describe the principles of fluorescence in situ hybridization (FISH).

- Interphase nuclei of interest are typically placed a microscope slide, either by touch prep or by blood drop. Tagged fluorescent probes bind specific DNA sequences on intact chromosomes prepared from interphase nuclei.
  · Fusion FISH: 2 probes come together to give specific color (translocations).
  · Break apart FISH: 2 probes are together in wild type/normal cells (color A); when translocation occurs, they separate (color B).
- The labeled probes are then visualized as colored signals on the prepared slides using fluorescent microscopy.

144. Give examples of clinical applications of FISH.

- Detection of:
  · Trisomy 13, 18, and 21 in prenatal testing (FISH is used for chromosome counting).
  · DiGeorge syndrome.
  · Chromosome aneuploidy in cancers.
  · Deletions or amplifications in cancers.
  · Cancer specific translocations (UroVysion for urothelial carcinoma).
  · *ERBB2* (formerly *HER2/neu*) (breast cancer).
  · 1p/19q co-deletion (gliomas).
  · Lymphomas and sarcomas (see specific translocations at the end of this chapter).

145. Describe the principles of comparative genomic array–based microarrays (CGH-based microarrays).

- CGH-based microarrays compare DNA content from 2 differentially labeled genomes.
- The 2 genomes, a test (or patient), and a reference (or control) — each labeled with a different dye — are co-hybridized onto a solid support (usually a glass microscope slide), on which cloned or synthesized DNA fragments have been immobilized.
- Arrays have been built with a variety of DNA substrates that may include oligonucleotides, cDNAs, or bacterial artificial chromosomes (BACs).

146. List the steps involved in CGH-based microarrays.
- Label genomic DNA from diseased tissue and control tissue with a different dye.
- Affix microarray DNA gene probes to slide (microarray).
- Hybridize genomic DNA on the slide.
- Compare levels of fluorescence with specific genes.

147. Give examples of clinical applications of CGH-based microarrays.
- Detection of aberrant chromosomal abnormalities in children.
- Tumor molecular classification (e.g., reclassification of breast cancer based on microarray gene expression, lymphoma classification).
- Definition of origin of metastatic tumor.
- Prediction of disease behavior or response to therapy.
- Prognosis (i.e., defining different prognostic groups).
- Study of pathogenesis.

148. What is a major limitation of CGH-based microarrays?
CGH arrays cannot detect balanced translocations or inversions because these techniques are hybridization techniques. If the DNA content does not change, the signal remains the same and the translocation is therefore undetectable.

149. Describe the technical processes for electron microscopy.
- Fixation and processing.
  - Fix tissue in glutaraldehyde.
  - Apply osmium tetroxide postfix.
  - Dehydrate tissue in a graded series of ethanols.
  - Infiltrate tissue with EM epoxy resin.
- Embedding.
  - Embed tissue in a mold.
- Sectioning.
  - Heat resin-infiltrated tissue and harden into blocks.
  - Cut sections with a microtome (60–90 µm thick).
  - Collect sections onto specimen grids.
- Microscopy.
  - Image specimens under electron microscope.
  - Obtain digital images.

150. List examples of clinical applications of electron microscopy.
- Pediatric pathology — storage diseases, cilia (primary ciliary dyskinesia), small blue cell tumors, others.
- Renal pathology — basement membrane change, identifying deposits.
- Adult tumors — carcinomas, sarcomas, neuroendocrine tumors, melanoma.
- Infections — viral (severe acute respiratory syndrome), parasites, bacteria (Whipple disease), others.
- Neuropathology — tauopathies, cerebral autosomal-dominant arteriopathy with subcortical infarcts and leukoencephalopathy (CADASIL: deposits in blood vessels), metabolic storage diseases.

151. Describe the principles of flow cytometry.
- Label cells with specific dyes.
  - Note: dyes can be attached to antibodies that detect specific proteins (such as cell lineage markers) or they can bind directly to cellular components (such as DNA or lipids).
- Measure the fluorescence of the dyes after exposure to a laser — fluorescence occurs as the cells, in a liquid medium, "flow" past the laser.
  - Note: cell size and number can also be determined.

152. Describe the value of flow cytometry in diagnosis.
- Cell marker/cell type analysis, as in detection of leukemia/lymphoma (CD antigens).
- Cell size analysis, as in defining lymphoma types.
- DNA ploidy analysis, as in molar pregnancy.
- Cell cycle analysis (G1, S, G2, M phases of cell cycle).

153. Describe the principles of DNA hybridization.
- The DNA strand complementary to a gene of interest is labeled (e.g., with a radioactive or fluorescent tag) to create a probe.
- The specimen DNA is denatured in situ, or isolated, and transferred to a membrane/slide.
- The specimen DNA is incubated with the labeled probe at a specific hybridization temperature (determined by the type of probe).
- Excess probe is washed off and an image is produced using an appropriate detection method.

154. List 3 applications of DNA hybridization in laboratory diagnostics.
- Southern blot DNA mutational analysis.
- Comparative genomic hybridization.
- FISH for detection of gene amplification, rearrangements, or translocations.

155. In addition to FISH and conventional cytogenetics, what is the best test to detect the translocation of *SYT* given a stable chimeric transcript?
Polymerase chain reaction (PCR).

156. Describe how to make a tissue microarray, and its clinical and research applications.
- Procedure:
  - Selected specimens are taken from a donor block of selected tissue with a punch.
  - An array block is made by transferring the core to a blank wax block. Immunohistochemistry stains using selected antibodies can be performed on these tissue arrays.
- Applications:
  - Comparing protein expression across multiple tissues for expression profiling, or to determine protein expression across multiple tumor types.

157. List 2 advantages of chromogenic in situ hybridization (CISH) over FISH.
- No loss of signal over time.
- No need for a fluorescent microscope.

158. List 3 strategies used to detect certain translocations.
- RT-PCR if there is a stable fusion product.
- DNA hybridization (in situ or Southern blot).
- Next generation DNA sequencing.

159. What component of the Epstein-Barr virus (EBV) is tested by CISH?
EBER1/EBER2 (EBV encoded snRNA).

160. What is the major feature that separates standard DNA sequencing from next-generation sequencing (NGS)?
- Quantity:
  - Traditional DNA sequencing (i.e., Sanger sequencing) sequences only 1 specific DNA target at a time.
  - NGS massively sequences multiple DNA targets or locations in parallel and simultaneously.

161. What are the main steps of traditional Sanger sequencing?
- The double-stranded DNA (dsDNA) is combined with: primers, DNA polymerase, DNA nucleotides, and chain-terminating dideoxy nucleotides (ddNTP).
- The mixture is heated to denature the dsDNA.
- The mixture is cooled to a temperature where the primers will anneal with the single-stranded DNA (ssDNA).
- The temperature is raised so that the DNA polymerase will synthesize DNA with the nucleotides.
- The extension is permanently stopped by the random insertion of a ddNTP.
- This cycle is repeated until each base pair position has a ddNTP which ends the extension.
- At this step, multiple methods exist to determine which ddNTP is present at the 3′ end position of each fragment.
  - The most common method is via microfluidics — i.e., capillary electrophoresis, in which a specific fluorescent tag is attached to each ddNTP type (adenine, guanine, thymine, cytosine).
  - Fragments of the same size will have the same ddNTP at the 3′ end, and will migrate along the gel capillary at the same rate.
  - A sequence of fluorescent signal is then generated starting from the smallest fragments (5′ prime end) to the longest fragment (3′ end).

162. What are the main steps of next-generation sequencing (NGS)?
- NGS uses many technologies, but follows similar general steps.
- Library preparation:
  - DNA is fragmented at random locations.
  - 5′ and 3′ adapters are ligated to the fragments of DNA.
  - The ligated fragments of DNA are amplified through PCR.
- Cluster generation:
  - The amplified ligated fragments of DNA are massively amplified according to the method used, creating clusters of DNA strands.
- Massively parallel sequencing:
  - These clusters of DNA strands are sequenced according to the method used.
- Data analysis:
  - The sequences are aligned to a reference genome.
  - Genetic alterations are determined through bioinformatics.
  - The variant calling step correlates each genetic alteration with a predicted clinical impact.

163. What are some of the clinical utilities of NGS sequencing?
- Diagnostic purposes:
  - Identification of diagnostic mutations in difficult-to-diagnose disease states (i.e., mutational analysis of myelodysplastic syndrome and myeloproliferative neoplasms).
  - Identification of the origin of occult primary metastases through common genetic alterations.
  - Whole genome sequencing for the identification of constitutional mutations in children (i.e., inherited diseases).
- Prognostic purposes:
  - Profiling of multiple genes simultaneously in solid and hematological neoplasia.

Note: NGS can detect mutations, deletions, amplifications, chromosomal rearrangements, gene expression, epigenetic changes, and other types of genetic alterations by varying the reagents or the bioinformatric algorithms.

164. What is CRISPR and how does it work? List 2 applications of CRISPR.
- CRISPR stands for **c**lustered **r**egularly **i**nterspaced **s**hort **p**alindromic **r**epeats — DNA sequences found through the genome. The repeats originate from genetic sequences of prior infectious agents that were integrated into the genome. They can generate an adaptative immune response to some agents, notably phages and plasmids.
- Briefly, the steps include:
  - The CRISPR sequence is transcribed into CRISPR RNA (crRNA), also referred to as guide RNA (gRNA).
  - gRNAs recognize very specific DNA sequences and direct CRISPR-associated genes (Cas) endonucleases to cleave these sequences.

- Applications include:
  - Genome editing in research, which integrates genetic sequences by homologous recombination into the DNA breaks created by the Cas9 endonuclease, after gRNA guidance. This can be used to create transgenic cell and mouse lines.
  - Genome editing in clinical trials, which inserts nonmutated gene sequences in patients with inherited diseases.
  - Genome editing in plant research trials, which creates genetically modified organisms to increase crop growth and yield.
- Ethical oversight is warranted asCRISPR can also be used to remove "undesired traits" in human embryos, reminiscent of eugenics.

165. What are the 3 classic classes of genetic diseases?
- Mutations.
- Chromosomal aberrations.

- Multigenic disorders.

166. Name 4 categories of nonclassical hereditary genetic diseases.
- Trinucleotide repeat diseases.
- Mitochondrial genetic diseases.

- Genetic imprinting diseases.
- Gonad mosaicism diseases.

167. Define a missense and a nonsense mutation.
- Missense: the mutation in the nucleic acid causes a change to the codon.

- Nonsense: the mutation in the nucleic acid causes a stop codon.

168. What are classic features of autosomal dominant disease?
- A significant proportion of cases do not have affected parents or siblings, due to a de novo mutation.
- The penetrance is sometimes incomplete.

- The age of onset is often later in life (compared to recessive disease).

169. What are classic features of autosomal recessive diseases?
- Parents are often not affected, but siblings are.
- Siblings have 1 chance out of 4 to develop the disease (most of the time).
- If 1 allele is rare in the population, the genetic abnormality is probably due to a consanguineous relationship.
- The phenotype is often uniform among affected individuals.

- Complete penetrance is more frequent.
- The age of onset is earlier.
- Multiple generations can be silent until 1 generation is particularly affected.
- Autosomal recessive diseases are often metabolic diseases.

170. What are classic features of X-linked hereditary diseases?
- Males do not transmit the disease to their boys.
- All girls of the affected parent are carriers.
- Boys of carrier mothers have 1 chance out of 2 to be affected.

- Women can sometimes be affected (for example, inherited glucose-6-phosphate dehydrogenase deficiency can cause hemolytic anemia in women exposed to some medications).

171. Describe the metabolism and transport of cholesterol in normal homeostasis.
- The liver secretes very low density lipoprotein (VLDL) into systemic circulation.
- When a VLDL particle reaches the capillaries of adipose tissue or muscle, it is cleaved by a lipase, which creates an intermediate density lipoprotein (IDL).

- Fifty percent of IDLs are rapidly take up by hepatocytes and are recycled to generate VLDL.
- The remaining IDLs, which are not taken up by the liver, are the converted to low density lipoprotein (LDL).

172. What causes aneuploidy?
- Nondisjunction: the chromosomes do not separate during the anaphase.

- Anaphase lag: 1 copy of the chromosome is stuck outside the nuclei.

173. What is the genetic abnormality of DiGeorge syndrome? List its symptoms.
- The genetic abnormality is deletion of 22q11.2.
- Symptoms include:
  - "CATCH-22" abnormalities: **c**ardiac defects; **a**bnormal facies; **t**hymic hypoplasia, which leads to immune deficiency; **c**left palate; and **h**ypocalcemia, which leads to **h**ypoplasia of the parathyroid glands.
  - Others: schizophrenia, bipolar disorder, attention deficit hyperactivity disorder.

174. What is the difference between a hermaphrodite and a pseudohermaphrodite?
- In hermaphrodism, individuals possesses ovaries and testicles.
- In pseudohermaphrodism, there is a divergence between the sexual phenotype and the gonad sex.
- Masculine pseudohermaphrodism: individuals have testicles and female genital organs.
- Female pseudohermaphrodism: individuals have ovaries and a penis.

175. What is the prototypical mitochondrial gene disease?
Hereditary optic neuropathy of Leber, which is a neurodegenerative disease with progressive loss of central vision.

176. What is heteroplasmy?
- The presence of mutant and wide-type mitochondrial individual DNA in the same individual.
- This is possible because the mitochondria possess thousands of copies of DNA and mutations can only affect a subset of copies.

Immunohistochemistry and Special Stains

177. Describe the principles of the unlabeled antibody peroxidase-antiperoxidase (PAP) method of immunohistochemical testing.
- Primary antibody recognizes epitope of interest (e.g., rabbit IgG).
- Linking antibody recognizes primary Ab (anti-rabbit IgG).
- An anti-peroxidase antibody from the same species as the primary antibody (e.g., rabbit anti-peroxidase), complexed with peroxidase, is incubated to allow a colorimetric detection.
- Peroxidase polymerizes diaminobenzidine into a pigment that stains tissue.

178. What is the histochemical stain for acid mucopolysaccharides? Describe the biochemistry for how it stains.
Alcian blue: copper-based dye that binds electrostatically to negatively charged (acidic) mucopolysaccharides to impart a blue color.

179. Describe the biochemical mechanism of silver stains (for argyrophilic and argentaffin cells) and their applications in histopathology.
- Silver stains tissues at sites of reduction of silver ions.
- Argyrophilic cells: the reducing agent is light or an external substance. Example: Grimelius stain for neuroendocrine cells.
- Argentaffin cells: the reducing substance is in the tissue that is stained. Example: Masson-Fontana stain for melanin.

180. Describe the biochemical mechanism of the periodic acid-Schiff (PAS) stain and its applications in histopathology.
- Principle: periodic acid and Schiff reagent interact with diols on carbohydrates (glycogen, glycoproteins, proteoglycans) resulting in a red stain.
- Application: identifying glycogen producing tumors, and staining of basement membranes, mucin, and fungal walls.

181. List 5 histochemical methods (stains) and indicate the diagnostic value of each method.
- Gram stain: used to identify bacteria; gram positive bacteria stain purple/blue and gram-negative bacteria stain red.
- Grocott stain: silver stain used to detect fungi.
- Ziehl–Neelsen: used to identify mycobacteria, such as *M. tuberculosis*.
- PAS/Alcian blue: detects acidic and neutral mucin.
- Congo red: detects amyloid protein.

Diseases of the Immune System

182. What is the function of the Langerhans cell? What unique cytoplasmic structure can be seen on electron microscopy?
- Function: antigen presentation in the skin.
- Immunohistochemistry: CD1a, Langherin, S100.
- Cytoplasmic structure: identified by the presence of Birbeck granules in the cytoplasm on electron microscopy.

183. What are the functions of mast cells?
- Degranulation and release of preformed allergic mediators from granules in response to allergens (immediate hypersensitivity).
- Release of eicosanoids (thromboxane, PGD2, leukotrienes) for late phase allergic response.

184. Describe the structure of an IgG molecule.
- Y-shaped structure with variable domain regions at the top of the Y's arms and the Fc domain at the base.
- 2 heavy chains and 2 light chains with 4 disulfide bonds stabilizing the structure.

185. What causes chronic granulomatosis disease (CGD)?
- Cause: a genetic defect in the phagocyte oxidase enzyme in neutrophils (NADPH oxidase).
  - The defect is either X-linked or autosomal recessive.
  - CGD patients are prone to bacterial infections.
- Process (which occurs in intracellular phagocytic vacuoles):
  - NADPH oxidase is required for the respiratory burst in neutrophils activated by bacteria.
- The generation of reactive oxygen species requires formation of a multiprotein complex (NADPH oxidase) that reduces oxygen to superoxide anion and forms H_2O_2.
- H_2O_2 is broken down by myeloperoxidase to generate hypochlorite and halides to kill bacteria.

186. Erythroblastosis fetalis is seen in what type of hypersensitivity reaction?
- Antibody mediated (type II) hypersensitivity reaction.
- The IgM/IgG binds to red blood cells and triggers phagocytosis or lysis from formation of the complement membrane attack complex.

187. List 5 gross morphological features of diabetes mellitus.
- Blood vessels (macrovascular): atherosclerosis of aorta (large and medium-sized blood vessels), peripheral vascular disease (with ischemic ulcers, gangrenous necrosis of lower extremities), hypertension (hyaline arteriolosclerosis), coronary artery atherosclerosis (with myocardial infarction), renal artery stenosis, stroke.
- Kidneys: nephrosclerosis of kidneys (due to glomerulosclerosis, arteriosclerosis, pyelonephritis).
- Eyes: retinopathy, glaucoma, cataracts.
- Skin: cellulitis, infections, ulcers due to peripheral neuropathy.
- Bladder: dysfunctional bladder with incontinence due to autonomic neuropathy.

188. List 5 clinical features in untreated diabetes.
- Diabetic retinopathy.
- Diabetic peripheral neuropathy.
- Diabetic foot necessitating amputation.
- Diabetic nephropathy.
- Atherosclerotic cardiovascular disease.

189. List 4 common causes of death in diabetes patients.
- Stroke.
- Myocardial infarction.
- Infection/sepsis.
- Renal failure.

190. Define amyloid and amyloidosis.
- Amyloid: a pathologic proteinaceous substance composed of a heterogeneous group of fibrillar proteins that share the ability to aggregate into an insoluble, cross β-pleated sheet tertiary conformation. It can be deposited in the extracellular space of various tissues and organs of the body in a wide variety of clinical settings.
  - With electron microscopy (EM), seen as a 7.5–10 nm diameter fiber. (See electron microscopy section in this chapter.)
  - With X-ray crystallography, seen as a β-pleated sheet.
- Amyloidosis: abnormal accumulation of amyloid proteins, which are resistant to degradation and get deposited in various organs, causing systemic disease.

191. List the types of amyloid and their associated clinical conditions.

TYPE OF AMYLOID	ASSOCIATED DISEASE/CONDITION
SYSTEMIC AMYLOIDOSIS	
• Primary amyloidosis 　· Amyloid light chain (AL).	• All types of systemic primary amyloidosis are associated with: 　· Multiple myeloma and other monoclonal plasma cell proliferations. 　· Chronic inflammatory conditions.
• Secondary amyloidosis 　· Amyloid associated protein (AA). 　· Transthyretin (ATTR). 　· β_2-microglobulin (A-β_2-m).	• All types of systemic secondary amyloidosis are associated with: 　· Systemic senile amyloidosis. 　· Hemodialysis (for chronic renal failure).
HEREDITARY AMYLOIDOSIS	
• Amyloid associated protein (AA). • Transthyretin (ATTR).	• All types of hereditary amyloidosis are associated with: 　· Familial Mediterranean fever. 　· Familial amyloidotic neuropathies.
LOCALIZED AMYLOIDOSIS	
• APP (A*b*). • Calcitonin (A Cal). • Islet amyloid peptide (AIAPP). • Atrial natriuretic factor (AANF).	• All types of localized amyloidosis are associated with: 　· Alzheimer disease. 　· Medullary carcinoma of thyroid. 　· Type 2 diabetes.

192. List the microscopic features of amyloidosis and the special stains for detecting amyloidosis.
- Microscopic features:
  - Eosinophilic, pink waxy accumulation in the extracellular space.
- Special stains:
  - Congo red stain shows apple green birefringence.
  - Thioflavin T shows yellow color.
  - Methyl/crystal violet shows a red-purple stain for amyloid on blue normal background).

193. How is amyloidosis diagnosed clinically?
- Abdominal fat pad aspiration (most frequent when the disease is clinically suspected).
- Biopsies: rectum, tongue, gingiva (when the disease is clinically suspected).
- Organ-specific biopsies (when a targeted form of amyloidosis is suspected or as an incidental finding).
- Serum and urine electrophoresis.
- Imaging/scintigraphy.

194. List types of ANCA and associated diseases.
- c-ANCA (antibody against proteinase 3, anti-PR3): Wegener granulomatosis.
- p-ANCA (antibody against myeloperoxidase, anti-MPO): Churg-Strauss syndrome, microscopic polyangiitis, ulcerative colitis, primary sclerosing cholangitis, rheumatoid arthritis, and polyarteritis nodosa (PAN).

195. What causes hypercalcemia in sarcoidosis?
- Serum angiotensin-converting enzyme is elevated in up to 75% of untreated sarcoidosis patients.
  - This leads to elevation of serum calcium levels due to extrarenal production of calcitriol by activated macrophages in the kidney (independent of PTH).
  - This leads to increased intestinal absorption of calcium with serum hypercalcemia and hypercalciuria.
- The same mechanism can also lead to hypercalcemia in other granulomatous disorders including tuberculosis.

196. What methods can you use to diagnose sarcoidosis?
- Pulmonary imaging: chest X-ray, computed tomography (CT) scan, positron emission tomography (PET) scan, radionuclide scan.
- Skin biopsy (naked granulomas).
- Nasal mucosal biopsy.
- Tonsil and lymph node biopsy.
- Biopsies of other involved organs (liver, spleen, bone marrow, muscle).

197. What are the 3 roles of innate immunity?
- Inflammation.
- Antiviral effect.
- Activation of humoral immunity.

198. Name 3 pattern recognition receptors.
- Toll-like receptors (TLR).
  - Activate production of cytokines and interferons.
- Nucleotide-binding oligomerization domain-like receptors.
  - In inflammasomes, cleave the precursor to IL-1.
  - Detect a large variety of cellular products and microorganisms.
- Lectin.
  - Recognizes fungal glycans.

199. Name 5 types of lymphocytes and describe their roles.
- B lymphocytes: neutralization of microbes, phagocytosis, and complement activation.
- Helper T lymphocytes: activation of macrophages, inflammation, and activation of T and B lymphocytes.
- Cytotoxic T lymphocytes: killing of infected cells.
- Regulatory T lymphocytes: suppression of immune response.
- NK cells: killing of infected cells.

200. List 4 characteristics of dendritic cells that allow them to perform their role in antigen presentation.
- Localization under the epithelium.
- TLR and lectin receptors.
- Migration toward zones rich in T lymphocytes in the lymph nodes.
- Strong expression of major histocompatibility complexes (MHCs) and other molecules that activate T lymphocytes.

201. List 3 roles of macrophages.
- Antigen presentation.
- Phagocytosis of microorganisms.
- Phagocytosis of microorganisms which are opsonized by IgG or C3b.

202. What is the role of NK cells and what are their receptors?
- Role: elimination of cells infected by viruses or tumoral cells.
- Receptors: CD16 and CD56.

203. What are the 4 classes of hypersensitivity reactions?
- Immediate, type 1 (e.g., anaphylaxis, allergies, asthma).
  - Production of IgE (implicates mastocytes).
  - Production of vasoactive amines and other mediators.
  - Later recruitment of inflammatory cells.
- Antibody-mediated, type 2 (e.g., autoimmune hemolytic anemia, Goodpasture syndrome, Graves disease, myasthenia gravis, ANCA vasculitis, pemphigus vulgar).
  - Production of IgM and IgG, which targets cells and induces:
    › Opsonization, phagocytosis.
    › Destruction of cells and tissues by complement activation and inflammation.
    › Inactivation or activation of cells.
- Immune complex-mediated, type 3 (e.g., lupus, serum sickness, PAN).
  - Deposition of immune complexes in the circulation or in situ.
  - Recruitment of leukocytes and activation of complement.
- Cellular, type 4.
  - Release of cytokines via CD4, which induce inflammation and cytotoxicity (delayed type).
    › Typical pathologies: TB skin test, tuberculosis, contact dermatitis, rheumatoid arthritis, inflammatory bowel disease (IBD).
  - Cytotoxicity due to T lymphocytes.
    › Typical pathologies : type 1 diabetes, viral infections, graft rejection.

204. Describe the pathophysiology of GVHD.

T cells derived from a bone marrow transplant recognize the recipient (host) as foreign tissue and mount an immune response, typically targeting the skin, mucosa, liver, or GI tract.

205. Describe the characteristic histomorphology of GVHD.

TISSUE	ACUTE GVHD (10–50 DAYS AFTER TRANSPLANT)	CHRONIC GVHD (> 100 DAYS AFTER TRANSPLANT)
Skin	• Grade 0: no changes. • Grade 1: vacuolar alteration of the epidermal/dermal junction. • Grade 2: dyskeratotic keratinocytes. • Grade 3: partial separation of the epidermis from dermis. • Grade 4: complete separation of the epidermis from dermis.	• Lichenoid GVHD or sclerodermoid GVHD.
Colon	Always rule out CMV infection with immunohistochemistry. • Grade 1: increased epithelial cell apoptosis (mainly crypts). • Grade 2: with crypt abscess. • Grade 3: necrosis of individual crypts. • Grade 4: complete destruction of mucosal lining.	• Ischemic changes from fibrosis. • Crypt loss.

(continued on next page)

(continued from previous page)

TISSUE	ACUTE GVHD (10–50 DAYS AFTER TRANSPLANT)	CHRONIC GVHD (> 100 DAYS AFTER TRANSPLANT)
Liver	• Severe presents as portal/periportal inflammation with extension into hepatic parenchyma and hepatocyte necrosis. • Resembles chronic hepatitis.	• Bile duct damage and loss. • Portal tract inflammation. • Fibrosis. • Endothelialitis with lifting of endothelial cells from the portal veins or hepatic veins.
Esophagus	• Similar to skin, desquamation. • Submucosal fibrosis.	
Stomach	• Glandular destruction. • Apoptotic debris.	

206. List clinical criteria that help diagnose systemic lupus erythematosus (SLE) according to the 2012 revised classification.
- Acute cutaneous lupus: malar rash, photosensitivity.
- Chronic cutaneous lupus: discoid rash.
- Nonscarring alopecia.
- Oral or nasal ulcers.
- Joint disease: nonerosive synovitis of 2 or more peripheral joints.
- Serositis: pleuritis (pleuritic pain or rub), pericarditis.
- Renal disorder: proteinuria or red cell casts.
- Neurologic disorder.
- Hemolytic anemia, leukopenia, lymphopenia or thrombocytopenia.

207. Name 6 immunological criteria that can help diagnose SLE according to the 2012 revised classification.
- Abnormal antinuclear antibody (ANA) titer.
- Abnormal anti-dsDNA antibody titer.
- Presence of anti-Sm antibody.
- Presence of antiphospholipid antibody based on: abnormal IgG or IgM anti-cardiolipin antibodies; positive lupus anticoagulant test; or false positive serologic test for syphilis confirmed by negative T pallidum.
- Low complement (C3, C4 or CH50).
- Direct Coombs test.

208. What are the antibodies associated with Sjögren syndrome?
- Rheumatoid factors.
- ANA.
- Anti-SSA.
- Anti-SSB.

209. Which organs does Sjögren syndrome affect?
- Lacrimal and salivary glands.
- Sometimes: GI tract, respiratory organs, and vagina.

201. What biopsy do you perform to diagnose Sjögren syndrome? What are the findings?
- Biopsy: lip biopsy, to evaluate the minor salivary glands.
- Findings: periductal and perivascular lymphocytic infiltrate.
  · Findings in chronic disease:
    › Lymphoid follicles with germinal centers (possible).
  › Obstructive changes due to hyperplasia of the epithelium in the ducts.
  › Atrophy, fibrosis, hyalinization, and fatty replacement.

211. What are the physiological processes associated with scleroderma?
- Autoimmunity.
- Vascular injury.
- Fibrosis.

212. Which organs does scleroderma affect? List 1 finding per organ.
- Skin: fibrosis of the derma and increased dense collagen.
- GI tract: atrophy and fibrosis of the muscularis, especially the esophagus with achalasia.
- Synovium: synovitis and fibrosis.
- Kidneys: vascular injury with intimal thickening.
- Lungs: pulmonary hypertension.
- Heart: pericarditis and fibrosis.

213. What are the 2 main classes of primary immune deficiency?
- Defects in leukocyte function: leukocyte adhesion deficiency, Chediak-Higashi syndrome, chronic granulomatous disease, myeloperoxidase deficiency.
- Defects in the complement system: C2 deficiency, C4 deficiency, C3 deficiency, deficiency of complement regulatory proteins.

214. How is severe combined immunodeficiency (SCID) inherited?
- X-linked transmission.
- Autosomal recessive transmission.

215. How is Bruton agammaglobulinemia inherited?

X-linked transmission.

216. What 5 adult groups in North America are at high risk of developing AIDS?

- Homosexual or bisexual men.
- Intravenous drug users.
- Hemophiliacs.
- Blood transfusion recipients.
- Heterosexual individuals in contact with 1 of the prior high-risk groups.

217. Where are the 2 main forms of HIV located geographically?

- Type 1: North America, Europe, and central Africa.
- Type 2: West Africa and India.

218. Describe the components of HIV.

- A central core containing: a major capsid protein (p24); the nucleocapsid protein p7/p9; 2 RNA copies; and protease, reverse transcriptase, and integrase.
- A matrix layer of protein p17.
- Glycoproteins on the viral envelop: gp120 and gp41.

219. List 3 major immune dysfunctions caused by AIDS.

- Lymphopenia.
- Dysfunction of T cells.
- Alteration of function of T cells.
- Activation of B cells.
- Alteration in the function of monocytes and macrophages.

220. List opportunistic infections in HIV and AIDS patients.

- Cryptosporidium, Isospora.
- Pneumocystis jiroveci.
- Toxoplasmosis.
- Candida.
- Cryptococcus.
- Coccidioidomycosis.
- Histoplasmosis.
- Atypical mycobacterium, such as Mycobacterium avium-intracellulare.
- Cytomegalovirus, varicella-zoster virus (also herpes simplex virus, but his is less common).

Neoplasia

221. What are the 4 main categories of genes implicated in carcinogenesis?

- Protooncogenes.
- Tumor suppressors.
- Apoptosis regulators.
- DNA repair genes.

222. What is a driver mutation?

The mutation that led to the acquisition of the malignant phenotype.

223. Name 2 epigenetic alterations implicated in carcinogenesis.

- DNA methylation.
- Histone modification.

224. What are the hallmarks of cancer?

- Sustained proliferative signals.
- Evasion of growth suppression.
- Evasion of immune destruction.
- Limitless replication.
- Tumor-promoting inflammation.
- Invasion of tissue and metastasis.
- Sustained angiogenesis.
- Genome instability and mutations.
- Resistance to cell death.
- Deregulation of cellular energetics.

225. What are the main pathways regulating oncogenic growth?

- Tyrosine kinase receptor-driven pathway.
- G-protein coupled receptor-driven pathway.
- JAK-STAT.
- Wnt.
- Notch.
- Hedgehog.
- TGF-β-SMAD.
- NF-κβ.

226. Name at least 2 protooncogenes from the following classes.

- Growth factors: *PDGFRB, HST1, FGF3, TGFA, HGF*.
- Growth factor receptors: *EGFR, HER, FLT3, RET, PDGFRB, KIT, ALK*.
- Proteins involved in signal transduction: *KRAS* (other *RAS*), *ABL, BRAF, NOTCH1, JAK2*.
- Nuclear regulatory proteins: *MYC, NMYC*.
- Cell cycle regulators: *CDK4, CCND1*.

227. Name 2 tumor suppressors from the following classes.
- Inhibitors of mitogenic signaling pathways: *APC, NF1, NF2, PTCH, PTEN, SMAD2, SMAD4*.
- Inhibitors of cell cycle progression: *RB, CDKN2A*.
- Inhibitors of progrowth programs of metabolism and angiogenesis: *VHL, STK11, SDHB, SDHD*.
- Inhibitors of invasion and metastasis: *CDH1*.
- Enablers of genomic stability: *TP53*.
- DNA repair factors: *BRCA1, BRCA2, MSH2, MLH1, MSH6*.
- Unknown mechanisms: *WT1, MEN1*.

228. List the functions of p53 in the normal cell cycle.
- p53 thwarts neoplastic transformation by 3 interlocking mechanisms:
  · Activation of temporary cell cycle arrest (quiescence) and induction of DNA repair.
  · Induction of permanent cell cycle arrest (senescence).
  · Triggering of programed cell death (apoptosis).

229. Describe the role of p53 in human carcinogenesis.
- It acts as the "guardian of the genome." It functions at the G1/S cell checkpoint.
- It senses DNA damage and induces DNA repair; p53 mutation leads to accumulation of DNA damage.
- It induces cell senescence or apoptosis; p53 mutation leads to immortalization of the cell via defective apoptosis.
- p53 mutation leads to aneuploidy via centrosome destabilization and multipolar mitotic spindle.

230. What are the clinical implications of testing p53 mutations?
- Confirming cancer diagnosis: lung, colon, breast.
- Identifying cancer subtypes, such as triple negative breast cancer and high grade serous carcinoma of the mullerian tract.
- Suggesting the mechanism of carcinogenesis: Li-Fraumeni syndrome equates with sarcomas, brain tumors, leukemias, osteosarcomas.
- Predicting the response to chemotherapy and radiotherapy.

231. List 5 common oncogenic viruses with an associated malignant neoplasm for each.
- EBV — Burkitt lymphoma, Hodgkin lymphoma, nasopharyngeal carcinoma.
- Human herpesvirus-8 (HHV-8) — Kaposi sarcoma.
- HPV (16, 18, 6, 11) — squamous cell carcinoma and adenocarcinoma of the cervix.
- Human T cell leukemia virus — T cell leukemia/lymphoma.
- Hepatitis B and C virus (HBV, HCV) — hepatocellular carcinoma.

232. List at least 4 neoplasms associated with EBV.
- Burkitt lymphoma.
- B-cell lymphoma.
- Nasopharyngeal carcinoma.
- Posttransplant lymphoproliferative disorder.
- Lymphomatoid granulomatosis.
- Plasmablastic lymphoma.
- Peripheral T-cell lymphoma.
- Classic Hodgkin lymphoma.
- NK T-cell lymphoma.
- Angioimmunoblastic lymphoma.
- Primary effusion lymphoma (coinfection with HHV-8).
- Smooth muscle tumors in immunosuppressed patients.

233. List at least 4 methods for detecting EBV in neoplasms.
- Quantitative or qualitative PCR — viral load (number of viral particles) or absence/presence of virus.
- EBER — small nuclear RNAs, imitates latent stage of infection.
- Peripheral smear — atypical lymphocytes (lymphocytosis).
- Monospot test — positive.
- Immunohistochemical staining — latent membrane protein 1.

234. Describe the role of EBV in associated neoplasms.
- Infection with EBV leads to expression of *EBNA1, EBNA2*, and *LMP-1* (oncogene).
- *EBNA2* increases transcription of cell cycle proteins (cyclin D).
- *LMP1* activates *NFKB* and *JAK/STAT* pathways.
- *NFKB* enters nucleus leading to transcription of cell cycle proteins (proliferation).
- *LMP1* prevents apoptosis by increased expression of *BCL2* (immortalization).
- Translocation (8,14) leads to c-Myc translocation in Burkitt lymphoma.

235. What nonneoplastic disorders are associated with EBV?
- Mononucleosis — sore throat, fever, lymphadenitis.
- Fever of unknown origin.
- Generalized rash.
- Splenomegaly.
- EBV hepatitis.
- Meningitis.
- Pneumonia.
- Encephalitis.
- Oral hairy leukoplakia.

236. Define oncogene.

Oncogene: a gene found in chromosomes of cancer cells which, when expressed, may directly or indirectly contribute to tumor cell growth, immortalization, dedifferentiation, and metastatic potential.

237. What is the function of oncogenes in normal cells?
- The normal gene counterpart in a cell is called a proto-oncogene.
- When mutated or abnormally expressed, the proto-oncogene contributes to cancer growth and is called an oncogene.

238. What are some of the roles of oncogenes in carcinogenesis?
- Can be antiapoptotic.
- Can be defective DNA repair proteins that cause accumulation of mutated or damaged DNA.
- Can result in increased cell motility and metastasis.
- Can cause growth factor receptors to become constitutively active without need for growth factors.
- Can cause continuous cell cycling or prevent cell cycle arrest.
- Can cause dedifferentiation.
- Can cause abnormal mitosis, resulting in chromosomal imbalance.
- Can induce telomerase expression and overcome cellular senescence.

239. Name 1 gene that underlies changes in oncometabolism in cancer cells.

IDH (isocitrate dehydrogenase): its loss of function catalyzes the production of 2-hydroxyglutarate, which in turn inhibits epigenome regulatory enzymes.

240. List at least 5 neoplasms encountered in patients with AIDS.
- Kaposi sarcoma (HHV-8).
- CNS lymphoma (HIV-associated lymphomas, EBV-driven lymphomas).
- Systemic lymphomas (diffuse large B-cell lymphoma and Burkitt lymphoma).
- Plasmablastic lymphoma.
- Primary effusion lymphoma.
- Squamous cell carcinoma of anus (males).
- Cervical cancer (females).
- Hepatocellular carcinoma (in individuals coinfected with HBV and/or HCV).
- Lung cancer.
- Melanoma.
- Hodgkin lymphoma.
- Carcinomas associated with the head and neck.

241. Describe the relationship between malignancy and thrombosis.
- Malignancies can cause a hypercoagulable state. The most commonly accepted theory for this is that CD142 (factor III or tissue factor) expressed on tumor cells induces thrombin formation.
- Pancreatic and bronchogenic carcinoma can cause the Trousseau phenomenon with secretion of mediators that promote thrombosis (also called migratory thrombophlebitis).

242. List 3 examples of chromosomal changes in cancer.
- Translocation — *BCR-ABL* in CML.
- Deletion — 3p in lung cancer, 1p/19q in oligodendroglioma.
- Amplification — 3q in lung cancer, *ERBB2* in breast cancer, N-myc in neuroblastoma.

243. What are oncofetal antigens and what is their clinical significance?
- Oncofetal antigens refer to tissue antigens that are expressed during early development but are lost in adulthood.
- Clinical significance: commonly re-expressed in malignancies (e.g., α-fetoprotein in hepatocellular carcinoma or carcinoembryonic antigen in colon adenocarcinoma).

244. Indicate the genes that are altered in each of the cancers listed below.
- Mantle cell lymphoma: IgH-cyclin D1.
- Follicular lymphoma: IgH/*BCL2*.
- Chronic myeloid leukemia: *BCR-ABL* fusion gene.
- Gastrointestinal stromal tumor: *c-KIT* gene (CD117), PDGFRA.

245. List 3 syndromes due to abnormality of DNA repair and give an example of an associated neoplasm.
- Fanconi anemia: colorectal cancer.
- Ataxia telangiectasias: lymphomas and leukemias.
- Xeroderma pigmentosum: melanoma and squamous cell carcinomas.

246. List 3 tumors that may be treated with tyrosine kinase receptor inhibitors.
- Gastrointestinal stromal tumor — treated with imatinib mesylate.
- Chronic myeloid leukemia — treated with imatinib.
- *EGFR* positive nonsmall cell lung cancer — treated gefitinib and erlotinib.
- *ERBB2* positive breast carcinoma — treated with herceptin.

247. List at least 2 genetic mutations that predict poor response to *EGFR* inhibitor therapy.
- *KRAS* mutation.
- *BRAF* mutation.
- *ALK* translocation.

248. List at least 3 tumors associated with *BRAF* V600E mutations.
- Melanoma.
- Papillary thyroid cancer (all variants).
- Anaplastic thyroid cancer.
- Ameloblastoma.
- Hairy cell leukemia.
- Subset of GIST.

249. List at least 5 reportable lung biomarkers.
- *EGFR*.
- *ALK*.
- *K-ras*.
- *RET*.
- *ROS1*.
- *MET*.
- *ERBB2*.
- *BRAF*.

250. List the components of the *RAS* kinase pathway in order.
Receptor tyrosine kinase > *RAS* > *RAF* > *MEK* > transcription factor (e.g., *FOS/JUN*).

251. Name 3 factors that influence where circulating tumor cells arrest and eventually form a metastatic deposit.
- Location and vascular drainage of the primary tumor.
- Tropism of particular kinds of tumor cells for specific tissues.
- Escape from tumor dormancy.

252. What types of tumor neoantigens induce an antitumor response?
- Neoantigens produced from genes bearing passenger and driver mutations.
- Overexpressed or abnormally expressed normal cellular proteins.
- Tumor antigens produced by oncogenic viruses.

253. Name 3 mechanisms of cancer immune evasion by tumors.
- Failure to produce tumor antigen, such as a tumor cell variant that has lost antigen.
- Mutations in *MHC* genes or genes needed for antigen processing.
- Production of immunosuppressive proteins or expression of inhibitory cell surface proteins.

254. What are CAR T cells? How can they be used to treat cancers?
- CAR T cells are cytotoxic T lymphocytes that are artificially engineered ex vivo to produce chimeric antigen receptors (CARs) against surface antigens expressed by certain tumors.
- They have shown great efficacy in certain lymphoid malignancies (acute lymphoblastic leukemia in adults, diffuse large B-cell lymphoma, multiple myeloma, and mantle cell lymphoma).
- Clinical trials are underway for solid tumors.
- A possible iatrogenic complication is the cytokine release syndrome similar to the systemic inflammation response syndrome (SIRS).

255. List examples of immune checkpoint inhibition treatment.
- CTLA-4 blockade (ipilimumab, tremelimumab).
- PD-1 blockade (pembrolizumab, nivolumab, cemiplimab).
- PD-L1 blockade (atezolizumab, avelumab, durvalumab).

256. List the main steps involved in immune checkpoint inhibition treatment.
- CTLA-4 blockade:
  · A dendritic cell presents a tumor peptide antigen with its MHC receptor.
  · When B7 (on an antigen-presenting cell [APC]) and CTLA4 (on a CD8+ T cell) are bound (no so-called costimulation), the CD8+ T cell is not activated since the costimulatory signal (CD28-B7) is not engaged. This constitutes a "brake" on the immune system.
  · When CTLA-4 is blocked by a synthetic antibody, CD28 (on a T cell) may bind to B7 (on an APC), which provides a costimulatory signal. This primes the cytotoxic T cell to kill tumor cells, having released the "brakes on the immune system."
- PD-1 or PD-L1 blockade:
  · A tumor cell presents its antigen bound to MHC to a cytotoxic CD8+ T cell, through its T-cell receptor.

(continued on next page)

- PD-1 (on the T cell) and PD-1 ligand (PD-L1) are bound, providing an inhibitory "do not kill me" signal to the T cell.
- Blocking with a synthetic antibody (either PD-1 [on a T cell] or PD-1 ligand [on a tumor cell]) removes this

inhibitory signal and allows the CD8+ T cell to become activated and release its cytotoxic granules, resulting in killing of the tumor cell.

257. List reasons that some tumors do not respond to checkpoint inhibitor therapies.
- Some tumors do not express PD-L1.
- Some tumors have exhausted PD-1-positive CD8+ T-cell infiltrates.

258. Which tumoral genomic alteration predicts a good response to checkpoint inhibition therapy?
- Tumors with a high neoantigen burden, such as tumors with deficiencies in mismatch repair proteins, have a good response. It is theorized that dysfunctional repair of tumors cells generates neoepitopes, which are then recognized by the immune system.
- Immune checkpoint therapy is often used for tumors that are mismatch-repair deficient and high in microsatellite instability, even across histologic types.

259. What are the main principles of scoring PD-L1 immunohistochemistry (IHC) assays?
- Each antibody clone must be stored in specific conditions, used according to specific protocols, and processed in a specific IHC autostainer.
- Each new antibody must be validated per regulation.
- Scoring must be performed by a specifically trained pathologist.

260. List 4 genetic defects that may lead to genomic instability and give 1 example of each.
- Dysfunction of DNA mismatch repair proteins: Lynch syndrome.
- Dysfunction of nucleotide excision repair factors: xeroderma pigmentosum (UV radiation).
- Dysfunction of homologous recombination repair factors: Bloom syndrome, ataxia telangiectasia, Fanconi anemia, familial breast cancer.
- Dysfunction of DNA polymerase: subsets of certain cancers such as endometrial carcinomas (*POLE* mutated) and colon cancers.

261. Name 4 risk factors for cancer.
- Infections.
- Smoking.
- Alcohol.
- Poor diet.
- Obesity.
- Particular obstetrical history (few pregnancies).
- Exposure to environmental carcinogens.
- Inflammatory bowel disease.
- Heredity.
- Immunosuppression.

262. What is the Warburg effect?
- The Warburg effect is the propensity of tumoral cells to generate ATP from glycolysis rather than oxidative phosphorylation.
- It is paradoxical, because oxidative phosphorylation generates more ATP.

263. Describe the theory that explains the propensity of tumoral cells to generate ATP through glycolysis instead of oxidative phosphorylation.
- The glycolysis pathway produces more metabolites used in the synthesis of cellular components.
- Signaling pathways used by protooncogenes (PIK3CA, tyrosine receptors, MYC) have been shown to increase the expression of enzymes responsible for glycolysis. Tumor suppressors have been shown to do the opposite.

264. What are the main pathways underlying angiogenesis?
- Hypoxia due to exaggerated growth causes stabilization of HIF1-α, which activates VEGF and bFGF.
- Oncogenic mutations and antitumor suppression can also increase angiogenesis on their own.

265. Name 1 epigenetic regulation gene in mutated in rhabdoid tumors.
SNF5.

266. What is the effect of type B ultraviolet (UVB) radiation on DNA?
It causes cross-linking and the formation of pyrimidine dimers.

267. Which genetic syndrome predisposes individuals to skin melanoma due to deficient DNA repair of radiation injury to the skin?
Xeroderma pigmentosum.

Environmental and Nutritional Diseases

268. What is the most important cause of reduced health in the world?
Malnutrition.

269. What is the main cause of death in developed countries? What environmental factors lead to it?
- Cardiovascular disease is the main cause of death.
- It is partially caused by smoking, hypertension, hyperlipidemia, and alcohol.

270. What mechanisms have led to increased new emerging infections?
- Development of new pathogenic variants (e.g., drug resistance).
- Zoonotic pathogens due to increased proximity of humans to animal habitats.
- An increase in the incidence of an already present pathogen (e.g., due to climate change).

271. List some direct effects of climate change on health.
- Exacerbation of cardiovascular and pulmonary disease.
- Increase in food infections and due to nonpotable water.
- Increase in disease vectors and changes in their geographical distribution.
- Malnutrition through reduced agricultural production.

272. What is a xenobiotic?
It is an exogenous chemical substance that can be absorbed through inhalation, ingestion, or through the skin.

273. What superfamily of enzymes is mostly responsible for metabolizing xenobiotics? What are their 2 main phases?
- Superfamily: CYP450.
- Phase 1: hydrolysis, reduction, oxidation. This solubilizes the xenobiotic.
- Phase 2: glucoronidation, sulfation, methylation, conjugation. This facilitates their elimination.

274. What are the 6 main atmospheric pollutants?
- Carbon monoxide.
- Sulfur dioxide.
- Nitric oxide.
- Ozone.
- Carbon dioxide.
- Particles which are smaller than 10 μm.

275. Describe the effect of irradiating the whole human body.

LEVEL OF IRRADIATION	EFFECTS
2–10 Sv	• Bone marrow destruction (leucopenia, infections, nausea and vomiting, fatigue). • Skin burns/rash; some patients have desquamation of skin, mucosal sloughing, and ulceration (oral, head and neck, esophagus).
10–20 Sv	• Damage to small bowel: severe diarrhea, nausea and vomiting, fatigue.
> 50 Sv	• Damage to brain: coma and convulsions.

Notes
100 rads = 1 Sv = 1 Gy (gray)
rad = radiation absorbed dose
Sv = sieverts

276. List the classifications of burns and describe how to estimate their severity.
- Classifications:
  - First degree (partial thickness).
  - Second degree (superficial and deep).
  - Third degree (full thickness).
- Methods of estimating burn severity:
  - "Rule of Nines" — estimates body percentage as follows: each arm 9%, anterior torso 18%, posterior torso 18%, each leg 18%, head and neck 9%.
- Severe burn (requires burn unit) — characterized by facial burns, perineal burns, circumferential extremity burns, burns that cross joints, inhalation injury, partial thickness burn with total body surface area (TBSA) > 10%, any full thickness (third degree) burns in any age group.

277. Which types of vitamins are affected by pancreatic insufficiency?
- Fat-soluble vitamins (vitamins A, D, E, and K).
- See chapter 9.

278. List fat-soluble vitamins, their physiological function, and diseases that result from deficiency.

• See chapter 9.

VITAMIN (FAT SOLUBLE)	FUNCTION	DISEASES FROM DEFICIENCY
Vitamin A (retinol)	• Vision. • Formation of teeth/bones. • Embryogenesis. • Epithelium formation. • Infection resistance. • Hematopoiesis.	• Night blindness (early). • Blindness (late). • Corneal dryness. • Infections. • Squamous metaplasia.
Vitamin D (calciferol)	• Calcium absorption from intestines. • Phosphate adsorption.	• Bone defects: rickets/osteomalacia, osteoporosis.
Vitamin E	• Antioxidant.	• Spinocerebellar degeneration/ataxia. • Muscle weakness and myopathies. • Retinopathies. • Immune response.
Vitamin K	• Cofactor for factors II, VII, IX and X in coagulation cascade.	• Bleeding.

279. List fat-insoluble vitamins, their physiological function, and diseases that result from deficiency.

VITAMIN (FAT INSOLUBLE)	FUNCTION	DISEASES FROM DEFICIENCY
Vitamin B_1 (thiamine)	• Coenzyme in decarboxylation reactions.	• Beriberi. • Wernicke-Korsakoff syndrome.
Vitamin B_2 (riboflavin)	• Enzyme cofactor (think ribose).	• Angular cheilitis • Oral ulcers. • Stomatitis. • Corneal ulcers. • Sore throat. • Photophobia.
Vitamin B_3 (niacin)	• NADH and NADPH formation.	• Pellagra — dementia, dermatitis, diarrhea, necklace lesions of lower neck, hyperpigmentation, thick skin, delirium.
Vitamin B_6 (pyridoxine)	• Serotonin, dopamine, norepinephrine, epinephrine synthesis.	• Cheilosis. • Glossitis. • Dermatitis. • Peripheral neuropathy. • Depression, anxiety.
Vitamin B_{12} (cobalamin)	• DNA/folate synthesis.	• Megaloblastic pernicious anemia. • Posterior lateral spinal cord degeneration.
Vitamin C (ascorbic acid)	• Collagen hydroxylation. • Redox reactions.	• Scurvy — malaise, lethargy, skin spots, scorbutic gums, bleeding mucous membranes.
Folate	• Essential for DNA synthesis.	• Megaloblastic pernicious anemia. • Neural tube defects. • Cognitive decline. • Poor memory. • Pregnancy complications.
Pantothenic acid	• Required for the synthesis of coenzyme A.	• Very rare: numbness and painful burning and tingling in the feet.

280. List the pathological features of vitamin B_{12} deficiency.

• Autoimmune gastritis with pernicious anemia.
• Inadequate vitamin B_{12} intake (e.g., vegans, alcoholics).
• Terminal ileum damage such as resection.
• Crohn disease with loss of small bowel (ileum).
• Intestinal bacterial overgrowth.
• Fish tapeworm infestation.

281. Describe the pathological features of vitamin B$_{12}$ deficiency.
- Peripheral neuropathy: degeneration of dorsal and lateral spinal columns (ataxia, weakness, paraplegia).
- Macrocytic anemia: leukopenia with macropolymorphonuclear neutrophils; giant platelets and precursors.
- Atrophy and intestinal metaplasia of stomach (pernicious anemia).

282. Describe the synthesis of vitamin D.
- 7-dehydrocholesterol interacts with UVB in the skin to form vitamin D$_3$.
- D3 is processed in the liver by 25-hydroxylase to form 25-OH D$_3$.
- 25-OH D$_3$ is processed in the kidney by 1-alpha-hydroxylase to form 1,25 dihydroxy vitamin D.

283. Describe the biological effects of vitamin D.
- Increases calcium and phosphate absorption in the gut.
- Induces bone mineralization.
- Suppresses parathyroid hormone (PTH) secretion.

284. List 4 occupations that have increased risk of lead poisoning.
- Lead miners.
- Plumbers.
- Welders.
- Battery recycling workers.

285. List the organ systems affected by lead poisoning and their clinical presentations.
- CNS: decreased IQ, peripheral neuropathy, behavioral changes, coma.
- Bone: lead lines in the epiphysis.
- Hematopoietic system: microcytic anemia, basophilic stippling sideroblasts.
- Kidney: proximal tubular damage (Fanconi syndrome).
- GI tract: diffuse abdominal pain, gingiva lead line.

286. Name 6 organs at risk of developing cancer in smokers and 6 chronic diseases associated with smoking.
- Organs at risk of cancer: oropharynx, larynx, esophagus, trachea, bronchus, lung, liver, stomach, pancreas, kidney, ureter, colon, rectum, cervix, bladder.
- Chronic diseases: stroke, blindness, cataracts, age-related macular degeneration, orofacial clefts (maternal smoking), periodontitis, aortic aneurysm, atherosclerosis, coronary artery disease, COPD, pneumonia, tuberculosis, diabetes, reduced fertility, ectopic pregnancy, hip fractures, erectile dysfunction, rheumatoid arthritis, decreased immune function.

287. What syndrome is associated with vaping, and what histological changes does it involve?
- Syndrome: vaping-induced acute lung injury.
- Histology: changes associated with acute lung injury, from organizing pneumonia to diffuse alveolar damage (DAD); airway-centered foamy macrophages and pneumocytes; bronchiolitis; intraalveolar fibrin.

288. List 2 conditions that arise from severe acute malnutrition.
- Marasmus: depletion of the somatic protein compartment due to a diet severely low in calories. The visceral compartment is spared, which leaves serum albumin levels unaffected.
- Kwashiorkor: protein deficiency that is more severe than the total reduction in calories from malnourishment. The visceral protein compartment is depleted, leading to hypoalbuminemia and edema. Kwashiorkor has characteristic skin lesions (hypo- and hyperpigmentation, desquamation) and enlarged fatty liver.

289. What is a pathognomonic autopsy finding of anorexia nervosa death?
Gelatinous transformation of the bone marrow.

290. Name 4 hormones that modulate food intake and energy expenditure through the hypothalamic circuits that regulate energy balance.
- Leptin released by adipocytes.
- Ghrelin released by parietal cells.
- Insulin released by β cells.
- Peptide gamma-gamma released by L cells from the small intestine.

291. What are the 3 main systems in alcohol metabolism?
- Alcohol dehydrogenase (ADH).
- Microsomes (CYP2E1).
- Peroxisomes (catalase).

292. What organs are acutely affected by alcohol intake?
- Central nervous system.
- GI tract.
- Liver.

293. What organs are chronically affected by chronic alcohol intake?
- Liver: NASH.
- GI tract: gastritis, ulcers, varices.
- Central nervous system: thiamin deficiency, Korsakoff dementia, peripheral neuropathies.
- Cardiovascular: alcoholic cardiomyopathy.
- Pancreas: chronic pancreatitis.
- Pregnancy: fetal-alcohol syndrome.
- Oncology: oral, esophageal, hepatic, breast cancers, and others.

294. List the 6 main classes of illicit drugs and their molecular targets. Give 1 example of each.

DRUG CLASS	MOLECULAR TARGETS	EXAMPLE
Opioids	µ opioid receptor (agonist)	Heroin
Sedative-hypnotics	$GABA_A$ receptor (agonist)	Barbiturates
Psychomotor stimulants	Dopamine transporter (antagonist) or serotonin receptor (toxicity)	Cocaine
Phencyclidine-like drugs	NMDA glutamate receptor channel (antagonist)	Ketamine
Cannabinoids	Cannabinoid receptor type 1 (agonist)	Marijuana
Hallucinogens	Serotonin 5-HT$_2$ receptors (agonist)	Mescaline

295. What are the complications of opioid intoxication?
- Sudden death.
- Lungs: pulmonary edema, septic emboli, opportunistic infections, and foreign body granulomas.
- Infections: skin, subcutaneous, cardiac valve, liver, and pulmonary.
- Skin: abscess, cellulitis, ulceration, scarring at injection sites.
- Kidneys: amyloidosis, focal and segmental glomerulosclerosis.

296. What are the most significant complications for burn patients?
- Hypovolemic shock.
- Infection and sepsis.
- Respiratory burns due to inhalation.

Miscellaneous

297. Define sensitivity and specificity.
- Sensitivity (SN): measurement of the rate of positive tests in patients who actually have a condition.
  - Negative results in highly sensitive tests mean the condition is not present (SNOUT: sensitive tests rule out a condition when negative).

$$SN = \frac{true\ positive}{true\ positive + false\ negative}$$

- Specificity (SP): the ability of a test to identify negative results in patients who do not actually have a condition.
  - Positive results in highly specific tests mean the condition is present (SPIN: specificity rules in a condition when positive).

$$SP = \frac{true\ negative}{true\ negative + false\ positive}$$

298. Define negative and positive predictive value.
- Positive predictive value (PPV): the ability of a test to identify true positives (condition present) among many positive tests.
- Negative predictive value (NPV): the ability of a test to identify true negatives (condition not present) among many negative tests.

299. Create a table to illustrate the meaning of sensitivity (SN), specificity (SP), positive predictive value (PPV), and negative predictive value (NPV).

	CONDITION + (PRESENT)	CONDITION – (ABSENT)	
Test +	A	B	PPV
Test –	C	D	NPV
	SN	SP	

$$SN = \frac{A \ or \ (true+)}{A+C \ (condition+)}$$

$$PPV = \frac{A \ or \ (true+)}{A+B \ (test+)}$$

$$SP = \frac{D \ or \ (true-)}{B+D \ (condition-)}$$

$$NPV = \frac{C \ or \ (true-)}{C+D \ (test-)}$$

300. What are the 4 steps of digital slide scanning?
- Image acquisition (scanning): "capture."
- Storage of images: "save."
- Editing images: "edit."
- Displaying images: "view."

301. List 3 types of whole slide imaging (WSI).
- Brightfield scanning: reproduces standard light microscopy.
- Fluorescent scanning: scans fluorescently labeled slides such as FISH or fluorescence IHC.
- Multispectral scanning: scans across the spectrum of light at each wavelength.

302. List 4 benefits of WSI.
- Quick retrieval for biopsy or resection comparison.
- Efficient presentation during tumor boards.

303. Based on the 2021 guidelines of the College of American Pathologists, what are the main steps for validating a digital pathology platform for clinical use?
- Include a sample set of at least 60 diverse cases per application (i.e., H&E, frozen sections, hematology, cytology).
- The validation study should represent a real-world clinical practice, and be carried out by each individual pathology laboratory planning to use a WSI system.
- Evaluate if all the tissue present on the glass slide is included in the digital scanned image.
- Digital slides can be viewed in a random or nonrandom order.
- Calculate concordance between scanned slides and glass slides for the same pathologist. Calculating interobserver variability is not recommended.
- Allow an interval of at least 2 weeks after having seen either the digital or glass slides set, before seeing the other set.
- Document how the WSI system was validated.

304. Define the following terms: *artificial intelligence, machine learning, deep learning algorithms, artificial neural network.*
- Artificial intelligence (AI): an umbrella term in which intelligence is demonstrated by machines. Intelligence is generally described as the capacity for logic, understanding, reasoning, planning, thinking, and problem-solving (among other features).
- Machine learning: a subset of AI in which the machine learns through experience.
- Deep learning algorithms: a form of machine learning based on artificial neural networks.
- Artificial neural network: a computation system that mimics the biology of animal brains, and is generally composed of multiple "layers" of connections (input layer, output layer, and hidden layers).

305. Name 3 forms of artificial neural networks used in biomedical image analysis.
- Convolutional neural networks.
- Recurrent neural networks.
- Generative adversarial networks.

306. List examples of AI applied to tasks in pathology.
- Low level tasks: detection and/or segmentation of objects in a microscopy field for automated estimations (mitotic count, positive IHC cell count).
- Higher level tasks: predicting diagnoses and prognosis from image patterns within a microscopy field.

CHECKLISTS

HEMATOPOIETIC CHECKLIST (MALIGNANCY TO GENETIC ALTERATION)

Acute lymphoblastic leukemia/lymphoma (B cell: B-ALL)

FAVORABLE:
- Hyperdiploidy.
- t(12;21) or *ETV6–RUNX6* fusion.

INTERMEDIATE:
- Normal karyotype.
- t(5;14) or *IL3-IGH* fusion.
- t(1;19) or *TCF3-PBX1* fusion.

UNFAVORABLE:
- Hypoploidy.
- t(9;22) or *BCR–ABL* fusion.
- Complex abnormalities.

Acute myeloid leukemia (AML)

FAVORABLE:
- t(8;21).
- t(15:17).
- inv(16).
- t(16;16).

UNFAVORABLE:
- 3q abnormalities.
- Inv(3).
- Del(5q).
- t(6;11).
- t(9;22).
- Complex karyotype.

Acute promyelocytic leukemia with t(15;17) (APML)

t(15;17)(q24;q21) or *PML-RARA* fusion 15-*PML* (promyelocytic leukemia).

Note: more favorable prognosis than other AML.

ALK+ anaplastic large cell lymphoma

t(2;5) 2-*ALK*, *NPM-ALK* fusion.

ALK– anaplastic large cell lymphoma

t(6;7) *IRF4-DUSP22* fusion (similar prognosis to ALK+).
t(3;3) *TBL1XR1-TP63* fusion.

Burkitt lymphoma

Endemic, sporadic, immunodeficiency-associated (HIV).
t(8;14) *IGH-MYC*.
t(2;8) *IGK-MYC*.
t(8;22) *IGL-MYC*.

Chronic myeloid leukemia, BCR-ABL1 positive

t(9;22) 9-*ABL*, 22-*BCR* (Philadelphia chromosome).

Diffuse large B-cell lymphoma, NOS

30% have *BCL6* (chromosome 3) translocation.
20–30% have t(14;18) involving *BCL2* (same as follicular lymphoma).
10% *MYC* rearrangement.

Follicular lymphoma

t(14;18) 14-*IgH*, 18-*BCL2*.

Mantle cell lymphoma

t(11;14) 11-*BCL1*, 14-*IgH*.

Marginal zone lymphoma

t(11;18).
t(14;18).
t(1;14) translocations for extranodal MZL (EMZL).

Gastric EMZL: Helicobacter pylori

Salivary gland EMZL: Sjögren syndrome.
Thyroid EMZL: Hasmimoto thyroiditis.
Cutaneous EMZL: Borrelia burgdoferi.
Small intestinal EMZL: *Campylobacter jejuni*.

Polycythemia rubra vera

JAK2 V617F mutation activating JAK-STAT signaling.
JAK2 exon 12 insertions and deletions.
Chronic neutrophilic leukemia
Colony stimulating factor 3R (*CSF3R*) mutation.

Essential thrombocytosis

JAK2 V617F mutations activating *JAK*-STAT signaling.
CALR mutations.

Primary myelofibrosis

JAK2 V617F mutations.
CALR mutations.
MPL mutations.

Mastocytosis

c-KIT mutations (D816V common).

SOLID TUMORS CHECKLIST (TUMOR TO GENETIC ALTERATION)

Adenoid cystic carcinoma
t(6;9) *MYB-NFIB*.
t(8;9) MYBL1-NFIB.

Alveolar soft part sarcoma
t(X;17) *ASPL-TFE3* gene fusion, PASD+ intracytoplasmic crystals.

Angiomatoid fibrous histiocytoma
EWSR1-CREB1.

Angiomyolipoma
TSC1 or *TSC2* loss.

Atypical rhabdoid tumor
SMARCB1 (INI) loss, same in renal or extrarenal.

Breast carcinoma
BRCA1 (17q21) (*ER–, PR–, HER2+*).
BRCA2 (13q12.3) (*ER+, HER2–*).
CDH1 gene: lobular carcinoma (E-cadherin protein).
Other germline mutations: *TP53, PALB2, PTEN, STK11, ATM, CHEK2*.
ER/PR — positive if > 1% of cells have nuclear staining.
ERBB2 (criteria may vary) — see the most recent guidelines from the College of American Pathologists.

CIC-rearranged sarcoma
CIC-DUX4.

Clear cell sarcoma (malignant melanoma of soft parts)
t(12;22) *EWS-ATF1* fusion.
t(2;22) *EWSR1-CREB1* fusion.

Clear cell sarcoma of the GI tract
Same fusions.

Clear cell sarcoma of the kidney
YWHAE-NUTM2.
BCOR tandem duplication.

Clear cell carcinoma (salivary glands)
t(12;22) *EWSR1-ATF1*.

Colorectal carcinogenesis
ADENOMA PATHWAY:
- Normal colon: first hit *APC* (5q21).
- Mucosa at risk, second hit: methylation abnormalities (*APC*, β-catenin).
- Adenomas: *KRAS* (12p12), inactivation of *TP53*, LOH at 18q21 involving *SMAD2* and *SMAD4*, overexpression *COX-2*.
- Carcinoma: telomerase and other cancer genes.

MISMATCH REPAIR PATHWAY:
- Normal colon: inherited or somatic mutations of mismatch repair genes (*MLH1, MSH2, MSH6, PMS1, PMS2*).
- Sessile serrated adenoma: second allele altered by LOH mutation or promoter methylation.
- Carcinoma: *TGFBR2, BAX, BRAF, TCF4, IGF2R*, others.

Congenital infantile fibrosarcoma
t(12;15) *ETV6-NTRK3* fusion.

Congenital mesoblastic nephroma, cellular type
Same fusion.

Desmoplastic small round cell tumor
t(11;22) *EWSR1-WT1*.

Dermatofibrosarcoma protuberans (DFSP)
t(17;22) COL1A1-PDGFB.

Endometrial adenocarcinoma
FOUR MOLECULAR SUBTYPES:
- Ultramutated/*POLE* tumors (DNA polymerase ε).
- Hypermutated/MSI tumors (microsatellite instable).
- Copy number low/MSS (microsatellite stable).
- Copy number high/serous-like tumors (*TP53*).

Endometrial stromal sarcoma
t(7;17) *JAZF1-SUZ12* (low grade endometrial stromal sarcoma).
t(10;17) *YWHAE-NUTM2A/B* (high grade endometrial stromal sarcoma).

Epithelioid hemangioendothelioma (EHE)
t(1;3): WWTR1-CAMTA1.
t(X;11): *YAP1-TFE3*.

Ewing sarcoma/primitive neuroectodermal tumor
t(11;22)(q24;q12) 11-*FLI1*, 22-*EWSR1*, most common fusion.
5' end of *EWSR1* joined to 3'end of: *ETS* gene family (*FLI1, ERG, ETV1, ETV4, FEV*).
Less commonly, 5' *FET* family gene can be *FUS* or *TAF15* instead of *EWSR1*.

Extraskeletal myxoid chondrosarcoma
t(9;22) EWSR1-NR4A3.
t(9;17) TAF15-NR4A3.

Gastrointestinal stromal tumor
Most: *c-KIT* mutation.
Some: *PDGFRA, BRAF* V600E (rare).
Pediatric GIST: SDH deficient.

Germ cell tumors
Isochromosome (12p) (germ cell neoplasia in situ associated [GCNIS-associated]).

Inflammatory myofibroblastic tumor (IMT)
ALK (most common).
ROS1 or *RET* fusions.

Liposarcoma
Myxoid liposarcoma: t(12;16) *FUS-DDIT3* (common) or *EWSR1-DDIT3* (rare).
Dedifferentiated liposarcoma and well-differentiated liposarcoma: *MDM2* amplification.
Pleomorphic liposarcoma: complex karyotype.

Low grade fibromyxoid sarcoma (Evans tumor)
t(7;16): *FUS-CREB3L2* (common).
t(11;16): *FUS-CREB3L1* (rare).

Melanoma (dysplastic nevus syndrome/heritable melanoma syndrome)
p16INK4A/CDNK2 (9p21) deletion.
BRAF V600E,K,R,D.
NRAS Q61, G12, G13.
KIT mutations.
TERT promoter mutations.

Mesenchymal chondrosarcoma
t(8;8): HEY1-NCOA2.

Metanephric adenoma
BRAF V600E mutation.
MiT family translocation renal cell carcinoma (RCC).
TFE3 rearrangements with multiple possible n' partners (*ASPSCR1*, *PRCC*, *PSF*, *NONO*, *MALAT1*).

Mucoepidermoid carcinoma
t(11;19): *CRTC1-MAML2*.
t(11;15): *CRTC3-MAML2*.

Myoepithelial tumor of soft tissue
t(19;22): EWSR1-ZNF444.
t(6;22): EWSR1-POU5F1.
t(1;22): EWSR1-PBX1.

Neuroblastoma
FAVORABLE:
- Schwannian stroma.
- *EPHB6*, *EFNB2*, *EFNB3*, *NTRK1*, *CD44*.

UNFAVORABLE:
- Diploidy, near-diploidy, near-tetraploidy.
- *MYCN* amplification.
- *TERT* rearrangements.
- *ATRX* mutations.
- 17q gain, 1p loss.

Nodular fasciitis
t(17;22): *MYH9-USP6* (same fusion also seen in aneurysmal bone cyst).

NUT carcinoma
t(15;19) *BRD4-NUT*.
t(9;15) *BRD3-NUT*.

Oligodendroglioma
Balanced loss of 1p/19q.
IDH1/2 mutations.
CIC and *FUBP1*: poor prognosis.

Pancreatic carcinoma
Very common: *KRAS* (12p), *p16/CDKN2A* (9p), *TP53* (17p), *SMAD4* (18q).
Common: AKT2, GATA6, FGFR, ATM.

Parathyroid adenoma
CDC73 mutation (tumor suppressor).
CCND1/Cyclin-D1 overexpression.
MEN1 inactivation (tumor suppressor).
RET mutation (MEN2A patients).

PEComa
TFE3 rearrangements or amplification (Xp11).

Pilocytic astrocytoma
KIAA1549-BRAF.

Renal cell carcinoma (papillary type)
Trisomy of chromosomes 7 and 17, loss of Y.
MET mutation (familial).
BAP1, SETD2, RID2, KEAP1.

Pleomorphic adenoma
PLAG1 or *HMGA2* rearrangements.

Renal cell carcinoma (clear cell type)
VHL mutations or chromosome 3p losses.
Chromosome 5q gains.
PBMR1, SETD2, BAP1, FHIT.

Renal cell carcinoma (chromophobe)
TP53, *PTEN*, *PIK3-AKT-mTOR* pathway genes mutations.
Hypodiploid DNA.

Rhabdomyosarcoma (alveolar type)
t(2;13) *PAX3-FOXO1* (more common, unfavorable prognosis).
t(1;13) *PAX7-FOXO1* (less common, favorable prognosis).

Rhabdomyosarcoma (embryonal)
Loss of 11p15, no translocations.

Secretory carcinoma (mammary analogue secretory carcinoma)
t(12;15) *ETV6-NTRK3*.
t(10;12) *ETV6-RET*.

Sclerosing epithelioid fibrosarcoma
t(11;22) EWSR1-CREB3L1.
t(7;16) FUS-CREB3L2.

Solitary fibrous tumor (SFT)
NAB2-STAT6.

Synovial sarcoma
t(X;18) *SSX* gene (*SSX1*, *SSX2*, or *SSX4*) fused to *SS18* (formerly *SYT*).

Thyroid carcinoma

FOLLICULAR:
- RAS family of oncogenes mutation.
- t(2;3) fusion of PAX-8 and PPARγ.
- TERT promoter mutation.
- Familial forms: PTEN (PTEN-hamartoma tumor syndrome), PRKAR1A (Carney complex), WRN (Werner syndrome), GNAS1 (McCune-Albright syndrome).

PAPILLARY:
- BRAF V600E mutation (most common).
- RE-PTCH1 or RET/NCOA4 gene fusions.
- RAS mutations (HRAS, KRAS, NRAS).

MEDULLARY:
- RET proto-oncogene mutation (MEN2A or MEN2B).

ANAPLASTIC:
- ATC loss and TP53 mutation.
- BRAF V600E mutation or RAS (NRAS, KRAS, HRAS).

NONINVASIVE FOLLICULAR THYROID NEOPLASM WITH PAPILLARY-LIKE NUCLEAR FEATURES (NIFTP):
- Absence of BRAF, TERT or RET mutations and rearrangements.
- RAS (NRAS, KRAS, HRAS) mutations.

CHECKLIST OF GENETIC ALTERATIONS COMMON TO SEVERAL TUMORS

ALK
Inflammatory myofibroblastic tumor.
ALK+ anaplastic large cell lymphoma.
Lung adenocarcinoma.
Neuroblastoma.
Spitz nevus.

BAP1
Malignant mesothelioma.
Uveal melanoma.
Cutaneous melanoma.

BRAF mutations
Papillary thyroid carcinoma.
Malignant melanoma.
Colorectal carcinoma.
Langerhans histiocytosis.
Erdheim-Chester disease.
Hairy cell leukemia.

BRAF fusions
Pilocytic astrocytoma.
Pancreatic acinar cell carcinoma.
Spitz nevus and spitzoid melanoma.
Lung adenocarcinoma.

BCOR
Clear cell sarcoma of the kidney.
Endometrial stromal sarcoma.
Round cell carcinoma with *BCOR* alterations.

BCR-ABL
Chronic myeloid leukemia.
B-ALL.
AML with *BCR-ABL* fusion.

ETV6
Infantile fibrosarcoma.
Congenital mesoblastic nephroma.
Secretory carcinoma of the breast, or its salivary gland counterpart.

EWSR1
Ewing sarcoma (*FLI1*, *ERG*, others).
Extraskeletal myxoid chondrosarcoma (*NR4A3*).
Desmoplastic small round cell tumor (*WT1*).
Myoepithelial tumor of soft tissue (*ZNF444*, *POU5F1*, *PBX1*).
Myxoid liposarcoma (*DDIT3*).
Clear cell sarcoma of soft tissue (*ATF1*).
Clear cell sarcoma of salivary gland (*ATF1*).
Angiomatoid fibrous histiocytoma (*CREB1*, *ATF1*).
Primary pulmonary myxoid sarcoma (*CREB1*).
Sclerosing epithelioid fibrosarcoma (*CREB3L1*).

FUS
Angiomatoid fibrous histiocytoma (*FUS-ATF1*).
Low grade fibromyxoid sarcoma (*FUS-CREB3L1/2*).
Sclerosing epithelioid fibrosarcoma (*FUSB-CREB3L2*).
Myxoid liposarcoma (*FUS-DDIT3*).

KIT
GIST.
Malignant melanoma.
Mastocytosis.

MET
Papillary renal cell carcinoma.
Lung carcinoma.

MYC (c-Myc)
Burkitt lymphoma.
Plasmablastic lymphoma.
Diffuse large B cell lymphoma.
Double-hit lymphoma.

MYC (n-Myc)
Neuroblastoma.

NTRK
Secretory carcinoma of the salivary gland.
Secretory breast carcinoma.
Congenital infantile fibrosarcoma.
Malignant melanoma.
Congenital mesoblastic nephroma.

RET
Medullary thyroid carcinoma (activating mutation).
Hirshprung disease (inactivating mutation).
Lung adenocarcinoma (fusion).
Papillary thyroid carcinoma (fusion).

SMARCA4 (BRG1)
SMARCA4-deficient thoracic sarcoma.
Small cell carcinoma of the ovary (hypercalcemic type).
SMARCA4-deficient undifferentiated uterine sarcoma
  ("malignant rhabdoid tumor of the uterus").

SMARCB1 (INI)
Rhabdoid tumors (renal and extrarenal, including
  atypical rhabdoid tumor of the brain).
Epithelioid sarcoma.
Myoepithelial carcinoma of soft tissue.
Medullary carcinoma of the kidney.

TFE3
Renal cell carcinoma with Xp11.2.
Alveolar soft part sarcoma.
PEComas.

WT1
Wilms tumor.
Desmoplastic small round cell tumor.

UNCLASSIFIED GENETIC ALTERATIONS CHECKLIST

Alkaptonuria (ochronosis)
Lack homogentisic oxidase.
Accumulation of homogentisic acid.
Black urine, black pigmentation of ears/nose/cheeks,
  arthropathy.

Celiac disease
HLA-B8, HLA-DQ2.

DM type 1
HLA-DR3 or HLA-DR4.

Familial hypercholesterolemia
Low density lipoprotein receptor mutation.

Hirschsprung disease
RET mutation.
Others: GDNF, SOX10, EDN3, EDNRB.

Rheumatoid arthritis
HLA-DR4 or HLA-DR1 (*DRB1* genes).

Seronegative spondyloarthropathies
HLA B27.
Reactive arthritis.
Ankylosing spondylitis.
Psoriasis associated with spondylitis.
IBD associated with spondylitis.

SYNDROMES CHECKLIST

Angelman syndrome
Deletion of *UBE3A* in the **maternally** derived chromosome (paternal chromosome is imprinted/inactivated).
Intellectual disability, ataxia, microcephaly, seizures and inappropriate laughter.

Prader-Willi syndrome
Series of genes deleted in 15q11–13 in the **paternally** derived chromosome, active *UBE3A* gene.
Loss of SNORP family of genes function (encode noncoding RNAs).

Ataxia-telangiectasia (ATM: DNA repair after radiation injury — 11q22.3)
Cerebellar dysfunction.
Recurrent infection (no thymus).
Lymphoid malignancy.
Telangiectasias (especially conjunctival).
Hypoplastic gonads.

Autoimmune polyendocrinopathy syndromes
Type 1: autosomal recessive, AIRE gene, hypoparatyroidism, adrenal insufficiency, hypogonadism, vitiligo, candidiasis.
Type 2: autosomal dominant, adrenal insufficiency and hypothyroidism or type I diabetes.
IPEX (immunodysregulation polyendoencrinopathy enteropathy X-linked syndrome): X-linked recessive, *FOXP3* gene, diabetes and diarrhea.

Autosomal dominant (adult) polycystic kidney disease
PKD1 (16p).
PKD2 (4q).

BAP1 hereditary cancer predisposition syndrome (BAP1)
Uveal and cutaneous melanoma.
Mesothelioma.
Clear cell renal cell carcinoma.

Beckwith-Wiedemann syndrome (Wilms tumor 2 locus — 11p)
Triad: macroglossia, abdominal wall defects, macrosomia.
Macrosomia involves: liver, spleen, pancreas, adrenals, heart, kidneys.
Renal medullary cysts.
Wilms and other primitive tumors.

Birt-Hogg-Dubé syndrome (BHD)
Renal carcinoma (clear cell, chromophobe, papillary).
Renal oncocytomas or hybrid chromophobe/oncocytoma tumors.
Cutaneous fibrofolliculomas and acrochordons.
Pulmonary cysts and spontaneous pneumothorax.

BRCA1 (DNA repair, 17q21)
Breast carcinoma (medullary, poorly differentiated), *ER/PR–*, *ERBB2–* (triple negative).
Ovarian carcinoma (high grade serous carcinoma).
Also prostate, colon, and pancreas carcinomas.

BRCA2 (DNA repair, 13q12.3)
Breast carcinoma, (histology similar to sporadic): ER–/HER2–; or ER+/HER2–; or HER2+.
Ovarian carcinoma (high grade serous carcinoma).
Prostate, pancreas, stomach, primary peritoneal.
Male breast cancer incidence higher in *BRCA2* than *BRCA1*.

Carney syndrome/complex (PRKAR1A)
Spotty pigmentation (lentiginoses) of the lips, conjunctiva, genital mucosa.
Psammomatous melanotic schwannoma.
Pigmented epithelioid melanocytoma (*PRKAR1A*-inactivated melanocytoma).
Endocrine overactivity (primary pigmented nodular adrenal cortical hyperplasia, Cushing disease, GH pituitary adenoma).
Myxomatosis: cutaneous, mucosal, breast and cardiac.
Large cell calcifying Sertoli cell testicular tumor.

Carney triad (SDHC promoter hypermethylation)
Pulmonary hamartoma.
GIST.
Paraganglioma/pheochromocytoma.

Carney-Stratakis syndrome (SDHB, SDHD, SDHC, SDHA)
Familial paraganglioma.
GIST.
SDH-deficient renal cell carcinoma.
Pituitary adenoma.

Cowden/PTEN hamartoma tumor syndrome (PTEN — 10q23)
Germline *PTEN* mutation.
Mucocutaneous: multiple trichilemmomas, acral keratoses, oral mucosal fibromas.
Breast: carcinoma.
Thyroid: multinodular goiter, thyroid carcinoma.
Endometrium: endometrial carcinoma.
GI tract: hamartomatous polyps of stomach, colon and esophagus.

Cystic fibrosis
Cystic fibrosis transmembrane conductance receptor (7q31.2); chloride channel.
Most common mutation: F508del.
Lungs, pancreas, GI system, hepatobiliary system, genitourinary system.

Chromosome 22q11.2 deletion syndrome

Congenital heart defects.
Abnormalities of the palate.
Facial dysmorphism.
Developmental delay.
T-cell immunodeficiency and hypocalcemia.

Note: now encompasses DiGeorge syndrome and velo-cardio-facial syndrome.

Denys-Drash syndrome (WT1 — 11p)

Gonadal dysgenesis.
Nephrotic syndrome → renal failure.
Wilms tumor.

DICER1 syndrome

Pleural or pulmonary blastoma.
Cystic nephroma.
Sertoli-Leydig cell tumor of the ovary.
Multinodular goiter.
Pituitary blastoma.

Down syndrome (trisomy 21)

CNS: mental defficiency.
Facial features: epicanthic folds, flat facial profile, abundant neck skin.
Extremities: simian crease, hypotonia, gap between first and second toes.
Cardiac: congenital heart defects (septal defects).
GI: intestinal stenosis, umbilical hernia, Hirschsprung.
Predisposition to leukemia.
Infections d/t abnormal immune responses.
Premature Alzheimer disease.

Edwards syndrome (trisomy 18)

CNS: prominent occiput, mental retardation.
Dysmorphisms: micrognathia, low set ears, short neck, overlapping fingers.
Cardiac: congenital heart defects.
Renal: horseshoe kidney.
MSK: limited hip abduction, rocker bottom feet.

Ehlers-Danlos syndrome

Defects in conversion of type I procollagen to collagen.
2 forms: arthrochalasia type (COL1A1, COL1A2) and dermatosparaxis type (ADAMTS2).

Familial atypical multiple mole melanoma syndrome (CDKN2A)

Hundreds of nevi, dysplastic nevi, melanoma.
Pancreatic adenocarcinoma.

Fragile X syndrome

Xq27.3 (FMR-1 protein) — CGG repeats, transcriptional silencing.

Gaucher disease

Glucocerebrosidase deficiency (lysosomal storage disease).
Accumulation of glucocerebroside in lysosomes of histiocytes.
3 clinical subtypes: type I: chronic nonneuronpathic form.
Type II: acute neuronopathic (in pediatric population).
Type III: intermediate form between types I and II.

Gorlin syndrome/nevoid basal-cell syndrome (PTCH1)

Basal cell carcinomas (2 or more before age 20).
Odontogenic keratocyst of the jaw.
Ovarian fibroma.
Medulloblastoma.
Congenital malformations and skeletal anomalies.

Hemochromatosis

HFE (chromosome 6) C282Y mutation.
HFE regulates hepcidin.

Huntington disease

4p16.3 (Huntington protein) — CAG repeats, toxic gain of function.

Hyper-IgM syndrome

CD40L (on T cells, Xq26).
CD40 (on B cells) mutation; can't class switch from production of IgM antibodies to the IgG, IgA or IgE.

Marfan syndrome

Defect in fibrillin-1: glycoprotein scaffolding for elastin deposition in the extracellular matrix (15q21.1).
Fibrillin-1 controls bioavailability of TGF-β.
Skeletal anomalies, ocular changes, cardiovascular lesions, aortic dissection.

Mucopolysaccharidoses

Deficiency of enzymes that degrade mucopolysaccharides.
11 recognized variants, which include Hurler syndrome and Hunter syndrome (X-linked).
Hepatosplenomegaly, skeletal deformities, valvular lesions and subendothelial arterial deposits, lesions in the brain.

Niemann-Pick disease

Sphingomyelinase deficiency leads to lysosomal accumulation of sphingomyelin.
Type A: severe pediatric form with neurologic involvement.
Type B: organomegaly but no central nervous system involvement.

Polyposis syndromes (GI)

CLASSIC FAMILIAL ADENOMATOUS POLYPOSIS (FAP)
(*APC* — 5Q21):
- > 100 adenomas in the colon.
- Congenital hypertrophy of retinal pigment epithelium.

ATTENUATED FAP (*APC*):
- < 100 adenomas in the colon.

GARDNER SYNDROME (*APC*):
- FAP with extraintestinal manifestations.
- Osteomas, thyroid and desmoid tumors, skin cysts.

TURCOT SYNDROME (*APC*):
- FAP and medulloblastoma and glioblastoma.

MUTYH-ASSOCIATED POLYPOSIS (*MUTYH*)
- > 100 adenomas and gastric and duodenal polyps.

IgG4-related disease
Lymphadenopathy (mediastinal, intraabdominal, axillary).
Orbital disease (orbital inflammatory pseudotumor).
Sclerosing sialadenitis (lacrimal gland, parotid, submandibular gland).
IgG4-related sclerosing cholangitis.
IgG4-related autoimmune pancreatitis.
Retroperitoneum fibrosis (infrarenal aorta soft tissue or retroperitoneal lymph nodes).
Hereditary hemorrhagic telangiectasia (Osler-Weber-Rendu syndrome):
- Multiple small aneurysmal telangiectasias: skin, cerebral, pulmonary, hepatic, GI.
  › Epistaxis, hemoptysis, GI/GU bleeding.
  › Mutations in ENG and ACVRL1 genes.

Hereditary nonpolyposis colon cancer (Lynch syndrome: mismatch repair, MSH2, MLH1, MSH6, or PMS2)
Colorectal carcinoma.
Small bowel carcinoma.
Endometrial carcinoma.
Ovarian carcinoma.
Pancreatobiliary carcinoma
Urothelial carcinoma, upper tract.

Hereditary leiomyomatosis and renal cell carcinoma (fumarate hydratase)
Papillary renal cell carcinoma (type 2).
Leiomyomas (uterus and skin).
Hyperparathyroidism-jaw-tumor syndrome (*CDC73*).

Hyperparathyroidism-jaw tumor syndrome (HRPT2)
Ossifying fibromas.
Parathyroid adenomas and carcinomas.
Hyperparathyroidism.
Higher incidence of different renal and uterine tumors.

Juvenile polyposis syndrome (SMAD4, BMPRIA, PTEN)
Juvenile polyps.
Carcinomas of stomach, small intestine, colon, pancreas.
Congenital malformations, clubbing.

Klinefelter syndrome (47,XXY in 80%, remainder mostly mosaics — e.g., 46,XY/47,XXY)
Eunuchoid body habitus.
Failure of male secondary sexual characteristics, atrophic testes (hypogonadism).
Gynecomastia, increased risk of breast carcinoma and autoimmune diseases.
Male infertility (reduced spermatogenesis).
High FSH and estrogen levels; low testosterone levels.

Li-Fraumeni syndrome (TP53, CHEK2)
Soft tissue sarcoma (rhabdomyosarcoma, embryonal rhabdomyosarcoma, leiomyosarcoma, etc.).
Osteosarcoma.
Breast carcinoma.
Carcinoma of colon, pancreas, adrenal cortex, kidney, lung, prostate.
Leukemia.
Lymphoma.
CNS tumors.

Maffucci syndrome
Somatic mutations of *IDH1/2*.
Multiple hemangiomas.
Multiple enchondromas (endochondromatosis).
Risk of chondrosarcoma and angiosarcoma.

McCune-Albright syndrome
Café-au-lait spots.
Polyostotic or monostotic fibrous dysplasia.
Autonomous endocrine function (precocious puberty, Cushing syndrome, hyperthyroidism, growth hormone excess).
GI anomalies (fundic gland polyps, gastric heterotopia, gastric hyperplastic polyps).
Mosaic loss of *GNAS1* (nonmosaic loss is embryonic-lethal).

MEN1 (MEN1 — 11q11–13)
Pituitary adenomas.
Pancreatic endocrine tumors (especially pancreatic polypeptide secreting).
Parathyroid hyperplasia/adenoma.
Duodenal gastrinomas (Zollinger-Ellison syndrome), carcinoid tumors. thyroid/adrenocortical adenomas.

MEN2A (*RET* activating mutation — 10)
Medullary thyroid carcinoma.
Pheochromocytoma.
Parathyroid hyperplasia.

MEN2B (RET mutation different from MEN2A)

Includes all of MEN2A plus:
- Neuromas/gangliomas in GI tract, etc.
- Marfanoid habitus.
  - **No** parathyroid hyperplasia.

Muscular dystrophy (Xp21 — dystrophin gene deletions)

Duchenne: earlier onset, more severe, cardiac involvement, kyphoscoliosis, progressive respiratory muscle weakness and failure.

Becker: later onset, less severe, cardiac involvement, infertility.

Muir-Torre syndrome (MLH1 or MSH2)

Form of Lynch syndrome, autosomal dominant.
Benign/malignant sebaceous tumors.
GI or genitourinary (GU) tract adenocarcinoma.

Neurofibromatosis type 1 (von Recklinghausen syndrome) (NF1, neurofibromin: downregulates p21 — 17)

CNS:
- CNS tumors (schwannomas, meningiomas, optic gliomas).
- Reduced intelligence.

EYES:
- Lisch nodules (2 or more).
- Optic nerve glioma.

SKIN:
- Neurofibromas (2 or more, or 1 plexiform neurofibroma).
- Malignant peripheral nerve sheath tumors (MPNSTs).
- Café-au-lait spots (6 or more).
- Bilateral axillary or inguinal freckling.

BONES:
- Sphenoid dysplasia.
- Tibial bowing or thinning of long bone cortex with pseudoarthrosis.

OTHER:
- Pheochromocytoma.
- Duodenal neuroendocrine tumor (carcinoid).

Neurofibromatosis type 2/Merlin syndrome (NF2, merlin: tumor suppressor — 22)

Bilateral or unilateral acoustic/vestibular schwannoma.
CNS meningioma (2 or more).
Ependymoma.
Juvenile subcapsular cataract, retinal hamartoma.
Peripheral polyneuropathy.
Café-au-lait-spots but less frequently than NF1 patients.

Nevoid basal cell carcinoma syndrome (PTCH1: development — 9q22.3) (Gorlin)

SKIN:
- Multiple BCCs < 20 years old.
- Pits of palms and soles.

CNS:
- Medulloblastoma.

ENT:
- Odontogenic keratocysts of the jaw.

GENITOURINARY:
- Bilateral calcified ovarian fibromas.

Patau syndrome (trisomy 13)

Microcephaly, mental retardation.
Microphthalmia.
Cleft lip, cleft palate and holoprosencephaly.
Polydactyly and simian crease.
Cardiac defects (PDA, ASD and/or VSD).
Omphalocele.
Renal defects (polycystic kidney, hydronephrosis, horseshoe kidney).
Rocker bottom feet.

PEComa family of tumors

Renal angiomyolipoma.
Lymphangiomyomatosis of lung and lymph nodes.
Clear cell/sugar tumor of lung.
Association with tuberous sclerosis.
Dual expression of melanocytic and myogenic markers.

Peutz-Jeghers syndrome (STK11)

Melanotic pigmentation of skin (hands and feet) and mucosa (lentiginoses).
Arborizing hamartomatous polyps: (most to least frequent): small intestine, colon, stomach.
Polyps also present in: bladder, renal pelvis, bronchus, nose, gallbladder.
Adenoma malignum of cervix.
Carcinomas in pancreas, breast, lung, ovary (sex cord tumor with annular tubules, mucinous tumors), testis (Sertoli cell tumor), uterus.

POEMS syndrome

Rare paraneoplastic plasma cell disorder:
- **P**olyneuropathy.
- **O**rganomegaly.
- **E**ndocrinopathy.
- **M**onoclonal gammopathy.
- **S**kin changes.

Retinoblastoma (RB1 tumor suppressor gene — 13q14)

Retinoblastoma.

Secondary cancer: pinealoblastoma, osteosarcoma, soft tissue sarcoma, melanoma, Hodgkin lymphoma, breast carcinoma.

Rhabdoid tumor predisposition syndrome (SMARCB1 [INI], SMARCA4 [BRG1])
Small cell carcinoma of the ovary, hypercalcemic type.
Malignant rhabdoid tumors (renal and extrarenal).
Cranial rhabdoid tumors (atypical rhabdoid tumor).

Sturge-Weber syndrome (GNAQ gene- 9q21.2)
Leptomeningeal angiomatous masses.
Facial port-wine stain.
Mental retardation.
Seizures.
Hemiplegia.
Skull radiopacities.
Glaucoma.
Pheochromocytoma.

Succinate dehydrogenase-deficient renal cell carcinoma (SDHB, SDHC, SDHD, SDHA)
Renal cell carcinoma with characteristic histology.
Pheochromocytoma/paraganglioma.
GIST.
Pituitary adenoma (as part of Carney-Stratakis syndrome).

Tay-Sachs disease
Alpha-subunit of hexosaminidase enzyme (HEXA) complex mutation on chromosome 15.
Accumulation of GM2-gangliosides in many tissues, mostly neurons and the retina. Cherry-red spot in the macula.

Tuberous sclerosis (TSC1 hamartin — 9q34, TSC2 tuberin — 16p13.3)

SKIN:
- Cutaneous angiofibroma.
- Ash-leaf macules.
- Shagreen patch.
- Ungual or periungual fibroma.

CNS:
- Seizures, epilepsy.
- Mental retardation.
- Cortical tubers.
- Subependymal giant astrocytoma (SEGA), subependymal nodule (SEN).

THORACIC:
- Cardiac rhabdomyoma.
- Lymphangioleiomyomatosis (PECOMA) of the lung.

EYES:
- Retinal hamartoma.

KIDNEYS:
- Renal angiomyolipoma.
- Renal cysts.
- Polycystic kidney disease.

Turner syndrome (45,X)
Three genetic mechanisms:
- Classic: 45,X.
- Defective second X chromosome (isochromosome, deletion, or ring chromosome).
- Mosaic type.

Short stature (due to *SHOX* gene haploinsufficiency).
Lymphedema of neck, hands, feet.
Webbing of neck.
Congenital heart disease (aortic coarctation).
Broad chest, widely spaced nipples.
Failure of breast development.
Infantile external genitalia.
Ovaries atrophic and fibrous (streak ovaries).
Primary amenorrhea.

Von Hippel-Lindau (VHL — 3p)
Hemangioblastoma in cerebellum, brainstem, eye (retinal hemangioblastoma).
Renal cell carcinoma, clear cell type.
Pheochromocytoma.
Pancreatic endocrine tumor (PanNET) and pancreatic cysts.
Endolymphatic sac tumor.

WAGR syndrome (Wilms tumor 1 and PAX6 — 11p13)
Wilms tumor.
Aniridia.
Genital anomalies and gonadoblastoma.
Mental retardation.

X-linked agammaglobulinemia of Bruton
BTK (B cell tyrosine kinase) mutation.
Failure of maturation of B cell precursors.

Xeroderma pigmentosum (nucleotide excision repair genes)
Melanoma.
Nonmelanoma skin carcinomas (basal and squamous cell carcinoma).
CNS tumors (medulloblastoma, glioblastoma, spinal cord astrocytoma, schwannoma).

ELECTRON MICROSCOPY CHECKLIST

Active protein synthesis
Abundant granular ER (ribosomes).

Adenocarcinomas
Lumens, intracellular lumens.
Microvilli.
Mucigen granules.
Glycogen.
Prominent Golgi.
Intermediate filaments (juxta nuclear).
Interdigitating cell membranes, cell junctions, rare cilia, basal lamina.

Alveolar soft part sarcoma
Rhomboid crystals (also PAS positive).

Amyloid
Nonbranching fibrils, indefinite length, diameter approximately 7.5–10 nm.

Carcinoid tumor
Dense core bodies, neurosecretory granules.

Clear cell carcinomas (e.g., kidney, vagina)
Abundant glycogen and/or lipid (both in RCC).
Lumen, microvilli, junctional complex.

Ewing sarcoma
Prominent pools of cytoplasmic glycogen.

Glucagonoma
Granules with closely apportioned membranes, dense round center.
Granular cell tumor.
Lysosomes.

Glomerulonephritides

TYPE	CHARACTERISTICS
Poststreptococcal	Subepithelial humps.
Goodpasture syndrome	GBM disruptions, fibrin, no deposits.
RPGN	GBM wrinkling, disruptions. No deposits (unless immune complex type).
Membranous	Subepithelial deposits.
Minimal change	Loss of foot processes, no deposits.
FSGS	Loss of foot processes, epithelial denudation.
MPGN type I	Subendothelial deposits.
MPGN type 2	Dense deposits.
IgA nephropathy	Mesangial and paramesangial dense deposits.
Alport	Split of GBM, thin GBM, "bread crumb" degeneration.
Diabetic glomerulosclerosis	Massive increase in mesangial matrix, thickened GBM (> 300–350 nm) and Bowman capsule.
Crescentic GN	+/− deposits, crescents, disrupted GBM.
Lupus	Mesangial deposits (type I, II). Mesangial and subendothelial deposits (type III, IV).
Chromophobe RCC	Microvesicles.

IHC of basal/myoepithelial cells
Prostate basal cells: K903+, p63+, CK5/6+, S100−, SMA−.
Breast myoepithelial cells: SMA+, p63+, S100+.
Salivary gland myoepithelial cells: SMA+, S100+.

Insulinoma
Membrane bound granules.
Dense, paracrystalline, often rectangular core.
Distinct halo separates core from membrane.

Irreversible cell injury
Mitochondria markedly swollen, contain amorphous densities.
Cell membranes disrupted.
Dense pyknotic nucleus.

Langerhans cell histiocytosis
Birbeck granules with characteristic periodicity and dilated terminal end.

Leiomyosarcoma
Myofilaments.
Smooth muscle derivation.

Medullary thyroid carcinoma
Membrane bound, electron dense granules.

Melanoma
Premelanosomes.
Melanosomes.

Neuroendocrine tumors (APUDomas) (e.g., carcinoid, islet cell tumors, medullary thyroid carcinoma, pituitary adenomas)
Neurosecretory type granules.
Microfilaments, cell junctions, basal lamina.

Oncocytic neoplasms (e.g., Hurthle cell tumor, oncocytoma, Warthin tumor)
Lots of mitochondria with stacked lamelliform cristae that lack matrix granules.
Intercellular junctions, lumens (microvilli).

Pheochromocytoma (1220)
Membrane bound secretory granules, distinct halo.

Pulmonary adenocarcinoma versus mesothelioma
Adenocarcinoma: short, plump microvilli.
Mesothelioma: numerous, long, slender microvilli in gaps between cells (3 long:1 wide).

Reversible cell injury
Microvilli lost.
Blebs, extrude into lumen.
Mitochondria slightly dilated.

Rhabdomyosarcoma/rhabdomyoma
Actin (6 nm) filaments, myosin (15 nm) fibrils in parallel arrays.
Sarcomeres, glycogen, primitive cell junctions, external lamina.

Schwannoma
Complexly entangled long cell processes.
Intermediate filaments, microtubules, long spacing collagen.

Smooth muscle tumors
Actin microfilaments, interspersed fusiform dense bodies.
Plasmalemmal attachment plaques, pinocytic vesicles.

Squamous cell carcinoma/squamous metaplasia
Cytokeratin filaments (tonofilaments), filopodia (fingerlike cell processes).
Well-developed desmosomes, primitive cell junctions.

Steroid producing tumors
Prominent smooth endoplasmic reticulum.
Mitochondria with tubulovesicular cristae.

Vascular tumors (EC origin)
Weibel-Palade bodies.
Bundles of intermediate filaments, tight and primitive cell junctions.
Pinocytotic vesicles.

Acknowledgment
The authors would like to acknowledge the contributions of Drs. Davide Salina and Adrian H. Box to the earlier editions of this chapter, which were a prominent framework for this new edition. Their work and effort are greatly appreciated.

Bibliography
Amin MB, Edge S, Greene F, et al, editors. AJCC cancer staging manual. 8th ed. New York: Springer; 2017

Evans AJ, Brown RW, Bui MM, et al. Validating whole slide imaging systems for diagnostic purposes in pathology: guideline update from the College of American Pathologists in collaboration with the American Society for Clinical Pathology and the Association for Pathology Informatics. Arch Pathol Lab Med. 2022;146(4);440-50. doi: 10.5858/arpa.2020-0723-CP

Gao Zu-hua. Gross pathology of common diseases. Edmonton (AB): Brush Education Inc., 2020.

Goldblum JR, Lamps LW, McKenney JK, et al. Rosai and Ackerman's surgical pathology. 11th ed. Philadelphia: Elsevier; 2017.

Kumar V, Abbas AK, Aster J. Robbins and Cotran pathologic basis of disease. 10th ed. Philadelphia: Elsevier; 2020.

Longacre TA, editor. Mills and Sternberg's diagnostic surgical pathology. 7th ed. Philadelphia (PA): Wolters Kluwar; 2022.

Rekhtman N, Baine MK, Bishop JA. Quick reference handbook for surgical pathologists. 2nd edition. New York: Springer; 2019.

WHO Classification of Tumours Editorial Board. WHO classification of tumours. 5th ed. Vol. 1, Digestive system tumours. Lyon (France): IARC; 2019.

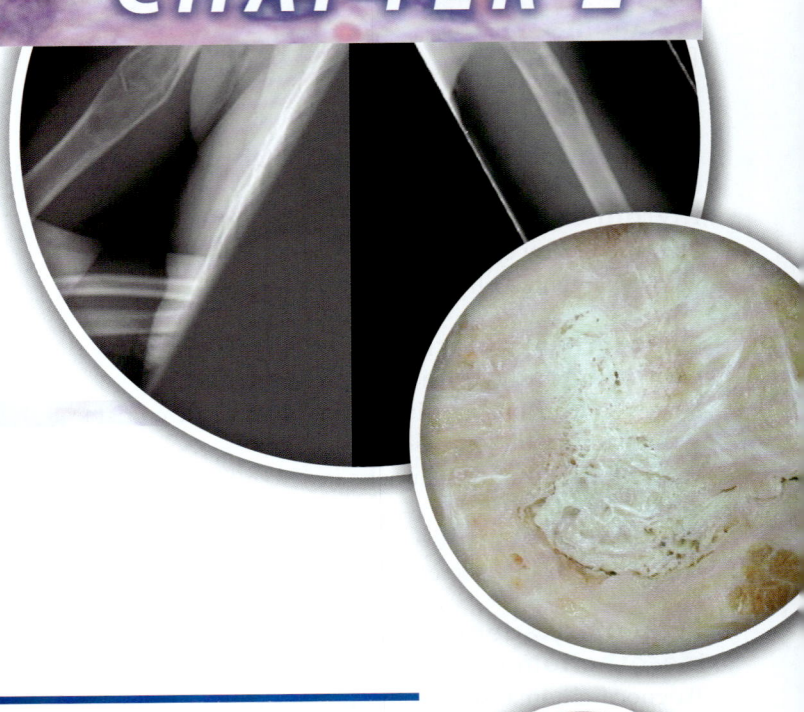

CHAPTER 2

Bone & Soft Tissue Pathology

BIBIANNA PURGINA

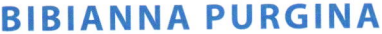

Bone and Soft Tissue Pathology Exam Essentials

MUST KNOW

Nonneoplastic bone and soft tissue

High-yield topics include:
- Bone:
  - Osteopenia/osteoporosis.
  - Paget disease of bone.
    - Stages.
    - Microscopic features.
    - Complications.
  - Hyperparathyroidism and renal osteodystrophy.
  - Osteonecrosis (avascular necrosis).
  - Causes and risk factors.
  - Osteomyelitis.
    - Definitions of sequestrum, involucrum.
    - Microscopic features.
    - Pyogenic osteomyelitis (most common bacteria in adults, IV drug users, neonates, sickle cell patients).
    - Mycobacterial osteomyelitis.
- Joints:
  - Osteoarthritis.
    - Gross and microscopic features.
  - Rheumatoid arthritis.
  - Seronegative spondyloarthropathies.
  - Infectious arthritis.

- Crystal-induced arthritis.
  - Gout versus pseudogout.
  - Types of crystals and their appearance.
  - Specimen handling.
- Synovial cysts and ganglion cysts.

World Health Organization (WHO) classification of bone and soft tissue tumors

Since soft tissue tumors may exist anywhere, adopt the WHO's lineage-based approach. For each lineage, you should be able to list at least 1 to 2 classic examples.
- Soft tissue:
  - Adipocytic tumors.
    - Use of terminology of atypical lipomatous tumor versus well-differentiated liposarcoma.
    - Behavior of deep-seated liposarcoma.
  - Fibroblastic and myofibroblastic tumors.
    - Differential diagnosis and ancillary workup for various entities in this category.
  - So-called fibrohistiocytic tumors.
  - Vascular tumors.
    - Exams often include questions regarding the classification of Kaposi sarcoma and its associated virus.

- Pericytic (perivascular) tumors.
- Smooth muscle tumors.
- Skeletal muscle tumors.
- Gastrointestinal stromal tumor.
- Chondroosseous tumors.
- Peripheral nerve sheath tumors.
  › Neural tumors are particularly high yield: they may appear on slides and in questions about associated syndromes.
- Tumors of uncertain differentiation.
  › Knowledge of molecular alterations for most of the tumors in this category.
- Undifferentiated small round cell sarcomas of bone and soft tissue.
- Bone:
  - Chondrogenic tumors.
  - Osteogenic tumors.
  - Fibrogenic tumors.
  - Vascular tumors of bone.
  - Osteoclastic giant cell-rich tumors.
  - Notochordal tumors.
  - Other mesenchymal tumors of bone.
  - Hematopoietic neoplasms of bone:
    › Hematolymphoid tumors will be covered in the hematopathology section.

AJCC and College of American Pathologists (CAP) protocols

Bone and soft tissue AJCC and CAP protocols are infrequently examined. Focus on key elements such as:
- Particular requirements for grossing and factors that affect FNCLCC (Fédération Nationale des Centres de Lutte Contre le Cancer) grade or tumor stage.
- Subtypes of sarcoma that should not be graded with the FNCLCC protocol.
- Subtypes of sarcoma for which CAP and AJCC staging is unreliable (i.e., solitary fibrous tumor).
- The importance of radiologic findings, anatomic site, and clinical behavior in assessing behavior and malignant potential of bone tumors.
- Types of surgeries that can be performed for bone and soft tissue tumors.
- How anatomic location affects which CAP or AJCC protocol is used.
- Mode of spread for sarcomas and how it differs from carcinomas.
  - Most sarcomas spread via the blood to lung and other sites. You should be able to list:
    › Subtypes of sarcoma that preferentially spread to lymph nodes.
    › The subtype of sarcoma that preferentially spreads to another soft tissue site.

Molecular pathology

You need to know the role of ancillary testing (including molecular techniques) in establishing the diagnosis for soft tissue tumors. In addition, you should memorize certain translocations because they are frequently examined. Key topics include:
- Ancillary studies for sarcomas such as cytogenetics, fluorescence in situ hybridization (FISH), electron microscopy, polymerase chain reaction (PCR), and next-generation sequencing (NGS), including tissue sampling techniques.
- Translocation or molecular changes in:
  - Ewing sarcoma.
  - Alveolar soft part sarcoma.
  - Clear cell sarcoma.
  - Desmoplastic small round cell tumor.
  - Dermatofibrosarcoma protuberans.
  - Rhabdoid tumor.
  - Alveolar rhabdomyosarcoma.
  - Solitary fibrous tumor.
  - Synovial sarcoma.
  - Infantile fibrosarcoma.
  - Inflammatory myofibroblastic tumor.
  - Liposarcoma.
- Tumors associated with commonly translocated genes (e.g., *EWSR1*, *FUS*): you should be able to name 3 to 5 tumors.

Genetic and syndromic conditions

- Some syndromes, whose manifestations may include bone and soft tissue tumors, are commonly examined, including:
  - Carney complex.
  - Beckwith-Wiedemann syndrome.
  - McCune-Albright syndrome.
  - Neurofibromatosis type 1 (NF1).
  - Neurofibromatosis type 2 (NF2).
  - Tuberous sclerosis.
- Commonly examined inherited diseases affecting collagen and connective tissues include:
  - Marfan syndrome.
  - Ehlers-Danlos syndrome.
  - Osteogenesis imperfecta.
  - Alport syndrome.
  - Achondrogenesis.

MUST SEE

- You need to know entities suitable for practical gross examination, including:
  - Osteoarthritis.
  - Synovial chondromatosis.
  - Loose bodies (joint mice).
  - Implant-related changes in the synovium.
  - Avascular necrosis of the femoral head.
  - Femoral neck fracture.
  - Toe with gout.
  - Osteoma (enostosis, torus).
  - Osteoid osteoma in the tibia (classic location).

- Osteochondroma.
- Osteosarcoma.
- Enchondroma of small bones of hands/feet.
- Central chondrosarcoma.
- Retroperitoneal dedifferentiated liposarcoma.
- Intramuscular myxoma.
- Schwannoma.
- Plexiform neurofibroma.
- You also need to know entities suitable for practical slide examination (simple H&E diagnosis with appropriate clinical history and classic anatomic site), including:
  - Nonneoplastic lesions:
    › Ganglion cyst.
    › Osteoarthritis.
    › Rheumatoid arthritis: pannus and/or rheumatoid nodule.
    › Tophaceous gout.
    › Pseudogout.
    › Osteomyelitis.
    › Osteonecrosis (avascular necrosis in femoral head, scaphoid).
    › Detritic synovitis (implant-associated synovitis).
    › Femoral neck fracture with osteopenia.
  - Soft tissue lesions:
    › Adipocytic tumors.
      » Conventional lipoma; angiolipoma; myelolipoma; spindle cell or pleomorphic lipoma; hibernoma; atypical lipomatous tumor or well-differentiated liposarcoma; dedifferentiated liposarcoma (provided the residual well-differentiated component is present and/or retroperitoneal in location); myxoid liposarcoma.
    › Fibroblastic and myofibroblastic tumors.
      » Nodular fasciitis, proliferative and ischemic fasciitis, elastofibroma (in periscapular location), palmar fibromatosis, desmoid fibromatosis, dermatofibrosarcoma protuberans, solitary fibrous tumor.
    › So-called fibrohistiocytic tumors.
      » Tenosynovial giant cell tumor (localized and diffuse), deep fibrous histiocytoma, giant cell tumor of soft tissue.
    › Vascular tumors.
      » Lobular capillary hemangioma (also known as pyogenic granuloma), papillary endothelial hyperplasia (Masson tumor), hemangioma, Kaposi sarcoma, epithelioid hemangioendothelioma (only if exhibiting classic histology and in the liver), angiosarcoma.
    › Pericytic (perivascular) tumors.
      » Glomus tumor, myofibroma, and myopericytoma.
    › Smooth tumors.
      » Leiomyoma, leiomyosarcoma.
    › Skeletal muscle tumors.
      » Rhabdomyoma, embryonal rhabdomyosarcoma, conventional alveolar rhabdomyosarcoma.
    › Gastrointestinal stromal tumor.
    › Peripheral nerve sheath tumors.
      » Granular cell tumor; schwannoma (and subtypes: ancient, cellular); cutaneous neurofibroma; plexiform neurofibroma; malignant peripheral nerve sheath tumor (MPNST) (only if history of NF1 or arising from a major nerve trunk).
    › Tumors of uncertain differentiation.
      » Intramuscular myxoma, biphasic synovial sarcoma, alveolar soft part sarcoma.
    › Undifferentiated small round cell sarcomas of bone and soft tissue.
      » Ewing sarcoma.
  - Bone tumors:
    › Chondrogenic tumors.
      » Bizarre parosteal osteochondromatous proliferation, synovial chondromatosis, osteochondroma, enchondroma, chondroblastoma, chondrosarcoma (low grade and mesenchymal), dedifferentiated chondrosarcoma (if residual low grade component is present on slide).
    › Osteogenic tumors.
      » Osteoma, osteoid osteoma, osteoblastoma, osteosarcoma variants.
    › Fibrogenic tumors of bone difficult to test on practical slide exam.
    › Vascular tumors of bone.
      » Hemangioma of bone, angiosarcoma of bone.
    › Osteoclastic giant-cell-rich tumors.
      » Aneurysmal bone cysts (ABCs). Be aware of secondary ABCs that may arise in association with other primary bone tumors. Be able to identify these 2 lesions: fibrous dysplasia with secondary ABC) and giant cell tumor of bone.
    › Notochordal tumors.
      » Conventional chordoma.
    › Other mesenchymal tumors of bone.
      » Adamantinoma of long bones, fibrous dysplasia, metastatic carcinoma to bone with classic histology.
    › Hematopoietic neoplasms of bone.
      » Plasmacytoma or plasma cell neoplasm, Langerhans cell histiocytosis, Rosai-Dorfman disease.

MUST DO
- For most of the tumors outlined in the Must See section, you should be comfortable generating a differential diagnosis and listing relevant additional ancillary studies.

- Fibroblastic and myofibroblastic tumors are difficult to diagnose on H&E alone, so you should be able to formulate a differential diagnosis and outline the ancillary workup.
- Topics suitable for **written** examination and/or **oral** examination include:
  · Approach to a poorly differentiated tumor, including:
    › Spindle cell pattern.
      » Pediatric age group versus older patients.
    › Epithelioid cell pattern.
    › Pleomorphic pattern.
    › Small round blue cell pattern.
      » Small round blue cell tumor: differential diagnosis and appropriate work up for tumors arising in children versus adults.
    › Biphasic or mixed patterns.
    › Myxoid pattern.
  · Perivascular epithelioid cell tumor (PEComa) in various sites, their syndromic association and prognosis.
  · Kaposi sarcoma: classification, pathogenesis, and how to differentiate it from angiosarcoma.
  · Tumors with:
    › *EWSR1* translocation.
    › *FUS* translocation.
    › *SMARCB1/INI1* loss.
  · Gastrointestinal stromal tissue versus gastric schwannoma.
  · Nonvascular tumors that are often CD34 positive (be able to list 3 to 5).
  · Indications for molecular testing.
  · Osteosarcoma versus fracture.
  · Chondrosarcoma versus enchondroma.
  · Dedifferentiated chondrosarcoma versus chondroblastic osteosarcoma.
  · Grading and staging of bone tumors.
  · Joint revision surgery and frozen section.
- You should be able to independently gross and describe the grossing protocol for:
  · Benign arthroplasty for degenerative joint disease.
  · Femoral head and hip arthroplasty done for pathologic fracture.
  · Synovial joint tissue, including hardware removal.
  · Resection of bone and/or soft tissue for malignancy.
  · Curettage or resection of benign bone and soft tissue lesions.
  · Limb and digit amputations for benign reasons.
  · Limb and digit amputations for malignancy.
  · Skin resections for soft tissue masses.
- You should be able to describe and handle fresh specimens and frozen sections of:
  · Synovial tissue for neutrophil count.
  · Bone biopsy for metabolic diseases.
  · Joint tissue for crystal arthropathies.
- You should be able to take tissue from an oncologic resection for special studies such as FISH, molecular studies, flow cytometry, and electron microscopy.

MULTIPLE CHOICE QUESTIONS

1. What is the most common primary malignancy of bone?
  a. Chondrosarcoma.
  b. Multiple myeloma.
  c. Osteosarcoma.
  d. Metastatic carcinoma.

Answer: b

Note: metastatic carcinoma is not a primary malignancy of bone.

2. Which of the following statements is **not** true regarding an aneurysmal bone cyst?
  a. It can affect any bone.
  b. It is considered a reactive phenomenon.
  c. It can produce a "blow out" appearance on X-ray.
  d. Local recurrence is common.

Answer: b

3. Causes of osteomalacia include all of the following **except**:
  a. Hyperphosphatemia.
  b. Vitamin D deficiency.
  c. X-linked hypophosphatemia.
  d. Malabsorption.

Answer: a

4. The most common type of collagen found in bone is:
  a. Type X collagen.
  b. Type II collagen.
  c. Type I collagen.
  d. Type V collagen.

Answer: c

5. All of the following fractures are classic for nonaccidental injury in a child (i.e., child abuse) **except**:
  a. A "bucket handle" fracture of the proximal tibial metaphysis.
  b. Complex skull fractures.
  c. "Greenstick" fractures of the bones of the forearm.
  d. "String of pearls" rib fractures in paravertebral gutters.

Answer: c

6. What is the prognosis for a patient with a granular cell tumor?
  a. Excellent.
  b. Intermediate, because local recurrences are common.
  c. Late metastases may occur.
  d. Good, but risk of malignant transformation is about 5%.

Answer: a

7. Which combination of immunohistochemical stains is expected in chordoma?
   a. Cytokeratin AE1:3+, EMA+, S100−.
   b. S100+, EMA+, cytokeratin AE1:3−.
   c. Brachyury+, S100+, cytokeratin AE1:3+.
   d. Brachyury−, vimentin+, cytokeratin AE1:3+.

   Answer: c

8. Which of the following statements does **not** describe chondromyxoid fibroma of the bone?
   a. It is a locally aggressive tumor.
   b. It occurs most often in the diaphysis.
   c. Chromosome 6 abnormalities are frequent.
   d. It is SOX9 positive.

   Answer: b

9. The most common causative organism of osteomyelitis in children older than 1 year is:
   a. *Staphylococcus aureus*.
   b. Anaerobic bacteria.
   c. *Haemophilus influenzae*.
   d. Gram-negative organisms.

   Answer: a

10. Risk factors for/associations with rheumatoid arthritis include all of the following **except**:
    a. Major histocompatibility complex (MHC) Class II antigens (DR).
    b. Higher incidence in those of Blackfoot and Pima descent.
    c. Female gender.
    d. MHC Class I antigens.

    Answer: d

11. High grade bone sarcomas metastasize most commonly to which site?
    a. Lymph nodes.
    b. Liver.
    c. Lung.
    d. They do not commonly metastasize to distant sites (local recurrence only).

    Answer: c

12. Approximately how much bone mass must be lost before a routine X-ray will show signs of osteopenia?
    a. 80%.
    b. 10%.
    c. 40%.
    d. 20%.

    Answer: c

13. Ochronosis (alkaptonuria) may result in all of the following findings at postmortem **except**:
    a. Chondromalacia patella.
    b. Black discoloration of the tracheal rings.
    c. Nephrolithiasis.
    d. Vertebral ankylosis.

    Answer: a

14. What is the most common cause of prosthetic joint failure?
    a. Aseptic loosening.
    b. Infection.
    c. Hypersensitivity (allergy) to materials.
    d. Breakage/failure of implant.

    Answer: a

15. Which of the following bone tumors demonstrates immunohistochemical staining with cytokeratin(s)?
    a. Adamantinoma.
    b. Osteofibrous dysplasia.
    c. Chordoma.
    d. All of the above.

    Answer: d

16. What is the most common site for Langerhans cell histiocytosis (eosinophilic granuloma) of bone?
    a. Spine.
    b. Skull (calvarium).
    c. Humerus.
    d. Pelvis.

    Answer: b

17. Which cytogenetic abnormality typifies low grade fibromyxoid sarcoma?
    a. t(12;16).
    b. t(X;18).
    c. t(9;22).
    d. t(7;16).

    Answer: d

18. Which clinical finding is **not** associated with nodular fasciitis?
    a. It occurs commonly in children.
    b. Rapid growth is often seen.
    c. It is found in the subcutaneous tissue.
    d. It may be related to trauma.

    Answer: a

19. The FNCLCC (Fédération Nationale des Centres de Lutte Contre le Cancer) grading system for soft tissue sarcoma:
    a. Includes tumor size as a parameter.
    b. Predicts local recurrence rate.
    c. Predicts likelihood of distant metastasis.
    d. Provides information on tumor extent.

    Answer: c

20. FNCLCC grading is **not** recommended for which of the following soft tissue sarcomas?
    a. Synovial sarcoma.
    b. Alveolar soft part sarcoma.
    c. Myxoid liposarcoma.
    d. Extraskeletal Ewing sarcoma.

    Answer: b

21. Alveolar soft-part sarcoma demonstrates which of the following ultrastructural features?
    a. Weibel-Palade bodies.
    b. Rhomboidal crystals.
    c. Birbeck granules.
    d. Paranuclear aggregates of intermediate filaments.

    Answer: b

22. Desmoid fibromatosis are associated with an abnormality in which cellular pathway?

a. ERBB2 (formerly HER2/neu).

b. Fibroblast growth factor receptor (FGFR).

c. c-KIT signaling.

d. Adenomatosis polyposis (APC)/β-catenin.

Answer: d

23. Which of the following combinations of immunohistochemical markers might be positive in a leiomyosarcoma?

a. Desmin, actin, (focal) cytokeratin.

b. Desmin, c-KIT, caldesmon.

c. Caldesmon, actin, S100 protein.

d. Calretinin, desmin, actin.

Answer: a

24. Which virus may be implicated in the formation of smooth muscle tumors?

a. Polyoma virus.

b. Human papilloma virus (HPV).

c. Human herpes virus 8 (HHV-8).

d. Epstein-Barr virus.

Answer: d

25. What is the appropriate treatment for an atypical neurofibroma?

a. Radiation followed by wide excision.

b. Curettage.

c. Chemotherapy, radiotherapy, and wide excision.

d. Local excision with a thin margin.

Answer: d

26. A palisading granuloma with central mucin deposition is most characteristic of:

a. Necrobiosis lipoidica.

b. Fungal infection.

c. Granuloma annulare.

d. Rheumatoid nodule.

Answer: c

27. Lyme disease is associated with all of the following **except**:

a. Erythema nodosum.

b. Borrelia burgdorferi.

c. Transmission via arthropods.

d. Synovitis.

Answer: a

28. The Carney complex includes all of the following **except**:

a. Superficial angiomyxomas.

b. Involvement of the Rb locus on chromosome 17.

c. Spotty pigmentation of the skin.

d. Endocrine overactivity.

Answer: b

29. The most common site of (extramammary) myofibroblastoma is:

a. Paratesticular region.

b. Lymph nodes.

c. Kidney.

d. Inguinal region.

Answer: d

30. All of the following are subtypes of rhabdomyoma **except**:

a. Embryonal type.

b. Adult type.

c. Genital type.

d. Fetal type.

Answer: a

31. Which of the following abnormalities characterizes dermatofibrosarcoma protuberans (DFSP)?

a. t(11;22).

b. t(11;17).

c. Supernumerary ring chromosomes.

d. Trisomy 12.

Answer: c

32. Which of the following rhabdomyosarcoma subtypes is not a poor prognosis subtype?

a. Pleomorphic rhabdomyosarcoma.

b. Embryonal rhabdomyosarcoma.

c. Alveolar rhabdomyosarcoma.

d. *MYOD1*-mutant spindle cell/sclerosing rhabdomyosarcoma.

Answer: b

33. Which of the following soft tissue sarcomas does **not** typically demonstrate an *EWSR1* gene fusion?

a. Infantile fibrosarcoma.

b. Clear cell sarcoma.

c. Desmoplastic small round cell tumor.

d. Extraskeletal myxoid chondrosarcoma.

Answer: a

34. Which of the following genetic syndromes are not associated with osteosarcoma?

a. Li-Fraumeni syndrome.

b. Werner Syndrome.

c. Retinoblastoma syndrome.

d. McCune-Albright syndrome.

Answer: d

35. Which of the following soft tissue tumors would not demonstrate loss of staining with SMARCB1 (INI1)?

a. Epithelioid sarcoma.

b. Malignant rhabdoid tumor.

c. Epithelioid malignant peripheral nerve sheath tumor (MPNST).

d. Epithelioid angiosarcoma.

Answer: d

36. Which of the following primary bone lesions do **not** typically occur in the epiphysis?

a. Giant cell tumor of bone.

b. Clear cell chondrosarcoma.

c. Chondroblastoma.

d. Nonossifying fibroma.

Answer: d

37. Which soft tissue tumor often metastasizes to other soft tissue sites?

a. Well-differentiated liposarcoma.
b. Epithelioid schwannoma.
c. Myxoid liposarcoma.
d. Solitary fibrous tumor.

Answer: c

38. Which benign adipocytic tumor is characterized by numerous true lipoblasts?

a. Chondroid lipoma.
b. Hibernoma.
c. Myelolipoma.
d. None of the above: true lipoblasts are diagnostic of well-differentiated liposarcoma.

Answer a

39. Which subtype of rhabdomyosarcoma occurs most commonly occurs in the head and neck?

a. Alveolar.
b. Pleomorphic.
c. Embryonal.
d. Spindle/sclerosing.

Answer: c

40. Nonspecific, strong, and diffuse cytoplasmic staining can be seen in formalin-fixed, paraffin-embedded (FFPE) tissue with which myogenic marker?

a. Myoglobin.
b. Myogenin.
c. Desmin.
d. MyoD1.

Answer: d

41. Nuclear β-catenin immunoreactivity may be seen in which of the following tumors?

a. Deep fibromatosis.
b. Synovial sarcoma.
c. Solitary fibrous tumor.
d. All of the above.

Answer: d

42. A 30-year-old woman presents with an enlarging mass involving the body of the mandible. Biopsy demonstrates a high grade malignant cartilaginous tumor. Your preferred diagnosis is:

a. Chondroblastic osteosarcoma.
b. Sarcomatoid carcinoma.
c. Chondrosarcoma.
d. Metastatic chondrosarcoma.

Answer: a

43. Which of the following syndromes is **not** associated with chondrosarcoma?

a. Maffucci syndrome.
b. Gardner syndrome.
c. Ollier syndrome.
d. Multiple osteochondromas.

Answer: b

SHORT ANSWER QUESTIONS

Soft Tissue Pathology
General Considerations

44. What is the most common site of a soft tissue sarcoma?

Most sarcomas (75%) of sarcomas are located in extremities.

45. What distance is considered to be an "adequate" resection margin in a soft tissue sarcoma?

2 cm.

46. When submitting tissue from a soft tissue tumor for cytogenetic and molecular studies, how much tissue is required? How are the specimens stored, and how are they shipped?

- Most molecular studies, including polymerase chain reaction (PCR), next-generation sequencing (NGS), and fluorescence in situ hybridization (FISH), can be performed using FFPE tissues. If tumor is identified on a routine H&E slide and deemed adequate (in general > 0.3 cm area of viable tumor on the slide is considered adequate), the tumor can then be microdissected from the block. If the slide shows only tumor, curls from the block can be performed.

- Cytogenetics requires a 1 cm³ sample, which is snap frozen in a plastic vial.
  · Frozen tissue should be stored at −70°C.
  · Frozen tissue should remain frozen and therefore should be shipped on dry ice.
- Note that fresh tissue can also be stored and shipped in media such as RPMI.

47. List 3 clinical parameters helpful in distinguishing benign from malignant soft tissue tumors.

- Rate of growth.
- Tumor size (> 5 cm).
- Depth: superficial/above fascia versus deep/below fascia).

48. Describe the FNCLCC (Fédération nationale des centres de lutte contre le cancer) grading system for soft tissue sarcomas.

- The FNCLCC grade is based on the assessment of 3 independent prognostic factors:
  - Differentiation.
  - Necrosis.
  - Mitotic activity (count per 10 high power fields).
- A score is assigned to each parameter and the scores are added to produce a tumor grade.
- The most challenging component is assigning a differentiation score.

49. List at least 3 sarcomas for which grading is less informative than the histologic type of tumor.

- Grading is less informative for these sarcomas:
  - Epithelioid sarcoma.
  - Alveolar soft part sarcoma.
  - Ewing sarcoma.
  - Clear cell sarcoma.
  - Rhabdomyosarcoma.
- Controversies also exist around grading of malignant peripheral nerve sheath tumor and angiosarcoma.

50. Outline the American Joint Committee on Cancer (AJCC) staging system* for soft tissue sarcoma of the trunk and extremities.

Primary tumor (T):

TX: primary tumor cannot be assessed.

T0: no evidence of primary tumor.

T1: tumor ≤ 5 cm in greatest dimension.

T2: tumor > 5 cm and ≤ 10 cm in greatest dimension.

T3: tumor > 10 cm and ≤ 15 cm in greatest dimension.

T4: tumor > 15 cm in greatest dimension.

Regional lymph nodes (N):

N0: no regional lymph node metastasis or unknown lymph node status.

N1: regional lymph node metastasis.

Distant metastasis (M):

M0: no distant metastasis.

M1: distant metastasis.

*This chapter uses the eighth edition of the AJCC staging manual.

Case Scenario

A biopsy from a large soft tissue paravertebral mass in a 2-year-old male demonstrates a "small round blue cell tumor."

51. List the top 4 entities in your differential diagnosis given the clinical information.

- Ewing sarcoma/primitive neuroectodermal tumor (PNET).
- (Metastatic) neuroblastoma.
- Malignant lymphoma/leukemia.
- Alveolar rhabdomyosarcoma.

52. How would your differential diagnosis change if the biopsy with small round blue cell tumor morphology were from a 65-year-old patient? From a 25-year-old patient?

- 65-year-old:
  - Neuroendocrine tumor/carcinoma (i.e., Merkel cell carcinoma).
  - Melanoma.
  - Lymphoma.
  - Sarcoma (less likely).
- 25-year-old:
  - Alveolar rhabdomyosarcoma.
  - Ewing sarcoma/primitive neuroectodermal tumor (PNET).
  - Melanoma.
  - Lymphoma/leukemia.
  - Carcinoma (less likely).

53. What immunohistochemical stains would be most helpful in distinguishing the entities in question 51?

- CD99 (O13).
- CD45 (leukocyte common antigen: LCA), terminal deoxynucleotidyl transferase (TdT).
- Synaptophysin, chromogranin, or glial fibrillary acidic protein (GFAP).
- Desmin, actin, or MyoD1/myogenin.

54. List 3 ancillary lab tests that might be helpful in making a diagnosis of Ewing sarcoma/PNET. Specify the abnormality you would be testing for in each example.

- Conventional cytogenetics for t(11;22).
- FISH for *EWSR1*.
- NGS and/or PCR for *EWSR1-FLI1* fusion or other transcripts (e.g., *EWSR1-ERG* fusion).

Case Scenario

A 60-year-old man presents with a rapidly growing nodule in his cheek. Excisional biopsy demonstrates a hypercellular spindle cell proliferation with scattered atypical spindle cells. There are readily identified mitoses and necrosis.

55. What is your main differential diagnosis?

- Sarcomatoid carcinoma (spindle cell squamous cell carcinoma) (arising from the skin or buccal mucosa).
- Spindle melanoma.
- Spindled salivary gland tumor.
- True spindled sarcoma (i.e., leiomyosarcoma).
- Other: although the nodule is most likely malignant, consider nonmalignant entities like nodular fasciitis.

56. What steps would you perform to distinguish the entities in your differential diagnosis?

- Review imaging findings (identify imaging characteristics of the lesion).
- Review clinical findings — Are there overlying skin or mucosal changes? Is there ulceration?
- Check for a prior history of carcinoma or skin procedures (i.e., liquid nitrogen removal of skin lesions).
- Sarcomatoid carcinoma:
  · Closely assess overlying skin/mucosa for dysplasia.
  · Submit more sections/cut deeper sections to identify a focus of residual conventional squamous cell carcinoma.
  · Obtain immunohistochemical stains for epithelial markers performed on several blocks:
    › Cytokeratin-5 (CK5), cytokeratin 34 beta E12 (Ck43βE12 [ker903]), p40, pancytokeratin.
- Spindle melanoma:
  · Closely assess overlying skin for an atypical melanocytic proliferation.

- Obtain immunohistochemical stains for melanocytic markers:
  › S100 protein, SOX10, human melanoma black 45 (HMB45), Melan-A.
    » In desmoplastic melanoma, SOX10 is the most reliable marker.
- Spindle salivary gland tumor:
  · Most often it is the myoepithelial cells that may have a spindled morphology.
  · In addition to S100 protein and SOX10 (which are also myoepithelial markers), add muscle-specific actin (MSA), smooth muscle actin (SMA), and calponin.
- True sarcoma:
  · Assess morphologic clues for lineage (i.e., eosinophilic spindle cells with cigar-shaped nuclei arranged in intersecting fascicles for leiomyosarcoma).
  · In addition to the above immunohistochemical stains, you may consider adding desmin, h-caldesmon, CD34, and ERG.

Adipocytic Tumors

57. Which adipocytic tumor may be fluorodeoxyglucose (FDG) avid on positron emission tomography (PET)?

- Hibernoma.
- Hibernomas, which are tumors of brown fat, are metabolically active, and may be incidentally found during PET scans performed for tumor staging.

58. Which adipocytic tumor can present as multiple painful subcutaneous lesions? Describe its histologic features.

- Angiolipoma.
  · Angiolipoma is in the category of painful lesions covered by the mnemonic BEGAL CO: **b**lue rubber bleb nevus, **e**ccrine spiradenoma, **n**eurilemmoma/**n**euroma, **g**lomus tumor, **a**ngiolipoma/**a**ngioleiomyoma/**a**ngiosarcoma, **l**eiomyoma, **c**utaneous endometriosis/**c**alcinosis cutis, **o**steoma cutis.

- Histologic features:
  · These tumors have a mixture of mature adipose tissue and branching capillaries, some of which contain fibrin thrombi.
  · Vascularity is more prominent at the periphery of lobules.
  · Proportion of capillaries is variable.

59. What is a lipoblast?

Lipid-containing mono- or multivacuolated immature adipocyte in which the vacuole(s) scallop or indent the nucleus.

60. List 3 potential mimics of lipoblasts.
- Brown fat.
- Fat atrophy.
- Lochkern cells.
- Histiocytes/foreign body giant cells.
- Signet-ring cell carcinoma.

61. Describe common features of spindle cell lipoma and pleomorphic lipoma.
- About 80% occur in the posterior neck and upper back.
- They represent a histologic spectrum.
  - Spindle cell lipoma:
    - Variable mixture of short spindle cells and adipocytes.
    - "Low fat" or "fat free" variants with < 5% fat.
    - Ropey, wire-like collagen, variable myxoid stroma.
    - Possible hemangiopericytoma-like vessels (pseudoangiomatous variant).
- Pleomorphic lipoma:
  - All of the features listed above in spindle cell lipoma, along with:
    - » Floret-like multinucleated giant cells.
    - » Pleomorphic spindle cells.
- Spindle cells and floret cells are CD34 positive.

62. Describe the histologic features required for the diagnosis of liposarcoma.
- Atypical lipomatous tumor/well-differentiated liposarcoma (ALT/WDLPS):
  - This consists of lobules of fat separated by fibrous septae.
  - It often has thick-walled vessels.
  - Large atypical, hyperchromatic cells are preferentially found in fibrous septae and within the vessel walls.
  - Lipoblasts are **not** required for the diagnosis.
- Dedifferentiated liposarcoma:
  - This may have a residual ALT/WDLPS component with progression to (usually) a nonlipogenic sarcoma of variable histologic grade.
  - There is typically an abrupt transition between the dedifferentiated component and the residual well-differentiated component.
- Dedifferentiation may occur in the primary or in recurrence.
- A residual well-differentiated component may not be identified.
- Rarely, the high grade (dedifferentiated) component may be lipogenic.
- Pleomorphic liposarcoma:
  - This is a high grade, typically pleomorphic, undifferentiated sarcoma with nonspecific immunohistochemical findings.
  - The diagnostic feature is the lipoblast.
    - The lipoblast may be multivacuolated or univacuolated.

63. What is the differential diagnosis for a tumor demonstrating a pleomorphic sarcoma pattern (also known as MFH-like pattern)?
- Pleomorphic sarcoma with specific lineage proven by immunohistochemistry (IHC) — i.e., pleomorphic leiomyosarcoma.
  - Pleomorphic leiomyosarcoma demonstrates smooth muscle differentiation via IHC.
- Dedifferentiated sarcoma (i.e., dedifferentiated liposarcoma).
- Pseudosarcoma (i.e., sarcomatoid carcinoma, melanoma, anaplastic large cell lymphoma, etc.).
  - Pseudosarcomas may also include benign soft tissue lesions that can mimic sarcoma including ischemic fasciitis, ancient schwannoma, and nodular fasciitis.
- Undifferentiated pleomorphic sarcoma.
  - When the above 3 have been eliminated, you are left with an undifferentiated pleomorphic sarcoma.

64. List at least 4 indications for molecular testing, specifically FISH testing for *MDM2* amplification, in adipocytic tumors.
- Recurrent "lipomas."
- Deep lipomas (below fascia) without atypia > 15 cm.
  - Deep extremity lesions > 10 cm in patients more than 50 years of age.
- Adipocytic tumors with equivocal cytologic atypia.
- Retroperitoneal or intraabdominal adipocytic tumors lacking cytologic atypia.
- Special clinical situations as directed by treating clinicians.[1]

65. List the most common sites of liposarcoma.
- Retroperitoneum.
- Thigh; buttock (more often than arm); trunk or abdomen.
- Scrotum/groin.

66. What are the 3 main histologic subtypes of a well-differentiated liposarcoma?
- Adipocytic (lipoma-like).
- Sclerosing.
- Inflammatory.

67. List the clinical, microscopic, and cytogenetic features of the myxoid subtype of liposarcoma.

DIAGNOSTIC CATEGORY	FEATURES
Clinical	• Young to middle-aged adults (fourth to fifth decades). • Large deep tumors (> 10 cm). • Most often involve thigh, buttock, knee, and lower leg. • Retroperitoneal lesions (these most often represent metastasis).

Microscopic	• Lobulated tumor of uniform, small, and bland round oval cells with ill-defined cytoplasm that typically condense at the periphery of the lobules.
	• Univacuolar (signet ring-type) lipoblasts.
	• Myxoid matrix with or without cystic change and a prominent plexiform pattern of thin-walled capillaries.
	• Mitoses and necrosis — rare.
	• High grade myxoid liposarcoma (formerly round cell liposarcoma):
	  · Diminished myxoid matrix.
	  · Obscured vasculature.
	  · Increased nuclear grade.
	  · Increased mitotic activity.

Cytogenetics	• t(12;16)(q13;p11)(*FUS/DDIT3*) more common than t(12;22)(*EWSR1/DDIT3*).

68. What percentage of hypercellularity (also known as round cell change) in myxoid liposarcoma is associated with a poor prognosis?

5%.

69. Myxoid liposarcoma may be treated with neoadjuvant therapy. What common histologic features are seen in a treated myxoid liposarcoma?

• Maturation into mature (white) adipose tissue.
• Stromal hyalinization.
• Marked decrease in cellularity.

70. Give the current classification of liposarcoma, along with a brief description of the prognosis.

• Well-differentiated liposarcoma/atypical lipomatous tumor.
  · Prognosis:
   › This has no metastatic potential without dedifferentiation.
   › Prognosis depends on location:
    » Peripherally located tumors (i.e., extremities, trunk):
     »» This is cured by complete local excision (margins clear).
     »» Atypical lipomatous tumor terminology is more appropriate in these locations.
    » Deep tumors (e.g., retroperitoneum, mediastinal):
     »» This has a greater potential for progression through dedifferentiation.
     »» Well-differentiated liposarcoma terminology is more appropriate in these locations.
     »» These recur locally and repeatedly.
     »» Death can be due to local effects (i.e., obstruction).
     »» Death can result from metastasis following dedifferentiation (up to 20% in retroperitoneal tumors).

• Dedifferentiated liposarcoma.
  · Prognosis:
   › 40% of dedifferentiated liposarcomas recur locally and the mortality rate is ~30%.
   › Distant metastasis occurs in 15–20% of cases.
   › The most important prognostic factor is anatomic location.

   › Retroperitoneal location is associated with worst prognosis.

• Myxoid liposarcoma.
  · Prognosis:
   › Prognosis depends on histologic grade (i.e., percentage of hypercellularity [round cell component]:
    » Low grade myxoid liposarcoma:
     »» This confers an intermediate prognosis with a propensity for local recurrence (12–25% of cases).
     »» Distant metastasis can develop years after initial diagnosis.
    » Higher grade tumors (> 5% hypercellularity):
     »» These have higher rates of metastasis and death from disease.

• Pleomorphic liposarcoma.
  · Prognosis:
   › The local recurrence and metastatic rate is 30–50%.
   › The 5-year survival rate is about 60%.

• Myxoid pleomorphic liposarcoma.
  · Prognosis:
   › This is an aggressive tumor with high recurrence rate, frequent metastasis (lung, bone, soft tissue), and poor overall survival.
   › Note that this tumor is extremely rare; typically occurs in children and adolescents; has histologic features of myxoid liposarcoma and pleomorphic liposarcoma; and lacks a characteristic molecular alteration.

Fibroblastic and Myofibroblastic Tumors

NODULAR FASCIITIS

71. List the 3 most common sites of nodular fasciitis. What age group is most often affected? What is a typical presentation of nodular fasciitis?
- Sites: upper extremity, trunk, and head and neck.
- Age group: young adults (usually).
- Typical presentation: rapidly growing lesion of short duration.

72. Name 2 subtypes of nodular fasciitis. Which of these subtypes most often occurs in infants (younger than 2 years)?
- Subtypes include intravascular fasciitis and cranial fasciitis.
- Cranial fasciitis most often occurs in infants.

73. List 5 microscopic features of nodular fasciitis.
- It has loose, myxoid stroma with microcystic changes and areas of hypercellularity.
- It has plump, spindled fibroblasts/myofibroblasts with tapering cytoplasmic processes (tissue culture), arranged in a storiform or fascicular pattern.
- It may be mitotically active, but mitoses are normal and there is no significant nuclear pleomorphism.
- It is well-defined but focally infiltrative.
- Extravasated red blood cells (RBCs) may be present.
- Other findings include osteoclast-like giant cells, inflammatory cells, and hyalinization/fibrosis in longer-standing lesions.

74. What is the characteristic molecular finding in nodular fasciitis?
MYH9-USP6 gene fusion.

75. Name at least 3 entities that may enter into the differential diagnosis of nodular fasciitis.
- Fibromatosis (desmoid).
- Dermatofibrosarcoma protuberans.
- Low grade myofibroblastic sarcoma.
- Benign fibrous histiocytoma.

ISCHEMIC FASCIITIS

76. Define ischemic fasciitis.
Ischemic fasciitis is a pseudoneoplastic, reactive fibroblastic proliferation that is related to age and ischemic conditions.

77. Give the typical clinical presentation of ischemic fasciitis.
- It occurs in elderly individuals (~80 years old), who are often bedridden.
- It has a predilection for soft tissue overlying bony prominences (hip, shoulder, back, chest wall).
- Skin overlying the lesion (based in subcutis) is hyperemic.

78. Identify the histologic features that allow distinction of ischemic fasciitis from soft tissue sarcoma.

HISTOLOGIC FEATURE	ISCHEMIC FASCIITIS	SARCOMA
Presence of necrosis	• Central fibrinous cavity surrounded by capillaries.	• Coagulative necrosis.
Cytological atypia	• Mild.	• Moderate, marked.
Mitotic activity	• Mild–moderate, rarely atypical mitoses.	• Moderate–high, atypical mitoses common.
Other	• Zones of "arcade-like" capillary proliferation.	

ELASTOFIBROMA

79. Which age group is commonly affected by elastofibroma? What is the most common anatomic site?
- The elderly are commonly affected.
- The most common site is the lower scapula (thoracic wall).

DERMATOFIBROSARCOMA PROTUBERANS

80. List at least 2 gross features of dermatofibrosarcoma protuberans (DFSP).
- Early skin lesion is plaque-like, indurated, and fibrous.
- It may also form a sharply circumscribed pigmented nodule on the skin or in the dermis; can appear with multiple nodules that protrude from the skin surface.
- On sectioning, it is firm, fibrous and gray-white with or without a whorled appearance.

81. List at least 4 histologic findings of DFSP.
- Involves dermis and subcutaneous adipose tissue.
- Shows infiltrative pattern into fat ("string of pearls"); grows along fibrous septae ("honeycomb" pattern).
- Does not show epidermal hyperplasia.
- Shows relatively bland, uniform fibroblasts arranged in a storiform pattern.
- Lacks significant atypia, necrosis, high mitotic rate, and secondary elements (e.g., foam cells).
- May show collagen trapping, myxoid change, or vascular myointimal proliferation.

82. What immunohistochemical stains can differentiate DFSP from dermatofibroma?
- Dermatofibroma is typically positive for FXIIIa and negative for CD34.
- DFSP is uniformly positive for CD34 and negative for FXIIIa.

83. What is the prognosis for a patient with DFSP?
- DFSP is considered a low grade sarcoma.
- The prognosis is excellent if completely excised with clear margins.
- Local recurrence rate is high if incompletely excised.
- Rarely, DFSP can develop into fibrosarcoma. If low grade, this carries a small risk of distant metastases (~5%). If high grade (resembling undifferentiated pleomorphic sarcoma), the prognosis is poor.

84. Describe the common features of malignant (sarcomatous) transformation in DFSP.
- Sarcomatous transformation is most often represented by fibrosarcomatous transformation.
- There is typically an abrupt transition from a storiform arrangement of spindle cells to fibrosarcoma (herring-bone) arrangement of spindle cells of variable atypia.
- There is often a loss of CD34 staining in fibrosarcomatous areas.

FIBROMATOSIS

85. Name the 3 types of superficial fibromatosis.
- Palmar (also known as Dupuytren contracture).
- Plantar (also known as Ledderhose disease).
- Penile (also known as Peyronie disease).

86. Which syndrome can be associated with desmoid fibromatosis?
Gardner syndrome/familial adenomatous polyposis.

87. What is the most common site for desmoid fibromatosis?
Extremities.

88. List at least 1 etiologic, nongenetic factor associated with desmoid fibromatosis.
- Recent or current pregnancy.
- Prior trauma or surgery in region of desmoid fibromatosis.

INFLAMMATORY MYOFIBROBLASTIC TUMOR

89. What is the most common site of inflammatory myofibroblastic tumor?
Intraabdominal soft tissues.

90. Describe the 3 histologic patterns of inflammatory myofibroblastic tumor.
- Myxoid pattern:
  · Plump myofibroblasts in an edematous, myxoid background, with abundant blood vessels and mixed inflammatory cell infiltrate.
  · Mimics granulation tissue or reactive process.
- Hypercellular pattern:
  · Hypercellular spindle cell proliferation in a compact fascicular pattern with variable myxoid and collagenous stroma and inflammatory infiltrate.
- Hypocellular fibrous pattern:
  · Hypocellular spindle cell proliferation in a hyalinized collagenous stroma and scant inflammatory cell population.
  · Mimics fibromatosis.

91. What percentage of inflammatory myofibroblastic tumor is immunoreactive for ALK?
- 50–60% of cases.

· There is a strong correlation of ALK immunoreactivity with *ALK* gene rearrangements.

92. Name the subtype of inflammatory myofibroblastic tumor that has a more aggressive clinical course.
Epithelioid inflammatory myofibroblastic sarcoma.

93. Describe the prognosis of an extrapulmonary inflammatory myofibroblastic tumor.
- It has a 25% recurrence rate.
- Inflammatory myofibroblastic tumors that are negative for anaplastic lymphoma kinase (ALK) have higher rates of metastasis.

- Epithelioid inflammatory myofibroblastic sarcoma has a more aggressive clinical course.

SOLITARY FIBROUS TUMOR

94. Describe the histologic features of solitary fibrous tumor and name 2 morphologic variants.
- Solitary fibrous tumor is a well-delineated, unencapsulated tumor composed of ovoid-to-spindled fibroblastic cells with pale-to-eosinophilic cytoplasm.
- Tumor cells are arranged in a "patternless pattern":
  · Alternating collagenized and hypercellular areas are present.
  · Thick bands of hyalinized/keloidal collagen with "cracking" are present.
- The tumor may be myxoid.

- There are hemangiopericytoma-like (HPC-like) vessels with or without perivascular hyalinization.
- Solitary fibrous tumor has 2 morphologic variants:
  · Giant cell solitary fibrous tumor (formerly giant cell angiofibroma), which has multinucleate stromal cells and pseudovascular spaces.
    › This often involves the orbit.
  · Fat-forming solitary fibrous tumor, which has prominent adipocytic component.

95. Name 1 highly specific immunohistochemical stain for solitary fibrous tumor, and 1 sensitive, but not specific, immunohistochemical stain for solitary fibrous tumor. Describe their staining patterns.
- Specific immunostain: STAT6 (nuclear).
- Sensitive, not-specific immunostain: CD34 (cytoplasmic).

· Others include BCL-2 and CD99, and immunostains for epithelial membrane antigen (EMA) and SMA (for which these tumors are variably positive).

96. What is the characteristic cytogenetic abnormality found in solitary fibrous tumor?
Recurrent *NAB2-STAT6* gene fusion (inv12 [q13q13]) is implicated in almost all solitary fibrous tumor (benign and malignant).

97. Describe the behavior of solitary fibrous tumor and any features that may be associated with a worse outcome.
- Typically, these tumors have an indolent course.
- Metastasis occurs in 5–25% of cases.
  · Metastasis is difficult to predict based on histology.
  · Conventional grading systems (i.e., FNCLCC) and sarcoma staging systems (i.e., AJCC) are poorly applicable to solitary fibrous tumor.

· Risk stratification models exist that assesses clinical and histologic features to predict behavior.
- Features associated with a worse outcome include older age (older than 55), larger tumor size, increased mitoses, and tumor necrosis.

LOW GRADE FIBROMYXOID SARCOMA (EVANS TUMOR)

98. List at least 3 microscopic features of a low grade fibromyxoid sarcoma. What is the most common molecular alteration?
- Microscopic features:
  · Bland spindle cells (translocation sarcoma — uniform spindle cells with minimal atypia).
  · Alternating myxoid and fibrous areas ("tiger stripe").

· Prominent arching vessels.
· Collagen rosettes (30% of cases).
- Most common genetic alteration:
  · Gene fusion of *FUS-CREB3L*.

99. Low grade fibromyxoid sarcoma is closely related to, and overlaps with, which other sarcoma?
Sclerosing epithelioid fibrosarcoma.

100. Name 1 sensitive and specific immunohistochemical stain for low grade fibromyxoid sarcoma.
MUC4.

101. List 2 possible causes of adult fibrosarcoma.
- Previous irradiation.
- Implanted foreign material.

102. List the diagnostic features of adult fibrosarcoma.
- Immunohistochemical and molecular diagnosis of exclusion.
- Hypercellular, atypical spindle cell proliferation arranged in a herringbone or fascicular architecture.
- Variable collagen production.
- Fibroblastic (focal myofibroblastic) differentiation.

So-called Fibrohistiocytic Tumors

103. Describe the characteristic histologic features of a tenosynovial giant cell tumor.
- Consists of variable proportions of mononuclear cells, osteoclast-like (multinucleated) giant cells, foamy macrophages, inflammatory cells, hemosiderin deposition and stromal fibrosis/collagenization.
- Localized-type tenosynovial giant cell tumor (also known as giant cell tumor of tendon sheath): lobulated and well circumscribed.
- Diffuse-type tenosynovial giant cell tumor (also known as pigmented villonodular synovitis):
  · Infiltrative features, arranged in diffuse, expansile sheets.
  · Cleft-like spaces.
  · Osteoclast-like giant cells that may be more difficult to identify (sparse).
- Malignant tenosynovial giant cell tumor:
  · Increased mitoses including atypical forms, necrosis.
  · Enlarged nuclei with nucleoli.
  · Spindling of mononuclear cells.
  · Occasionally, areas that resemble a myxofibrosarcoma or undifferentiated pleomorphic sarcoma.

104. What is the prognosis of diffuse-type tenosynovial giant cell tumor?
- The local recurrence rate is 40–60%.
- Multiple recurrences may compromise joint function.
- Very rare cases may develop metastatic disease to lungs or lymph nodes.

105. Describe the microscopic features of giant cell tumor of soft tissue. What is the prognosis of this tumor?
- This tumor arises in the superficial soft tissues of the extremities. Microscopically, it is similar to giant cell tumor of bone.
- Microscopic features include:
  · Multinodular proliferation of osteoclast-like giant cells and mononuclear cells in a richly vascular stroma.
  · Hemosiderin-laden macrophages.
  · Mitotically active.
  · Vascular invasion (~30% of tumors).
- It has a local recurrence rate of 12%; metastasis is very rare.

Vascular Tumors

106. What is the causative agent of Kaposi sarcoma?
Human herpesvirus 8 (HHV-8), also known as Kaposi sarcoma–associated herpesvirus.

107. List the 4 clinical-epidemiological types of Kaposi sarcoma. Identify the corresponding clinical groups, location of lesions, and disease course for each group.

TYPE	CLINICAL GROUPS	LESION LOCATION	DISEASE COURSE
Classic (indolent)	• Elderly males of eastern European, Ashkenazi Jewish or Mediterranean descent.	• Skin of lower legs.	• Indolent.
Endemic (African)	• Non-HIV infected children and middle-aged men from equatorial Africa.	• Skin of extremities. • Possibly viscera (lymph nodes in children).	• Indolent, protracted course in adults. • Lymphadenopathic form in African children: aggressive.

(continued on next page)

TYPE	CLINICAL GROUPS	LESION LOCATION	DISEASE COURSE
Iatrogenic	• Immunosuppressed individuals (e.g., solid organ transplant patients).	• Skin of lower legs. • Possibly viscera.	• Unpredictable: may resolve upon withdrawal of immunosuppressive therapy.
AIDS associated	• HIV-1 individuals.	• Widespread involvement of skin: face, lower extremities, genitalia. • Widespread involvement of viscera: lungs, G/I tract, lymph nodes, oral mucosa.	• Aggressive.

108. Describe the clinical presentation of epithelioid hemangioendothelioma.
- Common sites of involvement are soft tissue, lung, and liver.
- The tumor may be solitary or multifocal:
  - Solitary: skin and soft tissue lesions.
  - Multifocal: viscera and bone.

109. Name 1 genetic alteration identified in epithelioid hemangioendothelioma.
- *WWTR1-CAMTA1* gene fusion (more common).
- *YAP1-TFE3* gene fusion.

110. List at least 3 microscopic features of epithelioid hemangioendothelioma.
- Cords or nests of epithelioid cells.
- Cytoplasmic vacuolization (may contain red blood cells).
- Myxochondroid or hyaline stroma.
- Minimal atypia, infrequent mitoses.

111. List at least 3 risk factors for angiosarcoma.
- Postradiation.
- Long-standing lymphedema.
- Implanted foreign material.
- Areas of prior trauma.
- Heterologous component of another sarcoma (i.e., malignant peripheral nerve sheath tumor).
- Maffucci syndrome, neurofibromatosis, Klippel-Trenaunay syndrome.

112. List at least 4 diagnostic features of angiosarcoma.
- Vasoformative or sheet-like growth of endothelial cells.
- Multilayering of endothelial cells.
- Variable endothelial cell atypia.
- Increased mitoses with or without necrosis.
- Expression of vascular markers including ERG (nuclear), CD34 (variable), CD31 (membranous).
  - Epithelioid angiosarcoma may demonstrate keratin and EMA expression.
  - Strong MYC expression is present in lymphedema-associated and postradiation angiosarcoma.

113. *MYC* gene amplifications occur in which angiosarcomas?
- Postradiation angiosarcoma.
- Lymphedema-associated angiosarcoma.

114. List at least 1 other tumor in the "intermediate" vascular category, 2 in the "benign" vascular category, and 1 in the "malignant" vascular category.
- Intermediate:
  - Locally aggressive:
    › Kaposiform hemangioendothelioma.
  - Rarely metastasizing:
    › Retiform or composite hemangioendothelioma; papillary intralymphatic angioendothelioma; pseudomyogenic (epithelioid-sarcoma-like) hemangioendothelioma; Kaposi sarcoma.
- Benign: hemangioma, epithelioid hemangioma, lymphangioma, angiomatosis.
- Malignant: epithelioid hemangioendothelioma, angiosarcoma of soft tissue.

Pericytic Tumors

115. Define pericytic tumor.
Tumors composed of both vessels and perivascular myoid cells (pericytes).

116. Which lesions represent true hemangiopericytic tumors?
- Myopericytoma.
- Myofibroma(tosis) (infantile hemangiopericytoma).
- Glomus tumor.
- Angioleiomyoma (vascular leiomyoma).
- Sinonasal-type hemangiopericytoma (glomangiopericytoma).

117. What is the classic location for a glomus tumor?

The subungual region of a finger or toe.

118. List 2 histological features that are needed to make a diagnosis of "malignant" glomus tumor.

- Marked cytologic atypia in the presence of mitotic activity.
- The presence of atypical mitoses.

119. Describe the pattern of staining of collagen IV in glomus tumor. List at least 2 other helpful immunohistochemical stains.

- Collagen IV immunohistochemical staining pattern: pericellular staining (highlights basement membrane material produced by lesional cells).
- Other helpful immunohistochemical stains: SMA and MSA (glomus tumor stains positive); CD34 (glomus tumor shows focal or absent staining).

120. Describe the clinical features of myofibroma.

- A subset of these tumors is familial.
- They may present as solitary or multicentric (myofibromatosis) lesions.
  - Solitary lesions typically involve skin and muscle.
- Multiple lesions typically involve skin, viscera, muscle, and bone.
- They occur in patients of all ages, commonly infants (congenital) and children.

121. Describe the microscopic and immunohistochemical features of myofibroma.

- Superficial lesions tend to be circumscribed; deep lesions are more infiltrative.
- The lesions are nodular or multinodular with a biphasic pattern of light and dark staining areas:
  - Light areas: periphery; plump myoid spindle cells arranged in short fascicles or whorls.
  - Dark areas: center; oval-spindle cells with dark nuclei.
- The lesions have a hemangiopericytoma-like vascular pattern.
- IHC features include:
  - SMA positive, variable MSA staining.
  - Negative for desmin, h-caldesmon, keratins, and neural markers.

122. Name the lesion that exists on a morphologic spectrum with myofibroma.

Myopericytoma.

123. List the microscopic features of myopericytoma.

- Bland, myoid spindle cells.
- Multilayered, concentric pattern of spindle cells around vessels.
- Hemangiopericytoma-like vascular pattern may or may not be present.

Smooth Muscle Tumors

124. Leiomyomas involving the retroperitoneum are most common in which patients?

Women of perimenopausal age.

125. Which immunohistochemical stains are often positive in leiomyoma of the retroperitoneum-abdominal cavity but negative in leiomyoma of somatic soft tissue?

Estrogen receptor (ER) and progesterone receptor (PR) stains.

126. Which large blood vessel most often gives rise to leiomyosarcoma?

Inferior vena cava.

127. Name at least 1 predisposing factor for leiomyosarcoma.

- Li-Fraumeni syndrome.
- Hereditary retinoblastoma.
- Radiation exposure.

128. Which immunohistochemical stains are helpful in diagnosing leiomyosarcoma?

- Myogenic markers (i.e., SMA, desmin, or h-caldesmon).
  - In all cases (100%), at least 1 myogenic marker is positive.
- In more than 70% of cases, leiomyosarcoma is positive for more than 1 myogenic marker.
- Positivity for 2 myogenic markers is supportive.

129. What are the most important prognostic factors for leiomyosarcoma?

- Grade.
- Location.
- Tumor size.

Skeletal Muscle Tumors

RHABDOMYOMA

130. Name 1 syndrome that fetal rhabdomyoma may be associated with. Name the corresponding genetic mutation.

Basal cell nevus syndrome, which is an autosomal dominant disorder with mutations in the *PTCH1* gene (there are also a few reported cases in Birt-Hogg-Dubé syndrome, which is an autosomal dominant disorder with mutations in the *FLCN* gene).

131. List the most common sites of adult rhabdomyoma. Which patients are most often affected?

- The most common sites are the oral cavity and the superficial soft tissues of the head and neck (20% are multifocal); they most often arise from the branchial musculature (third and fourth branchial arches), thus they are restricted to the head and neck.
- It is more common in men (3M:1F) and the mean age is ~50 years.

132. Describe the histologic features of adult rhabdomyoma.

- Skeletal muscle tumor that consists of:
  - Large round/polygonal cells with abundant clear-to-eosinophilic cytoplasm and centrally or peripherally located nuclei.
  - PAS positive due to high intracytoplasmic glycogen.
  - Cross striations (possible).

RHABDOMYOSARCOMA

133. Give the current World Health Organization (WHO) classification of rhabdomyosarcoma and list the most common locations and cytogenetic abnormality of each type.

WHO CLASSIFICATION	AGE GROUP	LOCATION	CYTOGENETIC ABNORMALITIES
Embryonal rhabdomyosarcoma — includes botryoid and anaplastic variants.	• Most often diagnosed in children < age 10. • ~20% are diagnosed in patients > age 20.	• Head and neck — orbit, oropharynx, nasopharynx and sinuses, tongue, middle ear/auditory canal. • Genitourinary system — urinary bladder, prostate, paratesticular soft tissues. • Biliary tract. • Extremities rare.	• No consistent/recurrent cytogenetic translocations identified.
Alveolar rhabdomyosarcoma — Includes solid variants.	• Peak age: 10–25; median age: 16.	• Most common in the extremities. • Also found in paranasal sinuses (ethmoid sinus), paraspinal soft tissue, perineal region.	• t(2;13) (*PAX3/FOXO1*) or t(1;13) (*PAX7/FOXO1*).
Pleomorphic rhabdomyosarcoma.	• Elderly; sixth and seventh decades of life (mean age 72).	• Most common in deep soft tissues of the lower extremities.	• Highly complex karyotypes. • No consistent/recurrent translocation identified.

Spindle cell/sclerosing rhabdomyosarcoma.	• Infants, children, and adults.	• Most common in head and neck, followed by extremities.
		• Pediatric population: spindle variant most common in paratesticular region, followed by head and neck.
			• Infantile spindle RMS (< 1 year of age).
			  · *CITED2* and *NCOA2* fusions.
			  · Skeletal muscle development/regulation.
			  · Favorable prognosis.
			• *MYOD1*-mutation.
			  · Regulates muscle cell differentiation.
			  · Aggressive, poor prognosis.

134. Compare the incidence of rhabdomyosarcoma in children and adolescents versus adults.

- Rhabdomyosarcoma is the most frequent soft tissue sarcoma in children and adolescents (it accounts for 8% of childhood cancers and 40.2% of pediatric sarcomas; nearly one-half of patients are < 5 years).
- In contrast, rhabdomyosarcoma is a very rare sarcoma in adults (1.7% of adult sarcomas).

135. What is the most common subtype of rhabdomyosarcoma?

Embryonal rhabdomyosarcoma (accounts for 50–70% of rhabdomyosarcoma).

136. List at least 2 syndromes associated with embryonal rhabdomyosarcoma.
- Costello syndrome.
- Neurofibromatosis type 1 (NF1).
- Noonan syndrome.
- Uterine embryonal rhabdomyosarcoma is associated with *DICER1* syndrome.

137. List 2 microscopic features of embryonal rhabdomyosarcoma and describe the unique histologic feature of the botryoid variant.
- Microscopic features: primitive mesenchymal cells (rhabdomyoblasts) in varying stages of myogenesis (undifferentiated small cells in a prominent myxoid matrix to terminally differentiated cells with striations ["strap cell," "spider cell," and "tadpole cell" describe the same entity]; alternating zones of dense and loosely cellular areas, prominent myxoid matrix.
- Botryoid variant: subepithelial condensation of cells (cambium layer) with underlying paucicellular myxoid stroma (other than the cambium layer, it is histologically identical to conventional embryonal rhabdomyosarcoma).

138. What is the most common head and neck site for alveolar rhabdomyosarcoma?
Ethmoid sinus.

139. Compare the staining of myogenin in alveolar rhabdomyosarcoma and embryonal rhabdomyosarcoma.
- Myogenin most often is strong and diffuse in alveolar rhabdomyosarcoma.
- Myogenin most often demonstrates rare or focal staining in embryonal rhabdomyosarcoma.

140. Describe the microscopic features of a typical (conventional) alveolar rhabdomyosarcoma and solid pattern alveolar rhabdomyosarcoma.

TYPICAL ALVEOLAR RHABDOMYOSARCOMA	SOLID PATTERN ALVEOLAR RHABDOMYOSARCOMA
• "Small round blue cells" surrounded by fibrovascular septae. • "Alveolar" growth pattern. • Differentiating rhabdomyoblasts (uncommon). · Rarely, wreath-like giant cells with rhabdomyoblastic differentiation (helpful clue if present).	• Lack a fibrovascular stroma. • Variable rhabdomyoblastic differentiation (often little). • Areas with clear cell morphology (possible).

141. Describe the microscopic features of spindle cell/sclerosing rhabdomyosarcoma.
- Spindle cell rhabdomyosarcoma and sclerosing rhabdomyosarcoma exist on a morphologic spectrum.
- Microscopic features:
  · Spindle cell variant: fascicles and/or whorls of spindle cells with brightly eosinophilic cytoplasm; it may have terminally differentiated rhabdomyoblasts with striations.
- Sclerosing variant: tumor cells separated by eosinophilic and hyalinizing fibrous stroma (mimicking osteoid); and focal microalveolar or pseudovascular structures.

142. Describe the common immunohistochemical staining pattern for MyoD1 and myogenin in spindle cell/sclerosing rhabdomyosarcoma.
- Spindle cell/sclerosing rhabdomyosarcoma often exhibits strong positivity for MyoD1 with focal or even absent myogenin expression.
- Desmin may on occasion exhibit a dot-like pattern of staining in this variant.

143. Arrange the subtypes of rhabdomyosarcoma according to excellent prognosis, good prognosis, and poor prognosis.

EXCELLENT PROGNOSIS	GOOD PROGNOSIS	POOR PROGNOSIS
• Infantile spindle rhabdomyosarcoma (in patients aged < 1 year) with *NCOA2* or *CITED2* fusion.	• Embryonal rhabdomyosarcoma. • Spindle cell/sclerosing rhabdomyosarcoma with no known genetic abnormality.	• Alveolar rhabdomyosarcoma. • *MYOD1*-mutant spindle cell/sclerosing rhabdomyosarcoma. • Pleomorphic rhabdomyosarcoma.

144. List at least 4 prognostic factors in children with rhabdomyosarcoma.

- Histologic classification — infantile spindle rhabdomyosarcoma with an *NCOA2* or *CITED2* fusion has the best outcome.
- Age and tumor stage — this is most important in embryonal rhabdomyosarcoma; younger (ages 1–9) is better.
- Site of origin — orbital and paratesticular tumors do better; extremity and parameningeal tumors do worse.
- Alveolar subtype — cases with a *PAX7/FOX01* gene fusion have a better outcome than those with a *PAX3/FOX01* gene fusion.

Gastrointestinal Stromal Tumors (GISTs)

145. What is the cell of origin in GISTs?

The interstitial cell of Cajal ("pacemaker" cell of the gastrointestinal tract).

146. Describe the pathophysiology of the majority of sporadic GISTs.

Most (80%) of sporadic GISTs demonstrate a mutation in the *KIT* protooncogene, which leads to constitutive activation of the KIT-dependent signaling pathways and cell proliferation.

147. List the 3 most important prognostic factors in GISTs.

- Tumor size (2, 5, 10 cm cut-offs).
- Mitotic rate (mitoses per 5 mm^2 area: ≤ to 5 is low grade, > 5 is high grade).
- Site (stomach > small intestine).

148. List 3 immunohistochemical stains you would expect to be positive in a spindle cell GIST.

- CD117 (c-kit).
- DOG-1 (Ano-1).
- CD34.

Chondro-osseous Tumors

149. What is the most common location of a soft tissue chondroma?

80% occur in the fingers.

150. How would you distinguish juxtaarticular chondroma from a soft tissue chondroma?

Soft tissue chondromas lack attachment to the underlying bone.

151. What is the etiology of extraskeletal osteosarcoma?

- Five percent to 10% are associated with prior radiation.
- Most develop de novo.

152. List important diagnostic considerations that must be excluded prior to diagnosing an extraskeletal osteosarcoma.

- A sarcomatoid carcinoma with heterologous differentiation (heterologous component is an osteosarcoma).
- Dedifferentiated sarcoma with heterologous osteosarcoma comprising the dedifferentiated component.
- Sarcoma with heterologous differentiation (i.e., MPNST with heterologous osteosarcoma).

Peripheral Nerve Sheath Tumors
NEUROFIBROMA

153. What is the most common peripheral nerve sheath tumor?

Neurofibroma.

154. List 3 clinical features of neurofibromatosis type 2 (NF2).

- Multiple schwannomas before the age of 30.
- Bilateral vestibular (eighth cranial nerve) schwannomas.
- Gliomas (e.g., ependymoma of the cervical spinal cord).
- Multiple meningiomas.

155. List at least 3 clinical features of NF1.

- Café-au-lait spots.
- Lisch nodules (iris hamartoma).
- Nonossifying fibroma.
- Skeletal abnormalities: severed scoliosis, sphenoid wing dysplasia, tibial bowing.

156. Which soft tissue lesion is highly suggestive of NF1 syndrome?

Plexiform neurofibroma.

157. Name 5 macroscopic forms of neurofibroma.

- Cutaneous neurofibroma.
- Diffuse neurofibroma.
- Localized intraneural neurofibroma.
- Plexiform intraneural neurofibroma.
- Massive diffuse soft tissue neurofibroma.

158. The term "bag of worms" describes the macroscopic features of which type of neurofibroma.

Plexiform neurofibroma.

159. List features suggestive of malignant transformation (into an MPNST) of neurofibroma in an NF1 patient.

- Clinical features include:
  - Growing nodule in the setting of stable tumor.
  - Increased PET scan activity.
- Microscopic features include:
  - Nuclear atypia.
  - Increased cellularity.
- Mitotic activity.
- Fascicular architecture (rather than haphazard architecture).
- Zonal necrosis.
- Note that H3K27me3 (and p16) expression may be lost in MPNST.

160. Define atypical neurofibroma (also known as atypical neurofibromatous neoplasm of uncertain biological potential).

- Two or more of the following features must be present:
  - Cytologic atypia.
  - Loss of neurofibroma architecture: either on H&E or loss of CD34 expression.
- Increased cellularity.
- Mitotic rate < 3 per 10 high-power fields (HPFs).

SCHWANNOMA

161. List at least 3 typical features of a conventional schwannoma.

- It is an encapsulated spindle cell neoplasm with alternating cellularity.
  - Antoni A — hypercellular/compact.
  - Antoni B — hypocellular/loose, myxoid.
- It typically has nuclear palisading and may have Verocay bodies.
- Thick-walled hyalinized blood vessels are typically present.
- It demonstrates strong diffuse staining with S100 protein.

162. Give the percentage of schwannomas that arise as sporadic tumors.

The vast majority of schwannomas (90%) are sporadic and solitary.

163. List at least 3 subtypes of schwannoma. Describe the major difference(s) between these and conventional schwannoma.

- Ancient schwannoma: this is a conventional schwannoma with degenerative atypia consisting of large, scattered bizarre nuclei; it often has ischemic changes and/or stromal hyalinization.
- Plexiform schwannoma: these grow as plexiform or multinodular tumors (involving a nerve plexus or multiple nerve fascicles); unlike conventional schwannoma, they lack a thick capsule and hyalinized blood vessels.
- Microcystic/retiform schwannoma: this is the rarest subtype, which is most common in gastrointestinal tract; stroma is myxoid or fibrillary with microcystic areas and a retiform growth pattern; Verocay bodies and hyalinized blood vessels are not prominent.
- Cellular schwannoma: these are more cellular than conventional schwannoma, composed of Antoni A areas only; cells may be arranged in whorls; Verocay bodies are not seen; cells are hyperchromatic and may contain mitoses.
- Epithelioid schwannoma: this may arise in the setting of schwannomatosis; it consists of a mutlilobulated growth of eosinophilic epithelioid cells with round nuclei and small/inconspicuous nucleoli; there are occasional nuclear pseudoinclusions; it may have conventional areas; 40% show loss of SMARCB1/INI1 nuclear expression by immunohistochemistry.

164. List 5 worrisome histologic features of cellular schwannoma.

- Increased cellularity.
- Hyperchromatic nuclei.
- Mitotic activity (< 4/10 HPFs).
- Bone erosion or destruction (may be present).
- Focal necrosis (up to 10%).

165. How would you distinguish cellular schwannoma from MPNST?

	CELLULAR SCHWANNOMA	MPNST (SPINDLED)
S100 protein	Strong, diffuse staining for S100 protein is present.	Staining for S100 protein demonstrates rare/focal tumor cells (~50% of MPNSTs are positive for S100 protein).
Ki 67	Hot spots have up to 20% tumor cell staining.	There is typically > 20% tumor cell staining.
H3K27me3 and p16	Retained staining is present.	Loss of staining may be demonstrated.
Necrosis	Focal.	Zonal.
Other features	It may have conventional features focally (hyalinized blood vessels, subcapsular lymphocytes, etc.).	Cells adjacent to necrotic areas tend to be more atypical.

PERINEURIOMA

166. Describe the characteristic immunohistochemical staining profile for perineurioma.
- EMA positive.
- Often positive for claudin-1 and glucose transporter 1 (GLUT1).
- Negative for S100 protein, SOX10, and GFAP.

GRANULAR CELL TUMOR

167. Define granular cell tumor.

S100 positive Schwann cell-related neoplasm with pink granular cytoplasm rich in lysosomes.

168. What is the most common site of granular cell tumors?

Tongue.

169. Describe the histologic features of granular cell tumors. Name the associated histologic features that may be seen in the overlying skin or squamous mucosa.
- Histologic features:
  - This is an unencapsulated tumor consisting of sheets or nests of epithelioid or polygonal tumor cells with eosinophilic granular cytoplasm.
    › Pustuloovoid bodies of Milian are large eosinophilic granules within the cytoplasm.
    › Angulated bodies are larger glassy condensations in the cytoplasm.
  - Tumor cells may have indistinct cytoplasmic borders imparting a syncytial growth pattern.
  - Tumor cells are diffusely dispersed in a collagenous matrix.
  - Intimate association with muscle cells and/or small nerves is frequent.
  - In the tongue, it may form a checkerboard pattern with entrapped skeletal muscle bundles.
  - Nuclei vary from small hyperchromatic to medium-sized with open chromatin and distinct nucleoli.
  - Nuclear pseudoinclusions and focal atypia may occur.
- Associated histologic features that may be seen in overlying skin or mucosa: overlying mucosa or skin may demonstrate pseudoepitheliomatous hyperplasia (30–60%).

170. List the criteria associated with malignancy in granular cell tumors.
- The criteria include:
  - Necrosis.
  - Spindling of tumor cells.
  - Vesicular nuclei with large nucleoli.
  - Mitoses (> 2/10 HPFs x200).
  - High nuclear-cytoplasmic ratio.
  - Pleomorphism.
- Tumors with > 3 criteria are classified as malignant.
- Tumors with 1 or 2 criteria are classified as atypical.
- Tumors with focal nuclear pleomorphism alone are classified as benign.

MALIGNANT PERIPHERAL NERVE SHEATH TUMOR (MPNST)

171. What percentage of MPNST is associated with NF1? Compare the age of incidence of sporadic MPNSTs versus those associated with NF1.
- Percentage associated with NF1: 25–30%.
- Age range:
  - Sporadic MPNST: mean age fifth decade.
  - NF1: mean age third to fourth decade.

172. List the 2 most common ways in which MPNSTs may arise.
- They may arise de novo from peripheral nerves (major nerve trunk).
  - The most common major nerve trunk affected is the sciatic nerve.
- They may arise from malignant transformation of a benign nerve sheath tumor (more often from a neurofibroma than a schwannoma).
  - An epithelioid MPNST most likely arises from an epithelioid schwannoma.

173. Compare the S100 protein, H3K27me3, and SMARCB1/INI1 immunohistochemical staining pattern for epithelioid MPNST versus conventional MPNST.

	CONVENTIONAL MPNST	EPITHELIOID MPNST
S100 protein	• About 50% of cases are positive, usually on focal patchy/ isolated cells.	• Strong diffuse staining is demonstrated.
H3K27me3	• A loss of nuclear staining may be demonstrated, particularly in high grade tumors or radiation-induced MPNST.	• Retained nuclear staining is demonstrated.
SMARCB1/INI1	• Retained nuclear staining is demonstrated.	• About 70% loss of nuclear staining is demonstrated.

174. Name at least 1 tumor, other than MPNST, that may demonstrate loss of staining with H3K27me3 immunohistochemical marker.
- H3K27me3 is specific for MPNST.
  - It is a useful immunohistochemical marker to distinguish MPNST from other soft tissue sarcomas and spindle cell melanoma.
- Loss of staining (nuclear) also seen in:
  - High grade glial tumors.
  - Radiation-induced angiosarcoma of breast.
  - Dedifferentiated chondrosarcoma.

175. List at least 5 malignant nerve sheath tumors according to the 2020 WHO classification of soft tissue tumors.
- Conventional malignant peripheral nerve sheath tumor.
- Epithelioid malignant peripheral nerve sheath tumor.
- Malignant peripheral nerve sheath tumor with rhabdomyoblastic (skeletal muscle) differentiation (also known as malignant triton tumor).
- Malignant granular cell tumor.
- Malignant melanotic nerve sheath tumor.
- Ectomesenchymoma (this is exceedingly rare: a biphasic sarcoma with areas of rhabdomyosarcoma mixed with neuronal/neuroblastic areas).

Tumors of Uncertain Differentiation
INTRAMUSCULAR MYXOMA

176. Name 2 entities that may enter in the differential of a myxoma and how you would distinguish these entities.

	MICROSCOPIC CLUES	NUCLEAR PLEOMORPHISM?	DISTINCT VASCULAR PATTERN?	ANCILLARY TESTS
Intramuscular myxoma	• Hypocellular. • Entrapped muscular bundles at periphery, imparting a checkerboard appearance. • Atrophic skeletal muscle bundles.	• No. · Atrophic skeletal muscle bundles may mimic pleomorphic tumor cells at low power.	• No.	• S100–, MUC4–.
Myxoid nerve sheath tumor	• Focal conventional areas or features (i.e., hyalinized thick-walled blood vessels).	• No; may have degenerative atypia.	• No.	• S100+.
Myxoid liposarcoma	• Uniform round-to-oval cells with scattered lipoblasts (univacuolar type most common).	• No.	• Yes, delicate plexiform vascular pattern.	• DDIT3 gene fusions.
Low grade fibromyxoid sarcoma (Evans tumor)	• Alternating myxoid and fibrous areas ("tiger stripe" appearance). • Bland uniform spindle cells.	• No.	• Prominent arching vessels.	• MUC4+. • FUS gene fusions.

DEEP (AGGRESSIVE) ANGIOMYXOMA

177. What are the clinical features of deep (aggressive) angiomyxoma?

The tumor involves the deep soft tissue of the pelvis and perineal region in women.

178. List at least 3 microscopic features of deep (aggressive) angiomyxoma. What is the common immunohistochemical staining profile of this tumor?

- Microscopic features include:
  - An ill-defined boundary.
  - Hypocellular myxoid lesion with bland spindle cells.
- Collections of myoid bundles (smooth muscle cells) near blood vessels.
- Medium-sized hyalinized vessels.
- IHC is positive for desmin, ER, HMGA2, and PR, and often positive for CD34 and SMA (myoid bundles).

ATYPICAL FIBROXANTHOMA

179. What is the typical presentation of atypical fibroxanthoma?

Fast-growing, solitary, ulcerated nodule on sun-damaged skin of the head and neck in elderly white patients (more common in males than females).

180. List requisite histologic features for the diagnosis of atypical fibroxanthoma.

- Atypical fibroxanthomas by definition:
  - Lack subcutaneous invasion (they must be **above** the fascia).
- Lack tumor necrosis.
- Lack lymphovascular and/or perineural invasion.
- Lack staining with keratins, S100 protein, and SOX10.

PHOSPHATURIC MESENCHYMAL TUMOR

181. Name 1 clinical condition frequently associated with phosphaturic mesenchymal tumor.

Osteomalacia — associated with hypophosphatemia and elevated fibroblast growth factor 23 (FGF23) levels in the serum.

TRANSLOCATION SARCOMAS

182. Describe the typical histologic features common to most translocation sarcomas.

- Typically, they have:
  - Uniform lesional cells with minimal nuclear atypia.
  - A variable mitotic rate, but normal-appearing mitotic figures.
- The tumorigenic event is translocation, and, therefore, lesional cells are chromosomally stable: they have no atypical mitotic figures; no significant nuclear pleomorphism.

183. List the characteristic translocations and molecular events in 5 soft tissue tumors.

TUMOR TYPE	TRANSLOCATION	MOLECULAR EVENTS
Alveolar soft part sarcoma	• t(X;17)(p11;q25).	• *TFE3-ASPL* fusion.
Desmoplastic small round cell tumor	• t(11;22)(p13;q12).	• *EWSR1-WT1* fusion.
Angiomatoid fibrous histiocytoma	• t(12;16)(q13;q11). • t(12;22)(q13;q12).	• *FUS-ATF1* fusion. • *EWSR1-ATF1* fusion.
Clear cell sarcoma	• t(12;22)(q13;q12).	• *EWSR1-ATF1* fusion.
Ewing sarcoma/PNET	• t(11;22)(q24;q12).	• *EWRS1* fusions (most common: *EWSR1-FL11* fusion.
Dermatofibrosarcoma protuberans	• t(17;22)(q21;q13).	• *COL1A1-PDGFB* fusion.
Liposarcoma, well-differentiated	• Ring chromosome 12.	• Amplification of *MDM2, CDK4*, etc.
Liposarcoma, Myxoid/round cell	• t(12;16)(q13;p11). • t(12;22)(q13;q12).	• *TLS-DDIT3* fusion. • *EWSR1-DDIT3* fusion.
Low grade fibromyxoid sarcoma	• t(7;16)(q33;p11).	• *FUS-CREB3L2* fusion.
Synovial sarcoma	• t(X;18)(p11;q11).	*SS18-SSX1/SSX2/SSX4* fusions.
Rhabdoid tumor	• Deletion of 22 q.	• *1N1* inactivation.
Solitary fibrous tumor	• Inversion chromosome 12.	• *NAB2-STAT6*.

184. Describe the clinical features (age, site, presentation) of synovial sarcoma.

CLINICAL CATEGORY	CLINICAL FEATURES
Age	• Most common in young adults (median age: 30 years old); almost 80% occur patients less than 50 years of age. • Rare in children and the elderly.
Presentation	• Typically presents as a painful swelling. • Slow rate of growth can give the wrong clinical impression of a benign tumor.
Site	• 70% arise in the deep soft tissue of the upper and lower extremities (juxtaarticular locations). • 15% arise in the trunk. • Less than 10% arise in the head and neck.

185. Identify the classic features of a biphasic synovial sarcoma on light microscopy. List 3 microscopic subtypes of synovial sarcoma.

Classic light microscopic features of biphasic synovial sarcoma	• The tumor contains both neoplastic spindle cells and epithelial cells. • Spindle cells: · Are hyperchromatic, ovoid, uniform, and relatively bland. · Are tightly packed in sheets or fascicles (may have a herringbone or palisading architecture and a hemangiopericytoma-like vascular pattern). • Epithelial cells: · Are well-formed glandular structures lined by cuboidal or columnar epithelium containing PAS positive secretions. · May also form solid sheets. • Stroma: · May contain collagen, myxoid areas, calcification, or ossification. · May have mast cells (common). · May have mitoses (normal-appearing) and necrosis (variable). · May be cystic.
Subtypes	• Biphasic (20–30%). • Monophasic spindle cell (50–60%): · Cellular, monotonous spindle cells that are arranged in fascicles/sheets. · Presence or absence of alternating hyper- and hypocellular areas ("marbled" appearance). · Hemangiopericytoma-like vascular pattern. · Occasional (normal) mitoses; necrosis rare. • Poorly differentiated (uncommon): · 3 histologic patterns: (1) large cell or epithelioid pattern; (2) small cell pattern; and (3) high grade spindle pattern. · Hemangiopericytoma-like vascular pattern. · Frequent mitoses and necrosis.

186. List the immunohistochemical markers you would expect to be positive in a synovial sarcoma.
- Positive markers include EMA and focal cytokeratins (CK7, CAM5.2, or CK8/18, etc.), TLE-1 (nuclear), vimentin, variable CD99, and nuclear β-catenin (in most cases).
- EMA more often expressed than keratins.
- Calretinin, BCL-2, S100 protein, and CD56 may be positive, but are nonspecific.

187. What is the characteristic cytogenetic abnormality found in synovial sarcoma?
Reciprocal translocation t(X;18)(p11;q11), resulting in an *SS18- SSX1/2/4* fusion.

EPITHELIOID SARCOMA

188. List the 2 types of epithelioid sarcoma and their most common locations.
- Classic (distal) type: typically involves upper extremity, acral sites.
- Proximal-type: typically involves deep soft tissue of the pelvic region (perineal, genital, inguinal), buttock, or hip.

189. Name at least 3 entities that may enter into the differential diagnosis of epithelioid sarcoma and describe how you would distinguish between these entities using IHC.

ENTITY	IHC			
	SMARCB1/INI1	EPITHELIAL MARKERS (KERATINS AND EMA)	CD34	S100 PROTEIN
Epithelioid sarcoma	• Loss of staining.	• Positive.	• > 50% positive.	• Negative.
Necrobiotic granulomas (including necrotizing infectious granuloma, rheumatoid nodule, granuloma annulare, and necrobiosis lipoidica)	• Retainedstaining.	• Negative. • Macrophages: CD68 positive.		
Epithelioid MPNST	• Loss of staining (~70% of cases).	• Keratins: almost always negative. • EMA: possibly positive.	• Negative or focal CD34.	• Positive (strong, diffuse).
Malignant melanoma	• Retained staining.	• Typically negative (may be rarely positive).		• Positive (typically strong, diffuse). • Also positive for other melanocytic markers including HMB45, Melan-A.
Epithelioid angiosarcoma	• Retained staining.	• Positive.	• Positive.	• Negative.

190. What is the characteristic immunohistochemical staining profile for a classic epithelioid sarcoma?
- SMARCB1/INI1 shows loss of nuclear expression.
- Expression of epithelial markers (cytokeratins and EMA) is present.
- More than 50% express CD34.

ALVEOLAR SOFT PART SARCOMA

191. What is the most common location of an alveolar soft part sarcoma?
Deep soft tissues of the distal extremities.

192. Describe the characteristic histologic features of alveolar soft part sarcoma. Name 1 histochemical stain and 1 immunohistochemical stain that helps with diagnosis.
- Characteristic histologic features: alveolar nests of large polygonal tumor cells with granular eosinophilic cytoplasm, vesicular nuclei, and prominent nucleoli.
- Histochemical stain: PAS, which highlights crystals.
- Immunohistochemical stain: TFE3 nuclear staining corresponding to *TFE3* gene rearrangements.

CLEAR CELL SARCOMA

193. List at least 3 clinical features of clear cell sarcoma.
- Affects primarily young adults (peak incidence in third or fourth decade).
- Presents as a mass involving the deep soft tissue of the extremities (foot/ankle account for ~50% of cases).
- Often arises adjacent to, or as part of tendons and aponeuroses.
- Is slightly more common in females.
- Frequently involves lymph nodes.

194. Describe at least 3 morphological features of clear cell sarcoma.
- It grows in a nested or fascicular pattern, with thin collagenous bands dividing groups of cells.
- Tumor cells are large and epithelioid, with prominent nucleoli and clear or pale eosinophilic cytoplasm.
- Mitotic rate is low.
- Wreath-like multinucleated giant cells are seen.
- Tumor cells may contain melanin (may need a Masson-Fontana stain to highlight).

195. Identify a clue in each of the following 4 categories that would help differentiate clear cell sarcoma (CCS) from malignant melanoma: clinical, histological features, IHC, molecular.

	CLINICAL	HISTOLOGICAL	IHC	MOLECULAR
Malignant melanoma	• History or presence of a malignant melanoma.	• Marked cytological atypia, high mitotic rate.	• CD117+	• *BRAF* mutations present. • *EWSR1* fusions absent.
CCS	• No history or evidence of a malignant melanoma.	• Less cytological atypia, lower mitotic rate.	• CD117−	• *BRAF* mutations absent. • *EWSR1* fusions present.

196. Name 1 other soft tissue sarcoma that shares the same gene fusions as clear cell sarcoma.

Angiomatoid fibrous histiocytoma.

PERIVASCULAR EPITHELIOID CELL TUMOR (PECOMA)

197. What feature is common to all tumors in the PEComa group?

The presence of an HMB45 positive smooth muscle-like element.

198. What is the name of the PEComa found most often in the kidney? Describe the (inherited) disease commonly associated with this lesion. What 3 elements are seen histologically?

• Name: angiomyolipoma.
• Association: tuberous sclerosis complex (TSC) — 20% of angiomyolipomas occur in patients with TSC, which is inherited in an autosomal dominant pattern, although often occurs as a new mutation. TSC includes (in addition to angiomyolipoma) pulmonary lymphangioleiomyomatosis; cardiac rhabdomyoma; subependymal astrocytic nodules; angiofibromas with or without seizure disorder and cognitive impairment.
• 3 elements: lipomatous, vascular, smooth muscle-like cells (HMB45 positive).

199. What pathological features suggest malignant behavior in a PEComa tumor?

• Marked nuclear atypia/pleomorphism.
• Infiltrative growth.
• Size > 5 cm.
• Coagulative necrosis.
• Mitoses > 1/50 HPFs.

200. List 3 features of a *TFE3*-rearranged PEComa.

• Alveolar growth pattern.
• Epithelioid morphology, mild atypia, rare mitoses.
• Lack of spindle cells and lack of smooth muscle marker expression.
• Younger patients without a history of tuberous sclerosis complex.

Undifferentiated Small and Round Cell Sarcomas of Bone and Soft Tissue

EWING SARCOMA

201. Describe at least 4 morphological features of Ewing sarcoma and the typical immunohistochemical findings.

• Microscopic features:
  · Uniform small cells have powdery chromatin and scant-to-clear cytoplasm.
  · Clear cells contain intracytoplasmic glycogen.
  · Tumor cells are arranged in lobules/sheets with minimal stroma, delicate vessels; lobules are separated by delicate fibrous septae.
  · Pseudorosettes (Homer Wright): tumor cells arranged around neurofibrillary cores, and (rarely) true rosettes (Flexner-Wintersteiner), may be present.
• IHC:
  · Positive for CD99 (membranous), FLI1 (nuclear).
  · Positive for synaptophysin, chromogranin, neuron-specific enolase (NSE), S100, and low molecular weight cytokeratin (LMWCK).

202. Name 1 favorable prognostic factor for Ewing sarcoma.

Complete pathologic response to neoadjuvant chemotherapy.

Bone Pathology: Nonneoplastic
General Considerations

203. Describe the handling and processing of a bone biopsy specimen for metabolic bone disease.

- Note tetracycline administration: 2 cycles of tetracycline are given 12 days apart; 5 mm core of trabecular bone is obtained (commonly from the ilium) 7 days later.
- Fix the specimen in 70% alcohol (to preserve tetracycline label).
- Do not decalcify.
- Embed in plastic (glycol or methyl methacrylate).

- Prepare 5–10 micron sections cut and stained with H&E, von Kossa (or Goldner, modified trichrome) — for measurement of mineralized bone versus osteoid.
- Do other stains as needed: aluminum, iron stains.
- Cut unstained sections for visualization of the tetracycline under the fluorescent microscope (tetracycline labeling). Mineralization dynamics such as calcification rate, bone formation rate, and mineralization rate can then be evaluated.

204. Outline how you would handle an intraoperative consultation for a possible prosthetic joint infection.

- Freeze a representative section from each submitted fragment (to reduce sampling error) from the periprosthetic fibrous membrane (not the superficial fibrinous exudate).

- Count neutrophils located in the periprosthetic fibrous tissue and not in surface fibrin or within the lumens of the capillaries.
- Five or more neutrophils in each of 3 HPFs suggests a periprosthetic joint infection.

205. Describe the significance of neutrophils in periprosthetic tissues.

- Low neutrophil counts are unlikely to be infection.
- High neutrophil counts may be due to infection or inflammatory processes.

· Clinical benchmarks are important to determine infectious etiology.
· In inflammatory processes, increased neutrophils may arise in the setting of rheumatoid arthritis and crystal-induced arthritis.

OSTEOGENESIS IMPERFECTA

206. What is the basic defect in osteogenesis imperfecta?

An abnormality in type I collagen.

207. List 3 other nonosseous abnormalities that may be present in a patient with OI.

- Blue/gray sclera.
- Ligamentous and/or skin laxity.
- Deafness or hearing loss.

- Abnormal dentition.
- Cardiovascular abnormalities (aortic and mitral valve incompetence).

208. Identify 3 other conditions (apart from OI) that may explain multiple fractures of varying ages in a child.

- Other congenital/developmental bone diseases (juvenile idiopathic osteoporosis, Cole-Carpenter syndrome, Bruck syndrome, achondrogenesis).

- Hypophosphatemia.
- Nonaccidental injury (child abuse).

OSTEOPETROSIS

209. Define osteopetrosis.

Genetic disease characterized by reduced bone resorption due to impaired formation or function of osteoclasts leading to diffuse symmetric skeletal sclerosis.

210. Compare severe and mild forms of osteopetrosis.

- Severe infantile osteopetrosis:
  · It is autosomal recessive.
  · In utero fractures may occur, and it has high rates of postpartum mortality due to fractures, hydrocephaly, and anemia.
  · Infants that survive will have cranial nerve defects (deafness, facial paralysis, optic atrophy), repeated severe infections due to leukopenia, and hepatosplenomegaly due to extramedullary hematopoiesis.

- Mild form of osteopetrosis:
  · It is autosomal dominant.
  · Patients have a history of repeated fractures.
  · It may not be detected until adolescence or early adulthood (incidentally discovered on routine X-rays).
  · Patients may have mild cranial nerve deficits and anemia.

OSTEOPOROSIS

211. Define osteopenia and osteoporosis.
- Osteopenia: decrease in bone mass.
- Osteoporosis: an acquired decrease in bone mass, which weakens the microarchitecture of the bone and makes it prone to spontaneous fracture.

212. List at least 5 common causes of osteoporosis or conditions associated with osteoporosis.
- Primary:
  - Idiopathic.
  - Postmenopausal.
  - Senile.
- Secondary:
  - Endocrine disorders:
    › Estrogen deficiency, acromegaly, adrenocortical insufficiency, hypo- or hyperthyroidism, hyperparathyroidism, hypopituitarism, type 1 diabetes mellitus.
- Gastrointestinal disorders:
  › Hepatic insufficiency, malnutrition or malabsorption (low calcium and/or vitamin D, etc.).
- Medications:
  › Corticosteroids, alcohol, anticonvulsants, chemotherapy, heparin.
- Miscellaneous:
  › Infiltrative marrow diseases: malignant lymphoma/leukemia, myeloma, Gaucher disease, extensive metastatic disease.
  › Inactivity, immobilization (osteopenia of disuse).
  › Smoking.
  › Caucasian, female, lean body build.

Note: postmenopausal and senile types are the most common forms of osteoporosis.

213. List at least 3 common sites of fracture in osteoporosis.
- Vertebrae — spinal compression fractures (thoracic and lumbar).
- Femur — head or neck.
- Distal radius — Colles fracture.
- Proximal humerus.

214. List at least 2 histologic features of osteoporosis.
- Normal bone is decreased in quantity.
- Lamellar bone trabeculae in the cancellous compartment lose their connections to each other and become thin and perforated.
- Postmenopausal type: there may be increased osteoclastic activity.
- Senile type: the cortex is thinned, and Haversian systems are enlarged such that the cortex mimics the appearance of cancellous bone.

PAGET DISEASE OF BONE

215. Define Paget disease of bone.
A localized skeletal disorder characterized by the activation of osteoblasts and osteoclasts, resulting in the abnormal remodeling of bone.

216. List at least 4 clinical symptoms of Paget disease of bone.
- The disease may be asymptomatic.
- Most cases are polyostotic (involve more than 1 site); 15% of cases are monostotic.
- Bone symptoms include pain (may be warmth and tenderness at site), arthritis, fracture, deformity (leontiasis ossea, "saber shin," etc.).
- Neurological symptoms include cranial or spinal nerve compression, deafness, brainstem or cerebellar dysfunction.
- Cardiac symptoms include high output heart failure (vascular marrow stroma; seen in polyostotic Paget disease), cardiac hypertrophy.
- Other symptoms include hypercalcemia, nephrolithiasis.

217. List 3 stages of Paget disease of bone and their corresponding histologic findings.
- Initial lytic phase:
  - This is characterized by increased osteoclast activity (osteoclasts are large and multinucleate [> 100 nuclei] and may contain prominent inclusion-like nucleoli) and bone resorption (scalloped bone surface).
- Mixed phase (active, ongoing disease):
  - Osteoclasts persist and osteoblasts now line the bone trabeculae surface.
- Disorganized remodeling of bone is present, which involves:
  › Increased osteoclast and osteoblast activity with osteoclastic and osteoblastic activity on the same side of the bone trabeculae (both bone formation and bone resorption), which leads to thick and thin trabeculae.
  › Newly formed bone (woven or lamellar) with irregular and wavy cement lines (start to appreciate mosaic pattern).
  › Marrow fat replaced with loose connective tissue with numerous blood vessels.

(continued on next page)

- Inactive, "burned out" disease:
  - Cellular activity decreases and mosaic pattern is prominent.

- Woven bone is replaced and all bone is lamellar type.
- Fibrovascular marrow is replaced by normal fatty marrow.

218. What is the pathogenesis of Paget disease of bone?
- Some (10%) can be inherited as an autosomal dominant trait (chromosome 18q mutations of the gene encoding sequestosome 1/p62: *SQSTM1* gene mutation).

- It may be initiated by a virus — e.g., RSV, paramyxovirus (measles), parainfluenza type 3, canine distemper.

219. Which bones are most commonly affected in Paget disease?
- Pelvis.
- Vertebrae and sacrum.

- Femur.
- Skull.

220. List 2 tumors that may arise in the setting of Paget disease of bone.
- Benign:
  - Giant cell tumor.
  - Giant cell reparative granuloma.
  - Extraosseous hematopoietic tissue masses.

- Malignant:
  - Secondary sarcoma (most often in polyostotic Paget disease): osteosarcoma or fibrosarcoma; the tumor is high grade and rapidly fatal.

OSTEOMALACIA

221. Define osteomalacia.

Impaired mineralization of bone that results in accumulation of osteoid (nonmineralized bone).

222. Contrast osteomalacia and osteoporosis.
- Osteomalacia is the accumulation of nonmineralized bone (osteoid).

- Osteoporosis is when the total bone mass is decreased; however, the mineral content of the bone is normal.

223. Name a tumor associated with osteomalacia (tumor-induced osteomalacia). What is the associated biomarker?
- Tumor: phosphaturic mesenchymal tumor.
- Associated biomarker: increased production of FGF-23 (associated with tumor-induced osteomalacia and phosphaturic mesenchymal tumor).

- This biomarker can be detected in the serum or ancillary tests for FGF-23, which can be performed on the tumor directly.

224. List at least 2 microscopic features of osteomalacia in children and in adults.
- Children (rickets):
  - Growth plates (where abnormality is particularly focused) that are thickened and poorly defined due to the failure of cartilage cells to mature.
  - Irregular tongues of cartilage that project into the metaphysis.
  - Enlargement and widening of the osteochondral junction.
  - Microfractures due to overgrowth of capillaries and fibroblasts in the osteochondral zones.
  - Skeletal deformities (in bones that form via enchondral ossification).

- Adults:
  - Wide osteoid seams surrounding disorganized bone trabeculae.
  - Irregular junction between the osteoid seams and mineralized bone.
  - Increased bone volume (often).
  - Normal (unaffected) contour of bone.
  - Weakened bone that is prone to gross or microfractures.
    › Femoral neck, vertebral bodies.

225. List 3 skeletal changes seen in a child with rickets.
- Frontal bossing of the skull.
- Chest deformities including:
  - "Rachitic rosary": overgrowth of cartilage or osteoid at the osteochondral junction of ribs.

- Pigeon breast deformity: anterior protrusion of sternum.
- Bowing of legs.
- Lumbar lordosis.

226. List at least 3 causes of osteomalacia.
- Osteomalacia is due to vitamin D disturbance (i.e., deficiency, abnormal metabolism, or calcium deficiency) caused by:
  - Poor intake: inadequate vitamin D, calcium, or phosphate (dietary deficiency, malabsorption, total parenteral nutrition, lack of exposure to sunlight).

- Renal disorders leading to decreased synthesis of vitamin D and/or phosphate depletion.
- Rare inherited disorders.
- Drugs (phenytoin, isoniazid, rifampin, phenobarbital).
- Hepatobiliary disease (binding by bile acids).
- Phosphaturic mesenchymal tumor.

HYPERPARATHYROIDISM

227. List at least 3 skeletal manifestation of untreated primary hyperparathyroidism.
- Osteoporosis.
- Brown tumor of hyperparathyroidism.
- Osteitis fibrosa cystica.
- Growth retardation.

228. List 3 microscopic features seen in the bone in the setting of untreated hyperparathyroidism.
- Dissecting osteitis: osteoclasts tunneling through bone trabeculae ("railroad tracks").
- Brown tumor of hyperparathyroidism: bone loss with microfractures leading to hemorrhage, hemosiderin deposition, increased osteoclastic activity, increased macrophages, and cystic degeneration.
- Osteitis fibrosa cystica: increased osteoclastic activity, peritrabecular fibrosis, and Brown tumors.

RENAL OSTEODYSTROPHY

229. Define renal osteodystrophy.
Skeletal changes that occur in the setting of long-standing chronic renal failure.

230. List 4 manifestations of renal osteodystrophy.
- Osteopenia/osteoporosis.
- Osteomalacia.
- Secondary hyperparathyroidism.
- Formation of Brown tumor in bone.

231. Describe the serum levels of calcium, phosphate, and parathyroid hormone (PTH) in the setting of renal osteodystrophy.
- Hypocalcemia.
- Hyperphosphatemia.
- Elevated PTH levels.

FRACTURES

232. Describe at least 3 clinical types of bone fractures.
- Simple fracture: bone fracture in which the overlying skin is intact.
- Compound fracture: bone fracture that communicates with the skin surface.
- Comminuted fracture: fragmented bone fracture.
- Displaced bone fracture: lack of alignment between the ends of the bone.
- Stress fracture: a fracture that develops in a bone that is subjected to repeated loads, usually in the setting of increased physical activity.
- Greenstick fracture: a fracture that extends partially through bone, occurs in soft bones of infants and young children.
- Pathologic fracture: a fracture that occurs in the setting of a bone weakened by an underlying disease (i.e., metastatic tumor).

233. Name at least 3 carcinomas that commonly metastasize to bone and state whether they typically present with lytic or blastic (sclerotic) lesions.
- Breast carcinoma: lytic lesions.
- Thyroid carcinoma: lytic lesions.
- Renal cell carcinoma: lytic lesions.
- Lung carcinoma: lytic lesions.
- Prostate carcinoma: predominantly blastic lesions.

234. Name at least 1 metastatic carcinoma that may present with metastases to the small bones of the hands or feet.
- Lung (most common).
- Kidney.
- Colon.

Note: metastases most often involve the axial skeleton.

AVASCULAR NECROSIS

235. List 3 common sites of avascular necrosis of bone. Why does this condition occur most frequently at these particular sites?
- Sites: femoral head, proximal scaphoid, posterior talus (more often than tibia, lunate, navicular).
- Reason: tenuous blood supply — these areas have limited or no collaterals/overlapping blood supply or have an end arterial blood supply.

236. List at least 6 risk factors or associations for avascular necrosis of bone.
- Trauma.
- Corticosteroid use.
- Alcoholism.
- Gaucher disease.
- Hypercoagulable states — thrombomodulin deficiency, protein C or S deficiency.
- Sepsis/infection.
- Vasculitis.
- Idiopathic.
- Dysbarism (Caisson disease).
- Radiation.
- Chronic pancreatitis.
- Sickle cell disease.

237. Describe the classical X-ray appearance of early osteonecrosis in the femoral head.
- No changes initially (possible) — i.e., normal.
- Preserved joint space — cartilage remains viable.
- Cystic and sclerotic changes; subchondral fracture changes the contour of the joint.
- Subsequent collapse of the infarcted area — lucent area ("crescent sign").

238. Describe the characteristic gross appearance of avascular necrosis in the femoral head.
- Wedge-shaped area of pale yellow necrotic bone below the articular cartilage.
- Overlying articular cartilage that often lifts away from the bone.
- Presence or absence of hyperemic band below the necrotic foci.
- Presence or absence of collapse of the femoral head with distortion of surface cartilage and associated severe degenerative changes.

OSTEOMYELITIS

239. Name a pathogen implicated in osteomyelitis unique to IV drug users.
Pseudomonas aeruginosa.

240. Individuals with sickle cell disease are prone to osteomyelitis caused by which pathogen?
Salmonella.

241. List 3 ways a bacterial pathogen may reach the bone and cause osteomyelitis.
- Hematogenous spread.
- Direct extension from an infected contiguous site.
- Foreign body implant.

242. Which pathogen is most often implicated in pyogenic osteomyelitis?
Staphylococcus aureus.

243. In the setting of osteomyelitis, define sequestrum, involucrum, and Brodie abscess.
- Sequestrum: a fragment of dead bone that is separated from its surrounding bone in the setting of osteomyelitis.
- Involucrum: reactive woven bone that forms around necrotic sequestrum.
- Brodie abscess: an intraosseous abscess often within the cortex and surrounded by reactive bone (often seen in subacute osteomyelitis).

244. Which bone region is affected in Garré sclerosing osteomyelitis?
Jaw bones.

245. List 4 complications of osteomyelitis.
- Pathologic fracture.
- Infective endocarditis.
- Sepsis.
- Long-term complications:
  · Reactive systemic (secondary) amyloidosis.
  · Squamous cell carcinoma in draining sinus tracts.
  · Secondary sarcoma.

246. Describe the most common pathway of infection for mycobacterial osteomyelitis.
- Hematogenous spread in the setting of active visceral disease during primary infection.
- Direct extension (e.g., a pulmonary focus from the rib and into vertebrae from lymph nodes).

247. How often is the spine involved in mycobacterial osteomyelitis?
40%.

248. List 1 complication of tuberculous spondylitis (Pott disease).

- Mycobacterial infection spreads from the intervertebral discs to infect multiple vertebra and adjacent soft tissue, leading to destruction of the intervertebral discs and vertebrae.
- This leads to:
  - Compression fractures that cause scoliosis and/or kyphosis.
  - Neurologic deficits due to compression of nerve and/or spinal cord.

249. In congenital syphilis, where in the bone do the spirochetes concentrate?

- Areas of endochondral ossification (osteochondritis).
- Periosteum (periostitis).

250. Which bones are most often involved in acquired syphilis?

Nose, palate, skull, and extremities.

251. Describe saber shin in the setting of skeletal syphilis.

In congenital syphilis, it represents massive reactive periosteal bone formation along the anterior and medial surface of the tibia leading to sharp anterior bowing of the tibia.

252. Describe the typical histologic features of skeletal syphilis and mycobacterial osteomyelitis.

- Skeletal syphilis:
  - Necrotic bone associated with edematous granulation tissue with abundant plasma cells and neutrophils.
  - Spirochetes, which can be identified via immunohistochemical or silver stains.
- Presence or absence of gumma.
- Mycobacterial osteomyelitis:
  - Necrotic bone with necrotizing granulomas.
  - Mycobacterium, which can be identified via special stains.

Joint Disorders

OSTEOARTHRITIS

253. Estimate the incidence of osteoarthritis in the following populations: 20-year-olds, 40-year-olds, and 70-year-olds.

- 20-year-olds: 5%.
- 40-year-olds: 30–40%.
- 70-year-olds: 70–80%.

254. List at least 4 classic radiological features of osteoarthritis.

- Joint space narrowing (loss of cartilage).
- Osteophyte formation.
- Subchondral pseudocysts (geodes) and sclerosis.
- Joint enlargement.
- Varus deformity.

255. Describe at least 4 gross findings of osteoarthritis.

- Cartilage pitting, scoring, fibrillation, and erosion.
- Eburnation and sclerosis of underlying bone.
- Osteophyte.
- Subchondral pseudocyst.
- Deformity of bone (flattening, enlargement).
- Secondary osteonecrosis.
- Tenosynovium with degenerative and reactive changes including proliferative synovitis and chondroid metaplasia (grossly mimicking cartilage).

256. Name common pathogens associated with infection of prosthetic joints.

- Acute infections: *S. epidermidis* and *S. aureus*.
- Late infections: gram-negative bacilli.

RHEUMATOID ARTHRITIS

257. List at least 3 histologic features of rheumatoid arthritis involving the joint.

- Synovial cell hyperplasia and proliferation.
- Dense chronic inflammatory cell infiltrates consisting of lymphocytes and plasma cells.
  - Frequent lymphoid follicles.
- Surface fibrin deposition with formation of "rice" bodies.
- Formation of rheumatoid pannus.
  - Mass of edematous synovium with abundant chronic inflammatory cells and granulation tissue.
- Erosion into articular surface by the rheumatoid pannus, along with increased osteoclastic activity leading to bone destruction.

258. Compare the gross features of a joint with advanced rheumatoid arthritis to a joint with advanced osteoarthritis.

RHEUMATOID ARTHRITIS	OSTEOARTHRITIS
• Abundant synovial pannus. • Fibrous ankylosis in joint space. • Bone ankyloses fusing bones crossing joint space. • Articular cartilage erosion.	• Subchondral sclerosis. • No ankylosis. • Osteophyte and/or bony spur formation. • Articular cartilage thinning (eburnation in most severe) and fibrillations. • Presence or absence of subchondral cyst(s).

SERONEGATIVE SPONDYLOARTHROPATHIES

259. List at least 3 common features of seronegative spondyloarthropathies.
- Pathologic changes seen in the ligamentous attachments rather than within the synovial tissue.
- Involvement of sacroiliac joints.
- Absence of rheumatoid factor.
- Association with human leukocyte antigen B27 (HLA-B27).

260. Name at least 2 examples of seronegative spondyloarthropathies.
- Ankylosing spondylitis.
- Psoriatic arthritis.
- Reactive arthritis.
- Enteritis associated arthritis.

261. Which patients are most often affected by reactive arthritis? Name 2 commonly associated pathogens.
- Reactive arthritis most commonly affects young men, usually in their 20s and 30s.
- It may affect HIV infected individuals.
- More than 80% of cases are HLA-B27 positive.
- Autoimmune reaction is initiated by prior infection of genitourinary tract by *Chlamydia* or the gastrointestinal tract (*Salmonella, Yersinia, Shigella, Campylobacter*).

CRYSTAL-INDUCED ARTHRITIS

262. How do you differentiate gout crystals from pseudogout (calcium pyrophosphate dihydrate deposition: CPPD) in tissue sections?

CRYSTAL TYPE	SHAPE	COLOR (ON H&E)	APPEARANCE UNDER POLARIZED LIGHT (ALIGNED IN PARALLEL WITH RED COMPENSATOR)	GIANT CELL AND/ OR GRANULOMATOUS RESPONSE
Gout	• Long, needle-like. • "Haystack" appearance when clumped together.	• Brown or amorphous white (if dissolved).	• Negative birefringence: yellow.	• Common.
CPPD	• Square or rhomboidal.	• Magenta.	• Weakly positive birefringence: blue or white.	• Occasional.

263. How do you handle a fresh specimen in which there is a suspicion of gout, and why?
Sodium urate is soluble in the water component of formalin preparations and in H&E staining (water bath steps), so to preserve crystals, touch preps fixed in 100% alcohol are preferred and an unstained slide is covered with a glass coverslip.

264. List at least 3 findings you might expect to see at autopsy in a patient with gout.
- Gouty tophi (soft tissue collections of urate): toes, fingers, ear, elbow.
- Nephrolithiasis.
- Uric acid deposits in synovium, menisci (white, chalky/paste-like nodules).
- Joint deformities from longstanding gout.

265. List at least 3 nongenetic associations or risk factors for the development of gout.
- Diabetes.
- Hypertension.
- Lymphoproliferative disease.
- Obesity.
- Diet high in purines (especially red meats) and/or alcohol.
- Renal insufficiency.
- Hyperparathyroidism.
- Medications (diuretic therapy).
- Hypothyroidism.

266. Describe the typical appearance of CPPD on a plain X-ray of the knee.

A linear, radio-opaque deposition is seen in the joint space, corresponding to CPPD dehydrate deposition within the menisci.

267. List 2 routine specimens where CPPD crystals are often seen.
- Knee arthroplasty specimens.
- Intervertebral discs.

GANGLION AND SYNOVIAL CYSTS

268. Compare and contrast ganglion and synovial cysts.
- Both ganglion and synovial cysts are expansile, fluid-filled cysts arising around joints (most often wrists, knees, and feet).
- Ganglion cyst:
  · Is characterized by cystic or myxoid degeneration of fibroconnective tissue surrounding joints.
  · Is composed of uni- or multilocular cysts.
  · Lacks true cell lining.
  · Has no communication with joint space.
- Synovial cyst:
  · Arises from herniated synovium through a joint capsule or enlargement of a bursa.
  · Has true cell lining of cyst consisting of synovial cells that may be hyperplastic.
  · Is filled with synovial fluid.
  · Communicates with joint space.

Bone Pathology: Neoplastic
Grading

269. In a postchemotherapy resection specimen of Ewing sarcoma of bone, describe how you grade the "treatment effect."
- The treatment effect is based on an assessment of tumor necrosis as follows:
  · Grade 1: 0% necrosis (no chemotherapy effect).
  · Grade 2A: < 50% necrosis (partial or low chemotherapy effect).
  · Grade 2B: 50–95% necrosis (partial or high chemotherapy effect).
  · Grade 3: 96–99% necrosis (scattered foci of viable tumor only).
  · Grade 4: 100% necrosis (no residual viable tumor).

270. List the required elements of a bone tumor resection report.
- Specimen type (e.g., distal femur).
- Procedure (e.g., marginal resection).
- Tumor site (e.g., appendicular skeletal, spine, etc.).
- Tumor location and extent (e.g., metaphysis, tumor involves joint, etc.).
- Tumor size (greatest dimension).
- WHO classification of histologic type (e.g., osteosarcoma, conventional).
- Necrosis (macroscopic or microscopic).
- Histologic grade (if appropriate).
- Margins (all margins < 2 cm should be listed).
- Regional lymph nodes and status.
- Pathologic staging (pTNM).
  · pT based on anatomic site (different pT staging for tumor site).
- Ancillary studies (required only if applicable).
- Treatment effect.
- Data elements not required for accreditation:
  · Mitotic rate (reported per 10 HPFsx, x40 objective).
  · Lymphovascular invasion.
  · Additional pathologic findings.
  · Radiographic findings (if available).
  · Preresection treatment.
  · Comments.

271. List at least 5 gross characteristics of a primary bone tumor that should be included in the gross description of a pathology report.
- Tumor size (3 dimensions).
- Appearance — color, bone and/or cartilage formation.
- % tumor necrosis.
- Location of tumor in bone:
  · Surface (periosteal) versus intramedullary versus intracortical.
  · Region of bone — epiphysis, metaphysis, and/or diaphysis.
- Erosion of cortex and/or cortical breakthrough with soft tissue extension.
- Extension through epiphyseal plate.
- Extension into joint space.
- Skip metastases in bone.
- Distance from margin.
- Relationship to adjacent structures.
- Vascular involvement.

Chondrogenic Tumors

BIZARRE PAROSTEAL OSTEOCHONDROMATOUS PROLIFERATION

272. What is the most common location for bizarre parosteal osteochondromatous proliferation?
Small bones of the hands and feet.

273. List at least 3 microscopic features of bizarre parosteal osteochondromatous proliferation.
- Variable mixture of cartilage with mildly atypical chondrocytes, bone, and fibrous tissue.
- Exophytic bone and cartilage growth with intact underlying cortex.
- So-called blue bone (even after decalcification).
- Absence of atypical mitoses and nuclear hyperchromasia.

ENCHONDROMA

274. Compare and contrast enchondroma versus chondrosarcoma using clinical, radiological, and microscopic findings.

TUMOR TYPE	CLINICAL FINDINGS	RADIOLOGICAL FINDINGS	MICROSCOPIC FINDINGS
Enchondroma	• Patients are young to middle-aged adults (20–40 years old). • Not painful unless a fracture occurs.	• Small (< 5 cm). • Peripheral: tubular bones of hands, feet. • No erosion or penetration of cortex.	• Mildly cellular. • No significant atypia (small, round nuclei with small nucleoli). • No mitoses. • Pushing border (no invasion into haversian system).
Chondrosarcoma	• Patients are older adults (50–70 years old). • Often painful (night pain).	• Large (> 5 cm). • Central, metaphyseal: pelvis > long bones (femur, humerus) > ribs. • Cortical erosion or destruction (+/− soft tissue extension).	• Hypercellular. • Cytological atypia: enlarged, hyperchromatic nuclei, numerous binucleate chondrocytes. • Mitoses +/− necrosis. • Permeation of host bone. • > 20% myxoid matrix.

OSTEOCHONDROMA

275. Describe the characteristic gross appearance of an osteochondroma.
- This is a mushroom-shaped exostosis from the bone surface, usually at the end of a long tubular bone, near the growth plate.
- Bone at stalk base merges with cortical bone and the medullary cavities are in continuity.
- The bone is covered by a cartilage cap of variable thickness.

276. What is the prognosis of an osteochondroma?
- Osteochondromas stop growing at skeletal maturity (growth plate closure).
- Nearly all are cured with simple excision.
- Oteochondromas progress to (secondary peripheral) chondrosarcoma rarely in sporadic cases (1%) and more often in the setting of multiple hereditary exostosis (~5%).
- Cartilage cap thickness must be assessed and documented.
- Cartilage cap thickness of > 2.0 cm in adults is worrisome for progression to chondrosarcoma.

CHONDROBLASTOMA

277. In which part of the bone do chondroblastomas typically arise?
Chondroblastomas affect young patient and typically arise in the epiphysis or apophysis of the long bones (around the growth plate).

278. List 3 histological features of chondroblastoma.
- Sheets of round/polygonal cells with round/oval nuclei with grooves and eosinophilic cytoplasm.
- Pericellular "chicken wire" calcifications.
- Foci/nodules of more mature-appearing chondroid tissue.
  - True basophilic hyaline cartilage rare.
- Osteoclast-like giant cells (common).
- Mitoses (frequent, but never atypical).
- (Secondary) aneurysmal bone cyst-like changes (in approximately one-third of cases).

279. Which immunostain may be helpful in diagnosing chondroblastoma?
- DOG1 may be focally positive (seems to be clone dependent).
- S100 protein is positive.

CHONDROMYXOID FIBROMA

280. What is the most common location of a chondromyxoid fibroma?

This lesion is most often metaphyseal involving the proximal tibia or distal femur.

281. List at least 3 histologic features of chondromyxoid fibroma.
- It is well-demarcated from surrounding bone.
- Lobules spindle/stellate cells are seen in a chondromyxoid background.
- Cells condense at the periphery of lobules.
- Osteoclast-like giant cells, if present, are often at the periphery of lobules.
- Coarse calcifications are present in approximately one-third of cases.
- (Secondary) aneurysmal bone cyst-like changes occur in 10% of cases.

SYNOVIAL CHONDROMATOSIS

282. What is the most common site of synovial chondromatosis?

The knee joint.

283. List features that would help distinguish synovial chondromatosis from peripheral low grade conventional chondrosarcoma.
- Synovial chondromatosis may demonstrate atypia with enhanced cytologic detail of chondrocytes and easily identified binucleate chondrocytes.
- Features that favor a peripheral low grade conventional chondrosarcoma include:
  - Loss of chondrocyte clustering.
- Significant nuclear atypia with enlargement, pleomorphism, and hyperchromasia.
- Numerous mitoses including atypical forms.
- Infiltration of underlying bone.

CHONDROSARCOMA

284. Classify cartilaginous tumors of bone.
- Benign:
  - Osteochondroma, chondroma (enchondroma/periosteal chondroma), osteochondromyxoma, subungual exostosis, bizarre parosteal osteochondromatous proliferation (BPOP, also known as Nora lesion), synovial chondromatosis.
- Intermediate (locally aggressive):
  - Chondromyxoid fibroma.
  - Atypical cartilaginous tumor/conventional chondrosarcoma grade 1.
- Intermediate (rarely metastasizing):
  - Chondroblastoma.
- Malignant:
  - Conventional chondrosarcoma grade 2 or grade 3.
    - › Primary (no preexisting lesion).
    - › Secondary:
      - » (Preexisting) osteochondroma (peripheral).
      - » (Preexisting) multiple enchondromata (Ollier disease, Maffucci syndrome).
      - » Synovial chondromatosis: extraordinarily rare.
  - Variants:
    - › Dedifferentiated chondrosarcoma (grade 3).
    - › Mesenchymal chondrosarcoma (grade 3).
    - › Clear cell chondrosarcoma (grade 1).
    - › Periosteal chondrosarcoma.

285. What are the risk factors for the development of chondrosarcoma?
- Multiple enchondromatosis syndromes (Maffucci syndrome, Ollier disease); 40% or more transform to chondrosarcoma.
  - Ollier disease and Maffucci syndrome are rare, congenital, nonhereditary skeletal disorders characterized by multiple enchondromas.
- In Maffucci syndrome, patients also present with multiple hemangiomas.
- Hereditary multiple osteochondromas (*EXT1* gene abnormalities).

286. List the general criteria for malignancy in central chondroid tumors.
- Architecture:
  - Permeation of bone or extension beyond periosteum.
  - Disorganized arrangement of malignant cartilage lobules.
- Increased cellularity.
- "Enhanced" cytologic detail (normal chondrocytes have minimal cytoplasm and small, dark [pyknotic] nuclei).
  - Readily apparent cytoplasm.
  - Visible nuclear membranes and chromatin distribution; visible nucleoli.
- More than occasional binucleate chondrocytes.

(continued on next page)

Note: criteria are best applied to central cartilaginous tumors. It is problematic when applied to cartilaginous tumors on the surface of bone, in soft tissue, and in the small bones of the hands and feet.

287. List criteria for grading central chondrosarcoma.

GRADE	HISTOLOGIC FEATURES
Grade 1	Atypical chondrocytes with small dark nuclei; multiple nuclei per lacuna; mild-to-moderate cellularity; absent mitoses; predominantly hyaline matrix.
Grade 2	Atypical chondrocytes, moderate-sized, with more vesicular nuclei; < 2 mitoses/10 HPFs; greater cellularity; matrix more myxoid.
Grade 3	Greater cellularity; atypical chondrocytes with pleomorphic nuclei; 2 or more mitoses/10 HPFs; myxoid or spindled matrix (peripheral spindling).

Note: low grade: grade 1 and 2 (includes clear cell chondrosarcoma [grade 1]); high grade: grade 3 and dedifferentiated chondrosarcoma (includes mesenchymal chondrosarcoma [grade 3]).

Note: a central conventional chondrosarcoma with a predominantly myxoid matrix represents a chondrosarcoma of higher grade.

PERIOSTEAL CHONDROSARCOMA

288. Define periosteal chondrosarcoma.

Periosteal chondrosarcoma arises on the surface of the bone, typically the metaphyseal region of long tubular bones, in close association with the periosteum, and invades the underlying cortex or is > 5 cm in size.

CLEAR CELL CHONDROSARCOMA

289. List at least 3 microscopic features of clear cell chondrosarcoma.

- Sheet-like proliferation of tumor cells with ample clear to eosinophilic cytoplasm, well-defined cytoplasmic borders, centrally placed nuclei.
- Mild atypia and rare mitoses.
- Lack of chondroid matrix — unless associated with conventional chondrosarcoma (~50% cases).
- Irregularly shaped trabeculae of immature woven bone with osteoclast-like giant cells.
- (Secondary) aneurysmal bone cyst-like changes (common).
- Intracytoplasmic glycogen, which are highlighted by PAS or PAS plus diastase (PASD) histochemical stains.

MESENCHYMAL CHONDROSARCOMA

290. What percentage of mesenchymal chondrosarcomas are extraosseous in location?

40%.

291. List 3 histologic features of mesenchymal chondrosarcoma.

- Mesenchymal chondrosarcoma is a high grade biphasic tumor consisting of:
  - Low grade (hyaline) conventional chondrosarcoma.
  - An undifferentiated small round blue cell component with HPC-like vessels.
- The undifferentiated component is positive for CD99 and SOX9.

292. Name the gene fusion seen in mesenchymal chondrosarcoma.

HEY1-NCOA2 fusion.

DEDIFFERENTIATED CHONDROSARCOMA

293. Define dedifferentiated chondrosarcoma.

- This is a highly malignant variant of chondrosarcoma.
- It develops in 10–15% of central conventional chondrosarcomas.
- It has sharply demarcated areas of a low grade chondrosarcoma and a dedifferentiated component that consists of a noncartilaginous high grade sarcoma.
  - The dedifferentiated component is most commonly an undifferentiated pleomorphic sarcoma or osteosarcoma.

Osteogenic Tumors

OSTEOMA

294. Define osteoma.
- This is a benign lamellar or cortical-type bone tumor on the surface of bone.
- If it arises in the medullary cavity, it is diagnosed as a bone island.

295. Which anatomic sites are most often affected by osteoma?
- It most often develops in bone formed via membranous ossification.
- The most common sites are calvarium, facial, and jaw bones.

OSTEOID OSTEOMA

296. Describe the typical clinical presentation of osteoid osteoma.
- Patients are typically young males — condition peaks in second decade.
- They present with severe, sharp, localized pain.
- The pain is worse at night, and relieved by acetylsalicylic acid (ASA) or nonsteroidal antiinflammatory drugs (NSAIDs).

297. What are the expected findings for osteoid osteoma on (plain) X-ray?
- Small, circumscribed lesion (~1 cm).
- Intracortical.
- Common locations: shaft of femur, tibia, distal humerus, fingers.
- Presence of a nidus (lytic area) surrounded by sclerosis; possible presence of a central area of ossification (targetoid appearance).

298. Describe the histologic correlate of a nidus.
- Vascular fibro connective tissue containing thin, regularly distributed trabeculae of benign osteoid rimmed by plump osteoblasts.
- Outer rim of densely sclerotic bone.
- Possible presence of a central focus of ossified bone.

299. A lesion with the same histologic appearance, but measuring > 2 cm, should be given what diagnosis?
Osteoblastoma.

OSTEOBLASTOMA

300. Compare and contrast osteoid osteoma and osteoblastoma.

	OSTEOID OSTEOMA	OSTEOBLASTOMA
Clinical features/symptoms	• Male-to-female ratio 3:1. • Age: teens and early 20s. • Extreme pain at night relieved by NSAIDs.	• Progressive pain not resolved with NSAIDs. • 20% recurrence rate.
Imaging features	• Radiolucent or ossified nidus with a radiolucent halo, surrounded by sclerotic reactive cortical bone.	• Lytic lesion with intralesional ossification. • Possible presence of (secondary) aneurysmal bone cyst-like changes (expansile growth).
Size	• < 2.0 cm.	• > 2.0 cm.
Sites of origin	• Predilection for appendicular skeleton. • Involvement of tibia or femur (50% of cases). • Cortex much more commonly involved than the medullary cavity.	• Posterior spine (laminae and pedicles).
Histologic features	• Nidus that consists of irregular trabeculae of variably mineralized woven bone. • Osteoblastic rimming and osteoclasts. • Loose, fibrovascular stroma. • Thick, sclerotic bone that surrounds nidus.	• Features of osteoid osteoma, plus: · Cement lines (pagetoid reversal lines). · (Secondary) aneurysmal bone cyst-like changes/ intralesional hemorrhage (common). · Degenerative atypia (rarely present).
Treatment	• Radiofrequency ablation (most often); curettage.	• Curettage or en bloc resection.

LOW GRADE CENTRAL OSTEOSARCOMA

301. List at least 2 entities that are frequently in the differential diagnosis of low grade central osteosarcoma.

- Fibrous dysplasia.
- Desmoplastic fibroma (if bone formation is not appreciated).
- Low grade fibrosarcoma.

302. Name an immunohistochemical test and a molecular test that can help diagnosis a low grade central osteosarcoma.

- MDM2 and/or CDK4 immunohistochemical stains.
- FISH for *MDM2* amplification.

303. List microscopic features of low grade central osteosarcoma.

- Mild to moderately cellular fascicles of mildly atypical spindle cells set in a fibrous stroma.
- Long, thick trabeculae of immature woven bone in a parallel arrangement; rarely lamellar bone, which may have cement lines (Pagetoid reversal lines).
- Permeation of host bone.
- Cortical breakthrough with soft tissue extension (possible).
- Dedifferentiation in primary or recurrent lesion in up to about one-third of cases.
  - Dedifferentiated areas may consist of undifferentiated pleomorphic sarcoma, fibrosarcoma or high grade osteosarcoma.

304. Describe the prognosis of low grade central osteosarcoma.

- There is good prognosis for tumors removed with wide resection and clear margins (> 80% survival rate).
- Tumors removed with curettage, or that have positive margins, have high recurrence.
- Dedifferentiated tumors have a worse prognosis.

CONVENTIONAL OSTEOSARCOMA

305. Describe the classical clinical presentation of osteosarcoma.

- Typical patient is a young male, age 10–20, large stature.
- Patient presents with pain, followed by mass, followed by pathological fracture.
- There is a large, aggressive tumor in the metaphysis of long bones — distal femur (30%) or proximal tibia (15%) are most common.

306. Identify at least 3 important prognostic factors for osteosarcoma.

- Tumor response to neoadjuvant chemotherapy for appendicular osteosarcoma (most important prognosticator).
- Location — in order of most to least favorable outcome: parosteal, periosteal, conventional intramedullary.
- Site — extremity is more favorable than axial.
- Surgical margin status — complete resection has more favorable outcomes.
- Tumor stage.
- Grade — low grade is more favorable than high grade (conventional osteosarcomas are high grade).
- Histologic subtype — small cell has a worse prognosis; low grade central osteosarcoma and chondroblastic osteosarcoma have a better prognosis.

307. What percentage of tumor necrosis is considered a good response to neoadjuvant chemotherapy in osteosarcoma?

≥ 90%.

308. List at least 3 common radiologic features of osteosarcoma.

- Aggressive periosteal reaction in the form of:
  - Sunburst appearance.
  - Codman triangle: periosteal lifting.
  - Lamellated (onion skin) reaction.
- Medullary and cortical bone destruction.
- Permeative growth with an ill-defined "fluffy" or "cloud-like" tumor matrix ossification/calcification.
- Soft tissue mass.

309. List the 3 most common histologic patterns of conventional osteosarcoma.

These are classified based on their predominant matrix:

- Osteoblastic osteosarcoma (most common; accounts for ~80% cases).
- Chondroblastic osteosarcoma.
- Fibroblastic osteosarcoma.

310. Describe the common histologic features of conventional osteoblastic osteosarcoma.
- Identification of neoplastic immature woven bone (osteoid) is a requisite for diagnosis.
  - No minimum amount is required.
  - The osteoid may be mineralized, imparting a basophilic appearance.
- Neoplastic osteoid is intimately associated with the tumor cells.
- Tumor cells often demonstrate nuclear pleomorphism and mitoses, including atypical forms.
- Osteoblastic rimming is absent.
  - Lack of osteoblastic rimming distinguishes it from reactive new bone formation often seen in a fracture, or adjacent to osteonecrosis or osteomyelitis).
- Variable organization of the osteoid is present.
  - Osteoid may be arranged in delicate strands ("filigree"); or coarse, lace-like patterns; or thickened, irregular trabeculae.

311. Describe how to distinguish chondroblastic osteosarcoma from chondrosarcoma.
- Chondrosarcoma:
  - This consists of malignant cartilage only.
    › Exception: if dedifferentiated chondrosarcoma is present, the dedifferentiated component may consist of osteosarcoma.
      » The 2 malignant components (dedifferentiated component and residual chondrosarcoma component) demonstrate an abrupt transition.
      » No mixing or transition occurs between the 2 components.
      » The residual chondrosarcoma component is typically low grade.
  - Mutations of *IDH1* and *IDH2* are present.
- Chondroblastic osteosarcoma:
  - This consists of malignant cartilage (chondrosarcomatous component) and malignant bone (osteosarcomatous component).
  - The 2 malignant components are intimately mixed together with a smooth transition between them.
  - The chondrosarcomatous component is invariably high grade.
  - Mutations of *IDH1* and *IDH2* are absent.

312. Describe the histologic features of telangiectatic osteosarcoma and name 1 radiologic mimic.
- This is a rare high grade variant of conventional osteosarcoma, composed of loculated, blood-filled or empty spaces lined by pleomorphic tumor cells.
- Atypical mitoses are frequent.
- Osteoid formation is often focal.
- The differential diagnosis includes aneurysmal bone cyst (it mimics aneurysmal bone cyst radiologically and at low power examination).
  - To differentiate, examine the cyst walls for pleomorphic tumor cells and neoplastic osteoid.

313. Describe the histologic features of small cell osteosarcoma. Explain how to distinguish this entity from entities commonly in the differential diagnosis.
- Small cell osteosarcoma is composed small tumor cells with round-to-oval nuclei and little cytoplasm. The tumor cells are associated with lace-like osteoid.
- A focal hemangiopericytoma-like vascular pattern may be present.
- The differential diagnosis commonly includes Ewing sarcoma and mesenchymal chondrosarcoma.
  - Molecular testing distinguishes them: small cell osteosarcoma demonstrates the absence of *HEY1-NCOA2* fusion or *EWSR1* rearrangements.

SURFACE OSTEOSARCOMAS (INCLUDING PAROSTEAL OSTEOSARCOMA, PERIOSTEAL OSTEOSARCOMA, AND HIGH GRADE SURFACE OSTEOSARCOMA)

314. What is the most common location of parosteal osteosarcoma?
Along the bone surface on the posterior aspect of the distal femur (~70%).

315. What genetic alteration is frequently identified in parosteal osteosarcoma?
MDM2 amplifications detected by FISH or by IHC for MDM2 expression (and positivity for CDK4 immunostain).

316. List entities in the differential diagnosis of parosteal osteosarcoma.
- Reactive periostitis.
- Juxtacortical myositis ossificans.
- Desmoplastic fibroma.
- Fibrous dysplasia.

317. Briefly compare the microscopic features of parosteal and periosteal osteosarcoma.

- Parosteal osteosarcoma:
  - This is a low grade spindle cell tumor with woven bone trabeculae often arranged in a parallel fashion.
  - The tumor arises on surface of bone, below the periosteum.

- Periosteal osteosarcoma:
  - This is an intermediate grade chondroblastic osteosarcoma on the surface of the bone, below the periosteum.

318. Compare the treatment and prognosis of parosteal, periosteal, and high grade surface osteosarcoma.

	PAROSTEAL OSTEOSARCOMA	PERIOSTEAL OSTEOSARCOMA	HIGH GRADE SURFACE OSTEOSARCOMA
Treatment	• Wide surgical excision with clear margins is curative. • Chemotherapy is needed for dedifferentiated tumors.	• Wide surgical resection is needed. • Chemotherapy does not appear to influence outcomes.	• Neoadjuvant chemotherapy is needed, followed by wide surgical resection.
Prognosis	• Incompletely excised tumors recur locally. • These tumors (unless dedifferentiated) have excellent prognosis: 90% survival at 5 years. • Dedifferentiated tumors have poor prognosis.	• Marrow involvement may predict more aggressive behavior. • Assessment of postneoadjuvant chemotherapy tumor necrosis is not predictive of outcome. • This has better prognosis than conventional osteosarcoma, but not as good as parosteal osteosarcoma.	• Overall 5 year survival is ~60%. • Assessment of postneoadjuvant chemotherapy tumor is predictive of outcome. • Localized disease has a more favorable prognosis. • Metastases and recurrence are poor prognosticators.

SECONDARY OSTEOSARCOMA

319. List at least 3 clinical settings in which secondary osteosarcoma may arise.

- Postradiation (strongest risk factor).
- Paget disease of bone.
- Fibrous dysplasia.
- Bone infarction.
- Chronic osteomyelitis.
- Orthopedic implants (rare).

320. Describe the clinical features of secondary osteosarcoma.

- Secondary osteosarcomas are:
  - Invariably high grade.
  - Clinically more aggressive than primary osteosarcoma.
  - Most likely to arise in older patients.

Fibrogenic Tumors

321. List 2 entities in the differential diagnosis of desmoplastic fibroma of bone.

- Desmoplastic fibroma of bone is an extremely rare primary bone tumor that morphologically resembles desmoid-type fibromatosis.

- In order to diagnose desmoplastic fibroma of bone, you must exclude:
  - Fibrous dysplasia (*GNAS* mutations).
  - Low grade central osteosarcoma (*MDM2* amplifications).

Vascular Tumors

322. Name 2 common anatomic sites where hemangioma of bone may develop.

- Vertebral bodies (~10% of the adult population).
- Craniofacial bones.

Malignant Vascular Tumors

323. Explain how to distinguish an epithelioid hemangioendothelioma of bone from epithelioid hemangioma of bone and angiosarcoma of bone.

EPITHELIOID HEMANGIOMA OF BONE	EPITHELIOID HEMANGIOENDOTHELIOMA OF BONE	ANGIOSARCOMA OF BONE
• Lobular architecture that infiltrates bone trabeculae.	• Solid mass with no vasoformation.	• Lack of lobular architecture; presence of numerous extravasated red blood cells.
• Presence of epithelioid endothelial cells n the center of the lobules; presences of small capillaries with flat endothelial cells at the periphery of lobules (often).	• Epithelioid and spindle cells arranged in cords in a myxohyaline stroma.	• Epithelioid atypical endothelial cells with vesicular nuclei and prominent nucleoli, which are mitotically active.
• Vascular lumen lined by epithelioid cells in a "tombstone" arrangement.	• Intracytoplasmic lumina which may contain fragmented on intact red blood cells.	• Intracytoplasmic lumina which may contain fragmented or intact red blood cells.
• Rearrangement of *FOS* or *FOSB* in most cases.	• *WWTR1-CAMTA1* fusion more commonly seen than *YAP1-TFE3* fusion.	• No characteristic molecular alteration.

324. List 1 microscopic difference between classic epithelioid hemangioendothelioma (*WWTR1-CAMTA1* fusion) and epithelioid hemangioendothelioma with *YAP1-TFE3* fusion.

- Myxohyaline stroma minimal or absent.
- Epithelioid cells with abundant cytoplasm with a feathery appearance.

Osteoclastic Giant Cell-Rich Tumors

ANEURYSMAL BONE CYST

325. List at least 1 characteristic radiologic feature of aneurysmal bone cyst.
- Multicystic lesion with fluid-fluid levels.
- Lytic, expansile lesion with well-defined margins.

326. What are the most common locations for aneurysmal bone cyst?
- Metaphyses of long bones — femur, tibia, and humerus.
- Posterior elements of vertebral bodies lead to nerve compression.

327. Aneurysmal bone cyst-like changes (formerly known as secondary aneurysmal bone cyst) can be seen in a variety bone tumors. List at least 3 primary bone tumors that are often complicated by aneurysmal bone cyst-like changes.
- Giant cell tumor of bone.
- Osteoblastoma.
- Chondroblastoma.
- Fibrous dysplasia.
- Others (less often): malignant bone sarcomas, most often osteosarcoma; clear cell chondrosarcoma.

328. List at least 3 microscopic features of aneurysmal bone cyst.
- This is a well-circumscribed, multiloculated blood-filled cyst.
- The cyst walls contain cellular proliferation of bland fibroblasts with scattered osteoclast-type giant cells.
- Reactive woven bone is lined by osteoblasts and frequently follows the contours of the cyst wall.
- Normal mitoses are frequent.

329. Name the most common molecular alteration in aneurysmal bone cyst.
USP6 gene rearrangement (in classic and solid variant; not detected in gnathic giant cell reparative granulomas).

GIANT CELL TUMOR OF BONE

330. Identify the part of the bone most commonly affected by giant cell tumors.
Epiphysis (around the growth plate).

331. Describe the gross appearance of giant cell tumors of bone.
- Circumscribed; may erode cortex +/– pathological fracture.
- Moderate size (4–8 cm).
- Soft, hemorrhagic, gritty.

332. List 3 characteristic histologic features of giant cell tumors of bone.

- They have numerous evenly distributed, multinucleated giant cells — may have > 50 nuclei. These are reactive and not the neoplastic component.
- The stromal cell component has 2 types of cells: (1) macrophage-like osteoclast precursors (nuclei identical to those in the giant cells), (2) plump, uniform mononuclear cells with poorly defined cytoplasm (may have "naked" nuclei). The latter are derived from primitive mesenchymal cells and are the proliferative cells in the tumor.
- Mitoses and hemorrhage/hemosiderin are common.
- They do not contain bone, but reactive bone may be seen around the periphery.
- They may have (secondary) aneurysmal bone cyst-like changes.
- Lymphatic invasion may be identified.

333. List 2 histologic changes that may be seen in a giant cell tumor of bone treated with denosumab.

- Substantial new bone formation, particularly at the periphery of the lesion.
- Depletion of the osteoclast-like giant cells.

334. List 3 other entities in the differential diagnosis of giant cell tumors of bone.

- Giant cell reparative granuloma.
- "Brown tumor" of hyperparathyroidism.
- Other tumors with a giant cell component (chondroblastoma, giant cell–rich osteosarcoma).
- Chondroblastoma.
- Solid variant of aneurysmal bone cyst.

335. Outline how to distinguish giant cell tumor of bone from solid aneurysmal bone cyst and giant cell rich osteosarcoma.

GIANT CELL TUMOR OF BONE	SOLID ANEURYSMAL BONE CYST	GIANT CELL RICH OSTEOSARCOMA
• Epiphyseal often extends to articular surface; distal femur and proximal tibia are the most common sites.	• Metaphyses, and small bones of the hands and feet, are the most common sites.	• Metaphyses near the growth plates are the most common sites.
• Osteoclast-like giant cells are more evenly distributed and larger with numerous (> 50) nuclei (compared to solid aneurysmal bone cyst).	• Osteoclast-like giant cells are unevenly distributed and are smaller (fewer nuclei) (compared to giant cell tumor of bone).	• Nonneoplastic osteoclast-type giant cells are scattered throughout the tumor. Nuclear pleomorphism and brisk mitoses, with atypical forms, are common.
• Less fibrotic stroma is present.	• Stroma fibrotic is present.	• Malignant osteoid is identified in association with atypical tumor cells.
• *H3F3A* gene mutations are present. H3.3 G34W IHC is a reliable surrogate marker.	• *USP6* gene rearrangement is present.	• This has no characteristic molecular alteration.

NONOSSIFYING FIBROMA

336. Describe the classic clinical, radiologic, and microscopic features of a nonossifying fibroma.

- Clinical features:
  - These occur in skeletally immature individuals, with peak incidence during the teenage years.
  - It manifests as a metaphyseal lesion in the cortex.
  - Small tumors are asymptomatic and incidentally found. Larger tumors may be painful due to microfractures, or they may cause pathologic fractures.
- Radiographic appearance:
  - The lesions involve the cortical bone; they are well defined, lobulated, and radiolucent with scalloped, sclerotic borders.
  - They run parallel with the long axis of bone.
- Microscopic features:
  - The lesions have bland spindle cells in a storiform pattern with scattered osteoclast-like giant cells.
  - Occasional mitoses are present.
  - Reactive changes are present, including foamy macrophages and hemosiderin deposition.

337. Name at least 1 genetic syndrome associated with nonossifying fibroma.

- Neurofibromatosis type 1.
- Jaffe-Campanacci syndrome (multifocal lesions may be seen).
- Oculoectodermal syndrome (multifocal lesions may be seen).

Notochordal Tumors

CONVENTIONAL CHORDOMA

338. What is the most common site of conventional chordoma?

Sacrum.

339. Name 1 genetic syndrome that may be associated with chordoma arising in children.

Tuberous sclerosis.

340. List at least 3 microscopic features of conventional chordoma.

- Cords of tumor cells are embedded within a myxoid matrix and arranged in lobules separated by fibrous septae.
- Tumor cells have:
  - Prominent cytoplasmic borders.
  - Abundant eosinophilic cytoplasm.
- Physaliferous cells: tumor cells with intracytoplasmic vacuoles.
- Atypia may be heterogeneous: low grade (uniform tumor cells and occasional mitoses) to high grade (nuclear pleomorphism and frequent mitoses).
- Necrosis is frequent and may be extensive.

341. Describe the classic immunohistochemical staining profile of conventional chordoma.

- It is cytokeratin positive.
- It is often positive for EMA and S100 protein.
- Nuclear expression of brachyury (marker of notochord differentiation) is highly specific for chordoma.

342. Describe the microscopic features of chondroid chordoma in relation to conventional chordoma.

- Neoplastic cells of chondroid chordoma are identical to conventional chordoma.
- The matrix resembles neoplastic hyaline cartilage (rather than myxoid stroma).

343. Outline how to distinguish chordoma from a chondrosarcoma.

CHORDOMA	CHONDROSARCOMA
• Lobular arrangement of cells with thin fibrous septae is seen.	• No fibrous septae are present.
• Tumor cells are arranged in cords.	• Tumors cells are not arranged in cords.
• Tumor cells have abundant eosinophilic cytoplasm and physaliferous cells.	• Tumor cells have minimal cytoplasm.
• Tumor cells are immunoreactive for cytokeratins, brachyury, EMA, and often S100 protein.	• Tumor cells are immunoreactive for S100 protein, and negative for cytokeratins and brachyury. • Note: EMA immunoreactivity may be seen in ~20% of chondrosarcomas.

DEDIFFERENTIATED CHORDOMA

344. Define dedifferentiated chordoma and describe a characteristic immunohistochemical finding.

- Dedifferentiated chordoma has sharply demarcated areas of conventional chordoma, and dedifferentiated areas that may consist of an undifferentiated pleomorphic sarcoma or osteosarcoma.
- Dedifferentiated areas often demonstrate a loss of brachyury immunohistochemical staining.

POORLY DIFFERENTIATED CHORDOMA

345. What is the most common location and age group for poorly differentiated chordoma?

- Skull base; sacrum (rare).
- Children.

346. Describe the histologic features of poorly differentiated chordoma.

- This tumor lacks physaliferous cells and consists of tightly packed small epithelioid cells with increased nuclear-cytoplasmic ratios and irregular nuclei.
- The tumor cells may have a rhabdoid morphology.
- The tumor cells are arranged in irregular nests and sheets set in a more fibrous background.
- Geographic necrosis is present.

347. What is the characteristic immunohistochemical staining profile of poorly differentiated chordoma?

- This tumor is immunoreactive for cytokeratin and brachyury, and variably positive for S100 protein.
- It demonstrates loss of staining with SMARCB1 (INI1).
- Malignant rhabdoid tumors will enter the differential diagnosis of a tumor showing SMARCB1 (INI1) loss of staining, particularly in pediatric patients.

Other Mesenchymal Tumors of Bone

ADAMANTINOMA OF LONG BONES

348. What are the most common clinical and radiographic features of adamantinoma?

- Clinical features:
  - It presents in the second to third decades.
  - The most common sites are the tibia and fibula (tibia is more common).
    - › Be cautious about diagnosing adamantinoma in a site other than the tibia or fibula.
  - Multifocality is common and 10% of patients have additional lesions in the ipsilateral fibula.
- It is a locally aggressive or malignant tumor.
- Radiographic features:
  - It is a cortical-medullary based lesion in the diaphyseal region.
  - It has mixed lytic/blastic appearance.
  - It has a soap-bubble appearance.

349. Describe the characteristic microscopic appearance of adamantinoma of long bones.

- Classic adamantinoma:
  - This is a biphasic tumor with:
    - › A prominent epithelial component (tubular, squamous, basaloid, or spindle-shaped), which can be highlighted with epithelial markers.
    - › A bland fibroosseous component.
- Osteofibrous dysplasia-like adamantinoma:
  - The bland osteofibrous component is predominant.
- The tumor has small epithelial clusters that are often difficult to see by light microscopy (visible with immunohistochemical stains for epithelial markers).
- Note that osteofibrous dysplasia-like adamantinoma is a lesion distinct from osteofibrous dysplasia, which also occurs in the tibial cortex.
  - › Osteofibrous dysplasia has no clusters of epithelial cells; epithelial markers are typically completely negative, but rare single cell staining for epithelial markers is allowed.

OSTEOFIBROUS DYSPLASIA

350. Describe how to distinguish osteofibrous dysplasia from fibrous dysplasia.

- Compared to fibrous dysplasia, osteofibrous dysplasia:
  - Has a stroma that is less cellular.
  - Has woven bone with prominent osteoblastic rimming.
- Is a cortical-based lesion in the tibia, rather than a lesion in the medullary cavity.
- Lacks *GNAS* mutations.

SIMPLE BONE CYST

351. Describe simple bone cyst.

- It was formerly known as unicameral bone cyst.
- It is an intramedullar unilocular cyst lined by a fibrous membrane and filled with serous or serosanginous fluid.
- It has no cyst-lining cells.
- Fibrin-like deposits or cementum-like material are often seen on the cyst surface or within the cyst wall.

FIBROUS DYSPLASIA

352. Describe the gross appearance of fibrous dysplasia involving a rib.

- Fusiform expansion of the bone.
- Thinned cortex.
- Replacement of bone with firm, white/gray tissue.
- Presence or absence of cyst(s) (i.e., [secondary] aneurysmal bone cyst-like changes) and/or cartilage.
- Presence or absence of fracture through lesion.

353. Classify 3 clinical forms of fibrous dysplasia of bone.

- Monostotic (most common form).
- Polyostotic, monomelic — 1 extremity or side of body.
- Polyostotic, polymelic — diffuse involvement.

354. Briefly explain how fibrous dysplasia develops.

- It is caused by postzygotic activating missense mutations in *GNAS* gene.
- The phenotype depends on the timing of the mutation:
  - Mutation during embryogenesis procures McCune-Albright syndrome with polyostotic fibrous dysplasia.
- Mutation after skeletal formation results in monostotic fibrous dysplasia.

355. What is the characteristic radiologic appearance of fibrous dysplasia?
- Ground-glass appearance.
- Well-defined lesion.

356. Describe the microscopic features of fibrous dysplasia of bone.
- This is a well-circumscribed, intramedullary lesion.
- It has variable amounts of fibrous and osseous tissue.
- The osseous component consists of irregular, curvilinear trabeculae of typically woven bone with inconspicuous osteoblasts.
- Rarely, there may be psammomatous or cementum-like deposits (most often in jaw lesions).
- The fibrous component consists of bland fibroblastic spindle cells.
- Possible secondary features include aneurysmal bone cyst-like changes, foam cells, osteoclast-like giant cells, myxoid change, and a cartilaginous component.

357. Identify at least 1 syndrome that may be associated with fibrous dysplasia of bone.
- McCune-Albright syndrome — precocious puberty or other endocrine abnormalities, café-au-lait skin pigmentation.
- Mazabraud syndrome — intramuscular myxomas.

358. List 3 complications of fibrous dysplasia of bone.
- Pathological fracture.
- Deformity +/− cosmetic problems.
- (Secondary) aneurysmal bone cyst-like changes.
- Malignant transformation — rare.

Hematopoietic Neoplasms of Bone
LANGERHANS CELL HISTIOCYTOSIS

359. Define Langerhans cell histiocytosis.
- This is clonal proliferation of dendritic cells expressing a Langerhans cell phenotype, which most often involves bone but may also involve lymph nodes, skin, and lung.
- It can be uni- or multifocal, and may affect a single system (usually bone) or multiple systems.

360. What is the characteristic immunohistochemical staining profile of Langerhans cell histiocytosis?
Often expresses CD1A, langerin (CD207), S100 protein, and CD68.

361. Describe the characteristic microscopic appearance of Langerhans cell histiocytosis.
- This consists of oval cells with grooved/indented nuclei, fine chromatin, and abundant, slightly eosinophilic cytoplasm.
- The background typically contains eosinophils, macrophages (which can include osteoclast-type giant cells in bone), neutrophils, and lymphocytes.

362. What is the characteristic ultrastructural (electron microscopy) finding in Langerhans cell histiocytosis?
Cytoplasmic Birbeck granule (tennis-racket shape).

ERDHEIM-CHESTER DISEASE

363. What are the most common sites of involvement of Erdheim-Chester disease?
- More than 90% of cases involve long bone (symmetrical osteosclerosis of long bones).
- Other sites include retroperitoneum, central nervous system (20–50% cases), lungs, cardiovascular system, and skin.
- Involvement of central nervous system and cardiovascular system is associated with worse outcomes.

364. What is the characteristic immunohistochemical staining profile of Erdheim-Chester disease?
Expresses CD68, CD163, and CD14, and is negative for langerin (CD207) and CD1A.

365. Describe the characteristic microscopic appearance of Erdheim-Chester disease.
- Foamy macrophages associated with variable numbers of Touton giant cells, small lymphocytes, plasma cells, and neutrophils.
- Variable amount of fibrous tissue.

Soft Tissue Pathology

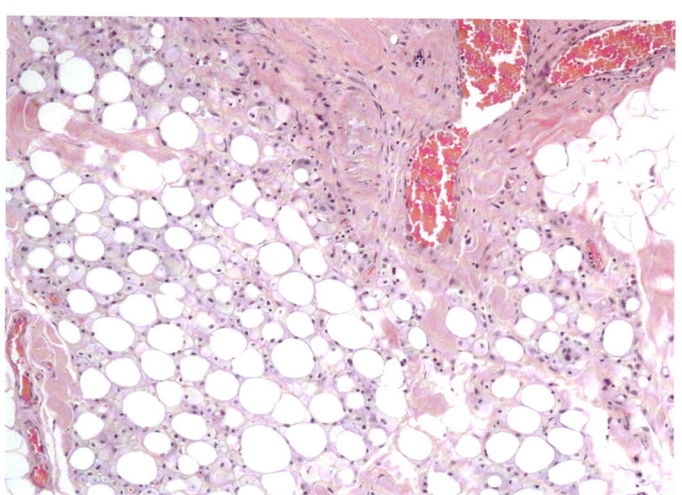

IMAGE 2.1 Fat necrosis contains numerous foamy histiocytes often admixed with variable amounts of inflammatory cells (H&E, x10).

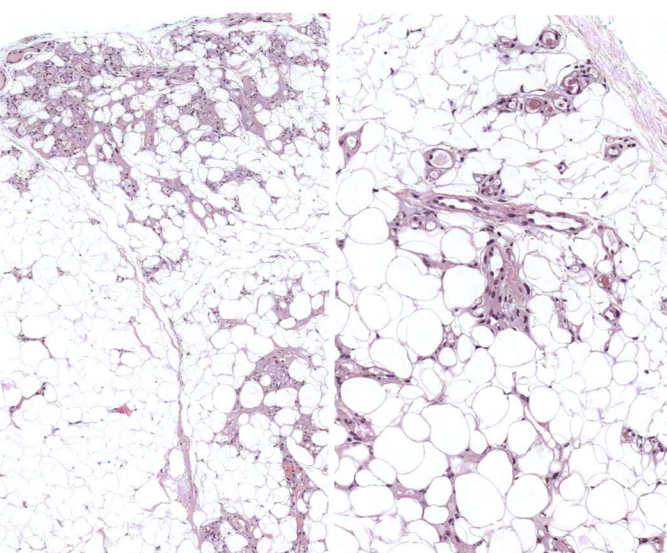

IMAGE 2.3 Angiolipoma. Left: the image shows characteristic lobules of mature adipose tissue intermingled with small capillaries that tend to concentrate at the periphery of the lobules (H&E, x10). Right: the capillaries often contain fibrin thrombi.

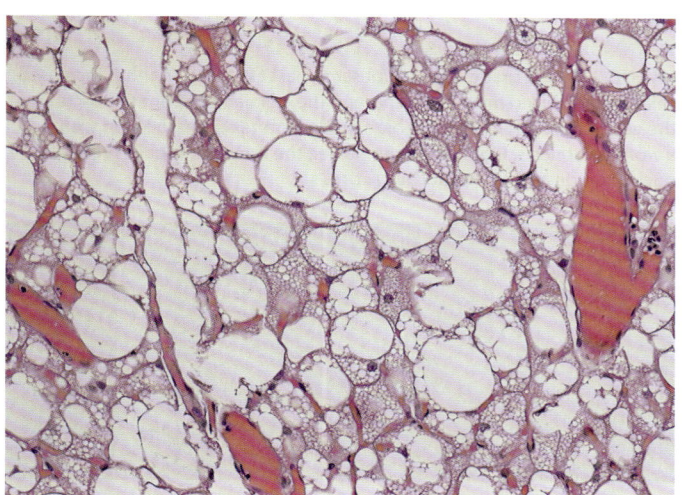

IMAGE 2.2 Hibernoma is characterized by variable amounts of brown fat and mature adipose tissue (white fat). Brown fat adipocytes contain a small central, bland nucleus and multivacuolated cytoplasm containing lipid droplets (H&E, x20).

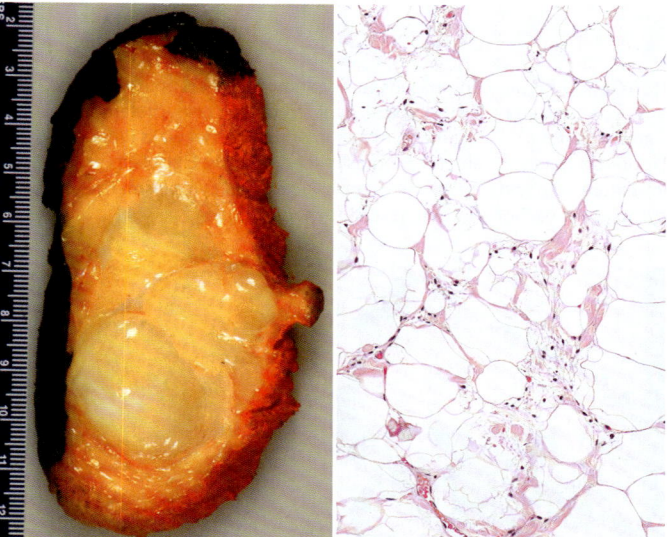

IMAGE 2.4 Spindle cell lipoma is an encapsulated tumor of mature adipose tissue that most often occurs in the upper back/neck. Left: note that the tumor is well-defined and composed of mature adipose tissue with fibrous septae. Right: spindle cell lipoma is characterized by short, ovoid spindle cells, ropey collagen, and a variable amount of fat (H&E, x20).

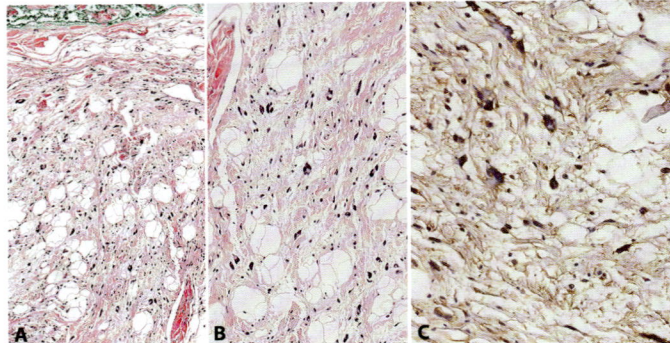

IMAGE 2.5 Pleomorphic lipoma. Image A (H&E, x10) and image B (H&E, x20): in addition to the features of spindle cell lipoma, pleomorphic lipoma contains scattered floret-like multinucleated cells and atypical spindle cells. Image C: CD34 highlights the spindle cells and floret-like cells.

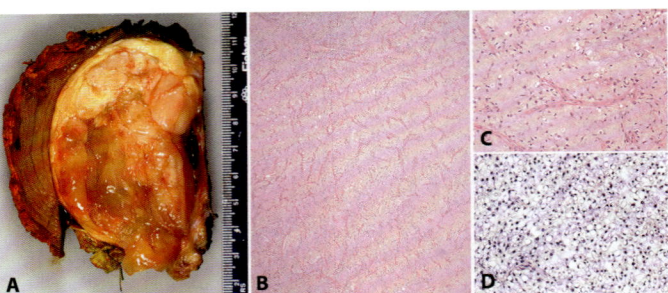

IMAGE 2.8 Conventional myxoid liposarcoma. Image A: this gross image shows myxoid liposarcoma involving the thigh (most common location). On cut section, note the pale, glistening gross surface with areas of necrosis. Image B: at low power, note the striking plexiform vascular pattern. Images C and D: in these higher power images, the tumor is hypocellular with a mix of bland oval cells and lipoblasts (image D with univacuolated lipoblasts).

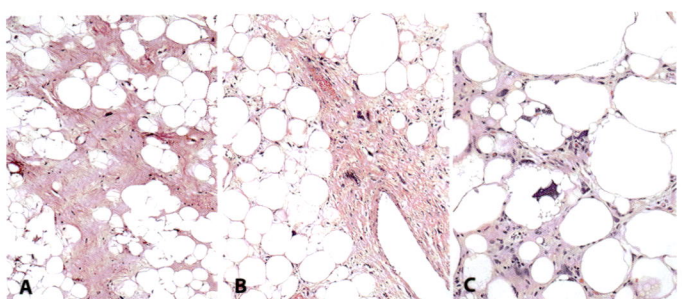

IMAGE 2.6 Atypical lipomatous tumor and well-differentiated liposarcoma are characterized by large atypical, hyperchromatic cells, preferentially found in fibrous septae (image A) and in or near vessel walls (image B). Lipoblasts (image C) are not a requisite for diagnosis. Lipoblasts are immature adipocytes with uni- or multivacuolated cytoplasm. The cytoplasmic vacuoles indent or scallop the nucleus.

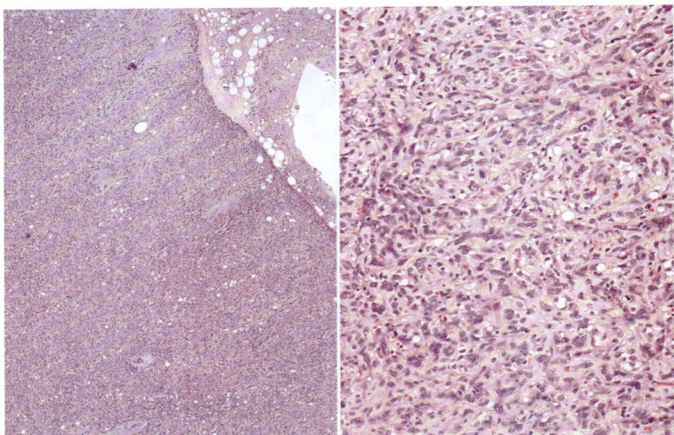

IMAGE 2.9 High grade myxoid liposarcoma. Left: this tumor has increased cellularity, reduced myxoid stroma, and the cellular component obscures the vasculature. More than 5% high grade features are associated with a worse prognosis. Right: at higher power, the tumor cells have higher nuclear grade and are mitotically active.

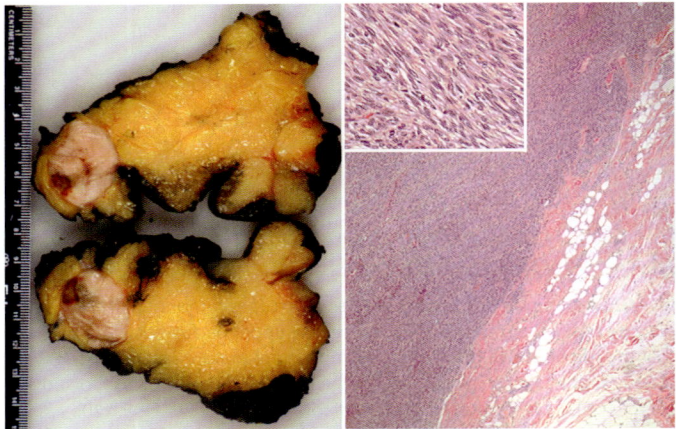

IMAGE 2.7 Dedifferentiated liposarcoma. Left: these are gross images demonstrating the abrupt transition between the dedifferentiated component and the residual well-differentiated component. Note that, grossly, it may be impossible to distinguish between normal fat and a (residual) well-differentiated liposarcoma. It is crucial to sample the adjacent grossly normal-appearing fat with any resected high grade sarcoma, particularly in the retroperitoneum. Right: a low power view shows the abrupt transition between the dedifferentiated component and the residual well-differentiated liposarcoma. Inset: the dedifferentiated component consists of an undifferentiated spindle sarcoma.

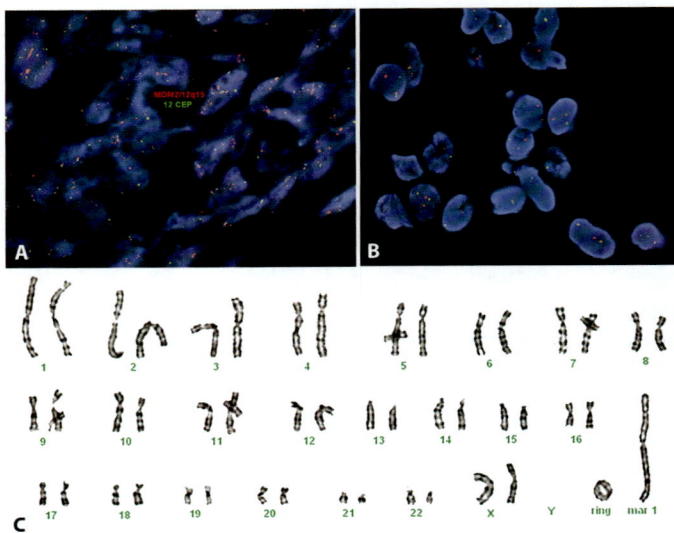

IMAGE 2.10 Differentiated liposarcoma. Image A: fluorescence in situ hybridization (FISH) demonstrates *MDM2* amplification. Image B: a FISH *DDIT3/FUS* break-apart probe is shown in a myxoid liposarcoma. Image C: this is a karyotype of an atypical lipomatous tumor (ALT). Ring and/or marker chromosomes are present, distinguishing between an ALT and a benign lipoma.

Image C courtesy of Dr. Lisa M. Defrancesco, University of Calgary.

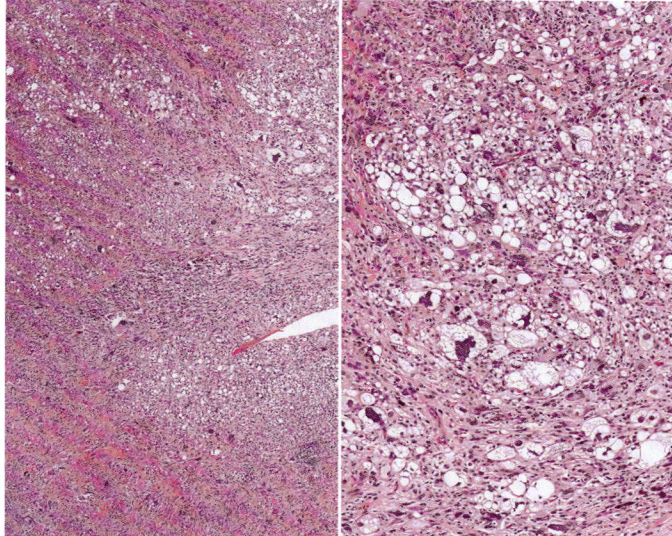

IMAGE 2.11 Pleomorphic liposarcoma. Left: low power (H&E, x4) view of a pleomorphic liposarcoma which is an otherwise undifferentiated pleomorphic sarcoma with numerous, defining scattered lipoblasts. Unlike other variants of liposarcoma, there are no characteristic molecular alterations. Right: a higher power view of the defining multivacuolated lipoblasts (H&E, x10).

Right image courtesy of Dr. Lisa M. Defrancesco, University of Calgary.

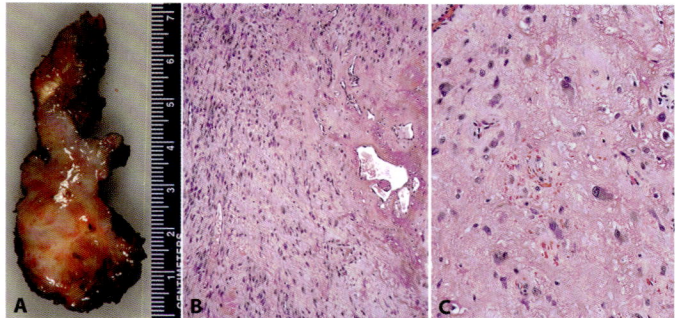

IMAGE 2.13 Ischemic fasciitis. Image A: ischemic fasciitis grossly is a white fibrous to tan-yellow lesion which may have central necrosis or cystic change. Image B: this low power view demonstrates a zonal appearance with fibrinoid necrosis surrounded by proliferation fibroblasts and myofibroblasts, some of which have a ganglion cell-like appearance. Image C: a higher power view demonstrates polygonal fibroblasts and myofibroblasts with a ganglion cell-like appearance.

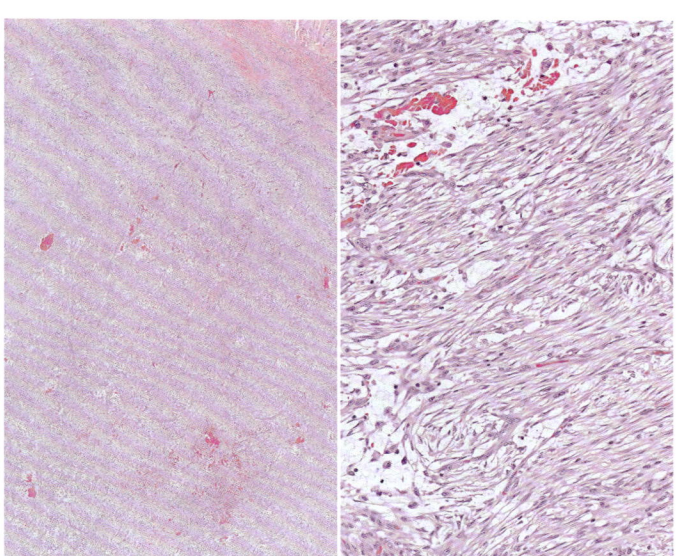

IMAGE 2.12 Nodular fasciitis. Left: nodular fasciitis is a well-defined, focally infiltrative spindle cell proliferation of myofibroblasts with cellular and myxoid areas. Right: plump myofibroblasts with tapering cytoplasmic process and extravasated red blood cells without hemosiderin are some of the characteristic features of nodular fasciitis (H&E, x20).

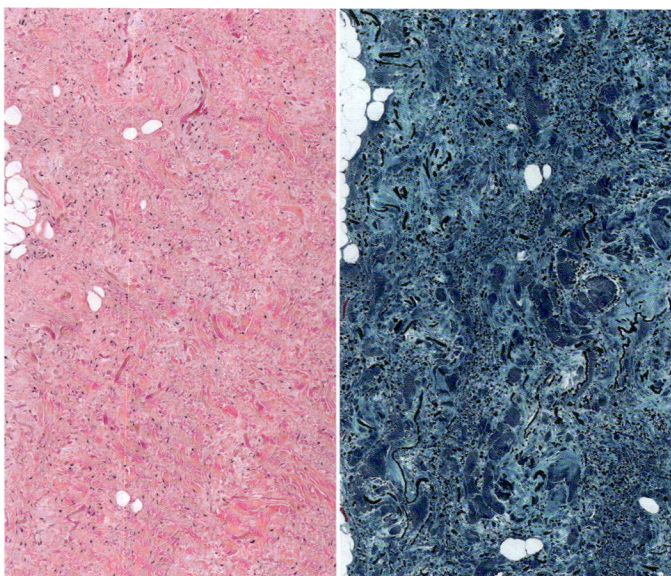

IMAGE 2.14 Elastofibroma is a lesion that occurs almost exclusively in elderly patients. Left: it is composed of fibrocollagenous tissue with abnormal, fragmented elastic fibers that resemble beads on a string (H&E, x10). Right: these fragmented elastic fibers can be highlighted by an elastic stain (Verhoeff elastic stain, x10).

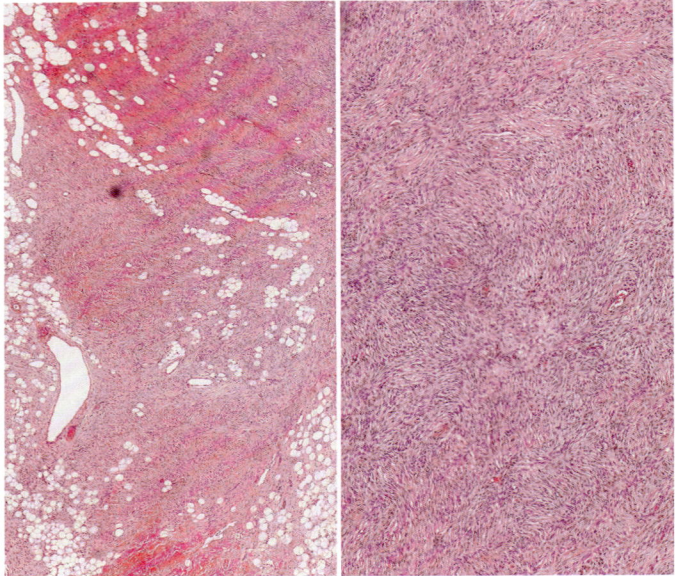

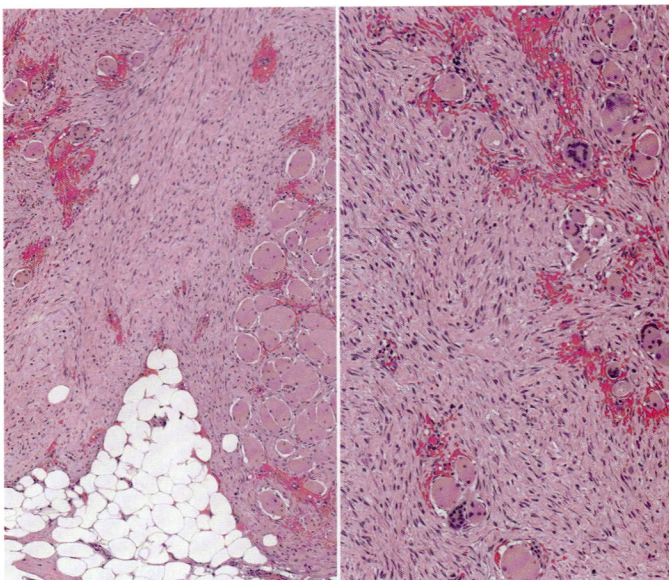

IMAGE 2.15 Left: the image shows dermatofibrosarcoma protuberans (DFSP) with a honey-comb pattern of fat infiltration (H&E, x4). Right: the image shows a hypercellular, storiform arrangement of spindle cells (H&E, x10). DFSP is an intermediate grade sarcoma that may progress to a high grade sarcoma. Most often the high grade sarcoma consists of a fibrosarcoma and demonstrates loss of staining with CD34.

IMAGE 2.17 Deep fibromatosis (desmoid tumor). Left: deep fibromatosis consists of a proliferation of bland fibroblasts and collagen that infiltrates surrounding tissue (H&E, x10). Right: bland fibroblasts entrap skeletal muscle bundles (H&E, x20).

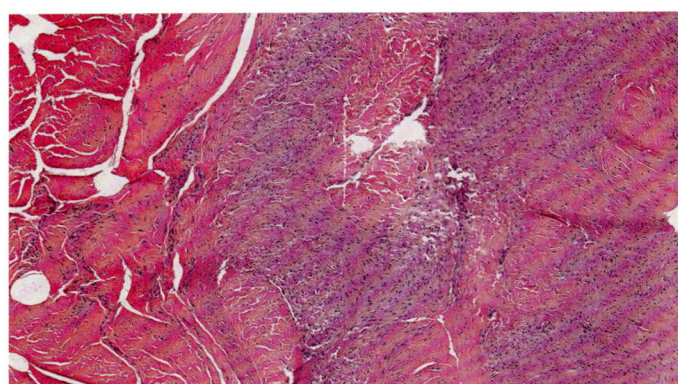

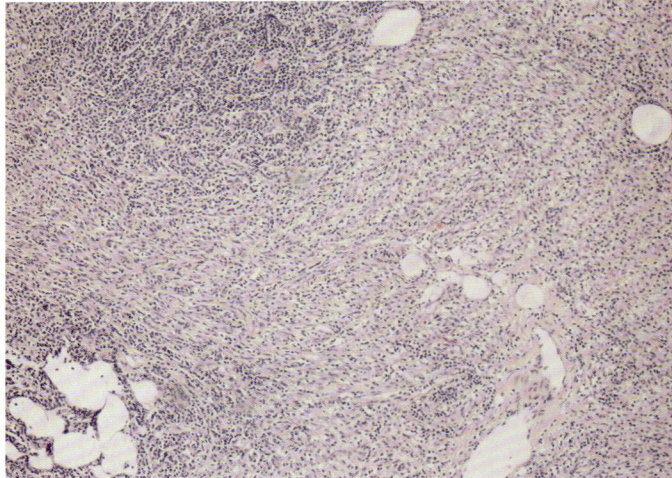

IMAGE 2.16 Palmar fibromatosis is an ill-defined cellular proliferation of uniform, plump fibroblasts and myofibroblasts involving the fascia. Older lesions are often less cellular with dense collagen (H&E, x10).

IMAGE 2.18 Inflammatory myofibroblastic tumor consists of myofibroblasts and inflammatory cells. Approximately 60% will be immunoreactive for ALK protein (not shown).

Courtesy of Dr. Denis Gravel, University of Ottawa.

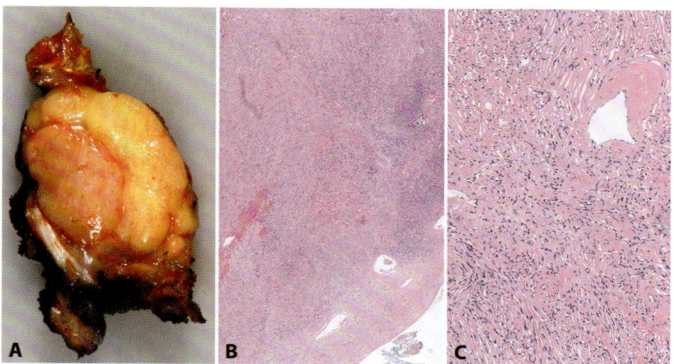

IMAGE 2.19 Solitary fibrous tumor. Image A: this well-defined, firm, white mass, adjacent to fat, represents a solitary fibrous tumor. Image B: the image shows a well-defined proliferation of fibroblasts with hypercellular and less cellular areas, arranged in a so-called "patternless pattern," and ectatic, hemangiopericytoma-like blood vessels (H&E, x4). Image C: higher power demonstrates bland fibroblasts and "cracking" artifact between the thick collagen and spindle cells. Focal perivascular hyalinization may be seen. STAT6 (specific) and CD34 are positive in solitary fibrous tumor (H&E, x20).

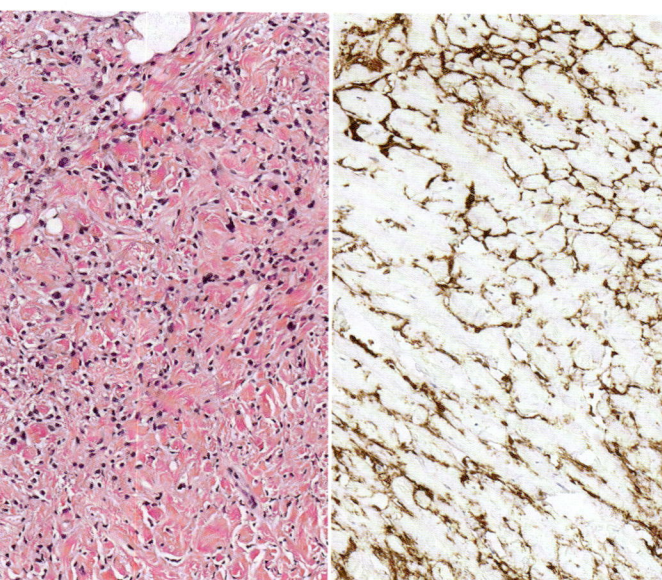

IMAGE 2.21 Sclerosing epithelioid sarcoma is a tumor closely related to low grade myxoid sarcoma. Left: the image shows proliferation of bland epithelioid tumor cells arranged in cords and embedded within a densely collagenous stroma (H&E, x20). Tumor cells may also be arranged in nests (not shown) Right: the image shows strong, diffuse staining with MUC4 (x20).

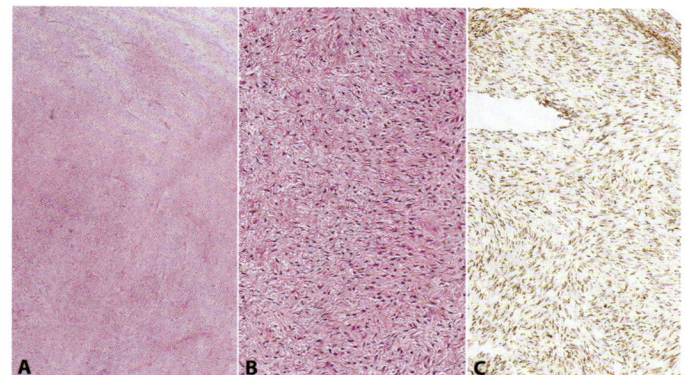

IMAGE 2.20 Low grade fibromyxoid sarcoma. Image A: at low power (H&E, x2), low grade fibromyxoid sarcoma is characterized by alternating myxoid and cellular areas, imparting a "tiger-stripe" appearance and arching blood vessels. Image B: the spindle cells are bland and uniform in appearance, mimicking the appearance of fibromatosis or perineurioma (H&E, x20). Image C: MUC4 is sensitive and specific marker for low grade fibromyxoid sarcoma (H&E, x20).

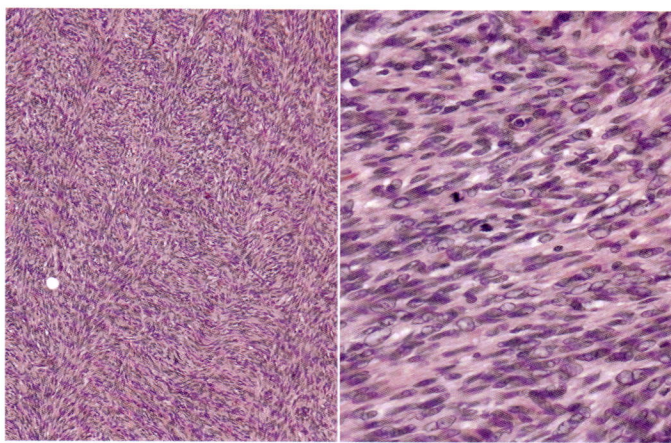

IMAGE 2.22 Adult fibrosarcoma. Low (left) and high (right) power views of an adult fibrosarcoma show a hypercellular proliferation of atypical spindle cells, often in a herringbone pattern, and easy-to-identify mitoses, often including atypical forms.

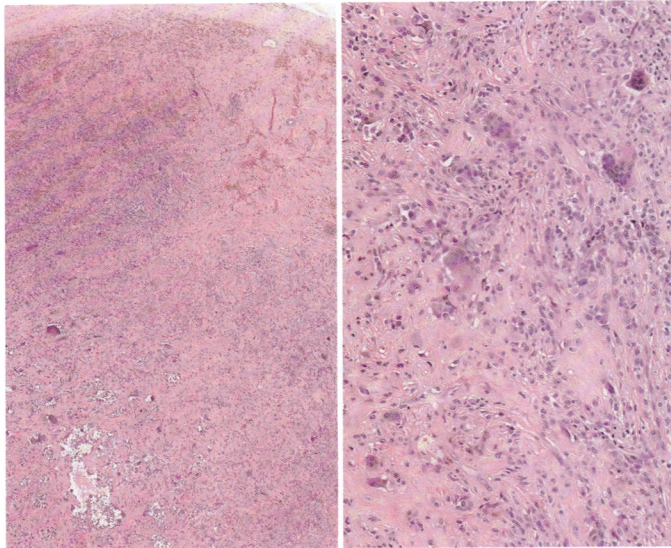

IMAGE 2.23 Tenosynovial giant cell tumor, localized type (also called giant cell tumor of tendon sheath). Low (left, H&E, x4) and high (right, H&E, x20) power views of a tenosynovial giant cell tumor, localized type demonstrate a variable mixture of mononuclear cells, osteoclast-like giant cells, and hemosiderin deposition.

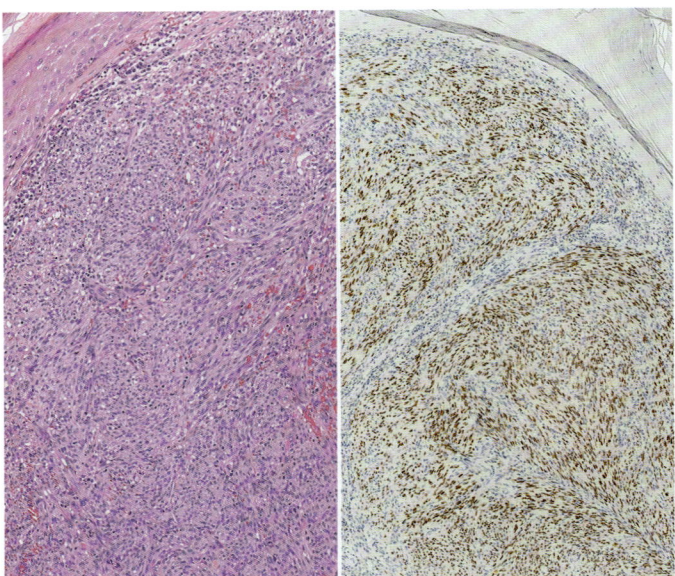

IMAGE 2.25 Kaposi sarcoma. Left: Kaposi sarcoma has variable amounts of spindle cells, blood vessels, and extravasated red blood cells (H&E, x10). Right: the spindle cells demonstrate diffuse nuclear staining with HHV-8 (x10).

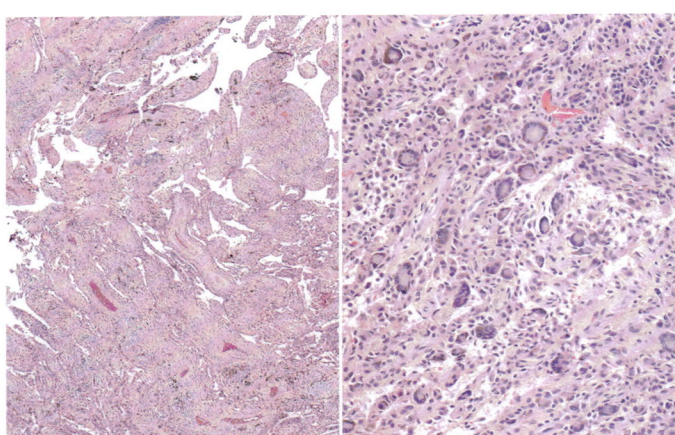

IMAGE 2.24 Tenosynovial giant cell tumor, diffuse type (also called pigmented villionodular synovitis). Low (left) and high (right) power views of a tenosynovial giant cell tumor, diffuse type, demonstrate proliferative synovium with mononuclear cells, osteoclast-like giant cells, hemosiderin deposition, and large clefts. The amount of giant cells is variable and, when minimal, the diagnosis can be challenging.

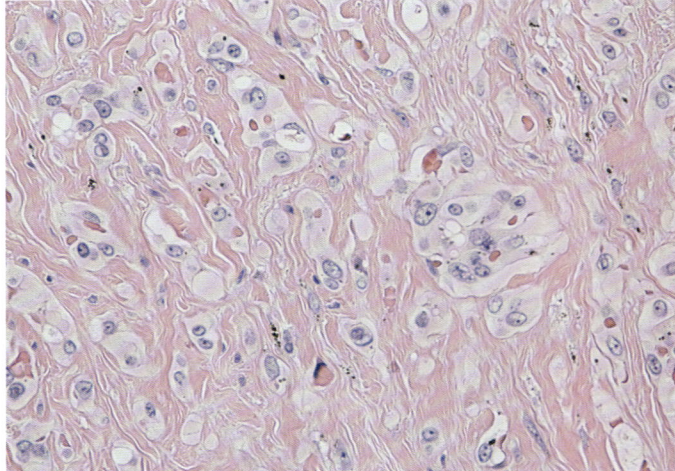

IMAGE 2.26 Epithelioid hemangioendothelioma consists of large endothelial cells arranged in nests and cords with eosinophilic cytoplasm. It is embedded in a myxohyaline stroma. Some tumor cells have intracytoplasmic vacuoles representing vascular lumina which may contain red blood cells.

Courtesy Dr. Denis Gravel, University of Ottawa.

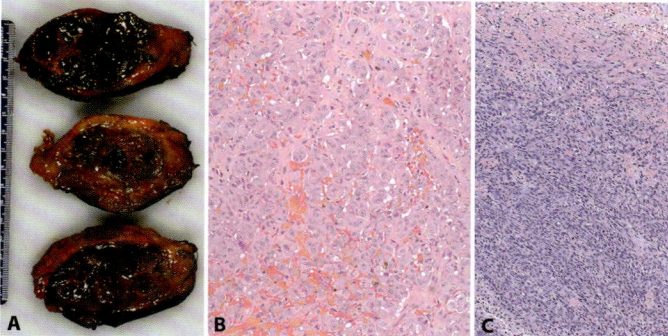

IMAGE 2.27 Image A: this is a gross image of an epithelioid angiosarcoma with a hemorrhagic appearance. Image B: this shows an epithelioid angiosarcoma with atypical epithelioid tumor cells arranged in sheets and nests. Epithelioid angiosarcoma may express epithelial markers. Image C: Conventional angiosarcoma consists of atypical spindle endothelial cells forming irregular anastomosing vascular channels. Numerous mitoses are seen.

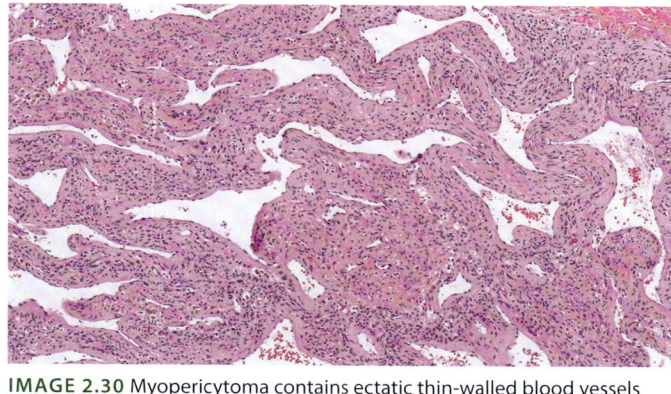

IMAGE 2.30 Myopericytoma contains ectatic thin-walled blood vessels with a perivascular arrangement of plump spindle myoid cells.

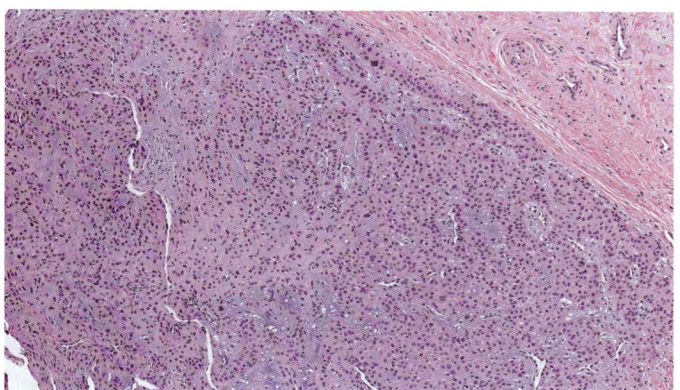

IMAGE 2.28 Glomus tumor consists of branching capillaries surrounded by uniform glomus cells arranged in a myxohyaline stroma. The glomus cells are epithelioid with indistinct cytoplasmic borders and may be arranged in nests, sheets, or trabeculae. Glomus tumors are positive for actins, collagen IV (pericellular staining pattern, H&E, x10) and demonstrate variable staining with CD34 (not shown).

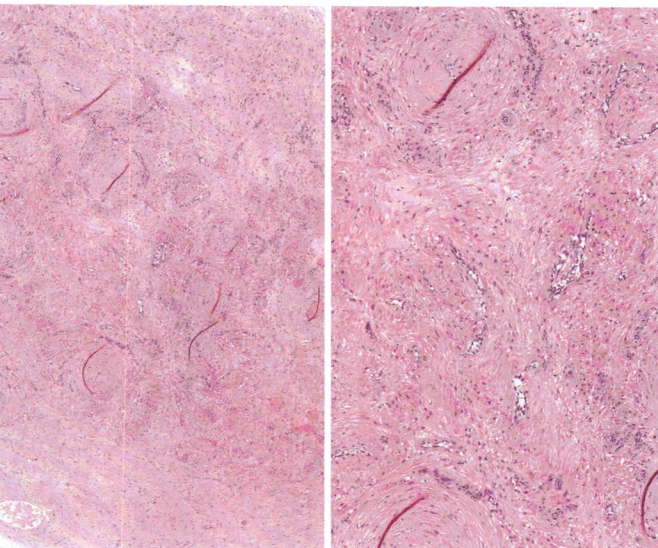

IMAGE 2.31 Angioleiomyoma (also called vascular leiomyoma). A low-power view (left, H&E, x4) and a high-power view (right, H&E, x10) of angioleiomyoma show well-circumscribed nodules consisting of fascicles of smooth muscle surrounding variably size blood vessels. On occasion, there may be central degenerative changes.

IMAGE 2.29 Myofibroma demonstrates a nodular or multinodular growth pattern with a biphasic appearance consisting of a peripheral zone with plump, myoid cells, and a central zone with immature, hyperchromatic cells and hemangiopericytoma-like vessels (compressed in this example).

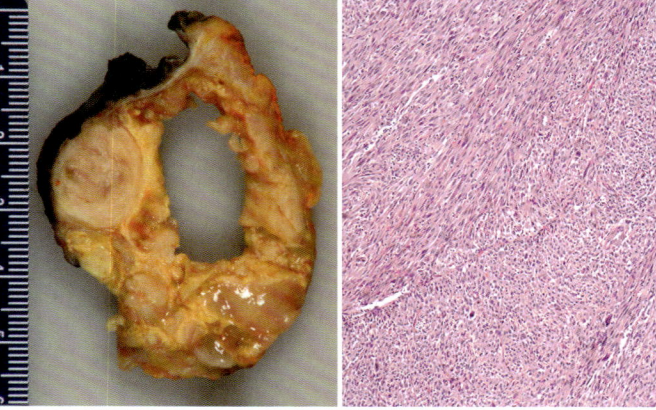

IMAGE 2.32 Leiomyosarcoma. Left: this is a gross image of a multifocal leiomyosarcoma involving the ankle. Cut section demonstrates a firm, white whorled surface. Right: leiomyosarcoma consists of atypical eosinophilic spindle cells arranged in intersecting fascicles with mitoses, often including atypical forms (not shown) and necrosis (not shown).

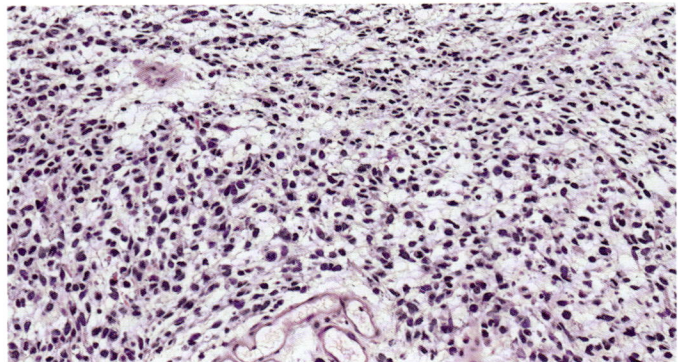

IMAGE 2.33 Embryonal rhabdomyosarcoma. The image shows conventional embryonal rhabdomyosarcoma consisting of small round and spindle cells representing primitive mesenchymal cells in various stages of skeletal muscle differentiation, embedded in a myxoid stroma (H&E, x20). Terminally differentiated strap cells may be present (not shown).

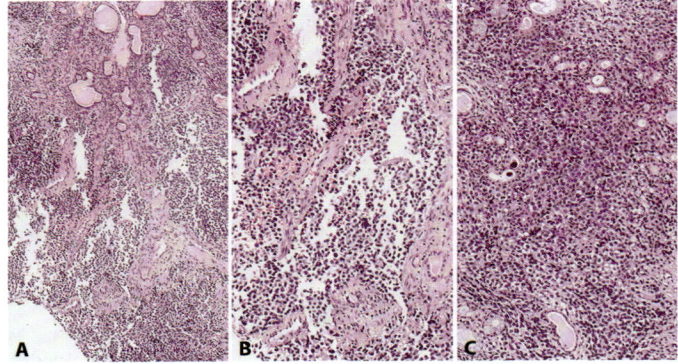

IMAGE 2.34 Alveolar rhabdomyosarcoma. Image A (H&E, x10): this shows conventional alveolar rhabdomyosarcoma involving the ethmoid sinus (most common head and neck site) and infiltrating between mucoserous glands. Tumor cells are arranged in nests that are discohesive in the center, imparting an alveolar growth pattern. Image B (H&E, x20): at higher power, there are round blue cells associated with fibrovascular septae. Terminally differentiated rhabdomyoblasts are uncommon. Image C (H&E, x20): this shows solid variant of alveolar rhabdomyosarcoma with focal clear cell change. The presence of clear cell change makes Ewing sarcoma a strong diagnostic consideration that is resolved with molecular testing.

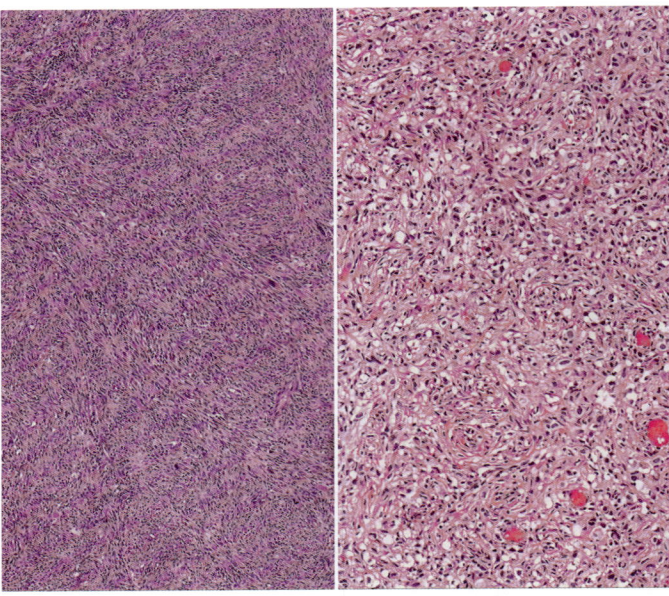

IMAGE 2.35 Spindle/sclerosing rhabdomyosarcoma. Left: the image shows a fascicular arrangement of atypical eosinophilic spindle cells with scattered, terminally differentiated rhabdomyoblasts (H&E, x10). Right: the image shows a sclerosing area with tumor cells separated by eosinophilic, hyalinizing fibrous stroma (mimicking osteoid) (H&E, x10).

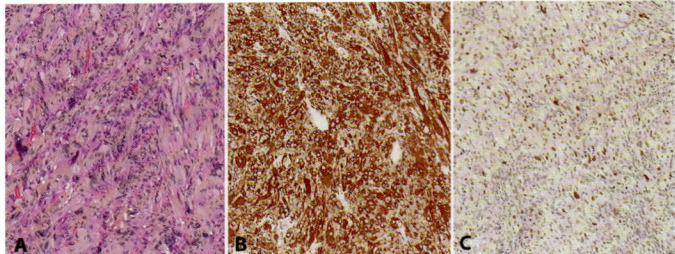

IMAGE 2.36 Pleomorphic rhabdomyosarcoma, which most often occurs in the distal extremity of elderly patients, consists of pleomorphic spindle cells with brightly eosinophilic cytoplasm (image A, H&E, x10). The tumor cells are positive for desmin (image B) and myogenin (image C), confirming the diagnosis.

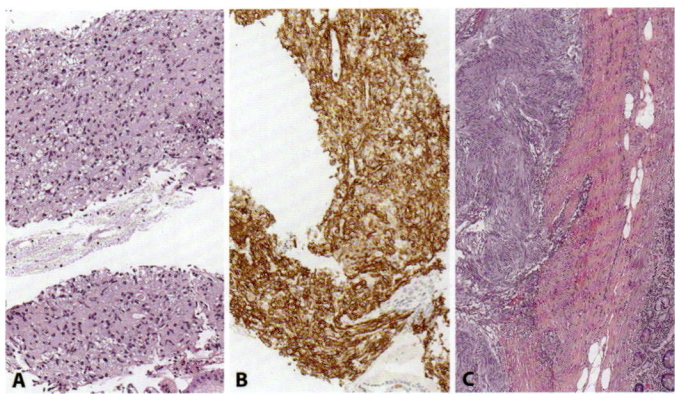

IMAGE 2.37 Gastrointestinal stromal tumor (GIST) can have variable morphologic appearances and mimic the appearance of other soft tissue lesions including schwannoma and smooth muscle tumors. Image A: core biopsy of a gastric GIST shows bland spindle cells set in a loose stroma. Image B: CD117 is diffusely positive. Image C (H&E, x7): this shows another example of a gastric GIST, which at low power morphologically resembles a schwannoma. However, it lacks the characteristic lymphoid cuff of gastric schwannoma and shows staining with S100 protein. In addition, the spindle cells were diffusely positive for CD117 and DOG-1 (not shown), confirming the diagnosis of GIST.

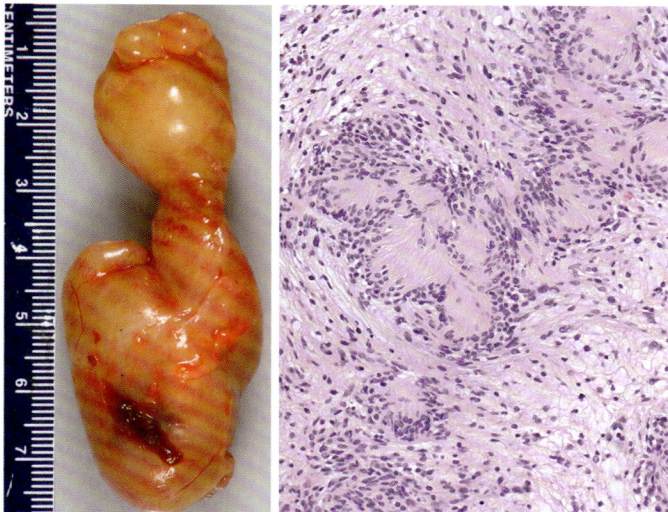

IMAGE 2.38 Left: this schwannoma distorts the nerve in a globoid, eccentric manner. Right: schwannomas are encapsulated spindle cell lesions with alternating cellular (Antoni A) and myxoid (Antoni B) areas. The spindle cells often demonstrate nuclear palisading and Verocay bodies may be seen, as depicted in this image.

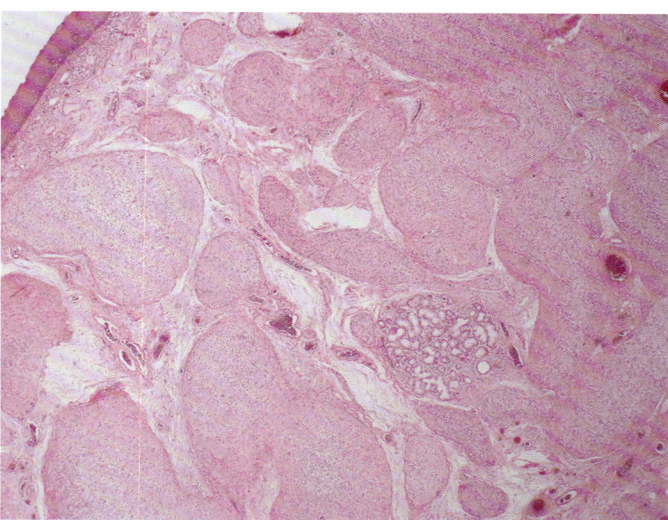

IMAGE 2.40 Plexiform neurofibroma involving the parapharyngeal space is a multinodular lesion involving numerous nerve fascicles that are surrounded by perineurium. The multinodularity imparts a "bag-of-worms" appearance.

Courtesy of Dr. Akeesha Shah, Cleveland Clinic.

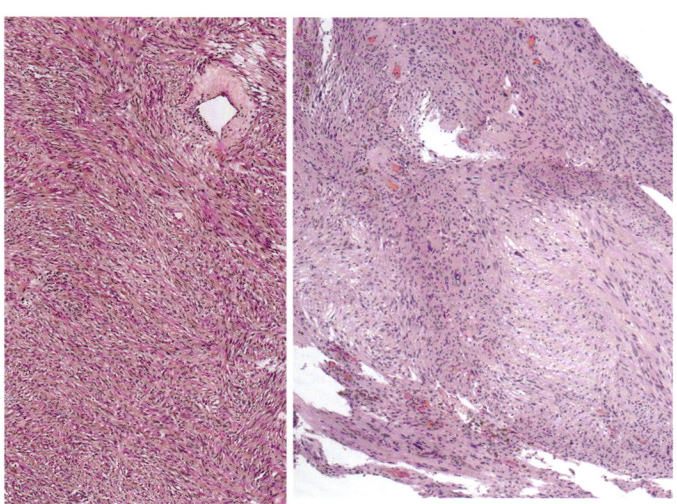

IMAGE 2.39 Left: cellular schwannoma is composed almost exclusively of Antoni A (hypercellular) tissue without Verocay bodies. The increased cellularity, mitoses, and (rarely) small foci of necrosis is concerning for a malignant peripheral nerve sheath tumor. However, strong diffuse staining with S100 protein, along with other features of typical schwannoma, are reassuring. Right: this image shows ancient schwannoma. In addition to the features of conventional schwannoma, ancient schwannoma is characterized by scattered bizarre-appearing nuclei that are considered degenerative. Other degenerative features may be seen, including central ischemic changes, hemorrhage, and hyalinization.

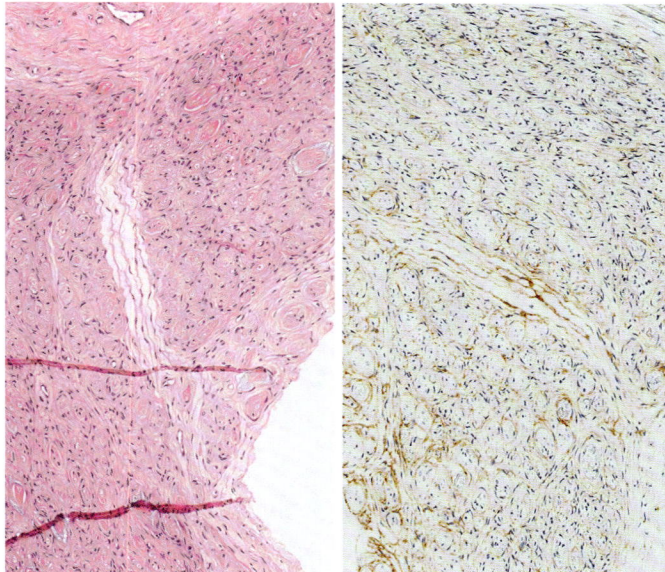

IMAGE 2.41 Intraneural perineurioma. Left: the image shows a multilayered proliferation of perineurial cells around a central axon, forming an onion-bulb-like shape (H&E, x20). Right: EMA immunostain highlights the "onion bulbs" composed of perineurial cells (x20).

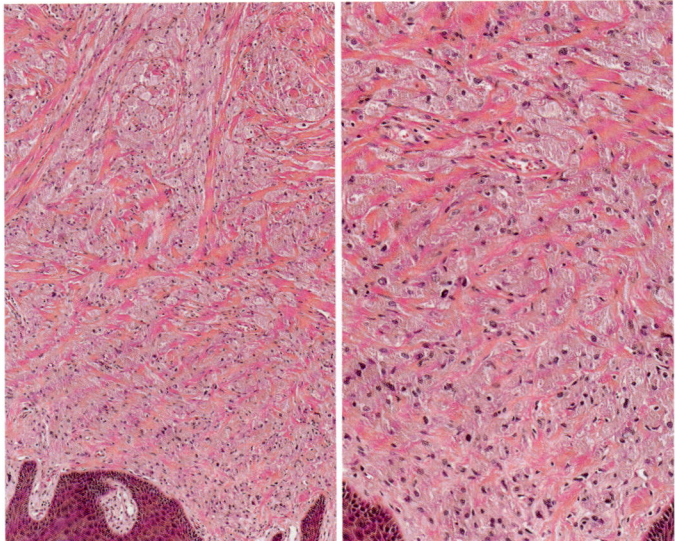

IMAGE 2.42 Granular cell tumor is an ill-defined lesion consisting of large epithelioid-to-polygonal cells with finely granular eosinophilic cytoplasm due to the accumulation of lysosomes. In anatomic sites with an overlying squamous epithelium, granular cell tumor may be associated with pseudoepitheliomatous hyperplasia, which can mimic a squamous cell carcinoma. Left: H&E, x10. Right: H&E, x20.

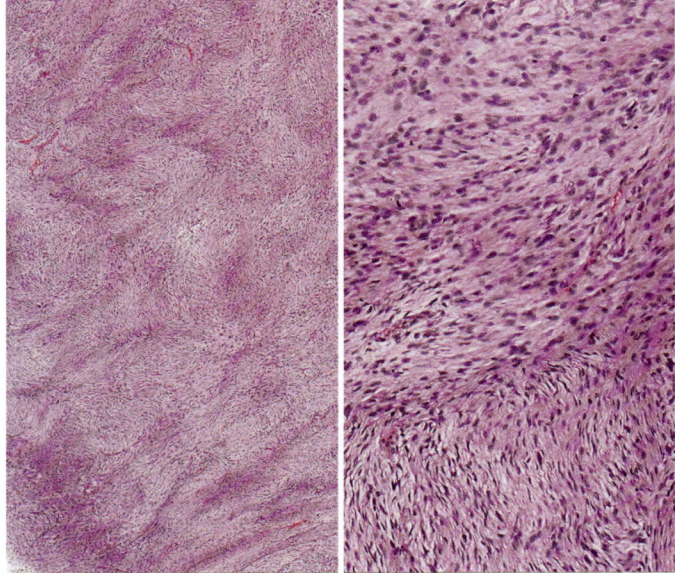

IMAGE 2.43 Malignant peripheral nerve sheath tumor. Left (H&E, x4): at low power, alternating cellular and myxoid areas imparts a marbled effect. Right (H&E, x20): at higher power, the spindle cells have wavy or buckled nuclei. There are scattered pleomorphic tumor cells and numerous mitoses.

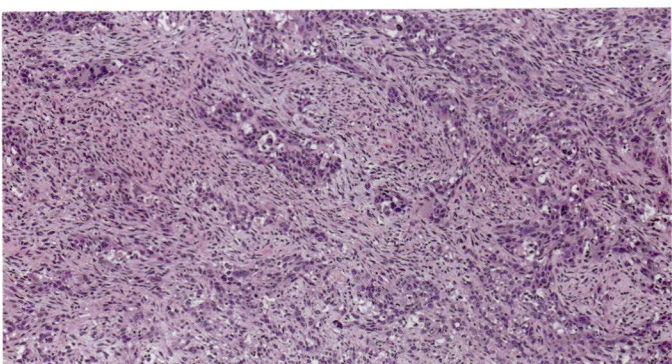

IMAGE 2.44 Malignant peripheral nerve sheath tumor with glandular differentiation (also called glandular MPNST) is a very rare variant of MPNST with glandular differentiation, with or without mucus, that almost always arises in NF1 patients. The glandular elements will stain with epithelial markers (not shown) (H&E, x10).

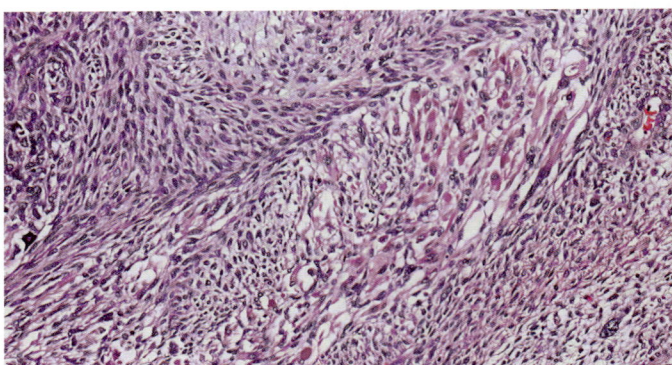

IMAGE 2.45 MPNST with rhabdomyoblastic (skeletal muscle) differentiation (malignant triton tumor) will contain scattered rhabdomyoblasts with eosinophilic cytoplasm, eccentric nucleus, and may have cross-striations (H&E, x20). These rhabdomyoblasts can be highlighted with skeletal muscle immunohistochemical stains.

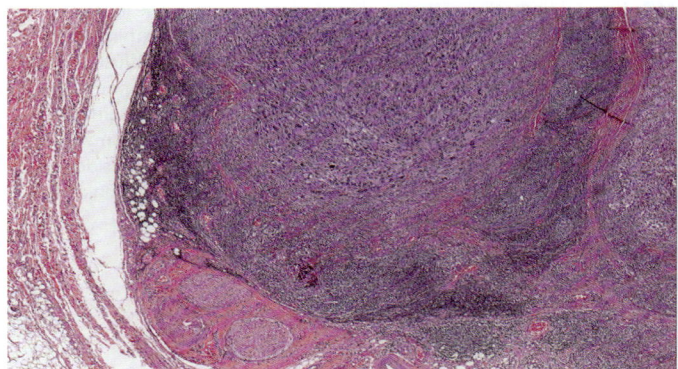

IMAGE 2.46 Epithelioid MPNST arising from a large nerve trunk. It is characterized by epithelioid cells with eosinophilic cytoplasm (H&E, x4). Unlike conventional MPNSTs, epithelioid MPNST demonstrate strong diffuse staining with S100 protein (not shown). This subtype most often arises from schwannomas.

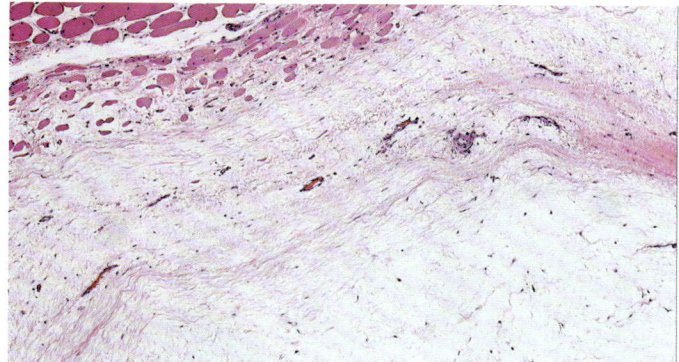

IMAGE 2.47 Intramuscular myxomas are most common in the musculature of the thigh. These are hypocellular myxoid lesions with bland spindle cells and indistinct vasculature. At the periphery, the skeletal muscle bundles often show a checker-board pattern and may demonstrate atrophy (H&E, x10).

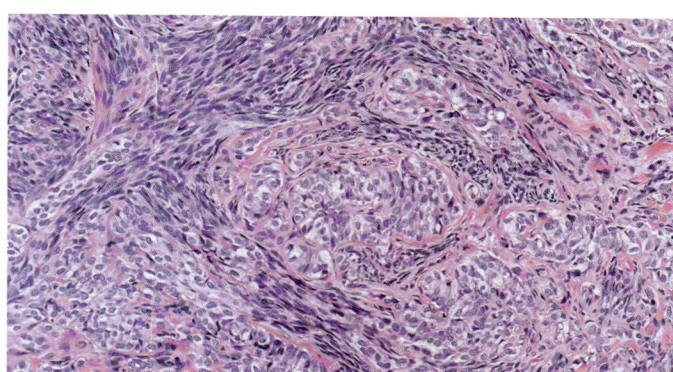

IMAGE 2.50 Biphasic synovial sarcoma consists of a spindle cell component admixed with an epithelial component (H&E, x20).

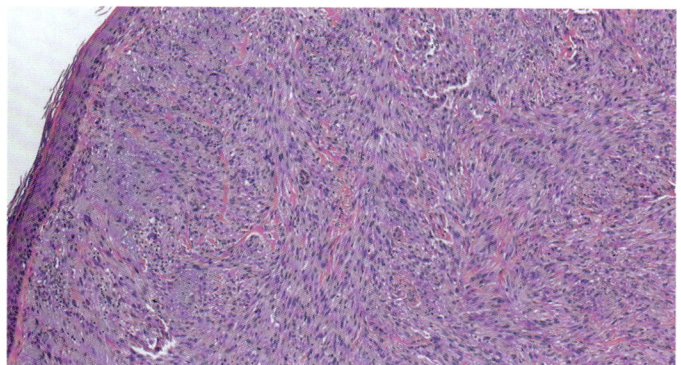

IMAGE 2.48 Atypical fibroxanthoma is a well-defined nodule confined to the dermis, abutting the epidermis, in skin demonstrating solar elastosis (sun damage). The lesion is composed of spindled-to-epithelioid tumor cells in haphazard or fascicular pattern (H&E, x10).

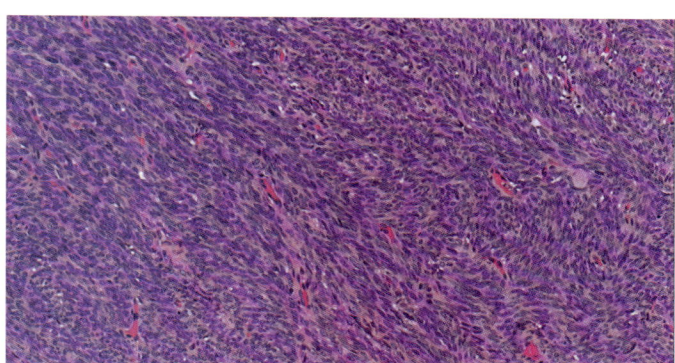

IMAGE 2.51 Monophasic spindle synovial sarcoma consists of a uniform population of spindle cells with minimal atypia arranged in fascicles, often with a hemangiopericytoma-like vascular pattern (H&E, x20).

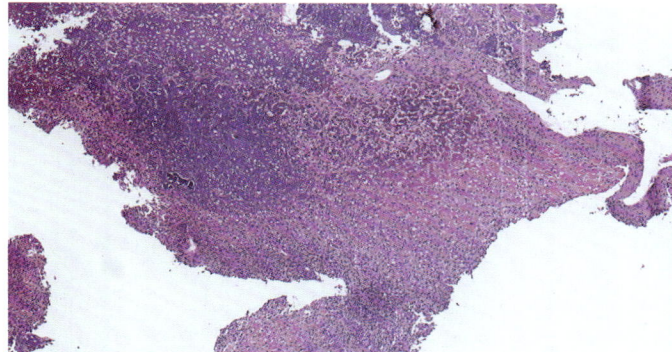

IMAGE 2.49 Phosphaturic mesenchymal tumor, a tumor with a strong association with osteomalacia, consists of variable amounts of short spindle cells, osteoclast-like giant cells, hemangiopericytoma-like vessels, and grungy calcifications (H&E, x8).

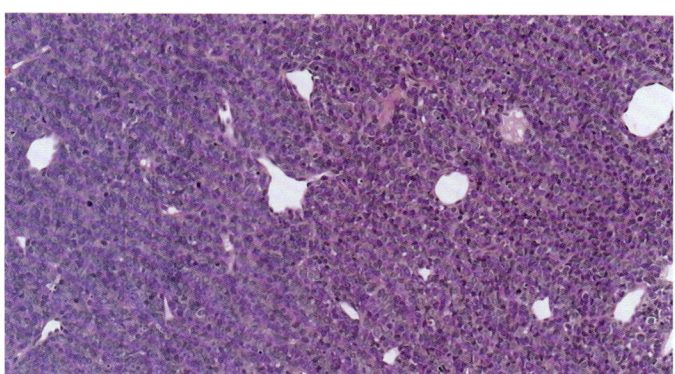

IMAGE 2.52 The image shows a poorly differentiated synovial sarcoma consisting of small round cells with scattered mitoses and apoptotic debris. The hemangiopericytoma-like vascular pattern is well-preserved in this example (H&E, x20).

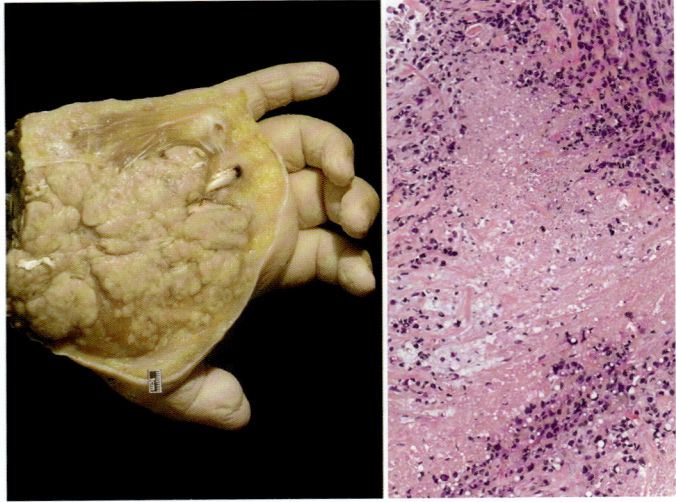

IMAGE 2.53 Epithelioid sarcoma. Left: gross image of an epithelioid sarcoma involving the right hand. Right: discohesive epithelioid tumor cells with central necrosis, mimicking the appearance of a necrobiotic, palisading granuloma (H&E, x20).

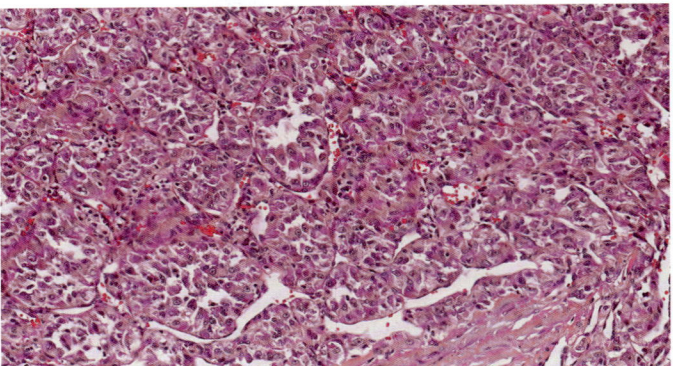

IMAGE 2.55 Alveolar soft part sarcoma of the thigh consists of large, round-to-polygonal tumor cells with abundant eosinophilic granular cytoplasm, vesicular nuclei, and prominent nucleoli. The tumor cells are arranged in nests that are separated by thin-walled sinusoidal vascular channels.

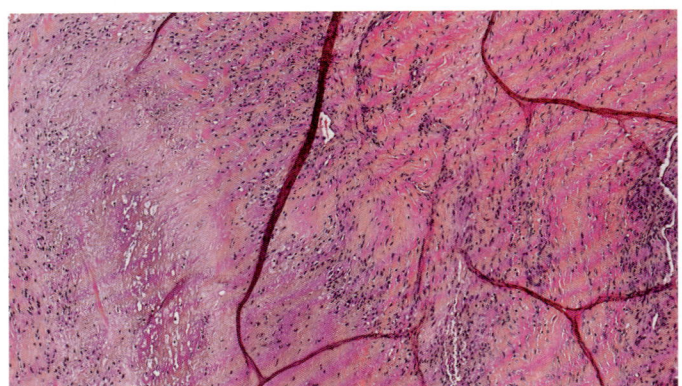

IMAGE 2.54 Rheumatoid nodules are characterized by palisading and necrotizing granulomata with central fibrin (H&E, x10).

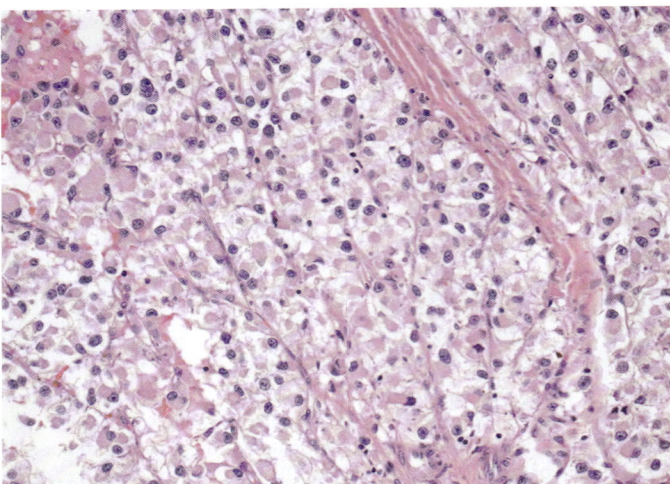

IMAGE 2.56 Clear cell sarcoma demonstrates nests of epithelioid-to-plump spindle cells with prominent nuclei and eosinophilic-to-clear cytoplasm, separated by thin fibrous septae.

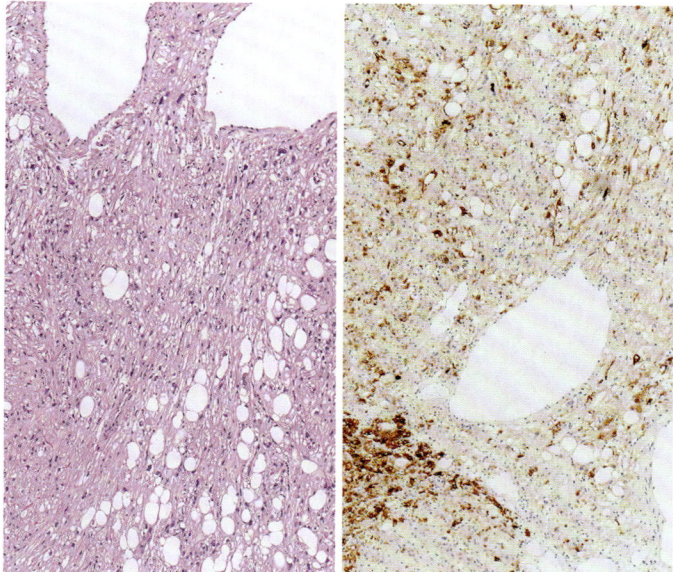

IMAGE 2.57 Classic angiomyolipoma subtype of PEComa. Left: the image shows a mixture of abnormal thick-walled blood vessels, smooth muscle and adipose tissue. There is a characteristic perivascular pattern of growth with spindle cells radially arranged around blood vessels. PEComas coexpress smooth muscle and melanocytic markers (H&E, x10). Right: the image shows Melan-A staining of the smooth muscle and adipocytic cells (x8.2).

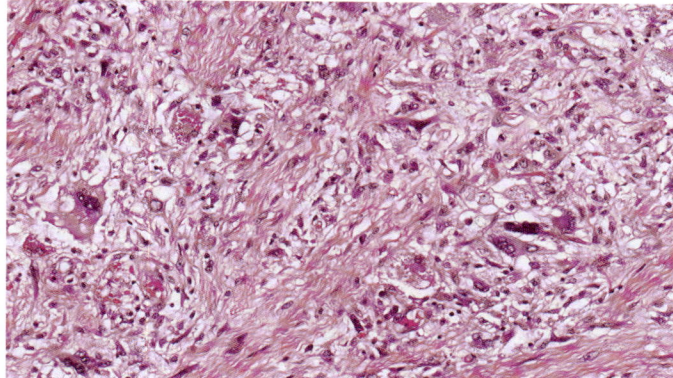

IMAGE 2.59 Undifferentiated pleomorphic sarcoma is a high grade tumor with no differentiating features on gross examination, microscopy, or ancillary studies (H&E, x20).

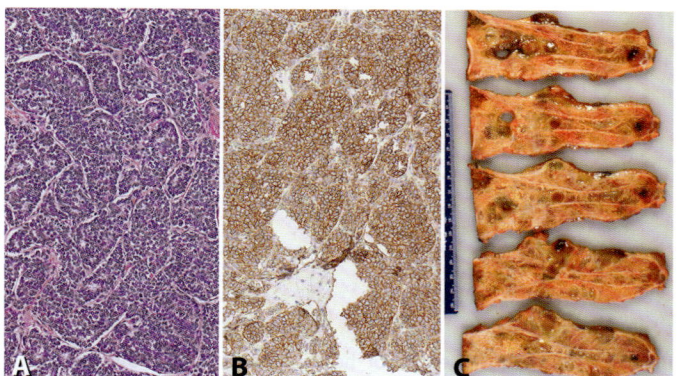

IMAGE 2.58 Image A: this shows a Ewing sarcoma with uniform round cells arranged in nests with neuroectodermal differentiation (H&E, x20). Image B: this shows diffuse, crisp membranous staining with CD99 (x20). Image C: this shows a Ewing sarcoma involving the pelvis, after neoadjuvant therapy. On cut sections, note the striking periosteal reaction nearly completely enveloping the native bone.

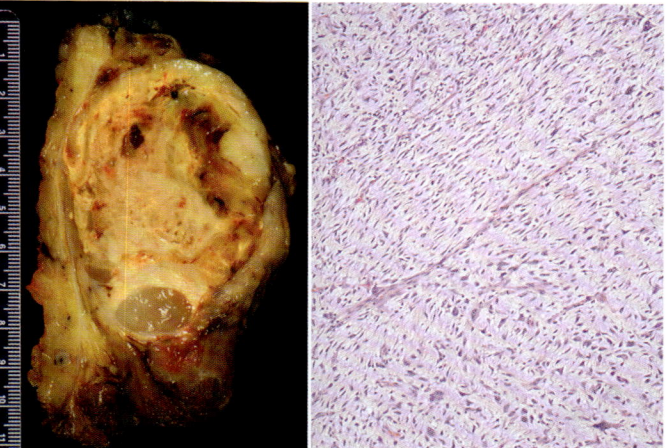

IMAGE 2.60 Myxofibrosarcoma. Left: the image shows a high grade myxofibrosarcoma involving the thigh with extensive tumor necrosis and focal myxoid areas. Right: myxofibrosarcoma is characterized by pleomorphic tumor cells set in a myxoid stroma with curvilinear blood vessels.

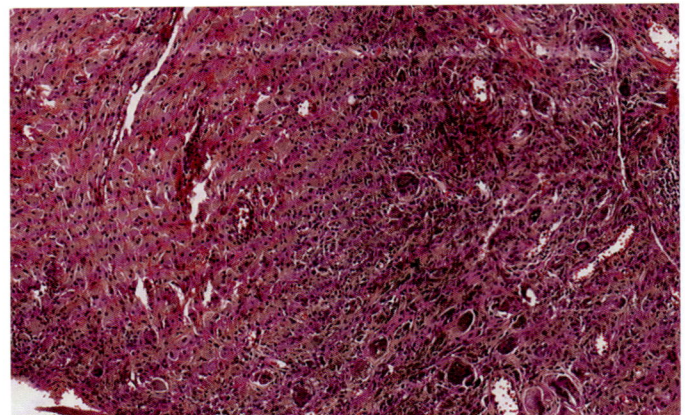

IMAGE 2.61 Detritic synovitis consists of sheets of macrophages, including macrophages containing prosthetic debris, and foreign body giant cells in dense fibrous tissue (H&E, x20).

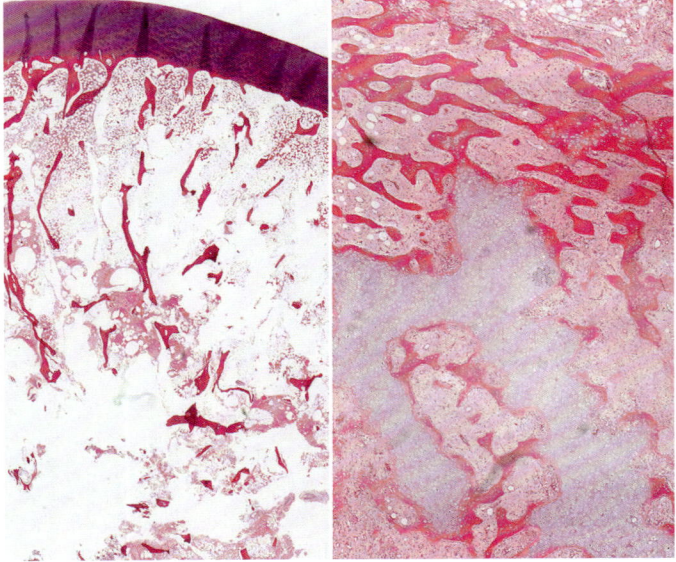

IMAGE 2.62 Left: the image shows osteopenia in the setting of a femoral neck fracture in a patient with osteoporosis. Note the thin trabeculae of lamellar bone that have lost their interconnections (H&E, x1). Right: the image shows a primary fracture callus consisting of a mixture of hypercellular lobules of cartilage, hypervascular tissue, and disorderly bone. Primary fracture callus tends to be more abundant in unstable areas and can mimic a sarcoma. Helpful features to exclude a sarcoma include maturation of the elements, lack of significant atypia, and no atypical mitoses.

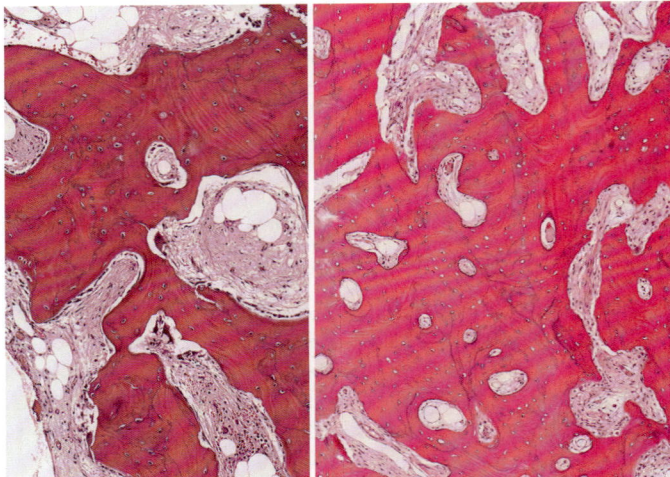

IMAGE 2.63 Paget disease of bone. Left: in the mixed phase of Paget disease, the variably thin and thick trabeculae have a disorganized arrangement of osteoclasts and osteoblasts. In this example, the reversal or cement lines are prominent, imparting a mosaic pattern (H&E, x20). Right: in the osteosclerotic phase of Paget disease, the sclerotic bone trabeculae are variably thin and thick with the characteristic mosaic pattern.

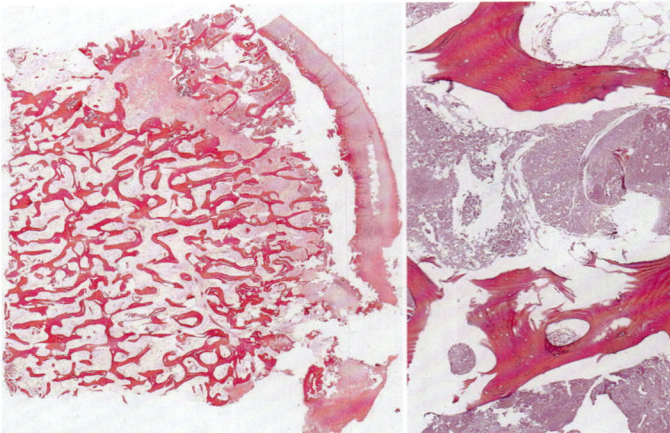

IMAGE 2.64 Avascular necrosis of the femoral head. Left: the image shows osteonecrosis of the femoral head with a wedge-shaped area of necrosis below the cartilage (H&E, x0.5). Right: at higher power, the lacunae are empty and the marrow fat is necrotic. Calcium salts are often seen in the necrotic fat (H&E, x10).

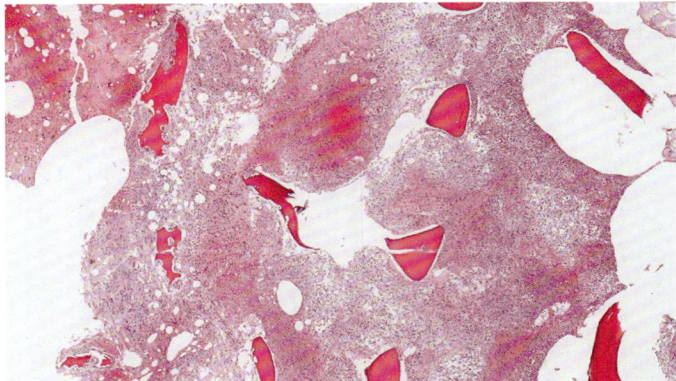

IMAGE 2.65 Acute (pyogenic) osteomyelitis involving a metatarsal bone (H&E, x4). There is diffuse acute inflammation associated with necrotic bone demonstrating remodelling changes including scalloping of the bone contour secondary to osteoclast activity.

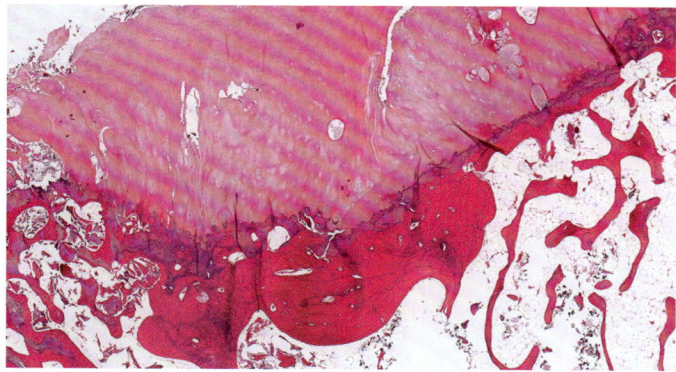

IMAGE 2.66 Osteoarthritis. The image shows osteoarthritis of the femoral head with thinning of the articular cartilage along with fissures and clefts (H&E, x4). The chondrocytes focally demonstrate cloning. The subchondral bone is sclerotic. In areas where the cartilage is completely worn off (eburnation), microfractures can develop and subchondral cysts will form (not shown).

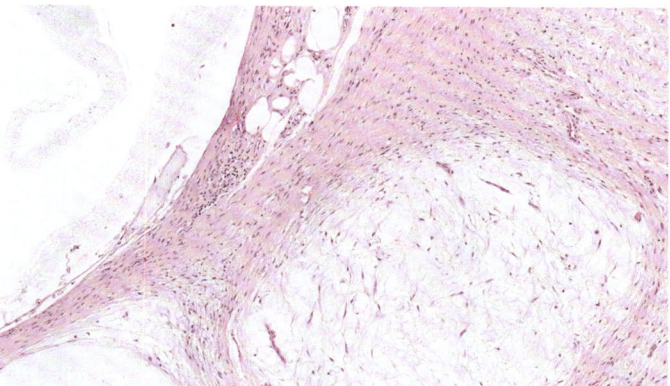

IMAGE 2.68 Ganglion cyst (H&E, x10). Ganglion cysts typically arise within the soft tissues surrounding a joint, and on occasion may arise within bone. A ganglion cyst is a fibrous-walled cyst lacking a cell lining and filled with clear mucinous fluid. Often, there is extensive myxoid change with the fibrous tissue surrounding the cyst.

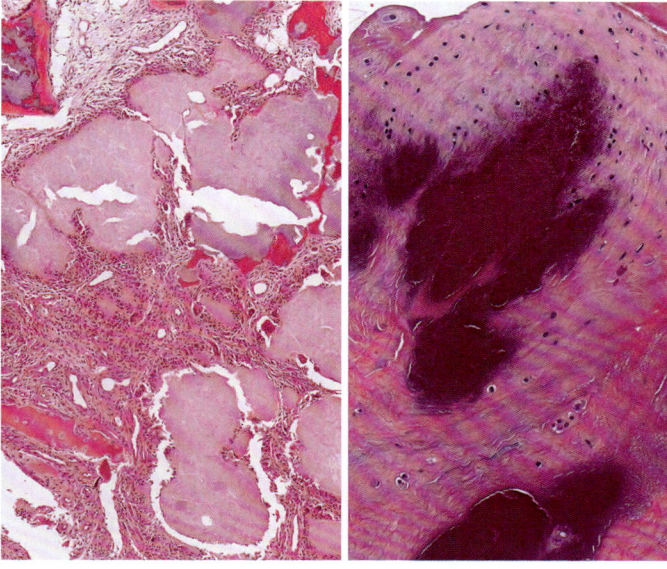

IMAGE 2.67 Gout and pseudogout. Left: the image shows tophaceous gout involving the toe and eroding into bone (H&E, x10). On routine sections, the actual crystals within the tophi have been dissolved and can no longer be seen. Surrounding the nodular deposits of sodium urate, there is an associated histiocytic and foreign body giant cell reaction. Acute inflammatory cells may also be seen. Right: the image shows secondary pseudogout (calcium pyrophosphate dehydrate deposition) involving the synovium of a knee with severe osteoarthritis. There are clusters of purple-appearing rhomboid crystals on routine stains that may be associated with a histiocytic or foreign body giant cell reaction (not shown). Under polarized light, the crystals are weakly positively birefringent. Note the synovial tissue has other degenerative features including chondroid metaplasia. There is surface fibrin deposition.

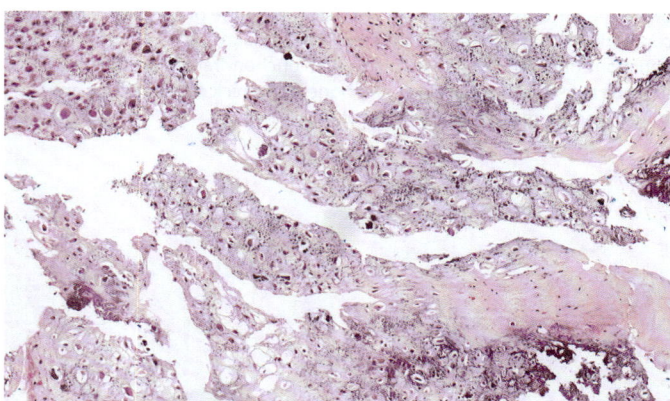

IMAGE 2.69 Bizarre parosteal osteochondromatous proliferation consists of variable amounts of cartilage, bone, and fibrous tissue. The cartilage often looks atypical, with increased numbers of chondrocytes with abundant cytoplasm and vesicular nuclei, and easy-to-identify binucleate forms. Basophilic bone ("blue bone") is characteristic (H&E, x10).

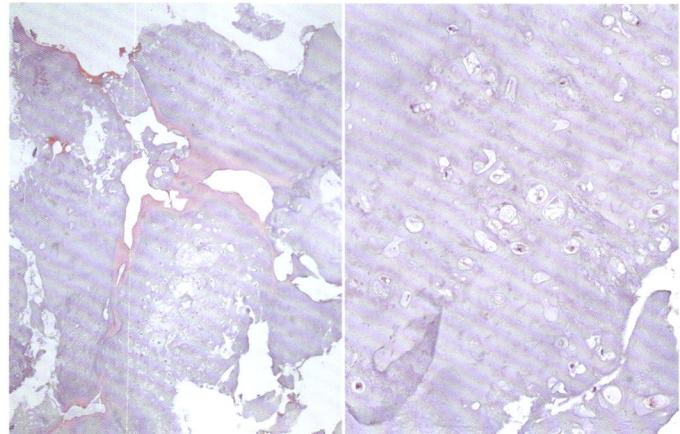

IMAGE 2.70 Enchondroma of the femur. Left: the low power view demonstrates a lobular proliferation of hypocellular hyaline cartilage. The lobules often have peripheral ossification, which is a sign a slow growing tumor. Right: at higher power, the chondrocytes of enchondroma, particularly in long tubular bones, demonstrate little to no atypia. In the small bones of the hands and feet, enchondromas tend to be more cellular with enhanced cytologic detail and binucleate chondrocytes.

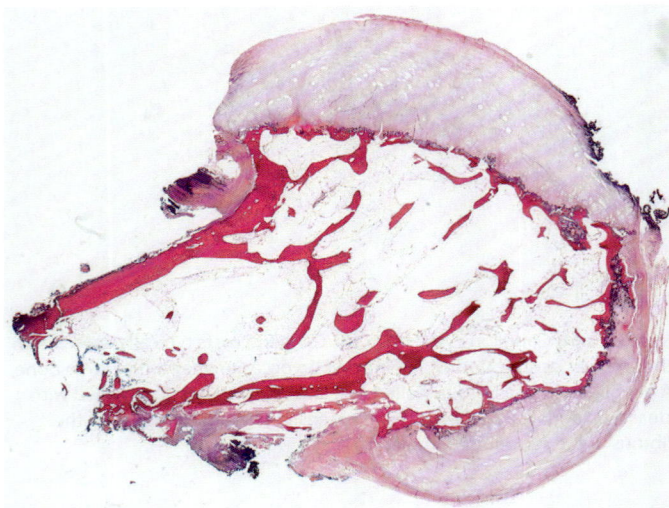

IMAGE 2.71 Osteochondroma (H&E, x0.8). The base of the stalk is in continuity with the underlying cortex. The cartilage cap consists of perichondrium and hyaline cartilage, with enchondral ossification at the interface between cartilage and bone. Very thick cartilage caps are concerning for malignant transformation.

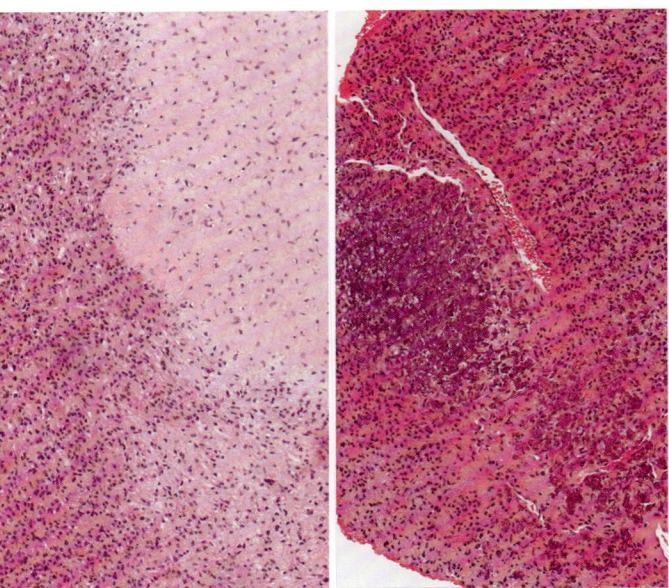

IMAGE 2.73 Chondromyxoid fibroma (CMF) of the pelvis. Left (H&E, x20): CMF demonstrates a lobular pattern with spindled or stellate cells in a chondromyxoid background. The lobules demonstrate hypocellular centers, with features similar to hyaline cartilage, and hypercellular peripheries. Often, osteoclast-like giant cells are seen at the periphery of the lobules. Right (H&E, x20): CMF may contain areas with coarse calcifications, most often seen in flat bone.

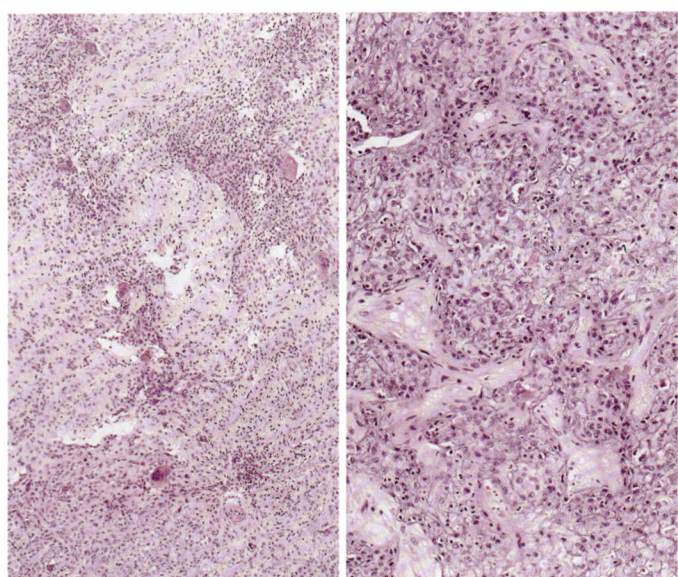

IMAGE 2.72 Chondroblastoma consists of oval cells with nuclear grooves and eosinophilic cytoplasm, arranged in sheets. Pericellular "chicken wire" calcification is a characteristic feature. Osteoclast-like giant cells and islands of chondroid matrix are also seen. Left: x10. Right: x20.

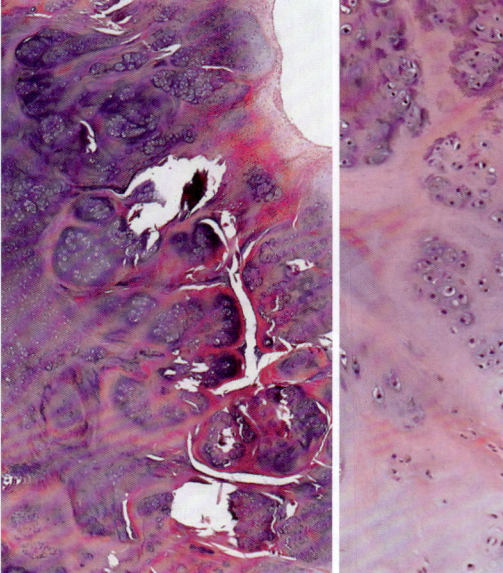

IMAGE 2.74 Synovial chondromatosis. Left (H&E, x4): synovial chondromatosis consists of multiple lobules of hyaline-type cartilage arising in the synovium. Note the residual synovial tissue in the upper left corner. Some examples may demonstrate peripheral ossification of the lobules. Right (H&E, x20): at higher power, synovial chondromatosis often demonstrates mild nuclear atypia. A diagnosis of malignancy requires infiltration of adjacent bone, increased mitoses (including atypical forms), and nuclear pleomorphism. A reassuring feature is the preservation of chondrocyte clustering.

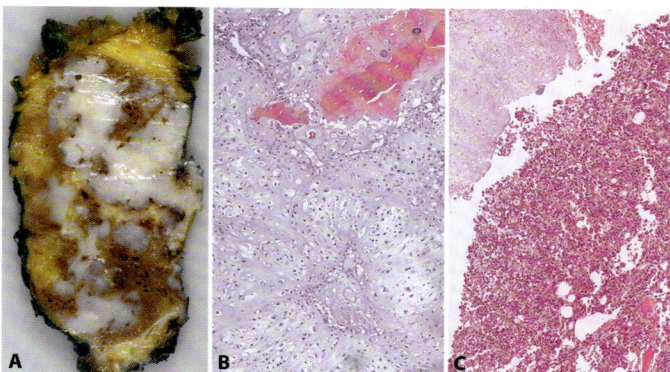

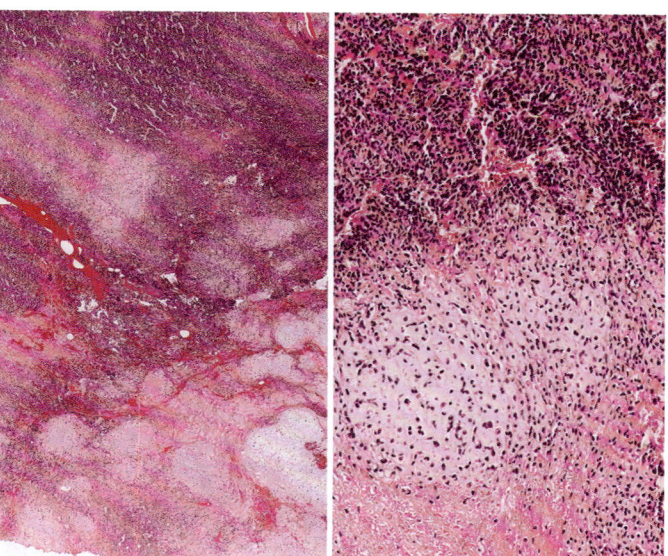

IMAGE 2.75 Conventional chondrosarcoma involving the pelvis. Image A: this gross image demonstrates a multilobulated tumor with a translucent bluish-grey cut surface. Image B (H&E, x20): conventional chondrosarcoma consists of lobules of hypercellular cartilage infiltrating bone The atypical chondrocytes have enhanced cytologic detail with more abundant cytoplasm and vesicular nuclei. Binucleate chondrocytes are easy to identify. Higher grade conventional chondrosarcoma has greater nuclear pleomorphism, increased mitoses, and the chondroid matrix may appear more myxoid with peripheral spindling. Image C (H&E, x10): this shows dedifferentiated chondrosarcoma demonstrating an abrupt transition from a residual focus of low grade conventional chondrosarcoma (bottom left) and high grade pleomorphic sarcoma.

IMAGE 2.77 Mesenchymal chondrosarcoma. Left (low, H&E, x4) and right (intermediate power, H&E, x20): the images show a biphasic tumor consisting of a low grade chondrosarcoma (hyaline type) juxtaposed to a small round blue cell tumor, often with focal hemangiopericytoma-like vascular pattern.

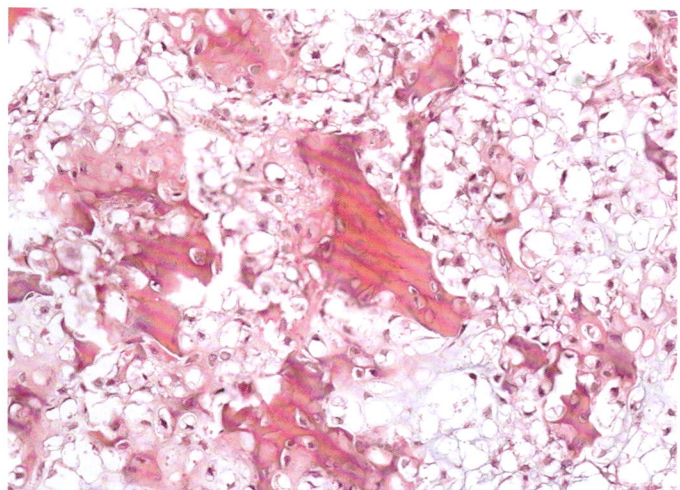

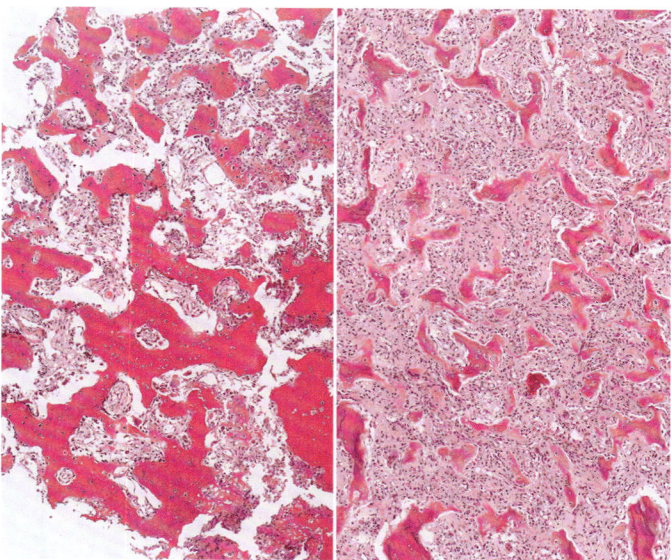

IMAGE 2.76 Clear cell chondrosarcoma involving the femoral head. It is characterized by a sheet-like proliferation of large tumor cells with ample clear-to-eosinophilic cytoplasm, well-defined cytoplasmic borders, and small centrally located nuclei. Often there are irregularly shaped trabeculae of immature woven bone. Clear cell chondrosarcoma typically lacks a chondroid matrix unless it is associated with a conventional chondrosarcoma.

IMAGE 2.78 Osteoid osteoma and osteoblastoma. Left (H&E, x10): the image shows an osteoid osteoma involving the tibial cortex. Osteoid osteoma consists of a nidus composed of immature woven bone lined by osteoblasts set in a vascular stroma. At the periphery of the nidus, there is transition to sclerotic bone (not shown). Right (H&E, x10): the images shows an osteoblastoma involving the posterior elements of T3. Osteoblastoma also consists of a nidus composed of immature woven bone trabeculae lined by 1 or more layers of plump osteoblasts and scattered osteoclast-type giant cells. The intervening stroma appears loose and contains dilated vascular spaces.

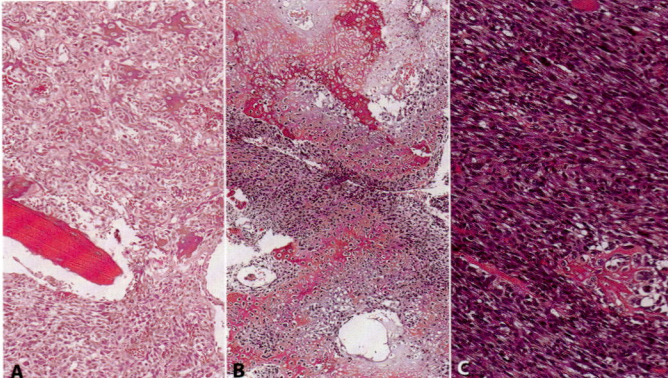

IMAGE 2.79 Conventional osteosarcoma. Image A: this shows an osteoblastic osteosarcoma consisting of immature woven bone (osteoid) arising from atypical spindle cells, and infiltrating and destroying native bone (H&E, x20). Image B: this shows a chondroblastic osteosarcoma consisting of high grade malignant cartilage intimately mixed with malignant osteoid (H&E, x10). Image C: this shows a fibroblastic osteosarcoma consisting of atypical spindle cells in fascicular pattern with focal filigree osteoid (H&E, x20).

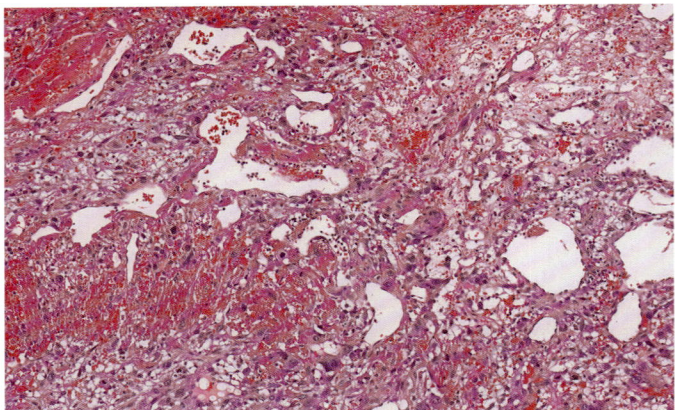

IMAGE 2.80 Telangiectatic osteosarcoma consists of cystic spaces that may contain blood. The cyst walls are of variable thickness and contain pleomorphic tumor cells. Mitoses, including atypical forms, are numerous (H&E, x20). Osteoid formation is usually only focal and can be difficult to identify and may be absent on a biopsy specimen.

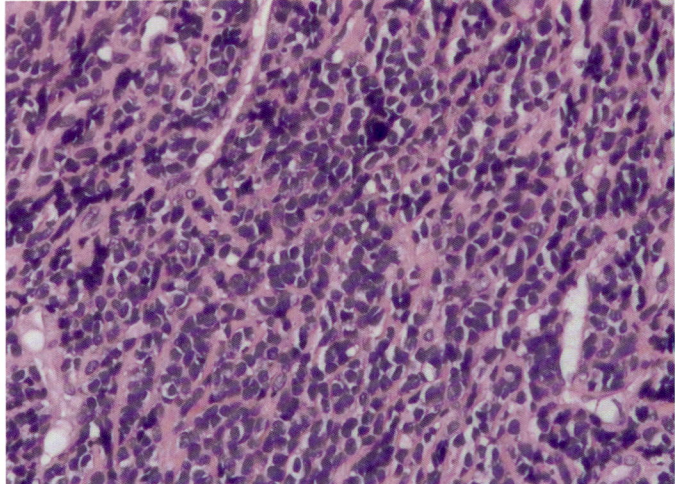

IMAGE 2.81 Small cell osteosarcoma consists of small round cells with minimal cytoplasm intimately associated with lace-like osteoid (H&E, x20). It is important to distinguish from Ewing sarcoma as well as the undifferentiated component of mesenchymal chondrosarcoma, especially on biopsy. Molecular testing can distinguish between these entities.

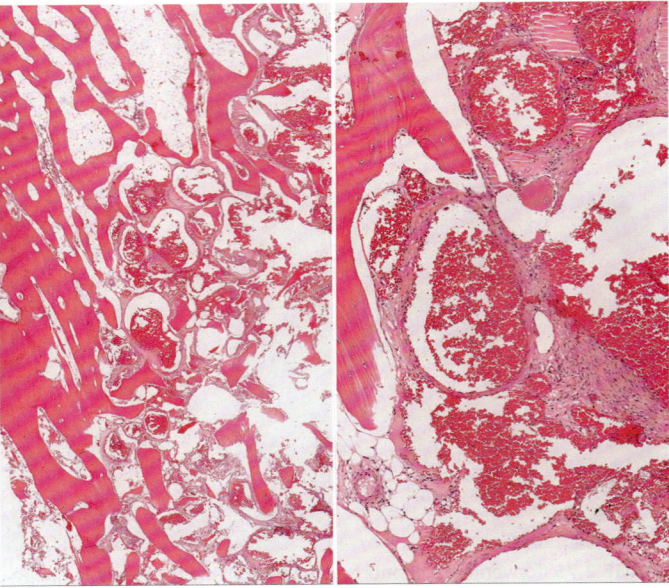

IMAGE 2.82 Hemangioma of bone. Left: (H&E, x2), right (H&E, x10): hemangioma of bone consists of a proliferation of thin-walled blood vessels, lined by bland endothelial cells. The vessels permeate through the marrow spaces and surrounding the bone trabeculae.

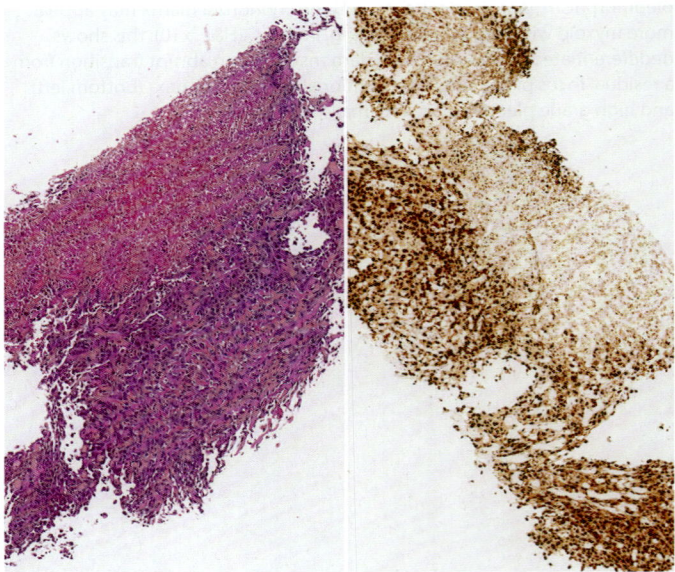

IMAGE 2.83 Left (x10): epithelioid angiosarcoma of bone may grow in solid nests, mimicking the appearance of metastatic carcinoma. The tumor cells have eosinophilic cytoplasm and vesicular nuclei with prominent nucleoli. Mitoses are numerous, including atypical forms (not shown). The tumor cells are often associated with extravasated red blood cells and hemosiderin deposits. Necrosis may be present. Right (x10): angiosarcoma of the bone will be immunoreactive for endothelial markers, including ERG.

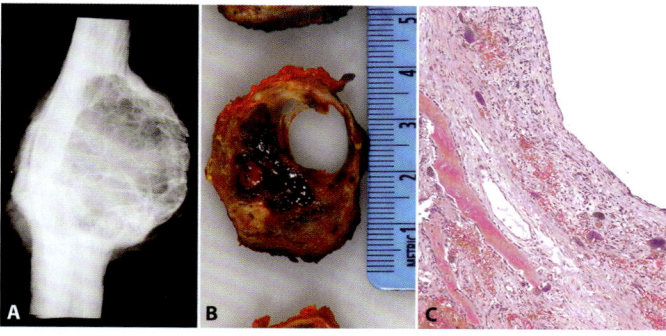

IMAGE 2.84 Aneurysmal bone cyst (ABC) involving the fibula. Image A: this specimen radiograph demonstrates a lytic, expansile lesion with well-defined margins. On imaging studies, fluid-fluid levels are characteristic. Image B: on cut section, ABC is a well-defined, multiloculated lesion with blood-filled cystic spaces separated by sponge-like septae. Solid areas and peripheral reactive bone may be seen. Image C: microscopically, ABC contains blood-filled cystic spaces separated by fibrous septa composed of moderately cellular proliferation of bland fibroblasts and scattered osteoclast-like giant cells. Within the fibrous septae, reactive woven bone, lined by osteoblasts, often follows the contour of the septae or cyst wall.

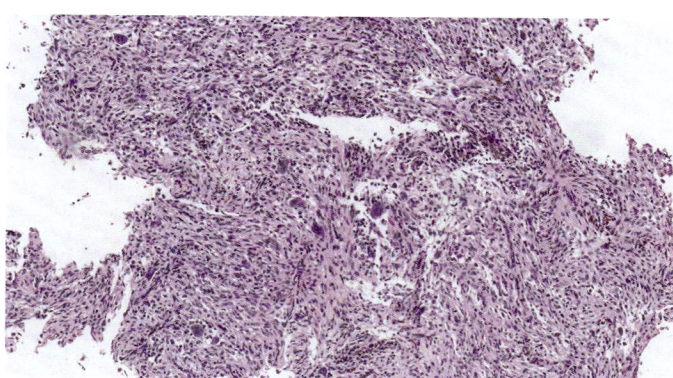

IMAGE 2.86 Nonossifying fibroma consists of a cellular spindle cell stroma with scattered osteoclast-like giant cells, lymphocytes, and focal hemosiderin deposition. Often the spindle cells are arranged in a storiform pattern and foamy macrophages are present. Nonossifying fibroma may be confused with other giant cell rich neoplasms of bone; however, the clinical and radiographic features are characteristic (H&E, x10).

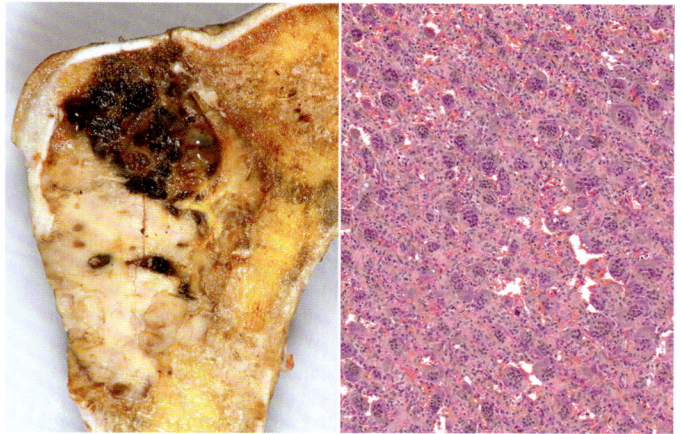

IMAGE 2.85 Giant cell tumor (GCT) of bone involving the distal femur. Left: typically, GCT is located at the end of a long bone, and is well-defined and eccentric in location. The surrounding cortex is thinned and focally disrupted. Viable tumor is hemorrhagic in appearance. The creamy-yellow and white areas typically correspond to xanthomatous change and fibrosis. Right: GCT consists of evenly dispersed osteoclast-like giant cells and mononuclear cells. The nuclear features of the mononuclear cells are identical to the osteoclast-like giant cells. Normal osteoclasts usually contain around 10 to 12 nuclei. The osteoclast-like giant cells of GCT have many nuclei, some with even more than 50.

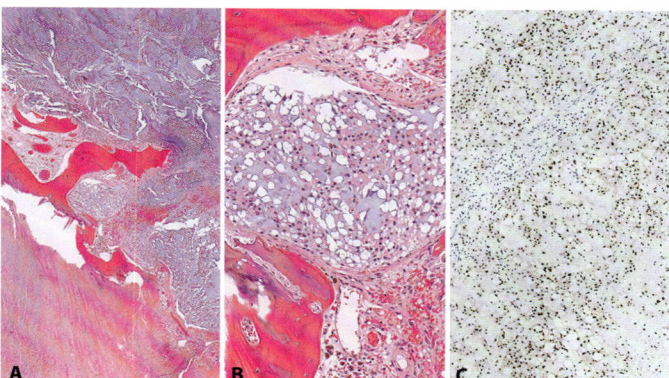

IMAGE 2.87 Conventional chordoma involving the sacrum. Image A: this lower power view demonstrates a lobulated myxoid tumor with corded tumor cells within the bone (H&E, x4). Image B: at intermediate power, some of the tumor cells are multivacuolated, representing physaliferous cells (H&E, x20). Image C: brachyury is a highly specific immunostain for chordoma and demonstrates a nuclear pattern of staining. Loss of staining can follow prolonged fixation and/or excessive decalcification (x10).

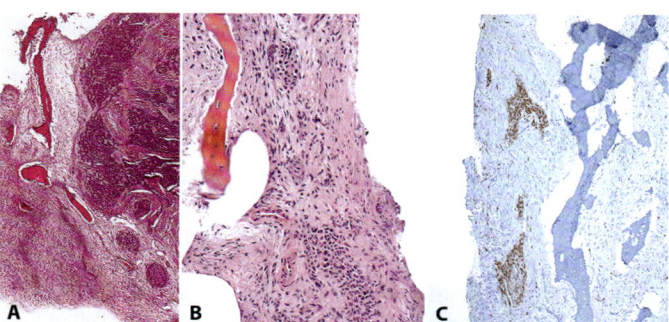

IMAGE 2.88 Image A: classic adamantinoma is a biphasic tumor consisting of epithelial structures admixed with a bland osteofibrous component (H&E, x8.6). Image B: osteofibrous dysplasia-like adamantinoma consists of a predominantly bland osteofibrous component with focal epithelial elements that are often difficult to identify on routine stains. Image C: pancytokeratin immunostain highlights small nests of epithelial cells.

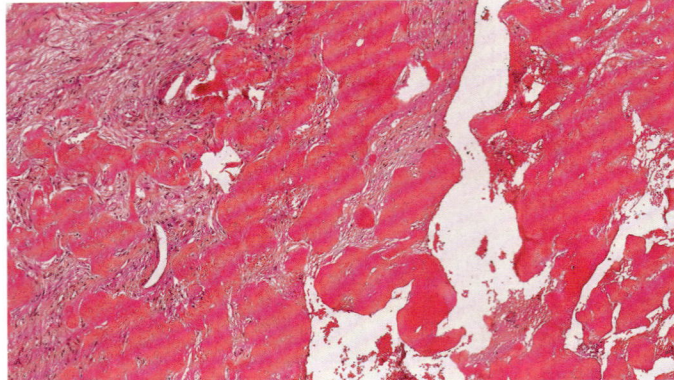

IMAGE 2.89 Simple bone cyst is a cyst composed of fibrous tissue that lacks a cell lining. Often there are fibrin-like deposits within the cyst wall, which may mineralize and resemble cementum or bone. Simple bone cysts can be associated with hemosiderin, cholesterol clefts, and chronic inflammation (H&E, x10).

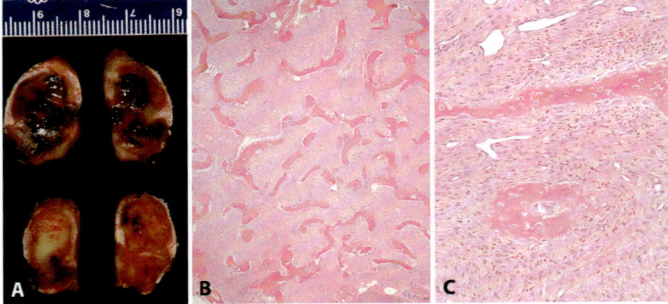

IMAGE 2.90 Fibrous dysplasia involving the rib. Image A: note the fusiform expansile lesion with aneurysmal bone cyst-like changes on the cut cross-section of rib. Image B: this shows curvilinear trabeculae of immature woven bone set in a background of a bland spindle cell proliferation. Image C: this high power view demonstrates the bland spindle stroma and Sharpey-like fibers associated with woven bone trabeculae.

Acknowledgment

I would like to thank Dr. Lisa DiFrancesco for her outstanding contribution to the previous editions of this chapter. I also would like to thank Dr. Zuzanna Gorski for taking the time to review this chapter.

Reference

1. Clay MR, Martinez AP, Weiss SW, et al. MDM2 amplification in problematic lipomatous tumors: analysis of FISH testing criteria. Am J Surg Pathol. 2015;39(10):1433-9. doi: 10.1097/PAS.0000000000000468

Bibliography

Amin MB, Edge S, Greene F, et al, editors. AJCC cancer staging manual. 8th ed. New York: Springer; 2017.

Bullough PG. Orthopaedic pathology. 5th ed. Maryland Heights (MO): Mosby, Inc.; 2010.

Clay MR, Martinez AP, Weiss SW, et al. MDM2 amplification in problematic lipomatous tumors: analysis of FISH testing criteria. Am J Surg Pathol. 2015;39(10):1433-9. doi: 10.1097/PAS.0000000000000468

Demicco EG, Wagner MJ, Maki RG, et al. Risk assessment in solitary fibrous tumors: validation and refinement of a risk stratification model. Mod Pathol. 2017;30(10):1433-42. doi: 10.1038/modpath.2017.54

Fanburg-Smith JC, Meis-Kindblom JM, Fante R, et al. Malignant granular cell tumor of soft tissue: diagnostic criteria and clinicopathologic correlation.

Am J Surg Pathol. 1998 Jul;22(7):779-94. doi: 10.1097/00000478-199807000-00001

Folpe AL, Neilsen GP. Bone and soft tissue pathology. 2nd ed. North York (ON) Elsevier Canada; 2022.

Goldblum JR., Folpe AL, Weiss SW. Enzinger and Weiss's soft tissue tumors. 7th ed. North York (ON): Elsevier Canada; 2020.

Jo VY, Fletcher CD. Nuclear β-catenin expression is frequent in sinonasal hemangiopericytoma and its mimics. Head Neck Pathol. 2016;11(2):119-23. doi: 10.1007/s12105-016-0737-2

Klein MJ, Bonar SF, Freemont T, et al. Non-neoplastic diseases of bones and joints. Washington, DC: American Registry of Pathology, Armed Forces of Pathology; 2011.

Laurini JA, Antonescu R, Cooper K, et al; Cancer Committee, College of American Pathologists. Protocol for the examination of specimens from patients with tumors of bone (Version: Bone Resection 4.0.1.0) [Internet]. College of American Pathologists; 2020 Feb. Available from www.cap.org.

Laurini JA, Cooper K, Fletcher CDM, et al; Cancer Committee, College of American Pathologists. Protocol for the examination of specimens from patients with tumors of soft tissue (Version: Soft Tissue Resection 4.0.2.0) [Internet]. College of American Pathologists; 2020 Feb. Available from www.cap.org.

Makise N, Sekimizu M, Konishi E, et al. H3K27me3 deficiency defines a subset of dedifferentiated chondrosarcomas with characteristic clinicopathological features. Mod Pathol. 2019;32(3):435-45. doi: 10.1038/s41379-018-0140-5

Mentzel T, Kiss K. Reduced H3K27me3 expression in radiation-associated angiosarcoma of the breast. Virchows Arch. 2018;472(3):361-68. doi: 10.1007/s00428-017-2242-8

Miettinen M, editor. Modern soft tissue pathology: tumors and non-neoplastic conditions. Cambridge, UK: Cambridge University Press; 2016.

Prieto-Granada CN, Wiesner T, Messina JL, et al. Loss of H3K27me3 expression is a highly sensitive marker for sporadic and radiation-induced MPNST. Am J Surg Pathol. 2016;40(4):479-89. doi: 10.1097/pas.0000000000000564

Rudzinski ER, Bahrami A, Parham DM, et al; Cancer Committee, College of American Pathologists. Protocol for the examination of resection specimens from pediatric patients with rhabdomyosarcoma (Version: Rhabdomyosarcoma Resection 4.0.0.0) [Internet]. College of American Pathologists; 2019 Feb. Available from www.cap.org.

Rudzinski ER, Pawel B, Bahrami A, et al; Cancer Committee, College of American Pathologists. Protocol for the examination of resection specimens from pediatric patients with Ewing sarcoma (Version: Ewing Sarcoma Resection 4.0.0.0) [Internet]. College of American Pathologists; 2019 Feb. Available at www.cap.org.

WHO Classification of Tumors Editorial Board. WHO classification of tumours, 5th ed. Vol. 3, Soft tissue and bone tumours. Lyon (France): IARC; 2020.

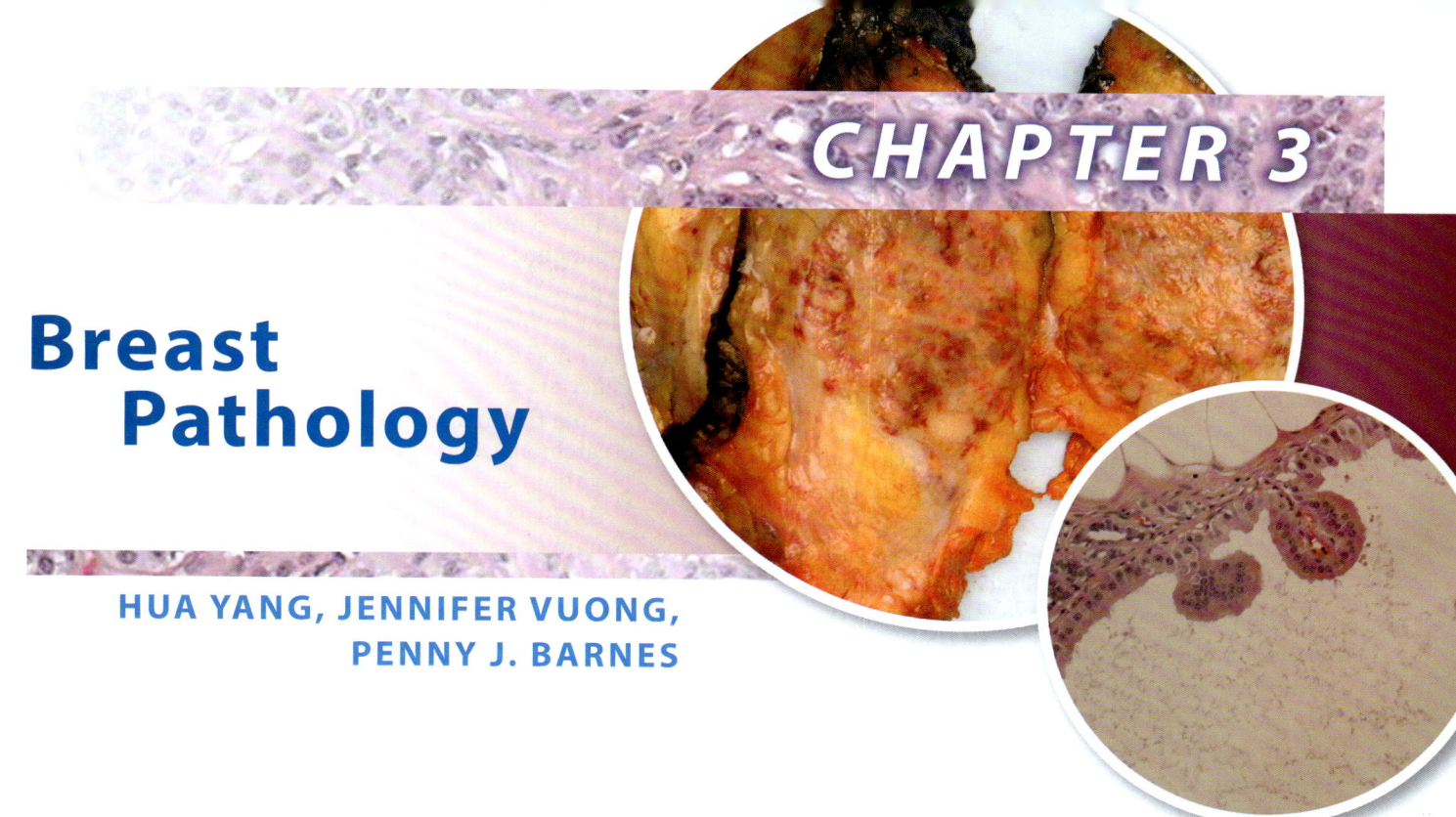

CHAPTER 3

Breast Pathology

HUA YANG, JENNIFER VUONG, PENNY J. BARNES

Breast Pathology Exam Essentials

MUST KNOW

World Health Organization (WHO) classification, 5th edition, 2019

- The WHO classification provides a comprehensive list of benign and malignant neoplasms. The main entities to review include:
  - Benign epithelial proliferations and precursors.
  - Sclerosing lesions, adenomas, epithelial-myoepithelial tumors and papillary neoplasms.
  - Noninvasive lobular neoplasia.
  - Ductal carcinoma in situ (DCIS).
  - Invasive and microinvasive carcinoma, including special types.
  - Rare and salivary gland-type tumors.
  - Neuroendocrine neoplasms.
  - Tumors of the nipple.
  - Fibroepithelial lesions, mammary hamartoma.
  - Mesenchymal tumors, hematolymphoid tumors.
  - Genetic tumor syndromes.
- You should understand the clinical aspects of diagnosis and management of breast diseases including:
  - Clinical and radiologic features of common breast lesions.
  - Importance of clinical-pathologic correlation of breast core biopsy and cytopathology.
  - Techniques for core biopsy and fine-needle aspiration (FNA) sampling of breast lesions.
  - Management of breast lesions found on biopsy; be aware of atypical lesions that might be difficult to separate from benign lesions on small biopsy alone.
- You should know how to differentiate benign proliferative glandular lesions from carcinoma, and how to diagnose them individually based on morphologic clues and immunohistochemistry (IHC) workup. Benign proliferative glandular lesions include:
  - Adenosis, sclerosing adenosis, apocrine adenosis.
  - Microglandular adenosis.
  - Radial scar and complex sclerosing lesion.
  - Tubular, lactating, apocrine, ductal, and pleomorphic adenomas.
  - Relative risks of malignancy for various benign and atypical lesions.
- You should know how to differentiate benign from atypical lesions among intraductal and papillary lesions, and the morphologic clues and IHC workup that help to differentiate each lesion. Benign lesions in this category include:
  - Usual ductal hyperplasia (UDH) versus atypical ductal hyperplasia (ADH) and DCIS.
  - Diagnostic criteria for low grade DCIS versus ADH.
  - Types and nuclear grading of DCIS.
  - Columnar cell change/hyperplasia and flat epithelial atypia (FEA).

- Papilloma versus papilloma with ADH or DCIS versus papillary DCIS.
- Variants of papillary carcinoma.
- Invasive breast carcinoma is often tested and is a high-yield topic to review:
  - Nottingham grading.
  - Special types of invasive carcinoma.
  - Types of invasive carcinoma that can mimic benign lesions, and vice versa.
  - Relative prognosis of different types of carcinoma and typical biomarker profile.
  - Molecular classification of invasive breast carcinoma.
  - Molecular and genetic diseases related to breast cancer.
  - Protocols for biomarker testing in breast cancer from the American Society of Clinical Oncology (ASCO) and the College of American Pathologists (CAP).
- You should also review lobular neoplasia:
  - Molecular changes leading to lobular neoplasia.
  - Morphology of ALH, LCIS, and invasive lobular carcinoma.
  - How to separate ALH and classic LCIS from DCIS.
  - Variants of LCIS: pleomorphic and florid.
  - Immunoprofile of lobular neoplasia.
  - Prognosis and management of various lobular lesions found on biopsy and excision.
- Review fibroepithelial lesions (phyllodes tumor is often examined):
  - Fibroadenoma versus benign phyllodes tumor.
  - Grading of phyllodes tumor.
  - Gross appearance of various fibroepithelial lesions.
  - Clinical management of phyllodes tumor.
- The exam may include slides of mesenchymal and miscellaneous lesions of the breast. Although many of these occur in various body sites, others are more "breast centric":
  - Myoepithelial IHC markers, and their staining pattern in various breast lesions.
  - Pseudoangiomatous stromal hyperplasia (PASH).
  - Benign mesenchymal lesions (see the Must See section in this chapter for a complete list).
  - Sarcomas, particularly angiosarcoma of the breast.
  - Nipple and skin tumors of the breast.
  - Mammary Paget disease, including immunoprofile and differential diagnosis.
  - Gynecomastia in males.
  - Lymphomas of the breast (pay attention to breast implant-associated anaplastic large cell lymphoma [BIA-ALCL]).
  - Metastases to the breast (e.g., melanoma, carcinoma from another site [lung, ovary, renal cell carcinoma])

AJCC and College of American Pathologists (CAP) protocols

- AJCC and CAP protocols for breast are excellent, up-to-date resources; some of the content within the

DCIS resection and invasive carcinoma resection protocols overlap. Note that there is a new protocol for resection specimens with phyllodes tumor of the breast (2022).
- The DCIS resection protocol has the following components:
  - Type of breast resection.
  - How to measure the size and extent of DCIS.
  - Radiologic and clinical features of DCIS, mammary Paget disease, and indolent papillary carcinomas.
    › Note that mammary Paget disease, solid papillary carcinoma, and encapsulated papillary carcinoma without associated conventional invasion are staged as pTis due to their favorable behavior.
  - Architectural patterns of DCIS.
  - Nuclear grading of DCIS.
  - Surgical margins.
  - Sentinel lymph node sampling.
    › You should know the criteria for isolated tumor cells versus micro versus macrometastasis.
  - Hormone testing in DCIS.
- The invasive carcinoma protocol has the following important elements:
  - Type of breast resection.
  - Radiologic and clinical features of invasive carcinomas.
  - Tumor type (including ductal no special type [NST], lobular, and special types).
  - How to measure the size and extent of invasive tumor.
  - How to report multifocal breast cancer.
  - Nottingham grading.
  - Pathological staging (pT) criteria, with attention to findings that qualify as pT4 disease.
  - Criteria for extensive intraductal component (EIC positive).
  - Effect of neoadjuvant treatment on characteristics of breast cancer and nodal disease and reporting criteria (ypT, ypN).
  - Lymph nodes: isolated tumor cells versus micrometastasis versus macrometastasis.
- The breast biomarker protocol is very important and may be tested in the written part of the exam. Furthermore, this protocol includes quality assurance (QA) issues in IHC and molecular tests, which may be assessed in the oral part. ASCO-CAP guidelines for hormone receptor and HER2 testing in breast cancer are important to review for the following details:
  - Scoring criteria for estrogen receptor (ER), progesterone receptor (PR), and HER2 IHC.
  - Fluorescence in situ hybridization (FISH), silver in situ hybridization (SISH), and dual in situ hybridization (DISH) criteria for *HER2* gene amplification.
  - Preanalytic specimen handling issues.

- Technical (analytic) issues that may affect IHC, resulting in false-negative and false-positive results.
- Types of on slide controls, internal controls.
- Review molecular recurrence score assays. Be aware of the clinical utility of multigene recurrence score assays such as the Oncotype DX test, a proprietary assay. The assays quantify mRNA levels in breast cancer cells dissected from formalin fixed paraffin embedded (FFPE) tumor blocks. The assays are weighted toward genes related to cell proliferation, ER, and *HER2*. These tests are used to help predict the magnitude of benefit of systemic chemotherapy for patients with early stage ER-positive/HER2-negative invasive breast cancer. The greatest value of these assays is the identification of patients with low recurrence scores due to slowly growing, hormone-responsive tumors: these patients can be spared cytotoxic chemotherapy.
- Review handling of postneoadjuvant treatment (post-NAT) specimens.
  - Grossing protocol, which includes: reviewing previous imaging for tumor size, multifocality, and location pre-NAT; and sampling of tumor bed.
  - Assessment of ypT and ypN stage.
  - Residual cancer burden (RCB) calculation, which includes the following pathologic features required for RCB assessment:
    › Primary tumor area in 2 largest dimensions.
    › Overall cancer cellularity as a percentage of the primary tumor area.
    › Percentage of cancer that is in situ disease.
    › Number of lymph nodes positive for metastasis.
    › Size of the largest lymph node metastasis.
- The MD Anderson Center has an online resource for RCB calculation (www.mdanderson.org).
- Repeat biomarkers if they are negative on previous core biopsy and/or if the tumor morphology differs in the resection specimen.

Nonneoplastic breast diseases

Fewer nonneoplastic diseases are high yield exam topics. Topics to review include:
- Infectious mastitis, including cystic neutrophilic granulomatous mastitis (usually *Corynebacterium* infection).
- Diabetic mastopathy and lymphocytic mastitis.
- Pregnancy-related changes, such as lactating adenoma, mastitis.
- Duct ectasia.
- Squamous metaplasia of lactiferous ducts (SMOLD).
- Implant-associated issues, including complications of ruptured implants.
- Benign lesions that mimic malignancy: fat necrosis, collagenous spherulosis.
- IgG4-related disease.

Genetic and syndromic conditions

- As with lung, GI tract, and brain tumors, molecular alterations related to breast cancer have become a hot topic. You should study molecular alterations and molecular testing in breast cancer, including the following inherited syndromes with breast cancer: *BRCA1/2*, Li-Fraumeni cancer syndrome, Cowden disease, Peutz-Jeghers syndrome.
  - Always study these syndromes in conjunction with other chapters to know manifestations in various organs.
  - Know the basics of what each gene does, especially *BRCA* genes.
- Also review Stewart-Treves syndrome (chronic lymphedema-associated angiosarcoma).

Breast core biopsy issues

Key topics include:
- Radiologic-pathologic correlation (this is essential).
- Breast Imaging Reporting and Data System (BI-RADS) scoring.
- Calcifications: calcium pyrophosphate and oxalate crystals.
- The importance of multidisciplinary meetings to resolve discordant findings.

MUST SEE

- Review the main breast lesions, which are listed here in the same order as the modified WHO classification:
  - UDH.
  - Columnar cell lesions: columnar cell change and hyperplasia, and FEA.
  - ADH.
  - Sclerosing adenosis.
  - Apocrine adenosis/adenoma.
  - Microglandular adenosis.
  - Radial scar/complex sclerosing lesion.
  - Tubular adenoma.
  - Lactating adenoma (fibroadenoma with lactational change).
  - Ductal adenoma (sclerosed intraductal papilloma).
  - Pleomorphic adenoma.
  - Adenomyoepithelioma.
  - Intraductal papilloma.
  - Intraductal papilloma with ADH and DCIS.
  - Papillary variant of DCIS.
  - Encapsulated papillary carcinoma (EPC).
  - Solid papillary carcinoma.
  - Invasive papillary carcinoma.
  - ALH, lobular carcinoma in situ (LCIS).
  - DCIS.
  - Mammary Paget disease.
  - Nipple adenoma.
  - Microinvasive carcinoma (definition).

- Invasive carcinoma of no special type, with Nottingham grades (1, 2, 3).
- Invasive lobular carcinoma (classic and pleomorphic variants).
- Tubular carcinoma.
- Cribriform carcinoma.
- Mucinous carcinoma.
- Metaplastic carcinoma (including variants).
- Invasive micropapillary carcinoma.
- Inflammatory carcinoma (clinical diagnosis).
- Salivary gland type carcinomas.
- Neuroendocrine neoplasms.
- Hamartoma.
- Fibroadenoma.
- Phyllodes tumor: benign, borderline, and malignant grades.
- Nodular fasciitis.
- PASH.
- Myofibroblastoma.
- Fibromatosis.
- Granular cell tumor.
- Hemangioma, atypical vascular lesion and angiosarcoma.
- Lipoma and liposarcoma.
- Lymphoma: diffuse large B cell lymphoma (DLBCL), MALT lymphoma.
- BIA-ALCL.
- Gynecomastia.
- The main nonneoplastic lesions include the following:
  - Acute mastitis.
  - Granulomatous mastitis (GM), including cystic neutrophilic GM.
  - Diabetic mastopathy.
  - Lymphocytic mastopathy.
  - Lactating adenoma.
  - Duct ectasia.
  - Amyloidosis.
  - Silicone granuloma.
  - Fat necrosis.
  - Collagenous spherulosis.
  - IgG4-related disease.
- Disorders of development:
  - Juvenile papillomatosis.
  - Gynecomastia.
  - Hamartoma.

MUST DO

- For each of the tumors outlined in the Must See section, you should be comfortable generating a differential diagnosis and listing relevant ancillary studies such as histochemistry and IHC staining.

- When studying in groups, work through:
  - QA measures for breast biomarkers (preanalytic, analytic, and postanalytic variables).
  - What to do if you cannot find calcifications on a slide, or if you cannot find the mass or core biopsy tract marker grossly in a large breast excision or mastectomy.
  - Safe disposal of radioactive seeds.
  - Equivocal and uncertain diagnoses on biopsies (e.g., fibroepithelial lesions with cellular stroma, papillary lesions, microglandular adenosis).
  - Radiologic-pathologic correlation, especially for breast core biopsy and FNA cytology.
- You should be able to describe the grossing protocols for key specimens, and independently gross them, including:
  - Breast core biopsies.
  - Lumpectomy, including those with guide wire or radioactive seed.
  - Mastectomy for malignancy, including those with radioactive seed.
  - Mastectomy for benign reasons (often nipple sparing), such as prophylaxis, gender-affirming.
  - Lumpectomy or mastectomy after neoadjuvant chemotherapy.
  - Reduction mammoplasty.
  - Optimal fixation duration and cold-ischemic time for breast specimens.
  - Use of specimen radiography to look for calcifications, biopsy clips.
  - Skin resections from breast.
  - Sentinel and nonsentinel lymph node grossing.
  - Explanted breast prosthesis storage guidelines.
  - Sampling of capsulectomies associated with explanted breast prostheses, including cases with a concern for BIA-ALCL (+/- lymphoma protocol).
- You should be able to describe and handle fresh specimens and frozen sections of specimens, including:
  - Skin margins from mastectomy.
  - Sentinel and nonsentinel lymph node sampling (frozen section, intraoperative imprint cytology).
  - Triaging of breast implant seroma fluid concerning for BIA-ALCL for cytopathology and ancillary studies.
  - Orienting and inking margins of large breast specimens: slice specimens in 5–10 mm slices ("bread loaf" slices) and fix in a large volume of fresh neutral buffered 10% formalin within 60 minutes of resection.
- Know when to avoid frozen section of breast lesions, such as small lesions < 10 mm in size, nipple lesions (nipple adenoma may be misdiagnosed as invasive carcinoma on frozen section).

MULTIPLE CHOICE QUESTIONS

1. The following types of invasive breast cancer, when matched for stage, deliver a better prognosis **except**:

a. Mucinous carcinoma.

b. Tubular carcinoma.

c. Solid papillary carcinoma.

d. Invasive micropapillary carcinoma.

e. Encapsulated (intracystic) papillary carcinoma.

Answer: d

2. The following breast lesions have a similar relative risk of developing invasive breast cancer **except**:

a. Papilloma.

b. Radial scar.

c. Florid hyperplasia.

d. Sclerosing adenosis.

e. Apocrine metaplasia.

Answer: e

3. Pseudoangiomatous stromal hyperplasia (PASH) is a benign proliferation of which cell type?

a. Myoepithelial cells.

b. Smooth muscle cells.

c. Fibroblasts.

d. Myofibroblasts.

e. Lymphatic endothelial cells.

Answer: d

4. The cells lining the slit-like spaces in mammary PASH express the following markers **except**:

a. CD31.

b. Vimentin.

c. Actin.

d. Estrogen receptor (ER).

e. CD34.

Answer: a

5. The following pathologic features of invasive breast carcinoma have strong independent prognostic value **except**:

a. Nottingham grade.

b. Lymph node status.

c. Lymphovascular invasion.

d. Tumor size.

e. Tumor necrosis.

Answer: e

6. Based on molecular phenotypes, breast carcinoma can be classified into the following types **except**:

a. Luminal A.

b. Luminal B.

c. HER2+.

d. Basal-like.

e. Medullary.

Answer: e

7. After surgical excision, adjuvant treatment decisions for invasive breast carcinoma are heavily based on the following pathologic indices **except**:

a. Tumor size.

b. Nottingham grade.

c. Nuclear grade of ductal carcinoma in situ (DCIS).

d. HER2 status.

e. Presence of lymphovascular invasion.

Answer: c

8. According to the current AJCC staging system,* which of the following cases qualifies as pN1?

a. 1 node positive for macrometastases (macromets), 2 nodes positive for micrometastases (micromets), 1 node positive for isolated tumor cells (ITCs).

b. 2 nodes positive for micromets, 1 node positive for ITCs.

c. 1 node positive for macromets, 2 nodes positive for micromets, 1 node positive for ITCs.

d. 3 nodes positive for macromets, 1 node positive for ITCs.

e. All of the above.

Answer: e

*This chapter uses the eighth edition of the AJCC staging manual.

9. The following immunohistochemical markers can be used to highlight myoepithelial cells in breast tissue **except**:

a. Smooth muscle myosin heavy chain (SMMHC).

b. Calponin.

c. Cox2.

d. p63.

e. Actin.

Answer: c

10. The most helpful combination of immunohistochemical markers to help distinguish florid usual ductal hyperplasia from atypical ductal hyperplasia (ADH) is:

a. Calponin and ER.

b. p63 and smooth muscle myosin heavy chain (SMMHC).

c. Gross cystic disease fluid protein (GCDFP) and mammaglobin.

d. CK5/6 and ER.

e. HER2 and ER.

Answer: d

11. Current literature recommends consideration of excisional biopsy for the following lesions diagnosed on core needle biopsy **except**:

a. Microglandular adenosis.

b. Spindle cell lesion.

c. Columnar cell hyperplasia.

d. Pleomorphic lobular carcinoma in situ.

e. Flat epithelial atypia with atypical duct hyperplasia.

Answer: c

12. The following histologic features may help to distinguish benign from malignant phyllodes tumors **except**:

a. Leaflike architecture.

b. Degree of nuclear atypia.

c. Mitotic rate.

d. Infiltrative growth.

e. Degree of cellularity.

Answer: a

13. The following statements are true regarding breast fibromatosis **except**:

a. Proliferation of myofibroblastic cells.

b. Positive nuclear expression of β-catenin.

c. Association with trauma.

d. Association with Gardner syndrome.

e. Responds to hormonal therapy.

Answer: e

14. Granular cell tumors of the breast typically express the following markers **except**:

a. Neuron specific enolase (NSE).

b. Vimentin.

c. S100.

d. CD68.

e. ER.

Answer: e

15. The neoplastic cells in mammary Paget disease are often positive for the following markers **except**:

a. Epithelial membrane antigen (EMA).

b. Carcinoembryonic antigen (CEA).

c. HMB45.

d. CK7.

e. HER2.

Answer: c

16. Flat epithelial atypia (FEA) is associated with a higher incidence of the following lesions **except**:

a. Atypical ductal hyperplasia (ADH).

b. Lobular carcinoma in situ (LCIS).

c. Tubular carcinoma.

d. Metaplastic carcinoma.

e. Atypical lobular hyperplasia (ALH).

Answer: d

17. Compared to high grade ductal carcinoma in situ (high grade DCIS), low grade DCIS is more often positive for the following tests **except**:

a. ER.

b. Progesterone receptor (PR).

c. HER2.

d. Cyclin D1.

e. Near diploidy.

Answer: c

18. Which of the following clinical presentations has the highest association with invasive breast carcinoma?

a. Mammographic calcification.

b. Palpable mass.

c. Lumpiness or asymmetry.

d. Pain.

e. Nipple discharge.

Answer: b

19. The following breast lesions have no increased relative risk of subsequent breast cancer **except**:

a. Cysts.

b. Duct ectasia.

c. Mild epithelial hyperplasia.

d. Apocrine change.

e. Radial scar.

Answer: e

20. Risk factors for the development of breast carcinoma include all of the following **except**:

a. Increased breast density.

b. Ethnicity.

c. Breast implants.

d. Hormone replacement therapy.

e. Alcohol consumption.

Answer: c

21. Which of the following syndromes corresponds to postmastectomy angiosarcomas?

a. Rosen-Finch.

b. Von Hippel-Lindau.

c. Stewart-Treves.

d. Li-Fraumeni.

e. McCune-Albright.

Answer: c

22. Which of the following biomarker profiles is common in BRCA1 associated breast cancers?

a. ER−, PR−, HER2−, CK5/6+.

b. ER−, PR−, HER2+, CK5/6−.

c. ER+, PR+, HER2−, CK5/6−.

d. ER+, PR+, HER2+, CK5/6+.

e. ER+, PR+, HER2−, CK5/6+.

Answer: a

23. Which of the following is not a histologic feature of diabetic mastopathy?

a. Keloidal like stromal fibrosis.

b. Usual epithelial hyperplasia.

c. Lymphocytic ductitis.

d. Lymphocytic lobulitis.

e. Lymphocytic vasculitis.

Answer: b

24. Which of the following favors a diagnosis of ADH over low grade DCIS?

a. Associated lymphocytic response.

b. Partial involvement of ducts with mildly atypical ductal cells measuring 1 mm.

c. Punched out round spaces within the duct lumen.

d. "Roman arch" orientation of cells around spaces.

e. High grade cytologic atypia.

Answer: b

25. Which of the following should generate the most concern for false results when interpreting ER/PR immunohistochemistry?

a. No immunohistochemical staining noted on the negative external control tissue.

b. Nuclear staining of cervix stromal cells noted on external control tissue.

c. No staining noted in some of the normal internal control duct epithelial cells.

d. No staining noted in an invasive lobular carcinoma, Nottingham grade 2.

e. Heterogeneous staining noted in the tumor.

Answer: d

26. Extensive intraductal component (EIC positive) is defined as:

a. DCIS involving at least 25% of the area of the invasive carcinoma and extending beyond the area of invasive carcinoma.

b. DCIS involving 25% or more of the specimen.

c. DCIS involving 25% or more of the core biopsy samples.

d. DCIS involving > 1 quadrant of the breast.

e. DCIS present and directly involving > 1 surgical margin.

Answer: a

27. What is the name of cytologically bland clear cells found in the epidermis of the nipple that are CK7 positive, CD138 negative, and HER2 negative?

a. Tavassoli cells.

b. The organ of Chivietz.

c. The organ of Zuckerkandl.

d. The organ of Corti.

e. Toker cells.

Answer: e

28. Which of the following, if present, would indicate a better prognosis for patients with invasive ductal carcinoma, no special type (NST)?

a. Invasive tumor necrosis.

b. Perineural invasion.

c. High Ki 67 index.

d. High Oncotype DX score (50).

e. High percentage of tubule formation (> 75%).

Answer: e

29. Which of the following is true regarding sentinel lymph nodes and breast cancer?

a. A single cluster of tumor cells < 0.2 mm in size would be classified as isolated tumor cells.

b. There is no difference in prognosis between patients that have sentinel node micrometastases versus those with macrometastases.

c. Frozen section analysis has a sensitivity of 70–90% for detecting micrometastases.

d. The likelihood of nonsentinel nodes containing macrometastases if the sentinel node is negative is between 10 and 15%.

e. Immunohistochemistry should be performed routinely on all breast sentinel lymph node biopsies.

Answer: a

30. An invasive breast carcinoma is considered HER2 positive with the following results, **except**:

a. Strong complete membranous staining of > 10% of cells with HER2 immunohistochemistry (IHC).

b. HER2/CEP17 ratio of 1.8 and an average of 4 HER2 signals/cell (HER2 fluorescence in situ hybridization [FISH]).

c. HER2/CEP17 ratio of 3.0 and > 6 HER2 signals/cell (HER2 FISH).

d. HER2/CEP17 ratio of 2.1 and > 4 HER2 signals/cell (HER2 FISH).

e. HER2/CEP17 ratio of 1.5 and > 6 HER2 signals/cell (HER2 FISH).

Answer: b

31. Regarding radiation-associated angiosarcoma, which statement is **false**?

a. It is associated with amplification of the MYC gene.

b. It typically occurs in the irradiated skin.

c. It has an indolent prognosis.

d. It typically shows expression of ERG and CD31 IHC.

e. It may be preceded by an atypical vascular lesion.

Answer: c

32. Which statement is correct about HER2 testing for breast cancer?

a. Both the invasive and in situ components are scored with HER2 in situ hybridization (ISH).

b. HER2 positivity is virtually always seen in ER negative tumors.

c. HER2 testing can be optimally performed in decalcified bone metastasis specimens.

d. A HER2/CEP17 ratio ≥ 2.0 is considered amplified if the mean HER2 copy/cell count is ≥ 4.0.

e. A HER2/CEP17 ratio ≥ 2.0 is considered amplified if the mean HER2 copy/cell count is < 4.0.

Answer: d

33. Which statement is correct about ductal carcinoma in situ (DCIS)?

a. DCIS usually presents symptomatically.

b. Determination of nuclear grade is an important prognostic factor.

c. Most cases of high grade DCIS show ER expression.

d. DCIS is usually multicentric.

e. HER2 testing is routinely assessed for DCIS.

Answer: b

34. Which statement about fibroadenoma is **incorrect**?

a. Fibroadenoma is most common in adolescent girls and women under 35 years.

b. Fibroadenoma is hormone sensitive and may grow rapidly during pregnancy.

c. Fibroadenoma should be excised following core biopsy diagnosis.

d. Complex fibroadenoma is associated with a minimal increase in relative breast cancer risk.

e. Most fibroadenomas do not recur following surgical excision.

Answer: c

35. Which statement about myofibroblastoma is **incorrect**?

a. It is treated by surgical excision, with no tendency to recur.

b. Myofibroblastoma occurs equally in women and men.

c. It has similar morphologic, IHC, and molecular alterations as spindle cell/pleomorphic lipoma and cellular angiofibroma.

d. It typically expresses desmin, CD34, ER, and PR.

e. It may have a high mitotic rate and infiltrative margins.

Answer: e

36. Which statement about encapsulated papillary carcinoma (EPC) is **true**?

a. It is a papillary neoplasm with myoepithelial cells lining papillary fronds.

b. It most commonly occurs in young women.

c. In the absence of conventional invasive carcinoma, it has a favorable prognosis.

d. It is usually HER2 IHC positive (3+).

e. Tumor cell nests within the fibrous capsule are staged as invasive carcinoma.

Answer: c

37. Which statement about breast implant-associated anaplastic large cells lymphoma (BIA-ALCL) is **false**?

a. Most patients present with a unilateral seroma around their implant > 1 year after implantation.

b. Cytopathologic evaluation of the breast implant seroma fluid is not helpful for diagnosis.

c. It is associated with textured implants, not smooth devices.

d. The neoplastic cells are CD30 positive and anaplastic lymphoma kinase (ALK) negative.

e. Surgical management includes removal of the implant and surrounding capsule.

Answer: b

38. Which statement is **false** regarding breast specimen handling and reporting following neoadjuvant chemotherapy treatment (NAT)?

a. Biomarker studies are never repeated, because they will have been performed on the previous core biopsy.

b. Tumor size for pathological staging (ypT) is based on the size of the largest contiguous cluster of residual tumor cells.

c. Complete pathologic response (pCR) is defined as complete eradication of invasive carcinoma post-NAT and is most commonly seen following treatment of HER2 positive and triple negative (TN) invasive breast carcinoma.

d. Residual lymphovascular invasion is not considered pCR to treatment.

e. If residual carcinoma is not identified, definite treatment-related changes and biopsy site changes must be identified and documented before reporting pCR.

Answer: a

SHORT ANSWER QUESTIONS

Proliferative Breast Lesions

39. Describe 5 features of sclerosing adenosis that distinguish it from an invasive ductal carcinoma (e.g., tubular carcinoma).

- Lobulated clustered arrangement (retention of the lobular architecture versus haphazard distribution of tubules).
- Compressed (and distorted) tubular lumens (versus open angulated tubules).
- Fibrous stroma compressing tubules (versus desmoplastic stroma).
- Tubules lined by 2 layers of cells (luminal epithelial and outer myoepithelial).
- Tubules invested by basement membrane (highlighted by periodic acid-Schiff stain).

40. Describe the characteristic features of microglandular adenosis (MGA).

- Haphazard proliferation of small round tubules.
- Tubules have open lumens.
- Tubules lined by single layer of epithelial cells (absent myoepithelial cell layer).
- Lumen contains colloid-like secretory material.
- Dense fibrous stroma.
- Multilayered basement membrane on electron microscopy.
- Epithelial cells are positive for S100 and cytokeratins; lack expression of ER and PR.

41. What is the clinical significance of MGA and how should it be managed?

- MGA may be mass forming or associated with microcalcifications, but it is often detected incidentally.
- MGA is a benign proliferation, but atypical forms and carcinomas (triple negative) arising with MGA can occur.
- It may be a nonobligate precursor of basal-type breast carcinoma.
- MGA should be excised with clear margins.

42. List common benign proliferative breast lesions and the relative risk of developing invasive carcinoma related to each entity.

EPITHELIAL BREAST LESIONS	RELATIVE RISK OF DEVELOPING INVASIVE BREAST CARCINOMA
• Nonproliferative changes: · Duct ectasia. · Cysts. · Apocrine change. · Mild epithelial hyperplasia. · Fibroadenoma without complex features.	• 1.0 (3% lifetime risk).
• Proliferative changes without atypia: · Moderate to florid hyperplasia. · Sclerosing adenosis. · Papilloma. · Complex sclerosing lesion. · Fibroadenoma with complex features.	• 1.5–2.0 (5–7% lifetime risk).
• Proliferative disease with atypia: · Atypical ductal hyperplasia. · Atypical lobular hyperplasia.	• 4.0–5.0 (13–17% lifetime risk, bilateral).
• Carcinoma in situ: · Lobular carcinoma in situ. · Low grade ductal carcinoma in situ.	• 8–10 (~25–35% lifetime risk; bilateral for LCIS).

43. What are the histologic features of a radial scar?

- Stellate configuration (flower head).
- Central elastosis and fibrosis.
- Entrapped distorted ductules in the central scar.
- Dilated ductules at the periphery with various patterns of epithelial hyperplasia.
- Tubules lined by 2 layers of cells (luminal epithelial and outer myoepithelial).
- IHC for some myoepithelial markers may be aberrant (negative) in the ducts within the central nidus of radial sclerosing lesions.

44. What is the clinical significance of a radial scar?
- A radial scar is a benign mimic of cancer.
- The relative risk of subsequent breast carcinoma is 1.5–2 x baseline population.
- Management of radial scar/complex sclerosing lesion detected by mammography remains controversial. Lesions with associated epithelial atypia should be excised.

45. Describe the characteristic histologic features of usual ductal hyperplasia (UDH).
- Architectural features:
  - Peripheral elongated clefts.
  - Intraductal secondary spaces irregular in size, shape and location.
  - Streaming (cells arranged in parallel bundles).
  - Tufts and mounds projecting into the lumen.
  - Irregularly shaped/twisted bridges (long axis of nuclei are parallel to the long axis of the bridge).
- Cellular features:
  - 2 cell types (epithelial and myoepithelial).
  - Nuclei oval, normochromatic, overlapping with indistinct nucleoli.
  - Indistinct cell borders — nuclei seem to lie in a syncytial mass.
  - Apocrine metaplasia, foamy macrophages common.
  - Absence of necrosis (usually).
- IHC: heterogeneous expression of ER and CK5/6 (mosaic pattern).

46. List 8 features that differentiate epithelial hyperplasia from low grade DCIS.

FEATURE	EPITHELIAL HYPERPLASIA	LOW GRADE DCIS
Secondary spaces	• Irregular, slit-like, mainly peripheral.	• Regular, rounded, rigid.
Streaming	• Present.	• Absent.
Bridges	• Orientation of long axis of nuclei: parallel to bridges.	• Orientation of long axis of nuclei: perpendicular to bridges (resembling Roman arches).
Cell types	• Polymorphous.	• Monomorphous.
Cell margins	• Indistinct.	• Well defined.
Nuclei	• Overlapping; normochromatic; indistinct nucleoli.	• Evenly spaced; low grade atypia (mild nuclear enlargement, hyperchromasia).
Apocrine metaplasia	• Focally present (or absent).	• Absent.
Necrosis	• Usually absent.	• Present or absent.

47. Which immunostains can be used to differentiate UDH from atypical ductal hyperplasia (ADH) and low grade DCIS?
- High molecular weight keratins (CK5/6, 34BE12) are positive (mosaic pattern) in UDH, and negative in ADH and low grade DCIS.
- ER will be patchy (mosaic pattern) in UDH, and diffusely positive in ADH and low grade DCIS.

48. What is the definition of atypical ductal hyperplasia (ADH)?

ADH is an epithelial proliferative lesion with cytological and architectural features similar to low grade DCIS but it is less developed in extent (it has partial involvement of multiple duct spaces or uniformly involved duct spaces, but the lesion measures no more than 2–3 mm in contiguous extent).

49. List 4 benign breast conditions whose histology may be confused with that of invasive breast carcinoma.
- Complex sclerosing lesion (radial scar).
- Sclerosing adenosis.
- Microglandular adenosis.
- Sclerotic papilloma, especially in core biopsies.

50. Name 2 malignant lesions that can mimic collagenous spherulosis.
- Adenoid cystic carcinoma.
- DCIS, cribriform pattern.

51. List the World Health Organization (WHO) classification of columnar cell lesions.
- Columnar cell change.
- Columnar cell hyperplasia.
- Flat epithelial atypia (FEA).

52. What is the clinical significance of columnar cell lesions (CCLs)?
- They are often detected mammographically due to associated luminal calcifications.
- CCLs are regarded as nonobligate precursors of ADH, low grade DCIS, and low grade invasive carcinomas.
- The need for surgical excision of FEA diagnosed by core biopsy is uncertain and requires radiologic-pathologic correlation.
- Clear margins for FEA (or any CCL) are not required.

53. List 2 clinical and 4 histologic features of a nipple adenoma.
- Clinical features:
  - Nipple discharge.
  - Swelling of the nipple with or without erosion.
- Histologic features:
  - Well circumscribed.
- Haphazardly arranged, proliferating tubular structures.
- Myoepithelial layer surrounding the proliferative tubules.
- Varying degrees of epithelial hyperplasia.
- Fibrous stroma.
- Areas of papillary architecture (possible).

Practical Issues

54. A core biopsy for calcifications does not show any calcifications in the sections. Explain briefly the next steps that you would take to resolve the issue.
- Check the accompanying specimen radiographs for calcifications.
- Use polarized light to search for calcium oxalate crystals.
- Cut deeper levels x3.
- If calcifications are still not seen, take X-rays of the block.
- If the X-rays show calcifications, cut the block at the level of the calcifications.
- If the X-rays do not show calcifications, have the specimen radiographs and block X-rays reviewed by radiology to confirm the presence or absence of calcifications in the respective images. This can be done at multidisciplinary rounds.
- If the specimen radiograph has confirmed calcifications, but the slide sections and block X-rays do not, then report as calcifications not seen in slide sections or block X-rays. Calcifications may have fallen out during block trimming.

55. A mastectomy specimen suspicious for malignancy is received in the lab. You cannot find a mass. How do you handle the specimen?
- Check if patient identification is correct (at least 2 identifiers should match).
- Check if the correct side of the breast was operated on.
- Look up the pertinent imaging studies for the size and location of the mass.
- Check to see if there was a previous core biopsy or placement of a biopsy marker.
- If you still cannot identify the mass or previous biopsy site/marker, have a specimen radiograph done to localize any abnormalities for sectioning.
- If you can still not identify the lesion, take random samples of the 4 quadrants and map them. Focus sections on the area in the breast where the abnormality was initially suspected.
- If any of the samples are positive histologically, go back and take more samples from that specific quadrant.
- If none of the samples are positive, submit the entire specimen serially, with mapping.

56. What are indications for synoptic reporting based on types of specimens?
- The following types of breast specimens and procedures may be reported using the College of American Pathologists (CAP) checklist for resection specimens:
  - Excisions +/– wire localization (palpable lesions or not).
  - Total mastectomy.
- The following types of specimens should not be reported using the CAP checklist:
  - Very small incisional biopsies (including core needle biopsies).
  - Reexcision specimens after the definitive resection.

57. List relevant clinical information that is important for pathologists in making a diagnosis of breast cancer.
- Patient information:
  - Family history of breast or ovarian cancer and/or *BRCA1* or *BRCA2* germline mutation.
  - Current pregnancy or lactation.
  - Prior breast biopsy or surgery (including implants).
  - Prior breast cancer diagnosis (type, location in breast, date of diagnosis).
  - Prior treatment that could affect the breast:
    › Radiation.
    › Chemotherapy.
  - Hormonal therapy (e.g., tamoxifen, aromatase inhibitors, or oral contraceptives).
  - Systemic diseases that may affect the breast (e.g., collagen vascular disease, sarcoidosis, Wegener granulomatosis).
- Specimen information:
  - Type of lesion sampled:
    › Palpable mass.
    › Nipple discharge.
    › Nipple lesion (e.g., scaling crust).
- Imaging findings:
  - Mammographic or ultrasound mass: shape of mass (irregular, circumscribed, ill defined, cystic, or solid).
  - Mammographic calcifications, and their extent and location.
  - Mammographic architectural distortion.
  - Prior core needle biopsy site, with or without a clip/biopsy site marker, with or without residual radiologic or clinical lesion.
  - Lesion detected on magnetic resonance imaging (MRI).

(continued on next page)

- Type of specimen:
  - Excision without wire localization.
  - Excision with wire localization — for these specimens, the specimen radiograph with an interpretation should be available to the pathologist.
- Nipple duct excision.
- Total mastectomy.
- Lymph node specimen.

Epidemiology

58. What are the risk factors for developing breast cancer, including genetic factors?
- Female sex.
- Age — peak age 75–80 years.
- Age at first live birth (nulliparous or > 35 years at first birth).
- Age at menarche/menopause — menarche younger than 11 years and late menopause.
- Breast feeding — decreases risk.
- Carcinoma of the contralateral breast.
- Estrogen exposure (postmenopausal hormone replacement therapy).
- High breast density.
- First degree relatives with breast cancer.
- Genetic factors (germ-line mutations):
  - BRCA1.
  - BRCA2.
  - CHEK2.
  - Li-Fraumeni syndrome.
- History of atypical hyperplasia in previous biopsy.
- Race/ethnicity — in order of highest to lowest risk: non-Hispanic whites, African-Americans, Asian/Pacific islanders, Hispanics.
- Radiation exposure.

Ductal Carcinoma In Situ (DCIS)

59. List 6 histologic subtypes of DCIS.
- Solid.
- Cribriform.
- Micropapillary.
- Comedo.
- Flat.
- Papillary.

Note: nuclear grade and the presence of necrosis are more predictive of clinical outcome, although architectural pattern is traditionally reported. Pure micropapillary DCIS is more commonly multicentric.

60. How do you grade DCIS?
- Low grade: well-defined cell membranes, uniform nuclear and cell size and shape, rare mitosis, punched out appearance of lumen with polarization of cells around. Arcades and bridges uniform in thickness with rigid contours. Necrosis unusual but possible. Calcifications frequent.
- High grade: cells with large pleomorphic nuclei, coarse chromatin, prominent nucleoli, frequent mitosis, frequent central comedo necrosis (necrosis can be so extensive that only 1 layer of atypical cells is left at periphery of duct: clinging DCIS). Desmoplasia and angiogenesis can be seen in stroma.
- Intermediate grade: cells do not fulfill the criteria of either low grade or high grade. Some intermediate grade lesions grow in patterns mimicking UDH (irregular architecture, streaming).

61. What histologic features should be included in a report of DCIS?
- Nuclear grade: I, II, III.
- Necrosis: absent, punctate, comedo.
- Pattern: cribriform, solid, micropapillary, papillary, comedo.
- Size of the largest focus (cm).
- Microinvasion: present/absent.
- Distance to resection margins or involvement of resection margin(s) and extent of involvement.
- Calcification: intraluminal, stromal, in benign breast tissue.

62. List required reporting elements for DCIS in the College of American Pathologists (CAP) checklist.
- Procedure.
- Lymph node sampling.
- Specimen laterality.
- Tumor site (optional).
- Size (extent) of DCIS.
- Histologic type.
- Architectural patterns (optional).
- Nuclear grade.
- Necrosis.
- Margins.
- Treatment effect (optional): response to presurgical (neoadjuvant) therapy.
- Lymph nodes (required only if lymph nodes are present in the specimen).

(continued on next page)

- Pathologic staging (pTNM).
- Additional pathologic findings (optional).
- Ancillary studies (optional).

- Microcalcifications (optional).
- Clinical history (optional).
- Comment (optional).

63. What goals should inform specimen sampling of excisions for DCIS?

- The clinical or radiologic lesion for which the surgery was performed must be examined microscopically.
- If DCIS, lobular carcinoma in situ (LCIS), or atypical hyperplasia is identified, all fibrous tissue should be examined.
- All other gross lesions noted in the specimen must be sampled.
- The margins must be evaluated for involvement by DCIS.

- For specimens with a known diagnosis of DCIS (e.g., by prior core needle biopsy), it is highly recommended that the entire specimen be examined using serial sequential sampling to exclude the possibility of invasion, to completely evaluate the margins, and to aid in determining extent.
- If an entire excisional specimen or grossly evident lesion is not examined microscopically, it is helpful to note the approximate percentage of the specimen or lesion that has been examined.

64. In the setting of DCIS, how should resection margins be reported?

- If margins are sampled with perpendicular sections, the pathologist should report the distance from the DCIS to the closest margin, when possible.
- The color of ink, and designated margin(s) that is (are) positive should be documented.

- If DCIS is present at the margin, the extent of margin involvement should be reported:
  · Focal (e.g., DCIS at the margin in a < 1 mm area in 1 block).
  · Minimal/moderate (between focal and extensive).
  · Extensive (e.g., DCIS at the margin in an area ≥ 15 mm or in 5 or more low power fields and/or in 8 or more blocks).

65. What is the clinical significance of different extents of DCIS?

- Size < 2 cm: in most women, breast conservation with wide negative margin can be achieved.
- Size 2–4 cm: in some women, wide negative margin may be difficult to achieve with breast-conserving surgery.

- Size > 4 cm: in some women, breast conservation with wide negative margins may be impossible to achieve.

66. How do you measure the extent of DCIS?

- If DCIS is present in only 1 block, use the size on the slide as the tumor extent.
- If DCIS involves > 1 block in sequential sampling, the size can be determined from the location of the involved blocks.
- If DCIS involves > 1 block in nonsequential sampling, use the number of blocks containing DCIS to estimate

the extent: the number of blocks multiplied by 0.4 cm (thickness of tissue per block) equals the approximate extent.
- If DCIS involves 2 opposing margins, use the distance between these margins as the tumor extent.

67. How do you report DCIS that involves nipple skin only?

If there is no underlying invasive carcinoma or DCIS, the classification is DCIS — i.e., Tis (Paget).

68. Should ER status be reported for DCIS?

- ER testing for cases of newly diagnosed DCIS (without associated invasion) is recommended by the American Society of Clinical Oncology (ASCO) and CAP to determine the benefit of endocrines therapies to reduce the risk of future breast cancer. PR testing for DCIS is optional.

- In some centers, hormone receptor IHC is done upon clinician request and not reflexively.
- The same quality assurance (QA) measures apply as per ER/PR assessment for invasive breast carcinoma.

Regional Lymph Node Assessment

69. How should axillary lymph nodes be examined and reported?

- Examine:
  · Grossly involved nodes, which may have 1 or more sections submitted for microscopic evaluation.
  · All other lymph nodes (should be thinly sectioned (2 mm or thinner) and entirely submitted for microscopic evaluation).

  · Note that a single H&E section from each lymph node block is considered sufficient for routine evaluation.
  · Use of Keratin IHC should be considered for the assessment of lymph nodes in cases of invasive lobular carcinoma.
- Report:
  · The total number of lymph nodes examined, including sentinel lymph nodes.

(continued on next page)

- The number of nodes with metastases.
  - › Only nodes with micro- and macrometastases are included for the total number of involved nodes for pN classification. Nodes with isolated tumor cells only are not included in this count.
- The greatest dimension of the largest metastatic focus.
- Additional studies, if performed (i.e., additional H&E levels or immunohistochemical studies).

- Presence of extranodal tumor extension, because it may be associated with a higher frequency of axillary recurrence.
- Note that:
  - › Classification based solely on sentinel lymph node biopsy is designated "(sn)" for "sentinel node" — e.g., pN0(i+)(sn). If 6 or more lymph nodes are removed the "(sn)" modifier should not be used.
  - › Isolated tumor cells (ITCs) are defined as single tumor cells or small cell clusters ≤ 0.2 mm and numbering < 200 cells.

70. What is the clinical importance of finding isolated tumor cells in the lymph node in patients with DCIS?
- Almost all tumor cells present in lymph nodes of patients with DCIS are isolated tumor cells or the cells may be artifactually displaced from a previous procedure.
- Isolated tumor cells detected in cases of DCIS have not been shown to have prognostic importance.
- Consider whether an occult focus of invasion has been missed: block more tissue, obtain deeper levels.

71. What should be done if lymph node metastasis is found in a patient with DCIS?
If a larger metastasis is found, additional tissue sampling, review of slides and deeper levels should be performed to determine if an area of occult invasion is present.

Invasive Ductal Carcinoma (IDC)

72. List 7 special types of invasive breast carcinoma.
- Lobular.
- Tubular.
- Mucinous.
- Cribriform.
- Invasive micropapillary.
- Carcinoma with apocrine differentiation.
- Metaplastic.

73. Describe briefly the criteria used to grade IDC.
- The Nottingham grading system is internationally used to grade IDC. It assigns points to 3 criteria: percentage of tumor with tubule formation, number of mitotic figures, and nuclear pleomorphism.
- The Nottingham grade is based on the total points:
  - Grade 1: 3–5 points.
  - Grade 2: 6–7 points.
  - Grade 3: 8–9 points.

CRITERION	POINTS
Percentage of tumor with tubule formation · Counting only those tubules with clear central lumina. · With overall appearance of the tumor taken into consideration.	• 1 point: > 75%. • 2 points: 10–75%. • 3 points: < 10%.
Number of mitotic figures · Counting 10 HPFs (x40 objective comparable to a field diameter of 0.44 mm) in the most active areas.	• 1 point: ≤ 5. • 2 points: 6–11. • 3 points: > 11. If the field diameter is 0.55 mm: • 1 point: ≤ 8. • 2 points: 9–17. • 3 points: > 17.
Nuclear pleomorphism (variation in size and shape of nuclei)	• 1 point: minimal. • 2 points: moderate. • 3 points: marked (> 2 times the size of a benign epithelial cell nucleus).

74. List 10 prognostic factors and 3 predictive factors commonly employed for breast carcinoma.

PROGNOSTIC — ASSESSES OUTCOME AT THE TIME OF DIAGNOSIS.	PREDICTIVE — ASSESSES LIKELIHOOD OF RESPONSE TO A GIVEN THERAPY.
• Invasive carcinoma versus in situ disease. • Distant metastases. • Axillary lymph node metastases. • Size of the primary tumor. • Skin invasion with ulceration/inflammatory carcinoma. • Nottingham grade. • Lymphovascular invasion. • Histologic subtype. • ER and PR status. • HER2 status.	• ER. • PR. • HER2.

Note: ER, PR, and HER2 are both prognostic and predictive factors.

75. List 5 histologic subtypes of invasive breast carcinoma that indicate a better prognosis than invasive ductal carcinoma, no special type (NST).
- Mucinous carcinoma.
- Papillary.
- Tubular.
- Cribriform.
- Adenoid cystic.

76. If a sentinel node is negative on frozen section and positive on permanent section, what would you do?
- Document in the final report that the sentinel lymph node is positive on permanent sections, and comment on whether it was a sampling issue (not present in the frozen) or an interpretive issue (isolated cells, or a difficult-to-identify histologic subtype) as the reason for reporting the frozen sections as negative.
- Make sure that the pathologist who has reported the frozen is aware of the discrepancy.
- Contact the surgeon directly to relay the change in node status and document this communication in your report.

77. If a sentinel lymph node is reported as positive, what is the expected treatment?
- Axillary lymph node dissection (ALND) historically would be the most common treatment for macrometastases (> 2 mm) and micrometastasis (> 0.2–2 mm and/or > 200 cells). Currently, axillary radiation therapy has been shown to be an acceptable alternative for limited nodal disease in clinical trials. As a result, treatment may vary by institution, surgeon, and patient factors.
  - Isolated tumor cells in the sentinel node are treated as node negative — pN0 (i+) (sn).

78. What findings should be reported in the case of a positive lymph node?
- Number of nodes involved out of the total number examined.
- Size of the largest metastatic deposit.
- Presence/absence of extracapsular extension.
- Histologic subtype of metastasis and whether it resembles the identified primary tumor.

79. What information would you include in your histologic report of breast carcinoma?
- Tumor size.
- Histologic type.
- Lymph node status.
- Nottingham grade.
- Lymphatic-vascular invasion.
- Margin status.
- ER/PR, HER2 status.
- Presence and type of associated in situ carcinoma.
- Size and extent of in situ component.
- Nipple involvement (Paget disease).
- Skin involvement.
- Skeletal muscle involvement.
- Pathologic stage (T and N status).

80. What are the major molecular subtypes of breast cancer? Compare the subtypes for the following factors: genetic, biologic, immunoprofile, and clinical.
- Major molecular subtypes:
  - ER positive, *HER2* negative (luminal).
  - Low proliferation (luminal A).
  - High proliferation (some luminal B).
  - *HER2* positive (some luminal B).
  - ER negative, *HER2* negative (basal-like).
- Comparison of subtypes (see the table that follows).

FACTOR	ER+ HER2– (LOW PROLIFERATION)	ER+ HER2– (HIGH PROLIFERATION)	HER2	BASAL-LIKE
Gene expression pattern	• High expression of normal luminal profile (LMWCK) and hormone receptors. • HER2 expression negative.	• Expression of normal luminal profile (LMWCK), with weak to moderate expression of hormone receptors.	• High expression of HER2 on chromosome 17. • Approximately 50% ER+ usually low positive when positive. • TP53 mutation common.	• High expression of basal epithelial profile (HMWCK). • Low expression of both hormone receptors and HER2. • TP53 mutation common.
Biologic features	• ~50%. • Slow growing.	• ~15%. • Higher grade.	• ~20%. • High grade, high proliferation index, high node positive.	• ~15%. • High proliferation index.
IMMUNOPROFILE				
ER/PR	• ER/PR: positive.	• ER positive may be low. • PR: low positive or negative.	• ER low positive 50%. • PR: negative.	• ER/PR: negative.
HER2	• HER2: negative. • Ki 67 < 14%.*	• HER2: negative. • Ki 67 > 14%.*	• HER2: positive.	• HER2: negative (triple negative).
CLINICAL FEATURES				
Response to therapy	• Good response to hormonal therapy.	• Response to hormonal therapy not as good, but better response to chemotherapy.	• Responds to anti-HER therapies and anthracycline-based chemotherapy.	• Responds to platinum based chemotherapy.
Prognosis	• Good.	• Not as good.	• Poor.	• Poor.

*Note: high and low proliferation rate cutoffs are laboratory specific based on the methodologies used.

81. What are the features of breast carcinoma associated with *BRCA1*?
- Poorly differentiated.
- Syncytial growth pattern (medullary pattern).
- Pushing margins.
- Prominent stromal lymphocytic response.
- ER/PR negative.
- HER2 negative.
- High proliferating index (Ki 67) and mitotic count.
- CK5/6+, EGFR+.

Note: ~15% of tumors associated with *BRCA1* are medullary-pattern carcinomas.

82. What are the pathologic features of secretory carcinoma?
- This is an invasive carcinoma with intracytoplasmic secretory vacuoles and extracellular eosinophilic secretions.
- It is frequently associated with *ETV6-NTRK3* fusion.
- Tumor cells typically express CEA (polyclonal), S100, mammaglobin, SOX10, MUC4.
- Tumor cells are typically negative for ER, PR and HER2 (may have weak ER and PR expression).

83. What are the morphologic features and prognosis of invasive micropapillary carcinoma?
- Morphologic features include clusters of invasive tumor cells surrounded by clear spaces; the tumor cell clusters have a reversed cell polarity (inside-out pattern).
- The tumor frequently has lymphatic-vascular invasion and nodal disease, therefore it is associated with a worse prognosis than IDC, NST.
- It is usually ER and PR positive (triple negative in 15–20% of cases).
- It is often HER2 IHC 2+ with a basal-lateral staining pattern requiring reflex *HER2* ISH; it is variably *HER2* ISH positive.

84. List the WHO classification of metaplastic breast carcinoma.
- Low grade adenosquamous carcinoma.
- Fibromatosis-like metaplastic carcinoma.
- Spindle cell carcinoma.
- Squamous cell carcinoma.
- Metaplastic carcinoma with heterologous mesenchymal differentiation.
- Mixed metaplastic carcinoma.

85. What are the typical features of male breast cancer?

- Male breast cancer is rare; it is histologically similar to postmenopausal female breast carcinoma.
- It is associated with hormonal imbalance leading to excess estrogen (e.g., hepatic cirrhosis, Klinefelter syndrome).
- Mutations of *BRCA2* are more frequent than *BRCA1* in male breast cancer.

- It is usually invasive ductal carcinoma, NST; and ER and PR positive.
- Specimen handling and reporting are identical to female breast cancer.

Lobular Neoplasia

86. What are the differentiating features of atypical lobular hyperplasia (ALH) and lobular carcinoma in situ (LCIS)?

- See table below.
- The common feature is the proliferation of generally uniform discohesive cells with poorly defined cell borders, within the acini. The degree of distension and distortion of the acini, and the number of acini within a lobular unit and total number of lobules involved, differentiate ALH and LCIS.

	ALH	LCIS
Acini	• Not distended or distorted.	• Distended and distorted.
Lumen	• Present.	• Absent.
Pagetoid spread	• Usually absent.	• Along terminal ducts.
Lobular involvement	• Partial involvement of the acini within a TDLU.	• More than half of the acini within a TDLU. • > 1 TDLU involved. • Enlarged acini possibly showing confluence, with little intervening stroma (macroacini).
Cellular composition	• Variable cell types.	• Monomorphous cells.

Abbreviation: TDLU: terminal ductal lobular unit.

87. What are the histologic types/patterns of LCIS?

- Classic.
- Pleomorphic.

- Florid (may form a mass).

88. What are the clinical implications of classic LCIS?

- Some (20–30%) patients develop invasive carcinoma, after long-term follow-up of 30 years.
- This increased risk applies to both breasts (slightly greater on the ipsilateral side of the biopsy).
- The invasive carcinoma can be either ductal or lobular type.
- The relative risk increases from 4.9 after 1 biopsy to 16.1 after a second biopsy shows LCIS.

- From WHO:
  - If classic LCIS on core:
    - › Close, long-term follow-up.
    - › Excision when pathologic-radiology discordance.
  - If pleomorphic LCIS or florid LCIS is present:
    - › Excision.

89. What is the clinical management of LCIS?

- Classic LCIS at margins is not reported nor an indication for reexcision (WHO). The patient requires lifelong follow-up (breast screening), with or without tamoxifen.
- It is important to report pleomorphic LCIS and florid LCIS at the margins because clinicians may choose to reexcise the lesion.

- Reexcision can be considered in cases of strong family history, patient apprehension, and where prolonged follow-up cannot be ensured.
- Excision is recommended if LCIS does not account for mammographic abnormality or if something else was found that is usually excised (e.g., ADH).

90. What are 2 architectural and 3 cytological features of classic invasive lobular carcinoma (ILC)?

- Architectural features:
  - Single file pattern.
  - Targetoid pattern — neoplastic cells invade the stroma of residual ducts in concentric fashion.

- Cytologic features:
  - Small uniform cells with bland nuclei.
  - Lack of cohesiveness.
  - Presence of intracellular mucin droplets.

91. What are the histologic (architectural) variants of ILC?

- Classic.
- Alveolar.
- Tubulolobular.
- Mixed.
- Solid.

92. What are the cytologic variants of ILC?

- Pleomorphic.
- Signet ring.
- Histiocytoid.
- Apocrine.
- Mixed.

93. Name 2 associated genetic abnormalities of ILC.

- Loss of heterozygosity (LOH) on 16q — site of E-cadherin and β-catenin genes.
- LOH at 11q13.

94. What pattern of ER/PR/HER2 results do you expect in classic ILC?

- ER/PR: positive.
- HER2: negative.

95. Name the immunohistochemical (IHC) markers used to differentiate LCIS from low grade DCIS. What is the expected pattern of staining?

- E-cadherin: membranous staining in DCIS, absent/aberrant in LCIS (except at the periphery of the acini where the residual lining cells can be positive).
- HMWCK (34βE12): positive in LCIS (perinuclear pattern), negative in DCIS.
- p120 catenin: membranous staining in DCIS, diffuse cytoplasmic in LCIS.
- β-catenin: membranous staining in DCIS, diffuse cytoplasmic in LCIS.

Papillary Lesions

96. Classify papillary lesions of the breast.

- Papilloma (solitary central duct and multiple peripheral duct papillomas).
- Papilloma with ADH or DCIS.
- Papillary DCIS.
- Encapsulated papillary carcinoma.
- Solid papillary carcinoma (in situ and invasive).
- Invasive papillary carcinoma.

97. What are the features of an atypical papilloma (papilloma with ADH), and how do you differentiate between a papilloma with ADH, and DCIS arising in a papilloma?

- A papilloma with ADH is defined by:
  - Papilloma with focal proliferation of mildly atypical epithelial cells, often with loss of myoepithelial cells in these areas.
  - – and –
  - Areas of solid, cribriform, or micropapillary proliferation of uniform, monomorphous atypical cells, < 3 mm in extent.
- DCIS arising in a papilloma is defined by:
  - Involvement of areas of solid, cribriform, or micropapillary proliferation of uniform, monomorphous atypical cells, ≥ 3 mm in size.
  - Use of CK5/6 and ER can be helpful in the evaluation of the atypical epithelial proliferations.

Note: in DCIS, there is preservation of myoepithelial cells in the peripheral duct lining.

98. List 4 features that can differentiate an intraductal papilloma from an encapsulated papillary carcinoma.

FEATURE	BENIGN PAPILLOMA	ENCAPSULATED PAPILLARY CARCINOMA
Fibrovascular cores	• Well developed, arborizing.	• Delicate.
Lining cells (of the fibrovascular cores)	• 2 cell types. • Often areas of apocrine change.	• 1 cell type. • Atypical epithelial cells, often with hyperchromatic and elongated nuclei.
Peripheral duct lining	• Presence of myoepithelial cells.	• Absence of myoepithelial cells.
Clinical features	• Nipple discharge. • Mammographic mass, may be palpable.	• Usually presents as a mass.

99. What is the current recommended management for a papillary lesion diagnosed on core needle biopsy?

If there is radiologic concordance and the lesion appears benign on core needle biopsy, some surgeons will recommend clinical follow-up. In some centers, conservative local excision may be recommended for benign intraductal papillomas.

100. What are the pathologic features of solid papillary carcinoma?

- This is an in situ and/or invasive carcinoma with a solid growth pattern with delicate fibrovascular cores.
- It frequently shows neuroendocrine differentiation.
- It expresss ER and PR, and is negative for HER2.
- Unless there is associated conventional invasion (infiltrative tumor with jagged contours, stromal desmoplasia or fat infiltration), these tumors are typically indolent and staged as pTis, regardless of whether a myoepithelial layer is identified.

Paget Disease

101. What is the differential diagnosis of mammary Paget disease?

- Bowen disease.
- Malignant melanoma in situ.
- Toker cell hyperplasia.

102. How would you differentiate Paget disease from the differentials listed in question 101?

IHC	PAGET DISEASE	BOWEN DISEASE	MELANOMA IN SITU	TOKER CELL HYPERPLASIA
Mucin	+/−	−	−	−
CK7	+	−	−	+
Cam5.2	+	−	−	+/−
EMA	+	−	−	−
HMWCK	−	+	−	−
HMB45	−	−	+	−
HER2	+	−	−	−

103. Describe the staging of Paget disease.

- Paget disease of the nipple that is not associated with underlying parenchymal in situ or invasive carcinoma is staged as pTis (Paget).
- Paget disease associated with carcinoma in the breast parenchyma is staged according to the size and characteristics of the invasive disease.

104. What prognosis is associated with Paget disease? What is the treatment?

- Prognosis: this is determined by the prognostic variables of the associated carcinoma.
- Treatment: local excision of nipple and subareolar tissue is an option.

Mesenchymal Lesions

105. Classify mesenchymal tumors of the breast.

- Stromal tumors of the breast can be classified as:
  · Biphasic tumors:
    › Fibroadenoma.
    › Phyllodes tumor.
- Pure mesenchymal tumors according to tissue of origin, and whether primary or secondary (metastatic to the breast) — see table that follows.

BENIGN	MALIGNANT
• Fibroblastic and myofibroblastic tumors: · Myofibroblastoma. · Pseudoangiomatous stromal hyperplasia (PASH). · Nodular fasciitis. · Fibromatosis.	• Inflammatory myofibroblastic tumor (low malignant potential).
• Adipocytic tumors: · Lipoma. · Angiolipoma.	• Liposarcoma.
• Smooth muscle tumors: · Leiomyoma.	• Leiomyosarcoma.
• Neural origin: · Granular cell tumor. · Neurofibroma. · Schwannoma.	
• Vascular lesions: · Hemangiomas. · Angiomatosis. · Atypical vascular lesion.	• Angiosarcomas: primary, postradiation, post–radical mastectomy.

106. Describe the gross and histologic characteristics of a phyllodes tumor.

GROSS CHARACTERISTICS	HISTOLOGIC CHARACTERISTICS
• Well-circumscribed and firm. • Cut surface: gray-white, solid with cystic areas, with fleshy leaflike processes that protrude into the cystic spaces.	• 2 key features: · Stromal hypercellularity (pronounced in the periductal areas). · Expansile stroma and benign glandular/epithelial elements. • Leafy architecture (often seen but not required for diagnosis).

107. List 7 histologic features that help differentiate benign and malignant phyllodes tumors.

- Increased stromal mitotic activity — 5/10 high power fields (HPFs) indicates borderline malignancy; in the absence of any worrisome features listed below, 10/10 HPFs is significant.
- Marked stromal hypercellularity.
- Marked atypia of the stromal cells.
- Stromal overgrowth —epithelial elements are absent in at least 1 low power (x4) field.
- An infiltrating margin (versus a pushing margin).
- Tumor necrosis.
- Presence of malignant heterologous elements even in the absence of other criteria.

108. How would you differentiate a phyllodes tumor from a fibroadenoma?

- The most helpful features supporting the diagnosis of phyllodes tumor include:
  · An expansile, hypercellular and mitotically active spindled stroma.
  · Leaflike architecture — note that this alone in the absence of a hypercellular stroma does not qualify the lesion as a phyllodes tumor.

109. What is the recommended treatment for phyllodes tumor?

- The recommended treatment for malignant phyllodes tumor is local excision with a wide margin (at least 1 cm) of normal tissue (presence of tumor at the resection margin is a major determinant of local recurrence).
- If benign phyllodes tumor is excised without a wide margin, clinical follow-up with prompt excision of any recurrence is an option.
- Borderline phyllodes tumor ideally should be excised with a wide margin.

110. How would you word your diagnosis in a core needle biopsy where you cannot differentiate a cellular fibroadenoma from a benign phyllodes tumor?

- Wording: Fibroepithelial lesion with cellular stroma.
  - As the stromal cellularity can be variable within a tumor and the margins cannot be assessed, the differential between a fibroadenoma and a benign phyllodes tumor should be deferred to the resection specimen. (Note: a malignant phyllodes tumor can be diagnosed on core needle biopsy.)

  – or –

- Wording: Fibroepithelial lesion with increased stromal cellularity. Recommend excision for further evaluation of the lesion.

111. How do you differentiate malignant phyllodes tumor from sarcomatoid (metaplastic) carcinoma?

- Sample the lesion well to look for epithelial lined clefts.
- With IHC testing, stromal cells of phyllodes tumor are typially negative for epithelial markers such as AE1/AE3, CAM 5.2, CK5/6, and p63, and positive for CD34 and BCL-2.
- A broad panel of epithelial markers should be employed to exclude metaplastic carcinoma in the workup of a spindle cell breast neoplasm, including high molecular weight keratins and p63.

Note: malignant phyllodes tumor can show focal expression of keratins and p63; this can lead to misdiagnosis in core biopsies.

112. What other mesenchymal elements or metaplasias can be found in phyllodes tumor?

Others include adipose, osseous, chondroid, smooth muscle, and rhabdomyoblastic elements. Any of these can show a malignant component. (Presence of malignant stromal elements other than fibromyxoid and well-differentiated liposarcoma indicate a worse prognosis.)

Lymphomas

113. Classify lymphomas of the breast.

- Primary breast lymphoma (PBL).
- Disseminated lymphoma with breast involvement.
- Recurrent lymphoma.
- Breast implant associated anaplastic large cell lymphoma (BIA-ALCL).

114. What are the clinical features of lymphomas?

- Lymphomas comprise 0.13% of all breast malignancies.
- Unilateral PBLs affect elderly women.
- Some (20%) of PBLs are bilateral.
- Bilaterality is synchronous in 13%; tends to occur in young women with onset during puberty, pregnancy, or lactation (many are Burkitt lymphomas).

115. What are the most common types of lymphomas seen in the breast?

- Most are non-Hodgkin lymphomas of B cell lineage.
  - Most common: diffuse large B cell.
  - Burkitt lymphoma in bilateral cases.
  - Uncommon, but may be detected by screening mammography: extranodal marginal zone lymphoma; mucosa-associated lymphoid tissue (MALT) lymphoma; follicular and mantle cell lymphoma.

116. What are the clinical and pathologic features of BIA-ALCL?

- BIA-ALCL is a rare, recently recognized form of anaplastic large cell lymphoma (ALCL) that is CD30 positive and ALK-negative, and associated with breast implants.
- BIA-ALCL usually develops 7–10 years after placement of a textured surface implant, possibly related to chronic inflammation and/or bacterial infection.
- Most patients present with a late (> 1 year after implantation), spontaneous, unilateral, capsule-confined seroma; they may have pain, capsular contraction, and/or skin rash; symptomatic clinical findings may be misdiagnosed as implant rupture.

117. How should specimens from patients with clinical concern for BIA-ALCL be handled?

- Seroma fluid specimens should be taken for: 1) cytopathology, ideally with cell block preparation (postfixed in formalin) for potential IHC studies; 2) flow cytometry; and 3) culture and sensitivity (if sufficient fluid).
  - Look for medium to large atypical pleomorphic lymphocytes often with multinucleation, prominent nucleoli, and cytoplasmic vacuoles; atypical nuclei are 1.5–5 times larger than mature lymphocytes.
  - IHC is positive for CD30 and MUM-1, and negative for ALK; CD3 and CD2 are variable, CD43 and CD4 are usually expressed.
- Capsulectomy specimens must be sampled thoroughly and mapped, with the sections blocked on edge to determine the extent of capsular invasion (T stage).
- Lymph nodes and capsular masses should be submitted fresh for lymphoma protocol.

Breast Biomarkers

118. Which breast tumors should be tested for hormone receptors and HER2?
- All primary invasive breast carcinomas.
- All recurrent breast carcinomas.
- All metastatic breast carcinomas.

119. Which markers are currently optional?
- Ki 67.
- Multigene expression assays.
- Programmed death ligand 1 (PD-L1).

120. What percentage of breast carcinomas should be ER positive?
Approximately 80%.

121. What percentage of breast carcinomas should be HER2 positive?
Approximately 10–20%.

122. List 2 clinical uses of HER2 testing.
- Prognostic marker — HER2 overexpression is associated with a worse prognosis.
- Predictive marker — predicts sensitivity to anti-HER2 therapy, such as trastuzumab and anthracycline-based chemotherapy.

123. What 2 methods are commonly used for HER2 testing and how do you interpret the results?
- Methods:
  · IHC to detect protein overexpression.
  · In situ hybridization to detect gene amplification: FISH, CISH, or silver in situ hybridization (SISH).
- Interpretation:
  · Interpret data from both methods according to ASCO/CAP guidelines (see tables that follow).

IHC

INTERPRETATION	FINDING
Positive: 3+	Complete, intense circumferential membrane staining in > 10% of invasive tumor cells.
Equivocal: 2+	Incomplete and/or weak to moderate circumferential membrane staining in > 10 of invasive tumor cells; or complete, intense, circumferential membrane staining in ≤ 10% of invasive tumor cells. • Order reflex in situ hybridization on same specimen-, or a new test on a new specimen, if available, (IHC or in situ hybridization).
Negative: 1+	Incomplete, faint/barely perceptible membrane staining in > 10% invasive tumor cells.
Negative: 0	No staining, or incomplete, faint/barely perceptible membrane staining in ≤ 10% invasive tumor cells.

IN SITU HYBRIDIZATION: DUAL PROBE ASSAY

INTERPRETATION	CRITERIA
Group 1 Positive (amplified)	HER2/CEP17 ratio ≥ 2.0. – **and** – Average HER2 copy number ≥ 4.0 signals/cell.
Group 2 Nonamplified, *additional workup required	HER2/CEP17 ratio ≥ 2.0. – **and** – Average HER2 copy number < 4.0 signals/cell.
Group 3 Amplified, *additional workup required	HER2/CEP17 ratio < 2.0. – **and** – An average HER2 copy number ≥ 6.0 signals/cell.
Group 4 Nonamplified, *additional workup required	HER2/CEP17 ratio < 2.0. – **and** – An average HER2 copy number ≥ 4.0 and < 6.0 signals/cell.
Group 5 Negative, nonamplified	HER2/CEP17 ratio < 2.0. – **and** – An average HER2 copy number < 4.0 signals/cell.

*Additional workup: if IHC is 3+, the tumor is considered HER2 positive. If the tumor is not HER2 IHC 3+, additional ISH workup includes a seconded blinded observer to rescore the case and/or a new ISH test on a new specimen or block if consensus is not reached.

124. What preanalytic variables need to be recorded and reported as per ASCO and CAP guidelines?

- Cold ischemia time.
- Duration of fixation.
- Type of fixative.
- Treatment of tissue that can potentially alter immunoreactivity (i.e., decalcification).
- Status of internal and external controls.
- Adequacy of sample for evaluation.
- Primary antibody clone used.
- Regulatory status.

125. How do you report ER and PR status?

- If positive:
  - Percentage of cells with nuclear positivity (either specific or with a range).
- Average intensity of staining.
- If negative:
  - Status of internal control (staining or not).

126. What is the cutoff for positivity of ER and PR?

1%.

Note: if there is nuclear staining of ER in 1–10% of invasive tumor cells, this should be reported as "low positive." These cases are a challenge for test reproducibility. A low positive ER assessment should result in steps to adjudicate the result, such as blinded review by a seconded pathologist and repeat testing of another block or specimen.

127. What is the Allred score?

The Allred score is a method of quantifying ER and PR positivity. It combines the percentage of positive cells and the intensity of staining. The 2 types of scores are added for a final score of 8 possible values. Scores 0, 1, and 2 are considered negative. Scores 3 to 8 are considered positive.

PERCENTAGE OF POSITIVE CELLS	PROPORTION SCORE
0	0
< 1	1
1–10	2
11–33	3
34–66	4
> 67	5

INTENSITY OF STAINING	INTENSITY SCORE
None	0
Weak	1
Intermediate	2
Strong	3

128. What is the H-score?

The H-score is a method of quantifying ER and PR positivity. It is determined by multiplying the percentage of positive cells by each intensity. Theoretically, there are 300 possible values. In this system, < 1% positive cells is considered a negative result.

CELL SIGNAL	PERCENTAGE OF CELLS	CALCULATION
No signal = 0	A%	$A \times 0 = 0$
Weak signal = 1	B%	$B \times 1 = B$
Moderate signal = 2	C%	$C \times 2 = 2C$
Strong signal = 3	D%	$D \times 3 = 3D$
Total score		$B + 2C + 3D$

129. A breast IHC quality assurance program determines that the ER stain in your lab is insensitive. List at least 6 factors that can affect the results of ER and PR testing.

- Exposure of tumor cells to heat (e.g., carcinomas transected by using cautery during surgery).
- Delay in fixation (i.e., prolonged cold ischemic time), which may result in antigenic degradation. Specimens should be placed in 10% neutral buffered formalin within 1 hour of removal from the patient. Large breast excisions should be oriented, inked, incised and placed in fresh formalin within 1 hour of excision.

(continued on next page)

- Under- or overfixation. Fixation for at least 6 hours in buffered formalin is recommended, and prolonged fixation may also diminish immunoreactivity. Fixation of 12–72 hours is best.
- Type of fixative: ER is degraded in acidic fixatives such as Bouin's solution and B-5 (these should be avoided); formalin should be buffered to ensure a pH range between 7.0 and 7.4.
- Quality, freshness, and concentration of antibody — 3 clones commonly used: 6F11, SP1, and EP1. The platform should be considered when choosing a clone.

- Nonoptimized method of antigen retrieval.
- Decalcification, which may result in loss of immunoreactivity.
- Method of antigen retrieval.
- Dark hematoxylin counterstain obscuring faintly positive diaminobenzidine (DAB) staining.

130. List reasons for a false positive ER or PR, or HER2 result.
- Use of an impure antibody that cross-reacts with another antigen.
- Edge artifact: usually seen in core biopsies, where cells near the edges of the tissue stain stronger than those in the center, possibly because antibody pools at the sides. Specimens with stronger staining at the edge of the tissue should be interpreted with caution.
- Misinterpretation of entrapped normal cells or of an in situ component as invasive carcinoma. High grade DCIS is often HER2 positive. In cases with extensive DCIS relative to invasive carcinoma (particularly microinvasive carcinoma),

HER2 scoring may mistakenly be done on the DCIS component. Care must be taken to score only the invasive component.
- Analysis by an image analysis device that mistakenly counts overstained nuclei.
- Cytoplasmic positivity, which can obscure nuclear or membrane staining and make interpretation difficult.
- Overstaining (strong membrane staining of normal cells), which may be due to improper antibody titration (concentration too high).

131. Name factors that can affect the ability to obtain results for HER2 testing by FISH.
- Prolonged fixation in formalin (> 1 week).
- Fixation in nonformalin fixatives.
- Procedures or fixation involving acid that may degrade DNA (decalcification).
- Insufficient protease treatment of tissue.

132. What are 2 important issues that need to be addressed by a pathologist on the H&E or HER2 IHC slide prior to FISH testing?
- Identification of the invasive carcinoma and of the area to be scored.
- Identification of DCIS. In some cases, DCIS will show gene amplification whereas the associated invasive cancer will not. The FISH analysis must be performed on the invasive component only.

133. Why is the routine use of Ki 67 for breast carcinoma not currently recommended?
- Lack of consensus on scoring.
- Lack of consensus on definition of low versus high expression.
- Lack of an appropriate cut point for positivity.
- Lack of consensus on which part of the tumor should be tested (leading edge, hot spot, average).
- Paucity of data on effect of preanalytic variables (ischemic time, length of fixation, antigen retrieval).

IMAGES: BREAST PATHOLOGY

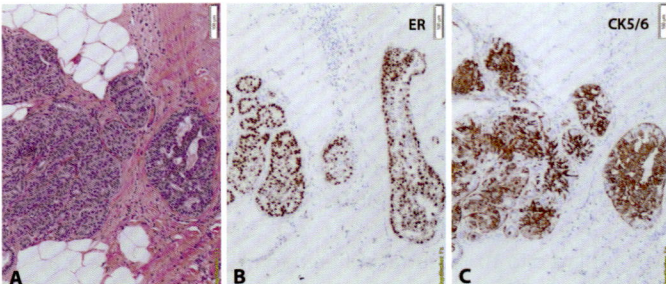

IMAGE 3.1 Usual ductal hyperplasia (UDH). Image A (H&E): this lesion consists of a cohesive proliferation of epithelial cells with haphazard streaming orientation. Image B: ER IHC has a mosaic pattern in UDH, and strong and diffuse positivity in ADH and low grade DCIS. Image C: UDH cells typically retain CK5/6 positivity; the feature is useful to distinguish from ADH.

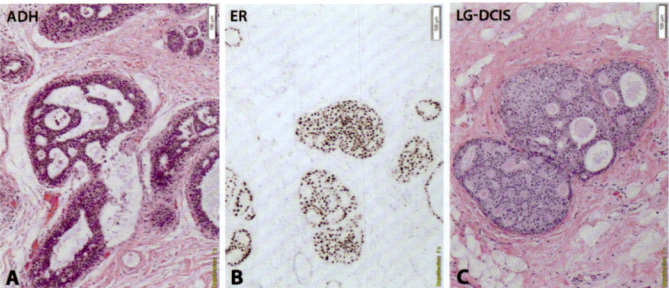

IMAGE 3.2 ADH (image A) versus low grade DCIS (image C), cribriform pattern. ADH shows similar cytologic and architectural features to low grade DCIS, but with a lesser extent of ductal involvement. ER (image B) is diffusely positive in both.

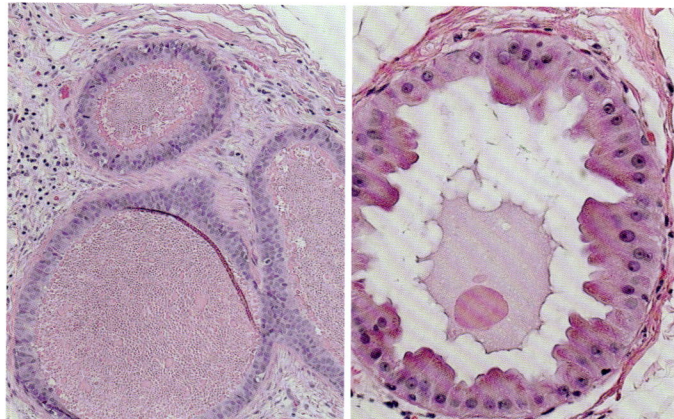

IMAGE 3.3 Flat epithelial atypia versus apocrine epithelium. Left: the image shows flat epithelial atypia (FEA) (H&E, x40). The glands within the columnar cell lesion are distended with luminal secretions. The cells may pile up and lose their regular orientation. The cells are round and monomorphic with eosinophilic cytoplasm and prominent apical tufts. Right: the image shows apocrine epithelium. Unlike FEA, the cells are basally oriented with abundant vesicular cytoplasm (H&E, x200).

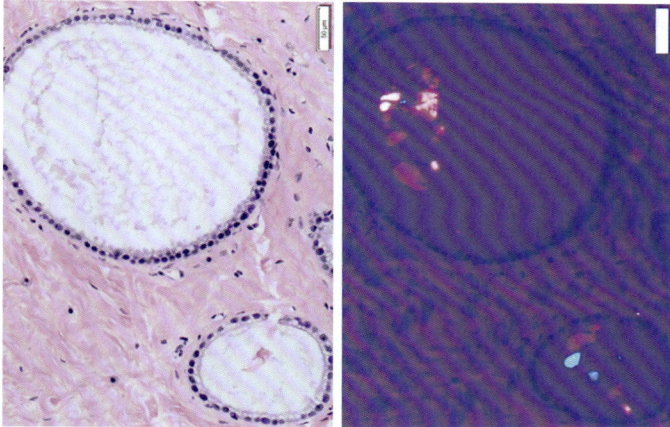

IMAGE 3.4 Calcium oxalate crystals. This is a form of calcification in breast tissue that is associated with benign breast lesions, often apocrine cysts. It is visible with polarized light.

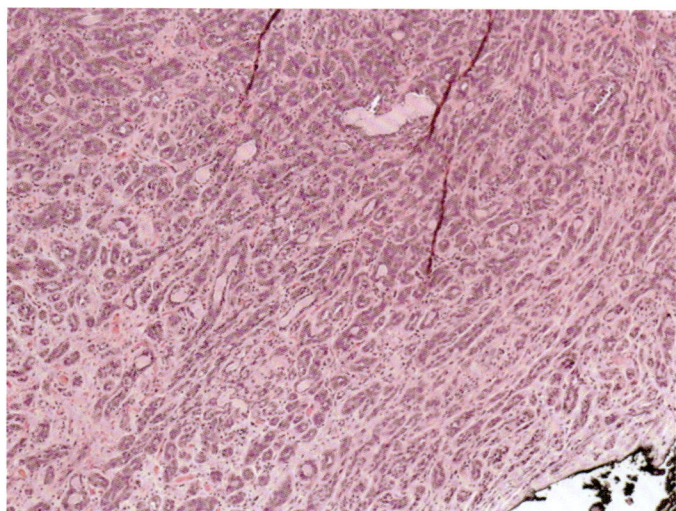

IMAGE 3.5 Sclerosing adenosis. This lesion consists of enlarged lobular units with tubular structures that are compressed by stromal collagen. The presence of myoepithelial cells can help distinguish this lesion from invasive carcinoma (H&E, x40).

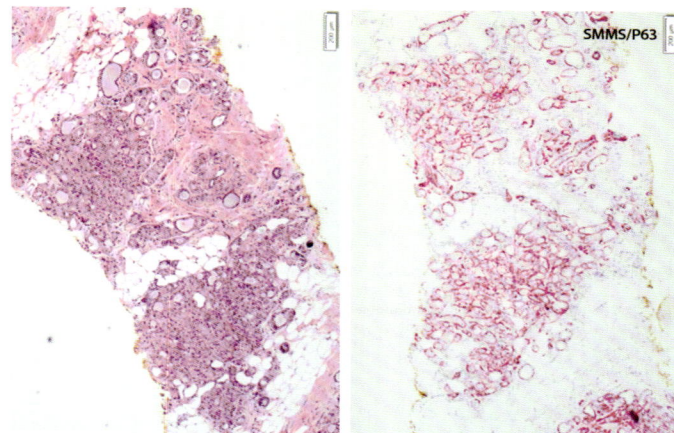

IMAGE 3.6 Apocrine adenosis. This consists of a proliferation of crowded glands with cells that have abundant eosinophilic cytoplasm, round nuclei, and central nucleoli. Myoepithelial cells are retained around the glands.

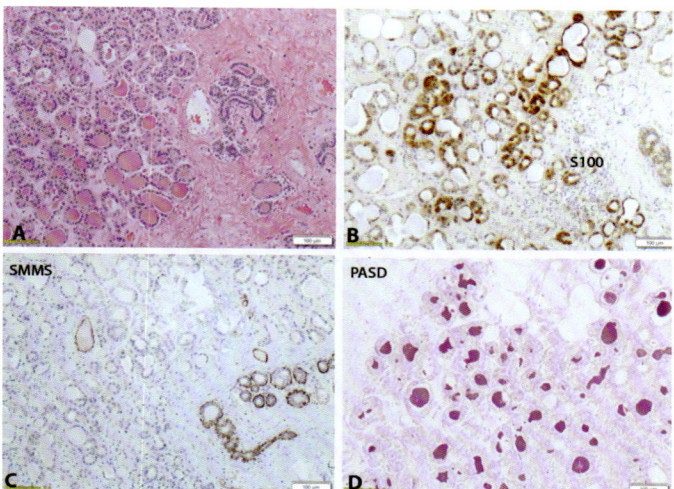

IMAGE 3.7 Microglandular adenosis (MGA). Image A (H&E): this benign lesion mimics an invasive ductal carcinoma by the absence of myoepithelial cells (image C). It consists of small round uniform glands with eosinophilic secretions haphazardly infiltrating into stroma or fat. These lesions are S100 positive (image B), and ER and PR negative. The secretions are PAS-D positive (image D).

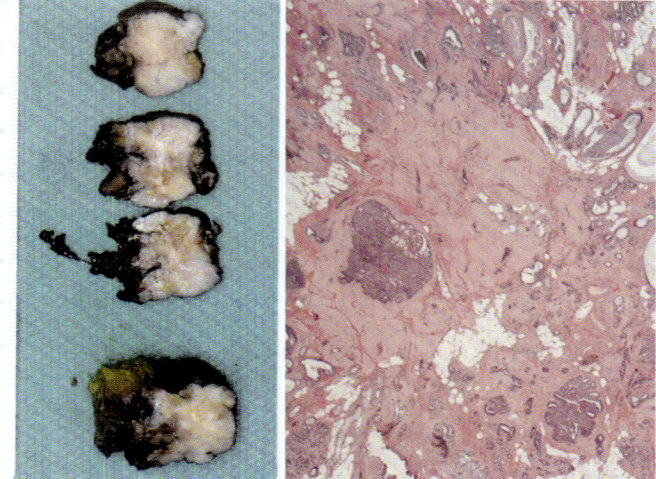

IMAGE 3.8 Complex sclerosing lesion. Left: gross examination shows a dense fibrous irregular mass with poorly defined borders. Right: histologically, the lesion is composed of central dense fibrous scar surrounded by irregularly compressed or dilated ducts with variable degrees of usual epithelial hyperplasia (H&E, x40).

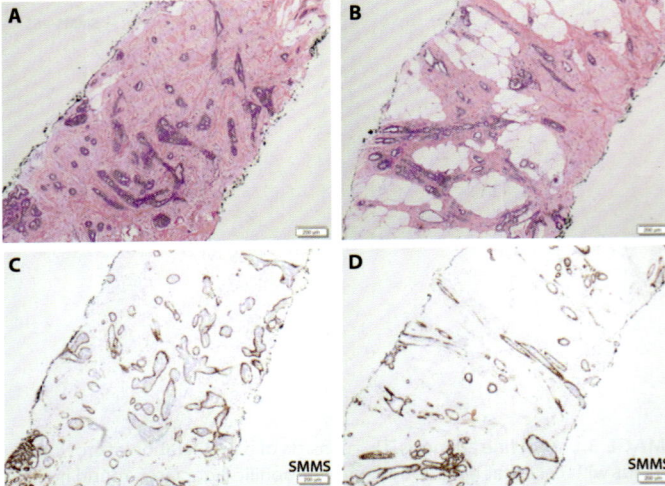

IMAGE 3.9 Complex sclerosing lesion with UDH. Histology shows ducts with UDH between bands of fibroelastotic stroma. Myoepithelial layers are retained. By definition, a complex sclerosing lesion is > 1 cm. If < 1 cm, it is termed a radial scar. Images A and B: H&E, x100. Images C and D: smooth muscle myosin heavy chain (SMMS) stain, x100.

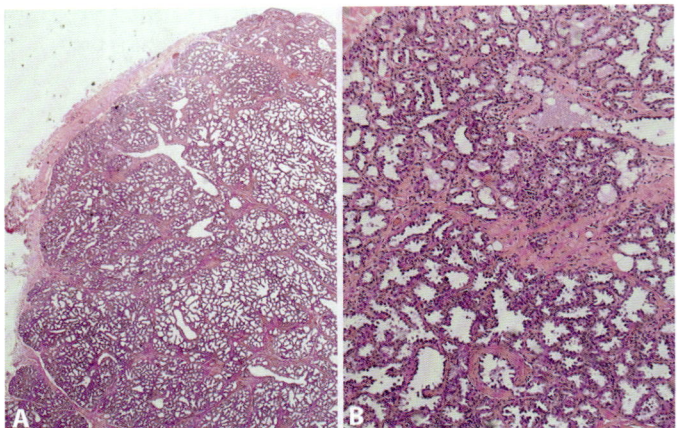

IMAGE 3.10 Lactating adenoma. There is physiologic hyperplasia of ducts and lobules. The glands are dilated with secretions. The luminal cells have lactational changes: hobnail morphology, prominent nucleoli, normal nuclear-cytoplasmic ratios, and vacuolated cytoplasm. Left: H&E, x40. Right: H&E, x100.

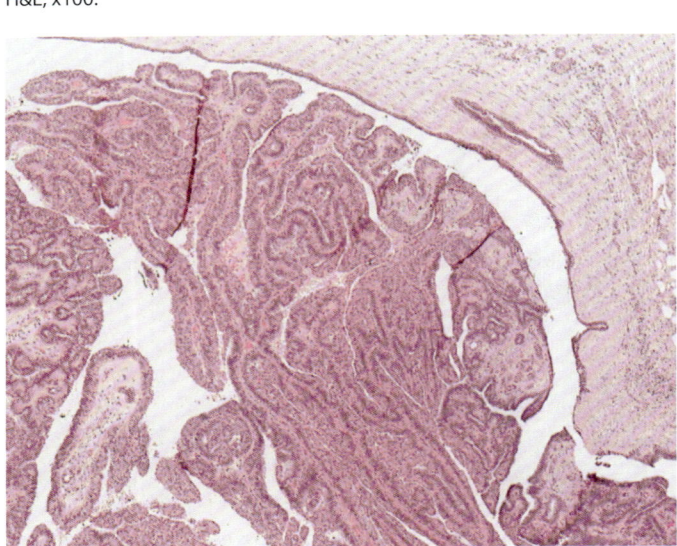

IMAGE 3.11 Intraductal papilloma without atypia. This lesion consists of an intraductal arborescent structure with fibrovascular cores lined by a myoepithelial and an epithelial layer. The periphery of the duct space is lined by a myoepithelial layer (H&E, x100).

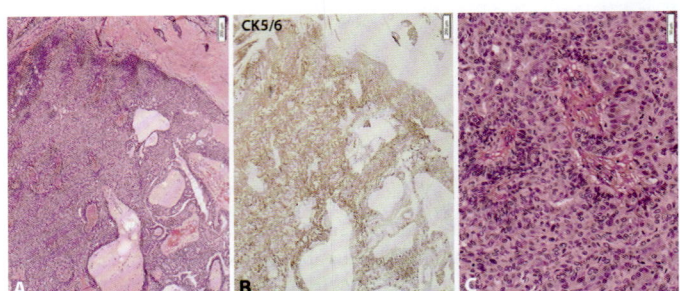

IMAGE 3.12 Intraductal papilloma with extensive UDH. Images A and C: fibrovascular cores are present with a florid epithelial proliferation. Image B: CK5/6 IHC has a mosaic pattern, supporting involvement by UDH.

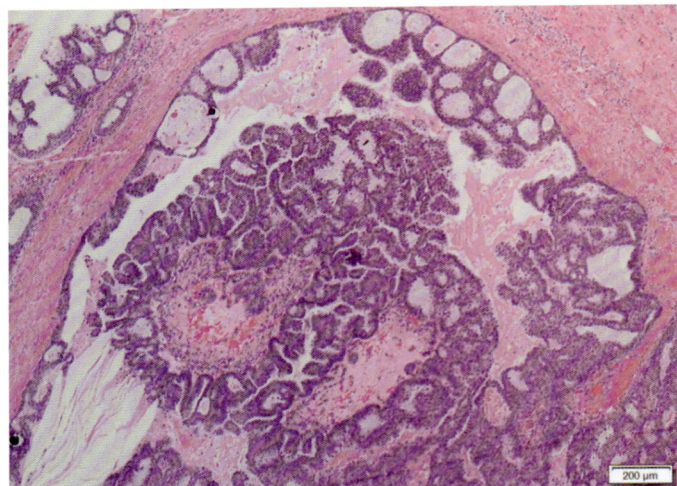

IMAGE 3.13 Papillary DCIS. Histology shows a papillary lesion with fibrovascular cores and a proliferation of monomorphous atypical epithelial cells forming rounded secondary spaces. Myoepithelial cells are present at the periphery of the expanded duct, but they do not line the papillary fronds (H&E, x100).

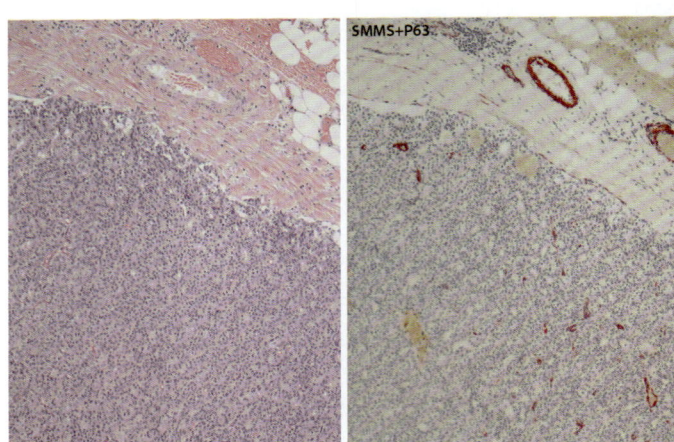

IMAGE 3.14 Encapsulated papillary carcinoma. This excision specimen shows an encapsulated atypical papillary proliferation that lacks myoepithelial cells within and at the periphery of the lesion. Left: H&E, x100. Right: SMMS with p63, x100.

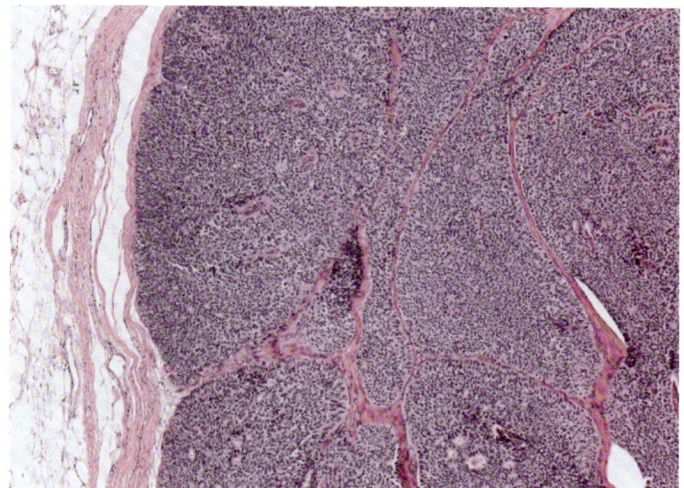

IMAGE 3.15 Solid papillary carcinoma. This tumor consists of expansile nodules with a solid growth of atypical epithelial cells with delicate inconspicuous fibrovascular cores. The lesion lacks myoepithelial cells lining the fibrovascular cores; presence of a myoepithelial layer at the periphery is variable. The tumor often shows neuroendocrine differentiation. ER IHC is strongly positive (H&E, x100).

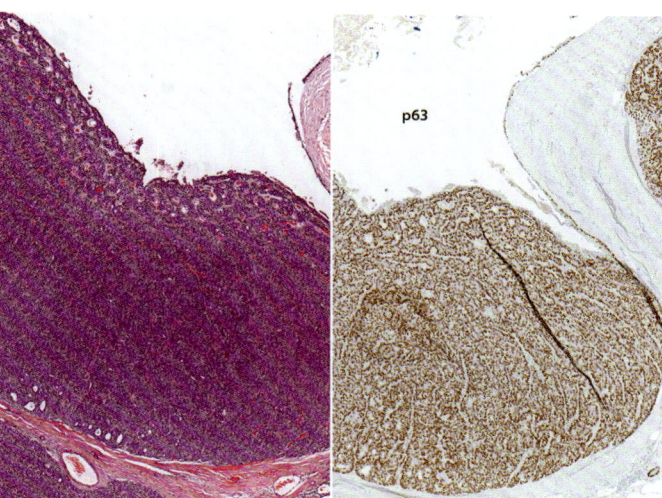

IMAGE 3.17 Adenomyoepithelioma. This is a well-delineated lesion composed of a proliferation of epithelial and myoepithelial cells. P63 highlights proliferative myoepithelial cells around the tubules. Left: H&E. Right: p63 IHC.

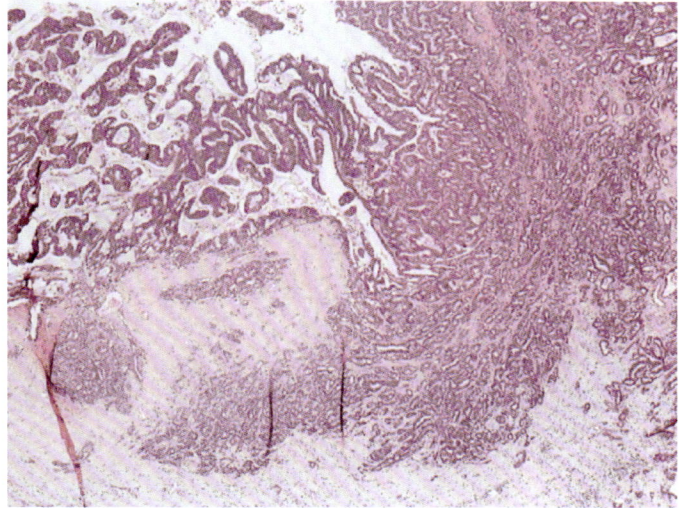

IMAGE 3.16 Invasive papillary carcinoma. There is invasive growth with papillary architecture. Myoepithelial cells are absent at the periphery of the lesion and along the papillary fronds. This lesion is rare and should be differentiated from metastases from other sites (H&E, x40).

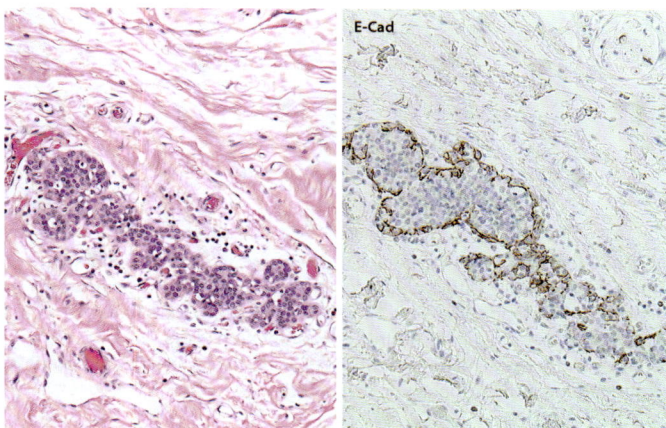

IMAGE 3.18 Atypical lobular hyperplasia (ALH). ALH is a lobulocentric proliferation of discohesive monomorphous epithelial cells with occasional cytoplasmic vacuoles. ALH expands < 50% of a terminal ductal lobular unit. E-cadherin IHC expression is aberrant. Left: H&E, x100. Right: E-cadherin, x100.

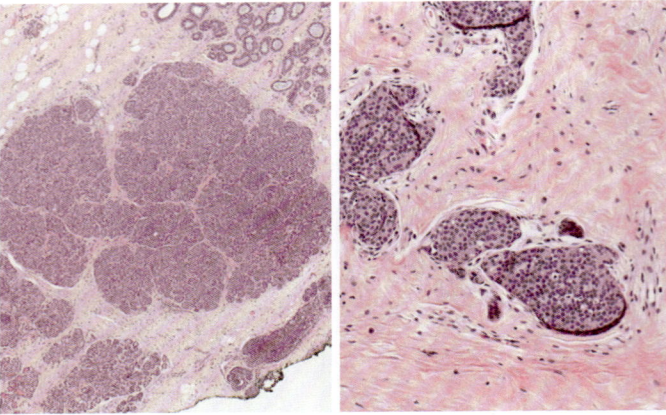

IMAGE 3.19 Lobular carcinoma in situ (LCIS). The terminal ductal lobular units are expanded by a discohesive proliferation of small uniform cells with round nuclei with homogenous chromatin. More than 50% of a terminal ductal lobular unit should be distorted and expanded to qualify as LCIS. Left: H&E, x40. Right: H&E, x100.

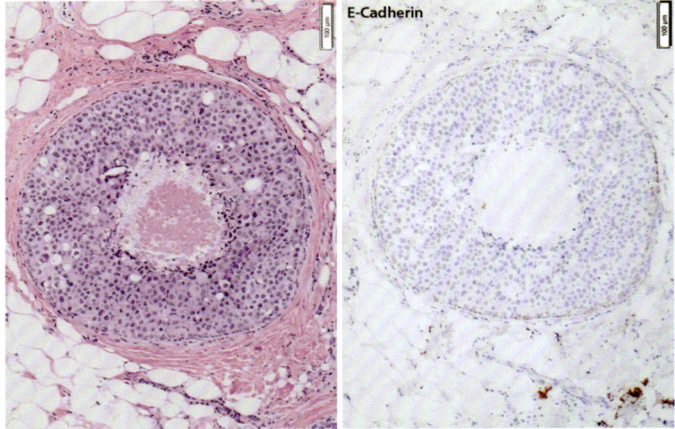

IMAGE 3.20 Pleomorphic lobular carcinoma in situ (PLCIS). Histology shows in situ disease with high grade nuclear atypia and central necrosis mimicking high grade DCIS (left: H&E). However, tumor cells have aberrant expression of E-cadherin IHC (right), consistent with PLCIS. The biologic behavior and surgical management of PLCIS are similar to DCIS, although data regarding biologic behavior are limited.

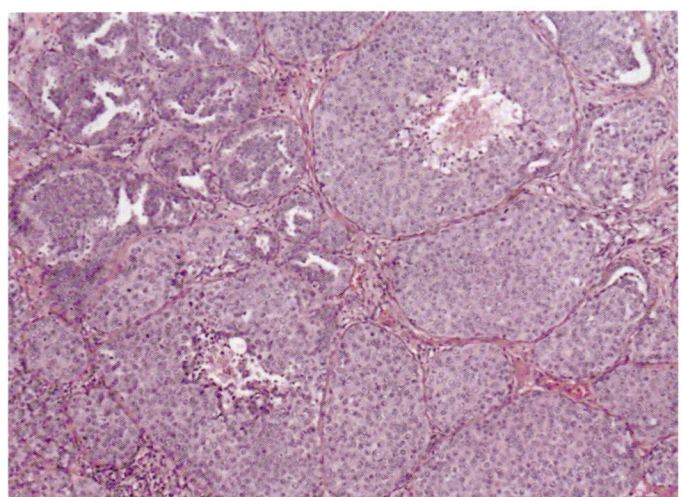

IMAGE 3.21 Florid LCIS. This variant of LCIS is defined by its architectural features, which are classic LCIS cells with marked distention of terminal ductal lobular units (TDLUs) or ducts, creating a confluent mass-like architecture, or with comedo necrosis and calcifications (H&E, x 200).

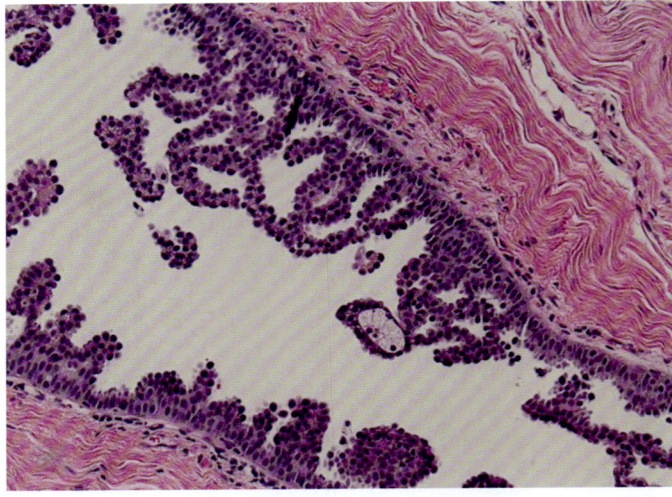

IMAGE 3.22 Micropapillary ductal carcinoma in situ (DCIS), low nuclear grade. The lesion consists of thin strands of monomorphic cells without fibrovascular cores (H&E, x200).

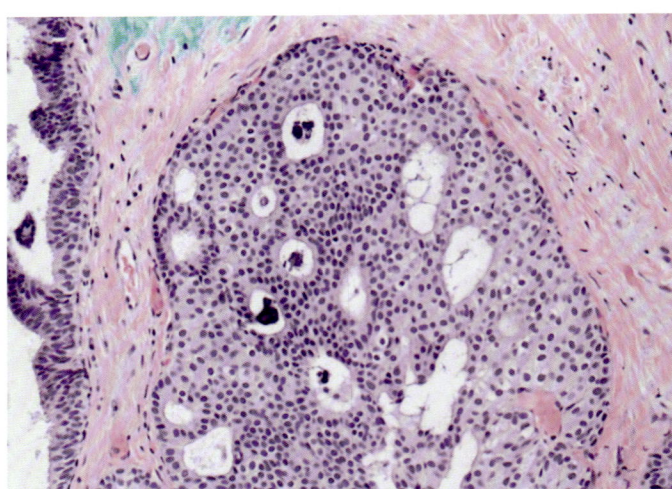

IMAGE 3.23 Ductal carcinoma in situ (DCIS). This lesion shows low nuclear grade and cribriform pattern (H&E, x200).

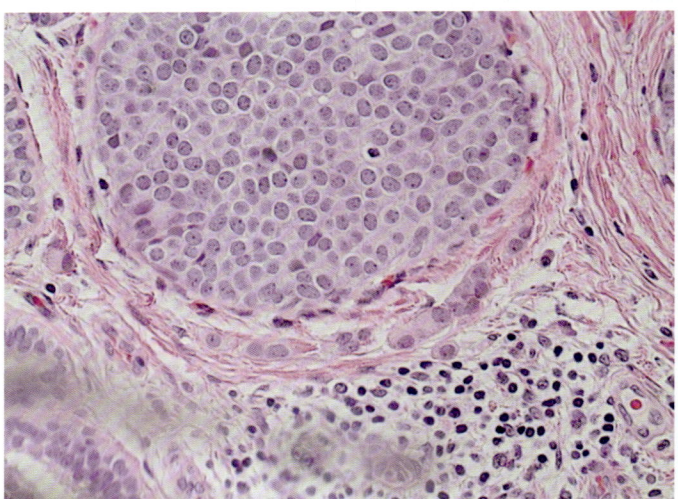

IMAGE 3.24 DCIS, intermediate nuclear grade with microinvasion. There are single pattern invasive cells adjacent to DCIS, measuring < 1 mm (H&E, x200).

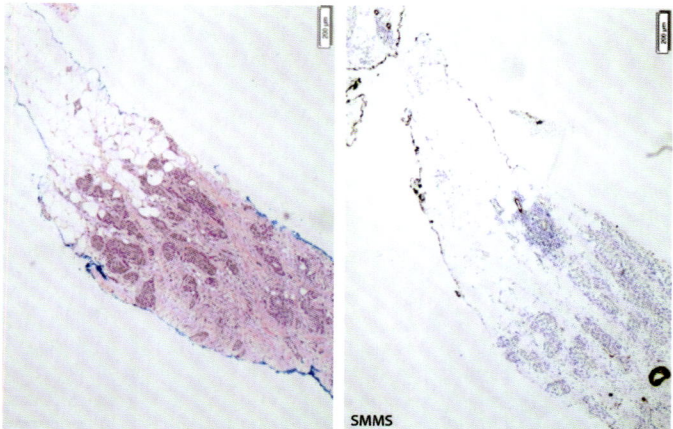

IMAGE 3.25 Invasive breast carcinoma of no special type. Biopsy shows irregular disorganized tumor nests/tubules infiltrating stroma and fat. The loss of myoepithelial cells on SMMS stain confirms the diagnosis. Left: H&E. Right: SMMS IHC.

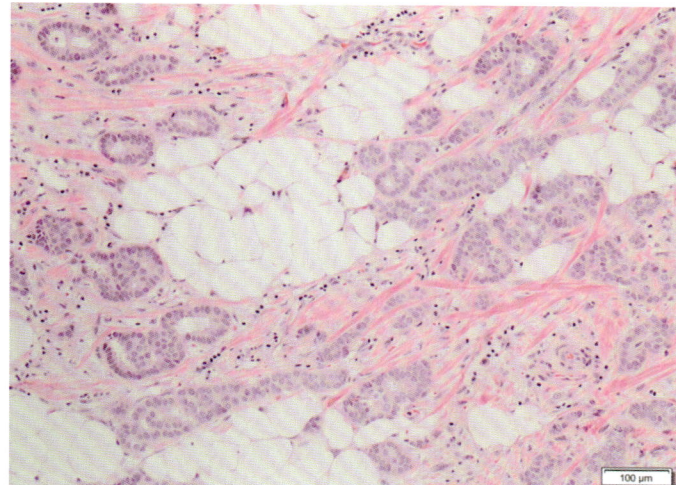

IMAGE 3.26 Invasive ductal carcinoma, Nottingham grade I. This lesion shows well-formed tubules (> 75%) with mild cytological atypia (H&E, x200).

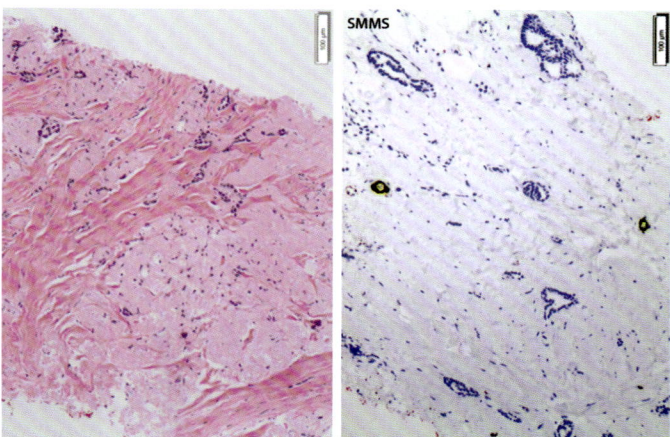

IMAGE 3.27 Invasive tubular carcinoma. Mammogram showed a mass possibly representing a radial scar. Histology shows a well-differentiated invasive carcinoma, Nottingham grade I, with open angulated tubules; myoepithelial cells are absent. Left: H&E. Right: SMMS IHC.

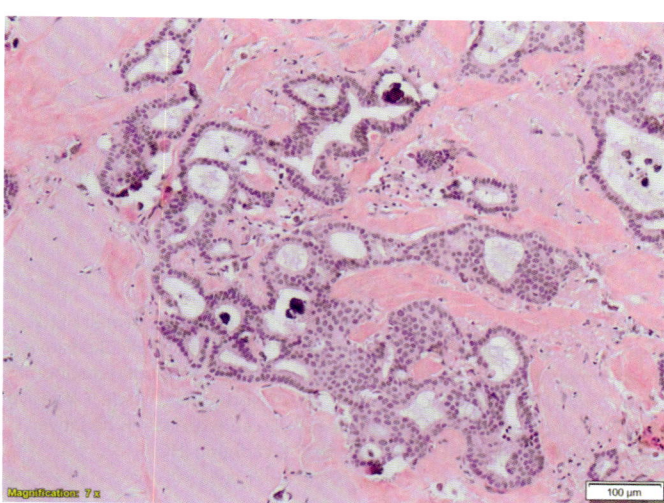

IMAGE 3.28 Invasive cribriform carcinoma. This well-differentiated invasive tumor forms rounded spaces resembling DCIS, cribriform pattern. These are usually Nottingham grade I tumors. Myoepithelial markers can be used to distinguish this invasive carcinoma from DCIS (H&E, x200).

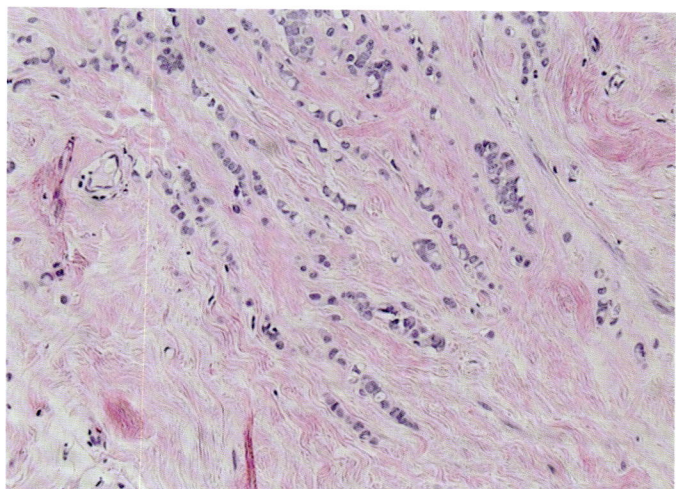

IMAGE 3.29 Invasive lobular carcinoma, classic type. The cells are discohesive, often in single files. The cells have scant cytoplasm and have low-intermediate grade nuclear atypia. A few signet ring cells may be seen. E-cadherin is aberrant. Lobular carcinomas are typically ER/PR positive and HER2 negative (H&E, x200).

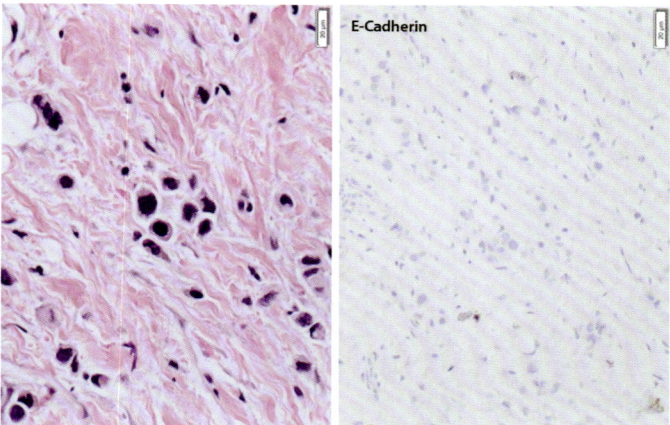

IMAGE 3.30 Pleomorphic invasive lobular carcinoma (PILC). This biopsy specimen shows single tumor cells with high grade nuclear atypia infiltrating the stroma singly or in linear files. Tumor cells are negative for E-cadherin immunohistochemical staining. Left: H&E. Right: E-cadherin IHC.

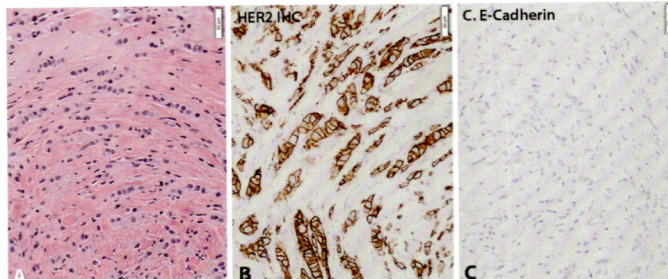

IMAGE 3.31 HER2 positive invasive lobular carcinoma. The overall HER2 positive rate in invasive breast carcinoma is ~12–18%. Most HER2 positive breast tumors are high grade ductal carcinoma. Invasive lobular carcinoma can be (rarely) HER2 positive, as in this case of Nottingham grade II, invasive lobular carcinoma. HER2 IHC is positive (3+). E-cadherin stain is negative. Image A: H&E. Image B: HER2 IHC. Image C: E-cadherin IHC.

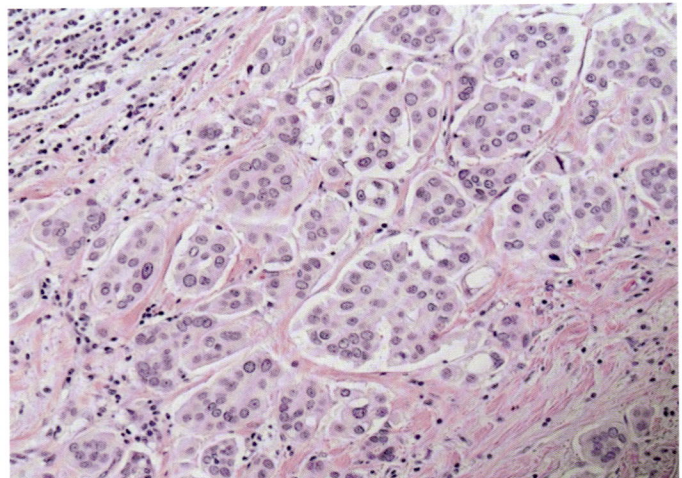

IMAGE 3.32 Invasive micropapillary carcinoma. The invasive tumor nests are oriented in clusters with clear spaces around them. There are no true fibrovascular cores. The cells have reverse polarity with the apex of the cells facing outward rather than toward the lumen. This subtype is associated with more frequent lymph node metastases and lymphovascular invasion (H&E, x200).

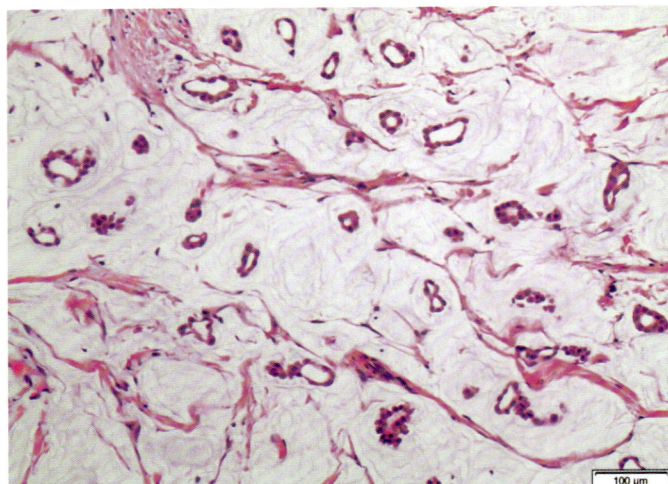

IMAGE 3.33 Invasive mucinous carcinoma. This tumor consists of clusters of malignant cells that are suspended in abundant extracellular mucin. In order to qualify as "mucinous carcinoma," the tumor must have Nottingham grade I features and pure mucinous morphology (H&E).

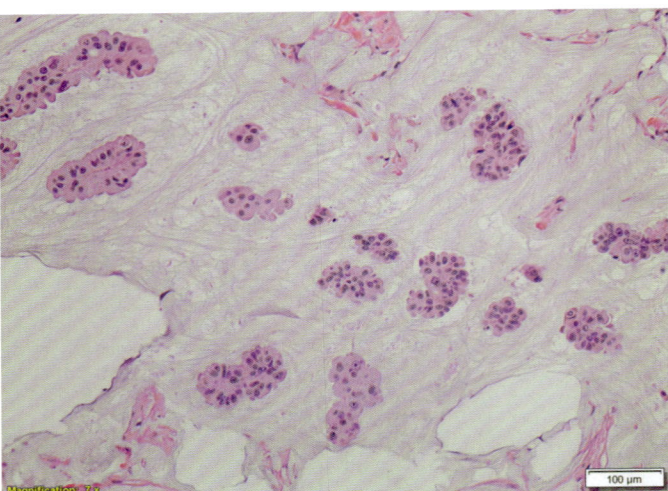

IMAGE 3.34 Mucinous micropapillary carcinoma. This rare entity has higher grade nuclear atypia than pure mucinous carcinoma, often with lymphovascular invasion and lymph node metastases (H&E).

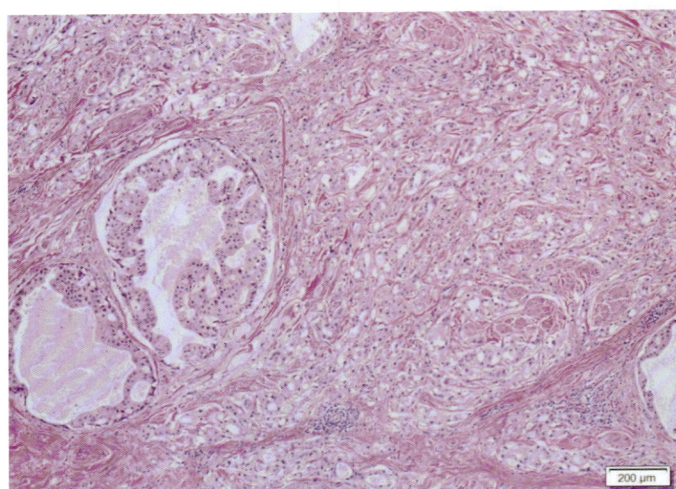

IMAGE 3.35 Carcinoma with apocrine differentiation. The tumor cells have abundant eosinophilic or vacuolated cytoplasm, round nuclei, and prominent nucleoli. Androgen receptor (AR) is often expressed; ER and PR are typically negative (H&E).

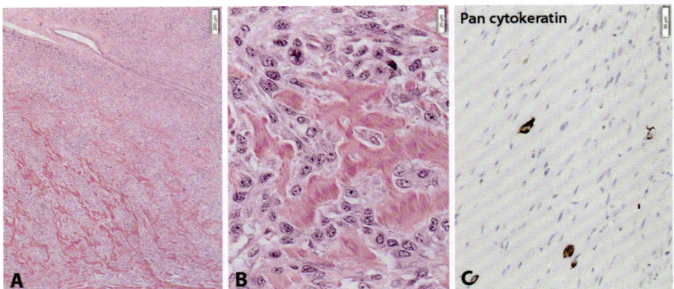

IMAGE 3.36 Metaplastic carcinoma with extensive osteosarcomatous differentiation. This mastectomy shows poorly differentiated carcinoma with extensive osteosarcomatous differentiation. Isolated pancytokeratin positive cells are demonstrated indicating that this is more likely a carcinoma than a sarcoma. Images A and B: H&E. Image C: Pankeratin.

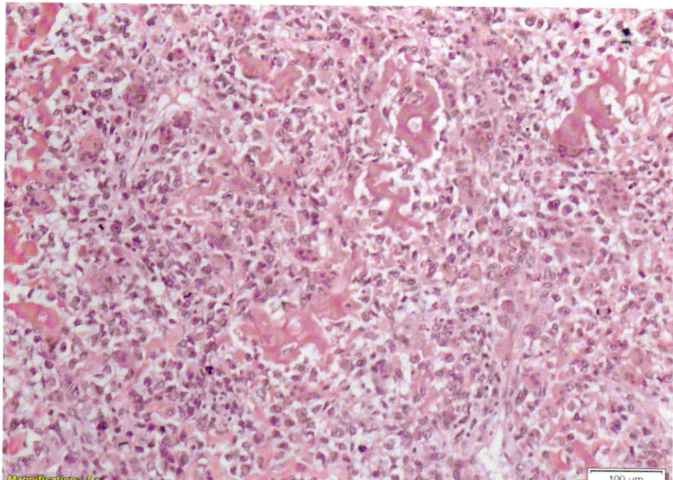

IMAGE 3.37 Metaplastic carcinoma with osteoclast-like giant cells. Note the pink acellular matrix between the tumor cells (H&E).

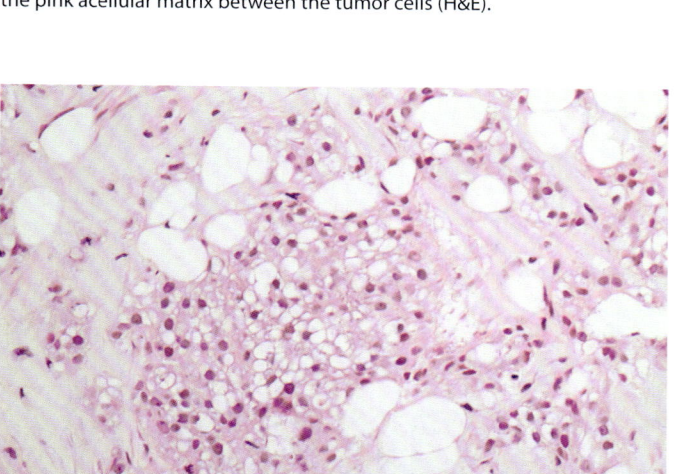

IMAGE 3.38 Acinic cell carcinoma. This tumor can show a variety of architectural patterns. Note the eosinophilic cytoplasmic granules (H&E).

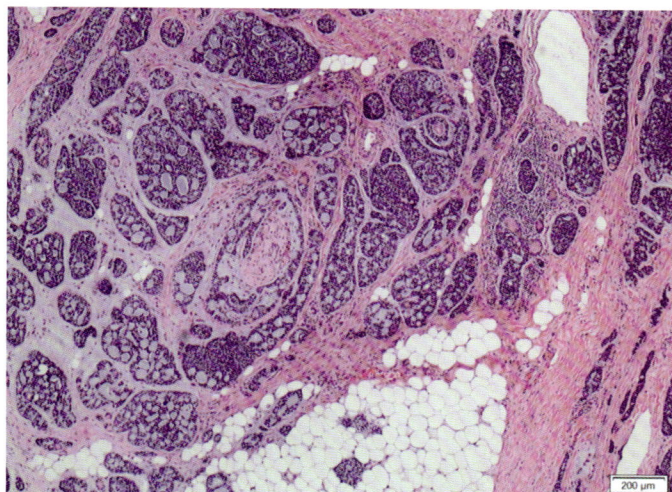

IMAGE 3.39 Adenoid cystic carcinoma. This lesion consists of epithelial and myoepithelial cells classically arranged in cribriform or tubular architecture. The tumor is often c-KIT positive, and ER, PR, HER2 triple negative (H&E).

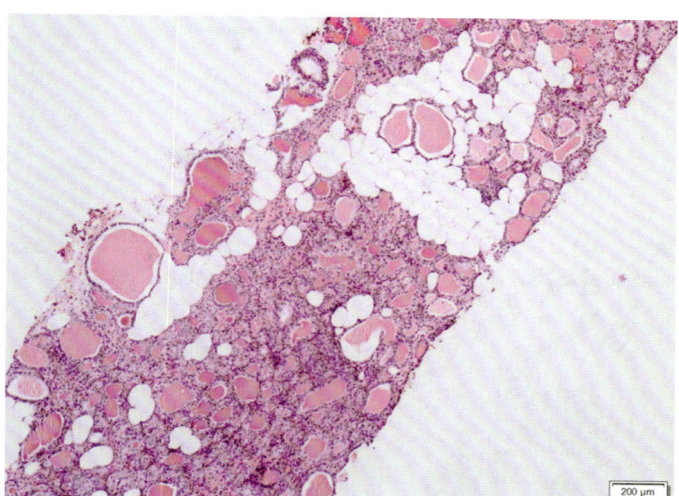

IMAGE 3.40 Cystic hypersecretory carcinoma. This lesion forms cysts containing eosinophilic secretions that resemble thyroid colloid. The secretions often retract from the epithelium to create a smooth, scalloped margin (H&E). Tumor cells can express S100 protein.

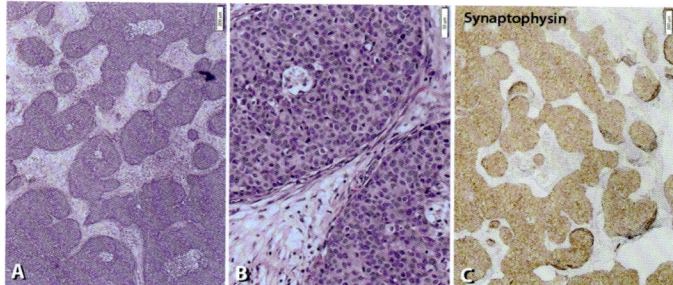

IMAGE 3.41 Primary neuroendocrine tumor of the breast. This lesion consists of solid nests and trabeculae. The cytoplasm is granular and the nuclei have "salt and pepper" chromatin. This tumor needs to be differentiated from a metastatic neuroendocrine tumor. Synaptophysin is positive. The presence of DCIS is helpful in determining if it is a breast primary. Images A and B: H&E. Image C: synaptophysin IHC.

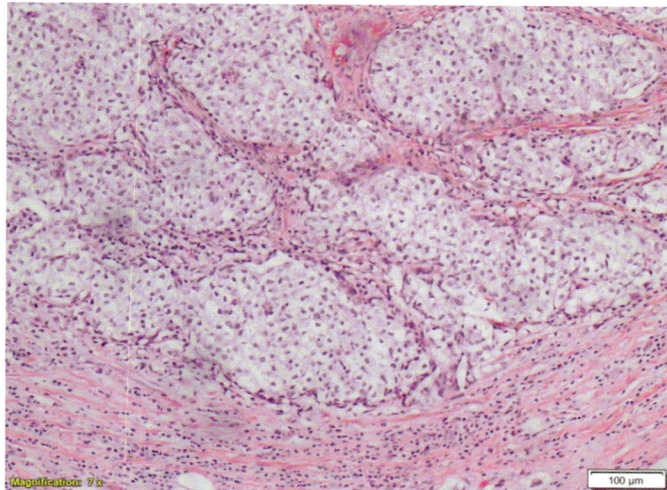

IMAGE 3.42 Invasive ductal carcinoma with clear cell differentiation. Renal cell carcinoma should be excluded with this type of morphology (H&E).

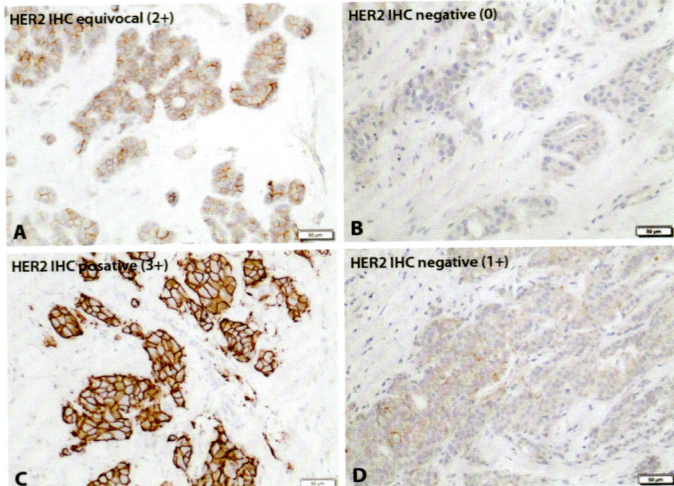

IMAGE 3.43 HER2 IHC scoring system. In cases with IHC equivocal results (2+), reflex SISH or FISH testing should be performed (HER2 IHC).

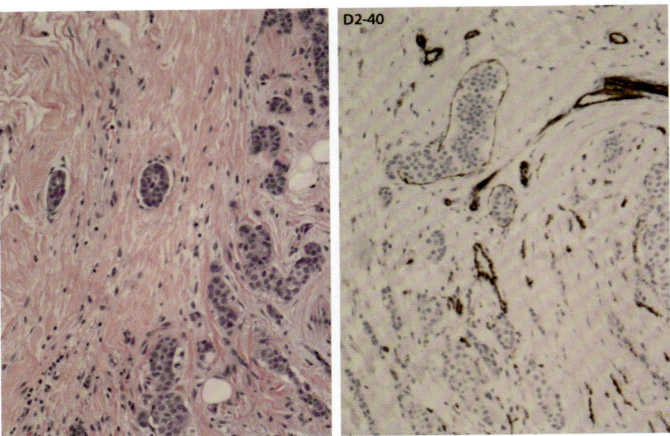

IMAGE 3.45 Lymphovascular invasion. Histology shows tumor cells in lymphatic spaces. This is a poor prognostic factor for invasive carcinoma. D2-40 stains endothelial cells in a sharp linear fashion. D2-40 also stains myoepithelial cells, but the staining is less discrete. Left: H&E, x100. Right: D2-40 IHC, x100.

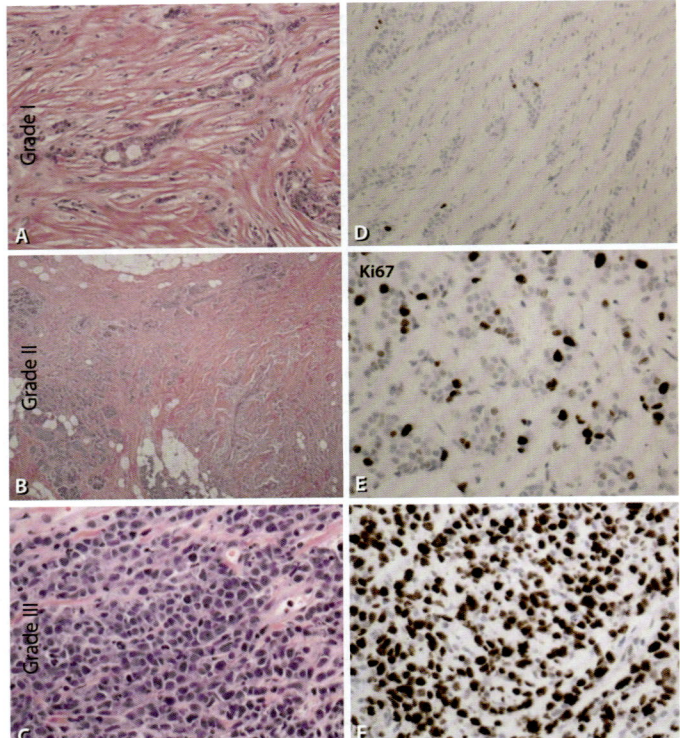

IMAGE 3.44 Ki 67 index. Ki 67 can be used as a predictive marker for invasive carcinoma. It correlates well with tumor grade, with higher grade tumors having higher Ki 67 index. Left panel: H&E. Right panel: Ki 67 IHC.

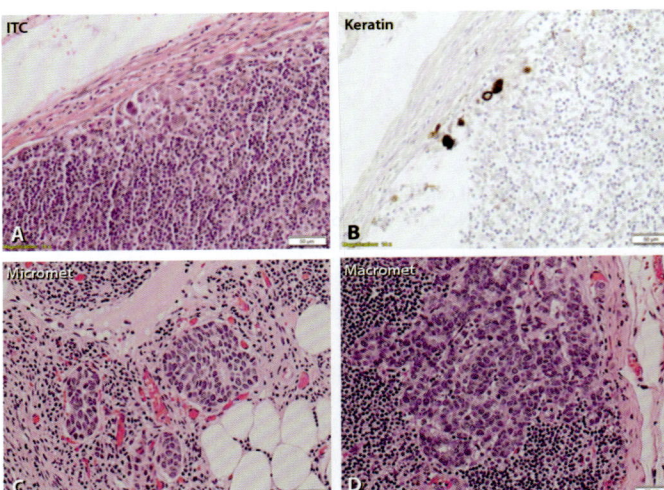

IMAGE 3.46 Lymph node metastases. Image A (H&E) and Image B (keratin IHC): isolated tumor cells (ITCs) are defined by contiguous tumor cells < 0.2 mm or < 200 cells per single cross-section. Image C (H&E): micromets are defined by contiguous tumor deposit ≥ 0.2 to < 2 mm and/or > 200 cells on single cross-section. Image D (H&E): macromets are ≥ 2 mm. ITCs are difficult to detect. Keratin can be performed when there is suspicion of ITCs.

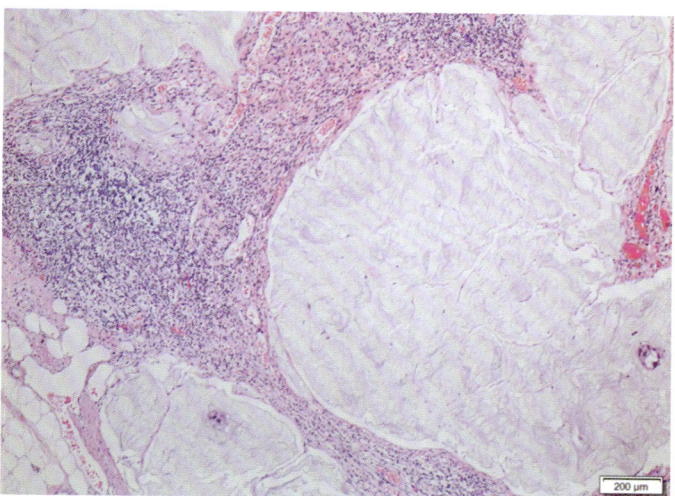

IMAGE 3.47 Post neoadjuvant therapy, lymph node. Histology shows a lymph node with mucin and few residual tumor cells indicating partial pathologic response (pPR) to treatment (H&E).

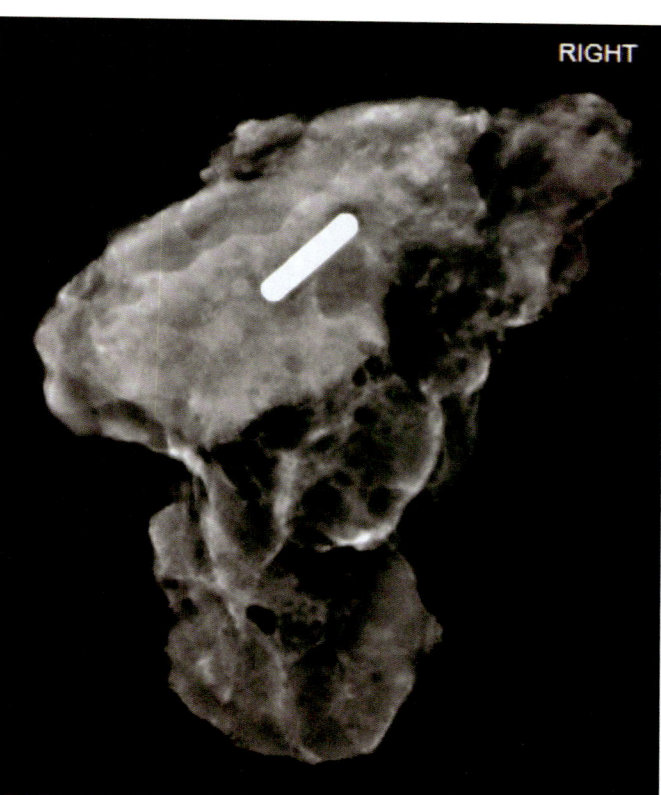

IMAGE 3.49 Radioactive seed-labeled axillary lymph node in an 86-year-old female. X-ray shows a radioactive seed embedded in surgically removed axillary contents.

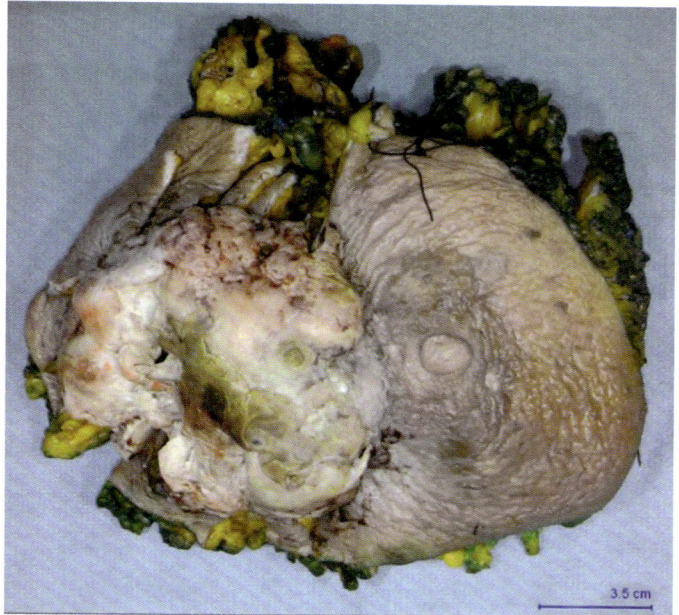

IMAGE 3.48 Skin invasion. Invasive ductal carcinoma with full epidermal ulceration upstages the carcinoma to pT4b regardless of tumor size.

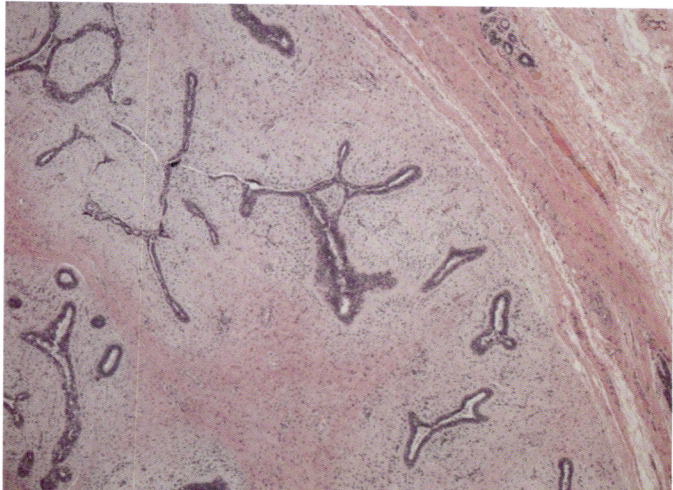

IMAGE 3.50 Fibroadenoma. Histology shows a well-circumscribed mass composed of both benign epithelial and intralobular-type stromal proliferations (H&E, x20).

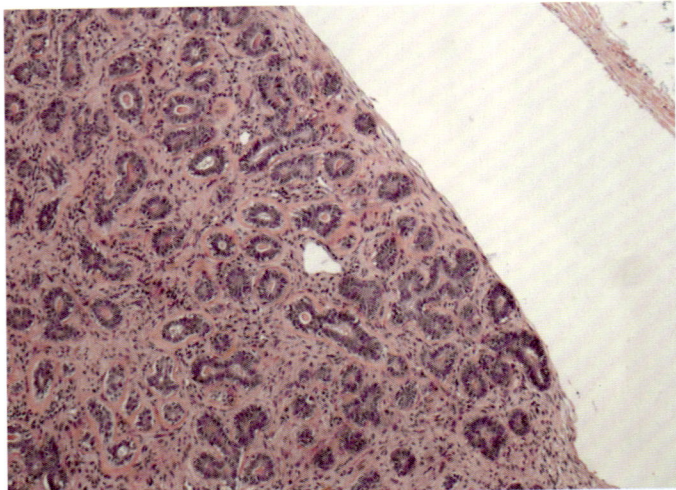

IMAGE 3.51 Breast tubular adenoma. Histology shows a fibroepithelial lesion with uniform, closely packed tubules lined by an attenuated myoepithelial layer. Compared to a fibroadenoma, there is much less stroma (H&E, x200).

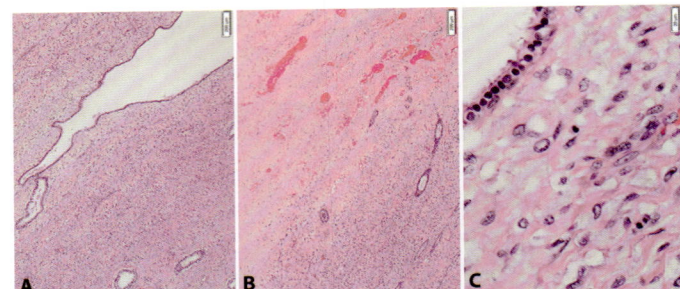

IMAGE 3.54 Malignant phyllodes tumor. Histology shows leaflike structures with stromal overgrowth, hypercellularity, necrosis, stromal pleomorphism, and increased mitotic activity (H&E).

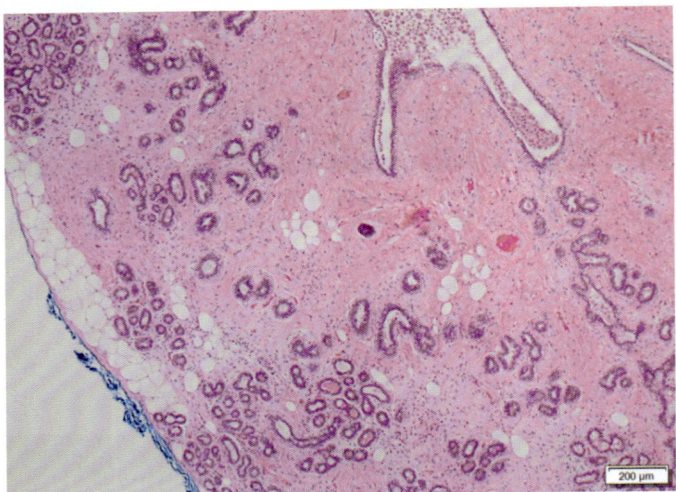

IMAGE 3.52 Breast hamartoma. Histology shows a well-circumscribed nodule composed of disorganized benign ductal and lobular structures mixed with adipose tissue. Breast hamartomas may also show other stroma components other than fat, including smooth muscle, hyaline cartilage, and pseudoangiomatous stromal hyperplasia (H&E).

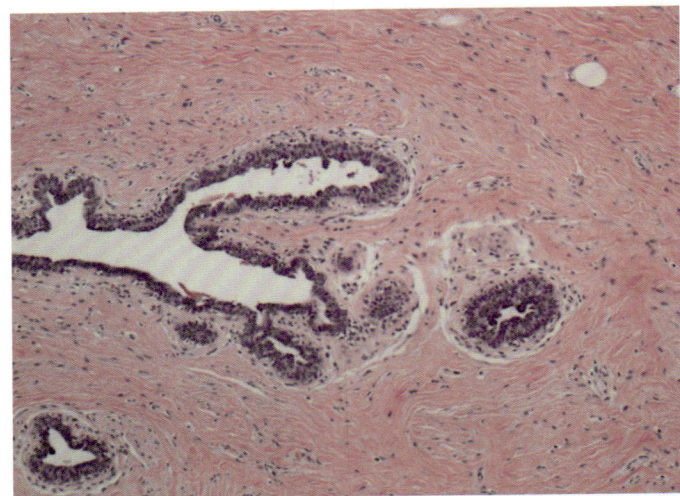

IMAGE 3.55 Gynecomastia in a 42-year-old male, with a history of prolonged steroid use and breast enlargement. This excision specimen shows male breast histology composed of mammary ducts and no lobules. Ductal epithelium exhibits typical gynecomastoid hyperplasia showing tapered projections in the background of dense fibrous stroma (H&E, x100).

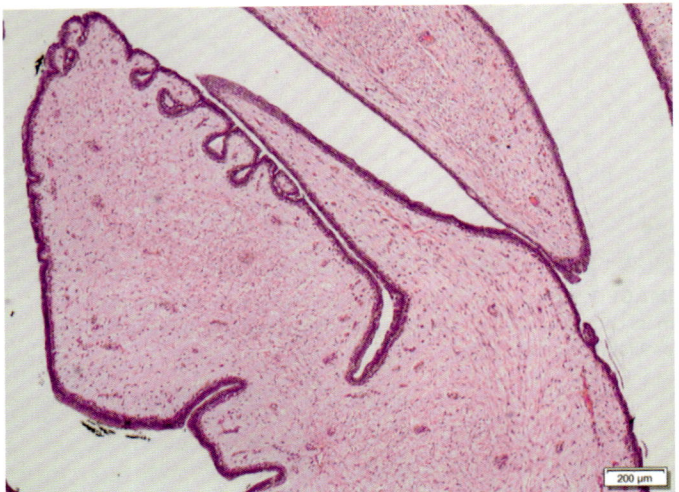

IMAGE 3.53 Benign phyllodes tumor. Resection shows a tumor with leaflike architecture and expansile stroma. The stroma cells are not atypical and there is minimal mitotic activity (H&E).

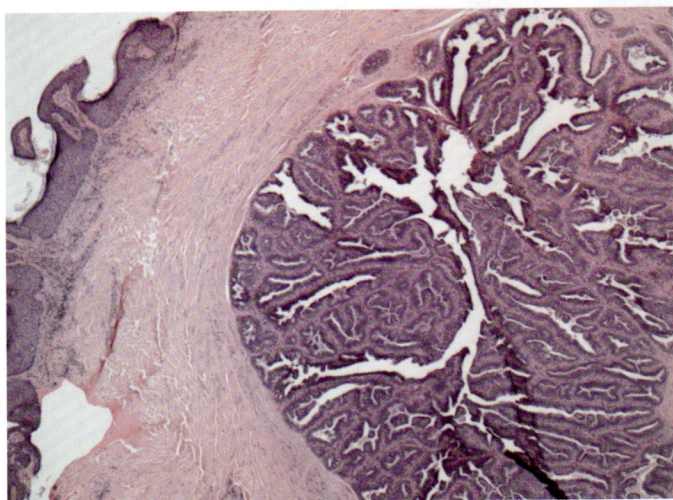

IMAGE 3.56 Nipple adenoma. This lesion consists of a nonencapsulated ductal proliferation of epithelial and myoepithelial cells deep to the nipple (H&E, x100).

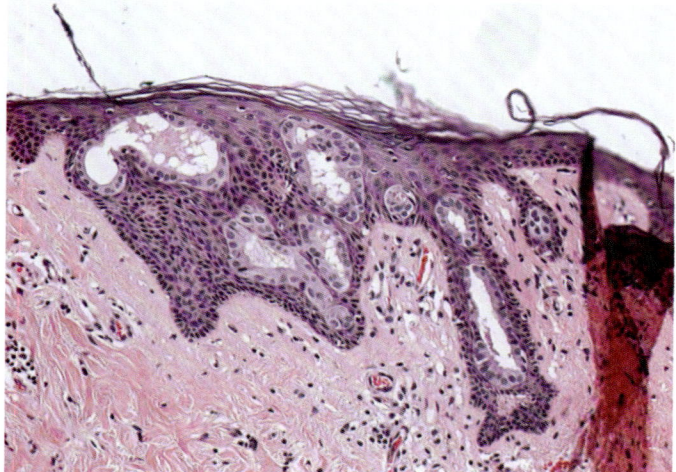

IMAGE 3.57 Paget disease of the breast. There are malignant cells with pale cytoplasm and large nuclei in the epidermis of the nipple. This is usually associated with underlying invasive carcinoma or DCIS. Paget disease is staged as in situ disease. In rare cases, Paget cells can form glands, as in this case (H&E, x200).

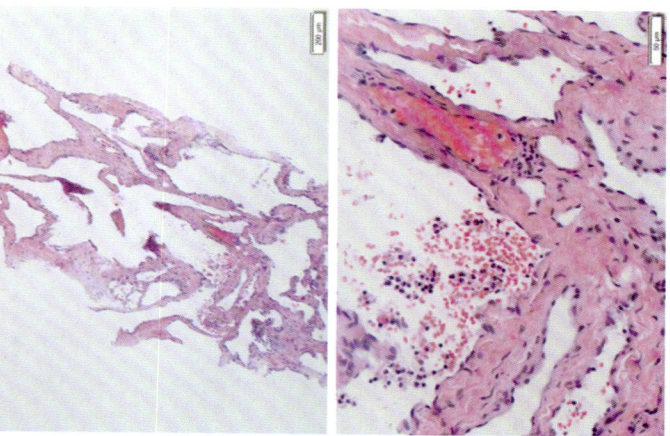

IMAGE 3.60 Cavernous hemangioma. This biopsy specimen shows a benign lesion consisting of large vascular spaces (H&E).

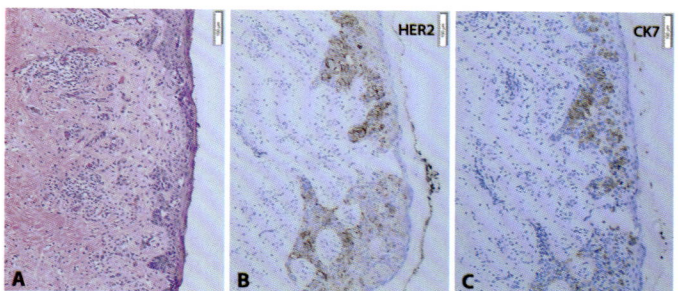

IMAGE 3.58 Paget disease of the breast with dermal microinvasion. Histology shows malignant cells in the epidermis. Small clusters of malignant cells have invaded into the underlying dermis. CK7 can highlight the malignant cells. Paget cells are often HER2 positive. Image A: H&E. Image B: HER2 IHC. Image C: CK7 IHC.

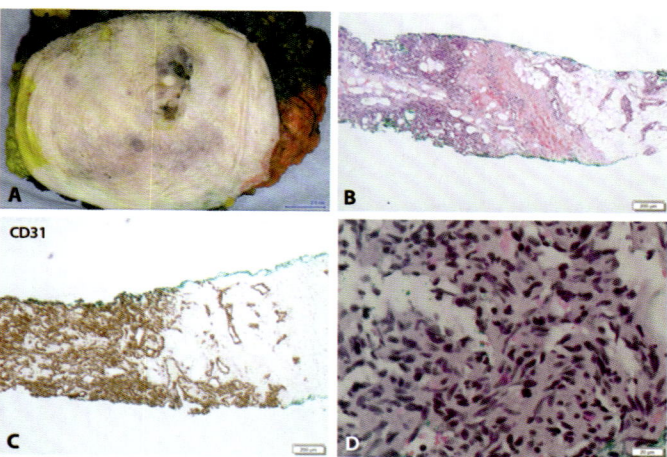

IMAGE 3.61 Angiosarcoma. This gross picture shows a red violaceous and poorly circumscribed mass. Histology shows high grade malignant neoplasm with poorly defined vascular spaces and atypical hobnailed cells which express ERG, CD34, and CD31. Images B and D: H&E. Image C: CD31 IHC.

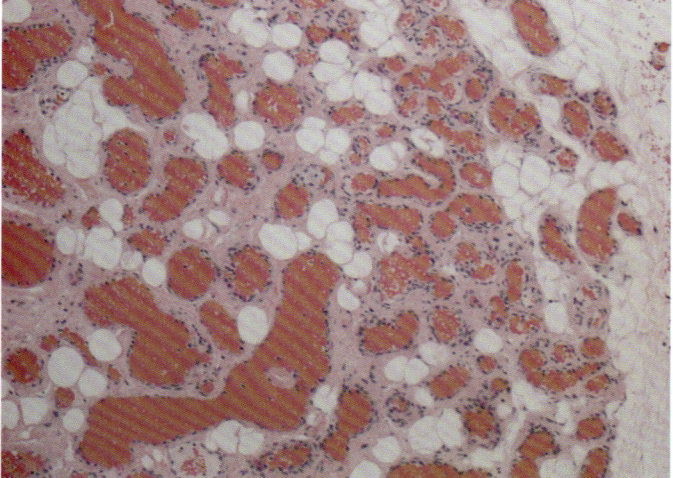

IMAGE 3.59 Cavernous hemangioma. Histology shows dilated vascular structures with a bland endothelial lining. Benign vascular tumors are uncommon deep in the breast parenchyma. Low grade angiosarcoma needs to be excluded (H&E, x40).

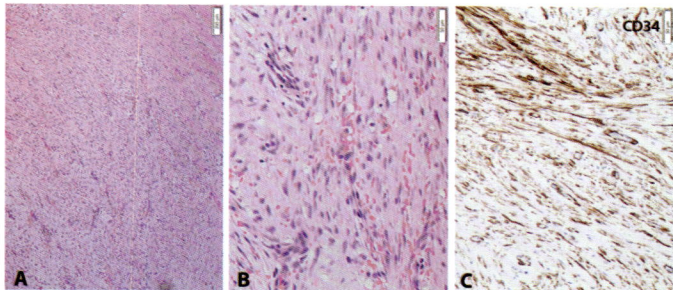

IMAGE 3.62 Nodular fasciitis. Histology shows a lesion with bland stellate spindle cells with a tissue culture–like appearance. Extravasated erythrocytes are present. CD34 IHC is positive. Images A and B: H&E. Image C: CD34 IHC.

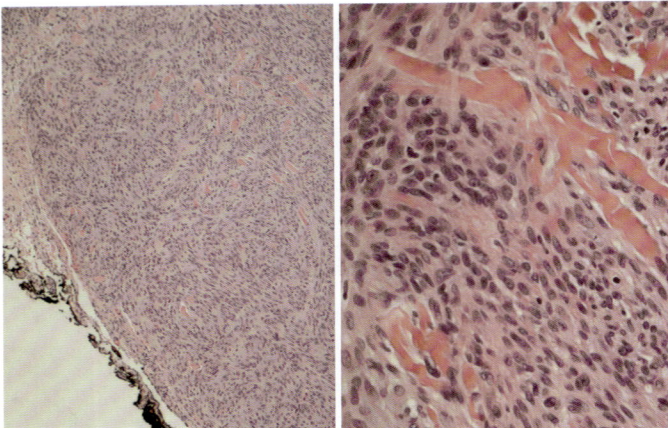

IMAGE 3.63 Myofibroblastoma. Low power shows a well-circumscribed cellular mass. High power shows bland spindle cell proliferation admixed with coarse hyalinized collagen bands. Myofibroblastoma has several morphologic variants. Tumor cells are often positive for desmin, CD34, BCL-2, and ER. Left: H&E, x40. Right: H&E, x200.

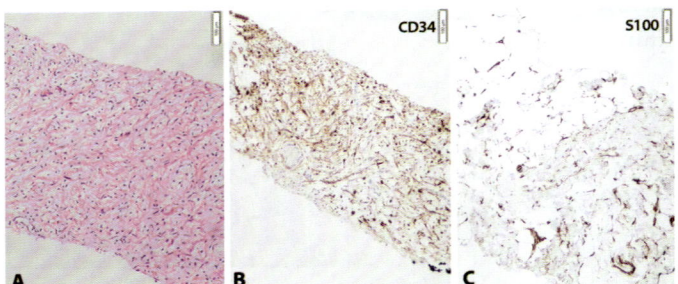

IMAGE 3.64 Neurofibroma/schwannoma. Histology shows a bland spindle cell lesion that is S100 and CD34 positive. Image A: H&E. Image B: CD34 IHC. Image C: S100 IHC.

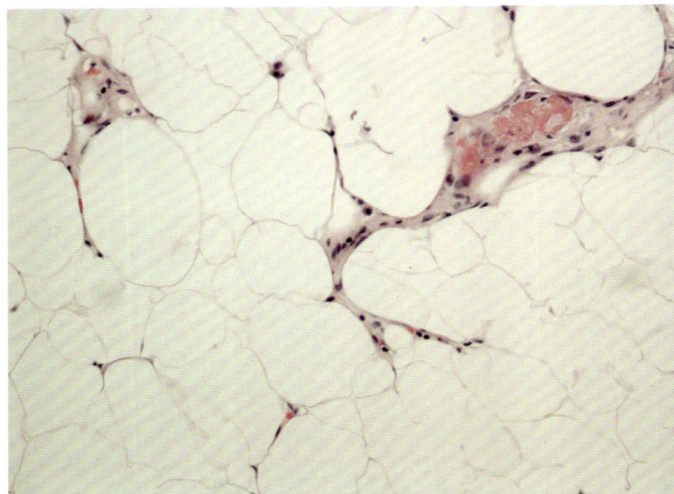

IMAGE 3.65 Angiolipoma. Histology shows a well-circumscribed lesion composed of mature adipose tissue and benign vessels with fibrin thrombi (H&E, x40).

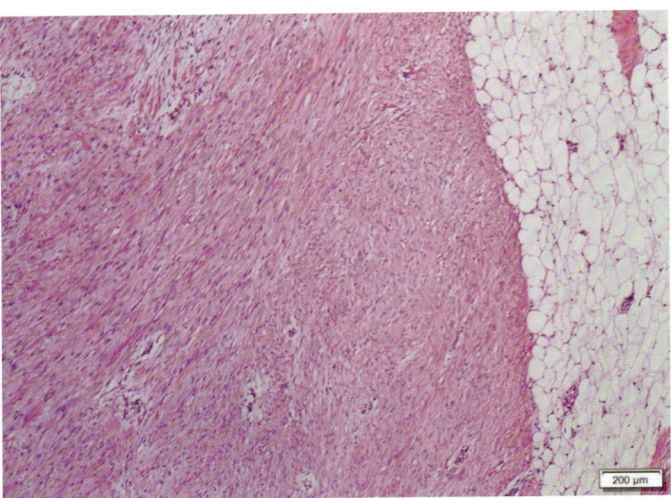

IMAGE 3.66 Fibromatosis in a 34-year-old female with a palpable breast nodule. Histology shows an infiltrative proliferation of long fascicles of interlacing bland spindle cells with variable collagen extending into the fat. ß-catenin IHC shows positive nuclear expression.

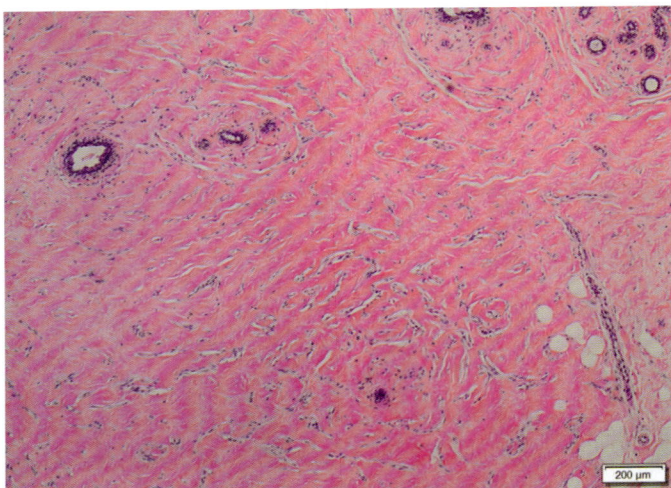

IMAGE 3.67 Pseudoangiomatous stroma hyperplasia (PASH). This biopsy specimen shows complex slit-shaped spaces in dense collagenous stroma. The spaces have spindled cells that resemble, but are not, endothelial cells (H&E).

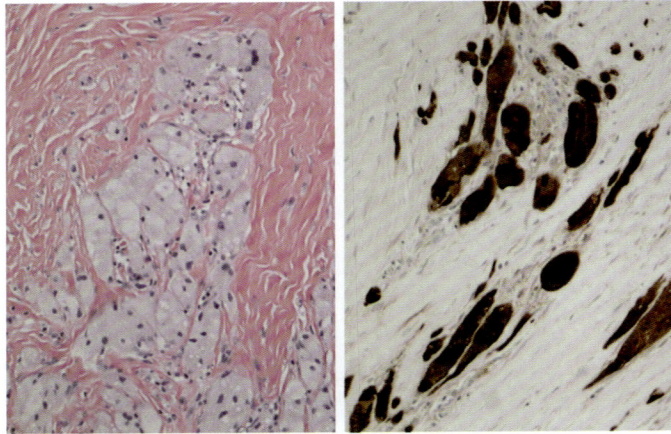

IMAGE 3.68 Granular cell tumor. This excisional biopsy specimen shows characteristic polygonal cells with large amounts of pale granular cytoplasm and bland small nuclei. Tumor cells are positive for S100 stain. Left: H&E, x100. Right: S100, x100.

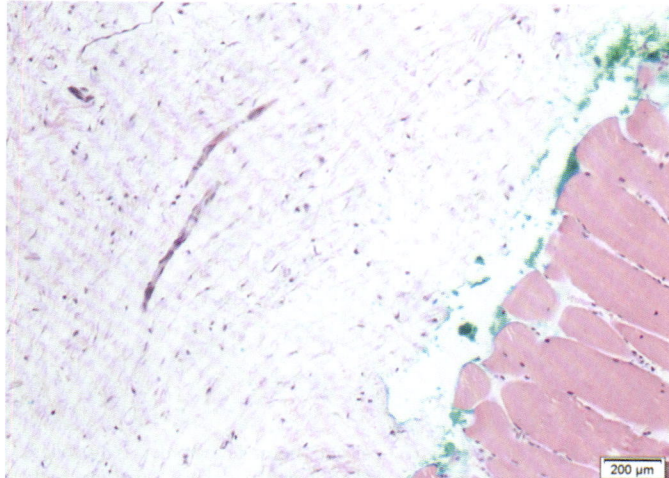

IMAGE 3.69 Intramuscular myxoma in a 50-year-old female. Ultrasound showed a 2.8 cm indeterminate solid hypoechoic nodule in the deep aspect of the left breast, possibly within the pectoralis muscle. Histology shows a hypocellular and slightly basophilic myxoid matrix with few bland spindle cells without mitotic activity (H&E).

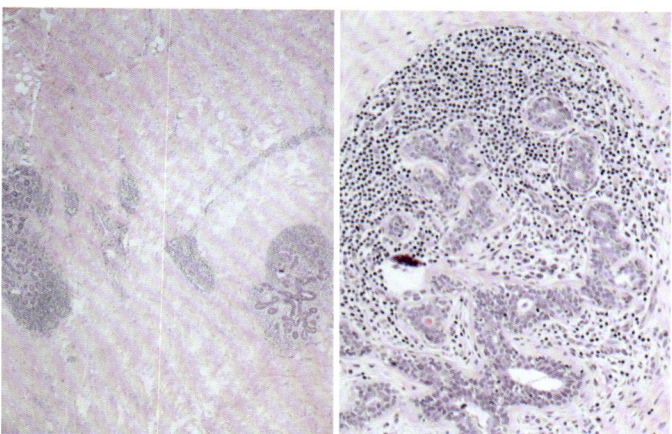

IMAGE 3.72 Lymphocytic mastitis with no diabetic history. This lumpectomy shows terminal ductal lobular unit centric lymphocytic mastitis with mixed reactive lymphocytic infiltration. This type of lesion can be mass forming and may be autoimmune related. Left: H&E, x20. Right: H&E, x100.

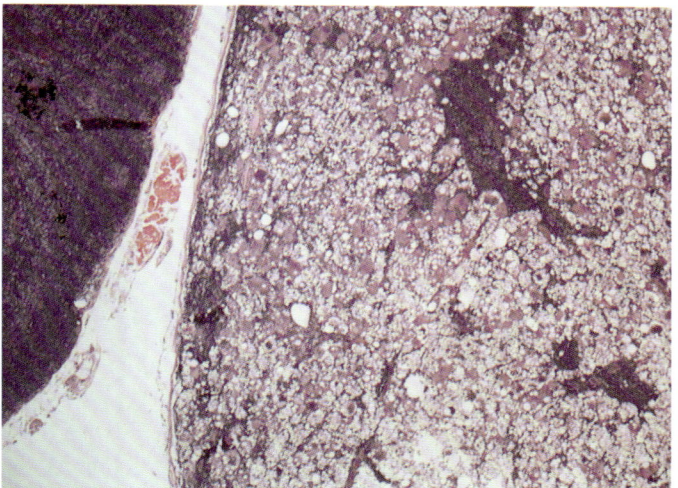

IMAGE 3.70 Extensive silicone reaction in a 45-year-old female with silicone-injection-type breast augmentation, now with enlarged axillary lymph nodes. This excisional biopsy specimen shows extensive giant cell reaction to silicone material in the lymph nodes (H&E, x20).

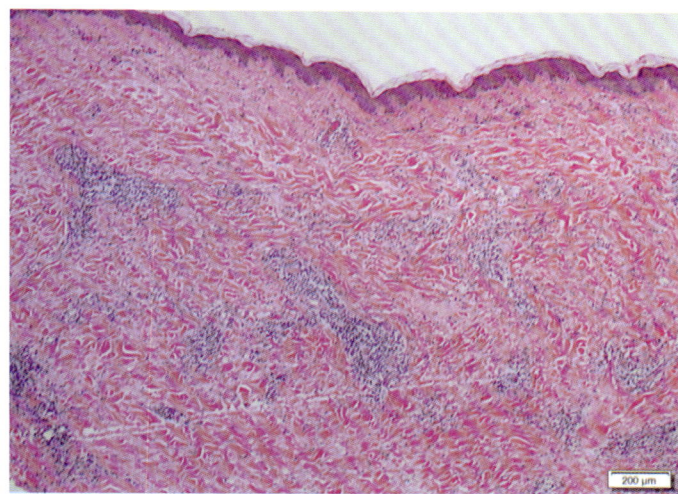

IMAGE 3.73 Inflammatory morphea in a 69-year-old female with a history of breast radiation. Histology shows superficial and deep perivascular lymphoplasmacytic infiltrates with deep dermal fibrosis (H&E).

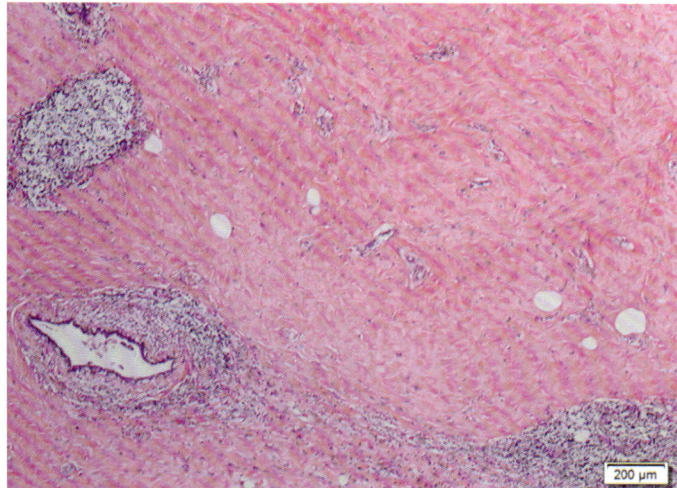

IMAGE 3.71 Diabetic mastopathy. This biopsy specimen shows periductal, perilobular, and perivascular lymphocytic infiltrates with a background of dense stromal fibrosis (H&E).

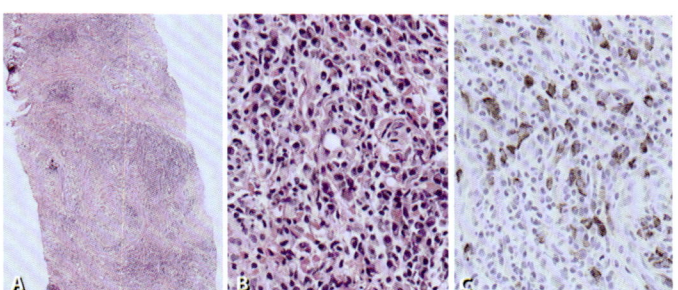

IMAGE 3.74 Mass-forming IgG4-related breast disease. This core biopsy specimen shows inflammatory reaction composed of mixed inflammatory cells. IgG4 stain shows significantly increased IgG4 positive plasma cells. Image A: H&E, x20. Image B: H&E, x200. Image C: IgG4 IHC, x200.

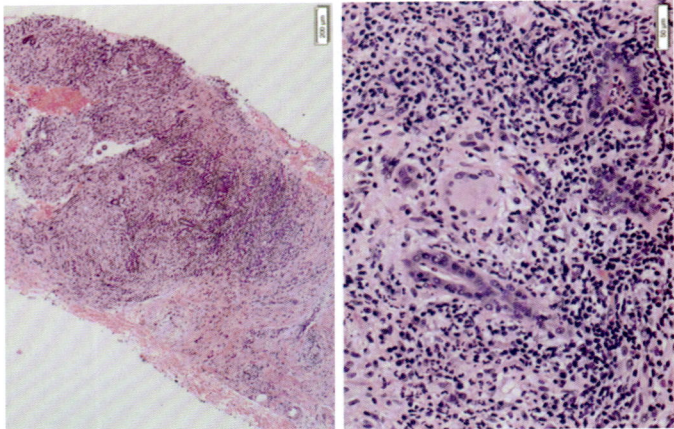

IMAGE 3.75 Idiopathic suppurative granulomatous mastitis in a patient with a clinical history of chronic nipple discharge and skin fistula formation, not responding to antibiotic treatment. Core biopsy H&E slides show suppurative granulomatous inflammation with many microabscesses and multinucleated giant cells. Special stains for microorganisms were negative. Tissue for culture and sensitivity should be suggested for any further biopsy or excision (H&E).

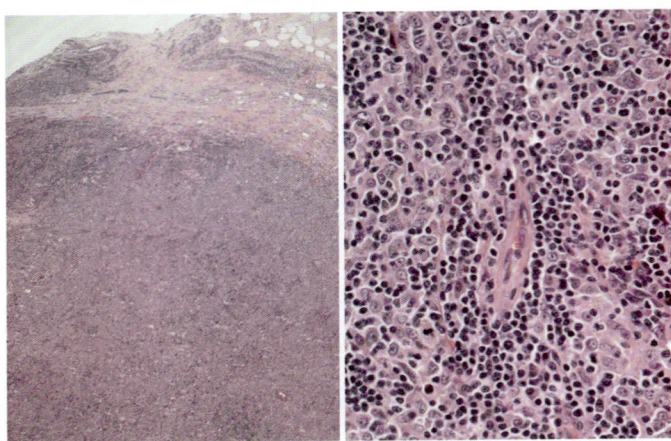

IMAGE 3.78 T-cell lymphoma. T-cell lymphoma of the breast is much less common than B-cell lymphoma and often rich in vascular structures. Left: H&E, x10. Right: H&E, x200.

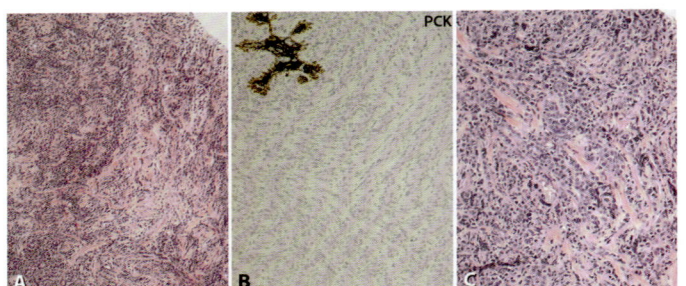

IMAGE 3.76 Diffuse large B-cell lymphoma. Histology shows highly atypical lymphoid cells with crushing artifact. Pankeratin stain is negative, demonstrating the nonepithelial nature of the cells. Image A: H&E, x40. Image B: Pankeratin IHC, x100. Image C: H&E, x100.

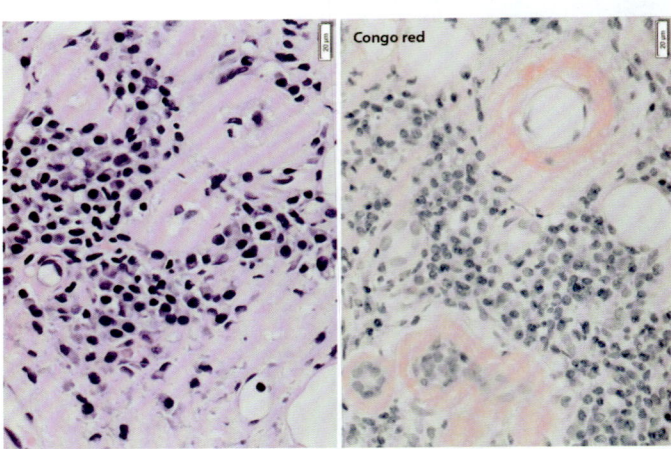

IMAGE 3.79 Amyloidosis. This biopsy specimen shows pink amorphous amyloid deposits, particularly in vessel walls associated with a mixed lymphocytic reaction. Congo red stain shows salmon pink appearance. The patient had a history of Sjögren syndrome and atypical plasmacytosis. Left: H&E. Right: Congo red stain.

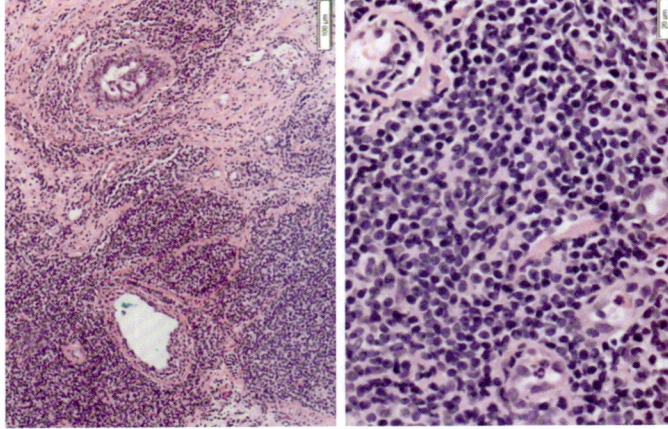

IMAGE 3.77 MALT lymphoma. Histology shows an atypical monomorphic population of plasmacytoid lymphocytes (H&E).

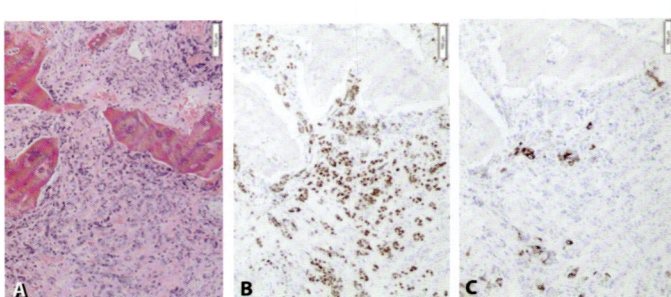

IMAGE 3.80 Metastatic breast carcinoma to the bone. Histology shows a poorly differentiated high grade tumor infiltrating bone. Positive GATA3 and mammoglobin expression support the diagnosis. Left: H&E. Image B: GATA3 IHC. Image C: mammoglobin IHC.

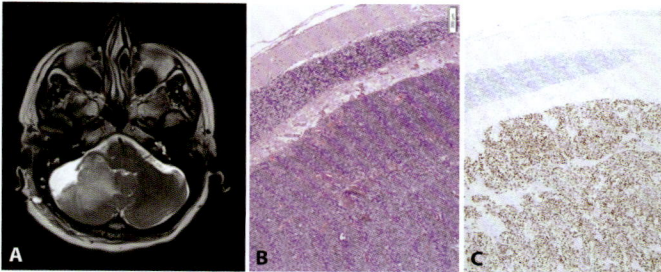

IMAGE 3.81 Brain metastasis in a 50-year-old female with a history of breast cancer. Image A: this MRI shows a right cerebellar mass. Image B (H&E) and Image C (GATA3 IHC): histology shows a poorly differentiated mass that is GATA3 positive.

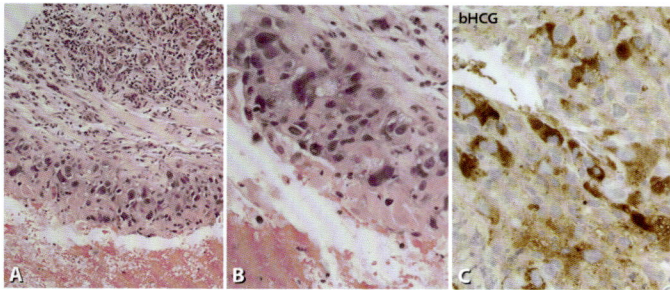

IMAGE 3.82 Metastatic choriocarcinoma. Image A (H&E, x100) and Image B (H&E, x200): the resected tumor shows markedly atypical pleomorphic cells with extensive hemorrhage. Image C: the tumor cells stained positive for β-HCG (x200).

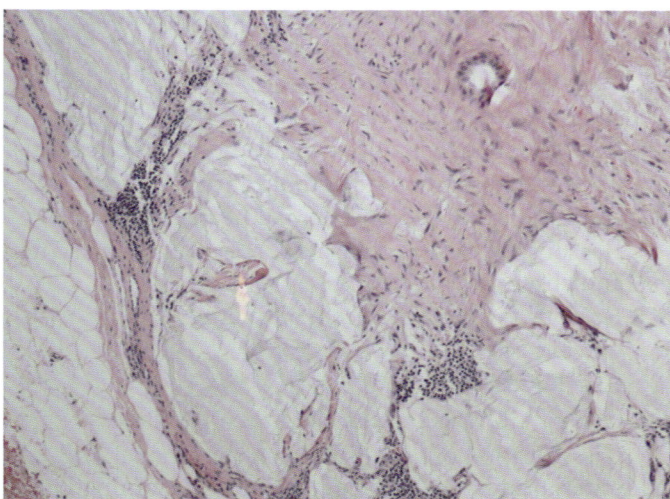

IMAGE 3.83 Metastatic appendiceal mucinous carcinoma. This is a differential diagnosis when considering a primary breast mucinous carcinoma (H&E, x100).

Bibliography

Allison KH, Hammond MEH, Dowsett M, et al. Estrogen and progesterone testing in breast cancer: American Society of Clinical Oncology/College of American Pathologists guideline update. Arch Pathol Lab Med. 2020;144(5):545–563. doi: 10.5858/arpa.2019-0904-sa

Amin MB, Edge S, Greene F, et al, editors. AJCC cancer staging manual. 8th ed. New York: Springer; 2017.

Fitzgibbons PL, Bartley AN, Connolly JL, et al; Cancer Biomarker Reporting Committee, College of American Pathologists. Template for reporting results of biomarker testing of specimens from patients with carcinoma of the breast (Version: Breast Biomarkers 1.4.0.0) [Internet]. College of American Pathologists; 2020. Available from www.cap.org.

Fitzgibbons PL, Connolly JL, Bose S, et al; Cancer Committee, College of American Pathologists. Protocol for the examination of resection specimens from patients with ductal carcinoma in situ (DCIS) of the breast (Breast DCIS Resection 4.3.0.1) [Internet]. College of American Pathologists; 2020 February. Available from www.cap.org.

Fitzgibbons PL, Connolly JL, Bose S, et al; Cancer Committee, College of American Pathologists. Protocol for the examination of resection specimens from patients with invasive carcinoma of the breast (Version: Breast Invasive Resection 4.4.0.0) [Internet]. College of American Pathologists; 2020. Available from www.cap.org.

Goldblum JR, Lamps LW, McKenney JK, et al, editors. Rosai and Ackerman's surgical pathology. 11th ed. Philadelphia (PA): Elsevier; 2018.

Hicks DG, Lester SC. Diagnostic pathology: breast. 2nd ed. Philadelphia (PA): Elsevier; 2016.

Kumar V, Abbas AK, Aster J. Robbins and Cotran pathologic basis of disease. 10th ed. North York (ON): Elsevier Canada; 2020.

Longacre TA, editor. Mills and Sternberg's diagnostic surgical pathology. 7th ed. Philadelphia (PA): Wolters Kluwar; 2022.

Wolff AC, Hammond MEH, Allison KH, et al. Human epidermal growth factor receptor 2 testing in breast cancer: American Society of Clinical Oncology/College of American Pathologists clinical practice guideline focused update. Arch Pathol Lab Med. 2018;142(11):1364–1382. doi: 10.5858/arpa.2018-0902-sa

World Health Organization. WHO classification of tumors. 5th ed. Vol. 2, Breast tumours. Lyon (France): IARC Press; 2019.

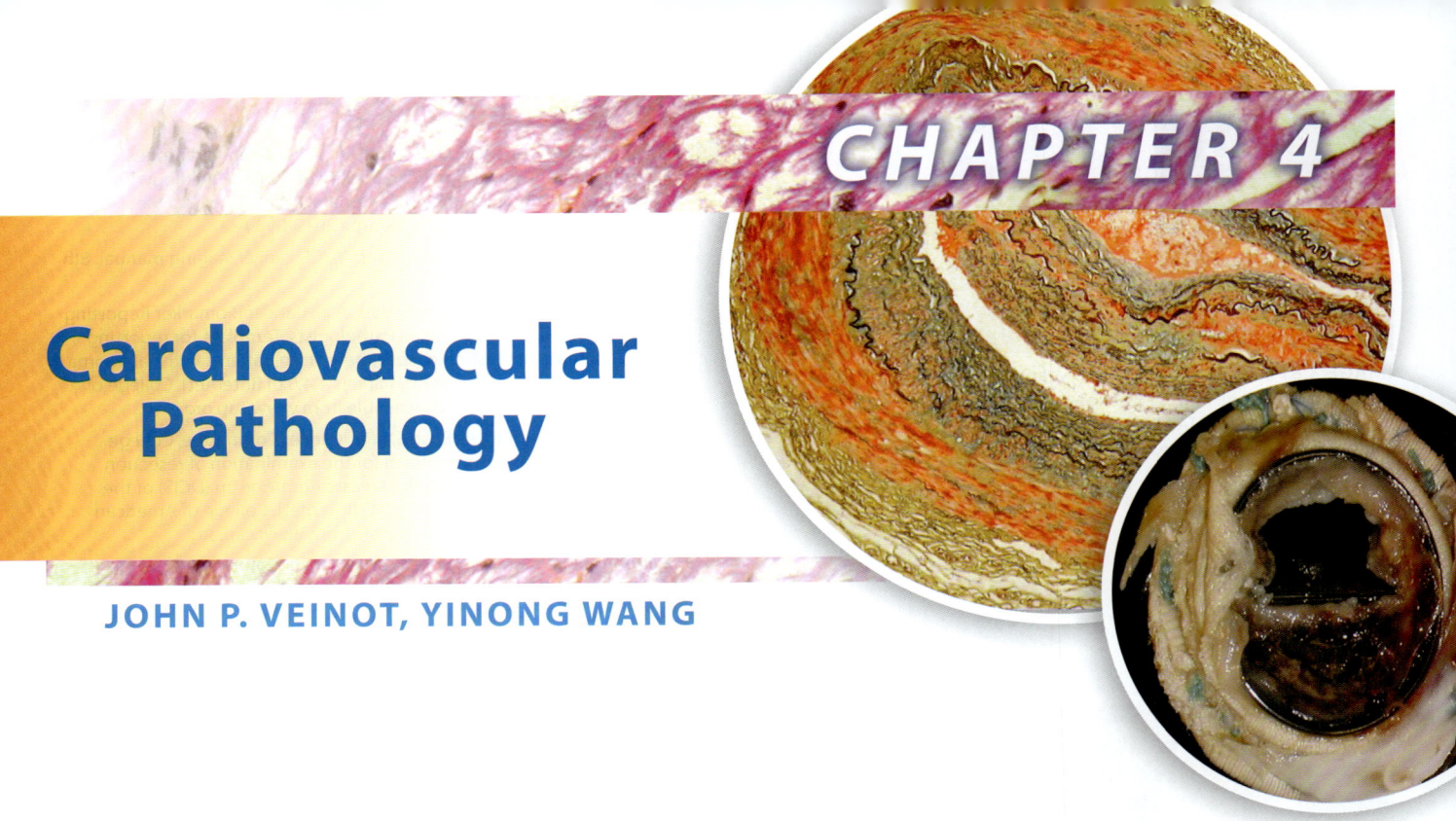

CHAPTER 4

Cardiovascular Pathology

JOHN P. VEINOT, YINONG WANG

Cardiovascular Pathology Exam Essentials

MUST KNOW

World Health Organization (WHO) classification

- The WHO classification of tumors of the heart is contained within the thoracic organ book. In general, tumors of the heart are very rare, and most of them are non-epithelial lesions that have overlap with other organs. Since we are focusing on lesions that are more "cardiac centric," the number of entities is quite limited:
  - Rhabdomyoma (especially those associated with tuberous sclerosis complex [TSC]).
  - Myxoma.
  - Papillary fibroelastoma.
  - Mediastinal and cardiac teratoma.
  - Cardiac lymphoma.
  - Metastasis to the heart.
  - Lesions of the pericardium (e.g., solitary fibrous tumors, sarcoma, mesothelioma).
- See chapter 2 (Bone and Soft Tissue Pathology) for benign and malignant vascular lesions.
- Note that the AJCC and College of American Pathologists (CAP) protocol for cardiac tumors has been discontinued as of 2017.

Nonneoplastic disease

- Key topics in cardiac-centric diseases include:
  - Anatomy of the heart, including valves, coronary vessels, and the regions they supply.
  - Clinical symptoms and ECG findings in stable and unstable plaque.
  - Clinical symptoms of left versus right heart failure.
  - How gross and microscopic findings in myocardial infarction (MI) change post MI, and the anatomic location of MI based on the vessel affected.
  - Short- and long-term complications of MI.
  - Dilated and constrictive cardiomyopathy, including causes, symptoms, and complications.
  - Common left heart valvular disease, including causes, findings, and complications.
  - Causes of valvular vegetations.
  - Various causes of myocarditis.
  - Causes, symptoms, and complications of pericarditis.
  - Causes, symptoms, and complications of arrhythmia.
  - Indications for endomyocardial heart biopsy.
  - Reasons for cardiac transplant rejection in the acute and chronic setting.
  - Reasons for valve replacement failure.
  - Sarcoidosis.
  - Amyloidosis.
- Key topics in vascular-centric diseases include:
  - Classification of vasculitis using the Chapel Hill criteria, and, for each type, diagnostic examinations, associated clinical symptoms, and findings in other organs.
  - Atherosclerosis: risk factors, steps, and complications.

- Dissection, causes, risk factors, symptoms, and gross and microscopic findings.
- Berry and other forms of aneurysm.
- Ancillary stains such as trichrome and elastic stain.

Genetic and syndromic conditions

The diseases in this category are mostly congenital or inherited rather than syndromic per se. The most likely context for exam questions is sudden cardiac death, or cardiovascular pathology associated with syndromes that affect other organs. You should also review the chapters on forensic pathology and pediatric pathology for related cardiovascular pathology. Key topics include:
- Hypertrophic obstructive cardiomyopathy (HOCM).
- Arrhythmogenic right ventricular cardiomyopathy (ARVC).
- Long and short QT.
- Marfan syndrome.
- Congenital bicuspid aortic valves.
- Pediatric congenital heart defects such as atrial septal defect, ventricular septal defect, tetralogy of Fallot, transposition of great vessels.
- TSC and cardiac rhabdomyoma.

MUST SEE

High-yield images include:
- Common tumors:
  - Rhabdomyoma (especially in context of TSC).
  - Cardiac myxoma.
  - Papillary fibroelastoma.
  - Other benign mesenchymal tumors (e.g., lipoma, fibroma, hemangioma, schwannoma, granular cell tumor).
  - Cardiac lymphomas.
  - Metastasis.
  - Mesothelioma.
- Common valvular changes:
  - Mitral valve in rheumatic disease.
  - Bicuspid aortic valve.
  - Degenerative calcific aortic valve.
  - Vegetations and endocarditis including infective endocarditis (IE), nonbacterial thrombotic endocarditis (NBTE), and Libman-Sacks endocarditis.
- Common myocardial changes:
  - Various anatomic locations and stages of MI.
  - HOCM.
  - Dilated cardiomyopathy.
  - ARVC.
  - Heart in hypertension.
  - Dilated cardiomyopathy.
  - Myocardial aneurysm.
  - Papillary muscle rupture.
  - Fibrinous pericarditis.

- Metastatic lymphoma and carcinoma.
- Coronary artery bypass graft.
- Gaucher disease.
- Myocarditis.
- Amyloidosis.
- Sarcoidosis.
- Cardiac allograft rejection.
- Common vascular changes:
  - Atherosclerosis, especially of coronary vessel.
  - Stable and unstable plaques.
  - Monckeberg calcification.
  - Abdominal aortic aneurysm.
  - Aortic plaques.
  - Thoracic aneurysm.
  - Berry aneurysm.
  - Dissections.
  - Renal stenosis.
  - Coarctation.
  - Giant cell arteritis in temporal artery biopsy.
  - Granulomatosis with polyangiitis (GPA) and eosinophilic granulomatosis with polyangiitis (EGPA) in kidney and lung.
  - Leukocytoclastic vasculitis in skin.
  - HSP in skin and kidney.
  - Dissection and aneurysm.

MUST DO

- When studying in groups, work through:
  - How to proceed if a person has died of a suspected cardiac cause, and autopsy reveals a particular finding or reveals no anatomical findings.
  - How to obtain DNA during autopsy to test for channelopathy.
  - Defining sudden cardiac death, classifying causes, and detailing autopsy findings and ancillary workup.
  - Critical values related to vasculitis, transplant rejection, and so on.
  - MI in detail, including risk factors, autopsy findings, microscopic findings, complications, and differential diagnosis.
- You should be able to describe the grossing protocol for key specimens, and independently gross key specimens, including:
  - Cardiac valves removed for degenerative changes.
  - Cardiac valves removed for infective and noninfective endocarditis.
  - Cardiac masses found in autopsy.
  - Endocardial biopsies.
  - Temporal artery biopsies.
  - Thrombi and plaques removed during, for example, endarterectomy.
  - Cardiac explant, including removal of cardiac devices.
  - Autopsy removal of heart.

- You should be able to describe and handle fresh and frozen sections of key specimens. Handling procedures include:
  - Taking tissue from biopsy, resection, or autopsy for special studies such as fluorescence in situ hybridization (FISH), molecular studies, flow cytometry, or electron microscopy.
  - Special handling of biopsy specimens for suspected vasculitis, including procedures for immunofluorescence and electron microscopy (also see chapter 10, Genitourinary and Renal Pathology).

MULTIPLE CHOICE QUESTIONS

1. What is the most likely age of the myocardial infarction in Figure 4.1?
- a. 4–8 hours.
- b. 12–24 hours.
- c. 3 days.
- d. 7 days.
- e. 14 days.

Answer: c

2. Which of the following are complications of acute myocardial infarction?
- a. Ventricular free wall rupture.
- b. Aortic dissection and rupture.
- c. Thrombus in a heart chamber.
- d. Petechial rash.
- e. Answers a and c only.
- f. All of the above.

Answer: e

3. Ventricular rupture in acute myocardial infarction most commonly occurs:
- a. 1 day after onset.
- b. 3–7 days after onset.
- c. 2 weeks after onset.
- d. 1 month after onset.
- e. 3 months after onset.

Answer: b

4. All of the following cause systolic left ventricle dysfunction **except**:
- a. Coronary heart disease (CHD).
- b. Hypertension.
- c. Idiopathic dilated cardiomyopathy.
- d. Alcoholic cardiomyopathy.
- e. Aortic and mitral valvular disease.
- f. Hypertrophic cardiomyopathy (HCM).

Answer: f

5. Polymyalgia rheumatica occurs in which type of vasculitis?
- a. Takayasu arteritis.
- b. Churg-Strauss syndrome (eosinophilic granulomatosis with polyangiitis).
- c. Buerger disease (thromboangiitis obliterans).
- d. Polyarteritis nodosa.
- e. Giant cell (temporal) arteritis.
- f. Wegener granulomatosis (granulomatosis with polyangiitis).
- g. Microscopic polyarteritis.

Answer: e

6. The differential diagnosis for restrictive cardiomyopathy includes the following **except**:
- a. Amyloid cardiomyopathy.
- b. Hemochromatosis.
- c. Radiation.
- d. Sarcoidosis.
- e. Metastatic tumor.
- f. Constrictive pericarditis.
- g. Dilated cardiomyopathy.

Answer: g

7. Cardiac angiosarcoma most commonly occurs in which part of the heart?
- a. Left ventricle.
- b. Right ventricle.
- c. Right atrium.
- d. Left atrium.
- e. Ventricular septum.

Answer: c

8. Figure 4.2 shows a microscopic image of a skin biopsy specimen from a 35-year-old man with skin rashes. What is the most likely diagnosis?
- a. Giant cell arteritis.
- b. Churg-Strauss (eosinophilic granulomatosis with polyangiitis): allergic stage.
- c. Wegener granulomatosis (granulomatosis with polyangiitis).
- d. Polyarteritis nodosa.
- e. Henoch-Schönlein purpura.

Answer: b

9. Figure 4.3 is a gross image of the resected bicuspid aortic valve of a 38-year-old man. What is the most likely diagnosis?
- a. Degenerative calcific aortic stenosis.
- b. Rheumatic heart disease.
- c. Acute infectious endocarditis.
- d. Nonbacterial thrombotic endocarditis.
- e. Libman-Sacks endocarditis.

Answer: a

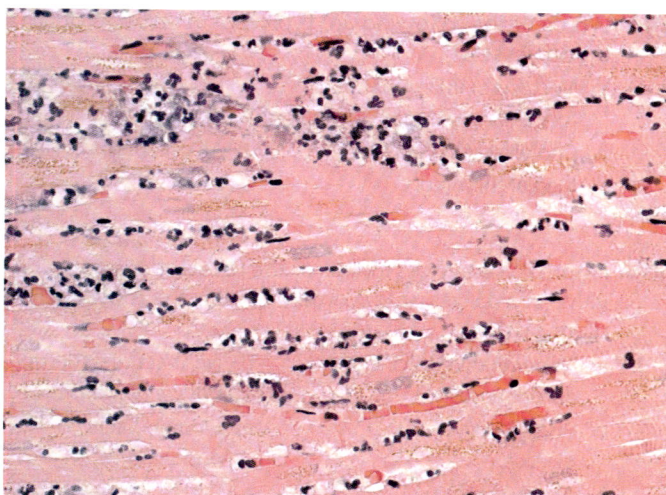

FIGURE 4.1

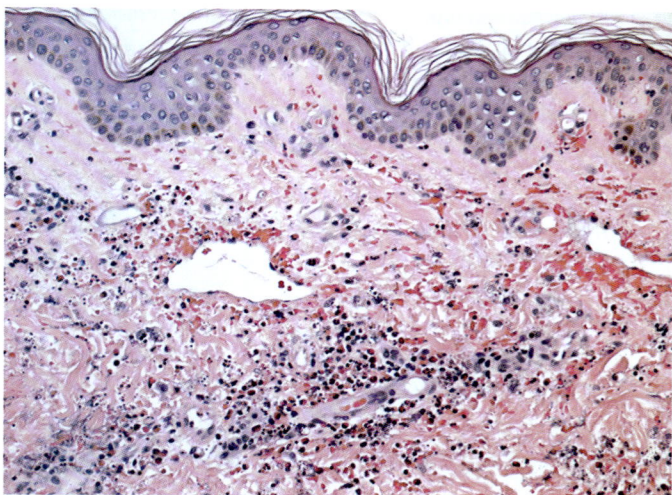

FIGURE 4.2

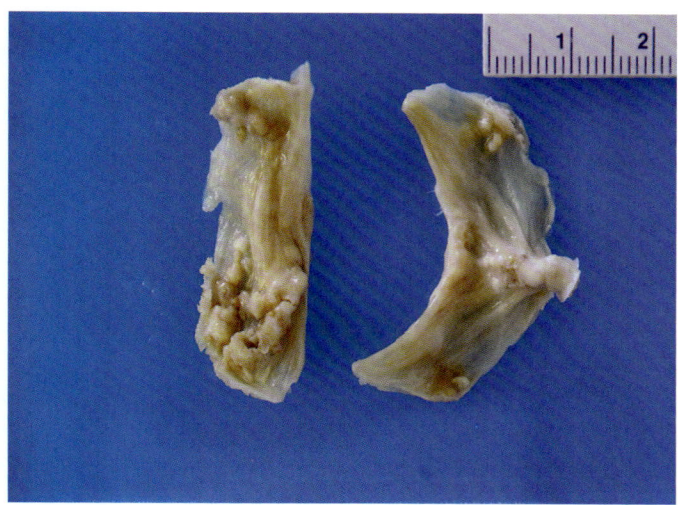

FIGURE 4.3

10. What are common gross changes observed in excised rheumatic mitral valves?

a. Chordal rupture.

b. Leaflet perforations from inflammation.

c. Leaflet and chordal fibrosis.

d. Verrucous endocarditis.

e. Necrotizing granulomas.

Answer: c

11. Figure 4.4 is a microscopic image from a mass resected from the left atrium of a 52-year-old man. Which of the following statements is **not** true regarding this neoplasm?

a. About 10% of these tumors are associated with Carney syndrome.

b. This tumor is the most common primary cardiac tumor in adults.

c. It arises most commonly from the right atrium.

d. The tumor cells often express calretinin and CD34.

e. Gland formation and extramedullary hematopoiesis can be found in this lesion.

Answer: c

12. A 32-year-old female with a history of cocaine use presented with purpura of the lower legs. Figure 4.5 shows a skin biopsy specimen of the purpura. What is the most likely diagnosis?

a. Polyarteritis nodosa.

b. Leukocytoclastic vasculitis.

c. Wegener granulomatosis (granulomatosis with polyangiitis).

d. Giant cell arteritis.

e. Buerger disease.

Answer: b

13. Figure 4.6 is a microscopic image of a temporal artery biopsy specimen from a 65-year-old woman with vision changes. What is your diagnosis?

a. Giant cell arteritis.

b. Churg-Strauss (allergic) vasculitis (eosinophilic granulomatosis with polyangiitis).

c. Wegener granulomatosis (granulomatosis with polyangiitis).

d. Polyarteritis nodosa.

e. Henoch-Schönlein purpura.

Answer: a

14. What are common clinical manifestations of active temporal arteritis?

a. Jaw pain after chewing.

b. Hematuria.

c. Generalized aches and pains.

d. Nodules on legs.

e. Answers a and c only.

f. All of the above.

Answer: e

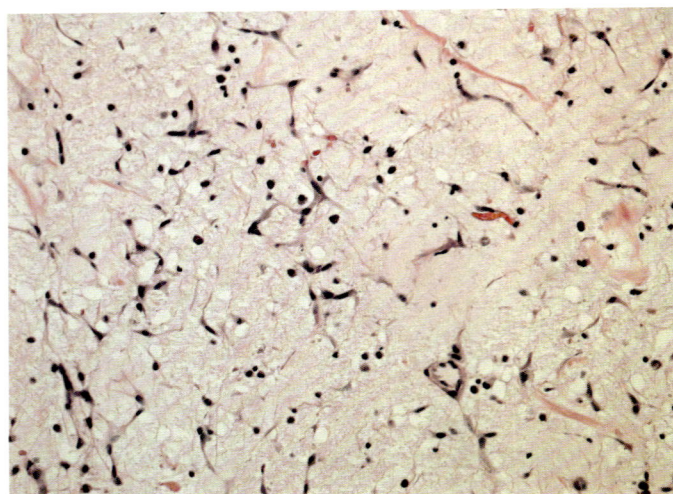

FIGURE 4.4

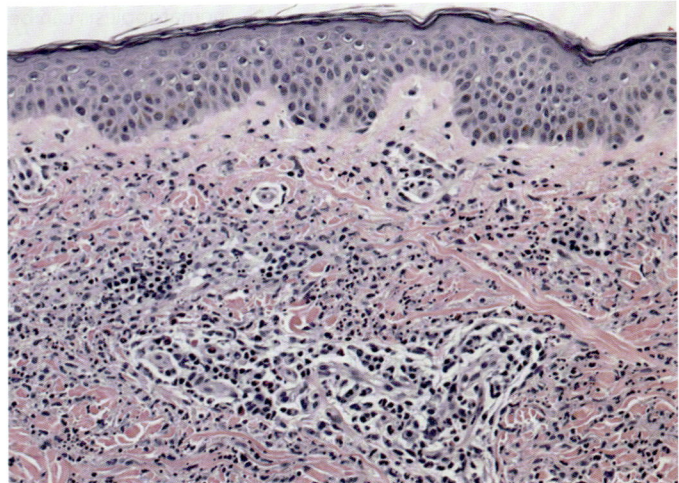

FIGURE 4.5

15. Which of the following are typical of atherosclerotic blood vessels?

   a. Necrosis of inflammatory cells in plaque.

   b. Cholesterol crystals.

   c. Medial thinning.

   d. Fibrinoid necrosis of the media.

   e. All except d.

Answer: e

16. Figure 4.7 is a gross image of the resected mitral valve of a 45-year-old woman. What is the most likely diagnosis?

   a. Degenerative calcific aortic stenosis.

   b. Rheumatic valve disease.

   c. Acute infectious endocarditis.

   d. Nonbacterial thrombotic endocarditis.

   e. Libman-Sacks endocarditis.

Answer: b

17. Aschoff bodies in an endomyocardial biopsy specimen of a 27-year-old woman indicate a diagnosis of:

   a. Acute rheumatic heart disease.

   b. Chronic rheumatic heart disease.

   c. Chagas disease.

   d. Lyme disease.

   e. Toxoplasma myocarditis.

Answer: a

18. An endomyocardial biopsy shows myocyte hypertrophy, myocyte disarray, and interstitial fibrosis. These features are:

   a. Specific for hypertrophic cardiomyopathy.

   b. Specific for dilated cardiomyopathy.

   c. Specific for restrictive cardiomyopathy.

   d. Nonspecific changes.

   e. Specific for systemic arterial hypertension.

Answer: d

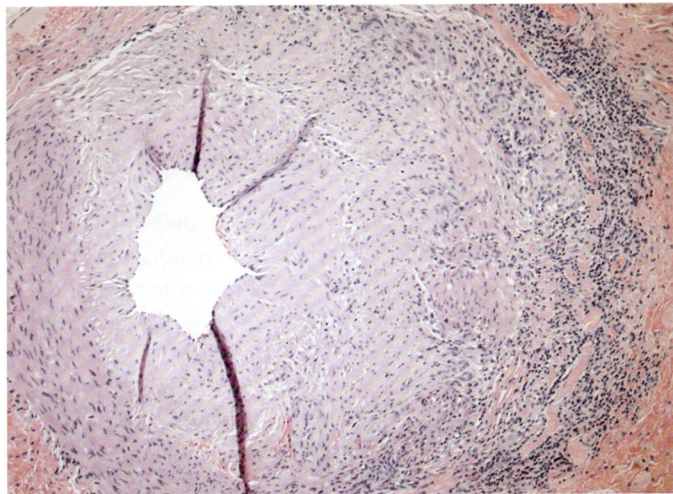

FIGURE 4.6

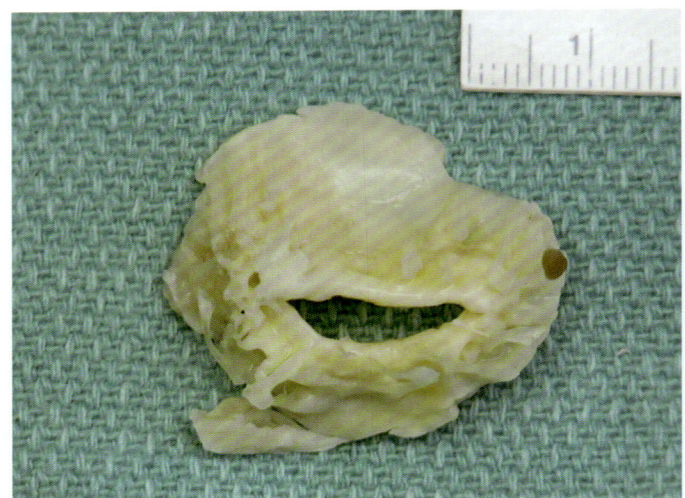

FIGURE 4.7

19. A 25-year-old man presents with progressive exercise intolerance. Auscultation discloses a harsh systolic ejection murmur. Echocardiography shows asymmetric left ventricular hypertrophy. The right ventricle wall is also thickened. The most likely etiology of his heart abnormalities is:

a. Gene mutations in the β-myosin heavy chain.
b. Chronic alcohol abuse.
c. Cardiac amyloid deposits.
d. Hypertension.
e. Deposition of iron (hemochromatosis).

Answer: a

20. The most common cause of myocarditis is:

a. *Streptococcus viridans*.
b. Coxsackievirus A.
c. *Aspergillus*.
d. *Borrelia burgdorferi*.
e. *Trypanosoma cruzi*.

Answer: b

21. A teenage girl has a blackout during exercise. She is referred to a cardiologist who orders an electrocardiogram (ECG). The ECG shows left ventricular hypertrophy and abnormal Q waves. An echocardiogram reveals left ventricular and septal hypertrophy, a small left ventricle, and reduced septal excursion. The septum has a ground-glass appearance. She then dies suddenly. Microscopically, the septum on trichrome stain shows myofiber disarray. Which of the following conditions is she most likely to have had?

a. Rheumatic heart disease.
b. Viral myocarditis.
c. Systemic lupus erythematosus.
d. Hypertrophic cardiomyopathy.
e. Diabetes mellitus.

Answer: d

22. A middle-aged woman has had decreasing exercise tolerance for several years. She is found to have decreased cardiac output with diminished diastolic filling on echocardiography. The heart seems normal sized. Which of the following pathologic findings would best explain this condition?

a. Dilated cardiomyopathy.
b. Rheumatic heart disease.
c. Chronic alcoholism.
d. Coxsackievirus B infection.
e. Constrictive pericarditis.

Answer: e

23. Which of the following can mimic restrictive cardiomyopathy?

a. Amyloidosis.
b. Dilated cardiomyopathy.
c. Constrictive pericarditis.
d. All of the above.
e. Answers a and c only.

Answer: e

24. The dominant coronary artery:

a. Is most commonly the right coronary artery.
b. Supplies the majority of the left ventricle.
c. Gives rise to the posterior descending artery.
d. All of the above.
e. Answers a and c only.

Answer: e

25. Coronary plaque rupture and thrombosis are common features of:

a. Acute myocardial infarction.
b. Chronic stable angina pectoris.
c. Sudden cardiac death.
d. All of the above.
e. Answers a and c only.

Answer: a

26. Circumferential subendocardial myocardial infarction is commonly associated with:

a. Coronary atherosclerosis.
b. Mitral regurgitation.
c. Hypotensive episodes.
d. Coronary artery spasm.
e. Coronary ostial stenosis.

Answer: c

27. Rupture of which of the following could complicate an acute **subendocardial** myocardial infarct?

a. Ventricular free wall.
b. Left ventricular papillary muscle.
c. Ventricular septum.
d. All of the above.
e. Answers a and c only.

Answer: b

28. When a person dies suddenly from a "heart attack," the most likely cause is:

a. Rupture of the heart.
b. Congestive heart failure.
c. Angina.
d. Coronary artery thrombus.
e. Cardiac arrhythmia.

Answer: e

29. Left sided heart failure frequently leads to right sided heart failure because:

a. The basic underlying disease usually involves both heart chambers.
b. Poor perfusion of the right coronary system results from the left ventricular failure.
c. The enlarged left ventricle partially obstructs the pulmonary veins.
d. The enlarged left ventricle partially obstructs the pulmonary arteries.
e. Increased pulmonary arterial pressure strains the right ventricle.

Answer: e

30. Which of the following manifestations of left heart failure may be apparent during autopsy?

a. Heavy lungs.
b. Congested spleen.
c. Congested liver.
d. Ascites.
e. Leg edema.

Answer: a

31. Which is **not** a characteristic of chronic peripheral venous insufficiency?

a. Brown skin discoloration.
b. Toe ulcers.
c. Edema.
d. Bullae.
e. Ulcers above ankle medially.

Answer: b

32. Mitral stenosis, in most instances, is a result of:

a. Bacterial infective endocarditis.
b. Nonbacterial thrombotic endocarditis.
c. Rheumatic fever sequelae.
d. Endocardial fibroelastosis.
e. Congenital anomaly of the valve.

Answer: c

33. Complications of a chronic true postmyocardial infarct left ventricular aneurysm include all of the following **except**:

a. Arrhythmias.
b. Systemic emboli.
c. Cardiac rupture.
d. Mural thrombus.
e. Congestive heart failure.

Answer: c

34. Atherosclerotic aneurysms most commonly occur in the:

a. Ascending aorta.
b. Carotid arteries.
c. Aortic arch.
d. Superior mesenteric artery.
e. Abdominal aorta.

Answer: e

35. Dissection of the aorta may be complicated by all of the following conditions **except**:

a. Aortic regurgitation.
b. Hemopericardium and tamponade.
c. Splenic emboli.
d. Coronary artery occlusion.
e. Stroke (cerebral infarction).

Answer: c

36. Dilated cardiomyopathy may be associated with all of the following **except**:

a. Lymphocytic myocarditis.
b. Peripheral eosinophilia.
c. Chronic alcoholism.
d. Peripartum state.
e. Familial transmission.

Answer: b

37. Endomyocardial biopsy may be indicated for the diagnosis of:

a. Myocarditis.
b. Myocardial infarction.
c. Amyloidosis.
d. Answers a and c only.
e. Answers a and b only.

Answer: d

38. Which of the following are elastic arteries?

a. Aorta.
b. Renal artery.
c. Carotid artery.
d. All of the above.
e. Answers a and c only.

Answer: e

39. Which of the following is true regarding Takayasu disease?

a. It involves the aorta only.
b. It may involve the pulmonary arteries.
c. It affects mainly women over the age of 50 years.
d. It may affect the popliteal arteries.
e. All of the above.

Answer: b

40. Which of the following groupings correctly pairs a disease with the vessels it affects?

a. Giant cell arteritis — muscular and elastic arteries only.
b. Classic polyarteritis nodosa (PAN) — muscular arteries, veins, and capillaries.
c. Buerger disease — leg arteries only.
d. Buerger disease — leg arteries, veins, and capillaries.
e. Answers a and c only.
f. All of the above.

Answer: a

41. Possible outcomes for a congenitally bicuspid aortic valve include:

a. Aortic stenosis.
b. Aortic regurgitation.
c. Infective endocarditis.
d. All of the above.
e. Answers a and c only.

Answer: d

42. Acute fibrinous pericarditis often occurs in combination with:

a. Atrioventricular conduction block.
b. Mitral regurgitation.
c. Myocarditis.
d. Pulmonary hypertension.
e. Coronary artery spasm.

Answer: c

43. A common noninfectious underlying cause of acute pericarditis is:

a. Acute stroke.
b. Chronic obstructive pulmonary disease.
c. Liver failure.
d. Renal failure.
e. Asthma exacerbation.

Answer: d

44. An elderly woman with long-standing systemic arterial hypertension has an aortic valve replacement and an ascending aortic aneurysm resection. What did microscopy of the aorta tissue most likely show?

a. Thrombus.
b. Medial degeneration.
c. Calcification of the media.
d. Adventitial granulomas.
e. Acute dissection.

Answer: b

45. An elderly woman has surgery for a rupturing abdominal aortic aneurysm. Histologically, which of the following is a clue that the aneurysm may be an infected mycotic aneurysm?

a. Large collections of macrophages.
b. Large collections of neutrophils.
c. Fragmentation of the elastic in the media.
d. Amorphous necrotic debris.
e. Recent thrombus.

Answer: b

46. A 58-year-old man had a cardiac transplant 10 years ago. He presents with increasing heart failure. The most likely cause is:

a. Acute cellular rejection.
b. Chronic vascular rejection.
c. Hyperacute rejection.
d. Infective endocarditis.
e. Fibrinous pericarditis.

Answer: b

47. Endomyocardial biopsy is a specific diagnostic modality for which of the following diseases?

a. Hypertrophic cardiomyopathy.
b. Hemochromatosis.
c. Aortic stenosis.
d. Systemic arterial hypertension.
e. Diabetes mellitus myocardial disease.

Answer: b

48. The most common tumor that involves the heart is:

a. Carcinoid tumor.
b. Fibroma.
c. Angiosarcoma.
d. Metastatic tumor.
e. Myxoma.

Answer: d

49. Which cardiac valve is often involved in carcinoid heart disease?

a. Aortic valve.
b. Mitral valve.
c. Tricuspid valve.
d. Pulmonary valve.
e. Tricuspid and pulmonary valves.

Answer: e

50. Carcinoid syndrome occurs in:

a. All patients with gastric carcinoid tumor.
b. Patients with hepatic metastasis of carcinoid tumor.
c. All patients with lung carcinoid tumor.
d. All patients with appendix carcinoid tumor.

Answer: b

51. Which immunohistochemical marker is useful in diagnosis of antibody-mediated rejection (AMR) in cardiac transplantation?

a. CD1a.
b. S100.
c. C4d.
d. AE1/AE3.

Answer: c

52. Which of the following is true regarding the diagnostic criterion for moderate acute cellular rejection in cardiac transplantation?

a. At least 1 focus of myocyte damage associated with lymphocytic infiltration.
b. At least 2 foci of myocyte damage associated with lymphocytic infiltration.
c. Diffuse lymphocytic infiltration without myocyte damage.
d. Endothelial damage such as endothelial cell swelling and endothelial cell pyknosis/karyorrhexis.

Answer: b

53. Which of the following is the most common clinical manifestation in patients with clinically evident cardiac sarcoidosis?

a. Congestive heart failure.
b. Complete heart block.
c. Pericardial effusion.
d. Ventricular tachycardia.

Answer: b

54. Causes of coronary artery dissection include:

a. Aortic dissection.
b. Spontaneous dissection with pregnancy.
c. Dissection following coronary intervention.
d. Pacemaker insertion.
e. Answers a, b, and c.

Answer: e

55. Sarcoidosis of the heart is histologically characterized by:

a. Nonnecrotizing epithelioid granulomas and fibrosis.
b. Diffuse giant cell inflammation with myocyte necrosis.
c. Necrotizing granulomas and fibrosis.
d. Interstitial myocardial inflammation with eosinophils and little myocyte damage.
e. Giant cells and macrophages with emperipolesis.

Answer: a

56. Pulmonary artery and pulmonary trunk sarcomas can include:

a. Leiomyosarcoma.
b. Osteosarcoma.
c. Chondrosarcoma.
d. Myxosarcoma.
e. All of the above.

Answer: e

57. Primary cardiac sarcomas may clinically present with:

a. Pericardial effusion and pericardial constriction.
b. Arrhythmias.
c. Metastases.
d. Heart failure and valve-obstruction-like symptoms.
e. All of the above.

Answer: e

58. Segmental necrotizing arteritis, resembling polyarteritis nodosa in appearance, may be seen in which diseases?

a. Granulomatosis with polyangiitis (Wegener granulomatosis).
b. Rheumatoid arthritis.
c. Systemic lupus erythematosus.
d. All of the above.
e. Answers a and c only.

Answer: d

59. The pathological finding diagnostic of myocardial perforation at endomyocardial biopsy is:

a. Fat by itself.
b. Fat attached to myocardium.
c. Inflammatory cells.
d. Mesothelial cells.
e. Fat with arterioles.

Answer: d

60. Which of the following statements about spontaneous coronary artery dissection is correct?

a. It is more common in males than females.
b. It is more common in females than males.
c. It shows no sex preference.
d. Pregnancy (during or after) is a particular risk factor.
e. Answers b and d.

Answer: e

SHORT ANSWER QUESTIONS

61. List the modifiable and nonmodifiable risk factors for atherosclerosis.

- Modifiable: fat intake, exercise, smoking, dental hygiene, homocystinemia, diabetes mellitus type 2.
- Nonmodifiable: age, sex, family history, genetics (hypercholesterolemia), diabetes mellitus type 1, coagulation abnormalities, primary systemic arterial hypertension.

62. How does atherosclerosis develop?

- Response to injury hypothesis:
  · Endothelial injury causing increased vascular permeability, leukocyte adhesion, and thrombosis.
  · Accumulation of lipoprotein in the vessel wall.
  · Monocyte adhesion to the endothelium followed by migration into the intima, and transformation into macrophages and foam cells.
  · Platelet adhesion.
- · Factors released for smooth muscle cell and macrophage recruitment.
- · Smooth muscle cell proliferation and extracellular matrix production, lipid accumulation extracellularly and intracellularly.
- · Inflammatory cell infiltration.
- · Metalloproteinase release.
- · Plaque complication — cap rupture, thrombus adherence, possible stenosis or embolism.

63. List at least 5 benign vascular neoplasms.

- Hemangioma.
- Angiofibroma.
- Pyogenic granuloma (lobular capillary hemangioma).
- Glomus tumor.
- Lymphangioma.

64. List several examples of immune complex vasculitis.

- Systemic lupus erythematosus vasculitis.
- IgA Henoch-Schönlein purpura.
- Cryoglobulin vasculitis.
- Drug hypersensitivity.
- Rheumatoid vasculitis.

65. How are vasculitides classified?

- Based on the caliber of blood vessel involved, vasculitides are classified as follows:
  · Large vessel vasculitis.
    › Giant cell arteritis.
    › Takayasu arteritis.
  · Medium vessel vasculitis.
    › Polyarteritis nodosa.
    › Kawasaki disease.
  · Small vessel vasculitis.
    › Microscopic polyangiitis.
    › Wegener granulomatosis (granulomatosis with polyangiitis).
    › Churg-Strauss syndrome (eosinophilic granulomatosis with polyangiitis).
    › Henoch-Schönlein purpura.

66. Classify and discuss acquired valvular disease of the left heart.

DATA CATEGORY	MITRAL STENOSIS	MITRAL REGURGITATION	AORTIC STENOSIS	AORTIC REGURGITATION
Etiology (most common)	• Postinflammatory scarring (rheumatic heart disease).	• Mitral valve prolapse (myxomatous degeneration).	• Senile calcification.	• Aortic dilation.
Pathophysiology	• Left atrial enlargement. • Atrial fibrillation.	• Left atrial enlargement. • Left ventricular hypertrophy. • Atrial fibrillation.	• Left ventricular hypertrophy.	• Left ventricular hypertrophy. • Dilated aorta.
Gross characteristics	• Leaflet thickening and commissural fusion. • Shortening, thickening, and fusion of the chordae tendineae.	• Hooding of mitral leaflets. • Leaflets are enlarged, redundant, thickened, and rubbery. • Chordae are elongated, thinned, and occasionally ruptured.	• Calcification within cusps.	• Cusps are from near normal to thickened and calcified, with commissural fusion, depending on the cause.
Microscopic features	• Diffuse fibrosis and neovascularization.	• Attenuation of fibrosa, marked thickening of the spongiosa with myxomatous material.	• Fibrosis. • Calcification.	• From near normal to fibrosis, calcification.

67. What are common causes of failure of cardiac valve prostheses?
- Thrombosis/thromboembolism.
- Prosthetic valve endocarditis.
- Structural deterioration: wear, fracture, cuspal tear, calcification.
- Nonstructural dysfunction: granulation tissue, suture or tissue entrapment, paravalvular leak.

68. What are characteristic features of cardiac lesions of rheumatic fever?
- Acute rheumatic fever:
  · Diffuse pancarditis and Aschoff bodies.
  · Verrucae: vegetations (1–2 mm) due to fibrinoid necrosis within cusps or tendinous cords.
- MacCallum plaques: subendocardial lesions, exacerbated by regurgitant jets, can induce irregular thickenings in the left atrium.
- Chronic rheumatic fever: valvular leaflet or cusp thickening; commissural fusion; shortened, fused, and thickened chordae tendineae; "fish mouth" mitral valve orifice.

69. What is the difference between borderline myocarditis and active myocarditis?
- Borderline: inflammation but no myocyte necrosis.
- Active: inflammation and myocyte necrosis.

70. What would you do and what recommendations would you make with a diagnosis of borderline myocarditis?
- Cut through the block to make sure you have not missed the myocyte necrosis.
- Stain the adjacent sections.
- Recommend a repeat biopsy or follow-up biopsy to the clinician (usual procedure).

71. What features of endomyocardial biopsies differentiate between dilated, hypertrophic, and restrictive cardiomyopathies?
- There are none: all show fibrosis and hypertrophy.
- Disarray can be a normal finding of endomyocardial right ventricular biopsies, and thus not specific for hypertrophic cardiomyopathy.

72. What are the main causes of aortic valve insufficiency and stenosis?
- Insufficiency:
  · Valve: infective endocarditis, rheumatic valve disease, congenitally bicuspid valve.
  · Aorta: aortic aneurysm, annular dilation (many causes including age and congenital heart disease), aortic dissection, aortitis.
- Stenosis:
  · Age related degeneration: calcific degenerative.
  · Congenitally bicuspid valve.
  · Postinflammatory disease: rheumatic valve disease.

73. What are the components of the mitral valve apparatus that are necessary for valve competence?

- Annulus.
- Leaflets.
- Chordae.
- Left ventricular papillary muscles.
- Left ventricle myocardium.

74. In congenital heart disease, the atrioventricular valves (tricuspid and mitral) may be switched to the other side of the heart. Name specific anatomical features that are useful for distinguishing between these 2 valves.

- Septal attachments are present on the tricuspid valve (none on the mitral valve).
- Mitral and atrioventricular valves are continuous: no continuity of tricuspid valve and pulmonary valve due to the infundibular septum.
- Mitral valve has a higher point of insertion on the ventricular septum.
- Mitral valve has 2 leaflets, tricuspid valve has 3 leaflets.

75. List the 4 major anatomic abnormalities of tetralogy of Fallot.

- Ventricular septal defect.
- Overriding aorta.
- Pulmonary stenosis.
- Right ventricular hypertrophy.

76. List examples of systemic or cardiac conditions associated with aortic dissection.

- Congenitally bicuspid aortic valve.
- Systemic arterial hypertension.
- Trauma:
  · Iatrogenic at surgery.
  · Iatrogenic at cardiac catheterization.
- Nonpenetrating blunt chest injury.
- Pregnancy.
- Connective tissue disease — Ehlers-Danlos, Marfan syndromes.
- Giant cell aortitis.

77. List the complications of acute aortic dissection.

- Myocardial infarction.
- Coronary artery dissection.
- Aortic rupture.
- Aortic valve insufficiency.
- Stroke.
- Visceral ischemia.
- Hemopericardium and cardiac tamponade.

78. What are complications of atherosclerotic plaques?

- Thrombosis.
- Plaque rupture.
- Plaque hemorrhage.
- Aneurysm.
- Embolism (thrombus and atheromatous debris).
- Plaque erosion.
- Vessel rupture.

79. You are looking at a surgical report on a piece of aorta removed at the time of a valve replacement and ascending aortic aneurysm resection. Unexpectedly, the specimen has giant cell inflammation. What should you do to work up the case?

- Get a patient history — check for tuberculosis (TB), infections.
- Consider syphilis — get past history, request serology. Note that stains for bacteria are mostly not useful.
- Check if cultures were done in the operating room. Any known infection?
- Check for any systemic disease — rheumatoid arthritis, ankylosing spondylitis, autoimmune, other vasculitis.
- Specify serology tests for rheumatoid factor, antinuclear antibodies (ANA), antineutrophil cytoplasmic antibody (ANCA).
- Call the clinician or surgeon for any critical value.

80. What is stunned myocardium versus hibernating myocardium?

- Stunned:
  · Post–myocardial infarction, noncontractile.
  · Reversible with time.
- Hibernating:
  · Chronic ischemia related (adenosine triphosphate depletion), "myocytolysis."
  · Noncontractile.
  · Reversible with revascularization.

81. Molecular testing at autopsy generally includes testing for which conditions?

- Hypertrophic cardiomyopathy.
- Arrhythmogenic cardiomyopathy.
- QT segment — long QT and short QT.
- Brugada syndrome.
- Catecholaminergic polymorphic ventricular tachycardia (CPVT).

Pericarditis

82. List several causes of constrictive pericarditis.
- Radiation.
- Tuberculosis.
- Cardiac surgery.
- Tumor involvement — secondary or primary tumors.

83. Pericarditis associated with a myocardial infarct can develop early or later. What are the clinical signs and symptoms of pericarditis? What is the pathogenesis of the pericarditis that develops later?
- Clinical signs: chest pain, dyspnea, fever/chills, weakness, occasional S1 + S2 decrease, friction rub, effusion on chest X-ray and/or echocardiogram, ST elevation, decreased QRS amplitude.
- Pathogenesis of later pericarditis: Dressler syndrome (autoimmune).

84. List several causes of fibrinous pericarditis.
- Viral pericarditis/myocarditis.
- Drugs and medications.
- Uremia.
- Collagen vascular disease.
- Trauma.
- Tumor, primary and secondary.
- Myocardial infarct.

Carcinoid Heart Diseases

85. Describe clinical manifestations of carcinoid heart disease:
- Valvular heart disease: tricuspid regurgitation, pulmonary regurgitation, or pulmonary stenosis.
- Coronary artery vasospasm: serotonin can cause vasoconstriction.
- Arrhythmias.
- Carcinoid tumor metastasis directly to the myocardium.
- Episodes of skin flushing, cramps, nausea, vomiting, and diarrhea.

86. Why is right-sided heart failure common in carcinoid heart disease?
Carcinoid heart disease does not spare the right side of the heart; the left side of the heart is spared because the lungs metabolize the vasoactive substances.

87. What are characteristic pathological findings of carcinoid heart disease?
- Endocardial plaques (fibromuscular thickenings) on the inside surfaces of the cardiac chambers and valves.
  - Most commonly involved: right ventricle, tricuspid valve, and pulmonary valve.
- Occasionally involved: venae cava, pulmonary artery, and coronary sinus.

Prosthetic Valves and Grafts

88. List some of the complications of bioprosthetic and mechanical prosthetic heart valves.
- Bioprostheses and mechanical prostheses:
  - Prosthesis size mismatch (valve usually too small).
  - Incorrect surgical position.
  - Suture impingement on disc.
  - Paravalvular leak.
  - Coronary artery ostial occlusion by valve ring.
  - Infective endocarditis.
  - Fibrous pannus.
- Bioprostheses:
  - Leaflet degenerative changes with fibrosis and calcification.
  - Leaflet tears and perforations with degeneration.
- Mechanical prostheses:
  - Cloth wear.
  - Ball or disc emboli or erosion.
  - Ball degeneration and cracking.
  - Stent creep.
  - Thrombosis.

89. List the regions that require thorough examination in assessing a coronary artery bypass graft.
- Bypass graft ostium anastomosis at aorta.
- Bypass graft body.
- Distal anastomosis.
- Distal coronary artery.
- Proximal native coronary artery.
- Coronary artery ostium.

Temporal (Giant Cell) Arteritis

90. List 4 key clinical features of temporal arteritis.
- Vasculitis involving the temporal artery and the aorta are present.
- It is more commonly found in older patients with a variety of symptoms including headaches, fatigue, fever, and vision loss.
- It is often associated with polymyalgia rheumatica.
- Ophthalmic artery involvement may result in irreversible blindness.

91. List 3 histologic features of temporal arteritis.
- Granulomatous inflammation with destruction of the internal elastic lamina.
- Mixed inflammatory cell infiltrate consisting of lymphocytes, eosinophils, and macrophages.
- Healed stage: collagenous scar and neovascularization of the vessel wall.
- Intimal proliferation.
- Medial fibrosis.

92. How do you process temporal artery biopsy specimens?
- A segment (generally 2–3 cm) of the superficial temporal artery is biopsied to evaluate giant cell arteritis.
- The artery should be placed in the cassette and tissue processed.
- The artery should then be cut into small cross-sections and embedded.
- Multiple levels are needed.

93. What is the clinical significance of a temporal artery biopsy with negative results?
- Because of the segmental nature of giant cell arteritis, biopsies may produce negative results.
- Negative biopsies do not rule out the disease.
- Glucocorticoid treatment should be started as soon as a diagnosis of giant cell arteritis is strongly suspected. Even after treatment, the sequelae of inflammation will be evident.

Mitral Valve Prolapse

94. List 4 key clinical features of mitral valve prolapse.
- It most commonly occurs in young women.
- It is often an incidental finding with a midsystolic click on auscultation.
- It is associated with Marfan syndrome.
- Complications include infective endocarditis, mitral insufficiency, ventricular arrhythmia.

95. List some pathological features of mitral valve prolapse (myxomatous degeneration of the mitral valve).
- Interchordal ballooning (hooding) of the mitral leaflets.
- Enlarged, redundant, thick, and rubbery leaflets.
- Elongated and thinned tendinous cords — occasionally ruptured.
- Annular dilatation.
- Microscopic features: attenuated fibrosa layer of the valve and thickened spongiosa layer with myxomatous degeneration.

96. List some clinical complications of mitral valve prolapse.
- Mitral valve regurgitation.
- Arrhythmias.
- Endocarditis.
- Chordae tendinae rupture.
- Embolism (stroke).

97. What is the pathogenesis of mitral valve prolapse?
Degenerative (myxomatous) disease.

Angiosarcoma

98. List 3 clinical features of angiosarcoma.
- It often occurs in older adults; it may affect patients receiving radiation therapy for breast cancer (rare).
- It most commonly occurs in the skin, soft tissue, breast, and liver.
- It is characterized by rapid growth, leading to ulcers and hemorrhage.

99. List some histologic features of angiosarcoma.
- Anastomosing vascular channels lined by atypical endothelial cells with frequent mitotic figures and necrosis.
- Possible presence of all degrees of differentiation, from those that are obviously vascular to undifferentiated tumors.

100. List 3 causes of angiosarcoma.
- Vinyl chloride.
- Radiation.
- Lymphedema.

101. What is the immunohistochemical profile of angiosarcoma?
Tumor cells are positive for CD31, CD34, and factor VIII.

Endocarditis

102. How do you classify endocarditis?

INFECTIVE ENDOCARDITIS (IE)	NONINFECTIVE ENDOCARDITIS
• Native valve endocarditis. • Prosthetic valve endocarditis, early and late. • Intravenous drug abuse endocarditis.	• Nonbacterial thrombotic endocarditis (NBTE). • Endocarditis of systemic lupus erythematosus (Libman-Sacks disease). • Verrucous endocarditis — acute rheumatic fever.

103. List some gross and microscopic features of each type of endocarditis.

TYPE OF ENDOCARDITIS	GROSS FEATURES	MICROSCOPIC FEATURES
Acute IE	• Bulky, irregular, friable vegetations on the valve cusps. • Valve destruction. • Abscess.	• Fibrin. • Inflammatory cells. • Bacteria or other organisms. • Destruction of the valve.
Healing IE	• Smaller, friable vegetations.	• Granulation tissue at the base of the vegetations. • Chronic inflammatory cells.
Rheumatic heart disease	• A row of small, warty vegetations along the lines of closure of the valve.	• Aschoff bodies. • Anitschkow cells. • Fibrin. • Inflammatory cells.
NBTE	• Small, bland vegetations, usually attached at the line of valve closure.	• Bland thrombus. • No inflammatory reaction. • No valve damage.
Libman-Sacks	• Small or medium-sized vegetations on either or both sides of the valve.	• Fibrin. • Cellular debris. • Inflammatory cells. • No polymorphs, usually.

104. List several predisposing conditions of infective endocarditis.
- Rheumatic heart disease.
- Myxomatous mitral valve.
- Bicuspid aortic valve.
- Prosthetic (artificial) valves.

105. How do you grossly evaluate an aortic valve?
- Assess the number of recognizable cusps, their size, and their consistency.
- If there is an abnormality of the cusps, describe the distribution, surface, and location of the abnormality.
- If there is any commissural fusion, describe the relationship of the cusps.
- Describe any vegetations.
- Submit representative sections taken from the free edge to the annulus.

106. You are doing an autopsy on a patient with endocarditis. What do you look for?
- Vegetations on aortic valve and mitral valve.
- Vegetations on pulmonary valve and tricuspid valve for IV drug abusers.
- Any valve abnormalities such as perforation or indentation, or ruptured chordae.
- Ring abscess.
- Septic emboli: skin (Janeway lesions, Osler nodes), brain, kidney, and other organs.

Systemic Lupus Erythematosus (SLE)

107. List 3 risk factors for SLE.
- Young women.
- Ethnicity: African-Americans, Hispanics, and Asians.
- Family history.

108. What are possible SLE triggers?
- Cold temperature.
- Fatigue.
- Stress.
- Chemicals.
- Sunlight.
- Certain drugs.

109. List 3 cardiac manifestations of SLE.
- Pericarditis.
- Myocarditis.
- Endocarditis: noninfective Libman-Sacks endocarditis.

Berry Aneurysms

110. List 3 systemic conditions associated with berry aneurysms.
- Autosomal dominant polycystic kidney disease.
- Systemic arterial hypertension.
- Atherosclerosis.

111. What are the histologic features of berry aneurysms?
- They exhibit deficiency of elastic and muscle tissue with dilatation (thinning) of the vessel wall.
- The arterial wall adjacent to the neck of the aneurysm shows intimal thickening and attenuation of the media.
- Smooth muscle and intimal elastic lamina do not extend into the neck and are absent from the aneurysm sac itself, which is made of thickened hyalinized intima and a covering of adventitia.

112. List 4 common causes of subarachnoid hemorrhage.
- Head trauma.
- Rupture of an intracranial berry (saccular) aneurysm.
- Vascular malformations.
- Tumors.

Wegener Granulomatosis (Granulomatosis With Polyangiitis)

113. What are the clinical findings of Wegener granulomatosis?
- Persistent pneumonitis with bilateral nodular and cavitary infiltrates.
- Chronic sinusitis, mucosal ulcerations of the nasopharynx.
- Renal disease including hematuria and proteinuria.

114. List 3 histologic features of Wegener granulomatosis.
- Acute necrotizing granulomas of the respiratory tract.
- Necrotizing or granulomatous vasculitis affecting small to medium-sized vessels.
- Renal disease: focal necrotizing and crescentic glomerulonephritis.

115. List 3 common sites involved in Wegener granulomatosis.
- Upper and lower respiratory tract.
- Kidney.
- Peripheral vessels.

116. Which ANCA subtype is associated with Wegener granulomatosis?
c-ANCA (PR3-ANCA).

117. List 2 pathogenetic causes of Wegener granulomatosis.
- Hypersensitivity.
- Immunologic mechanism: immune complexes.

118. List 2 major differentials of Wegener granulomatosis.
- Sarcoidosis: nonnecrotizing granulomas without vasculitis, negative ANCA.
- Polyarteritis nodosa (PAN): varying stages of vasculitis of small to medium-sized arteries.

Churg-Strauss (Allergic) Vasculitis (Eosinophilic Granulomatosis With Polyangiitis)

119. List at least 4 clinical features of Churg-Strauss vasculitis.
- It is associated with asthma, allergic rhinitis, lung infiltrates, and peripheral hypereosinophilia.
- Skin lesions are present: urticaria and palpable purpura.
- It typically occurs in young adults.
- It is positive for p-ANCA (MPO-ANCA).
- It may present with gastrointestinal tract bleeding.
- It may present with renal disease (focal and segmental glomerulosclerosis).
- It may present with cardiomyopathy (which accounts for half of the deaths from the syndrome).

120. What are the histologic characteristics of Churg-Strauss vasculitis (eosinophilic granulomatosis with polyangiitis)?
- Presence of effects in small sized arteries and veins (typically).
- Necrotizing vasculitis with eosinophilic infiltrate and granulomatous reaction.

Sudden Cardiac Death (SCD)

121. What is sudden cardiac death?
Unexpected death from cardiac causes that occurs without symptoms or within 1–24 hours of symptom onset.

122. List possible causes of SCD.
- Ischemic heart disease — coronary artery disease is the leading cause (80–90% of cases).
- Congenital structural or coronary arterial abnormalities.
- Aortic valve stenosis.
- Mitral valve prolapse.
- Myocarditis.
- Dilated or hypertrophic cardiomyopathy.
- Pulmonary hypertension.
- Hereditary or acquired abnormalities of the cardiac conduction system.
- Isolated left ventricular hypertrophy, due to systemic arterial hypertension or unknown causes.

123. When should a pathologist consider doing a conduction system examination, or referring a cardiac patient for conduction system examination?
- Sudden death with normal heart examination.
- Cardiomyopathies.
- Atrioventricular block including complete heart block.
- Certain arrhythmias where conduction system abnormalities are noted (e.g., accessory pathways).
- Sarcoidosis.
- Conduction problems post aortic valvular surgery.
- After cardiac arrhythmia ablation procedures (e.g., accessory pathways or atrial flutter).

124. What signs at autopsy reflect heart failure?
- Right heart failure:
  - Ascites.
  - Organomegaly (especially liver and spleen).
  - Peripheral edema.
  - Stasis dermatitis.
- Left heart failure:
  - Pleural effusions.
  - Heavy lungs.
  - Pulmonary edema.

Kaposi Sarcoma (KS)

125. How is KS classified?
- Classic Kaposi sarcoma: eastern European and Mediterranean males.
- Endemic Kaposi sarcoma: people indigenous to central Africa.
- Epidemic Kaposi sarcoma: HIV patients.
- Kaposi sarcoma in iatrogenic immunocompromised patients: transplant patients.

126. List some clinical features of KS.
- Patients have erythematous to violaceous cutaneous lesions (macular, patch, plaque, nodular, and exophytic).
- The cutaneous lesions can be solitary, localized, or disseminated.
- KS can involve the oral cavity, lymph nodes, and viscera.

127. List the histologic features of KS.
- Slit-like spaces, extravasated red blood cells, plasma cells.
- Proliferation of spindle shaped cells arranged as short fascicles, and diffuse proliferation of blood vessels.
- Later stage: greater degrees of cytological atypia, high mitotic rate.

128. What causes KS?
Human herpesvirus 8 (HHV-8) is responsible for all varieties of Kaposi sarcoma.

129. What is the differential diagnosis of KS?
- Benign vascular proliferations: targetoid hemosiderotic hemangioma, fibrous histiocytoma.
- Angiosarcoma.

Endocarditis

130. List 4 intracardiac complications of endocarditis.
- Valvular destruction.
- Paravalvular destruction/abscess.
- Valvular incompetence.
- Sinus of valsalva aneurysm.

131. List some common causative organisms of endocarditis in drug abusers.
- *Staphylococcus aureus.*
- *Staphylococcus epidermidis.*

132. What 4 possible features of endocarditis would suggest a worse prognosis?
- Acute endocarditis (*Staphylococcus aureus*).
- Heart failure.
- Intravenous drug abuse (often left- and right-sided disease).
- Prosthetic valve infection.
- Fungal endocarditis.
- Complications with ring or root abscesses or fistulas.

Aortic Dissection

133. List some common causes of aortic dissection.
- Inherited syndromes (Marfan, Loeys-Dietz, and Ehlers Danlos syndromes).
- Systemic arterial hypertension.
- Trauma.
- Infection.

134. What is the pathogenesis of aortic dissection?
Aortic dissection occurs when a tear of the intima of the aortic wall causes dissection of blood between and along the laminar planes of the media.

135. Describe the classification of aortic dissection.
- Stanford classification:
  · Type A: involves either ascending aorta only, or both the ascending and descending aorta.
  · Type B: involves the descending aorta only (usually distal to left subclavian artery origin).
- DeBakey classification:
  · I: involves ascending aorta and rest of aorta.
  · II: involves ascending aorta only.
  · III: arises after the ascending aorta.

136. List some clinical features of aortic dissection.
- Severe pain — usually back pain.
- Dyspnea.
- Limb pain from ischemia.
- Organ or visceral pain from infarction or ischemia.
- Stroke signs.

137. What are the effects of chronic systemic arterial hypertension on the heart, and on the large and small blood vessels?
- Heart: left ventricular hypertrophy, cardiac myocyte hypertrophy, interstitial myocardial fibrosis.
- Large blood vessels: increased atherosclerosis, aortic dissection, aortic aneurysms.
- Small blood vessels: retinopathy, nephrosclerosis, acute and chronic renal failure, cerebral infarct, and hemorrhage.

Antineutrophil Cytoplasmic Antibody (ANCA)

138. What is ANCA?
- Antineutrophil cytoplasmic antibody.
  - Acts against antigens in the cytoplasm of neutrophil granulocytes and monocytes.
- Mostly comprises IgG antibodies.
- Is particularly associated with systemic vasculitis.

139. List the 2 most common subtypes of ANCA.
- Most common subtypes: p-ANCA (MPO-ANCA) and c-ANCA (PR3-ANCA).
- p-ANCA (MPO-ANCA): perinuclear antineutrophil cytoplasmic antibody.
  - Staining pattern: perinuclear.
  - Target antigen: myeloperoxidase.
- c-ANCA (PR3-ANCA): cytoplasmic antineutrophil cytoplasmic antibody.
  - Staining pattern: diffuse, granular, cytoplasmic.
  - Target antigen: proteinase 3.

140. If a patient is positive for ANCA, what caliber or types of vessels could be affected by ANCA associated vasculitis?
- Small arteries, arterioles, venules, veins, and capillaries.
- Rarely large elastic arteries.

141. What is the clinical significance of positive ANCA?
- ANCA is associated with 3 primary diseases:
  - Wegener granulomatosis: c-ANCA.
  - Microscopic polyangiitis: p-ANCA.
  - Glomerulonephritis: p-ANCA.
- ANCA is also found in other diseases, such as Churg-Strauss syndrome (eosinophilic granulomatosis with polyangiitis) (p-ANCA), ulcerative colitis, and ankylosing spondylitis.

142. How is ANCA measured?
Generally with enzyme-linked immunosorbent assay (ELISA) and indirect immunofluorescence.

Immune Complex Mediated Vasculitis

143. What is the pathogenesis of noninfectious vasculitis?
- The main pathogenesis is initiated by:
  - Immune complex deposition within a vessel wall.
  - Antineutrophil cytoplasmic antibodies (ANCAs).
  - Antiendothelial cell antibodies.

144. List 5 examples of immune complex vasculitis.
- Essential cryoglobulinemic vasculitis: cryoglobulins, associated with hepatitis C.
- Hypersensitivity vasculitis (leukocytoclastic vasculitis): medications/drugs.
- Henoch-Schönlein purpura: IgA-containing immune complexes.
- Lupus vasculitis.
- Rheumatoid vasculitis.

Cardiac Myxoma and Neoplasms

145. List most common primary cardiac neoplasms in adults.
- Myxoma.
- Papillary fibroelastoma.
- Rhabdomyoma.

146. List most common primary cardiac neoplasms in children.
- Rhabdomyoma.
- Fibroma.
- Sarcoma.

147. What is the origin of myxoma tumor cells?
Probably primitive multipotential mesenchymal cells.

148. Cardiac myxoma is most commonly located in which part of the heart?
Left atrial septum near the fossa ovalis.

149. What are the gross and microscopic features of cardiac myxoma?
- Gross:
  - Appearance varies from a soft, gelatinous, and papillary mass to a firm, smooth surface.
  - Cut surface shows a variegated appearance with areas of hemorrhage and degenerative changes.
  - Calcification is present.
- Microscopic:
  - "Myxoma" cells are stellate, ovoid, or polygonal with inconspicuous nucleoli, eosinophilic cytoplasm, and indistinct borders.
  - Cells may form rings, ribbons, glandular structures, and cords.
  - There is a background of myxoid and loose fibrous tissue with scattered lymphocytes, hemosiderin laden macrophages, and a capillary network.

150. List the immunohistochemistry characteristics of cardiac myxoma.
"Myxoma" cells are often positive for CD34 and calretinin.

Primary Cardiomyopathies

151. How are primary cardiomyopathies classified?

CARDIOMYOPATHY TYPE	DILATED CARDIOMYOPATHY	HYPERTROPHIC CARDIOMYOPATHY	RESTRICTIVE CARDIOMYOPATHY

Etiology	• 30–40% gene mutations.
	• Others:
	  · Myocarditis.
	  · Toxic (e.g., alcohol).
	  · Peripartum.
	  · Idiopathic.
		• 100% gene mutations in sarcomere (actin, β-myosin heavy chain, troponin I/T, a-tropomyosin).
		• Autosomal dominant inheritance.
			• Amyloidosis.
			• Sarcoidosis.
			• Endomyocardial fibrosis.
			• Loeffler endomyocarditis.
			• Endocardial fibroelastosis.
			• Radiation.
			• Metabolic diseases.
			• Idiopathic.

Pathophysiology	• Ventricular systolic dysfunction.	• Diastolic dysfunction.	• Diastolic dysfunction.
Gross features	• 4 chamber dilation. • Bilateral ventricular hypertrophy or thinning. • Mural thrombi. • Endocardial fibrosis.	• Left ventricular hypertrophy. • "Banana-like" configuration of left ventricular cavity. • Asymmetric septal hypertrophy. • Endocardial thickening of the aortic outflow tract and the anterior mitral leaflet.	• Amyloidosis: firm, rubbery, thick walls. • Sarcoidosis: firm, parenchymal scarring (fibrosis).
Microscopic features	• Variable myocyte hypertrophy. • Interstitial and endocardial fibrosis.	• Extensive myocyte hypertrophy. • Haphazard disarray of bundles of myocytes, individual myocytes, or myofibers. • Interstitial fibrosis.	• Amyloidosis: nodular and/or pericellular amyloid deposits (apple-green birefringence by polarization with Congo red stain), and myocyte atrophy. • Sarcoidosis: nonnecrotizing granulomatous inflammation and fibrosis. • Idiopathic: interstitial fibrosis.

Myocardial Contraction Band Necrosis (CBN)

152. What is the morphologic feature of CBN?
On H&E section, contraction bands are eosinophilic staining bands that cross the short axis of the myocyte.

153. What is the pathogenesis of CBN?
- Causes irreversible myocardial injury.
- May occur in the setting of reperfusion injury of the myocardium.
- Is mediated by fluctuations in calcium concentration causing sarcomere hypercontraction.
- Can be an artifact often seen in an endomyocardial biopsy specimen.

Endomyocardial Biopsy (EMB)

154. What is the role of endomyocardial biopsy?
- It remains the gold standard for surveillance of cardiac transplant rejection and for diagnosing myocarditis.
- It is often helpful for diagnosis or monitoring of primary cardiomyopathies, amyloidosis, sarcoidosis, drug toxicities, Fabry disease, endocardial fibrosis, and neoplasia.

155. What is the best way to approach an endomyocardial biopsy?
- Interpretation of EMB specimens: requires the patient's clinical information and an appropriate understanding of cardiovascular pathophysiology.
- Adequacy: requires ≥ 4 good pieces of myocardium.
- Evaluation: requires careful attention to each component of the biopsy specimen — endocardium, myocardium, interstitium, and vasculature.
- Final report: should include the biopsy site, type of biopsy, and clinically relevant information including diagnosis, grading scheme, and a detailed microscopic description.

156. What are the characteristic findings of arterial and venous diseases of the legs?
- Arterial disease: deep distinct ulcers, gangrene, muscular atrophy, hair loss, toenail thickening, mottling.
- Venous disease: congestion, varices, shallow medial malleolar ulcers, stasis dermatitis with skin flaking and brownish discoloration.

Case Scenario

A 50-year-old male, who is a heavy smoker with a prior history of lung carcinoma, presents with shortness of breath and increasing fatigue. The clinician suspects clinical tamponade, constrictive pericarditis, or restrictive cardiomyopathy.

157. What are the clinical manifestations of tamponade?
Decreased heart sounds, decreased pulse, and increased jugular venous pressure.

158. What would an endomyocardial biopsy specimen show?
- Constrictive pericarditis:
  - Specimens show atrophy of cardiac myocytes or normal myocardium.
- Restrictive cardiomyopathy:
  - Specimens show fibrosis, and myocyte hypertrophy and degeneration.
  - Causes include cardiomyopathic changes, storage disease, amyloid, drug toxicity.

159. Pericardial tap yields a bloody effusion. What should be done with the specimen?
- Cultures (routine and mycobacterial).
- Cytology (often with cell block).

Case Scenario

A 79-year-old man is diagnosed with calcific aortic stenosis.

160. What kind of calcification is calcific aortic stenosis?
It is dystrophic calcification, which occurs in degenerated or necrotic tissue, and it is also active calcification with cholesterol, inflammation, and fibrosis very similar to atherosclerosis.

161. List at least 3 examples of dystrophic calcification.
- Leiomyoma.
- Calcification of a postinfarct ventricular aneurysm.
- Hyalinized scar.
- Tumor necrosis.
- Old granuloma.
- Fat necrosis.

162. What are 5 key gross features of rheumatic heart disease?
- Acute rheumatic fever may show small verrucous vegetations along the lines of valve closure.
- MacCallum patch may be evident: a thickening of the left atrial endocardium proximal to the base of the posterior mitral valve leaflet.
- The leaflets are thickened and show commissural fusion.
- The chordae are thickened, shortened, and fused.
- Fibrosis and calcification create a "fish mouth" orifice of the mitral valve.

Case Scenario

A previously healthy 40-year-old man dies suddenly.

163. List at least 3 possible causes for this sudden death, excluding cardiomyopathy.
- Mitral valve prolapse.
- Ischemic heart disease.
- Congenital structural abnormalities.
- Abnormalities of coronary arterial origin or arterial course.
- Aortic valve stenosis.
- Arrhythmia (hereditary or acquired).

164. List the 3 common types of cardiomyopathy.
- Dilated cardiomyopathy.
- Hypertrophic cardiomyopathy.
- Restrictive cardiomyopathy.

Case Scenario

A patient dies of diastolic heart disease with a history of constriction or restriction.

165. What gross and microscopic features do you look for in the heart?
- A thickened pericardium with/without necrosis.
- Dilated atria with normal sized ventricles.

166. What clinical history would this case prompt you to ask for?
Obtain a clinical history for hematological disorders, systemic arterial hypertension, amyloidosis, and hemochromatosis — e.g., myeloma, monoclonal gammopathy of uncertain significance (MGUS), renal disease, diabetes mellitus, bronze skin color, easy bleeding, and chronic infection (especially TB).

167. Are any special stains required on your heart sections for this case?
- Iron stain for hemochromatosis.
- Congo red, sulfated Alcian blue for amyloid detection.

Case Scenario

A young teenager dies during exercise.

168. What are the important causes to rule out in the investigation?
- Consider the probability that it is a cardiac related death.
- Consider HCM, anomalous coronary artery insertion, undiagnosed congenital heart disease.
- Check for pneumothorax.
- Do toxicology.
- Get a history to see if commotio cordis is a possibility.

169. Is there anything special to do at autopsy?
- Freeze blood, heart, and spleen tissue for possible molecular testing.
- Consider referral of heart for detailed cardiac pathology examination.

College of American Pathologists (CAP) Protocol for Examining and Reporting Tumors of the Heart

170. What are the main histologic types of malignant tumors of the heart?
- Angiosarcoma.
- Epithelioid hemangioendothelioma.
- Undifferentiated pleomorphic sarcoma.
- Fibrosarcoma.
- Myxoid fibrosarcoma.
- Rhabdomyosarcoma.
- Leiomyosarcoma.
- Osteosarcoma.
- Synovial sarcoma.
- Liposarcoma.
- Lymphoma (not included in this protocol; use heme protocol).
- Pericardial tumors:
  · Malignant mesothelioma.
  · Germ cell tumors.

171. What elements should be reported?

- Specimen procedure.
- Specimen integrity.
- Specimen laterality.
- Tumor site.
- Tumor size.
- Histologic type.

- Histologic grade.
- Tumor extension.
- Margins.
- Treatment effect.
- Lymphovascular invasion.

172. How are cardiac tumors graded?

Since most tumors are sarcoma, the FNCLCC (Fédération Nationale des Centres de Lutte Contre le Cancer) grading system is used.

- Tumor differentiation:
  - Score 1: sarcomas closely resembling normal adult mesenchymal tissue (e.g., low grade leiomyosarcoma).
  - Score 2: sarcomas for which histologic typing is certain (e.g., myxoid fibrosarcoma).
  - Score 3: undifferentiated, angiosarcoma.
- Mitotic count:
  - Score 1: 0–9 mitoses per 10 high power field (HPF).*
  - Score 2: 10–19 mitoses per 10 HPF.

- Score 3: ≥ 20 mitoses per 10 HPF.
- Tumor necrosis:
  - Score 0: no necrosis.
  - Score 1: < 50% tumor necrosis.
  - Score 2: ≥ 50% tumor necrosis.
- Histologic grade:
  - Grade 1: total score 2, 3.
  - Grade 2: total score 4, 5.
  - Grade 3: total score 6, 7, 8.

*Note: 1 HPF measures 0.1734 mm².

173. What is the pTNM staging for tumors of the heart?

There is no published staging system for primary cardiac tumors.

IMAGES: CARDIOVASCULAR PATHOLOGY

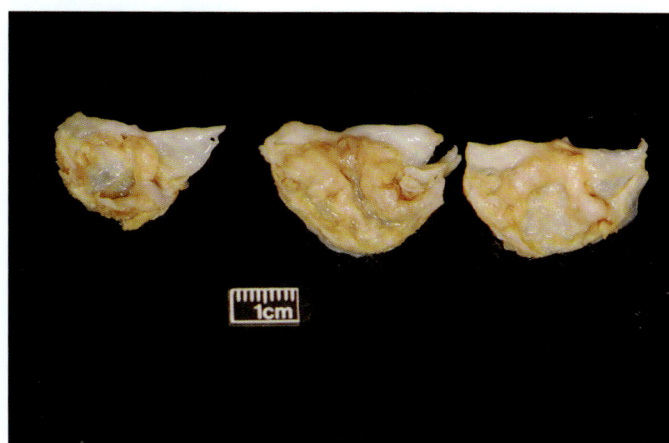

IMAGE 4.1 Excised aortic valve with age related degeneration showing 3 cusps with focal calcification. This is the most common cause of surgically excised aortic valve stenosis.

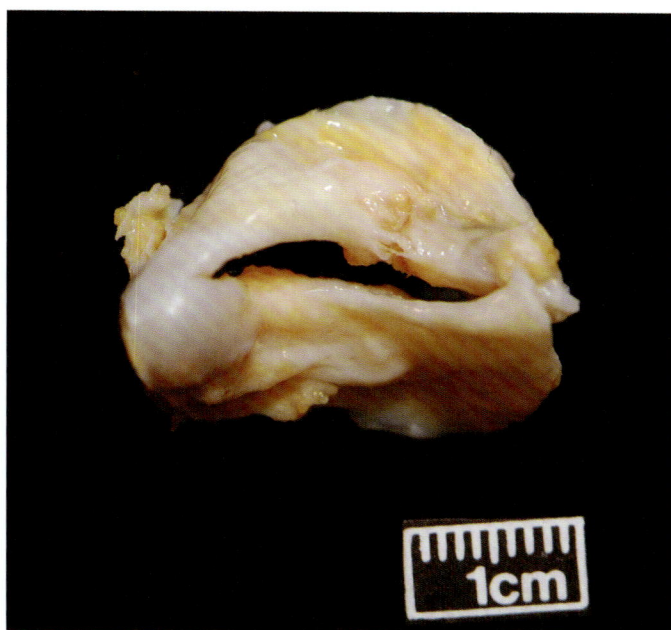

IMAGE 4.2 Congenitally bicuspid aortic valve with fibrosis and calcification. Only 2 cusps are present.

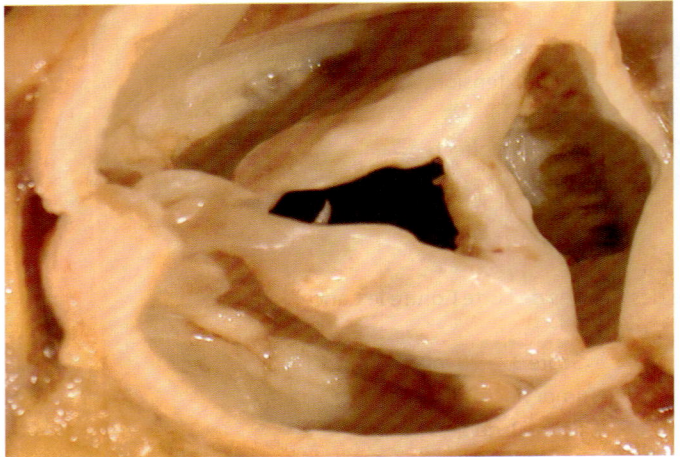

IMAGE 4.3 Rheumatic aortic valve stenosis. The image shows 3 cusps with commissural fusion.

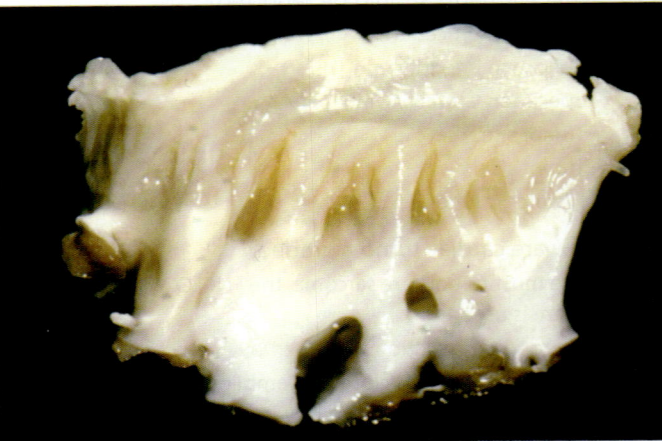

IMAGE 4.6 Rheumatic mitral valve stenosis. The image shows severe thickening and fusion of the chordae.

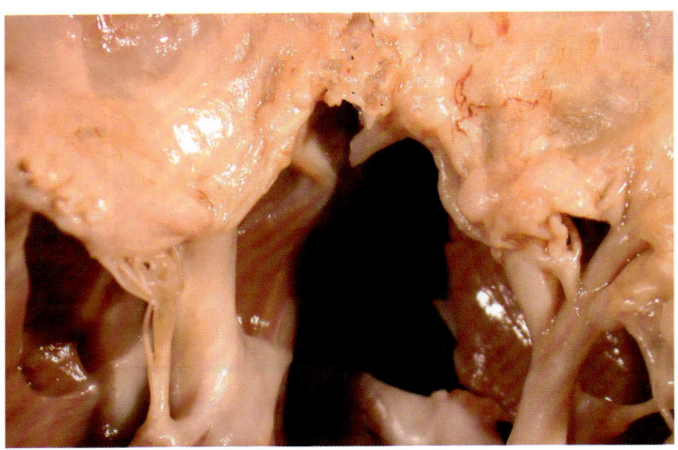

IMAGE 4.4 Tricuspid valve in a patient with carcinoid disease. The image shows fibromuscular plaques which thicken and distort the leaflets and chordae.

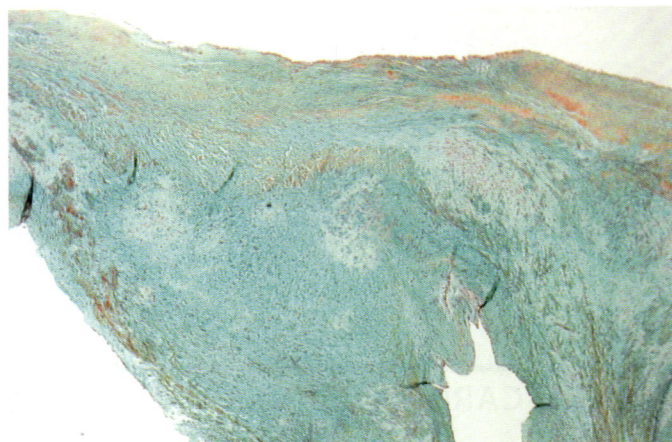

IMAGE 4.7 Myxomatous mitral valve. The image shows abundant bluish ground substance in the valve spongiosa layer, making the valve prone to prolapse (Movat pentachrome, x20).

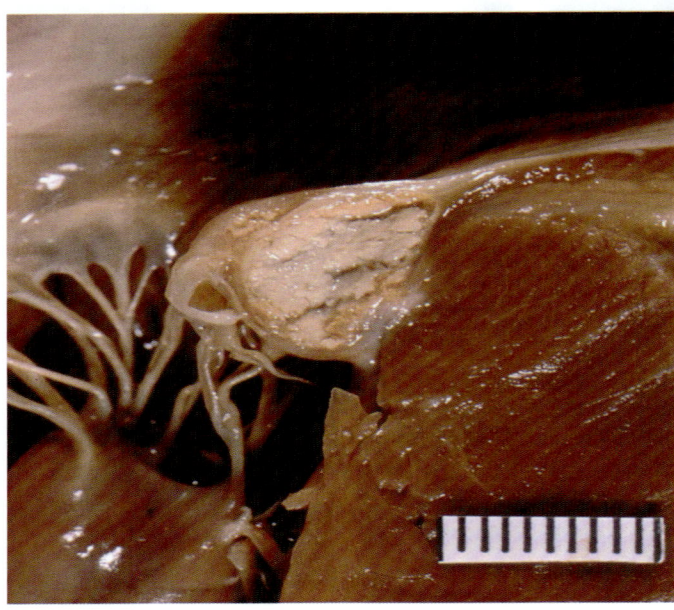

IMAGE 4.5 Mitral annular calcification.

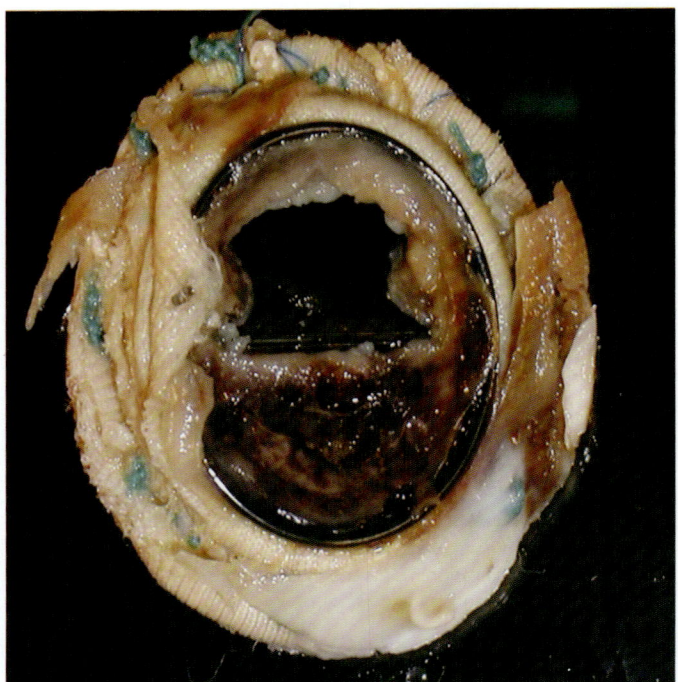

IMAGE 4.8 Mechanical bileaflet prosthesis with thrombosis. This common complication with mechanical prostheses justifies anticoagulation therapy.

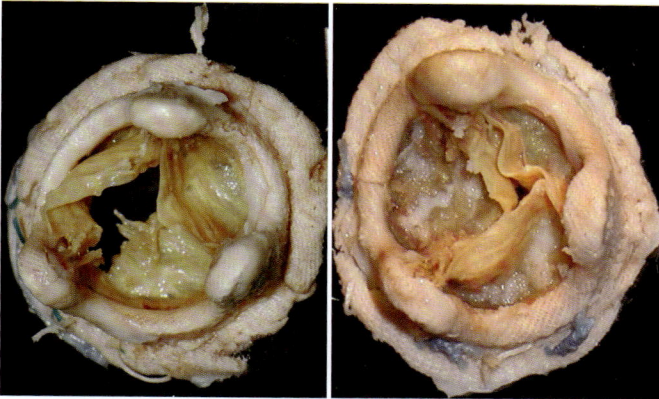

IMAGE 4.9 Bioprosthetic porcine valve. Left: degeneration and cusp tears. Right: cusp degeneration and calcification. These are the common cause of failure of these bioprosthetic valves.

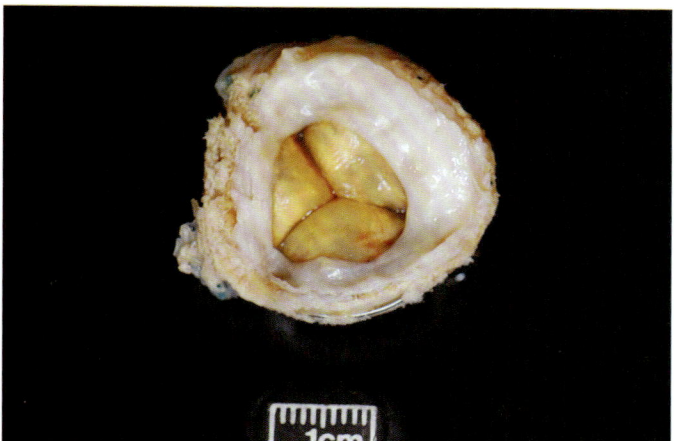

IMAGE 4.10 Excised bioprosthetic heart valve with white pannus material over the valve inflow indicating pannus related prosthesis stenosis.

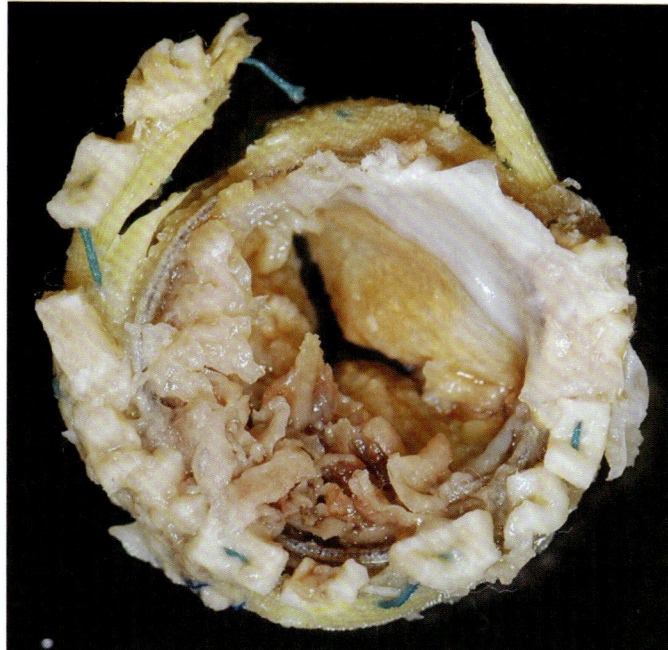

IMAGE 4.11 Excised cardiac valve bioprosthesis with infective endocarditis. Note the tan infected thrombus over the valve cusps and ring.

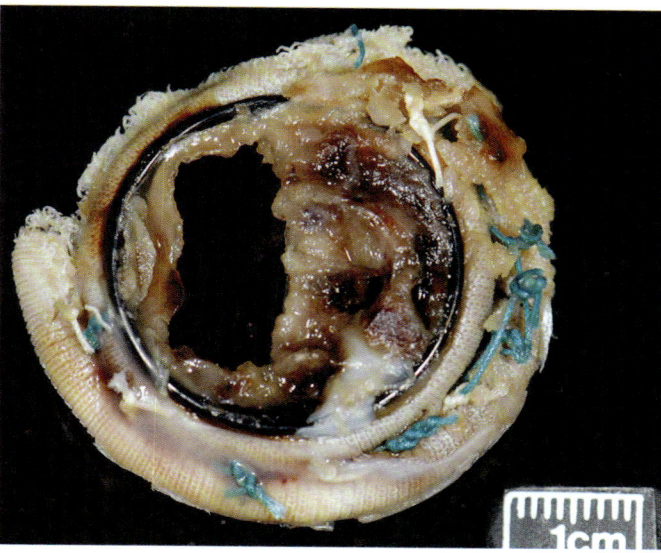

IMAGE 4.12 Mechanical heart valve prosthesis with thrombosis. The discs become immobile, resulting in stenosis.

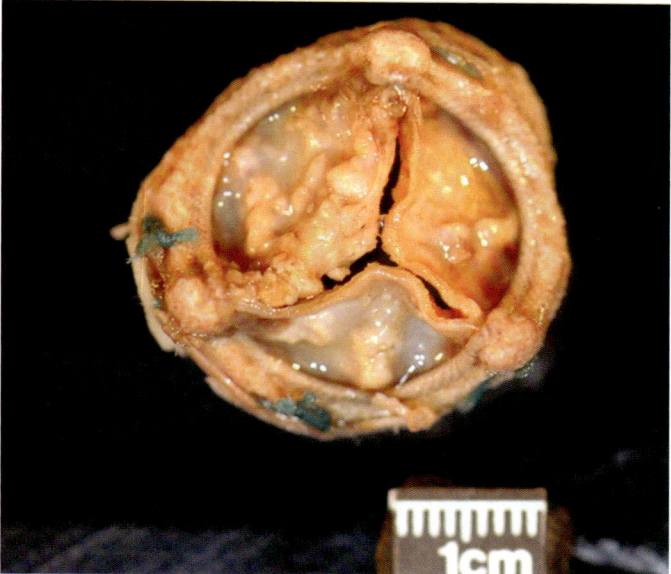

IMAGE 4.13 Bioprosthesis with degeneration calcification indicating bioprosthetic valve stenosis.

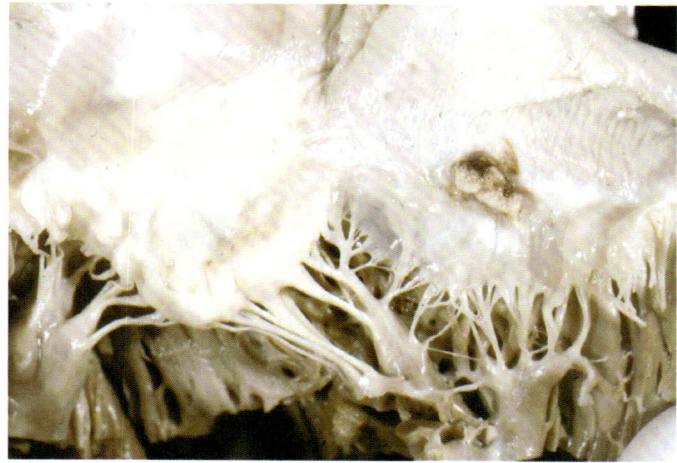

IMAGE 4.14 Mitral valve with nonbacterial thrombotic endocarditis (marantic). The thrombus is always located along the line of valve closure and there is no underlying valve destruction.

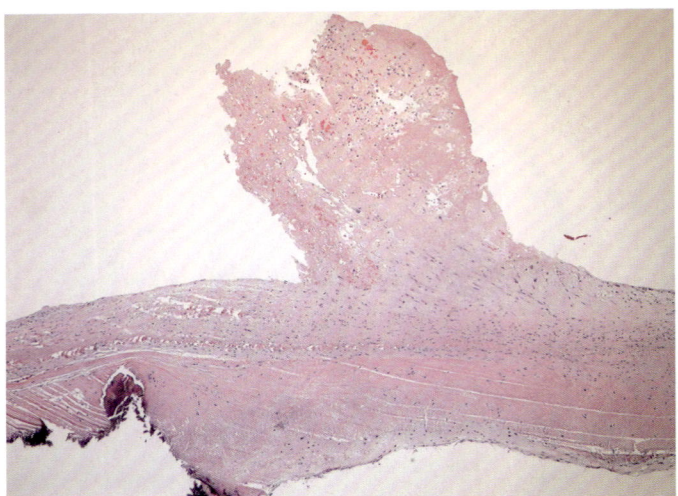

IMAGE 4.15 Aortic valve with NBTE (nonbacterial thrombotic endocarditis). The vegetation consists of platelets, fibrin, and rare inflammatory cells. NBTE is often seen in patients who are in a hypercoagulable state, including terminal malignancy, antiphospholipid syndrome, systemic lupus erythematosus (SLE), disseminated intravascular coagulation (DIC), etc. (H&E, x40).

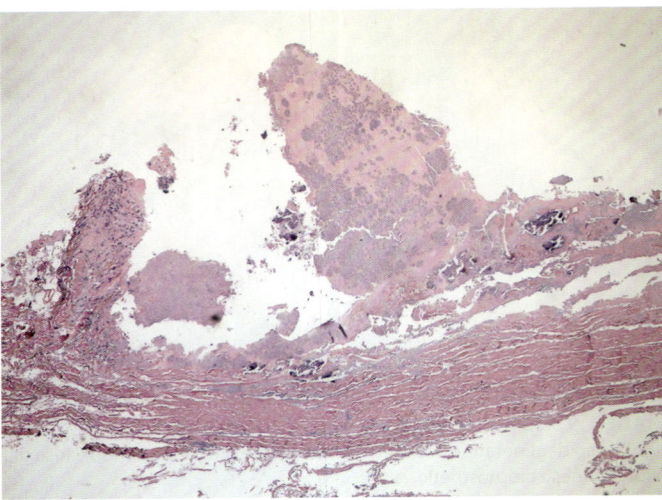

IMAGE 4.18 Bioprosthetic valve with bacterial endocarditis. The bacterial vegetation is composed of fibrin, inflammatory cells, and bacterial colonies (H&E, x40).

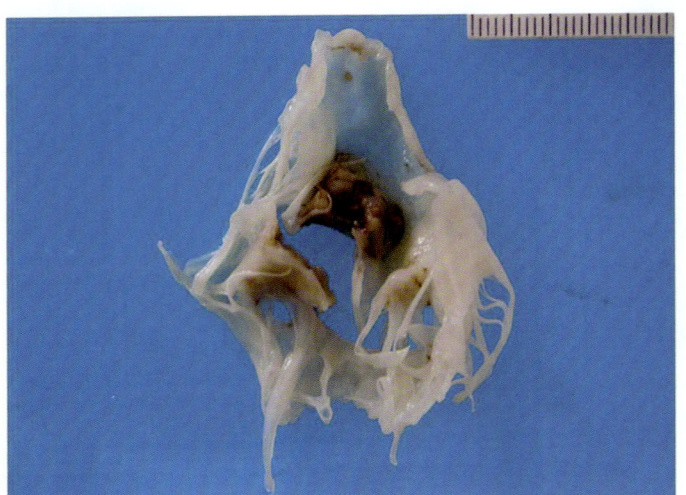

IMAGE 4.16 Mitral valve with acute bacterial endocarditis. The image shows a large friable vegetation.

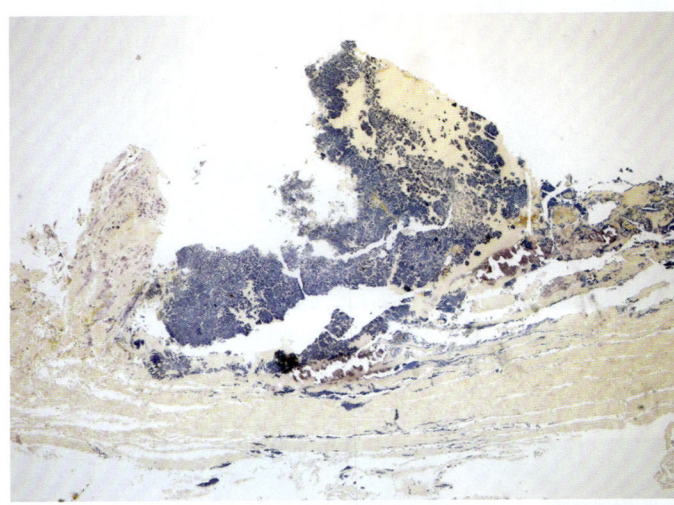

IMAGE 4.19 Bioprosthetic valve with bacterial endocarditis. The bacterial vegetation is composed of fibrin, inflammatory cells, and gram-positive cocci (Gram stain [blue], x40).

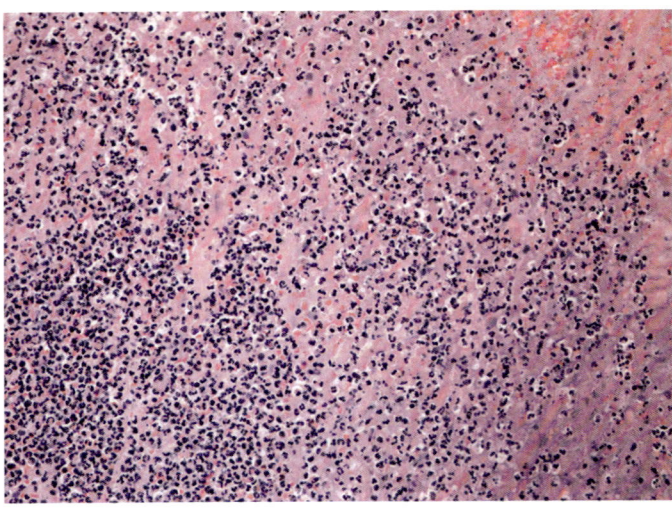

IMAGE 4.17 Mitral valve in acute bacterial endocarditis. The image shows extensive acute inflammatory cells and fibrin (H&E, x20).

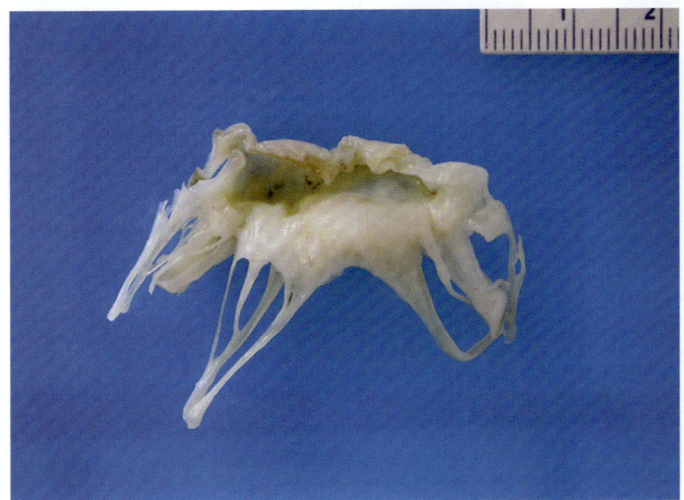

IMAGE 4.20 Mitral valve prolapse shows valve myxomatous degeneration, thickening and hooding of leaflet, and elongated thin chordae.

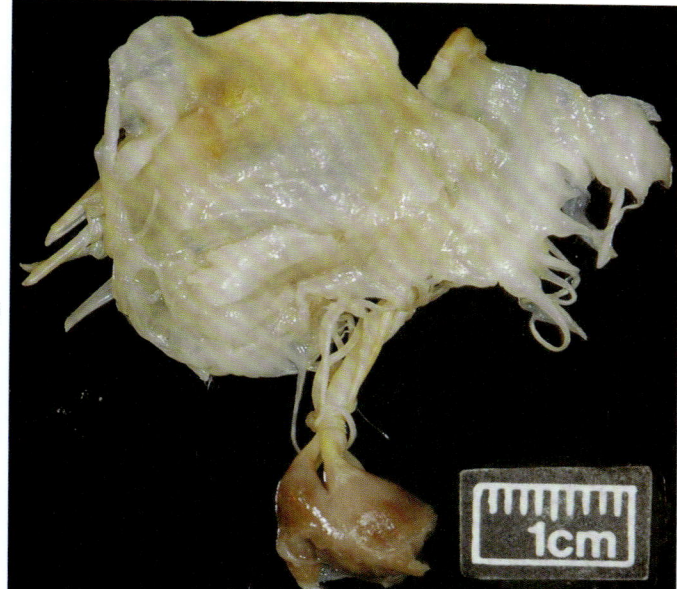

IMAGE 4.21 Excised ruptured papillary muscle and mitral valve. Note that the chordae are tangled and twisted.

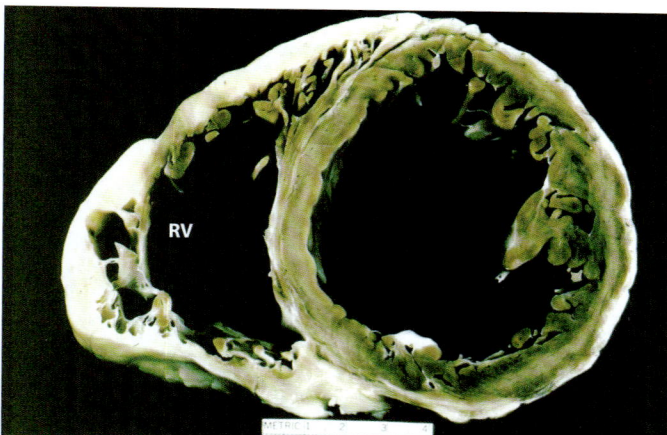

IMAGE 4.24 Arrhythmogenic cardiomyopathy. The right ventricle (RV) wall is nearly all replaced by fat.

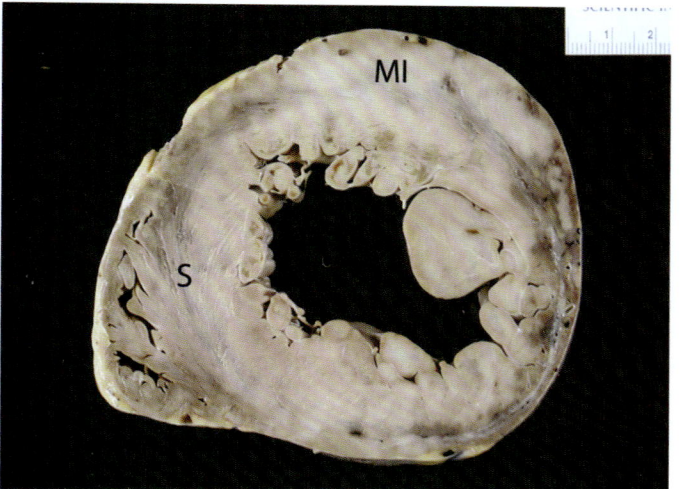

IMAGE 4.22 Hypertrophic cardiomyopathy. The image shows asymmetric septal hypertrophy (S) and a focus of remote myocardial infarction (MI).

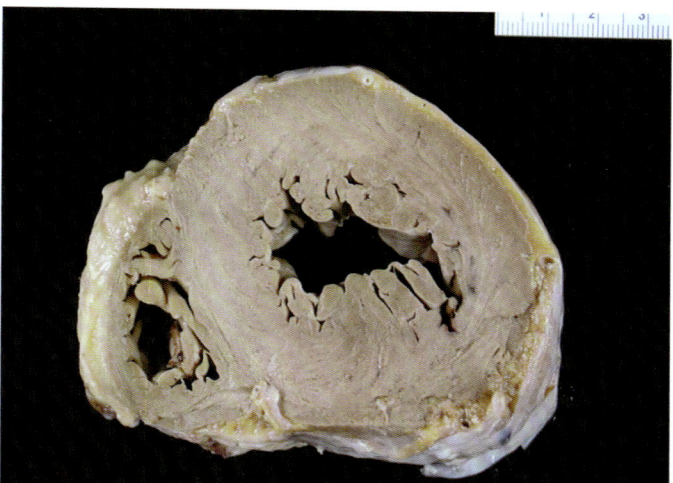

IMAGE 4.25 Heart in systemic arterial hypertension. The image shows concentric left ventricular hypertrophy.

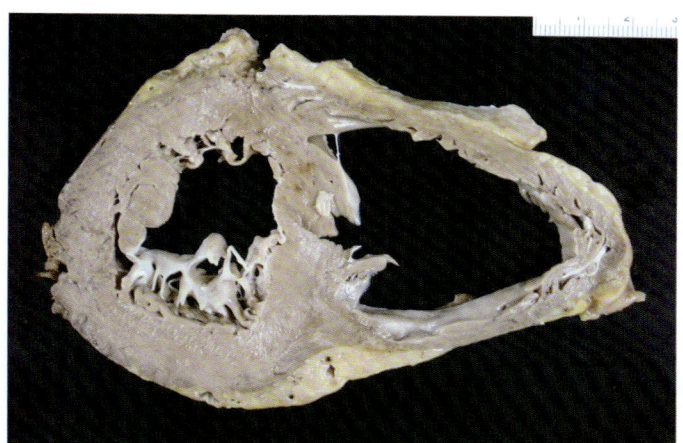

IMAGE 4.23 Dilated cardiomyopathy shows markedly dilated left and right ventricles.

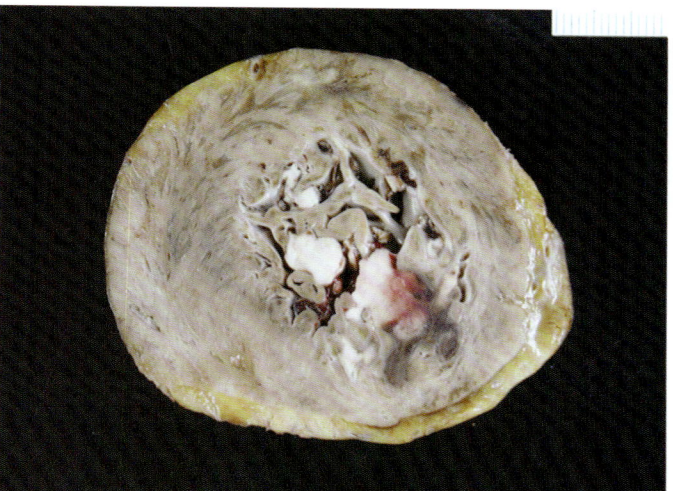

IMAGE 4.26 Acute myocardial infarction with a mural thrombus in the left ventricle.

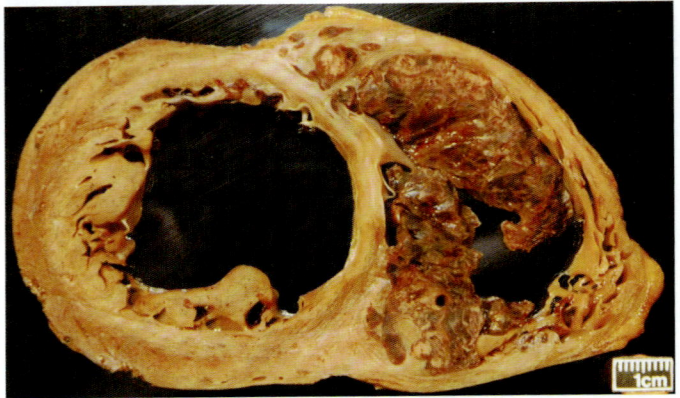

IMAGE 4.27 Dilated heart with biventricular dilation and extensive right ventricular mural thrombus.

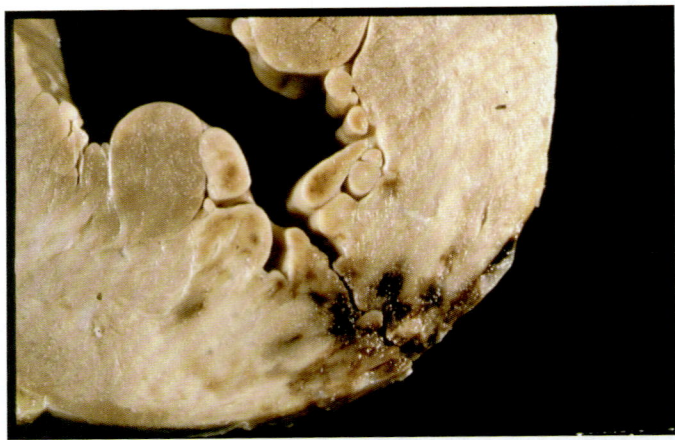

IMAGE 4.30 Recent myocardial infarct with transmural necrosis and free wall rupture.

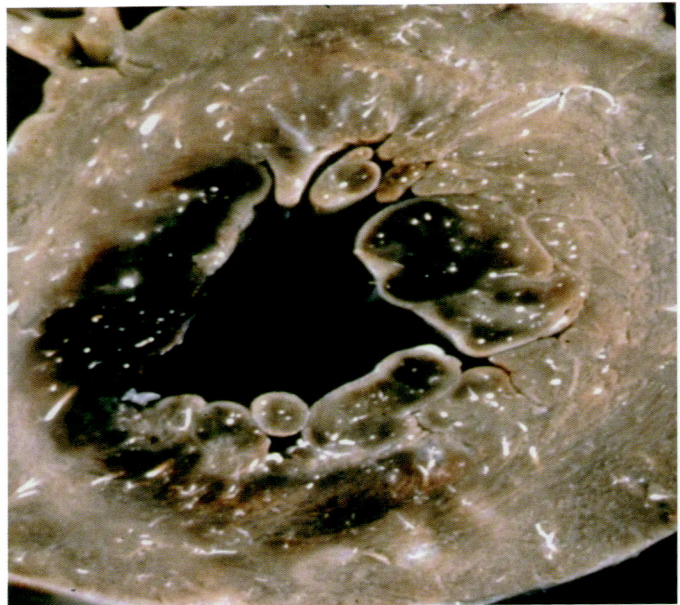

IMAGE 4.28 Recent circumferential subendocardial myocardial infarct. The white streaks are due to postmortem angiography material.

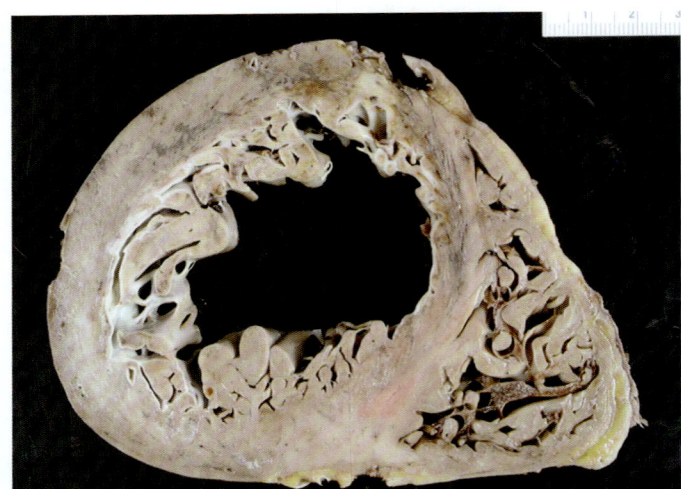

IMAGE 4.31 Acute and remote myocardial infarction shows necrosis and mottling in the anterior wall and anterior septal wall, and fibrosis in the lateral wall.

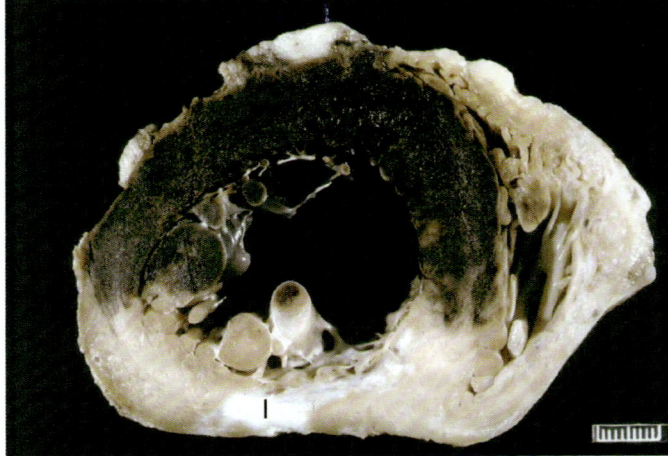

IMAGE 4.29 Recent anteroseptal myocardial infarct with severe reperfusion hemorrhage. There is also an old inferior infarct with a white scar (I).

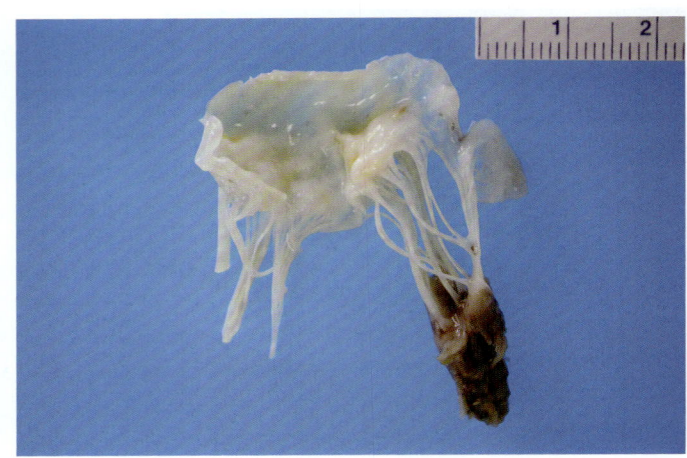

IMAGE 4.32 Ruptured papillary muscle of mitral valve, gross image.

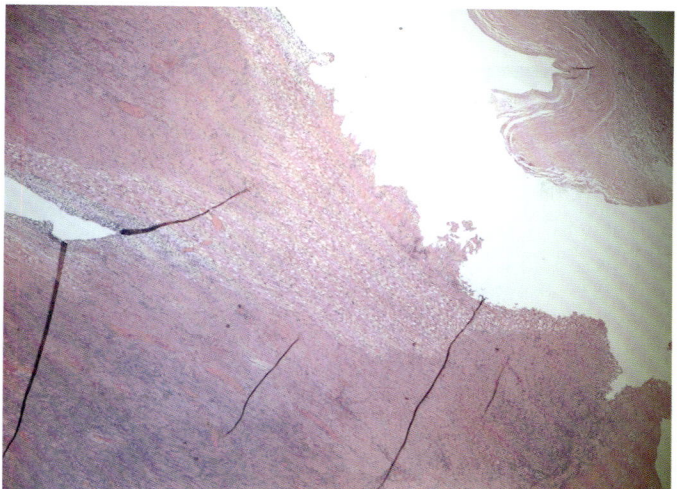

IMAGE 4.33 Ruptured papillary muscle of mitral valve, acute myocardial infarction (H&E, x20).

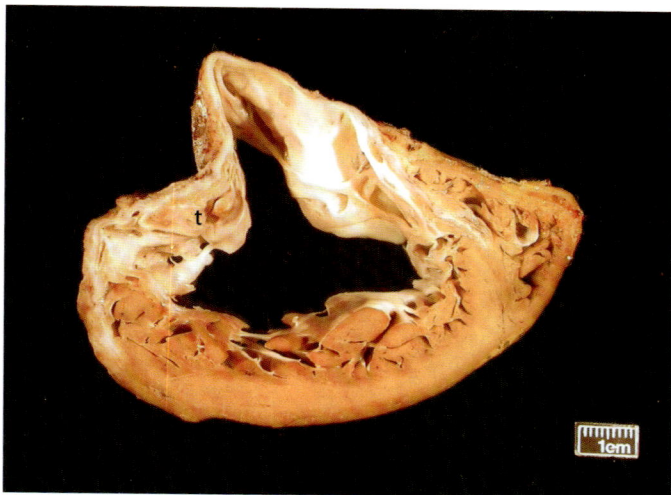

IMAGE 4.36 Old transmural anterior myocardial infarct. The image shows fibrosis and aneurysmal thinning. The inner endocardial surface has brown thrombus (t).

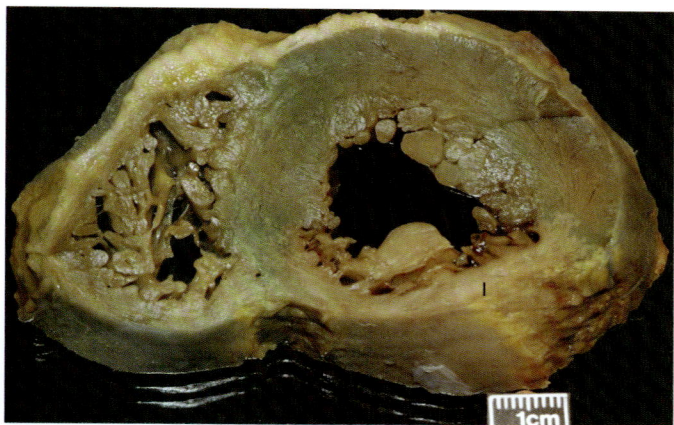

IMAGE 4.34 Healing transmural myocardial infarct (I). Note the wall thinning and pale discoloration of the myocardium. White fibrotic scar has not formed yet.

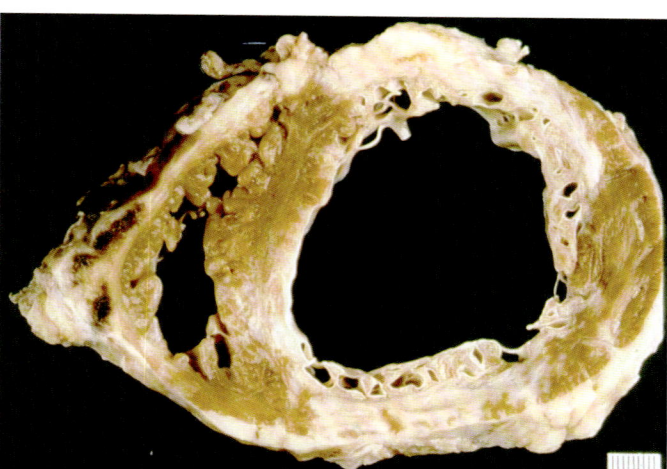

IMAGE 4.37 Severe ischemic heart disease with multiple old myocardial infarcts with white fibrous scars.

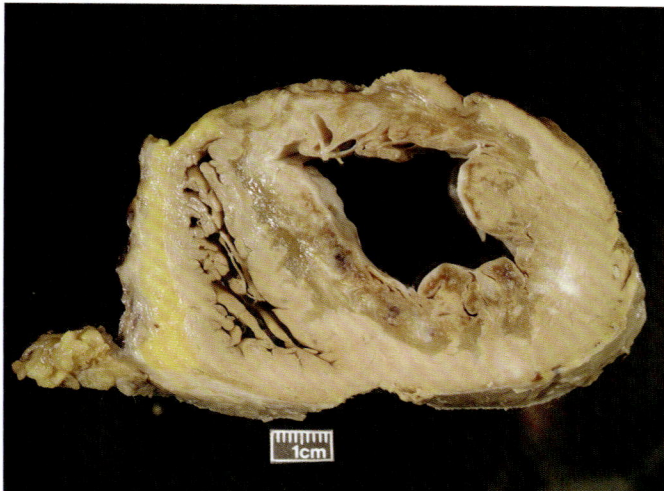

IMAGE 4.35 Cross-section of heart. The image shows a dark circumferential healing myocardial infarct.

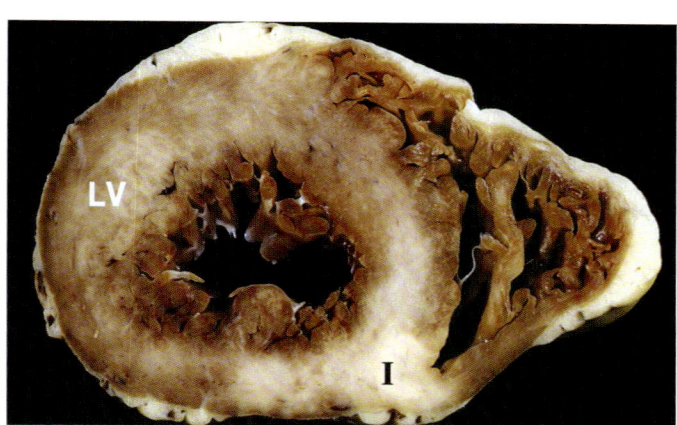

IMAGE 4.38 Cross-section of a heart with giant cell myocarditis. White scars represent fibrosis involving the left ventricle (LV), especially the inferior wall (I).

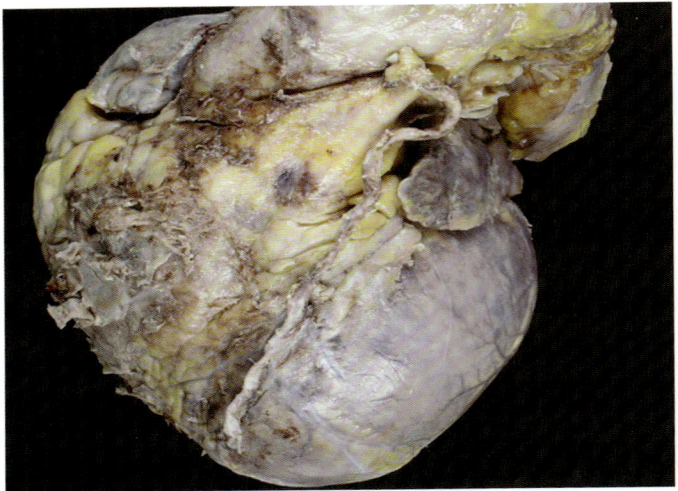

IMAGE 4.39 Postoperative pericarditis. The image shows fibrinous deposits in the pericardium.

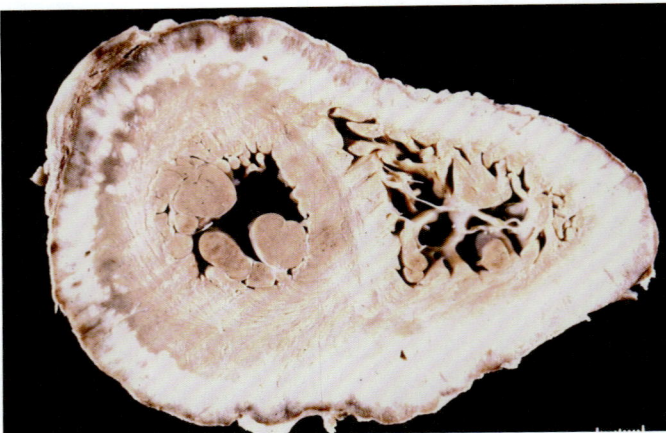

IMAGE 4.42 Cross-section of a heart. The image shows extensive involvement by pericardial lymphoma (white infiltrating tissue).

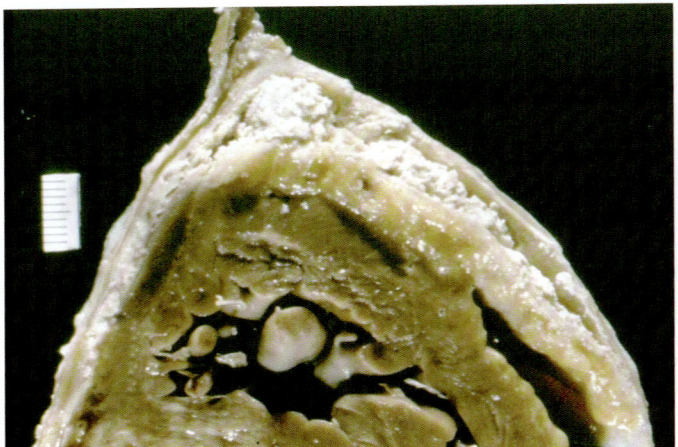

IMAGE 4.40 Caseous pericardial necrosis in a patient with tuberculosis.

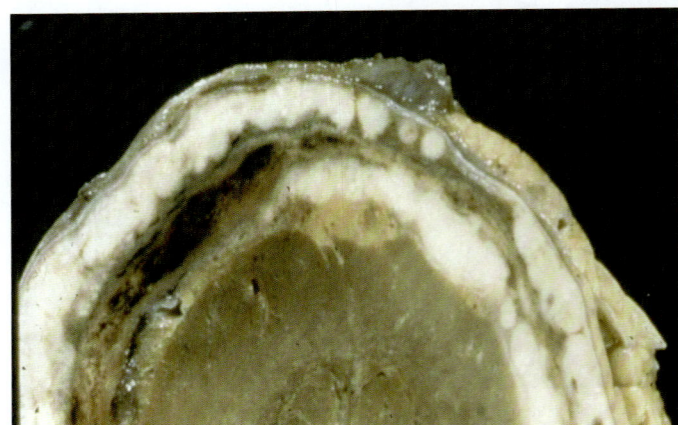

IMAGE 4.43 Metastatic carcinoma in the pericardium. The image shows whitish tumor deposits in both the parietal outer layer and the epicardial visceral layer.

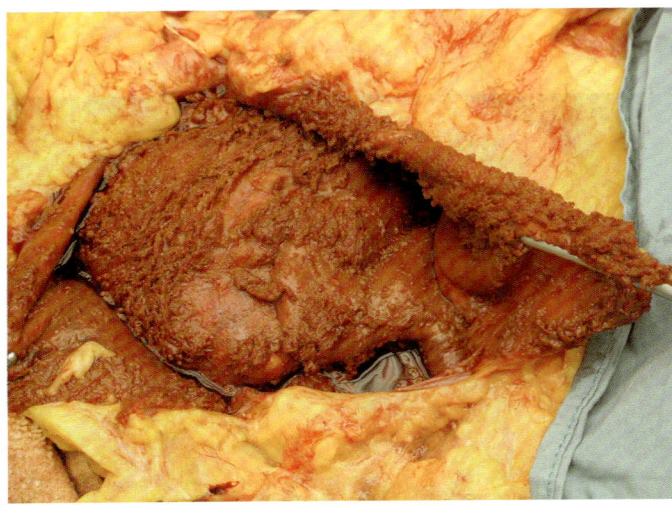

IMAGE 4.41 Opened pericardium showing fibrinous pericarditis.

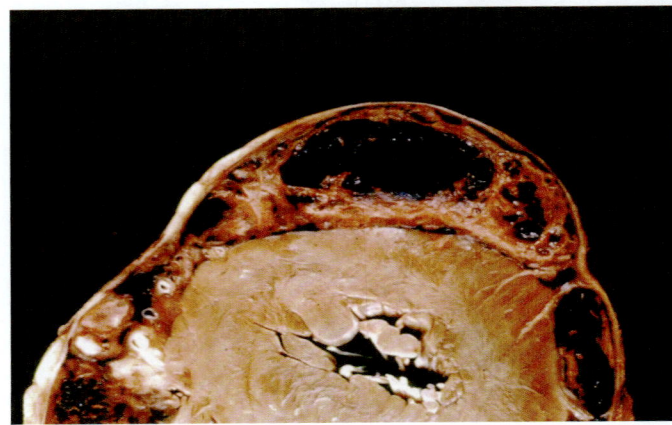

IMAGE 4.44 Cardiac angiosarcoma. The image shows a hemorrhagic and solid tumor mass predominantly involving the pericardial space.

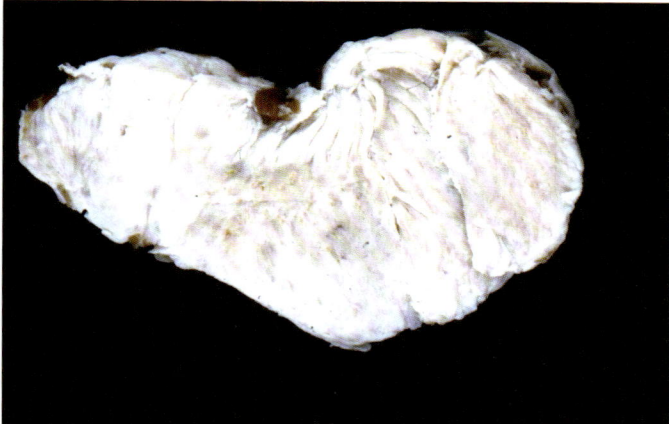

IMAGE 4.45 Cardiac fibroma. This is a rare benign fibrous tumor of the heart.

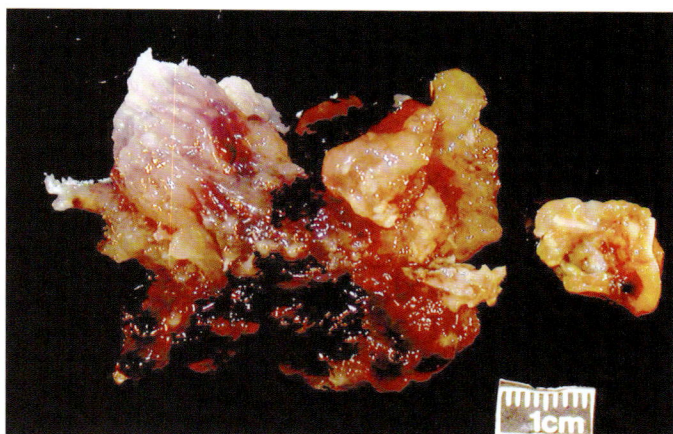

IMAGE 4.48 Excised cardiac myxoma from the left atrium. This tumor is often very gelatinous and friable.

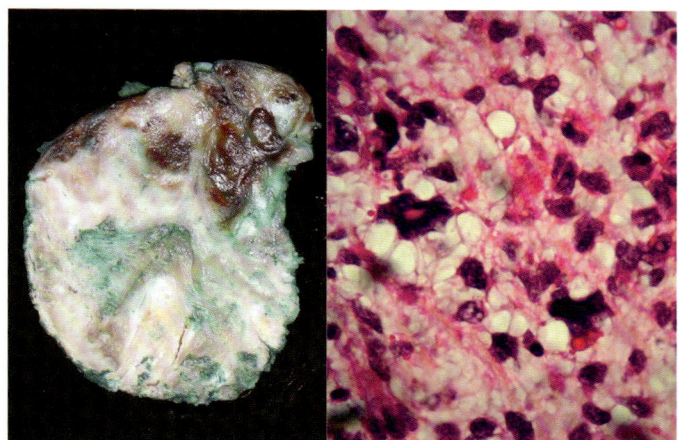

IMAGE 4.46 Cardiac sarcoma. Left (gross): necrosis and hemorrhage. Right (histology): atypical malignant cells (H&E, x200).

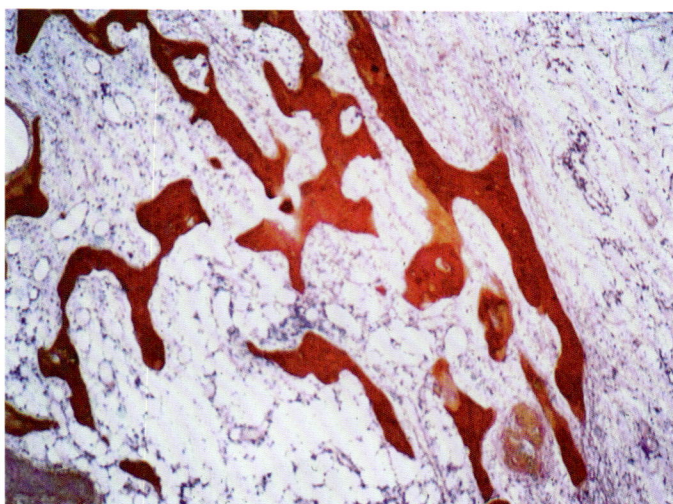

IMAGE 4.49 Cardiac myxomas may contain hemorrhage, glands, or bone (H&E, x20).

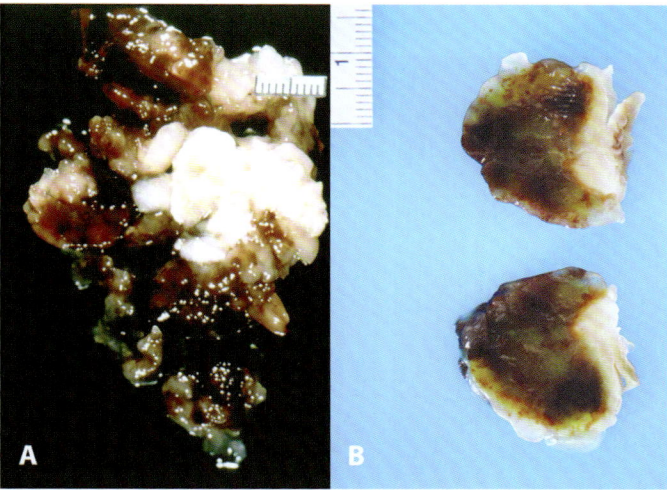

IMAGE 4.47 Cardiac myxoma (2 cases). Left (case A): a gelatinous soft lobulated tumor. Right (case B): a tumor with a hemorrhagic and gelatinous appearance.

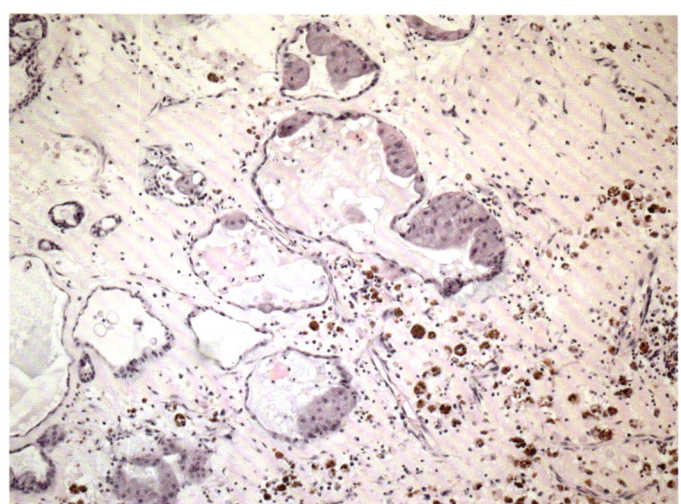

IMAGE 4.50 Myxoma with benign mucinous glands, myxoma cells, and hemosiderin laden macrophages (H&E, x100).

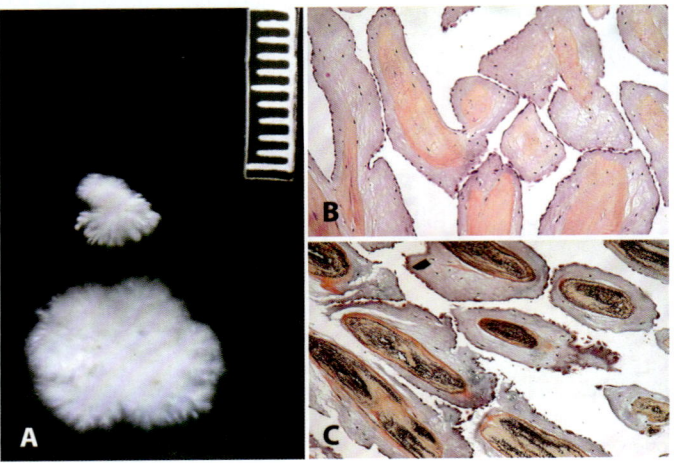

IMAGE 4.51 Image A: numerous fronds, photographed in water. Image B: fibroelastic fronds (H&E, x20). Image C: fibroelastic fronds (elastic stain, x20).

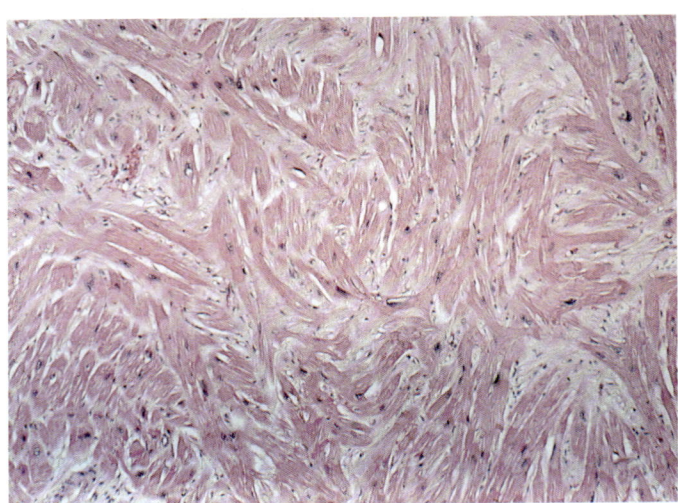

IMAGE 4.54 Hypertrophic cardiomyopathy. The image shows cardiomyocyte disarray (H&E, x40).

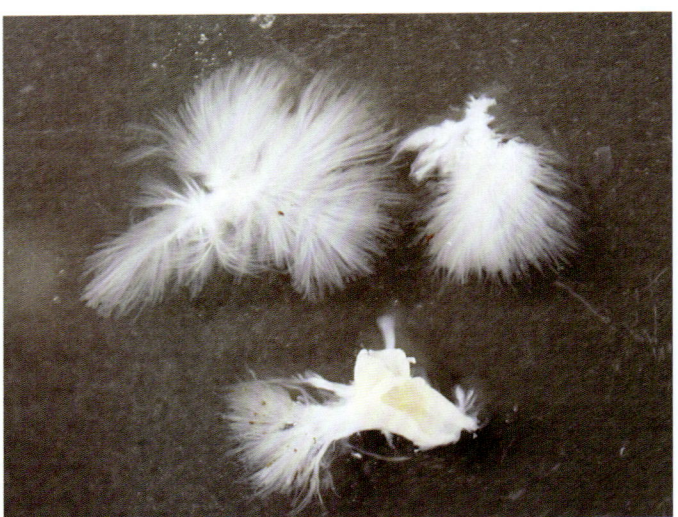

IMAGE 4.52 Papillary fibroelastoma. Its gross appearance resembles sea anemone with numerous delicate papillary fronds.

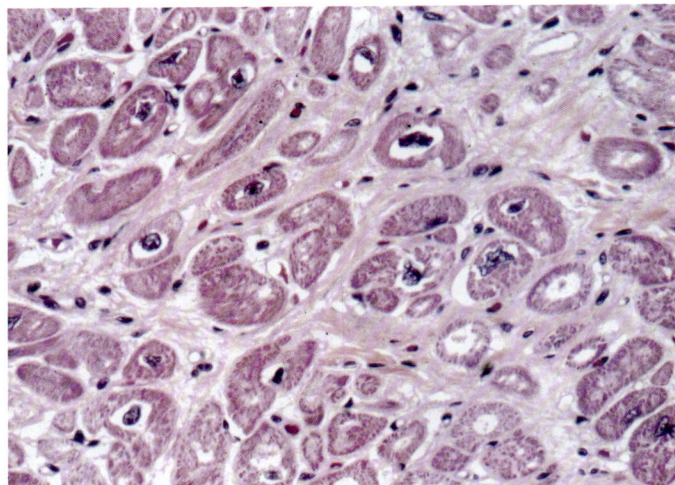

IMAGE 4.55 Dilated cardiomyopathy. The image shows enlarged hypertrophic myocytes with large nuclei, perinuclear clearing, and interstitial fibrosis (H&E, x200).

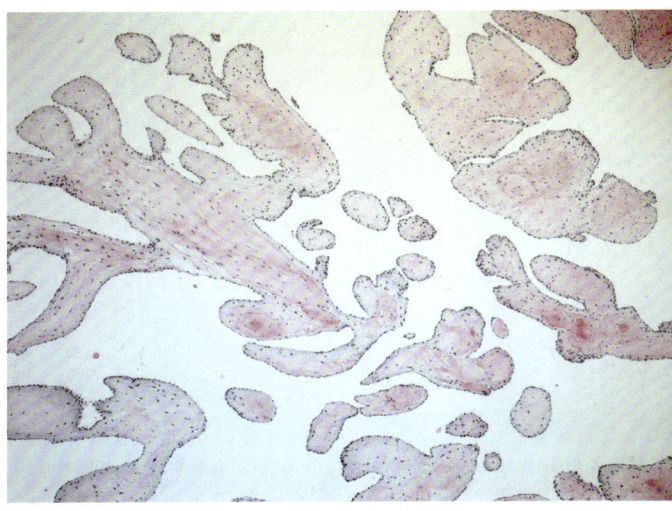

IMAGE 4.53 Papillary fibroelastoma. The image shows fibroelastic cores covered by a monolayer of endothelial cells (H&E, x40).

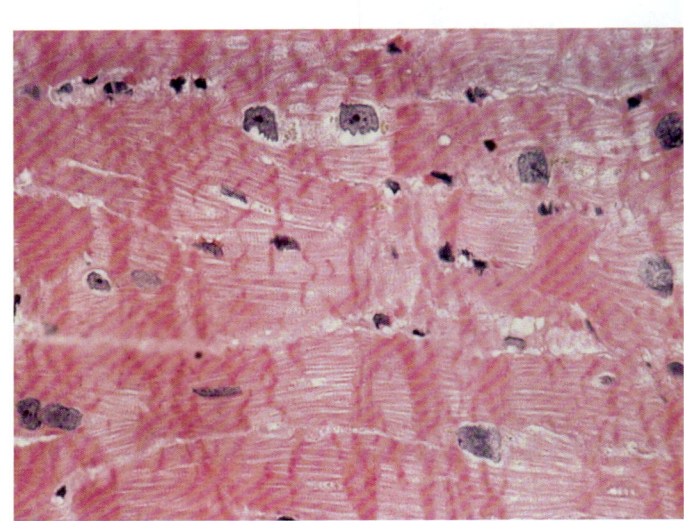

IMAGE 4.56 Myocardial contraction bands (H&E, x400).

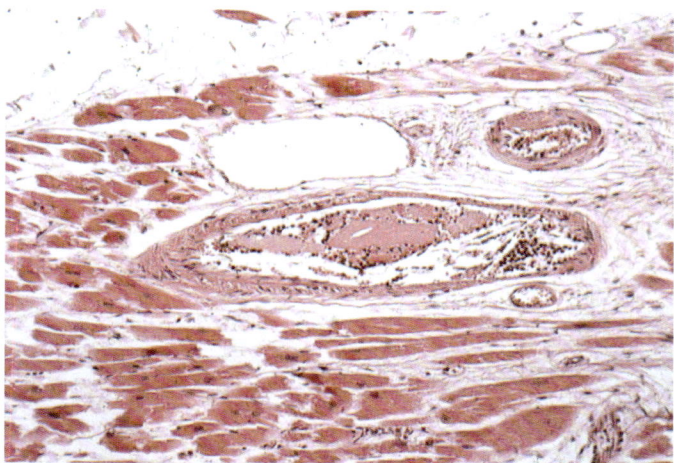

IMAGE 4.57 Myocardium with atheroembolic debris inside small arterioles (H&E, x40).

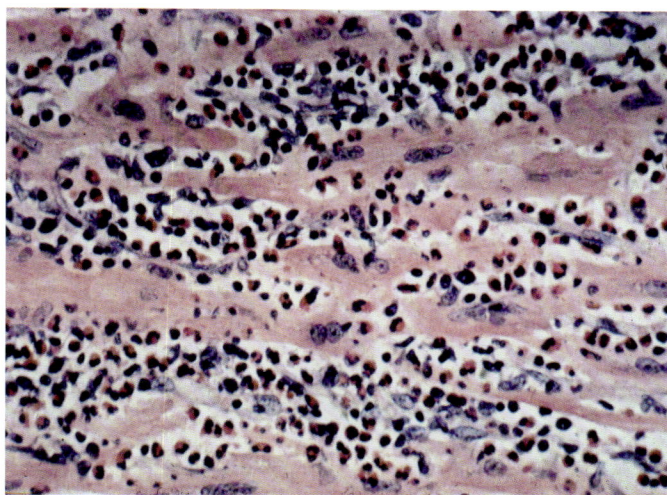

IMAGE 4.60 Eosinophilic myocarditis. The image shows myocyte damage and eosinophil infiltration (H&E, x100).

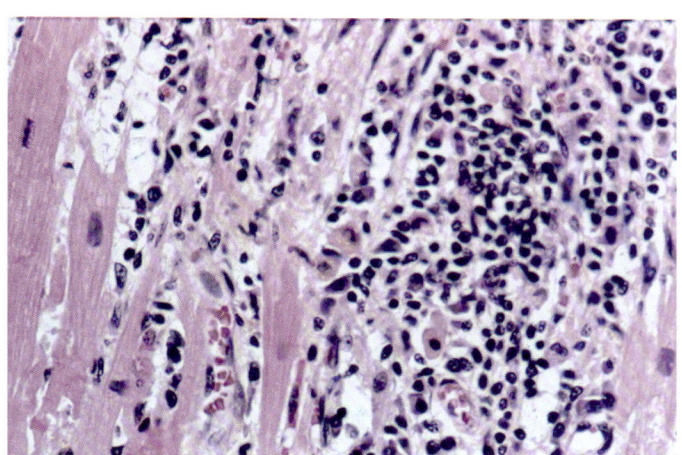

IMAGE 4.58 Myocarditis. The image shows lymphoplasmacytic infiltration with myocyte destruction (H&E, x200).

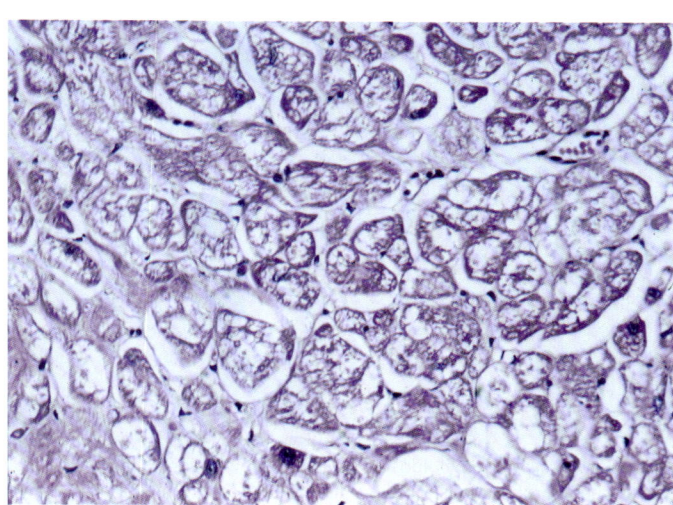

IMAGE 4.61 Chloroquine drug cardiotoxicity. The image shows vacuolated cardiomyocytes (H&E, x200).

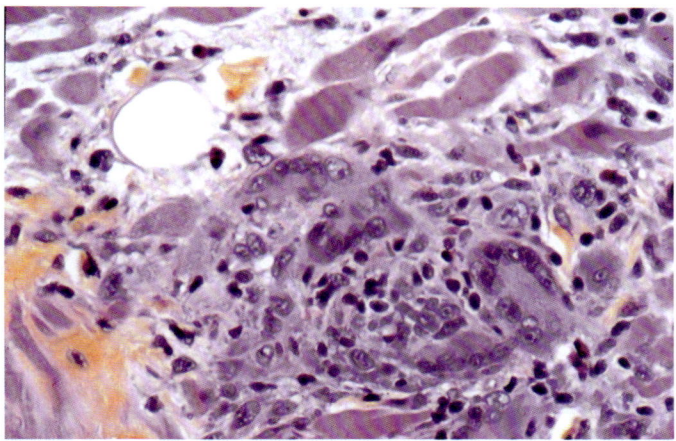

IMAGE 4.59 Giant cell myocarditis. The image shows giant cells and myocyte destruction (H&E, x200).

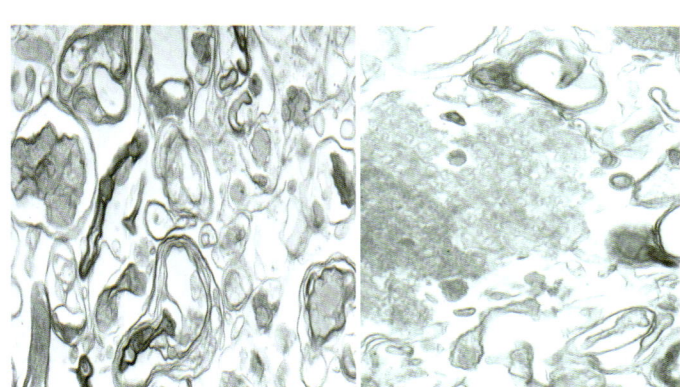

IMAGE 4.62 Chloroquine cardiotoxicity on electron microscopy. Left: curvilinear bodies. Right: myelinosomes.

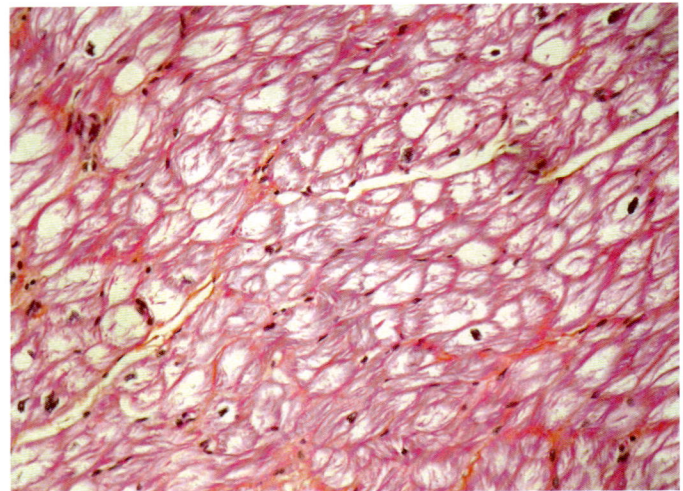

IMAGE 4.63 Glycogen storage disease. The image shows diffuse myocardial vacuolation (H&E, x100).

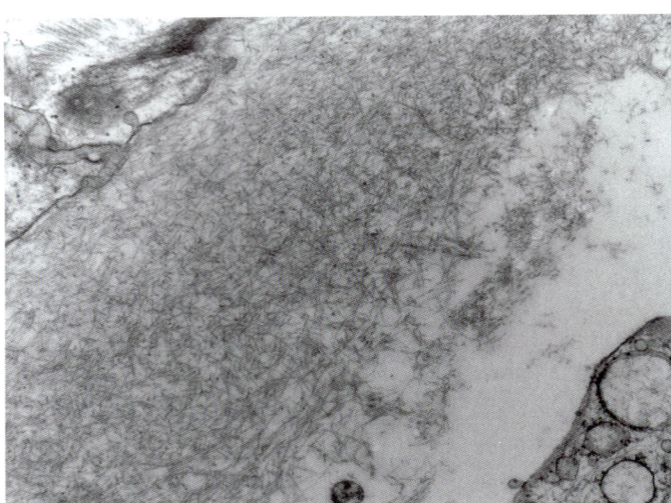

IMAGE 4.66 Electron microscopy (x12 000) of cardiac amyloid. The image shows a loose meshwork of linear, 7.5–10 nm in diameter nonbranching fibrils.

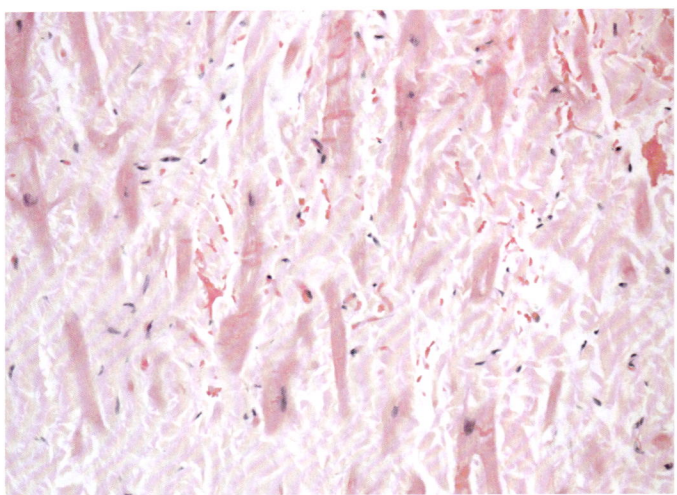

IMAGE 4.64 Cardiac amyloidosis. The image shows pericellular and interstitial amorphous eosinophilic material (H&E, x40).

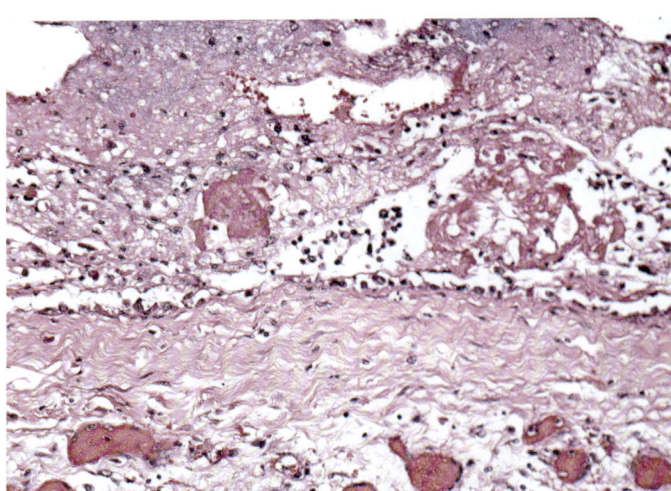

IMAGE 4.67 Organizing fibrinous pericarditis (H&E, x40).

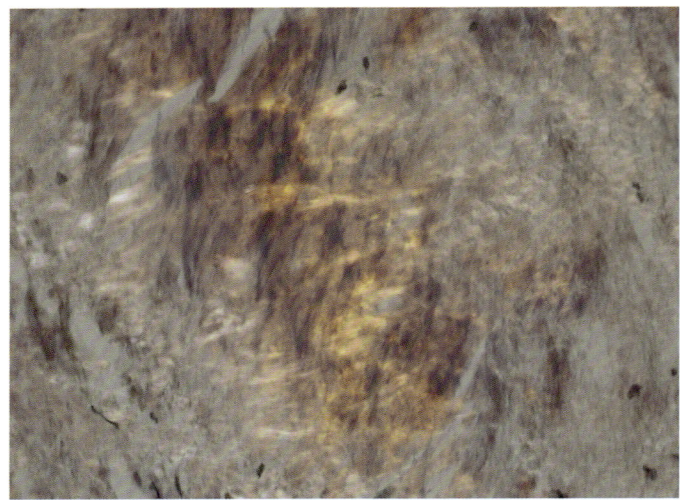

IMAGE 4.65 Cardiac amyloidosis. The image shows apple-green birefringence under polarized light (Congo red stain, x40).

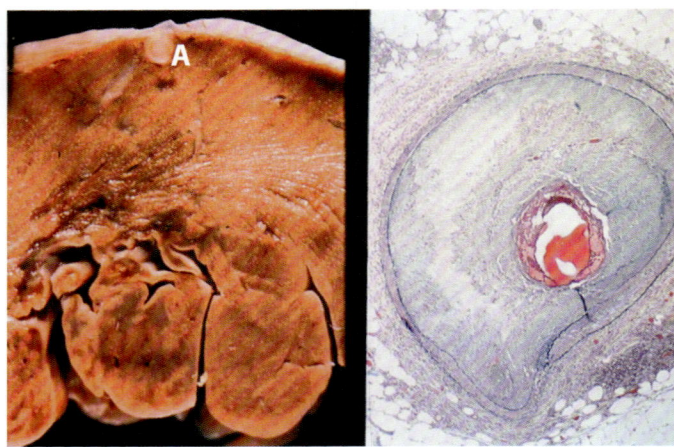

IMAGE 4.68 Cardiac allograft vascular disease. Left (gross): a narrowed artery (A) which has caused a subendocardial myocardial infarct. Right (histology): the artery with concentric disease and severe narrowing.

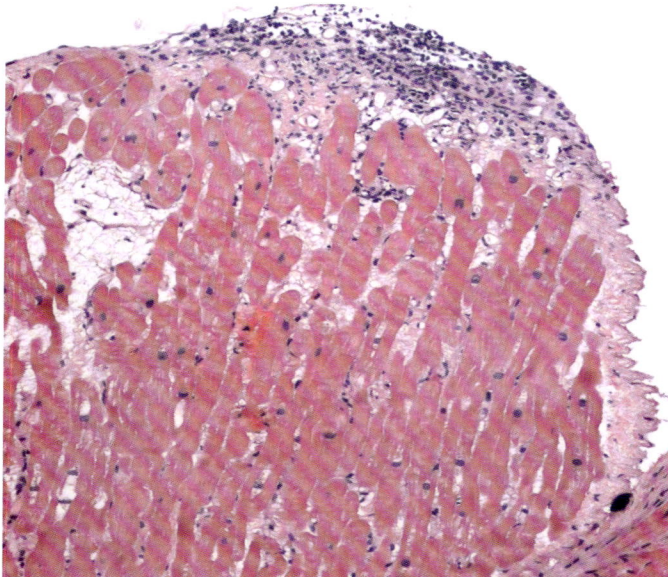

IMAGE 4.69 Transplant endomyocardial biopsy. The image shows an endocardial Quilty nodule (H&E, x40).

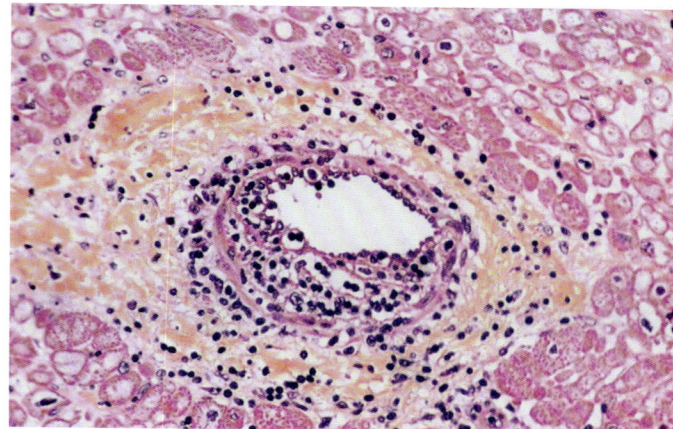

IMAGE 4.72 Cardiac allograft vascular disease extends into the small intramyocardial vessels. This is early disease, still with many lymphocytes (H&E, x100).

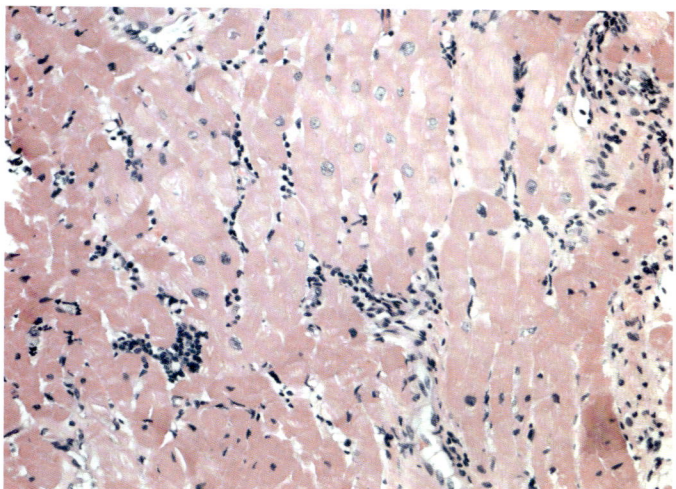

IMAGE 4.70 Cardiac allograft with acute cellular rejection, International Society for Heart and Lung Transplantation (ISHLT) grade 1R. The image shows interstitial and perivascular lymphocytic infiltration (H&E, x40).

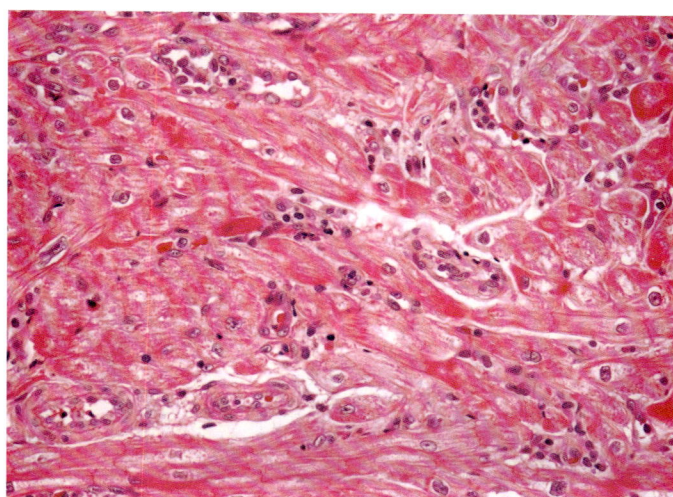

IMAGE 4.73 Antibody mediated cardiac allograft rejection. The image shows prominent endothelial cells, congestion, and intravascular adherent macrophages (H&E, x100).

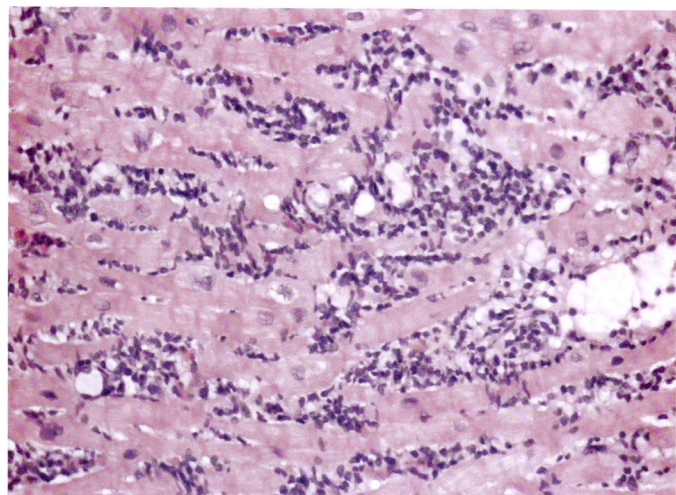

IMAGE 4.71 Severe cardiac allograft cellular rejection, ISHLT grade 3R. The image shows extensive inflammation and multifocal myocyte injury (H&E, x40).

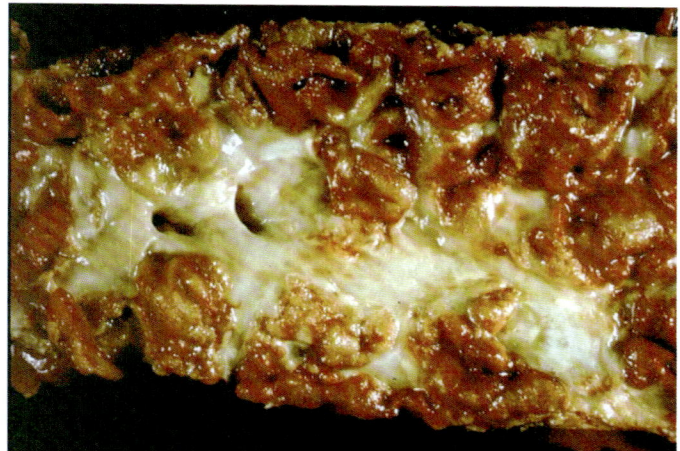

IMAGE 4.74 Atherosclerotic aorta with numerous complicated plaques and overlying red thrombus. Some mesenteric artery ostia are visible.

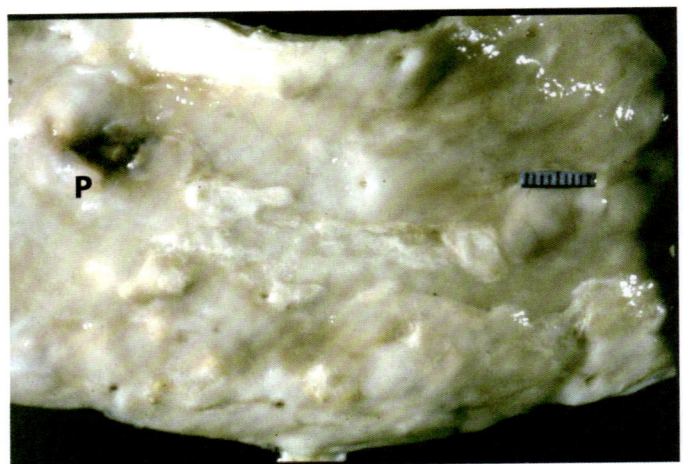

IMAGE 4.75 Aorta with a complicated plaque (P) and numerous fibrous intimal plaques.

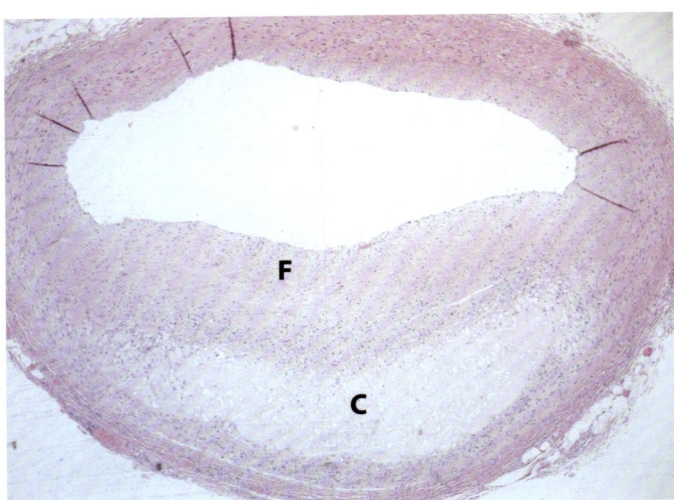

IMAGE 4.78 Coronary artery atherosclerosis. The image shows atheromatous plaque with fibrous cap (F) and necrotic (largely lipid) core (C) (H&E, x4).

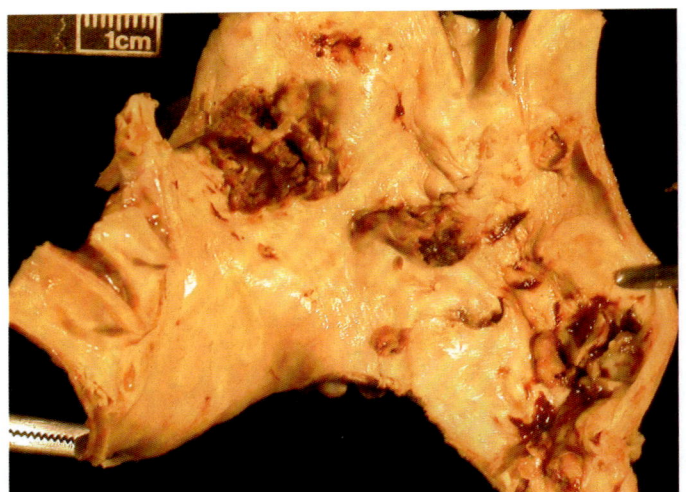

IMAGE 4.76 Atherosclerotic aortic arch. The image shows numerous complicated atherosclerotic plaques.

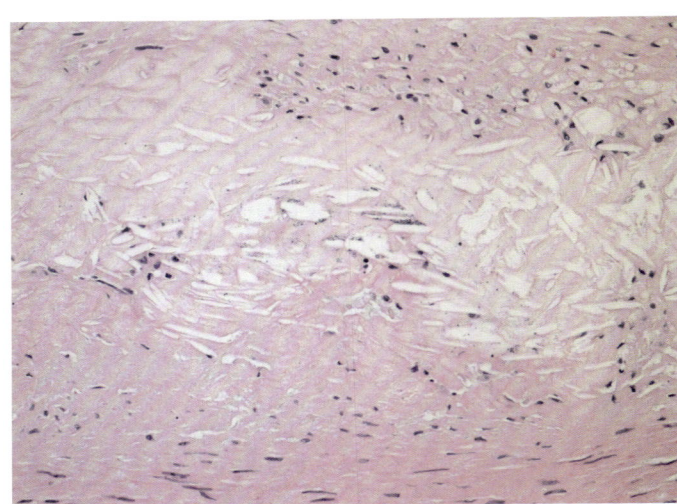

IMAGE 4.79 Coronary atherosclerosis. The image shows an atherosclerotic plaque with cholesterol clefts and inflammatory cells (H&E, x20).

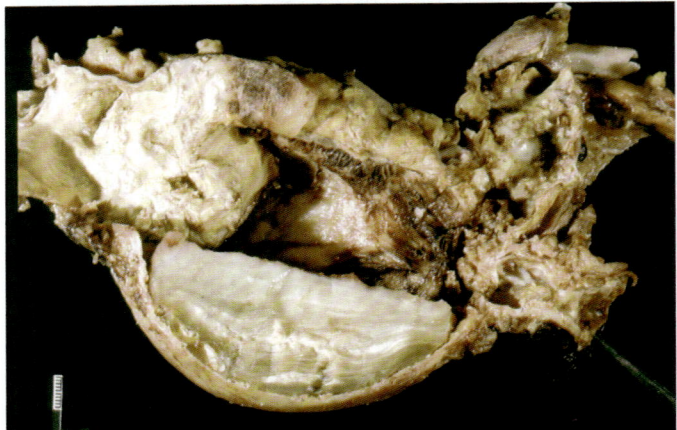

IMAGE 4.77 Atherosclerotic abdominal aortic aneurysm. The image shows pale old thrombus on top of complicated atheroma.

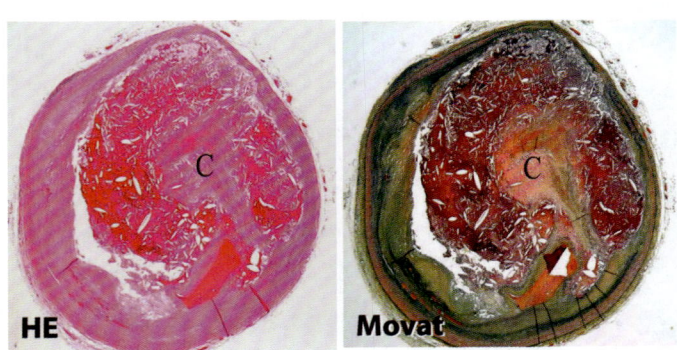

IMAGE 4.80 Coronary artery with ruptured plaques. C: plaque cap (H&E, Movat, x4).

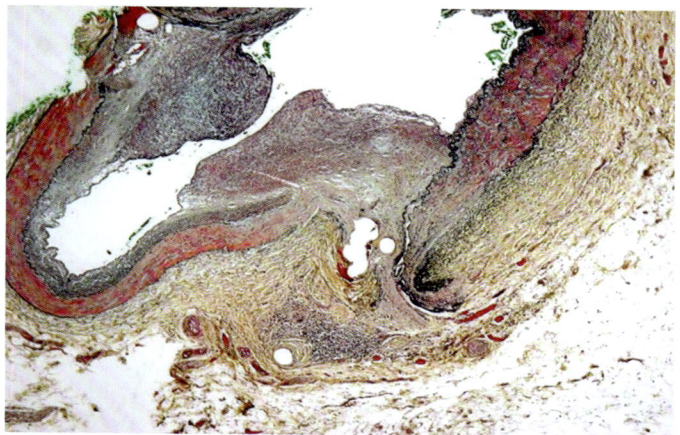

IMAGE 4.81 Coronary artery bypass grafting (CABG) arterial-arterial anastomosis with muscular coronary artery on the left and the internal thoracic artery on the right. The clear holes are from the sutures (elastic stain, x4).

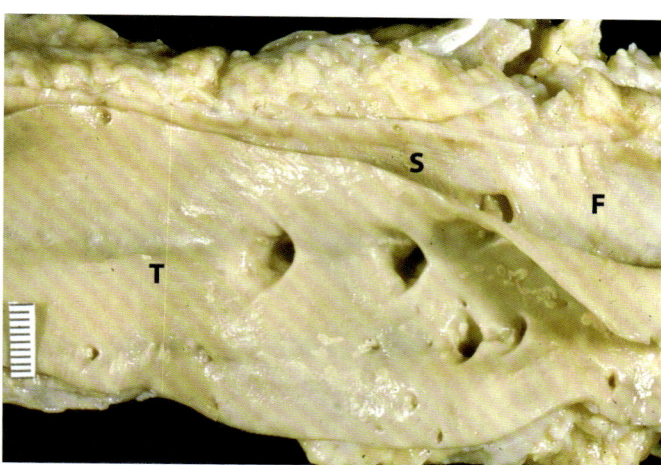

IMAGE 4.84 Opened aorta shows dissection and splitting (S) of the media forming a true lumen (T) and a false lumen (F).

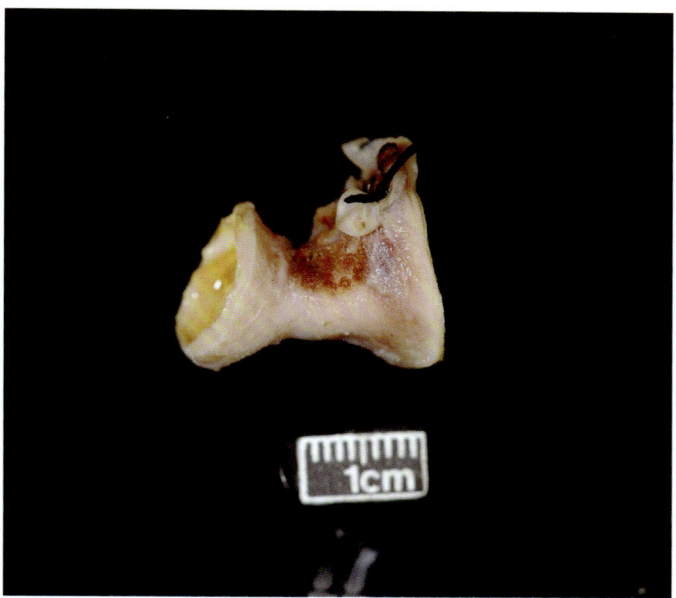

IMAGE 4.82 Aortic coarctation, excised.

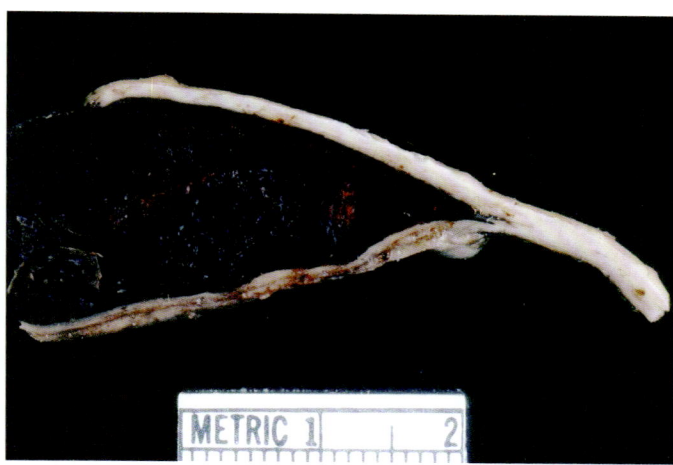

IMAGE 4.85 Aorta dissection shows blood clot splitting the aorta media.

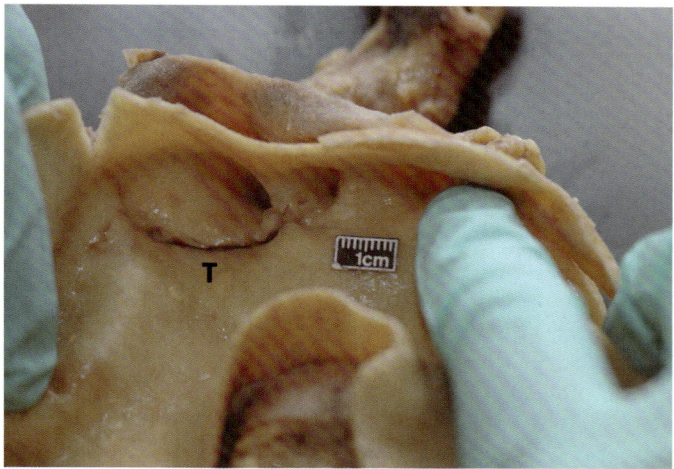

IMAGE 4.83 Opened aortic arch from a patient with aortic dissection demonstrating the entry tear (T) of the dissection.

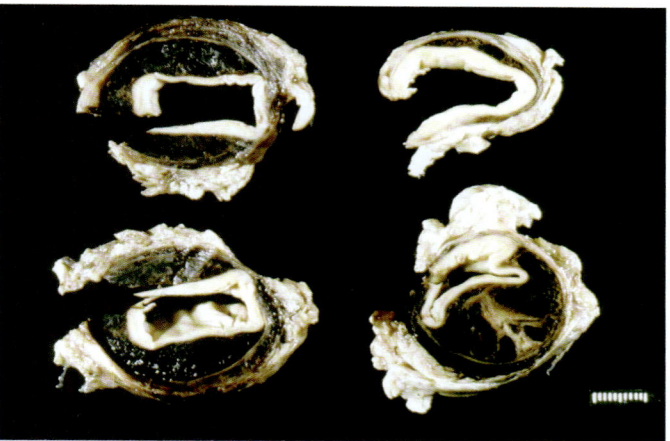

IMAGE 4.86 Cross-sections of the aorta demonstrate a large dissection with a blood clot in the false lumen compressing the inner aorta.

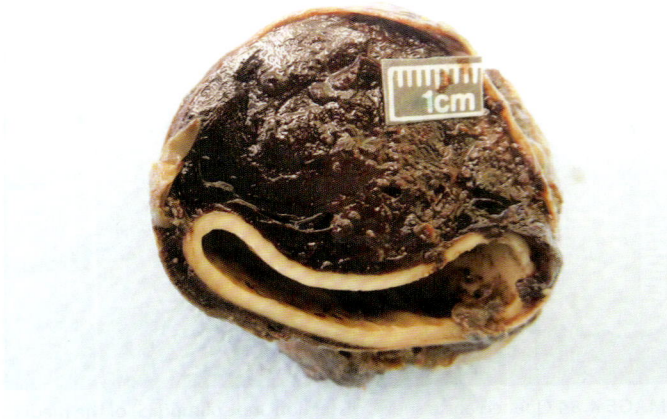

IMAGE 4.87 Cross-section of aorta with large aortic dissection.

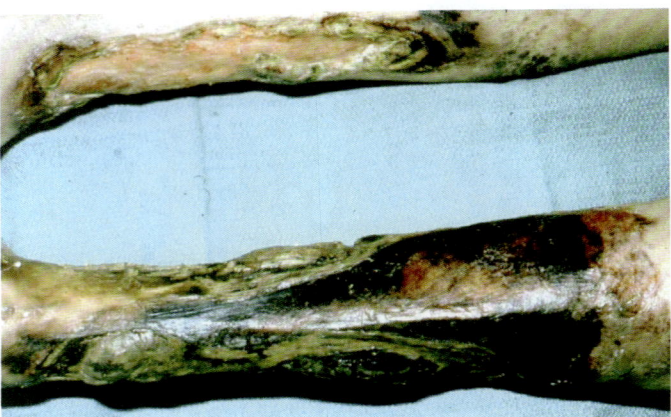

IMAGE 4.90 Legs with arterial vascular disease show gangrenous necrosis and deep ulcers.

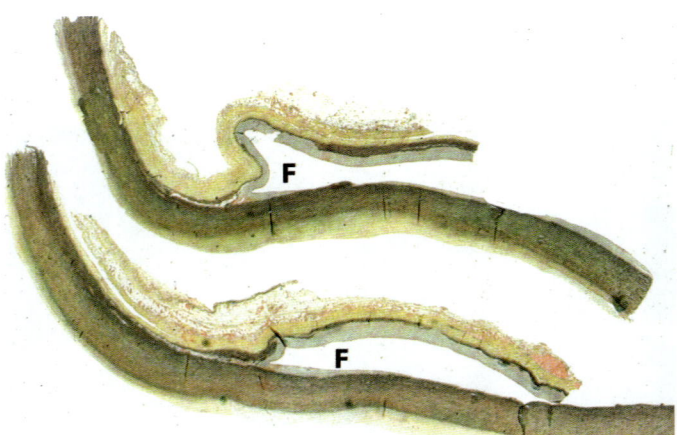

IMAGE 4.88 Histology of 2 pieces of aorta with aortic dissection. The false lumen in each piece is noted (F) (elastic stain, x4).

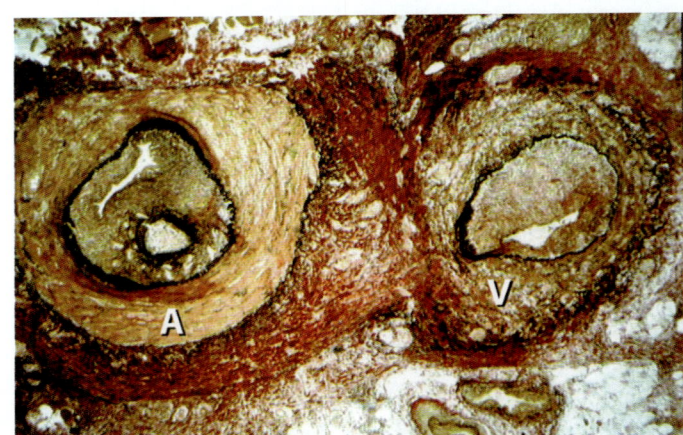

IMAGE 4.91 Buerger disease (thromboangiitis obliterans) shows obliteration of both medium-sized arteries (A) and veins (V). This disease is strongly associated with smoking (elastic stain, x4).

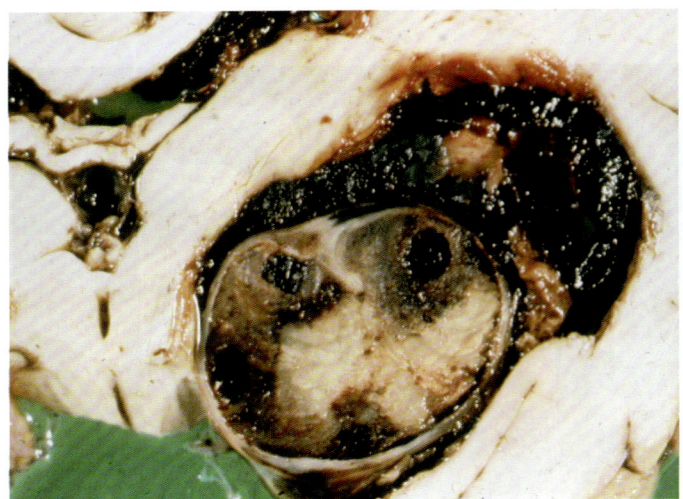

IMAGE 4.89 Brain with a ruptured giant berry aneurysm.

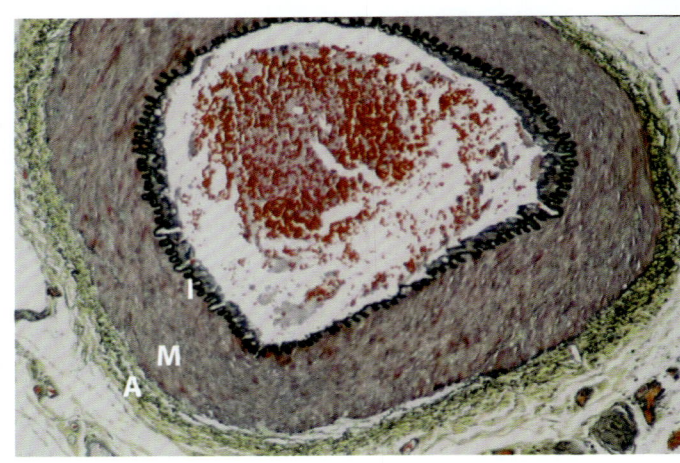

IMAGE 4.92 Histology of a normal muscular artery with intima (I), media (M), and adventitia (A) (elastic stain, x4).

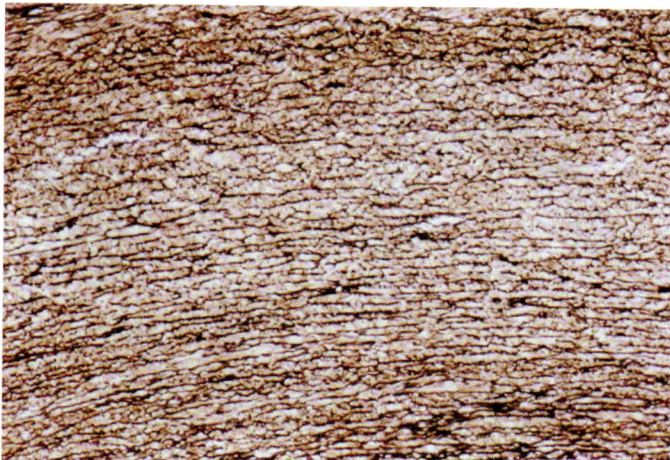

IMAGE 4.93 Histology of a normal elastic artery shows numerous elastic lamellae (elastic stain, x10).

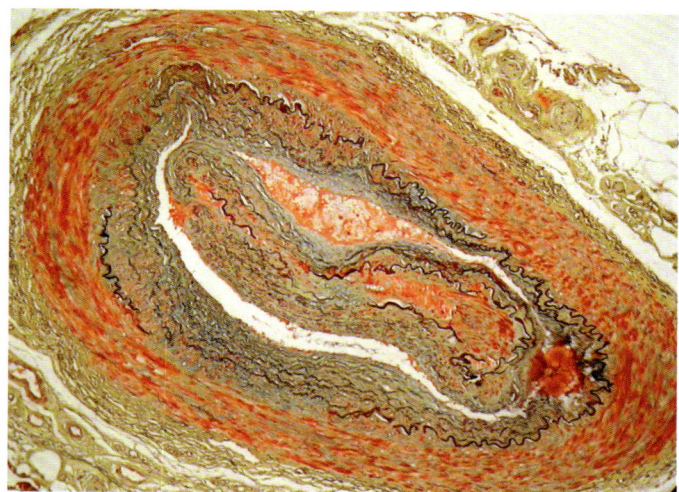

IMAGE 4.96 Intussusception of an artery inside an adjacent segment. This can be confused with thrombosis unless an elastic stain is done (elastic stain, x10).

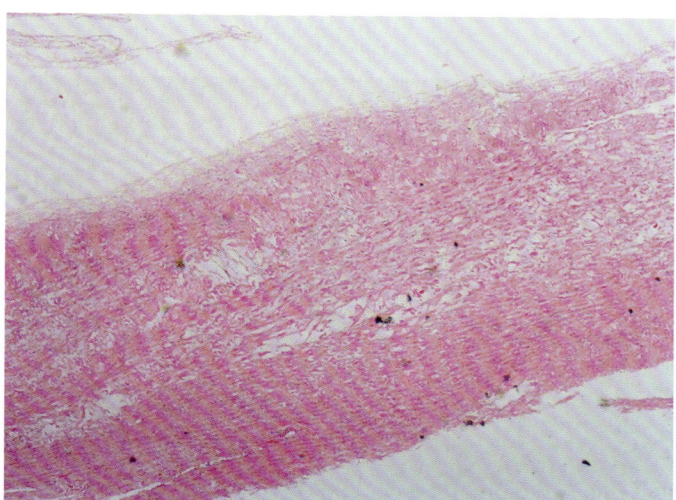

IMAGE 4.94 Marfan syndrome. The image shows aortic medial cystic degeneration (H&E, x4).

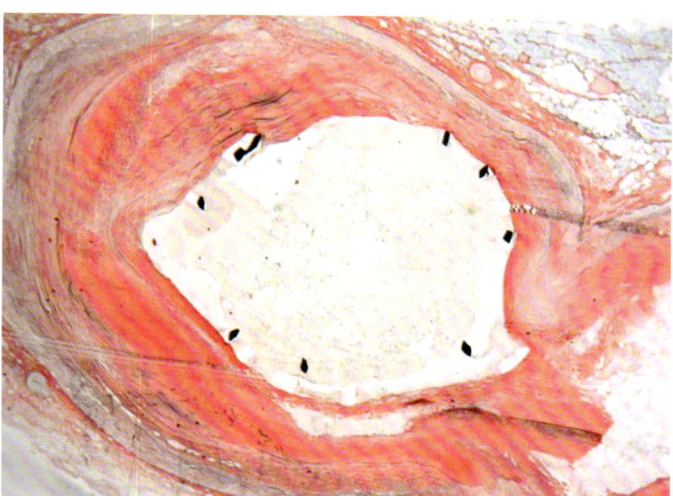

IMAGE 4.97 Stented atherosclerotic artery. Metal stent struts are visible holding the artery open (elastic stain, x4).

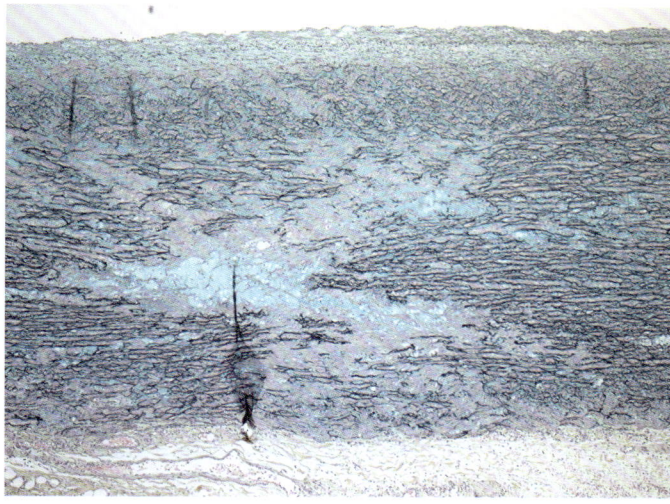

IMAGE 4.95 Aortic aneurysm with cystic medial degeneration. The aortic wall shows elastic fiber fragmentation and separation of the elastic fibromuscular elements by "cystic" spaces (Musto-Movat stain, x40).

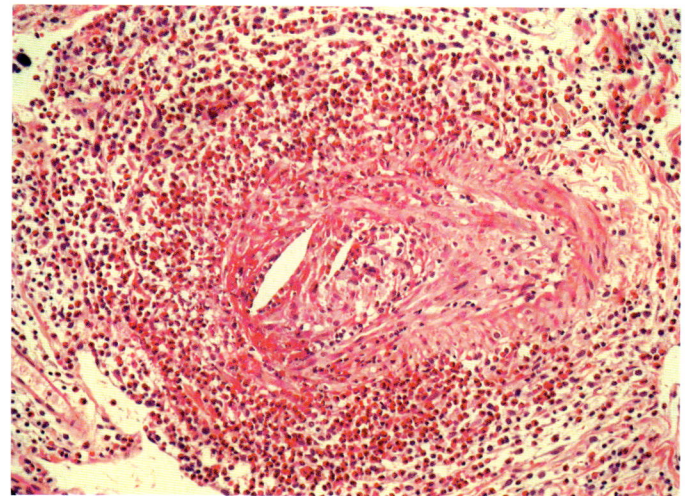

IMAGE 4.98 Atheroembolism causing eosinophilic arteritis. Note cholesterol crystals (H&E, x40).

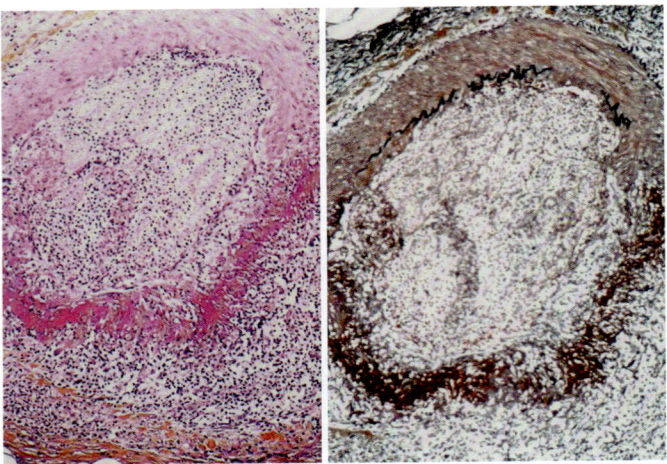

IMAGE 4.99 Segmental necrotizing arteritis with fibrinoid necrosis in a patient with Wegner granulomatosis (granulomatosis with polyangiitis). The upper part of the artery is unaffected. Left: H&E, x20. Right: elastic stain, x20.

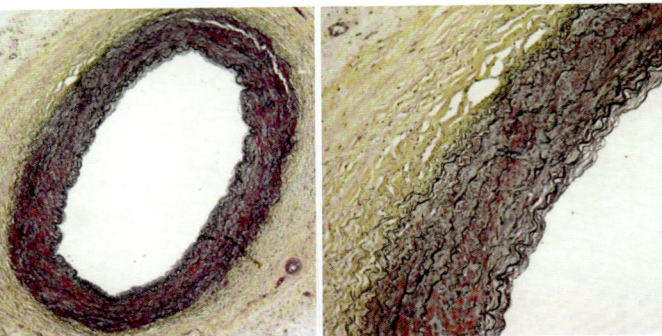

IMAGE 4.102 Internal thoracic artery grafts (mammary arteries) are small elastic type arteries with elastic lamellae. These are commonly used for coronary artery bypass grafting and have superior results as compared to venous grafts. Left: elastic stain, low power. Right: elastic stain, higher power.

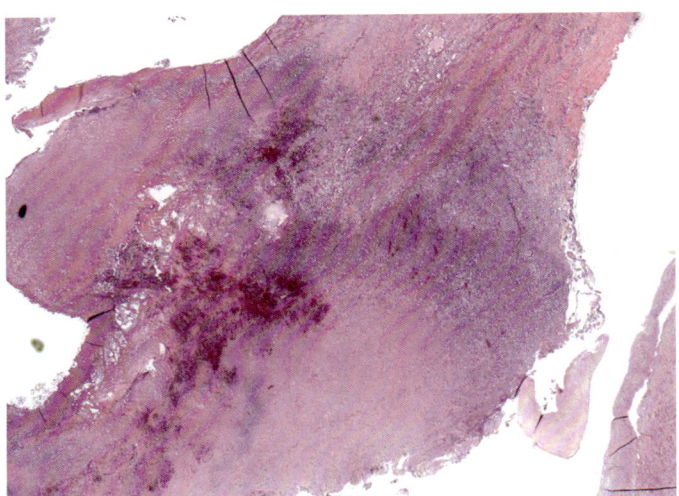

IMAGE 4.100 Mycotic bacterial aneurysm. The image shows a femoral artery with destructive necrosis (H&E, x10).

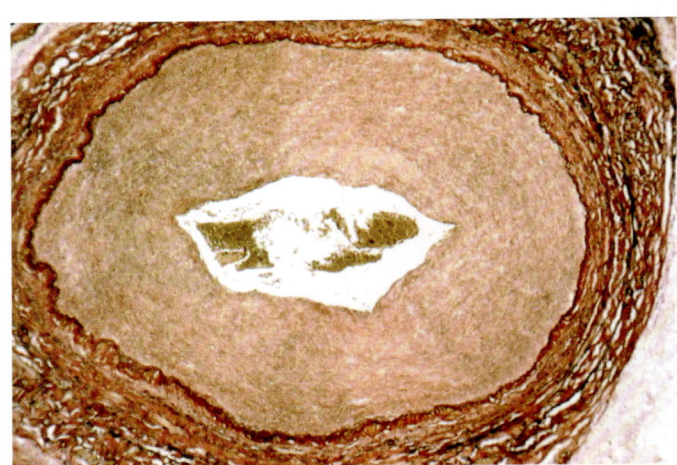

IMAGE 4.103 Vein graft shows fibrous intimal hyperplasia, which is a common cause of graft stenosis (elastic stain, x10).

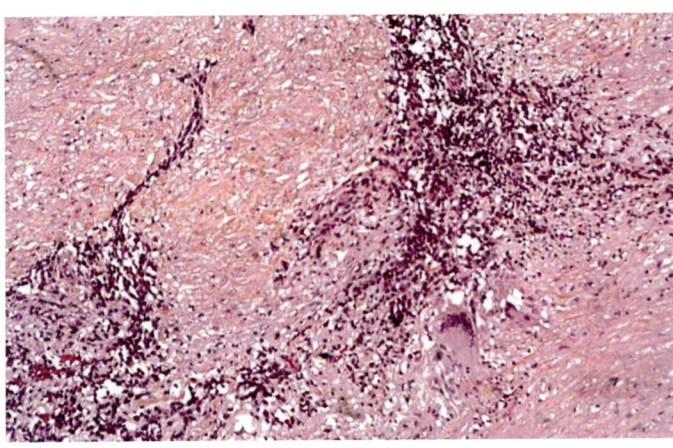

IMAGE 4.101 Giant cell aortitis. The image shows destruction of the vessel wall by inflammatory cells including giant cells (H&E, x40).

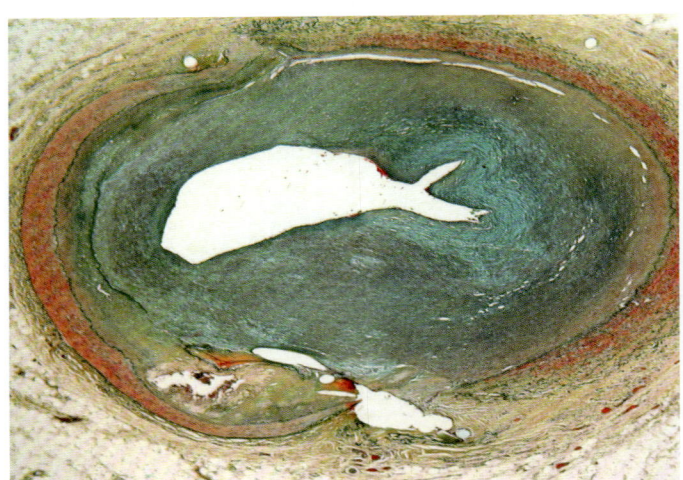

IMAGE 4.104 CABG arterial vein graft anastomosis with artery on left and vein on right. There is considerable fibrointimal hyperplasia (FIH) narrowing the anastomosis (elastic stain, x10).

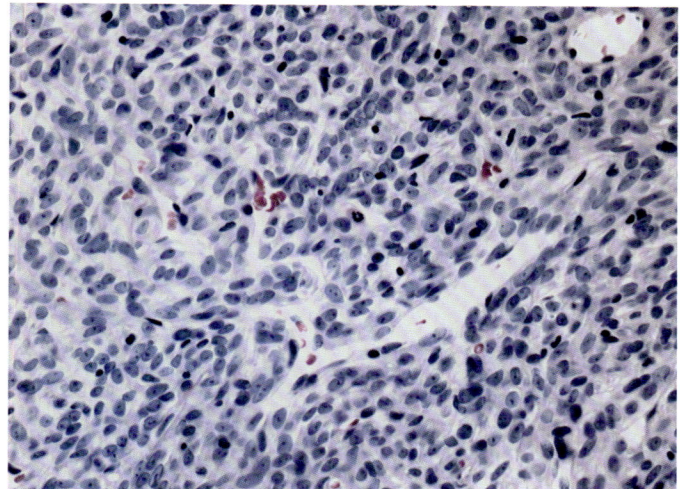

IMAGE 4.105 Hemangiopericytoma. The image shows thin-walled branching ("staghorn") vessels surrounded by round to oval pericytes (H&E, x100).

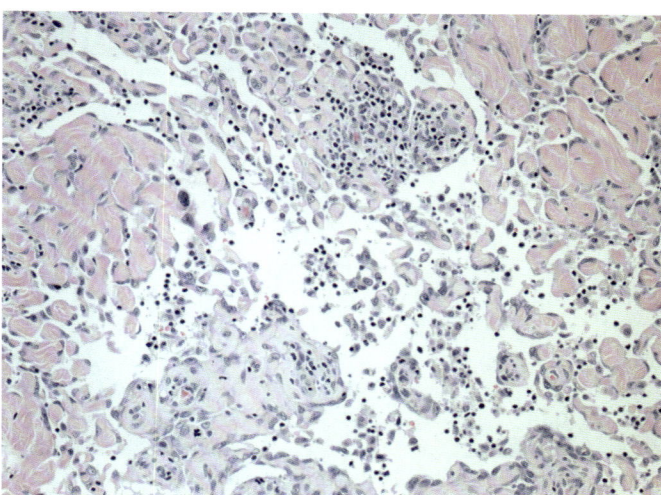

IMAGE 4.108 Angiosarcoma. The image shows irregular vascular channels lined by endothelial cells with pleomorphic hyperchromatic nuclei (H&E, x20).

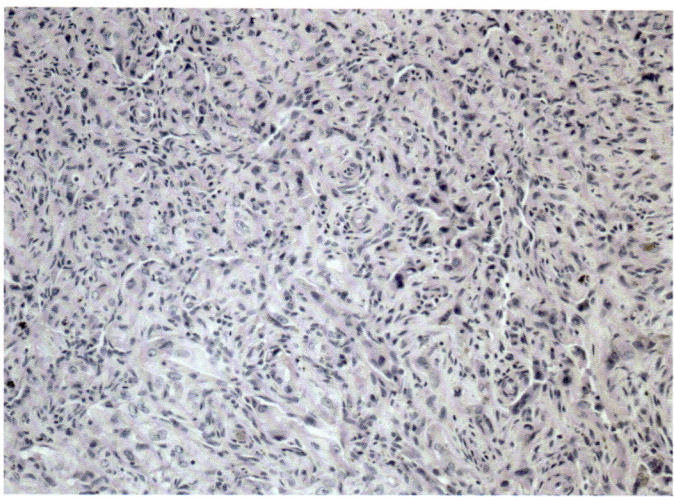

IMAGE 4.106 Epithelioid hemangioendothelioma. The image shows cords of epithelioid cells forming irregular vascular channels (H&E, x40).

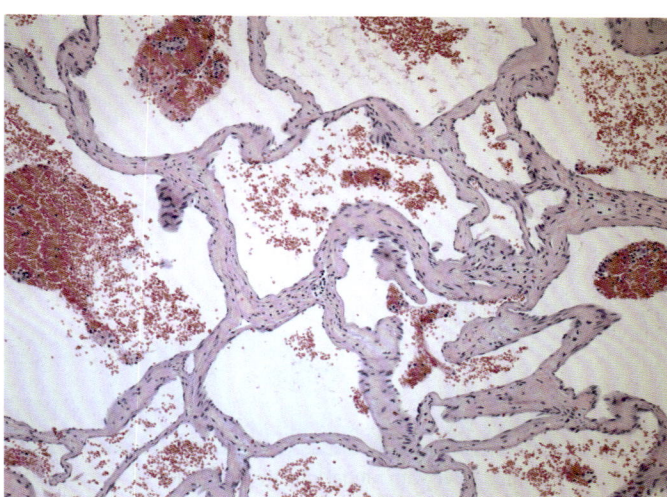

IMAGE 4.109 Cavernous hemangioma. The image shows spongelike spaces lined by benign endothelial cells (H&E, x20).

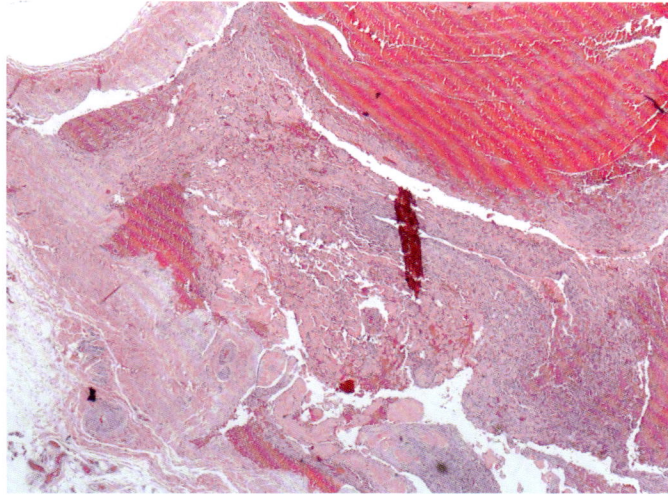

IMAGE 4.107 Masson tumor (intravascular papillary endothelial hyperplasia). The image shows papillary projections lined by endothelial cells (H&E, x20).

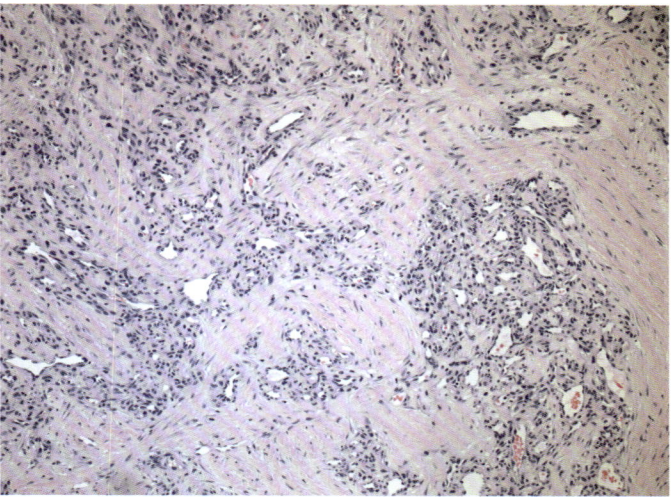

IMAGE 4.110 Pyogenic granuloma (lobular capillary hemangioma). The image shows lobular vascular proliferation with inflammation (H&E, x10).

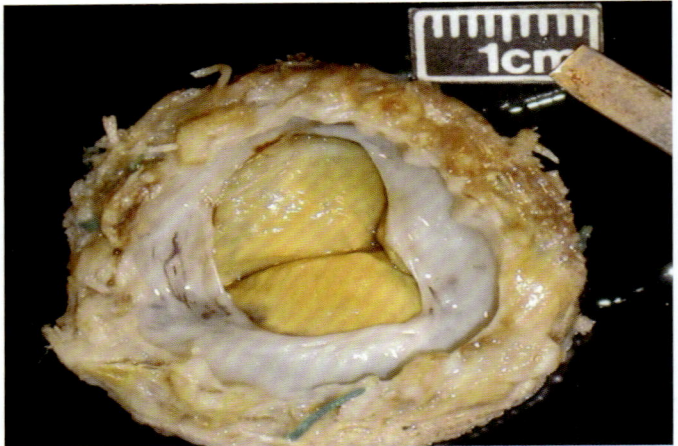

IMAGE 4.111 Bioprosthesis with white pannus material obstructing valve inflow.

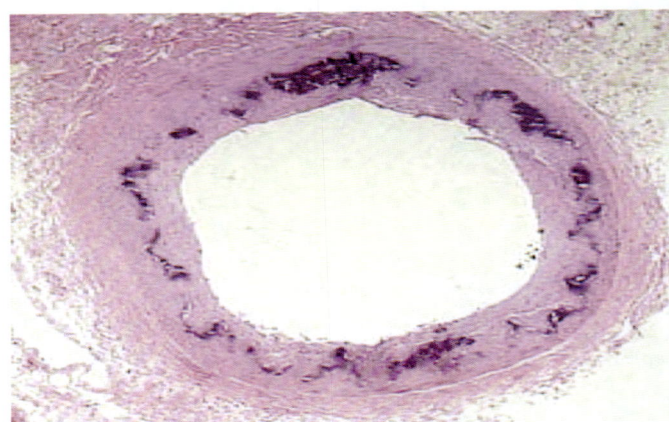

IMAGE 4.114 Monckeberg medial calcinosis with purple calcification near the internal elastic lamina and in the media. This is commonly seen in limb vessels and easily confused with atherosclerosis (H&E, x4).

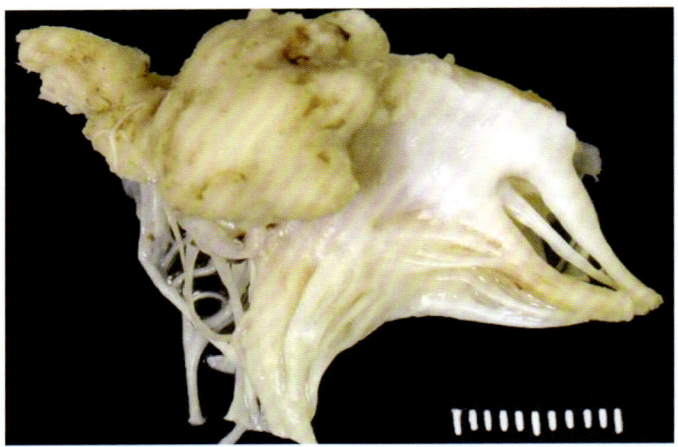

IMAGE 4.112 Mitral valve with fungal infective endocarditis. The image shows a large fungal vegetation.

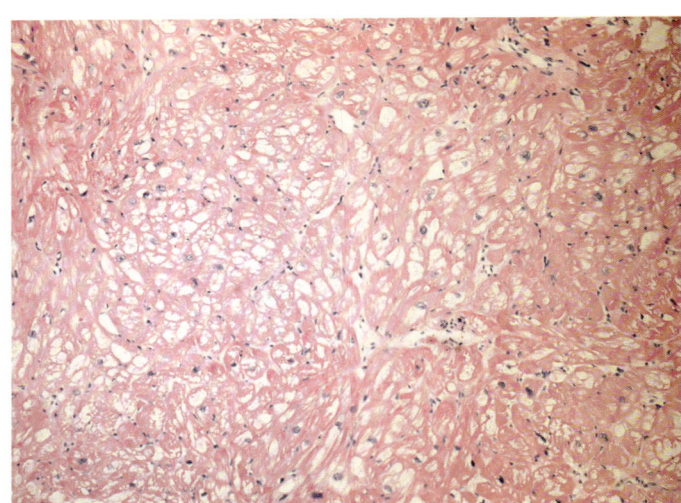

IMAGE 4.115 Fabry disease. The cardiac biopsy shows myocyte vacuolization (H&E, x100).

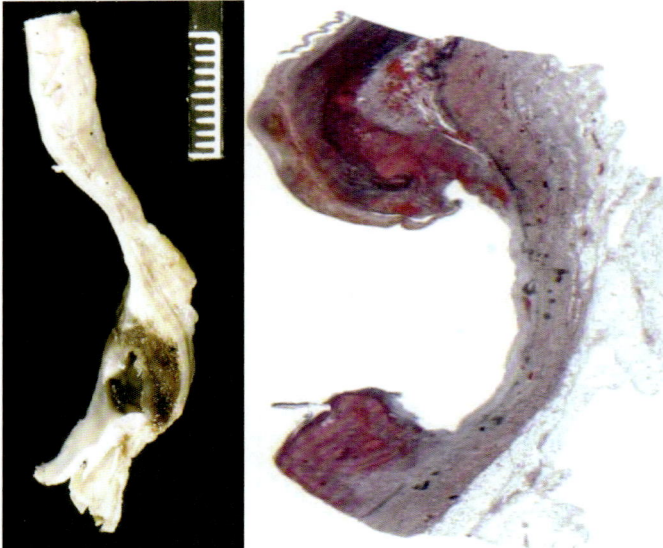

IMAGE 4.113 Penetrating aortic ulcer. Left (gross): a deeply erosive plaque which can cause rupture and dissection. Right (histology): a deeply ulcerated atherosclerotic plaque eroding through almost the full thickness of the vessel wall (elastic stain, x4).

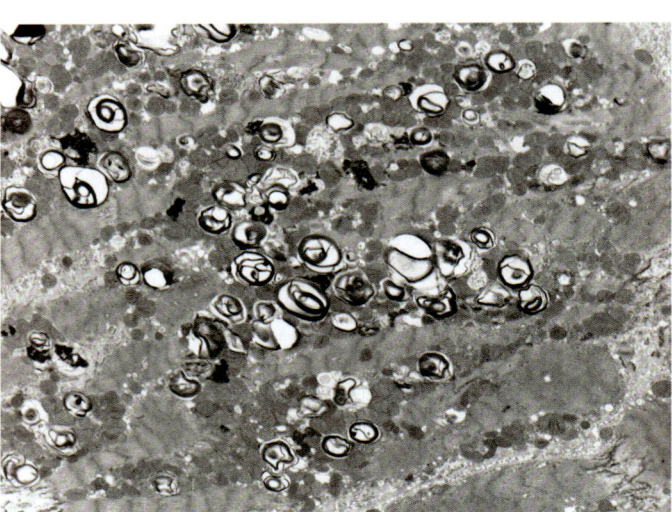

IMAGE 4.116 Fabry disease. Electron microscopy (x2000) shows lamellar inclusion bodies in the myocyte.

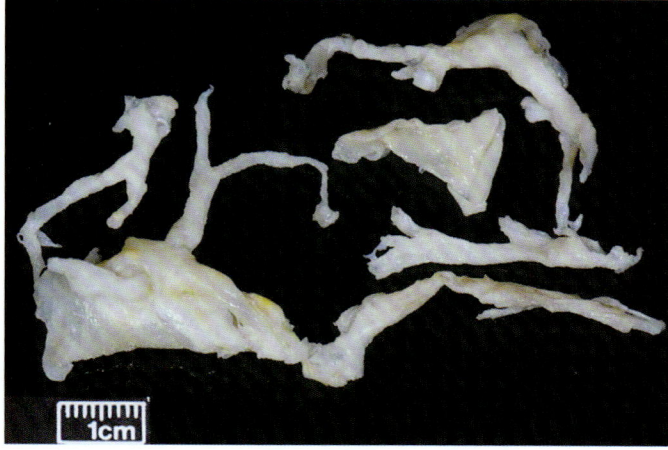

IMAGE 4.117 Pulmonary artery thromboendarterectomy specimens. These endarterectomy specimens were surgically removed from patients with chronic thromboembolic pulmonary hypertension.

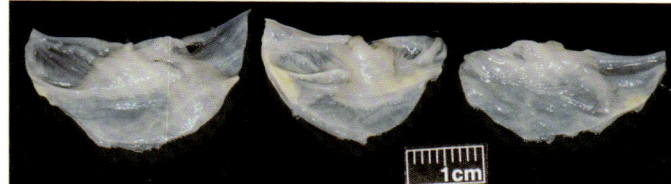

IMAGE 4.120 Aortic valve myxomatous changes consistent with chronic valvular insufficiency. The valve is thin, semitranslucent, and stretched. A common cause of this change is aortic root dilatation, where the valve is not longer competent.

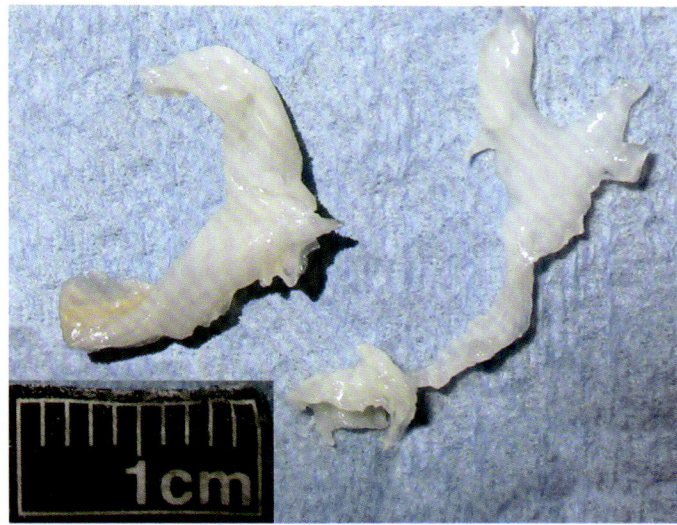

IMAGE 4.118 Subaortic membrane. This is the most common cause of subaortic stenosis. These may be surgically removed, but often the valve is damaged and membrane may recur.

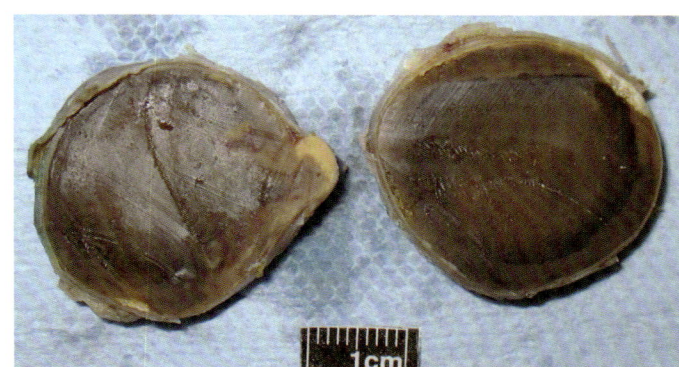

IMAGE 4.121 Arteriovenous fistula aneurysm, thrombosed. These fistulas are created for dialysis. Due to repetitive trauma to the wall with fibrosis, the fistula weakens and aneurysm is common. Thrombosis or infection may occur.

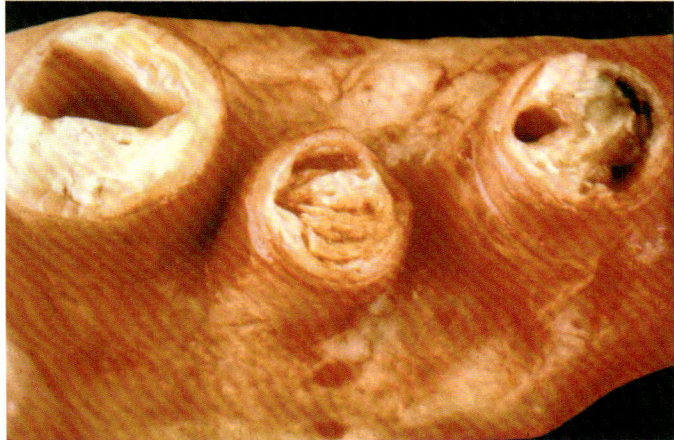

IMAGE 4.119 Aortic arch vessel atherosclerosis. The arch vessels are narrowed by soft atheromas; the right vessel has plaque hemorrhage, a complication.

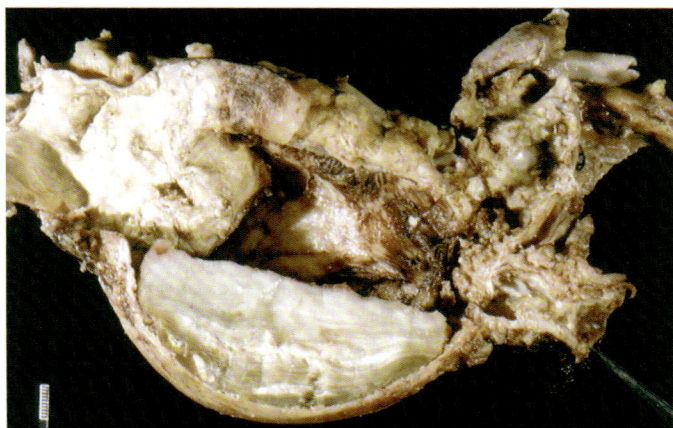

IMAGE 4.122 Atheromatous abdominal aortic aneurysm. This contains abundant laminated thrombus.

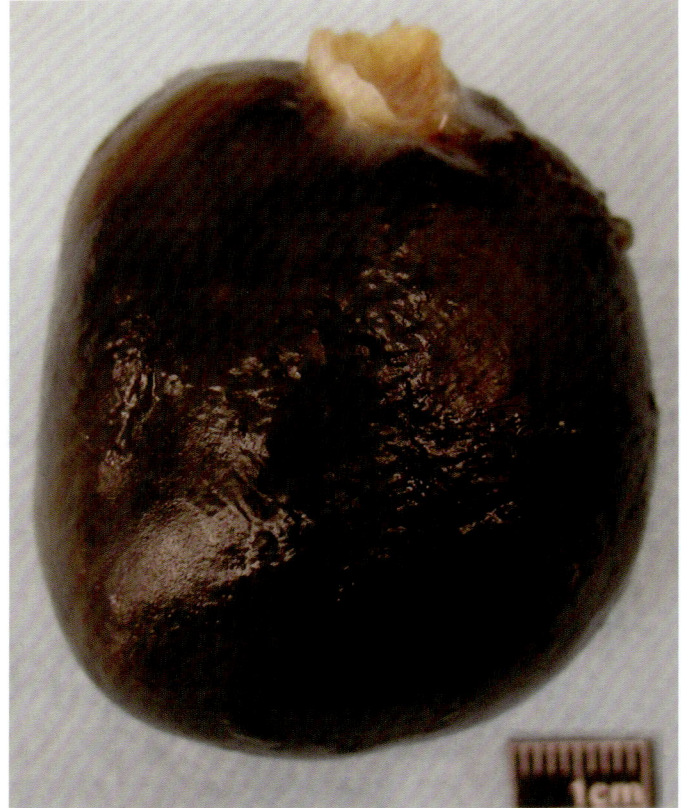

IMAGE 4.123 Cardiac myxoma, right atrium. Cardiac myxoma is the most common benign cardiac tumor. It may occur in any chamber, but left atrium is most common. This myxoma is dark colored probably because of hemorrhage, a common degenerative change in these tumors, along with fibrosis and calcification.

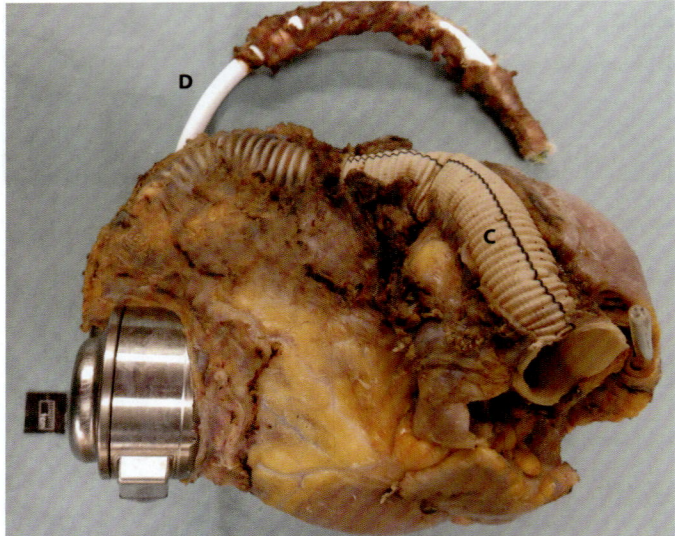

IMAGE 4.125 Heart with ventricular assist device. The heart has been removed for transplantation. The patient had previously had an assist device, which is the metal device at the apex. This pump moves blood from the left ventricle through a graft conduit (C) into the aorta. The white line is the drive line (D), containing wires that connect the device to the battery, which the patient wears on the outside. This line may become infected.

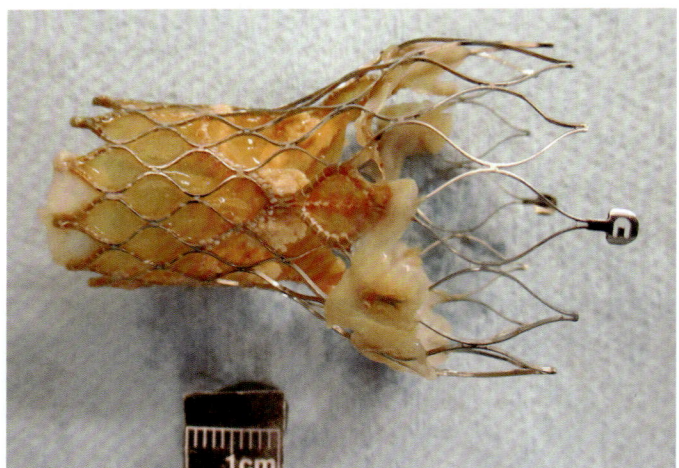

IMAGE 4.124 Corvalve — explanted transcatheter aortic valve implantation (TAVI). This is a transcutaneous aortic valve that may be placed peripherally or through the chest. It is a bioprosthetic valve surrounded by a metal stent that expands to keep the valve in place. No open heart surgery is required to place this valve, but it still has the complications of a bioprosthetic valve. This valve shows some fibrous intimal material on the metal stent, and the valve shows fibrosis and calcification.

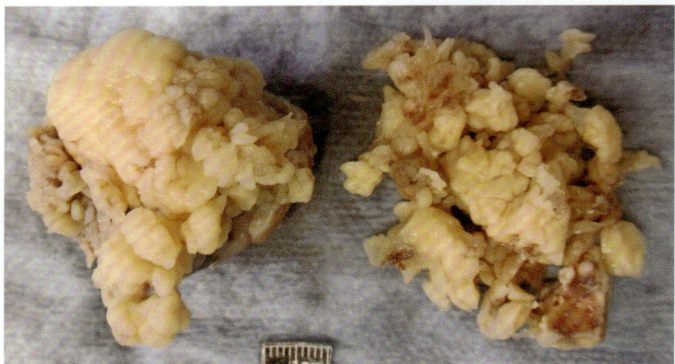

IMAGE 4.126 Left atrial myxoma. This is a multilobulated, polypoid, benign cardiac tumor. Its most common location is the left atrium. Thrombus or tumor may embolize causing symptoms.

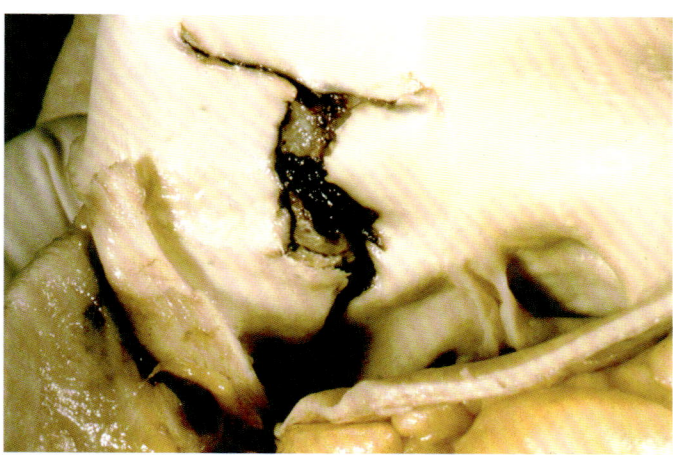

IMAGE 4.127 Aortic dissection intimal tear. This is the most common location for an entry tear in a type A aortic dissection; the tear may extend retrograde and also damage the integrity of the aortic valve apparatus.

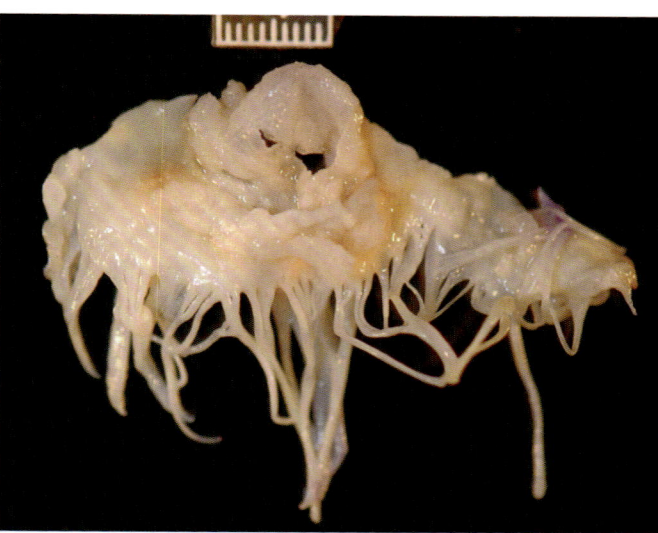

IMAGE 4.129 Mitral valve infective endocarditis perforated aneurysm. This anterior mitral leaflet has infective endocarditis from bacteria. The infection has caused weakening of the leaflet and an outpouching aneurysm, which is ruptured. This would produce a defect and mitral insufficiency.

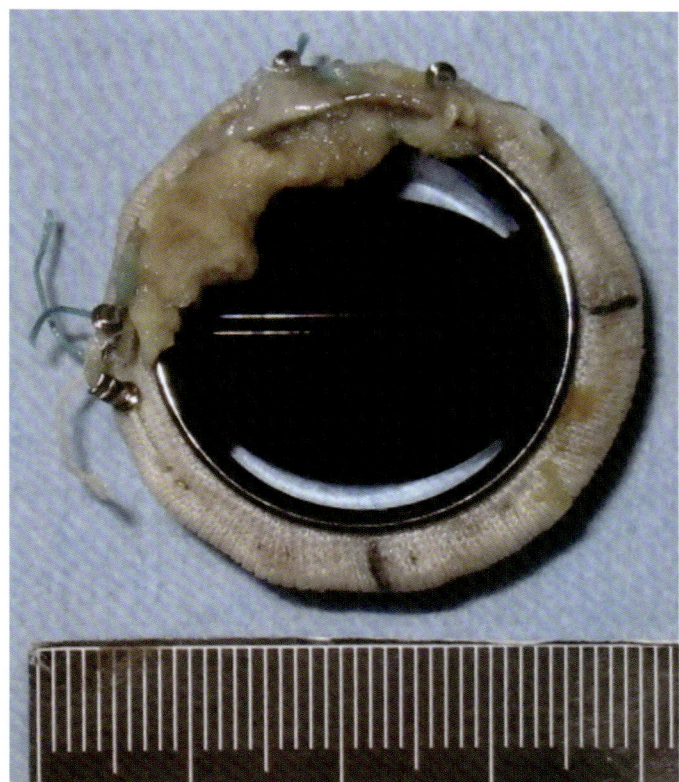

IMAGE 4.128 Mechanical valve prosthesis with thrombus. This mechanical prosthesis shows deposit of thrombus on 1 of the prosthetic leaflets. This may become infected. This also may result in valve stenosis due to leaflet immobility. Thrombolysis is indicated, as this may be an emergent situation.

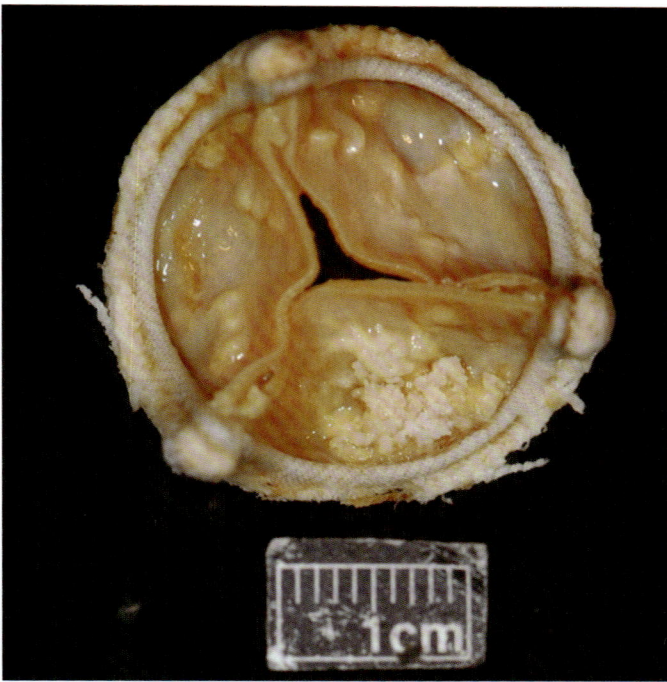

IMAGE 4.130 Pericardial valve prosthesis with degeneration. This pericardial bioprosthetic valve has leaflet degenerative changes with fibrosis and calcification. The leaflets may become stenotic and rigid. More commonly, the leaflets tear and the valve becomes regurgitant.

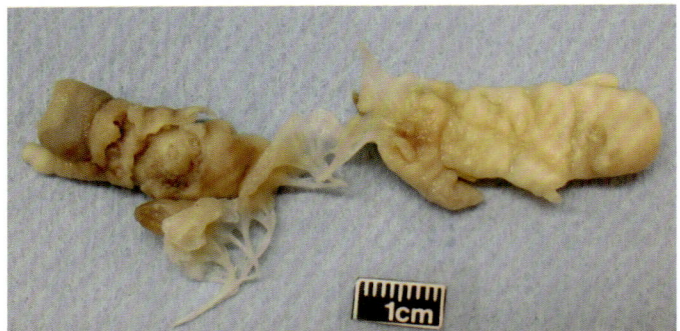

IMAGE 4.131 Tricuspid valve infective endocarditis. The tricuspid valve may be infected with bacteria or fungal endocarditis. Common causes include interventional lines or intravenous drug use.

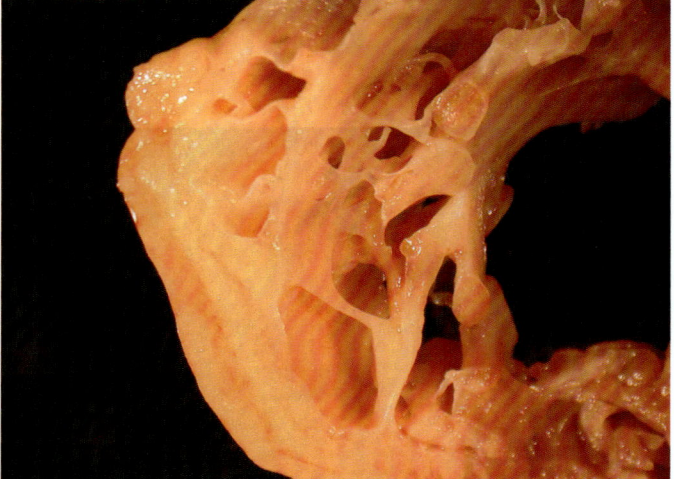

IMAGE 4.132 Arrhythmogenic cardiomyopathy right ventricle lateral wall fat. There is little myocardium remaining, as the ventricular wall has been replaced by yellow fat.

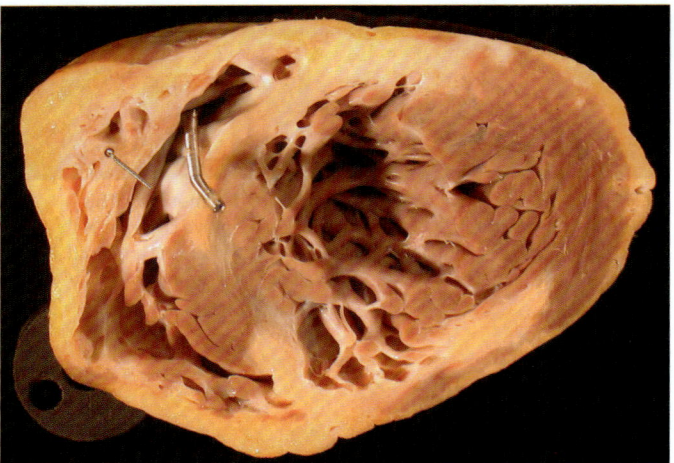

IMAGE 4.133 Arrhythmogenic cardiomyopathy biventricular involvement, cross-section of heart. Both ventricles are partially replaced by yellow fat, especially the thinner right ventricle on the left side of the image.

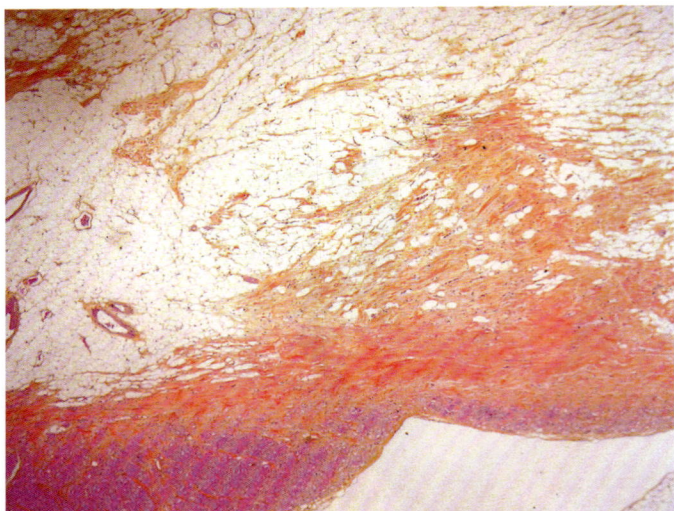

IMAGE 4.134 Arrhythmogenic cardiomyopathy microscopic fatty replacement. Almost the entire wall of the ventricle has been replaced by fat and fibrous tissue; all that remains is myocardium in the inner trabeculae at the lower part of the image (HPS, x4).

Bibliography

Buja LML, Butany J, editors. Cardiovascular pathology. 5th ed. Cambridge (MA): Academic Press; 2022.

Butnor KJ, Beasley MB, McKenna RJ, et al; Cancer Committee, College of American Pathologists. Protocol for the examination of specimens from patients with primary malignant tumors of the heart (Version: Heart 3.0.0.0) [Internet]. College of American Pathologists; 2009 Oct [accessed 2015 Jul 1]. 7 p. Available from www.cap.org.

Cunningham KS, Veinot JP, Butany J. An approach to endomyocardial biopsy interpretation. J Clin Pathol. 2006;59(2):121–9. Medline:16443725. doi: 10.1136/jcp.2005.026443

Kumar V, Abbas AK, Aster JC. Robbins and Cotran pathologic basis of disease. 10th ed. North York (ON): Elsevier Canada; 2020.

Lester SC. Manual of surgical pathology. 3rd ed. Philadelphia (PA): Elsevier Saunders; 2010.

Longacre TA, editor. Mills and Sternberg's diagnostic surgical pathology. 7th ed. Philadelphia (PA): Wolters Kluwar; 2022.

Reddy VB, David O, Spitz DJ, et al. Gattuso's differential diagnosis in surgical pathology. 4th ed. Philadelphia (PA): Elsevier; 2021.

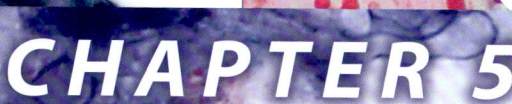

CHAPTER 5

Cytopathology

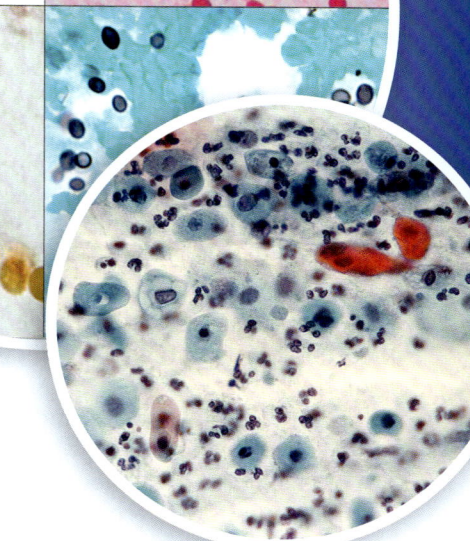

YONCA KANBER, IVAN CHEBIB, MANON AUGER

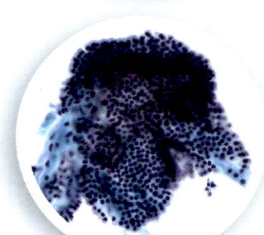

Cytopathology Exam Essentials

MUST KNOW

Classification schemes

High-yield topics include:
- Commonly accepted reporting systems for various organs:
  · The Bethesda system for reporting cervical cytology.
  · The Bethesda system for reporting thyroid cytopathology (including noninvasive follicular thyroid neoplasm with papillary-like nuclear features [NIFTP]).
  · The Paris system for reporting urine cytology.
  · The Milan system for salivary gland cytopathology.
  · The Papanicolaou Society of Cytopathology system for reporting pancreaticobiliary cytology.
  · The Papanicolaou Society of Cytopathology system for reporting respiratory cytology.
  · The International Academy of Cytology Yokohama system for reporting breast fine needle aspiration cytopathology.
  · The international system for serous fluid cytopathology.
- Other types of cytopathology specimens (not covered above):
  · Cerebrospinal fluid (CSF).
  · Esophageal brushing.
  · Lung, including sputum, bronchoalveolar lavage, aspiration of lung masses and lymph nodes (including EBUS [endobronchial ultrasound] and

EUS [endoscopic ultrasound]) guided FNAs.
  · Breast implant-associated effusion.
  · Liver.
  · Kidney.
  · Anus.
  · Lymph nodes.
- The parts of the each reporting system relevant to cytology:
  · Indications for performing cytology.
  · Methods of gathering samples.
  · Cytologic preparation techniques, including cell block preparation.
  · Adequacy criteria.
  · Factors that make samples inadequate.
  · Diagnostic categories and thresholds.
  · The findings of a "normal" specimen.
  · Differential diagnosis and mimics in each category, including benign mimics.
  · Appropriate ancillary workup.
  · Possible quality-assurance-related issues.

Cytology quality assurance (QA)

High-yield topics include:
- The process by which a cytology specimen is collected, prepared, and analyzed, and results are reported.

- Fixatives, dyes, and preparation methods used for cytology, and the advantages and disadvantages of each.
- The advantages of using cytology to make a diagnosis in contrast to other methods such as biopsy.
- Preanalytic, analytic, and postanalytic factors that can cause false-positive and false-negative results.
- The role of cytotechnologists and their limitations in scope of practice.
- The benefits and risks of using cytology as a screening or diagnostic tool.
- Common QA practices in cytology, including retrospective screening, prospective screening, various forms of correlation, and QA indicators and acceptable levels in particular diagnostic categories or rates of discrepancy.
- Common causes of discrepancies, including technologist-pathologist and cytology-histology discrepancies.
- The process, advantages, and disadvantages of rapid on-site evaluation (ROSE) of specimens.
- The diagnoses in cytology that qualify as critical values, and how to report them.

MUST SEE

Review the following common findings:
- Cervical cytology:
  · Negative for intraepithelial lesion or malignancy (NILM), with normal superficial, intermediate, and basal cells.
  · NILM, with metaplastic squamous cells.
  · NILM, with endocervical cells.
  · NILM, with atrophic changes.
  · NILM, with endometrial cells, including exodus, as well as endometrial cells in women older than 45.
  · NILM, with infectious changes including herpes simplex virus (HSV), cytomegalovirus (CMV), *Candida*, *Actinomyces*, *Trichomonas*, and bacterial vaginosis.
  · NILM, radiation and repair related changes.
  · Low grade squamous intraepithelial lesion (LSIL).
  · High grade squamous intraepithelial lesion (HSIL).
  · Invasive squamous cell carcinoma (keratinizing and nonkeratinizing).
  · Adenocarcinoma in situ (AIS).
  · Invasive adenocarcinoma.
  · Endometrial adenocarcinoma.
- Thyroid cytology:
  · Benign follicular nodule.
  · Cystic change.
  · Repair, and Hürthle cell change.
  · Hashimoto thyroiditis.
  · Follicular neoplasm, Hürthle cell neoplasm.
  · Papillary thyroid carcinoma and variants.
  · Medullary carcinoma.
  · Anaplastic carcinoma.

- Urine cytology:
  · Negative for high grade urothelial carcinoma (NHGUC), with normal umbrella cells.
  · NHGUC, with ileal conduit changes.
  · NHGUC, with *Polyomavirus*.
  · Positive for high grade urothelial carcinoma (PHGUC).
- Salivary gland cytology:
  · Pleomorphic adenoma.
  · Adenoid cystic carcinoma.
  · Warthin tumor.
  · Mucoepidermoid carcinoma.
  · Acinic cell carcinoma.
- CSF cytology:
  · Acute meningitis.
  · Metastatic carcinoma and melanoma.
  · *Cryptococcus*.
- Esophageal brush cytology:
  · Herpes esophagitis.
  · Squamous cell carcinoma.
  · *Candida* esophagitis.
- Lung and lymph node cytology:
  · Normal bronchial brush, sputum, and aspirate of lymph node.
  · Creola body.
  · Charcot-Leyden crystals.
  · Ferruginous body.
  · Organisms, including *Aspergillus*, *Mucor*, *Pneumocystis*, *Coccidioides*, *Cryptococcus*, and *Blastomyces*.
  · Lipoid pneumonia.
  · Reserve cell hyperplasia.
  · Pulmonary hamartoma.
  · Carcinoid tumor and small cell carcinoma.
  · Squamous cell carcinoma.
  · Adenocarcinoma.
  · Nonnecrotizing granulomatous lymphadenitis (e.g., sarcoidosis).
  · Metastatic carcinoma and melanoma to lymph node.
- Mesothelial lined cavity (pleural, pericardial, peritoneal) cytology:
  · Benign mesothelial cells.
  · Reactive mesothelial cells.
  · Infection with abundant neutrophils.
  · Malignant mesothelioma.
  · Metastatic carcinoma such as lung, breast ("cannonballs"), and gynecologic.
- Breast and implant-associated effusion cytology:
  · Fibrocystic change.
  · Fibroadenoma.
  · Mammary carcinoma, including lobular carcinoma.
  · Effusion-associated anaplastic large cell lymphoma.
- Liver and pancreas cytology:
  · Metastatic adenocarcinoma.
  · Pancreatic ductal adenocarcinoma.

- Pancreatic pseudocyst (and associated cytology fluid biochemistry findings).
- Kidney cytology:
  - Clear cell renal cell carcinoma (RCC).
- Anal cytology:
  - LSIL.
  - HSIL.
  - Squamous cell carcinoma.
- Lymph node cytology:
  - Small and large B-cell lymphoma.
  - Metastatic carcinoma and melanoma.
  - Granulomatous lymphadenitis (e.g., sarcoidosis).

MUST DO

- For each of the diagnostic categories outlined in the Must See section, you should be comfortable generating a differential diagnosis and listing additional studies (e.g., histochemical or immunohistochemical stains). Pay special attention to equivocal and positive categories.
- You should have practical experience with preparation of cytology samples, including:
  - The flow of a cytology specimen from accessioning to interpretation to reporting, and areas where QA is done.
  - The common ways to collect a specimen, and factors that may affect the adequacy and quality of the specimen collected.
  - The various staining and preparation methods for a specimen, and their advantages and disadvantages.
  - The various forms of QA in cytology, and how they differ from histopathology, including diagnostic discrepancies.
  - Findings that constitute critical values, and how to deal with them.
- You should be able to advise for triaging of fresh cytology specimens for flow cytometry, microbiology, and other ancillary studies.

MULTIPLE CHOICE QUESTIONS

1. Which cell types may be considered in the cell count for adequacy of a cervical smear, according to the Bethesda system for reporting cervical cytology?*

a. Mature squamous cells.

b. Mature squamous and squamous metaplastic cells.

c. Mature squamous and endocervical cells.

d. Mature squamous metaplastic and endocervical cells.

e. All cells on the smear.

Answer: b

*This chapter uses the third edition of the Bethesda system for reporting cervical cytology.

2. Which of the following should be considered **satisfactory** for a cervical smear, according to the Bethesda system?

a. Liquid based cytology cervical smear with approximately 1000 squamous cells.

b. Conventional cytology cervical smear with approximately 4000 squamous cells.

c. Liquid based cytology cervical smear with approximately 5000 mature squamous cells, but without endocervical glandular or squamous metaplastic cells.

d. Cervical smear with approximately 80% of squamous cells obscured by blood or inflammation.

e. Cervical smear specimen received without patient identification.

Answer: c

3. According to the Bethesda system, the minimum cellularity adequacy criteria for a cervical smear can be lowered in all the following special circumstances **except**:

a. Radiation to cervix/pelvic region.

b. Chemotherapy.

c. Hysterectomy or trachelectomy.

d. Pregnancy.

e. Atrophic vaginitis.

Answer: d

4. What minimum percentage of squamous cells must be obscured by inflammation or blood for an interpretation of "unsatisfactory" in a cervical smear, according to the Bethesda system?

a. 25%.

b. 50%.

c. 75%.

d. 100%.

e. Any percentage.

Answer: c

5. According to the Bethesda system, which of the following statements **best** characterizes the minimum criteria for an adequate transformation zone sample?

a. Abundant mucus.

b. No such criteria exist.

c. At least 5 well-preserved endocervical or squamous metaplastic cells.

d. At least 10 well-preserved endocervical or squamous metaplastic cells.

e. At least 20 well-preserved endocervical or squamous metaplastic cells.

Answer: d

6. A cervical smear from a 40-year-old female contains rare groups of benign-appearing endometrial cell clusters. Which category in the Bethesda system should be used to reflect this finding?

a. Negative for squamous intraepithelial lesion or malignancy.
b. Atypical endometrial glandular cells, not otherwise specified.
c. Atypical glandular cells, favor neoplastic.
d. Adenocarcinoma, endometrial.
e. Other (endometrial cells in a woman ≥ 45 years).

Answer: a

7. A cervical smear from a 45-year-old female contains rare groups of benign-appearing endometrial cell clusters. Which category in the Bethesda system should be used to reflect this finding?

a. Negative for squamous intraepithelial lesion or malignancy.
b. Atypical endometrial glandular cells, not otherwise specified.
c. Atypical glandular cells, favor neoplastic.
d. Adenocarcinoma, endometrial.
e. Other (endometrial cells in a woman ≥ 45 years of age).

Answer: e

8. According to the guidelines of the Canadian Society of Cytopathology, which of the following screened cervical smears in a low-risk population can be signed out by a cytotechnologist without pathologist review?

a. All smears.
b. All smears with the exception of atypical squamous cells of uncertain significance (ASC-US) or worse findings.
c. "Negative for squamous intraepithelial lesion or malignancy" smears with the exception of repair.
d. "Negative for squamous intraepithelial lesion or malignancy" smears including repair.
e. None.

Answer: c

9. According to the Bethesda system, atypical repair should be reported in which of the following categories?

a. Negative for squamous intraepithelial lesion or malignancy.
b. ASC-US.
c. Low grade squamous intraepithelial lesion (LSIL).
d. High grade squamous intraepithelial lesion (HSIL).
e. Atypical squamous cells; cannot rule out HSIL (ASC-H).

Answer: b

10. According to the Bethesda system, which of the following is the appropriate interpretation of a conventional cervical smear consisting of 8000–12 000 anucleate squamous cells?

a. Negative for intraepithelial lesion or malignancy (NILM).
b. ASC-US.
c. ASC-H.
d. LSIL.
e. Unsatisfactory.

Answer: e

11. All of the following statements concerning lower uterine segment (LUS) sampling in cervical cytology are true **except**:

a. LUS is a cause of false positive diagnoses (for HSIL or atypical glandular cells) in cervical cytology.
b. LUS typically presents as large, flat hyperchromatic groups.
c. LUS should be reported in the category "endometrial cells present."
d. LUS is due to direct sampling instead of spontaneous exfoliation of endometrial cells.
e. The correct interpretation of such a finding is NILM.

Answer: c

12. All of the following statements concerning tubal metaplasia in cervical cytology are true **except**:

a. Single ciliated cells in isolation are sufficient for the designation.
b. It is a pitfall for endocervical adenocarcinoma in situ (AIS).
c. Presence of cilia and/or terminal bars is characteristic.
d. The correct interpretation is NILM.
e. Increased nuclear to cytoplasmic ratio may be present.

Answer: a

13. All the following can cause perinuclear halos **except**:

a. *Trichomonas* infection.
b. Nonspecific inflammation.
c. LSIL.
d. Navicular cells.
e. Decidual cells.

Answer: e

14. Which of the following is **not** a feature of cervical AIS on cervical smear?

a. Hyperchromasia.
b. Macronucleoli.
c. Rosettes.
d. Feathering.
e. Mitotic figures.

Answer: b

15. All the following are often encountered in cervical smears from patients with an intrauterine device (IUD) **except**:

a. Actinomyces.
b. ASC-US-like epithelial cells.
c. ASC-H-like epithelial cells.
d. AGC, endometrial-like glandular cells (AGC: atypical glandular cells).
e. Prominent nucleoli.

Answer: b

16. In which phase of the menstrual cycle do you expect to see abundant *Lactobacilli* with cytolysis?

a. Luteal phase.
b. Follicular phase.
c. Menstrual phase.
d. Transitional phase.
e. Perimeno-pausal phase.

Answer: a

17. Strawberry coloring of the cervix and vagina is a classic sign of what infection?

a. Bacterial vaginosis.
b. Trichomonas vaginalis.
c. Candida albicans.
d. Leptothrix.
e. Chlamydia.

Answer: b

18. An NILM smear from a 30-year-old female is noted to have filamentous microorganisms arranged in clumps ("cotton balls"). The underlying source of this finding is:

a. Bacterial vaginosis.
b. Human papillomavirus (HPV) infection.
c. A foreign body, such as an IUD.
d. Chlamydia.
e. Trauma.

Answer: c

19. What is the name of the organism described as "cotton balls" in the previous question?

a. Actinomyces.
b. Nocardia.
c. Candida.
d. Leptothrix.
e. Lactobacilli.

Answer: a

20. The so-called "blue blobs" that can cause false positive diagnoses are characteristically seen in which of the following contexts?

a. LSIL.
b. HSIL.
c. Pregnancy.
d. Follicular cervicitis.
e. Atrophic vaginitis.

Answer: e

21. A shift in vaginal flora is associated with all of the following **except**:

a. Clue cells.
b. Fishy-smelling vaginal discharge.
c. Pelvic inflammatory disease.
d. Birth defects.
e. Postoperative gynecologic infections.

Answer: d

22. According to the Bethesda system, all of the following options are available for the interpretation of glandular lesions in cervical smears **except**:

a. Atypical endometrial cells, not otherwise specified (NOS).
b. Endometrial cells, favor neoplastic.
c. Atypical endocervical cells, NOS.
d. Atypical endocervical cells, favor neoplastic.
e. Endocervical AIS.

Answer: b

23. What is the recommended initial workup following an interpretation of a cervical smear as ASC-H?

a. Repeat cervical cytology in in 3 months.
b. Colposcopy.
c. Reflex HPV testing.
d. Cytology and HPV testing (cotesting).
e. Hysterectomy.

Answer: b

24. According to the Bethesda system, the minimum cellularity adequacy criteria for a conventional anal smear is:

a. 500–1000 nucleated squamous cells.
b. 1000–2000 nucleated squamous cells.
c. 2000–3000 nucleated squamous cells.
d. 4000–5000 nucleated squamous cells.
e. 8000–12 000 nucleated squamous cells.

Answer: c

25. A fine needle aspiration (FNA) lung biopsy specimen contains rigid, septate hyphae, with 45-degree branching. Name the most likely pulmonary infection.

a. *Aspergillus.*
b. Mucormycosis.
c. *Cryptococcus.*
d. Blastomycosis.
e. Histoplasmosis.

Answer: a

26. An FNA lung biopsy specimen contains yeasts that are 5–10 micrometers (µm) with narrow-based budding, and that have a thick mucicarmine positive capsule. Name the most likely pulmonary infection.

a. *Aspergillus.*
b. Mucormycosis.
c. *Cryptococcus.*
d. Blastomycosis.
e. Histoplasmosis.

Answer: c

27. An FNA lung biopsy specimen contains yeasts that are 10–20 µm with broad-based budding. Name the most likely pulmonary infection.

a. *Aspergillus.*
b. Mucormycosis.
c. *Cryptococcus.*
d. Blastomycosis.
e. Histoplasmosis.

Answer: d

28. An FNA lung biopsy specimen contains yeasts that are 5 µm, predominantly within granulomata. Name the most likely pulmonary infection.

a. *Aspergillus.*
b. Mucormycosis.
c. *Cryptococcus.*
d. Blastomycosis.
e. Histoplasmosis.

Answer: e

29. Which of the following statements about histoplasmosis is true?

a. The causative agent is mostly encountered in the southwestern states of the USA.

b. The vast majority of cases are asymptomatic in immunocompetent hosts.

c. The causative agent is acquired by drinking contaminated water.

d. The lung is a rare site of involvement.

e. Disease only occurs in immunosuppressed patients.

Answer: b

30. A 64-year-old male with a history of cigarette smoking presents with hypercalcemia and a lung mass on subsequent workup. An FNA biopsy of the lung mass is performed. What is the most likely histologic subtype of this lung mass?

a. Pulmonary hamartoma.

b. Carcinoid tumor.

c. Small cell carcinoma.

d. Adenocarcinoma.

e. Squamous cell carcinoma.

Answer: e

31. A 61-year old male with a history of cigarette smoking presents with progressive proximal muscle weakness, diagnosed as Lambert-Eaton myasthenic syndrome. On workup, he is found to have a lung mass. An FNA biopsy of the lung mass is performed. What is the most likely histologic subtype of this lung mass?

a. Pulmonary hamartoma.

b. Carcinoid tumor.

c. Small cell carcinoma.

d. Adenocarcinoma.

e. Squamous cell carcinoma.

Answer: c

32. A 52-year-old female with no history of cigarette smoking or asbestos exposure presents with an incidentally found nodule with a ground-glass appearance on computed tomography (CT) scan of the chest. An FNA biopsy is performed and interpreted as malignant. What is the most likely histologic subtype of this lung mass?

a. Small cell carcinoma.

b. Adenocarcinoma.

c. Squamous cell carcinoma.

d. Large cell carcinoma.

e. Sarcomatoid carcinoma.

Answer: b

33. Which diagnostic terminology is recommended for a pulmonary nonsmall-cell carcinoma with no obvious cytomorphologic glandular or squamous differentiation, and that is positive for thyroid transcription factor-1 (TTF-1) and negative for p40?

a. Nonsmall-cell carcinoma, favour squamous cell carcinoma.

b. Nonsmall-cell carcinoma, favour adenocarcinoma.

c. Squamous cell carcinoma.

d. Adenocarcinoma.

e. Adenosquamous carcinoma.

Answer: b

34. Which predictive biomarker testing is recommended, as a minimum, for an adenocarcinoma of pulmonary origin?

a. *EGFR*, *KRAS*, and *MET*.

b. *EGFR*, *BRAF*, and *RET*.

c. *EGFR*, *ALK*, and *ROS1*.

d. *ALK*, *ROS1*, and *NRAS*.

e. *ROS1*, *BRAF*, and *NTRK1*.

Answer: c

35. Which of the following is **false** regarding NUT carcinoma?

a. It is a poorly differentiated neoplasm.

b. It lacks glandular differentiation.

c. Its differential diagnosis includes small cell carcinoma,

lymphoma, and germ cell tumors.

d. NUT protein expression is characteristic.

e. It is mainly located in the periphery of the lung.

Answer: e

36. What cells must be seen to designate a mediastinal lymph node sample as adequate when obtained by endobronchial ultrasound–guided (EBUS) FNA?

a. Endobronchial cells and/or cartilage.

b. Endobronchial cells and/or pulmonary macrophages.

c. Lymphocytes and/or malignant cells.

d. Squamous cells and/or smooth muscle cells.

e. Squamous cells and/or cartilage.

Answer: c

37. A 73-year-old male smoker with a long history of asbestos exposure presents with a malignant pleural effusion. Which of the following immunohistochemical profiles most strongly suggests primary pulmonary adenocarcinoma?

a. Calretinin+, MOC-31+, WT-1+, Ber-EP4+, CK5/6+.

b. Calretinin+, MOC-31+, WT-1+, Ber-EP4−, CK5/6+.

c. Calretinin+, MOC-31−, WT-1−, Ber-EP4−, CK5/6+.

d. Calretinin−, MOC-31+, WT-1−, Ber-EP4+, CK5/6−.

e. Calretinin−, MOC-31−, WT-1−, Ber-EP4−, CK5/6−.

Answer: d

38. Which of the following malignant pleural effusion morphologies is most consistent with metastatic breast ductal adenocarcinoma?

a. Large hollow spherical ("cannonball") aggregates.

b. Abundant signet ring cells.

c. Picket-fence arrangement of columnar cells.

d. Papillary fragments with psammoma bodies.

e. Small cell clusters floating in mucinous background.

Answer: a

39. Which of the following is **not** a limitation of breast FNA?

a. Distinguishing invasive ductal from intraductal carcinoma.

b. Distinguishing papilloma from low grade papillary carcinoma.

c. Distinguishing fibroadenomas

d. Distinguishing mucocele from colloid carcinoma.

e. Distinguishing fibrocystic change from fat necrosis.

from benign phyllodes tumors.

Answer: e

40. Which of the following would **not** be present with spindle cell cytomorphology on breast FNA?

a. Lobular breast carcinoma.

b. Metaplastic breast carcinoma.

c. Malignant phyllodes tumor.

d. Fibromatosis.

e. Angiosarcoma.

Answer: a

41. All the following statements are true concerning lactating adenoma **except**:

a. The cytoplasm of the cells is vacuolated.

b. The nucleoli are inconspicuous.

c. It constitutes a known cause of false positive diagnoses.

d. It can have numerous single epithelial cells and/or stripped nuclei.

e. The cytological features can overlap with those of fibroadenoma.

Answer: b

42. According to the Bethesda system for reporting thyroid cytopathology,* what is the approximate risk of malignancy for a thyroid FNA specimen interpreted as atypia of undetermined significance (AUS)?

a. 0–3%.

b. 5–15%.

c. 10–30%.

d. 20–35%.

e. > 35%.

Answer: c

*This chapter uses the second edition of the Bethesda system for reporting thyroid cytopathology.

43. According to the Bethesda system for reporting thyroid cytopathology, what is the recommended upper limit for diagnosing AUS in a cytopathology laboratory?

a. 5%.

b. 10%.

c. 15%.

d. 20%.

e. 25%.

Answer: b

44. Which subtype of AUS in thyroid cytopathology is associated with the highest risk of papillary thyroid carcinoma in follow-up?

a. AUS, Hürthle cell type.

b. AUS, with architectural atypia.

c. AUS, with nuclear/cytological atypia.

d. AUS, lymphoid type.

e. AUS, NOS.

Answer: c

45. According to the Bethesda system for reporting thyroid cytopathology, which of the following is the most appropriate management recommendation for a thyroid FNA interpreted as AUS?

a. Clinical follow-up.

b. Yearly follow-up with ultrasound and FNA.

c. Immediate repeat FNA.

d. Repeat FNA, molecular testing, or lobectomy.

e. Total thyroidectomy.

Answer: d

46. According to the Bethesda system for reporting thyroid cytopathology, what are the adequacy criteria for a solid thyroid nodule sampled by FNA?

a. 4 groups of well-visualized follicular cells with ≥ 10 cells/group.

b. 4 groups of well-visualized follicular cells with ≥ 20 cells/group.

c. 6 groups of well-visualized follicular cells with ≥ 10 cells/group.

d. 6 groups of well-visualized follicular cells with ≥ 20 cells/group.

e. 10 groups of well-visualized follicular cells with ≥ 10 cells/group.

Answer: c

47. A 50-year-old male has a cystic parotid gland mass. The cyst has abundant, thick, brown (motor-oil-like) contents on FNA biopsy. What is the most likely diagnosis?

a. Pleomorphic adenoma.

b. Warthin tumor.

c. Lymphoepithelial cyst.

d. Mucoepidermoid carcinoma.

e. Cystic squamous cell carcinoma.

Answer: b

48. A 70-year-old male with a solid well-circumscribed neck mass undergoes FNA biopsy. Aspiration reveals an abundant pure population of oncocytes arranged in small clusters and single cells. What is the most likely diagnosis?

a. Oncocytoma.

b. Oncocytic carcinoma.

c. Warthin tumor.

d. Oncocytic mucoepidermoid carcinoma.

e. Acinic cell carcinoma.

Answer: a

49. Which of the following salivary gland lesions is most likely to result in a false negative aspirate?

a. Mucoepidermoid carcinoma.

b. Adenoid cystic carcinoma.

c. Acinic cell carcinoma.

d. Lymphoepithelial carcinoma.

e. Squamous cell carcinoma.

Answer: a

50. What type of lymphoma is diagnosed almost exclusively by cytology?

a. Follicular lymphoma.

b. Anaplastic large cell lymphoma.

c. Nodular lymphocyte predominant Hodgkin lymphoma.

d. Primary effusion lymphoma.

e. Burkitt lymphoma.

Answer: d

51. Which virus needs to be detected in a sample before a diagnosis of primary effusion lymphoma can be given?

a. Human immunodeficiency virus (HIV).

b. Human herpes virus 8 (HHV-8).

c. Epstein-Barr virus (EBV).

d. Cytomegalovirus (CMV).

e. Simian polyoma virus 40 (SV-40).

Answer: b

52. What immunophenotype would be most consistent with the diagnosis breast-implant-associated anaplastic large cell lymphoma (BIA-ALCL)?

a. CD68+, CD3–, CD20–, CD30–, ALK–.

b. CD68–, CD3–, CD20–, CD30+, ALK–.

c. CD68–, CD3+, CD20–, CD30+, ALK+.

d. CD68–, CD3, CD20+, CD30–, ALK–.

e. CD68–, CD3–, CD20–, CD30–, ALK–.

Answer: b

53. Which of these statements about BIA-ALCL is true?

a. The majority of effusions associated with breast implants that occur less than a year after implantation are caused by this condition.

b. The majority of effusions associated with breast implants that occur more than a year after implantation are caused by this condition.

c. This condition appears to be associated with smooth-textured breast implants.

d. This condition is usually considered an indolent disease with good prognosis, but a subset of patients have more aggressive disease.

e. This is an aggressive disease with poor prognosis in the majority of patients.

Answer: d

54. An 86-year-old male with a liver mass, seen on abdomen CT scan, undergoes FNA biopsy of the lesion. Cytology shows a cellular smear composed of cohesive groups of tall columnar cells in a "picket fence" arrangement, and acini with central and background necrotic debris. Which of the following is the most likely diagnosis?

a. Hepatocellular carcinoma.

b. Cholangiocarcinoma.

c. Metastatic colorectal carcinoma.

d. Metastatic breast carcinoma.

e. Epithelioid angiosarcoma.

Answer: c

55. A 56-year-old male with a liver mass in the background of cirrhosis, seen on abdomen CT scan, undergoes FNA biopsy of the lesion. Cytology shows a cellular smear composed of cohesive and single polygonal cells. Which of the following would most strongly suggest a diagnosis of hepatocellular carcinoma?

a. Strong HepPar-1 positivity.

b. Background of cirrhosis as seen on abdomen CT scan.

c. Thickened trabeculae lined by endothelial cells.

d. Lack of bile duct epithelium in the background.

e. Clinical history and serology consistent with hepatitis C infection.

Answer: c

56. A 64-year-old female with a cystic pancreatic head mass, seen on abdomen CT scan, undergoes an endoscopic ultrasound-guided FNA of the cystic lesion. Cytology shows rare bland mucinous epithelial cells and thick mucin. Which of the following would most strongly suggest a neoplastic mucinous neoplasm?

a. Elevated carcinoembryonic antigen (CEA) on cyst fluid analysis.

b. Elevated amylase on cyst fluid analysis.

c. Low CEA and amylase on cyst fluid analysis.

d. Presence of hemosiderin laden macrophages.

e. Ultrasound evidence of a dilated main pancreatic duct.

Answer: a

57. An FNA specimen from a solid, well-circumscribed pancreatic mass shows loosely cohesive and single epithelioid and plasmacytoid cells with round nuclei. Which of the following entities is **not** in the differential diagnosis?

a. Well-differentiated ductal adenocarcinoma.

b. Well-differentiated pancreatic neuroendocrine tumor.

c. Solid pseudopapillary neoplasm.

d. Acinar cell carcinoma.

e. Metastatic renal cell carcinoma (RCC).

Answer: a

58. An FNA specimen of a submucosal mass located in the stomach shows spindle cells. Which of the following immunoprofiles is consistent with a diagnosis of gastrointestinal stromal tumor (GIST)?

a. DOG1–, C-KIT–, desmin+, S100–, SOX10–.

b. DOG1+, C-KIT+, desmin–, S100–, SOX10–.

c. DOG1–, C-KIT–, desmin-, S100+, SOX10+.

d. DOG1–, C-KIT–, desmin–, S100–, SOX10–.

e. DOG1–, C-KIT–, desmin–, S100+, SOX10–.

Answer: b

59. A 51-year-old female is found to have metastatic adenocarcinoma to the cerebrospinal fluid (CSF) with no known primary cancer. What is the most likely occult primary site?

a. Breast.

b. Lung.

c. Stomach.

d. Colon/rectum.

e. Ovary.

Answer: b

60. According to the Paris system for reporting urinary cytopathology (2016), the main aim of urine cytology is to detect:

a. Microhematuria.

b. Urinary tract infections.

c. Papillary urothelial neoplasm of low malignant potential (PUNLMP).

d. Low grade urothelial carcinoma.

e. High grade urothelial carcinoma.

Answer: e

61. An 86-year-old male is found to have a renal mass. Numerous malignant cells with oncocytic features are found on FNA biopsy. Cytogenetics reveals trisomy 7, 16, and 17. What is the most likely diagnosis?

a. Oncocytoma.

b. Chromophobe RCC.

c. Conventional (clear cell) RCC with granular cells.

d. Papillary RCC.

e. Adrenocortical carcinoma.

Answer: d

62. According to the international system for serous fluid cytopathology, which of the following entities does **not** fall into the AUS category?

a. Cells from a borderline ovarian tumor.

b. Atypical groups of cells in a sample with no cell block.

c. Groups of cells with nuclear atypia.

d. Groups of cells with architectural atypia.

e. Markedly atypical cells with high nuclear-cytoplasmic ratios and prominent nucleoli in groups with community border and intracytoplasmic mucin.

Answer: e

63. According to the international system for serous fluid cytopathology, which effusion sample does **not** fall into the nondiagnostic category?

a. Pleural fluid exclusively composed of acute inflammatory cells.

b. Pleural fluid showing marked air-drying artifact with poor cellular visualization.

c. Peritoneal fluid of 100 mL with very scant mesothelial cells.

d. A thick preparation with poorly visualized cells.

e. Pericardial fluid sample showing 2 different cell populations (mesothelial and atypical glandular cells).

Answer: e

64. Which of the following statements is **false** with regard to malignant mesothelioma in effusion cytology?

a. It typically presents as a hypercellular sample with numerous morules, papillary fragments, and single cells.

b. Overt nuclear abnormalities such as nuclear enlargement, irregular nuclear membranes, and clear pleomorphism can be present.

c. The cells show a mesothelial immunophenotype: WT-1+, calretinin+.

d. Loss of BAP-1 expression supports the diagnosis of malignant mesothelioma.

e. Lack of homozygous deletion of p16/*CDKN2a* by fluorescence in situ hybridization (FISH) definitely excludes a diagnosis of malignant mesothelioma.

Answer: e

SHORT ANSWER QUESTIONS
Cervical Cytology

65. What is the specimen quantitative adequacy criterion for liquid based cytology of nonatrophic cervical smears, according to the Bethesda system for reporting cervical cytology?

5000 well-visualized squamous cells.

66. What is the specimen quantitative adequacy criterion for conventional cytology of nonatrophic cervical smears, according to the Bethesda system?

8000–12000 well-visualized squamous cells.

67. What cells can be included when counting cells for adequacy, according to the Bethesda system?

Mature nucleated squamous cells and squamous metaplastic cells.

68. What kinds of squamous cells are normally present in a 30-year-old female with a cervical smear interpreted as negative for intraepithelial lesion or malignancy?

- Superficial, intermediate, metaplastic.
- Parabasal and basal cells — exceptionally rare.

69. How many endocervical cells/squamous metaplastic cells must be present for a cervical smear to be considered adequate, according to the Bethesda system?

Endocervical cells and metaplastic squamous cells, representing a sampling of the transition zone, are not required for an adequate smear. Their presence/absence can be recorded in a quality indicator section.

70. What kinds of inflammatory cells can be seen in a cervical smear interpreted as negative for intraepithelial lesion or malignancy?

- Neutrophils.
- Lymphocytes, including follicular cervicitis.
- Rarely plasma cells.
- Histiocytes.

71. What are the classic features of human herpesvirus 2 (HSV-2) infection of the vagina/cervix?

- Mnemonic: "3M" (**m**ultinucleation, **m**argination, and **m**olding).
- Intranuclear inclusions (eosinophilic) or intranuclear clearing (ground-glass appearance).

72. What may account for multinucleated cells in cervical smears?

- Reactive endocervical changes (most common).
- Conditions that produce multinucleate giant histiocytes (atrophy, granuloma).
- HPV changes (ASC-US and LSIL) and, rarely, benign squamous changes.
- Radiation related cellular changes.
- Human herpesvirus (HSV) infection.
- Syncytiotrophoblast in pregnancy.

73. What findings can be considered reactive/reparative squamous changes?

- Nuclear enlargement (up to 2 times larger than a normal intermediate cell nucleus).
- Nonspecific, ill-defined small perinuclear halos.

74. What are the cytological features favoring metastatic adenocarcinoma over endocervical adenocarcinoma in a cervical smear?

- Clean background (i.e., no tumor diathesis).
- Rare malignant cells (unless direct extension).
- No AIS in background.

75. What are the major categories of the Bethesda system for reporting cervical cytology?

- NILM.
- Other.
- Epithelial cell abnormality.
- Other malignant neoplasms, specify.

76. What are the categories of squamous epithelial cell abnormalities in the Bethesda system for reporting cervical cytology?

- Atypical squamous cells (ASC).
  - Atypical squamous cells of undetermined significance (ASC-US).
  - Atypical squamous cells, cannot exclude HSIL (ASC-H).
- Low grade squamous intraepithelial lesion (LSIL).
- High grade squamous intraepithelial lesion (HSIL).
- Squamous cell carcinoma.

77. What are categories of glandular epithelial cell abnormalities in the Bethesda system for reporting cervical cytology?

- Atypical:
  - Endocervical cells, NOS.
  - Endometrial cells, NOS.
  - Glandular cells, NOS.
  - Endocervical cells, favor neoplastic.
  - Glandular cells, favor neoplastic.
- Endocervical AIS.
- Adenocarcinoma:
  - Endocervical.
  - Endometrial.
  - Extrauterine.
  - NOS.

78. What is the differential diagnosis of LSIL?

- Reactive changes.
- Small perinuclear halos in nonspecific reactive changes and in infections such as *Trichomonas* and *Candida*.
- Nuclear enlargement in perimenopausal patients.
- Multinucleation in reactive endocervical cells, HSV, histiocytes, syncytiotrophoblasts.

79. What is the differential diagnosis of HSIL?

Any cause of "hyperchromatic crowded groups" (HCG) enters the differential diagnosis, such as squamous metaplasia, atrophy, IUD, endometrial cells, LUS, follicular cervicitis, or endocervical AIS.

80. What features distinguish squamous cell carcinoma from HSIL?

- Macronucleoli.
- Tumor diathesis.
- Keratinization with unusual cell morphology (tadpole cells) — beware of keratinizing HSIL as a mimic.

81. Glandular cells that occur in a posthysterectomy patient may be secondary to what conditions?

- Recurrent adenocarcinoma of the cervix or endometrium.
- Metastatic adenocarcinoma.
- Primary adenocarcinoma of the vagina — rare.
- Glandular metaplasia — possibly radiation induced.
- Vaginal adenosis.
- Supracervical hysterectomy.
- Fallopian tube prolapse.
- Vaginal endometriosis/endosalpingiosis.

82. What are the features of endocervical AIS?

- Columnar cells.
- Crowded cells with pseudostratification.
- Nuclear enlargement.
- Nuclear hyperchromasia.
- Mitoses.
- Apoptosis.
- Rosettes.
- Feathering.
- Absent or inconspicuous nucleolus.

83. What features differentiate invasive adenocarcinoma from AIS?

- Tumor diathesis.
- Prominent nucleoli.
- Rounding of nucleus with increased cytoplasm.

84. What are the features of endometrial adenocarcinoma?

- Rounded cells.
- Nuclear hyperchromasia.
- Prominent nucleoli.
- Vacuolated cytoplasm.
- Intracytoplasmic neutrophils.
- Clear background (lack of diathesis).

85. What are the cytological features of sampling from the LUS?

- Large, cellular hyperchromatic crowded groups composed of 2 cell types: glandular and stromal cells.
- Branching glands and "tubules" can be seen within the large sheets.
- Glandular cells may be columnar and may mimic AGC or AIS.

Note: recognition of the endometrial stroma is key to distinguishing LUS from AGC or other diagnostic pitfalls (for false positive diagnoses).

Lung Cytology

86. What are the sampling techniques for acquiring cytology specimens from the lower respiratory tract?
- Sputum.
- Bronchial brushing.
- Bronchial washing.
- Bronchiolo-alveolar lavage (BAL).
- Percutaneous FNA biopsy with either CT or ultrasound guidance.
- Endobronchial ultrasound-guided FNA biopsy (EBUS-FNA).
- Endoscopic ultrasound-guided FNA biopsy (EUS-FNA) for sampling mediastinal lymph nodes in the context of staging for lung cancer.

87. What is the adequacy criterion for sputum samples?
The presence of easily identifiable pulmonary macrophages (there is no specific recommended number).

88. What are the cytologic features of *Pneumocystis jiroveci* (formerly *carinii*) pneumonia?
- Foamy proteinaceous material on Papanicolaou stain, shaped as alveolar casts.
- Cup- and crescent-shaped organisms on Grocott silver stain.
- Dots within cysts.

89. The cytological features of alveolar proteinosis resemble those of *Pneumocystis jiroveci* pneumonia. What cytologic features distinguish them?
- The acellular material is seen more diffusely in the background of the smears in alveolar proteinosis (rather than in focal/discrete agglomerates in *Pneumocystis jiroveci*).
- The material is positive for periodic acid-Schiff (PAS) stain, but negative for silver stain in alveolar proteinosis (whereas *Pneumocystis jiroveci* is positive for silver stain).

90. What are the cytologic features of small cell carcinoma?
- Cells 2–3 times the size of a lymphocyte.
- Predominantly single cells with small, loosely cohesive aggregates.
- Hyperchromatic evenly dispersed finely granular chromatin.
- Very high nuclear-cytoplasmic ratio.
- Nuclear molding.
- Indistinct nucleoli.
- Abundant mitoses.
- Abundant apoptosis.
- Abundant necrosis.
- Nuclear debris and crush artifact.
- Paranuclear blue bodies — on Wright-Giemsa stain.

91. What is the differential diagnosis of small cell carcinoma?
- Reserve cell hyperplasia (because the cells can also exhibit hyperchromasia, high nuclear-cytoplasmic ratio, and nuclear molding).
  - Note that, unlike small cell carcinoma, the cells in reserve cell hyperplasia are smaller (i.e., the same size as the nuclei of normal endobronchial cells, whereas cells from small cell carcinoma are larger than the nuclei of normal endobronchial cells), the cells are cohesive (i.e., no single cells), and there is no pyknosis or necrosis.
- Some variants of nonsmall-cell carcinoma (especially basaloid squamous cell carcinoma) and some adenocarcinomas.
- Lymphocytes and lymphomas.
- Typical and atypical carcinoid tumor.
- NUT carcinoma — small, round, blue cell tumors (e.g., neuroblastoma, Ewing sarcoma, and Wilms tumor).
- Pulmonary blastoma.

92. What are the cytologic features of a typical carcinoid?
- Predominantly single cells with small, loosely cohesive aggregates (may have rosette architecture).
- Epithelioid, plasmacytoid, or spindle cells.
- Coarsely granular cytoplasm.
- Evenly dispersed coarsely granular chromatin ("salt and pepper" chromatin).
- Inconspicuous nucleoli.
- Rare mitoses.
- No necrosis — focal necrosis is possible in atypical carcinoids, but these cannot be definitely diagnosed in cytologic material: histologic examination is required.

93. What are the cytologic features of well-differentiated squamous cell carcinoma?
- Large, round, or elongated cells ("tadpole" cells).
- Herxheimer spiral — tails of spiraling cytoplasm.
- Dense (waxy) orangeophilic cytoplasm on Papanicolaou stain.
- Dense blue cytoplasm ("robin's egg blue") on Wright-Giemsa stain.
- Pyknotic hyperchromatic nuclei with absent or inconspicuous nucleolus.
- Abundant keratin and anucleate keratinocytes.
- Squamous pearl formation.

94. What are the cytologic features of poorly differentiated squamous cell carcinoma?

- Cohesive three-dimensional groups.
- Elongated to spindle cells.
- Large cells.
- Coarse "chunky" chromatin.
- Multiple prominent nucleoli — usually (in contrast to well-differentiated squamous cell carcinoma, which has no or inconspicuous nucleoli).
- Single keratinized cells — rare, in background.

95. What are the cytologic features of adenocarcinoma?

- Cells arranged in honeycomb sheets, acini, papillae, and/or three-dimensional clusters.
- Eccentric or polarized nuclei.
- Very fine or vesicular light chromatin, when well differentiated.
- Large prominent single nucleoli, when well differentiated.
- Vacuolated (foamy) cytoplasm.
- Mucin vacuoles.

96. What is the importance of differentiating adenocarcinoma from other nonsmall-cell carcinoma?

EGFR, KRAS, ALK, and *BRAF* testing allows for the potential use of targeted therapy, such as with *EGFR* tyrosine kinase inhibitors.

97. List causes of false positive diagnoses in lung FNA cytology.

- Granulomatous inflammation.
- Radiation, chemotherapy.
- Lung abscess.
- Organizing pneumonia.
- Pulmonary infarct.

98. What are the diagnostic categories in the Papanicolaou Society of Cytopathology system for reporting respiratory cytology?

- Nondiagnostic.
- Negative (for malignancy).
- Atypical.
- Neoplastic:
  - Benign.
- Undetermined malignant potential.
- Suspicious (for malignancy).
- Malignant.

99. Which tumors fall into the neoplastic, benign category in the Papanicolaou Society of Cytopathology system for reporting respiratory cytology?

- Pulmonary hamartoma.
- Squamous papilloma.
- Granular cell tumor.
- Hemangioma.
- Sclerosing pneumocytoma.

100. In the Papanicolaou Society of Cytopathology system for reporting respiratory cytology, which tumors fall into the category of neoplasm–undetermined malignant potential?

- This category includes neoplasms whose cytomorphologic/histologic features cannot predict clinical behavior. Most of these are rare tumors. They include:
  - Epithelioid hemangioendothelioma.
  - Clear cell tumor of lung.
  - Sclerosing pneumocytoma.
- Primary pulmonary meningioma.
- Langerhans cell histiocytosis.
- Solitary fibrous tumor.
- Inflammatory fibroblastic tumor.
- Myoepithelial neoplasms.

Serous Fluid Cytology

101. What is the differential diagnosis of an eosinophilic effusion?

- Pneumothorax — including repeat thoracocentesis (the latter is the most common cause).
- Drug reaction.
- Parasitic infection.
- Pulmonary infarction.
- Vasculitis — including Churg-Strauss syndrome.
- Eosinophilic pneumonia.

102. What is the differential diagnosis of lymphocytic effusion?

- Nonspecific reaction (most common).
- Postsurgical reactive changes.
- Malignancy.
  - Lymphocytes are very commonly seen in the background of an effusion containing metastatic adenocarcinoma or other metastatic malignancy; it is very unusual to see a predominantly neutrophilic population in the context of a metastatic malignancy in fluids.
- Tuberculosis: especially in the absence of mesothelial cells.
- Lymphoma.

103. What is the most common cause of malignant pleural effusion?
- In men: lung carcinoma.
- In women: breast carcinoma.

104. What are the most common causes of malignant peritoneal effusion?
- In men: gastrointestinal (including pancreatic) carcinoma.
- In women: ovarian carcinoma.

105. What are the characteristic cytomorphologic features of metastatic adenocarcinoma in contrast to reactive mesothelial cells in effusions?
- Presence of two populations of cells.
- Large clusters and single cells.
- Smooth peripheral edges (common/communal border).
  - This is in contrast to scalloped borders in reactive mesothelial cells (however, beware of exception: any type of papillary carcinoma can also exhibit a scalloped border).
- Vacuolated cytoplasm — especially if containing mucin.
  - Be aware that degenerative, nonspecific vacuoles can also be seen in reactive mesothelial cells in long-standing effusions; those vacuoles would, however, be negative for mucin.

106. List 4 immunocytochemical stains useful in differentiating metastatic adenocarcinoma from reactive mesothelial cells in body fluid cytology.
- Mesothelial markers: calretinin, WT-1, CK5/6, D2-40.
- Glandular/adenocarcinoma markers: claudin 4, Ber EP4, MOC-31, B72.3, CEA, CD15.

107. List the differential diagnosis of psammoma bodies in effusions.
- Reactive mesothelial cells.
- Endosalpingiosis (terminal bars and cilia are definitively diagnostic).
- Metastatic serous carcinoma.
- Implants from serous neoplasms of low malignant potential from the female genital tract.

108. What are the cytomorphologic features of epithelioid mesothelioma?
- Large clusters of cells (typically > 75–100 cells/cluster) or numerous smaller clusters of cells (beyond the range seen in reactive conditions).
- Groups with scalloped contours.
- Single cell population (or spectrum without characteristic 2 cell population).
- Large cells — usually larger than benign mesothelial cells.
- Abundant cytoplasm with dense perinuclear cytoplasm and peripheral microvillous skirt.
- Intercellular windows.

109. List key causes of false positive diagnoses in effusion cytology.
- Visceral (e.g., lung) infarction.
- Acute or chronic inflammatory process.
- Prior treatment (surgery, radiation, chemotherapy).
- Reactive mesothelial cell proliferations (such as effusions in the setting of cirrhosis and renal dialysis).
- Pericardial effusions.

110. What are the diagnostic categories in the international system for serous fluid cytopathology?
- Nondiagnostic (ND).
- Negative for malignancy (NFM).
- Atypia of undetermined significance (AUS).
- Suspicious for malignancy (SFM).
- Malignant (MAL).
  - Primary.
  - Secondary.

111. Which ancillary tests are helpful in diagnosing malignant mesothelioma in effusion cytology when the morphologic features of overt malignancy are not present in mesothelial cells?
- Homozygous deletion of *CDKN2A* by FISH.
- Loss of *BRCA1*-associated protein 1 (BAP-1) expression by immunochemistry.
- Loss of methylthioadenosine phosphorylase (MTAP) expression by immunochemistry.

Breast Cytology

112. What are the diagnostic categories and their associated risk of malignancy in the International Academy of Cytology Yokohama system for reporting breast fine needle aspiration biopsy cytopathology?
- Insufficient/inadequate: 2.6–4.8%.
- Benign: 1.4–2.3%.
- Atypical: 13–15.7%.
- Suspicious: 84.6–97.1%.
- Malignant: 99–100%.

113. In the International Academy of Cytology Yokohama system for reporting breast FNA biopsy cytopathology, what are the management guidelines for the atypical and suspicious diagnostic categories?

- A triple test approach (clinical, imaging, pathology) is necessary for assessment of a breast lesion.
  - Atypical: review clinical and imaging findings:
    › If these are indeterminate or suspicious, a core needle biopsy (CNB) is necessary; if CNB is not available, a repeat FNA biopsy (FNAB) is recommended.
- › If these are benign, a repeat FNAB is recommended.
- Suspicious: follow-up is mandatory regardless of clinical and imaging findings:
  › Repeat sampling with CNB is ideal; if CNB is not available a repeat FNAB or excisional biopsy is recommended.

114. What are the cytologic features of fibroadenoma?

- Hypercellular smear.
- Three-dimensional epithelial cell clusters with branching staghorn-like structures.
- Many bipolar spindled and naked nuclei of myoepithelial cells in the background — very important.
- Myxoid to fibrous stromal fragments — although the diagnosis is made easier when present, these are not necessary for a diagnosis of fibroadenoma.
- Mild atypia possible, but the epithelial cells maintain regular spacing, fine chromatin, small nucleoli.

115. Can fibroadenomas (FAs) be accurately differentiated from phyllodes tumors on cytology?

- Benign phyllodes tumors cannot be easily differentiated from FAs — benign phyllodes tumors may have hypercellular stromal fragments, but FAs may as well.
- Malignant phyllodes tumors are easily distinguished from FAs by the presence of sarcomatous features, but they may be mistaken for metaplastic carcinoma or primary sarcoma of the breast.

116. Can intraductal papillomas and papillary carcinoma be distinguished on FNA?

- The classic teaching is not to distinguish them in cytologic material (i.e., histologic examination is necessary to make a reliable distinction).
- Markers of possible malignancy: complex architecture (cribriform or tubular architecture), lack of myoepithelial cells, or high grade atypia.

Note: the classic teaching is to sign out such cases as "papillary neoplasm" and ask for excision for subtyping.

117. What are the characteristic cytologic features of ductal carcinoma in FNA specimens?

- High cellularity.
- Single population of cells.
- Poorly cohesive/single epithelial cells with prominent single cell population.
- Atypical cells — enlarged irregular nuclei.
- Lack of myoepithelial cells.

Note: before making a definitive diagnosis of carcinoma in a breast FNA specimen, make sure that the single cells are not myoepithelial cells, macrophages, or apocrine metaplastic cells.

118. What are the cytologic features of lobular carcinoma?

- Variable cellularity — can be difficult to recognize if smear is hypocellular, and hypocellular smears are not uncommon due to stromal fibrosis surrounding linear arrays of infiltrating cells. This is why lobular carcinoma is a common cause of false negative diagnoses.
- Single cells, and cells arranged in small groups.
- Small nuclei with mild nuclear irregularity (when compared to ductal carcinoma).
- Minute nucleoli.
- Plasmacytoid cells.
- Cells with single intracytoplasmic vacuole containing targetoid mucin.

Note: the intracytoplasmic vacuoles are not pathognomonic of lobular carcinoma because they can also be seen in cases of ductal carcinoma; however, they tend to be less numerous in ductal carcinoma than in lobular carcinoma.

119. List the differential diagnosis of lymphocytes in breast FNA specimens.

- Intramammary lymph node (most common).
- Carcinoma with medullary features.
- Lymphoma.

120. List causes of false negative diagnoses in breast FNA specimens.

- In most cases, there is a sampling problem due to:
  · Poor sampling technique.
  · Necrosis.
  · Sclerosis.
  · Small size.
  · In situ lesions.
- Some false negative diagnoses are due to error of interpretation (underdiagnosis):
  · Lobular carcinoma.
  · Tubular carcinoma.
  · Adenoid cystic carcinoma.

121. List causes of false positive diagnoses in breast FNA specimens.
- Fibroadenoma.
- Fibrocystic changes.
- Papillary neoplasms and papillomatosis.
- Fat necrosis/repair.
- Lactating adenoma.
- Radiation induced atypia.

Thyroid Cytology

122. According to the Bethesda system for reporting thyroid cytopathology, what are the categories of interpretation for thyroid FNA specimens?
- Nondiagnostic/unsatisfactory.
- Benign.
- Atypical cells of undetermined significance or follicular lesion of undetermined significance.
- Follicular neoplasm or suspicious for a follicular neoplasm (includes follicular neoplasm, Hürthle cell type).
- Suspicious for malignancy.
- Malignant.

123. What are the adequacy criteria for thyroid FNA specimens under the Bethesda system?
- The adequacy criteria require at least 6 groups of benign follicular cells, each group composed of ≥ 10 cells.
- There are 3 special situations for which the above adequacy criteria are waived:
  · "Cyst fluid only" is a special category of nondiagnostic specimens.
- An FNA specimen containing very abundant colloid is considered diagnostic and benign.
- An FNA specimen exhibiting abundant lymphocytes (even in the absence of follicular cells) can be diagnosed as "benign and consistent with lymphocytic thyroiditis."

124. What are the cytologic features favoring a diagnosis of follicular neoplasm, Hürthle cell type over that of Hürthle cell metaplasia in the context of a nonneoplastic lesion?
- Predominant syncytial or microfollicular pattern and/or trabeculae (cords).
- Hypercellularity with a pure population of Hürthle cells.
- Scant colloid.
- Absence of lymphocytes.
- Transgressing blood vessels.

125. What are the cytologic features of a benign thyroid nodule on FNA?
- Predominantly flat sheets of follicular cells.
- Follicular cells with evenly spaced nuclei (honeycomb pattern).
- Small nuclei with coarse chromatin (without the nuclear features of papillary thyroid carcinoma).
- Abundant colloid in the background (but nonspecific).
- Oncocytes (Hürthle cells) in the background (but nonspecific).
- Cyst contents (macrophages) and cyst lining cells (but nonspecific).

126. What are the cytologic features of lymphocytic thyroiditis?
- Abundant lymphocytes in the background, typically corresponding to a polymorphous (rather than monotonous) lymphoid population.
- Germinal centers with tingible body macrophages.
- Presence of at least a few Hürthle cells (usually, but not essential).

Note: atypia in Hürthle cells in the background of lymphocytic thyroiditis is considered within the spectrum of benign changes in this condition. It is important not to overinterpret these reactive changes.

127. What are the cytologic criteria of a follicular neoplasm?
- Cellular smear.
- Predominantly microfollicular or syncytial architecture.
- Usually few single cells.
- Nuclei possibly enlarged and crowded, but without the nuclear features of papillary thyroid carcinoma.
- Colloid possibly present in the center of microfollicles, but no or little colloid in the background.

128. What are the cytologic features of papillary thyroid carcinoma (PTC)?
- Cellular smears.
- Cells arranged in syncytia, papillae, sheets.
- Nuclear changes of PTC:
  · Nuclear enlargement.
  · Nuclear irregularity (including nuclear membrane thickening, grooves).
  · Clear, finely granular (powdery) chromatin.
- · Micronucleoli (usually), peripherally located (attached to nuclear membrane).
- · Intranuclear cytoplasmic pseudoinclusions.
- Nuclear crowding with molding.
- Squamoid cytoplasm.
- Psammomatous calcifications.
- Thick, "bubble gum" colloid.
- Multinucleate giant cells.

Note: if only or mostly microfollicles are present in an FNA specimen, it is best diagnosed as follicular neoplasm even if some, but not all, diagnostic nuclear features of papillary carcinoma are present, as these may represent noninvasive follicular thyroid neoplasm with papillary-like features (NIFTP).

129. What are the benign differential diagnoses of papillary thyroid carcinoma?
- Lymphocytic thyroiditis.
- Cyst-lining cells.
- Previous FNA related changes.
- Radiation atypia.
- Hyperplastic nodule and follicular neoplasm (for follicular variant of PTC).

130. What are the cytologic features of medullary thyroid carcinoma (MTC)?
- Cellular smears.
- Cells arranged in loosely cohesive groups with abundant single cells.
- Nuclei eccentrically placed, giving the cells a plasmacytoid or epithelioid appearance.
- Coarsely granular chromatin without nucleoli ("salt and pepper" chromatin).
- Acellular fragments of amyloid possible in background.

Note: medullary thyroid carcinomas can exhibit many of the nuclear features of PTC; however, a predominant single cell pattern, while very common in MTC, is very unusual in PTC.

131. What are the differential diagnoses of oncocytic (Hürthle) cells in a thyroid FNA specimen?
- Multinodular goitre.
- Lymphocytic thyroiditis.
- Follicular neoplasm, Hürthle cell type.
- Papillary thyroid carcinoma (oncocytic or tall cell variants).
- Medullary thyroid carcinoma.
- Metastatic carcinoma (e.g., RCC).

132. What is the differential diagnosis of abundant lymphocytes on thyroid FNA?
- Lymphocytic thyroiditis.
- Lymph node aspirate.
- Lymphoma.
- Papillary thyroid carcinoma (Warthin-like, diffuse sclerosing variants).
- Medullary thyroid carcinoma (because of the single cell pattern of the neoplastic cells, which can mimic lymphocytes).

133. The cytological features of MTC and follicular neoplasm, Hürthle cell type (FNHCT) are very similar. List the immunocytochemical features that would help distinguish them.
- FNHCT:
  · Positive for TTF-1 and thyroglobulin.
  · Negative for calcitonin, chromogranin, synaptophysin, CD56, CEA.
- MTC:
  · Positive for TTF-1, calcitonin, chromogranin, synaptophysin, CD56, CEA.
  · Negative for thyroglobulin.

Salivary Gland Cytology

134. What are the diagnostic categories of the Milan system for reporting salivary gland cytopathology?
- Nondiagnostic.
- Nonneoplastic.
- AUS.
- Neoplasm.
· Benign.
· Salivary gland neoplasm of uncertain malignant potential (SUMP).
- Suspicious for malignancy.
- Malignant.

135. What are the cytologic features of pleomorphic adenoma?
- Cohesive "honeycomb" epithelial cells.
- Myoepithelial cells (spindled, plasmacytoid, epithelioid, clear cell).
- Chondromyxoid stroma with fibrillary and frayed edges.

136. What are the cytologic features of Warthin tumor?
- Abundant lymphocytes.
- Cohesive and single oncocytes.
  · Typically, these occur as a mixture of more abundant cuboidal oncocytes and less abundant columnar oncocytes.
- Abundant granular proteinaceous debris in the background.

137. What are the cytologic features of mucoepidermoid carcinoma, low grade?
- Mucus cells (mucin containing goblet-like cells).
- Epidermoid cells (squamoid cells).
- Intermediate cells (immature squamous-like cells).

138. What malignancy is the most common cause of a false negative diagnosis on salivary gland FNA?
Mucoepidermoid carcinoma, due to its characteristic cystic morphology and low grade cytologic features.

Note: acinic carcinoma is also often misdiagnosed as "normal salivary gland tissue" because of its bland cytology; however, it is overall a relatively infrequent cause of false-negative diagnoses, simply because it is a very rare neoplasm.

139. What are the cytologic features of adenoid cystic carcinoma?
- Cohesive groups of basaloid cells.
- Characteristic cluster of cells around distinct globules of acellular matrix.
- Acellular, amorphous matrix: metachromatic on Wright-Giemsa stain, colorless on Papanicolaou stain (this is in contrast to the matrix of pleomorphic adenoma, which has a characteristic fibrillary appearance).

140. What is the differential diagnosis of abundant oncocytic/oncocytoid cells on salivary gland FNA?
- Warthin tumor.
- Oncocytoma.
- Pleomorphic adenoma with oncocytic metaplasia.
- Mucoepidermoid carcinoma, oncocytic.
- Acinic cell carcinoma, oncocytic.
- Secretory carcinoma.
- Salivary duct carcinoma.
- Metastatic renal cell carcinoma.

141. What is the differential diagnosis of abundant lymphocytes on salivary gland FNA?
- Warthin tumor.
- Intraparotid lymph node.
- Chronic sialadenitis.
- Lymphoepithelial sialadenitis (LESA).
- Lymphoepithelial (HIV-associated) cyst.
- Acinic cell carcinoma.
- Lymphoepithelial carcinoma.
- Mucoepidermoid carcinoma (20%).
- Lymphoma.

142. What is the differential diagnosis of basaloid tumors on salivary gland FNA?
- Cellular pleomorphic adenoma (most common, due to sampling in the cellular epithelial portion with no or little sampling from the stromal component).
- Basal cell adenoma/adenocarcinoma.
- Adenoid cystic carcinoma.
- Epithelial-myoepithelial carcinoma.
- Myoepithelioma/myoepithelial carcinoma.
- Polymorphous adenocarcinoma.
- Basaloid carcinoma/basaloid squamous cell carcinoma.
- Basal cell carcinoma of skin.

143. Which immunocytochemical stains (surrogates for molecular alterations) are helpful in diagnosing salivary gland neoplasms?
- Pleomorphic adenoma and carcinomas ex pleomorphic adenoma: PLAG1, HMGA2+.
- Basal cell adenoma/adenocarcinoma: nuclear β-catenin+ and LEF-1+.
- Adenoid cystic carcinoma: MYB+.
- Acinic cell carcinoma: NR4A3+.
- Secretory carcinoma: pan-TRK+.

144. What is the recommended management for salivary gland FNAs diagnosed as AUS?
- Repeat FNA (if FNA was performed by palpation, consider ultrasound guided FNA).
- Clinical follow-up every 3 to 6 months.
- Imaging: contrast enhanced magnetic resonance imaging (MRI) or CT.
- Biopsy (core needle or open) or surgical resection if the clinical presentation is concerning for malignancy.

145. What is the recommended management for salivary gland FNAs diagnosed as SUMP?
- Parotid:
  · Preoperative imaging should be pursued to assess the neck.
  · Nerve sparing surgical resection is recommended (unless clinically not indicated).
  · Frozen section may be considered to better define the histologic classification and to determine if neck dissection is indicated.
- Submandibular gland (SMG):
  · Preoperative imaging and SMG resection in suprafascial plane are recommended.
  · Frozen section may be considered to better define the histologic classification and to determine if neck dissection is indicated.

Lymph Nodes

146. What are the cytologic features of reactive hyperplasia?
- Polymorphous lymphoid population with a predominance of small lymphocytes.
- Germinal center elements:
  - Centrocytes and centroblasts.
- Tingible body macrophages.
- Dendritic-lymphocytic and lymphohistiocytic aggregates.
- Immunoblasts.

147. What are the cytologic features of granulomatous lymphadenitis?
- Aggregates of epithelioid histiocytes +/– lymphocytes.
- Epithelioid histiocytes with elongated and spindle shaped nuclei (carrot shaped, boomerang shaped).
- Possible presence of background of necrosis.

148. Can "small cell" lymphomas be accurately diagnosed on FNA?
- FNA, in correlation with cell block immunohistochemistry and flow cytometry, can accurately subtype small cell lymphomas, based on appropriate sampling.
- The above answer is controversial and highly dependent on the following:
  - With cytomorphology alone, differentiating certain types of small cell lymphomas from nonneoplastic lymph nodes can be challenging — especially mucosa-associated lymphoid tissue (MALT) lymphomas and small lymphocytic lymphoma/chronic lymphocytic leukemia.
  - A negative smear may be due to sampling error (including partial node involvement).
  - Cytology is also limited by the increasingly complex histologic, immunohistochemical, and molecular characterization of lymphomas required for grading, staging, and prognosticating.
  - Although an excisional or core biopsy may be performed subsequently, FNA is a rapid triage for lymphoma versus nonlymphoid malignancy, and small cell versus large cell lymphoma. It also allows acquisition of material for initial immunohistochemistry, flow cytometry, and molecular testing.

149. What is in the differential diagnosis of "small cell" lymphoma?
- Reactive lymph node.
- Small cell carcinoma.
- Other small round blue cell tumors.
- Partial involvement of lymph node by lymphoma or metastasis.
- Hodgkin lymphoma with abundant reactive background.
- T cell rich, diffuse large B-cell lymphoma.

150. Can large cell lymphomas be accurately diagnosed on FNA?
- FNA is more accurate for large cell lymphomas than for "small cell" lymphomas.
- FNA, in correlation with cell block immunohistochemistry, can accurately subtype large cell lymphomas and Hodgkin lymphomas.
- Differentiation of large cell lymphomas from nonlymphoid malignancies can be done on cytomorphology alone.
- Even with large cell lymphomas, there are limitations to FNA, and a negative smear may again be due to sampling error (including partial node involvement), or to the presence of only a few malignant cells in the background of a large population of reactive lymphoid cells (T cell rich B-cell lymphoma, Hodgkin lymphoma).

151. What are the cytologic features of diffuse large B-cell lymphoma?
- Predominantly single cells — almost exclusively.
- Predominant population of large cells — typically (> 3 times the size of resting lymphocytes).
- Centroblast-like (multiple nucleoli) or immunoblast-like (single central nucleolus).

152. What are the cytologic features that differentiate large cell lymphomas from poorly differentiated nonlymphoid malignancies?
- Lymphoglandular bodies — fragments of cytoplasm in a background derived from benign lymph nodes and lymphoma (best seen on Wright-Giemsa stain).
- Single cell population without cellular cohesion — usually.
  - Note that the presence of dendritic-lymphocytic/lymphohistiocytic aggregates may be deceiving as they may appear as "cohesive" clusters mimicking epithelial clusters. In addition, certain nonlymphoid malignancies such as melanoma may exhibit a single cell pattern as lymphomas do.
- Monomorphous population of malignant cells — this is not the case for all lymphoma types.
- Very high nuclear-cytoplasmic ratio — usually.
- Pertinent negatives — e.g., lack of cytoplasm, mucin vacuoles, melanin pigment.

153. What is the classic differential diagnosis of lymphoma composed of lymphocytes of "intermediate" cell size?
- Burkitt lymphoma.
- Lymphoblastic lymphoma.
- Blastic variant of mantle cell lymphoma.

Hepatobiliary and Pancreas Cytology

154. What are the cytologic features of hepatocytes in FNA cytology?
- Large cells.
- Abundant granular cytoplasm.
- Large centrally placed nuclei with prominent nucleolus.
- Binucleate cells.
- Cells with intranuclear cytoplasmic pseudoinclusions.
- Cytoplasm contains pigment (lipofuscin, hemosiderin).

155. What are the benign liver nodules that can result in abundant, apparently normal hepatocytes on aspiration?
- Hepatocellular (liver cell) adenoma.
- Focal nodular hyperplasia.
- Cirrhosis and dominant regenerative nodules.
- Nodular regenerative hyperplasia.
- Normal background liver sampled when aspiration missed the nodule.

156. What are the cytologic features of hepatocellular carcinoma (HCC)?
- Hepatocytes arranged in thick trabeculae, clusters, nests, or sheets.
- Hepatocytes wrapped in flattened endothelial cells — characteristic, and important in differentiation between low grade HCC and benign hepatocytes.
- Higher nuclear-cytoplasmic ratio than normal hepatocytes.
- Possible mild nuclear atypia to high grade pleomorphism.
- Valuable for confirmation: background of hepatitis or cirrhosis (based on clinical history/imaging).

157. What is the differential diagnosis of hepatocellular carcinoma?
- Low grade HCC:
  · Hepatocellular (liver cell) adenoma.
  · Focal nodular hyperplasia.
  · Cirrhosis.
- High grade HCC:
  · Cholangiocarcinoma.
  · Metastatic adenocarcinoma.
  · Metastatic renal cell or adrenocortical carcinoma.

158. What are the cytologic features of cholangiocarcinoma?
- Cohesive 3-dimensional clusters and single cells.
- Glandular differentiation (eccentric nucleus, columnar shaped cells, thin vacuolated cytoplasm).
- High nuclear-cytoplasmic ratio.

Note: cytologically, the features of cholangiocarcinoma are similar to those of any other type of adenocarcinoma. Immunocytochemistry and clinical/radiological correlation are needed to distinguish cholangiocarcinoma from metastatic adenocarcinoma.

159. What are the cytologic features of pancreatic ductal adenocarcinoma?
- Cellular aspirates.
- Single cells (more common in higher grade carcinomas), and cells arranged in sheets.
- "Drunken honeycomb" arrangement of cells — cells lose their normal, evenly spaced honeycomb pattern, resulting in nuclear crowding, loss of polarity, pseudostratification.
- Nuclear irregularities — low grade adenocarcinoma may show irregular contours and grooves and pale chromatin that may resemble papillary thyroid carcinoma; high grade adenocarcinoma typically shows severe nuclear irregularities and hyperchromasia, chromatin clumping, and prominent nucleoli (features that are more obviously malignant).
- Nuclear pleomorphism and anisonucleosis within sheets (up to fourfold difference in nuclear size).
- Single malignant cells — look especially for these.

160. What is the differential diagnosis of low grade pancreatic ductal adenocarcinoma?
- Chronic pancreatitis.
- Stent associated atypia.
- Primary sclerosing cholangitis.
- Recent surgical instrumentation, such as endoscopic retrograde cholangiopancreatography (ERCP) or cholecystectomy.

161. What is the differential diagnosis of a predominantly single-cell pattern on cytology of a pancreatic mass?
- Acinar cell carcinoma.
- Well-differentiated pancreatic neuroendocrine tumor.
- Solid pseudopapillary neoplasm.
- Lymphoma (rarely primary).

162. What are the cytologic features of well-differentiated pancreatic neuroendocrine tumors?
- Cellular smears.
- Single cell pattern.
- Plasmacytoid cells.
- Granular cytoplasm.
- Coarsely granular chromatin ("salt and pepper" chromatin).
- Variable nucleoli — typically inconspicuous, but possibly conspicuous.

163. What are the cytologic features of pancreatic pseudocysts?
- Granular and inflammatory debris.
- Histiocytes.
- High amylase, low CEA on cyst fluid analysis — characteristic.

164. What is the differential diagnosis of mucinous epithelium on pancreatic cyst aspiration?
- Neoplastic mucinous cysts.
  · Intraductal papillary mucinous neoplasm (IPMN).
  · Mucinous cystic neoplasm (MCN).
- Pancreatic ductal adenocarcinoma with cystic degeneration.
- Contamination by gastric or duodenal epithelium.

165. If acinar cell carcinoma is suspected by cytomorphology in a pancreas FNA specimen, what ancillary cell block procedures could help confirm the diagnosis?
- PAS and PAS-diastase stain (positive in acinar cell carcinoma).
- Mucicarmine (negative in acinar cell carcinoma).
- Immunocytochemistry: positive for trypsin, BCL10, chymotrypsin.

166. What are the diagnostic categories of the Papanicolaou Society of Cytopathology system for reporting pancreatobiliary cytology?
- Nondiagnostic.
- Negative (for malignancy).
- Atypical.
- Neoplastic:
  · Benign.
- Other.
- Suspicious (for malignancy).
- Positive/malignant.

167. Which neoplasms fall into the diagnostic categories "neoplastic, benign" and "neoplastic, other" in the Papanicolaou Society of Cytopathology system for reporting pancreatobiliary cytology?
- Neoplastic, benign:
  · Serous cystadenoma — most commonly encountered neoplasm.
  · Other less common entities: neuroendocrine microadenoma (size < 0.5 cm), lymphangioma, cystic teratoma, and schwannoma.
- Neoplastic, other:
  · Well-differentiated pancreatic neuroendocrine tumors.
  · Solid pseudopapillary neoplasm.
  · Mucinous cysts (IPMN and mucinous cystic neoplasm).

168. What are the diagnostic criteria for a mucinous cyst based on the Papanicolaou Society of Cytopathology system for reporting pancreatobiliary cytology?
- Presence of mucin production: thick, extracellular, colloid-like mucin; inflammatory debris within mucin.
- Elevated cyst fluid CEA level (192 ng/ml is 80% accurate).
- Presence of mutations (*KRAS, GNAS, RNF43*).
- Presence of neoplastic cells (low grade versus high grade dysplasia).

169. Which neoplasms fall into the diagnostic category "malignant" in the Papanicolaou Society of Cytopathology system for reporting pancreatobiliary cytology?
- Adenocarcinoma.
- Acinar cell carcinoma.
- Poorly differentiated neuroendocrine carcinoma.
- Pancreatoblastoma.
- Metastasis.
- Lymphoma.

Kidney and Urine Cytology

170. What is the differential diagnosis of oncocytes on kidney FNA?
- Oncocytoma.
- Chromophobe RCC.
- Papillary RCC.
- Conventional (clear cell) RCC with prominent granular cells.
- Tubulocystic RCC.
- Succinate dehydrogenase deficient RCC.
- Hereditary leiomyomatosis RCC.
- Epithelioid angiomyolipoma (perivascular epithelioid cell tumor).
- Hepatocytes (inadvertent sampling of liver).

171. What are the cytologic features of clear cell (conventional) RCC?
- Cohesive groups.
- Large cells with abundant vacuolated thin cytoplasm.
- Round nuclei with prominent nucleoli — in higher grade RCC.
- Prominent thin-walled transgressing capillary network (and subsequently abundant blood in background).
- Intermixed inflammatory cells — especially neutrophils and hemosiderin-laden macrophages.
- Thin strands on Wright-Giemsa stain.

172. What are the cytologic features of high grade urothelial carcinoma?
- Single and small clusters of abnormal urothelial cells.
- According to the Paris system for reporting urine cytopathology: ≥ 10 abnormal cells (if fewer, categorize as "suspicious").
- Nondegenerated, nonsuperficial urothelial cells with increased nuclear-cytoplasmic ratio (≥ 0.7) with moderately to severely hyperchromatic nuclei, and with clumpy chromatin and/or irregular nuclear membranes.
- Possible presence of cercariform cells — cells with an elongated, nontapering cytoplasmic process that ends with a flat cytoplasmic edge.

173. What are the indications for urine cytology?
- Hematuria — most common.
- Patient being followed for treated urothelial carcinoma or carcinoma in situ.
- Patient at high risk of urothelial carcinoma.
  - Due to occupational chemical exposure.
  - Due to chemotherapeutic medications.

174. What is the differential diagnosis of urothelial cell clusters?
- Urolithiasis.
- Instrumented urine.
- Low grade urothelial papillary tumors (papilloma, PUNLMP, low grade papillary urothelial carcinoma).
- High grade urothelial carcinomas.

175. Can low grade urothelial carcinoma be accurately diagnosed on urine cytology?
- No, because there is too much overlap with reactive changes.
- The only scenario in which the diagnosis can be made reliably in urine cytology is when a true fibrovascular fragment is present.
- According to the Paris system, the main aim of urine cytopathology is to recognize high grade urothelial carcinoma (instead of the low grade urothelial neoplasms).
- Regardless, these lesions have a low risk of progression and are likely to be identified by cystoscopy and not urine cytology.

176. What features are diagnostic of low grade papillary urothelial neoplasm?
The only diagnostic feature is the presence of a true papillary fragment with a fibrovascular core.

177. What is the differential diagnosis of high grade urothelial carcinoma?
- Polyomavirus (decoy cells).
- Atypia in urolithiasis ("stone atypia").
- Ureter washing/brushing specimen.
- Chemotherapy/radiation atypia.
- Cervical or rectal carcinoma with bladder involvement.
- Prostate adenocarcinoma and renal cell carcinoma — rare.

178. When is the ideal time to take a sample for urine cytology?
3–4 hours after last urination.

179. What are the diagnostic categories in the Paris system for reporting urinary cytopathology (2016)?
- Negative for high grade urothelial carcinoma (HGUC).
- Atypical urothelial cells.
- Suspicious for high grade urothelial carcinoma.
- High grade urothelial carcinoma.
- Low grade urothelial neoplasia.
- Other malignancies: primary/secondary.

180. According to the Paris system,* what are the cytologic features of atypical urothelial cells?
- Both of the following:
  - Nonsuperficial urothelial cells.
  - Increased nuclear-cytoplasmic ratio (required): ≥ 0.5.
  – and –
- 1 of the following for nondegenerated cells, or more than 1 of the following for degenerated cells:
  - Hyperchromasia.
  - Irregular clumpy chromatin.
  - Irregular nuclear membranes.

*This chapter uses the 2016 edition of the Paris system.

181. According to the Paris system, what are the cytologic features of "suspicious for high grade urothelial carcinoma"?

- All of the following features:
  - Nonsuperficial and nondegenerated urothelial cells.
  - Increased nuclear-cytoplasmic ratio (required).
    › Generally ≥ 0.7 (should not be used with rigidity).
    › Take the specimen type and clinical setting into account.
  - Hyperchromasia (required).
    › Moderate to severe.
  › Compare to normal umbrella cell or intermediate cell nucleus.
  - Number of cells: 5–10 (quantitative).
  – and –
- 1 or both of the following features:
  - Irregular clumpy chromatin.
  - Irregular nuclear membranes.

182. List causes of false positive diagnoses in urinary cytology.

- Reactive umbrella cells.
- Lithiasis.
- Instrumentation.
- Inflammation.
- Radiotherapy, chemotherapy.
- Polyoma virus infection.
- Ileal bladder specimens.
- Cells from seminal vesicles.

183. List causes of false negative diagnoses in urinary cytology.

- Low grade urothelial papillary carcinoma.
- Obscuring by marked inflammation or blood.
- RCC.
- Prostatic carcinoma.

Cerebrospinal Fluid (CSF) Cytology

184. What are the cytologic features of leptomeningeal metastatic adenocarcinoma in CSF?

- Small clusters of cells and isolated single cells.
- Large cells with eccentric nuclei.
- Abundant cytoplasm with vacuolization, some containing mucin.

Note: breast carcinoma can exhibit linear arrangements.

185. How can you differentiate leukemia in CSF from peripheral blood contamination of CSF?

- CSF examination:
  - Peripheral blood contamination contains abundant erythrocytes in the background.
  - This is best seen on Wright-Giemsa stained cytocentrifuge specimens that have been air-dried. Fixing specimens with alcohol, for liquid based cytology, removes blood.
- Clinical history:
  - Patients in remission have peripheral blood that is negative for blasts.
- Hematology differential count:
  - This procedure assesses erythrocyte and blast concentrations in peripheral blood and CSF.
  - Formulas are used to predict CSF leukocyte concentration based on the differential cell counts (for erythrocytes and leukocytes) of CSF and of peripheral blood.
  - The calculated predicted value is compared to the CSF differential cell count to help assess for peripheral blood contamination.

186. List the following tumors from the highest to lowest likelihood of diagnosis in CSF: benign primary brain tumor, glioma, lymphoma/leukemia, medulloblastoma, metastasis.

- Lymphoma/leukemia.
- Medulloblastoma.
- Metastasis.
- Glioma.
- Benign primary brain tumor.

Screening and Quality Indicators in Cytology

187. What are the features of a good screening test?

- Identification of asymptomatic disease or risk factors.
- High sensitivity and preferably high specificity.
- Sensitivity to early stages of disease.
- Effective treatment available.
- Relatively simple.
- Low in cost.
- Safe and acceptable to patients.

188. List examples of cervical cytology quality assurance practices.

- Rescreening a subpopulation of NILM cervical smears — usually 10% reevaluated prospectively. Cases are from a mixture of randomly selected low-risk and high-risk populations.
- Rapid prescreening or rapid postscreening. These procedures are much more efficient than rescreening a subpopulation: using either procedure precludes random rescreening.
- Retrospective rescreening. In a patient with newly diagnosed HSIL, AIS, or carcinoma, this involves reviewing all of the patient's cervical smears interpreted as NILM from the previous 3 years (in Canada, but from the previous 5 years in the US).
- Correlating cytology and histology for biopsies with discrepant results.
- Reviewing cytotechnologist-cytopathologist discrepant results.
- Assessing laboratory performance via 1) the ratio of findings of atypical squamous cells to squamous intraepithelial lesion (ASC:SIL ratio; the upper limit is 3:1); and 2) correlating high-risk HPV results in ASC-US cases (if available; approximately 50% of ASC-US cases should be positive for high-risk HPV).

189. What are the possible causes of discrepancy during cervical cytology-histology correlation?

- Sampling error on cervical biopsy — e.g., no lesion seen at colposcopy, lesion seen but undersampled, biopsy embedded incorrectly (most common cause).
- Resolution/healing of lesion in interim between cervical smear and biopsy.
- Cytology interpretation error.
- Histology interpretation error.

190. What is the approximate breakdown of ASC-US and ASC-H interpretations in the ASC category?

- Approximately 90% should correspond to ASC-US.
- Approximately 10% should correspond to ASC-H.

IMAGES: CYTOPATHOLOGY

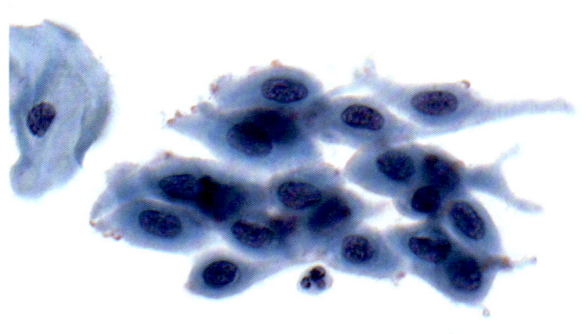

IMAGE 5.1 Cervical smear: squamous metaplastic cells, NILM (Papanicolaou, x400).

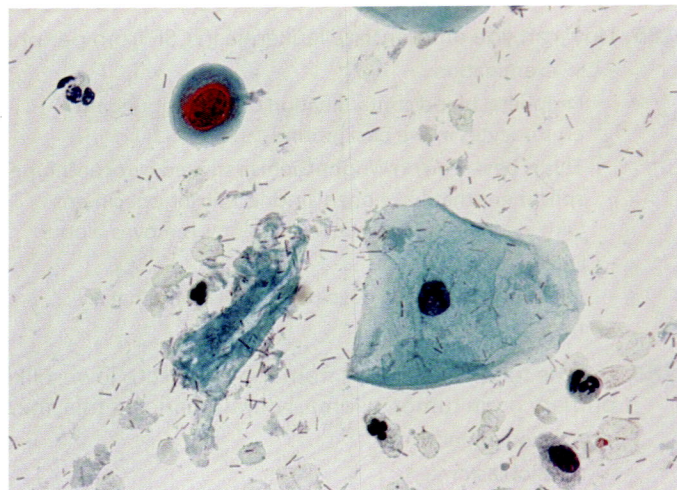

IMAGE 5.2 Cervical smear: 1 squamous metaplastic cell (smaller cell) and 1 intermediate squamous cell (larger cell; note the open chromatin of its nucleus) in a background of *Lactobacilli* (i.e., normal flora), NILM (Papanicolaou, x400).

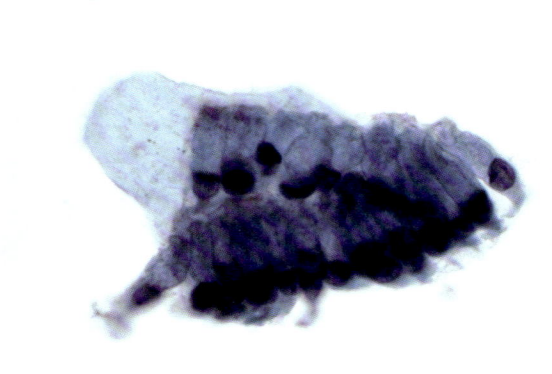

IMAGE 5.3 Cervical smear: normal endocervical cells (seen from the side), NILM (Papanicolaou, x400).

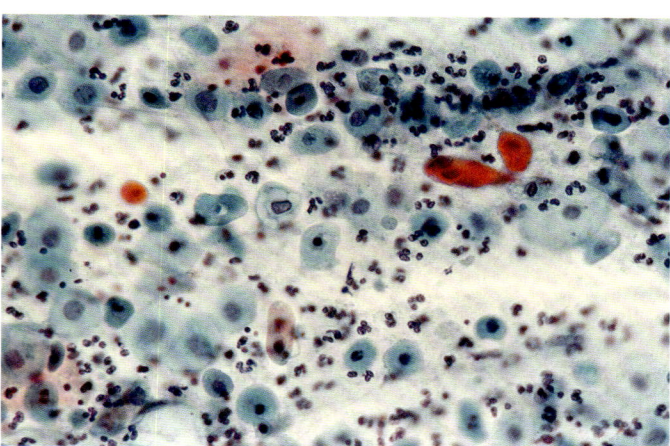

IMAGE 5.6 Cervical smear: atrophic vaginitis in a postmenopausal smear, NILM (Papanicolaou, x100).

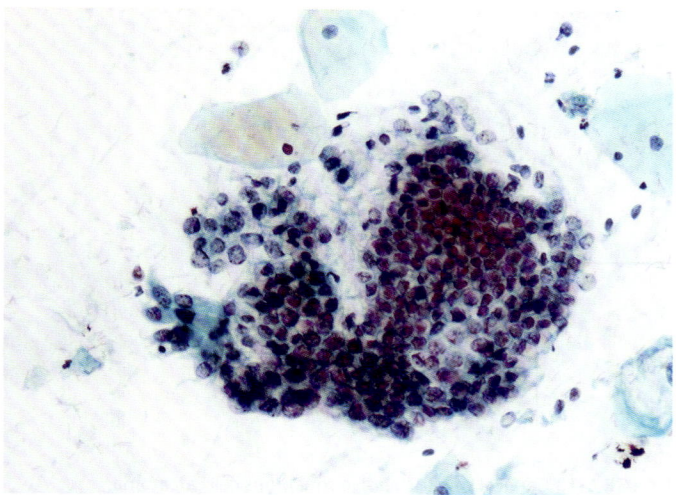

IMAGE 5.4 Cervical smear: normal endocervical cells (seen head-on with characteristic honeycomb arrangement), NILM (Papanicolaou, x200).

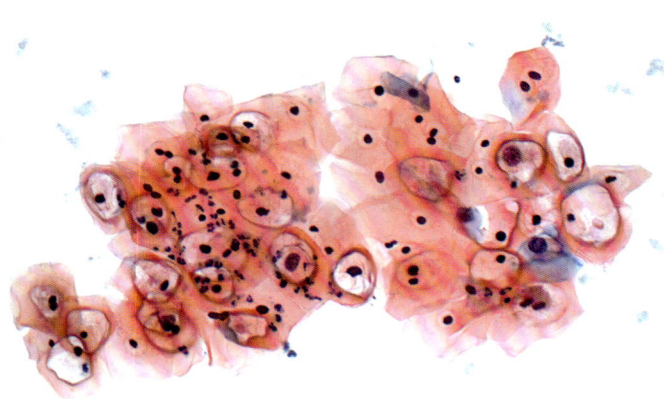

IMAGE 5.7 Cervical smear: koilocytes of low grade squamous intraepithelial lesion, LSIL (Papanicolaou, x200).

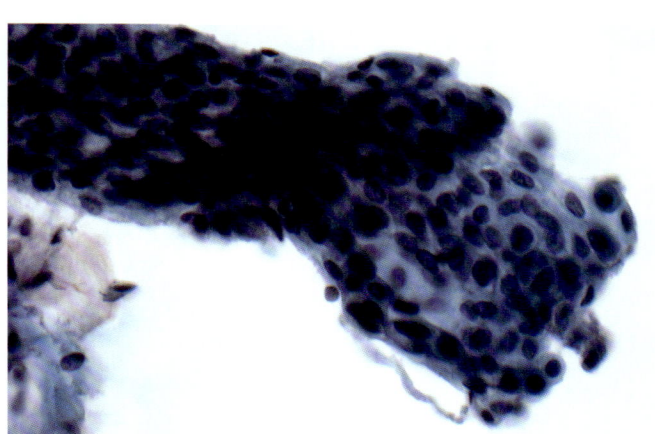

IMAGE 5.5 Cervical smear: group of parabasal cells in an atrophic postmenopausal smear, NILM (Papanicolaou, x400).

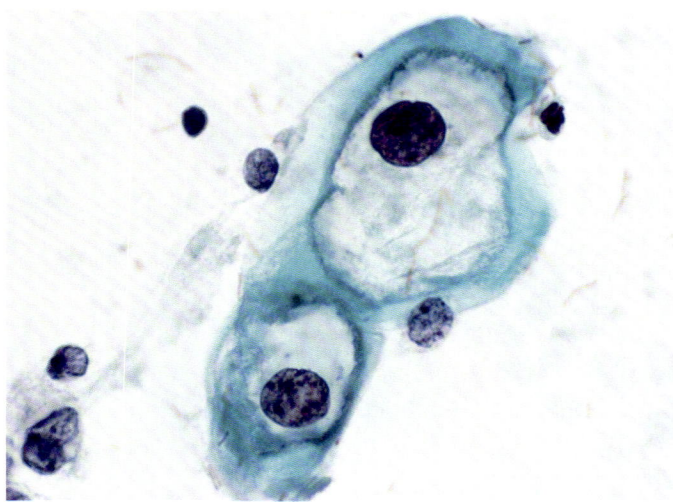

IMAGE 5.8 Cervical smear: koilocytes of low grade squamous intraepithelial lesion, LSIL (Papanicolaou, x600).

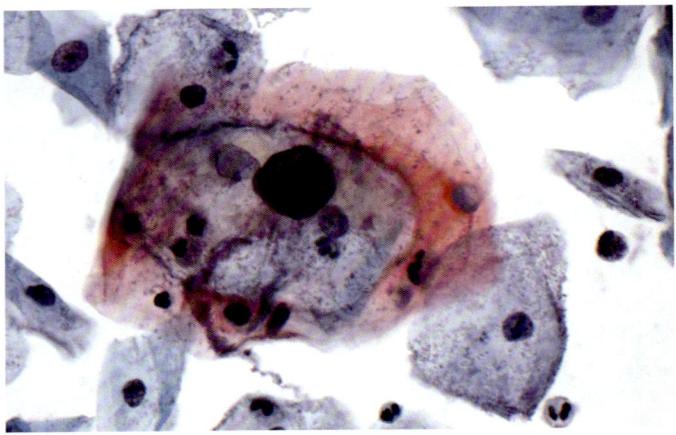

IMAGE 5.9 Cervical smear: low grade squamous intraepithelial lesion, LSIL (Papanicolaou, x400).

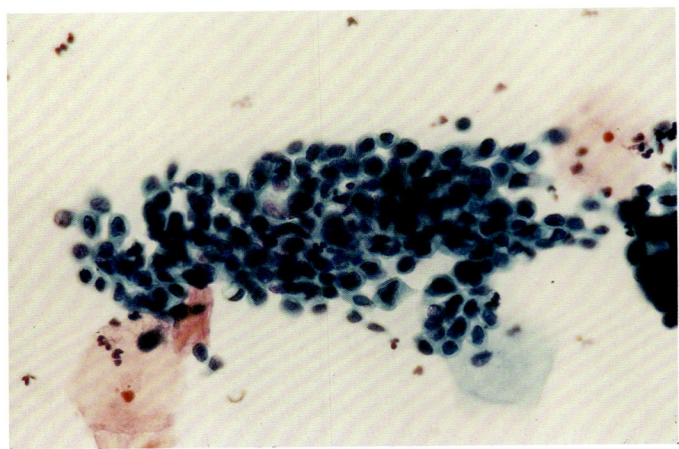

IMAGE 5.12 Cervical smear: high grade squamous intraepithelial lesion, HSIL in hyperchromatic crowded group (Papanicolaou, x200).

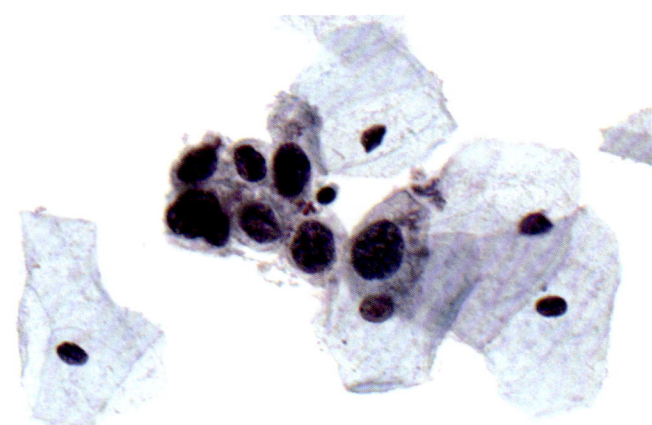

IMAGE 5.10 Cervical smear: high grade squamous intraepithelial lesion, HSIL (Papanicolaou, x400).

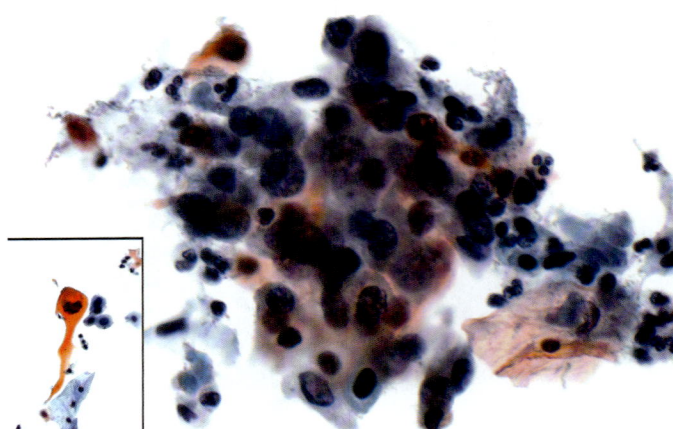

IMAGE 5.13 Cervical smear: invasive squamous cell carcinoma, keratinizing type. Inset: "tadpole" cell (Papanicolaou, x400).

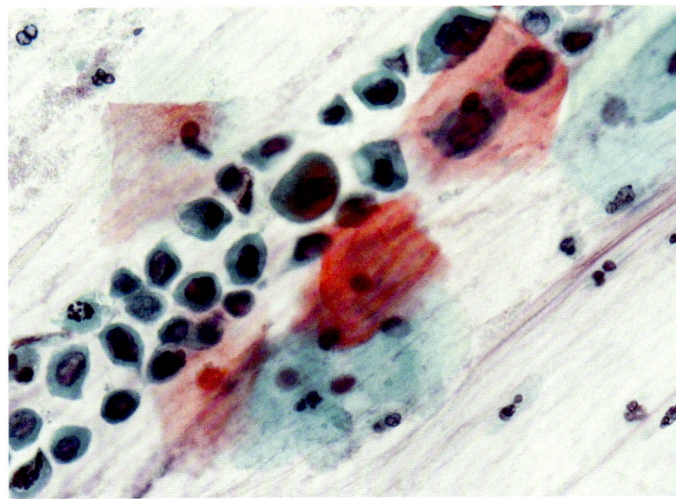

IMAGE 5.11 Cervical smear: high grade squamous intraepithelial lesion, HSIL (Papanicolaou, x200).

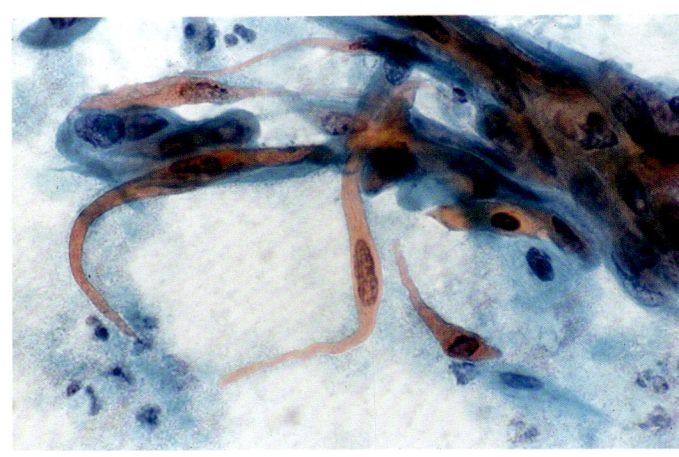

IMAGE 5.14 Cervical smear: invasive squamous cell carcinoma, keratinizing type (with "tadpole" cells) (Papanicolaou, x600).

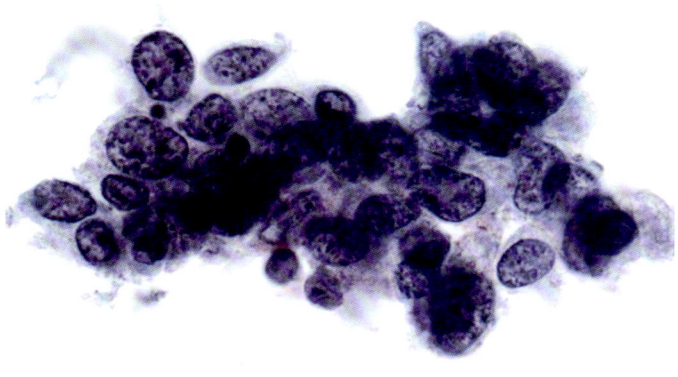

IMAGE 5.15 Cervical smear: invasive squamous cell carcinoma, nonkeratinizing type (Papanicolaou, x400).

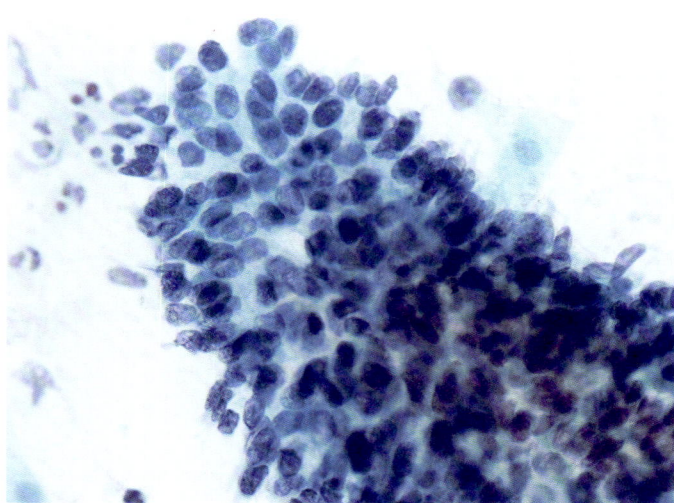

IMAGE 5.18 Cervical smear: adenocarcinoma in situ, AIS (Papanicolaou, x400).

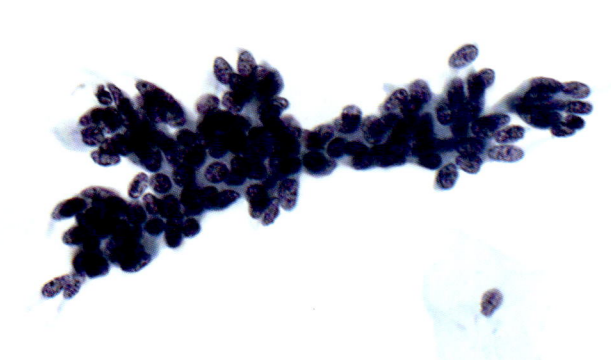

IMAGE 5.16 Cervical smear: adenocarcinoma in situ, AIS (Papanicolaou, x400).

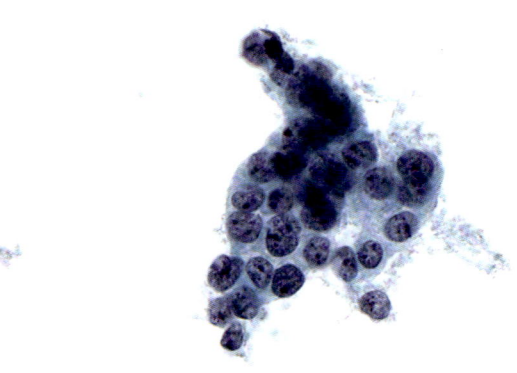

IMAGE 5.19 Cervical smear: endocervical adenocarcinoma (Papanicolaou, x400).

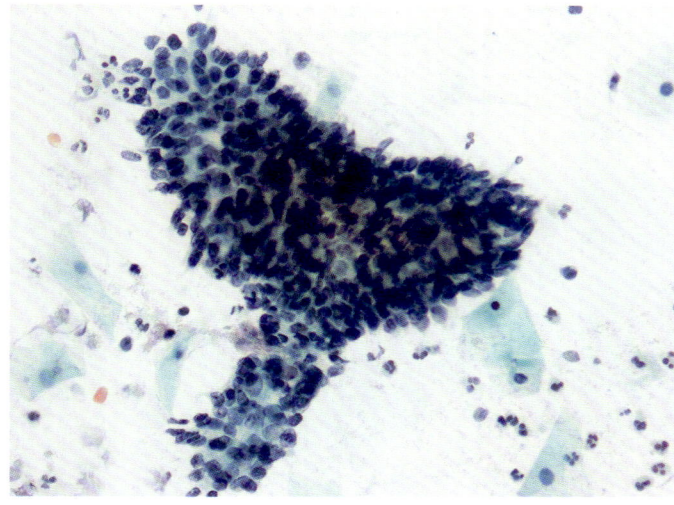

IMAGE 5.17 Cervical smear: adenocarcinoma in situ, AIS (Papanicolaou, x200).

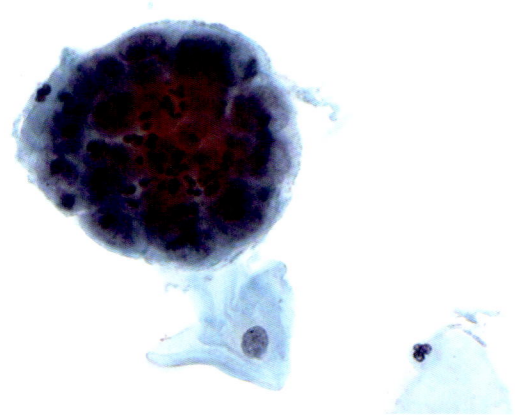

IMAGE 5.20 Cervical smear: endometrial endometrioid adenocarcinoma (Papanicolaou, x400).

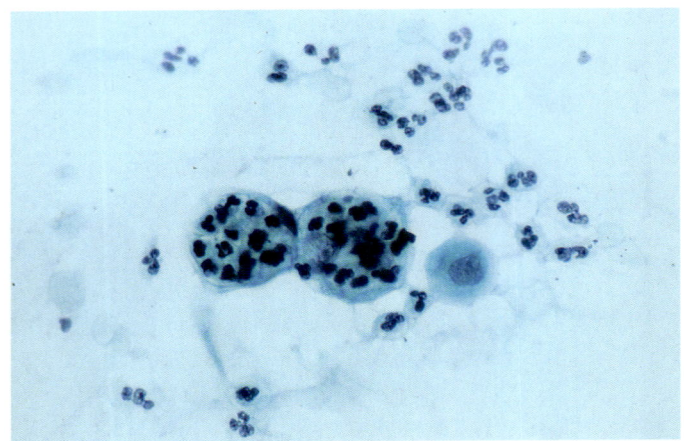

IMAGE 5.21 Cervical smear: endometrial endometrioid adenocarcinoma (Papanicolaou, x400).

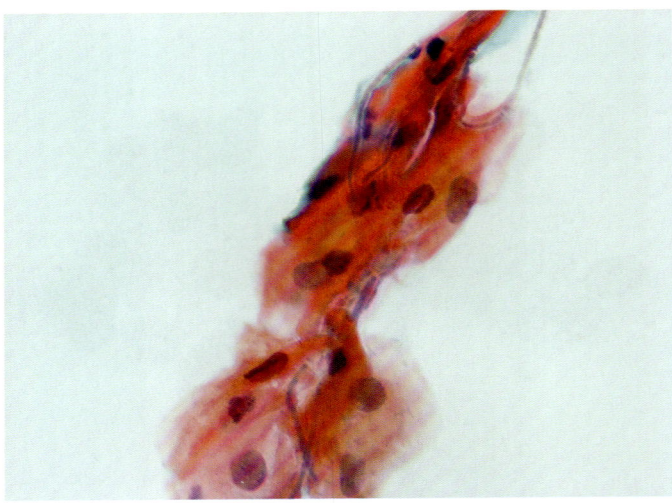

IMAGE 5.24 Cervical smear: *Candida spp.*, NILM (Papanicolaou, x400).

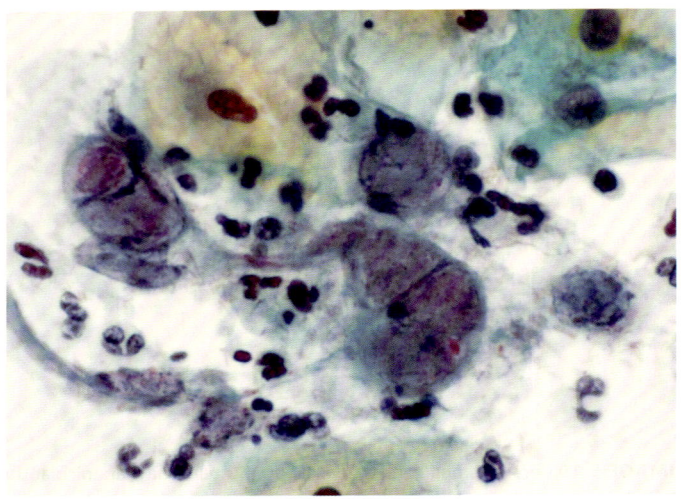

IMAGE 5.22 Cervical smear: herpes simplex infection, NILM (Papanicolaou, x400).

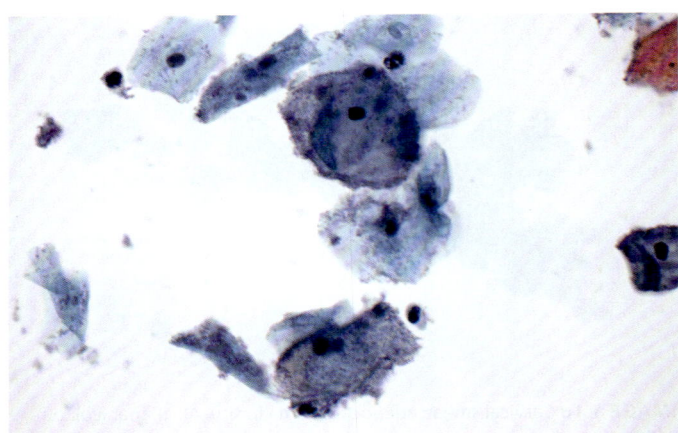

IMAGE 5.25 Cervical smear: clue cell (shift in vaginal flora), NILM (Papanicolaou, x400).

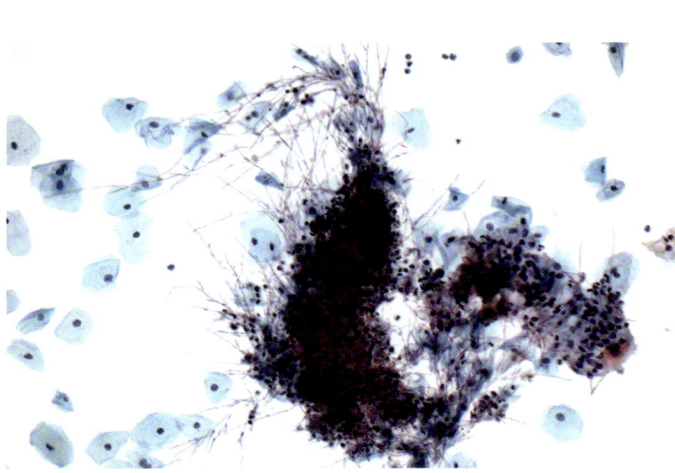

IMAGE 5.23 Cervical smear: *Candida spp.*, NILM (Papanicolaou, x100).

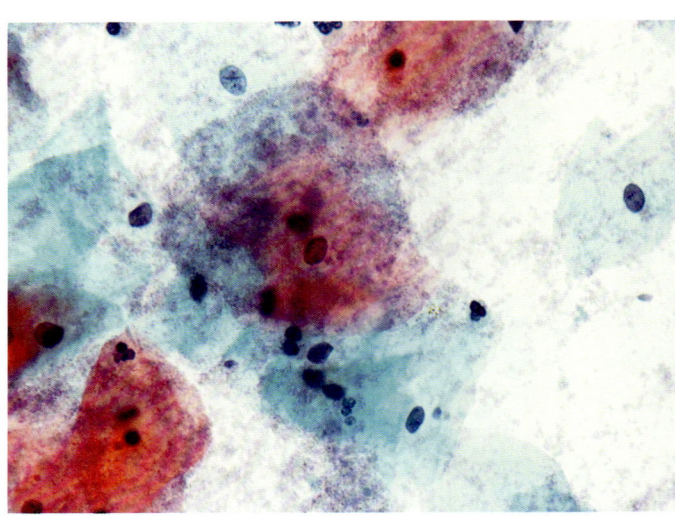

IMAGE 5.26 Cervical smear: shift in vaginal flora, NILM (Papanicolaou, x400).

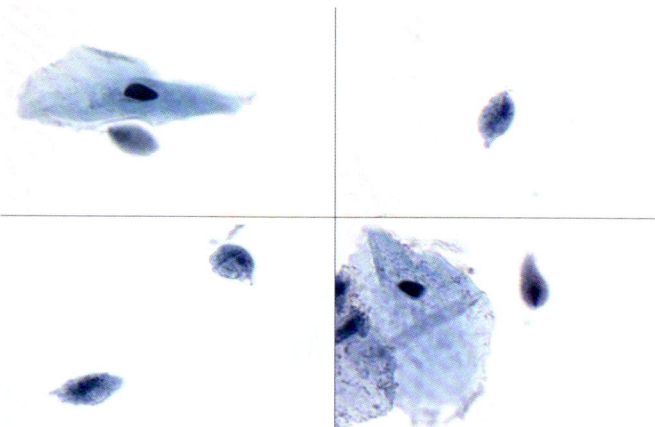

IMAGE 5.27 Cervical smear: *Trichomonas vaginalis* infection, NILM (all images: Papanicolaou, x400).

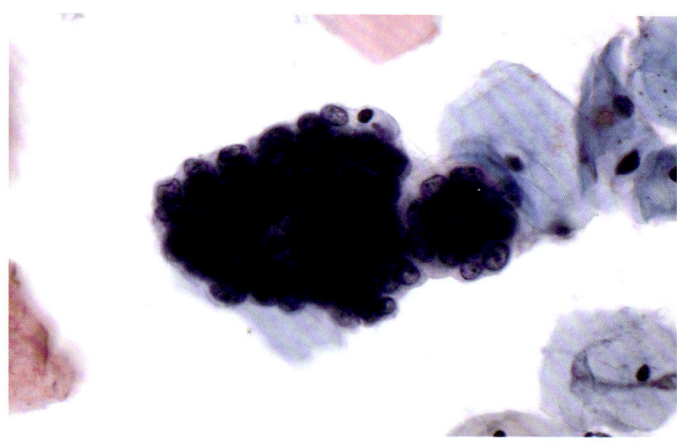

IMAGE 5.30 Cervical smear: exfoliated endometrial cells, NILM (Papanicolaou, x400).

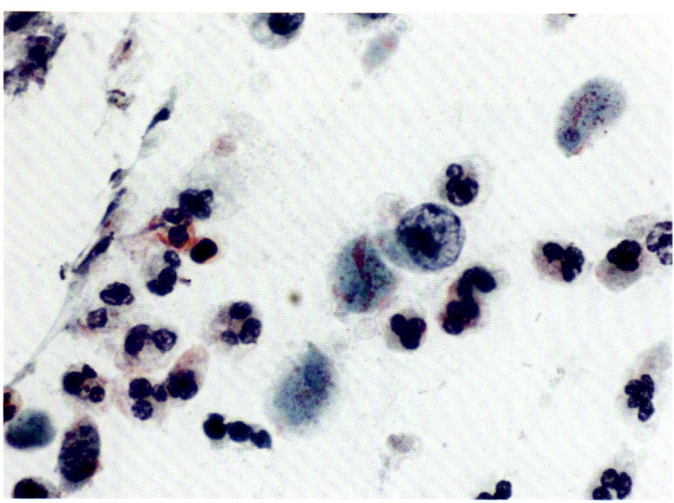

IMAGE 5.28 Cervical smear: *Trichomonas vaginalis* infection, NILM (Papanicolaou, x600).

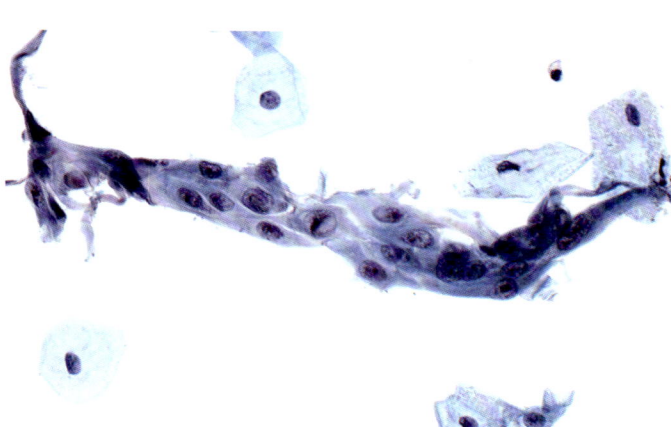

IMAGE 5.31 Cervical smear: reparative epithelium, NILM (Papanicolaou, x400).

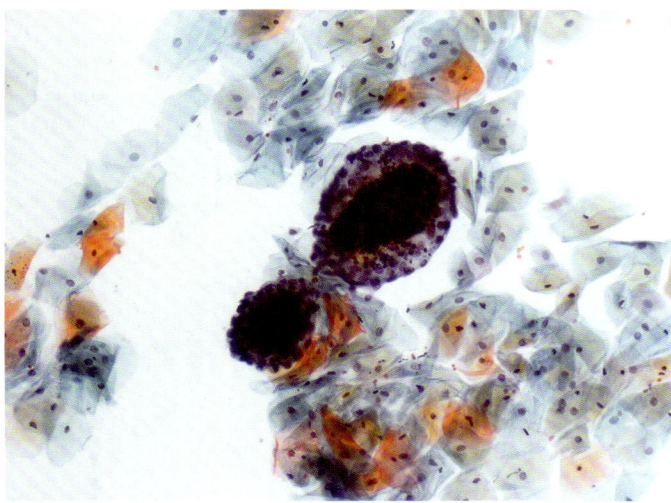

IMAGE 5.29 Cervical smear: a group of normal exfoliated endometrial cells (exodus) present in a background of superficial squamous cells (characterized by pyknotic nuclei) and of intermediate squamous cells (characterized by open chromatin), NILM (Papanicolaou, x100).

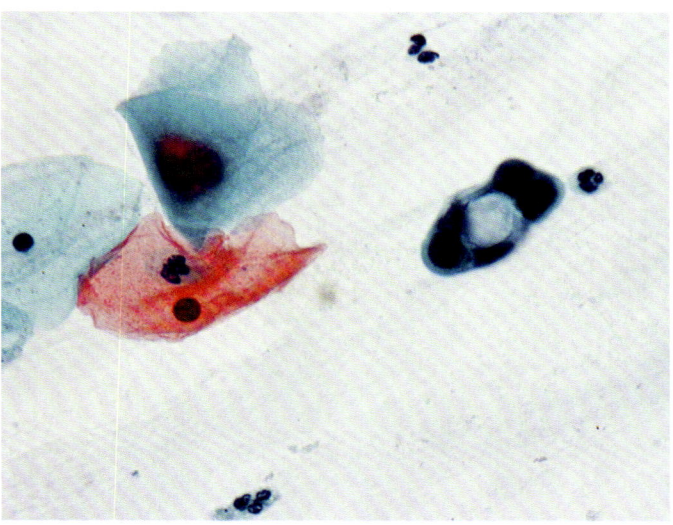

IMAGE 5.32 Cervical smear: reactive cellular changes associated with IUD, NILM (Papanicolaou, x400).

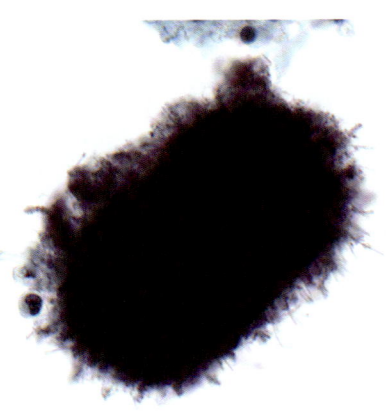

IMAGE 5.33 Cervical smear: *Actinomyces spp.* in a patient with IUD, NILM (Papanicolaou, x400).

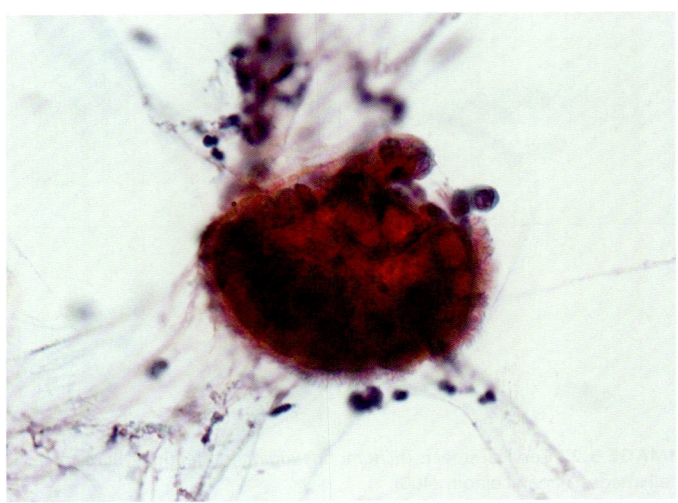

IMAGE 5.36 Bronchial wash: creola body (Papanicolaou, x400).

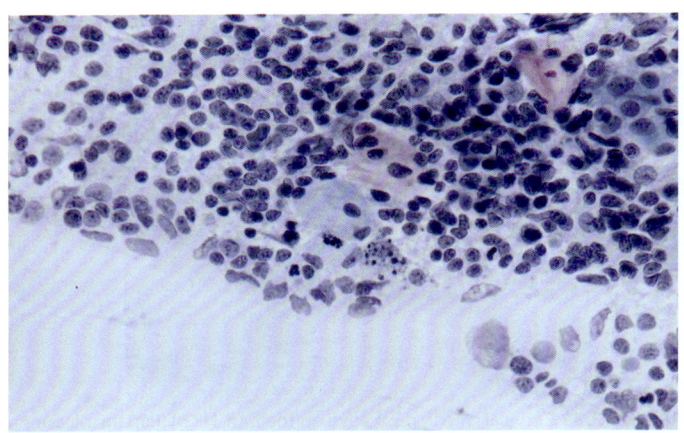

IMAGE 5.34 Cervical smear: follicular cervicitis, NILM (Papanicolaou, x200).

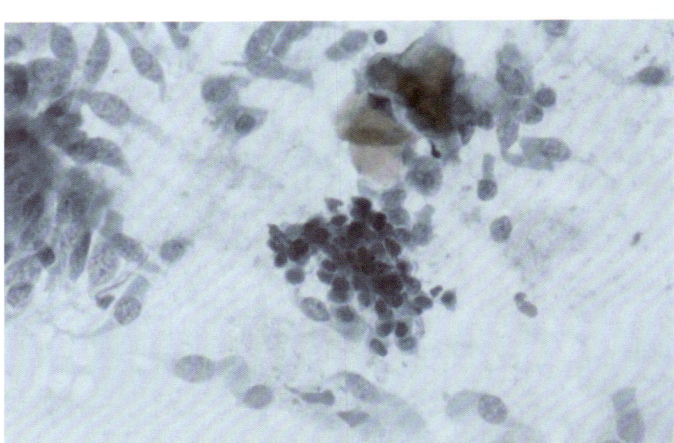

IMAGE 5.37 Bronchial brushing: reserve cell hyperplasia (Papanicolaou, x600).

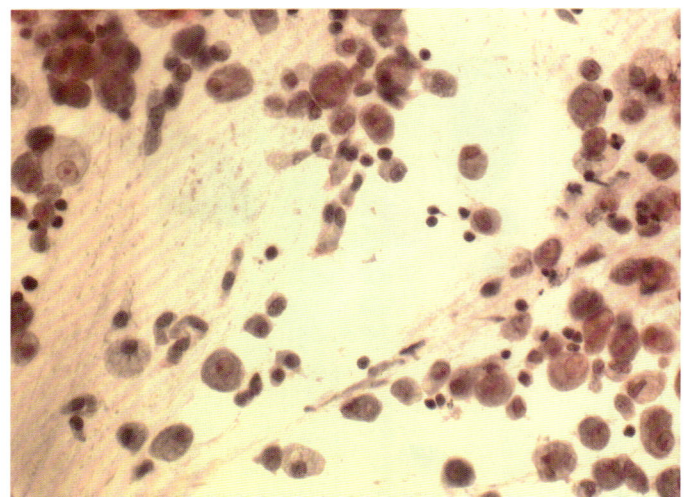

IMAGE 5.35 Bronchial brushing: normal endobronchial cells and pulmonary macrophages (Papanicolaou, x400).

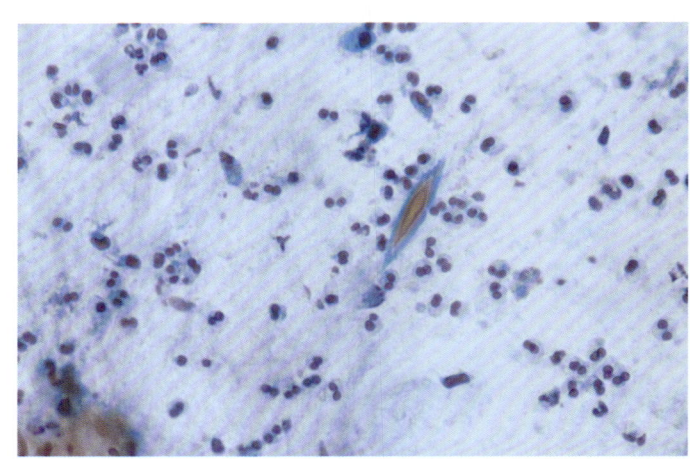

IMAGE 5.38 Bronchial wash: Charcot-Leyden crystals and eosinophils (Papanicolaou, x600).

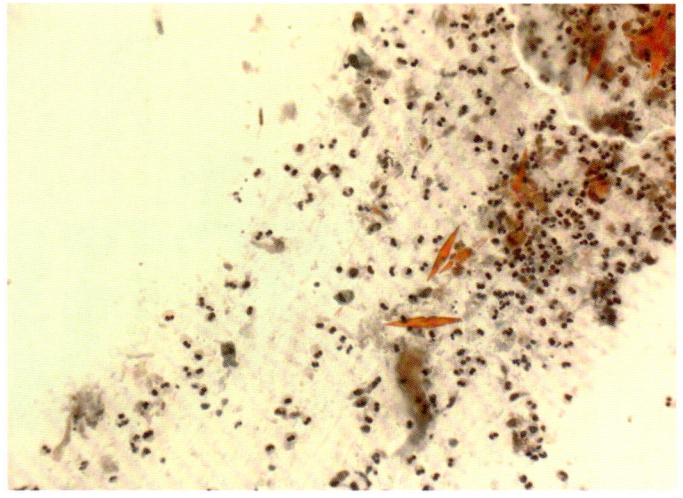

IMAGE 5.39 Bronchial washing: Charcot-Leyden crystals (Papanicolaou, x400).

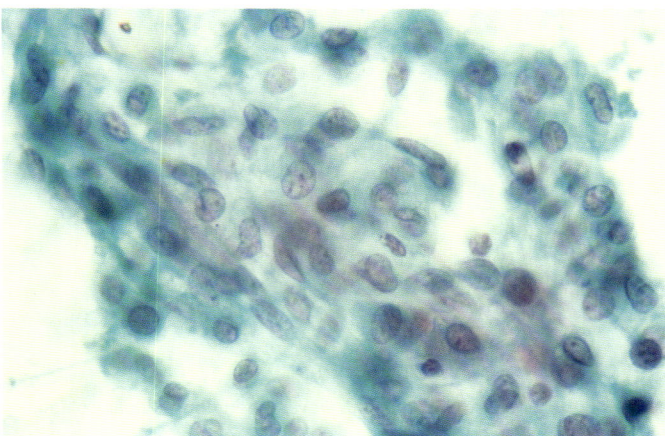

IMAGE 5.42 Lung FNA specimen: granuloma, nonnecrotizing (Papanicolaou, x600).

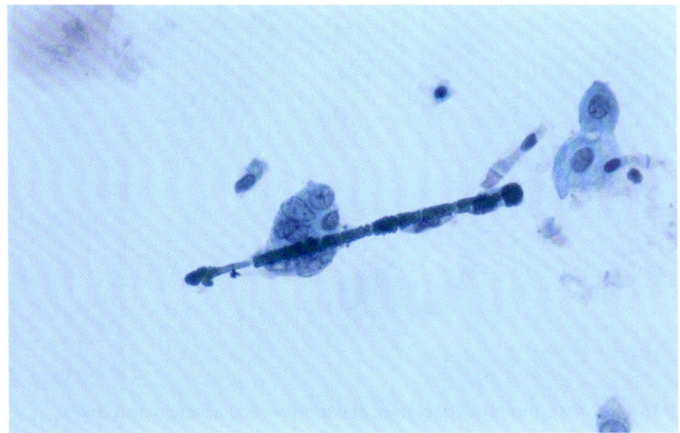

IMAGE 5.40 Bronchial wash: ferruginous body (Papanicolaou, x400).

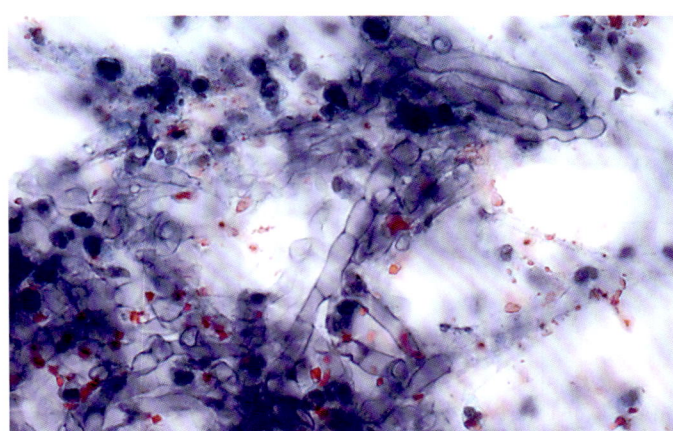

IMAGE 5.43 Lung FNA specimen: *Aspergillus* infection (Papanicolaou, x400).

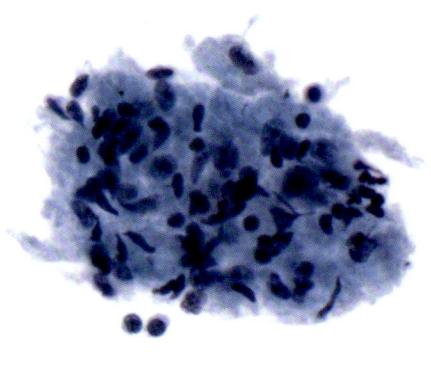

IMAGE 5.41 Pulmonary hilar lymph node FNA specimen: granuloma, nonnecrotizing (Papanicolaou, x400).

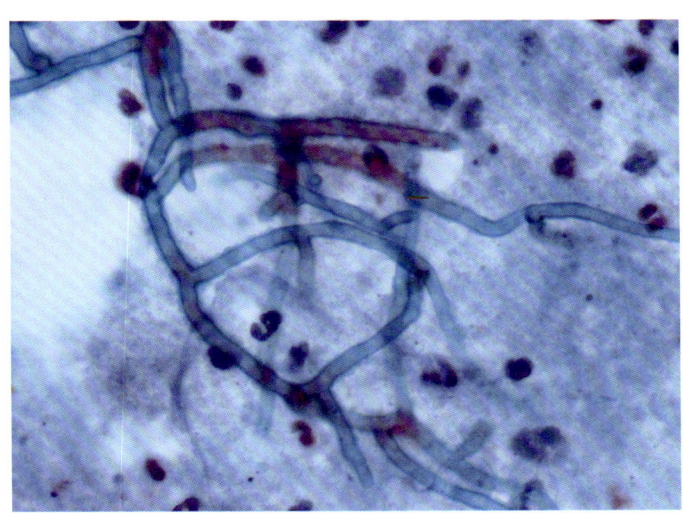

IMAGE 5.44 Bronchial wash: *Aspergillus* infection (Papanicolaou, x400).

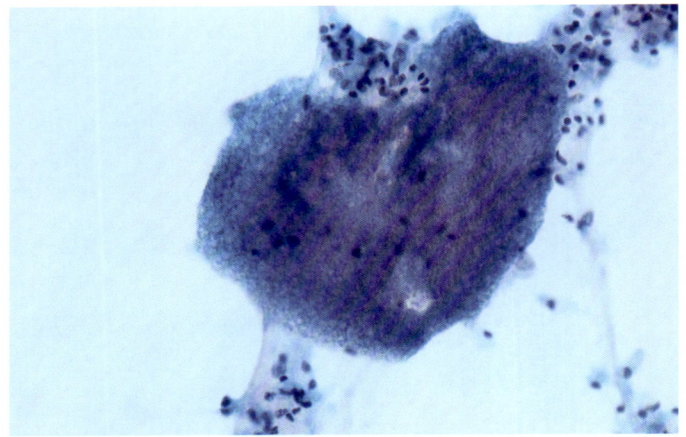

IMAGE 5.45 Lung BAL: *Pneumocystis jiroveci* pneumonia (Papanicolaou, x200).

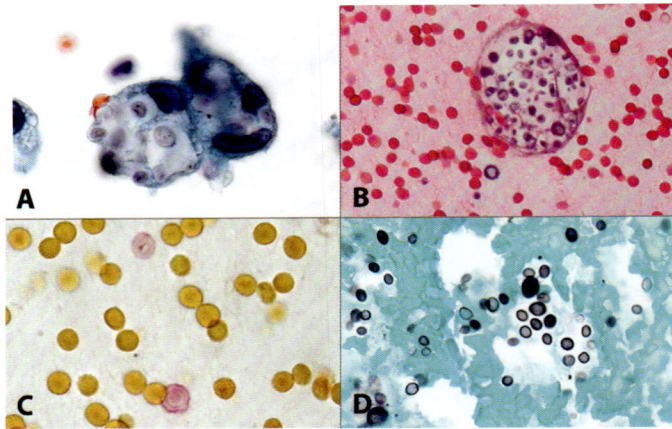

IMAGE 5.48 Lung FNA specimen: *Cryptococcus*. Image A: Papanicolaou, x400. Image B: H&E, x200. Image C: mucicarmine, x400. Image D: Grocott, x200.

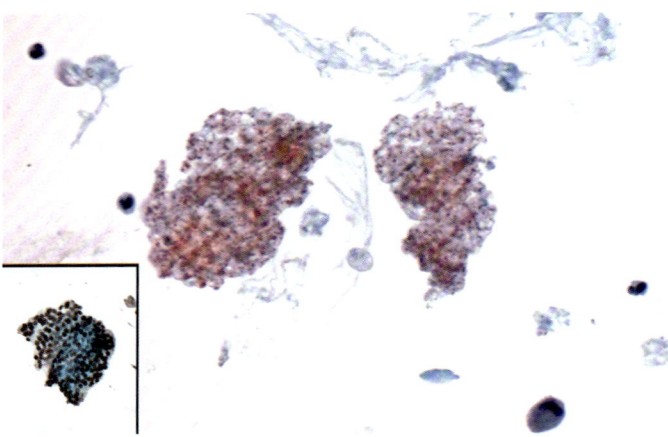

IMAGE 5.46 Lung BAL: *Pneumocystis jiroveci* pneumonia (Papanicolaou, x400). Inset: *P. jiroveci* organisms (Grocott stain, x200).

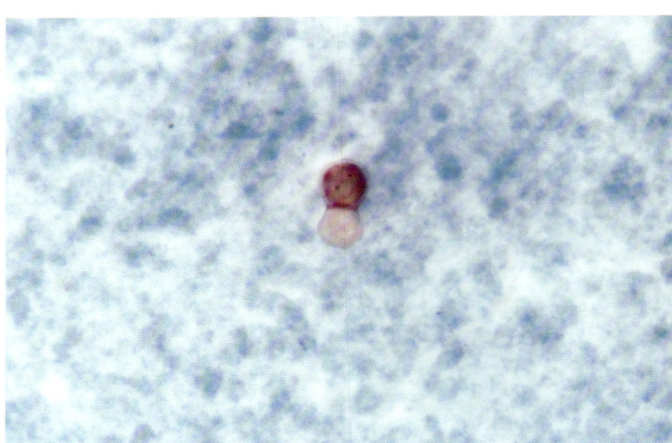

IMAGE 5.49 Lung FNA specimen: blastomycosis (Papanicolaou, x600).

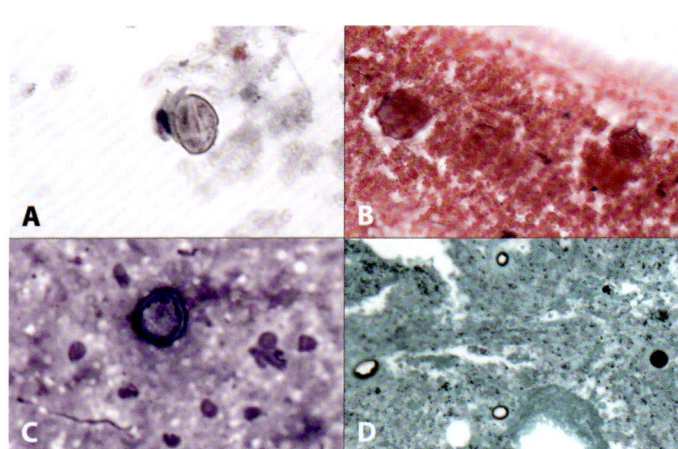

IMAGE 5.47 Lung FNA specimen: coccidioidomycosis. Image A: Papanicolaou, x400. Image B: H&E, x400. Image C: Wright-Giemsa, x400. Image D: Grocott, x200.

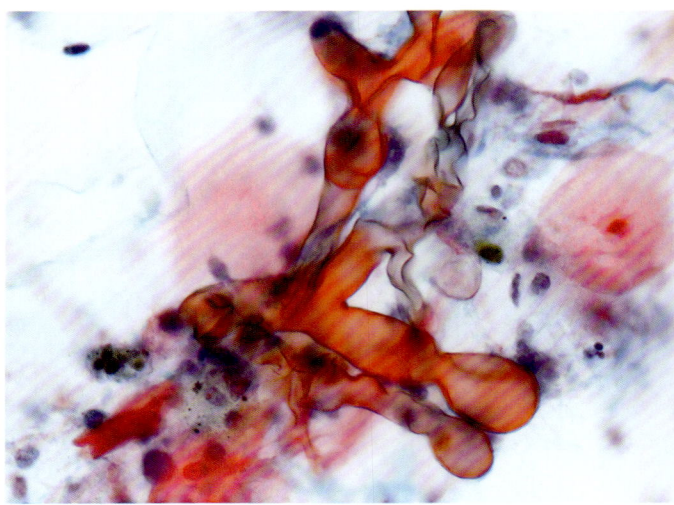

IMAGE 5.50 Lung FNA specimen: mucormycosis (Papanicolaou, x400).

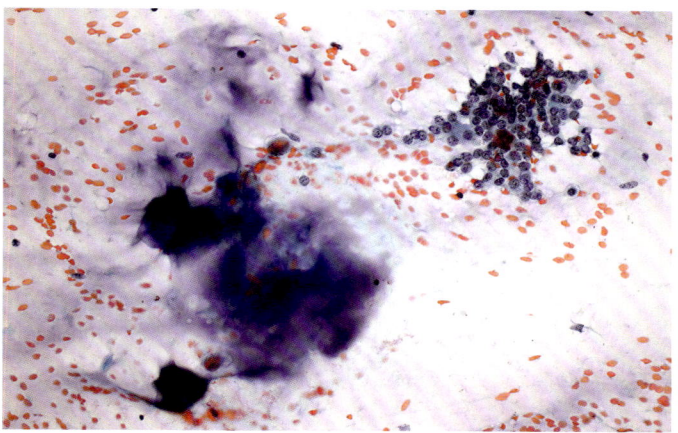

IMAGE 5.51 Lung FNA specimen: pulmonary hamartoma (Papanicolaou, x200).

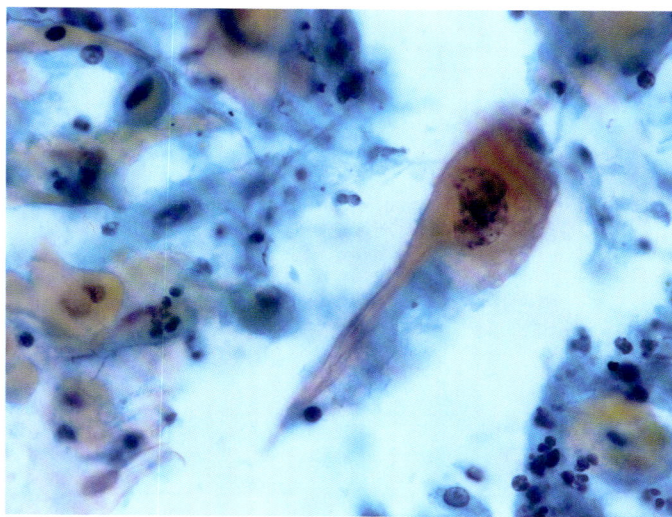

IMAGE 5.54 Lung FNA specimen: squamous cell carcinoma, well-differentiated/keratinizing type (Papanicolaou, x400).

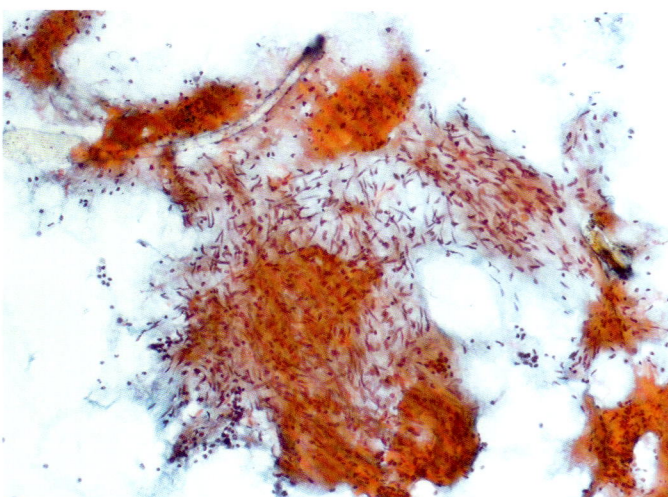

IMAGE 5.52 Lung FNA specimen: pulmonary hamartoma (Papanicolaou, x100).

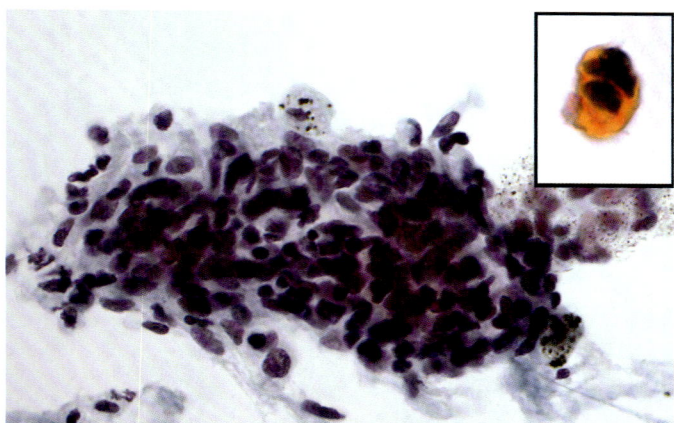

IMAGE 5.55 Lung FNA specimen: squamous cell carcinoma. Inset: malignant keratinized cell (Papanicolaou, x400).

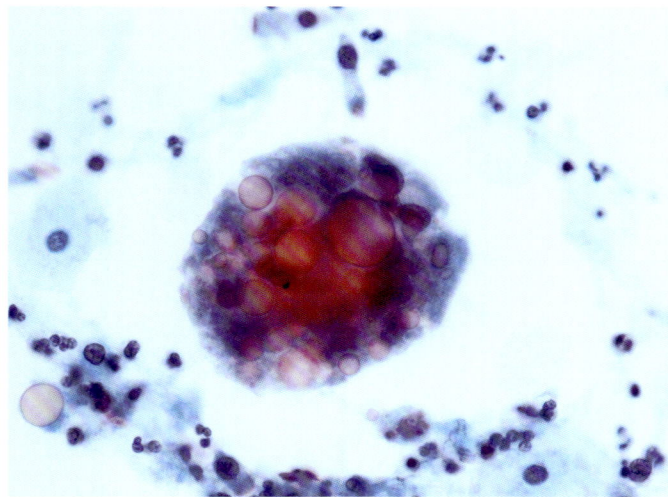

IMAGE 5.53 Lung FNA specimen: lipid pneumonia (Papanicolaou, x600).

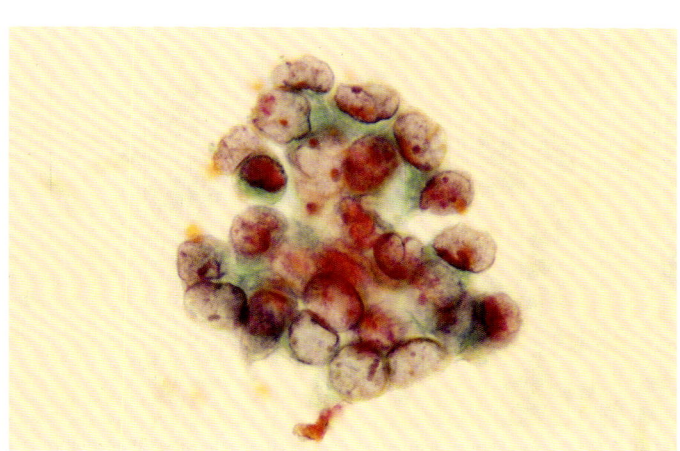

IMAGE 5.56 Lung FNA specimen: adenocarcinoma (Papanicolaou, x400).

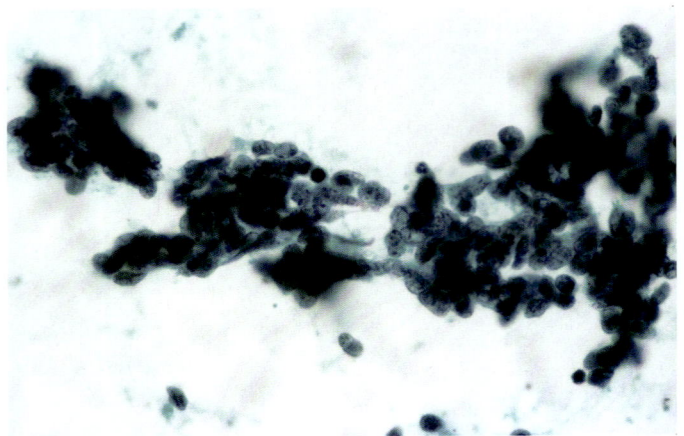

IMAGE 5.57 Lung FNA specimen: small cell carcinoma (Papanicolaou, x400).

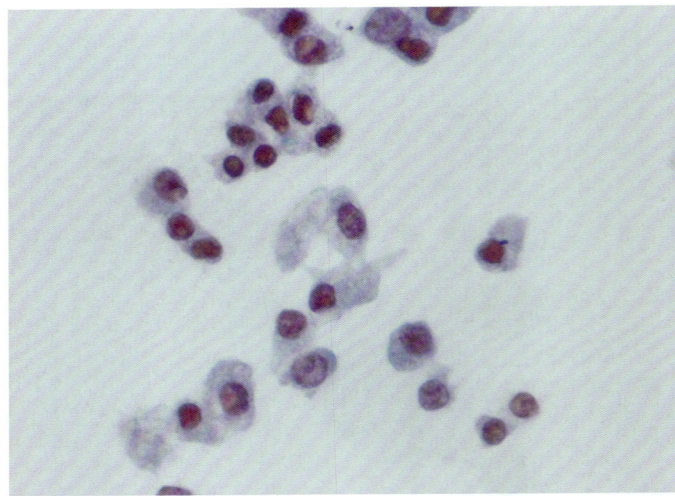

IMAGE 5.60 Lung FNA specimen: carcinoid tumor (Papanicolaou, x600).

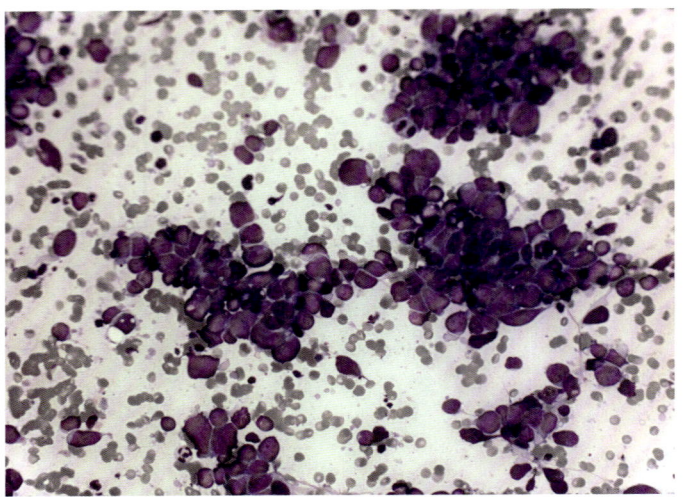

IMAGE 5.58 Lung FNA specimen: small cell carcinoma (Diff Quik, x400).

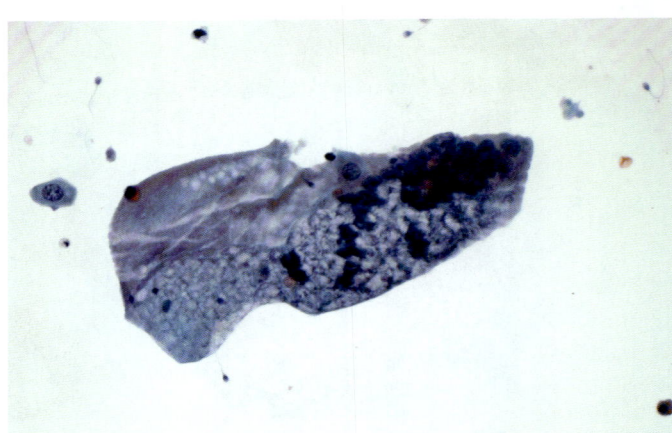

IMAGE 5.61 Urine: normal urothelial umbrella cell, negative for malignancy (Papanicolaou, x400).

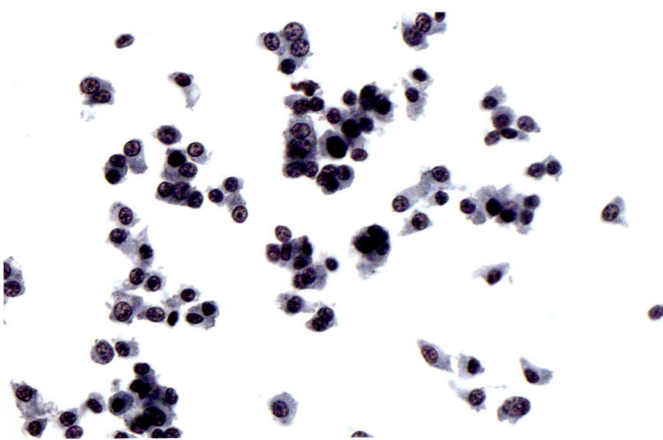

IMAGE 5.59 Lung FNA specimen: carcinoid tumor (Papanicolaou, x400).

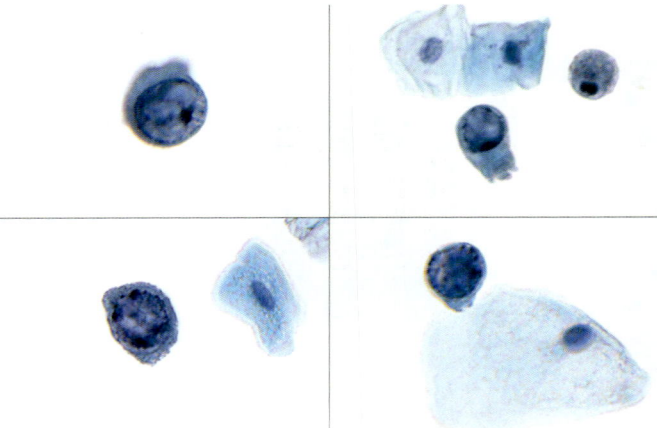

IMAGE 5.62 Urine: polyomavirus, negative for high grade urothelial carcinoma (all images: Papanicolaou, x400).

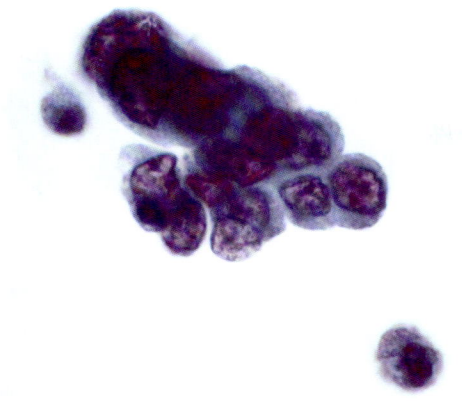

IMAGE 5.63 Urine from bladder wash: high grade urothelial carcinoma (Papanicolaou, x600).

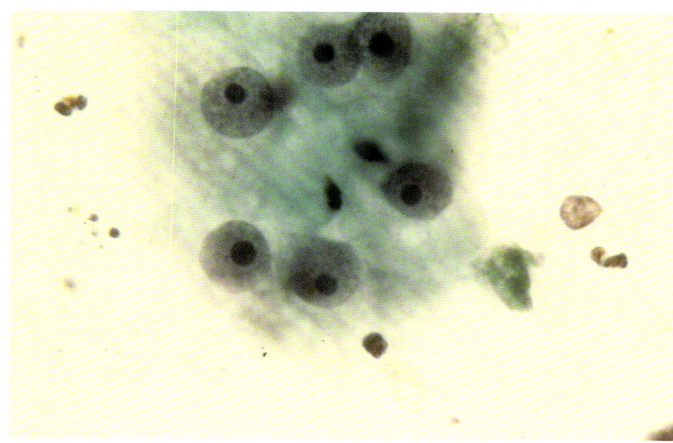

IMAGE 5.66 Kidney FNA specimen: renal cell carcinoma, clear cell type (Papanicolaou, x600).

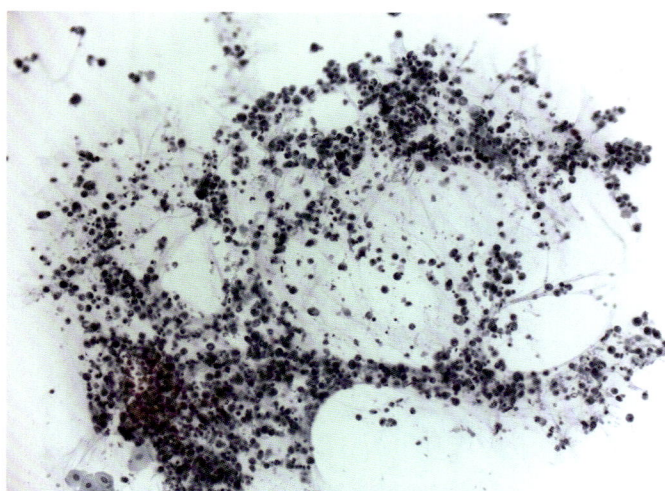

IMAGE 5.64 Urine from an ileal conduit: mucin and degenerated intestinal epithelial cells.

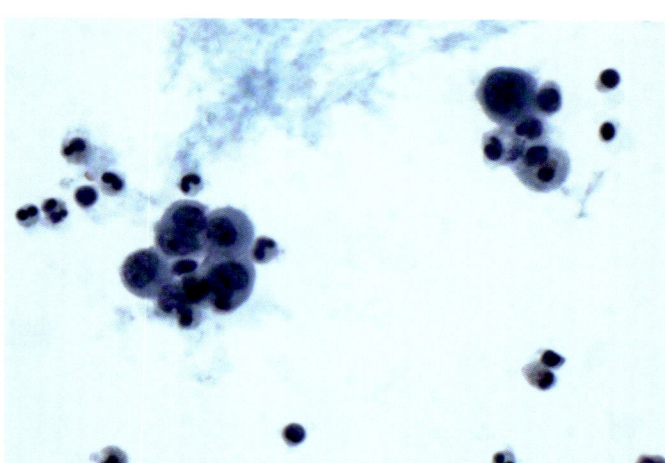

IMAGE 5.67 Pleural fluid: normal mesothelial cells (Papanicolaou, x400).

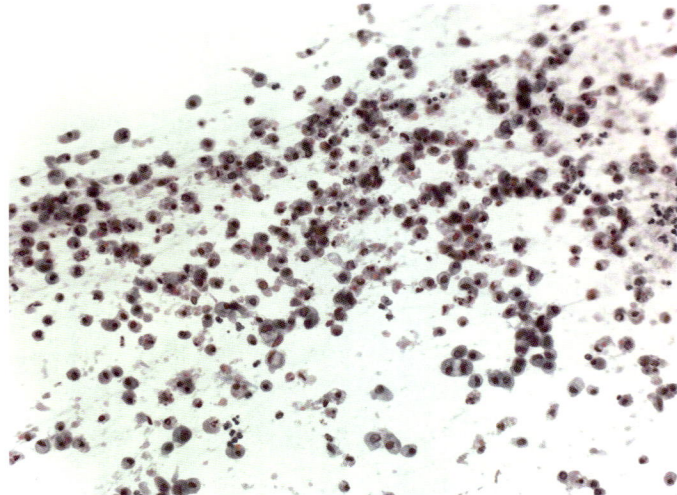

IMAGE 5.65 Urine from an ileal conduit: mucin and degenerated intestinal epithelial cells (Papanicolaou, x400).

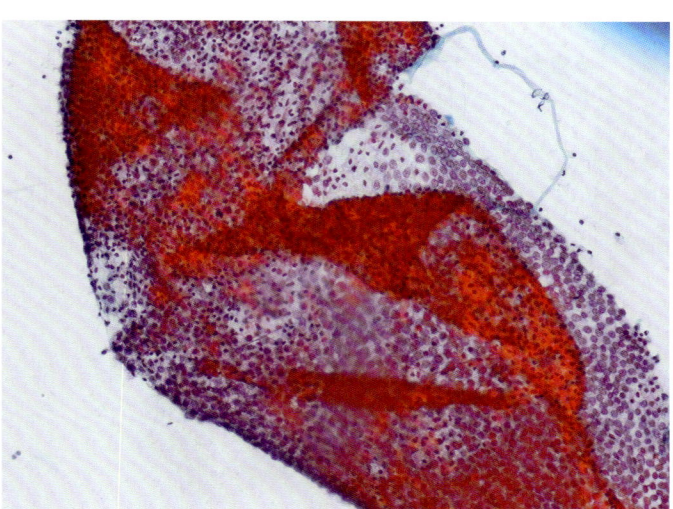

IMAGE 5.68 Peritoneal washing: normal mesothelial cells arranged in large folded sheets typical of peritoneal washings (Papanicolaou, x200).

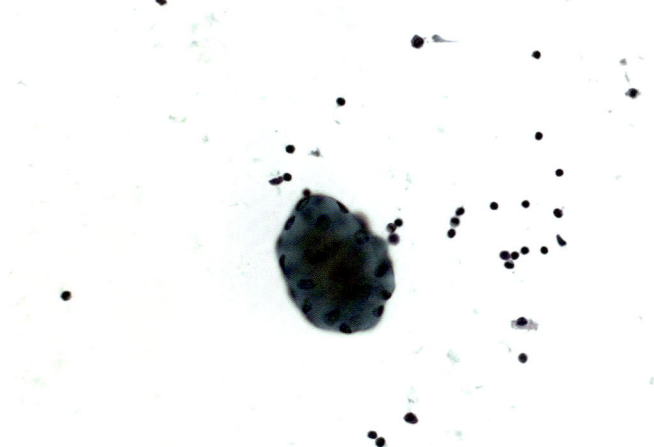

IMAGE 5.69 Peritoneal washing: collagen ball (Papanicolaou, x400).

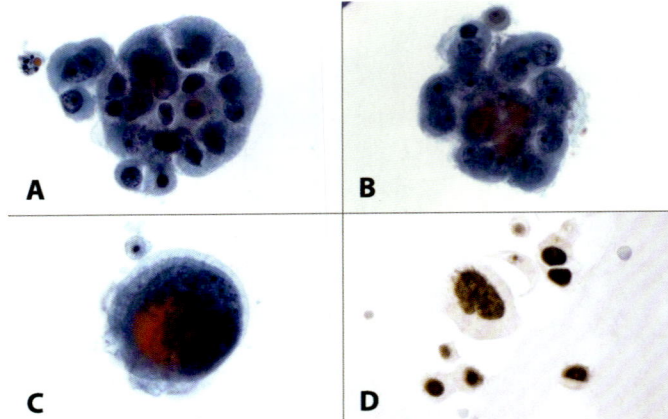

IMAGE 5.72 Pleural fluid: epithelioid mesothelioma. Images A, B, C: Papanicolaou, x400. Image D: WT-1, x200.

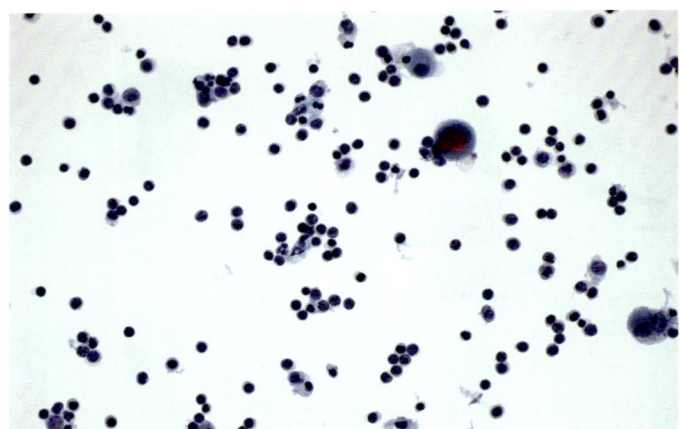

IMAGE 5.70 Pleural fluid: lymphocytic effusion (Papanicolaou, x200).

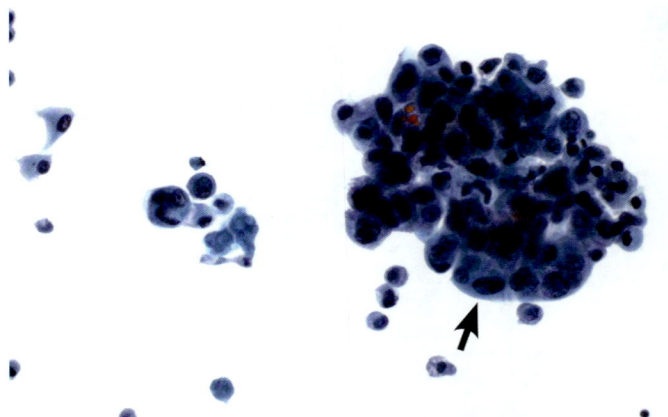

IMAGE 5.73 Pleural fluid: metastatic adenocarcinoma. Note: communal/smooth border, arrow (Papanicolaou, x400).

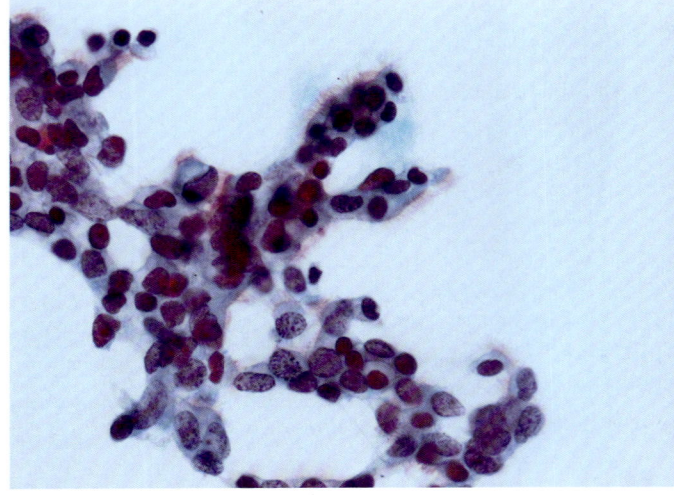

IMAGE 5.71 Peritoneal washing: endosalpingiosis. Note the presence of cilia (Papanicolaou, x400).

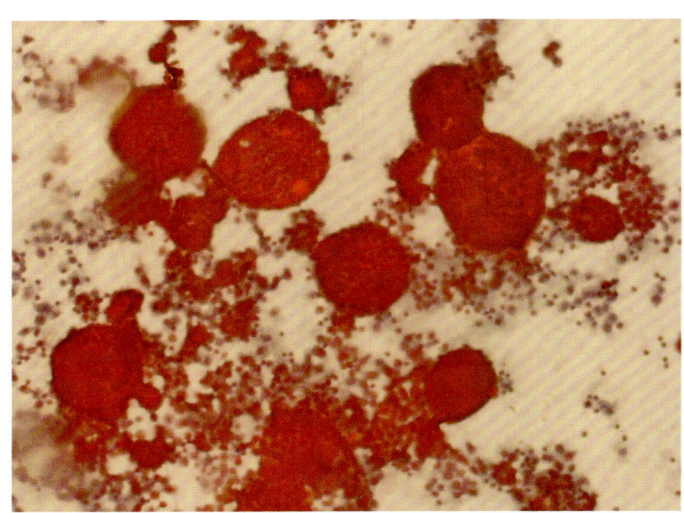

IMAGE 5.74 Pleural fluid: metastatic adenocarcinoma from a breast primary cancer. Note the "cannonball" arrangement (Papanicolaou, x100).

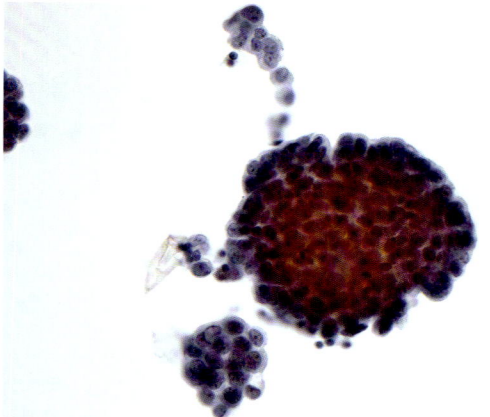

IMAGE 5.75 Peritoneal washing: high grade ovarian serous carcinoma (Papanicolaou, x200).

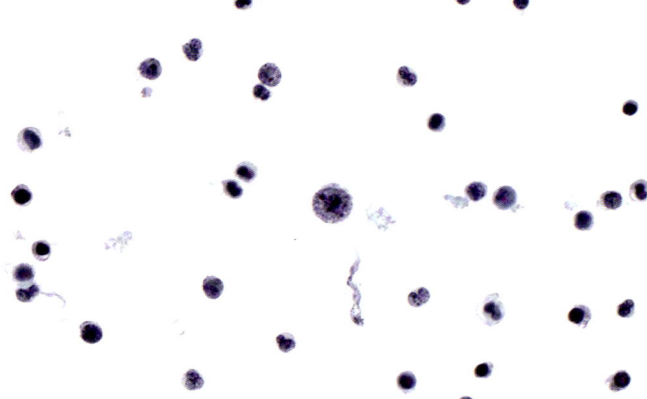

IMAGE 5.78 CSF: high grade B-cell lymphoma (Papanicolaou, x400).

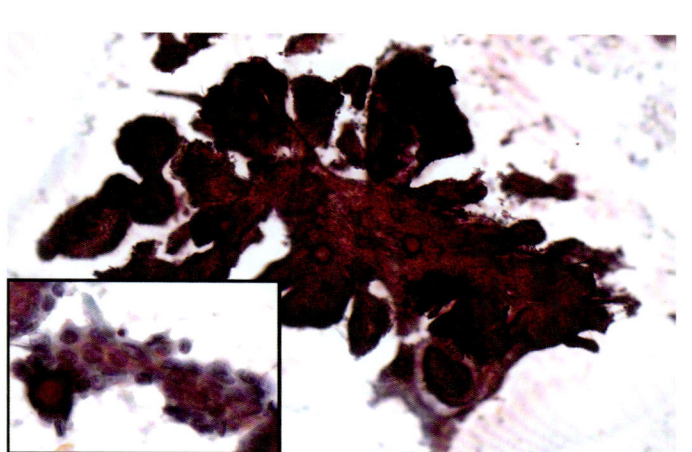

IMAGE 5.76 Peritoneal washing: low grade serous adenocarcinoma (Papanicolaou, x40). Inset: bland nuclear features and psammomatous calcification (Papanicolaou, x400).

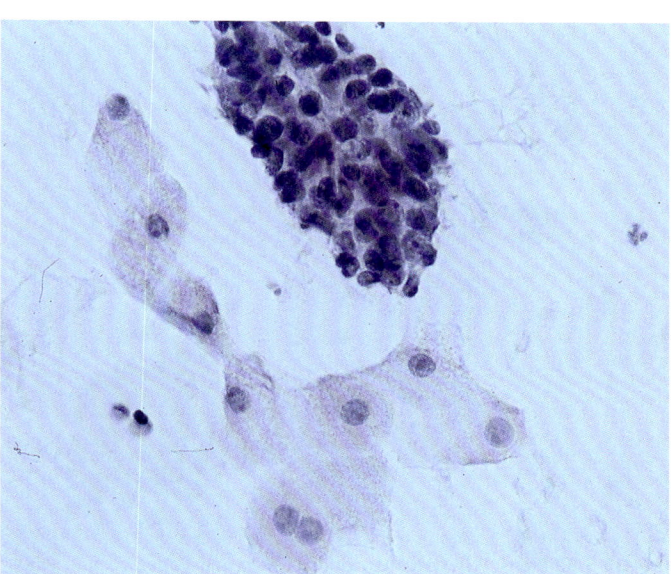

IMAGE 5.79 Breast FNA specimen: fibrocystic changes (Papanicolaou, x400).

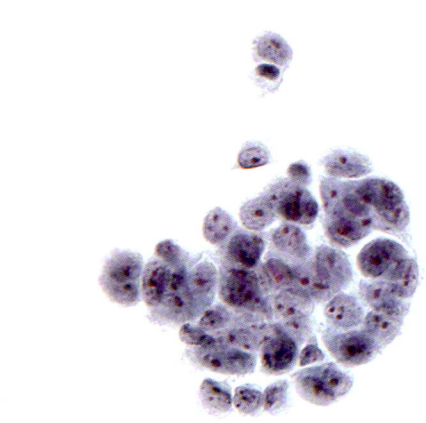

IMAGE 5.77 CSF: metastatic adenocarcinoma, breast primary (Papanicolaou, x400).

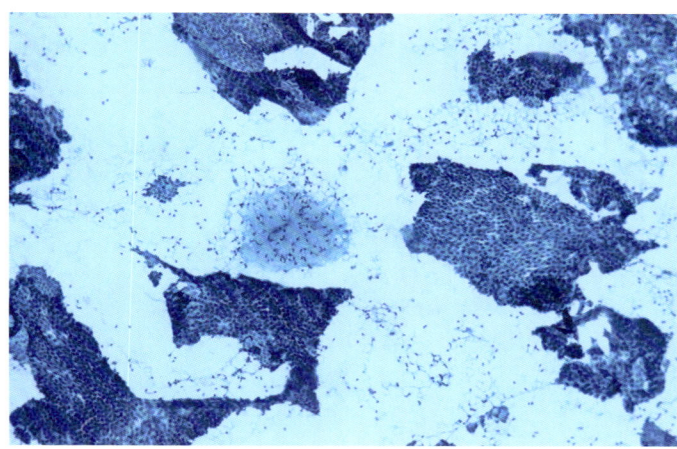

IMAGE 5.80 Breast FNA specimen: fibroadenoma (Papanicolaou, x100).

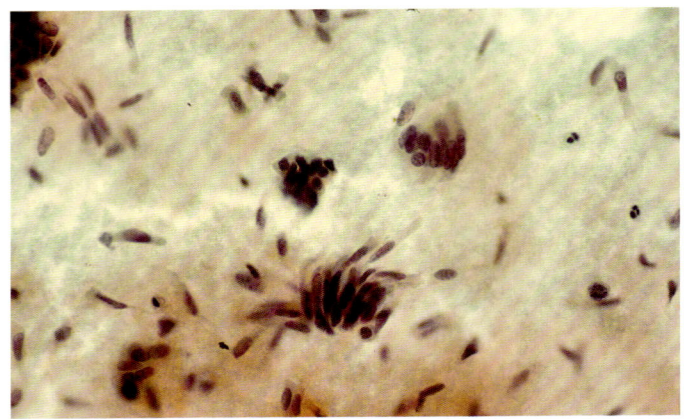

IMAGE 5.81 Breast FNA specimen: papillary neoplasm (Papanicolaou, x400).

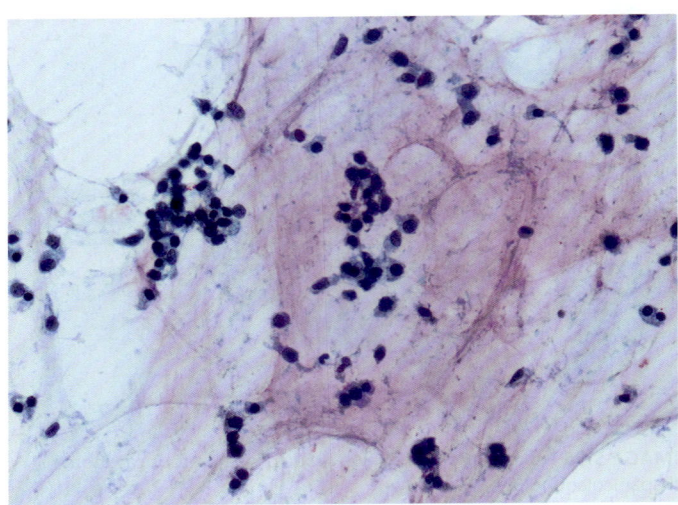

IMAGE 5.84 Breast FNA specimen: mucinous adenocarcinoma (Papanicolaou, x600).

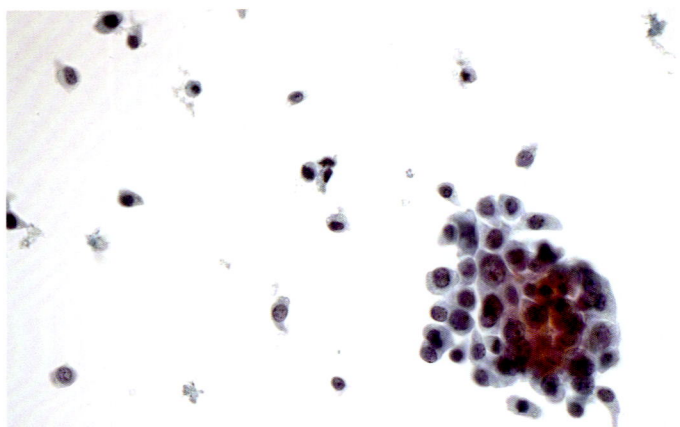

IMAGE 5.82 Breast FNA specimen: ductal carcinoma (Papanicolaou, x400).

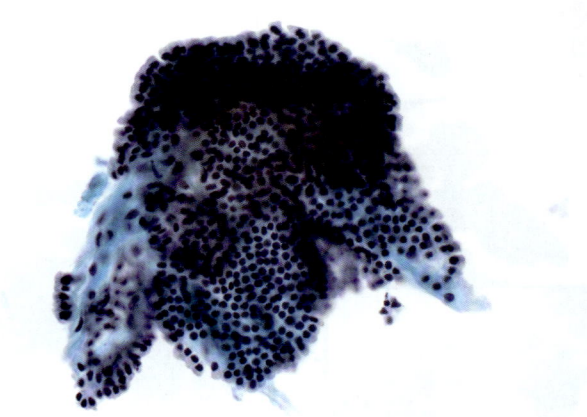

IMAGE 5.85 Thyroid FNA specimen: macrofollicular sheets, benign follicular nodule (Papanicolaou, x100).

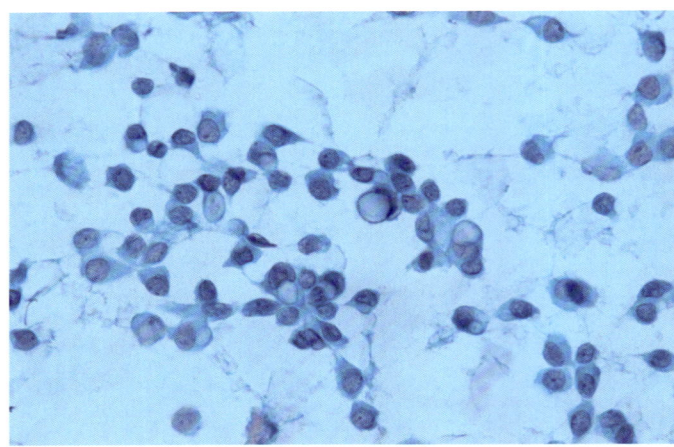

IMAGE 5.83 Breast FNA specimen: lobular carcinoma (Papanicolaou, x400).

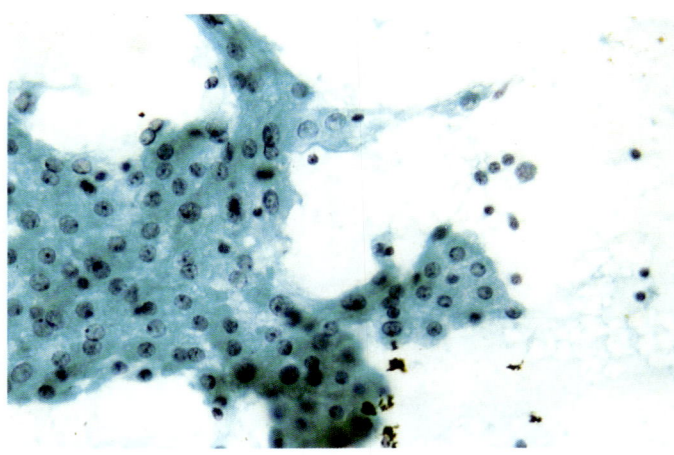

IMAGE 5.86 Thyroid FNA specimen: oncocytic (Hürthle) cells and lymphocytes, consistent with lymphocytic thyroiditis (Papanicolaou, x600).

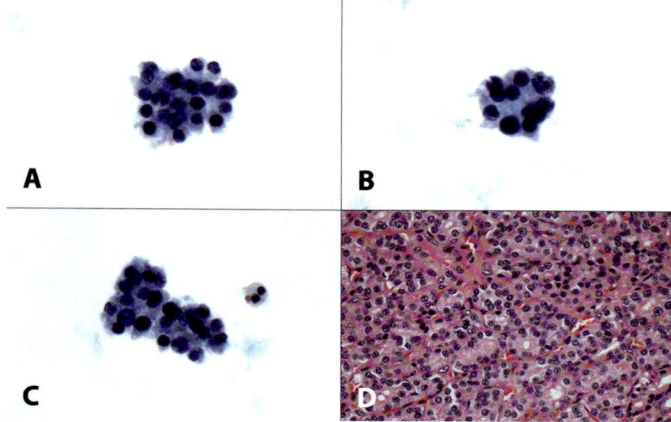

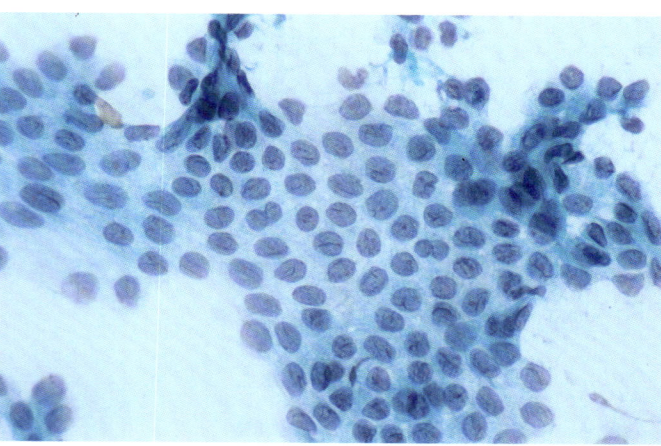

IMAGE 5.87 Thyroid FNA specimen: follicular neoplasm. Images A, B, C: Papanicolaou, x400. Image D: H&E, x200.

IMAGE 5.90 Thyroid FNA specimen: papillary thyroid carcinoma (Papanicolaou, x600).

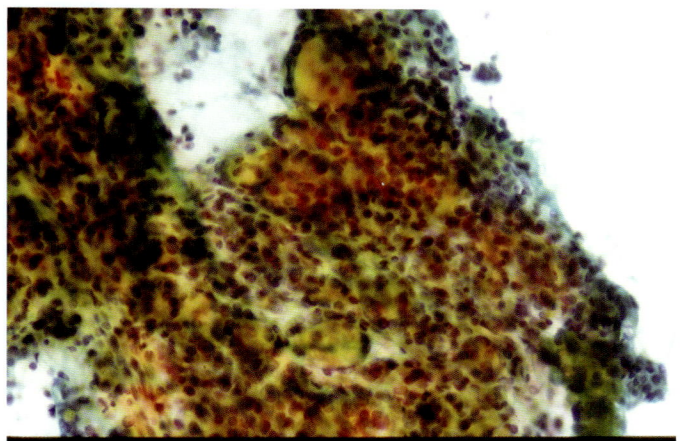

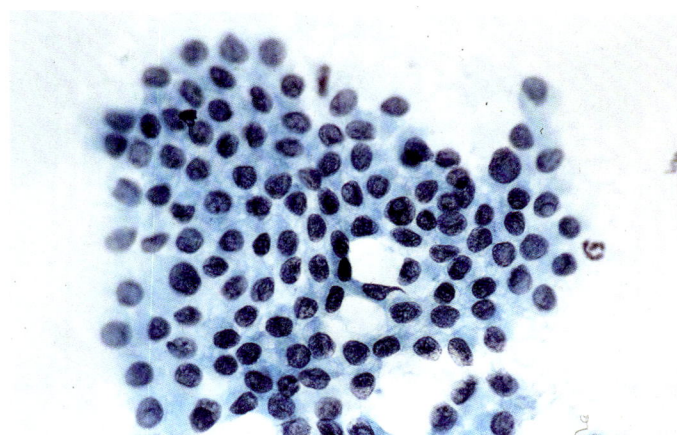

IMAGE 5.88 Thyroid FNA specimen: follicular neoplasm (Papanicolaou, x400).

IMAGE 5.91 Thyroid FNA specimen: papillary thyroid carcinoma (Papanicolaou, x600).

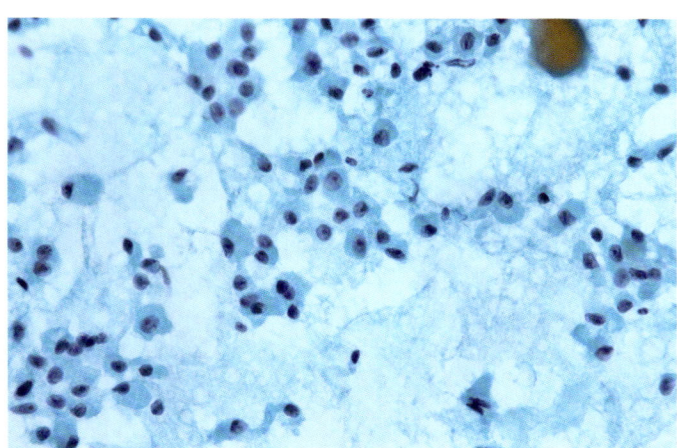

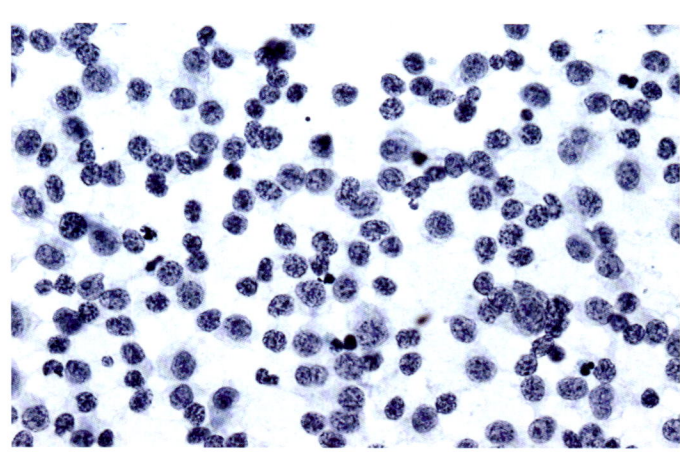

IMAGE 5.89 Thyroid, FNA specimen: follicular neoplasm, oncocytic (Hürthle) cell type (Papanicolaou, x200).

IMAGE 5.92 Thyroid FNA specimen: medullary thyroid carcinoma (Papanicolaou, x400).

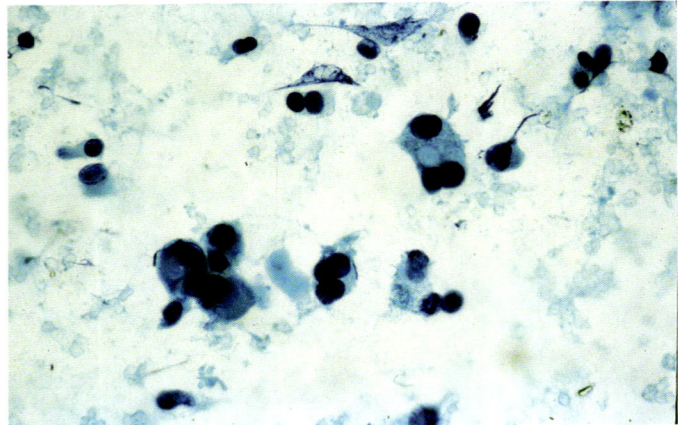

IMAGE 5.93 Thyroid FNA specimen: medullary thyroid carcinoma (Papanicolaou, x600).

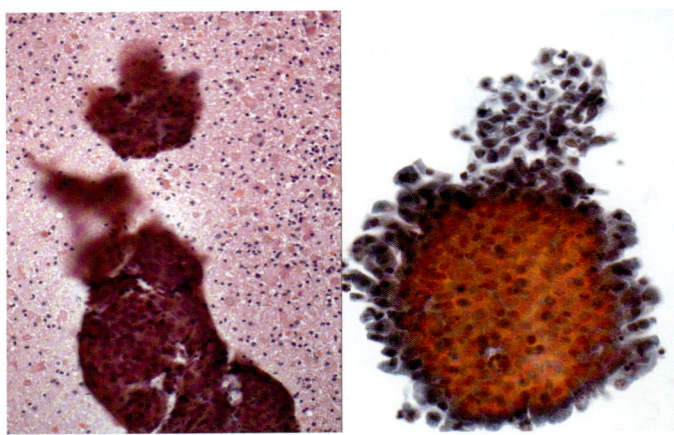

IMAGE 5.96 Salivary gland FNA specimen: Warthin tumor. Left: H&E, x100. Right: Papanicolaou, x200.

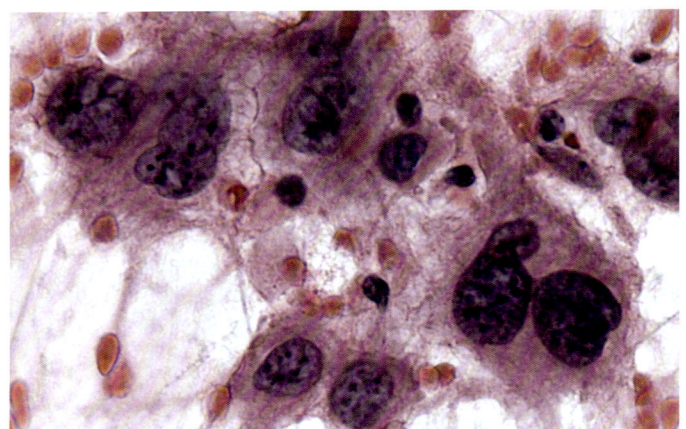

IMAGE 5.94 Thyroid FNA specimen: undifferentiated anaplastic thyroid carcinoma (H&E, x400).

Courtesy of Dr. Moosa Khalil, University of Calgary.

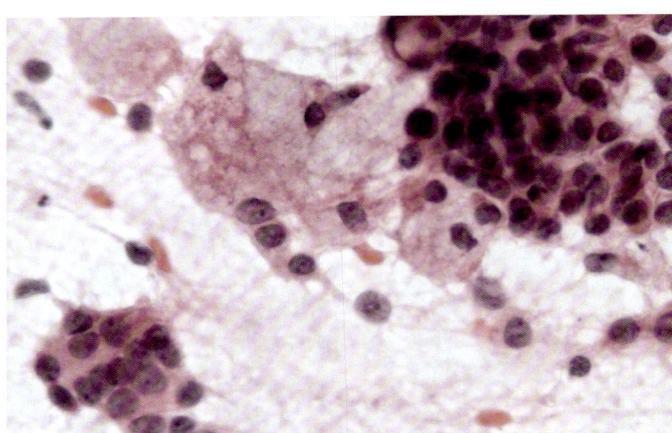

IMAGE 5.97 Salivary gland FNA specimen: mucoepidermoid carcinoma, low grade (H&E, x400).

Courtesy of Dr. Moosa Khalil, University of Calgary.

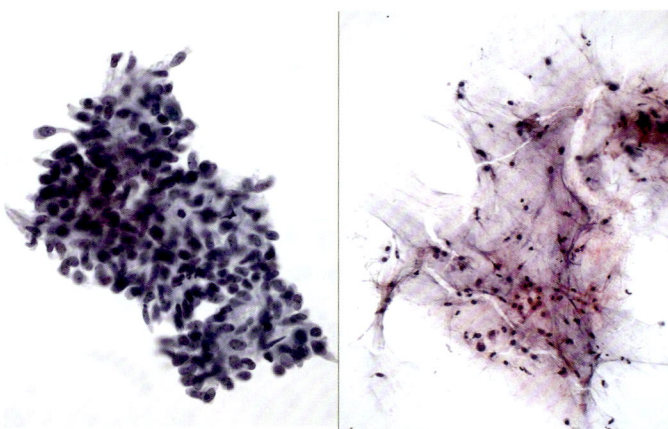

IMAGE 5.95 Salivary gland FNA specimen: pleomorphic adenoma (both images: Papanicolaou, x200).

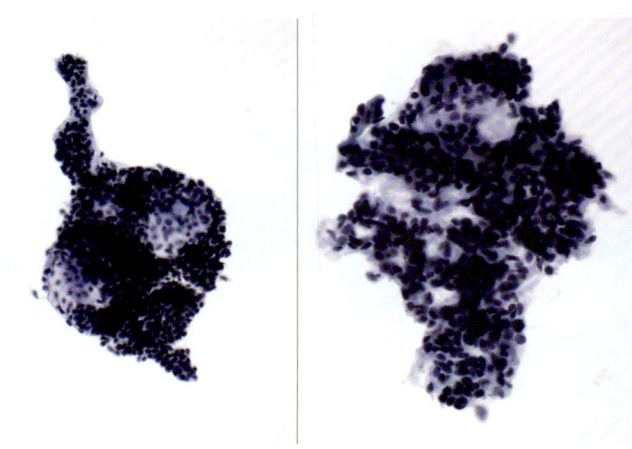

IMAGE 5.98 Salivary gland FNA specimen: adenoid cystic carcinoma (both images: Papanicolaou, x200).

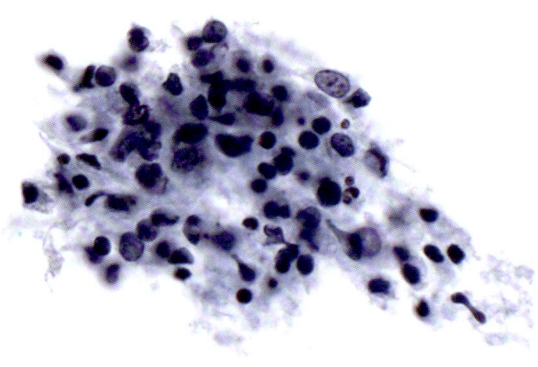

IMAGE 5.99 Lymph node (axillary) FNA specimen: germinal center of reactive lymphadenopathy (Papanicolaou, x400).

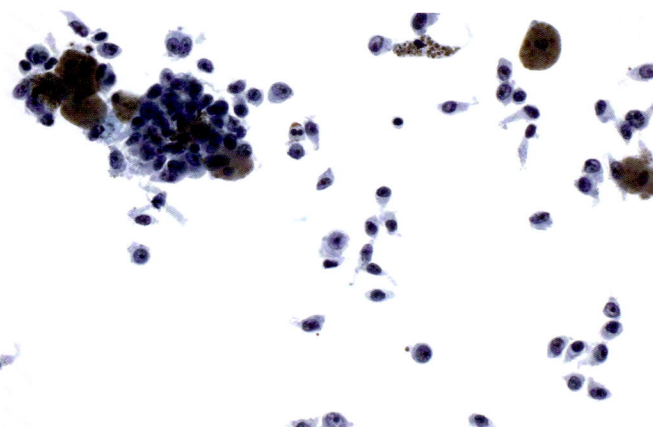

IMAGE 5.102 Lymph node (neck) FNA specimen: metastatic melanoma (Papanicolaou, x400).

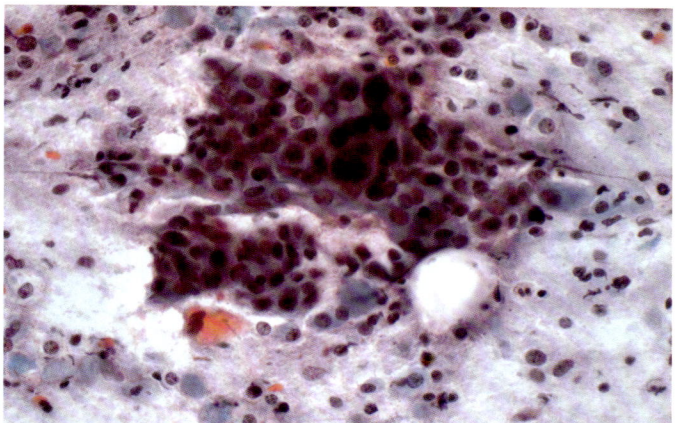

IMAGE 5.100 Lymph node (neck) FNA specimen: metastatic squamous cell carcinoma, cystic (Papanicolaou, x400).

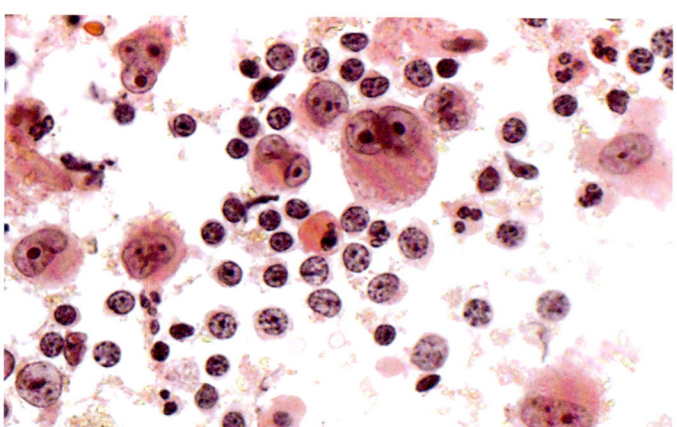

IMAGE 5.103 Lymph node (neck) FNA specimen: classical Hodgkin lymphoma (Papanicolaou, x400).

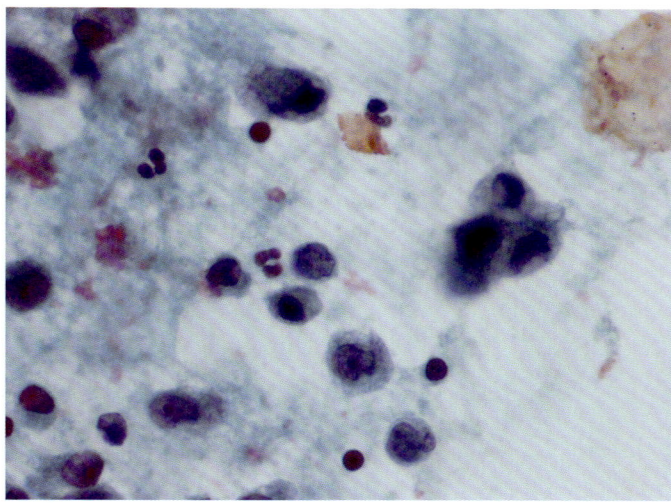

IMAGE 5.101 Lymph node (axillary) FNA specimen: metastatic adenocarcinoma (Papanicolaou, x600).

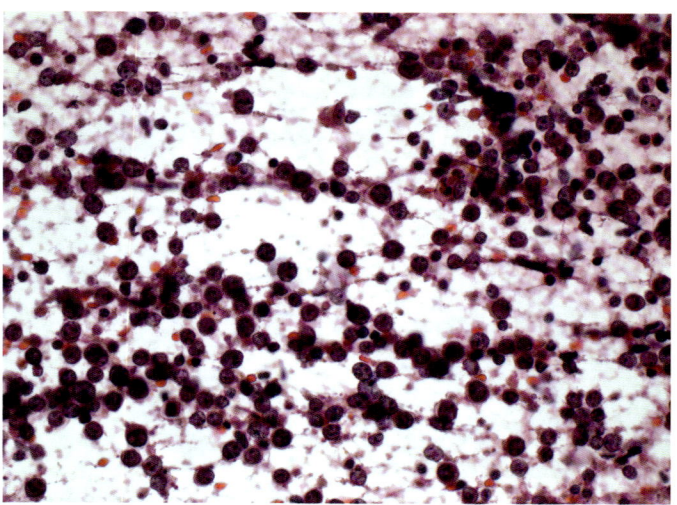

IMAGE 5.104 Lymph node (neck) FNA specimen: diffuse large B-cell lymphoma (H&E, x400).

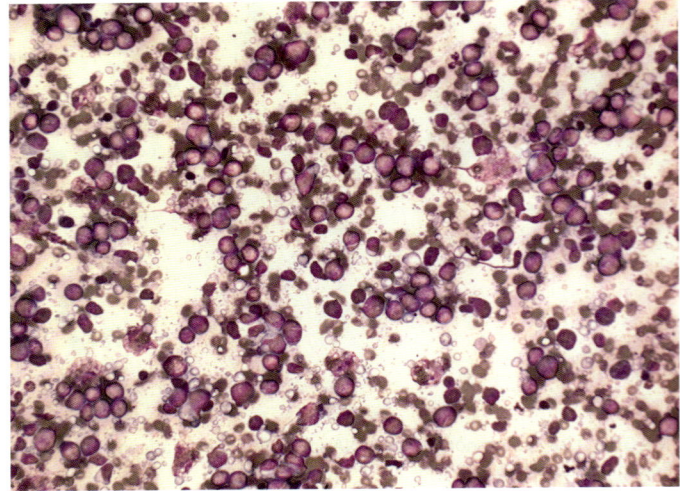

IMAGE 5.105 Lymph node (mediastinal) FNA specimen: diffuse large B-cell lymphoma. Lymphoglandular bodies are present (Diff Quik, x400).

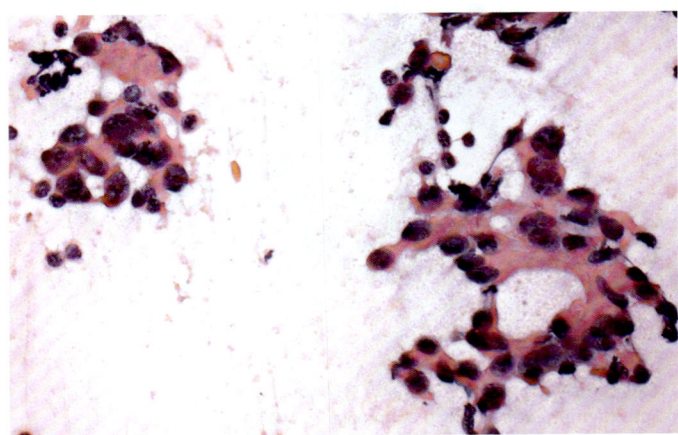

IMAGE 5.108 Liver FNA specimen: cholangiocarcinoma (Papanicolaou, x200).

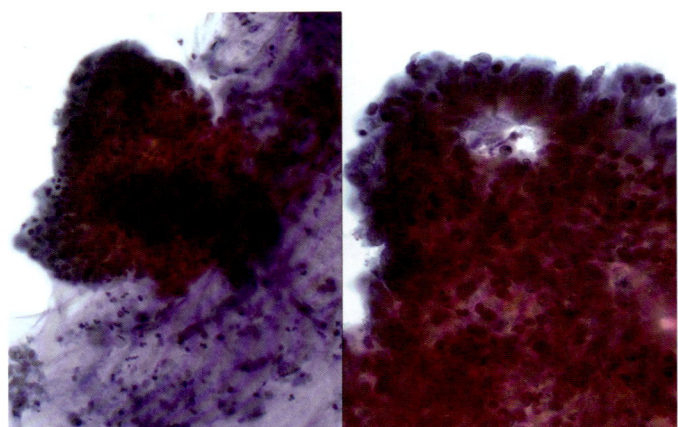

IMAGE 5.106 Liver FNA specimen: metastatic colorectal adenocarcinoma. Left: Papanicolaou, x100. Right: Papanicolaou, x400.

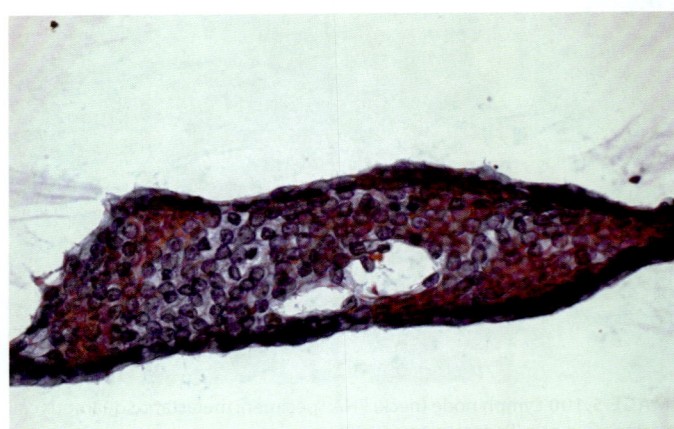

IMAGE 5.109 Pancreas FNA specimen: ductal adenocarcinoma (Papanicolaou, x200).

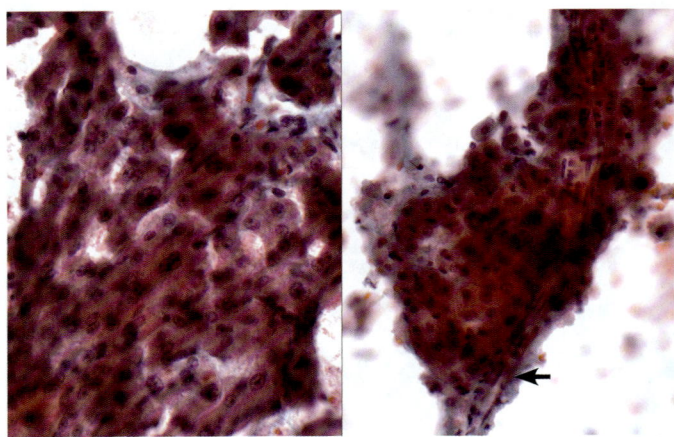

IMAGE 5.107 Liver FNA specimen: hepatocellular carcinoma with traversing blood vessel (arrow). Left: Papanicolaou, x400. Right: Papanicolaou, x200.

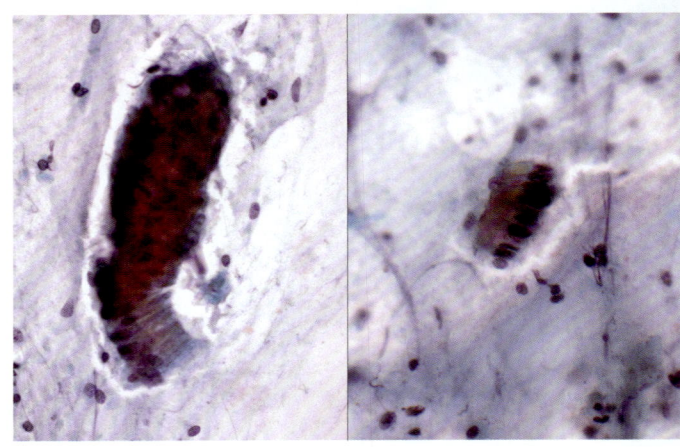

IMAGE 5.110 Pancreas FNA specimens showing mucinous cyst with low grade dysplasia (both images: Papanicolaou, x200).

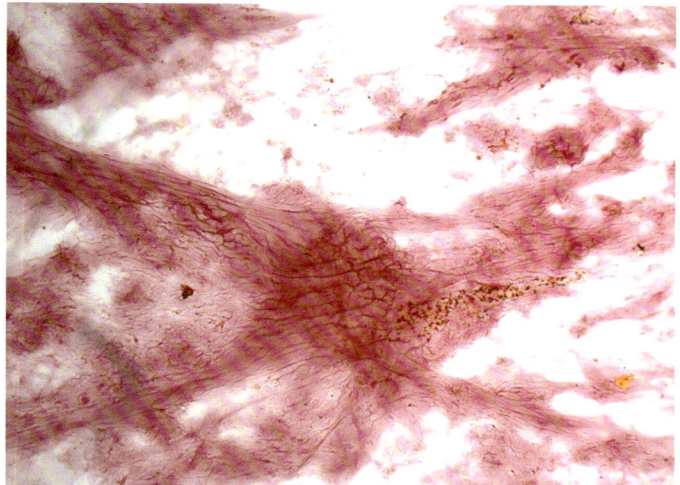

IMAGE 5.111 Pancreas FNA specimen: mucinous cyst. Thick, colloid-like mucin is present (Mucicarmine, x100).

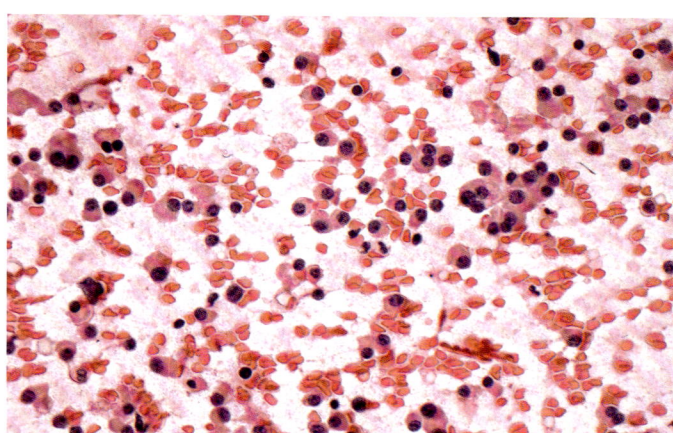

IMAGE 5.114 Pancreas FNA specimen: well-differentiated pancreatic neuroendocrine tumor (H&E, x200).

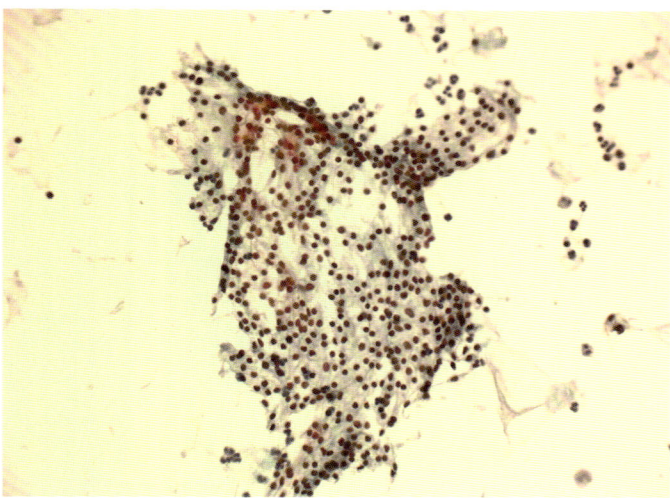

IMAGE 5.112 Pancreas FNA specimen: serous cystadenoma (Papanicolaou, x400).

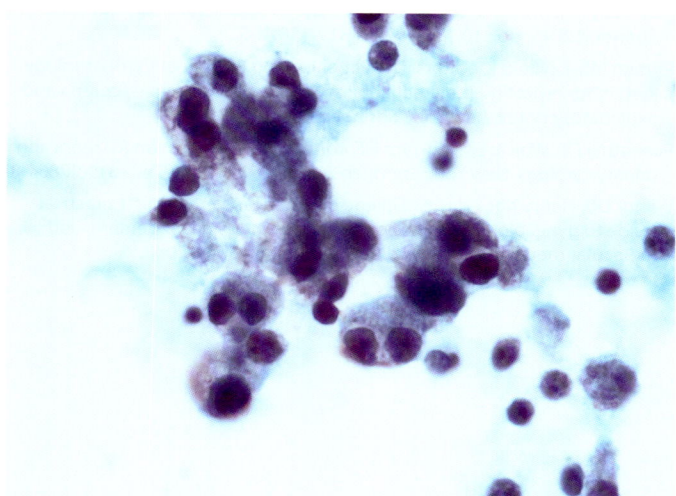

IMAGE 5.115 Pancreas FNA specimen: well-differentiated pancreatic neuroendocrine tumor (H&E, x600).

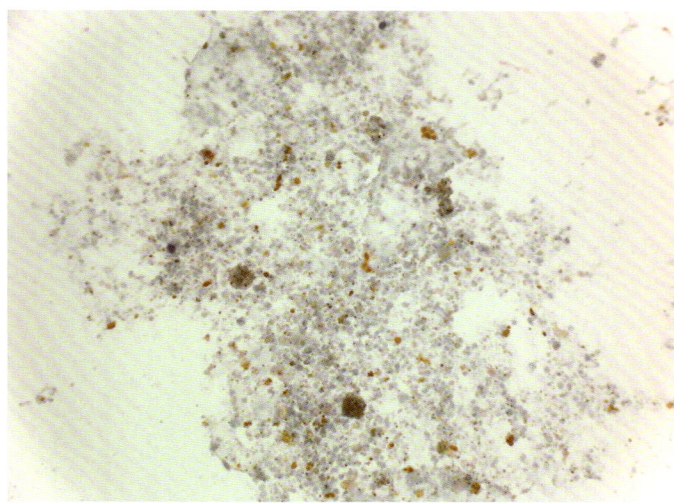

IMAGE 5.113 Pancreas FNA specimen: pseudocyst (Papanicolaou, x400).

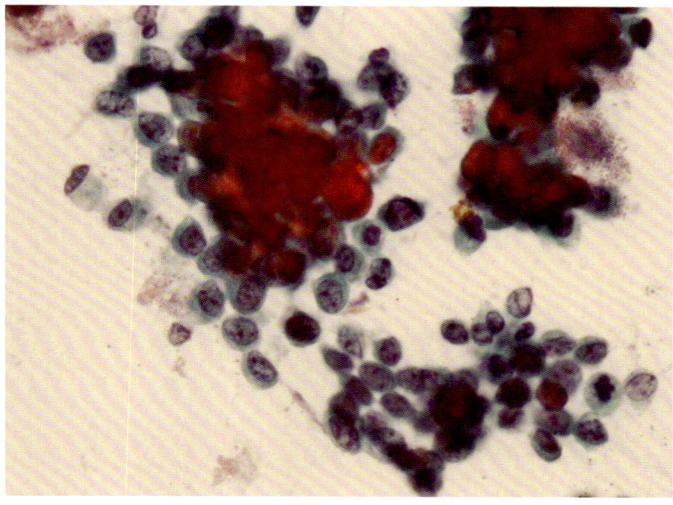

IMAGE 5.116 Bile duct brushing: adenocarcinoma (Papanicolaou, x400).

Bibliography

Ali SZ, Cibas ES, editors. The Bethesda system for reporting thyroid cytopathology: definitions, criteria and explanatory notes. 2nd ed. New York: Springer; 2018.

Canadian Society of Cytology. Canadian Society of Cytology guidelines for practice and quality assurance in cytopathology [Internet]. Canadian Society of Cytology; 1978 June [revised 2019 (5th rev. ed.); accessed 2021 March 7]. Available from: https://cytopathology.ca/wp-content/uploads/2019/04/CSC-cyto_guidelines-final-2019.-docx.pdf.

Chandra A, Crothers B, Iyama-Kurtycz D, et al, editors. The international system for serous fluid cytopathology. Cham (Switzerland): Springer; 2020.

Cibas ES, Ducatman BS, editors. Cytology: diagnostic principles and clinical correlates. 5th ed. Philadelphia (PA): Elsevier Saunders; 2021.

Faquin WC, Rossi ED, Baloch Z, et al, editors. The Milan system for reporting salivary gland cytopathology. Cham (Switzerland): Springer; 2018.

Field A, Raymond W, Schmitt F, editors. The International Academy of Cytology Yokohama system for reporting breast fine needle aspiration biopsy cytopathology. Cham (Switzerland): Springer; 2020.

Layfield LJ, Baloch Z, editors. The Papanicolaou Society of Cytopathology system for reporting respiratory cytology: definitions, criteria, explanatory notes, and recommendations for ancillary testing. Cham (Switzerland): Springer; 2019.

Nayar R, Wilbur DC, editors. The Bethesda system for reporting cervical cytology: definitions, criteria and explanatory notes. 3rd ed. New York: Springer; 2015. doi: 10.1007/978-3-319-11074-5

Pitman MB, Layfield L, editors. The Papanicolaou Society of Cytopathology system for reporting pancreaticobiliary cytology: definitions, criteria and explanatory notes. New York: Springer; 2015.

Rosenthal DL, Wojcik EM, Kurtycz DF, editors. The Paris system for reporting urinary cytology. New York: Springer; 2016. doi: 10.1007/978-3-319-22864-8

Wilbur DC, Henry MR, editors. College of American Pathologists practical guide to gynecologic cytopathology: morphology, management, and molecular methods. Northfield (IL): CAP Publications; 2008.

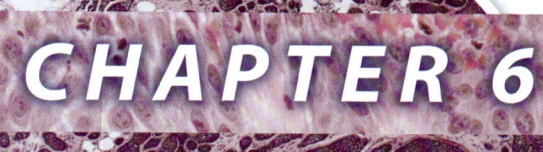

CHAPTER 6

Dermatopathology

THAI YEN LY, SYLVIA PASTERNAK, NOREEN M. WALSH

Dermatology Exam Essentials

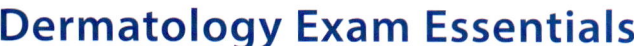

MUST KNOW

World Health Organization (WHO) classification

High-yield topics include:
- Keratinocytic and epidermal tumors:
  - Basal cell carcinoma (BCC) and variants.
  - Squamous cell carcinoma (SCC) and variants.
  - Merkel cell carcinoma.
  - Bowen disease and precursor lesions.
- Melanocytic tumors:
  - Conventional nevi.
  - Spitz nevi.
  - Nevi of special sites.
  - Dysplastic nevi (Clark nevi).
  - Malignant melanoma and common subtypes.
  - Desmoplastic melanoma.
  - *BAP1*-deficient melanocytic lesions.
  - Molecular changes in melanoma.
  - Familial melanoma.
- Appendageal tumors:
  - Eccrine, apocrine, follicular, and sebaceous.
- Hematolymphoid tumors:
  - Mycosis fungoides and Sezary syndrome.
  - Primary cutaneous low grade B-cell lymphomas (follicle center lymphoma, marginal zone lymphoma).
  - Large B-cell lymphoma, leg type.

- CD30-positive lymphoproliferative disorders.
- Soft tissue tumors:
  - Dermatofibroma and dermatofibrosarcoma protuberans (DFSP).
  - Atypical fibroxanthoma and pleomorphic dermal sarcoma.
  - Vascular tumors (hemangioma, Kaposi sarcoma, angiosarcoma).
  - Glomus tumor.
  - Neural tumors (schwannoma, neurofibroma).

AJCC and College of American Pathologists (CAP) protocols

High-yield topics include:
- Melanoma and Merkel cell carcinoma:
  - Pathological staging.
  - The importance of history, location, age, and clinical criteria (ABCDE criteria) for melanocytic tumors.
  - Risk factors for melanoma and Merkel cell carcinoma.
  - Optimal sampling methods for melanocytic tumors and limitations of small biopsies.
  - Characteristics and significance of microsatellite, satellite, and in-transit metastases.
  - The rationale for performing sentinel lymph node sampling.

 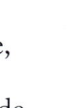

- Specimen handling of sentinel lymph nodes for potential metastatic melanoma and approach to microscopic examination.
- The role of ancillary testing (including molecular techniques) in establishing the diagnosis of skin tumors:
  · Histochemical and immunohistochemical stains for melanoma.
  · Immunofluorescence for bullous diseases (including salt-split skin technique).
  · Histochemical stains for common inflammatory conditions.
  · Various bacterial, spirochete, acid fast, and fungal stains.
  · Immunohistochemistry (IHC) for Merkel cell carcinoma.
  · IHC for differentiating spindle cell tumors.
  · IHC and T-cell receptor (TCR) studies for mycosis fungoides.

Nonneoplastic diseases

High-yield topics include:
- Ackerman's pattern approach to inflammatory dermatoses.
- Basic understanding of clinical manifestations of common inflammatory conditions (e.g., psoriasis, lichen planus, lupus erythematosus, dermatophytosis).
- Systemic diseases with associated skin manifestations, such as:
  · Psoriasis and psoriatic arthritis.
  · Dermatitis herpetiformis and celiac disease.
  · Pyoderma gangrenosum, erythema nodosum and inflammatory bowel disease (IBD).
  · Malar rash, discoid rash, photosensitivity, panniculitis, and lupus.
  · Panniculitis and α_1-antitrypsin deficiency.
  · Morphea and systemic sclerosis.
- Classification of bullous skin diseases based on level and mechanism of split.
- Vasculitides involving skin: etiology, clinical presentation, and histopathologic features.
- Granulomatous processes of the skin.

Genetic and syndromic conditions

Syndromes with skin findings are high-yield topics, including:
- Familial atypical multiple mole melanoma (FAMMM).
- Xeroderma pigmentosum.
- Gorlin syndrome.
- Peutz-Jeghers syndrome.
- Neurofibromatosis 1 and 2.
- Paraneoplastic syndromes.
- Tuberous sclerosis.
- Birt-Hogg-Dubé syndrome.
- Muir-Torre syndrome.
- Cowden disease.

MUST SEE

High-yield images include:
- Clinical images of skin findings in common syndromes:
  · Tuberous sclerosis: angiofibroma, shagreen patch, ash-leaf macules, subungual fibroma.
  · Muir-Torre syndrome: sebaceous carcinoma.
  · Birt-Hogg-Dubé syndrome: fibrofolliculoma, trichodiscoma, acrochordon.
  · Cowden disease: trichilemmoma, palmar pits.
- Histologic images of common tumors (make note of pathognomonic features, especially those that can be diagnosed at low to medium power):
  · Epidermal: benign (verruca, seborrheic keratosis), precursors (actinic keratosis, Bowen disease), SCC including variants, BCC including variants, keratoacanthoma.
  · Merkel cell carcinoma.
  · Melanocytic tumors: conventional nevi, Spitz nevi including variants, dysplastic (Clark) nevi, malignant melanoma (nodular, lentiginous, superficial spreading, lentigo maligna, desmoplastic).
  · Adnexal tumors: poroma, syringoma, cylindroma, hidradenoma, spiradenoma, syringocystadenoma papilliferum, mixed tumors, pilomatricoma, microcystic adnexal carcinoma, adenoid cystic carcinoma, sebaceous tumors.
  · Site-specific lesions: mammary and extramammary Paget disease, chondrodermatitis nodularis helicis.
  · Hematolymphoid tumors and/or disorders: mycosis fungoides, primary cutaneous low grade B-cell lymphomas, mastocytosis, CD30+ lymphoproliferative disorders, Langerhans cell histiocytosis, Rosai-Dorfman disease.
  · Soft tissue tumors: lipoma and variants, dermatofibroma, DFSP, smooth muscle tumors, glomus tumor, vascular tumors (benign and malignant), neurofibroma, perineurioma, granular cell tumor, schwannoma, malignant peripheral nerve sheath tumor (MPNST).
  · Tumors of uncertain origin: atypical fibroxanthoma, pleomorphic dermal sarcoma, epithelioid sarcoma, clear cell sarcoma, neurothekeoma.
- Histologic images of common inflammatory dermatoses:
  · Superficial perivascular:
    › Without epidermal changes: viral exanthem, drug reaction, urticaria, mastocytosis, insect bite.
    › With epidermal changes: vacuolar (erythema multiforme, Stevens-Johnson syndrome, toxic epidermal necrolysis, lupus); lichenoid (lichen planus, drug reaction, lupus, mycosis fungoides); spongiotic or psoriasiform (psoriasis, lichen simplex chronicus, fungus, chronic spongiotic dermatitis).
  · Superficial and deep perivascular: lupus, insect bite, drug reaction.

- Vasculitis: leukocytoclastic vasculitis, polyarteritis nodosa (PAN), granulomatosis with polyangiitis (GPA), eosinophilic granulomatosis with polyangiitis (EGPA).
- Nodular and diffuse: granulomatous (tuberculosis, sarcoid, granuloma annulare, rheumatoid nodule, necrobiosis lipoidica, foreign body), neutrophilic (Sweet syndrome, infection), lymphoid (leukemia, lymphoma, pseudolymphoma).
- Vesicular and pustular: subcorneal (pemphigus foliaceus, staphylococcal scalded skin syndrome, impetigo), intraepidermal (pemphigus vulgaris, Hailey-Hailey, Darier disease, Grover disease), subepidermal (bullous pemphigoid, dermatitis herpetiformis, porphyria).
- Peri and folliculitis: alopecia, lupus, acne, rosacea.
- Fibrosing: keloid, morphea, lichen sclerosus.
- Panniculitis: septal (erythema nodosum, morphea), lobular (lupus profundus, nodular vasculitis, pancreatitis), calciphylaxis.

___

MUST DO

- For each of the tumors outlined in the Must See section, be able to generate a differential diagnosis and immunohistochemical panel. Topics to practice include:
  - Differential for spindle cell tumors of the skin.

- Differential for small round blue cell tumors of the skin.
- Differential for painful lesions of the skin.
- Context and risk factors for cutaneous angiosarcoma.
- Mammary and extramammary Paget disease, differential diagnosis, and workup.
- For each of the inflammatory dermatoses outlined in the Must See section, know at least 2 other entities with similar histopathological features.
- Know entities with immunofluorescence (IF) findings:
  - Pemphigus vulgaris.
  - Bullous pemphigoid.
  - Dermatitis herpetiformis.
- Demonstrate knowledge and practical skills in gross handling of the following specimens:
  - Punch and shave biopsies.
  - Oriented and unoriented skin ellipses.
  - Reexcisional specimens for atypical lesions and malignancy (including melanoma).
  - Large resections with complex orientation.
  - Resections from special areas (e.g., nose, ear, lips, eyelids).
  - Sentinel lymph nodes for melanoma.
- Demonstrate knowledge and practical skills in specimen handling of the following **fresh** specimens:
  - Cutaneous lymphoma, with appropriate workup.
  - Bullous disease, including transport media for IF.

___

MULTIPLE CHOICE QUESTIONS

1. The following microscopic findings are true for cutaneous drug eruptions except:

a. Vacuolar interface change is a common feature.

b. Virtually any inflammatory reaction pattern is possible.

c. A mixed picture of different inflammatory reaction patterns is a clue.

d. The presence of eosinophils is a reliable and consistent feature.

e. A pseudolymphomatous pattern is possible.

Answer: d

2. All of the following are true for spongiotic dermatitis except:

a. Etiologic classification is possible on histopathology alone.

b. The acute, subacute, and chronic phases show different features.

c. Dermatophytosis is in the histopathologic differential diagnosis.

d. Lichenification is a common feature in chronic lesions.

Answer: a

3. All of the following are found in mycosis fungoides except:

a. Pautrier microabscesses.

b. Munro microabscesses.

c. Papillary dermal fibroplasia (chicken-wire pattern).

d. Epidermotropism of lymphocytes.

e. Usually, a predominance of CD4-positive over CD8-positive lymphocytes.

Answer: b

4. Net-like or intercellular immunofluorescence is seen in what inflammatory skin disease?

a. Lichen planus.

b. Bullous pemphigoid.

c. Linear IgA bullous dermatosis.

d. Pemphigus vulgaris.

e. Dermatitis herpetiformis.

Answer: d

5. All of the following are true about lichen planus **except**:

a. Pruritic flat-topped erythematous or violaceous papules are typical.
b. Wickham striae may be observed.
c. Wrists and ankles are common sites of involvement.
d. It may be associated with scarring alopecia.
e. Arthritis is a common association.

Answer: e

6. All of the following present with a subepidermal blister **except**:

a. Dermatitis herpetiformis.
b. Linear IgA bullous dermatosis.
c. Pemphigoid gestationis.
d. IgA pemphigus.
e. Porphyria cutanea tarda.

Answer: d

7. Which of the following is a fungal infection of the skin?

a. Pityriasis lichenoides et varioliformis acuta.
b. Pityriasis rosea.
c. Pityriasis versicolor.
d. Pityriasis rubra pilaris.
e. Pityriasis alba.

Answer: c

8. All of the following are true for pyoderma gangrenosum **except**:

a. Inflammatory bowel disease is a known association.
b. The histopathologic features are distinct and highly specific.
c. Clinical lesions consist of ulcers with undermined edges and violaceous borders.
d. It is a diagnosis of exclusion that requires careful clinical-pathologic correlation.
e. The histopathologic differential diagnosis often includes infection.

Answer: b

9. Nail pigmentation can be caused by all of the following **except**:

a. Hemorrhage into the nail plate.
b. Fungal infection.
c. Subungual melanoma.
d. Subungual nevus.
e. Subungual keratoacanthoma.

Answer: e

10. Which of the following is classified as a scarring alopecia?

a. Alopecia areata.
b. Alopecia due to trichotillomania.
c. Alopecia due to lupus erythematosus.
d. Androgenetic alopecia.
e. Syphilitic alopecia.

Answer: c

11. Which of the following is the most likely clinical scenario for Merkel cell carcinoma?

a. An 8-year-old with a raised nodule on the cheek.
b. A 19-year-old with a pigmented lesion on the calf.
c. A 45-year-old with a pearly papule on the forehead.
d. A 60-year-old with a flat, roughened lesion on the face.
e. A 75-year-old with a nodular lesion on the scalp.

Answer: e

12. All of the following stains are usually positive in Merkel cell carcinoma **except**:

a. CK20.
b. Synaptophysin.
c. Neurofilament.
d. Monokeratin.
e. Thyroid transcription factor-1 (TTF-1).

Answer: e

13. All of the following paired vesiculobullous disorders show similar or almost identical histopathological features **except**:

a. Porphyria cutanea tarda and pseudoporphyria.
b. Bullous pemphigoid and pemphigoid gestationis.
c. Bullous pemphigoid and epidermolysis bullosa acquisita.
d. Dermatitis herpetiformis and linear IgA dermatosis.
e. Pemphigus vulgaris and bullous lichen planus.

Answer: e

14. Which of the following is a genodermatosis?

a. Lichen planus.
b. Dermatitis herpetiformis.
c. Hailey-Hailey disease.
d. Grover disease.
e. Bowen disease.

Answer: c

15. Which of the following is **not** a feature of tuberous sclerosis?

a. Cortical tubers.
b. Lisch nodules.
c. Angiofibromas.
d. Shagreen patch.
e. Cardiac rhabdomyomas.

Answer: b

16. All of the following disorders typically present with annular skin lesions **except**:

a. Erythema multiforme.
b. Nummular eczema.
c. Granuloma annulare.
d. Subacute cutaneous lupus erythematosus.
e. Pretibial myxedema.

Answer: e

17. What is the most common antigen in pemphigus vulgaris?

a. Desmoplakin.
b. Desmoglein 1.
c. Desmoglein 3.
d. Desmoglein 4.
e. BpAg1.

Answer: c

18. Which of the following stains will **not** highlight mast cells?

a. Gomori methenamine silver (GMS).
b. C kit (CD117).
c. Leder stain.
d. Giemsa.
e. Tryptase.

Answer: a

19. A patient is diagnosed with Muir-Torre syndrome. Which of the following malignancies is linked with this syndrome?

a. Merkel cell carcinoma.
b. Sebaceous carcinoma.
c. Microcystic adnexal carcinoma.
d. Malignant melanoma.
e. Basal cell carcinoma.

Answer: b

20. Which of the following lesions does **not** show granulomatous inflammation in the skin?

a. Sarcoidosis.
b. Drug reaction.
c. Granuloma annulare.
d. Granuloma faciale.
e. Tuberculosis.

Answer: d

21. A patient develops a lesion on the arm after taking a certain drug. The lesion resolves but remains hyperpigmented. When the patient is exposed to the drug again, the lesion recurs in the same location. This history is most compatible with which diagnosis?

a. Fixed drug eruption.
b. Lichenoid drug reaction.
c. Drug induced lupus.
d. Interstitial granulomatous dermatitis.
e. Bullous drug reaction.

Answer: a

22. All of the following conditions may resemble lichen planus histopathologically **except**:

a. Lichenoid drug reaction.
b. Lichen simplex chronicus.
c. Lichenoid graft versus host disease (GVHD).
d. Mycosis fungoides.
e. Lichen planus–like keratosis.

Answer: b

23. Clear cells can be observed in all of the following **except**:

a. Clear cell acanthoma.
b. Trichilemmoma.
c. Gout.
d. Sebaceous carcinoma.
e. Metastatic renal cell carcinoma.

Answer: c

24. A 45-year-old HIV-positive patient presents with a generalized eruption of erythematous macules and papules with palmoplantar involvement and flu-like symptoms. The skin biopsy shows a psoriasiform and lichenoid dermatitis with plasma cells. Which of the following investigations is most pertinent in this setting?

a. Human herpesvirus 8 (HHV-8) immunohistochemistry.
b. Cytomegalovirus immunohistochemistry.
c. Human papillomavirus immunohistochemistry.
d. PAS diastase and herpes simplex virus (HSV) immunohistochemistry.
e. Silver stain and/or *Treponema pallidum* immunohistochemistry.

Answer: e

25. All of the following are true regarding epithelioid sarcoma **except**:

a. It is a variant of angiosarcoma.
b. It typically affects young patients.
c. It may present as a painless nodule on the distal extremities.
d. It may mimic a palisading granulomatous dermatitis on light microscopy.
e. It usually demonstrates an aggressive course.

Answer: a

26. Histopathologic mimics of pagetoid squamous cell carcinoma (Bowen disease) include all of the following except:

a. Melanoma in situ.
b. Paget disease.
c. Sebaceous carcinoma (intraepidermal component).
d. Psoriasis.
e. Clonal seborrheic keratosis.

Answer: d

SHORT ANSWER QUESTIONS

Lichen Planus

27. List the histopathological features of classic lichen planus.
- Confluent orthokeratosis without parakeratosis.
- Wedge shaped hypergranulosis.
- Epidermal acanthosis with saw-toothed rete ridges.
- Band-like lymphocytic infiltrate in the superficial dermis.
- Vacuolar degeneration of basal keratinocytes with necrotic keratinocytes (Civatte bodies) in epidermis and papillary dermis (colloid bodies).

28. Name 4 histopathological variants of lichen planus.
- Bullous lichen planus.
- Hypertrophic lichen planus.
- Lichen planopilaris.
- Atrophic lichen planus.

29. What are the immunofluorescence findings of lichen planus?
- Colloid bodies stain with IgM, occasionally with IgG, IgA, and C3.
- Fibrinogen deposits are present at the dermoepidermal junction.

Cutaneous Graft Versus Host Disease (GVHD)

30. List the types, timing, and histopathological manifestations of cutaneous GVHD.

TYPE	ONSET	HISTOPATHOLOGICAL FEATURES
Acute	Within first 3 months posttransplant (can be recurrent).	Vacuolar interface dermatitis.
Chronic (lichenoid)	Greater than 3 months posttransplant (often follows acute GVHD).	Lichenoid interface dermatitis.
Chronic (sclerodermoid)	Up to 18 months posttransplant.	Morphea-like fibrosing dermatitis.

31. Although it is not universally applied, what is the grading scheme for GVHD?
- Grade 1: basal vacuolar change.
- Grade 2: dyskeratotic keratinocytes; some associated with lymphocytes (satellite cell necrosis).
- Grade 3: subepidermal cleft and microvesicle formation.
- Grade 4: dermoepidermal split +/− epidermal necrosis.

Erythema Multiforme

32. What causes erythema multiforme?
- A variety of triggers have been implicated in the development of erythema multiforme, most commonly:
- Infection — especially herpes simplex, but also *Mycoplasma pneumoniae*.
- Drugs — e.g., nonsteroidal antiinflammatory drugs.

33. What are the histopathological findings in erythema multiforme?
- Early form: characterized by a vacuolar interface dermatitis — lymphocytes obscuring the dermoepidermal junction with vacuolar degeneration and necrosis/apoptosis of keratinocytes.
- More advanced form: characterized by bullous lesions with subepidermal vesiculation.
- Severe forms: resemble toxic epidermal necrolysis with marked epidermal necrosis.

Note: erythema multiforme is included in the spectrum of Stevens-Johnson syndrome and toxic epidermal necrolysis.

Lupus Erythematosus

34. Discuss the clinical variants and histopathological patterns of lupus skin disease.

VARIANT	SYSTEMIC DISEASE	CLINICAL SKIN LESION(S)	HISTOPATHOLOGICAL PATTERN
Cutaneous manifestations of active systemic lupus erythematosus (SLE)	+	• Malar rash.	• S PVD + vacuolar interface change.
	+	• More extensive photosensitive eruption.	• S or S&D PVD + vacuolar interface change.
	+	• Bullous systemic lupus erythematosus (rare).	• Subepidermal blister with neutrophils.
Subacute cutaneous lupus erythematosus (SACLE)	+ (usually mild)	• Annular or psoriasiform lesions (S~S).	• S PVD + vacuolar interface change.
Discoid lupus erythematosus (DLE)	+ or −	• Classically atrophic scaly plaques (S~S).	• S&D PVD + vacuolar interface change.*
	+ or −	• Scarring alopecia (occasionally).	• S&D PVD + vacuolar interface change.*
	+ or −	• Hypertrophic variant (rare) — exuberant verrucous hyperkeratotic lesions (S~S).	• S&D PVD + vacuolar interface change.**
Tumid lupus erythematosus	+ or −	• Erythematous nonscaly plaques (S~S).	• S&D PVD (without interface change).
Lupus profundus	+ or −	• Subcutaneous nodules (trunk/extremities).	• Lobular panniculitis.
OTHER			
• Vasculitis	+	• Palpable purpura.	• Small vessel vasculitis.
• Neonatal lupus (infant of mother with anti-Ro antibodies)	+ or − (mother)	• Transient eruption in neonatal period (resembles SACLE).	• S or S&D PVD + vacuolar interface change.

Abbreviations: S~S: sun-exposed sites; S&D PVD: superficial and deep perivascular dermatitis; S PVD: superficial perivascular dermatitis.
*The chronicity of DLE often results in a thinned hyperkeratotic epidermis with thickening of the subepidermal basement membrane. Moreover it frequently shows prominent periadnexal (as well as perivascular) inflammation, which results in follicular keratotic plugging and occasionally a scarring alopecia.
**The uncommon hypertrophic variant of DLE displays epidermal hyperplasia (instead of atrophy) with marked hyperkeratosis and can mimic squamous cell carcinoma clinically and histopathologically.

Note: the variants of cutaneous lupus erythematosus that involve the dermoepidermal junction may exhibit a "lupus band" (IgG and/or IgM and/or C3) on direct immunofluorescence.

35. Which histochemical stains may be useful in the diagnosis of lupus?
- Stains to highlight increased dermal mucin (e.g., Alcian blue, colloidal iron).
- Stains to highlight basement membrane thickening (e.g., PAS).

36. What is the significance and diagnostic value of the "lupus band" found on direct immunofluorescence?
- Incidence of positivity is related to lesion site and duration.
- The lupus band test has a high incidence of positivity in systemic lupus erythematosus (SLE), in both lesional and nonlesional sun-exposed skin.
- It has a lower incidence of positivity in SLE if nonlesional sun-protected skin is sampled.
- It may be falsely positive in chronically sun-exposed skin of normal controls (up to 30% of cases).

Vesiculobullous Diseases and Immunofluorescence

37. A clinician calls you about a patient with a bullous disease. What advice should you give about the site of the biopsy and the transport medium to use?
- Specify lesional skin for routine sections and perilesional skin for direct immunofluorescence (IF).
- Specify formalin fixation for the "routine sample" and normal saline or Michel's transport medium for the "immunofluorescence sample."
- Specify normal saline if transport time to the lab < 24 hrs.
- Specify Michel's transport medium if transport time to the lab > 24 hrs.
- Beware not to contaminate an immunofluorescence sample with formalin — even small amounts can lead to test failure (false negative IF).
- If the disease is focal, a shave biopsy (to include the whole blister) may be preferable to a punch biopsy for routine histopathology.

38. Which conditions require lesional (not perilesional) tissue for direct immunofluorescence (DIF)?

- Lupus.
- Vasculitis (new lesion < 24 hrs old).
- Lichen planus.

39. How are vesiculobullous diseases classified?

- Based on 3 features:
  - Location of the split (e.g., subepidermal, intraepidermal).
  - Mechanism of the split (e.g., intraepidermal spongiosis, acantholysis, ballooning).
- Presence or absence of dermal inflammatory infiltrate and composition (see "Algorithmic guide to diagnosis of inflammatory diseases of the skin" later in this chapter).

40. List 4 disorders characterized by intraepidermal acantholysis with relevant clinical and histopathological findings.

DISEASE	CLINICAL FEATURES	HISTOPATHOLOGICAL FEATURES	IMMUNOFLUORESCENCE FINDINGS	OTHER
Pemphigus vulgaris	• Middle-aged adults, cutaneous and oral involvement. • Fragile blisters that can be induced by rubbing normal skin (Nikolsky sign).	• Suprabasal acantholysis with retained lining ("tomb stoning") of basal keratinocytes. • Broad zone of acantholysis with involvement of follicular epithelium. • Mild mixed infiltrate.	• DIF: net-like or intercellular IgG +/– C3.	• Target antigen: desmoglein 3 (most common) and desmoglein 1.
Hailey-Hailey disease (benign familial pemphigus)	• Autosomal dominant genodermatosis, second to fourth decade of life. • Vesicles, erosions, and crusted lesions of mostly flexural skin.	• Acantholysis in a "dilapidated brick wall" pattern. • Minimal dyskeratosis. • Adnexal epithelium spared.	• Negative.	• Mutation of *ATP2C1* (3q21-q24).
Darier disease (keratosis follicularis)	• Autosomal dominant genodermatosis, first or second decade of life. • Pruritic, greasy, crusted papules and plaques on seborrheic areas of body — chest, scalp, back.	• Acantholysis with prominent dyskeratosis — formation of "corps ronds" and "grains."	• Negative.	• Mutation of *ATP2A2* (12q23-q24).
Grover disease (transient acantholytic dermatosis)	• Acquired disease of unknown etiology, middle-aged and elderly adults, males > females. • Small, pruritic polymorphic vesicles and papules, mostly affecting trunk.	• Focal acantholysis and variable dyskeratosis with different patterns: pemphigus-like, Hailey-Hailey-like, Darier-like, and spongiotic.	• Negative.	• Histopathologic clues to diagnosis: focal nature of changes and mixed patterns that mimic other acantholytic disorders.

41. List 6 disorders characterized by subepidermal blisters with relevant clinical and histopathological findings.

DISEASE	CLINICAL FEATURES	HISTOPATHOLOGICAL FEATURES	IMMUNOFLUORESCENCE FINDINGS	OTHER
Epidermolysis bullosa acquisita (EBA)	• Acquired form within group of predominantly inherited blistering disorders. • Adult onset with blisters, milia, and scarring.	• Usually cell poor blister.	• DIF: linear IgG and C3 along the basement membrane zone (BMZ). • Salt split skin: immune deposits localize to dermal side (floor) of blister.	• Target antigen is type VII collagen.
Porphyria cutanea tarda (PCT)	• Most common type of porphyria (disorder of porphyrin metabolism). • Blisters, milia, scarring, hypertrichosis. • Associated with liver disease (e.g., hepatitis C).	• Cell poor blister with projection of dermal papillae ("festooning") into blister cavity. • Eosinophilic, PAS+ basement membrane material ("caterpillar bodies") in blister roof. • Thick walled papillary dermal vessels containing hyalinized PAS+ material.	• DIF: IgG and C3 along the BMZ and within thickened papillary dermal vessels +/− IgM, fibrinogen.	• Pseudoporphyria related to renal disease and certain drugs is identical to PCT on light microscopy and direct immunofluorescence. • Clinical context aids in distinction.
Bullous pemphigoid (BP)	• Most common autoimmune blistering disorder. • Older adults, oral involvement uncommon. • Early lesions: +/− pruritic and/or urticarial; later lesions: tense bullae.	• Usually eosinophil-rich blister and dermal infiltrate; sometimes mixed with neutrophils; sometimes cell poor. • Eosinophilic spongiosis possible in early or urticarial phase.	• DIF: linear IgG and C3 along BMZ. • Salt split skin: deposits localize to epidermal side (roof) of blister.	• Target antigen is BPAg1 and BPAg2.
Pemphigoid (herpes) gestationis	• Pregnancy associated autoimmune disorder unrelated to herpes virus. • Development of pruritic vesicles, papules, and plaques — often periumbilical — in second or third trimester.	• Histopathologically indistinguishable from BP (see above). • Clinical context aids in distinction.	• DIF: linear C3 (most often) and IgG along BMZ.	• Target antigen is mainly BPAg2 but also BPAg1.
Dermatitis herpetiformis (DH)	• Chronic blistering disorder associated with gluten sensitive enteropathy. • Grouped pruritic papulovesicles, classically on the elbows, knees, and buttocks.	• Neutrophil-rich blisters and microabscesses at the tips of dermal papillae.	• DIF: granular IgA along the BMZ, with accentuation at the tips of dermal papillae.	• It is associated with HLA B8, HLA DR3, HLA DQW2, HLA DQ8.
Linear IgA dermatosis	• Heterogeneous disorder affecting children and adults. • Tense blisters in annular or "string of pearls" arrangement.	• Similar to DH (see above).	• DIF: linear IgA along the BMZ.	• It is associated with inflammatory bowel disease, lymphoproliferative disorders, and drugs (classically vancomycin).

Abbreviations: DIF: direct immunofluorescence.

Vasculitis

42. What are the histopathological features of leukocytoclastic vasculitis?
- Fibrinoid necrosis of small vessel walls with extravasated red blood cells.
- Angiocentric neutrophilic infiltrate with nuclear dust (karyorrhexis, leukocytoclasis).
- Direct immunofluorescence findings: dermal vessel staining with IgG, C3, (IgA in Henoch-Schönlein purpura), fibrinogen +/− IgM.
- Secondary changes: necrosis/ulceration of epidermis or subepidermal blister formation.

43. What are possible causes of leukocytoclastic vasculitis?
- Infection (bacterial, rickettsial, fungal, viral).
- Autoimmunity (immune complex diseases; antineutrophil cytoplasmic antibody–associated diseases, etc.).
- Drugs.
- Malignancies.
- Idiopathic (40%).

44. What are the clinical findings and histopathology of Sweet syndrome?
- Clinical findings:
  - Patients have sudden eruptions of painful plaques and papules on the face and extremities, often following an infection.
  - Fever and leukocytosis may be present.
- It is of unknown etiology, but is associated with malignancies (especially acute myeloid leukemia), autoimmune diseases, infection, and drugs.
- Histopathology:
  - Dense diffuse dermal neutrophilic infiltrate.
  - Subepidermal edema.
  - Usually no true vasculitis.

Psoriasiform Reaction Pattern

45. What are the histopathological features of plaque-type psoriasis?
- Regular acanthosis of the epidermis with elongated, club-shaped rete ridges and thinned suprapapillary plates.
- Prominent dilated capillaries in the papillary dermis.
- Confluent dry (without serum) parakeratosis overlying a diminished granular layer.
- Kogoj microabscesses: collections of neutrophils in the spinous layer.
- Munro microabscesses: mounds of parakeratosis with neutrophils.

46. Give a differential diagnosis for a biopsy showing psoriasiform epidermal hyperplasia.
- Psoriasis.
- Chronic eczematous (spongiotic) dermatitis.
- Pityriasis rubra pilaris.
- Lichen simplex chronicus.
- Mycosis fungoides.
- Infection (e.g., secondary syphilis).

Granulomatous Reactions in the Skin

47. List the patterns of granulomatous inflammation with relevant disease associations.

PATTERN	HISTOPATHOLOGY	EXAMPLES
Tuberculoid	• Nodules of epithelioid histiocytes with central necrosis and peripheral rim of lymphocytes.	• Tuberculosis, leprosy, rosacea.
Sarcoidal	• "Naked granulomata" (lack rim of lymphocytes and no necrosis).	• Sarcoidosis, berylliosis, zirconium granulomas, Crohn disease.
Foreign body	• Abundant irregularly distributed foreign-body giant cells.	• Suture granuloma, keratin, tattoo.
Xanthomatous	• Many foamy histiocytes.	• Xanthogranuloma, infections (leprosy, syphilis).
Suppurative and granulomatous	• Aggregations of neutrophils with interspersed histiocytes.	• Ruptured follicular cyst/unit, deep fungal infection, atypical mycobacterial infection.
Palisading	• Geographic pattern with histiocytic rims.	• Granuloma annulare, rheumatoid nodule, necrobiosis lipoidica.

48. Compare the clinical and histopathological features of granuloma annulare, rheumatoid nodule, and necrobiosis lipoidica.

DISEASE	CLINICAL FEATURES	HISTOPATHOLOGICAL FEATURES	OTHER
Granuloma annulare (GA)	• Common, asymptomatic dermatosis of unknown etiology. • Usually in young adults at acral sites, but other sites also possible. • Annular arrangement of skin colored papules.	• Usually focal involvement of the upper and mid reticular dermis. • Palisading histiocytes. • Increased dermal mucin (highlighted by Alcian blue or colloidal iron stains).	• Variants include the interstitial, generalized, deep/subcutaneous, and perforating forms of GA.
Rheumatoid nodule (RN)	• Associated with rheumatoid arthritis. • Over boney prominences of forearms, elbows, hands, feet, and knees.	• Usually located deep in the dermis and/or subcutis. • Palisading and sometimes serpiginous granulomas surrounding fibrinoid change. • Lack of significant dermal mucin (compared to GA).	• Subcutaneous GA (pseudorheumatoid nodule) can mimic RN histopathologically.
Necrobiosis lipoidica (NL)	• Associated with diabetes in a minority of cases. • Atrophic yellow plaques, typically on the shins.	• Usually diffuse dermal involvement and extending into the superficial subcutis. • Palisaded, interstitial or tiered inflammatory infiltrate with intervening sclerotic collagen ("layer cake" appearance). • Mixed infiltrate composed of histiocytes, lymphocytes, and plasma cells. • Lack of significant dermal mucin.	• NL sometimes cannot be distinguished from GA histopathologically.

49. A clinician suspects gout. What procedures do you suggest for the biopsy specimen?
Fixing the specimen in alcohol rather than formalin to preserve the crystals.

Panniculitis

50. List the histopathologic features of erythema nodosum.
- Predominantly septal panniculitis with some overflow into fat lobules.
  · Early phase: predominance of neutrophils.
  · Late phase: predominance of lymphocytes, eosinophils, and multinucleated giant cells with Miescher granulomas.
  · Chronic recurrent erythema nodosum: prominent septal fibrosis together with inflammatory cells.

51. List 5 conditions associated with erythema nodosum.
- Drug reaction (e.g., oral contraceptives).
- Infection.
- Sarcoidosis.
- Inflammatory bowel disease.
- Malignancy (e.g., hematolymphoid).

52. List 5 key causes of lobular panniculitis.
- Infection.
- Nodular vasculitis.
- Lupus profundus.
- Deficiency of α_1-antitrypsin.
- Pancreatic panniculitis.

Other Nonneoplastic Dermatopathological Conditions

53. What are the classic clinical and histopathological findings of fixed drug eruptions?
- Clinical:
  · Ovoid or annular erythematous lesions develop in response to exposure to a drug that resolve with hyperpigmentation and recur in the same location upon reexposure to the same drug.
  · Common sites include the lips, face, hands, and genitalia.
- Histopathology:
  · The typical appearance is that of a vacuolar interface dermatitis with necrotic/apoptotic keratinocytes, accompanied by a superficial and deep perivascular infiltrate containing lymphocytes and eosinophils.
  · Acute phase resembles erythema multiforme.
  · Pigment incontinence alone is observed in quiescent pigmented phase.

54. Describe pityriasis rosea.
- Self-limited papulosquamous eruption occurring most often in children and young adults.
- Characteristic progression: begins with a salmon colored, scaly "herald patch" on the trunk, and develops into multiple smaller scaly papules on the trunk and extremities in a "Christmas tree" pattern.
- Clinically similar to secondary syphilis.
- Histopathology: subacute spongiotic dermatitis (superficial perivascular lymphocytic infiltrate with mild spongiosis and acanthosis with overlying mounds of parakeratotic scale).

55. What is a cornoid lamella? In which dermatosis is it found?
- Cornoid lamella is an angulated pillar of parakeratosis arising from an epidermal invagination with loss of the granular layer and localized dyskeratosis.
- It is a characteristic feature of porokeratosis of which there are many clinical variants.
- In porokeratosis of Mibelli, it corresponds with the peripheral annular scale seen clinically.

56. What are the clinical and histopathological features of morphea?
- Clinical:
  - There are 3 main clinical forms: localized or plaque-like (most common), linear, and generalized.
  - Indurated plaques are present on the trunk and extremities, often with shiny white centers surrounded by a violaceous border.
- Histopathologic:
  - Early phase: features include superficial and deep perivascular and interstitial lymphoplasmacytic infiltrate; dermal fibrosis may be absent.
  - Late phase: features include thickened dermal collagen resulting in a biopsy specimen with "square edges," atrophy of adnexal structures with loss of periadnexal fat, diminished inflammation (ultimately the thickened dermal collagen may become atrophic).
- Changes may impinge on or extend into subcutis along septa (morphea profundus/deep morphea).
- There may be associated changes of lichen sclerosus.

57. Which conditions may result in a "normal appearing skin biopsy"?
- Dermatophytosis.
- A subtle pigmentary disorder (e.g., solar lentigo or vitiligo).
- Cutaneous amyloidosis.
- Urticaria.
- Ichthyosis.

58. What are the clinical and histopathological features of lichen sclerosus?
- Clinical: pruritic white plaques with a wrinkled appearance (epidermal atrophy) most commonly in the anogenital area of females.
- Histopathology: epidermal atrophy and hyperkeratosis with homogenized superficial dermal collagen and vacuolar degeneration of basal keratinocytes, with an associated perivascular lymphocytic infiltrate.

59. Name 4 common cysts in the skin and their characteristic histopathological features.

TYPE	HISTOPATHOLOGY
Follicular infundibular cyst (epidermoid or epidermal inclusion cyst)	• Lining is composed of stratified squamous epithelium with preserved granular layer. • Cyst contents consist of laminated keratin.
Trichilemmal cyst (pilar cyst)	• Lining is composed of stratified squamous epithelium displaying trichilemmal keratinization with no granular layer. • Cyst contents consist of dense, homogeneous keratin +/− calcification.
Steatocystoma (simplex or multiplex)	• Lining is composed of stratified squamous epithelium with corrugated eosinophilic lining (cuticle) with no granular layer. • Sebaceous lobules are within or near the cyst wall. • Cyst appears empty due to loss of sebaceous fluid during processing.
Hidrocystoma	• Lining is composed of simple cuboidal or columnar epithelium +/− decapitation secretion. • Cyst appears empty.

60. Name skin conditions to which AIDS patients are predisposed.
- Psoriasis.
- Seborrheic dermatitis.
- Eosinophilic folliculitis.
- Infections (herpes simplex, molluscum contagiosum, bacillary angiomatosis, mycobacteria, and others).
- Kaposi sarcoma.

61. What are the histopathological features of stasis dermatitis?
- Superficial and deep dermis shows neovascularization with a lobular proliferation of small vessels and a mild lymphocytic perivascular infiltrate.
- Adjacent dermis may contain extravasated erythrocytes and hemosiderin.
- Overlying epidermis may be acanthotic and shows spongiosis and hyperkeratosis.

62. List syndromes with cutaneous manifestations.
- Muir-Torre syndrome.
  · Autosomal dominant mutations in DNA mismatch repair genes (e.g., *MLH1*, *MSH2*) causing microsatellite instability.
  · Colon polyps, gastrointestinal carcinoma, endometrial carcinoma.
  · Sebaceous neoplasms, keratoacanthomas, and epidermal cysts.
- Birt-Hogg-Dubé syndrome.
  · Autosomal dominant mutation of folliculin gene (17p11.2).
  · Renal tumors of various types, pulmonary cysts, spontaneous pneumothorax.
  · Fibrofolliculomas, trichodiscomas, acrochordons.
- Cowden syndrome.
  · Autosomal dominant mutation of *PTEN* (10q23.3).
  · Hamartomatous lesions of multiple systems.
  · Benign and malignant lesions of thyroid and breast.
  · Trichilemmomas, palmar pits.
- Tuberous sclerosis.
  · Autosomal dominant mutations of *TSC1* (hamartin, 9q34) or *TSC2* (tuberin, 16p13).
  · Cortical tubers, renal angiomyolipomas, cardiac rhabdomyoma, pulmonary lymphangioleiomyomatosis.
  · Angiofibromas, shagreen patch, "ash leaf" macules, periungual fibromas.

63. What are some histopathological findings of dermatophyte infections?
- Biopsy specimens may look relatively normal.
- Findings include neutrophils in the cornified layer and "sandwich sign," in which organisms are "sandwiched" between normal and altered (parakeratotic or compact hyperkeratotic) stratum corneum.
- Epidermis may be psoriasiform.
- Some dermatophyte infections can be vesicular with prominent spongiosis.
- PAS stain highlights fungal forms (use PAS diastase stain to avoid PAS+ debris).

64. Name 3 common viral infections of the skin and list their histopathological findings.
- Herpes simplex and varicella-zoster virus.
  · Intraepidermal vesicle (acantholysis, ballooning degeneration, and apoptotic keratinocytes).
  · Ground-glass nuclei of keratinocytes with chromatin margination and eosinophilic nuclear inclusions (Cowdry type A), often multinucleate epithelial cells with "molded" nuclei.
  · Perivascular lymphohistiocytic inflammation (sometimes dense) +/− neutrophils.
- Human papilloma virus.
  · Acanthosis, papillomatosis, hyperkeratosis with parakeratosis overlying papillae.
  · Dilated blood vessels in dermal papillae.
  · Large, coarse keratohyalin granules in superficial keratinocytes — characteristic of some viruses, but not all.
- Molluscum contagiosum (pox virus).
  · Lobulated and often crateriform lesion.
  · Epidermal hyperplasia with eosinophilic "molluscum bodies" (Henderson-Patterson) in keratinocyte cytoplasm.

65. List the key variants of cutaneous viral warts and the most commonly associated type(s) of human papillomavirus (HPV).

VARIANT	HPV TYPE
Common wart (verruca vulgaris)	1, 2, 4.
Plantar wart (myrmecial wart)	1.
Flat/plane wart (verruca plana)	3, 5, 10.
Genital wart (condyloma acuminatum)	6, 11, 18.
Epidermodysplasia verruciformis	2, 3, 5, 8.

66. List some dermatologic conditions associated with significant morbidity and/or mortality, which thus require urgent recognition.
- Pancreatic panniculitis.
- Stevens-Johnson syndrome / toxic epidermal necrolysis.
- Staphylococcal scalded skin syndrome.
- Acute graft versus host disease.
- Calciphylaxis.
- Angioinvasive fungal infection.
- Pemphigus (including paraneoplastic pemphigus).
- Vasculitis.
- Hematological malignancies (leukemia cutis, blastic plasmacytoid dendritic cell neoplasm, etc.).

67. Define erythroderma and list possible causes.

- Clinically, erythroderma refers to generalized redness and scaling of the skin involving > 90% of the skin surface.

- Causes: psoriasis (common), atopic dermatitis (common), drug reaction (common), cutaneous T-cell lymphoma (mycosis fungoides, Sézary syndrome), pityriasis rubra pilaris, and others.

68. List conditions affecting the skin in which there are electron microscopic findings of diagnostic value.

- Amyloidosis: randomly arranged, nonbranching 6–10 nm diameter filaments.
- Langerhans cell histiocytosis: Langerhans cells with Birbeck granules.
- Fabry disease: lamellar inclusion bodies within endothelial cells, smooth muscle cells, fibroblasts, and macrophages; due to lipid deposition in lysosomes.

- Various forms of epidermolysis bullosa: different levels of split at the basement membrane zone.
- Merkel cell carcinoma: dense core granules within cytoplasm of tumor cells.
- Melanoma: melanosomes.
- Cerebral autosomal dominant arteriopathy with subcortical infarcts and leucoencephalopathy (CADASIL): electron dense, granular material in vascular smooth muscle cells.

Melanoma

69. What clinical findings are suggestive of melanoma?

- ABCDE mnemonic:
  - **A**symmetry.
  - **B**orders: irregular.
  - **C**olor variegation.
  - **D**iameter > 6 mm.
  - **E**volution: change in lesion.

70. By which procedure is a melanocytic lesion best evaluated? What are the limitations of alternate biopsy procedures?

- Complete excision that incorporates the full thickness of the lesion is best.
- Shaves may not include an intact base and may interfere with assessment of Breslow thickness.

- Punch biopsies impair assessment of important architectural features, such as lesion size, symmetry and circumscription.

71. Review the American Joint Committee on Cancer (AJCC) staging system for melanoma (8th edition) and list the microscopic features in the evaluation of primary melanoma that affect this staging system.

- Breslow thickness.
- Presence or absence of ulceration.

- Presence or absence of microsatellites.

72. How is depth of melanoma invasion measured?

- Measure from the top of the granular layer to the deepest broad base of the tumor (avoiding vertically oriented deep periadnexal extensions).

- If the epidermis is ulcerated, measure from the base of the ulcer to the base of the tumor.

73. List the Clark levels of melanoma invasion.

- Clark levels:
  - Level I: intraepidermal (in situ) tumor only.
  - Level II: invades papillary dermis to minimal degree.
  - Level III: expands and fills papillary dermis.
  - Level IV: invades reticular dermis.

  - Level V: invades subcutis.
- Significance: although important in previous staging schemes, Clark levels are not used in the current AJCC staging system. Rather, the Clark level is recorded as a characteristic of primary melanoma.

74. Why is ulceration important in melanoma staging?

- It is an established prognostic factor in tumors without metastasis.
- If ulceration is present, the T stage is upgraded from "a" to "b" for pT1 to pT4 tumors (e.g., pT3a upgrades to pT3b).

- It is associated with significantly worse prognosis and higher risk of metastasis.

75. How is ulceration defined?

- A combination of the following features:
  - Full-thickness epidermal defect (including absence of stratum corneum and basement membrane) not due to trauma or previous procedure.

  - Evidence of reactive changes (fibrin deposition, neutrophils).

76. Describe cutaneous microsatellite, satellite, and in-transit metastases in the context of clinical pathological staging of melanoma.

- Microsatellite metastases are microscopically determined; they are microscopic cutaneous and/or subcutaneous tumor deposits adjacent or deep to the primary melanoma as separated by normal tissue (i.e., absence of fibrosis or inflammation, which may suggest regression of intervening tumor).
- Satellite metastases are clinically determined: they are **clinically evident** cutaneous and/or subcutaneous tumor deposits within 2 cm of, but discontinuous from, the primary melanoma.
- In-transit metastases are clinically determined: they are **clinically evident** cutaneous and/or subcutaneous tumor deposits located > 2 cm from the primary melanoma in the region between the primary tumor and the nearest regional lymph nodes.
- The presence or absence of microsatellite, satellite, and in-transit metastases, irrespective of number or type of such lesions, impacts N-categorization.
- Microsatellite, satellite, and in-transit metastases are grouped together for staging purposes due to lack of substantial differences in survival outcome between the defined entities.

77. What are the basic management strategies for melanoma?

- Local excision.
- Sentinel lymph node biopsy +/− regional lymphadenectomy.
- Adjuvant therapies (e.g., interferon, *BRAF* inhibitors).

78. How is a sentinel lymph node defined? What is its significance?

- A sentinel lymph node is defined as the first node to receive lymphatic drainage from a primary tumor.
- There may be more than 1 sentinel node for some tumors (e.g., a lesion on the central back draining to both axillae).
- Metastatic involvement of a sentinel node increases the likelihood that other, more distant nodes may contain metastatic disease.
- Conversely, if sentinel nodes are negative, other regional nodes would be unlikely to contain metastasis.

79. How should sentinel lymph nodes be assessed for metastasis?

- They should **not** be assessed by frozen sections.
- Different protocols exist in different institutions.
- In general, small nodes are bisected and larger nodes are sectioned at 2–3 mm intervals.
- Serial sections should be cut to include H&E and immunostained sections (e.g., S100 protein, Melan-A/Mart1, SOX10, HMB45).
- The finding of a single melanoma cell in a node marks it as positive.
- Beware of misdiagnosing a capsular nevus as metastatic melanoma.
- Beware of misdiagnosing collections of pigmented macrophages as metastatic melanoma.

80. How can capsular nevi be distinguished from metastatic melanoma in lymph nodes?

	CAPSULAR NEVUS	METASTATIC MELANOMA
Location	• Benign nevus cells characteristically in nodal fibrous tissue such as capsule and trabeculae.	• Malignant melanocytes in the subcapsular sinus and nodal parenchyma.
Histopathology	• Small, uniform cells lacking significant cytologic atypia. • Absence of mitoses.	• Large atypical cells similar to the primary melanoma. • Prominent nucleoli. • Mitoses (possible).
Other	• S100+, SOX10+, MART1/Melan-A+. • Weak or negative staining for HMB45 and Ki 67.	• S100+, SOX10+, MART1/Melan-A+. • Frequent positive staining for HMB45 and Ki 67.

81. What are important features to remember in desmoplastic melanoma?

- It often occurs on the head and neck of older patients as a flesh colored nodule.
- It is frequently nonpigmented and may be mistaken for a scar histopathologically.
- It is sometimes associated with a subtle junctional proliferation of melanocytes.
- Presence of lymphoid aggregates at the periphery of the tumor is a clue to the diagnosis.
- It frequently shows perineural involvement and deep extension.
- It may be associated with elements of "conventional" melanoma.
- It stains with S100 and SOX10, but is typically negative for other melanocytic markers (Melan-A/MART1, HMB45).

82. List locations of primary melanoma other than the skin.
- Mucosa (oral, genital, and gastrointestinal tract).
- Eye.
- Meninges.

83. Name the gene mutation most frequently associated with melanoma.
- The most common is *CDKN2A*, which encodes p16 (chromosome 9p21) most often.
- *BRAF, NRAS, HRAS,* and *CKIT* mutations are also found in some melanomas.
- *GNAQ* and *GNA11* mutations are found in uveal melanoma.

Other Melanocytic Lesions

84. What is the utility of immunohistochemistry in the evaluation of melanocytic lesions?
- Lineage markers.
- Markers to highlight epidermal pattern of malignant proliferation.
- Markers to check for subtle dermal involvement by thin melanomas.
- Markers of proliferation rate.
- Markers to detect *BRAF* mutations in melanoma.

85. List the typical histopathological features of a Clark nevus or so-called "dysplastic nevus."
- Lentiginous proliferation of melanocytes singly and in nests involving the tips and sides of rete ridges with bridging of adjacent rete ridges.
- "Shoulder" phenomenon of extension of epidermal component beyond the dermal component.
- Papillary dermal fibrosis.
- Variable cytological features.
- Perivascular lymphohistiocytic infiltrate.

86. List variants of melanoma that may be mistaken for nevi or other benign lesions.
- Nevoid melanoma.
- Spitzoid melanoma.
- Desmoplastic melanoma.
- Blue nevus–like metastatic melanoma.

87. List benign melanocytic lesions that may be mistaken for melanoma.
- Spitz nevus.
- Combined nevi.
- Halo nevi.
- Recurrent or persistent nevi after biopsy or partial excision.
- Irritated or traumatized nevi.
- Nevi in pregnancy with increased mitotic rate.
- Nevi of special sites (acral, ear, genital, breast/milk line, flexural).

88. List the histopathological features of a "classical" Spitz nevus.
- Clinical context: usually young patients with a pink, dome-shaped papule on the head and neck.
- Microscopically small, symmetrical, and circumscribed proliferation of spindled or epithelioid melanocytes arranged in nests surrounded by clefts at the dermoepidermal junction, +/– a dermal component.
- Junctional, compound, or completely dermal.
- Spindled cells often vertically oriented as "hanging bananas" at the tips of acanthotic rete ridges.
- Intraepidermal Kamino bodies (collections of eosinophilic basement membrane material).
- Minimal pagetoid extension, maturation with extension into dermis, no mitoses at base.
- Epidermis often acanthotic with hypergranulosis and hyperkeratosis.

89. List molecular findings associated with Spitz nevi.
- *HRAS* aberrations.
- *BAP1* loss.
- Deletions in *6p23*
- Fusion or translocations involving tyrosine kinases (*ROS1, ALK, NTRK1* are less often than *BRAF, RET, MET, NTRK3*).

90. Describe typical features of spitzoid nevi with *BAP1* loss.
- These are typically dermal.
- They lack epidermal hyperplasia and Kamino bodies.
- They typically arise from common nevi showing a biphasic pattern with a component of small melanocytes adjacent to the spitzoid component (has large epithelioid melanocytes with abundant pale cytoplasm, in which multinucleated cells are common).
- Both types of melanocytes harbor *BRAF* mutations.
- Only the spitzoid component shows *BAP1* loss.

91. Which malignant tumors are associated with germline *BAP1* mutations?
- Uveal melanoma.
- Cutaneous melanoma.
- Mesothelioma.
- Renal cell carcinoma.

92. List the histopathological features of blue nevus.
- Common blue nevus:
  - Clinical context: blue papule or nodule often on the dorsal hand, foot, or face.
  - Small, wedge-shaped dermal aggregation of spindled and dendritic melanocytes in a fascicular pattern with admixed melanophages and, often, dermal fibrosis.
  - No junctional component.
  - HMB45-positive.
- Cellular blue nevus:
  - Clinical context: usually a larger lesion than common blue nevus, and usually on the scalp, buttock, or sacral region.
  - Dermal or subcutaneous fascicles of monomorphous spindled cells without prominent pigmentation.
  - Mitotic rate: low or zero.
  - HMB45-positive.

93. What histopathological features suggest a "congenital nevus"?
- Deep extension of melanocytes into dermis +/− subcutaneous fat.
- Extension of melanocytes along blood vessels and adnexal structures.
- Splaying of nevus cells between collagen bundles of the reticular dermis.

Squamous Cell Carcinoma

94. List clinical features of squamous cell carcinoma that are associated with an aggressive course.
- Tumors in immunosuppressed patients.
- Tumors of the lip, ear, vulva, perineum, and penis.
- Tumors arising in chronic ulcers, scars, and sinuses.

95. Which histopathological variants of squamous cell carcinoma are associated with an aggressive course?
- Acantholytic squamous cell carcinoma.
- Pseudovascular squamous cell carcinoma.
- Adenosquamous carcinoma.

96. List some benign lesions or conditions that can simulate squamous cell carcinoma on histopathology.
- Pseudoepitheliomatous hyperplasia associated with scar, ulcer, infection or granular cell tumor.
- Prurigo nodularis.
- Hypertrophic cutaneous lupus erythematosus.
- Hypertrophic lichen planus.
- Inverted follicular keratosis.
- Desmoplastic trichilemmoma.
- Modified verruca vulgaris.
- Proliferating pilar tumor.

Keratoacanthoma

97. What are the histopathological features of keratoacanthoma?
- It is an exophytic and endophytic crateriform epidermal lesion with papillomatosis and abundant keratin in the crater.
- It has glassy eosinophilic keratinocytes toward the center of nests and entrapment of elastic fibers in the periphery.
- It exhibits inflammation, usually including some eosinophils and neutrophilic microabscesses.
- It can simulate well-differentiated squamous cell carcinoma.

98. What is the "classic" clinical history of keratoacanthoma?
- A rapidly growing nodule on sun-exposed skin of elderly individuals, often with a cutaneous horn.
- Lesion that usually involutes over several months.

Merkel Cell Carcinoma

99. What factors are of oncogenetic importance in Merkel cell carcinoma?
- Risk factors include advanced age, chronic sun exposure, fair skin, and immunosuppression.
- Merkel cell polyomavirus-mediated oncogenesis occurs in approximately 80% of cases.
- Ultraviolet-mediated oncogenesis occurs in a minority of cases.

100. Which immunohistochemical stains can be used in the diagnosis of Merkel cell carcinoma?

- Synaptophysin, chromogranin positive.
- Paranuclear dot-like positivity with CK20 and CAM5.2.
- Dot-like positivity with neurofilament.

- Nuclear positivity with Merkel cell polyomavirus immunohistochemistry (CM2B4).
- Relevant negative markers: TTF-1, S100 protein, SOX10, HMB45, Melan-A, leukocyte common antigen (LCA), and other lymphocyte markers.

Basal Cell Carcinoma

101. What is nevoid basal cell carcinoma syndrome?

- It is an autosomal dominant condition, also known as Gorlin syndrome, caused by a mutation in *PTCH* on chromosome 9q22.
- Cutaneous findings include multiple basal cell carcinomas and palmar/plantar pits.

- Patients also develop odontogenic keratocysts, rib anomalies, and intracranial calcifications, and often have characteristic facies.

102. List key basaloid epithelial tumors that can simulate nodular basal cell carcinoma histopathologically.

- Basaloid squamous cell carcinoma.
- Merkel cell carcinoma.
- Trichoepithelioma.

- Trichoblastoma.
- Adenoid cystic carcinoma.
- Sebaceous carcinoma.

103. Which pathological features can help differentiate trichoepithelioma from basal cell carcinoma?

FEATURES	TRICHOEPITHELIOMA	BASAL CELL CARCINOMA
Perilesional clefts	Between stroma and normal dermis.	Between tumor and mucinous stroma.
Papillary mesenchymal bodies	Present.	Absent.
Keratin cysts and calcifications	Common.	Less common.
Mucinous stroma	Absent.	Common.
CK20+ Merkel cells	Present.	Uncommon.
BCL2	Peripheral positivity in lesion.	Diffuse positivity in tumor.
CK15	Positive.	Negative.

Kaposi Sarcoma (KS)

104. What are the 4 clinical settings of KS?

- Classic — occurs in elderly men of Mediterranean origin.
- African (endemic) — includes variants such as the lymphadenopathic subtype, which occurs predominantly in children with diffuse aggressive disease.

- AIDS associated (epidemic) — presents with multiple skin lesions and visceral involvement.
- Immunosuppressed/iatrogenic — may resolve with withdrawal of immunosuppression.

105. List the stages of KS and their histopathological findings.

- Patch:
  · Subtle proliferation of irregular thin walled vascular channels usually arising around preexisting blood vessels ("promontory sign") and adnexal structures in the dermis.
  · Hemosiderin, extravasated erythrocytes, and a lymphoplasmacytic infiltrate in a perivascular distribution.
- Plaque:

  · Diffuse infiltrate of small, sometimes slit-like vascular channels with spindle cells that may contain PAS positive eosinophilic globules (degenerated products of red blood cells).
- Nodule:
  · Diffuse confluent spindle cell proliferation with subtle vascular differentiation and erythrocyte extravasation.

106. What immunohistochemical stains may assist in KS diagnosis?

- Markers of blood vessel and lymphatic endothelium are positive: CD31, CD34, D2-40.

- Nuclear HHV-8 is regarded as diagnostic.

Mycosis Fungoides (MF)

107. What are the stages of mycosis fungoides?
- Patch.
- Plaque.
- Tumor.

108. What is the clinical evolution of mycosis fungoides?
- Chronic scaly patches develop mainly on doubly clothed areas of the body (e.g., buttocks, thighs, breast), usually in adults.
- Disease is slowly progressive, evolving to plaques/tumors (patients usually die of other causes).
- Mycosis fungoides may evolve to erythroderma.
- Lymph node and other organ involvement can occur.

109. What are some important points to be aware of when considering mycosis fungoides as a diagnosis?
- Careful clinicopathologic correlation is the single most important step.
- Histopathological features differ depending on the stage of the disease.
- The immunohistochemical findings in MF are usually of limited utility:
  - Findings usually include a predominance of CD4+ > CD8+ T-lymphocytes.
- Late stage lesions may show partial loss of pan T-lymphocyte markers (CD2, CD3, CD5).
- Molecular studies have also demonstrated limited utility:
  - Early lesions may contain too few neoplastic cells for analysis.
  - Clonal populations of T- lymphocyte have been identified in inflammatory conditions that enter the differential diagnosis for MF, including lichen planus, lichen sclerosus, and others.
  - Detection of the same clone in lesions from different sites over time is supportive of MF.

110. List the histopathological features of patch stage MF.
- Sparse lymphocytic infiltrate is present in the superficial dermis and extends into basal epidermis, often as a single file of cells (cells may have halos).
- There are increased lymphocytes within the epidermis in the absence of significant spongiosis.
- Pautrier microabscesses — clusters of atypical lymphocytes in the epidermis — are uncommon, but useful when present.
- Atypia is uncommon, but cells with angular and slightly enlarged hyperchromatic nuclei may be observed in the epidermis (less evident in the dermis).
- Papillary dermal collagen has a coarse chicken-wire pattern.

Spindle Cell Lesions in the Skin

111. List benign spindle cell lesions of the skin categorized by lineage with examples.
- Melanocytic cells (spindle cell nevus, blue nevus).
- Fibrohistiocytic cells (dermatofibroma).
- Myofibroblastic cells (cellular scar).
- Nerve sheath cells and axons (schwannoma, neurofibroma, neuromas).
- Endothelial cells (spindle cell hemangioma).
- Smooth muscle cells (leiomyoma).
- Perivascular cells (myofibroma).
- Mast cells (mastocytosis may sometimes display spindled cells).

112. List malignant spindle cell lesions of the skin.
- Melanoma.
- Squamous cell carcinoma.
- Atypical fibroxanthoma/pleomorphic dermal sarcoma.
- Leiomyosarcoma.
- Dermatofibrosarcoma protuberans.
- Malignant peripheral nerve sheath tumor.
- Kaposi sarcoma.
- Angiosarcoma.
- Metastasis or extension of deeper soft tissue tumor.

113. What immunohistochemical panels can be useful in the differential diagnosis of malignant spindle cell lesions on sun-damaged skin?
- Cytokeratin 5/6 (CK5/6), p63 and p40 for squamous cell carcinoma.
- S100, SOX10, Mart1/Melan-A, and HMB45 for melanoma.
- Desmin, α-actin, and calponin for leiomyosarcoma.
- ERG, CD31 and CD34 for angiosarcoma.
- CD31, CD34, D2-40 and HHV-8 for Kaposi sarcoma.
- CD34 for dermatofibrosarcoma protuberans (DFSP).
- CD10 and procollagen for atypical fibroxanthoma (AFX) and pleomorphic dermal sarcoma (these are usually a diagnoses of exclusion).
- S100 for malignant peripheral nerve sheath tumor.

114. What features can assist in distinguishing dermatofibroma (DF) and dermatofibrosarcoma protuberans (DFSP)?

- DFSP is usually larger (plaque-like) with deep extension into dermis and subcutis, with a lace-like pattern of adipose tissue infiltration. Cytology is uniform with usually mild cytologic atypia.
- DF is a smaller, poorly circumscribed dermal nodule that demonstrates peripheral "collagen trapping" and is associated with overlying epidermal hyperplasia. A heterogeneous cell population with multinucleated, pigmented, and foamy cells may be seen.
- DFSP is positive for CD34 and negative for factor XIIIA; DF is usually positive for factor XIIIA and rarely positive for CD34.
- DFSP shows t(17;22) *COL1A1-PDGFB* translocation.

115. How do you approach the diagnosis of a small round blue cell tumor in the skin?

- The most common tumors present as small round blue cell tumors in the skin include Merkel cell carcinoma, other undifferentiated primary cutaneous carcinomas (e.g., sebaceous carcinoma), melanoma, and hematolymphoid neoplasms.
- Rare entities such as primitive neuroectodermal tumors (PNETs) also occur.
- Metastases from a noncutaneous site must be excluded.
- Clinical history and immunohistochemistry are usually required to reach a diagnosis.

116. Compare the clinical and histopathological features of cutaneous sebaceous lesions.

	CLINICAL FEATURES	HISTOPATHOLOGICAL FEATURES
Sebaceous hyperplasia	• Benign. • Small, typically 1–3 mm. • Not associated with Muir-Torre syndrome (MTS).	• Prominent mature sebaceous lobules are connected to a common central follicular infundibulum. • Peripheral rim of basaloid germinative cells is 1 to 2 cells thick.
Sebaceous adenoma	• Benign. • Usually a small, solitary nodule of head and neck. • Typically larger than lesions of sebaceous hyperplasia. • Most common sebaceous tumor in MTS. • Concerning for MTS if: multiple lesions, young patient, site other than head and neck region, unusual configurations.	• Lesions are circumscribed and lobulated with connection to overlying epidermis. • Normal architectural relationship of sebaceous lobules to central follicular infundibulum is lost. • Peripheral rim of basaloid germinative cells may be > 2 cells thick. • Mature sebocytes are major cell type (< 50% of tumor cells are basaloid germinative cells). • Morphological heterogeneity can result in overlapping features with sebaceous hyperplasia and sebaceoma.
Sebaceoma	• Benign. • Variable in size (can be large). • Solitary lesion or multiple lesions that may arise in nevus sebaceous. • Usually head and neck skin, female predilection. • Possible association with MTS.	• Well circumscribed, uni- or multinodular, with infrequent connection to overlying epidermis. • Mature sebocytes are minor cell type (> 50% of tumor cells are basaloid germinative cells). • Conspicuous mitoses are possible, but atypical mitoses, and marked nuclear pleomorphism and tumor necrosis are absent. • Lesions may exhibit distinct morphological patterns: rippled, sinusoidal, carcinoid-like. • Morphological heterogeneity can result in overlapping features with sebaceous adenoma and sebaceous carcinoma.
Sebaceous carcinoma	• Malignant. • Variable in size (can be large). • Painless +/− ulceration. • Variants: periocular and extraocular. • Majority of cases: elderly patients; eyelid involvement (arising in meibomian glands); and face involvement. • Risk factors: immunosuppression, UV exposure, radiotherapy. • MTS association (minority of cases). • No MTS association in eyelid lesions. • Significant morbidity and mortality regardless of site (30–40% recurrence rate, 20–25% risk of distant metastasis, 10–30% risk of mortality).	• Lesions are poorly circumscribed with an asymmetrical, multinodular pattern, and +/− infiltrative peripheral margin. • There is a predominance of atypical basaloid cells with large and irregular vesicular nuclei. • Mature sebocytes and occasionally sebaceous ducts may be seen, in varying proportions. • Nuclear atypia can range from mild to severe. • Mitotic activity is variable, but usually frequent and with atypical forms. • Tumor necrosis is common, including comedo type. • Well-differentiated tumors can resemble sebaceous adenoma or sebaceoma. • Poorly differentiated tumors can be difficult (or impossible) to identify as of sebaceous lineage.

117. What is the classic clinical description of a glomus tumor?

- Painful nodule most commonly on the digits, especially subungual.
- Derived from modified smooth muscle cells involved in thermoregulation (Sucquet-Hoyer canal).

118. List painful cutaneous lesions.
- ANGEL mnemonic:
  - **A**ngiolipoma.
  - **N**euroma.
  - **G**lomus tumor.
  - **E**ccrine spiradenoma.
  - **L**eiomyoma.

119. What are settings in which patients may develop cutaneous angiosarcoma?
- Elderly patients: head and neck, no predisposing condition.
- Chronic lymphedema (e.g., Stewart-Treves syndrome).
- Postirradiation.

120. Describe 2 variants of lipoma seen in the skin.
- Angiolipoma: painful nodule, often on the forearms, composed of mature adipose tissue with admixed blood vessels containing fibrin thrombi.
- Spindle cell lipoma: lesion on the neck/shoulder of older men, composed of variable proportions of mature adipose tissue, CD34 positive spindled cells, and myxoid matrix, often with thick intervening "ropey" collagen and admixed mast cells.

121. Discuss mammary and extramammary Paget disease.

	MAMMARY PAGET DISEASE	EXTRAMAMMARY PAGET DISEASE
Location	• Mammary skin, usually nipple.	• Genital and perianal skin.
Histopathology	• Pale staining, single or grouped atypical cells within the epidermis (distinct from keratinocytes) +/− glandular structures.	• Virtually identical to mammary Paget disease.
Stains	• Positive for mucin. • Usually CK7+, *ERBB2*+, and often CEA+. • Negative for melanocytic markers.	• Virtually identical to mammary Paget disease. • Lower frequency of ERBB2-positivity. • Staining profile that may be similar to associated malignancy (e.g., CK20+ if related to underlying colon carcinoma).
Associated conditions	Underlying breast carcinoma.	Visceral malignancies of the GI or GU tract.

Abbreviations and notes: CEA: carcinoembryonic antigen; *ERBB2*: formerly HER2/neu; GI: gastrointestinal; GU: genitourinary.

122. List the histopathological features of epithelioid sarcoma.
- Multinodular proliferation of epithelioid or spindled cells demonstrating variable atypia and mitotic activity. Areas of geographical necrosis may impart a "palisading" appearance resembling a granulomatous process.
- Majority are positive for vimentin, cytokeratin, and epithelial membrane antigen (EMA) +/− CD34.
- Loss of nuclear *INI1* expression is observed in > 90% of cases.

123. Classify primary cutaneous lymphoma according to the World Health Organization (WHO) classification.*

CUTANEOUS T-CELL AND NK-CELL LYMPHOMAS	CUTANEOUS B-CELL LYMPHOMAS
• Mycosis fungoides. • Sézary syndrome. • Adult T-cell leukemia/lymphoma (HTLV-I). • Primary cutaneous CD30+ lymphoproliferative disorders: · Lymphomatoid papulosis. · Primary cutaneous anaplastic large cell lymphoma. • Other less common and provisional entities.	• Extranodal marginal zone lymphoma of mucosa-associated lymphoid tissue (MALT lymphoma). • Primary cutaneous follicle center lymphoma. • Primary cutaneous diffuse large B-cell lymphoma, leg type. • Intravascular large B-cell lymphoma.
	OTHER
	• Blastic plasmacytoid dendritic cell neoplasm.

*This chapter uses the 2018 update of the WHO and European Organization for Research and Treatment of Cancer (EORTC) classification.

124. List some inflammatory conditions in which the associated lymphoid infiltrate may contain CD30-positive lymphocytes.
- Molluscum contagiosum.
- Persistent arthropod bite reactions including nodular scabies.
- Drug eruptions.
- Viral warts.
- Herpes simplex.
- Herpes zoster.

Algorithmic Guide to Diagnosis of Inflammatory Diseases of the Skin: A Method Based on Pattern Analysis

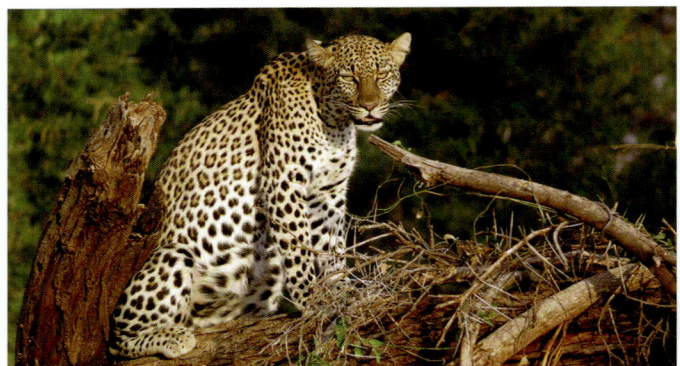

Leopard

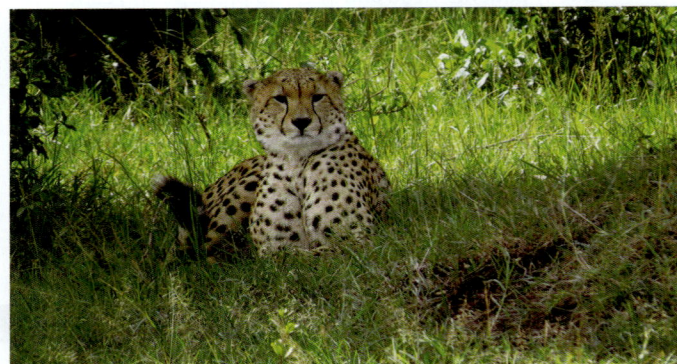

Cheetah

In nature, pattern analysis allows us to distinguish a leopard from a cheetah; in pathology, it enables us to differentiate inflammatory diseases of the skin.

This algorithmic outline of the 9 basic histopathological patterns of inflammatory skin disease is adapted from Dr. A. Bernard Ackerman's approach to diagnosis in his 1978 textbook *Histologic Diagnosis of Inflammatory Skin Diseases: A Method by Pattern Analysis*, supplements to that book, and later editions. It is designed as a practical guide to diagnosis of the more common inflammatory skin diseases and not as a replacement for traditional textbooks on this subject. The following points are emphasized:

1. To optimize the value of this scheme, the user is encouraged to:

   - Examine sections of skin without knowledge of the relevant clinical information.
   - Identify the morphological pattern of disease.
   - Construct a differential diagnosis based on microscopy.
   - Correlate the histopathological and clinical possibilities to reach a final diagnosis.

2. The lists are not totally comprehensive, and for additional information, refer to traditional dermatology textbooks (*Weedon's Skin Pathology, McKee's Pathology of the Skin with Clinical Correlation, Lever's Histopathology of the Skin*, and others).

3. A number of diseases are listed in different categories, reflecting the morphologic diversity of these conditions.

4. In some categories, neoplastic diseases (such as mycosis fungoides) that simulate inflammatory diseases are included in the lists.

5. Abbreviations used in the algorithms are listed below:

BMZ	basement membrane zone
BP	bullous pemphigoid
CLL	chronic lymphocytic leukemia
DIC	disseminated intravascular coagulation
GA	granuloma annulare
GVHD	graft versus host disease
LGV	lymphogranuloma venereum
LS&A	lichen sclerosus et atrophicus
NL	necrobiosis lipoidica
PAN	polyarteritis nodosa
PLEVA	pityriasis lichenoides et varioliformis acuta
PNH	paroxysmal nocturnal hemoglobinuria
PUPPP	pruritic urticarial papules and plaques of pregnancy
PV	pemphigus vulgaris
RA	rheumatoid arthritis
TB	tuberculosis
TTP	thrombotic thrombocytopenic purpura

Nine Basic Patterns of Inflammatory Skin Disease

1. Superficial perivascular dermatitis.
2. Superficial and deep perivascular dermatitis.
3. Vasculitis.
4. Nodular and diffuse dermatitis.
5. Intraepidermal vesicular and pustular dermatitis.
6. Subepidermal vesicular dermatitis.
7. Folliculitis and perifolliculitis.
8. Fibrosing dermatitis.
9. Panniculitis.

FIGURE 6.1 SUPERFICIAL PERIVASCULAR DERMATITIS

Without Epidermal Changes

Lymphohistiocytic

- drug eruption
- viral exanthem
- pigmented purpura (Schamberg disease)
- postinflammatory pigmentary alteration
- superficial gyrate erythema
- vitiligo
- erythrasma
- tinea versicolor

Mixed cell (eosinophils)

- urticaria
- urticarial allergic eruption
- drug eruption
- bullous pemphigoid (urticarial phase)
- pemphigoid gestationis (urticarial phase)
- pemphigus vulgaris (urticarial phase)
- PUPPP
- superficial arthropod bite reaction

Mast cells

- urticaria pigmentosa

With Epidermal Changes

Interface

Vacuolar

- erythema multiforme
- lupus
- dermatomyositis
- drug eruption
- GVHD (acute)
- bullous pemphigoid (urticarial)
- LS&A
- viral exanthem
- mycosis fungoides
- erythema dyschromicum perstans
- chronic radiation dermatitis

Lichenoid

- lichen planus
- drug
- lupus
- photodermatitis
- pigmented purpura (Gougerot-Blum)
- GVHD (chronic)
- lichen planus-like keratosis
- mycosis fungoides
- pityriasis lichenoides chronica
- lichen striatus

Spongiotic

- allergic contact dermatitis (acute)
- dyshidrotic dermatitis (acute)
- nummular dermatitis (acute)
- id reaction (acute)
- seborrheic dermatitis (acute)
- dermatophytosis (occasionally)
- prebullous phase of blistering disorders (e.g., BP, PV)

Spongiotic Psoriasiform

- allergic contact dermatitis (subacute)
- dyshidrotic dermatitis (subacute)
- nummular dermatitis (subacute)
- id reaction (subacute)
- seborrheic dermatitis (subacute)
- pityriasis rosea
- superficial gyrate erythema
- guttate parapsoriasis and digitate dermatosis

Psoriasiform

- allergic contact dermatitis (chronic)
- dyshidrotic dermatitis (chronic)
- nummular dermatitis (chronic)
- id reaction (chronic)
- seborrheic dermatitis (chronic)
- psoriasis
- lichen simplex chronicus
- pityriasis rubra pilaris
- mycosis fungoides
- dermatophytosis or candidiasis
- necrolytic migratory erythema

Psoriasiform/ Lichenoid

- 2° syphilis
- mycosis fungoides
- lichen striatus

FIGURE 6.2 SUPERFICIAL AND DEEP PERIVASCULAR DERMATITIS

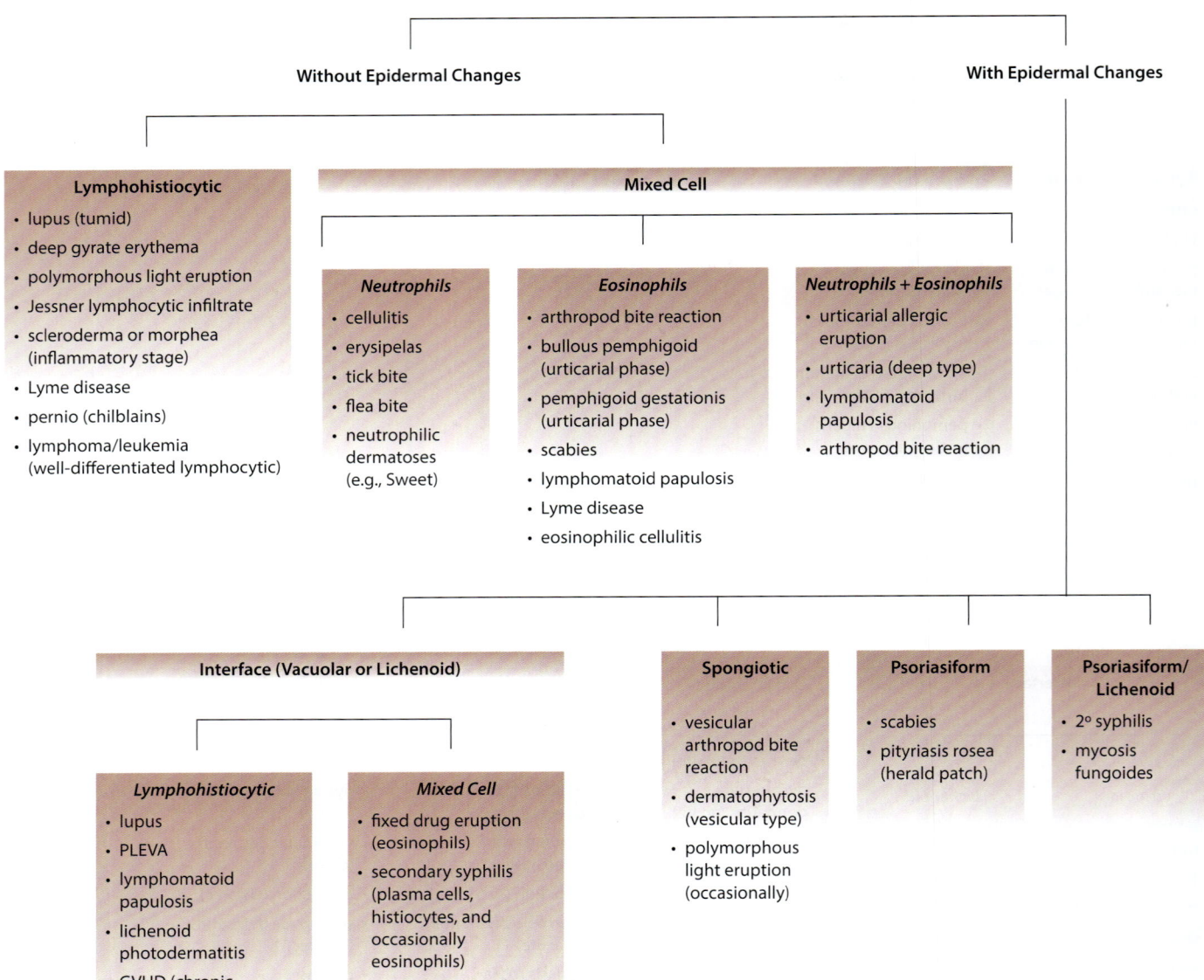

Without Epidermal Changes

With Epidermal Changes

Lymphohistiocytic

- lupus (tumid)
- deep gyrate erythema
- polymorphous light eruption
- Jessner lymphocytic infiltrate
- scleroderma or morphea (inflammatory stage)
- Lyme disease
- pernio (chilblains)
- lymphoma/leukemia (well-differentiated lymphocytic)

Mixed Cell

Neutrophils
- cellulitis
- erysipelas
- tick bite
- flea bite
- neutrophilic dermatoses (e.g., Sweet)

Eosinophils
- arthropod bite reaction
- bullous pemphigoid (urticarial phase)
- pemphigoid gestationis (urticarial phase)
- scabies
- lymphomatoid papulosis
- Lyme disease
- eosinophilic cellulitis

Neutrophils + Eosinophils
- urticarial allergic eruption
- urticaria (deep type)
- lymphomatoid papulosis
- arthropod bite reaction

Interface (Vacuolar or Lichenoid)

Lymphohistiocytic
- lupus
- PLEVA
- lymphomatoid papulosis
- lichenoid photodermatitis
- GVHD (chronic lichenoid)
- drug
- dermatophytosis
- lichen striatus
- actinic reticuloid
- mycosis fungoides

Mixed Cell
- fixed drug eruption (eosinophils)
- secondary syphilis (plasma cells, histiocytes, and occasionally eosinophils)

Spongiotic
- vesicular arthropod bite reaction
- dermatophytosis (vesicular type)
- polymorphous light eruption (occasionally)

Psoriasiform
- scabies
- pityriasis rosea (herald patch)

Psoriasiform/ Lichenoid
- 2° syphilis
- mycosis fungoides

FIGURE 6.3 VASCULITIS

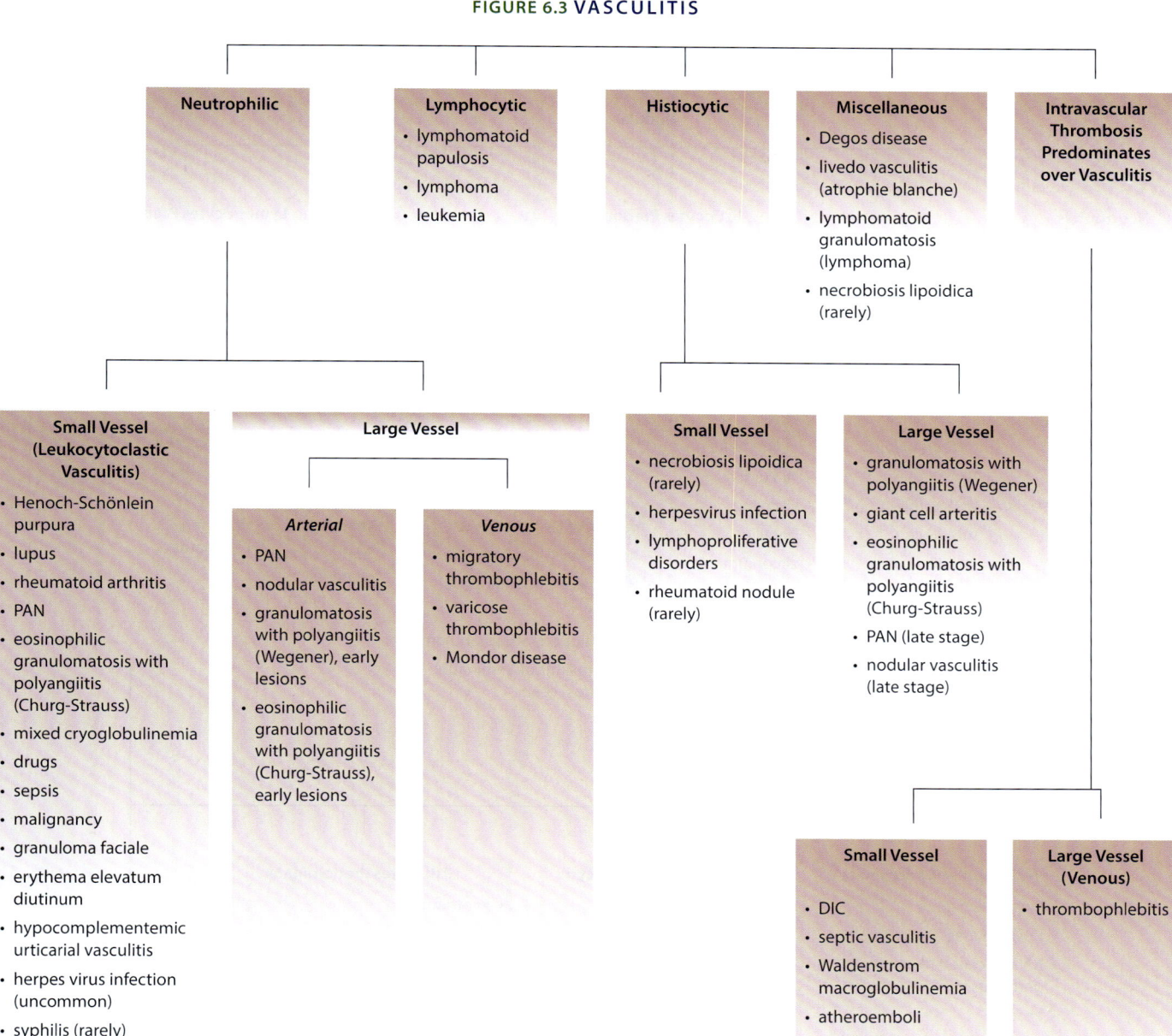

Neutrophilic

Lymphocytic
- lymphomatoid papulosis
- lymphoma
- leukemia

Histiocytic

Miscellaneous
- Degos disease
- livedo vasculitis (atrophie blanche)
- lymphomatoid granulomatosis (lymphoma)
- necrobiosis lipoidica (rarely)

Intravascular Thrombosis Predominates over Vasculitis

Small Vessel (Leukocytoclastic Vasculitis)
- Henoch-Schönlein purpura
- lupus
- rheumatoid arthritis
- PAN
- eosinophilic granulomatosis with polyangiitis (Churg-Strauss)
- mixed cryoglobulinemia
- drugs
- sepsis
- malignancy
- granuloma faciale
- erythema elevatum diutinum
- hypocomplementemic urticarial vasculitis
- herpes virus infection (uncommon)
- syphilis (rarely)
- leprosy (rarely)
- cutaneous Crohn disease
- cocaine/levamisole vasculopathy

Large Vessel

Arterial
- PAN
- nodular vasculitis
- granulomatosis with polyangiitis (Wegener), early lesions
- eosinophilic granulomatosis with polyangiitis (Churg-Strauss), early lesions

Venous
- migratory thrombophlebitis
- varicose thrombophlebitis
- Mondor disease

Small Vessel
- necrobiosis lipoidica (rarely)
- herpesvirus infection
- lymphoproliferative disorders
- rheumatoid nodule (rarely)

Large Vessel
- granulomatosis with polyangiitis (Wegener)
- giant cell arteritis
- eosinophilic granulomatosis with polyangiitis (Churg-Strauss)
- PAN (late stage)
- nodular vasculitis (late stage)

Small Vessel
- DIC
- septic vasculitis
- Waldenstrom macroglobulinemia
- atheroemboli
- cryoglobulinemia (type 1)
- purpura fulminans
- coumarin necrosis
- PNH
- TTP
- cocaine/levamisole vasculopathy

Large Vessel (Venous)
- thrombophlebitis

FIGURE 6.4 NODULAR AND DIFFUSE DERMATITIS

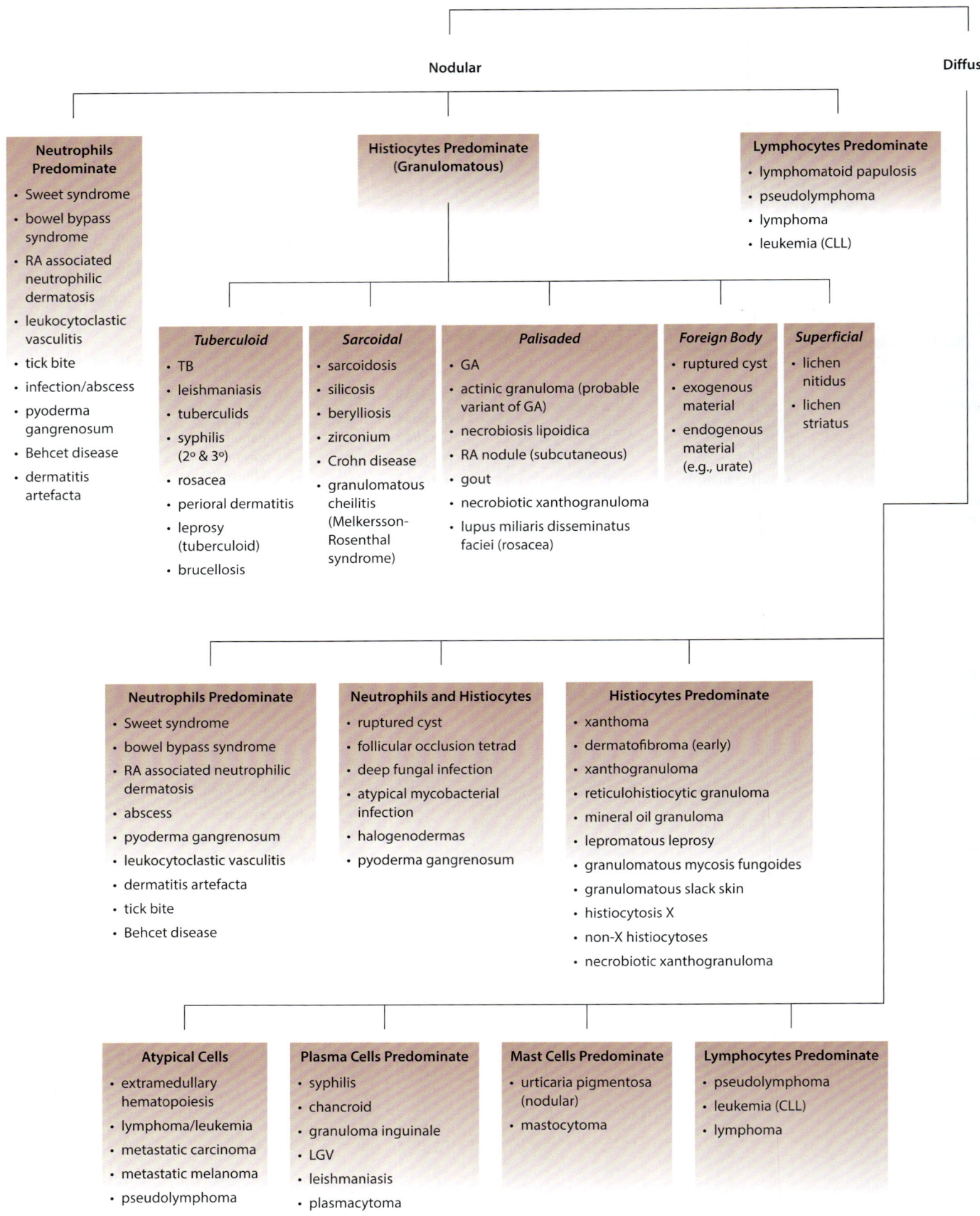

Nodular

Diffuse

Neutrophils Predominate
- Sweet syndrome
- bowel bypass syndrome
- RA associated neutrophilic dermatosis
- leukocytoclastic vasculitis
- tick bite
- infection/abscess
- pyoderma gangrenosum
- Behcet disease
- dermatitis artefacta

Histiocytes Predominate (Granulomatous)

Lymphocytes Predominate
- lymphomatoid papulosis
- pseudolymphoma
- lymphoma
- leukemia (CLL)

Tuberculoid
- TB
- leishmaniasis
- tuberculids
- syphilis (2º & 3º)
- rosacea
- perioral dermatitis
- leprosy (tuberculoid)
- brucellosis

Sarcoidal
- sarcoidosis
- silicosis
- berylliosis
- zirconium
- Crohn disease
- granulomatous cheilitis (Melkersson-Rosenthal syndrome)

Palisaded
- GA
- actinic granuloma (probable variant of GA)
- necrobiosis lipoidica
- RA nodule (subcutaneous)
- gout
- necrobiotic xanthogranuloma
- lupus miliaris disseminatus faciei (rosacea)

Foreign Body
- ruptured cyst
- exogenous material
- endogenous material (e.g., urate)

Superficial
- lichen nitidus
- lichen striatus

Neutrophils Predominate
- Sweet syndrome
- bowel bypass syndrome
- RA associated neutrophilic dermatosis
- abscess
- pyoderma gangrenosum
- leukocytoclastic vasculitis
- dermatitis artefacta
- tick bite
- Behcet disease

Neutrophils and Histiocytes
- ruptured cyst
- follicular occlusion tetrad
- deep fungal infection
- atypical mycobacterial infection
- halogenodermas
- pyoderma gangrenosum

Histiocytes Predominate
- xanthoma
- dermatofibroma (early)
- xanthogranuloma
- reticulohistiocytic granuloma
- mineral oil granuloma
- lepromatous leprosy
- granulomatous mycosis fungoides
- granulomatous slack skin
- histiocytosis X
- non-X histiocytoses
- necrobiotic xanthogranuloma

Atypical Cells
- extramedullary hematopoiesis
- lymphoma/leukemia
- metastatic carcinoma
- metastatic melanoma
- pseudolymphoma

Plasma Cells Predominate
- syphilis
- chancroid
- granuloma inguinale
- LGV
- leishmaniasis
- plasmacytoma
- marginal zone lymphoma with plasmacytic differentiation

Mast Cells Predominate
- urticaria pigmentosa (nodular)
- mastocytoma

Lymphocytes Predominate
- pseudolymphoma
- leukemia (CLL)
- lymphoma

FIGURE 6.5 INTRAEPIDERMAL VESICULAR AND PUSTULAR DERMATITIS

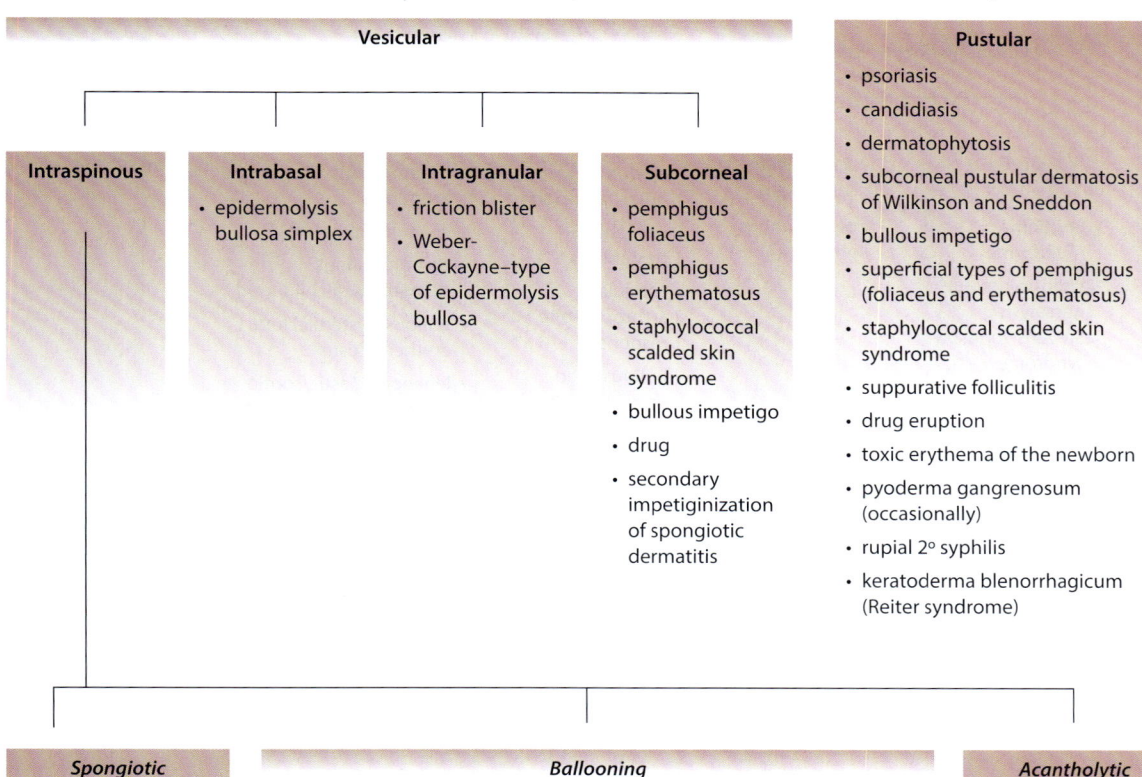

Vesicular

Intraspinous

Intrabasal
- epidermolysis bullosa simplex
- Weber-Cockayne–type of epidermolysis bullosa

Intragranular
- friction blister

Subcorneal
- pemphigus foliaceus
- pemphigus erythematosus
- staphylococcal scalded skin syndrome
- bullous impetigo
- drug
- secondary impetiginization of spongiotic dermatitis

Pustular
- psoriasis
- candidiasis
- dermatophytosis
- subcorneal pustular dermatosis of Wilkinson and Sneddon
- bullous impetigo
- superficial types of pemphigus (foliaceus and erythematosus)
- staphylococcal scalded skin syndrome
- suppurative folliculitis
- drug eruption
- toxic erythema of the newborn
- pyoderma gangrenosum (occasionally)
- rupial 2° syphilis
- keratoderma blenorrhagicum (Reiter syndrome)

Intra- and Subepidural Vesicular Dermatitis (Occasional Combined Pattern)
- erythema multiforme
- fixed drug eruption
- herpetic vesicles
- vesicular arthropod bites
- dermatophytosis
- acute spongiotic dermatitides, occasionally (contact, nummular, id, dyshidrotic)

Spongiotic
- allergic contact dermatitis
- nummular dermatitis
- id reaction
- dyshidrotic dermatitis
- dermatophytosis (occasionally)
- vesicular arthropod bite response
- prebullous phase of blistering disorders (e.g., BP and PV)

Ballooning

Viral
- herpesvirus infection
- vaccinia/variola
- milker's nodule
- orf
- hand, foot, and mouth disease

Deficiencies
- necrolytic migratory erythema (glucagonoma syndrome)
- pellagra
- acrodermatitis enteropathica
- zinc deficiency

Other
- immersion blister
- irritant contact dermatitis
- PLEVA (occasionally)

Acantholytic
- pemphigus (vulgaris and vegetans)
- Hailey-Hailey disease
- Darier disease
- Grover disease
- herpesvirus infection
- drug induced disorders (e.g., penicillamine)

FIGURE 6.6 SUBEPIDERMAL VESICULAR DERMATITIS

Little/No Inflammatory Infiltrate

- cell poor bullous pemphigoid
- cell poor pemphigoid gestationis
- epidermolysis bullosa (different types)
- porphyria cutanea tarda
- pseudoporphyria
- burn
- suction blister
- hypoxemic blister (including autolysis)
- pressure blister
- gas gangrene
- blister over scar
- bullous cutaneous amyloidosis
- bullous drug eruption (some)

Lymphohistiocytic Infiltrate

Superficial

- erythema multiforme
- toxic epidermal necrolysis/ Stevens-Johnson syndrome
- LS&A
- bullous graft-versus-host disease
- bullous lichen planus

Superficial and Deep

- polymorphous light eruption

Eosinophils Prominent

- bullous pemphigoid
- epidermolysis bullosa acquisita
- pemphigoid gestationis
- vesicular arthropod bite response
- bullous fixed drug eruption

Neutrophils Prominent

- dermatitis herpetiformis
- dermatitis herpetiformis–like drug eruption
- linear IgA dermatosis
- chronic bullous dermatosis of childhood
- bullous (systemic) lupus erythematosus
- leukocytoclastic/septic vasculitis
- cicatricial pemphigoid
- bullous pemphigoid (rarely)
- erysipelas
- erythropoietic protoporphyria
- bullous pyoderma gangrenosum
- bullous Sweet syndrome (occasionally)

Mast Cells Prominent

- bullous urticaria pigmentosa (mastocytosis)

FIGURE 6.7 PERIFOLLICULITIS AND FOLLICULITIS

Perifolliculitis

Predominantly Lymphocytic

- keratosis pilaris
- lichen spinulosus
- lichen planopilaris
- cutaneous lupus erythematosus
- scurvy
- folliculotropic mycosis fungoides
- pseudolymphomatous folliculitis

Predominantly Histiocytic

- acne rosacea
- perioral dermatitis
- acneiform 2° syphilis

Folliculitis

Spongiotic

- follicular spongiotic dermatitis
- atopic dermatitis
- seborrheic dermatitis
- Fox-Fordyce disease
- follicular mucinosis (may resemble follicular spongiosis)

Suppurative and Granulomatous

Noninfectious

- acne vulgaris (+ variants)
- perforating disorders (e.g., Kyrle disease)
- follicular occlusion tetrad (e.g., hidradenitis suppurativa)
- acne rosacea (occasionally)

Infectious

- fungal (dermatophytes or Candida)
- bacterial (e.g., Staphylococcus)
- syphilis
- viral (herpes)

Nonscarring Inflammatory Alopecia

- alopecia areata
- trichotillomania
- traction alopecia
- follicular mucinosis
- 2° syphilis

Scarring Inflammatory Alopecia

- lupus
- lichen planopilaris
- scleroderma (linear)
- sarcoidosis
- physical or chemical injury
- dissecting cellulitis (and any other long-standing suppurative folliculitis)

FIGURE 6.8 FIBROSING DERMATITIS

Fibrosis

Hypertrophic
- hypertrophic scar
- keloidal scar
- dermatofibroma (late)
- chronic lymphedema or venous stasis
- nephrogenic fibrosing dermopathy
- scleromyxedema

Atrophic
- atrophic scar
- striae distensae
- anetoderma
- poikilodermas
- acrodermatitis chronica atrophicans (Lyme disease, late)
- regression of preexisting lesion

Sclerosis

Hypertrophic
- scleroderma/morphea
- eosinophilic fasciitis
- chronic graft-versus-host-disease (sclerodermoid)
- scleredema of Buschke

Atrophic
- LS&A
- chronic radiodermatitis
- necrobiosis lipoidica
- morphea (end stage)
- atrophoderma of Pasini and Pierini (possible end stage of morphea)

Fibrohistiocytic Proliferation
- dermatofibroma
- late juvenile and adult xanthogranulomas
- nodular fasciitis
- histoid leprosy
- juxtaarticular node of syphilis (late stage)

FIGURE 6.9 PANNICULITIS

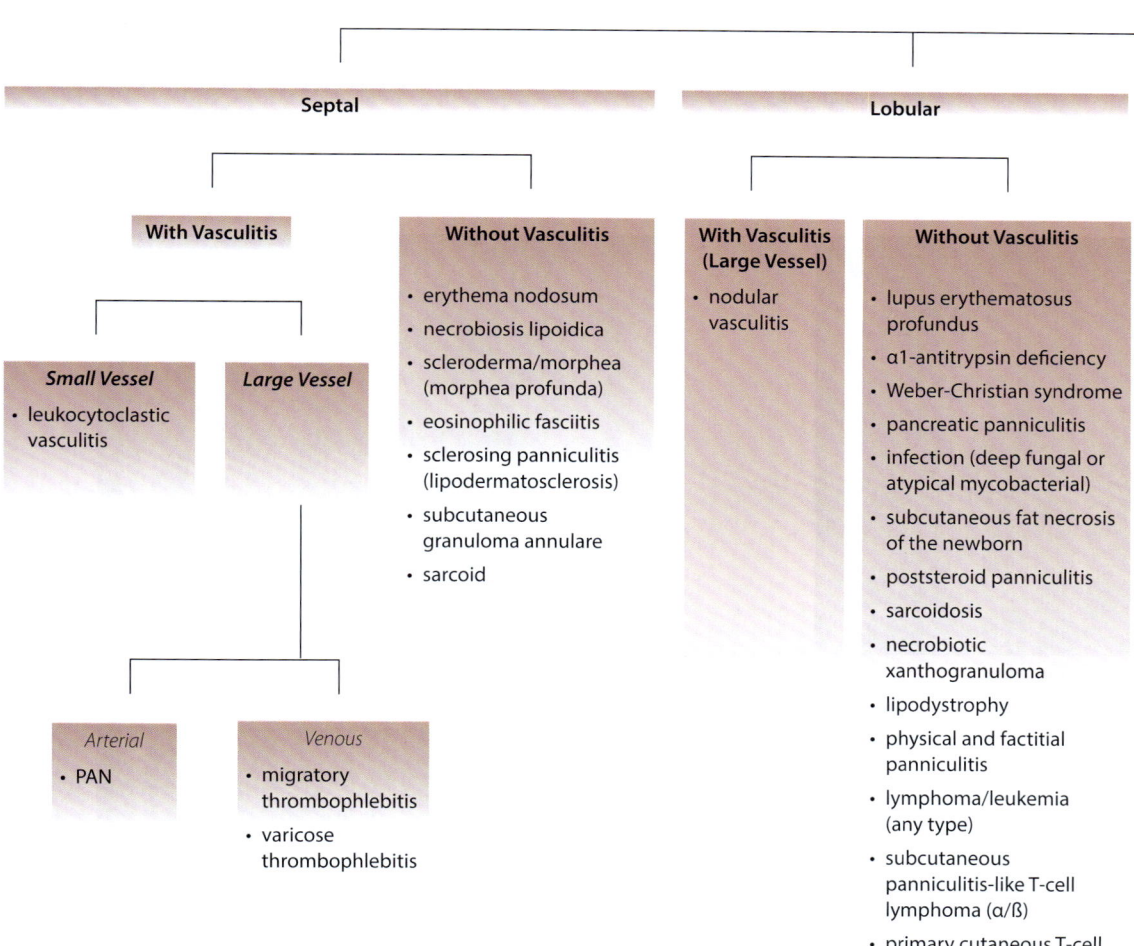

Septal

With Vasculitis

Small Vessel
- leukocytoclastic vasculitis

Large Vessel

Arterial
- PAN

Venous
- migratory thrombophlebitis
- varicose thrombophlebitis

Without Vasculitis
- erythema nodosum
- necrobiosis lipoidica
- scleroderma/morphea (morphea profunda)
- eosinophilic fasciitis
- sclerosing panniculitis (lipodermatosclerosis)
- subcutaneous granuloma annulare
- sarcoid

Lobular

With Vasculitis (Large Vessel)
- nodular vasculitis

Without Vasculitis
- lupus erythematosus profundus
- α1-antitrypsin deficiency
- Weber-Christian syndrome
- pancreatic panniculitis
- infection (deep fungal or atypical mycobacterial)
- subcutaneous fat necrosis of the newborn
- poststeroid panniculitis
- sarcoidosis
- necrobiotic xanthogranuloma
- lipodystrophy
- physical and factitial panniculitis
- lymphoma/leukemia (any type)
- subcutaneous panniculitis-like T-cell lymphoma (α/ß)
- primary cutaneous T-cell lymphoma (γ/δ)

Lobular and Septal
- subcutaneous granuloma annulare
- necrobiotic xanthogranuloma
- nodular vasculitis
- infection
- sclerosing panniculitis (lipodermatosclerosis)

FIGURE 6.10 SCHEMATIC STRUCTURAL APPROACH TO DIRECT IMMUNOFLUORESCENCE IN INFLAMMATORY SKIN DISEASE

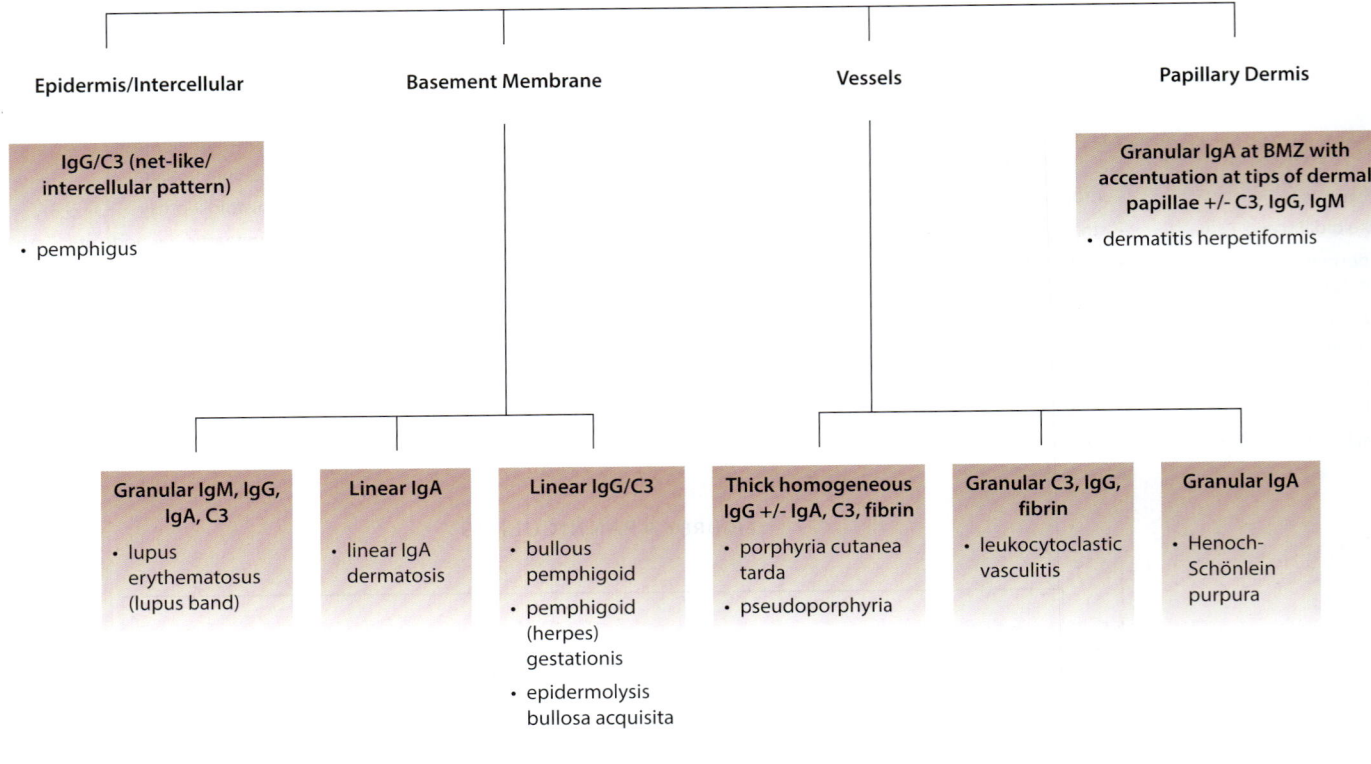

Epidermis/Intercellular

IgG/C3 (net-like/intercellular pattern)
- pemphigus

Basement Membrane

Granular IgM, IgG, IgA, C3
- lupus erythematosus (lupus band)

Linear IgA
- linear IgA dermatosis

Linear IgG/C3
- bullous pemphigoid
- pemphigoid (herpes) gestationis
- epidermolysis bullosa acquisita

Vessels

Thick homogeneous IgG +/- IgA, C3, fibrin
- porphyria cutanea tarda
- pseudoporphyria

Granular C3, IgG, fibrin
- leukocytoclastic vasculitis

Granular IgA
- Henoch-Schönlein purpura

Papillary Dermis

Granular IgA at BMZ with accentuation at tips of dermal papillae +/- C3, IgG, IgM
- dermatitis herpetiformis

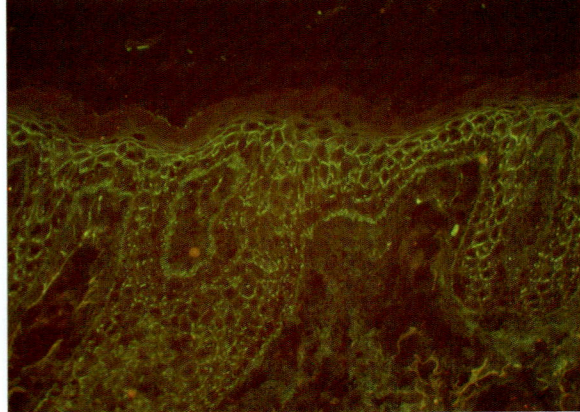

Pemphigus. Net-like/intercellular pattern of IgG.

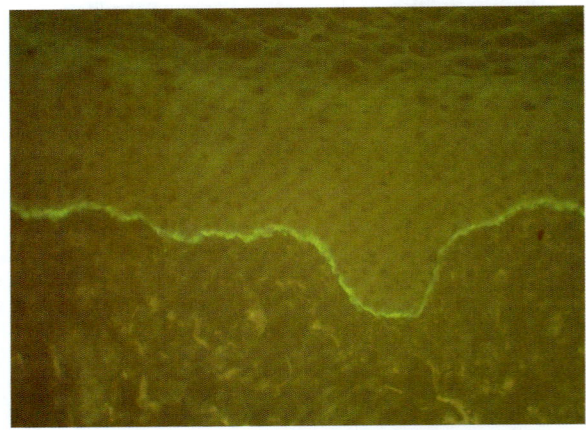

Bullous pemphigoid. Linear IgG deposition at the basement membrane zone.

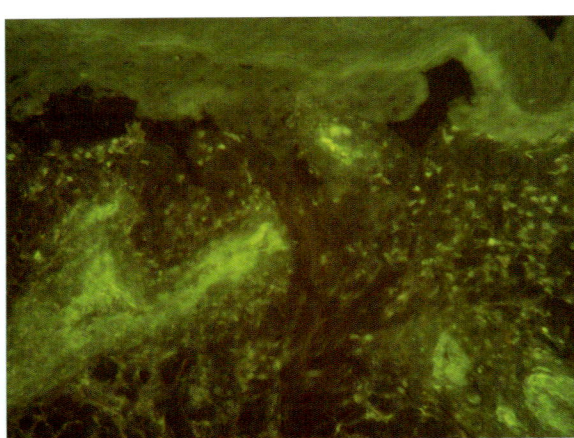

Vasculitis. Granular C3 deposition within dermal vessels.

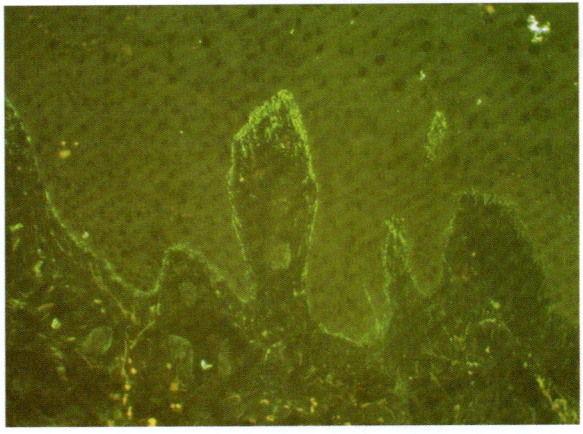

Dermatitis herpetiformis. Granular IgA deposition is concentrated at the tips of dermal papillae.

IMAGES: DERMATOPATHOLOGY

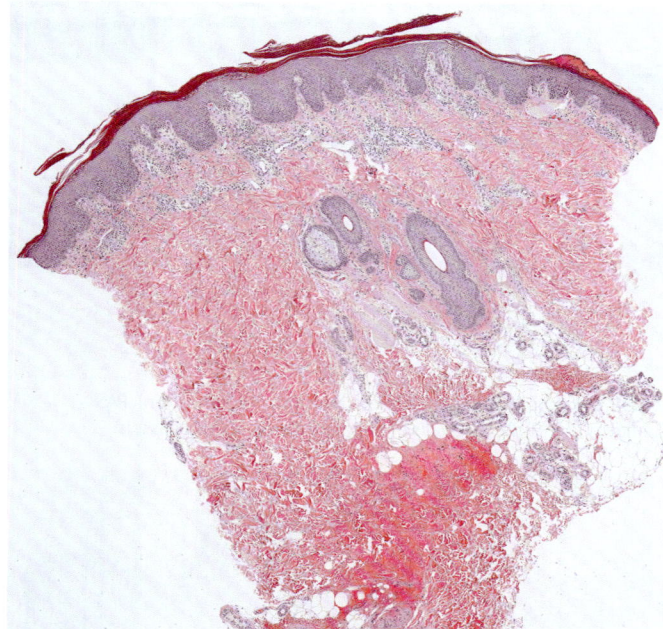

IMAGE 6.1 Psoriasis vulgaris (low magnification). Superficial perivascular lymphocytic inflammation with psoriasiform epidermal change is evident.

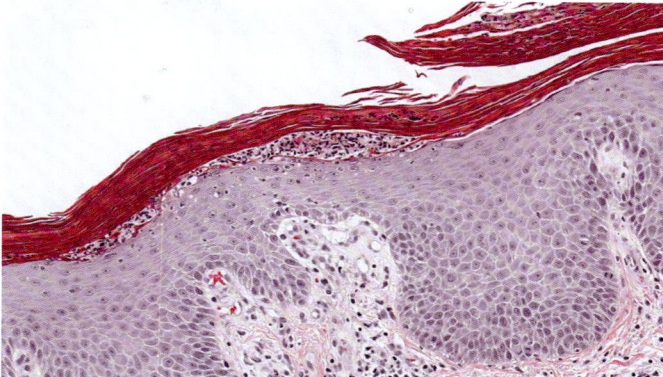

IMAGE 6.2 Psoriasis vulgaris (high magnification). The epidermal hyperplasia with suprapapillary thinning, hypogranulosis, confluent parakeratosis, and intracorneal pustules (Munro microabscesses) are typical of psoriasis, as is the dilatation of papillary dermal capillaries.

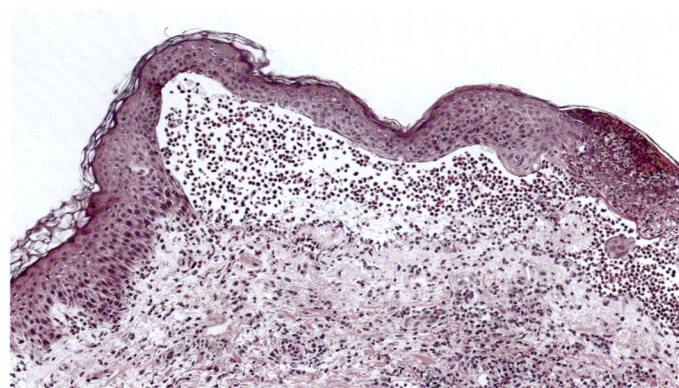

IMAGE 6.3 Bullous pemphigoid (medium magnification). A subepidermal blister is evident.

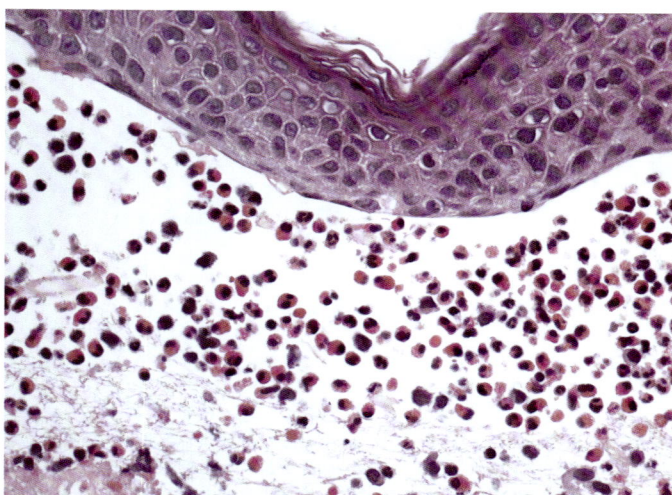

IMAGE 6.4 Bullous pemphigoid (high magnification). An eosinophil rich infiltrate spills into the blister cavity.

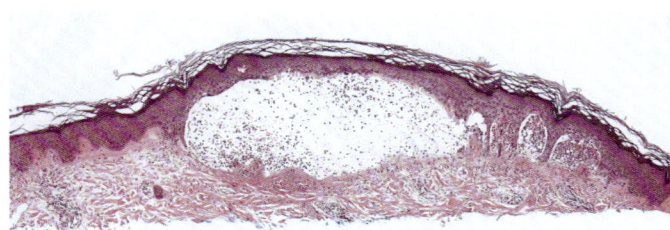

IMAGE 6.5 Dermatitis herpetiformis (low magnification). The image shows a subepidermal blister.

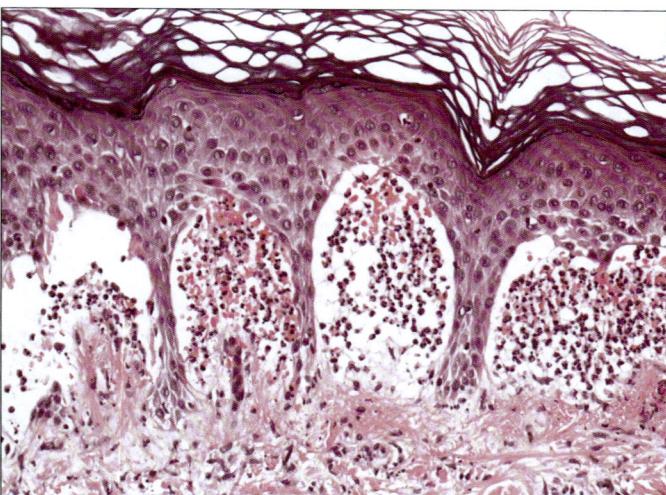

IMAGE 6.6 Dermatitis herpetiformis (high magnification). The image shows a neutrophil rich infiltrate in the papillary dermis and blister cavities.

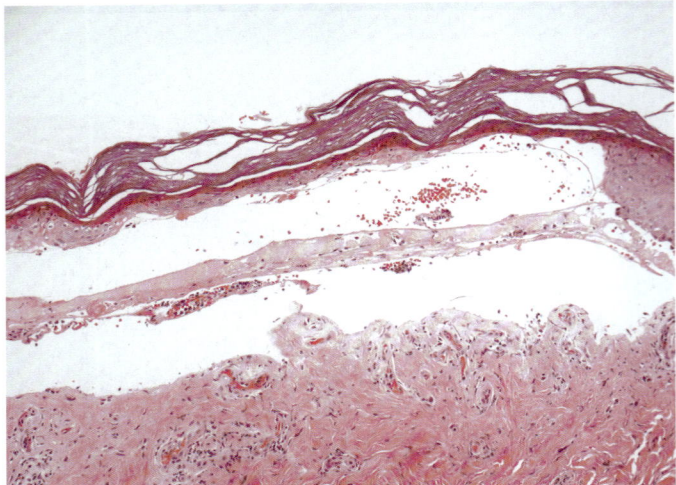

IMAGE 6.7 Porphyria cutanea tarda (medium magnification). The image shows a cell poor subepidermal blister with "festooning" of the papillary dermis at the base of the blister.

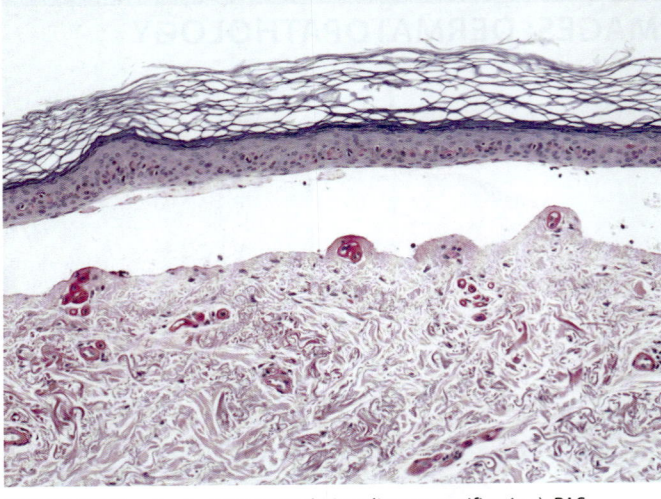

IMAGE 6.8 Porphyria cutanea tarda (medium magnification). PAS highlights the thickened walls of papillary dermal blood vessels.

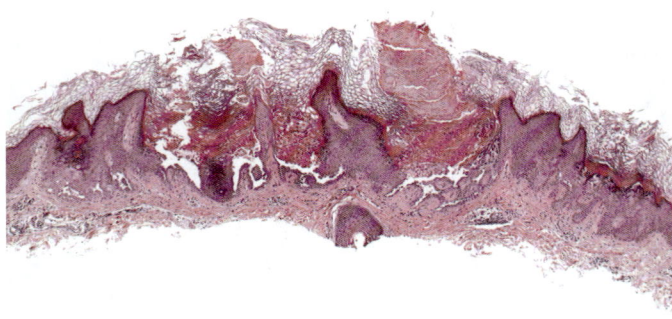

IMAGE 6.9 Darier disease (low magnification). A hyperkeratotic papule displaying intermittent foci of suprabasilar acantholysis is evident. This histopathological pattern represents focal acantholytic dyskeratosis.

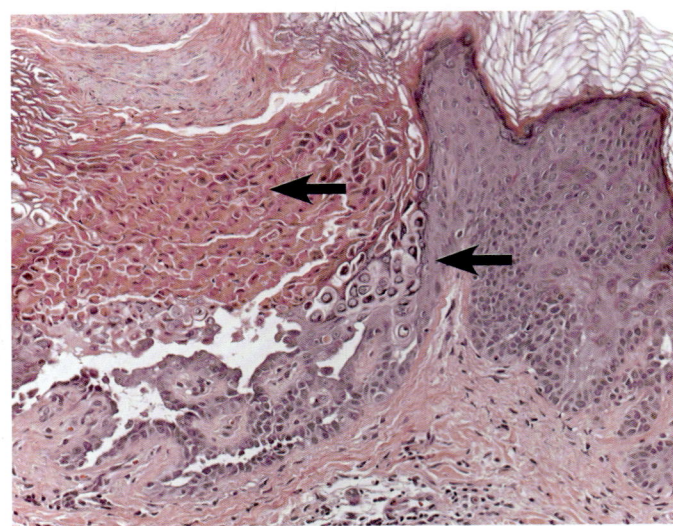

IMAGE 6.10 Darier disease (high magnification). Above and to the right of the suprabasal cleft there are dyskeratotic cells known as "corps ronds" (round cells with abundant cytoplasm, pyknotic nuclei and perinuclear halos) and "grains" (small cells with elongated nuclei resembling parakeratotic cells).

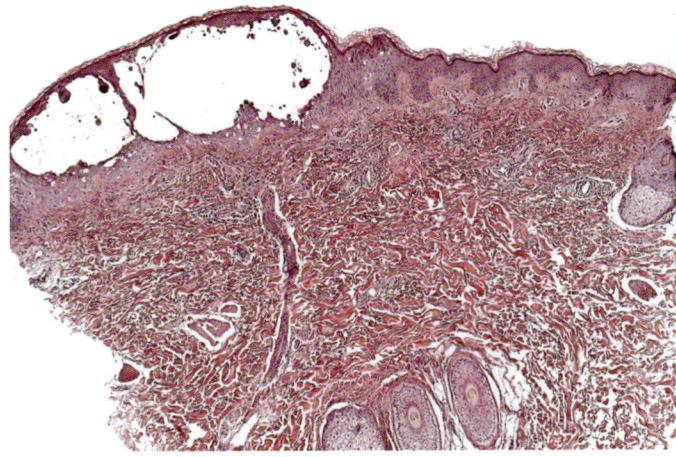

IMAGE 6.11 Herpetic vesicle (low magnification). An intraepidermal acantholytic vesicle is evident.

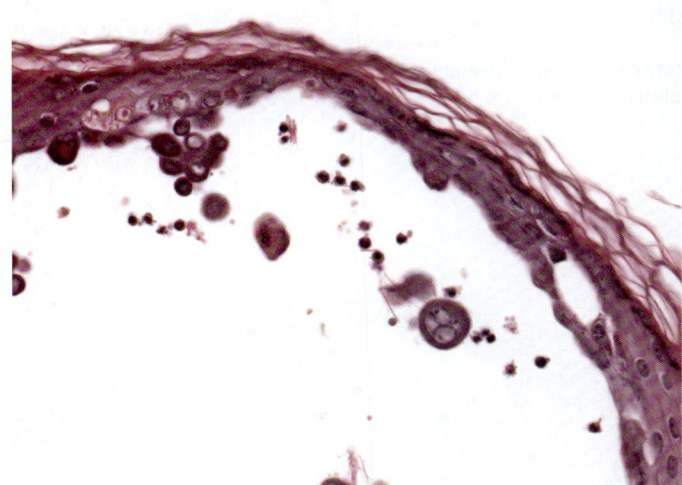

IMAGE 6.12 Herpetic vesicle (high magnification). Free-floating acantholytic cells are observed in the blister cavity, some displaying multinucleation and nuclear clearing (steel gray nuclei).

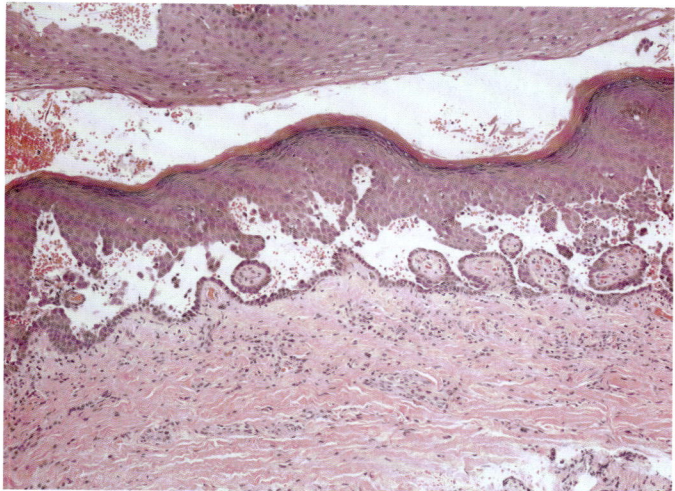

IMAGE 6.13 Pemphigus vulgaris (medium magnification). The image shows a suprabasal acantholytic blister with a "tombstone row" of residual basal keratinocytes.

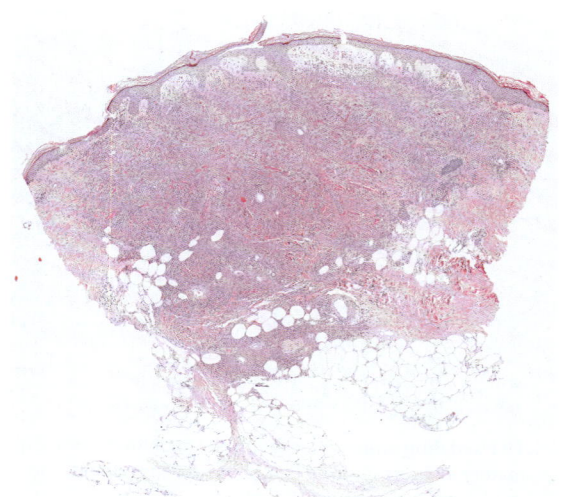

IMAGE 6.14 Sweet syndrome (low magnification). The dense diffuse cellular infiltrate throughout the reticular dermis and the prominent edema of the papillary dermis are characteristic.

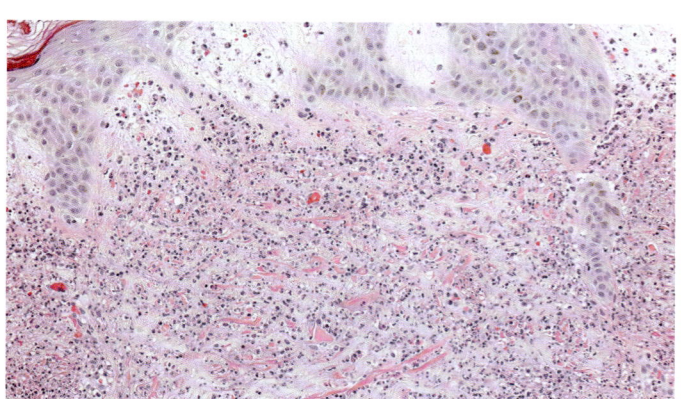

IMAGE 6.15 Sweet syndrome (medium magnification). The diffuse dermal infiltrate consists of neutrophils with leukocytoclasis, in the absence of vasculitis.

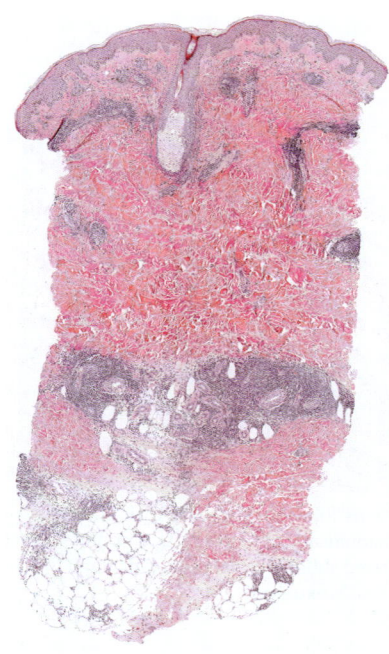

IMAGE 6.16 Arthropod bite reaction (low magnification). A superficial and deep perivascular infiltrate without epidermal change is the typical inflammatory pattern in this setting.

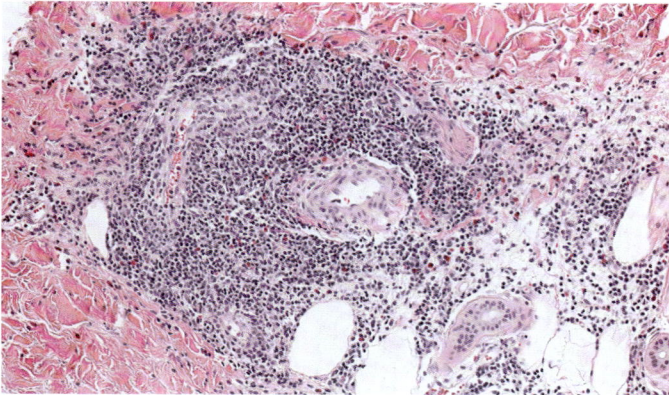

IMAGE 6.17 Arthropod bite reaction (high magnification). The perivascular infiltrate is mixed and typically contains abundant eosinophils.

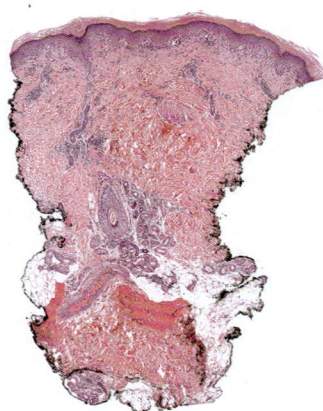

IMAGE 6.18 Fixed drug eruption (acute phase) (low magnification). A superficial and deep perivascular inflammatory infiltrate is accompanied by interface change.

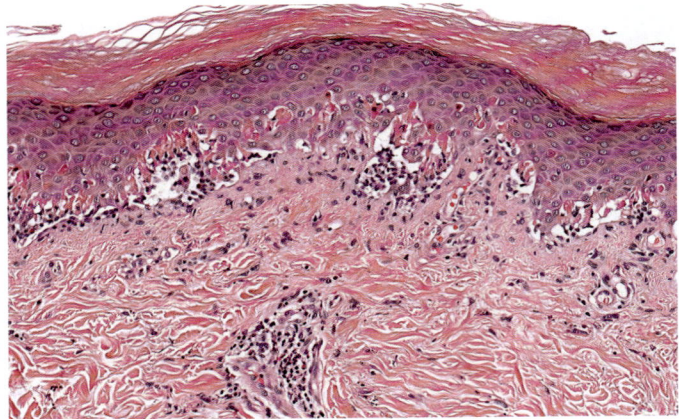

IMAGE 6.19 Fixed drug eruption (acute phase) (high magnification). The inflammatory infiltrate is mixed (lymphocytes, eosinophils, and neutrophils), and is associated with vacuolization and prominent apoptosis of basal keratinocytes.

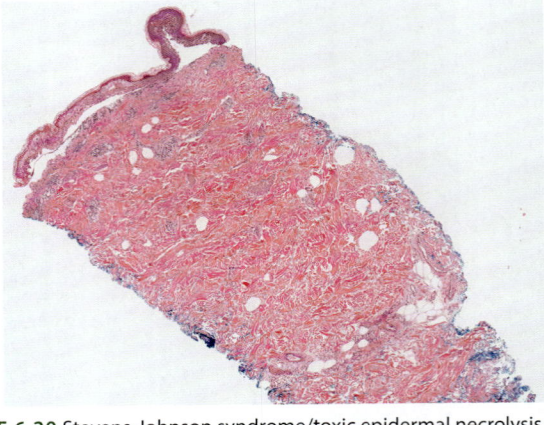

IMAGE 6.20 Stevens-Johnson syndrome/toxic epidermal necrolysis (low magnification). At this severe end of the erythema multiforme spectrum, sub-epidermal blister formation and confluent epidermal necrosis occur.

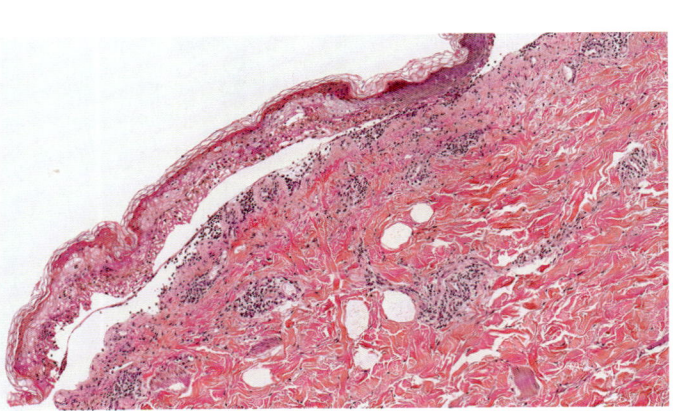

IMAGE 6.21 Stevens-Johnson syndrome/toxic epidermal necrolysis spectrum (high magnification). In this setting, confluent vacuolar interface change has facilitated subepidermal vesiculation and the degree of keratinocyte necrosis is extreme.

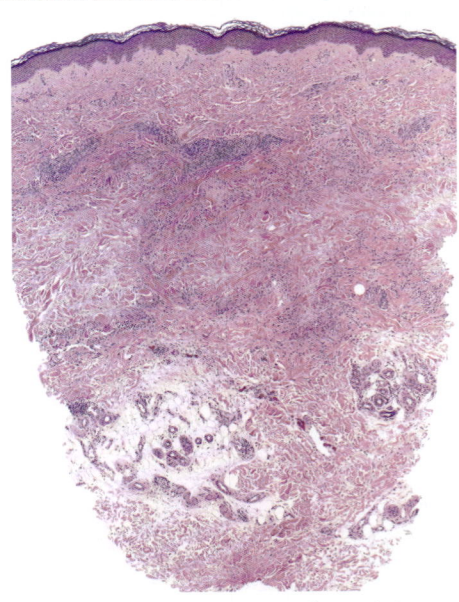

IMAGE 6.22 Granuloma annulare (low magnification). A central pale geographic zone in the dermis (representing a palisading granuloma) is accompanied by a perivascular lymphocytic infiltrate.

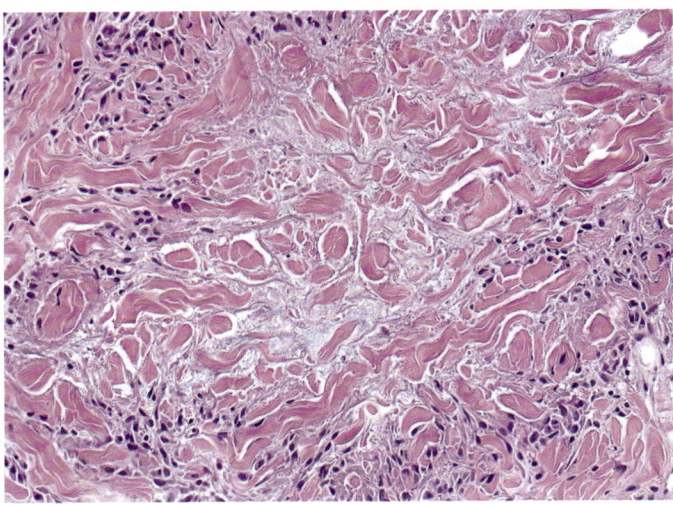

IMAGE 6.23 Granuloma annulare (high magnification). A palisade of histiocytes is observed at the periphery of the granuloma and centrally dermal collagen bundles are separated by interstitial mucin.

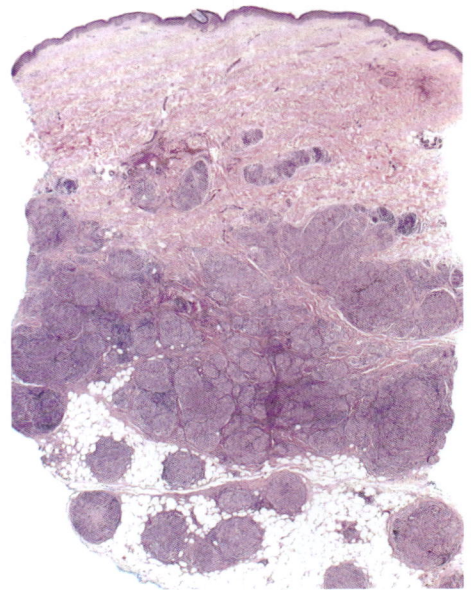

IMAGE 6.24 Sarcoidosis (low magnification). The deep dermis and subcutis exhibit confluent and discrete granulomata.

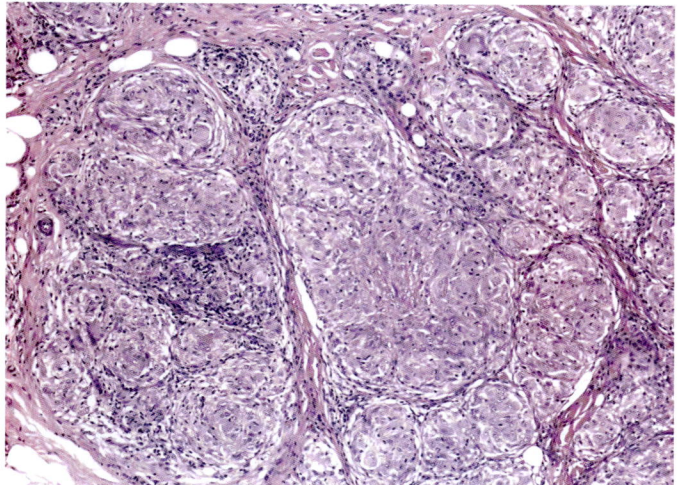

IMAGE 6.25 Sarcoidosis (high magnification). The naked, nonnecrotizing, epithelioid cell features of these granulomata are characteristic of sarcoidosis.

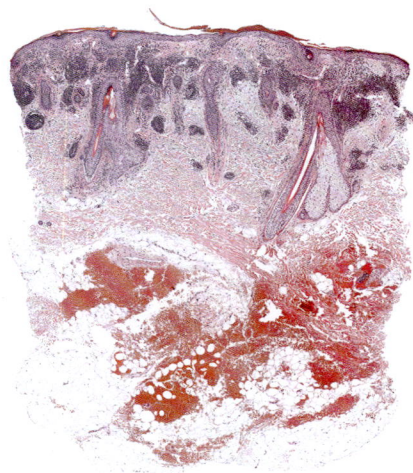

IMAGE 6.26 Cutaneous lupus erythematosus (low magnification). This punch biopsy of facial skin displays a dense superficial and deep perivascular and periadnexal lymphohistiocytic infiltrate, with a thinned epidermis and interface change.

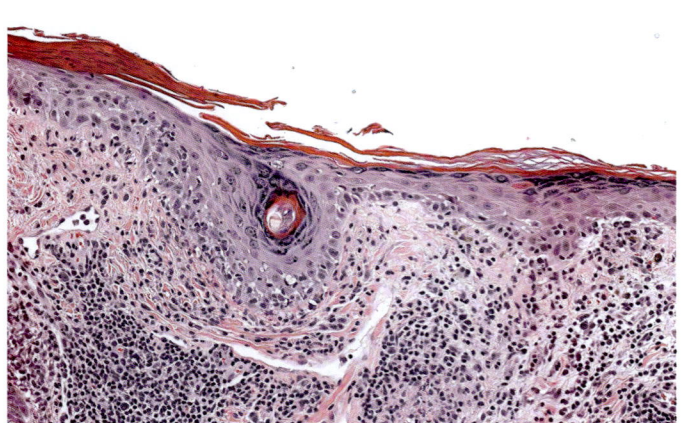

IMAGE 6.27 Cutaneous lupus erythematosus (high magnification). A vacuolar interface dermatitis is observed and the thinned epidermis displays hyper- and parakeratosis.

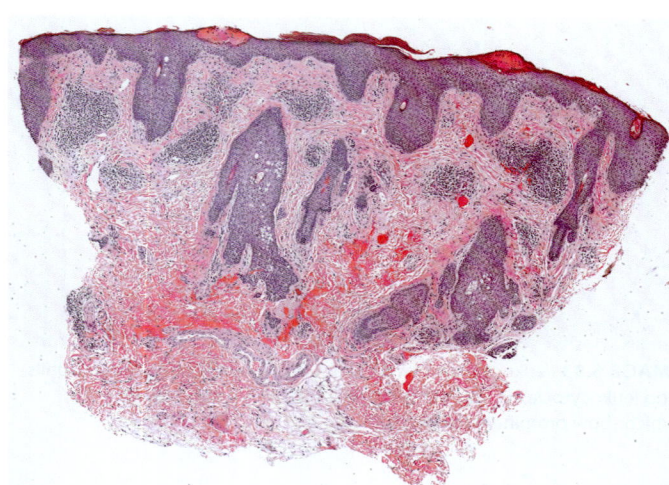

IMAGE 6.28 Subacute spongiotic dermatitis (low magnification). The biopsy features a superficial perivascular lymphohistiocytic infiltrate associated with epidermal changes.

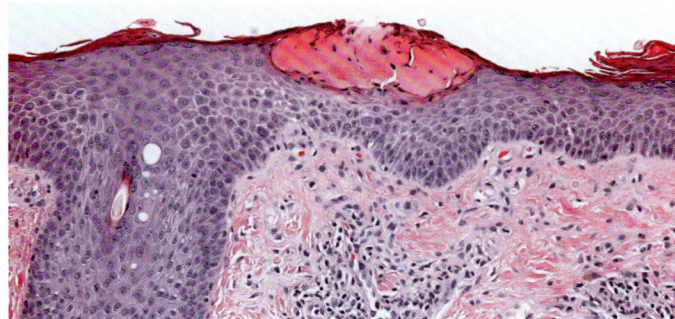

IMAGE 6.29 Subacute spongiotic dermatitis (high magnification). The epidermal changes include spongiosis (intercellular edema), intraepidermal vesicle formation due to loculated serum, mild acanthosis, and parakeratosis.

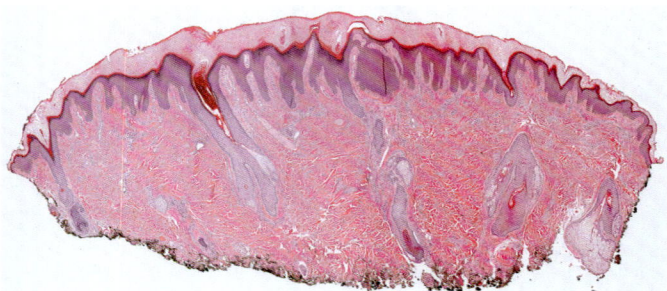

IMAGE 6.30 Lichen simplex chronicus (low magnification). The compact hyperkeratosis, hypergranulosis, and psoriasiform epidermal hyperplasia, in a pauci-inflammatory background, resemble palmar or plantar skin — yet hair follicles are present! Hence, a "hairy palm" appearance is a clue to lichen simplex chronicus.

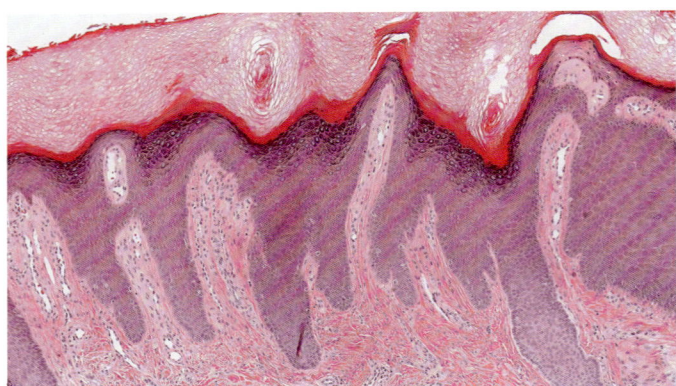

IMAGE 6.31 Lichen simplex chronicus (high magnification). In addition to the characteristic epidermal features, vertical streaking of collagen fibers, parallel to dilated capillaries, in the papillary dermis is typical of this entity.

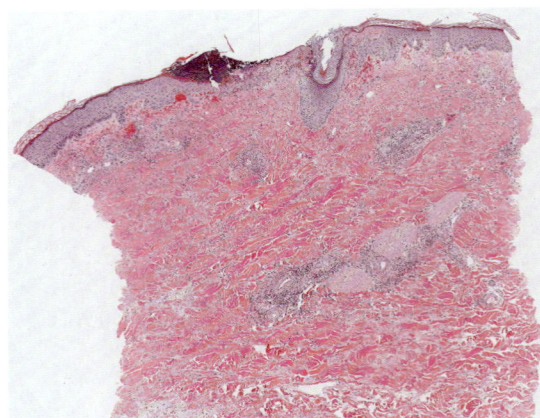

IMAGE 6.32 Leukocytoclastic vasculitis (low magnification). Angiocentric inflammation in the dermis is accompanied by interstitial hemorrhage and a focally crusted epidermis.

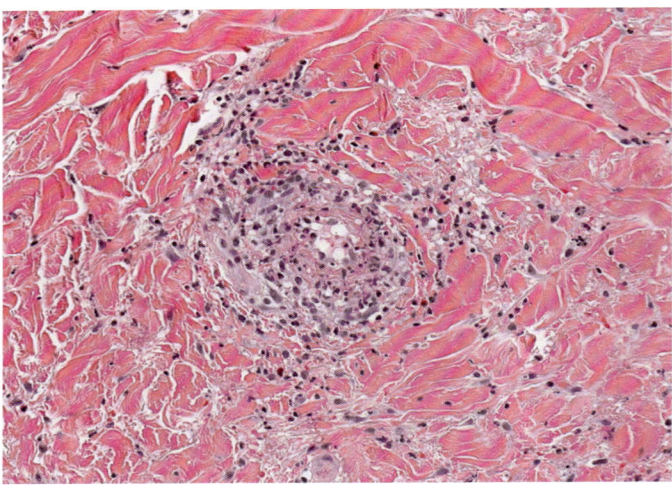

IMAGE 6.33 Leukocytoclastic vasculitis (high magnification). Neutrophils and leukocytoclastic fragments (nuclear dust) infiltrate capillary walls, which show prominent fibrinoid change.

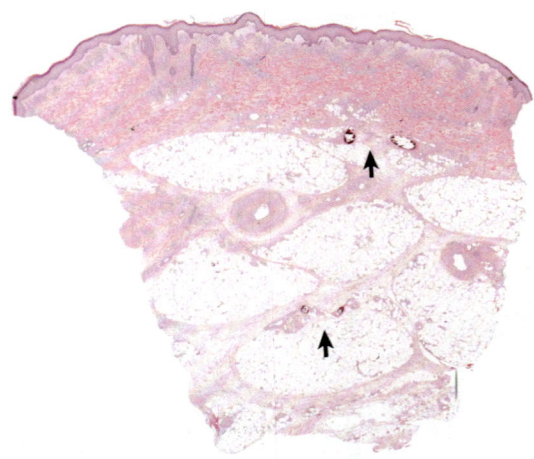

IMAGE 6.34 Calciphylaxis (low magnification). An incisional biopsy including a generous amount of subcutis is required in this setting and it reveals mural calcification of small vessels within the fat (black arrows).

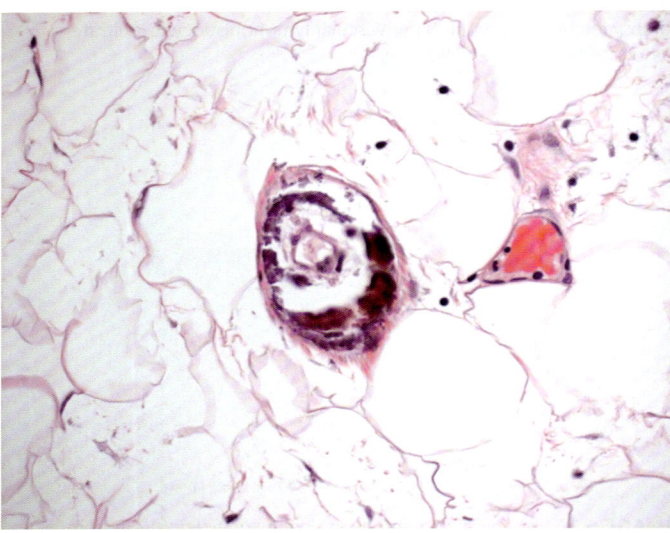

IMAGE 6.35 Calciphylaxis (high magnification). The circumferential calcification of small vessel walls, accompanied by pale or lucent intimal thickening and luminal stenosis are characteristic of calciphylaxis.

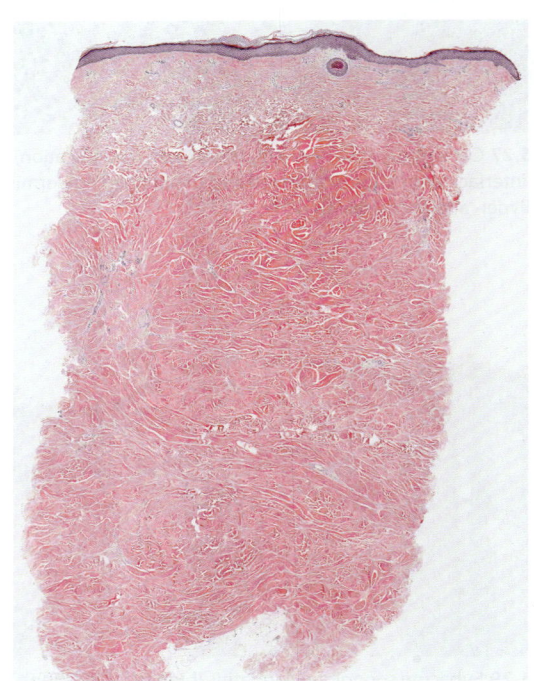

IMAGE 6.36 Morphea (low magnification). The late sclerosing phase of morphea depicted here shows a dense confluent pattern of dermal collagen, devoid of inflammation, with loss of adnexal structures. The collagen changes result in a biopsy with "square edges."

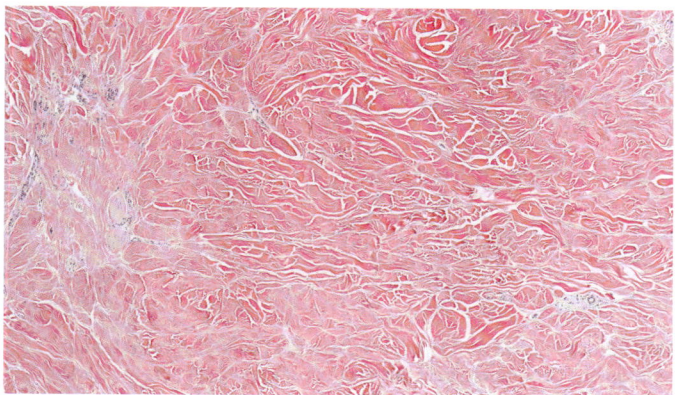

IMAGE 6.37 Morphea (high magnification). Collagen bundles in the reticular dermis are thickened and closely approximated to one another.

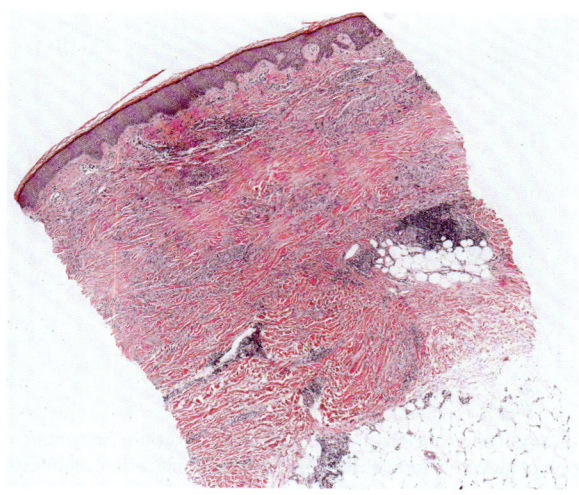

IMAGE 6.38 Necrobiosis lipoidica (low magnification). This pan-dermal process conveys a layered or tiered pattern of inflammation alternating with zones of altered collagen.

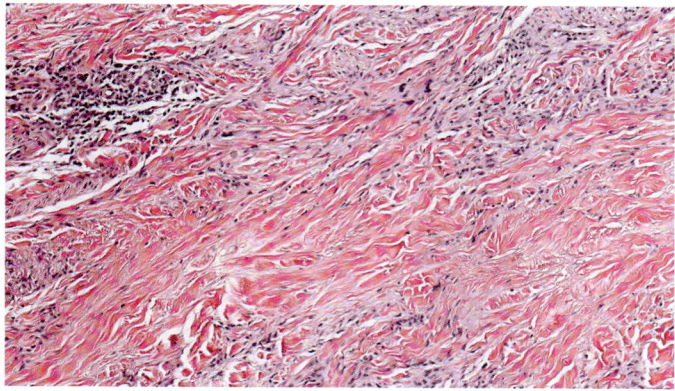

IMAGE 6.39 Necrobiosis lipoidica (high magnification). Interstitial granulomatous inflammation (with giant cells) encircles areas of altered collagen (in a vague palisaded pattern), and is accompanied by aggregates of lymphocytes and plasma cells.

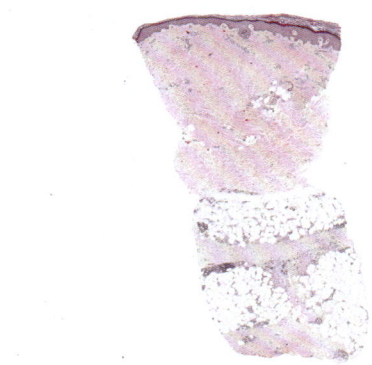

IMAGE 6.40 Erythema nodosum (low magnification). The image shows an abnormality in the subcutaneous fat characterized by septal thickening and inflammation (septal panniculitis).

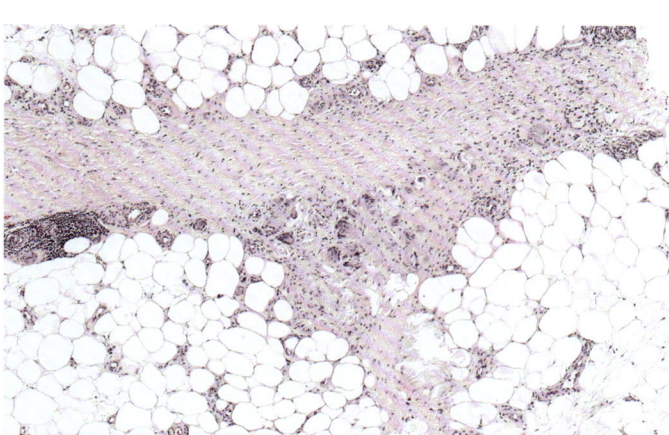

IMAGE 6.41 Erythema nodosum (high magnification). The fibrotic septal thickening is accompanied by granulomatous inflammation.

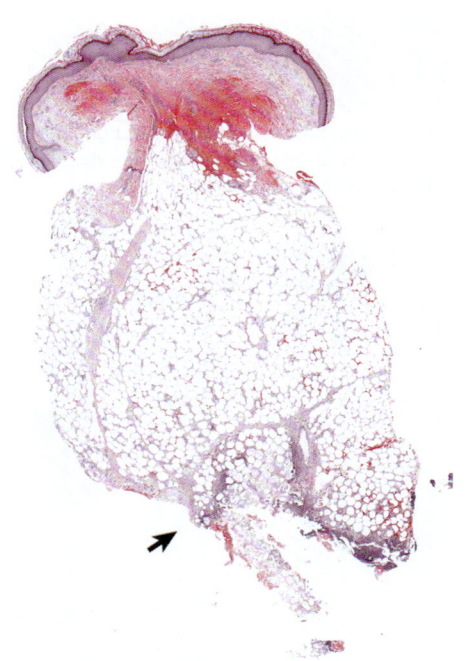

IMAGE 6.42 Pancreatic panniculitis (low magnification). Apart from the procedural artifacts superficially, the pathology lies in the deep subcutis (black arrow) and is characterized by a lobular panniculitis.

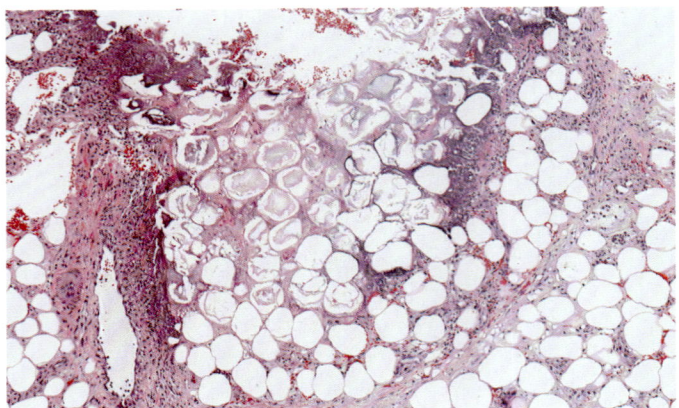

IMAGE 6.43 Pancreatic panniculitis (high magnification). Enzymatic digestion of fat within lobules has resulted in saponification, manifested by necrotic adipocytes or ghost cells (centrally) and deposition of basophilic calcium deposits (peripherally), with admixed neutrophils.

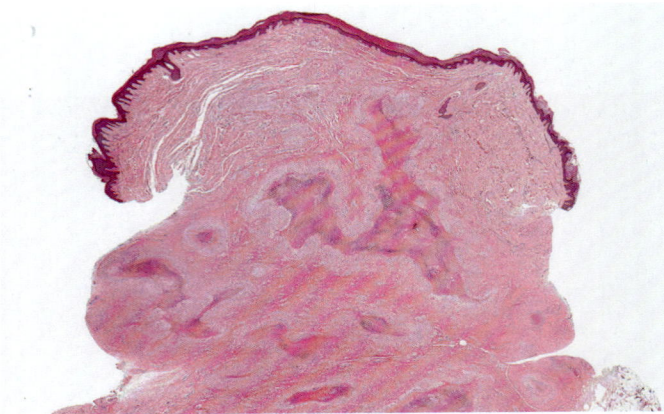

IMAGE 6.44 Rheumatoid nodule (low magnification). A collection of serpiginous geographic structures with eosinophilic centers (palisading granulomata) are observed in the deep dermis and subcutis.

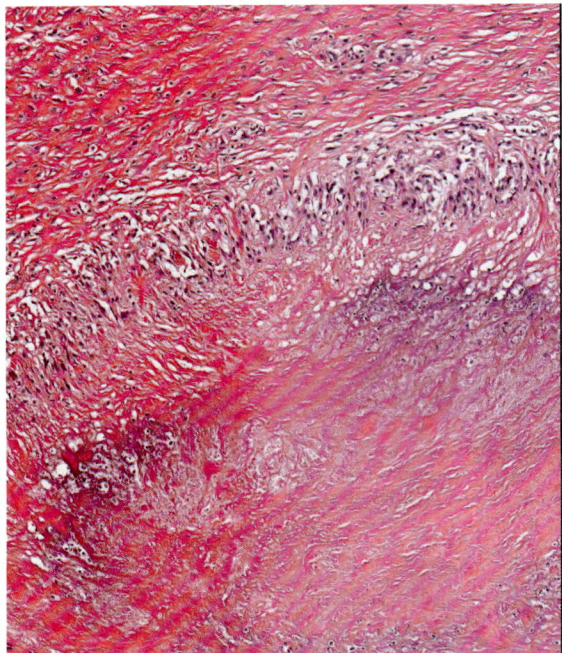

IMAGE 6.45 Rheumatoid nodule (high magnification). The periphery of the granulomata shows a rim of palisaded histiocytes and central eosinophilic amorphous fibrinous material.

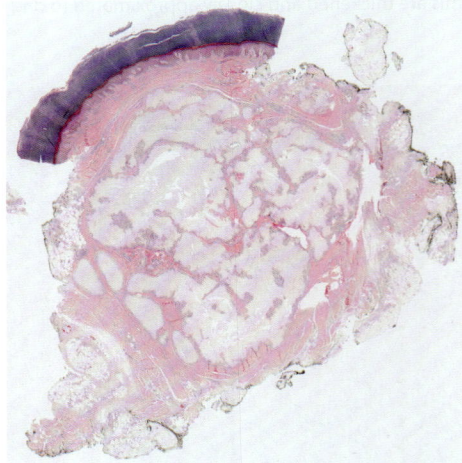

IMAGE 6.46 Gout (low magnification). Palisaded granulomatous inflammation surrounds pale amorphous material in the dermis of acral skin.

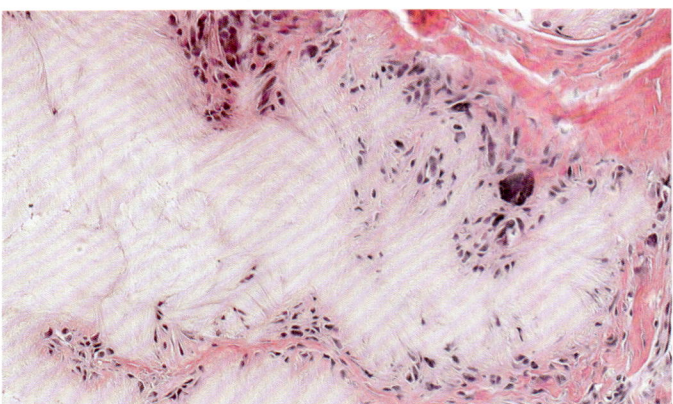

IMAGE 6.47 Gout (high magnification). The pale amorphous material represents deposits of uric acid. The prominent granulomatous response features multinucleated giant cells.

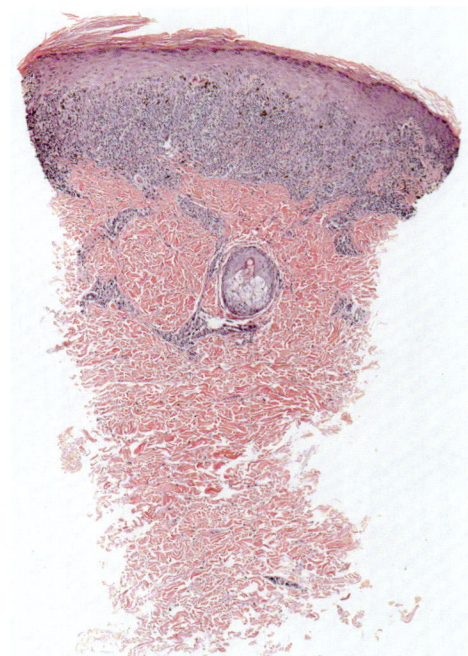

IMAGE 6.48 Lichen planus (low magnification). The biopsy shows a superficial perivascular lymphohistiocytic infiltrate with a band-like (lichenoid) pattern at the dermoepidermal junction. The interface zone is obscured and the epidermis displays hypergranulosis and hyperkeratosis.

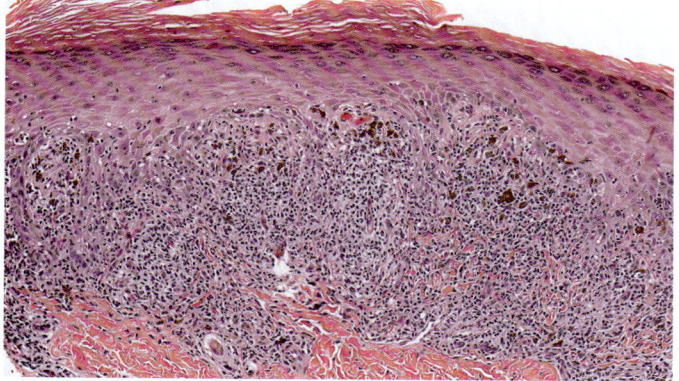

IMAGE 6.49 Lichen planus (high magnification). The epidermis shows sawtooth hyperplasia with focally wedge-shaped hypergranulosis and compact orthokeratosis. The interface inflammation is associated with apoptosis of basal keratinocytes (Civatte bodies).

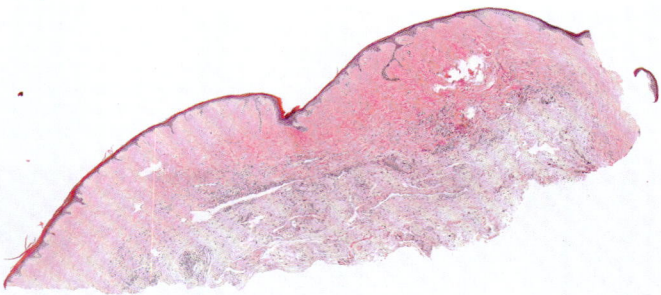

IMAGE 6.50 Lichen sclerosus (low magnification). There is expansion and replacement of the papillary dermis by hyalinized collagen beneath which a light band-like cellular infiltrate is evident.

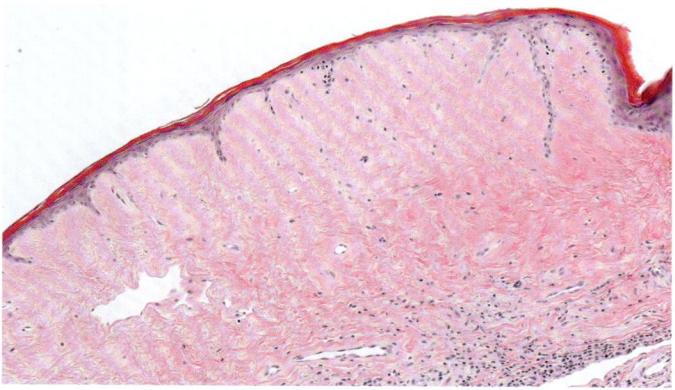

IMAGE 6.51 Lichen sclerosus (medium magnification). Overlying the zone of homogenous dermal sclerosis, epidermal atrophy with compact orthokeratosis is seen. The underlying inflammatory infiltrate consists of lymphocytes and plasma cells.

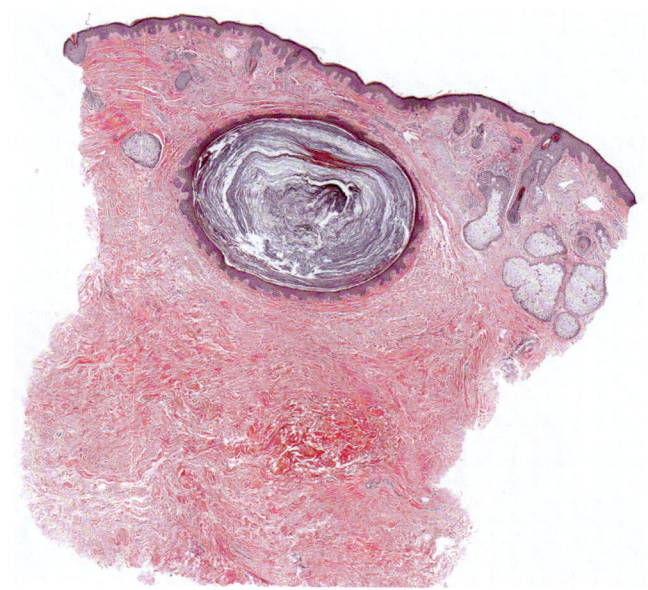

IMAGE 6.52 Epidermal (infundibular) cyst (low magnification). The unilocular, squamous-lined cyst contains abundant laminated keratin.

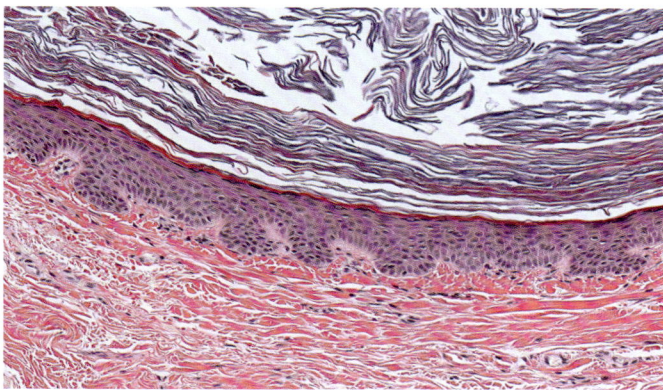

IMAGE 6.53 Epidermal (infundibular) cyst (high magnification). The squamous lining resembles normal epidermis (which has the same features as infundibular epithelium) with a granular layer.

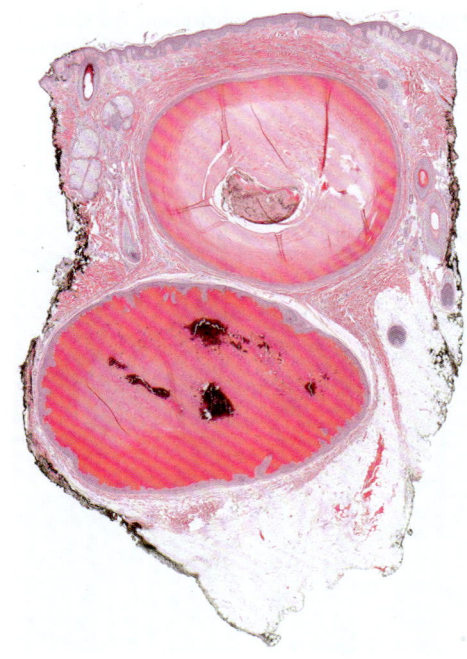

IMAGE 6.54 Trichilemmal (pilar) cysts (low magnification). The squamous-lined cysts contain homogeneous eosinophilic keratin with central calcifications.

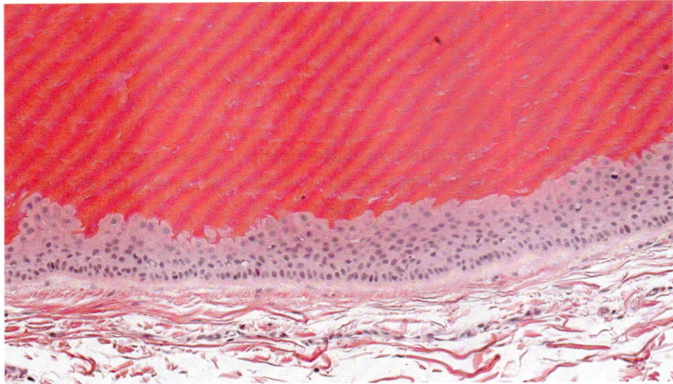

IMAGE 6.55 Trichilemmal (pilar) cyst (high magnification). The squamous lining demonstrates trichilemmal keratinization (plump, bloated cells gradually merging with luminal keratin) without a granular layer.

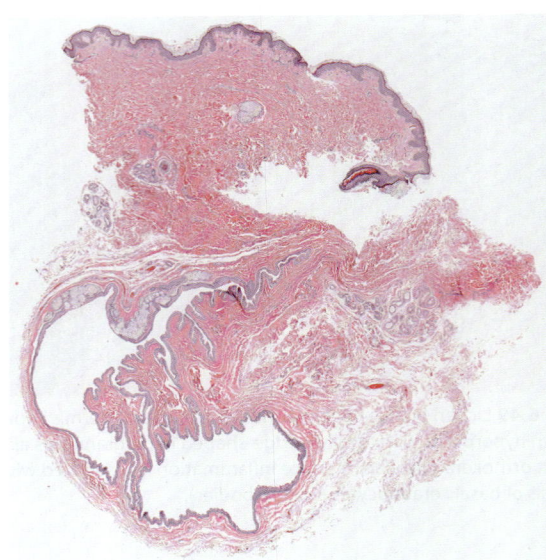

IMAGE 6.56 Steatocystoma (low magnification). The squamous-lined cyst features sebaceous lobules in its wall and the lumen is empty.

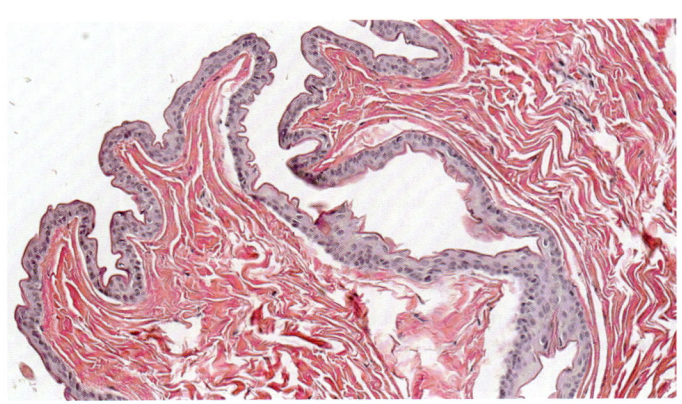

IMAGE 6.57 Steatocystoma (high magnification). The squamous lining exhibits a crenulated, eosinophilic cuticle on the luminal aspect, resembling that seen in the sebaceous duct.

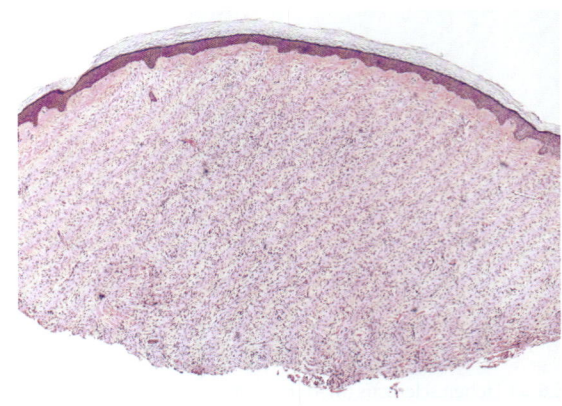

IMAGE 6.58 Neurofibroma (low magnification). A poorly circumscribed dermal nodule is observed.

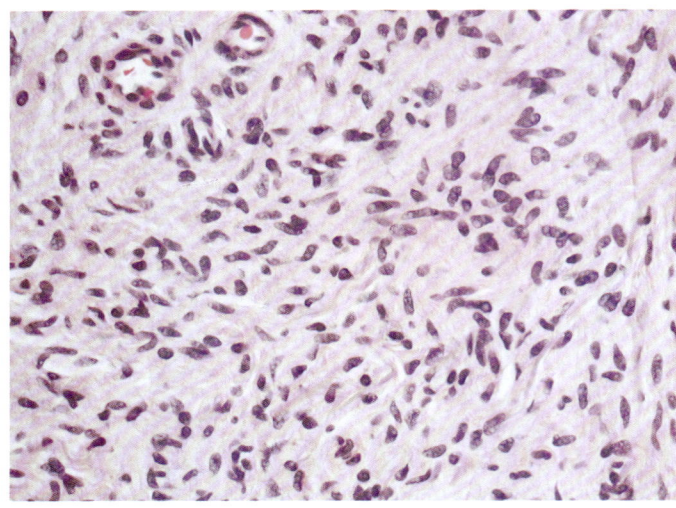

IMAGE 6.59 Neurofibroma (high magnification). The constituent spindle-shaped cells show "wavy" nuclei.

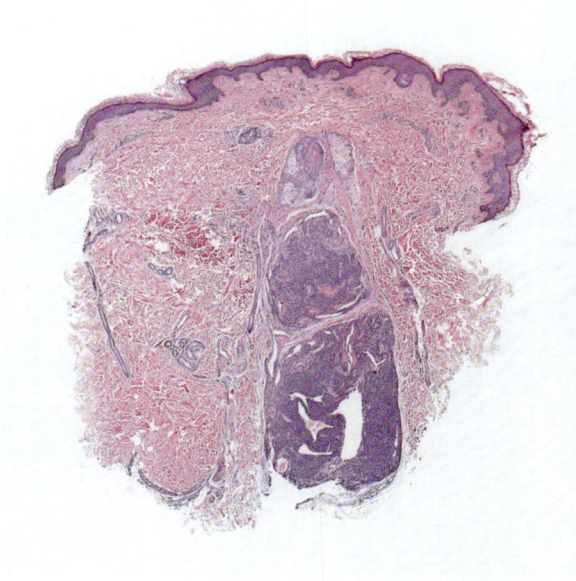

IMAGE 6.60 Glomus tumor (low magnification). A circumscribed, cellular, dermal tumor incorporates elongated (vascular) spaces.

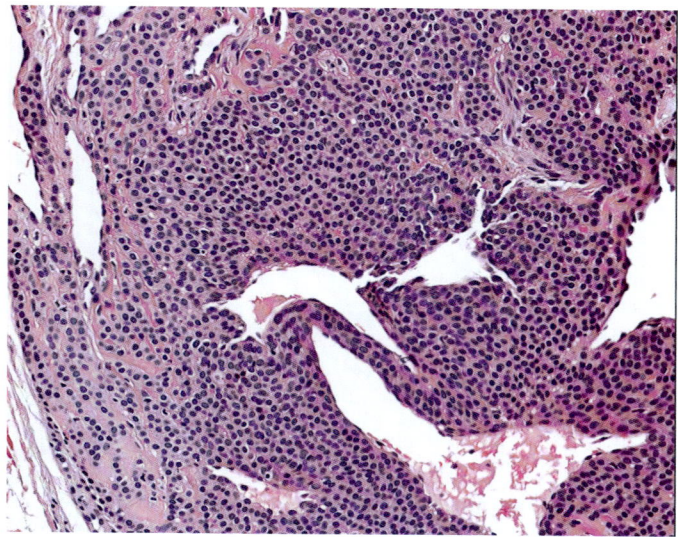

IMAGE 6.61 Glomus tumor (high magnification). The strikingly monomorphous epithelioid lesional cells (glomus cells) intimately surround vascular spaces.

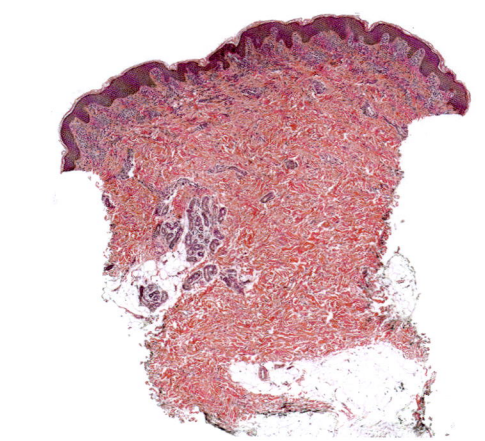

IMAGE 6.62 Urticaria pigmentosa (low magnification). A superficial perivascular and interstitial cellular infiltrate occupies the papillary dermis.

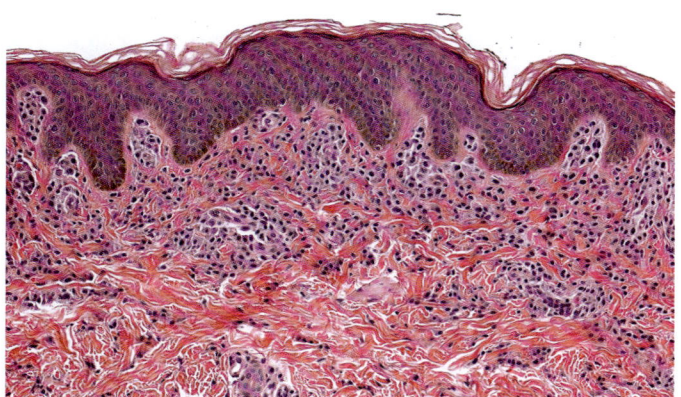

IMAGE 6.63 Urticaria pigmentosa (high magnification). The infiltrate is composed of a monomorphous population of mast cells with uniform round nuclei and gray cytoplasm (fried egg appearance). The overlying epidermis displays basal hyperpigmentation.

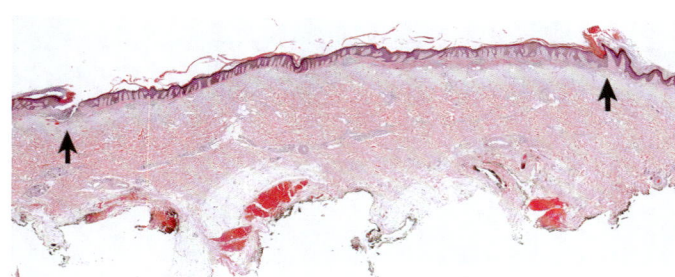

IMAGE 6.64 Porokeratosis (low magnification). At the periphery of this flat lesion, 2 "pillars" of keratin (cornoid lamellae) (black arrows) are seen to emanate from the surface, yielding a clue to the diagnosis.

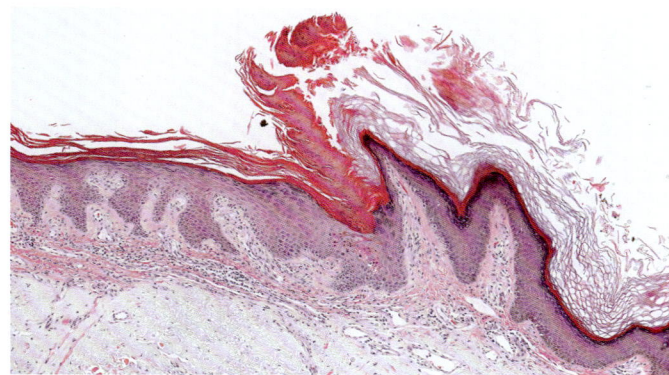

IMAGE 6.65 Porokeratosis (high magnification). This peripheral cornoid lamella consists of a pillar of parakeratin, which leans toward the center of the lesion and arises from an invaginated epidermis showing dyskeratotic keratinocytes and hypogranulosis.

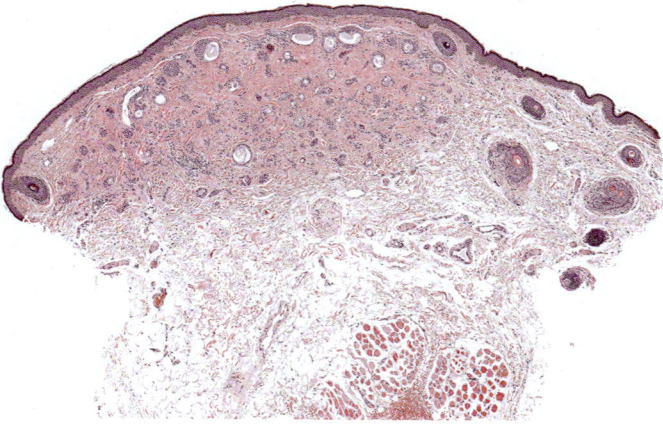

IMAGE 6.66 Syringoma (low magnification). A discrete, superficial, dome-shaped dermal papule is composed of ductal epithelial elements within a sclerotic stroma.

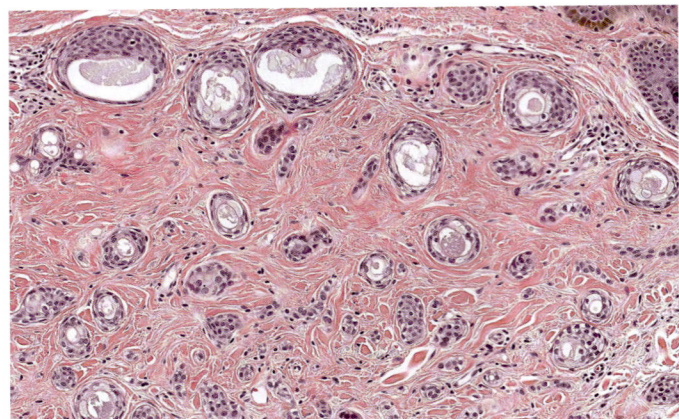

IMAGE 6.67 Syringoma (high magnification). The benign ductal elements (which sometime display a comma-shaped appearance) and a few cords of epithelial cells are present in a dense collagenous background.

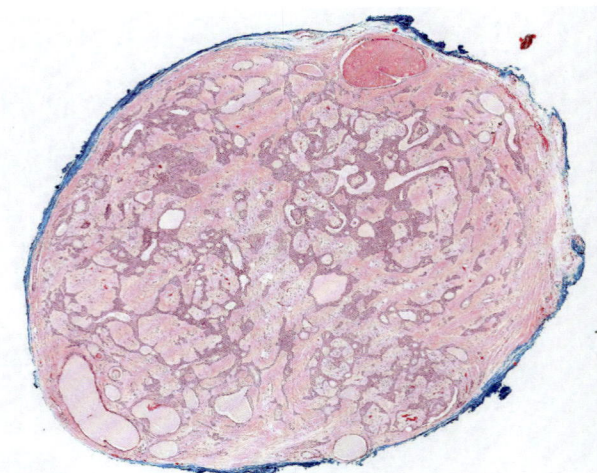

IMAGE 6.68 Benign mixed tumor (folliculo/sebaceous/apocrine-type) (low magnification). A circumscribed nodule is composed of a complex branching array of trabecular, ductal, and cystic epithelial elements embedded in a myxoid and fibrotic stroma.

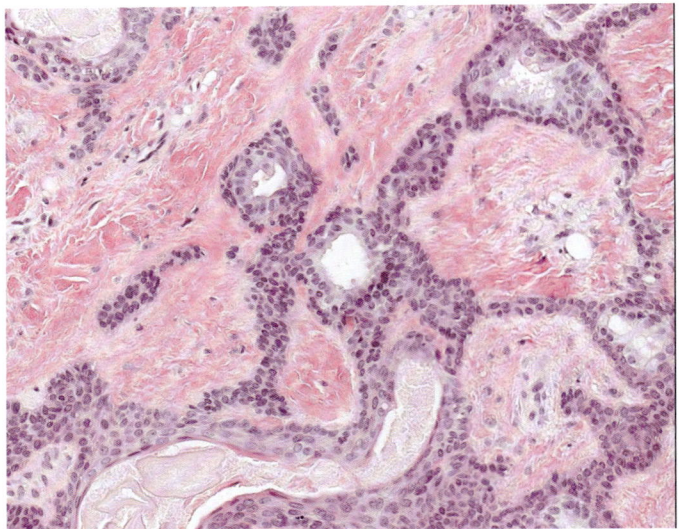

IMAGE 6.69 Benign mixed tumor (folliculo/sebaceous/apocrine-type) (high magnification). Ducts lined by apocrine-type epithelium (with apocrine snouts) connect with a squamous epithelial-lined (infundibular) structure.

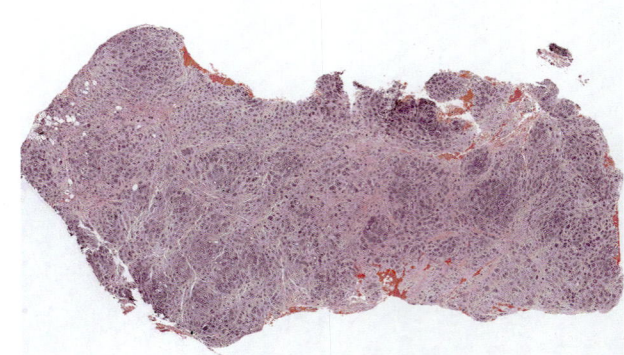

IMAGE 6.70 Benign mixed tumor (eccrine type) (low magnification). A circumscribed, lobulated, grayish nodule has "shelled out" of surrounding tissue.

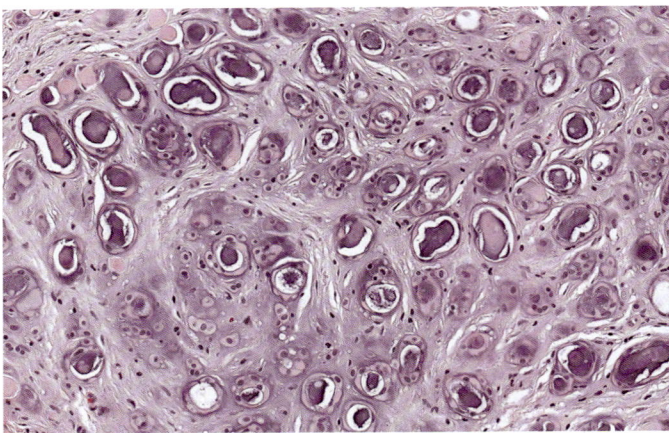

IMAGE 6.71 Benign mixed tumor (eccrine type) (high magnification). The tumor is composed of simple benign ducts containing luminal mucin, embedded in a myxoid stroma.

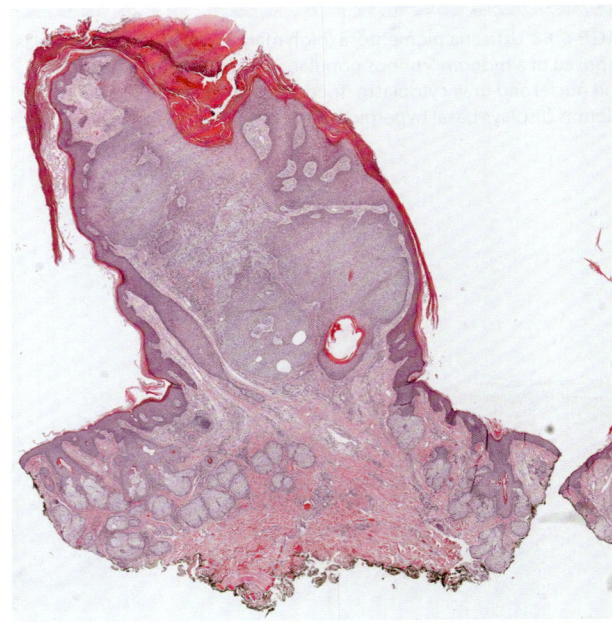

IMAGE 6.72 Desmoplastic trichilemmoma (low magnification). This exophytic, verrucous, crusted papule displays circumscribed lobules of pale cells in its core.

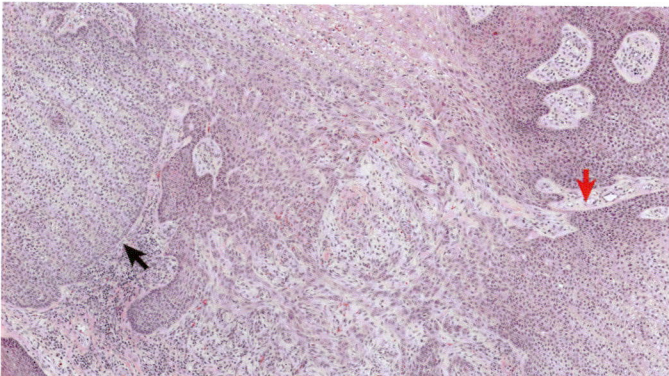

IMAGE 6.73 Desmoplastic trichilemmoma (medium magnification). The lobules are composed of pale vacuolated keratinocytes with peripheral nuclear palisading (black arrow) and a surrounding thickened basement membrane (red arrow). The lobular architecture is disrupted centrally and replaced by a pseudoinfiltrative pattern of lesional cells in a desmoplastic stroma. This feature (likely due to trauma) can lead to a mistaken diagnosis of invasive carcinoma.

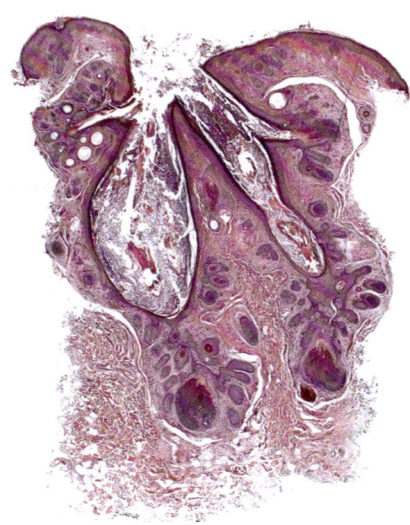

IMAGE 6.74 Trichofolliculoma (low magnification). The typical architecture of this tumor is evident and characterized by 1 or 2 central dilated follicular infundibular structures, from the walls of which radiate multiple small (vellus-type) follicles ("the pig and the piglets").

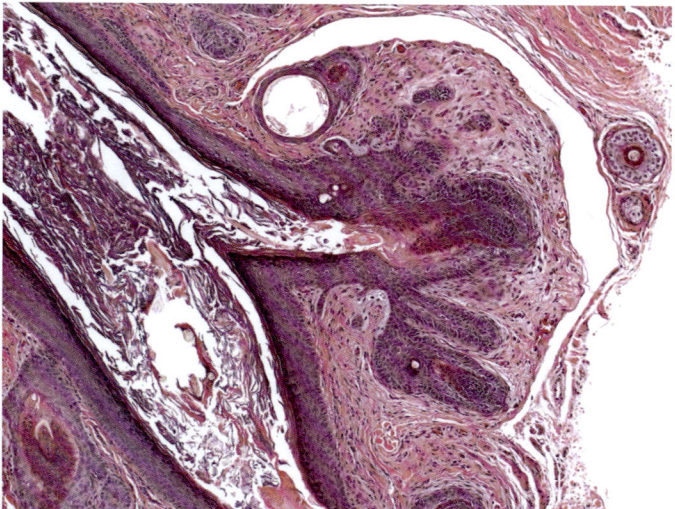

IMAGE 6.75 Trichofolliculoma (high magnification). A cluster of vellus-type follicles connected to the central infundibulum is surrounded by stroma reminiscent of the perifollicular connective tissue sheath.

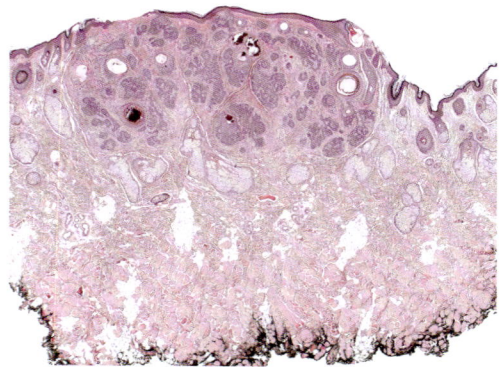

IMAGE 6.76 Trichoepithelioma (low magnification). This low-domed dermal papule represents a lobulated basaloid epithelial tumor with a substantial stromal component. Infundibular cysts, some calcified, are admixed with aggregations of basaloid epithelial cells displaying a "fenestrated" appearance.

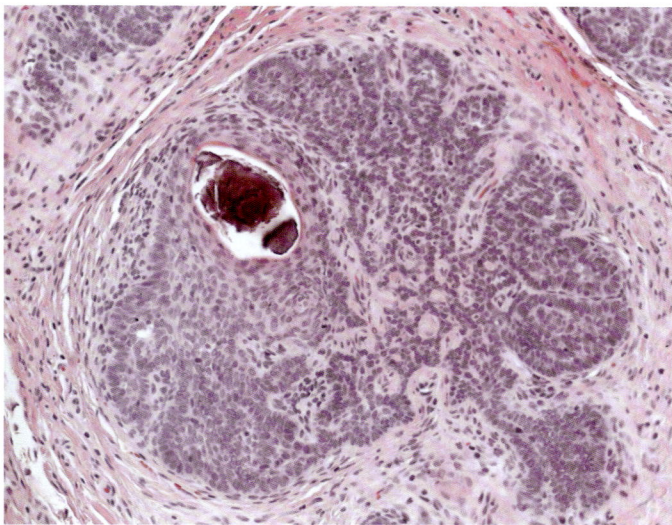

IMAGE 6.77 Trichoepithelioma (high magnification). The "fenestrated" pattern of basaloid cells is evident, with peripheral nuclear palisading and an accompanying cellular stroma reminiscent of follicular papillary mesenchyme. Calcifications are common.

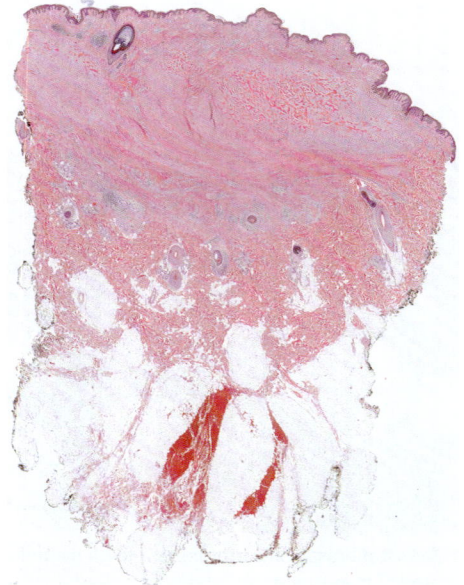

IMAGE 6.78 Keloid (low magnification). An ill-defined, paucicellular nodule occupies the upper half of the dermis.

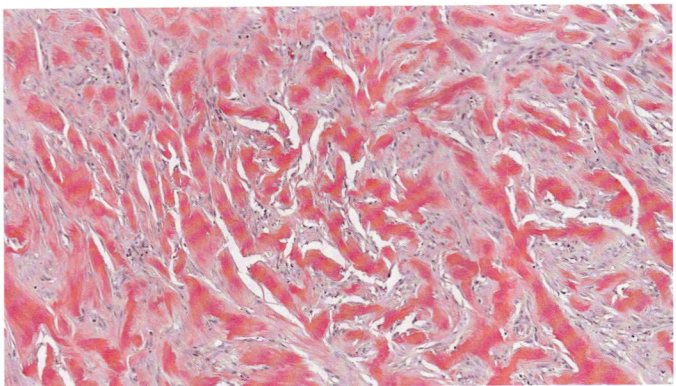

IMAGE 6.79 Keloid (high magnification). The nodule is composed of haphazardly arranged bundles of thickened, hypereosinophilic, "glassy" collagen (keloidal collagen) dispersed in a fibroblastic stroma.

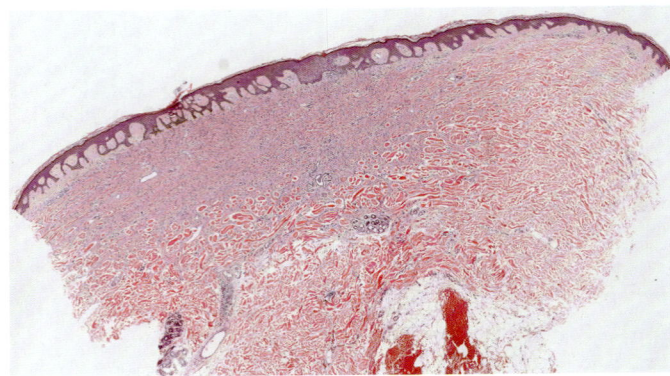

IMAGE 6.80 Dermatofibroma (low magnification). The lesion is characterized by a poorly circumscribed, cellular nodule in the dermis, with trapping of thick collagen bundles at the periphery and overlying epidermal hyperplasia.

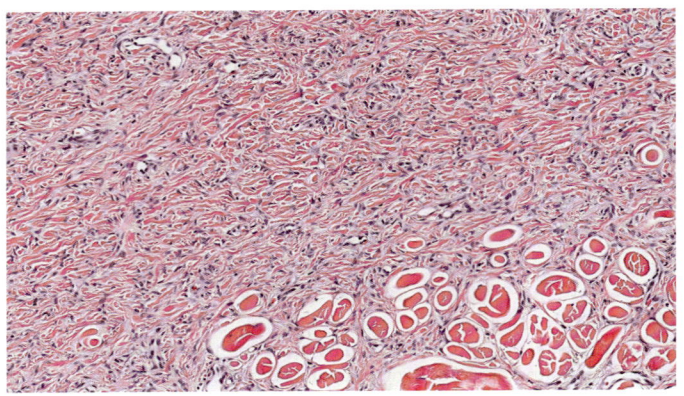

IMAGE 6.81 Dermatofibroma (high magnification). The bland spindled lesional cells are arranged in a vaguely storiform pattern and exhibit trapping of thick collagen bundles at the periphery.

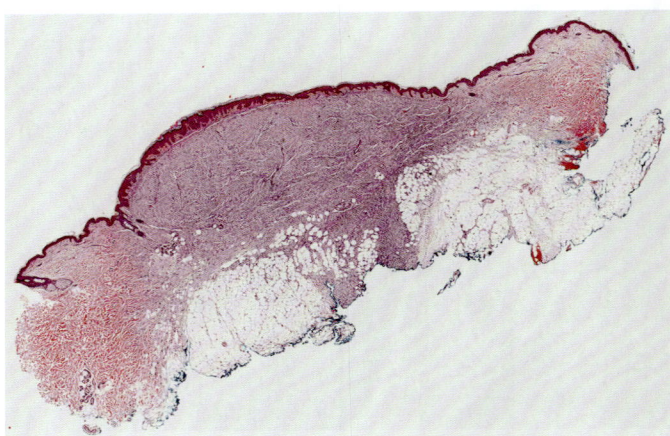

IMAGE 6.82 Dermatofibrosarcoma protuberans (low magnification). The image shows a poorly circumscribed cellular nodule expanding the dermis with lacelike pattern involvement of the subcutaneous fat.

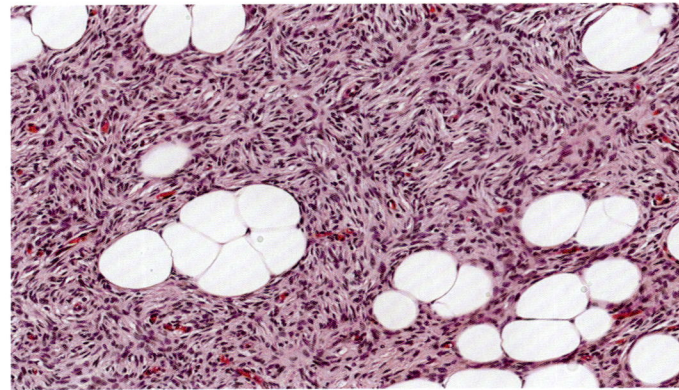

IMAGE 6.83 Dermatofibrosarcoma protuberans (high magnification). The lesion is composed of bland, monomorphous, spindle-shaped cells, which often display a storiform pattern. They surround and entrap adipocytes in the subcutis in a lacelike pattern.

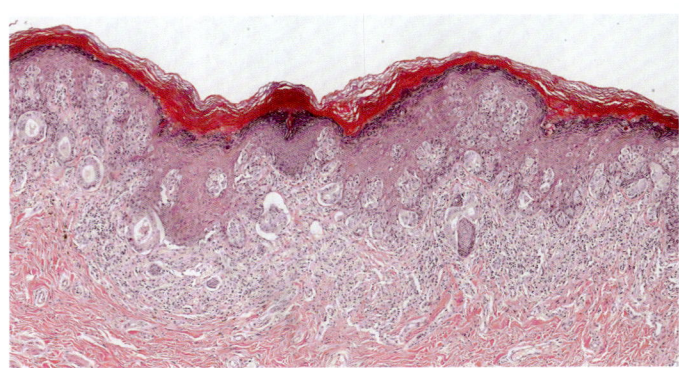

IMAGE 6.84 Paget disease (low magnification). There is a prominent intraepidermal proliferation of pale cells arranged as single cells and nests, with focal gland formation.

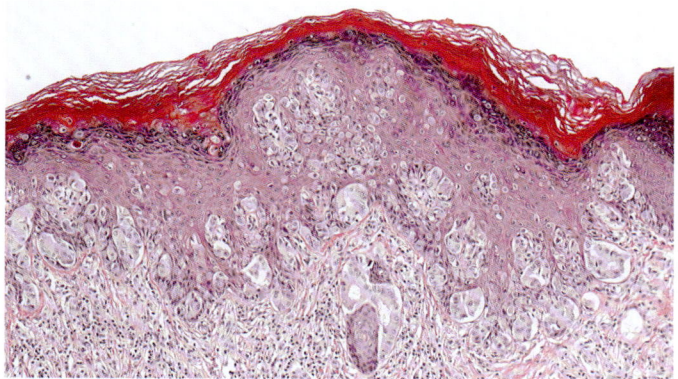

IMAGE 6.85 Paget disease (medium magnification). Atypical, pale, epithelioid cells are scattered in a pagetoid pattern among epidermal keratinocytes and focally form glandular acini (the latter helping to distinguish this process from melanoma in situ and pagetoid Bowen disease).

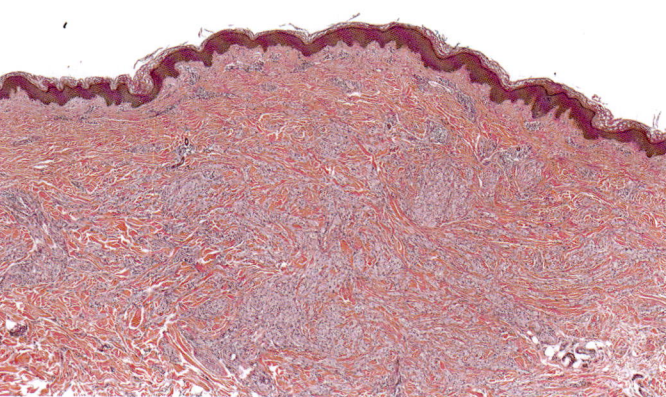

IMAGE 6.86 Granular cell tumor (low magnification). A poorly circumscribed, confluent proliferation of pale cells occupies the upper dermis.

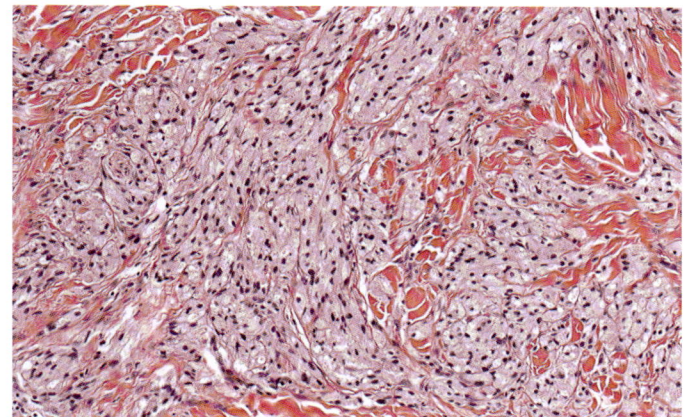

IMAGE 6.87 Granular cell tumor (high magnification). The large "histiocytoid" lesional cells (modified Schwann cells) display relatively small nuclei and abundant cytoplasm containing eosinophilic granules.

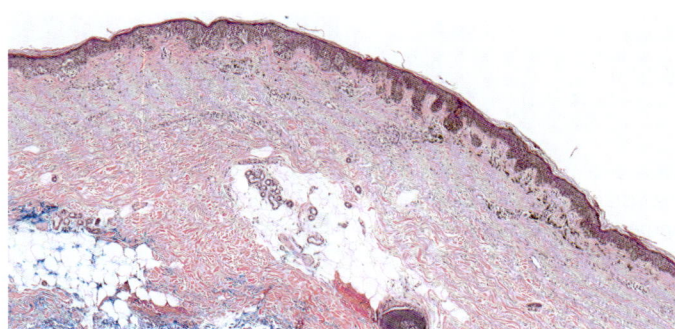

IMAGE 6.88 Melanoma in situ (low magnification). A broad, ill-defined, junctional proliferation of melanocytes is observed in sun-damaged skin. The distribution of nests is uneven and contiguous with zones where single cells predominate.

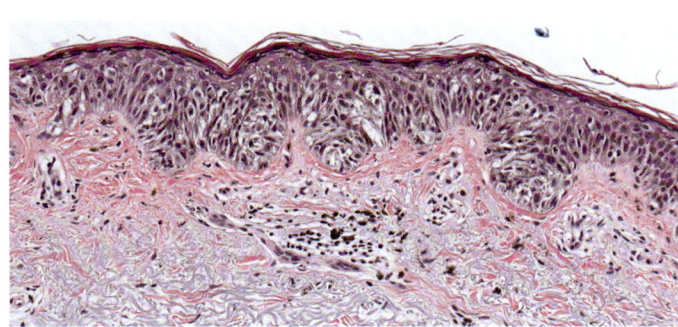

IMAGE 6.89 Melanoma in situ (high magnification). The junctional melanocytic proliferation is florid, disorganized and features large melanocytes in pagetoid pattern at all levels of the epidermis.

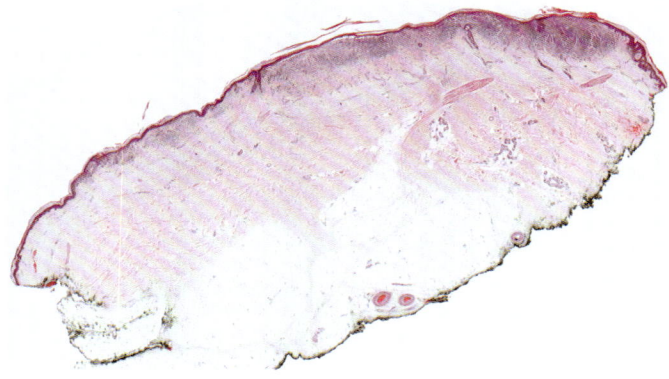

IMAGE 6.90 Malignant melanoma (low magnification). This broad, asymmetrical, variably cellular proliferation of melanocytes on sun-damaged skin exhibits architectural features of a malignant melanoma.

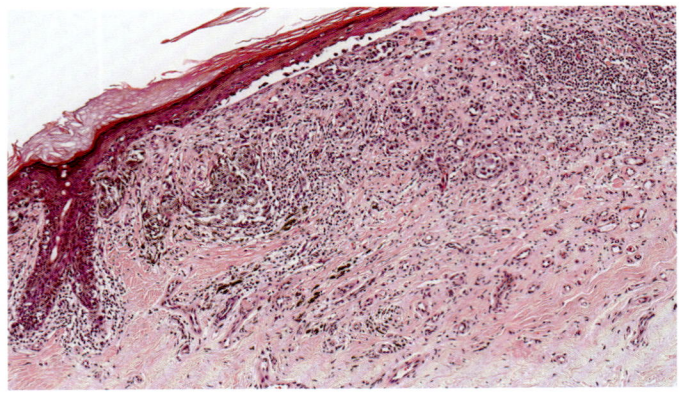

IMAGE 6.91 Malignant melanoma (medium magnification). The melanoma, with in situ and invasive components (best seen on the left), exhibits confluent cleft formation at the junction (a clue to melanoma) and is associated with regressive changes in the dermis (lymphocytic infiltrate, fibrosis, hypervascularity).

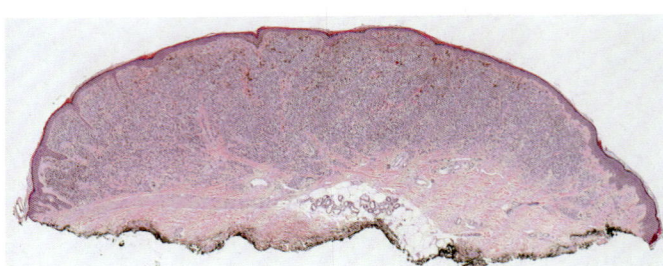

IMAGE 6.92 Nevoid malignant melanoma (low magnification). Although the dome-shaped architecture of this melanocytic lesion conveys an impression of benignancy, the sheetlike distribution of lesional cells in the dermis should raise the suspicion of melanoma.

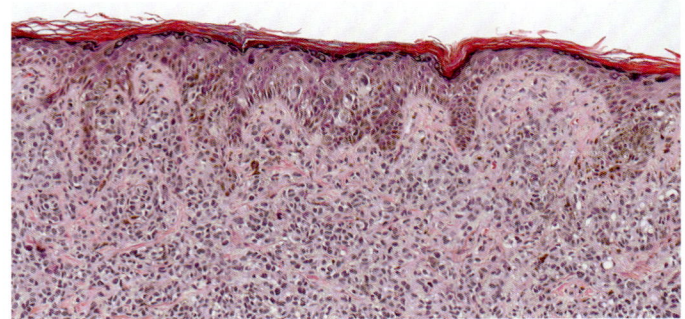

IMAGE 6.93 Nevoid malignant melanoma (medium magnification). Close inspection reveals a disorganized junctional proliferation of plump, atypical melanocytes indicative of melanoma in situ.

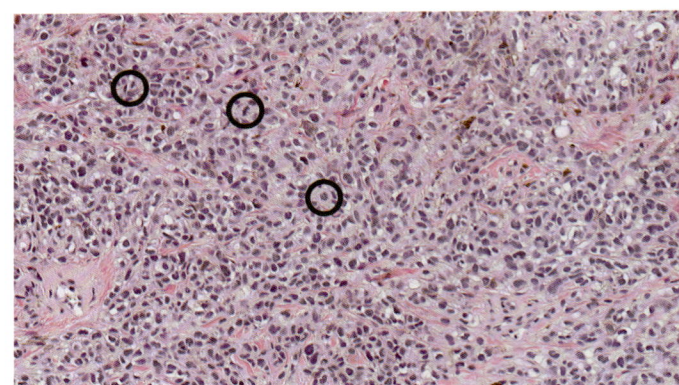

IMAGE 6.94 Nevoid malignant melanoma (high magnification). The dermal melanocytes, though relatively monomorphous, are atypical, with scattered mitotic figures (black circles) and show limited maturation with descent.

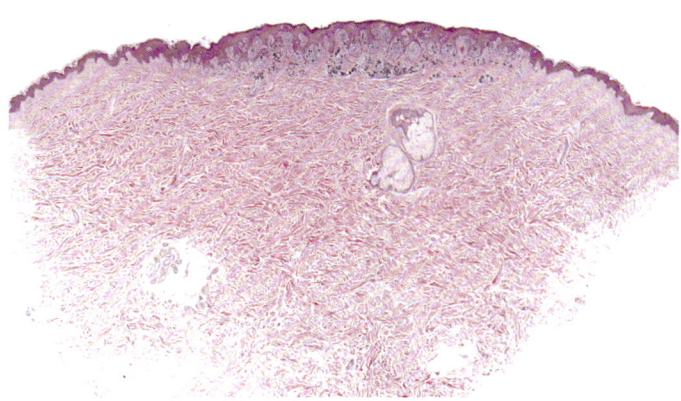

IMAGE 6.95 Spitz nevus (low magnification). This compound melanocytic neoplasm is small, symmetrical and well circumscribed, exhibiting the typical architecture of a nevus.

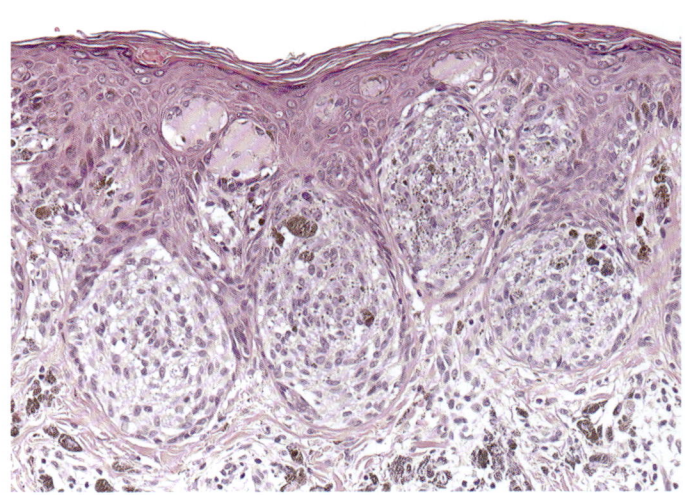

IMAGE 6.96 Spitz nevus (high magnification). Vertically oriented nests of plump spindle-shaped melanocytes are seen at the dermoepidermal junction and pink Kamino bodies are evident in the epidermis.

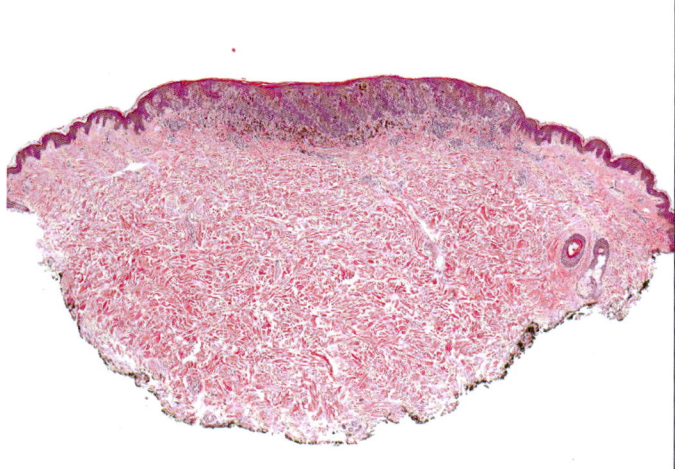

IMAGE 6.97 Spitz nevus (pigmented spindle cell variant/Reed nevus) (low magnification). This compound melanocytic neoplasm is small, symmetrical, and well circumscribed (i.e., exhibiting architectural features of a nevus).

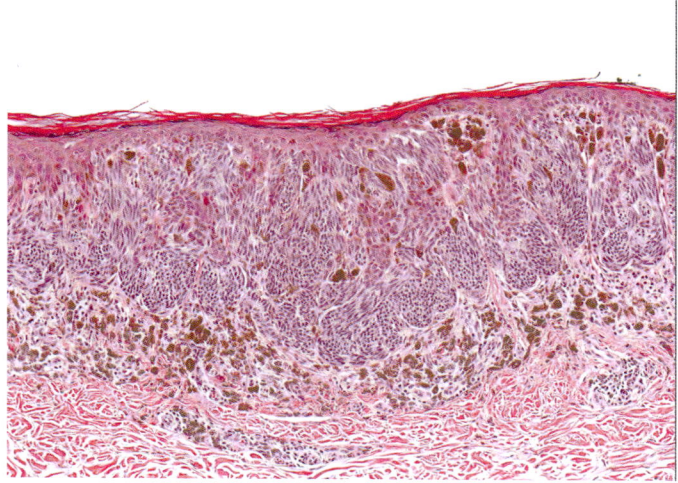

IMAGE 6.98 Spitz nevus (pigmented spindle cell variant/Reed nevus) (high magnification). Vertically oriented nests of spindled pigmented melanocytes at the dermoepidermal junction are seen to merge with smaller melanocytes in the papillary dermis, reflecting maturation with descent. There are abundant melanophages at the base.

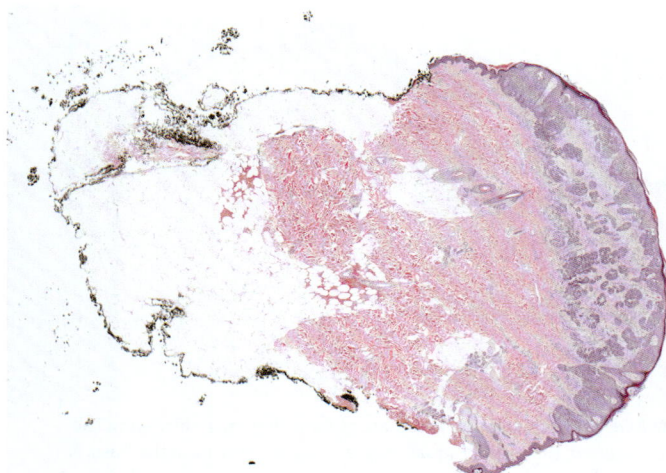

IMAGE 6.99 Spitz nevus with *NTRK1* gene fusion (low magnification). This small, symmetrical, well-circumscribed, melanocytic lesion, with junctional and dermal components, displays the typical architecture of a compound Spitz nevus.

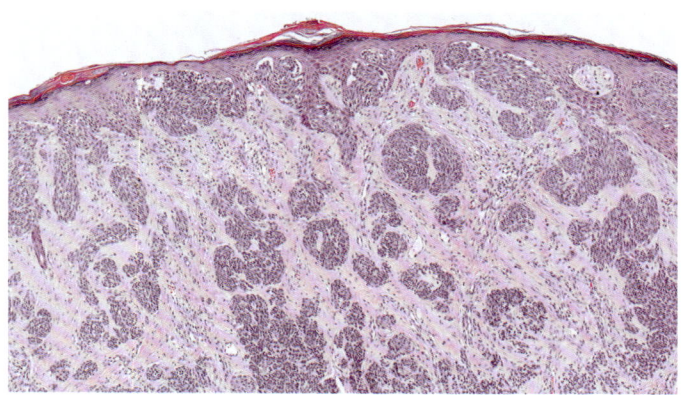

IMAGE 6.100 Spitz nevus with *NTRK1* gene fusion (medium magnification). Melanocytes are arranged as large nests and short fascicles.

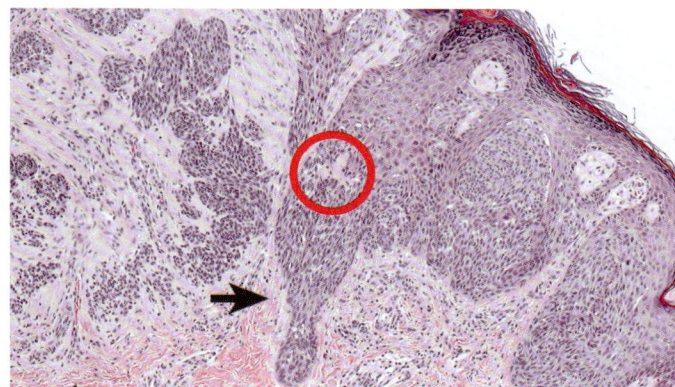

IMAGE 6.101 Spitz nevus with *NTRK1* gene fusion (medium magnification). Adnexal extension (black arrow) and Kamino bodies (red circle) are common features.

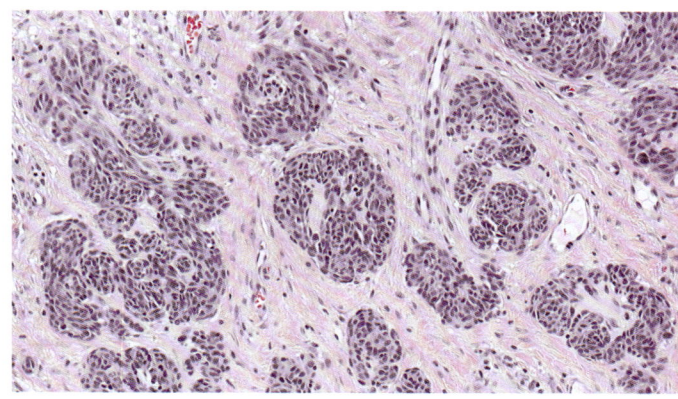

IMAGE 6.102 Spitz nevus with *NTRK1* gene fusion (high magnification). Constituent melanocytes are plump and epithelioid-to-spindled in shape.

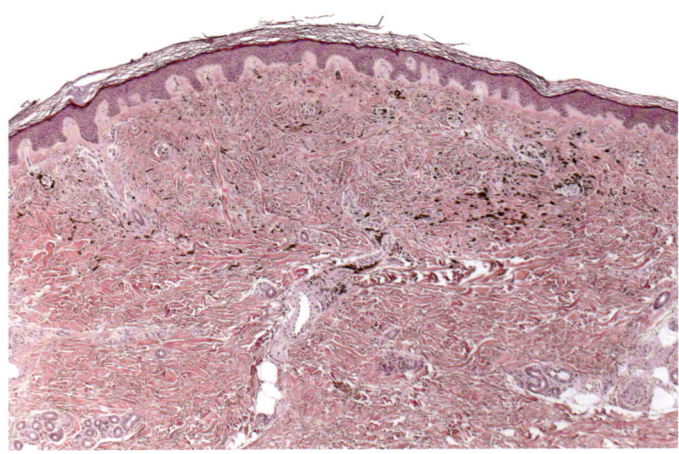

IMAGE 6.103 Common blue nevus (low magnification). The lesion is characterized by a low-domed dermal papule composed of pigmented cells.

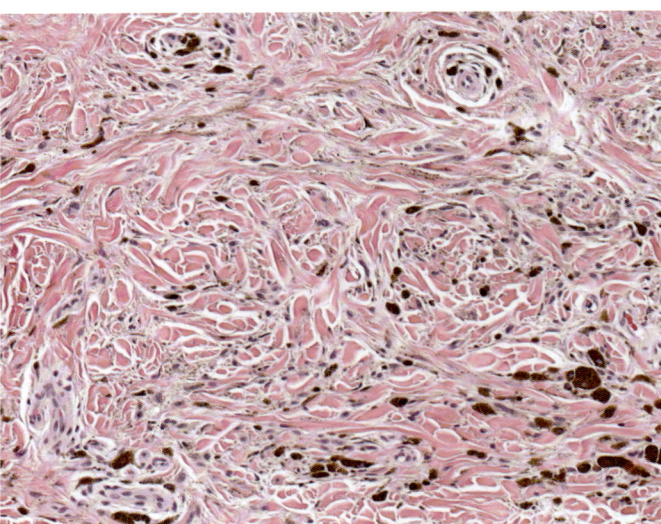

IMAGE 6.104 Common blue nevus (high magnification). An interstitial proliferation of lightly pigmented dendritic melanocytes is accompanied by heavily pigmented melanophages.

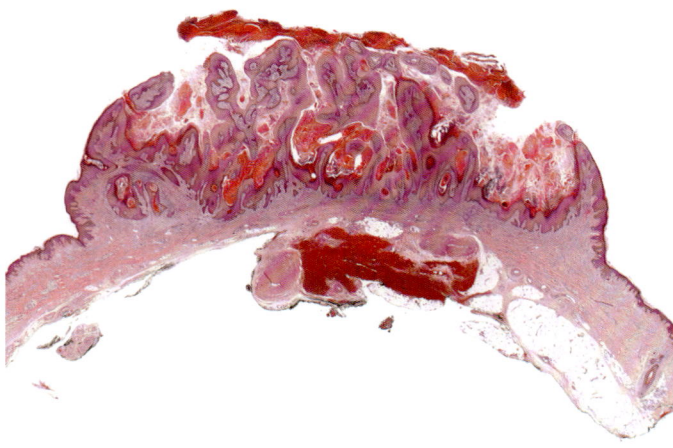

IMAGE 6.105 Established keratoacanthoma (low magnification). This crateriform, exo/endophytic proliferative squamous lesion (with papillomatosis and hyperkeratosis in its core) characterizes a mature keratoacanthoma.

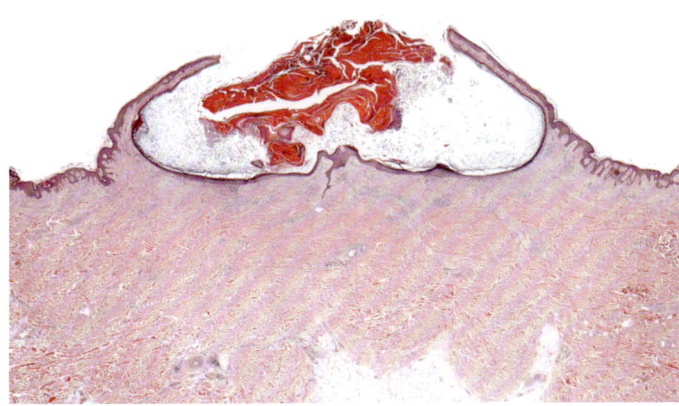

IMAGE 6.106 Involuting keratoacanthoma (low magnification). The cup-shaped, thin walled squamous lesion, with fibrosis at the base, is characteristic of the late (involutional) phase of a keratoacanthoma.

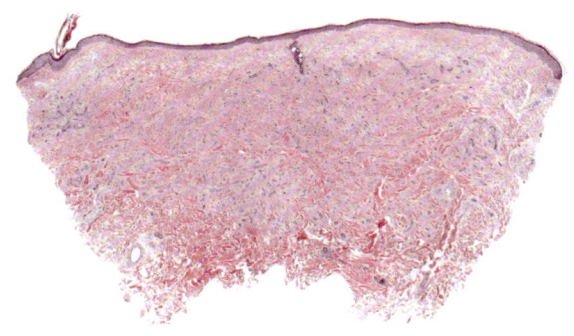

IMAGE 6.107 Basal cell carcinoma, morpheaform pattern (low magnification). A poorly circumscribed, interstitial infiltrate of epithelial cells occupies the dermis.

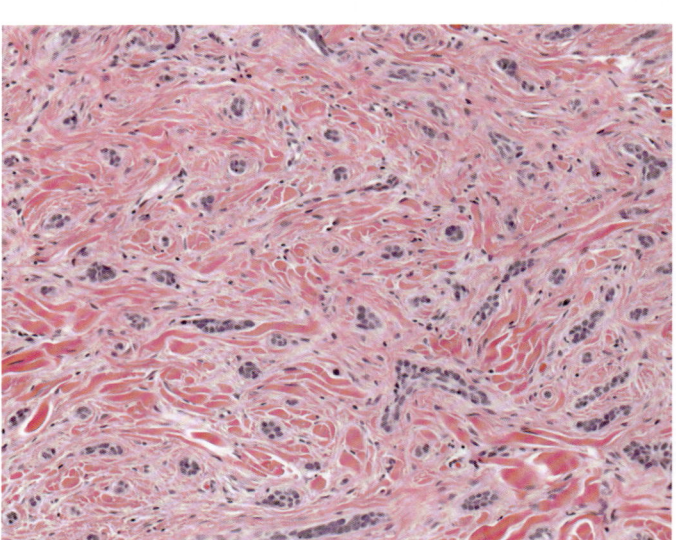

IMAGE 6.108 Basal cell carcinoma, morpheaform pattern (high magnification). The slender cords, trabeculae, and small nests of basaloid cells are embedded in a fibrotic stroma.

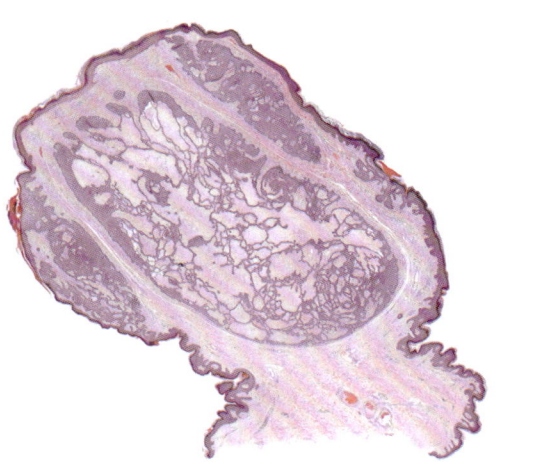

IMAGE 6.109 Basal cell carcinoma, fibroepithelial variant (fibroepithelioma of Pinkus) (low magnification). The typically polypoid architecture of the tumor is evident and its "fenestrated" proliferation of basaloid epithelium focally emanates from the base of the epidermis.

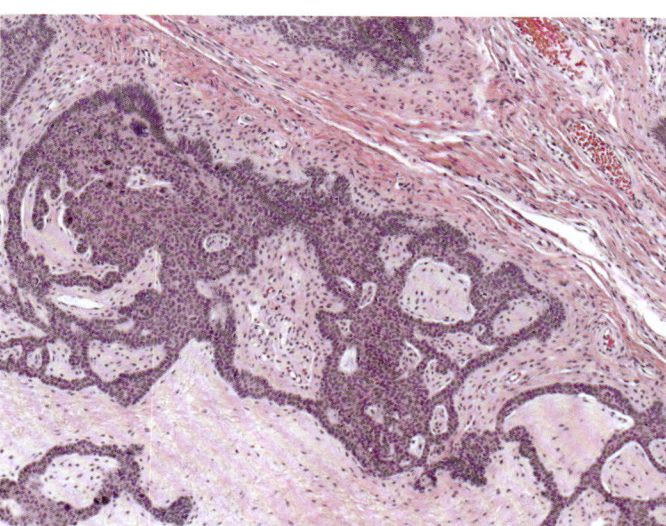

IMAGE 6.110 Basal cell carcinoma, fibroepithelial variant (fibroepithelioma of Pinkus) (medium magnification). The basaloid epithelium shows peripheral palisading and it is surrounded by a cellular stroma that mimics the papillary mesenchyme of a hair follicle.

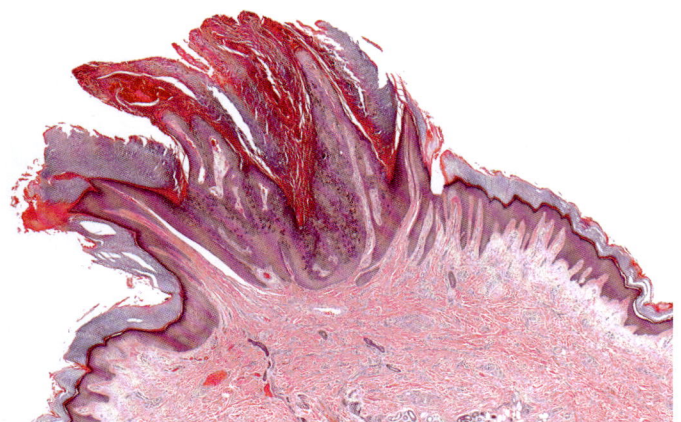

IMAGE 6.111 Verruca vulgaris (low magnification). This raised, papillomatous lesion features "in bending" of rete pegs at the base. Marked hyperkeratosis, parakeratosis, and hemorrhage surmount the papillomatous projections.

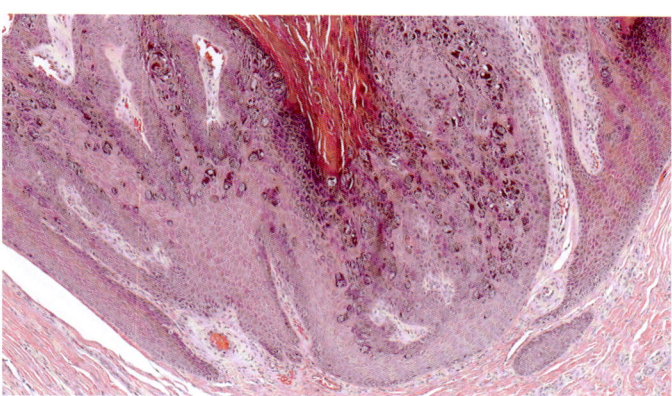

IMAGE 6.112 Verruca vulgaris (high magnification). A prominent granular cell layer, and vacuolated keratinocytes with enlarged and irregular keratohyalin granules (koilocytes,) are evident. There are dilated vessels in the dermal papillae.

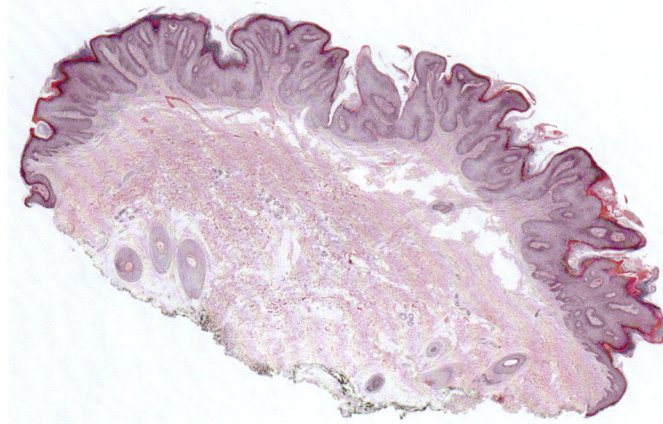

IMAGE 6.113 Condyloma acuminatum (low magnification). This type of HPV-related wart on genital skin typically displays a broad, mamillated silhouette.

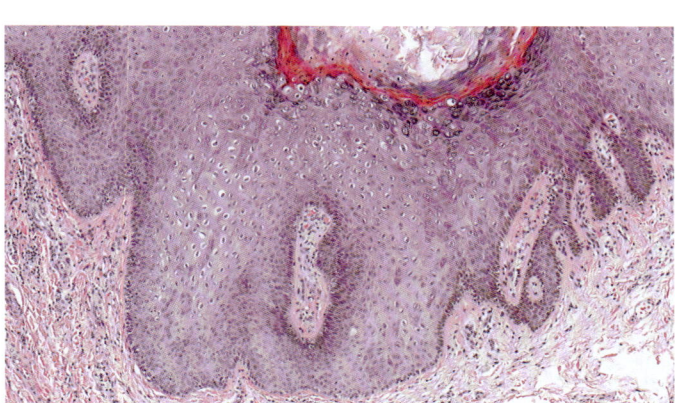

IMAGE 6.114 Condyloma acuminatum (high magnification). The hyperplastic epidermis displays characteristic vacuolated keratinocytes (koilocytes), hypergranulosis, hyperkeratosis, and parakeratosis.

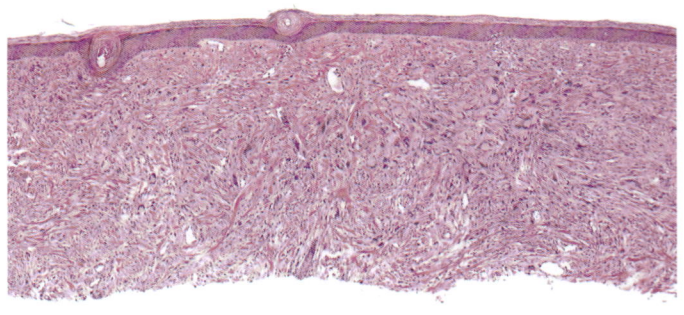

IMAGE 6.115 Atypical fibroxanthoma (low magnification). A pleomorphic spindle cell tumor occupies the entire dermis.

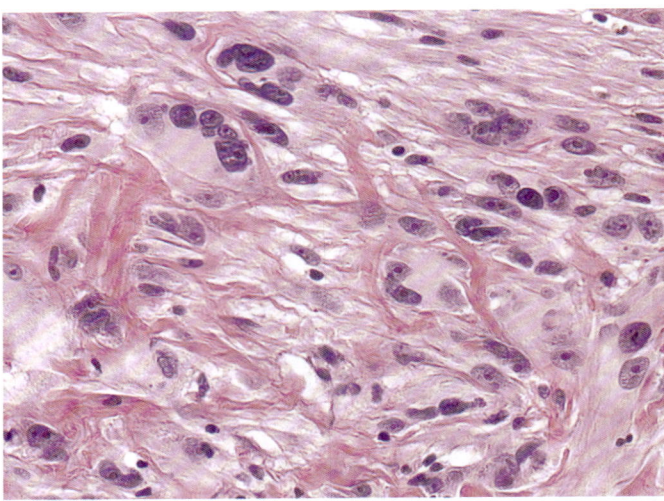

IMAGE 6.116 Atypical fibroxanthoma (high magnification). The striking cytological atypia and tumor giant cells characteristic of this entity are evident.

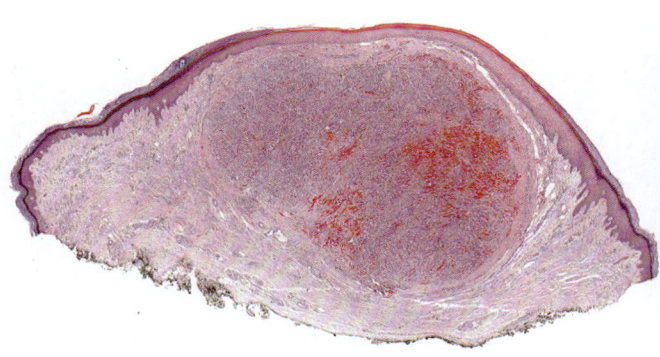

IMAGE 6.117 Kaposi sarcoma (low magnification). A cellular nodule with abundant hemorrhage expands the upper dermis.

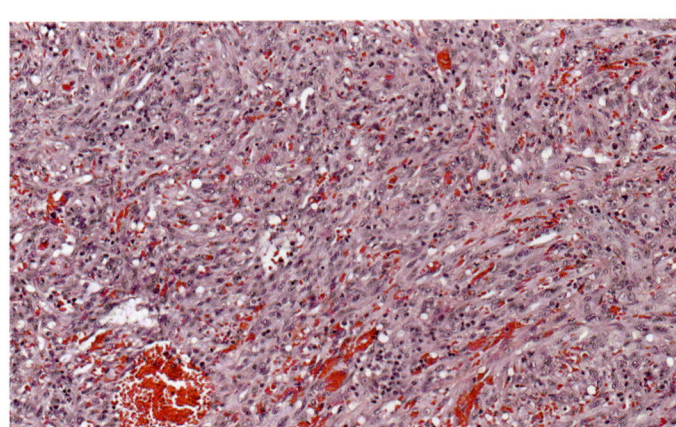

IMAGE 6.118 Kaposi sarcoma (high magnification). A proliferation of plump spindle-shaped cells incorporates occasional slit-like vascular spaces. Rounded vacuoles (representing intracytoplasmic lumina) are also present, some containing pale pink globules (degenerated red blood cells).

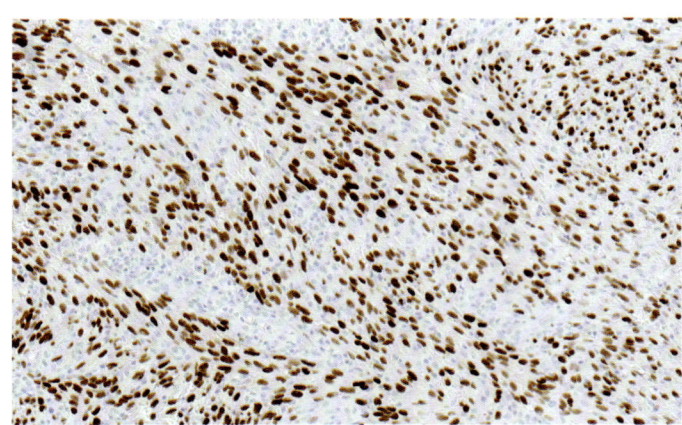

IMAGE 6.119 Kaposi sarcoma (immunohistochemical stain for HHV-8) (high magnification). Nuclear positivity of lesional cells for human herpesvirus 8 confirms the diagnosis of Kaposi sarcoma.

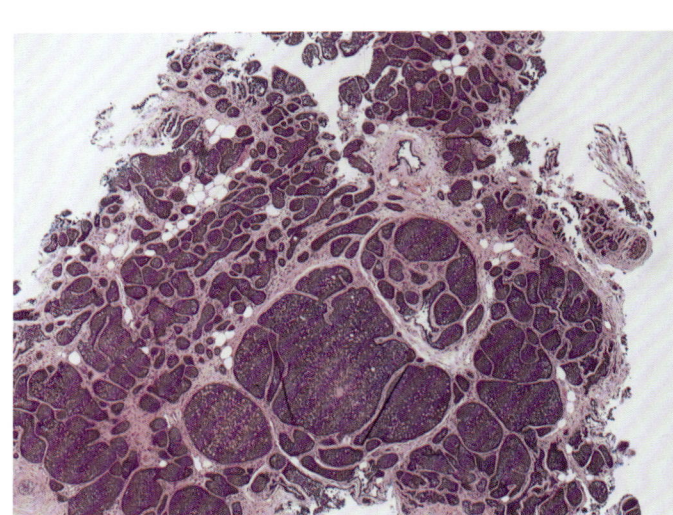

IMAGE 6.120 Cylindroma (low magnification). The images shows a multinodular tumor with a "jigsaw puzzle" arrangement of basaloid epithelial cells.

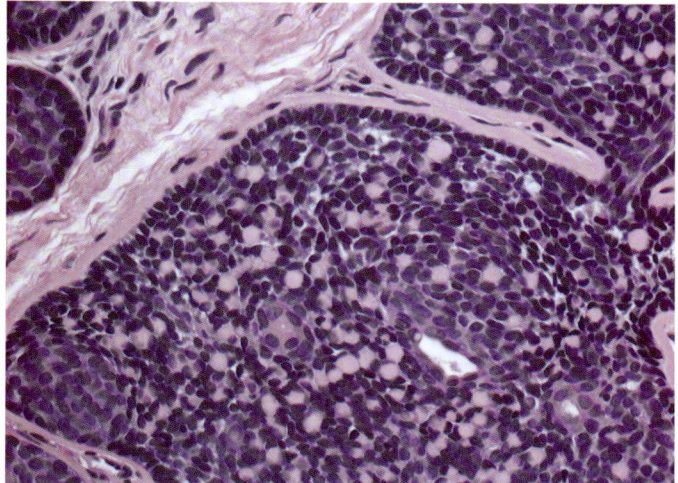

IMAGE 6.121 Cylindroma (high magnification). The tumor lobule is composed of small basaloid cells in a palisade at the periphery with larger cells centrally. A thickened basement membrane surrounds the lobule and eosinophilic globules are present between cells centrally.

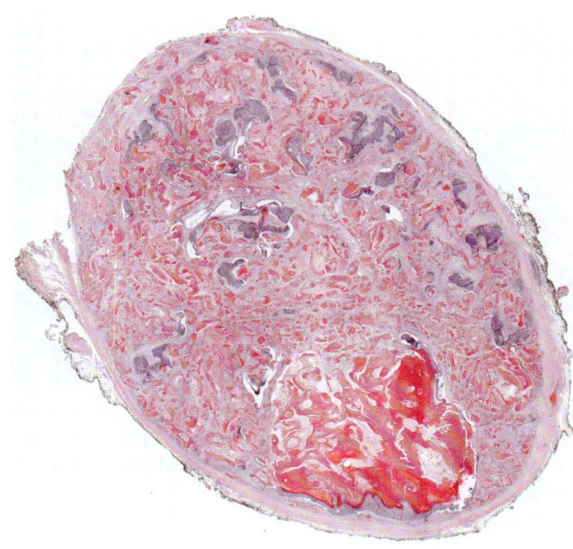

IMAGE 6.122 Pilomatricoma (low magnification). This circumscribed nodule, which appears to have "shelled out" of surrounding tissue, exhibits a variegated appearance, comprising islands of basaloid cells interspersed with zones of eosinophilic material.

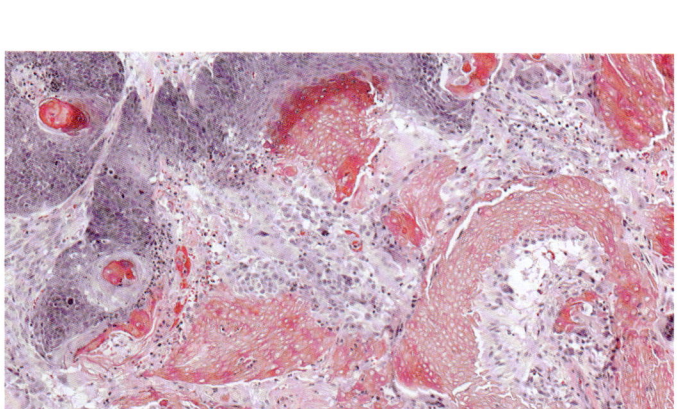

IMAGE 6.123 Pilomatricoma (high magnification). The islands of basaloid matrical cells merge with aggregations of eosinophilic ghost or shadow cells, representing a faulty attempt at hair shaft formation. This keratinous material typically elicits a foreign body–type granulomatous reaction.

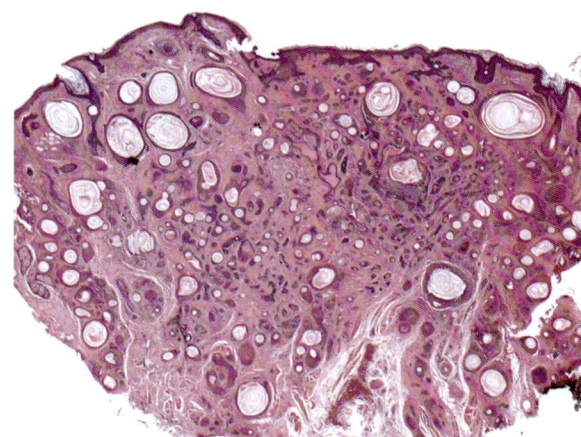

IMAGE 6.124 Microcystic adnexal carcinoma (low magnification). This indolent, morphologically bland, adnexal carcinoma of folliculo-sebaceous-apocrine lineage is characterized by a poorly circumscribed, complex array of trabecular, ductal, and microcystic structures. These usually extend into the deep dermis/subcutis and often display perineural involvement.

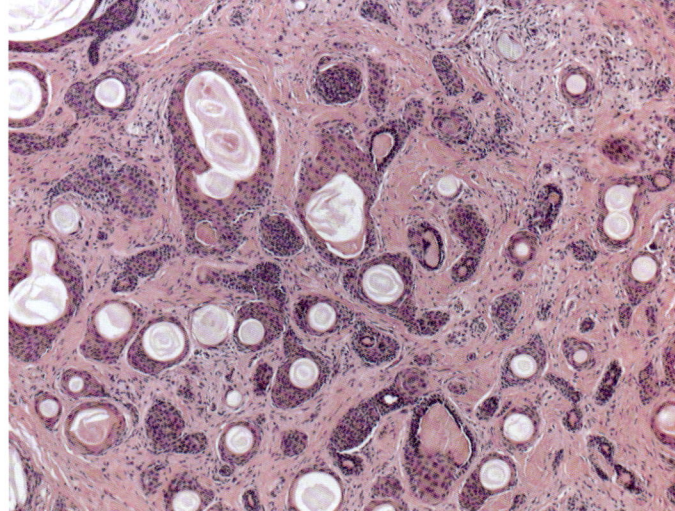

IMAGE 6.125 Microcystic adnexal carcinoma (high magnification). Apocrine-type ducts connect with infundibular structures; occasional comma-shaped ducts (resembling those of a syringoma) are evident.

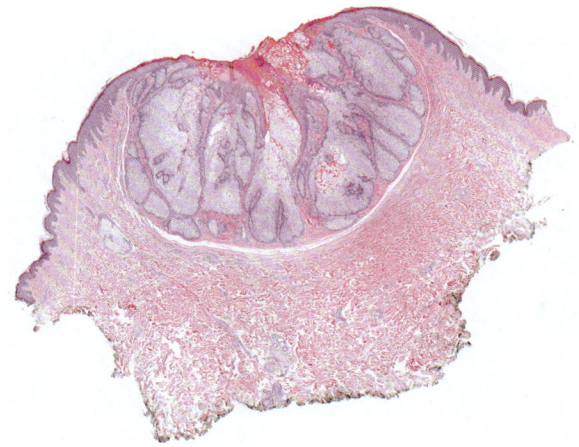

IMAGE 6.126 Sebaceous adenoma (low magnification). This lobulated, circumscribed, well-differentiated sebaceous tumor connects directly with the epidermis and the skin surface.

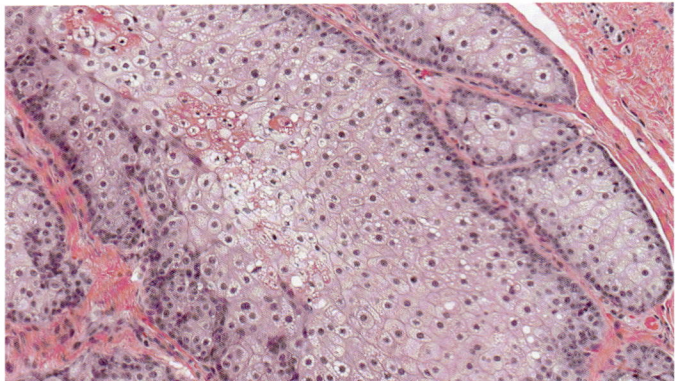

IMAGE 6.127 Sebaceous adenoma (high magnification). The lobules are composed of cells, with pale vesicular cytoplasm and scalloped nuclei, representing mature sebocytes. A thin rim of basaloid germinative cells is evident at the base.

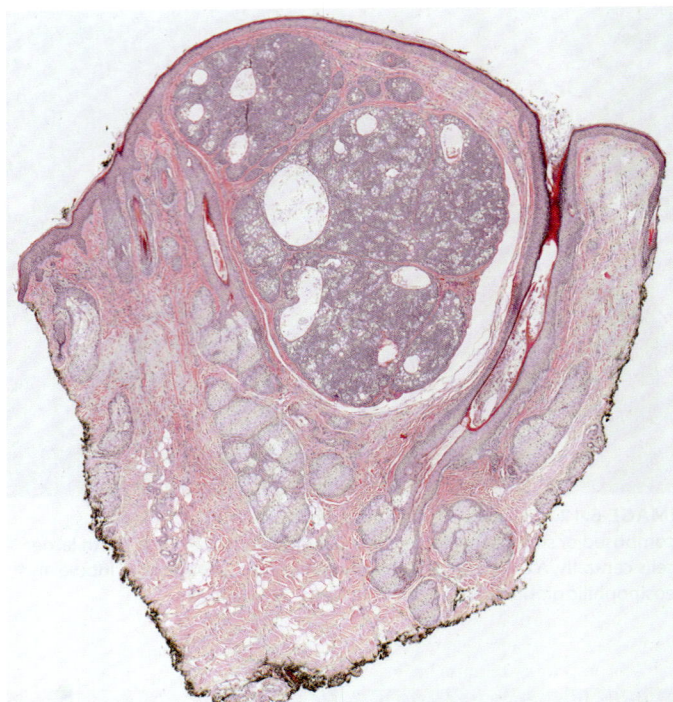

IMAGE 6.128 Sebaceoma (low magnification). Unlike sebaceous adenomas, which frequently open on to the surface of the skin, sebaceomas are typically manifested by 1 or more circumscribed dermal nodules.

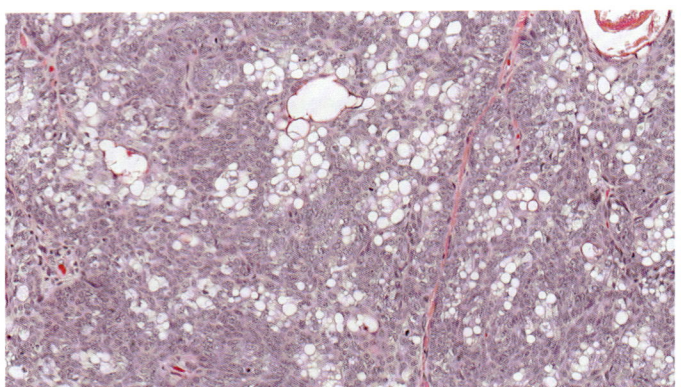

IMAGE 6.129 Sebaceoma (high magnification). Basaloid germinative cells predominate over mature vacuolated sebocytes, in contrast to proportions observed in sebaceous adenomas. A classic sebocyte with microvesicular cytoplasm and a scalloped nucleus is seen centrally. Sebaceous ducts, with eosinophilic cuticles, are also evident.

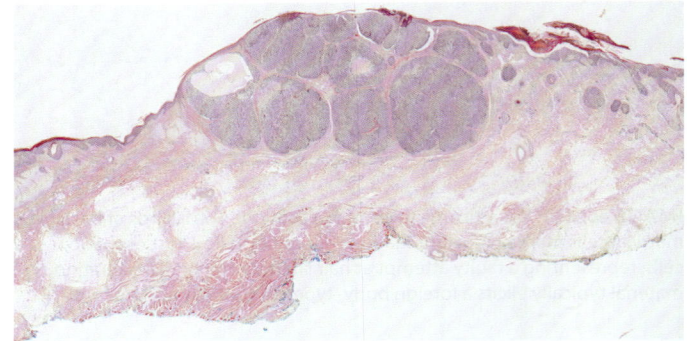

IMAGE 6.130 Sebaceous carcinoma (low magnification). There is an asymmetrical basaloid tumor, with a central focus of geographic eosinophilic necrosis, connected to the surface and exhibiting pagetoid involvement of the epidermis on the right side.

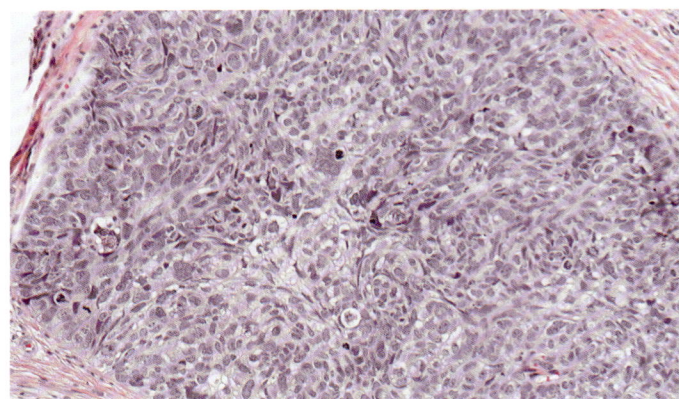

IMAGE 6.131 Sebaceous carcinoma (high magnification). The basaloid cells exhibit cytological atypia, with scattered mitotic figures. Some display sebocytic differentiation with cytoplasmic microvesiculation and scalloped nuclei.

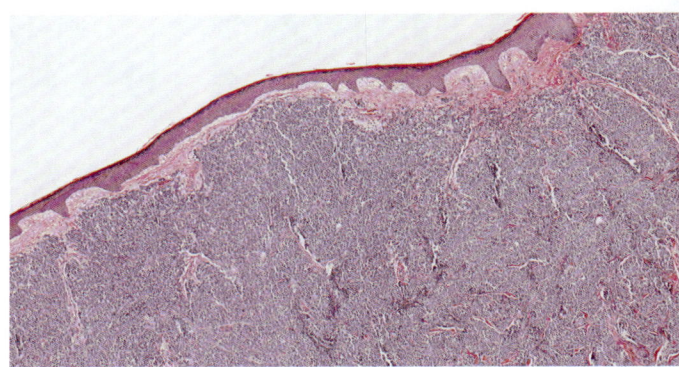

IMAGE 6.132 Merkel cell carcinoma (low magnification). This densely cellular dermal tumor is composed of "small blue round cells" arranged in sheets.

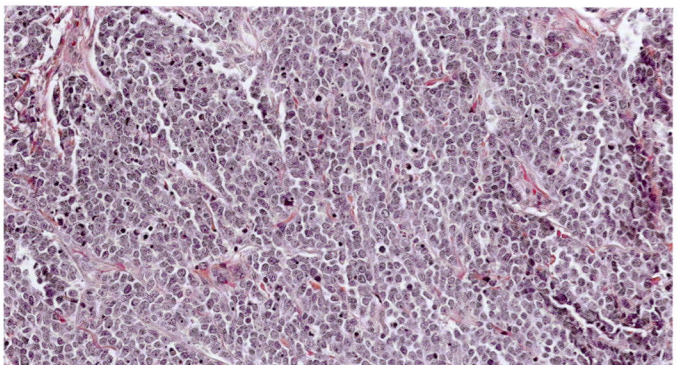

IMAGE 6.133 Merkel cell carcinoma (medium magnification). The neoplastic cells exhibit a high nuclear-cytoplasmic ratio, nuclei with a salt-and-pepper chromatin pattern, and inconspicuous nucleoli. Numerous mitoses and apoptosis of single cells are observed.

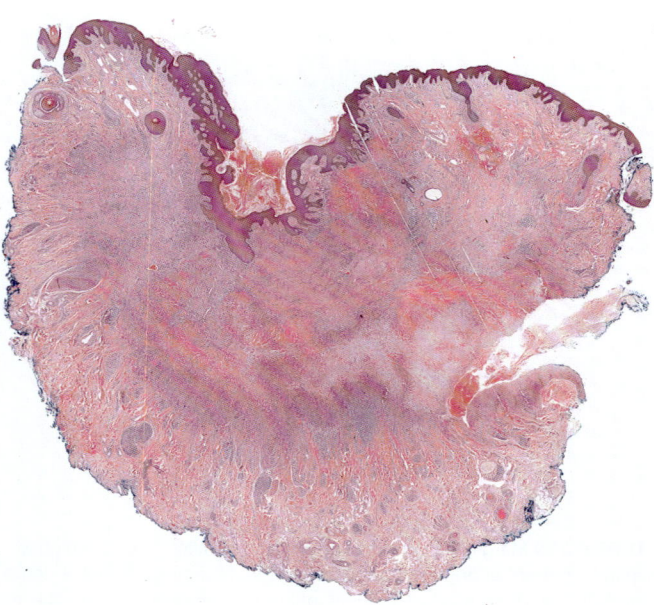

IMAGE 6.134 Epithelioid sarcoma (low magnification). This ill-defined dermal nodule is characterized by a cellular proliferation surrounding eosinophilic hypocellular zones (of necrosis), reminiscent of a palisading granulomatous process.

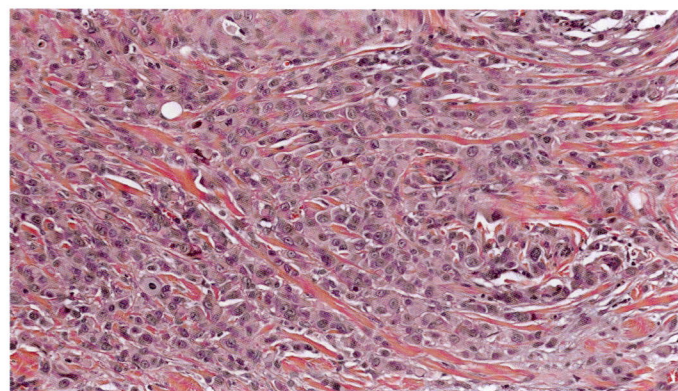

IMAGE 6.135 Epithelioid sarcoma (high magnification). The lesional cells exhibit atypical epithelioid features with eosinophilic cytoplasm and occasional mitoses.

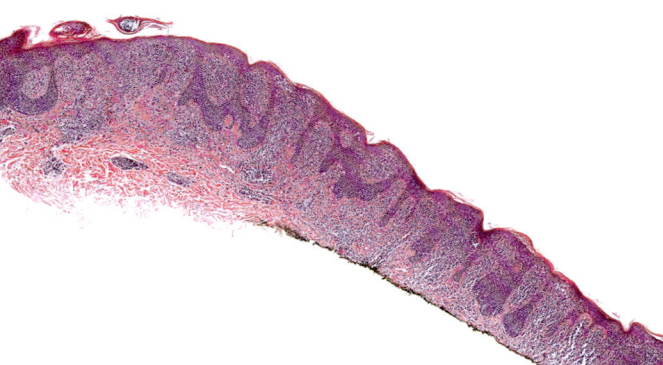

IMAGE 6.136 Mycosis fungoides (low magnification). A dense, patchy, lichenoid, lymphocytic infiltrate occupies the papillary dermis and partially obscures the base of a hyperplastic epidermis.

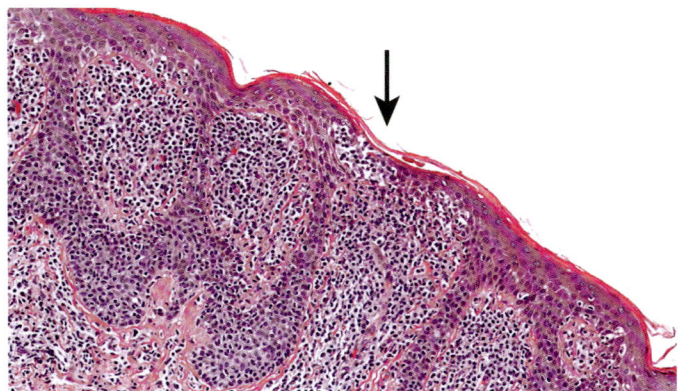

IMAGE 6.137 Mycosis fungoides (high magnification). Lymphocytes are seen to infiltrate the epidermis (epidermotropism) and form localized collections called Pautrier microabscesses (black arrow). The associated papillary dermal collagen is coarse, often displaying a chicken-wire pattern.

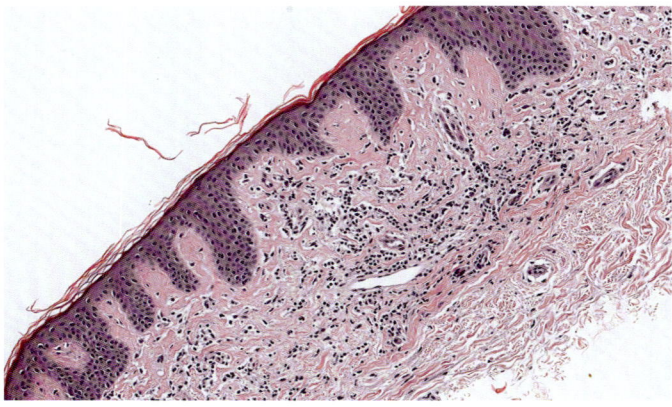

IMAGE 6.138 Mycosis fungoides (high magnification). Occasionally the manifestations of the disease are subtle, showing only a light lymphocytic infiltrate devoid of epidermotropism. The coarse chicken-wire pattern of papillary dermal collagen in this setting is a clue to the diagnosis.

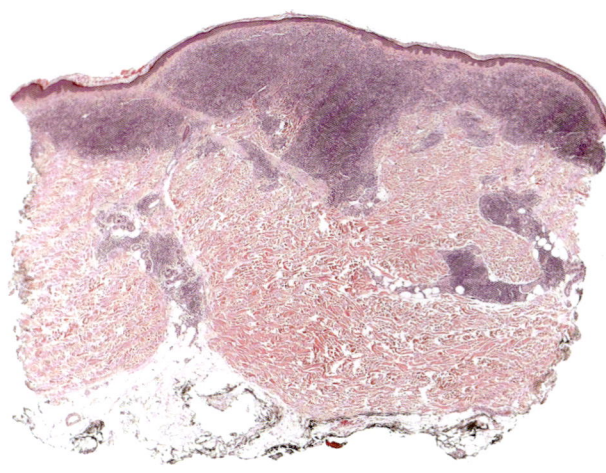

IMAGE 6.139 Marginal zone lymphoma (low magnification). This biopsy displays 1 pattern of primary cutaneous marginal zone lymphoma. A dense, superficial and deep, focally confluent infiltrate of lymphocytes and plasma cells is observed in the dermis, sparing the epidermis.

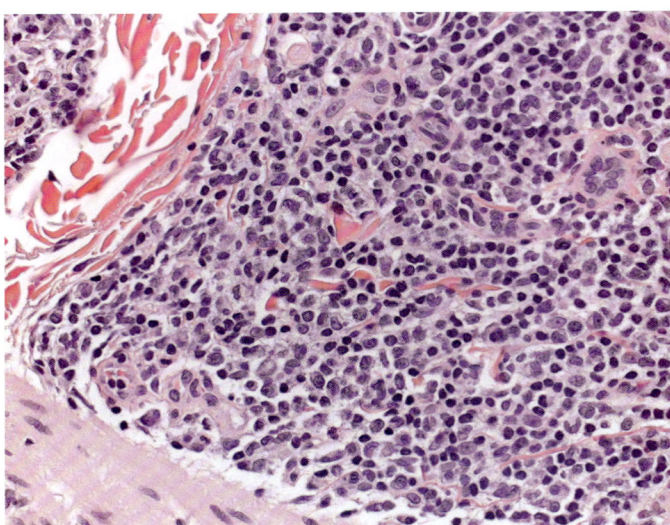

IMAGE 6.140 Marginal zone lymphoma (high magnification). Small benign lymphocytes are interspersed with medium-sized marginal zone cells displaying relatively abundant pale cytoplasm. The plasma cells in the infiltrate were monotypic on immunohistochemistry.

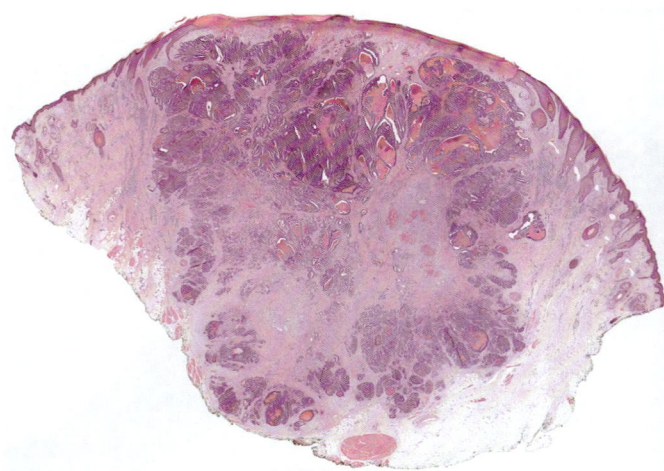

IMAGE 6.141 Metastatic colonic adenocarcinoma (low magnification). A well-defined, cellular nodule occupies the dermis and displays focal acinar structures filled with eosinophilic secretions.

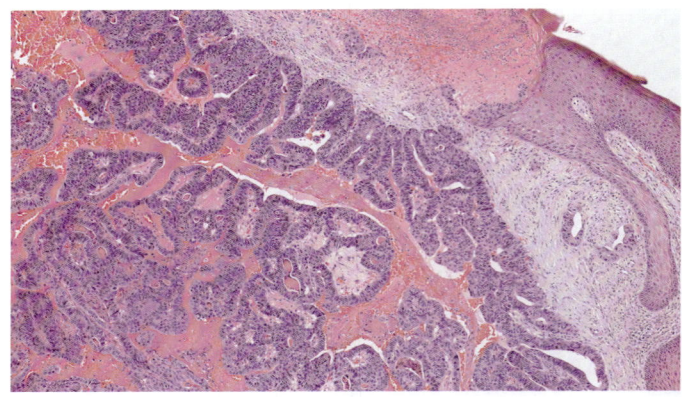

IMAGE 6.142 Metastatic colonic adenocarcinoma (medium magnification). The malignant glandular tumor displays a papillary pattern reminiscent of that seen in primary colonic adenocarcinoma. "Dirty necrosis" (i.e., necrosis with neutrophilic debris) is often present (not shown here).

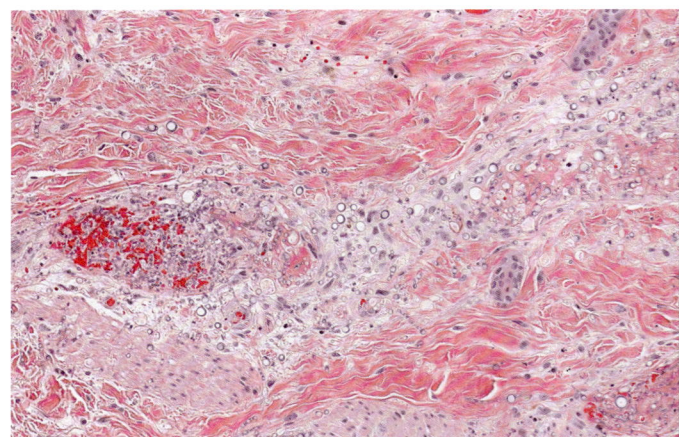

IMAGE 6.143 Angioinvasive fungal infection (medium magnification). In this case of disseminated *Fusarium* infection, a tangled mass of septate fungal hyphae and yeast-like forms fills a vascular lumen and spills into the surrounding dermis.

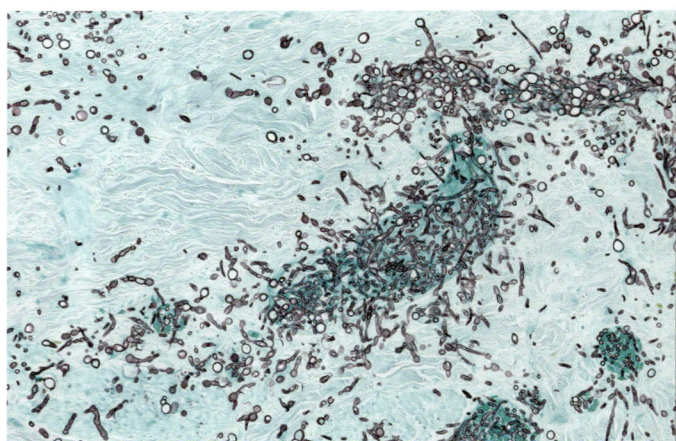

IMAGE 6.144 Angioinvasive fungal infection (medium magnification). A Gomori methenamine silver (GMS) stain highlights the *Fusarium* organisms and better illustrates their extent, distribution, and morphology.

Images of Select Infectious Organisms at High Magnification

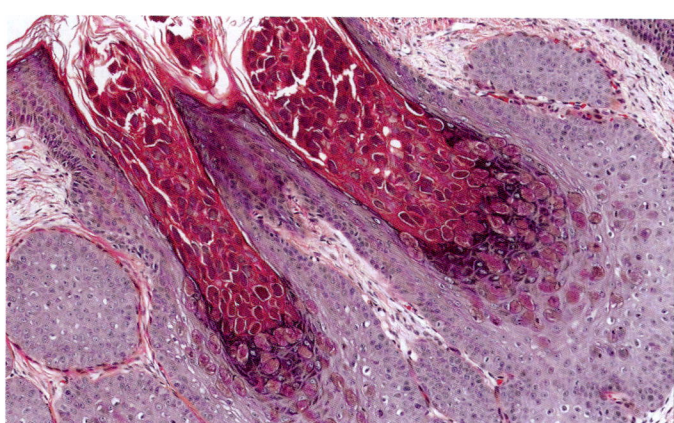

IMAGE 6.145 Molluscum contagiosum (medium magnification). The image shows a typical umbilicated papule displaying lobulated, endophytic epidermal hyperplasia with invaginations. Epidermal keratinocytes are expanded by collections of molluscum bodies (Henderson-Patterson bodies), which become increasingly eosinophilic superficially and the cells are ultimately shed into the invaginations.

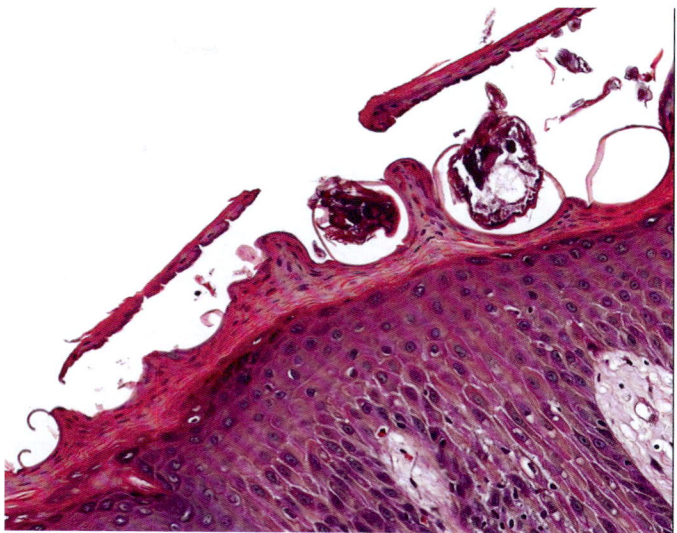

IMAGE 6.146 Scabies (medium magnification). A case of scabies displays eggs of the *Sarcoptes scabiei* mite within a fractured intracorneal burrow, along with "pink pigtails" (far left) representing the casings of eggs left behind after the mites have hatched.

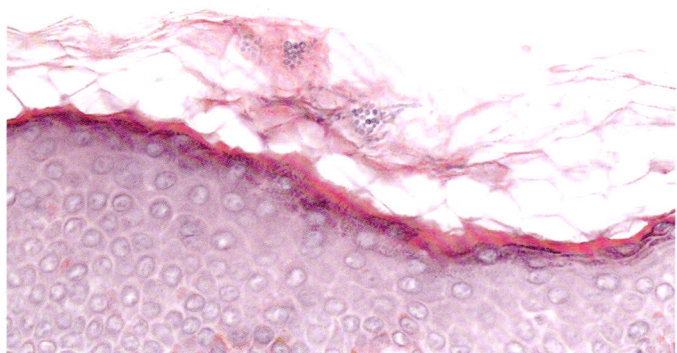

IMAGE 6.147 Tinea versicolor (high magnification). The images shows a case of tinea versicolor displaying budding yeasts and short hyphae ("spaghetti and meatballs") of the *Malassezia* genus. These can be highlighted by a PAS stain.

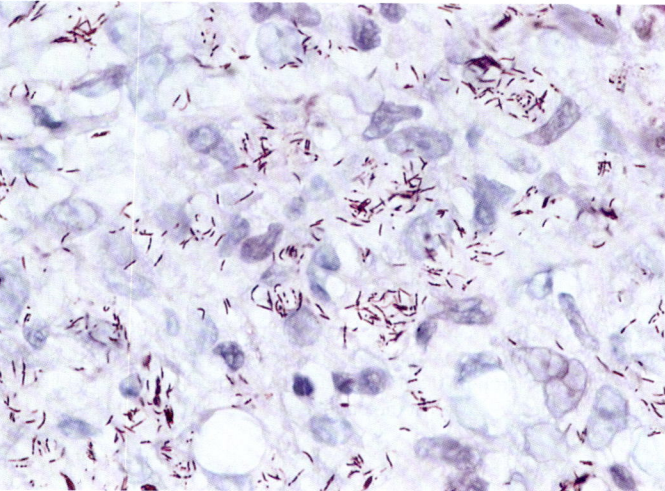

IMAGE 6.148 Lepromatous leprosy (high magnification). A Fite stain in a case of lepromatous leprosy shows abundant, intracytoplasmic, rod shaped, acid fast bacilli (Mycobacterium leprae) within macrophages.

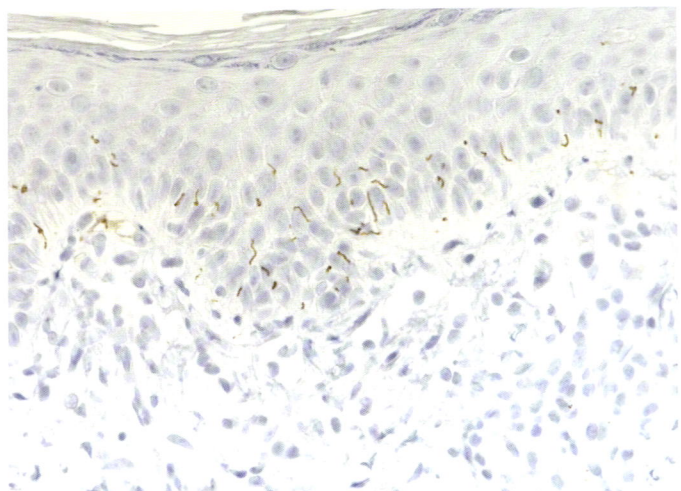

IMAGE 6.149 Syphilis (high magnification). Immunohistochemical stain for *Treponema pallidum* in a case of secondary syphilis displaying corkscrew-shaped spirochetes within the epidermis. The organisms may also be observed in the dermis, around blood vessels and in adnexal structures.

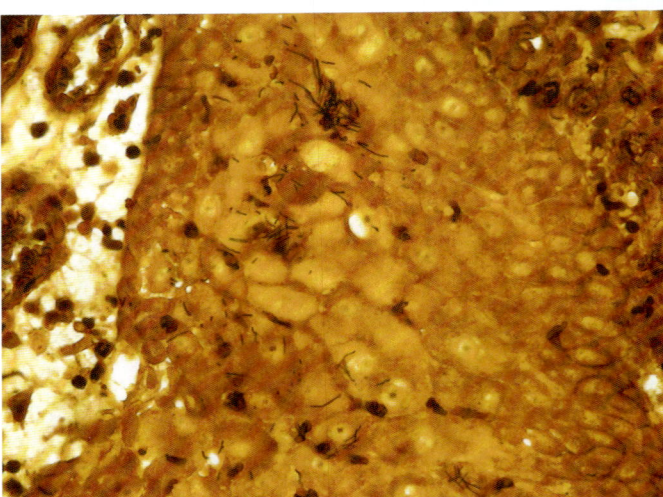

IMAGE 6.150 Syphilis (high magnification). Warthin-Starry stain for *Treponema pallidum* in a case of secondary syphilis displaying corkscrew-shaped spirochetes within the epidermis. The organisms may also be observed in the dermis, around blood vessels and in adnexal structures.

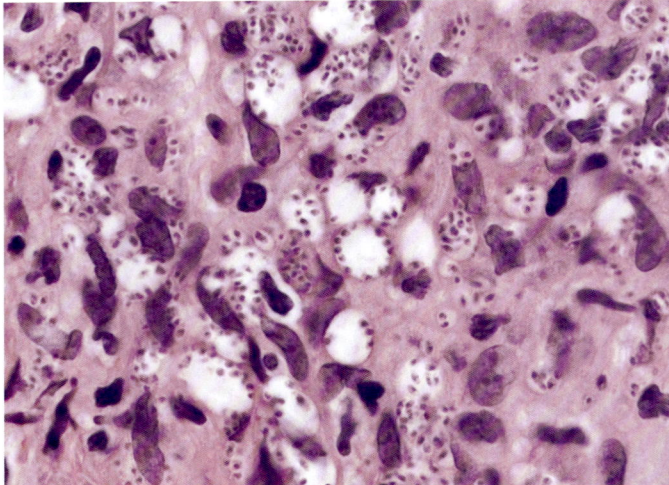

IMAGE 6.151 Leishmaniasis (high magnification). A lymphohistiocytic infiltrate in a case of leishmaniasis displays the intracytoplasmic round/oval parasites (2–4 microns in diameter) with an eccentrically located dot-like kinetoplast, focally arrayed at the periphery of the cell ("marquee sign").

Acknowledgments

We wish to acknowledge the excellent work done by the original authors of this chapter, Drs. Karen Naert and Duane Barber. The high quality of their initiative made it a privilege to supplement the material provided. We also thank Dr. E. Chang Jung and Mr. Stephen Whitefield who contributed some of the photomicrographs.

Bibliography

Ackerman AB. Histologic diagnosis of inflammatory skin diseases: a method by pattern analysis. Philadelphia (PA): Lea & Febiger; 1978.

Amin MB, Edge S, Greene F, et al, editors. AJCC cancer staging manual. 8th ed. New York: Springer; 2017.

Billings SD, Cotton J. Inflammatory dermatopathology: a pathologist's survival guide. New York: Springer; 2011. doi: 10.1007/978-1-60327-838-6

Busam KJ. Dermatopathology. In: Foundations in diagnostic pathology. Goldblum JR, editor. Philadelphia (PA): Saunders-Elsevier; 2010.

Calonje E, Brenn T, Lazar A, et al. McKee's pathology of the skin with clinical correlation. 5th ed. Oxford (UK): Elsevier; 2020.

Cerroni L. Skin lymphoma: the illustrated guide. 5th ed. Hoboken (NJ): Wiley-Blackwell; 2020.

Elder DE, editor. Lever's dermatopathology: histopathology of the skin. 12th ed. Philadelphia (PA): Wolters Kluwar; 2022.

Elder DE, Massi D, Scolyer RA, et al. WHO classification of tumours. 4th ed. Vol. 11, WHO classification of skin tumours. Lyon (France): IARC; 2018.

Elston DM, Stratman EJ, Miller SJ. Skin biopsy. Biopsy issues in specific diseases. J Am Acad Dermatol 2016;74:1-16. doi: 10.1016/j.jaad.2015.06.033

Ferreira I, Wiedemeyer K, Demetter P, et al. Update on the pathology, genetics and somatic landscape of sebaceous tumors. Histopathology 2020;76:640-9. doi: 10.111/his.14044

Patterson JW. Weedon's skin pathology. 5th ed. North York: Elsevier Canada; 2020.

Rapini R. Practical dermatopathology. 3rd ed. North York (ON): Elsevier Canada; 2021.

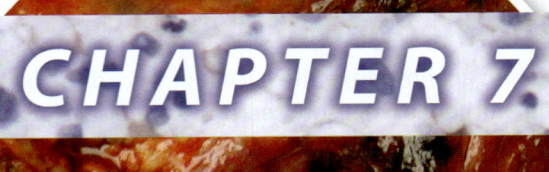

CHAPTER 7

Endocrine Pathology

MOOSA KHALIL, SYLVIA L. ASA

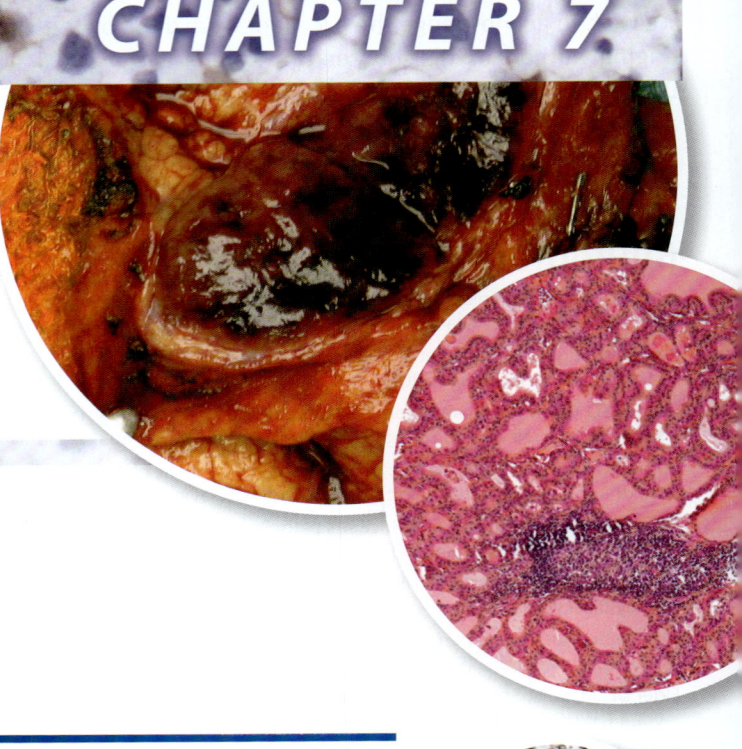

Endocrine Pathology Exam Essentials

MUST KNOW

You should be familiar with the scope of endocrine pathology, which includes endocrine organs, neuroendocrine cells in nonendocrine organs, and soft tissue throughout the body.[1] You should also be able to classify the diseases of these endocrine cells and tissues.

World Health Organization (WHO) classification

High-yield topics include:

- The approach to classification of tumors as listed in the fifth edition of the WHO classification of endocrine and neuroendocrine tumors (NETs), which specifically includes:
  · Pituitary gland.
  · Thyroid gland.
  · Parathyroid gland.
  · Adrenal cortex.
  · Adrenal medulla and extraadrenal paraganglia.
  · Neuroendocrine pancreas.
  · Neuroendocrine neoplasms in nonendocrine organs.
  · Inherited endocrine tumor syndromes.
- Cell lineage-based classification of pituitary NETs based on the WHO classification.
- General classification of thyroid tumors based on the WHO classification. Pay particular attention to the distinctions between encapsulated expansile carcinomas and infiltrative papillary thyroid carcinoma and its variants. You must be able to recognize features

of high grade carcinomas and dedifferentiation leading to poorly differentiated and anaplastic carcinoma.

- Classification of parathyroid tumors based on the WHO classification. You should be able to distinguish parathyroid hyperplasia from neoplasia, and to appreciate the importance of immunohistochemical biomarkers in the distinction of adenoma with degenerative features from carcinoma.
- Classification of adrenal cortical tumors based on the WHO classification. You should be able to distinguish adrenal cortical hyperplasia from neoplasia, and to appreciate the importance of immunohistochemical biomarkers in distinguishing adenoma from low grade adrenal cortical carcinoma and in recognizing high grade adrenal cortical carcinoma.
- Locations and diagnostic criteria of paragangliomas and the criteria for diagnosing metastatic paraganglioma.
- Classification of pancreatic neuroendocrine neoplasms based on the WHO classification, including the molecular and immunohistochemical features that distinguish well-differentiated NETs and poorly differentiated neuroendocrine carcinomas (NECs). In addition, pay attention to hormones that can be secreted by pancreatic NETs and their clinical presentations.
- Classification of neuroendocrine neoplasms at multiple body sites, including but not limited to upper

aerodigestive tract, lung, thymus, gastrointestinal tract, genitourinary tract, skin, and gonads, based on the WHO classification. The molecular and immunohistochemical features that distinguish NETs and poorly NECs is a critical component of this system.

- Genetic predisposition syndromes (fluency in these is important: the exam often includes them). Study the clinical symptoms, associated benign tumors, and associated malignant tumors of these syndromes, and the inheritance patterns, and gene defect or molecular mechanisms, for these syndromes. Key specific topics include:
  · Multiple endocrine neoplasia syndrome type 1 (MEN1), MEN2A, MEN2B, MEN4, and MEN5.
  · Hyperparathyroidism-jaw tumor (HPT-JT) syndrome.
  · Von Hippel-Lindau (VHL) syndrome.
  · Succinate dehydrogenase (SDH) deficiency–related syndromes.
  · Neurofibromatosis type 1 (NF1).
  · Carney complex.
  · McCune-Albright syndrome.
  · DICER1 syndrome.
  · Glucagon cell hyperplasia and neoplasia syndrome.
  · Familial hyperinsulinism syndrome.
  · Syndromic familial nonmedullary thyroid carcinoma.
  · Nonsyndromic familial nonmedullary thyroid carcinoma.

International Collaboration on Cancer Reporting (ICCR) and College of American Pathologists (CAP) protocols

For each of the endocrine ICCR and CAP protocols, focus on the elements that are important for prognostication. These include tumor type and grade, invasive features, and staging. For NETs in nonendocrine organs, you should understand how the anatomical location affects staging; in the pancreas and gastrointestinal tract, NETs have their own distinct protocols whereas NECs are usually staged in the same way as nonendocrine tumors. High-yield topics in particular include:

- For thyroid carcinomas of follicular cell derivation, the distinction between lymphatic and vascular invasion is critical. Lymphatic invasion correlates with locoregional lymph node metastasis that may increase morbidity but has no impact on mortality. In contrast, vascular invasion correlates with distant metastasis that increases disease-specific mortality.
- For thyroid carcinomas, the definition of extrathyroidal extension requires invasion into skeletal muscle to have prognostic significance; involvement of perithyroidal fibroadipose soft tissue does not increase risk.
- For many NETs, tumor grade is based on mitotic count and the Ki 67 labeling index. The methodology to perform these counts is clearly defined and you

should be familiar with the various acceptable methods. Mitotic counts are being recalibrated to mm^2 to increase accuracy and reproducibility, since high power fields vary from one microscope to another.

Special considerations

- Structure-function correlations are critical in endocrine pathology where signs and symptoms are due to hormone production as well as mass effects. Tumor cell function is as important as cell proliferation in many examples. Some tumors express hormones ectopically (a phenomenon incorrectly classified as "paraneoplastic" syndrome).
  · Follicular thyroid tumors with papillae are not all malignant. Well-circumscribed tumors with intrafollicular centripedal complex papillae lined by cells with bland basally oriented nuclei are benign tumors that are usually associated with clinical or subclinical hyperthyroidism (i.e., suppressed thyrotropin [TSH]).
  · You should be fluent in primary and secondary hyperparathyroidism, including causes, clinical symptoms, and pathologic findings, and the limitations of frozen section for intraoperative consultation.
  · For gastric NET, in addition to the above points, you should also know the various types of gastric NET and their associated risk factors (atrophic gastritis and MEN1).
  · For gastroenteropancreatic NETs, it is helpful to know the hormones that can be secreted and the clinical symptoms they can cause, including:
    › Calcitonin and diarrhea/flushing.
    › Gastrin and Zollinger-Ellison syndrome.
    › Insulin excess and hypoglycemia.
    › Glucagon excess and glucagonoma syndrome with necrolytic migratory erythema.
    › Serotonin and the carcinoid syndrome.
    › Vasoactive intestinal polypeptide (VIP), pancreatic polypeptide (PP), and Verner-Morrison syndrome (secretory diarrhea).
  · For pituitary tumors, you should be aware of the clinical features of:
    › Prolactin (PRL) excess, and amenorrhea and galactorrhea.
    › Growth hormone (GH) excess and acromegaly and gigantism.
      » Multiple additional effects of insulinlike growth factor 1 (IGF1) excess including acanthosis nigricans.
    › Adrenocorticotropic hormone (ACTH) and Cushing disease.
    › Antidiuretic hormone (ADH) and syndrome of inappropriate diuresis (SIAD).
  · For neuroendocrine neoplasms (NENs) at any site, ectopic production of any peptide hormone producing 1 of the syndromes listed above (most

commonly small cell lung carcinoma which is a pulmonary NEC).

- For paragangliomas, functional biochemistry correlates with genetic alterations; know the biochemical clusters.
- For adrenal tumors, clinical symptoms and biochemical findings related to hormones secreted can impact diagnosis; for example, a feminizing tumor in a male is malignant until proven otherwise.
- You should be fluent in the syndromes associated with adrenocortical hormone excess, including signs and symptoms, biochemical findings, and pathologic changes of Cushing syndrome (and its distinction from Cushing disease which is due to pituitary ACTH-dependent cortisol excess) and Conn syndrome.
- Some common paraneoplastic symptoms include:
  - Parathyroid hormone-related protein (PTHrP) and hypercalcemia.
  - Insulinlike substance and hypoglycemia.
  - Lambert-Eaton myasthenic syndrome.

Nonneoplastic diseases
- Inflammatory thyroid conditions are frequently seen in clinical practice. You should know the clinical symptoms, pathologic findings, differential diagnosis, and the molecular changes or syndromic associations of the following entities:
  - Hashimoto thyroiditis (including associated antibodies).
  - Graves disease.
  - De Quervain (giant cell or subacute) thyroiditis.
  - Riedel thyroiditis (now recognized to be IgG4-related disease). IgG4 disease, which is an emerging entity. You should know how the disease manifests in the head and neck, as well as other manifestations, including:
    › Kuttner tumor, Mikulicz disease, inflammatory orbital pseudotumor, and IgG4-related hypophysitis, previously known as "pituitary pseudotumor."
- You should know some of the common midline cysts and embryonic remnants (e.g., thyroglossal duct cyst; branchial cleft cyst and branchial cleft-like cysts of thyroid; dermoid and epidermoid cysts).

Molecular genetics and syndromic conditions
- The molecular bases of several endocrine tumors have been clarified. You should be aware of somatic alterations that define endocrine tumors.
  - Thyroid carcinomas of follicular cell derivation are divided into RAS-like neoplasms that tend to be expansile, delineated and follicular in architecture with subtle nuclear atypia (follicular carcinoma, follicular variant papillary carcinoma), and

BRAF-like neoplasms (BRAF V600E) that are infiltrative and papillary in architecture with florid nuclear atypia (papillary carcinoma).
  › Fusions also fall into these 2 categories (e.g., *PAX8-PPARgamma* is RAS-like whereas *RET* and *NTRK* fusions are BRAF-like).
- The aggressiveness of thyroid follicular cell-derived neoplasms is associated with additional *TERT* alterations and dedifferentiation with additional *PICK3CA* and *TP53* mutations.
- Medullary thyroid carcinoma is usually associated with *RET* mutations, less frequently *RAS* mutations.
- Adrenal cortical adenomas and carcinomas are associated with specific mutations that define function and aggressiveness.

- Endocrine diseases and tumors are frequently associated with syndromes due to germline mutations. You should focus on the syndromes outlined in the WHO classification. For each syndrome, it is a good idea to create a table with the genes implicated, organs affected, associated diseases, molecular changes, and mode of inheritance. Create a summary based on the following:
  - MEN1.
  - MEN2.
  - MEN4.
  - MEN5.
  - VHL.
  - NF1.
  - HPT-JT.
  - SDHx-related disease.
  - Carney complex.
  - McCune-Albright syndrome.
  - DICER1.
  - Syndromic thyroid cancer, including cribriform morular thyroid carcinoma with familial adenomatous polyposis (FAP).
  - Nonsyndromic thyroid cancer.
  - Polyendocrine autoimmune syndromes.

MUST SEE
High-yield topics include:
- Common radiologic investigations used in various endocrine organs, including:
  › Ultrasound and radiologic assessment of malignancy risk in thyroid.
  › Radioactive iodine uptake scan for metabolic thyroid disease.
  › Sestamibi scanning for parathyroid tumors (MIBI scans).
  › Octreotide and Ga68-DOTATATE positron emission tomographic (PET) scans for NET.
  › Fluorodeoxyglucose (FDG) PET scans for high grade malignancies.

- Gross and microscopic images of the following lesions and tumors:
  - Common pituitary lesions:
    - Pituitary NETs.
    - Craniopharyngioma.
    - Meningioma.
    - Pituicytoma.
    - Germ cell tumor.
  - Common thyroid lesions:
    - Various forms of thyroiditis including chronic lymphocytic thyroiditis; Graves disease; granulomatous thyroiditis including palpation thyroiditis and de Quervain thyroiditis; and IgG4 disease, or Riedel thyroiditis.
    - Follicular lesions, including follicular nodular disease, follicular adenoma, noninvasive follicular thyroid neoplasm with papillary-like nuclear features (NIFTP), and carcinoma, including variants such as oncocytic and clear cell types.
    - Papillary lesions, including Graves disease, follicular adenoma with papillary architecture, and papillary thyroid carcinomas (including multiple variants: hobnail, tall cell, columnar cell and oncocytic).
    - Solid and trabecular lesions of follicular cells, including hyalinizing trabecular tumor, solid and trabecular papillary carcinoma, poorly differentiated carcinoma (including oncocytic variants, known by the misnomer "Hürthle cell tumors").
      » Be aware of the differential diagnosis of medullary thyroid carcinoma.
    - Anaplastic carcinoma.
    - Thyroid lymphoma.
  - Common adrenal lesions:
    - Cortical hyperplasia, adenoma, and carcinoma.
    - Pheochromocytoma, neuroblastoma, and ganglioneuroma.
    - Myelolipoma.
    - Pseudocyst.
  - Common paragangliomas:
    - Pheochromocytoma.
    - Carotid body tumor.
      » Be aware of extraadrenal paraganglioma in the differential diagnosis of "paraaortic lymphadenopathy."
  - Common NETs (note their location and multifocal nature in gross images):
    - NET of the stomach, which are common in biopsies (be aware of the various types and their associations with other gastric pathologies [or not]).
    - NETs of small bowel, appendix, colon, and rectum (be aware of the distinction between incidental lesions in appendix and those that present with mass effects and hormonal syndromes).
    - Pancreatic NETs with various morphologies, hormonal products, and associated hormone syndromes.
  - Other related lesions:
    - Thyroglossal duct cyst.
    - Branchial cleft cyst.

MUST DO

- For each of the tumors outlined in Must See section, you should be comfortable generating a differential diagnosis and immunohistochemical panel.
- When studying in groups:
  - Practice generating differential diagnosis for thyroid tumors both on cytology as well as on histology.
  - Pay attention to high yield thyroid tumors such as papillary thyroid carcinoma (PTC), NIFTP, and medullary thyroid cancer (MTC).
  - Always discuss syndromic associations and molecular changes where relevant.
  - Generate a list of IgG4 disease related entities involving all endocrine glands.
  - Discuss grading and staging for NETs at all sites.
- You should be able to describe the grossing protocol for the following specimens, and independently gross them:
  - Thyroidectomy for benign diseases, and what to do if there isn't a dominant nodule.
  - Thyroidectomy for malignancies, and the definition of extrathyroidal extension.
  - Adrenalectomy for benign and malignant diseases.
  - Various gastrointestinal (GI) resections for NET, especially small bowel and gastric specimen.
- You should be able to describe and handle fresh specimens and frozen sections of the following specimens:
  - Parathyroid hyperplasia and adenoma.
  - Thyroid with nodule(s).

MULTIPLE CHOICE QUESTIONS

1. Figure 7.1 shows follicular nodular disease. Which of the following statements is **not** true about this disease?

a. It is of unknown etiology.

b. The nodules are both polyclonal and monoclonal.

c. It causes Plummer syndrome when there is associated infiltrative ophthalmopathy.

d. Serum T$_3$ and T$_4$ are usually normal and goiter develops when the gland enlarges.

e. Histologically, it shows cystic inactive follicles and areas of cellular active follicular epithelium.

Answer: c

2. Figure 7.2 is a photomicrograph of a thyroid nodule. Which of the following statements is true about this thyroid nodule?

a. Thyroid radioactive iodine uptake is diffusely increased.

b. Total thyroidectomy is the treatment of choice.

c. It may be associated with subclinical hyperthyroidism.

d. Levels of T$_3$ and T$_4$ may be normal but thyrotropin (TSH) is usually elevated.

e. It is a painful condition.

Answer: c

3. Which is true about the diffuse thyroid disorder in Figure 7.3?

a. Thyroid radioactive iodine shows a hot nodule.

b. It is an autoimmune disease.

c. It is associated with hypothyroidism.

d. Levels of T$_3$ and T$_4$ may be normal but thyrotropin (TSH) is usually elevated.

e. It is a painful condition.

Answer: b

4. Which of the following is **not** true about the thyroid neoplasm shown in Figure 7.4?

a. It has oncocytic cytology.

b. It has a thick fibrous capsule.

c. It has nuclear features that predict malignancy.

d. It has chromosomal copy number alterations.

e. It is benign.

Answer: c

5. Which statement is true about the thyroid neoplasm shown in Figure 7.5?

a. It has a BRAF-like molecular signature.

b. It has a high risk of distant metastatic disease.

c. It is associated with hyperthyroidism.

d. It has a RAS-like molecular signature.

e. It is associated with pheochromocytoma.

Answer: d

6. The oncocytic thyroid tumor in Figure 7.6 has the following feature:

a. It is composed of cells that take up radioactive iodine avidly.

b. It has a thick fibrous capsule.

c. It has a high risk of distant metastatic disease.

d. It has no molecular alterations.

e. It is benign.

Answer: c

7. The thyroid neoplasm in Figure 7.7 is associated with which of the following?

a. A BRAF-like molecular signature.

b. A high risk of distant metastatic disease.

c. Hyperthyroidism.

d. A RAS-like molecular signature.

e. Pheochromocytoma.

Answer: a

8. Figure 7.8 shows a photomicrograph of a thyroid disease. Which of the following statements is **not** true about this disease?

a. It has complex papillary architecture.

b. It has oncocytic cytology.

c. It has a BRAF-like molecular signature and may stain for *BRAF* V600E using the VE1 antibody.

d. It has a very high risk of extrathyroidal extension and recurrence.

e. It has a high risk of lymph node metastases.

Answer: d

9. What is the best diagnosis for the thyroid carcinoma shown in Figure 7.9?

a. Papillary carcinoma, classical variant.

b. Papillary carcinoma, hobnail cell variant.

c. Papillary carcinoma, tall cell variant.

d. Papillary carcinoma columnar cell variant.

e. Papillary carcinoma, cribriform variant.

Answer: b

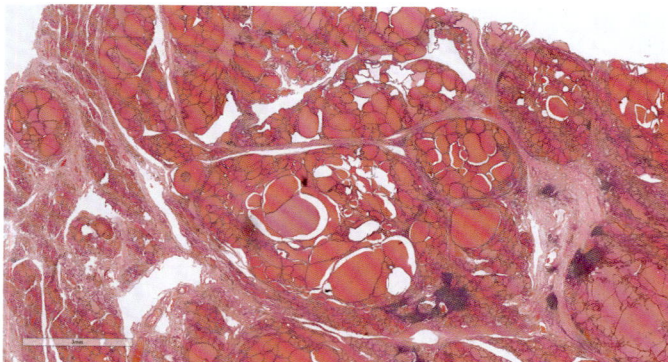

FIGURE 7.1 Thyroid follicular nodular disease. Follicular nodular disease is a proliferative disorder of thyroid follicular epithelium that is of unknown etiology.[2] The thyroid is distorted by nodules that vary in size and may be well delineated or poorly defined. The nodules are usually highly heterogeneous in architecture; there are areas of abundant colloid storage and flattened inactive epithelium admixed with cellular areas of active cuboidal follicular epithelium and even columnar follicular epithelium that can be quite cellular. As nodules grow, they become fibrotic and outgrow their blood supply, resulting in focal hemorrhage, scarring, and reactive atypia. The nodules are polyclonal and monoclonal, with no correlation between clonality and morphology. With enlarging nodules, goiter develops. These tumors may be associated with hypothyroidism, but usually the patients are euthyroid. Occasionally a nodule can be hyperfunctioning due to clonal mutation of *GNAS* or *TSHR*; these lesions give rise to clinical or subclinical hyperthyroidism, known as Plummer syndrome in this setting; there is no associated ophthalmopathy.

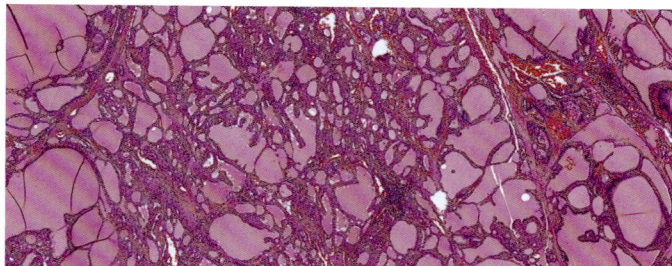

FIGURE 7.3 Thyroid Graves disease. This diffuse hyperplastic disorder of the thyroid is due to an autoimmune phenomenon that gives rise to antibodies that stimulate the thyrotropin (TSH) receptor.[2] This causes hyperthyroidism and suppresses pituitary thyrotropin (TSH). There is diffusely increased uptake of radioactive iodine on scan. The entire gland is composed of follicles that contain invaginations of follicular epithelium forming intrafollicular papillary structures; the follicular epithelium is generally columnar reflecting hyperfunction, and there is scalloping of the colloid where the follicular epithelial cell villi secrete enzymes to digest the colloid. Although this is an autoimmune phenomenon, inflammatory cells are usually scant and scattered in small clusters. Most patients are treated medically prior to surgery, and the effect of the medical therapy may reverse the characteristic features throughout the gland or in areas, with residual medically resistant foci of hypercellularity. This disease is not painful (unlike granulomatous or "subacute" thyroiditis) but may be associated with ophthalmopathy.

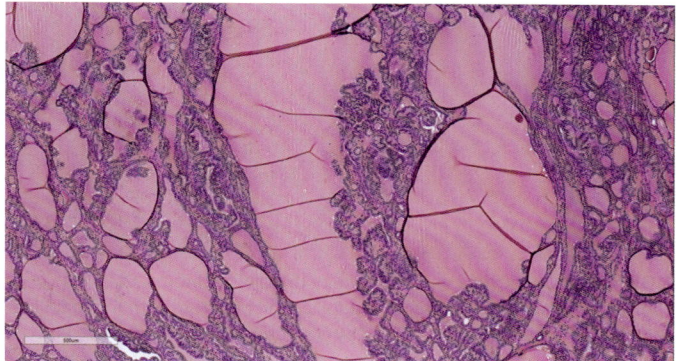

FIGURE 7.2 Thyroid follicular adenoma with papillary architecture ("papillary adenoma"). This thyroid nodule is well-delineated and noninvasive; it has papillary architecture, but the papillae are organized and arranged in a centripetal fashion within follicles.[2] The papillae are true papillae with fibrovascular cores lined by follicular epithelium; however, there are no nuclear features of papillary carcinoma. In the situation where a biopsy has been performed, there is extensive uptake of hemosiderin by the hyperactive follicular epithelial cells. The histological appearance is similar to that of Graves disease, but these are focal lesions with surrounding uninvolved parenchyma that may show involution or atrophy. These lesions are benign follicular adenomas that are hyperfunctioning due to clonal mutation of *GNAS* or *TSHR*; they give rise to clinical or subclinical hyperthyroidism. In patients with subclinical disease, levels of T3 and T4 may be normal, but thyrotropin (TSH) is suppressed; a radioiodine uptake scan identifies a hot nodule with suppressed parenchyma surrounding it. These lesions are treated with resection by lobectomy or isthmusectomy and do not require total thyroidectomy or postoperative radioactive iodine therapy. It is not painful (unlike granulomatous or "subacute" thyroiditis).

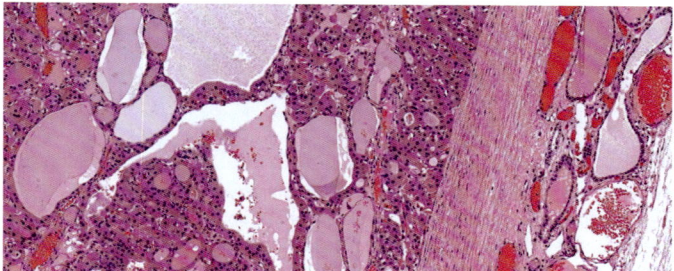

FIGURE 7.4 Oncocytic follicular thyroid adenoma. This neoplasm is composed of oncocytic follicular epithelial cells. It is well delineated and thickly encapsulated; there is no evidence of capsular invasion in multiple sections. The tumor cells have abundant granular eosinophilic cytoplasm consistent with oncocytic change, and they have bland, round, dark, uniform nuclei that may harbor bright red macronucleoli; however, they have no significant irregularity of contour and no grooves, and the chromatin is dark and evenly distributed. These are the features of a benign oncocytic follicular adenoma. All oncocytic lesions of the thyroid exhibit chromosomal copy number alterations and may have mitochondrial mutations.[3]

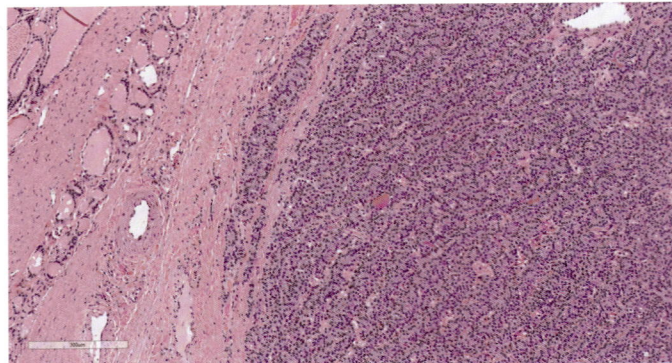

FIGURE 7.5 Minimally invasive follicular thyroid carcinoma. This tumor is a classical RAS-like follicular neoplasm: it has an expansile growth pattern rather than an infiltrative growth pattern, which is characteristic of BRAF-like carcinomas, and it has follicular and focally solid architecture.[4] The tumor cells have nuclear atypia; the nuclei are not uniform, and they are irregular in contour with focal crowding. There is superficial invasion into and through the capsule, but not widely into the surrounding parenchyma. Tumors of this type are low-risk carcinomas when they have only focal capsular invasion and no vascular invasion. They are not usually associated with functional alterations but present as mass lesions. They are not known to be part of familial syndromes.

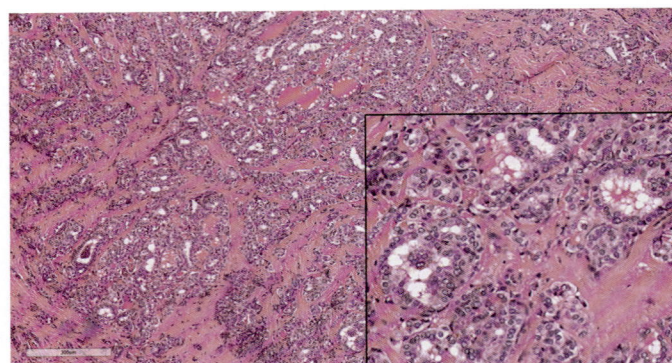

FIGURE 7.7 Infiltrative follicular variant papillary thyroid carcinoma. This infiltrative thyroid carcinoma has predominant follicular architecture but florid nuclear atypia, and careful examination will identify abortive papillae (inset). This lesion falls into the category of BRAF-like papillary thyroid carcinomas[4] in contrast to the expansile follicular lesions that are RAS-like. Like classical papillary carcinomas, they have stromal fibrosis and the nuclei are crowded, with striking irregularity of nuclear contours forming grooves and pseudoinclusions; the nuclear chromatin is very clear, mimicking Orphan Annie's eyes. They may have psammoma bodies. They have a high rate of lymphatic invasion, and metastases to locoregional lymph nodes are common. These lesions are not usually associated with functional changes or multiendocrine syndromes.

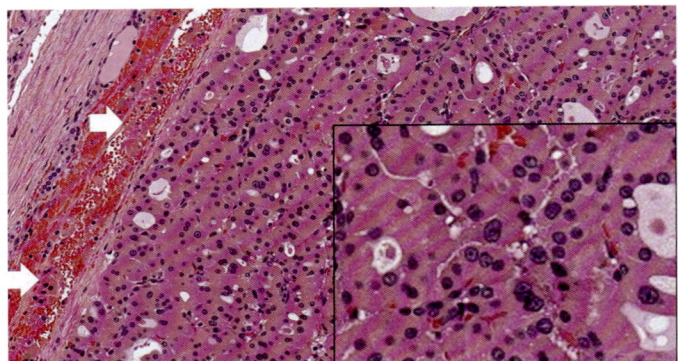

FIGURE 7.6 Angioinvasive oncocytic follicular thyroid carcinoma. This RAS-like thyroid follicular neoplasm is expansile and encapsulated with predominant follicular architecture. The tumor cells show marked nuclear atypia (inset); the nuclei are irregular in size and contour with focal overlap and molding, and there is peripheral margination of chromatin with focal clearing of the nucleoplasm. There are also prominent large nucleoli characteristic of oncocytes. Follicular neoplasms of this type (with or without oncocytic change) can be classified as follicular carcinoma or follicular variant papillary carcinoma; these 2 entities are almost identical and the distinction has been historical based on nuclear atypia.[5] When they are minimally invasive, they are low risk, but in this case, there are tumor cells in a vascular channel associated with thrombus (arrows). This feature indicates a high risk of distant metastatic disease. Oncocytic tumors often have chromosomal copy number alterations and may have mitochondrial mutations.[3] They tend to have lower iodine uptake than nononcocytic tumors and therefore may respond poorly to radioactive iodine therapy.

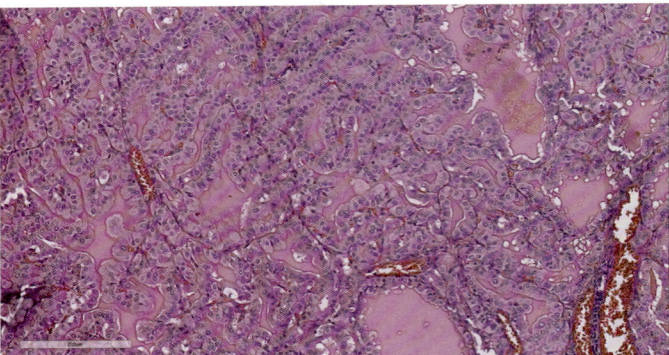

FIGURE 7.8 Oncocytic classical papillary thyroid carcinoma. Classical papillary carcinomas have complex papillary architecture with thin papillae containing fibrovascular cores lined by crowded follicular epithelial cells. The oncocytic variant shown here has oncocytic cytology, but still retains the florid nuclear features of papillary carcinoma with marked crowding. These tumors often have psammoma bodies. Like most classical papillary thyroid carcinomas, these tumors have *BRAF* V600E mutations that can be identified using immunohistochemistry (IHC) with the VE1 antibody.[3] Classical papillary thyroid carcinomas have a high incidence of lymph node metastasis, but the risk of extrathyroidal extension and recurrence is no higher in oncocytic variant tumors than any other classical papillary thyroid carcinoma.

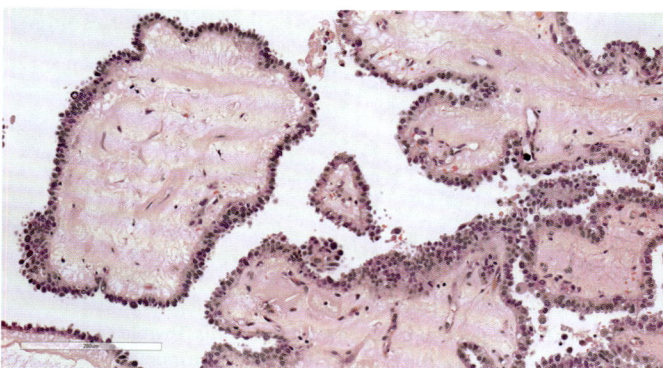

FIGURE 7.9 Hobnail variant papillary thyroid carcinoma. This variant of papillary thyroid carcinoma has classic complex papillary architecture and unusual cytology; the tumor cells have a hobnail appearance.[6–9] Tumors with this cytology in the majority of the tumor mass are more aggressive; however, this cytology is frequently seen as a focal change in papillae that are dilated and edematous as shown here. The prognostic implications of this remain to be proven.

10. Which of the following statements is **not** true about the thyroid tumor shown in Figure 7.10?

a. It is a BRAF-like thyroid cancer.

b. It is more common in younger patients.

c. It has a high risk of extrathyroidal extension.

d. It has a "tramtrack" appearance.

e. The tumor cells have a height-to-width ratio of at least 3:1.

Answer: b

11. Which of the following is true about the thyroid neoplasm shown in Figure 7.11?

a. *RET* protooncogene mutations are diagnostic of familial tumors.

b. Patients with MEN2A-associated tumors have a worse prognosis than those with MEN2B-associated tumors.

c. These tumors all feature abundant amyloid deposition.

d. Patients can present with diarrhea.

e. These tumors are treated with radioactive iodine.

Answer: d

12. Which statement is true about the thyroid carcinoma shown in Figure 7.12?

a. This papillary carcinoma is a high-risk disease.

b. It likely has only a *BRAF* V600E mutation.

c. It takes up radioactive iodine and is treated with success using that targeted therapy.

d. It may harbor an activating mutation of *CTNNB1*.

e. The necrosis is not a relevant feature.

Answer: a

13. Which of the following features is **not** consistent with the thyroid carcinoma shown in Figure 7.13?

a. PAX8 positivity.

b. TTF1 reactivity.

c. An associated differentiated follicular neoplasm.

d. Angioinvasion.

e. Amyloid with Congo red reactivity and apple-green birefringence.

Answer: e

14. Which statement is **false** about the anaplastic thyroid carcinoma (undifferentiated carcinoma) shown in Figure 7.14?

a. It may arise from well-differentiated carcinoma.

b. It may harbor a *BRAF* V600E mutation.

c. Inactivation of *TP53* is common in anaplastic carcinoma.

d. Histologically, it may resemble sarcoma.

e. The 5-year survival rate is approximately 40%.

Answer: e

15. Figure 7.15 shows thyroid carcinoma with angioinvasion. This tumor is characterized by all of the following **except**:

a. Tumor cells in vascular lumens.

b. Associated thrombus.

c. Tumor cells underlying intact endothelium.

d. A higher risk of distant metastatic disease.

e. Associated red blood cells in the vascular lumen.

Answer: c

16. Figure 7.16 shows cribriform morular thyroid carcinoma. Which of the following statements about this carcinoma is correct?

a. It is more common in males.

b. It is a variant of papillary thyroid carcinoma.

c. It is associated with Lynch syndrome.

d. It cannot be sporadic.

e. It harbors mutations that activate the WNT/β-catenin pathway.

Answer: e

17. Figure 7.17 shows primary hyperparathyroidism. The following statements are true about primary hyperparathyroidism **except**:

a. Parathyroid hyperplasia is the most common etiology.

b. It affects women more than men.

c. Parathyroid adenomas can be composed of chief cells, clear cells, or oncocytes.

d. *MEN1* gene mutations may occur in familial and in sporadic parathyroid adenomas.

e. It can be associated with osteitis fibrosa cystica.

Answer: a

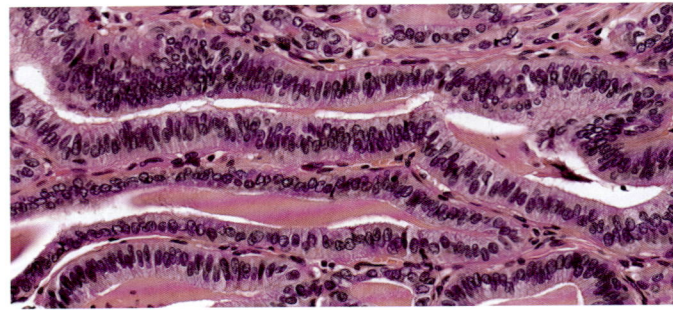

FIGURE 7.10 Tall cell papillary thyroid carcinoma. These aggressive thyroid carcinomas have a papillary architecture that is so complex it develops a "tramtrack" appearance.[10,11] The tumor cells have a height-to-width ratio that equals or exceeds 3:1. This striking elongation of the cells results in marked crowding and overlap of the nuclei; the nuclei are also elongated, but careful examination reveals irregularity of the nuclear membrane with grooves and pseudoinclusions. The tumors usually have a *BRAF* V600E mutation; they may also harbor additional mutations and often have a distinct epigenetic profile. Tumors of this type have more frequent extrathyroidal extension and behave aggressively. They are more common in older patients. Focal tall cell change of < 30% of the tumor mass does not qualify for this designation, but may be clinically relevant and should be documented.[12]

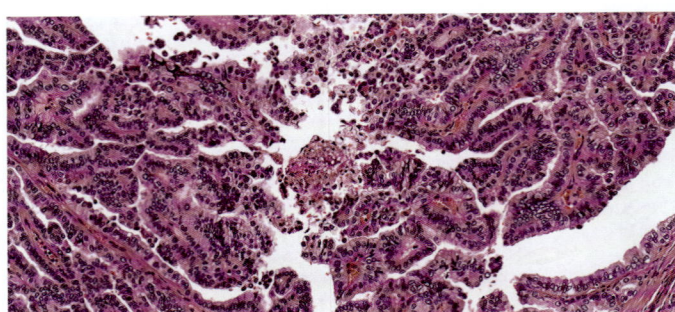

FIGURE 7.12 High grade papillary thyroid carcinoma. Thyroid carcinomas span a spectrum from low risk to highly aggressive carcinomas. In the middle are high grade malignancies. Papillary carcinoma is usually a relatively indolent carcinoma, but when it has necrosis and numerous mitoses, as in this case, it is an aggressive malignancy with a high risk of metastasis and radioactive iodine resistance.[15] Note the prominent complex papillary architecture and crowded cytology; the identification of necrosis should prompt a search for mitoses. These tumors usually have initial *BRAF* V600E mutations but also second genetic events, such as *TERT* promoter mutations, that account for more aggressive disease than typical papillary thyroid carcinomas. *CTNNB1* mutations are not characteristic of these lesions.

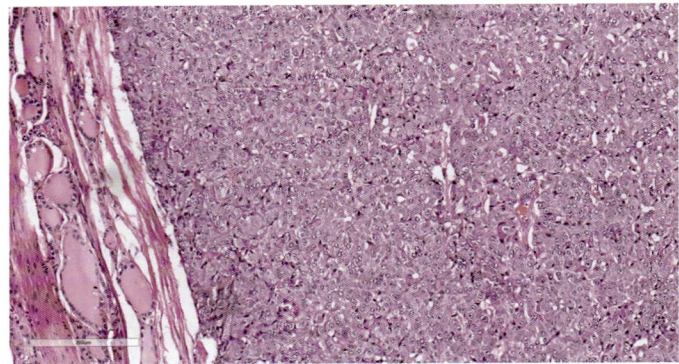

FIGURE 7.11 Medullary thyroid carcinoma. These tumors are derived from C cells and represent the neuroendocrine tumors (NETs) of thyroid. They are characterized by a solid nesting growth pattern and lack of defined cell borders. Some, but not all, medullary thyroid carcinomas have amyloid stroma due to deposition of a preprohormone of calcitonin.[13] Since amyloid is only found in about half of these tumors, it is important to think of this diagnosis in cases like the one shown here, in some cases that have papillary architecture due to breakdown of the solid nests, and in cases that have follicular architecture due to trapping of nontumorous elements. Medullary thyroid carcinomas may be familial when attributed to germline *RET* mutations, but sporadic tumors can harbor somatic *RET* mutations. Patients with MEN2A usually have a better prognosis, probably due to early detection. Calcitonin excess may cause diarrhea. These tumors do not concentrate iodine and are not treated with radioactive iodine. Grading has been proposed based on mitoses and necrosis.[14]

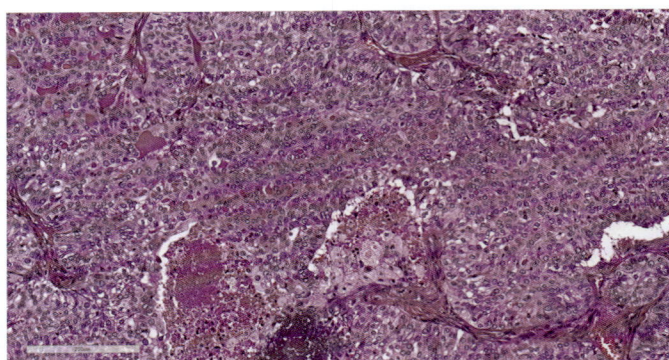

FIGURE 7.13 Poorly differentiated ("insular") thyroid carcinoma. Any differentiated thyroid carcinoma can progress to a high grade malignancy that has solid architecture, loss of cohesive growth, and necrosis. The most common scenario for the development of this so-called "insular" carcinoma is progression and dedifferentiation of a RAS-like carcinoma,[16] but BRAF-like papillary carcinomas can also develop into these poorly differentiated carcinomas that retain PAX8 positivity and positivity for thyroid transcription factor-1 (TTF1), but lose thyroglobulin expression[17] and have a high incidence of angioinvasion. These tumors mimic medullary thyroid carcinoma with their neuroendocrine "insular" architecture, but they are negative for insulinoma-associated protein 1 (INSM1), synaptophysin, and chromogranin, and for calcitonin, carcinoembryonic antigen (CEA), and amyloid.

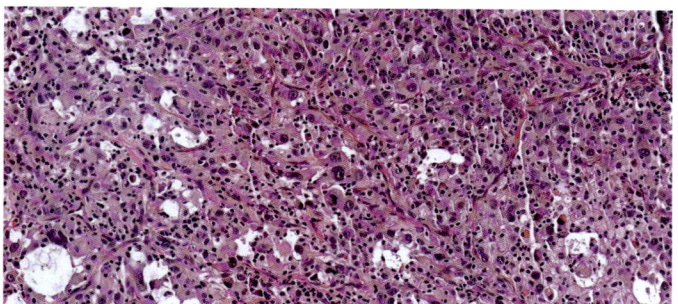

FIGURE 7.14 Anaplastic thyroid carcinoma. This is a diagnosis of exclusion, made when a thyroid malignancy has no features of differentiation. This anaplastic malignancy has prominent giant cells with bizarre nuclei, but these neoplasms can also have spindle cell morphology or may contain multinucleate giant cells that mimic sarcoma. Necrosis is usually readily identified and may be comedo-like or geographic in pattern. The tumor cells are usually negative for TTF1 and thyroglobulin, but there may be focal PAX8 positivity and focal keratin staining to distinguish them from sarcoma.[17] Careful examination and/or history will confirm a preexisting differentiated thyroid carcinoma; if that carcinoma was a papillary carcinoma, the anaplastic carcinoma may have a *BRAF* V600E mutation, and there will almost certainly be evidence of additional genetic alterations, most commonly a *TP53* loss of function event. These highly aggressive malignancies have a very rapid course and are usually lethal within 6 months to 1 year, however new targeted therapies are extending survival.

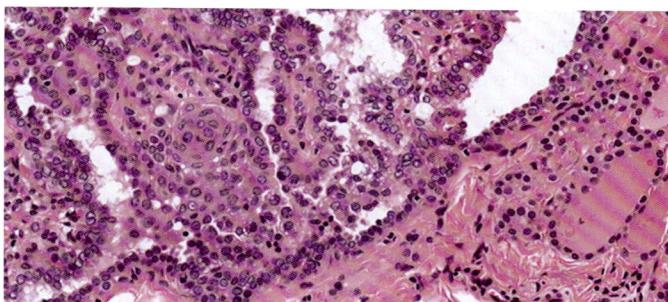

FIGURE 7.16 Cribriform morular thyroid carcinoma. This tumor resembles papillary thyroid carcinoma, but it is now recognized to be a distinct lesion with a specific mutational profile.[19] While it has complex papillary architecture, the tumor cells are often more columnar in pattern, and the tumors have characteristic morules of concentric squamoid epithelial cells (center of image). The tumor is most often due to germline *APC* mutation in patients with familial adenomatous polyposis (FAP) syndrome, but sporadic forms exist; there is a striking female predominance. The tumor cells do not express thyroglobulin or PAX8 and often are even focally negative for TTF1, proving that they are not likely to be of thyroid follicular differentiation. The morules show nuclear localization of β-catenin and express CD5 and keratin 5, suggesting possible thymic or ultimobranchial body derivation.[20]

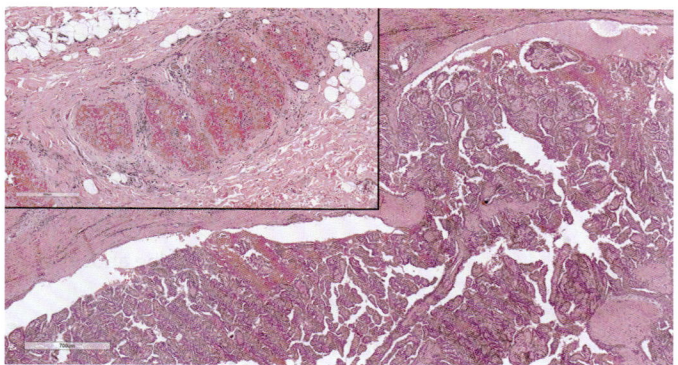

FIGURE 7.15 Angioinvasive papillary thyroid carcinoma. While many thyroid carcinomas can invade lymphatics and involve locoregional lymph nodes, this does not alter survival. In contrast, thyroid carcinomas with angioinvasion have a higher risk of distant metastasis that does impact survival. Angioinvasion must be clearly defined as the presence of tumor cells within vascular lumens associated with thrombus, that is a host response which clearly distinguishes true invasion from artefact.[18] Artefact is common in endocrine tissues that have fenestrated endothelium. It is important to recognize that tumor cells underlying intact endothelium indicates tumor invasion only into the capsule of the lesion; if it does not break through the endothelium, it is not true angioinvasion. The presence of red blood cells in the lumen can distinguish a vessel from a lymphatic channel without the need for special stains.

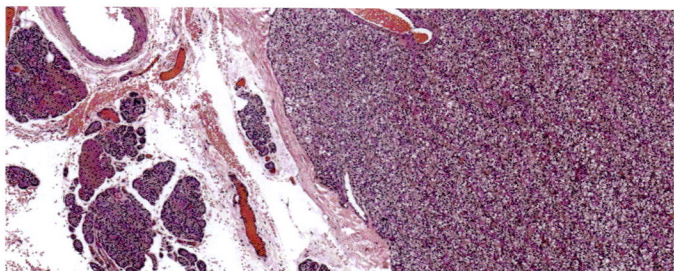

FIGURE 7.17 Primary hyperparathyroidism due to parathyroid adenoma. The most common cause of primary hyperparathyroidism is a solitary adenoma that can be composed of chief cells, clear cells, oncocytes, or a mix of cell types. These lesions are relatively well delineated but not always encapsulated; they are cellular and devoid of stromal fat. It is imperative to identify nontumorous parenchyma around the lesion to exclude the diagnosis of hyperplasia. Primary hyperparathyroidism is most common in women in the sixth to seventh decade.[21] It is common in patients with MEN1 and they develop multifocal adenomas involving multiple glands (this is mistakenly called "parathyroid hyperplasia"). *MEN1* gene mutations occur in sporadic adenomas.[22] Untreated, it can cause osteitis fibrosa cystica.

18. Figure 7.18 shows parathyroid carcinoma. Which statement is **false** about parathyroid carcinoma?

a. It can be associated with hyperparathyroidism jaw tumor (HPT-JT) syndrome.

b. A palpable neck mass may be present.

c. Associated bone and kidney disease is not uncommon.

d. The tumor is difficult to separate from the surrounding structures during surgery.

e. Positive immunohistochemical staining for parafibromin confirms the diagnosis.

Answer: e

19. Atypical parathyroid neoplasms (Figure 7.19) have fibrosis and pseudoinvasion, hemosiderin deposition, and focal necrosis. These features can be attributed to:

a. Ischemia.

b. Delayed fixation.

c. Previous biopsy.

d. Genetic predisposition.

e. Hypercalcemia.

Answer: c

20. Tertiary hyperparathyroidism (Figure 7.20) is due to:

a. A third genetic event in a parathyroid carcinoma.

b. Familial disease due to a mutation in the third *MEN* gene.

c. A neoplasm arising in the setting of secondary hyperplasia.

d. Malignancy arising in an adenoma.

e. Postbiopsy degeneration in an adenoma.

Answer: c

21. The pituitary tumor in Figure 7.21 was associated with Cushing disease. Which of the following is **not** true?

a. The tumor is composed of basophilic cells.

b. The tumor cells express TPIT.

c. The tumor cells are keratin negative.

d. The tumor cells are strongly PAS positive.

e. The nontumorous corticotrophs exhibit Crooke hyaline change.

Answer: c

22. Which of the following statements is correct about the pituitary tumor illustrated in Figure 7.22?

a. The tumor stains for *BRAF* V600E.

b. The tumor is associated with hypersecretion of growth hormone.

c. Staining for β-catenin is nuclear.

d. The tumor is positive for chromogranin.

e. This tumor is positive for synaptophysin.

Answer: c

23. The type of lung tumor illustrated in Figure 7.23 has all of the following features **except**:

a. It stains for INSM1, chromogranin, and hormones.

b. It is benign.

c. It can be part of multiple endocrine neoplasia types 1 and 4.

d. It can be associated with neuroendocrine cell hyperplasia.

e. It is also known as a carcinoid tumor.

Answer: b

24. Which of the following is true about gastric NETs (Figure 7.24)?

a. Type 1 enterochromaffin-like (ECL) cell tumors are more common in women with atrophic gastritis.

b. Type 3 tumors are usually multiple.

c. Type 4 tumors are usually solitary.

d. Type 2 tumors occur in a background of atrophic gastritis.

e. Type 2 tumors are more common in women.

Answer: a

25. Which statement is true about pancreatic NETs such as the one shown in Figure 7.25?

a. They may be associated with MEN1 syndrome.

b. They may develop in patients with von Hippel-Lindau (VHL) syndrome.

c. They are graded using mitotic count and Ki 67 labeling index.

d. They may secrete hormones or may be clinically nonfunctioning.

e. All of the above.

Answer: e

26. Duodenal neuroendocrine neoplasms (Figure 7.26) include all of the following **except**:

a. Gastrin-producing G-cell tumors.

b. Somatostatin-producing D-cell tumors.

c. Insulin-producing B-cell tumors.

d. Paragangliomas.

e. Composite ganglio-cytoma/ganglioneuroma and neuroendocrine tumor.

Answer: c

27. Small bowel NETs (Figure 7.27) do **not** usually present as which of the following:

a. Bowel obstruction.

b. Carcinoid syndrome.

c. Liver metastasis.

d. Lung metastasis.

e. Pelvic mass.

Answer: d

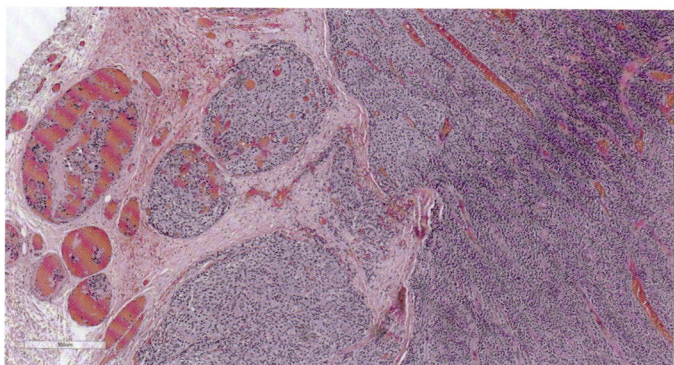

FIGURE 7.18 Parathyroid carcinoma. This malignancy can present as a severe primary hyperparathyroidism with bone and kidney manifestations but often there is a palpable neck mass. These are cellular and fibrotic tumors that the surgeon will identify as difficult to separate from the surrounding structures; this is due to the fibrosis and invasive tumor. The presence of unequivocal angioinvasion illustrated in the left of this figure (see definition in legend to Figure 7.15) confirms the diagnosis of malignancy. In questionable cases, the diagnosis can be made by showing loss of nuclear parafibromin, the tumor suppressor that is most commonly implicated in the pathogenesis of this carcinoma,[23] and other biomarkers.[24] Some patients with this disease have germline mutations of *CDC73* that encodes parafibromin; they develop a multisystem disease known as hyperparathyroidism jaw tumor syndrome.

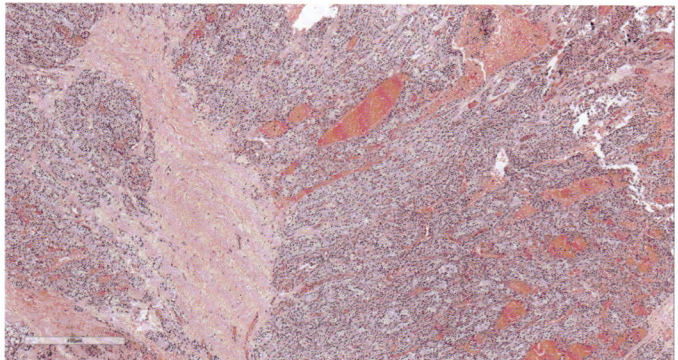

FIGURE 7.19 Atypical parathyroid neoplasm: adenoma with postbiopsy reactive changes. Parathyroid adenomas may be subjected to biopsy, either intentionally or because they are mistaken for or associated with a thyroid nodule. The effects of biopsy include fibrosis that can mimic invasion as shown here, hemosiderin deposition, and necrosis.[25,26] These worrisome features raise the possibility of carcinoma and have given rise to the diagnosis of "atypical" neoplasm. The judicious use of biomarkers can resolve this dilemma; when the tumor has intact parafibromin, BCL2, and p27, and is negative for galectin-3 and p53 overexpression, it is likely to be benign. There is no evidence that patient factors like hypercalcemia, or handling issues such as ischemia or delayed fixation, can cause these worrisome changes. Genetic predisposition does not cause atypical morphology.

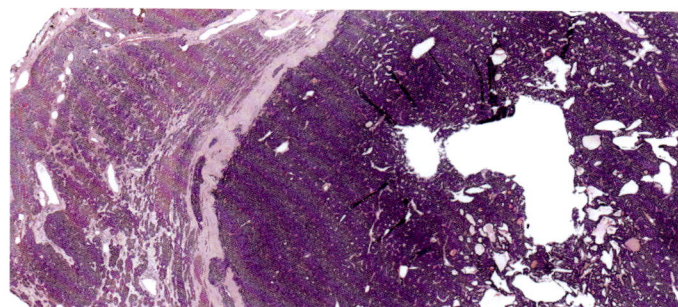

FIGURE 7.20 Tertiary hyperparathyroidism: adenoma arising in secondary hyperplasia. Patients with secondary hyperparathyroidism, most commonly due to renal failure, develop diffuse hyperplasia; all 4 glands are enlarged and cellular. With time, the glands can develop focal fibrosis and nodularity. However the emergence of a clonal autonomous neoplasm is the cause of tertiary hyperparathyroidism.[21] In this image, a cellular neoplasm is seen within a thick fibrous capsule with a surrounding hypercellular gland.

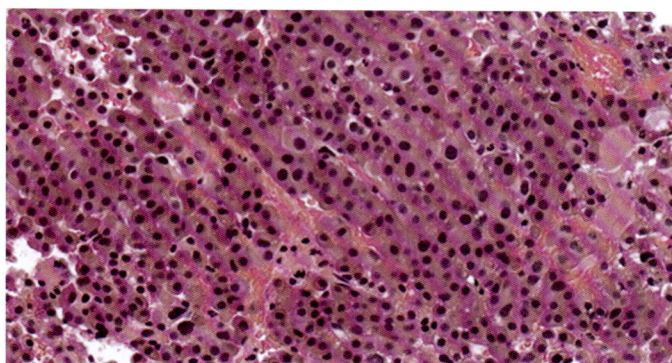

FIGURE 7.21 Densely granulated corticotroph tumor of the pituitary. This tumor has a classic basophilic appearance on H&E and the tumor cells are strongly positive with PAS stain since adrenocorticotropic hormone (ACTH) is a heavily glycosylated protein.[27–30] The tumor cells express nuclear TPIT and cytoplasmic ACTH. They are strongly positive for keratins and the nontumorous corticotrophs show evidence of suppression by the prolonged glucocorticoid excess with the accumulation of concentric whorls of pale pink hyaline cytoplasmic material that corresponds to keratin 18.[31]

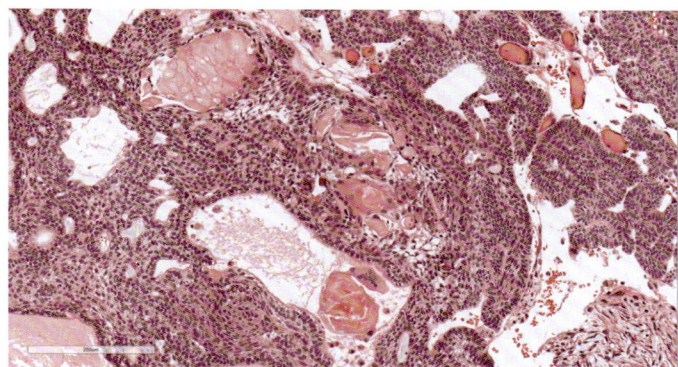

FIGURE 7.22 Adamantinomatous craniopharyngioma. Craniopharyngioma is a neoplasm that arises from remnants of Rathke pouch, an invagination of oral ectoderm of the roof of the mouth. The neoplasms can be composed of squamous epithelium, known as papillary craniopharyngioma, or they may resemble ameloblasts with stellate reticulum, "wet" keratin, and cystic spaces, giving rise to adamantinomatous craniopharyngiomas as shown here. The former are characterized by *BRAF* V600E mutations whereas the latter have mutations in *CTNNB1* that result in nuclear localization of β-catenin. These tumors are not hormonally active and cause hypopituitarism; they are negative for markers of neuroendocrine differentiation.[30,32]

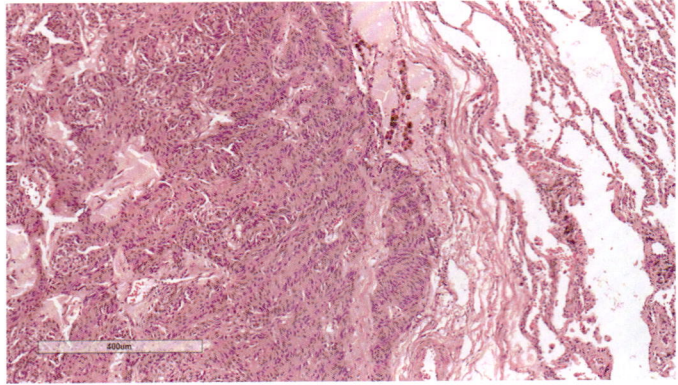

FIGURE 7.23 Well-differentiated pulmonary NET ("carcinoid tumor"). This tumor arises from the neuroendocrine cells of the respiratory mucosa and stains for neuroendocrine markers including INSM1, synaptophysin, and chromogranin; it may also express 1 or more of the known pulmonary hormones including calcitonin, calcitonin gene-related peptide (CGRP), bombesin, and serotonin.[33] There are 2 variants; central tumors tend to be more epithelioid, whereas peripheral tumors are often composed of spindle-shaped cells, as in this case. Peripheral tumors are more frequently hormonally active. These lesions are part of the spectrum of NETs that arise in MEN1 and MEN4. In some patients they are multifocal and are associated with neuroendocrine cell hyperplasia. Like all NETs, they are low grade malignancies that can give rise to metastatic disease.

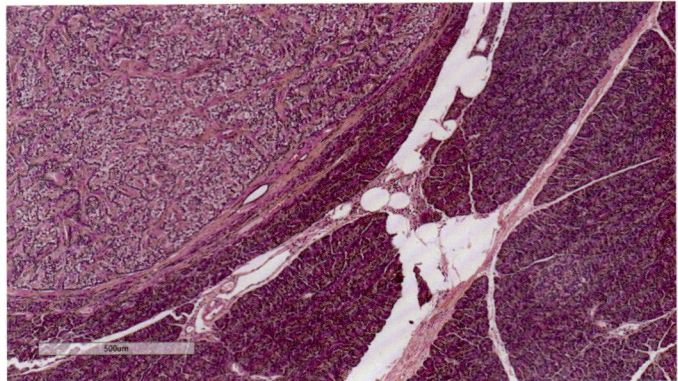

FIGURE 7.25 Pancreatic NET in MEN1. Pancreatic NETs are classified clinically as functional or nonfunctioning, but pathology shows hormone reactivity in the majority. They are graded based on mitotic counts and/or Ki 67 labeling index (G1, G2, and G3). They are distinguished from poorly differentiated high grade pancreatic neuroendocrine carcinomas based on morphology and expression of biomarkers that correlate with the different genetic basis of NETs versus neuroendocrine carcinomas (NECs): loss of menin or ATRX and expression of somatostatin receptor subtype 2 (SSTR2) supports a diagnosis of NET, whereas mutant p53, loss of retinoblastoma (RB), and negativity for SSTR2 support a diagnosis of NEC.[35] NETs are seen in patients with MEN1 or VHL syndrome, where they are often multifocal and are associated with abnormal islets that show disordered growth (dysplasia), microtumors, and peliosis.[36] Patients with VHL syndrome also develop serous proliferations and cysts, and their tumors are often oncocytic or composed of clear cells. The example illustrated is from a patient with multiple endocrine neoplasia type 1 and was among more than a dozen tumors identified in the pancreatic tail. Note also in the bottom right a large and irregular islet.

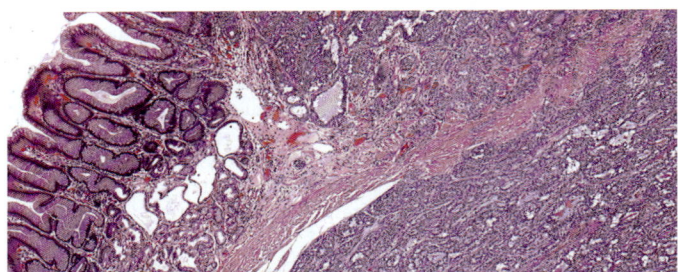

FIGURE 7.24 Gastric NET, type 4. There are multiple varieties of gastric NETs that are distinguished by cell type, morphology, and associated disorders.[34] The vast majority are composed of ECL cells that produce histamine (and pancreastatin). They stain for chromogranin. IHC for histamine is not routinely available; another biomarker is vesicular monoamine transporter 2 (VMAT2). Three types of ECL cell tumors are multifocal and considered to be secondary to an altered gastric acid environment: type 1 in patients with long-standing hypergastrinemia due to atrophic gastritis and achlorhydria; type 2 in patients with gastrinoma, usually in the setting of multiple endocrine neoplasia type 1 (MEN1); and type 4 in patients with defects of the proton pump. In contrast, type 3 lesions are solitary ECL cell NETs that occur sporadically in otherwise normal gastric mucosa. The example shown, type 4, is associated with dilated oxyntic glands containing inspissated secretory material, and lined by parietal cells with abundant eosinophilic and vacuolated cytoplasm in the peritumoral mucosa.

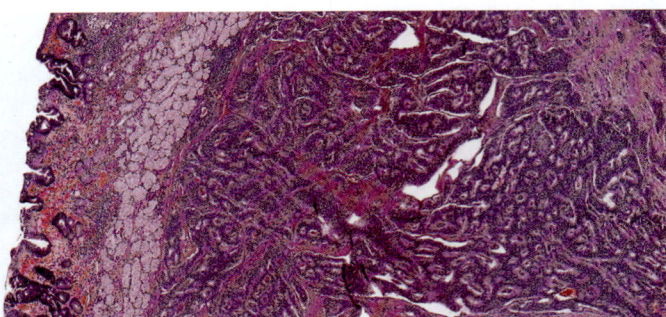

FIGURE 7.26 Duodenal gastrin-producing NET. Well-differentiated NETs arising in the duodenum can be hormonally active or clinically silent mass lesions[37]; they may secrete gastrin or somatostatin. Gastrinomas are frequently found in patients with MEN1 and duodenal somatostatinomas are common in patients with neurofibromatosis (less often in VHL syndrome and tuberous sclerosis). Occasional tumors contain pancreatic polypeptide. Unlike in the pancreas, insulinomas are not usually primary in this location. The example illustrated shows characteristic trabecular and pseudoglandular architecture, underlying Brunner glands, and infiltration through the muscularis propria. Another important entity is primary paraganglioma, which should always be considered in the differential diagnosis of a well-differentiated NET. A rare but interesting lesion that is found in the duodenum is a composite tumor composed of epithelial neuroendocrine cells, ganglion cells, and Schwann cells, representing a composite gangliocytoma/ganglioneuroma and neuroendocrine tumor (CoGNET); this lesion was previously called *gangliocytic paraganglioma* but has no relationship to paraganglia.[38]

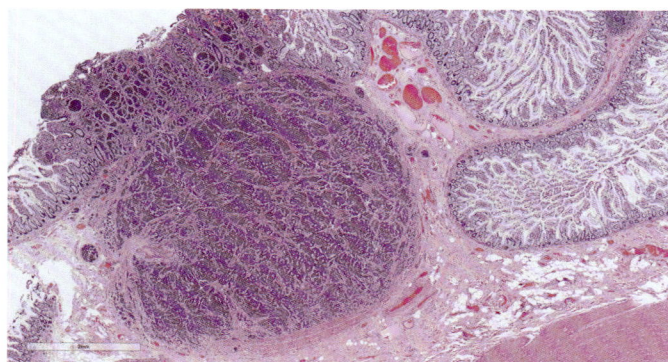

FIGURE 7.27 Small bowel enterochromaffin cell NET. The vast majority of small bowel NETs have a highly characteristic morphology.[2] They are composed of solid nests of basophilic cells that begin as small nodules in the mucosa, infiltrate to form larger nodules in the submucosa, and then infiltrate through the muscularis propria to involve the mesentery. They are usually relatively small primary tumors that present with complications of metastasis, including large mesenteric or pelvic masses that cause obstruction, liver metastasis, and carcinoid syndrome that is not manifest until the lesion has bypassed the liver's ability to inactivate serotonin in the portal circulation. Lung metastasis is exceptionally rare. These tumors express CDX2 and serotonin as well as the markers of neuroendocrine differentiation INSM1, synaptophysin and chromogranin; they are positive for keratins. They are graded by mitoses and/or Ki 67 as G1, G2, and G3 lesions.

28. The features of a rectal polyp that is classified as an L-cell tumor (Figure 7.28) include all of the following **except**:

a. A well-differentiated NET with low Ki 67 labeling index.

b. A characteristic morphology with concentric whorls of ribbons and trabeculae.

c. Immunoreactivity for glucagon, pancreatic polypeptide, and peptide YY (PYY).

d. Low risk of recurrence.

e. Biochemical surveillance by urinary 5-hydroxyindoleacetic acid (5-HIAA) levels.

Answer: e

29. The clinical management of the rectal lesion shown in Figure 7.29 includes which of the following?

a. Polypectomy with no need for further assessment.

b. Measurement of circulating pancreatic polypeptide levels.

c. Assessment by imaging using fluorodeoxyglucose positron emission tomography (FDG-PET).

d. Genetic testing for familial endocrine syndrome.

e. Biochemical surveillance by urinary 5-HIAA levels.

Answer: c

30. The adrenal lesion shown in Figure 7.30 has all of the following features **except**:

a. High incidence of genetic predisposition.

b. Positivity for INSM1, chromogranin, and GATA3.

c. Positivity for TTF1.

d. Association with medullary thyroid carcinoma.

e. Positivity for inhibin in some cases.

Answer: c

31. Which is the most valuable immunohistochemical profile for the neck lesion shown in Figure 7.31?

a. INSM1, chromogranin, S100, TTF1.

b. Chromogranin, GATA3, tyrosine hydroxylase, SDHB.

c. Chromogranin, S100, keratin.

d. Chromogranin, keratin, Ki 67.

e. Chromogranin, TTF1, CDX2 and Ki 67.

Answer: b

32. The differential diagnosis of the lesion shown in Figure 7.32 includes all of the following **except**:

a. Metastatic neuroendocrine carcinoma.

b. Metastatic small bowel NET.

c. Metastatic pituitary NET.

d. Metastatic paraganglioma.

e. Primary paraganglioma.

Answer: a

33. The clinical presentation of the patient with the adrenal lesion shown in Figure 7.33 was:

a. Cushing syndrome.

b. Conn syndrome.

c. Addison disease.

d. Hyperpigmentation.

e. Abdominal pain.

Answer: a

34. The patient with the adrenal lesion shown in Figure 7.34 had a history that included:

a. Cushing syndrome.

b. Cardiac myxoma.

c. Hyperaldosteronism.

d. a and b.

e. b and c.

Answer: d

35. The adrenal mass shown in Figure 7.35 can be proven to be adrenal cortical carcinoma with the following immunoprofile:

a. Vimentin and calretinin.

b. Steroidogenic factor 1 (SF1) and inhibin.

c. Melan-A and synaptophysin.

d. p53.

e. None of the above.

Answer: b

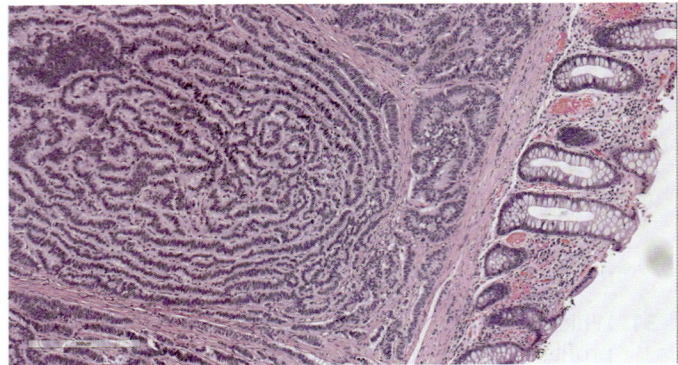

FIGURE 7.28 Rectal L-cell NET. A well-differentiated NET of the rectum that frequently presents as a rectal polyp is composed of L cells that express glucagon, pancreatic polypeptide, and PYY. These tumors have a characteristic histology with ribbons and trabeculae of cells forming concentric whorls. These are usually low grade with low Ki 67 labeling indices and they have a low risk of recurrence.[39–41] They do not express serotonin, therefore there is no value in surveillance by measuring the breakdown product of that hormone, 5-HIAA.

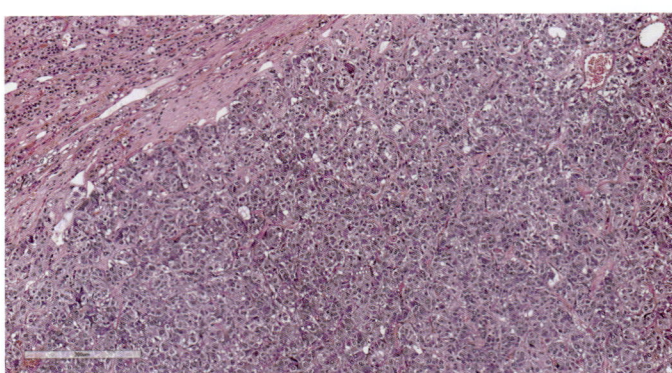

FIGURE7.30 Pheochromocytoma (intraadrenal paraganglioma). These nonepithelial NETs derive from the sympathetic paraganglion that is the adrenal medulla. They have a characteristic zellballen architecture with solid nests of chief cells in a highly vascular stroma. The chief cells stain for INSM1, synaptophysin and chromogranin and are negative for keratins. They express GATA3, and tyrosine hydroxylase.[43] TTF1 is negative. The tumors usually have sustentacular cells that stain for S100 (so do the tumor cells, but less intensely) as well as SOX10. These lesions have a high incidence of genetic predisposition; a large number of mutations have been documented and each is associated with a distinct syndrome.[44] The most common involve alterations in the hypoxia response pathways (SDH-related disease and VHL syndrome) and tumors in those patients can express inhibin, an important feature to note since it cannot be used to distinguish cortical from medullary lesions.[45] The kinase pathway tumors are exemplified by MEN2 in which pheochromocytoma is associated with medullary thyroid carcinoma.[46] All paragangliomas are considered to have malignant potential and, while there have been proposals for features that predict malignancy, this is no longer a relevant topic. Metastatic paragangliomas must be distinguished from multifocal primary disease in patients with genetic predisposition.

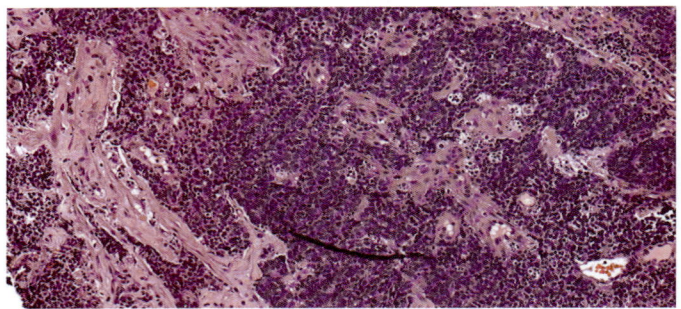

FIGURE 7.29 Rectal neuroendocrine carcinoma. The diagnosis of high grade poorly differentiated neuroendocrine carcinoma is made for tumors with solid nesting architecture, focal necrosis, and high cellularity (often small cell morphology but occasional large cell cytology) with numerous mitoses. This diagnosis should prompt assessment of the extent of disease, which is likely to have metastasized. These lesions may present as rectal polyps, but they often have lymph node spread at the time of diagnosis. These tumors are not usually hormonally active and do not express somatostatin receptors at high levels, therefore they are not best assessed by Ga68 DOTATATE scan; their high proliferative activity renders them detectable by FDG-PET scan.[42] Neuroendocrine carcinomas, unlike NETs, are not recognized to be manifestations of familial endocrine syndromes.

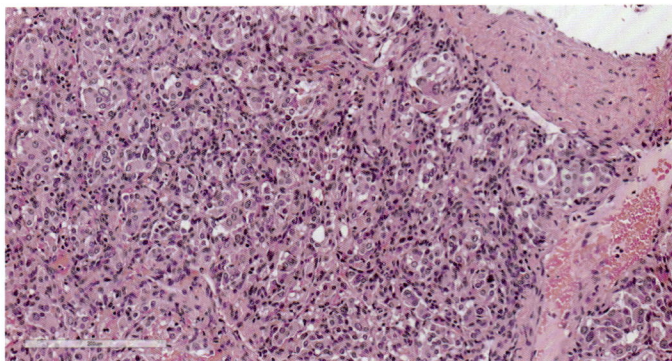

FIGURE 7.31 Carotid body paraganglioma. These nonepithelial NETs derive from the parasympathetic paraganglion that is the carotid body. The tumor has characteristic zellballen architecture and vascular stroma. The tumor cells, known as chief cells, stain for INSM1, synaptophysin, and chromogranin, and are negative for keratins. They express GATA3 and tyrosine hydroxylase. TTF1 and caudal-type homeobox 2 (CDX2) are negative. Sustentacular cells in paragangliomas, and most NETs, express nuclear SOX10, and nuclear and cytoplasmic S100. These lesions have a high incidence of genetic predisposition; a large number of mutations have been documented and each is associated with a distinct syndrome. The most common involve alterations in 1 member of the serine dehydratase (SDH) complex (SDHA, SDHB, SDHC, SDHD, and SDHAF) and any mutation results in destabilization of the complex, resulting in negative staining for SDHB.[47] Ki 67 may be helpful to predict the likelihood of recurrence or metastasis,[46] but these tumors are currently not graded.

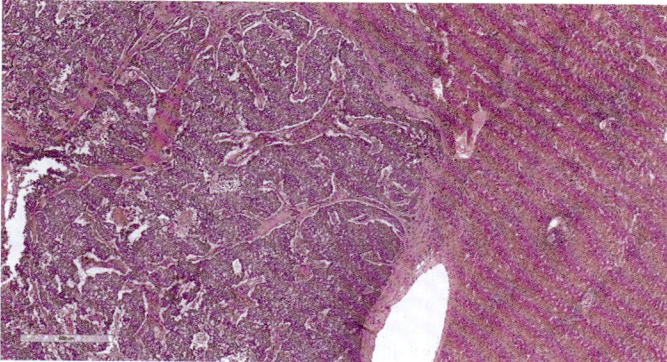

FIGURE 7.32 Liver with NET. The detection of a well-differentiated neuroendocrine neoplasm (NEN) in the liver should precipitate a careful workup, as the differential diagnosis is large. The differential diagnosis includes metastatic NET from almost any site, including pituitary gland, parathyroid gland, lung, thymus, gastroenteropancreatic system, gonads, and genitourinary system. It also includes paragangliomas that can metastasize to the liver, but may also arise as a primary lesion at that site.[48] This well-differentiated lesion cannot be considered for a diagnosis of metastatic NEC, since by definition NEC is a poorly differentiated high grade malignancy (usually small cell or large cell type).

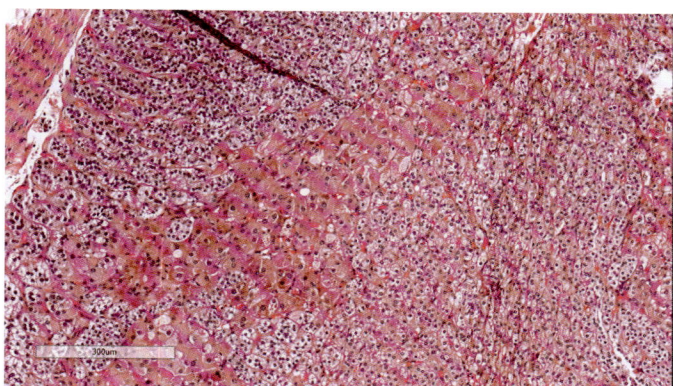

FIGURE 7.34 Primary pigmented nodular adrenocortical disease (PPNAD). This patient presented with Cushing syndrome, but the adrenal glands were not enlarged. The presence of microscopic nodules of pigmented cortical cells is a characteristic feature of Carney complex, in which germ-line mutation of *PRKAR1A* predisposes to increased cAMP levels in tissues that are dependent on 7-transmembrane domain G-protein-coupled receptors (e.g., the ACTH receptor in adrenal glands) with somatic knockout of the normal allele.[50,51] Patients with Carney complex also develop cardiac myxomas, hyperpigmentation of the skin (lentigines), and other forms of endocrine overactivity, including thyroid and pituitary hyperfunction. Aldosterone is dependent on ion channels rather than cAMP and is therefore not a part of this disorder.

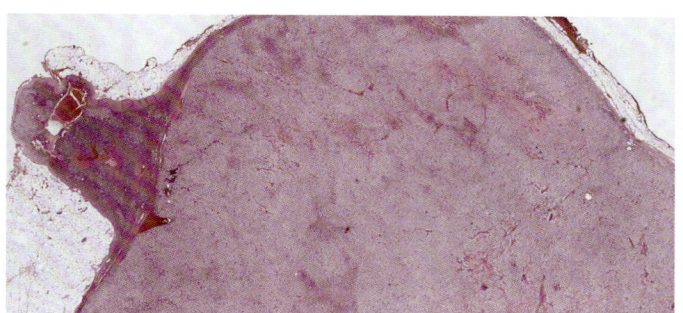

FIGURE 7.33 Adrenal cortical adenoma causing Cushing syndrome. The adrenal gland contains a well-differentiated adenoma composed of clear and compact cells. The diagnosis of adenoma is not difficult, but the atrophy of the adjacent gland is striking, with only medulla and clear cells at the periphery and no zona reticularis. This indicates hyperfunction by the lesion, resulting in pituitary suppression and reduced ACTH.[49] The pituitary suppression results in postoperative adrenal insufficiency that requires supplementation and gradual weaning. The pathologist should check the clinical story and ensure that clinical or subclinical Cushing syndrome was not missed by the treating team.

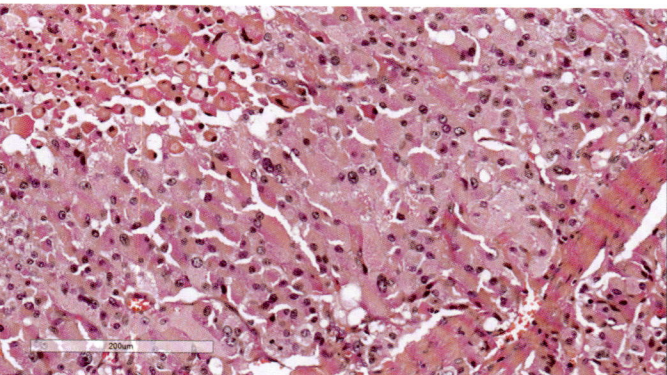

FIGURE 7.35 Adrenal cortical carcinoma. Adrenal cortical carcinomas generally come in 2 morphologic types.[52] Low grade lesions tend to be readily recognized as adrenal cortical neoplasms, but the challenge is to identify the atypical mitoses and vascular invasion that define them as malignant. The more common type is a high grade malignancy that must be proven to be of adrenal cortical origin, as in this case where the tumor cells are large, oncocytic, and focally rhabdoid, with discohesive growth and necrosis. In this situation, expression of nuclear SF1 and cytoplasmic inhibin are helpful to confirm adrenal cortical carcinoma and exclude a sarcoma or metastatic carcinoma. These tumors also express vimentin, calretinin, Melan-A, and synaptophysin, and they may have mutation of *TP53*, but none of these are specific for adrenal cortical carcinoma: they can be expressed by other lesions that can give rise to an adrenal mass (e.g., metastatic carcinomas and melanoma).[53]

36. The adrenal mass shown in Figure 7.36 is most likely to be:

a. An adrenal corti-
cal carcinoma.

b. A metastatic sarcoma.

c. A posttraumatic
pseudocyst.

d. A myelolipoma.

e. An infection.

Answer: c

37. Which of the following is true about the adrenal tumor in Figure 7.37?

a. This is an undif-
ferentiated adrenal
cortical neoplasm.

b. By immunohis-
tochemistry, the
neoplastic cells
are positive for
inhibin, Melan-A,
and chromogranin.

c. Amplification
of c-MYC is the
most frequent

molecular alteration
in these tumors.

d. According to the
International Neu-
roblastoma Pathol-
ogy Classification
(INPC), this tumor is
considered poorly
differentiated.

e. Tumors with MYCN
amplification have
good prognosis.

Answer: d

38. Which of the following is true about thyroglossal duct cyst?

a. It usually presents as
a lateral neck mass
in young adults.

b. It is derived from the
tracheal mucosa.

c. Papillary thyroid
carcinoma occurs
in approximately
3% of cases.

d. Medullary thyroid
carcinoma is the most
common malig-
nancy that develops
in this lesion.

e. Thyroid lobec-
tomy is curative.

Answer: c

Thyroglossal duct cyst is a developmental cyst derived from the thyroglossal duct remnants. It typically presents as a midline infrahyoid cystic mass with bimodal age distribution in the first and fifth decades. The cyst wall is lined by respiratory-type ciliated columnar epithelium and, to a lesser extent, stratified squamous epithelium. Thyroid gland follicles, minor salivary glands, and cartilage may be found in the cyst wall. Papillary thyroid carcinoma has been reported in approximately 3% of thyroglossal duct cysts. Medullary thyroid carcinoma, which is derived from the C cells, typically develops in the thyroid lobes (not in the midline). Sistrunk procedure is the standard surgical treatment of thyroglossal duct cyst. It entails en block resection of the cyst with the duct remnants and the middle third of the hyoid bone.[58]

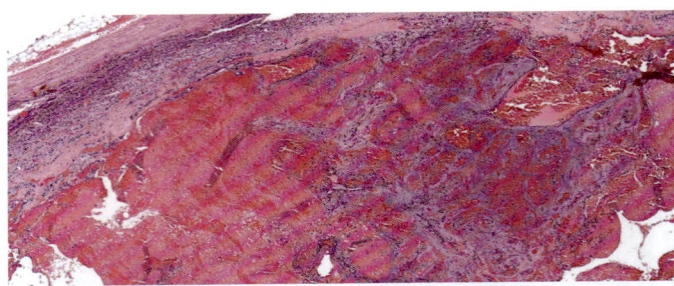

FIGURE 7.36 Adrenal pseudocyst. Large adrenal masses are usually discovered incidentally on imaging or palpation, but may cause pain and/ or gastrointestinal symptoms. Acute presentations may result from rupture, hemorrhage, or infection. The differential diagnosis includes adrenal cortical carcinoma, myelolipoma, metastatic malignancy, sarcoma, and a cystic lesion.[2] There are 4 main types of adrenal cysts that fall into this differential diagnosis: epithelial lined cysts that result from cystic degeneration of an adenoma, endothelial cysts, parasitic cysts, and pseudocysts. This is an example of a pseudocyst in which a wall composed of fibrotic tissue has no lining and is filled with hemorrhage in various stages of organization. These lesions often develop after an episode of trauma.

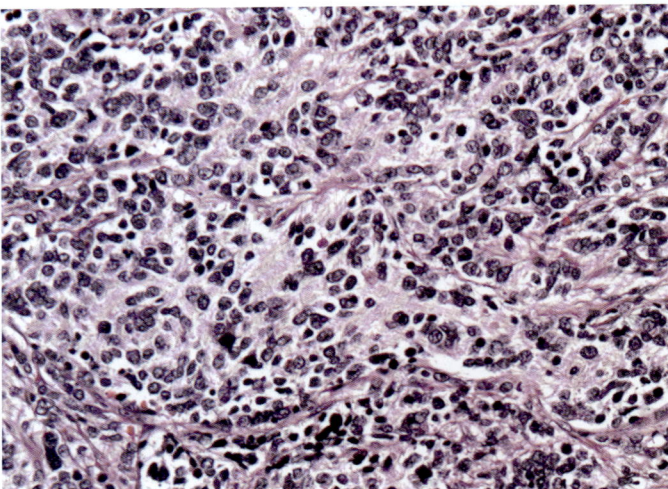

FIGURE 7.37 Adrenal neuroblastoma. Neuroblastoma is a peripheral neuroblastic tumor of neural crest origin. It is the most common neoplasm in infants. Tumors show significant size variation and can be unicentric or multicentric. Areas of hemorrhage and necrosis are typically seen on gross examination. Histologically, neuroblastomas can be "Schwannian stroma-poor" or "Schawnnian stroma-rich" (ganglioneuroblastoma). According to the INPC, stroma-poor neuroblastomas can be subclassified into undifferentiated, poorly differentiated, and differentiating subtypes. The undifferentiated subtype lacks the neuropil background and requires ancillary immunohistochemistry to distinguish it from other small blue cell tumors. Positive immunohistochemical stains include synaptophysin, chromogranin, PGP9.5, neurofilament protein, and neural crest markers such as tyrosine hydroxylase (TH) and PHOX2B. Poorly differentiated neuroblastoma is composed of neuroblasts in a background of neuropil with minimal ganglion cell differentiation (< 5%) while differentiating neuroblastomas exhibit > 5% ganglion cell differentiation. Amplification of MYCN is the most frequent molecular alteration (20% of cases) and is associated with aggressive biologic behavior.[54-57]

39. Noninvasive follicular thyroid neoplasm with papillary-like nuclear features (NIFTP) is characterized by all the following features **except**:

a. It is well circumscribed/encapsulated.

b. There is no capsular invasion or infiltration of the surrounding thyroid parenchyma.

c. The tumor has a predominantly follicular architecture

d. The neoplastic cells exhibit the nuclear features of papillary thyroid carcinoma.

e. Mutation in *NRAS* is the most frequent molecular alteration detected in these tumors.

with less than 10% papillary component.

Answer: c

Noninvasive follicular thyroid neoplasm with papillary-like nuclear features (NIFTP) is an indolent follicular cell-derived neoplasm. A subset of tumors previously classified as encapsulated follicular variant of papillary carcinoma, NIFTP is encapsulated/well demarcated with no capsular invasion, vascular invasion, or infiltration of the surrounding thyroid parenchyma. True papillae are typically rare or absent but some authors allow papillary architecture comprising up to 1% of the tumor. The neoplastic cells exhibit the nuclear features of papillary carcinoma usually in a multifocal distribution and, less frequently, in a diffuse manner. The nuclear features of papillary carcinoma in NIFTP are typically not as well developed as in classic papillary carcinoma. The presence of tumor necrosis, increased mitotic count (> 3 mitoses/2 mm^2), cytologic features of aggressive variants of papillary carcinoma (tall cell or hobnail), or a solid component that exceeds 30% of the tumor exclude the diagnosis of NIFTP. Molecular alterations in *RAS*, *PPAR gamma*, *THADA*, and *EIF1AX* have been reported in NIFTP. *NRAS* mutation is the most frequent molecular alteration. In contrast to classic papillary carcinoma, mutation in *BRAF* V600E is typically absent and if detected, the diagnosis of NIFTP should be excluded.[59–61]

40. Which of the following is **not** true about adrenal ganglioneuroma?

a. It is a circumscribed, firm, grey-white or yellow mass.

b. Metastases occur in approximately 10% of cases.

c. The mature subtype is composed of mature ganglion cells embedded in schwannian spindle cell stroma.

d. The maturing subtype may contain scattered differentiating neuroblasts/maturing ganglion cells.

e. Absence of distinct microscopic neuroblastomatous nests distinguishes the maturing subtype of ganglioneuroma from ganglioneuroblastoma.

Answer: b

Ganglioneuroma is a rare tumor of the adrenal medulla and extra adrenal paraganglia. Grossly, the tumor is a circumscribed grey-white or yellow-tan mass with no hemorrhage or necrosis. Microscopically, the mature subtype is composed of mature ganglion cells admixed with Schwann cells. The maturing subtype contains scattered differentiating neuroblasts (maturing ganglion cells) but no distinct microscopic nests of neuroblasts — a feature that distinguishes this tumor from ganglioneuroblastoma. Ganglioneuroma behaves in a benign manner and does not metastasize.[54,55,62]

41. The following features are characteristic of aldosterone-producing adrenal cortical adenoma **except**:

a. Imaging of the contralateral adrenal gland is usually normal.

b. The adrenal cortex away from the tumor is of normal thickness (not atrophic).

c. The vast majority of tumors are composed

of cells that resemble zona glomerulosa.

d. Laminated eosinophilic cytoplasmic inclusions may be identified in the tumor cells.

e. The tumor cells are positive for CYP11B2 by immunohistochemistry.

Answer: c

Primary hyperaldosteronism is the most common cause of secondary hypertension. Bilateral adrenal cortical hyperplasia is the most frequent cause of primary hyperaldosteronism (60–70% of cases) while solitary adenoma accounts for approximately 30–40% of cases. Imaging studies (CT) and selective adrenal vein sampling (to determine lateralization) are essential to distinguish bilateral from unilateral adrenal cortical disease in patients with hyperaldosteronism. Histologically, most aldosterone-producing adrenal cortical adenomas are lipid rich (resembling zona fasciculata) and the absence of associated adrenal cortical atrophy helps to distinguish these tumors from cortisol-producing adenomas. As many of the patients with hyperaldosteronism are treated preoperatively with spironolactone, the concentric laminated "spironolactone bodies" are often detected in the histologic sections of these tumors. Immunohistochemistry for CYP11B2 (aldosterone synthase) is also helpful to confirm the functional status of an aldosterone producing adenomas.[52,63]

42. Which of the following statements is not true about adrenal myelolipoma?

a. This tumor typically develops in in adults with myelofibrosis.

b. Most of the tumors are detected incidentally on imaging studies.

c. Approximately 10% of the tumors are associated with

congenital adrenal hyperplasia.

d. It may be associated with other adrenal tumors such as cortical adenoma.

e. The main differential considerations include lipoma and angiomyolipoma.

Answer: a

Adrenal myelolipoma is a benign neoplasm that is usually discovered as an incidental finding (6–16% of adrenal incidentalomas). Large tumors may cause compression of adjacent structures, or may rupture and cause abdominal hemorrhage. It can occur with other adrenal tumors and approximately 10% of cases are associated with congenital adrenal hyperplasia. Microscopically, myelolipomas are composed of adipose tissue and trilineage hematopoietic elements, resembling extramedullary hematopoiesis (EMH). However, in contrast to EMH, which is a diffuse process, myelolipoma is circumscribed and is not related to bone marrow disorders.[64]

SHORT ANSWER QUESTIONS

43. List autoimmune disorders that can be associated with autoimmune thyroiditis.
- Addison disease.
- Type 1 diabetes mellitus.
- Hypoparathyroidism.
- Vitiligo.
- Pernicious anemia.
- Connective tissue diseases (rheumatoid arthritis, systemic lupus erythematosus, Sjögren syndrome).
- Schmidt syndrome (Addison disease, diabetes, and hypothyroidism secondary to Hashimoto thyroiditis).

44. What are the endocrine manifestations of immunoglobulin G4 (IgG4) disease?
- Hypothalamic-pituitary involvement (formerly known as pituitary pseudotumor).
  - Mass lesion, headaches, visual disturbance, hypopituitarism, and diabetes insipidus.
- Thyroiditis (formerly known as Riedel thyroiditis).
  - Sclerosing thyroiditis, asymmetrical, extrathyroidal extension, obliterative vasculitis.

45. Describe the molecular alterations in thyroid carcinoma and their genotype-phenotype correlations.
- Differentiated thyroid cancer (DTC): *RAS* versus *BRAF* mutations, fusions as drivers, *TERT* and *STK11* in progression, *TP53* in anaplastic thyroid cancer (ATC).
- Medullary thyroid cancer (MTC): *RET* mutations, extracellular versus kinase mutations in MEN2A versus MEN2B, codon 918 mutations and *RAS* mutations in sporadic forms.

46. Discuss the variants of papillary thyroid carcinoma (PTC) and their clinical implications.
- Classical PTC (none).
- Encapsulated classical PTC (low risk).
- Infiltrative follicular variant PTC (none).
- Diffuse sclerosing PTC (more common in children, often high stage with metastasis at diagnosis).
- Oncocytic PTC (none).
- Warthin-like PTC (none).
- Clear cell PTC (none).
- Solid/trabecular PTC (more aggressive).
- Spindle cell PTC (uncertain).
- PTC with fibromatosis/fasciitis-like/desmoid-type stroma (none).
- Tall cell PTC (more aggressive).
- Hobnail PTC (more aggressive).
- Columnar cell (very aggressive).

47. Discuss the morphologic features of high grade thyroid carcinomas and their clinical relevance.
- Morphologic features:
  - Necrosis, mitoses, widely invasive growth, angioinvasion.
  - Two types: papillary and insular.
  - Immunohistochemical loss of thyroglobulin.
- Clinical relevance:
  - The features predict extensive local invasion, incomplete local resection; angioinvasion predicts distant metastasis.
  - Loss of thyroglobulin positivity is associated with lack of uptake of radioactive iodine and inability to monitor progression with circulating thyroglobulin levels.

48. Discuss the role of frozen sections in the management of thyroid disease.
- To identify parathyroid glands for sparing.
- To identify unexpected metastatic disease.
- **Not** to determine the nature of a thyroid nodule — that should be done preoperatively using biopsy.

49. Discuss the role of molecular testing in thyroid fine-needle aspiration (FNA) specimens.
- Not useful for benign or clearly malignant lesions.
  - Ancillary testing with IHC can be helpful for diagnosis of medullary thyroid carcinoma.
- Useful for borderline lesions (atypia of undetermined significance [AUS], follicular lesion of undetermined significance [FLUS]) where detection of a known driver mutation can alter diagnosis, and identification of a molecular alteration indicating aggressive behavior may determine the extent of surgery.

50. Discuss the role of frozen sections in the management of parathyroid disease.
- Frozen sections are used to identify parathyroid glands during surgery.
- Parathyroid hormone monitoring can be used to determine the successful identification and resection of the culprit gland.
- It is important to identify the hilum of the gland on gross examination to allow identification of normal tissue and confirmation of adenoma.

51. Classify hyperparathyroidism.

- Primary hyperparathyroidism, which is due to parathyroid adenoma(s) or carcinoma; multifocal disease is a feature of genetic predisposition.
- Secondary hyperparathyroidism, which is mainly due to renal failure, but can also be associated with inadequate dietary intake of calcium, steatorrhea, and vitamin D deficiency.
- Tertiary hyperparathyroidism, which occurs in a minority of renal-failure patients if parathyroid activity becomes autonomous.

52. Outline the classification of pituitary neoplasms.

- Adenohypophysial cell neoplasms: pituitary NETs (PitNETs, formerly "adenomas").
  - PIT1-lineage: somatotroph tumors; mammosomatotroph tumors; lactotroph tumors; thyrotroph tumors; mature plurihormonal and immature PIT-lineage tumors; acidophil stem cell tumors; and mixed somatotroph-lactotroph tumors.
  - TPIT-lineage: corticotroph tumors.
  - SF1-lineage: gonadotroph tumors.
  - Lineage-deficient: null cell tumors, unusual plurihormonal tumors.
  - Multiple synchronous PitNETs.
  - Metastatic PitNETs (formerly "pituitary carcinomas").
- Rathke cleft-derived neoplasms.
  - Pituitary blastoma.
  - Adamantinomatous craniopharyngioma.
  - Papillary craniopharyngioma.
- Posterior lobe and hypothalamic neoplasms.
  - Pituicytomas (including oncocytic and granular cell types).
  - Gangliocytomas.
  - Neurocytomas.
- Other tumors that occur in the sellar region.

53. List genetic syndromes associated with pancreatic NETs.

- MEN1/4: anterior pituitary NET, multiglandular parathyroid disease (multiple adenomas, known clinically as "hyperplasia"), pancreatic NET, adrenocortical tumors, other NETs.
  - MEN1/4 is associated with nesidiodysplasia and peliosis.
- VHL syndrome: hemangioblastoma of the central nervous system, clear cell renal cell carcinoma, pheochromocytoma/paragangliomas, pancreatic NET, endolymphatic sac tumor.
  - Pancreatic NETs are often oncocytic or clear cell.
  - VHL syndrome is associated with nesidiodysplasia and peliosis.
- Neurofibromatosis (NF1): café au lait macules, multiple neurofibromas (or plexiform neurofibroma), Lisch nodules (iris hamartoma), optic glioma, osseous lesions, pancreatic NETs, pheochromocytomas.
- Tuberous sclerosis: hamartomas of the central nervous system, giant cell astrocytoma, retinal glial hamartomas, renal angiomyolipoma, cutaneous angiofibromas, shagreen patches, ash-leaf patches, subungual fibromas, pancreatic NETs.

54. Discuss the common clinical presentations of small bowel NETs. Discuss the features that explain these presentations.

- Common clinical presentations include:
  - Small bowel obstruction due to intussusception or fibrosis from mesenteric masses.
  - Abdominal pain from mass or obstruction.
  - Weight loss.
  - Flushing and diarrhea.
- Carcinoid syndrome explains the flushing and diarrhea: the features indicate metastasis to or beyond the liver, since serotonin is metabolized in the liver and these tumors usually drain into the portal circulation.

55. Discuss the distinction between NETs and NECs. Give examples of both.

- Well-differentiated NETs versus small cell and large cell carcinomas (NECs) of lung, pancreas, gut, and genitourinary tract have distinct molecular events.
- NETs tend to have genetic alterations that target the epigenetic pathways; NECs tend to have mutations that are present in the corresponding exocrine carcinomas of the same organs.
- Prostate NECs are common, especially in hormone-resistant aggressive carcinomas.
- Skin NECs are represented by Merkel cell carcinoma.

56. Discuss the various familial syndromes associated with pheochromocytoma/paraganglioma (PPGL).

GENE	SYNDROME	MOST-COMMON PPGL LOCATIONS	ASSOCIATED LESIONS
RET	MEN2	Adrenal gland.	• Medullary thyroid carcinoma. • Parathyroid proliferations. • Mucocutaneous ganglioneuromas.
VHL	VHL	Adrenal gland & extraadrenal paraganglia.	• Clear cell renal cell carcinoma. • Hemangioblastomas. • NETs. • Pancreatic serous cystadenomas.
NF1	NF1	Adrenal gland & extraadrenal paraganglia.	• Neurofibroma and MPNST. • Ocular manifestations. • Duodenal NET.
SDHA	PGL5	Extraadrenal paraganglia, adrenal gland.	• Renal cell carcinoma. • Gastrointestinal stroma tumor. • Pituitary tumor.
SDHB	PGL4	Extraadrenal paraganglia: A&T, H&N.	• Renal cell carcinoma. • Gastrointestinal stroma tumor. • Pituitary tumor.
SDHC	PGL3	Extraadrenal paraganglia: H&N.	• Renal cell carcinoma. • Gastrointestinal stroma tumor.
SDHD	PGL1	Extraadrenal paraganglia, adrenal gland.	• Renal cell carcinoma. • Gastrointestinal stroma tumor. • Pituitary tumor.
SDHAF2	PGL2	Extraadrenal paraganglia: H&N.	• Unknown.
TMEM127	—	Adrenal gland & extraadrenal paraganglia.	• Renal cell carcinoma.
MAX	—	Adrenal gland & extraadrenal paraganglia.	• Unknown.
FH	HLRCC	Adrenal gland & extraadrenal paraganglia.	• Cutaneous and uterine leiomyoma. • Renal cell carcinoma.
EPAS1	PZS	Adrenal gland & extraadrenal paraganglia: A&T.	• Duodenal NET. • Polycythemia. • Ocular manifestations.
EGLN1	—	Adrenal gland & extraadrenal paraganglia: A&T.	• Polycythemia.
EGLN2	—	Adrenal gland & extraadrenal paraganglia: A&T.	• Polycythemia.
MDH2	—	Extraadrenal paraganglia: A&T.	• Unknown.
KIF1B	—	—	• Ganglioneuroma/neuroblastoma. • Leiomyosarcoma. • Lung adenocarcinoma.
MEN1	—	Adrenal gland & extraadrenal paraganglia: H&N.	• Parathyroid proliferations. • Pituitary tumor. • NETs.

Abbreviations: A&T: abdomen and thorax; H&N: head and neck; HLRCC: hereditary leiomyomatosis and renal cell carcinoma; MEN: multiple endocrine neoplasia; MPNST: malignant peripheral nerve sheath tumor; NET: neuroendocrine tumor; NF: neurofibromatosis; PGL: paraganglioma; PGL1 (also 2, 3, 4, 5): syndromes also known as Carney-Stratakis syndrome; PPGL: pheochromocytoma/paraganglioma; PZS: Pacak-Zhuang syndrome; VHL: von Hippel-Lindau syndrome.

57. Discuss the fundamental difference between the genetics of MEN1 and MEN2 that alters prophylaxis for cancer development.

• MEN1 is, like most heritable cancer syndromes, due to inheritance of a mutated tumor suppressor gene. This disease manifests when a "second hit," a somatic alteration, results in loss of the normal allele. There is no way to predict when and where that second event will occur, so screening is the usual approach to monitor patients with this disorder.

• In contrast, MEN2 is an exceptional example of inheritance of a mutated oncogene. Thus, it can be predicted that all patients with this disorder will develop the potentially lethal manifestation: medullary thyroid carcinoma. For this reason, guidelines have been developed that recommend prophylactic thyroidectomy at ages that vary based on the specific mutation, a feature that determines the likely age of onset of medullary thyroid carcinoma.[65]

58. Outline the various schemes that assess the risk of malignancy in adrenal cortical neoplasms.

CLASSIFICATION	WEISS (1984)	MODIFIED WEISS (2002)	WIENEKE CRITERIA (2003)	BISCEGLIA-WEISS (2004)	RETICULIN ALGORITHM (2009)	HELSINKI (2015)
RESTRICTION			PEDIATRIC	ONCOCYTIC		
Scoring pattern	≥ 3 malignant	≥ 3 malignant	> 3	1 major malignant 1–4 minor UMP	Altered reticulin with any 1 of the elements listed in this column, below	> 8.5 malignant
Tumor weight			> 400 g	> 200 g minor		
Tumor size			> 10.5 cm	> 10 cm minor		
Nuclear grade	Fuhrman nuclear grade (FNG) III or IV					
Mitotic rate > 5/50HPF	> 5/50 HPF	x2	> 15/20 HPF	Major	> 5/HPF	Number x3
Ki 67%		Unknown.				Number
Mitotic figures	Atypical mitosis	Atypical mitosis		Major		
Cytoplasm	Clear cells ≤ 25%	Clear cells ≤ 25% x2				
Architecture	Diffuse pattern > 30%					
Necrosis	Necrosis	Necrosis	Necrosis	Minor	Necrosis	x5
Vascular invasion	Venous invasion		Vascular invasion	Major	Vascular invasion	
Sinusoidal invasion	Sinusoidal invasion			Minor		
Capsular invasion	Capsular invasion	Capsular invasion	Capsular invasion	Minor		
Extraadrenal extension			Extraadrenal extension			

Modified and reprinted with permission from Innovative Science Press.

59. Discuss the various ways to obtain a Ki 67 labeling index and their accuracy.
- An accurate Ki 67 labeling index depends on identifying hot spots.
- You can eyeball the proportion of stained tumor cells versus the total number of tumor cells to estimate a Ki 67 score, but it will not provide an accurate score.
- A better method is to photograph and print the area of most intense staining, then count 500–2000 tumor cells and report the Ki 67 index as the percentage of positive tumor cells.
- Automated image analysis is also available and accurate.

60. A 65-year-old woman with primary hyperparathyroidism is undergoing parathyroidectomy. You are called to the operating room for intraoperative consultation. Discuss your approach to this case.
- The role of intraoperative consultation is to document parathyroid tissue as opposed to lymph node or other soft tissue nodules.
- The tissue should be carefully examined to identify the hilum of the gland, as that is where the nontumorous tissue is most likely to be found; the identification of nontumorous parenchyma is the ideal way to distinguish adenoma from hyperplasia.
- The critical role of intraoperative parathyroid hormone in ensuring resection of a culprit parathyroid gland should be emphasized with the surgeon.

61. A 62-year-old man has undergone thyroidectomy and you have received the specimen. Discuss how you would handle the gross inspection.
- Clarify the extent of surgery: know the definitions of a lobectomy, hemithyroidectomy, subtotal thyroidectomy, and total thyroidectomy. Define the components of the specimen.
- Weigh the specimen.
- Paint resection margins.
- Measure each component.
- Identify any surface nodules that may represent lymph nodes, parathyroids, or other relevant perithyroidal tissues.

(continued on next page)

- Section the lobe(s) carefully in the transverse plane and the isthmus in the sagittal plane.
- Document any lesions with respect to location, size, and appearance; describe the appearance of all tissue.

- Sample generously to ensure accurate assessment of each lesion, including careful evaluation of the capsule(s) of any nodules, and any lymph nodes, parathyroids, or other relevant perithyroidal tissues; use your judgement!

62. A neck lymph node is biopsied and contains a solid tumor with focal necrosis. The clinical history indicates that the patient has a thyroid mass. What is your approach to this lesion?

- Morphology is critical; does this look like a NET and is likely to be MTC? Is it a poorly differentiated tumor of follicular cell derivation? Is it anaplastic thyroid carcinoma? Could it be a paraganglioma or a metastatic carcinoma from elsewhere that is also involving the thyroid?

- IHC must be performed and probably in a stepwise fashion, starting with PAX8, TTF1, thyroglobulin, chromogranin, and CEA. Subsequent workup will depend on the outcome of the initial stains.

63. A liver biopsy specimen contains a lesion that is histologically consistent with metastatic neuroendocrine neoplasia. What is your approach?

- Confirm neuroendocrine differentiation: INSM1, synaptophysin, chromogranin.
- Ensure epithelial versus PPGL distinction: keratins.
- Establish NET versus NEC: morphology; Ki 67; if necessary, p53, RB, and SSTR IHC.

- Grade NET: Ki 67, mitoses.
- Determine site of origin: review history; use transcription factors and hormones wisely.
- Consider molecular IHC for genetic predisposition.

64. A 48-year-old woman has a lung mass that was biopsied and diagnosed as well-differentiated NET/carcinoid. You receive the lobectomy specimen. What are the main features you need to determine?

- Confirm lesional diagnosis: morphology, chromogranin, Ki 67, possibly other neuroendocrine markers (TTF1, calcitonin, serotonin, bombesin, CEA).

- Determine the extent of disease: lymph nodes, etc.
- Examine the nontumorous lung carefully for neuroendocrine cell hyperplasia.

65. A 29-year-old male has undergone distal pancreatectomy for a 2 cm neuroendocrine neoplasm. What are the main features that you must determine and report?

- Tumor size and location.
- Tumor type and grade (careful correlation with clinical data can uncover functionality).
- Lymph node status.

- Presence of other associated pathology: islet proliferations, dysplasia, peliosis; serous cystic lesions, etc. (given the young age, consider molecular IHC for genetic predisposition).

66. You receive an adrenalectomy specimen from a 50-year-old woman. The gland weighs 45 g and there is a dominant yellow nodule that is well delineated and homogeneous. The surrounding adrenal gland is atrophic. How would you handle this case?

- Immediately check the chart; if the clinical diagnosis was Cushing syndrome, proceed with routine handling.
- If the diagnosis does not include a history of Cushing syndrome, check the biochemistry to determine whether there was a proper workup.

- In any situation where the diagnosis of Cushing syndrome is unclear, contact the clinician to ensure that they are aware of the probable requirement for steroid coverage.

67. You receive a large hemorrhagic mass identified as "adrenal tumor." Describe your approach to the gross description and sectioning of this specimen.

- Check the clinical history for presentation, functionality.
- Weigh, measure, and paint the specimen.
- Carefully remove adherent fat, and weigh and measure the gland with the tumor.
- Examine serial sections for areas of necrosis, hemorrhage, and calcification.

- Sample all areas of the capsule, with particular focus on identifying areas of angioinvasion.
- Generously sample the tumor to include all areas of unusual morphology.
- Dissect periadrenal fat to identify and sample any lymph nodes.

68. You are grossing an ileocolectomy specimen and identify a large fibrotic mesenteric mass. What is the likely diagnosis and how will you confirm it?

- The most likely diagnosis is a mesenteric deposit of a small bowel NET.
- These are most commonly located in the terminal ileum; they can be very small and may be multiple.

- The pathologist must carefully examine the entire mucosa of the small bowel to the ileocecal valve to ensure identification of the primary tumor(s).
- Of course, all margins and lymph nodes must also be sampled, in addition to the dominant mesenteric mass.

69. You receive a biopsy of a para-aortic lymph node with a clinical diagnosis of "?metastatic carcinoma versus lymphoma." The initial H&E section shows a NET. Describe how you proceed.

- The differential diagnosis includes paraganglioma, which may be multiple in patients with genetic predisposition.
- Workup should include INSM1, chromogranin, and keratin(s).
- If the NET is keratin negative, GATA3, S100 (SOX10), and tyrosine hydroxylase will confirm paraganglioma; SDHB should be assessed as well as carbonic anhydrase (CAIX), and inhibin.
- If the NET is keratin positive, consider rectal or other pelvic NET; staining for SATB2 and PSAP points to the possibility of a rectal primary, and the case should be assessed for serotonin, PP, and/or glucagon expression.

IMAGES: ENDOCRINE PATHOLOGY

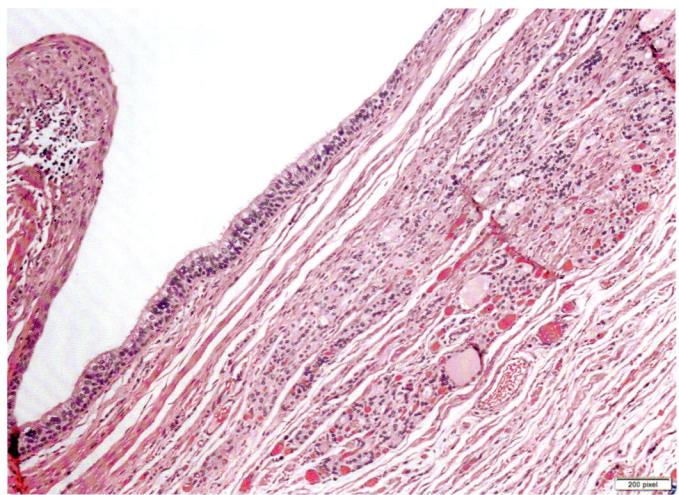

IMAGE 7.1 Thyroglossal duct cyst with thyroid follicles in the cyst wall. The cyst is lined by pseudostratified ciliated columnar epithelium (respiratory-type epithelium) and stratified squamous epithelium (upper left) (H&E, x100).

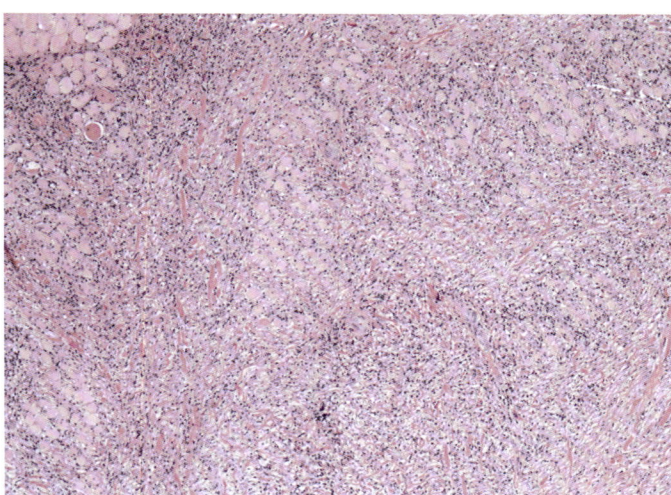

IMAGE 7.3 IgG4-related thyroiditis (previously known as Riedel thyroiditis). Note the inflammation and fibrosis involving perithyroidal skeletal muscle (H&E, x20).

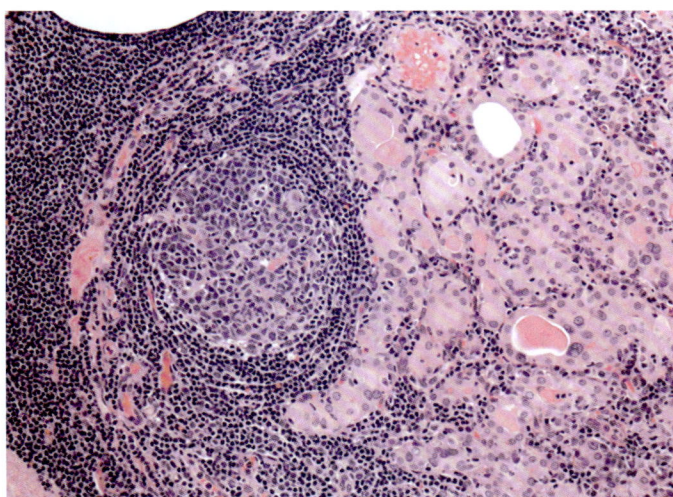

IMAGE 7.2 Chronic lymphocytic thyroiditis (Hashimoto thyroiditis). Note the dense lymphoplasmacytic infiltration of the thyroid parenchyma, with reactive germinal centers. Oncocytic metaplasia of the follicular epithelial lining is evident (H&E, x40).

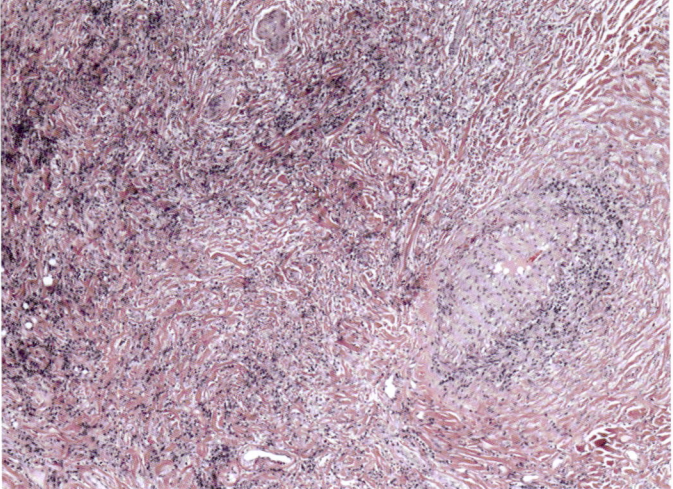

IMAGE 7.4 IgG4-related thyroiditis, showing obliteration of the thyroid parenchyma by lymphoplasmacytic infiltration and storiform fibrosis. Obliterative phlebitis is noted (lower right) (H&E, x40).

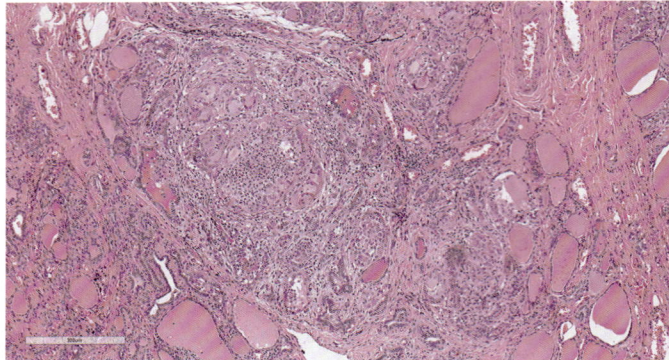

IMAGE 7.5 De Quervain thyroiditis. The thyroid is distorted by a heterogeneous mild chronic inflammatory process with prominent histiocytic infiltration that mainly involves follicles where foreign body giant cells are numerous.

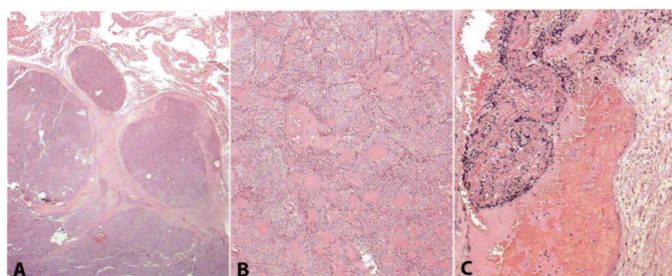

IMAGE 7.8 Image A: this follicular carcinoma is widely invasive with tumor nodules well beyond the tumor capsule. Image B: the tumor is composed of follicular epithelial cells that form follicles with colloid contents. Image C: tumor cells within a vascular channel form a thrombus with fibrin.

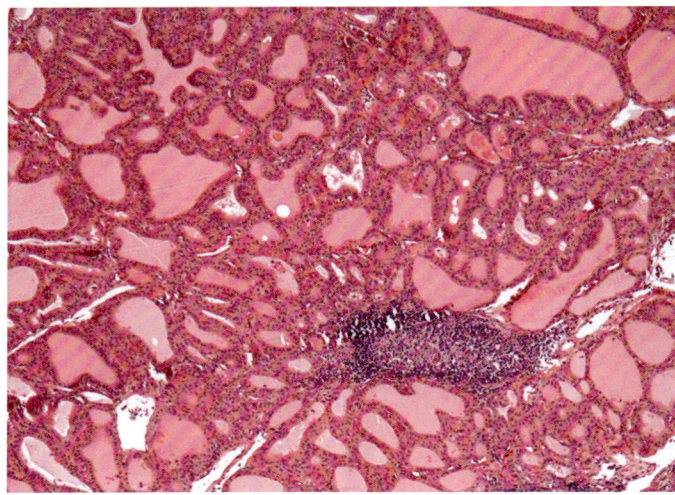

IMAGE 7.6 Graves disease. Note papillary hyperplasia of the follicular epithelium. Oncocytic metaplasia and focal lymphocytic infiltration are also present in this example (H&E, x40).

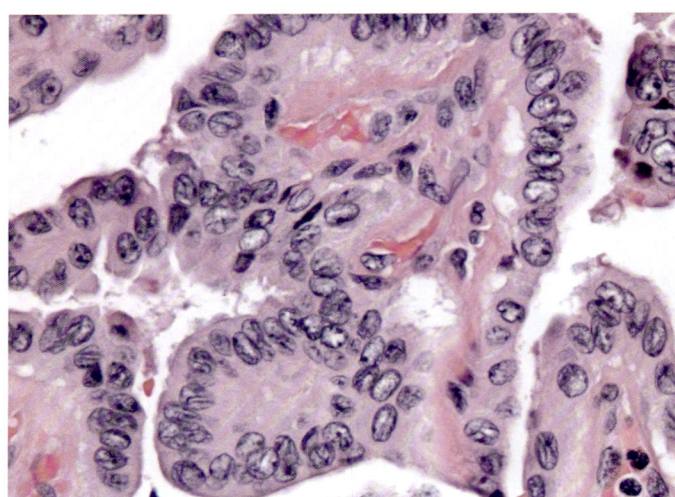

IMAGE 7.9 Papillary thyroid carcinoma. The image shows the typical appearance of this entity: papillary structures lined by epithelial cells with large, elongated, molded nuclei that exhibit nuclear membrane grooves and fine chromatin (H&E, x200).

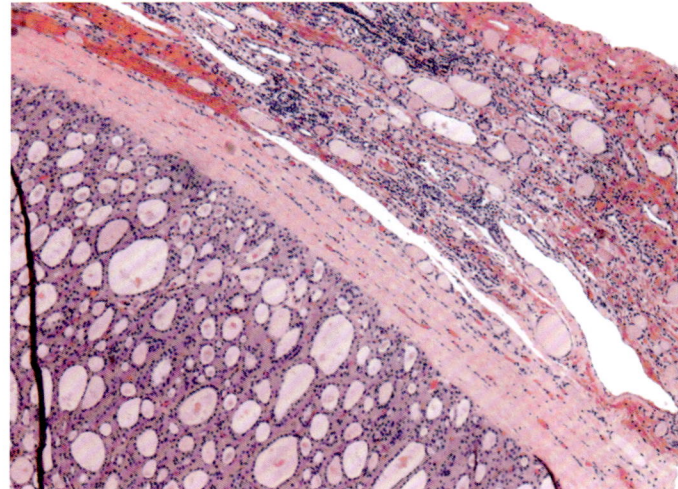

IMAGE 7.7 Oncocytic follicular adenoma. This is a solitary, encapsulated, architecturally distinct neoplasm composed of follicles that are lined by oncocytic epithelial cells that lack nuclear atypia. There is no capsular or vascular invasion. The background thyroid parenchyma shows lymphocytic thyroiditis (H&E, x20).

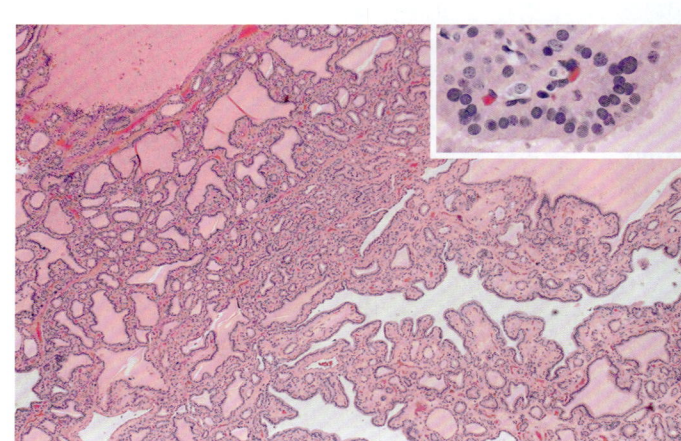

IMAGE 7.10 Papillary hyperplasia in a benign follicular nodule (H&E, x40). Note the absence of the nuclear features of papillary thyroid carcinoma (inset, x200).

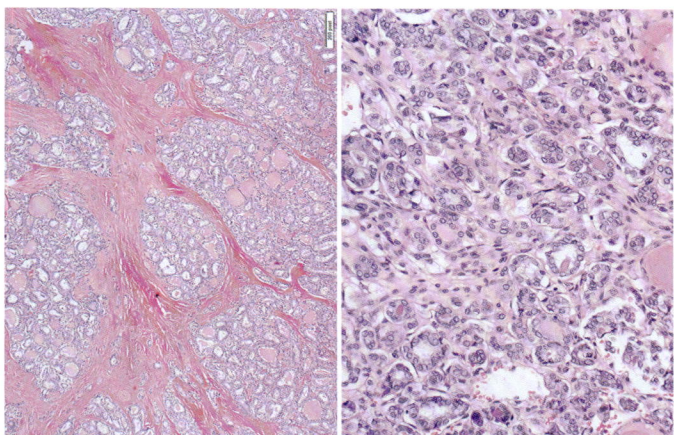

IMAGE 7.11 Image A: this tumor — a follicular variant of papillary thyroid carcinoma, infiltrative type — has follicular architecture and infiltrative growth pattern. No frankly complex papillary structures are seen, but there are small "abortive" papillae and elongated follicles and the nuclear atypia is so florid that it can be seen even at low magnification (H&E, x40). Image B: the neoplastic cells have enlarged, elongated, molded nuclei with nuclear membrane grooves and pale ground-glass chromatin (H&E, x200).

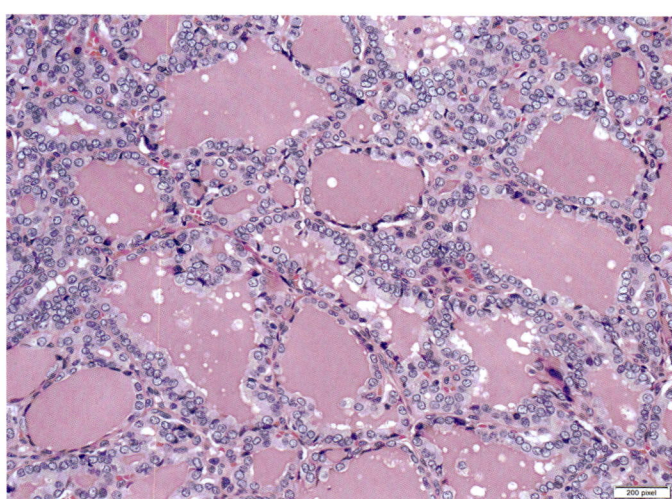

IMAGE 7.13 NIFTP. The epithelial lining of the neoplastic follicles has enlarged, elongated, crowded nuclei with nuclear membrane grooves and pale chromatin (H&E, x200).

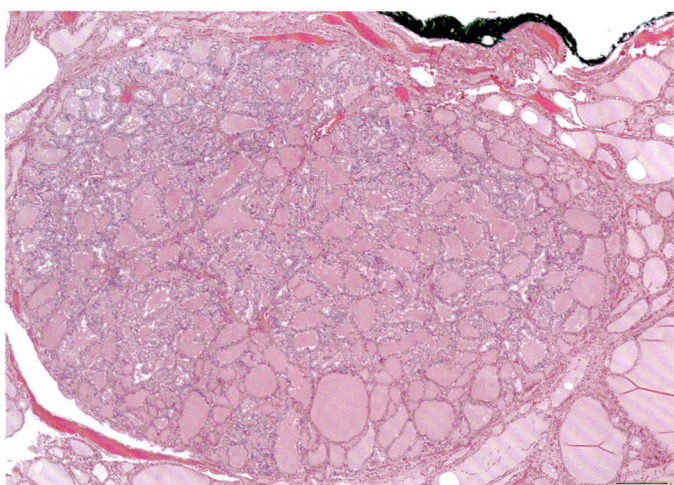

IMAGE 7.12 Nonivasive follicular thyroid neoplasm with papillary-like nuclear features (NIFTP). Circumscribed, follicular-patterned, expansile tumor with no invasion of the surrounding thyroid parenchyma or vascular invasion. No papillae, psammoma bodies or solid areas are noted. There is no necrosis or mitotic figures (H&E, x40).

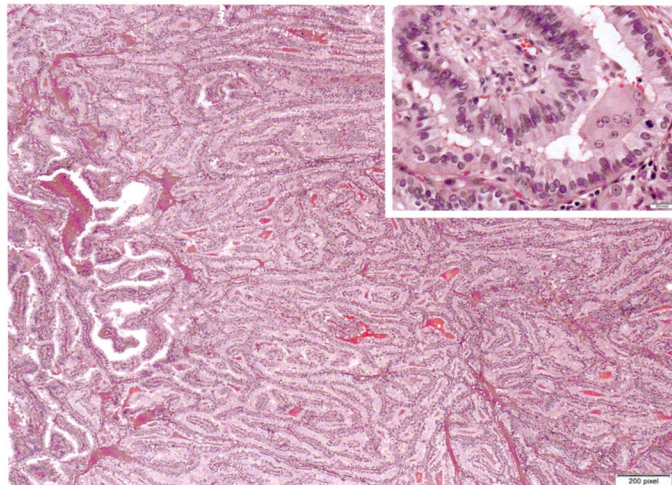

IMAGE 7.14 Tall cell papillary thyroid carcinoma with the characteristic "tram track" appearance on low power (H&E, x40). The neoplastic cells are tall and columnar, with a height-to-width ratio ≥ 3:1. These cells have eosinophilic cytoplasm and exhibit the nuclear features of papillary carcinoma (inset: H&E, x400).

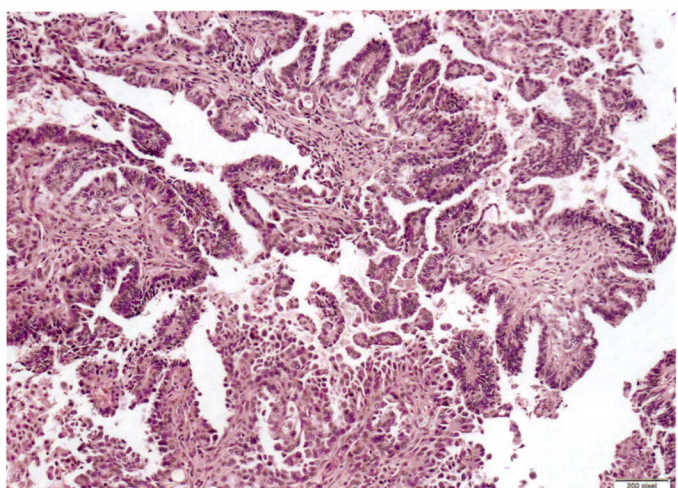

IMAGE 7.15 Hobnail papillary thyroid carcinoma (PTC). The tumor has micropapillary architecture (H&E, x100).

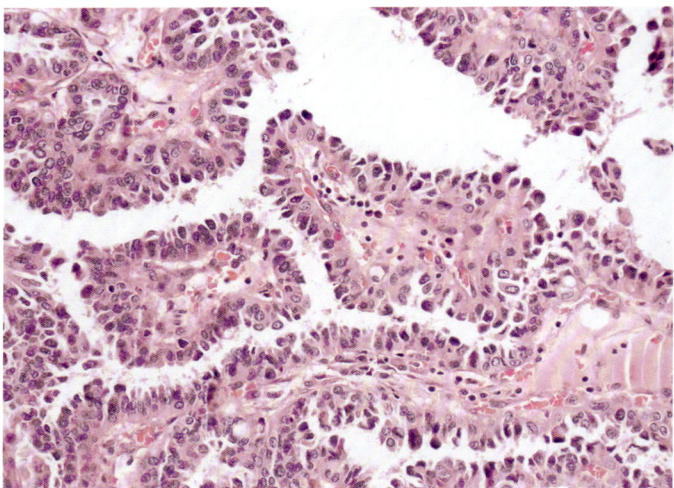

IMAGE 7.16 Hobnail PTC. The neoplastic cells are dyscohesive and have "hobnail" appearance (H&E, x200).

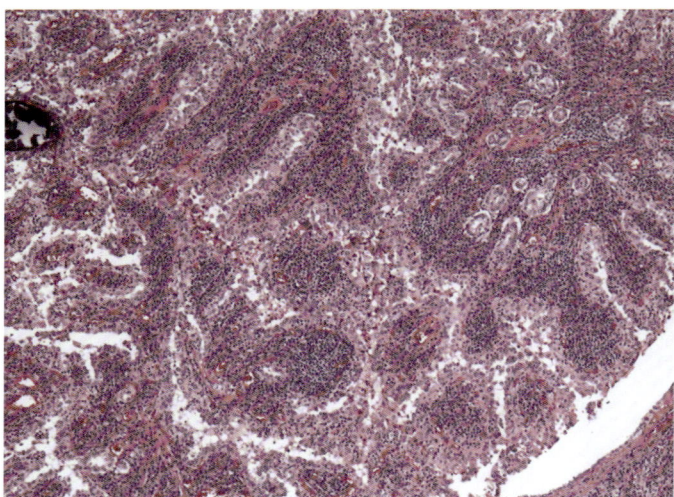

IMAGE 7.17 Warthin-like papillary carcinoma. Note the papillary architecture and the dense lymphoplasmacytic infiltration of the fibrovascular cores (H&E, x40).

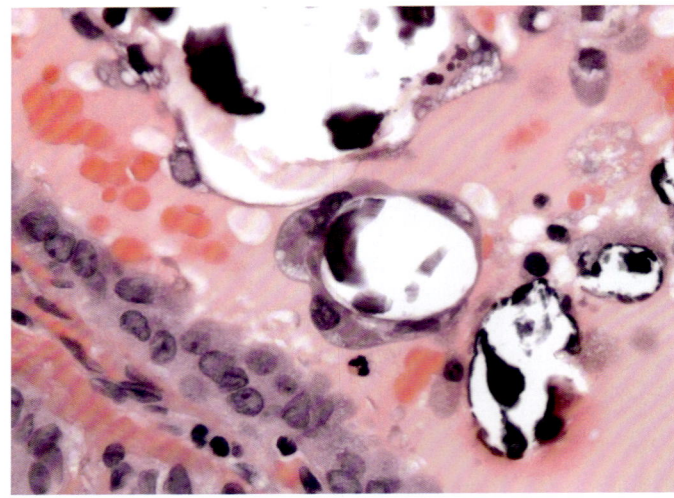

IMAGE 7.18 Cystic lymph node metastasis of papillary thyroid carcinoma. The nuclear features of PTC are evident in the neoplastic epithelium in the lower left. Note the fragmented psammoma bodies and abundant colloid in the background (H&E, x200).

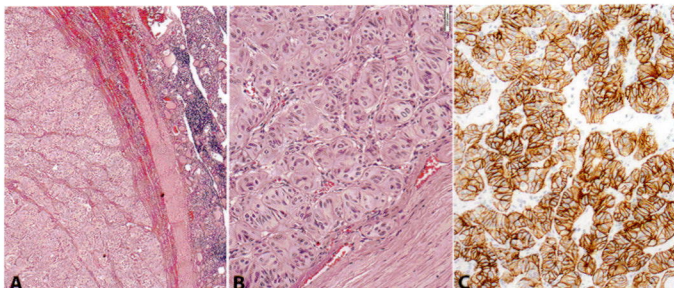

IMAGE 7.19 Hyalinizing trabecular tumor. Image A: the tumor has a fibrous capsule and trabecular architecture with scattered "empty follicles" (H&E, x40). Image B: the tumor cells are fusiform and are arranged perpendicular to the perimeter of the trabeculae. Their nuclei are elongated with nuclear membrane grooves and occasional pseudoinclusions. Note the hyalinized material within trabeculae (H&E, x200). Image C: immunohistochemical stain for Ki 67 (MIB 1) shows characteristic membranous staining pattern.

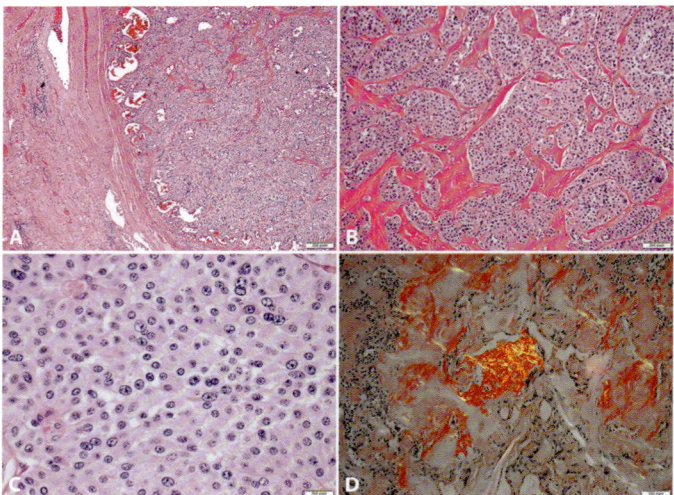

IMAGE 7.20 Medullary thyroid carcinoma. Image A: a circumscribed thyroid tumor is devoid of colloid and shows no follicular differentiation (H&E, x40). Image B: the tumor has solid/trabecular architecture (H&E, x100). Image C: the neoplastic cells have amphophilic cytoplasm and round-to-oval nuclei with stippled chromatin consistent with neuroendocrine differentiation (H&E, x400). Image D: this is a photomicrograph of a section of the tumor with Congo red stain viewed under polarized light. Note the apple-green birefringence of the amyloid deposits in the stroma.

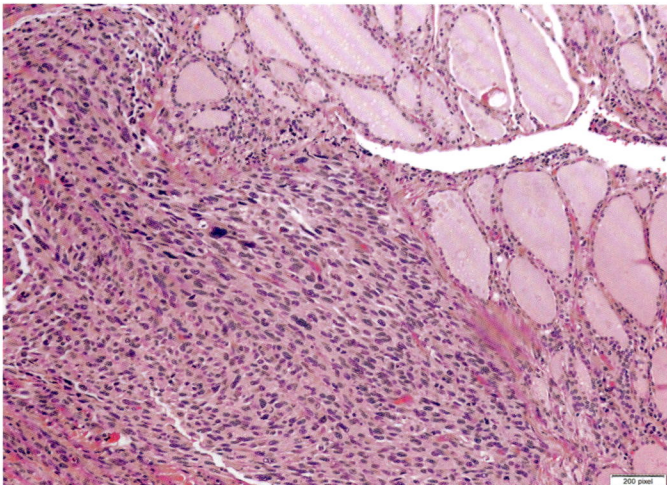

IMAGE 7.21 Anaplastic thyroid carcinoma with sarcomatoid (spindle cell) morphology. The tumor cells are positive for cytokeratin and p53 and they may be variably positive for PAX8, but are negative for thyroglobulin, calcitonin, and TTF1 (H&E, x200).

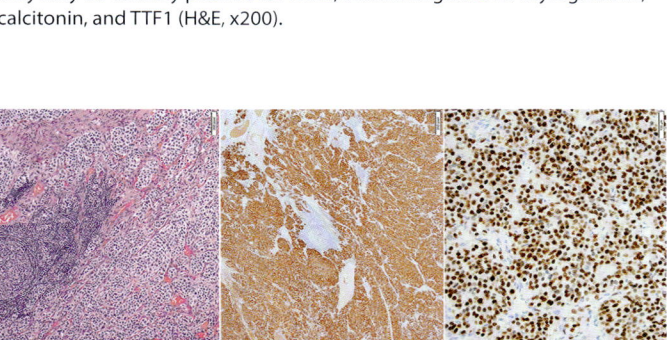

IMAGE 7.22 Metastatic paraganglioma in cervical lymph node. Image A: the tumor has nested architecture and prominent capillary network (H&E, x100). Image B: IHC shows the neoplastic cells are positive for tyrosine hydroxylase Image C: the neoplastic cells are also positive for GATA3.

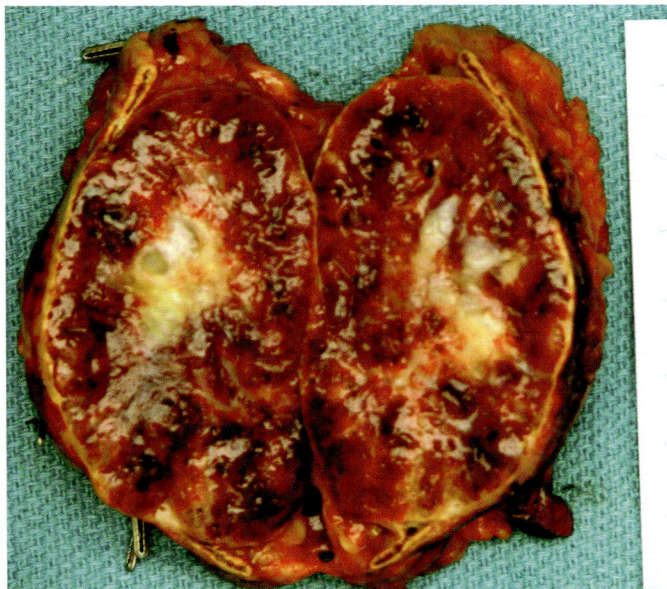

IMAGE 7.23 Adrenal pheochromocytoma. The tumor is circumscribed and is confined within the adrenal gland. The cut surfaces are pink-tan with areas of hemorrhage and cystic degeneration.

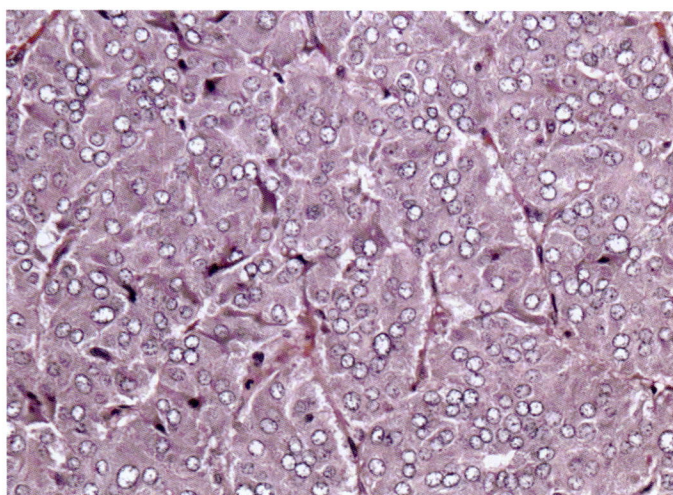

IMAGE 7.24 Pheochromocytoma. The tumor shows characteristic zellballen architecture. The tumor chief cells have abundant granular basophilic cytoplasm and exhibit moderate nuclear pleomorphism (H&E, x100).

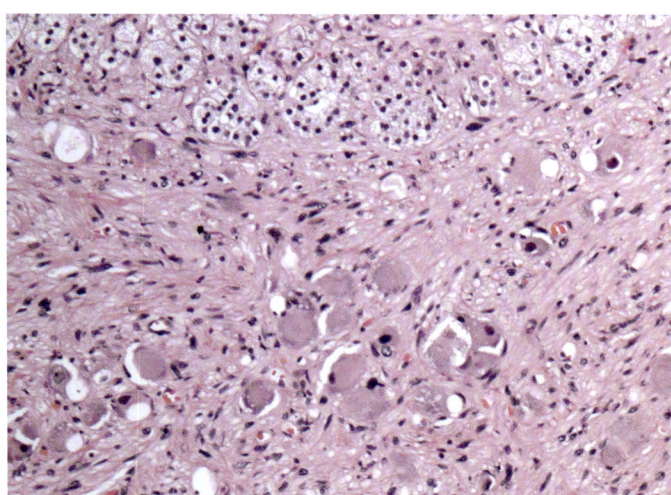

IMAGE 7.25 Adrenal ganglioneuroma. This photomicrograph shows an unencapsulated tumor composed of dispersed large ganglion cells in a background of Schwann cells. There is a residual island of adrenal cortical tissue at the top of the image (H&E, x40).

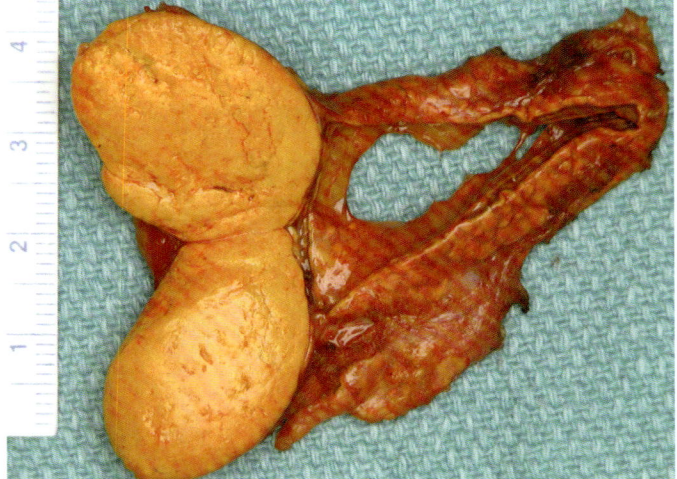

IMAGE 7.26 Adrenal cortical aldosteronoma in a patient with Conn syndrome. The cut surfaces show a solitary, circumscribed adrenal cortical tumor with a characteristic yellow-orange color.

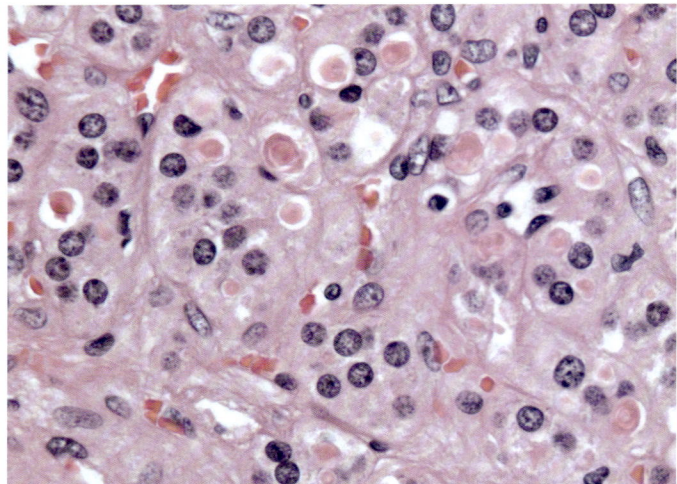

IMAGE 7.27 Section of adrenal cortical adenoma from a patient with Conn syndrome, who was treated with spironolactone. Note the intracytoplasmic laminated eosinophilic inclusions (spironolactone bodies) (H&E, x400).

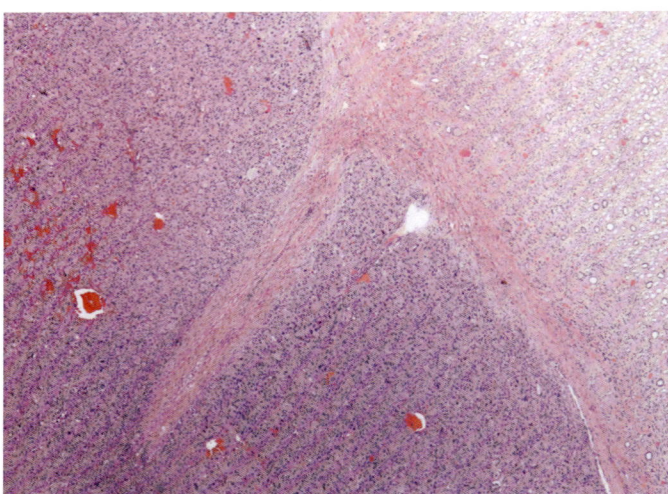

IMAGE 7.30 Adrenal cortical carcinoma invading adjacent kidney. Note the diffuse architecture and loss of the clear cell morphology (H&E, x40).

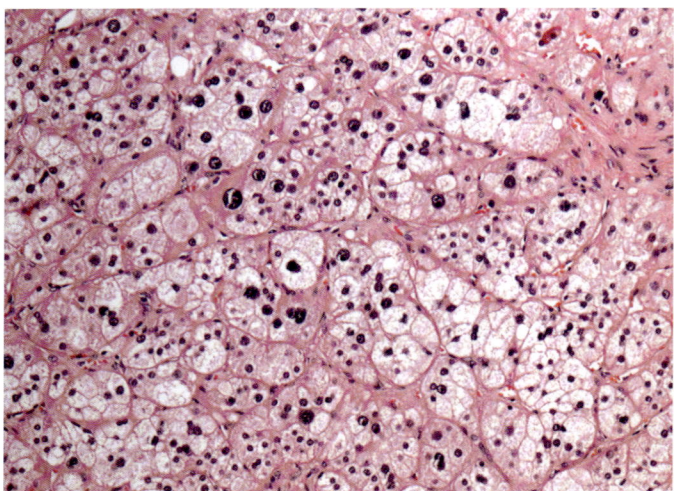

IMAGE 7.28 Adrenal cortical adenoma. This photomicrograph shows a cortical tumor with preserved alveolar architecture and clear cell morphology. There is no necrosis and no mitotic figures. Nuclear pleomorphism and hyperchromasia can be seen in benign cortical lesions (H&E, x200).

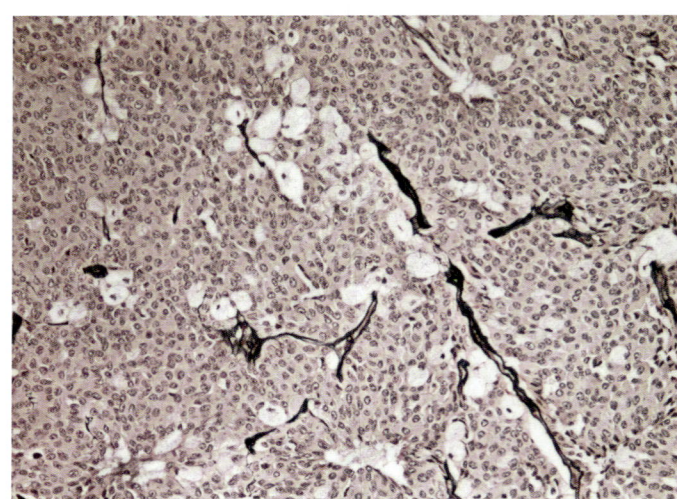

IMAGE 7.31 Adrenal cortical carcinoma with reticulin disruption (reticulin stain, x100).

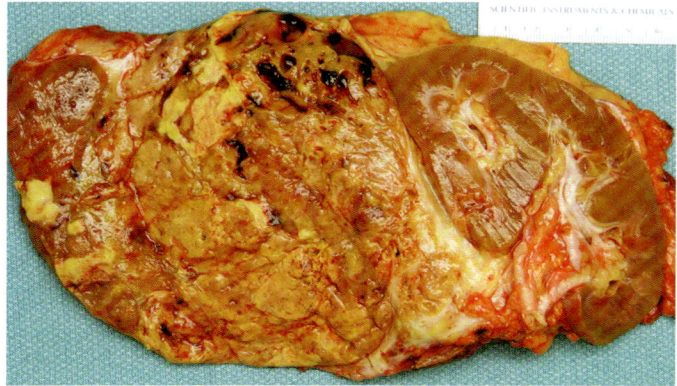

IMAGE 7.29 Gross image of adrenal cortical carcinoma. This tumor weighed > 750 g. Note the multinodular cut surface and areas of necrosis and hemorrhage.

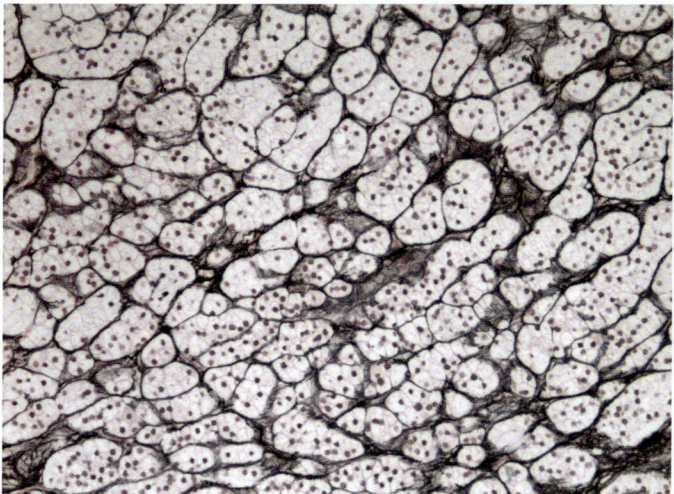

IMAGE 7.32 Benign adrenal cortical nodule with preserved reticulin pattern (reticulin stain, x100).

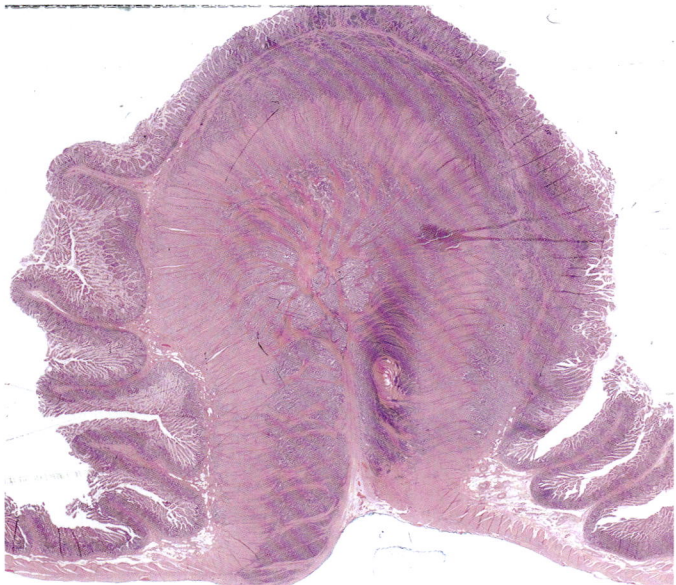

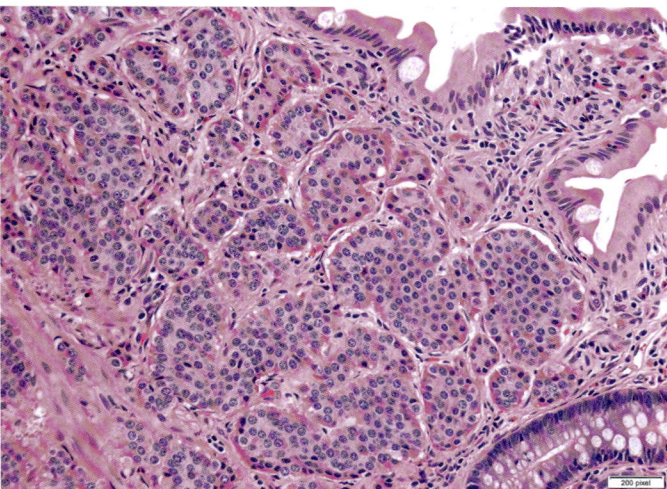

IMAGE 7.33 Ileal NET. Upper image: this low power photomicrograph shows a tumor infiltrating the entire thickness of the intestinal wall and is associated with dense serosal adhesions causing angulation of intestinal loop (H&E, x1). Lower image: the tumor has nested/trabecular architecture. The neoplastic cells have amphophilic cytoplasm and monotonous round nuclei with "salt and pepper" chromatin and inconspicuous nucleoli. Mitotic figures are rare (H&E, x100).

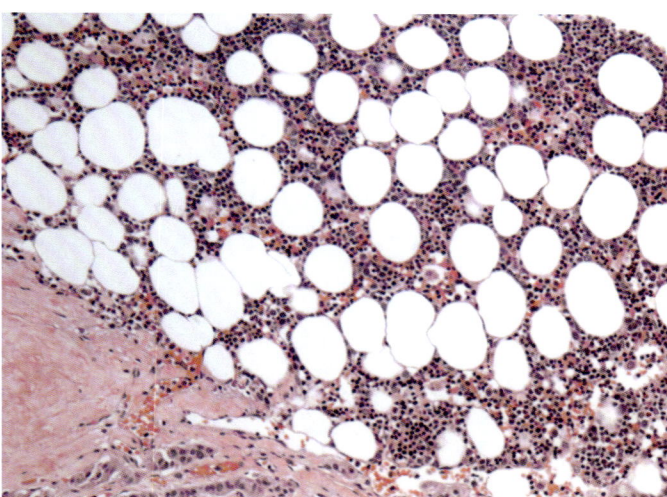

IMAGE 7.35 Adrenal myelolipoma. This section shows normal hematopoietic elements in adipose tissue, resembling bone marrow. Note the adrenal cortical tissue (lower left corner) (H&E, x20).

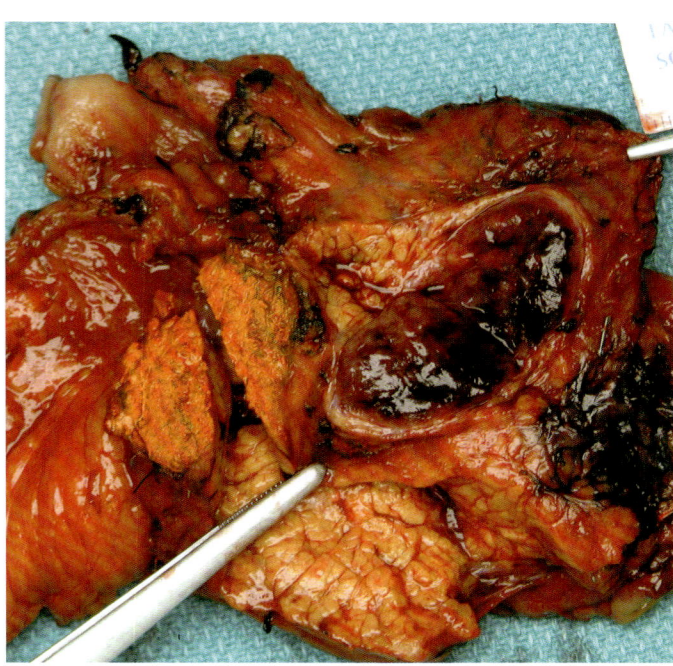

IMAGE 7.36 Pancreatic NET. Cut surfaces show a solitary circumscribed pink-tan tumor with areas of hemorrhage.

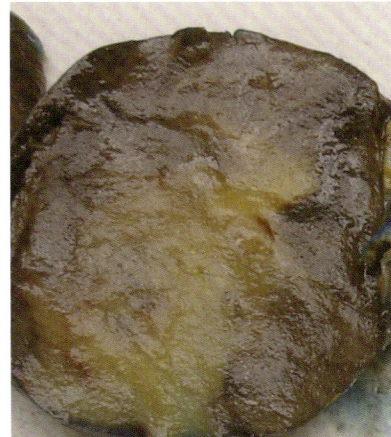

IMAGE 7.34 Adrenal myelolipoma. The cut surfaces of the tumor are brown-tan with yellow (fat) areas.

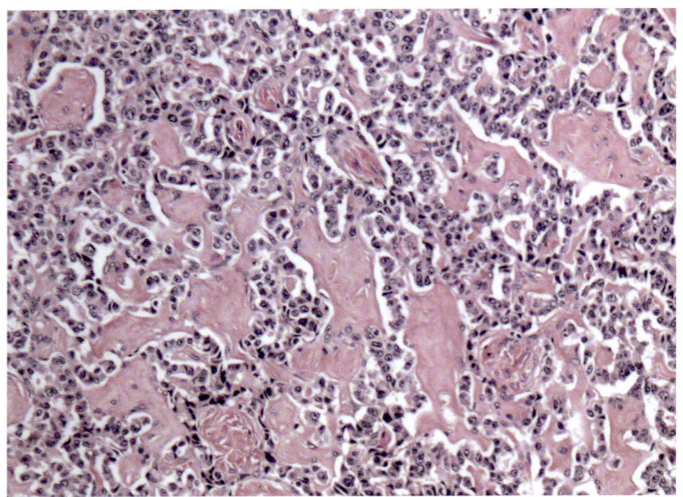

IMAGE 7.37 Pancreatic NET. This photomicrograph shows a tumor with organoid architecture and stromal sclerosis (H&E, x100).

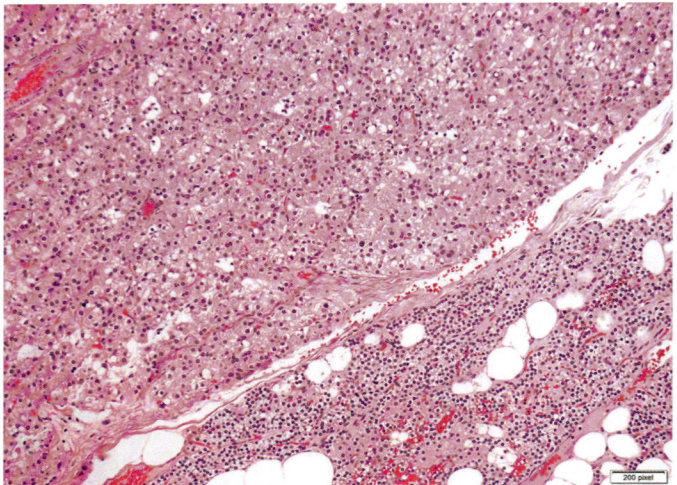

IMAGE 7.38 Parathyroid adenoma. The tumor has a delicate fibrous capsule, solid/trabecular architecture, and predominantly oncocytic cytomorphology. A rim of residual normal parathyroid tissue is seen (bottom right) (H&E, x100).

References

1. Asa SL, Mete O. Endocrine pathology: past, present and future. Pathol. 2018;50(1):111-18. doi: 10.1016/j.pathol.2017.09.003

2. Asa SL. Survival guide to endocrine pathology. Virginia: Innovative Pathology Press; 2020.

3. Asa SL, Mete O. Oncocytic change in thyroid pathology. Front Endocrinol. 2021;12:678119. doi: 10.3389/fendo.2021.678119

4. The Cancer Genome Atlas Research Network. Integrated genomic characterization of papillary thyroid carcinoma. Cell. 2014;159(3):676-90. doi: 10.1016/j.cell.2014.09.050

5. Asa SL. The evolution of differentiated thyroid cancer. Pathol. 2017;49(3):229-37. doi: 10.1016/j.pathol.2017.01.001

6. Watutantrige-Fernando S, Vianello F, Barollo S, et al. The hobnail variant of papillary thyroid carcinoma: clinical/molecular characteristics of a large monocentric series and comparison with conventional histotypes. Thyroid. 2018;28(1):96-103. doi: 10.1089/thy.2017.0248

7. Cameselle-Teijeiro JM, Rodriguez-Perez I, Celestino R, et al. Hobnail variant of papillary thyroid carcinoma: clinicopathologic and molecular evidence of progression to undifferentiated carcinoma in 2 cases. Am J Surg Pathol. 2017;41(6):854-60. doi: 10.1097/PAS.0000000000000793

8. Lubitz CC, Economopoulos KP, Pawlak AC, et al. Hobnail variant of papillary thyroid carcinoma: an institutional case series and molecular profile. Thyroid. 2014;24(6):958-65. doi: 10.1089/thy.2013.0573

9. Asioli S, Erickson LA, Sebo TJ, et al. Papillary thyroid carcinoma with prominent hobnail features: a new aggressive variant of moderately differentiated papillary carcinoma: a clinicopathologic, immunohistochemical, and molecular study of eight cases. Am J Surg Pathol. 2010;34(1):44-52. doi: 10.1097/PAS.0b013e3181c46677

10. Hernandez-Prera JC, Machado RA, Asa SL, et al. Pathologic reporting of tall-cell variant of papillary thyroid cancer: have we reached a consensus? Thyroid. 2017;27(12):1498-504. doi: 10.1089/thy.2017.0280

11. Dettmer MS, Schmitt A, Steinert H, et al. Tall cell papillary thyroid carcinoma: new diagnostic criteria and mutations in BRAF and TERT. Endocr Relat Cancer. 2015;22(3):419-29. doi: 10.1530/ERC-15-0057

12. Bongers PJ, Kluijfhout WP, Verzijl R, et al. Papillary thyroid cancers with focal tall cell change are as aggressive as tall cell variants and should not be considered as low-risk disease. Ann Surg Oncol. 2019;26(8):2533–39. doi: 10.1245/s10434-019-07444-2

13. Thomas CM, Asa SL, Ezzat S, et al. Diagnosis and pathologic characteristics of medullary thyroid carcinoma-review of current guidelines. Curr Oncol. 2019;26(5):338-44. doi: 10.3747/co.26.5539

14. Alzumaili B, Xu B, Spanheimer PM, et al. Grading of medullary thyroid carcinoma on the basis of tumor necrosis and high mitotic rate is an independent predictor of poor outcome. Mod Pathol. 2020;33(9);1690-1701. doi: 10.1038/s41379-020-0532-1

15. Hiltzik D, Carlson DL, Tuttle RM, et al. Poorly differentiated thyroid carcinomas defined on the basis of mitosis and necrosis: a clinicopathologic study of 58 patients. Cancer. 2006;106(6):1286-95. doi: 10.1002/cncr.21739

16. Volante M, Rapa I, Gandhi M, et al. RAS mutations are the predominant molecular alteration in poorly differentiated thyroid carcinomas and bear prognostic impact. J Clin Endocrinol Metab. 2009;94(12):4735-41. doi: 10.1210/jc.2009-1233

17. Baloch Z, Mete O, Asa SL. Immunohistochemical biomarkers in thyroid pathology. Endocr Pathol. 2018;29(2):91-112. doi: 10.1007/s12022-018-9532-9

18. Mete O, Asa SL. Pathological definition and clinical significance of vascular invasion in thyroid carcinomas of follicular epithelial derivation. Mod Pathol. 2011;24(12):1545-52. doi: 10.1038/modpath.2011.119

19. Cameselle-Teijeiro JM, Peteiro-Gonzalez D, Caneiro-Gomez J, et al. Cribriform-morular variant of thyroid carcinoma: a neoplasm with distinctive phenotype associated with the activation of the WNT/beta-catenin pathway. Mod Pathol. 2018;31(8):1168-79. doi: 10.1038/s41379-018-0070-2

20. Boyraz B, Sadow PM, Asa SL, et al. Cribriform-morular thyroid carcinoma is a distinct thyroid malignancy of uncertain cytogenesis. Endocr Pathol. 2021;32(3):327-35. doi: 10.1007/s12022-021-09683-0

21. Wilhelm SM, Wang TS, Ruan DT, et al. The American Association of Endocrine Surgeons guidelines for definitive management of primary hyperparathyroidism. JAMA Surg. 2016;151(10):959–68. doi: 10.1001/jamasurg.2016.2310

22. Juhlin CC, Erickson LA. Genomics and epigenomics in parathyroid neoplasia: from bench to surgical pathology practice. Endocr Pathol. 2021;32(1):17-34. doi: 10.1007/s12022-020-09656-9

23. Gill AJ, Clarkson A, Gimm O, et al. Loss of nuclear expression of parafibromin distinguishes parathyroid carcinomas and hyperparathyroidism-jaw tumor (HPT-JT) syndrome-related adenomas from sporadic parathyroid adenomas and hyperplasias. Am J Surg Pathol. 2006;30(9):1140-49. doi: 10.1097/01.pas.0000209827.39477.4f

24. Erovic BM, Harris L, Jamali M, et al. Biomarkers of parathyroid carcinoma. Endocr Pathol. 2012;23(4):221-31. doi: 10.1007/s12022-012-9222-y

25. Kim J, Horowitz G, Hong M, et al. The dangers of parathyroid biopsy. J Otolaryngol Head Neck Surg. 2017;46(1):4. doi: 10.1186/s40463-016-0178-7

26. Alwaheeb S, Rambaldini G, Boerner S, et al. Worrisome histologic alterations following fine-needle aspiration of the parathyroid. J Clin Pathol. 2006;59(10):1094-96. doi: 10.1136/jcp.2005.029017

27. Al Brahim NY, Asa SL. My approach to pathology of the pituitary gland. J Clin Pathol. 2006;59(12):1245-53. doi: 10.1136/jcp.2005.031187

28. Asa SL. Challenges in the diagnosis of pituitary neuroendocrine tumors. Endocr Pathol. 2021;32(2):222-27. doi: 10.1007/s12022-21-09678-x

29. Asa SL, Perry A. Tumors of the pituitary gland. Arlington, VA: ARP Press; 2020. (American Registry of Pathology, ed. AFIP atlas of tumor and non-tumor pathology, series 5; vol. 1).

30. Asa SL, Mete O. Immunohistochemical biomarkers in pituitary pathology. Endocr Pathol. 2018;29(2):130-36. doi: 10.1007/s12022-018-9521-z

31. Asa SL, Mete O. Cytokeratin profiles in pituitary neuroendocrine tumors. Hum Pathol. 2021;107:87-95. doi: 10.1016/j.humpath.2020.10.004

32. Goschzik T, Gessi M, Dreschmann V, et al. Genomic alterations of adamantinomatous and papillary craniopharyngioma. J Neuropathol Exp Neurol. 2017;76(2):126-34. doi: 10.1093/jnen/nlw116

33. Uccella S, La RS, Volante M, et al. Immunohistochemical biomarkers of gastrointestinal, pancreatic, pulmonary, and thymic neuroendocrine neoplasms. Endocr Pathol. 2018;29(2):150-68. doi: 10.1007/s12022-018-9522-y

34. La Rosa S, Solcia E. New insights into the classification of gastric neuroendocrine tumours, expanding the spectrum of ECL-cell tumours related to hypergastrinaemia. Histopathology. 2020;77(6):862-64. doi: 10.1111/his.14226

35. Asa SL, La RS, Basturk O, et al. Molecular pathology of well-differentiated gastro-entero-pancreatic neuroendocrine tumors. Endocr Pathol. 2021;32(1):169-91. doi: 10.1007/s12022-21-09662-5

36. Mete O, Asa SL. Precursor lesions of endocrine system neoplasms. Pathol. 2013;45(3):316-30. doi: 10.1097/PAT.0b013e32835f45c5

37. Vanoli A, La RS, Klersy C, et al. Four neuroendocrine tumor types and neuroendocrine carcinoma of the duodenum: analysis of 203 cases. Neuroendocrinology. 2017;104(2):112-25. doi: 10.1159/000444803

38. Okubo Y, Yokose T, Motohashi O, et al. Duodenal rare neuroendocrine tumor: clinicopathological characteristics of patients with gangliocytic paraganglioma. Gastroenterol Res Pract. 2016;2016:5257312. doi: 10.1155/2016/5257312

39. Lee SH, Kim BC, Chang HJ, et al. Rectal neuroendocrine and L-cell tumors: diagnostic dilemma and therapeutic strategy. Am J Surg Pathol. 2013;37(7):1044-52. doi: 10.1097/PAS.0b013e3182819f0f

40. Sohn JH, Cho MY, Park Y, et al. Prognostic significance of defining L-cell type on the biologic behavior of rectal neuroendocrine tumors in relation with pathological parameters. Cancer Res Treat. 2015;47(4):813-22. doi: 10.4143/crt.2014.238

41. Kim JY, Kim KS, Kim KJ, et al. Non-L-cell immunophenotype and large tumor size in rectal neuroendocrine tumors are associated with aggressive clinical behavior and worse prognosis. Am J Surg Pathol. 2015;39(5):632-43. doi: 10.1097/PAS.0000000000000400

42. Rindi G, Klimstra DS, Abedi-Ardekani B, et al. A common classification framework for neuroendocrine neoplasms: an International Agency for Research on Cancer (IARC) and World Health Organization (WHO) expert consensus proposal. Mod Pathol. 2018;31(12):1770-86. doi: 10.1038/s41379-018-0110-y

43. Juhlin CC. Challenges in paragangliomas and pheochromocytomas: from histology to molecular immunohistochemistry. Endocr Pathol. 2021;32(2):228-44. doi: 10.1007/s12022-021-09675-0

44. Turchini J, Cheung VKY, Tischler AS, et al. Pathology and genetics of phaeochromocytoma and paraganglioma. Histopathology. 2018;72(1):97-105. doi: 10.1111/his.13402

45. Mete O, Pakbaz S, Lerario AM, et al. Significance of alpha-inhibin expression in pheochromocytomas and paragangliomas. Am J Surg Pathol. 2021;45(9):1264-73. doi: 10.1097/PAS.0000000000001715

46. Fishbein L, Leshchiner I, Walter V, et al. Comprehensive molecular characterization of pheochromocytoma and paraganglioma. Cancer Cell. 2017;31(2):181-93. doi: 10.1016/j.ccell.2017.01.001

47. Menara M, Oudijk L, Badoual C, et al. SDHD immunohistochemistry: a new tool to validate SDHx mutations in pheochromocytoma/paraganglioma. J Clin Endocrinol Metab. 2015;100(2):E287-E291.

48. Asa SL, Ezzat S, Mete O. The diagnosis and clinical significance of paragangliomas in unusual locations. J Clin Med. 2018;7(9):280. doi: 10.3390/jcm7090280

49. Mete O, Asa SL. Morphological distinction of cortisol-producing and aldosterone-producing adrenal cortical adenomas: not only possible but a critical clinical responsibility. Histopathology. 2012;60(6);1015-16. doi: 10.1111/j.1365-2559.2011.04141.x

50. Groussin L, Cazabat L, Rene-Corail F, et al. Adrenal pathophysiology: lessons from the Carney complex. Horm Res. 2005;64(3):132-39. doi: 10.1159/000088586

51. Carney JA, Gordon H, Carpenter PC, et al. The complex of myxomas, spotty pigmentation, and endocrine overactivity. Medicine. 1985;64(4):270-83. doi: 10.1097/00005792-198507000-00007

52. Juhlin CC, Bertherat J, Giordano TJ, et al. What did we learn from the molecular biology of adrenal cortical neoplasia? From histopathology to translational genomics. Endocr Pathol. 2021;32(1):102-33. doi: 10.1007/s12022-021-09667-0

53. Mete O, Gucer H, Kefeli M, et al. Diagnostic and prognostic biomarkers of adrenal cortical carcinoma. Am J Surg Pathol. 2018;42(2):201-13. doi: 10.1097/PAS.0000000000000400

54. Shimada H, Ambros IA, Dehner LP, et al. Terminology and morphologic criteria of neuroblastic tumors: recommendations by the International Neuroblastoma Pathology Committee. Cancer. 1999;86;349-63. doi: 10.1002/(SIC)1097-0142(19990715)86:2<349::AID-CNCR20>3.0CO;2-Y

55. Mete O, Asa SL, Gill AJ, et al. Overview of the 2022 WHO Classification of Paragangliomas and Pheochromocytomas. Endocrine Pathol. 2022;33(1):90-114. doi: 10.1007/s12022-022-09704-6

56. Matsuino R, Gifford AJ, Fang J, et al. Rare MYC-amplified neuroblastoma with large cell histology. Pediatr Dev Pathol. 2018;21(5):461-66. doi: 10.1177/1093526617749670

57. Takita J. Molecular basis and clinical features of neuroblastoma. jma j. 2021;4(4):321-31. doi: 10.31662/jmaj.2021-0077

58. Thompson LDR, Herrera HB, Lau SK. A clinicopathologic series of 685 thyroglossal duct remnant cysts. Head Neck Pathol. 2016;10:465-74. doi: 10.1007/s12105-016-0724-7

59. Nikiforov YE, Seethala RR, Tallini G, et al. Nomenclature revision for encapsulated follicular variant of papillary thyroid carcinoma: a paradigm shift to reduce overtreatment of indolent tumors. JAMA Oncol. 2016;2(8):1023-29. doi: 10.1001/jamaoncol.2016.0386

60. Xu B, Serrette R, Tuttle M, et al. How many papillae in conventional papillary carcinoma? A clinical evidence-based pathology study of 235 unifocal encapsulated papillary thyroid carcinomas, with emphasis on the diagnosis of noninvasive follicular thyroid neoplasm with papillary-like nuclear features. Thyroid. 2019;12:1792-1803. doi: 10.1089/thy.2019.0328

61. Basolo F, Macerola E, Ugolini C et al. The molecular landscape of noninvasive follicular thyroid neoplasm with papillary-like nuclear features (NIFTP): a literature review. Adv Anat Pathol. 2017;24:252-58. doi: 10.1097/PAP0000000000000163

62. Xie Jing, Dai J, Zhou W and Sun F. Adrenal ganglioneuroma: features and outcomes of 42 cases in a Chinese population. World J Surg. 2018;42(8):2469-75. doi: 10.1007/s00268-018-4499-8

63. Mete O, Duan K. The many faces of primary aldosteronism and Cushing syndrome: a reflection of adrenocortical tumor heterogeneity. Front Med (Lausanne). 2018;5:54. doi: 10.3389/fmed.2018.00054

64. Decmann A, Perge P, Toth M, et al. Adrenal myelolipoma: a comprehensive review. Endocrine. 2018;59(1):7-15. doi: 10.1007/s12020-017-1473-4

65. Wells SA Jr., Asa SL, Dralle H, et al. Revised American Thyroid Association guidelines for the management of medullary thyroid carcinoma. Thyroid. 2015;25(6):567-610. doi: 10.1089/thy.2014.0335

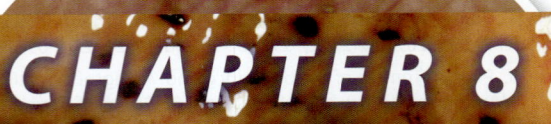

CHAPTER 8

Forensic Pathology

ALFREDO E. WALKER

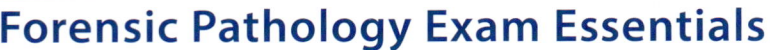

Forensic Pathology Exam Essentials

MUST KNOW

Basics of forensic medicine

Within this field, which is vast and contains a great amount of specialized knowledge, focus on common scenarios and topics. Some foundational topics include:

- Cause versus manner versus mechanism of death.
- Identifying the deceased.
- Determining time of death.
- Rigor and lividity.
- Decomposition types, related changes, and postmortem artifacts (e.g., tache noire).
- Endogenous and exogenous factors that may affect factors mentioned above.

Motor vehicle collision

This topic is common, both in practice and on the exam. Consider dividing injuries related to motor vehicle collisions by occupants of vehicles versus those hit by vehicles (e.g., pedestrians). High-yield topics include:

- Glass injuries (e.g., dicing from tempered glass versus laceration from sharp glass).
- Seatbelt bruising.
- Airbag injury.
- Steering wheel injury,
- Injuries due to ejection from vehicle.
- Pedestrian injuries (e.g., bumper fractures, head injury).

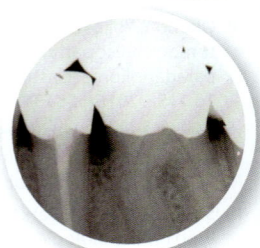

Toxin-related death

High-yield topics include:

- Ethanol- and alcohol-related death, including overdose and withdrawal.
- Complications of alcoholism and cirrhosis.
- Stimulants and depressants.
- Opioids.
- Drug trafficking–related death (e.g., rupture of drug sack in body cavity).
- Inhalation of drugs, toxins.
- Heavy metals.

Firearm and projectile death

High-yield topics include:

- Types of firearm and projectiles (e.g., arrow, spear).
- Entrance versus exit gunshot wounds.
- How distance and type of gun affect the appearance of gunshot wounds.

Heat- and electrical-related death

High-yield topics include:

- Electrocution, including lightning injury.
- Fire and explosion–related injury, including artifacts caused by fire and smoke-inhalation injuries.
- Hyper- and hypothermia.

Trauma

High-yield topics include:
- Fall from height.
- Brain hemorrhages due to head trauma.
- Blunt and sharp force trauma.
- Fractures, spinal injuries.

Cardiopulmonary death

High-yield topics include:
- Congenital heart diseases (e.g., tetralogy of Fallot).
- Hypertrophic cardiomyopathy.
- Atherosclerosis and coronary artery disease.
- Dissections and aneurysms.
- Valvular diseases.
- Endocarditis, myocarditis, pericarditis.
- Conduction disorders and causes of "normal appearing heart."
- Pulmonary embolism and other forms of embolism.
- Pneumonia.
- Asthma, chronic obstructive pulmonary disease (COPD).

Neuropathology

High-yield topics include:
- Aneurysm.
- Seizure, sudden unexpected death in epilepsy (SUDEP).
- Meningitis.
- Cerebral edema, herniation.
- Various brain hemorrhages.
- Primary and secondary neoplasms.
- Spinal cord injuries.

Infant death

High-yield topics include:
- Sudden infant death syndrome (SIDS), including inclusion and exclusion criteria.
- Child abuse.
- Scalding injury.
- Head trauma.
- Congenital and natural causes.

Asphyxia

High-yield topics include:
- Hanging versus ligature strangulation.
- Chemical asphyxia, such as carbon monoxide and cyanide.
- Positional asphyxia.
- Autoerotic asphyxia.
- Mechanical asphyxia.

Other death

High-yield topics include:
- Infections.
- Neoplasms.

- Diabetes (e.g., ketoacidosis, hypoglycemia).
- Thyroid abnormality.
- Pregnancy complications.
- Surgical and iatrogenic complications.
- Drowning.

Postmortem examination

High-yield topics include:
- The roles of those involved in death investigations: coroner, medical examiner, police, and others.
- Mandatory reporting to coroner.
- Indication for autopsy, and the role and limit of autopsy.
- Medical versus forensic autopsies.
- Preautopsy procedures, including safety precautions.
- Special circumstances in autopsy (e.g., infectious diseases, unidentified body).
- Chain of custody and collection of evidence.
- Special dissection techniques.
- Collection of body fluid and various samples.
- Use of ancillary studies (e.g., microbiology, radiology, molecular pathology).
- Reporting and documentation of autopsy findings.
- Confidentiality and record keeping.

MUST SEE
- Focus on common entities and those that have pathognomonic findings, including eponymous lesions. Some commonly tested gross findings include:
  - Basic forensics:
    › Identification techniques (e.g., radiology, medical devices, tattoos).
    › Livor, rigor.
    › Decomposition and postmortem artifacts, tache noire, drying artifact.
    › Insect and animal predation.
    › Adipocere, mummification, putrefaction.
  - Motor vehicle:
    › Bumper fracture.
    › Damage to car.
    › Dicing injury.
    › Seatbelt bruise.
    › Steering wheel abrasion.
  - Toxins:
    › Cirrhosis, jaundice, ascites, scleral icterus, cirrhosis, varices.
    › Intravenous (IV) drug use, track marks.
    › Body packing.
    › Drug paraphernalia.
    › Lead poisoning.
    › Carbon monoxide poisoning.
    › Cyanide poisoning.
    › Mouth frothing causes.

- Firearm:
  - › Types of guns and projectiles.
  - › Gunshot wounds (entrance, exit, various ranges) and knife wounds.
  - › Contact wounds, close-range wounds, and intermediate and long-range wounds.
- Heat and electrical:
  - › Ferning (Lichtenberg figures).
  - › Burned body.
  - › Soot in airway.
  - › Cherry-red lividity.
  - › Gastrointestinal ulcers in hypothermia.
- Trauma:
  - › Laceration, abrasion, incision, stab wound, contusions.
  - › Skull injury, periorbital bruise, hemotympanum, basilar skull fracture, temporalis bruising.
- Cardiopulmonary:
  - › Various causes of endocarditis, myocarditis, fibrinous pericarditis.
  - › Congenital heart disease, atrial septal defect (ASD), ventricular septal defect (VSD), tetralogy.
  - › Hypertrophic cardiomyopathy, arrhythmogenic cardiomyopathy.
  - › Myocardial infarction (old and new), free wall rupture, hemopericardium.
  - › Valvular stenosis and regurgitation, artificial valves.
  - › Berry aneurysm, abdominal aortic aneurysm, aortic dissection, aortic coarctation.
  - › Endocarditis, nodules.
  - › Pulmonary embolism (PE).
  - › Pneumonia.
  - › Asthma.
  - › COPD and complications of smoking.
  - › Pneumoconiosis.
- Neuropathology:
  - › Skull fractures.
  - › Cerebral edema, herniation, Duret hemorrhages.
  - › Meningitis.
  - › Tongue biting in seizure.
  - › Various brain hemorrhages.
  - › Gliomas, meningiomas, metastasis.
  - › Transection of spinal cord.
- Infant:
  - › Child abuse, rib fracture, bruises, skull fracture, retinal hemorrhage.
  - › Scalding injury.
- Asphyxia:
  - › Hanging, ligature strangulation, choking, smothering.
  - › Positional asphyxia.
  - › Autoerotic asphyxia.

- Although the forensic portion of the exam is mainly focused on gross images, occasionally either the quick slide or the oral exam includes some component of forensic pathology. Some of the commonly tested microscopic findings include:
  - › Cirrhosis, peptic ulcer.
  - › Injection of foreign material.
  - › Asthma.
  - › Soot deposition.
  - › Embolism, PE, bone marrow embolism.
  - › Hypertrophic cardiomyopathy, arrhythmogenic cardiomyopathy.
  - › Dissection, stenosis, aneurysms, atherosclerosis.
  - › Infective endocarditis.
  - › Various cardiac tumors.
  - › Duret hemorrhages.
  - › Infectious diseases, fungal, mycobacterial.

MUST DO
- For each of the items outlined in the Must Know and Must See sections, you should think about causes, mechanisms of death, and possible manners of death.
- You should be fluent in the actions to take before, during, and after performing an autopsy. You should also think about safety and quality assurance (QA) procedures.
- For preautopsy, you should be able to:
  - › Establish the identity of the deceased.
  - › Note consent, autopsy restrictions, and any issue with organ retention.
  - › Gather police information and medical history.
  - › Set up a workbench, don personal protection equipment (PPE), and implement safety measures.
  - › Take photographs and secure the chain of custody for evidence collected.
- For the autopsy, you should be able to:
  - › Remove a body from a body bag and take measurements.
  - › Document external findings.
  - › Remove the deceased's personal items.
  - › Document evidence of medical intervention.
  - › Open cavities and eviscerate of organs.
  - › Collect cultures, tissue, fluids, and samples.
  - › Perform special dissection techniques (e.g., Rokitansky dissection, dry neck, layered dissection).
  - › Dissect each organ and document the findings.
  - › Appropriately dispose of tissue and waste.
- For postautopsy, you should be able to:
  - › Dispose of the body in the appropriate manner.
  - › Document the preliminary findings.
  - › Report the findings to the pathologist and coroner.
  - › Ensure proper storage of tissue and evidence.

> Order ancillary studies (e.g., DNA, cultures, radiology).
> Examine microscopic sections of tissue.
> Using data from gross, microscopic, and ancillary studies, synthesize findings and come up with a final mechanism, cause, and manner of death.

> Write up the final pathology report.
> Answer any questions the coroner, police, or family have about the final report.

MULTIPLE CHOICE QUESTIONS

1. Lacerations of the skin differ from incised wounds in that lacerations can display of all the following features **except**:

a. A vital reaction.
b. Complete division of the tissues.
c. Ragged wound edges.
d. Irregular wound margins.
e. "Connective tissue bridges" across the depths of the wound.

Answer: b

2. Which of the following statements about skull fractures is false?

a. Linear fractures are usually caused by blunt impact over a broad area.
b. Skull fractures can directly cause death.
c. Bilateral periorbital hematomas (black eyes) can be caused by a backward fall
with impact of the occiput onto the ground.
d. Ring fractures occur in falls from a great height.
e. Hinge fractures run across the base of the skull.

Answer: b

3. An epidural (extradural) hematoma is a collection of blood in:

a. The space between the arachnoid mater and the cortical surface of the brain.
b. The space between the dura mater and the arachnoid mater.
c. The space between the internal surface
of the skull and outer surface of the dura mater.
d. The brain parenchyma, no matter the location.
e. The space between the scalp and the outer surface of the skull.

Answer: c

4. Which of the following statements is true about the development of both epidural and subdural hematomas in their pure state?

a. Both are associated with a lucid interval.
b. Both are due to venous bleeding.
c. Both are due to arterial bleeding.
d. Both can cause instantaneous death.
e. Both can cause immediate unconsciousness.

Answer: a

5. A periorbital hematoma (black eye) of the left eye can be caused by all of the following **except**:

a. A direct blow to the left eye.
b. Downward tracking of blood beneath the scalp from a blow to the forehead.
c. A backward fall onto the ground with impact of the back of the head.
d. A slap across the face.
e. Fractures of the orbital roofs.

Answer: d

6. Chronic subdural membranes are commonly associated with all of the following **except**:

a. Normal sized brains.
b. Dementia.
c. Chronic alcoholism.
d. Elderly patients.
e. Cerebral atrophy.

Answer: a

7. Which of the following statements about fire deaths is false?

a. A carboxyhemoglobin (COHb) concentration > 50% is considered fatal in a healthy individual.
b. Cyanide can be produced after death.
c. Cyanide cannot be produced after death.
d. Cigarette smoking can account for COHb concentrations up to 15%.
e. Deaths in flash fires can have low/absent COHb concentrations.

Answer: c

8. A 48-year-old alcoholic man with cirrhosis of the liver was found dead in the bathroom of his home with a large quantity of fresh blood on the floor. External examination at postmortem did not reveal any bleeding injury to explain his death. In the given scenario, which of the following is the most likely explanation of the blood at the scene?

a. An ulcer of the stomach.

b. An ulcer of the duodenum.

c. Esophageal varices.

d. Cancer of the lung.

e. Pulmonary tuberculosis.

Answer: c

9. A previously healthy 70-year-old woman died at home 2 weeks after she had been discharged from hospital following surgical treatment of a fracture of her left hip, which was sustained in a fall. The operation had gone well and she was encouraged to mobilize at home, but she had refused to get out of bed except for going to the toilet. Her left leg had become swollen and painful, but she did not seek medical attention. She then developed a sudden onset of shortness of breath shortly before she collapsed and died. Which of the following conditions is the most likely cause of death?

a. Bronchopneumonia.

b. Acute myocardial infarction.

c. Hemorrhagic stroke.

d. Pulmonary thromboembolism.

e. Fat embolism.

Answer: d

10. A 17-year-old national footballer collapsed and died during an international qualifying game. Postmortem examination did not find a cause of death and toxicological analysis was negative. The heart was examined by an experienced specialist cardiac pathologist, who reported that it was normal on both naked eye and microscopic examination. In the context of the above, which of the following is the most likely explanation of his death?

a. Viral myocarditis.

b. Long QT syndrome.

c. Hypertrophic cardiomyopathy.

d. Arrhythmogenic cardiomyopathy.

e. Hypertensive heart disease.

Answer: b

11. A 45-year-old obese diabetic and hypertensive man collapsed and died 5 days after he had complained of a sudden onset of crushing central chest pain while walking up a hill. He did not seek medical attention. What pathology in Figure 8.1 explains his death?

a. Amyloidosis.

b. Arrhythmogenic cardiomyopathy.

c. Acute myocardial infarction.

d. Myocarditis.

e. Myocardial fibrosis.

Answer: c

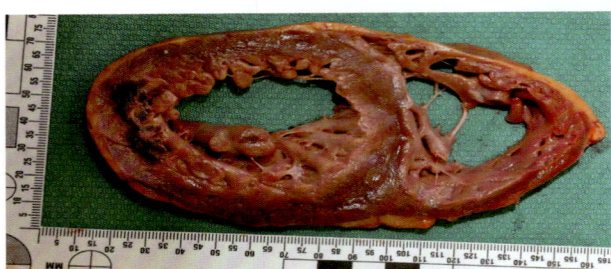

FIGURE 8.1

12. Which of the following findings is **not** a demonstrable postmortem finding of fatal acute stimulant drug abuse?

a. Thrombotic occlusion of a coronary artery.

b. Acute myocardial infarction.

c. Coronary artery dissection.

d. Intracerebral hemorrhage.

e. Coronary artery spasm.

Answer: e

13. The term *tache noire* refers to:

a. Retinal hemorrhages associated with blunt head trauma.

b. Horizontal linear discoloration of the sclera of the eyes due to postmortem drying.

c. Multiple small red-purple hemorrhages on the skin.

d. A charred area of the skin due to an electrical burn.

e. Skin changes associated with necrotic venom of a spider bite.

Answer: b

14. The charred body of a 25-year-old man is found in the burned rubble of an abandoned house. The police investigation revealed that the individual had gang affiliations and raised the possibility that he was killed prior to the fire. What findings indicate that the individual died as a result of the fire?

a. Absence of soot in the airways and low or absent COHb concentration.

b. Pugilistic stance.

c. Epidural hematoma.

d. Soot throughout the airways and elevated COHb concentration.

e. Multiple full- and partial-thickness skin splits.

Answer: d

15. The following asphyxial deaths are usually associated with an anatomically negative postmortem examination **except**:

a. Plastic bag asphyxia.
b. Infant smothering.
c. Traumatic asphyxia.
d. Helium inhalation.
e. Inhalation of nitrous oxide.

Answer: c

16. In cases of autoerotic asphyxiation, what is the manner of death?

a. Suicide.
b. Homicide.
c. Accident.
d. Undetermined.
e. Natural.

Answer: c

17. The "pugilistic position" is a pathological feature of which of the following cases?

a. Severely burned bodies.
b. Advanced decomposition.
c. Drowning.
d. Gunshot wounds.
e. Electrocution deaths.

Answer: a

18. Figure 8.2 shows sagittal sections of lung from an 85-year-old man who died after a 3-day history of a productive cough and fever. What pathology of the lung is apparent?

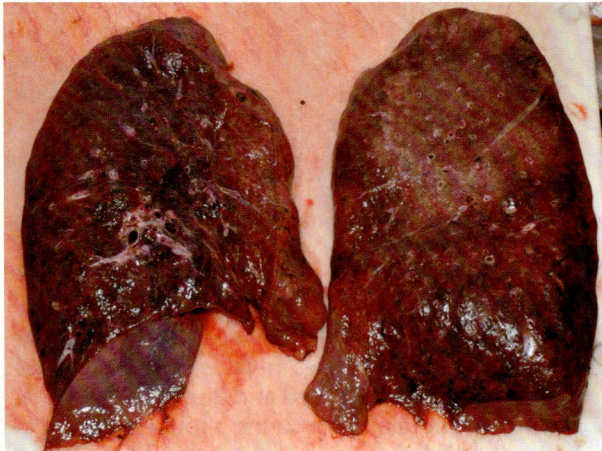

FIGURE 8.2

a. Bilateral bronchopneumonia.
b. Lobar pneumonia — left upper lobe.
c. Lobar pneumonia — right upper lobe.
d. Lobar pneumonia — left lower lobe.
e. Lobar pneumonia — right lower lobe.

Answer: c

19. A previously healthy 19-year-old male rugby player with no medical history collapsed and died during game and was found to have a heavier-than-expected heart weight with marked eccentric thickening of the interventricular septum. Which of the following conditions best describes the likely reason for this finding?

a. Hypertensive heart disease.
b. Hypertrophic cardiomyopathy.
c. Long QT syndrome.
d. Arrhythmogenic cardiomyopathy.
e. Hemochromatosis.

Answer: b

20. Arrhythmogenic (right ventricular) cardiomyopathy is **typically** associated with which of the following?

a. Marked fatty infiltration of the left ventricle grossly.
b. Fibrofatty change of the right ventricle on histological examination.
c. Disorganization of cardiac muscle cells (myocyte disarray) on histology.
d. Sudden death in the elderly.
e. Sudden death in middle age.

Answer: b

21. The ion channelopathies are a group of genetic disorders of the cardiac muscle ion channels associated with specific mutations of coding genes. The following are all ion channelopathies **except**:

a. Long QT syndrome.
b. Brugada syndrome.
c. Catecholaminergic polymorphic ventricular tachycardia (CPVT).
d. Wolff-Parkinson-White (WPW) syndrome.
e. Short QT syndrome.

Answer: d

22. Which of the following statements about sharp force injuries caused by knives is **false**?

a. A stab wound is a penetrating sharp force injury that is deeper than it is wide.
b. Defensive incised wounds commonly occur on the palms and forearms.
c. A 10 cm stab wound track of the abdomen could not have been caused by insertion of the full length of a 3.5 cm long blade.
d. The position of a lateral fishtail split in a stab wound indicates the position of the blunt back edge of the blade.
e. The width of the blade roughly corresponds to the length of the stab wound on the skin surface.

Answer: c

23. An 18-year-old female pedestrian was struck and killed by a standard-sized car while attempting to cross a road. Independent eyewitness accounts indicated that the car had run a red light while traveling above the speed limit in a 30 mph (50 kph) zone. On impact, the decedent was thrown into the air, landed on the hood and rolled over the roof of the car before coming to rest on the road behind the car. The car did not run over the body. The driver fled the scene. Examination of the scene revealed evidence of forceful braking of the car. A forensic postmortem examination identified bilateral blunt-impact bumper injuries of the legs at a distance of 20 inches (52 cm) above the heel. Consider the relationship of the height of the car bumper above flat ground (measured when the car is parked) to the height of the bumper-impact injuries of the legs. Which of the following statements is true?

a. The car bumper height must be slightly > 20 inches (52 cm).

b. The car bumper height must be half of 20 inches (52 cm).

c. The car bumper height must be the same as the height of the bumper injuries of 20 inches (52 cm).

d. The car bumper height must be slightly < 20 inches (52 cm).

e. The car bumper height must be 50% greater than the height of the bumper injuries of 20 inches (52 cm).

Answer: a

24. What pathology is depicted in Figure 8.3?

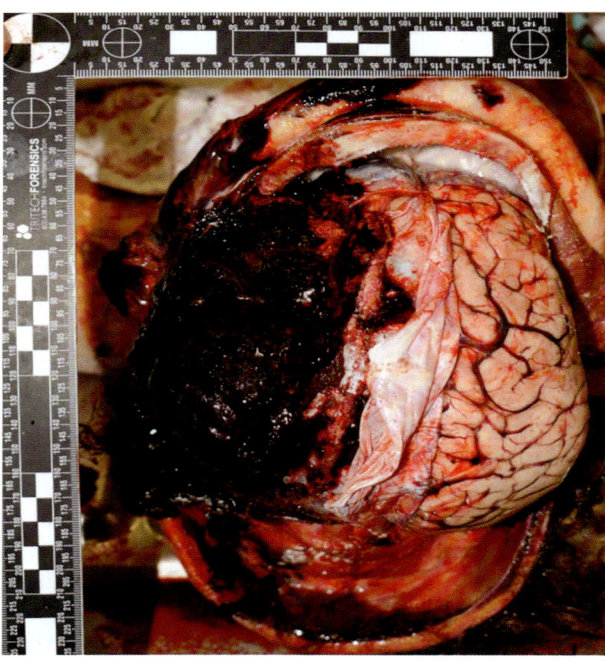

FIGURE 8.3

a. Acute left subdural hematoma.

b. Acute right subdural hematoma.

c. Acute left epidural hematoma.

d. Acute right epidural hematoma.

e. Left subarachnoid hemorrhage.

Answer: c

25. What underlying disease process should be the main consideration in Figure 8.4?

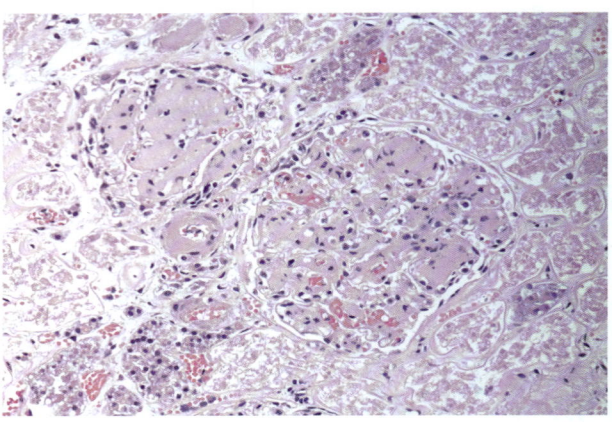

FIGURE 8.4

a. IgA nephropathy.

b. Amyloidosis.

c. Diabetes mellitus.

d. Hypertension.

e. Systemic lupus erythematous.

Answer: c

26. In a coroner's system of medicolegal death investigation in a province of Canada, which of the following documents must the forensic pathologist have in hand before a medicolegal postmortem examination can be performed?

a. A signed medical cause of death certificate.

b. Coroner's warrant for postmortem examination.

c. Consent form signed by the next of kin and properly witnessed.

d. Postmortem consultation request form signed by the treating physician.

e. A request from the investigating police service.

Answer: b

27. An obese 55-year-old man with a history of ischemic heart disease, diabetes mellitus, and uncontrolled hypertension, collapsed and died from an acute myocardial infarction during a robbery at his place of business after a gun was pointed in his face without the infliction of any physical injury. What manner of death must be ascribed in this scenario?

a. Suicide.

b. Natural.

c. Homicide.

d. Accident.

e. Undetermined.

Answer: c

28. A previously healthy 21-year-old freshman collapsed and died after attending a party during the first week of university. Acute dissection of the proximal segment of the anterior descending branch of his left coronary artery was identified at postmortem as the cause of death. From the options below, what specific toxicological analysis would you request?

a. Stimulant drugs.

b. Opioids.

c. Acetaminophen.

d. Barbiturates.

e. Ethanol.

Answer: a

29. The development of rigor mortis is the result of the postmortem depletion of what substance within skeletal muscle?

a. Glycogen.
b. Actin.
c. Myosin.
d. Adenosine triphosphate (ATP).
e. Calcium.

Answer: d

30. All of the following represent potential artifacts of cardiopulmonary resuscitation **except**:

a. Epidural hematoma.
b. Anterior rib fractures.
c. Hemorrhage into the pericardial fat.
d. Hepatic lacerations.
e. Conjunctival petechiae.

Answer: a

31. Which of the following is the **most** common location for fatal intracerebral hemorrhages secondary to systemic arterial hypertension?

a. Cingulate gyrus.
b. Basal ganglia.
c. Cerebellum.
d. Hippocampus.
e. Pons.

Answer: b

32. Dominance of coronary artery circulation is defined as the epicardial coronary artery which:

a. Has the largest caliber of all the coronary arteries.
b. Supplies the sinoatrial node.
c. Gives rise to the posterior descending artery.
d. Supplies the majority of the left ventricular myocardium.
e. Supplies the anterior wall of the left and right ventricles.

Answer: c

33. You perform an autopsy on a 54-year-old man with a history of chronic alcoholism, and identify the cause of death as upper gastrointestinal tract hemorrhage due to ruptured esophageal varices. Which of the following pathologic conditions **must** be present for this to be true?

a. Cirrhosis of the liver.
b. Erosive esophagitis.
c. Peptic ulcer disease.
d. Chronic pancreatitis.
e. Gastric antral vascular ectasia (GAVE).

Answer: a

34. The complications of cirrhosis of the liver include all of the following **except**:

a. Caput medusae.
b. Esophageal varices.
c. Hemorrhoids.
d. Duodenitis.
e. Portal hypertension.

Answer: d

35. Melena is associated with all of the following **except**:

a. Benign gastric ulcers.
b. Benign duodenal ulcers.
c. Diverticular disease.
d. Erosive gastritis.
e. Erosive esophagitis.

Answer: c

36. Which of the following is the **most** common **generic** location for berry aneurysm of the circle of Willis?

a. A vertebral artery.
b. A posterior cerebral artery.
c. An internal carotid artery.
d. The anterior communicating artery.
e. A middle cerebral artery.

Answer: d

37. In chronic intravenous drug users who develop infectious endocarditis as a complication of their drug abuse, which of the cardiac valves is **most** commonly affected?

a. Tricuspid valve.
b. Pulmonary valve.
c. Mitral valve.
d. Aortic valve.
e. The tricuspid and pulmonary valves equally.

Answer: c

38. A 31-year-old homosexual man with a recent diagnosis HIV died in hospital. He had presented in the ER with abdominal pain after ingesting an unknown liquid, and had exhibited progressive neurological deterioration over 3 hours (acute confusion and slurred speech) that was associated with metabolic acidosis. A hospital alcohol breath test for ethanol was negative, but urine toxicological screening was positive for a substance. Based on the section of kidney in Figure 8.5, what substance was ingested?

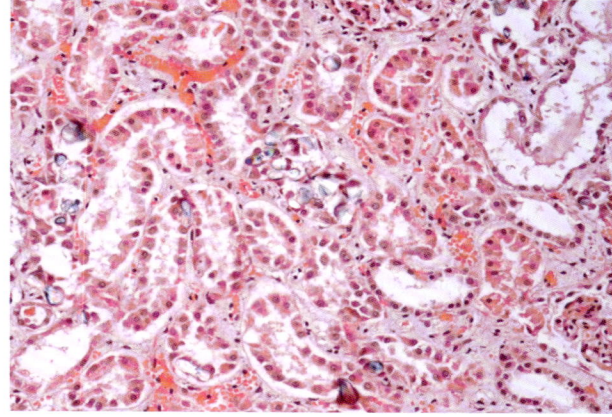

FIGURE 8.5

a. Sulphuric acid.
b. Methanol.
c. Ethylene glycol.
d. Fentanyl.
e. Cocaine.

Answer: c

39. A body that is recovered after a significant period of time from a cold, wet, and oxygen-depleted environment would be expected to show which type of decompositional change?

a. Adipocere formation.
b. Mummification.
c. Wet putrefaction.
d. Skeletonization.
e. Massive gaseous bloating of the face, abdomen and scrotum.

Answer: a

40. At autopsy, an elderly man with peripheral vascular disease is found to have infarction of the proximal two-thirds of his small intestine secondary to superimposed thrombotic occlusion of an artery on top of high grade atheromatous narrowing. Which artery was affected?

a. Superior mesenteric artery.

b. Celiac artery.

c. Inferior mesenteric artery.

d. A renal artery.

e. Splenic artery.

Answer: a

41. A female chronic alcoholic dies of upper gastrointestinal hemorrhage secondary to ruptured esophageal varices in the setting of cirrhosis of the liver. What is the **manner** of death?

a. Accident.

b. Natural.

c. Suicide.

d. Undetermined.

e. Homicide.

Answer: b

42. In a coroner's system in Canada, who is responsible for the official certification of both cause and manner of death in medicolegal autopsies?

a. Investigating coroner.

b. Medical examiner.

c. Forensic pathologist.

d. Provincial registrar general.

e. Medical chief of staff.

Answer: a

43. A previously fit and healthy 17-year-old boy of normal body mass index (BMI) who played competitive ice hockey, collapsed suddenly and died within minutes after finishing a shift during a junior hockey tournament. Of the following, which is **not** the most likely explanation of his death?

a. Hypertrophic obstructive cardiomyopathy.

b. Arrhythmogenic cardiomyopathy.

c. Catecholaminergic polymorphic

ventricular tachycardia.

d. Anomalous left coronary artery.

e. Atherosclerotic coronary artery disease.

Answer: e

44. You perform an autopsy on a 62-year-old man of unknown medical history who was witnessed to collapse and die while shoveling snow. Postmortem examination revealed a large hemopericardium secondary to a ruptured acute myocardial infarct of the lateral free wall of the left ventricle in the context of a right dominant coronary artery circulation. Which coronary artery must have been occluded to explain the acute myocardial infarct?

a. Anterior descending branch of the left coronary artery (LAD).

b. Acute marginal artery.

c. Right coronary artery (RCA).

d. Circumflex branch of the left coronary artery (LCX).

e. Posterior descending coronary artery.

Answer: d

45. A previously healthy 25-year-old woman collapsed and died while playing tennis. A complete autopsy shows no anatomical cause of death and the heart appeared grossly normal. The following ancillary investigations should be considered **except**:

a. Collection of blood and/or fresh tissue for targeted cardiac genetic testing.

b. Retention of the heart for cardiac pathology consultation.

c. Toxicological analysis of the blood for stimulant drugs.

d. Complete dissection of the heart by a junior resident.

e. Routine histological examination of the main organs.

Answer: d

46. A chronic alcoholic dies of acute ethanol toxicity (alcohol poisoning) after a weekend of recreational binge drinking. What is the **manner** of death?

a. Accident.

b. Natural.

c. Suicide.

d. Undetermined.

e. Homicide.

Answer: a

47. Identification of which of the following infectious diseases at autopsy mandates that you report the case to public health immediately (and will result in you having to take prophylactic antibiotics)?

a. *Klebsiella pneumoniae* bronchopneumonia.

b. Urosepsis secondary to *Enterobacter* species.

c. Respiratory syncytial virus (RSV) infection in an infant.

d. *Neisseria meningitides* meningitis.

e. Streptococcal bronchopneumonia.

Answer: d

48. Which of the following is **not** ascribed as the color of a fresh bruise?

a. Yellow.

b. Red.

c. Purple.

d. Blue.

e. Bluish purple.

Answer: a

49. Pink coloration of the skin at autopsy can be associated with each of the following **except**:

a. Carbon monoxide poisoning.

b. Cyanide poisoning.

c. Opioid toxicity.

d. Hypothermia.

e. Refrigeration of a body at 39.2°F (4°C).

Answer: c

50. Deaths in cases of autoerotic asphyxia are **typically** associated with all of the following **except**:

a. A secluded scene of death.

b. Female decedents.

c. Ligatures around the neck.

d. Pornographic material.

e. Male decedents.

Answer: b

51. The diatom test is an ancillary investigation that can be used in the investigation of deaths by:
a. Drowning.
b. Fire.
c. Firearms.
d. Strangulation.
e. Drug abuse.

Answer: a

52. Which of the following autopsy findings is not necessarily a sign that an individual was alive and breathing when a fire was started?
a. Soot in the esophagus.
b. Soot in the larynx, trachea and bronchial tree.
c. Soot in the buccal cavity only.
d. An elevated blood concentration of COHb.
e. Soot in the stomach.

Answer: c

53. Which of the following statements about fire deaths is **false**?
a. A COHb concentration > 50% is considered fatal in a healthy individual.
b. Cyanide cannot be produced after death.
c. Cigarette smoking can account for COHb concentrations up to 15%.
d. Deaths in "flash fires" tend to have low or absent COHb concentrations.
e. Self-immolation deaths tend to have low or absent COHb concentrations.

Answer: b

54. What is the range of fire for the entrance gunshot wound in Figure 8.6?

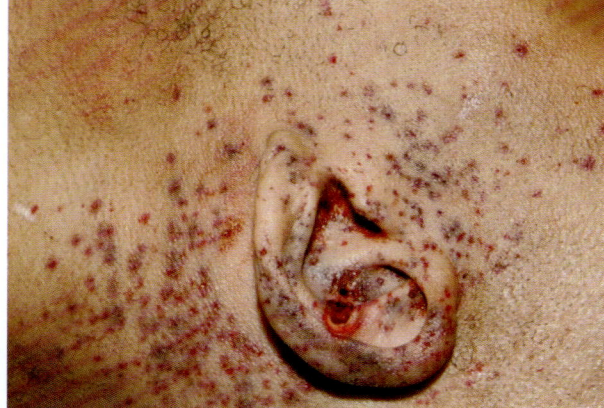

FIGURE 8.6
a. Indeterminate.
b. Contact.
c. Distant.
d. Intermediate.
e. Close contact.

Answer: d

55. The onset of rigor mortis can be delayed in all of the following contexts **except**:
a. Electrocution.
b. Emaciation.
c. Elderly individuals.
d. Very young individuals.
e. Lower ambient temperature.

Answer: a

56. The onset of rigor mortis can be hastened by all of the following contexts **except**:
a. Increased core body temperature at the time of death.
b. Increased physical activity shortly before death.
c. Electrocution.
d. Emaciation.
e. Higher ambient temperature.

Answer: d

57. Which of the following methods of identification is **not** scientific?
a. Comparison of tattoos.
b. Comparative DNA profiling.
c. Comparative forensic odontological examination.
d. Fingerprint comparison.
e. Comparison of ante-mortem and post-mortem radiographs.

Answer: a

58. Concerning gunshot wounds of the head, which of the following anatomical sites of entrance is not typical of self-infliction?
a. Occipital region.
b. Submental region.
c. Intraoral.
d. Temporal region.
e. Glabellar region/central forehead.

Answer: a

59. Which of the following statements is false about sharp force injuries caused by knives?
a. A stab wound is a penetrating incised wound that is deeper than its length on the skin surface.
b. Defensive incised wounds in homicidal stabbings commonly occur on the hands and forearms.
c. A 4 inch (10 cm) stab wound track of the abdomen could not have been caused by a 1.38 inch (3.5 cm) length blade.
d. Fatal self-inflicted incised wounds of the neck and forearms tend to be associated with the presence of more superficial incised wounds around them called tentative/hesitation injuries.
e. Fatal self-inflicted stab wounds are most commonly inflicted on the front of the left chest.

Answer: c

60. Each of the following pairs of compounds consists of a drug followed by its corresponding metabolite **except**:
a. Cocaine and benzoylecgonine (BE).
b. Methamphetamine and amphetamine.
c. 3, 4 - methylenedioxy-methamphetamine
(MDMA) and methylenedioxyamphetamine (MDA).
d. Carfentanil and fentanyl.
e. Heroin and morphine.

Answer: d

Case Scenario

Figure 8.7 shows a section of kidney from the postmortem of a 35-year-old man.

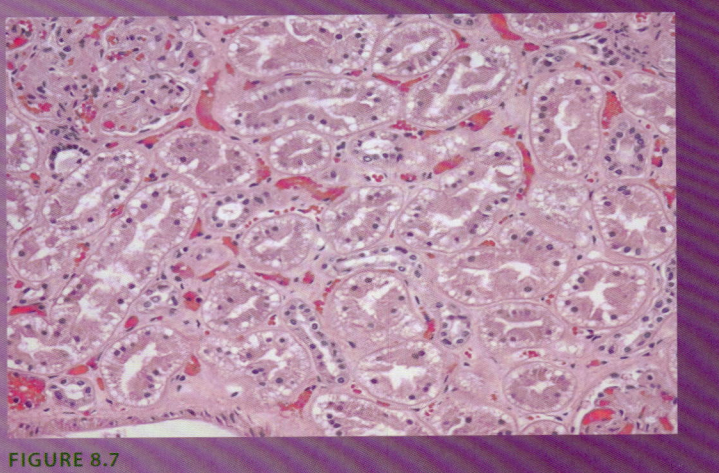

FIGURE 8.7

61. What descriptive finding is depicted in the proximal tubules of the kidney specimen in Figure 8.7?

Subnuclear vacuolation of the proximal tubular epithelium.

62. What substance is responsible for the appearance of the proximal tubules?

Accumulation of lipid droplets.

63. What histochemical stain can be employed to demonstrate your answer to the previous question? What type of specimen preparation is appropriate for this stain?

Any fat stain (e.g., oil red O stain) can be used, which is appropriate for fresh-frozen or formalin-fixed tissue, but not for processed tissue.

64. List 2 conditions associated with this lesion.

• Diabetic ketoacidosis.

• Alcoholic ketoacidosis.

Case Scenario

Figure 8.8 shows the buccal cavity of a 75-year-old male who was found dead in his garage after a recent diagnosis of stage 4 metastatic carcinoma of the prostate gland.

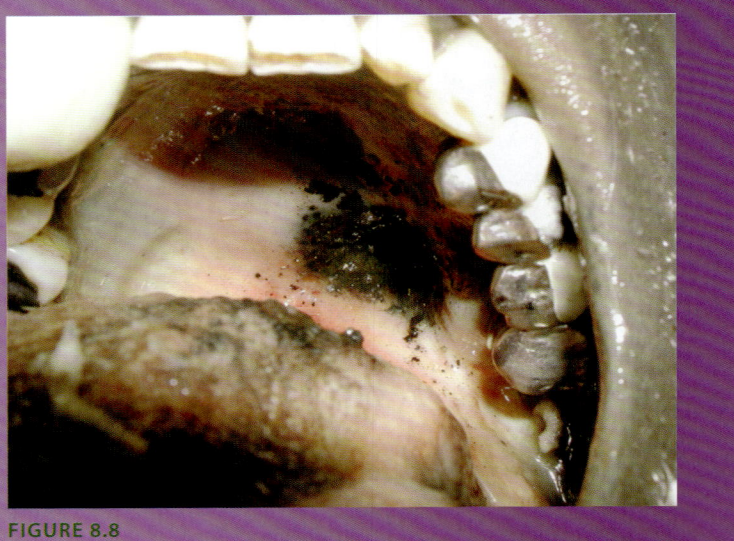

FIGURE 8.8

65. What is the cause of death and **likely** manner of death?
- Cause of death: intraoral gunshot wound of the head.
- Likely manner of death: suicide.

66. State 3 other regions of the head where this pathological finding would be consistent with the same manner of death.
- Submental region.
- Temporal (temple) region.
- Glabellar region of the forehead.

Case Scenario

Figure 8.9 shows a section of the left ventricle of a 72-year-old man with a clinical feature of restrictive cardiomyopathy.

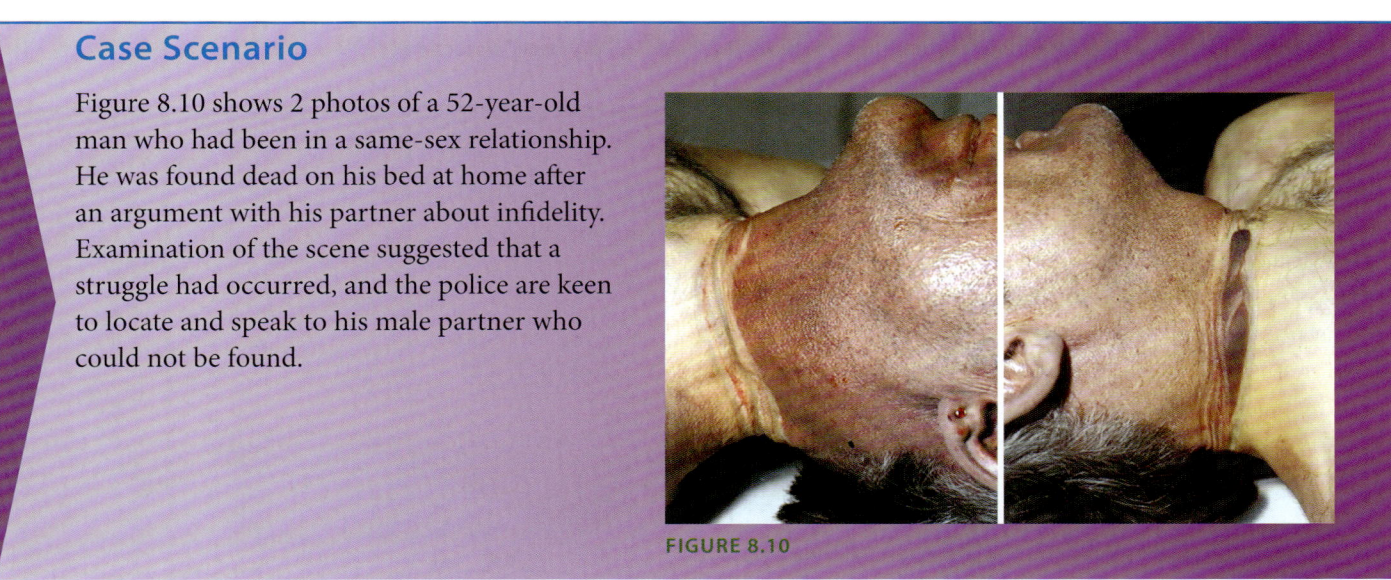

FIGURE 8.9

67. What is the main entity a pathologist should suspect?
Amyloidosis.

68. How would you confirm your suspected diagnosis?
Congo red stain.

Case Scenario

Figure 8.10 shows 2 photos of a 52-year-old man who had been in a same-sex relationship. He was found dead on his bed at home after an argument with his partner about infidelity. Examination of the scene suggested that a struggle had occurred, and the police are keen to locate and speak to his male partner who could not be found.

FIGURE 8.10

69. What is specific cause of death should be considered?
Ligature strangulation.

70. What is the suspected manner of death?
Homicide.

Case Scenario

Figure 8.11 shows the front of the neck of a 28-year-old woman, whose body was discovered at the residence of her estranged husband following unsuccessful attempts by relatives to contact her.

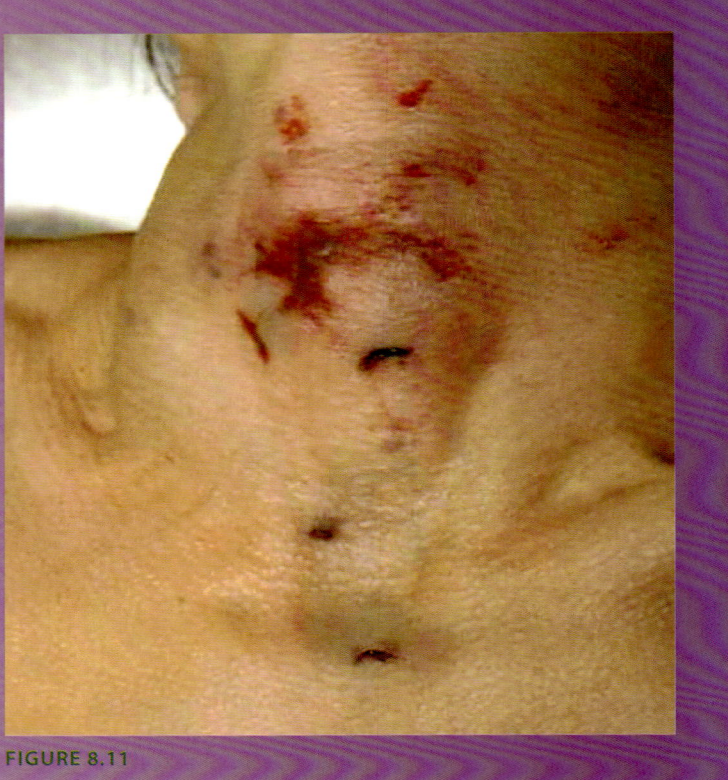

FIGURE 8.11

71. What specific cause of death should be considered?
Manual strangulation.

72. What specific pathological finding should the eyes be examined for?
Petechiae.

73. What special examination technique of the neck should be employed?
Layered dissection of the anterior neck structures in a bloodless field (i.e., "dry neck" dissection).

Case Scenario

Figure 8.12 shows a section of the opened colorectum of a 44-year-old woman who was admitted for emergent total abdominal hysterectomy and bilateral salpingo-oophorectomy after a diagnosis of left ovarian torsion. The procedure was uneventful, but the patient became ill in hospital between the first and second postoperative days, and progressively deteriorated over the next 7 days (sepsis with multiorgan failure and disseminated intravascular coagulation [DIC]) before she died, prior to having undergone the following sequential procedures:

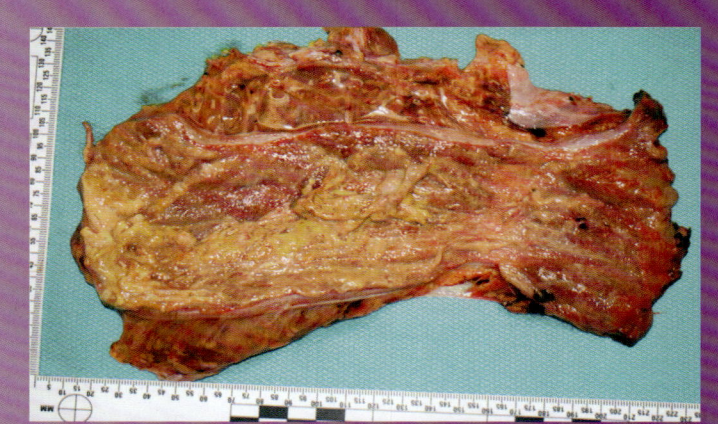

FIGURE 8.12

- A negative exploratory laparotomy for iatrogenic injuries or intraabdominal collections.
- Flexible sigmoidoscopy.
- An emergent subtotal colectomy and end ileostomy, which was indicated on postoperative day 5.

At postmortem, there was scleral icterus; features of DIC; a postsurgical appearance of the abdominal cavity (with no features of suppurative inflammation); and collections of serous fluid in the pericardial and pleural cavities. The intestinal tract consisted of 156 inches (397 cm) of small intestine and 12 inches (31 cm) of colorectum.

74. What pathology is depicted on the mucosal aspect of the colorectum?
Pseudomembranous colitis.

75. What is the etiology of this finding?
Infection with *Clostridium difficile*.

Case Scenario

The body of a 65-year-old woman was discovered on her basement floor at the bottom of a flight of stairs. Examination of the scene indicated that she had been taking a basket of laundry down into the basement after having had a few drinks.

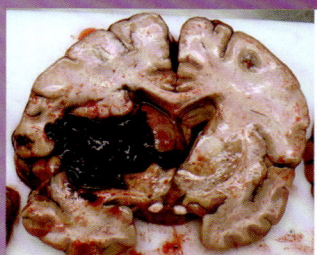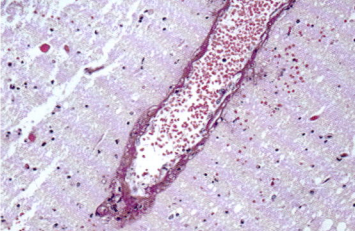

FIGURE 8.13

Figure 8.13 is a gross photo of the decedent's brain that depicts an intracerebral hematoma of the left basal ganglia and histology of the brain at the edge of the hematoma.

76. What is the manner of death?
Natural.

77. What is the underlying disease process?
Hypertension.

Case Scenario

Figure 8.14 is a histological image of a section of lung (x40) from a 52-year-old man who suffered a sudden cardiac death.

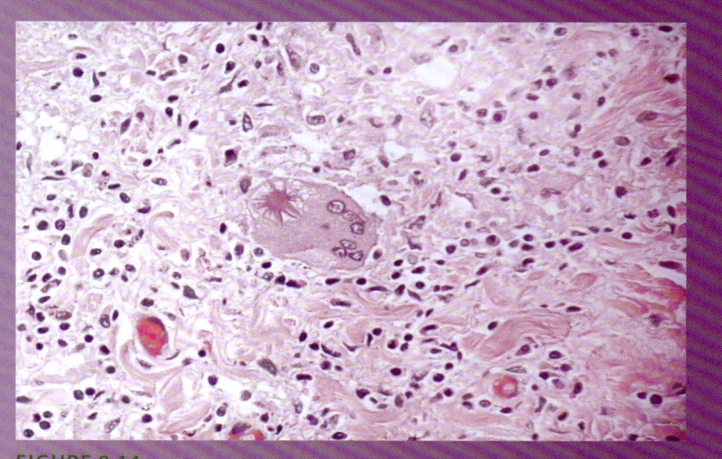

FIGURE 8.14

78. What finding is depicted in the center of Figure 8.14?
An asteroid body in a multinucleated giant cell.

79. Name the disease process that is typically associated with this finding.
Sarcoidosis.

Case Scenario

The body of a 22-year-old woman, with a recurrent history of domestic violence at the hands of her boyfriend, was found hanging from first floor bannister at her boyfriend's home. Given the history of domestic violence, the police were concerned about the death.

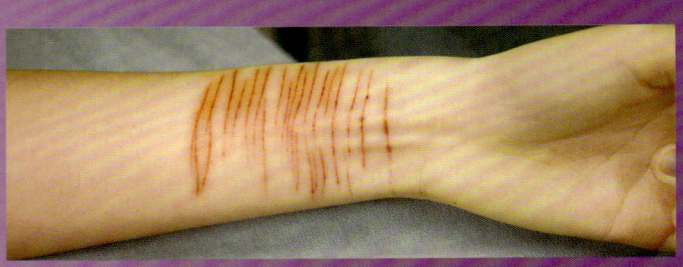

FIGURE 8.15

Scene examination established that the body was in full vertical suspension from bannister (by a length of torn bedsheet around the neck as the ligature) with the feet a few centimeters above the floor. There were no signs of a disturbance. A small box-cutter knife was on the stairs.

At postmortem examination, there was no congestion or cyanosis of the facial skin, and no petechiae of the facial skin, but a few conjunctival petechiae of the eyes. The neck exhibited an upwardly slanted, complete ligature mark that rose to an apical point of the left side of the back of the upper neck behind the left ear, where the knot of the noose was located, and was consistent with having been caused by the ligature around the neck. Injuries of the left forearm were also noted, as depicted in Figure 8.15.

80. What terminology can be used to describe what is shown?
Tentative/hesitation marks/wounds.

81. What manner of death would you advise the police is applicable?
Suicide.

Case Scenario

The body of a 56-year-old female chronic alcoholic was discovered in bed. Postmortem examination did not reveal any acute pathology or injury to explain her death. The single positive anatomical finding was an enlarged and heavier-than-expected liver with a golden yellow color, shown in Figure 8.16.

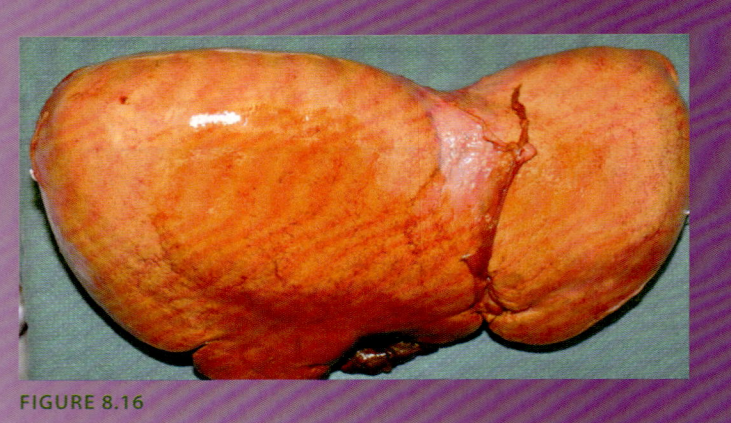

FIGURE 8.16

82. What probable cause of death should be strongly considered?
Alcoholic ketoacidosis.

83. What 2 specific ancillary investigations should be requested to support this?
• Blood ethanol concentration.
• ß-hydroxybutyrate (BHB) concentration (vitreous humor and/or blood).

84. Comment on the interpretation of the results of the 2 ancillary investigations that you have provided above.
Low/absent ethanol and elevated BHB will diagnose alcoholic ketoacidosis.

Case Scenario

Figure 8.17 shows the inside of the skullcap of an 87-year-old male with a history of frailty, dementia, and recurrent falls.

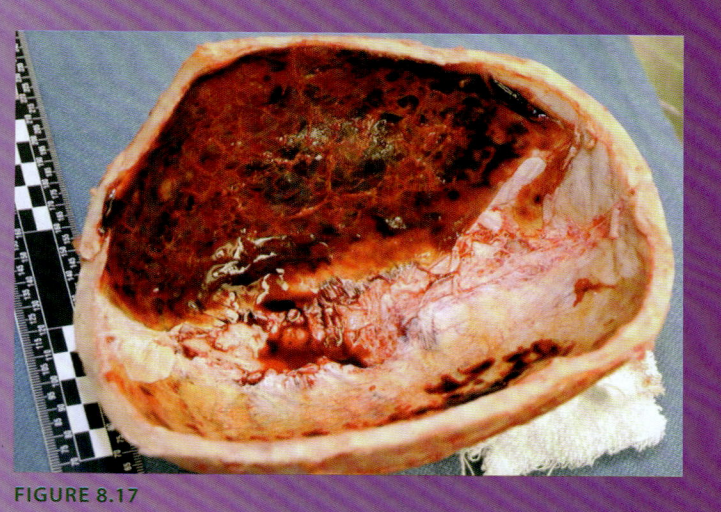

FIGURE 8.17

85. Name the intracranial lesion.

Chronic subdural hematoma.

86. Comment on the expected appearance and weight of the brain in relation to his age.

Cerebral atrophy with gyral atrophy and lower than expected weight.

Case Scenario

A 65-year-old male shopkeeper with a history of hypertension, non-insulin-dependent diabetes mellitus, and atherosclerotic coronary artery disease collapsed during a robbery after a loaded revolver was pointed at him. He died in the ICU 2 days later. Figure 8.18 shows his right coronary artery (left image) and transverse slice of his ventricular myocardium (right image).

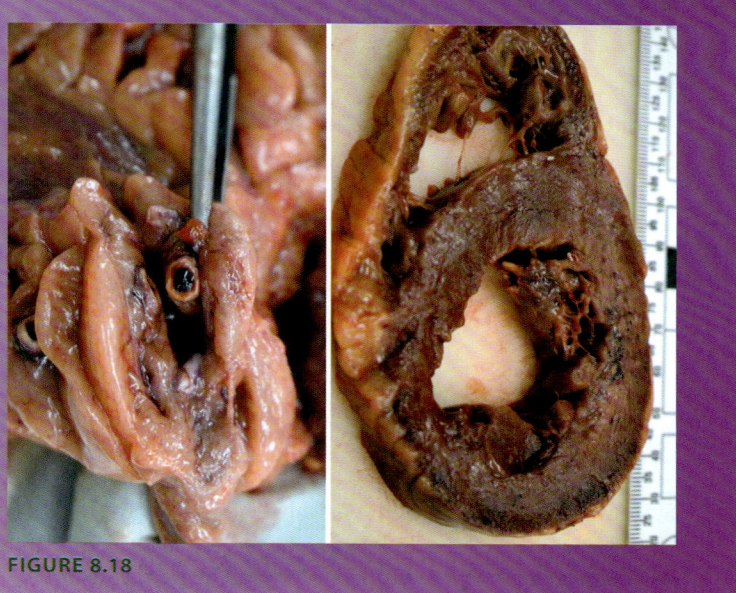

FIGURE 8.18

87. What pathologies are depicted in Figure 8.18?

• Acute thrombotic occlusion of right coronary artery.

• Acute myocardial infarction of the posterior wall of the left ventricle.

88. What is the manner of death?

Homicide.

Case Scenario

Figure 8.19 shows the body of a 19-year-old male with a history of schizophrenia who died at a house party.

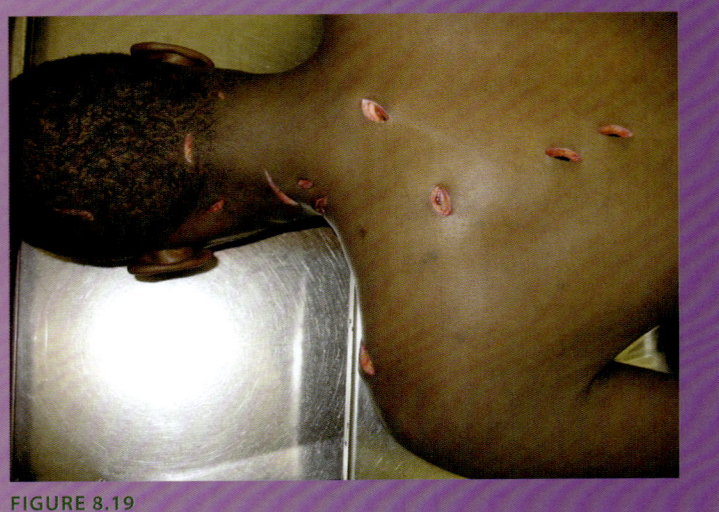

FIGURE 8.19

89. What injuries are depicted?
Multiple stab wounds.

90. State the likely manner of death.
Homicide.

Case Scenario

The body of a 52-year-old woman with a history of alcoholism and heavy cigarette smoking was recovered from fire in her residence. Figure 8.20 shows her laryngotracheobronchial tree.

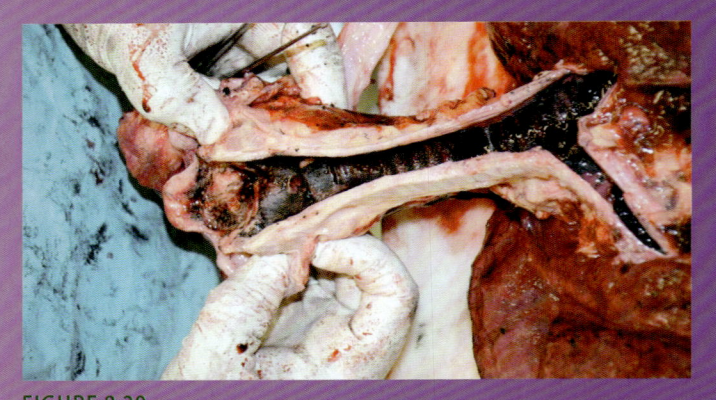

FIGURE 8.20

91. State whether the decedent was alive when the fire started and support your answer.
The decedent was alive at the start of the fire, as can be inferred from the present of soot throughout the laryngotracheobronchial tree, below the level of the vocal cords.

92. State 2 products of combustion that toxicologists can screen for in fire fatalities.
• Carbon monoxide (in the form of carboxyhemoglobin). • Cyanide.

Case Scenario

A previously well 23-year-old man with no medical history collapsed suddenly and died during a fight. He was found to have an enlarged, heavier-than-expected heart at postmortem examination with characteristic gross and microscopic features. Figure 8.21 shows a section of the anterior left ventricle (x200).

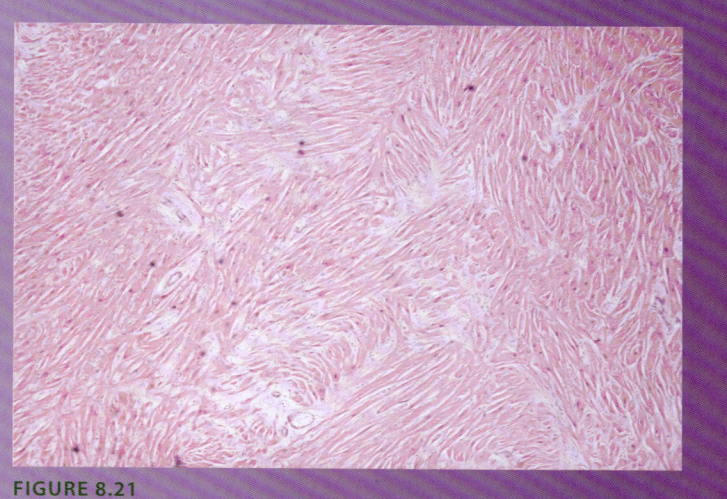

FIGURE 8.21

93. What is the likely diagnosis?
Hypertrophic cardiomyopathy.

94. Comment on the expected gross features of the left ventricle.
- Asymmetrical hypertrophy of the wall of the left ventricle with increased thickness of the interventricular septum.
- Endocardial impact lesion of the left ventricular outflow tract.

Case Scenario

Figure 8.22 shows the body of a 35-year-old man with no underlying medical conditions who was found dead in his bed.

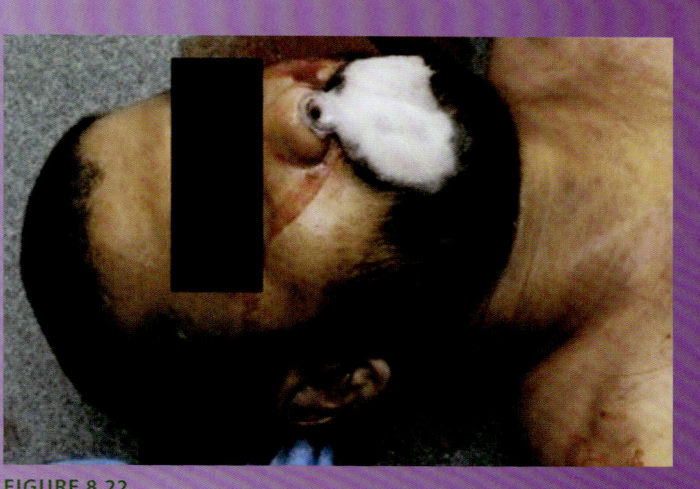

FIGURE 8.22

95. What cause of death should be most strongly considered?
Opioid toxicity.

96. What alternative cause of death should be considered had this body been recovered from a lake?
Drowning.

97. List 2 other causes of the diagnostic feature depicted in the image.
- Congestive cardiac failure.
- Epilepsy.

Case Scenario

A 32-year-old female chronic intravenous drug abuser, who would inject crushed pills, had developed progressive shortness of breath over some months with positive cardiac investigations. She decompensated acutely and died. Autopsy findings included:

- Height: 168 cm.
- Weight: 68 kg.
- Heart: 452 g — enlarged and globular.
- Lungs: left 678 g; right 876 g — marked congestion and edema.

Figure 8.23 shows a transverse section of the ventricles.

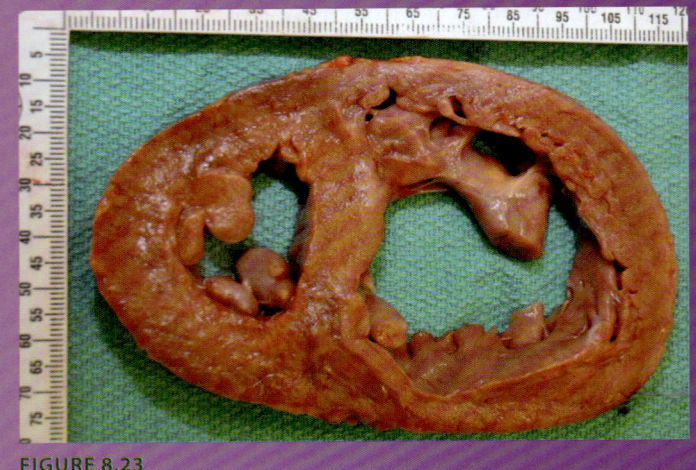

FIGURE 8.23

98. What pathology in depicted in Figure 8.23?
Right ventricular hypertrophy.

99. What terminology can be used to describe her proximate cause of death?
Acute cor pulmonale.

100. In the context of her history, what underlying pathological finding would be expected in her lungs?
Foreign body granulomatous inflammatory reaction centered on the pulmonary arterioles (i.e., "junkie's lung").

Case Scenario

The body of a 15-year-old female, who had a history of depression secondary being bullied at school over her weight, was found dead in her bedroom. Scene examination revealed a suicide note and an unknown clear liquid in a chemistry bottle, which appeared to have been ingested.

No anatomical cause of death was evident at autopsy. Toxicological analysis of the femoral venous blood identified **substance X** and its metabolite formic acid as the only positive findings as follows:

Femoral venous blood

Formic acid — 620 mg/L.
Substance X — 110 mg/100 mL.

101. What compound is **substance X**?
Methanol.

102. What major morbidity would have occurred if ingestion had not been fatal?
Blindness.

Case Scenario

Figure 8.24 shows a finding from a 29-year-old woman discovered dead in bed.

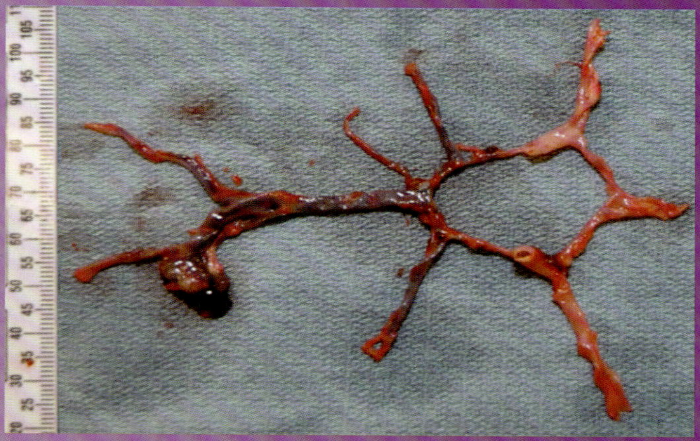

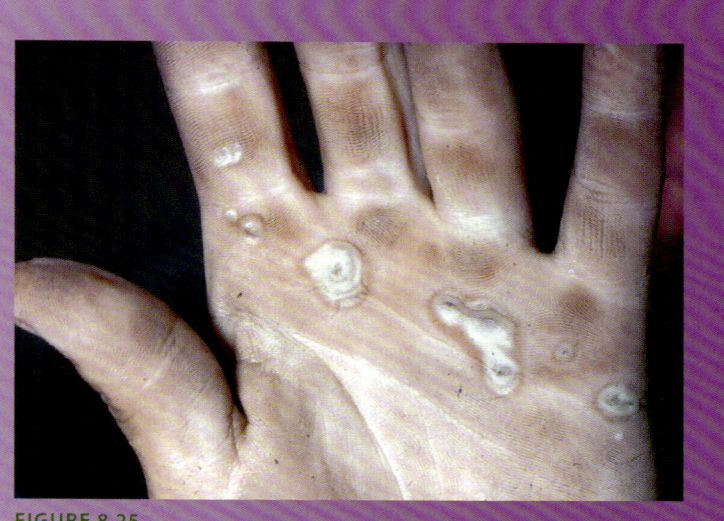

FIGURE 8.24

103. What lesion is depicted?
Berry aneurysm of the circle of Willis.

104. What pathological intracranial finding would be first observed at autopsy?
Basal subarachnoid hemorrhage.

105. What possible associated finding may be seen in the kidneys?
Polycystic disease (adult polycystic kidney disease).

Case Scenario

Figure 8.25 shows the left palm a healthy 35-year-old man. The man had been working in his garage with power tools and was discovered dead on garage floor in nonsuspicious circumstances. The lesions on the left palm were the only positive finding.

FIGURE 8.25

106. Define the lesions seen on his palm.
Electrocution/Joule marks.

107. What cause of death do they indicate?
Electrocution.

Case Scenario

Figure 8.26 shows the base of the skull of a 36-year-old male driver of a car that crashed into a concrete wall. The cause of death was multiple blunt force injuries.

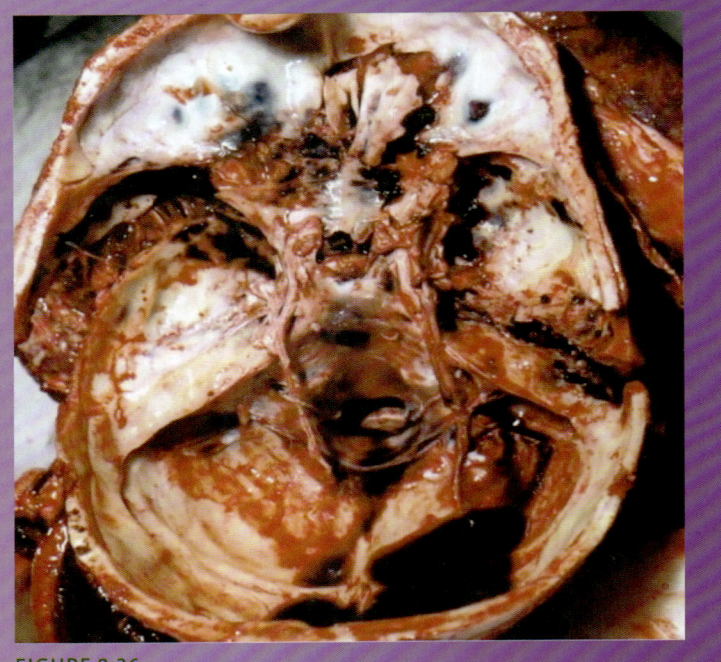

FIGURE 8.26

108. What is the main abnormality depicted in the image?

Hinge fracture across the base of the skull through the middle cranial fossae.

Case Scenario

Figure 8.27 is from the postmortem of a 52-year-old woman with a history of abdominal pain. It shows the opened abdomen with reflected mesentery.

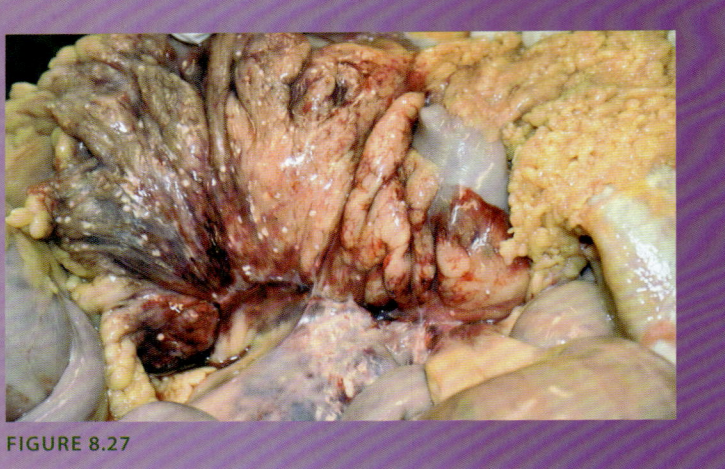

FIGURE 8.27

109. What pathological term describes the abnormality depicted in the mesentery?

Saponification.

110. What diagnosis does this abnormality indicate?

Acute pancreatitis.

111. List possible predisposing factors to this diagnosis.

- Alcohol abuse use.
- Gallstones.
- Scorpion venom.

Case Scenario

Figure 8.28 shows the heart of a 15-year-old boy who felt acutely short of breath while playing basketball and collapsed shortly after leaving the court. He was successfully resuscitated but died in hospital 2 days later.

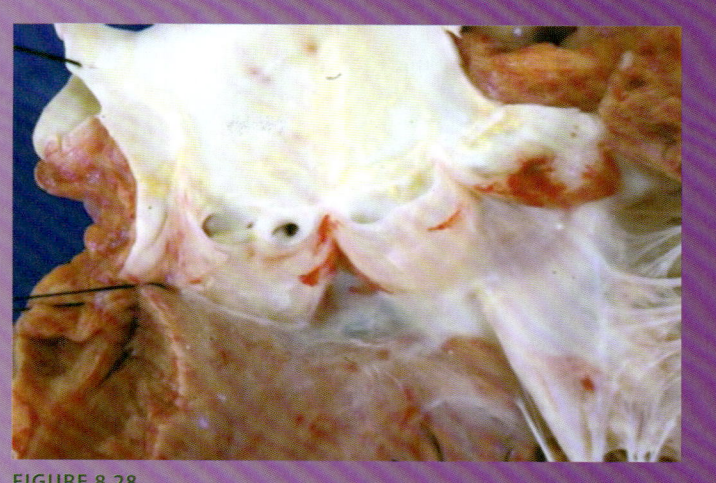

FIGURE 8.28

112. What is the underlying cause of death?
Anomalous left coronary artery.

Case Scenario

Figure 8.29 shows the body of a 42-year-old man who was found dead on the bedroom floor of his secured apartment in nonsuspicious circumstances.

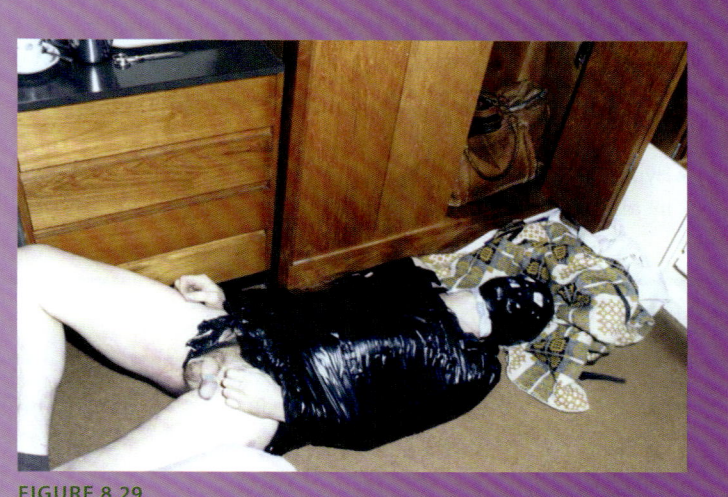

FIGURE 8.29

113. What cause of death should be considered?
Autoerotic asphyxia.

114. What supportive evidence is usually present on scene to support this cause of death?
Pornographic material.

115. What is the manner of death?
Accident.

Case Scenario

Figure 8.30 depicts the mucosal aspect of the stomach of a 54-year-old man.

FIGURE 8.30

116. What are these findings?

Superficial gastric erosions.

117. What eponymous name do they carry?

Wischnewski spots.

118. What pathophysiological process do they represent?

Agonal physiological stress.

119. List at least 3 types of death associated with this finding.

- Burn injury.
- Hypothermia.
- Increased intracranial pressure.

- Diabetic ketoacidosis.
- Alcoholic ketoacidosis.

IMAGES: FORENSIC PATHOLOGY*

*The images in this section are courtesy of Dr. Evan Matshes.

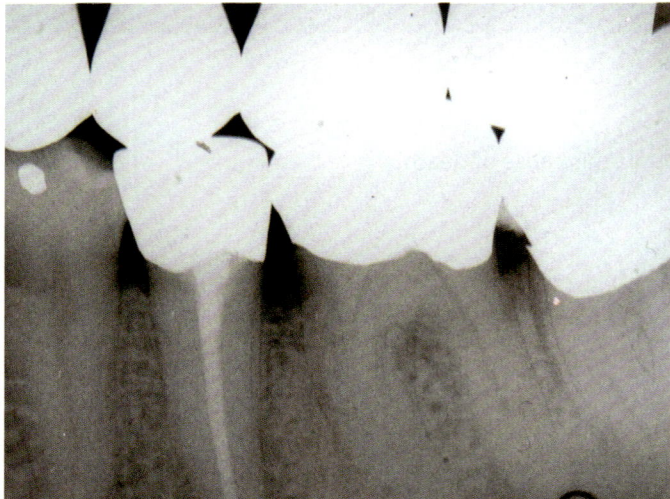

IMAGE 8.1 Dental radiograph. Dental radiography can be used for identification if antemortem dental radiography is available for comparison.

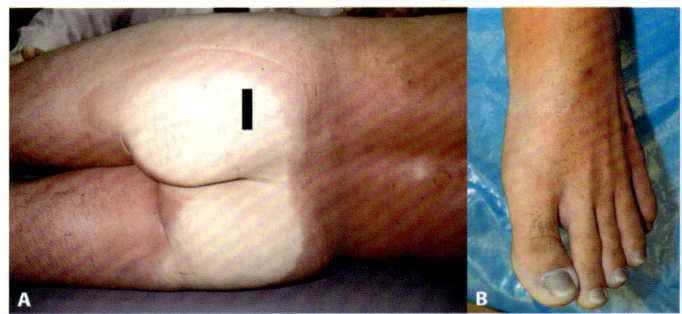

IMAGE 8.2 Lividity. Left: postmortem lividity is the settling of blood in dependent areas. Skin surfaces that are compressed are spared from lividity. Right: small capillaries can break and blood can leak out, causing small hemorrhages called Tardieu spots.

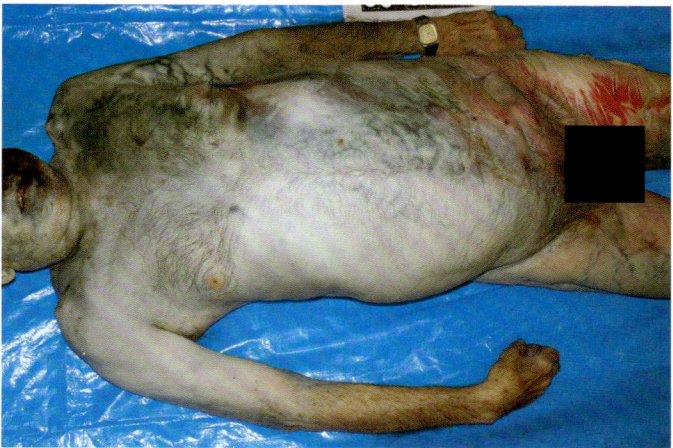

IMAGE 8.3 Putrefaction. Decomposition begins almost immediately after death and is characterized by greenish discoloration of the skin, skin slippage, and expulsion of purge fluid from body orifices. Marbling, the green discoloration of superficial vessels, is pictured here.

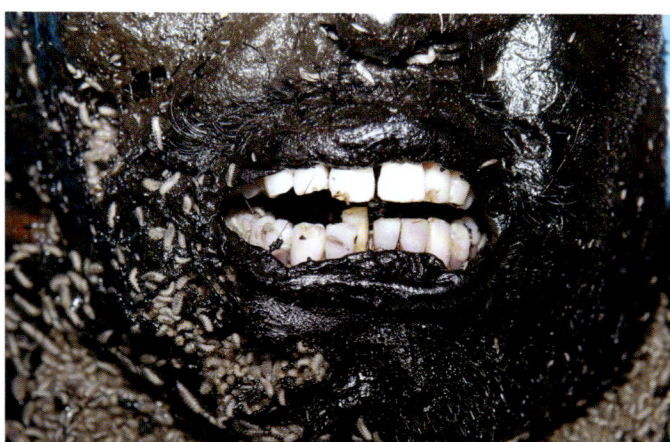

IMAGE 8.6 Postmortem insect activity. Maggots are seen here on the face of a decomposing body.

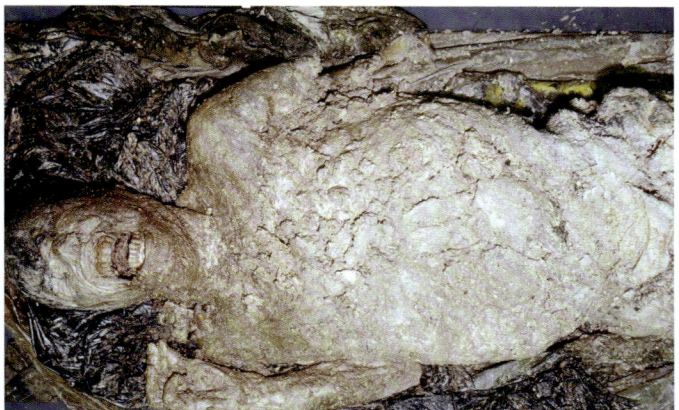

IMAGE 8.4 When bodies are kept in cool, damp environments, the fat can undergo saponification, creating a gray-white wax known as adipocere or grave wax.

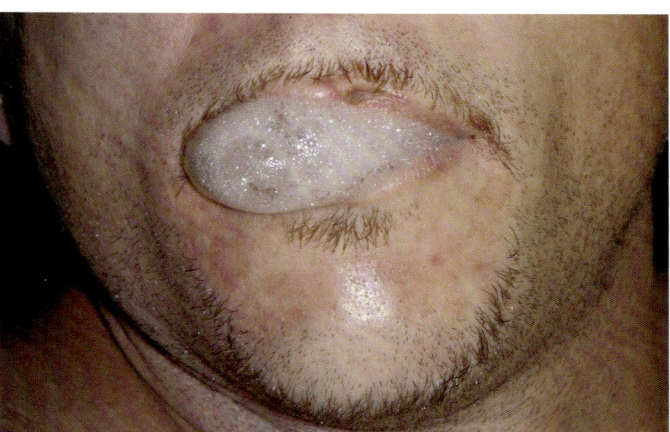

IMAGE 8.7 Froth expulsion. Froth can be noted coming from the mouth and nose in a variety of circumstances, including drowning, narcotic overdose, congestive heart failure, and epilepsy.

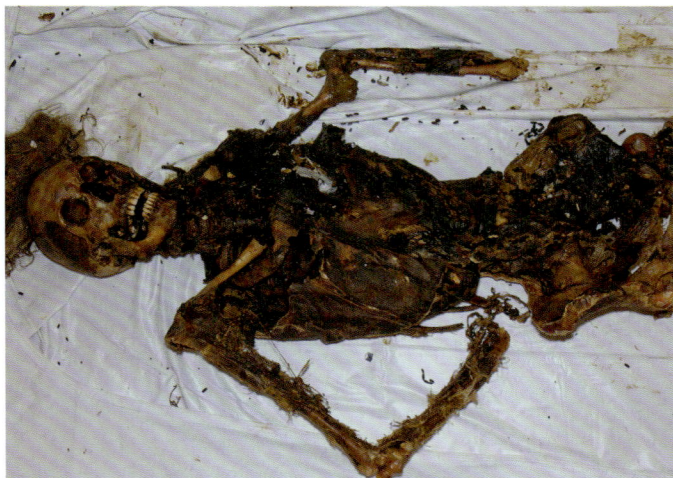

IMAGE 8.5 Mummification and skeletonization. When bodies are kept in dry environments, the skin becomes leathery and mummified. As the tissues break down, skeletonization can occur.

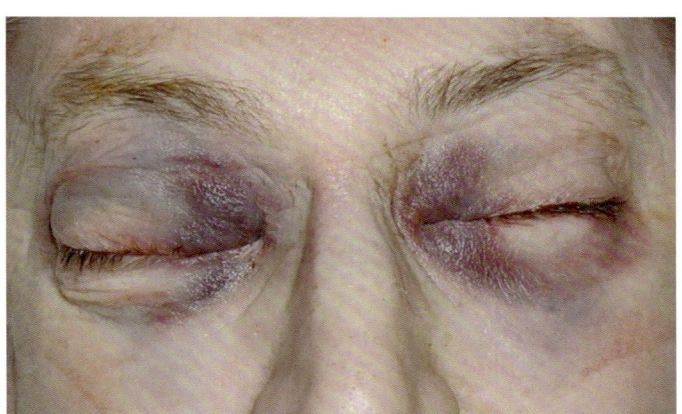

IMAGE 8.8 Periorbital hemorrhage. Periorbital hemorrhage can be seen with basilar skull and orbital plate fractures, but also after eye donation. The circumstances of death must be carefully considered before determining the nature of the finding and its significance.

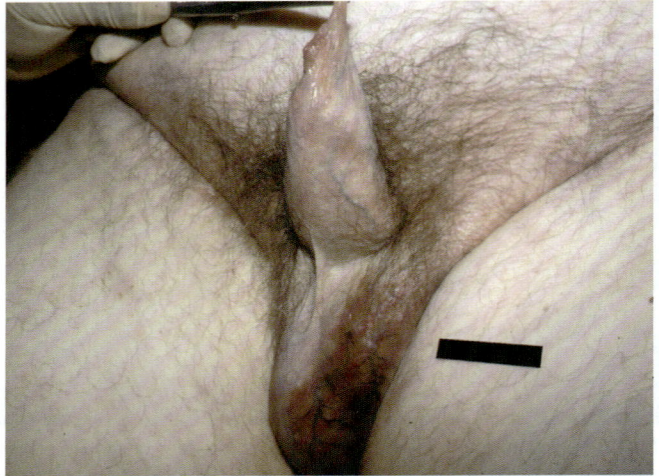

IMAGE 8.9 Postmortem drying. As the skin dries after death, it can mimic bruising or abrasion, particularly on the scrotum. This should not be confused with trauma.

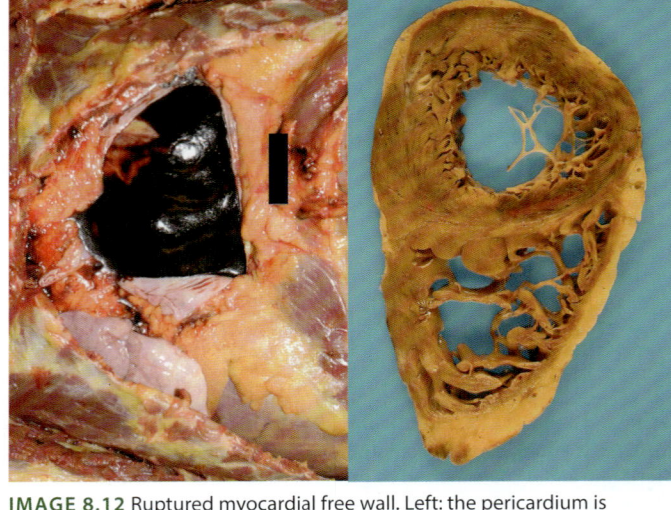

IMAGE 8.12 Ruptured myocardial free wall. Left: the pericardium is opened to reveal hemopericardium. Right: the heart was opened to reveal an acute myocardial infarction that had ruptured (adjacent nonruptured site pictured). Rupture of the papillary muscles or the interventricular septum can also occur as a consequence of acute myocardial infarction.

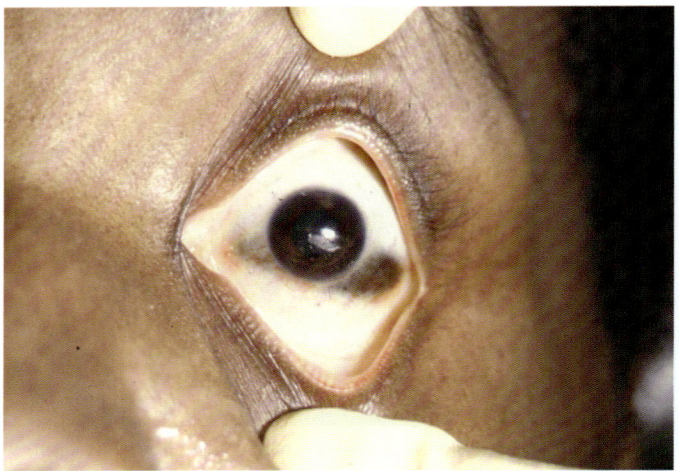

IMAGE 8.10 Tache noire. Scleral drying produces a dark band across the area exposed to air if the eyes are open after death.

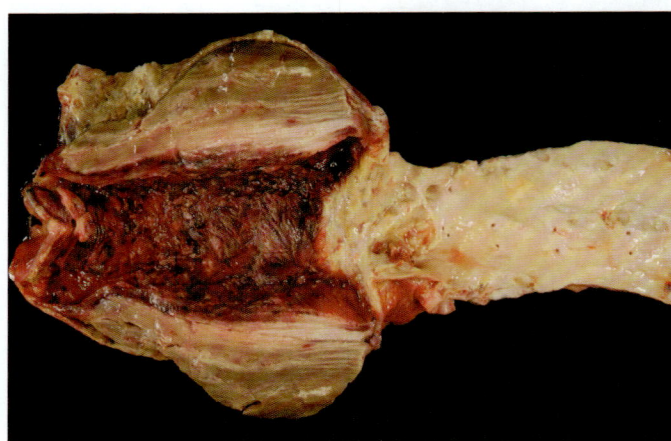

IMAGE 8.13 Abdominal aortic aneurysm. The aorta is opened to reveal the laminated thrombus and residual lumen of this aneurysm. The typical location is the distal aorta, between the renal arteries and the iliac bifurcation.

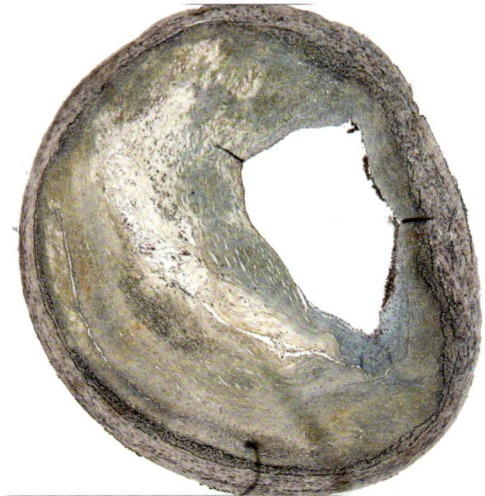

IMAGE 8.11 Coronary artery atherosclerosis. This cross section of a coronary artery shows significant luminal narrowing due to atherosclerosis (Musto stain).

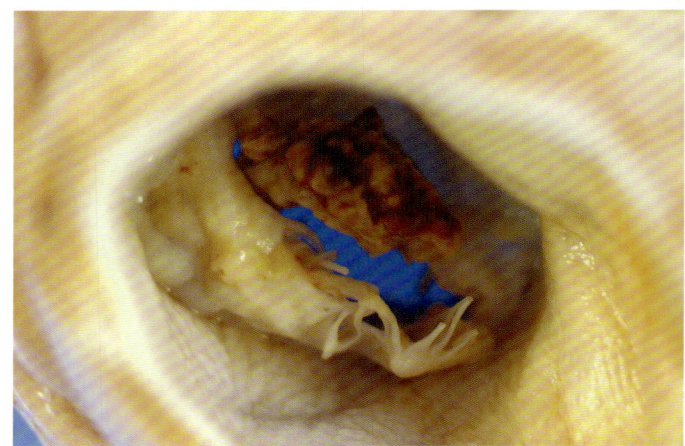

IMAGE 8.14 Aortic dissection. Hemorrhage around the aortic root, proximal aorta, and carotid arteries are associated with this aortic dissection.

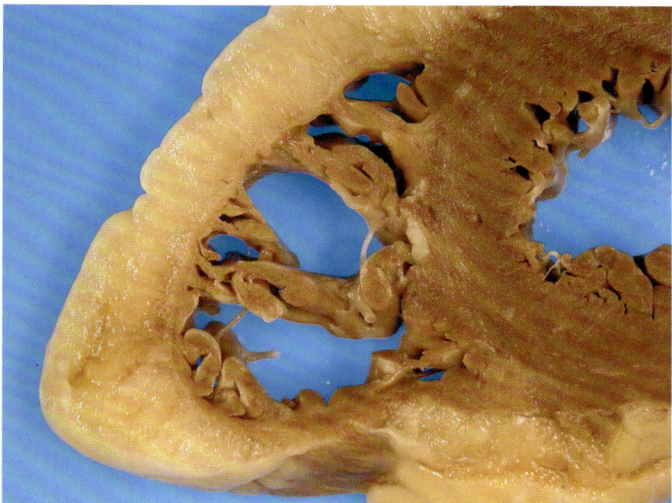

IMAGE 8.15 Arrhythmogenic right ventricular cardiomyopathy. The right ventricular myocardium is replaced with mature fat and fibrous tissue.

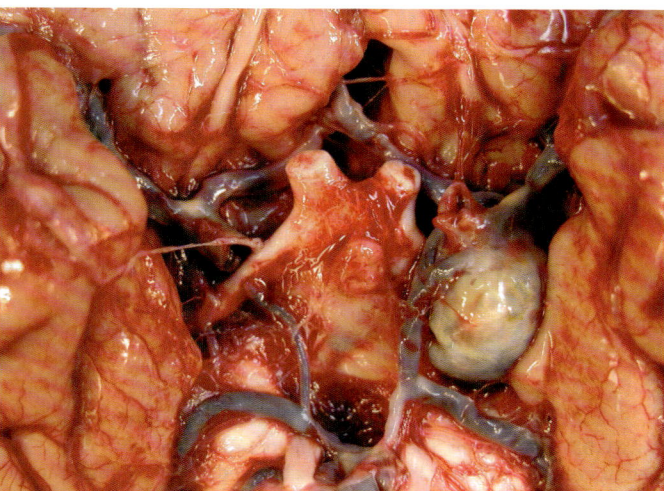

IMAGE 8.18 Berry aneurysm. The circle of Willis is shown here, with a relatively large berry aneurysm at the bifurcation of the internal carotid and the posterior communicating artery.

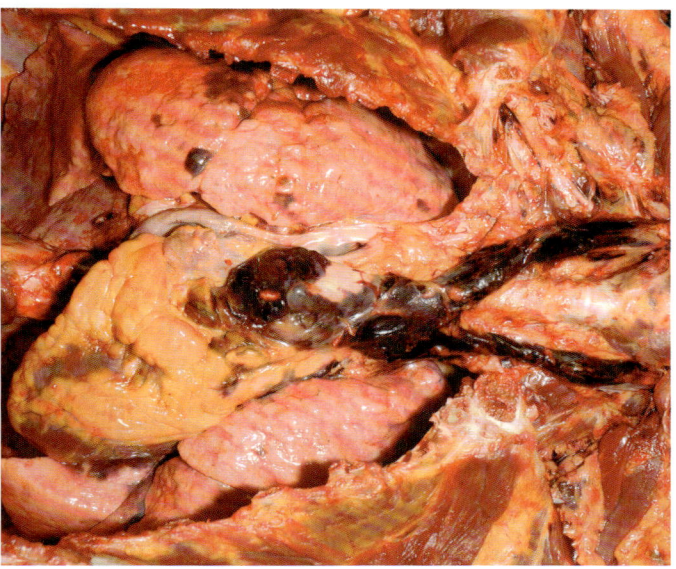

IMAGE 8.16 Infective endocarditis. This vegetation is destroying the normal valve and is extremely friable, both features of infective endocarditis.

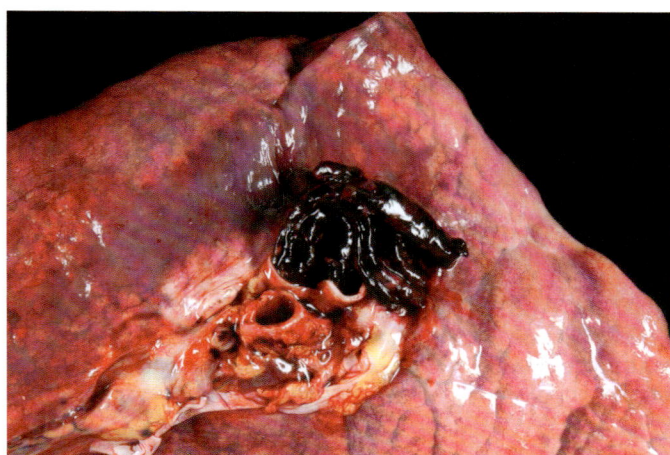

IMAGE 8.19 Pulmonary embolism. This large, slightly granular, thromboembolism occludes the pulmonary artery. Note the difference from postmortem settling of blood, which has a "chicken fat" appearance.

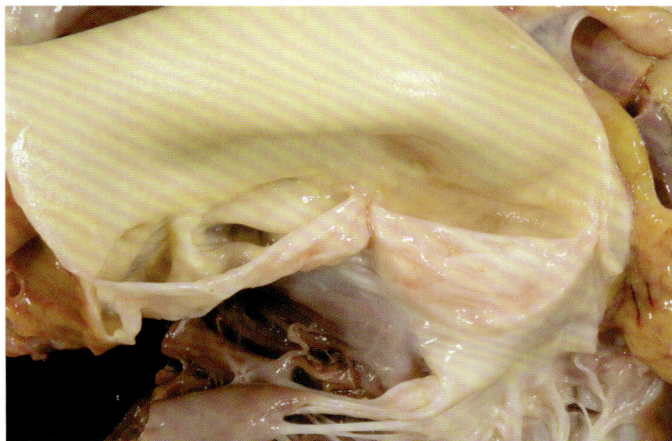

IMAGE 8.17 Bicuspid aortic valve. Look carefully at this valve and you will notice that there are only 2 cusps where there should be 3.

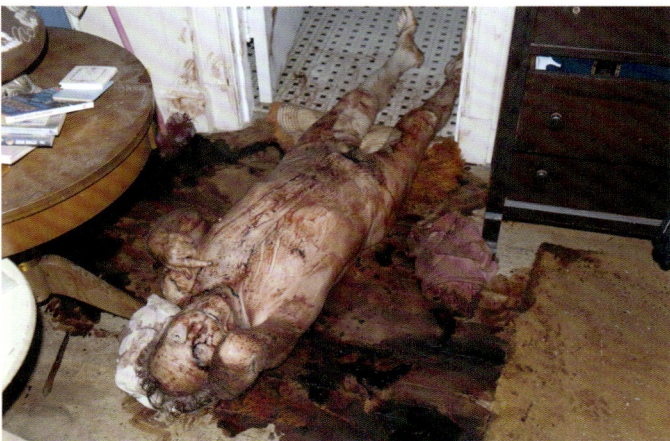

IMAGE 8.20 Ruptured esophageal varices. Blood soaked death scenes often indicate violence. Sudden deaths from esophageal varices can be dramatic and may involve extensive blood staining.

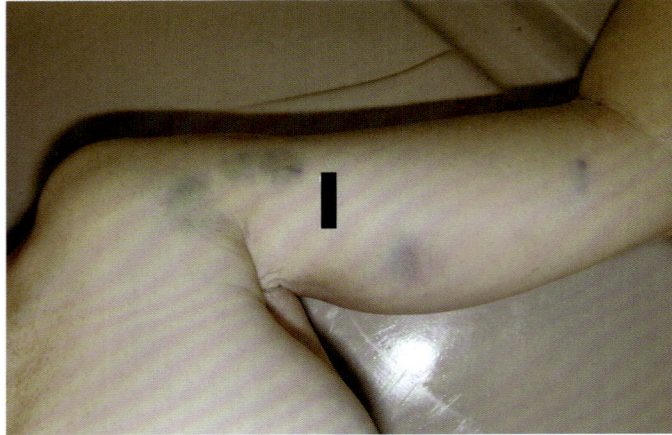

IMAGE 8.21 Contusions. These contusions, or bruises, are of varying shapes, sizes, and colors. Color is not a reliable predictor of contusion age.

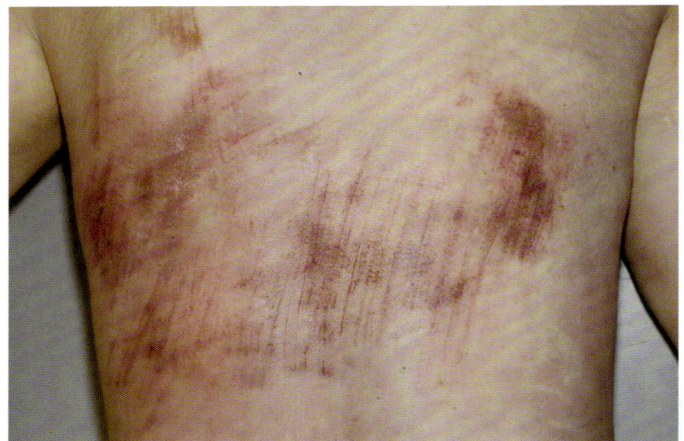

IMAGE 8.22 Abrasions. These scratches and scrapes are often associated with the body having been moved along an irregular surface, such as a road.

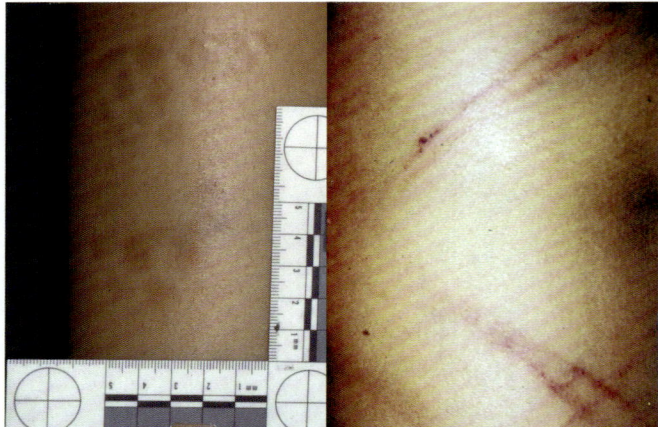

IMAGE 8.23 Patterned contusions and abrasions. These pictures illustrate the pattern left when an irregular or shaped object is forced against the skin and soft tissue. Left: the pattern of the sole of a shoe. Right: a classic "tram track" appearance of a long, narrow object. These features can be helpful in identifying the implement used to cause an injury.

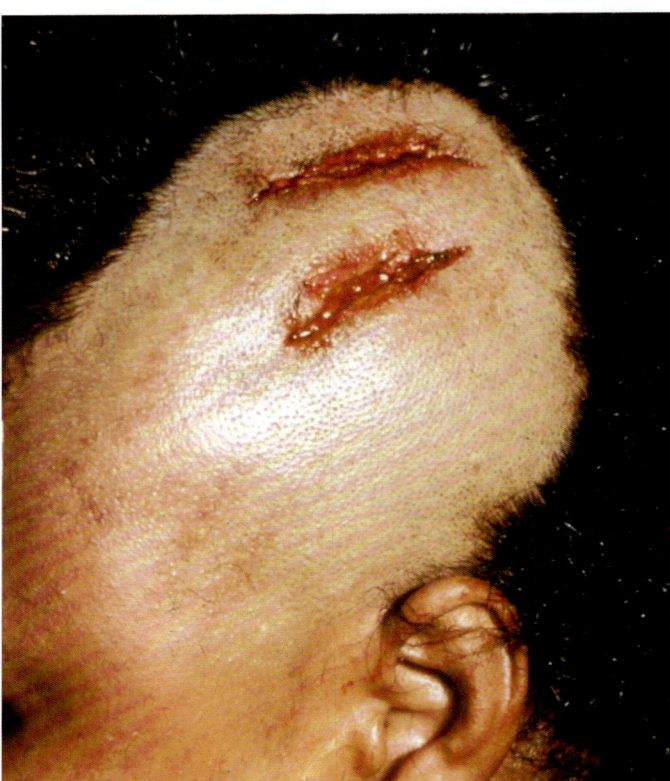

IMAGE 8.24 Laceration. The irregular tearing of the skin associated with blunt trauma leaves blood vessels and nerves bridging the wound.

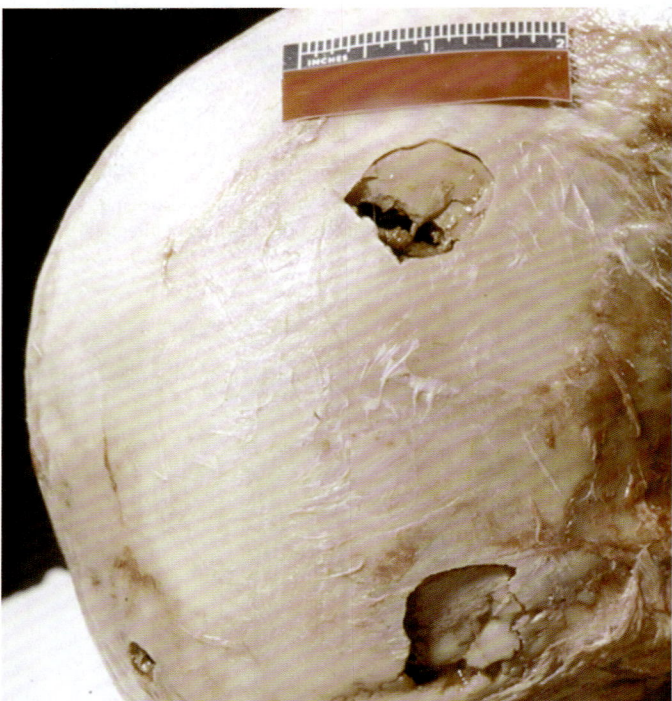

IMAGE 8.25 Depressed skull fracture. When the force of impact with an object is concentrated in a small area (such as an impact with a hammer), it can produce a depressed skull fracture. This finding can be helpful in determining the implement used to cause injury.

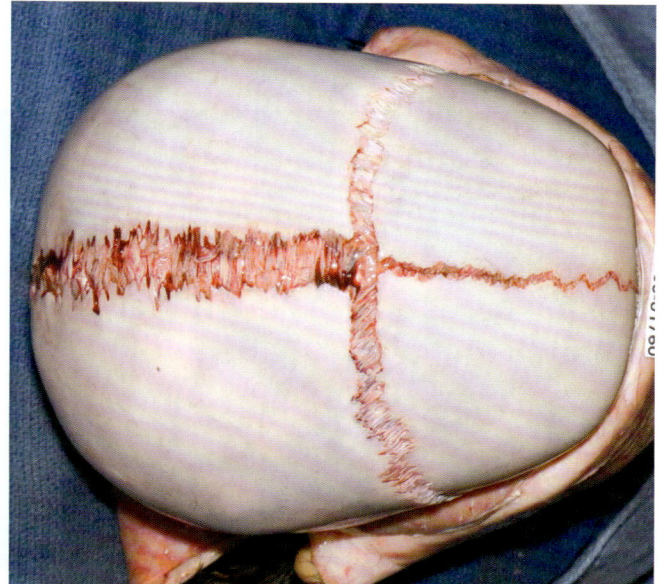

IMAGE 8.26 Diastatic fracture. Diastatic fractures occur when the fracture line transverses 1 or more sutures of the skull causing a widening of the suture. This particular example is that of a sutural diastasis, the splitting of sutures due to increased intracranial pressure. Notice the metopic suture.

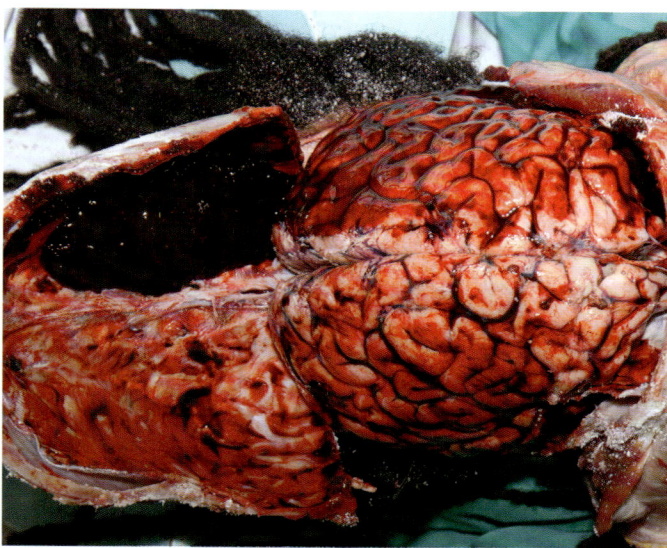

IMAGE 8.28 Subdural hemorrhage. Blood is located between the arachnoid layer and the dura, and can be washed off.

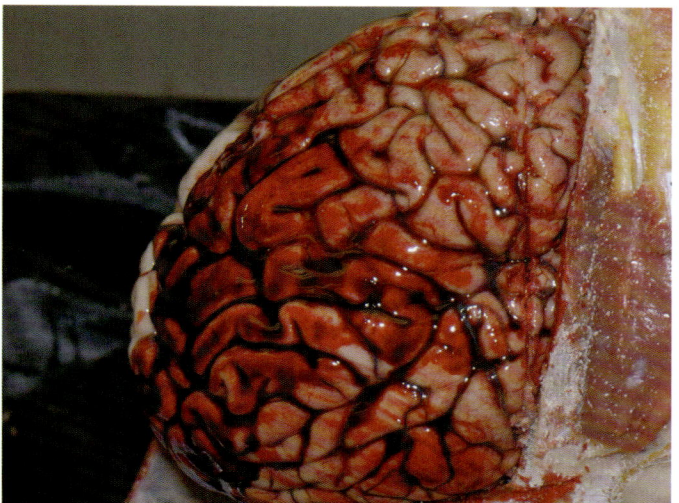

IMAGE 8.27 Subarachnoid hemorrhage. Blood is located underneath the delicate arachnoid layer. It does not wipe off the surface and does not cause mass effect.

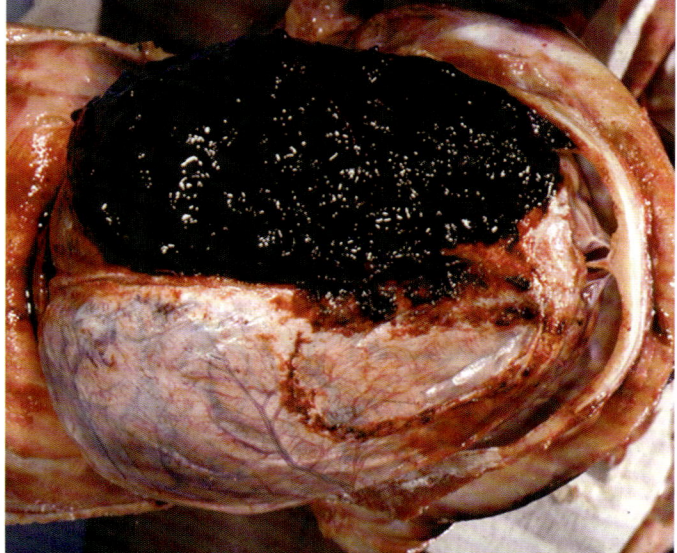

IMAGE 8.29 Epidural hemorrhage. Blood is located between the dura and the skull. Rapid accumulation of blood will cause mass effect.

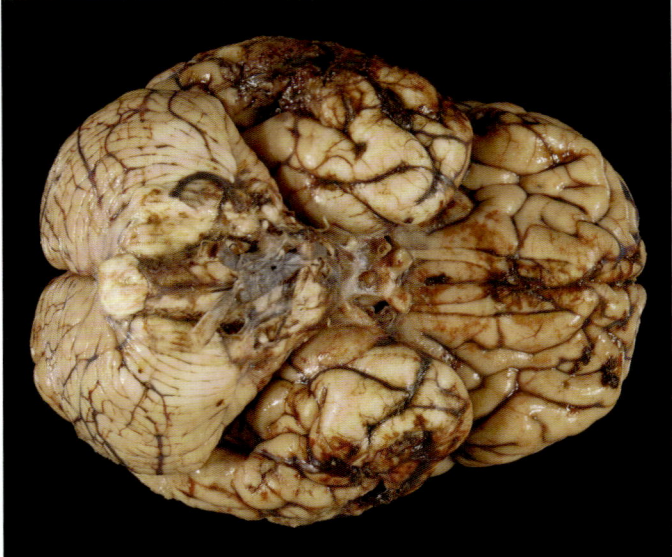

IMAGE 8.30 Coup and contrecoup contusions. Contusions on the brain surface have a slightly discolored appearance and often appear ragged. The coup contusion occurs at the site of impact and the contrecoup contusion occurs opposite to the site of impact.

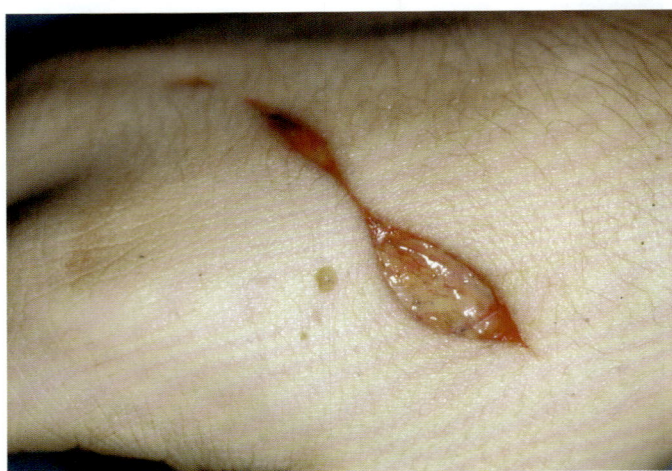

IMAGE 8.33 Incised wound. This is an incised wound: it is longer than it is deep and created by a sharp object (there is no abrasion around the wound edges and no tissue bridging).

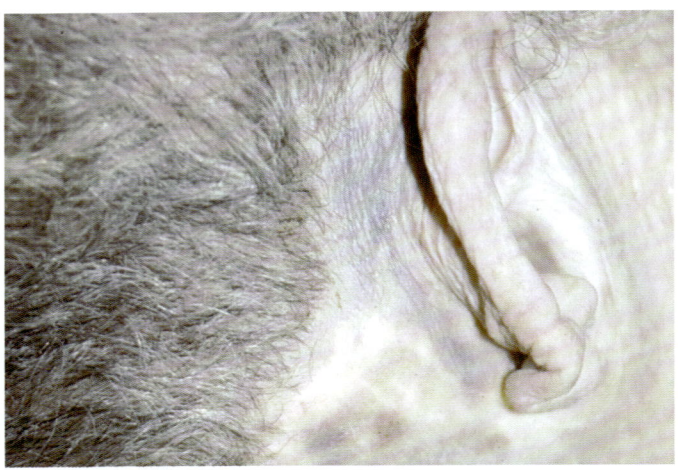

IMAGE 8.31 Battle sign. Battle sign, or mastoid ecchymosis, is an indication of a skull base fracture.

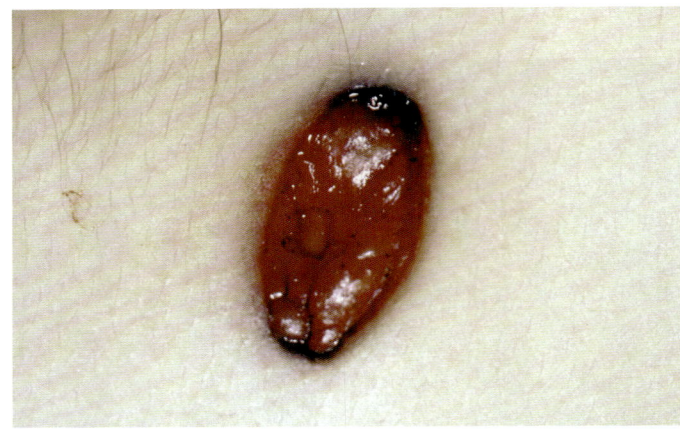

IMAGE 8.34 Stab wound. This stab wound is created by sharp force, and, in contrast to an incised wound, is deeper than it is long.

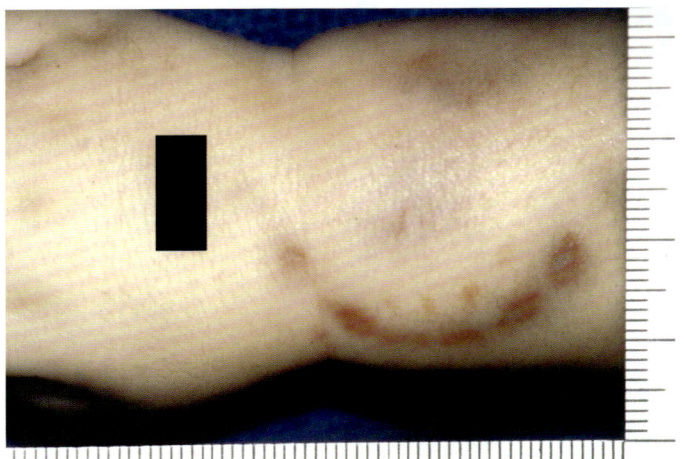

IMAGE 8.32 Bite mark. If a bite mark is identified on external exam, it is important to photograph it, swab it for DNA, and consult a forensic dentist.

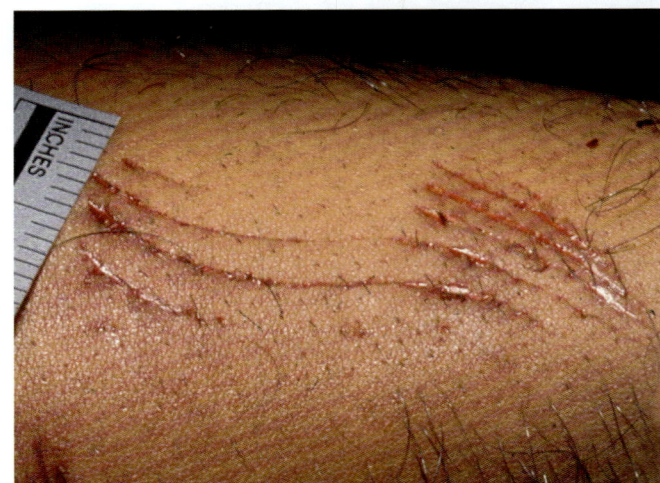

IMAGE 8.35 Serrated blade. Characteristics of a wound can provide information about the weapon that created it. In this case, the parallel scrapes at the edge of the wound indicate a serrated blade.

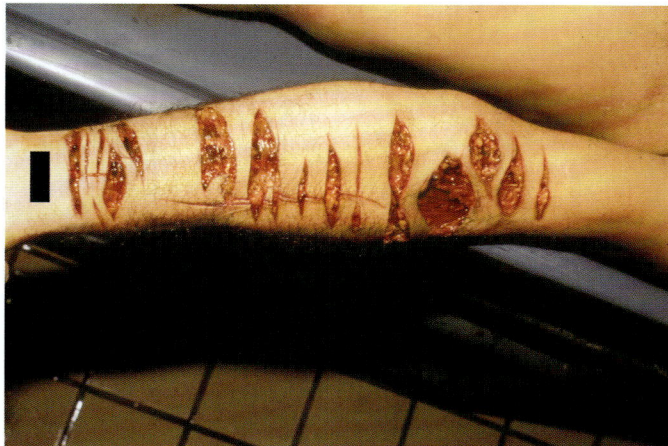

IMAGE 8.36 Hesitation marks. Hesitation marks are characteristically shallow incised wounds on the wrists, often associated with a lethal suicidal wound. This is a dramatic example of multiple, superficial, parallel incised wounds on the forearm and wrist.

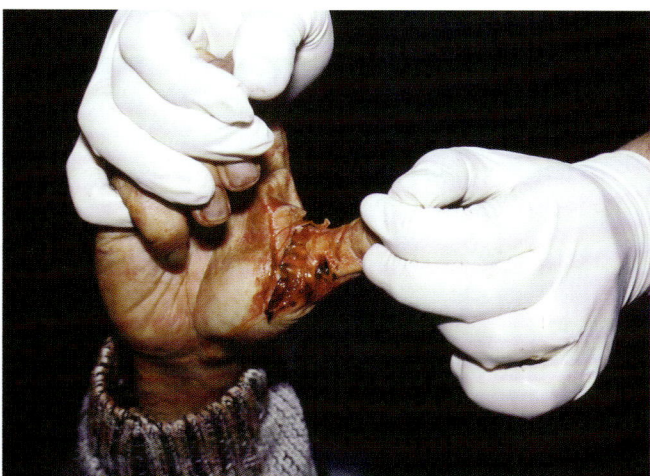

IMAGE 8.37 Defense wounds. While defense wounds can be found anywhere on a victim and have many forms, the classic finding is sharp injury to the palm of the hand and the fingers, caused when a victim tries to grab the knife or other weapon from their attacker.

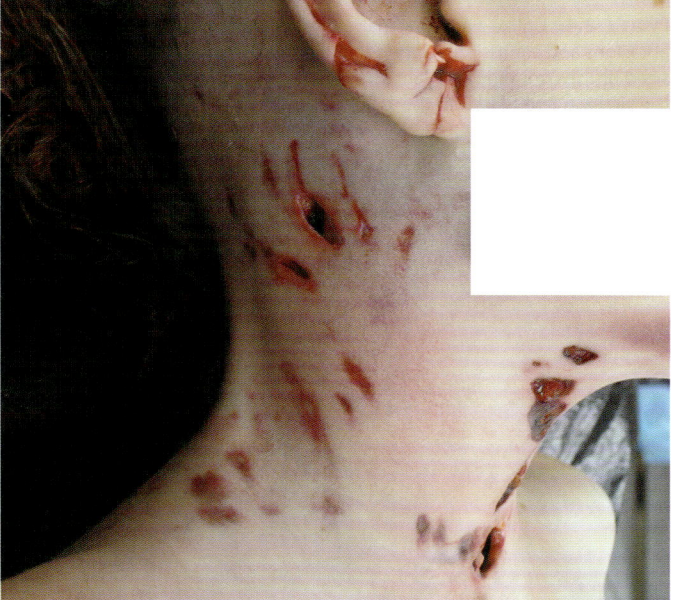

IMAGE 8.38 Dog bite. This constellation of sharp injuries (including puncture wounds) was caused by a dog attack.

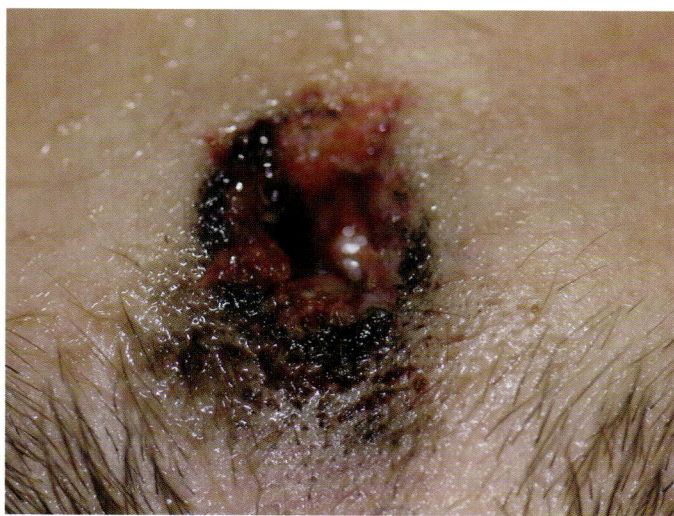

IMAGE 8.39 Contact entrance gunshot wound. The features of a contact gunshot wound include muzzle abrasion (not pictured here), and gray-black discoloration from the burned powder and tissue searing.

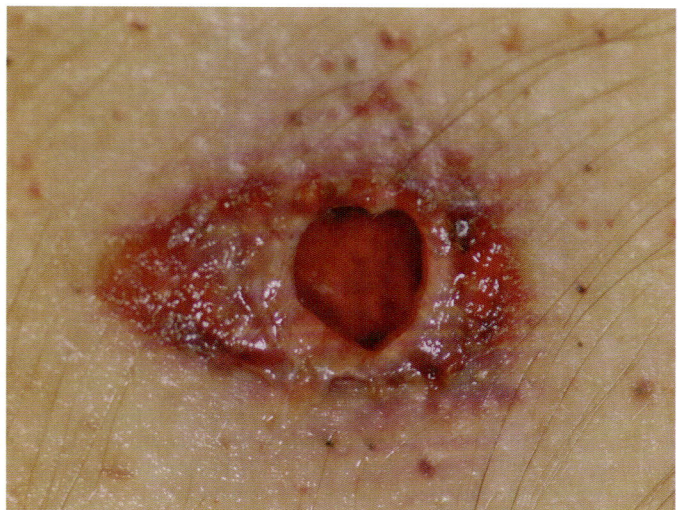

IMAGE 8.40 Close range entrance gunshot wound. As the muzzle is held back from the target, bits of unburned gunpowder abrade the skin around the entrance wound. This pattern is called stippling.

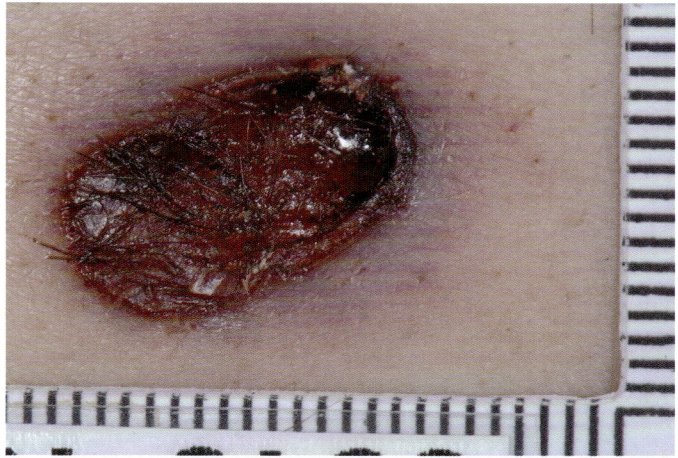

IMAGE 8.41 Distant entrance gunshot wound. This wound has no tissue searing, soot deposition, stippling, or muzzle abrasion. The range of fire is best labeled "indeterminate." While the appearance of this wound is consistent with "distant" gunshot wounds, this appearance also occurs in cases where there is an indeterminate target (such as clothing) between the muzzle and the skin.

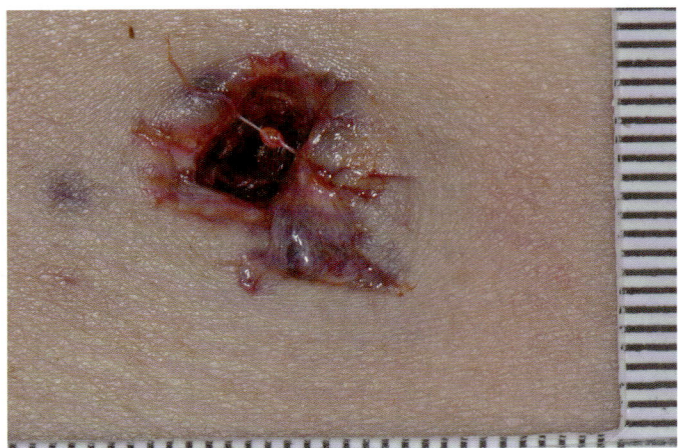

IMAGE 8.42 Exit gunshot wound. This exit is stellate, does not have soot or stippling, and the tissue can be seen protruding from the skin defect.

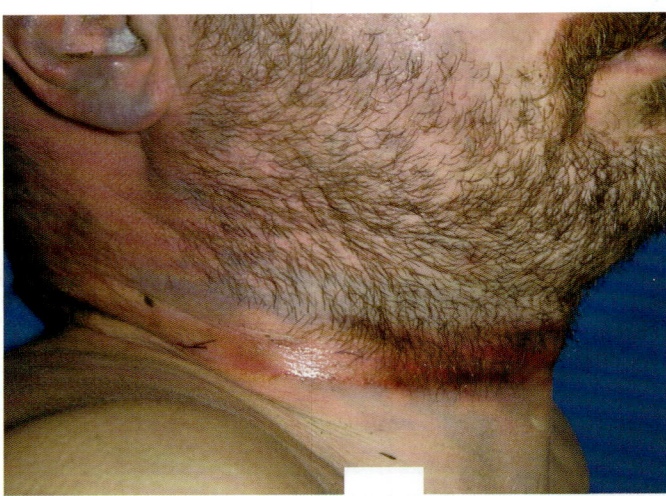

IMAGE 8.45 Ligature furrow. The indentation of the soft tissue of the neck from hanging forms a furrow or abrasion.

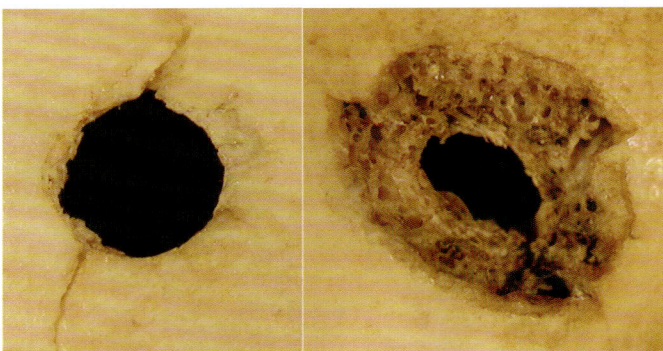

IMAGE 8.43 Bevelling. If the gunshot wound passes through the skull or other flat bone, the entrance and exit wounds can be sorted based on the configuration of the bevelling. Left: the entrance wound will have internal bevelling, where the internal defect is larger than the external defect. Right: the exit wound will have external bevelling, where the internal defect is smaller than the external defect.

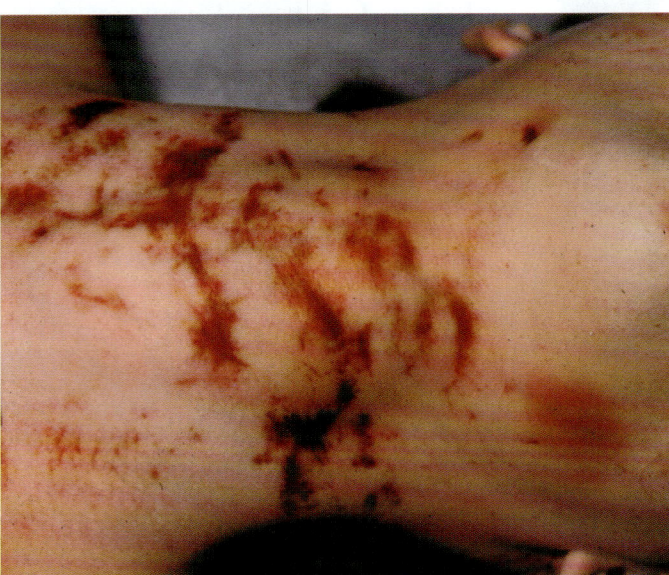

IMAGE 8.46 Unlike a ligature, manual strangulation may have multiple abrasions and contusions. Depending on the scenario, multiple fingertip-sized bruises from the assailant's fingers may be present, or scratches from the victim trying to loosen the assailant's grip may be present.

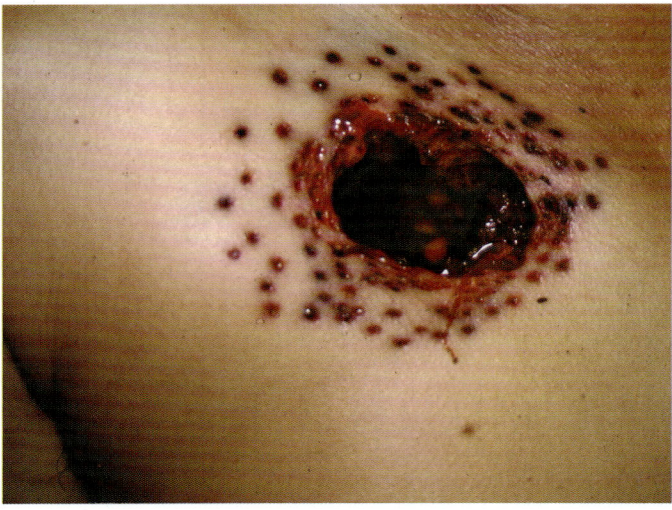

IMAGE 8.44 Shotgun wound. The shot in a shotgun wound from intermediate range makes a characteristic central cavity with a scatter of smaller wounds around it.

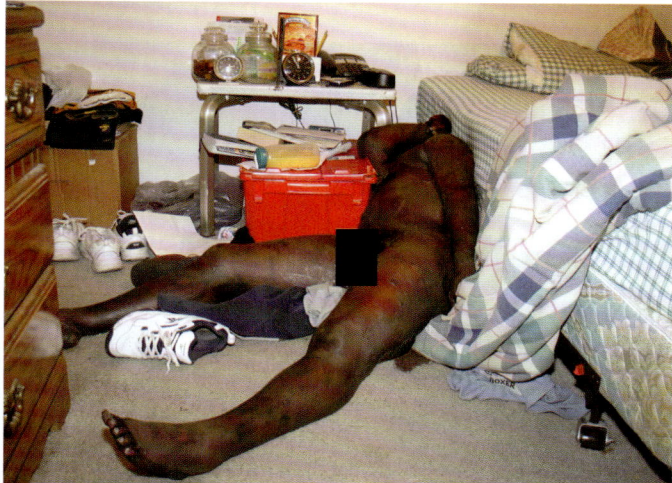

IMAGE 8.47 Positional asphyxia. When individuals get into positions where their ability to breathe is physically compromised, they can succumb to positional asphyxia. As seen here, this individual is stuck between the bed, and the nightstand and red box. Drugs, alcohol, or other obtunding factors can play a role in positional asphyxia.

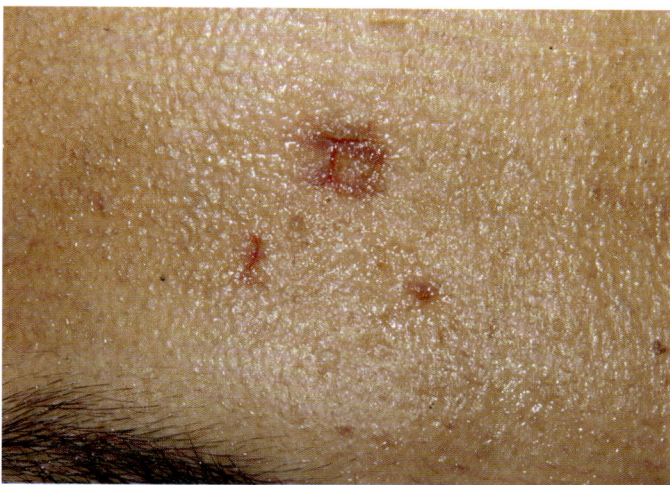

IMAGE 8.49 Dicing. This close-up view of the side of a driver's face shows a square abrasion that was caused by the shattered glass of the side windows in a vehicle, an injury called *dicing*. While the windshield will shatter, it will not fragment because of the type of glass or covering over it. Dicing injury can help determine the position of the decedent in the vehicle.

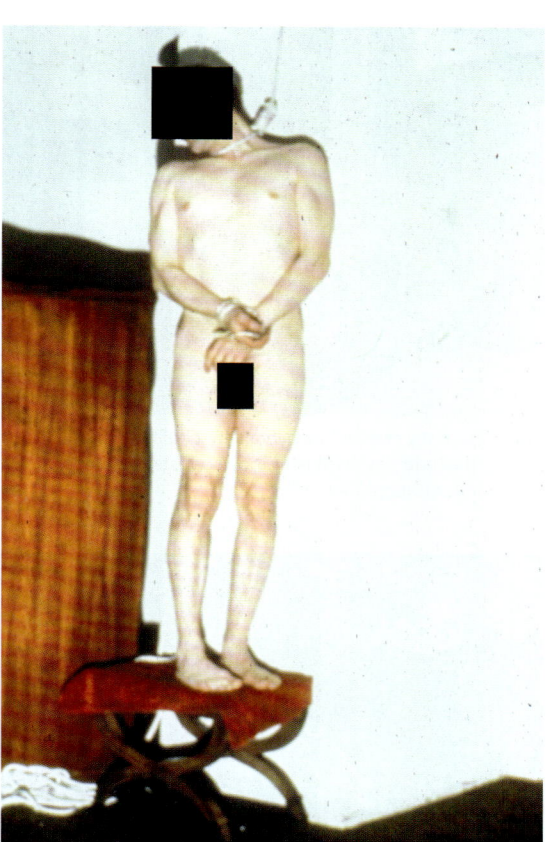

IMAGE 8.48 Autoerotic asphyxia. The features of autoerotic asphyxia usually include sexual paraphernalia around the body, a self-releasing ligature, and a secure location. Scene investigation is crucial to try to understand the intentions of the decedent.

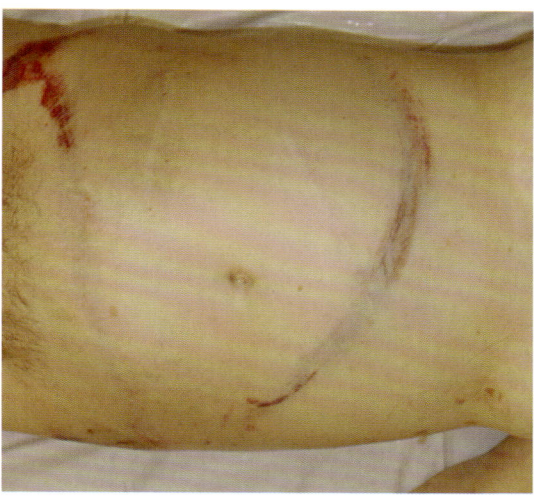

IMAGE 8.50 Abraded contusion from a seatbelt. This picture clearly shows the imprint of a seatbelt. Not only does this indicate that the seatbelt was in use, but it also helps determine the position of the decedent in the vehicle.

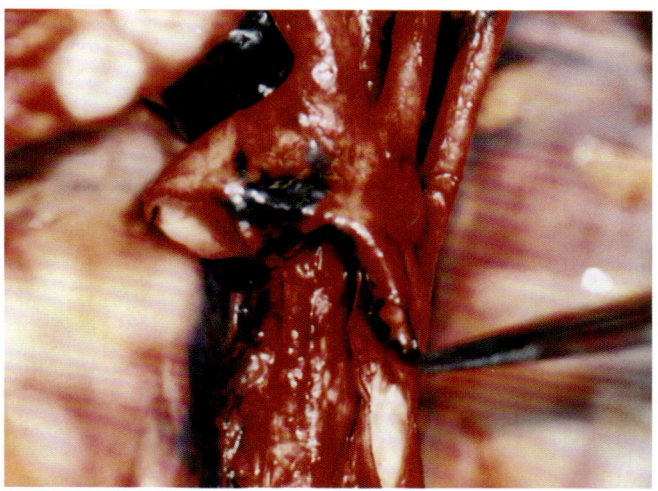

IMAGE 8.51 Aortic transection. The aorta is transected just distal to the left subclavian artery; the luminal surface is visible.

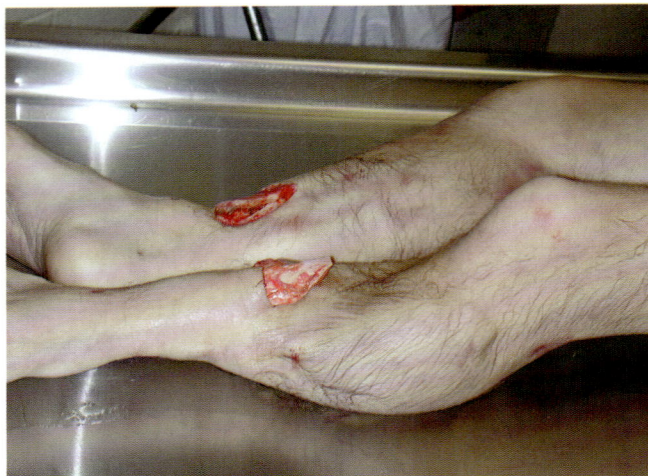

IMAGE 8.52 Bumper fractures. When a pedestrian is struck by a vehicle, characteristic fractures of the lower extremities result. The height of these fractures can help identify the type of vehicle, although care must be taken to incorporate the victim's footwear into the measurement.

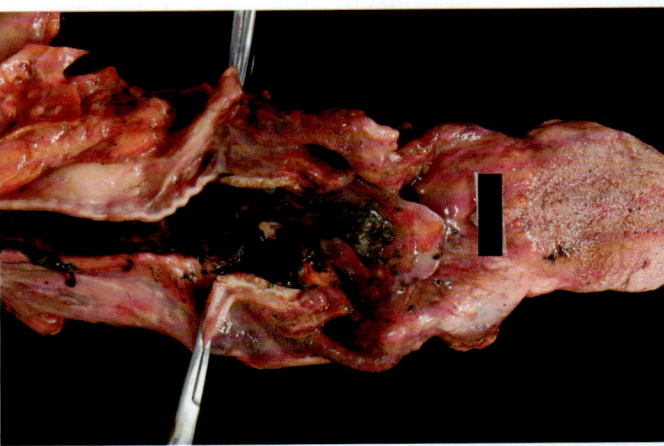

IMAGE 8.55 Soot in the airways. Soot in the airways, especially the distal airways, is an indication that the victim was alive at the time of the fire and inhaled products of combustion. Carbon monoxide levels are also helpful in making this determination.

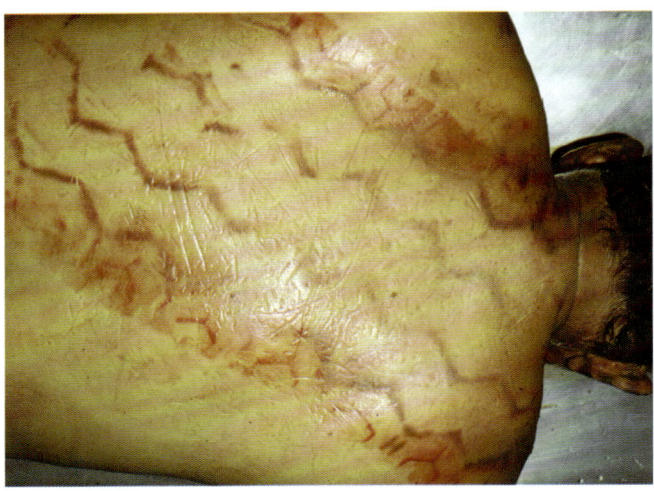

IMAGE 8.53 Tire tread abrasion. In this case, the tire tread is clearly evident on the decedent and can be used to match the wounds to a suspect vehicle.

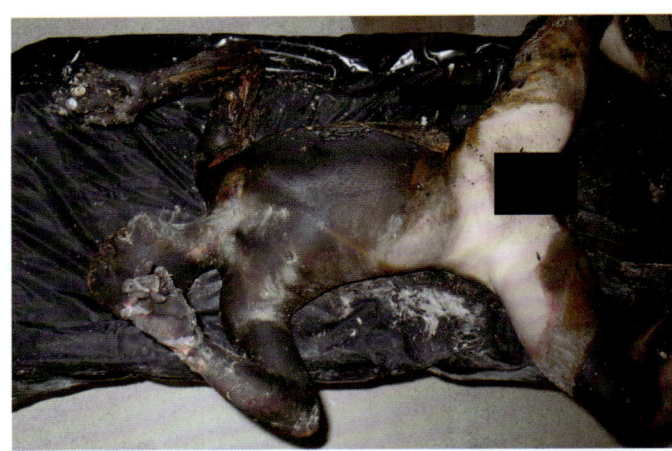

IMAGE 8.56 Pugilistic stance. The overall effect of heat on muscle proteins causes contracture and flexion at the elbows, wrists, and knees, causing a boxer's pose, or pugilistic stance.

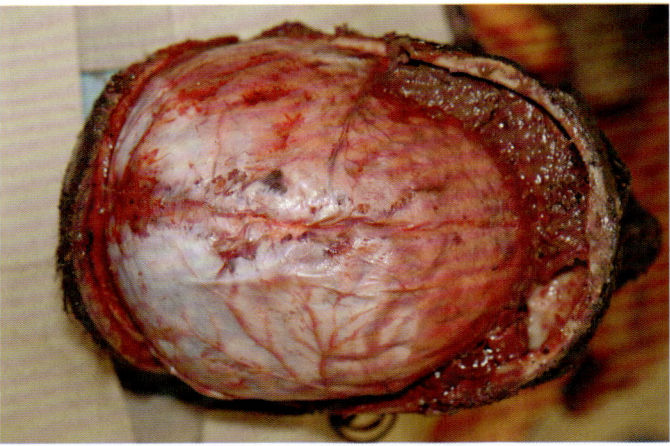

IMAGE 8.54 Postmortem epidural heat hematoma. This granular, brown epidural hematoma is an artifact of exposure to extreme heat. It must not be mistaken for an antemortem injury.

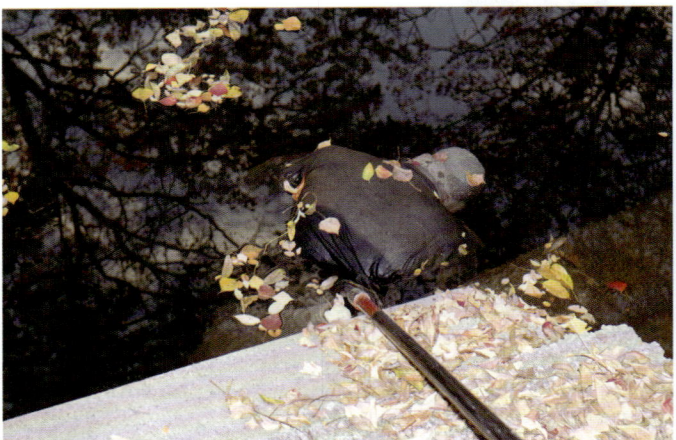

IMAGE 8.57 Body in water. Bodies in water pose a challenge to the forensic pathologist. The pathologist must determine if the water was the cause of death, as in drowning, or if the decedent ended up in the water after dying by another means. Regardless of the mechanism of the decedent's arrival in water, bodies in water can exhibit "washer woman" skin; abrasions on the hands, knees, and bony prominences due to dragging along the bottom of the water; and signs of crustacean or animal activity.

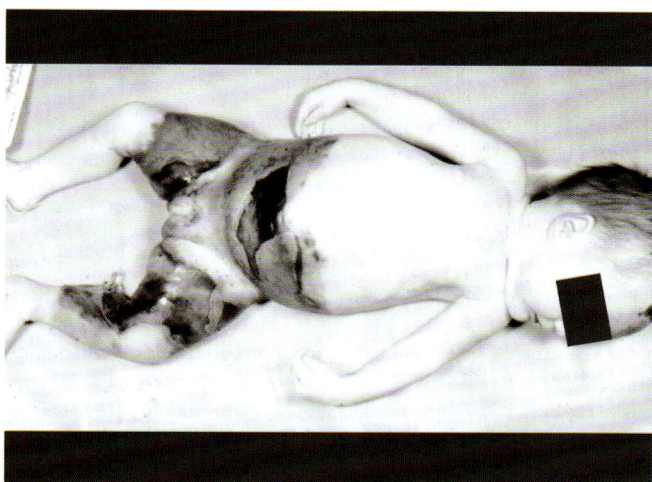

IMAGE 8.58 Scalding. When a child is placed in a bath that is too hot, the scalding pattern spares the skin folds and has a sharp demarcation from scalded skin to normal.

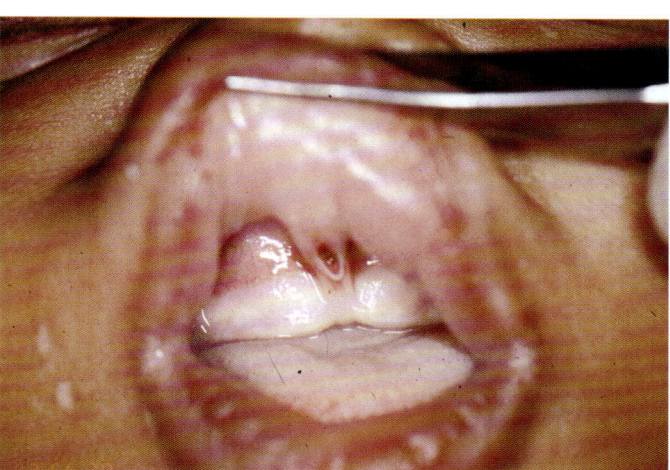

IMAGE 8.61 Torn frenulum. A torn maxillary frenulum is a finding of great concern to forensic pathologists. While the finding may have a benign explanation, the cause of this blunt injury (impact, pressure on the mouth, etc.) must be determined.

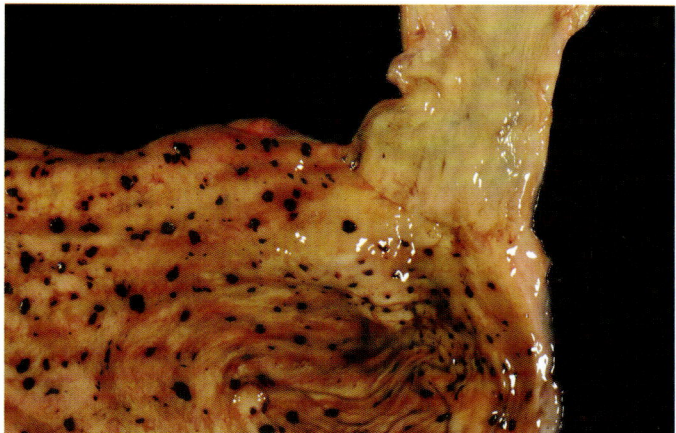

IMAGE 8.59 Wischnewski ulcers. Shallow, small gastric mucosal erosions are not pathognomonic of hypothermia, but are seen with some frequency in hypothermic deaths.

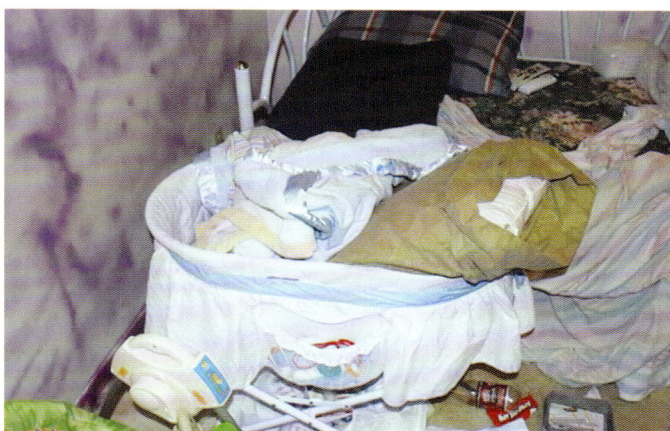

IMAGE 8.62 Unsafe sleep environment. Infants are at risk of asphyxia if there are many toys, blankets, and pillows in their sleep environment. Scene investigation of all child deaths is crucial.

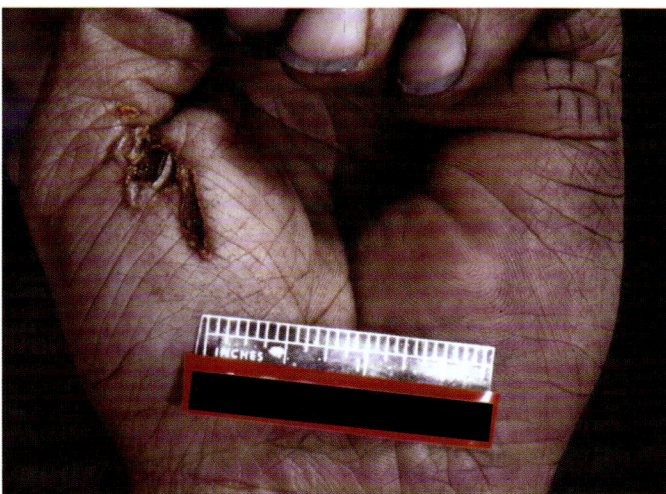

IMAGE 8.60 Electrical burn. This small charred skin defect is an electrical burn.

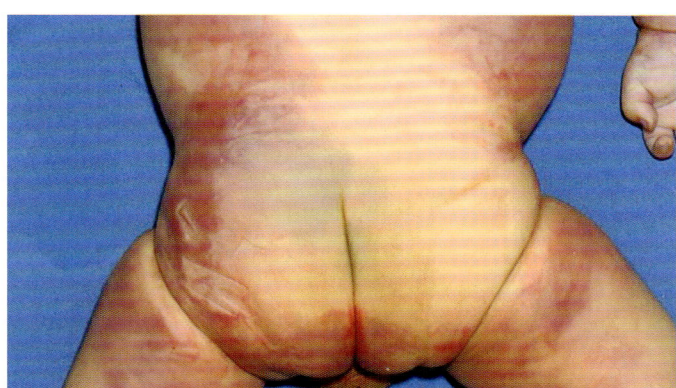

IMAGE 8.63 Mongolian spot. Commonly seen on the lower back or buttocks of infants of East Asian descent, this congenital birthmark caused by dermal melanocytosis can be seen in many ethnicities and should not be confused with a bruise. Mongolian spot and bruising can be easily distinguished by incising to examine for subcutaneous hemorrhage.

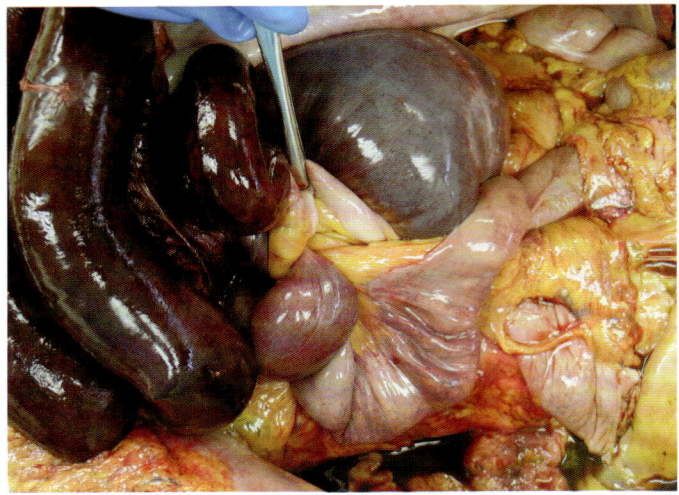

IMAGE 8.64 Volvulus. Volvulus is the twisting of a loop of intestine around its mesenteric attachment and is a cause of sudden death in neonates.

Bibliography

Dettmeyer RB. Forensic histopathology: fundamentals and perspectives. New York: Springer; 2011.

Di Maio VJM. Gunshot wounds: practical aspects of firearms, ballistics and forensic techniques. 3rd ed. Boca Rata (FL): CRC Press; 2015.

Di Maio VJM, Dana SE. Handbook of forensic pathology. 2nd ed. Boca Rata (FL): CRC Press; 2007,

Di Maio D, Di Maio VJM. Forensic pathology. 2nd ed. Boca Rata (FL): CRC Press; 2001.

Dolinak D, Matshes E, Lew EO. Forensic pathology: principles and practice. Cambridge (MA): Academic Press; 2005.

Kumar V, Abbas AK, Aster J. Robbins and Cotran pathologic basis of disease. 10th ed. North York (ON): Elsevier Canada; 2020.

Saukko P, Knight B. Knight's forensic pathology. 4th edition. Boca Rata (FL): CRC Press; 2016.

Shkrum M, Ramsay DA. Forensic pathology of trauma: common problems for the pathologist. Totowa (NJ): Humana Press; 2007.

Suvarna KS. Atlas of adult autopsy: a guide to modern practice. New York: Springer; 2016.

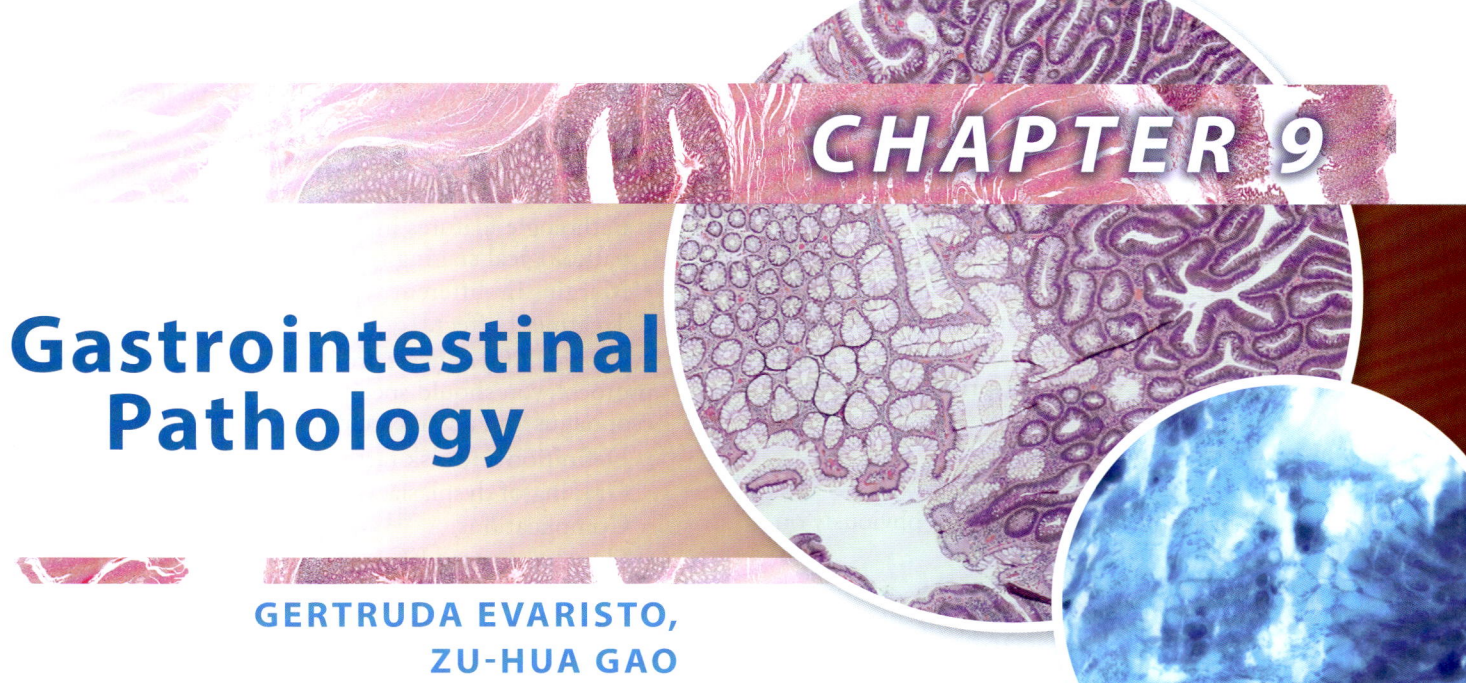

CHAPTER 9

Gastrointestinal Pathology

GERTRUDA EVARISTO, ZU-HUA GAO

Gastrointestinal Pathology Exam Essentials

MUST KNOW

World Health Organization (WHO) classification

- You should be familiar with the organs and anatomic sites that fall under the WHO classification of tumors of the digestive tract. For the luminal gastrointestinal (GI) tract, the WHO specifically includes tumors at the following locations:
  - Esophagus.
  - Esophagogastric junction (EGJ).
  - Stomach.
  - Small intestine and ampullary region.
  - Appendix.
  - Colon and rectum.
  - Anal canal.
- For the esophagus, both squamous and glandular lesions are equally important. EGJ tumors are included here since they are almost exclusively adenocarcinomas. For both, you should know the risk factors, clinical features, premalignant lesions, and malignant lesions associated with:
  - Squamous dysplasia.
  - Invasive squamous cell carcinoma.
  - Barrett esophagus and Barrett dysplasia.
  - Invasive adenocarcinoma of the esophagus and EGJ.
  - Common stromal tumor: leiomyoma.
- For the stomach, the focus is on adenocarcinoma. (Note that chapter 7 covers GI neuroendocrine tumors

[NETs] in more detail.) Gastric lesions include:

  - Nonadenomatous polyps: fundic gland polyp (FGP), hyperplastic polyp (HP), mucosa changes in Cronkhite-Canada syndrome, and Ménétrier disease.
  - Adenomatous polyps (pay special attention to intestinal type adenomas).
  - Invasive adenocarcinoma (pay special attention to histologic subtypes [including the Lauren classification], risk factors, and genetic factors including syndromes).
  - NETs: grading, types, especially those associated with autoimmune gastritis and Zollinger-Ellison syndrome.
  - Lymphomas, especially those associated with *Helicobacter pylori*.
  - Gastric gastrointestinal stromal tumors (GIST) (pay special attention to the differential diagnosis [e.g., schwannoma] and immunohistochemistry [IHC] workup).
- For the small bowel and ampulla, the emphasis is very similar to that of the stomach. High-yield topics include:
  - Adenomatous polyps.
  - Hamartomatous polyps.
  - Invasive adenocarcinoma (pay attention to those related to syndromes such as familial adenomatous polyposis [FAP]).

- NET and GIST, as above (for small bowel NET, review the carcinoid syndrome).
- For the appendix, a few special entities are relatively new to the classification and are worthwhile knowing, in addition to traditional tumors, including:
  - Low grade and high grade appendiceal mucinous neoplasms (LAMN and HAMN), as well as their distinction from benign mimickers (e.g., mucocele).
  - Serrated lesions and adenomatous polyps.
  - Goblet cell adenocarcinoma (formerly goblet cell carcinoid).
  - Invasive adenocarcinoma.
  - NET.
- For the colon and rectum, the focus is obviously on glandular lesions, including:
  - Adenomatous polyps.
  - Hamartomatous polyps.
  - Inflammatory bowel disease (IBD) associated dysplasia.
  - Invasive adenocarcinoma.
  - NET and GIST (pay special attention to the different morphology lower GI NET can undertake in contrast to upper GI NET).
- In contrast to the bowel, tumors of the anal canal are more commonly squamous lesions. Focus on:
  - Anatomy and landmarks of the anal canal.
  - Human papillomavirus (HPV) and anal squamous dysplasia (intraepithelial neoplasia).
  - Squamous cell carcinoma.
  - Lymph node drainage of the anal canal.
  - Approach to adenocarcinoma involving anal canal (primary versus secondary adenocarcinomas, including Paget disease).
- The WHO also lists several mesenchymal and hematolymphoid tumors of the luminal GI system. The exam tends to include these tumors in the practical section more than the written section. Important tumors include:
  - MALT lymphoma.
  - Mantle cell lymphoma (including presentation as lymphomatous polyposis).
  - Enteropathy associated T-cell lymphoma and celiac disease.
  - Mature B-cell lymphomas that occasionally involve the GI tract.
  - GIST.
  - Mesenchymal tumors that occur elsewhere (see the Must See section for an expanded list).

AJCC and College of American Pathologists (CAP) protocols

- For the esophagus, you should focus on epithelial tumors, specifically squamous cell carcinoma. Other tumors of the esophagus are occasionally tested, including mesenchymal tumors. While these tumors may commonly exist elsewhere in the body or the GI tract (e.g., GIST, granular cell tumor), you should be able to diagnose them by "thinking outside the box." For squamous cell carcinoma, you should know:
  - Epidemiology and risk factors.
  - Clinical presentation, including endoscopic findings.
  - Pathologic features including subtypes, grading, and pathological staging (pT staging).
  - Margins in different types of esophageal resections.
  - Treatment effect.
- Although EGJ cancers are included in the esophagus protocol, you should specifically focus on Barrett esophagus and adenocarcinoma, including:
  - Definition and risk factors for Barrett esophagus.
  - Grading of dysplasia.
  - Complications.
  - How to separate EGJ from gastric tumors anatomically.
- A wide array of stomach topics may be tested, including malignant and premalignant conditions. Some examples include:
  - Dysplasia and risk factors.
  - Hereditary gastric cancer.
  - Lauren versus WHO classification of gastric adenocarcinoma.
  - Definition of early gastric adenocarcinoma.
  - pT staging criteria.
  - Treatment effect.
  - Margins for different types of gastric resections.
  - HER2 testing (less important than breast cancer testing protocol).
- For the small bowel, you should review:
  - Adenomatous and hamartomatous polyps and associated syndromes.
  - GIST.
  - NET (duodenum and ampulla, jejunum and ileum).
  - General staging parameters for adenocarcinoma.
- Many tumors of the appendix are similar, but a few entities are unique. You should pay particular attention to:
  - LAMN and HAMN, including the concepts of pseudomyxoma peritonei and extravasation of mucin outside the appendix.
  - Goblet cell adenocarcinoma.
  - NET and neuroendocrine carcinomas.
  - pT staging criteria.
  - Margins for appendectomies.
- Colorectal polyps and adenocarcinomas are very frequently tested. Some examples include:
  - Location, size and microscopic features of adenomatous polyps, including their molecular pathways.
  - High grade dysplasia and malignant polyps, true versus pseudoinvasion.
  - Familial adenomatous polyposis, attenuated FAP, Turcot syndrome.
  - Lynch syndrome, microsatellite instability, Muir-Torre and Turcot syndromes.

- Serrated polyposis syndrome.
- The 3 molecular pathways of colon cancer development.
- Grading and pT staging factors.
- Margins in different types of colon resections.
- Evaluation of quality of resection in total mesorectal excision (TME) specimens.
- Tumor budding.
- Tumor deposit and its staging.
- Definition of isolated tumor cells, micrometastasis, and macrometastasis, and their staging.
- Mismatch repair (MMR) protein testing in colorectal cancer.
- Particular aspects of anal cancers are key topics, including:
  - Anatomical landmarks.
  - Lymph node drainage.
  - Grading and staging factors.
  - HPV and anal squamous dysplasia.
- The only CAP/AJCC protocol for mesenchymal tumors available is the protocol for GIST. It is important to know:
  - Histologic subtypes.
  - Histologic grading.
  - pT staging criteria (based on size only).
  - Risk assessment for progressive disease.
  - IHC for GIST.
  - Molecular analysis of key genes including *KIT*, *SDH*, *PDGFRA*.
  - Targeted treatment for GIST and treatment effects.
  - GIST predisposition syndromes: Carney triad, Carney-Stratakis syndrome, neurofibromatosis type 1 (NF1).

Nonneoplastic diseases

- The esophagus is a commonly tested topic. You should know the clinical symptoms, pathophysiology, endoscopic and pathologic findings, and differential diagnosis for commonly examined esophageal conditions, including:
  - Mechanical causes of obstruction.
  - Achalasia and motility disorders.
  - Eosinophilic esophagitis versus reflux esophagitis.
  - Other causes of eosinophilia in the GI tract.
  - Chemical and infectious esophagitis.
  - Varices, bleeding, perforation.
  - Congenital anomalies.
- For the stomach, stomach infections, inflammation, and ulcers are the most important topics. Focus on the same factors as for the esophagus. Specific examples include:
  - Causes of gastric and duodenal ulcers.
  - Features of benign versus malignant gastric ulcers.
  - Epidemiology and virulence mechanisms of *H. pylori*.

- How to diagnose *H. pylori* with invasive and noninvasive methods.
- Neoplastic and nonneoplastic complications of *H. pylori*.
- Chemical/reactive gastropathy and common causes.
- Autoimmune gastritis, including pathogenesis, classification, morphology, and IHC to confirm diagnosis.
- For the small bowel, celiac disease is the most important topic. You should also review infections, and other causes of intraepithelial lymphocytosis and architectural changes. Some topics include:
  - Clinical presentation, microscopic findings, and differential diagnosis of celiac disease.
  - Serology tests for celiac disease, including those done in cases of patients with immunoglobulin A (IgA) deficiency.
  - Nonneoplastic and neoplastic complications of celiac disease.
  - Other causes of malabsorption.
  - Other causes of intraepithelial lymphocytosis and/or architectural changes.
  - Common infections (e.g., *Giardia*, *Cryptosporidium*, Whipple disease, *Mycobacterium avium-intracellulare* [MAI]).
- The colon can have a wide array of nonneoplastic diseases. It should be an area of focus within the GI system. Some key topics include:
  - Microscopic colitis: lymphocytic colitis, collagenous colitis.
  - Pseudomembranous colitis.
  - Ischemic colitis pattern of injury.
  - Infectious colitis (bacterial, viral, parasitic).
  - Clinical, gross, and microscopic differences between Crohn disease and ulcerative colitis (UC).
  - GI and extraintestinal manifestations of IBD.
  - Assessment of dysplasia in IBD.
  - Skip lesions in UC.
  - Other colitides including diversion colitis, diverticular disease associated colitis, radiation colitis, and drug-induced colitis.
  - Causes of apoptotic colopathy pattern of injury (infection, medication, graft versus host disease, common variable immune deficiency [CVID], bowel prep artifact).
  - Mucosal prolapse, solitary rectal ulcer syndrome.

Genetic and syndromic conditions

- Genetic and syndromic conditions is an extremely important topic for the GI system. Here, the key is to separate hamartoma syndromes from carcinoma syndromes. For all the syndromes listed, you should know the gene, their function, mode of inheritance, associated lesions, and systemic manifestations.
- The hamartoma syndromes include:
  - Peutz-Jeghers syndrome.
  - Juvenile polyposis syndrome.

- Cowden syndrome.
- Cronkhite-Canada syndrome.
- Other minor ones include Gorlin syndrome, NF1, MEN2B and Birt-Hogg-Dubé syndrome.
- The carcinoma syndromes include:
  - FAP and attenuated FAP.
  - *MUTYH* (*MYH*) associated polyposis.
  - Lynch syndrome.
  - Muir-Torre syndrome.
  - Turcot syndrome.
  - Serrated polyposis.
  - Hereditary diffuse gastric cancer.

MUST SEE

The luminal GI system is a very high-yield topic. It can show up in the rapid slide segment of the exam, in the short answer questions, and in the oral component. High-yield topics include:

- Esophagus:
  - Achalasia.
  - Varices.
  - *Candida* esophagitis.
  - Eosinophilic esophagitis, including endoscopic findings.
  - Reflux esophagitis.
  - Chemical and pill esophagitis.
  - Herpes simplex virus (HSV) esophagitis.
  - Mallory-Weiss tear and Boerhaave syndrome.
  - Esophageal diverticula, atresia, and tracheoesophageal fistula.
  - Squamous cell carcinoma.
- EGJ:
  - Barrett esophagus.
  - Adenocarcinoma, including posttreatment.
- Stomach:
  - *H. pylori* gastritis.
  - Autoimmune atrophic gastritis.
  - Lymphocytic and eosinophilic gastritis.
  - Fundic gland polyps.
  - Hamartomatous polyps (e.g., Peutz-Jeghers syndrome, Cowden syndrome, juvenile polyposis, Cronkhite-Canada syndrome, tuberous sclerosis complex).
  - Polyps with dysplasia.
  - Intestinal and diffuse types of gastric adenocarcinoma.
  - Enterochromaffin-like (ECL) cell hyperplasia and NET.
  - GIST.
  - Other submucosal and mesenchymal lesions.
  - MALT lymphoma.
- Small bowel:
  - Celiac disease.
  - Giardiasis.
  - *Cryptosporidium*, *Microsporidia*, *Isospora*.
  - Whipple disease, MAI.
  - CVID.
  - Meckel diverticulum.
  - Hamartomatous polyps (e.g., Peutz-Jeghers syndrome, Cowden syndrome, juvenile polyposis, Cronkhite-Canada syndrome, tuberous sclerosis complex)
  - GIST.
  - NET.
- Colon, rectum, and anus:
  - Collagenous and lymphocytic colitis.
  - Pseudomembranous colitis.
  - Amyloidosis.
  - Infectious colitis (HSV, cytomegalovirus [CMV], *Entamoeba*, MAI, spirochetosis).
  - Ischemic colitis pattern of injury and pneumatosis intestinalis.
  - Crohn disease and UC.
  - IBD-associated dysplasia.
  - Extraintestinal manifestations of IBD.
  - Adenomas: tubular, villous, tubulovillous adenoma; sessile serrated lesion; traditional serrated adenoma.
  - High grade dysplasia, pseudo- and true invasion.
  - FAP, attenuated FAP.
  - Adenocarcinoma, various subtypes.
  - Tumor deposits.
  - Mucosal prolapse syndromes including solitary rectal ulcer syndrome.
- Appendix:
  - Mucocele.
  - LAMN and HAMN, including pseudomyxoma peritonei and extravasation of mucin outside the appendix.
  - Various colonic-type polyps that can also be found in the appendix.
  - Goblet cell adenocarcinoma.
  - NET and neuroendocrine carcinomas.
- Hematolymphoid and mesenchymal tumors:
  - MALT lymphoma and *H. pylori* gastritis.
  - Enteropathy associated T-cell lymphoma and celiac disease.
  - Other mature B-cell lymphomas that can involve the GI tract.
  - GIST, epithelioid and spindled types.
  - Leiomyoma.
  - Leiomyosarcoma.
  - Lipoma.
  - Schwannoma.

- Perineurioma.
- Ganglioneuroma.
- Fibromatosis.
- Inflammatory myofibroblastic tumor.
- Inflammatory fibroid polyp.
- Granular cell tumor.
- Solitary fibrous tumor.
- PEComa.
- Kaposi sarcoma.

MUST DO

- For each of the entities outlined in the Must See section, you should be comfortable generating a differential diagnosis and listing additional studies such as histochemical or immunohistochemical stains.
- When studying in groups, practice:
  - Comparing features of Crohn disease versus UC.
  - Comparing features of gastroesophageal reflux disease (GERD) versus eosinophilic esophagitis.
  - Comparing features of various hamartomatous polyps.
  - Comparing various spindle cell lesions in the GI tract.
  - Outlining the molecular pathways of various adenomatous polyps and adenocarcinoma.
  - Listing syndromes that predispose to colon adenocarcinoma, especially FAP and Lynch syndrome (pay special attention to this). Do not forget about MMR protein testing in Lynch syndrome.
  - Discussing landmarks in the anus and lymph node (LN) drainage of anal cancers.

- Discussing clinical and pathologic aspects of celiac disease.
- You should be able to describe the grossing protocol for key specimens, and independently gross them, including:
  - Biopsy, polypectomies, and mucosal resections from various locations within the luminal GI tract.
  - Esophagectomy.
  - EGJ resection.
  - Partial and total gastrectomy for both benign and malignant diseases.
  - Small bowel resection for both benign and malignant diseases.
  - Resection of mesenteric nodules and masses.
  - Appendectomy and right hemicolectomy for appendiceal lesions.
  - Hemicolectomy for colon cancer.
  - Total colectomy for benign indications such as IBD.
  - Total colectomy for malignancy, including multiple malignant polyps and tumors.
  - Total colectomy for FAP and various polyposis syndromes.
  - Low anterior resection and total mesorectal excision.
  - Ileostomies and various anastomoses from previous resections.
- You should be able to describe and handle fresh specimens and frozen sections of the following specimens:
  - Margins from prophylactic gastrectomy in cases of hereditary diffuse gastric cancer.
  - Mucosal margins from various oncologic resections.

MULTIPLE CHOICE QUESTIONS

1. In a patient with endoscopic evidence of replacement of squamous mucosa by glandular mucosa, a definitive diagnosis of Barrett esophagus can only be made when the esophageal biopsy shows:

a. Junctional mucosa.

b. Gastric cardia type mucosa.

c. Columnar cells with periodic acid-Schiff (PAS) positive mucin.

d. Goblet cells with acidic mucin.

e. Villous mucosa surface with low grade dysplasia.

Answer: d

2. Epidermal growth factor receptor (EGFR) inhibitors (cetuximab and panitumumab) are an effective therapy for EGFR positive colorectal cancer when:

a. The tumor is negative for both *KRAS* and *BRAF* mutations.

b. The tumor is positive for both *KRAS* and *BRAF* mutations.

c. The tumor is negative for *KRAS* mutation, but positive for *BRAF* mutation.

d. The tumor is negative for *BRAF* mutation, but positive for *KRAS* mutation.

e. The tumor is positive for *CDH1* mutation.

Answer: a

3. According to the 2020 update of the International Gastric Cancer Linkage Consortium practice guidelines, the criteria for testing for the *CDH1* mutation include:

a. Family history of 2 or more cases of gastric cancer, at least 1 confirmed to be diffuse-type gastric cancer.

b. Personal history of diffuse gastric cancer before age 50.

c. Diffuse-type gastric cancer in an individual with a personal or

  family history of cleft lip or cleft palate.

d. Personal history of diffuse-type gastric cancer and lobular breast cancer, both diagnosed before age 70.

e. All of above.

Answer: e

4. The following statements about colon cancer arising via the microsatellite instability pathway are true **except**:

a. Serrated polyps constitute the precursor lesion for the malignancy.

b. It is histologically characterized by right-sided location, Crohn-like peritumor lymphocytes, mucin production, poor differentiation, and signet ring cell features.

c. Cases arising in the setting of Lynch syndrome are due to germline mutation

  in 1 of the 4 mismatch repair genes (*MSH2, MLH1, MSH6* or *PMS2* genes) or the *EPCAM (TACSTD1)* regulatory gene.

d. *KRAS* and *BRAF* mutation never occur in this type of tumor.

e. Tumors with high microsatellite instability (MSI-H) respond to topoisomerase 1 inhibitor irinotecan therapy.

Answer: d

5. A 29-year-old female presents with weight loss, fatigue, and diarrhea. She undergoes endoscopy, and a biopsy specimen from the duodenum is obtained. After reviewing the microscopic findings, the patient is put on a special diet that excludes wheat and rye. She shows significant improvement after the change of diet. What is the characteristic histologic feature of her biopsy?

a. Cryptitis and crypt abscess.

b. Noncaseating granulomas.

c. Foamy macrophages in the lamina propria.

d. Villus shortening and intraepithelial lymphocytosis.

e. Gastric metaplasia of mucosal epithelium.

Answer: d

6. A 72-year-old male was treated within the last 2 weeks with tazobactam/piperacillin for community-acquired pneumonia. He develops severe diarrhea and the stool is positive for *Clostridium difficile* toxin. What histologic features would you expect to see in his colon biopsy?

a. Acute self-limited colitis.

b. Ischemic colitis.

c. Pseudomembranous colitis.

d. Caseating granulomas with mycobacterial infection.

e. Lymphocytic colitis.

Answer: c

7. A 60-year-old male presented with a 3-month history of dyspepsia, nausea, and weight loss. Examination by endoscopy showed a thickened gastric antral mucosa without an obvious mass. A biopsy specimen of the gastric mucosa showed diffuse lymphoplasmacytic infiltration. Some crypts were infiltrated by clusters of lymphocytes. There was no obvious crypt loss. Numerous *Helicobacter pylori* bacteria were found on the mucosal surface. The patient was treated with lansoprazole, amoxicillin, and clarithromycin for 2 weeks. On repeat biopsy after treatment, the lymphoplasmacytic infiltration has essentially disappeared. What is your diagnosis of the original biopsy?

a. Active gastritis.

b. Chronic gastritis.

c. Autoimmune gastritis.

d. Mucosa associated lymphoid tissue due to severe *H. pylori* infection.

e. Diffuse large B-cell lymphoma.

Answer: d

8. A 30-year-old male presents with dysphagia, specifically reporting the sensation of food being stuck after it is swallowed. Examination by endoscopy shows a series of rings along the entire length of the esophagus resembling a cat esophagus. A biopsy specimen from the middle portion of the esophagus is likely to show:

a. Predominantly neutrophilic inflammation.

b. Predominantly lymphocytic inflammation.

c. Predominantly eosinophilic inflammation.

d. Intestinal metaplasia.

e. Fungal infections such as *Candida*.

Answer: c

9. A 50-year-old male presents with progressive jaundice. On biopsy, the liver shows feature of primary sclerosing cholangitis. Which of the following entities in the gastrointestinal tract is likely to coexist with the liver disease?

a. Celiac disease.

b. Atrophic gastritis.

c. Crohn disease.

d. Ulcerative colitis.

e. Collagenous colitis.

Answer: d

10. A 5-day-old infant presents with vomiting and a distended abdomen. X-rays of the abdomen show marked colonic dilatation with a narrowed rectosigmoid segment. A biopsy specimen taken from the narrowed segment shows a complete absence of ganglion cells in the submucosa and in the muscle wall. The most likely diagnosis is:

a. Congenital colonic atresia.
b. Necrotizing enterocolitis.
c. Hirschsprung disease.
d. Down syndrome.
e. Idiopathic intestinal pseudoobstruction.

Answer: c

11. A 12-year-old boy presents with multiple colonic polyps. Histologically, all the polyps show an overgrowth of nondysplastic epithelium on an arborizing smooth muscle core. The branching smooth muscle seems to derive from the muscularis mucosae. All the following statements about this patient are correct **except**:

a. The patient is likely to have mucocutaneous pigmentations.
b. The patient is likely to have a germline mutation in the *STK11/LKB1* tumor suppressor gene.
c. The polyp has no risk of progression to malignancy.
d. If this patient were female, she would have an increased risk of breast cancer and gynecological malignancy.
e. He has an increased risk of testicular malignancy.

Answer: c

12. All the following statements regarding gastrointestinal stromal tumors (GIST) are true **except**:

a. The interstitial cell of Cajal is considered the cell of origin for the tumor.
b. A gain of function mutation in *KIT* or *PDGFR* gene may exist.
c. Only those tumors with a *KIT* mutation respond to Gleevec (imatinib) therapy.
d. Mitotic rate and tumor size are the 2 main features that determine the risk of aggressive behavior.
e. Histologic criteria for benign and malignant GIST are identical in different parts of the gastrointestinal tract.

Answer: e

13. An 18-month-old boy presents with acute abdominal pain resembling acute appendicitis. On surgery, the appendix is normal. At the antimesenteric side of the terminal ileum, a 5 cm blind pouch is found. The resected specimen shows ectopic gastric mucosa and ulceration of the mucosa within the pouch. Which of the following statements does **not** accurately describe the characteristics of this particular entity?

a. It occurs in approximately 2% of the population.
b. It is generally present within 2 feet of the ileocecal valve.
c. It is twice as common in males.
d. It is most often symptomatic by age 2.
e. Only 2% of patients are ever symptomatic.

Answer: e

14. A 35-year-old female undergoes an appendectomy for acute appendicitis. Within the tip of the resected appendix, there is a tumor composed of uniform nests of cells with "salt and pepper" chromatin. The tumor cells stain positive for synaptophysin. Which of the following statements regarding the tumor is correct?

a. The tumor is often associated with carcinoid syndrome.
b. It is the most common type of appendiceal neoplasm.
c. It is uncommon in children.
d. It has a worse prognosis for patients than the same type of tumor in other parts of the gastrointestinal tract.
e. Tumor size has nothing to do with the risk of metastasis.

Answer: b

15. A 19-year-old man has had abdominal pain and bloody diarrhea for 6 months. A biopsy specimen of the colon shows mucosal architectural alteration with chronic inflammation, deep lymphoid aggregates, and deep fissures extending into the muscularis propria. Multiple granulomas are identified within the lamina propria. Which of the following statements regarding this case is correct?

a. This condition is commonly associated with primary sclerosing cholangitis.
b. The majority of patients are positive for perinuclear antineutrophil cytoplasmic antibody (p-ANCA).
c. Resection of the diseased segment and anastomosis of the remaining healthy segments can cure the disease.
d. This is a disease exclusively involving the colon. The disease process does not usually involve other parts of the gastrointestinal tract.
e. Genetic factors are important in predisposing individuals to the disease.

Answer: e

16. All of the following are inherited hamartomatous polyposis syndromes **except**:
   a. Cowden syndrome.
   b. Familial juvenile polyposis.
   c. Peutz-Jeghers syndrome.
   d. Carney syndrome.
   e. Basal cell nevus syndrome.

Answer: d

17. The gross appearance of the gastric mucosa in Ménétrier disease resembles which of the following?
   a. Fundic gland polyps.
   b. Atrophic gastritis.
   c. Hyperplastic polyps.
   d. Zollinger-Ellison syndrome.
   e. Inflammatory fibroid polyps.

Answer: d

18. Patients with celiac disease are prone to which of the following types of lymphoma in the small intestine?
   a. Diffuse large B-cell lymphoma.
   b. T-cell lymphoma.
   c. Hodgkin lymphoma.
   d. Mucosa associated lymphoid tissue (MALT) lymphoma.
   e. Follicular lymphoma.

Answer: b

19. The most common site of amebic ulcers in the gastrointestinal tract is the:
   a. Duodenum.
   b. Ileum.
   c. Cecum or ascending colon.
   d. Transverse colon.
   e. Sigmoid colon and rectum.

Answer: c

20. Which of the following is the most common cause of segmental colitis confined to the sigmoid colon?
   a. Ulcerative colitis.
   b. Crohn colitis.
   c. Diverticular disease.
   d. Ischemic colitis.
   e. Cytomegalovirus (CMV) colitis.

Answer: c

21. In the American Joint Committee on Cancer (AJCC) staging manual,* esophagogastric junctional (EGJ) carcinoma is defined as:
   a. Carcinoma with the bulk of the tumor located at the EGJ.
   b. Carcinoma that involves EGJ, with its epicenter located within 2 cm of the EGJ and extending into the esophagus.
   c. Carcinoma that involves the EGJ, with its epicenter located within 5 cm into proximal stomach.
   d. Carcinoma located entirely above the EJG but within 5 cm of the EGJ.
   e. Carcinoma with epicenter located at the EGJ, irrespective of where the bulk of the tumor lies.

Answer: b

22. All the following entities can show increased epithelial apoptosis **except**:
   a. Active ulcerative colitis.
   b. Phospho soda bowel preparation.
   c. An organ transplant patient using mycophenolate mofetil (MMF).
   d. Patient using nonsteroidal antiinflammatory drugs (NSAIDs).
   e. Acute graft versus host disease (GVHD).

Answer: a

23. When evaluating a specimen of low anterior resection with total mesorectal excision (TME), which of the following statements is correct?
   a. A "complete" specimen means the mesorectal surface has no defects.
   b. A "complete" specimen can have defects < 5 mm deep.
   c. A "complete" specimen can have defects < 10 mm deep.
   d. A "complete" specimen can have some coning as long as the coned surface is smooth.
   e. If muscularis propria is exposed focally, the specimen should be called "near complete."

Answer: b

24. If invasive carcinoma was found in a pedunculated polyp, which of the following histological features is **not** important in planning further therapy?
   a. Histological grade of the invasive component.
   b. The depth of tumor invasion into the submucosa.
   c. The presence of vascular invasion.
   d. The presence of lymphatic invasion.
   e. The distance of the invasive component to the resection margin.

Answer: b

25. A 32-year-old woman presents to the emergency room with severe bloody diarrhea, abdominal pain, fever, and abdominal distention. On X-ray, dilated loops of bowel are identified, particularly in the transverse colon. The patient undergoes total colectomy and histological sections show diffuse mucosal ulceration, focal early fissuring ulcers, focal transmural inflammation, and relative sparing of the rectum. Which of the following diagnoses is most likely?
   a. Severe Crohn disease and colitis.
   b. Fulminant ulcerative colitis.
   c. Acute ischemic colitis.
   d. Pseudomembranous colitis.
   e. Severe infectious colitis by hemorrhagic *E. coli*.

Answer: b

*This chapter uses the eighth edition of the AJCC staging manual.

26. A 66-year-old white male presents with abdominal pain. On physical examination, he has multifocal peripheral lymphadenopathy and moderate splenomegaly. Colonoscopy reveals innumerable small polypoid lesions involving most of the colon. What is the most likely diagnosis on biopsy of the polyp?

a. MALT lymphoma.

b. Mantle cell lymphoma.

c. Multiple tubular adenomas.

d. Primary follicular lymphoma of the gastrointestinal tract.

e. Hyperplastic polyposis.

Answer: b

27. A screening endoscopy of a 65-year-old female with a 20-year history of Crohn disease reveals a slightly elevated 2 mm by 2 mm lesion at the descending colon. Histologically, the lesion is composed of colonic mucosa with focal low grade dysplasia. The lesion is completely resected. Specimens taken from the mucosa immediately adjacent to the lesion, as well as random specimens from the remaining colon and terminal ileum, all show nearly normal mucosa without evidence of active or chronic inflammation or flat dysplasia. According to the SCENIC international consensus statement, the most appropriate next step in the patient's management is:

a. Total colectomy.

b. Left hemicolectomy.

c. Repeat colonoscopy in 3–6 months.

d. Repeat colonoscopy in 1–3 years.

e. Increased dose of medication for Crohn disease.

Answer: c

28. The designation N1c in the AJCC staging manual indicates which of the following scenarios?

a. The deposit is > 3 mm.

b. The contours of the deposit are smooth.

c. The contours of the deposit are irregular.

d. > 4 lymph nodes contain metastatic cancer.

e. All sampled lymph nodes are negative, but there are tumor deposits in the subserosa, mesentery, or nonperitonealized pericolic, perirectal/mesorectal tissue.

Answer: e

29. The most important prognostic feature in a low grade appendiceal mucinous neoplasm is:

a. The grade of dysplasia in the tumor epithelium.

b. Whether there is mucin dissecting into the muscularis propria.

c. Whether there is mucinous epithelium in extraappendiceal mucin.

d. Whether the margin of resection is involved.

e. Whether the muscularis mucosae has been breached by mucinous epithelium.

Answer: c

30. Which of the following statements regarding the interpretation of microsatellite instability (MSI) immunohistochemistry data is **not** correct?

a. Lack of nuclear staining indicates a positive result for MSI testing.

b. Loss of expression of *MLH1* may be due to Lynch syndrome or methylation of the promoter region.

c. Eighty percent of sporadic *MLH1* loss has a *KRAS* mutation.

d. Loss of *MSH2* expression essentially always implies Lynch syndrome.

e. Loss of *MLH1* expression is the most common type detected.

Answer: c

SHORT ANSWER QUESTIONS

Nonneoplastic Disorders of the Esophagus

31. List the common causes of esophageal dysphagia.

- Eosinophilic esophagitis.
- Mechanical obstruction — esophageal rings, webs, stricture, scar.
- Achalasia — incomplete relaxation of the lower esophageal sphincter, increased tone of the lower esophageal sphincter, and aperistalsis of the esophagus.
- Secondary injury of vagus nerve — Chagas disease, diabetic autonomic neuropathy.
- Infiltrative disorders — e.g., malignancy, amyloidosis, or sarcoidosis.
- Lesions of dorsal motor nuclei.

32. List the diagnostic criteria of eosinophilic esophagitis (EoE).
- Clinical presentation of esophageal dysfunction/dysphagia.
- Compatible endoscopic findings (rings, furrows).
- Esophageal biopsies with ≥ 15 eosinophils per high power field (HPF).
- No other causes of symptoms and/or esophageal eosinophilia.

33. List 5 gastrointestinal tract disorders than can have extensive eosinophilic infiltration in the esophageal mucosa.
- Eosinophilic esophagitis.
- Reflux esophagitis.
- Allergic reaction to food or medication.
- Eosinophilic gastroenteritis.
- Parasitic infection.

34. List 5 esophageal causes of hematemesis.
- Varices (cirrhosis).
- Lacerations (Mallory-Weiss syndrome).
- Esophageal perforation (Boerhaave syndrome).
- Esophageal carcinoma.
- Esophagitis (pill, chemical, infection).

35. List common congenital anomalies of the esophagus.
- Tracheesophageal fistula.
- Atresia.
- Esophageal cysts.

Neoplasms of the Esophagus

36. Define Barrett esophagus.
- Barrett esophagus (American College of Gastroenterology definition): a change in the esophageal epithelium extending ≥ 1 cm proximally to the gastroesophageal junction (> 3 cm long segment, ≤ 3 cm short segment) that can be recognized on endoscopy and confirmed to have intestinal metaplasia by biopsy.
- In order to diagnose Barrett esophagus, 2 criteria must be met:
  · Endoscopic evidence of replacement of gray squamous mucosa by salmon-colored glandular mucosa.
  · Histologic evidence of intestinal metaplasia in the glandular mucosa.

37. Suggest 1 helpful histochemical stain for Barrett esophagus.
Alcian blue/periodic acid-Schiff (AB/PAS, pH 2.5) to highlight goblet cells.

38. Classify dysplasia in Barrett esophagus.
- Negative for dysplasia.
- Indefinite for dysplasia.
- Low grade dysplasia.
- High grade dysplasia.

39. What are the therapeutic implications of each category of Barrett esophagus according to the 2022 guidelines of the American College of Gastroenterology (ACG)?
- Negative for dysplasia: repeat endoscopy in 3–5 years.
- Low grade dysplasia: endoscopic eradication therapy or repeat endoscopy in 6 months.
- High grade dysplasia or intramucosal carcinoma: endoscopic eradication therapy.
- Indefinite for dysplasia: repeat endoscopy in 6 months.

40. List microscopic scenarios that qualify for a diagnosis of "indefinite for dysplasia."
- Insufficient cytologic atypia.
- Dysplasia-like epithelium in the background of marked inflammation or mucosal erosion.
- Subsquamous extension of "dysplastic-appearing glands."
- Dysplastic glands that mature to the surface.
- Technical issues (denuded surface epithelium, poor orientation, tangential sectioning, etc.).

41. List histologic features that differentiate low grade dysplasia (LGD) from high grade dysplasia (HGD).

FEATURE	LGD	HGD
Architecture	• Preserved crypt architecture or villiform surface.	• Architectural distortion: · Crowding. · Branching. · Budding. · Cribriforming.
Nuclei	• Preserved polarity. • Stratification. • Enlargement. • Hyperchromasia. • Crowding. • Less pleomorphic.	• Lack of polarity. • Stratification to luminal surface. • Prominent enlargement. • Irregular membrane contour. • More pleomorphism.
Cytoplasm	• Diminished mucin. • Dystrophic goblet cells.	• Mucin absent.

42. List 3 esophagus-preserving new modalities in the treatment of Barrett esophagus with high grade dysplasia or intramucosal carcinoma.
- Photodynamic therapy.
- Laser ablation.
- Endoscopic mucosectomy.

43. List 5 complications of Barrett esophagus besides malignancy.
- Reflux esophagitis and aspiration pneumonia.
- Esophageal stricture.
- Esophageal ulcer.
- Esophageal perforation.
- Esophageal bleeding.

44. List the 2 most common benign esophageal tumors.
- Squamous papilloma.
- Leiomyoma.

45. Identify 4 types of benign glands that mimic tumors on esophageal biopsy.
- Gastric cardia glands.
- Subepithelial mucous glands.
- Salivary glands.
- Heterotopic pancreatic glands.
- Other: embryonal remnants found in infants (ciliated), sebaceous glands.

46. Name 5 risk factors for esophageal squamous cell carcinoma.
- Alcohol and tobacco use.
- Caustic esophageal injury.
- Achalasia.
- Tylosis.
- Plummer-Vinson syndrome.
- Other: poverty, frequent consumption of very hot beverages, diets deficient in fruits or vegetables.

47. Which specific subtype of esophageal squamous cell carcinoma has been associated with human papillomavirus (HPV) infection and what is the role of HPV in the development of squamous cell carcinoma?
- Verrucous squamous cell carcinoma has been associated with HPV-51 and HPV-11.
- HPV is not considered as a substantial risk factor in squamous cell carcinomas of the esophagus.

Note: unlike the oropharyngeal basaloid squamous cell carcinoma, the basaloid squamous cell carcinoma of the esophagus is not associated with HPV infection.

48. Name 3 risk factors for adenocarcinoma of esophagus and EGJ.
- Gastroesophageal reflux disease.
- Smoking.
- *Helicobacter pylori* infection.

49. Define EGJ carcinoma according to the AJCC staging manual.

Adenocarcinoma with epicenter within 2 cm of EGJ and extending into the esophagus.

Note: squamous cell carcinoma that occurs at the EGJ is considered carcinoma of the distal esophagus, even if it crosses the EGJ.

50. List 3 predictive factors in esophageal and EGJ adenocarcinoma.

- *HER2* gene amplification and resulting overexpression of HER2 protein predict response to HER2targeted therapy, including trastuzumab.
- Microsatellite instability is a potential biomarker predicting response to immunotherapy, including pembrolizumab.
- PDL1 overexpression is a potential biomarker predicting response to immunotherapy, including pembrolizumab.

Nonneoplastic Disorders of the Stomach

51. List the 3 most common sites of peptic ulcer disease.

- First portion of duodenum (within 2 cm of pylorus).
- Lesser curvature of stomach, near incisura angularis (interface of body and antrum).
- Gastric antrum.
- Other sites include the gastresophageal junction (in the setting of GERD/Barrett esophagus); the mucosa adjacent to the anastomosis line in patients with gastrojejunostomy; the duodenum, stomach, or jejunum in patients with Zollinger-Ellison syndrome; and Meckel diverticulum containing ectopic gastric mucosa.

52. Name the most common cause of duodenal ulcers.

Helicobacter pylori infection.

53. Name the most common cause of gastric ulcers.

Helicobacter pylori infection.

54. What is a stress ulcer? Give 2 examples.

- Stress ulcers: stress related mucosal ulceration developing in individuals with shock, sepsis, or severe trauma.
- Most common:
- Cushing ulcer: gastric, duodenal, and esophageal ulcers arising in patients with intracranial disease.
- Curling ulcer: ulcers occurring in the proximal duodenum in patients with severe burns or trauma.

55. How do you differentiate benign from malignant gastric ulcers of the stomach?

FACTOR	BENIGN	MALIGNANT
Age	• Younger.	• Older.
History	• Longer.	• Shorter.
Pain	• Common.	• Less common.
Location	• Antrum or lesser curve.	• Cardia or body, greater curvature.
Ulcer base on radiology	• Outside gastric wall.	• Inside gastric wall.
Gross features	• Punched out with overhanging edges.	• Irregular with heaped up margins.
Mucosal folds	• Terminate at ulcer edge.	• Do not reach ulcer edge.

56. List 4 reasons for surgery in patients with peptic ulcers.

- Hemorrhage.
- Perforation.
- Obstruction.
- To exclude malignancy.

57. List 4 gastric disease processes associated with *H. pylori* infection.

- Chronic gastritis.
- Peptic ulcer disease.
- Gastric adenocarcinoma.
- Gastric MALT lymphoma.

58. List 4 methods to confirm *H. pylori* in biopsy tissue.

- Routine or special stains (Giemsa, Warthin-Starry, or Steiner) to identify bacteria in tissue sections.
- Culture of biopsy tissue.
- PCR to detect bacterial DNA.
- Immunohistochemistry.

59. What enzyme is involved in the breakdown of urea in *H. pylori*?
Urease.

60. How is *H. pylori* gastritis treated clinically?
- Proton pump inhibitor + amoxicillin + clarithromycin × 14 days.
- If penicillin allergy: proton pump inhibitor + metronidazole + clarithromycin × 14 days.
- If macrolide allergy or resistance: proton pump inhibitor + bismuth subsalicylate + metronidazole + tetracycline × 14 days.

61. What are the clinical indications for rebiopsy in a patient treated for *H. pylori* gastritis?
- Persistence of symptoms after medical treatment.
- To confirm eradication of bacteria.
- To exclude malignancy.
- To exclude other superimposed disease processes.

62. List 3 noninvasive tests for *H. pylori* infection.
- Urea breath test.
- Serum IgG antibody against *H. pylori*.
- Stool antigen.

63. List 4 other types of chronic gastritis in addition to *H. pylori* gastritis.
- Autoimmune gastritis.
- Eosinophilic gastritis.
- Lymphocytic gastritis.
- Granulomatous gastritis.

64. List 6 characteristic histologic features of autoimmune gastritis.
- Diffuse mucosal damage/atrophy of the oxyntic (acid producing) mucosa within the body and fundus. Minimal or no inflammation in the antral mucosa.
- Lymphocytes, macrophages, and plasma cells centered on deep gastric glands.
- Intestinal and pyloric metaplasia.
- Epithelial nuclear enlargement (megaloblastic change) due to vitamin B_{12} deficiency.
- Antral G cell hyperplasia.
- Enterochromaffin-like (ECL) cell hyperplasia in the fundus and body.

65. List 4 characteristic clinical features of autoimmune gastritis.
- Antibodies to parietal cells and intrinsic factor that can be detected in serum and gastric secretions.
- Reduced serum pepsinogen I concentration.
- Anemia due to vitamin B_{12} deficiency.
- Defective gastric acid secretion (achlorhydria).

66. List 3 common causes of granulomatous gastritis.
- Crohn disease.
- Sarcoidosis.
- Infections including mycobacteria, fungi, CMV, and *H. pylori*.

67. List 3 common causes of reactive gastropathy.
- Chemical injury.
- NSAID use.
- Bile reflux.

68. List 4 entities that can show giant cerebriform enlargement of the rugae on gross examination.
- Ménétrier disease.
- Zollinger-Ellison syndrome.
- Diffuse signet-ring type gastric carcinoma.
- Gastric lymphoma.

69. On biopsy, an endoscopically nodular gastric mucosa shows hyperplasia of mucous secreting foveolar epithelial cells. List 3 differential diagnoses.
- Reactive/chemical gastropathy.
- Hyperplastic polyp.
- Ménétrier disease.

Neoplasms of the Stomach

70. List 3 common types of gastric polyps.
- Adenomatous polyp.
- Hyperplastic polyp.
- Fundic gland polyp.

71. List the 2 main types of dysplasia in the stomach.
- Intestinal-type dysplasia (adenomatous type, type 1).
- Foveolar-type dysplasia (hyperplastic type, type 2).

72. List 3 types of gastric polyps that have risks of developing dysplasia.
- Hyperplastic polyp: greatest risk if size > 2 cm, age > 50.
- Fundic gland polyp in syndromic setting (FAP/GAPPS or other fundic gland polyposis syndromes).
- Juvenile polyp in patients with juvenile polyposis syndrome.

73. List 4 types of adenomatous polyp occurring in the stomach.
- Intestinal-type adenoma.
- Foveolar-type adenoma.
- Pyloric gland adenoma.
- Oxyntic gland adenoma.

74. Define early gastric carcinoma.
Carcinoma limited to the mucosa or submucosa regardless of nodal metastasis.

75. List the risk factors for recurrence in early gastric carcinoma.
- Vascular invasion.
- Poor differentiation.
- Presence of occult metastasis.

76. List the 4 molecular gastric carcinoma subtypes defined by the Cancer Genome Atlas (TCGA).
- Epstein-Barr virus (EBV) positive (9%).
- Microsatellite instability (MSI) (22%).
- Genomically stable (20%).
- Chromosomally unstable (50%).

77. For each TCGA molecular subtype of gastric carcinoma, list the associated histology, key molecular alterations, and the main biological pathways affected.

	EBV POSITIVE	MSI	GENOMICALLY STABLE	CHROMOSOMALLY UNSTABLE
Associated histology	• Gastric carcinoma with lymphoid stroma (medullary carcinoma).	• No specific histology, but more commonly intestinal type.	• Diffuse type.	• Intestinal type.
Key molecular alterations	• EBV-associated CIMP profile. • *PIK3CA* mutation. • *PDL1/2* overexpression. • *CDKN2A* silencing.	• Hypermutation. • *MSI*-associated gastric-CIMP profile. • *MLH1* silencing.	• *CDH1*, *RHOA* mutations. • *CLDN18-ARHGAP* fusion.	• *TP53* mutation.
Biologic pathways affected	• Immune cell signaling.	• Mitotic pathways.	• Cell adhesion.	• *RTK-RAS* activation.

Abbreviations: CIMP: CpG island methylator phenotype.

78. Which TCGA molecular subtypes are associated with better prognosis?
EBV positive and MSI gastric cancers are associated with better prognosis.

79. Name at least 2 genetic mutations that are associated with the development of diffuse type gastric adenocarcinoma.
- *CDH1*.
- *CTNNA1*.
- *BRCA2*.

80. List predictive biomarkers in gastric carcinoma.
- Established biomarkers:
  - *HER2* gene amplification and resulting overexpression of HER2 protein predict response to *HER2*-targeted therapy, including trastuzumab.
- Partly established biomarkers:
  - MSI is a potential biomarker predicting response to *PD1/PDL1*-targeted immunotherapy.
  - EBV positivity and associated amplification and increased expression of *PDL1* are potential biomarkers predicting response to PD1/PDL1-targeted immunotherapy.

81. List 3 distinct types of gastric neuroendocrine tumor.
- Type 1: associated with autoimmune chronic atrophic gastritis.
- Type 2: associated with multiple endocrine neoplasia type 1 (MEN1) and Zollinger-Ellison syndrome.
- Type 3: sporadic.

82. List the 2 most common lymphomas of the gastrointestinal tract.
- MALT lymphoma.
- Diffuse large B-cell lymphoma.

83. List at least 3 translocations that are associated with gastric mucosa associated lymphoid tissue (MALT) lymphoma and their common downstream molecule.

- Translocations:
  - t(11;18)(q21;q21) — most common translocation; predicts resistance to remission after *H. pylori* eradication with antibiotic therapy.
  - t(1;14)(p22;q32).
  - t(14;18)(q32;q21).
  - t(3;14)(p14;q32).
- Common downstream molecule:
  - NF-κB — transcription factor that promotes B cell growth and survival.

84. Describe the histologic and immunohistochemical characteristics of MALT lymphoma.

- Dense lymphoid infiltrate in the lamina propria.
- Small lymphoid cells, centrocyte-like cells, monocytoid cells, plasma cells.
- Lymphoepithelial lesion.
- Immunohistochemistry (IHC):
  - Positive: CD19, CD20, CD79a, CD43 (25%).
  - Negative: CD10, CD23, CD5, Bcl-6.
  - Monoclonality demonstrated by restricted expression of either κ or λ immunoglobulin light chain.

85. Why is it important to diagnose gastrointestinal stromal tumors (GISTs) and differentiate them from other types of gastrointestinal spindle cell neoplasms?

Because GISTs respond to targeted chemotherapy: imatinib and other tyrosine kinase inhibitors that block c kit and platelet derived growth factor receptor–α (PDGFRα).

86. What do we know about GISTs that differentiates them from other types of gastrointestinal spindle cell neoplasms?

- They derive from interstitial cells of Cajal located in the myenteric plexus.
- They have characteristic immunohistochemical features: positive for CD117 (95%), DOG1 (99%).
- They have distinct genetic mutations.
  - Most GISTs (~75%) have oncogenic, gain-of-function mutations of the gene that encodes the tyrosine kinase receptor KIT.
- ~10% of GISTs have mutations that activate a related tyrosine kinase, PDGFRα.
- In sporadic GISTs, KIT and PDGFRα gene mutations are mutually exclusive.
- Mutations, which cause loss of succinate dehydrogenase (SDH) function, are often inherited in the germline and confer an increased risk for GIST and paraganglioma (Carney-Stratakis syndrome).
- They respond to targeted chemotherapy.

87. List 4 syndromes associated with GISTs and their corresponding molecular alteration.

- Carney triad: SDH promoter methylation.
- Carney-Stratakis syndrome: germline *SDHB*, *SDHC*, and *SDHD* mutation.
- Neurofibromatosis type 1: germline *NF1* mutation.
- Familial GIST syndrome: germline *KIT* or *PDGFRα* mutation.

88. What is the Carney triad?

- A nonhereditary syndrome seen primarily in young females that includes:
  - Gastric GISTs.
  - Paraganglioma.
  - Pulmonary chondroma.

89. List 3 clinical characteristics associated with SDH-deficient GISTs.

- Occurs more commonly in females.
- Presents at a younger age.
- Arises almost exclusively in the stomach.

90. List key pathologic features associated with SDH-deficient GISTs.

- Multinodular/plexiform growth pattern.
- Epithelioid morphology.
- Lymphovascular invasion.
- Nodal metastases.
- Distant metastases (liver, peritoneum).

91. What are the prognostic parameters of GISTs?

- Tumor size.
- Mitotic rate.
- Anatomical site.

92. List at least 4 types of cells that stain positively for CD117.

- GIST cells or interstitial cells of Cajal.
- Mast cells.
- Germ cells.
- Melanocytes.

Nonneoplastic Disorders of the Small Bowel

93. List the 3 most commonly encountered chronic malabsorptive disorders in North America.
- Pancreatic insufficiency.
- Celiac disease.
- Crohn disease.

94. List 5 common causes of duodenal intraepithelial lymphocytosis with preserved villous architecture.
- *H. pylori* infection (gastritis).
- NSAID use.
- Early celiac disease or tropical sprue.
- Inflammatory bowel diseases (Crohn disease).
- Other immunological processes such as lymphocytic colitis, lymphocytic gastritis.

95. List 2 neoplastic and 3 nonneoplastic diseases associated with celiac disease.
- Neoplastic:
  · Enteropathy-associated T-cell lymphoma.
  · Intestinal adenocarcinoma.
- Nonneoplastic:
  · Dermatitis herpetiformis.
  · Lymphocytic gastritis.
  · Lymphocytic colitis.

96. In a patient with the classic clinical presentation and histology of celiac disease, but with negative serological testing for IgA antibodies against tissue transglutaminase or deamidated gliadin, what can you do to confirm the diagnosis?
- The patient most likely has IgA deficiency, which can be confirmed with IgA serology.
- Measuring serum IgG antibodies to tissue transglutaminase and deamidated gliadin can confirm the diagnosis of celiac disease.

97. What is the characteristic histology of celiac disease on duodenal biopsy?
- Increased intraepithelial CD8 positive T lymphocytes (intraepithelial lymphocytosis).
- Villous atrophy (blunted to flattened).
- Crypt hyperplasia.
- Increased lymphocytes and plasma cells in lamina propria.

98. What are the diagnostic criteria for celiac disease?
- Clinical features of malabsorption and/or iron deficiency anemia.
- Presence of serum IgA antibodies to gliadin (AGA-IgA), tissue transglutaminase (tTG-IgA) and endomysium (EMA-IgA), and IgG antibody to gliadin (AGA-IgG).
- Characteristic histology.
- Response to treatment with a gluten free diet.

99. What are the common complications of celiac disease?
- Malabsorption.
- Anemia.
- Chronic fatigue.
- Osteoporosis.
- Short stature.
- Lymphoma.

100. Describe the most common morphologic alterations in the small intestine in patients with AIDS.
- Crypt hypertrophy.
- Increased apoptotic enterocytes.
- Villous atrophy.
- Opportunistic infections.
- Neoplasms — Kaposi sarcoma, lymphoma.

Nonneoplastic Disorders of the Colon and Rectum

101. Define and classify microscopic colitis.
- Clinically: presents with chronic watery diarrhea, more commonly in middle-aged females.
- Endoscopically: shows normal colonic mucosa.
- Histologically: divided into collagenous colitis and lymphocytic colitis.

102. Describe the histologic characteristics of each subtype of microscopic colitis.

FEATURE	COLLAGENOUS COLITIS	LYMPHOCYTIC COLITIS
Intraepithelial lymphocytes	• Usually present.	• ≥ 20/100 enterocytes.
Subepithelial collagenous plate	• Thickened (> 10 µm).	• Normal.
Lamina propria mononuclear cells	• Increased.	• Increased.
Epithelial degeneration or sloughing	• Common.	• Less common.
Architectural changes	• Absent.	• Absent.
Apoptosis	• Absent.	• Absent.

103. Describe the etiology and pathogenesis of antibiotic associated colitis.
- Disruption of the normal colonic flora by antibiotics allows *Clostridium difficile* overgrowth.
- Toxins released by *C. difficile* cause epithelial damage, cytokine release, and apoptosis.
- The mechanisms that lead to the characteristic morphology of pseudomembranous colitis are incompletely understood.

104. What is a pseudomembrane? List 3 disease processes that can lead to the formation of pseudomembranes in the colonic mucosa.
- Pseudomembrane: an adherent layer of inflammatory cells and debris at sites of colonic mucosal injury.
- Can be caused by:
  - *C. difficile* associated colitis.
  - Ischemia.
  - Necrotizing infections.

105. How is pseudomembranous colitis diagnosed clinically?

Diagnosis of *C. difficile* associated colitis is usually accomplished by detection of *C. difficile* toxin, rather than culture, and is supported by the characteristic histopathology.

Ischemic Colitis

106. In adult patients, what are the common causes of bowel ischemia?
- Running or other strenuous exercise.
- Estrogen compounds; drugs that cause vasoconstriction.
- Hypoperfusion (mucosal or mural): cardiac failure, shock, dehydration.
- Vascular obstruction (transmural): severe atherosclerosis, aneurysm, hypercoagulable state, embolization of cardiac vegetation, or aortic atheroma.
- Vasculitis: polyarteritis nodosa, Henoch-Schönlein purpura, granulomatosis with polyangiitis.
- Mesenteric venous thrombosis (rare): mass, trauma, cirrhosis, hypercoagulation.

107. What is the most common site for bowel ischemia?
- Watershed zones: splenic flexure between superior and inferior mesentery artery.
- Less commonly, rectosigmoid colon.

Inflammatory Bowel Disease

108. Describe characteristic gross, histologic, and clinical features that allow pathologists to differentiate between ulcerative colitis and Crohn disease.

FEATURE	ULCERATIVE COLITIS	CROHN DISEASE
GROSS FEATURES		
Distribution	• Diffuse, colon only.	• Segmental, but anywhere along gastrointestinal tract.
Skip lesions	• Usually absent.	• Present.
Rectal involvement	• Present.	• Usually absent.
Terminal ileum	• Normal or "backwash ileitis."	• Often thickened and stenosed.
Strictures/fistulas	• Absent.	• Present.
Thickened bowel wall	• Absent.	• Present.
Mucosa	• Hemorrhagic appearance.	• Cobblestone-like and linear ulcers.
Mesenteric adipose tissue	• Normal.	• Possible extension over serosal surface (creeping fat).
HISTOLOGIC FEATURES		
Depth of inflammation	• Mucosa based.	• Transmural.
Mucosal ulcers	• Superficial, broad based.	• Deep, fissured.
Lymphoid hyperplasia	• Infrequent.	• Common.
Crypt abscesses	• Extensive.	• Focal.
Crypt architectural distortion	• Severe and widespread.	• Discontinuous.
Epithelioid granulomas	• Absent.	• Present.
Fissures and sinuses	• Absent.	• Present.
Submucosal fibrosis	• Absent.	• Present.
Neuronal hyperplasia	• Absent.	• Present.
Thickening of muscularis mucosa	• Absent.	• Present.
Serositis	• Absent.	• Present.
CLINICAL FEATURES		
Perianal fistula	• Absent.	• Can be present.
Fat/vitamin malabsorption	• No.	• Yes.
Recurrence after surgery	• No.	• Common.
Toxic megacolon	• Yes.	• No.
Primary sclerosing cholangitis	• More common.	• Less common.
p-ANCA	• Positive (75%).	• Mostly negative (only 10% positive).
Antibodies to *Saccharomyces cerevisiae*	• Negative.	• Positive.

109. List at least 5 extraintestinal manifestations in patients with inflammatory bowel disease (chronic ulcerative colitis or Crohn disease).

- Eyes: uveitis, episcleritis.
- Skin: granulomatous inflammation, erythema nodosum, pyoderma gangrenosum.
- Joints: ankylosing spondylitis, sacroiliitis, migratory polyarthritis.
- Biliary tree: primary sclerosing cholangitis (more common in ulcerative colitis).
- Lungs: bronchiectasis.
- Vascular: venous and arterial thromboembolism.

110. What is the classification of dysplasia in inflammatory bowel disease (IBD), and what are its therapeutic implications?

CLASSIFICATION	MANAGEMENT
GROSS CLASSIFICATION	
Visible dysplasia — polypoid dysplastic lesion (protrusion from mucosa into lumen)	• If completely removed and unifocal, continued surveillance.
Visible dysplasia — nonpolypoid dysplastic lesion (no protrusion above mucosa)	• If completely removed and unifocal, continued surveillance.
Invisible dysplasia — dysplasia identified on random biopsy without a visible lesion	• Referral to an endoscopist with expertise in IBD surveillance for individualized management.
MICROSCOPIC CLASSIFICATION	
Negative for dysplasia	• Continued surveillance.
Indefinite for dysplasia	• Follow-up colonoscopy within 3–6 months or sooner, depending on clinical suspicion.
Low grade dysplasia (visible)	• If completely removed and unifocal, continued surveillance.
Low grade dysplasia (invisible)	• Referral to an endoscopist with expertise in IBD surveillance. • Unifocal: individualized management. • Multifocal: colectomy.
High grade dysplasia (visible)	• If completely removed and unifocal, continued surveillance.
High grade dysplasia (invisible)	• Referral to an endoscopist with expertise in IBD surveillance. • Colectomy.

111. List 5 common reasons for making a diagnosis of indeterminate colitis.
- Fulminant colitis.
- Insufficient clinical and radiological information.
- Interpretation of a small biopsy — it is supposed to be diagnosed on a colectomy specimen.
- Failure to recognize unusual variants of Crohn disease or ulcerative colitis.
- Superimposed other disease processes.

112. List 3 reasons for a mucosal biopsy in a patient with ulcerative colitis.
- Assessment of disease activity.
- Surveillance of dysplasia.
- Exclusion of other superimposed disease processes.

113. How does adenocarcinoma arising in ulcerative colitis (UC) differ from "ordinary" adenocarcinoma?
- Colitis-associated colorectal carcinoma develops in an inflammation-dysplasia-carcinoma sequence, whereas conventional colorectal carcinoma develops in an adenoma-carcinoma sequence.
- Due to the lack of a preceding adenomatous polyp and inflammatory background, adenocarcinoma in UC can be difficult to detect early.
- The surface of a carcinoma can deceptively show only a low grade dysplasia in a disorganized crypt pattern.

114. List 2 sites of isolated skip lesions in UC (i.e., UC that is discontinuous from the rectum).
- Cecum (cecal patch).
- Appendix or periappendiceal patch.

Mucosal Prolapse

115. Give 3 examples of entities constituting mucosal prolapse syndromes.
- Solitary rectal ulcer syndrome.
- Inflammatory cloacogenic polyp.
- Colitis cystica profunda/polyposa.
- Others: inflammatory cap polyp, diverticular disease–associated polyps.

116. List 3 manifestations of solitary rectal ulcer syndrome.
- Rectal bleeding.
- Mucus discharge.
- Inflammatory lesion of the anterior rectal wall.
- Others: anorectal pain, abdominal cramps, tenesmus.

117. List 4 typical histologic features of solitary rectal ulcer syndrome.
- Lamina propria fibromuscular hyperplasia.
- Mixed inflammatory infiltrates.
- Mucosal surface erosion.
- Epithelial hyperplasia.

118. What is the most common site of angiodysplasia in the gastrointestinal tract?
Ascending colon and cecum.

Neoplasms of the Colon and Rectum

119. List 5 types of epithelial polyps and 5 types of nonepithelial polyps.
- Epithelial polyps:
  · Hamartomatous polyp.
  · Adenomatous polyp.
  · Hyperplastic polyp.
  · Sessile serrated lesion.
- Nonepithelial polyps:
  · Inflammatory fibroid polyp.
  · Intramucosal lipoma.
  · Mucosal schwannoma.
  · Submucosal leiomyoma.

120. List 3 histologic features of advanced adenoma.
- High grade dysplasia.
- Size > 1 cm.
- Villous architecture.

121. Describe how to handle and report a colonic polyp.
- Gross dissection:
  · Describe size and shape.
  · Identify stalk if present.
  · Paint deep margin.
  · Cut in 3 mm sections perpendicular to the deep margin.
- Report:
  · Type of specimen: polypectomy versus biopsy.
  · Type of polyp.
  · Type of adenoma (tubular, tubulovillous, villous).
  · Size.
  · Resection margin.
  · For those with submucosal invasion: presence/absence of high-risk features (high grade, lymphovascular invasion, positive margin) and the necessity of further therapy.

122. List 4 factors that increase the likelihood of concomitant carcinoma in colorectal adenoma.
- Greater number of polyps.
- Larger size (invasive cancer is seen in 0.5% of adenomas < 1 cm; 5% of adenomas 1–1.9 cm; 10–20% of adenomas > 2 cm; 40% of adenomas > 4 cm).
- Higher proportion of villous architecture.
- Higher proportion of high grade dysplasia.

123. Define a malignant polyp.
- Malignant polyp: an adenomatous polyp with adenocarcinoma invading through the muscularis mucosa and into the submucosa (pT1).
- The definition excludes:
  · Adenomas with high grade dysplasia (intraepithelial carcinomas).
  · Intramucosal carcinomas (invasive carcinoma limited to the lamina propria or invading no deeper than the muscularis mucosae).

124. List the pathologic parameters that must be reported for a malignant polyp.
- Histologic grade.
- Status of the resection margin.
- Lymphovascular invasion.

125. List key features of malignant polyps that are associated with adverse outcome.
- High grade carcinoma.
- Tumor ≤ 1 mm from the resection margin.
- Presence of lymphovascular invasion.

126. Differentiate true invasion from pseudoinvasion in a polypectomy specimen.

COMPARISON CATEGORY	TRUE INVASION	MISPLACEMENT
Pedunculated polyp	• No.	• Yes.
History of biopsy	• No.	• Yes.
Granulation tissue	• Absent.	• Present.
Surface ulcer or reepithelialization	• No.	• Yes.
Architecture	• Irregular, tortuous.	• Round, smooth, lobular.
Fresh hemorrhage or hemosiderin	• Absent.	• Present.
Lamina propria rim around the deep glands	• Absent.	• Present.
Mucin pools (if present)	• Irregular, more cellular. • Dysplastic glands in the mucin pool have a higher degree of dysplasia than the surface epithelium.	• Round, acellular. • Dysplastic glands in the mucin pool have the same degree of dysplasia as the surface epithelium.
Stromal desmoplasia	• Yes.	• No.
Individual dysplastic cells	• Present.	• Absent.
Aborted incomplete dysplastic glands	• Present.	• Absent.

127. Differentiate dysplasia associated with inflammatory bowel disease from sporadic adenoma.

PARAMETER	SPORADIC ADENOMA	IBD ASSOCIATED DYSPLASIA
Patient age	• Older.	• Younger.
Extent of IBD	• Focal.	• More extensive.
Activity of IBD	• Inactive.	• Active.
Duration of IBD	• Shorter < 10 years.	• Longer.
Polyp location	• Disease-free area (such as right colon for chronic UC).	• Diseased area (left colon for chronic UC).
Associated flat dysplasia	• Never.	• Occasional.
Inflammation in crypts and lamina propria	• Absent.	• Present.
Villous architecture	• Usually absent.	• Occasionally present.
Mixture of benign and dysplastic crypts at the surface of the polyp	• Usually absent.	• Usually present.
Top down dysplasia	• Present.	• Absent.
Bottom up dysplasia	• Absent.	• Present.
TP53	• Absent.	• Present.
APC, KRAS	• More common.	• Less common.
Nuclear β-catenin	• Prominent.	• Absent.
LOH of 3p	• Uncommon.	• Common.
LOH of CDKN2A (p16, chr 9)	• Rare.	• Common.

Abbreviations: LOH: loss of heterozygosity.

128. What are the 2 main genetic pathways leading to the development of colorectal adenocarcinoma? What is their associated precursor lesion?

- The classic adenoma-carcinoma sequence: conventional adenomas.
- The hypermutant pathway: serrated polyps.

129. What is intramucosal carcinoma?

- It is characterized by high grade histology, irregular glands, cribriform architecture, desmoplastic or inflamed stroma, but no invasion beyond muscularis mucosae.
- It is now classified in the high grade dysplasia category. However, it should be mentioned in the report, especially in biopsy, since most of these will end up having invasive carcinoma at the surgical resection.

130. Discuss the differences between colorectal cancers associated with Lynch syndrome and colon cancers associated with familial adenomatous polyposis (FAP) in terms of age of occurrence, gross findings in the colectomy specimen, histological findings, and findings in the stomach and duodenum.

FACTOR	COLORECTAL CANCERS ASSOCIATED WITH LYNCH SYNDROME	COLORECTAL CANCERS ASSOCIATED WITH FAP
Age of occurrence	• < 50 years of age (usually around 45 years of age).	• Approximately 30 years of age.
Gross findings in the colectomy specimen	• Usually < 15 polyps per patient. • Usually right sided lesions. • Multiple adenocarcinomas (possible).	• > 100 polyps carpeting the colectomy specimen. • Adenocarcinoma may be present.
Adenoma histology	• Mostly sessile serrated lesion. • Other types possible.	• Mostly tubular adenoma. • Occasionally with villous features.
Adenocarcinoma histology	• Poorly differentiated, medullary, mucinous, or signet ring cell type. • Tumor-infiltrating lymphocytes. • Crohn disease–like reaction.	• Adenocarcinomas similar in appearance to sporadic colorectal carcinoma.
Findings in the stomach and duodenum	• Gastric cancer. • Adenocarcinoma of duodenum.	• Fundic gland polyps. • Gastric adenomas. • Adenoma of ampulla of Vater. • Adenocarcinoma of duodenum (periampullary).

131. What is the most common location of sessile serrated lesion?
Cecum and ascending colon.

132. What are the characteristic histologic features that allow differentiation of sessile serrated lesion (SSL) from hyperplastic polyps (HP)?

HISTOLOGIC FEATURES	SSL	HP
Common location	• Right colon, appendix.	• Rectosigmoid colon.
Shape	• Flat.	• Pedunculated or raised.
Size	• > 0.5 cm.	• < 0.5 cm.
Cytological atypia	• Subtle.	• Absent.
Thickened subepithelial collagen band	• Absent.	• Present.
Basal crypt dilatation	• Present.	• Absent.
Horizontal crypts	• Present.	• Absent.
Basal crypt serration	• Present.	• Absent.
Activating mutation	• *BRAF*.	• *BRAF* (microvesicular HP) or *KRAS* (goblet cell-rich HP).

133. What molecular alteration in sessile serrated lesion is associated with development of dysplasia and invasive carcinoma?
CpG-island methylation.

134. Describe 3 characteristic histologic features of traditional serrated adenoma (TSA).
• Tall columnar cells with pencillate nuclei and eosinophilic cytoplasm.
• Slit-like crypt serration.
• Ectopic crypt formation.

135. What is the most common location of TSA? How does macroscopic morphology vary depending on polyp location?
• The most common location is distal colorectum (~70%).
• In distal colorectum, TSAs usually grow as large protuberant polyps.
• TSAs occurring in the proximal colon, which are a minority of TSAs, usually present as flat lesions.

136. What are the most common gene mutations in TSAs?
• *KRAS* is mutated in 50–70% of TSAs.
• *BRAF* is mutated in 20–40% of TSAs.

137. List the 5 mismatch repair associated genes that can be involved in the development of MSI-H tumors in the colon.
- MLH1.
- MSH2.
- MSH6.
- PMS2.
- EPCAM.

138. List 3 histologic subtypes of invasive carcinoma that can derive from the MSI pathway.
- Medullary adenocarcinoma.
- Mucinous adenocarcinoma.
- Signet-ring cell carcinoma.

139. List high-risk (poor prognostic) features of colorectal cancer.
- Poorly differentiated histology.
- High tumor stage.
- Lymphatic invasion.
- Intramural and extramural vascular invasion.
- Perineural invasion.
- High grade tumor budding.
- Tumor deposits.
- Bowel obstruction and perforation.
- Age < 40 years.

140. List 3 predictive biomarkers in colorectal carcinoma and explain their clinical significance.
- *RAS* genes (45–50% of colorectal cancers): mutations predict ineffectiveness of anti-EGFR (HER1) therapy.
- MSI (15% of colorectal cancers): presence predicts response to PDL1-targeted therapy and reduced effectiveness of fluorouracil-based chemotherapy.
- *BRAF* gene (10% of colorectal cancers): mutation may also predict ineffectiveness of anti-EGFR therapy (currently limited evidence).

141. Classify appendiceal carcinoma.
- Low grade mucinous neoplasm (LAMN).
- High grade mucinous neoplasm (HAMN).
- Adenocarcinoma, not otherwise specified (NOS).
- Mucinous adenocarcinoma.
- Signet-ring cell carcinoma.
- Carcinoma, undifferentiated, NOS.
- Goblet cell adenocarcinoma.

142. Classify appendix neuroendocrine neoplasms.
- Neuroendocrine tumor (NET), NOS:
  · NET grade 1.
  · NET grade 2.
  · NET grade 3.
- Neuroendocrine carcinoma (NEC), NOS:
  · Large cell NEC.
  · Small cell NEC.
- Mixed neuroendocrine-nonneuroendocrine neoplasm (MiNEN).

143. List common benign and malignant neoplasms in the appendix.
- Benign appendix tumors:
  · Serrated lesion: hyperplastic polyp, sessile serrated lesion.
- Malignant appendix tumors:
  · Appendiceal mucinous neoplasm.
  · Appendiceal adenocarcinoma.
  · Neuroendocrine tumor and carcinoma.
  · Goblet cell adenocarcinoma.
  · Mixed neuroendocrine-nonneuroendocrine neoplasm (MiNEN).

144. According to the North American Neuroendocrine Tumor Society guidelines, how is appendiceal neuroendocrine tumor managed based on its size?[1]

TUMOR SIZE	MANAGEMENT	JUSTIFICATION
< 1 cm	• Appendectomy if: · Completely excised. · No lymphovascular invasion (LVI). · No mesoappendix invasion.	• It is generally cured by complete local excision. • Risk of lymph node metastasis is 0–11%.
1–2 cm	• Right hemicolectomy if: · Incomplete excision or tumor involves the base of the appendix. · LVI or mesenteric lymph node involvement. · Mesoappendix invasion. · Grade 2 or 3.	• Risk of lymph node metastasis is 18–44%.
> 2 cm	• Right hemicolectomy.	• Risk of lymph node metastasis is 30–86%.

145. What histologic features distinguish HAMN from LAMN?

- Architecture: HAMN has a micropapillary pattern, cribriforming, and piling up of epithelial cells.

- Cytology: HAMN has unequivocal high grade epithelium with enlarged hyperchromatic and pleomorphic nuclei, numerous atypical mitotic figures, single cell necrosis, and sloughed necrotic epithelial cells in appendiceal lumen.

146. How does histologic grading of pseudomyxoma peritonei correspond to the classification of appendiceal mucinous neoplasm in the WHO classification?*

PSEUDOMYXOMA PERITONEI	APPENDICEAL MUCINOUS NEOPLASM
• Grade 1	• Low grade appendiceal mucinous neoplasm.
• Grade 2	• High grade appendiceal mucinous neoplasm. • Invasive mucinous adenocarcinoma without a signet ring cell component.
• Grade 3	• Signet-ring cell adenocarcinoma with numerous signet ring cells in mucin pools or infiltrating tissue.

*This chapter uses the fifth edition of the WHO classification of tumors of the digestive system.

Neoplasms of the Anal Canal

147. Classify epithelial tumors of the anal canal using the WHO classification.

- Benign epithelial tumors and precursors.
  · Squamous dysplasia or intraepithelial neoplasia (IEN), low grade.
  · Squamous dysplasia or intraepithelial neoplasia (IEN), high grade.
- Malignant epithelial tumors.
  · Squamous cell carcinoma, NOS.
    › Verrucous squamous cell carcinoma.
  · Adenocarcinoma, NOS.

- Neuroendocrine tumor (NET), NOS.
  › NET G1.
  › NET G2.
  › NET G3.
- Neuroendocrine carcinoma (NEC).
  › Large cell NEC.
  › Small cell NEC.
- Mixed neuroendocrine-nonneuroendocrine neoplasm (MiNEN).

148. List 5 risk factors for anal squamous cell carcinoma.

- HPV infection (most commonly HPV-16).
- Coinfection with other sexually transmitted infections.
- Anoreceptive intercourse.

- Cellular immunodeficiency.
- Smoking.

Familial Syndromes

149. List 4 syndromes that can be associated with mutations of the adenomatous polyposis coli, or *APC*, gene.

- FAP syndrome.
- Attenuated FAP syndrome.

- Gastric adenocarcinoma and proximal polyposis of the stomach (GAPPS).
- Turcot syndrome.

Note: the term *Gardner syndrome* is considered obsolete in the 5th edition of WHO classification as almost all patients with FAP have features of Gardner syndrome.

150. List 5 syndromes associated with increased risk for gastric carcinoma.

- Hereditary diffuse gastric cancer syndrome.
- Lynch syndrome.
- FAP and GAPPS.

- Peutz-Jeghers syndrome.
- Li-Fraumeni syndrome.

151. List at least 3 genetic syndromes with hamartomatous polyps other than FAP, their patterns of inheritance, and the genes involved.

SYNDROME	PATTERN OF INHERITANCE	GENES INVOLVED
Peutz-Jeghers syndrome	• Autosomal dominant.	• *STK11/LKB1*.
Juvenile polyposis	• Autosomal dominant.	• *SMAD4, BMPR1A*.
Cowden syndrome	• Autosomal dominant.	• *PTEN*.
Tuberous sclerosis	• Autosomal dominant.	• *TSC1, TSC2*.

152. Name at least 2 nongastrointestinal neoplasms in Peutz-Jeghers syndrome.
- Breast carcinoma.
- Cervical gastric-type mucinous adenocarcinoma.
- Sex cord tumor with annular tubules.
- Sertoli cell tumor of the testis or ovary.

153. List the main nongastrointestinal causes of death in patients with FAP.
- Perioperative complications.
- Desmoid tumors.
- Suicide.

154. Outline the Amsterdam II criteria for the clinical identification of families with Lynch syndrome.
- Amsterdam II criteria:
  · At least 3 relatives with any Lynch-syndrome-associated cancer (at least 1 of whom is a first-degree relative).
  · At least 2 successive generations affected.
- At least 1 relative diagnosed before age 50.
- Exclusion of FAP.
- Verification of tumors by pathological examination.

155. Outline the revised Bethesda guidelines for MSI testing in colorectal tumors.
- Revised Bethesda guidelines:
  · Colorectal cancer (CRC) in patients < 50 years.
  · Synchronous or metachronous colorectal tumor or other Lynch-syndrome-associated tumor.
  · CRC with MSI-H-associated histologic features in patients < 60 years.
- CRC in patients with:
  › At least 1 first-degree relative with a Lynch-syndrome-associated tumor, with 1 of the cancers being diagnosed < 50 years.
  › At least 2 first- or second-degree relatives with Lynch – syndrome-associated tumor, regardless of age.

156. Outline the clinical criteria for the diagnosis of serrated polyposis.
- Criterion 1:
  · At least 5 serrated lesions and/or polyps are located proximal to the rectum.
  · All are ≥ 5 mm in size and at least 2 are ≥ 10 mm in size.
- Criterion 2:
  · More than 20 serrated lesions and/or polyps of any size are distributed throughout colon.
  › At least 5 are located proximal to the rectum.

157. List 2 carcinomas associated with hereditary diffuse gastric cancer syndrome.
- Diffuse-type gastric carcinoma.
- Invasive lobular breast carcinoma.

Case Scenario

Your lab receives a colon specimen that has many bluish macrophages and small dot-like organisms (*Isospora*) on the surface epithelium, and apoptotic bodies.

158. What is your differential diagnosis?
- *Mycobacterium avium-intracellulare* complex (MAC).
- Whipple disease.
- Isosporiasis.

159. What are the causative organisms for each of the diagnoses listed in the previous question?
- MAC: *Mycobacterium avium* and *Mycobacterium intracellulare*.
- Whipple disease: *Tropheryma whippeli*.
- Isosporiasis: *Isospora belli*.

160. Describe the clinical circumstances in which individuals can get infected with *Mycobacterium avium-intracellulare* complex, *Tropheryma whippeli*, or *Isospora belli*.
- *Mycobacteria avium* complex: usually through disseminated infections in immunocompromised patients, particularly in AIDS patients and transplant recipients.
- *Tropheryma whippeli*: through exposure of a susceptible host to this bacterium ubiquitously present in the environment (why certain people get infected while most do not develop an infection is still unknown).
- *Isospora belli*: through ingestion of the parasite's oocytes in contaminated water by immunocompromised patients, in particular AIDS patients.

161. Describe stains that can aid diagnosis for this case.

- Whipple disease results in coarse, granular PAS positive inclusions in macrophages that have large vacuoles, whereas PAS stain in MAC reveals faintly positive bacilli in macrophages.
- *Isospora* can be identified on a Giemsa stain as ovoid forms.
- Acid fast stains are positive in MAC, but negative in Whipple disease.

162. When do AIDS patients get MAC infection?

The risk of acquiring MAC infection increases drastically when the CD4 count drops below 50 cells/mm^3.

163. What other infections in the bowel can AIDS patients get?

- Bacterial:
  - *Clostridium difficile.*
  - Spirochetosis.
  - *Neisseria gonorrhea.*
  - *Mycobacteria tuberculosis.*
- Parasitic:
  - *Giardia lamblia.*
  - *Entamoeba histolytica.*
  - *Cryptosporidia.*
  - *Microsporidia.*
  - *Toxoplasma.*
- *Blastocystis hominis.*
- Fungal:
  - *Histoplasma capsulatum.*
  - *Candida.*
  - *Pneumocystis jiroveci.*
  - *Aspergillus fumigatus.*
  - *Cryptococcus neoformans.*
- Viral:
  - Cytomegalovirus (CMV).
  - Herpes simplex virus (HSV).
  - Epstein-Barr virus (EBV).

164. What gastrointestinal neoplasms can immunocompromised patients get?

- Esophageal carcinoma.
- Colorectal carcinoma.
- Lymphoma.
- Burkitt lymphoma.
- Diffuse large B-cell lymphoma.
- Kaposi sarcoma.

Case Scenario

The slide from an esophagus specimen of a 60-year-old male shows Barrett esophagus.

165. What are the mimickers of Barrett esophagus?

- Pseudo–goblet cells — gastric cardia glandular epithelium with mucin retention.
- Columnar blue cells.
- Submucosa glands/drainage ducts.
- Intestinal metaplasia of cardia mucosa.

166. How does mucin stain help to confirm a diagnosis of Barrett esophagus?

- Alcian blue/PAS (pH 2.5) stains intestinal type acidic mucin blue.
- Neutral mucins such as those expressed in gastric mucosa stain magenta.

167. What are some predisposing factors for Barrett esophagus?

- Gastresophageal reflux disease (GERD).
- Factors that predispose to GERD:
  - Alcohol intake.
  - Smoking.
- Obesity.
- Pregnancy.
- Hiatal hernia.

Case Scenario

The slide from a stomach specimen of a 72-year-old male shows pale eosinophilic extracellular amorphous material.

168. What is your differential diagnosis?

- Amyloidosis.
- Elastosis.
- Collagen deposition.
- Scarring.
- Fibrin deposition.

169. How do you confirm the diagnosis of amyloidosis?
- Examination of section stained with Congo red under polarized light — should fluoresce apple green.
- Cresyl violet.
- Immunohistochemical stain for amyloid.
- Electron microscopy — shows 10 nm wide fibrils in a "haystack" arrangement.
- Mass spectrometry — distinguishes AL from AA, etc.

170. Classify types of amyloids and their associations with disease.
- AA: amyloid associated protein (secondary).
  - Chronic inflammatory states.
- AL: light chain (primary).
  - Plasma cell neoplasm.
- A-β.
  - Alzheimer disease.
- Transthyretin (hereditary).
- Familial amyloid polyneuropathies.
- Senile systemic amyloidosis.
- β_2-microglobulin (dialysis associated).
  - Patients on long-term dialysis.
- Atrial natriuretic factor.
  - Isolated atrial amyloidosis.

171. Where is amyloidosis usually seen in the gastrointestinal tract?
- Tongue.
- Stomach.
- Rectal mucosa.

172. From where would you recommend taking a specimen for amyloid?
- Abdominal fat pad aspiration (90% sensitivity).
- Rectal biopsy (80% sensitivity).
- Tongue.
- Stomach.

173. What is amyloid composed of?
- Misfolded proteins which self-associate and aggregate, being deposited as fibrils.
  - The proteins may be normal proteins produced in higher-than-normal quantities, or mutant proteins, both of which have tendencies to misfold.
- The aggregates are resistant to breakdown by endogenous mechanisms.
- The specific protein varies depending on the clinical scenario.

174. What is the structure of amyloid and its appearance on electron microscopy?
- Structure: ß-pleated sheet.
- Appearance on electron microscopy (EM): nonbranching fibrils measuring 7.5–10 nm in diameter forming a "haystack."

175. What do you do if the stains are negative, but you are strongly suspicious of amyloid? What do you tell the clinician?
- Ensure the Congo red sections are cut at 6 microns and check the positive control.
- Check the positive controls for your other stains, such as cresyl violet.
- Submit some tissue for EM.
- Tell the clinician your differential diagnosis and ask for a repeat biopsy, and ensure that other serological and urine tests for plasma proteins have been done.

176. What other history should be obtained?
- Family history of amyloidosis.
- History of plasma cell neoplasm.
- History of renal failure and dialysis.
- History of chronic inflammatory conditions such as rheumatoid arthritis or inflammatory bowel disease.

Case Scenario

The slide for a 60-year-old male shows pseudomembranous colitis.

177. What is your differential diagnosis?
- Pseudomembranous colitis.
- Inflammatory bowel disease.
- Ischemic colitis.
- Infectious colitis.

178. What is the workup for this case?
- Check laboratory studies such as stool *Clostridium difficile* toxin assay.
- Examine stool for ova and parasites.
- Check recent travel history.
- Check history for recent antibiotic use.
- Check risk factors for bowel ischemia: atherosclerosis, athletes.
- Proceed with special stains such as PAS for amoeba.

179. What clinical tests should be performed?

- Stool should be sent for:
  - *C. difficile* toxin assay.
- Ova and parasite examination.

180. How do you approach an infectious autopsy?

- Check the history for identification of infectious organisms and check all available microbiological studies including cultures, PCR studies, and ELISA tests.
- Follow institutional policies regarding biological hazards, communication, and management if available.
- Communicate with local health authorities if the disease is reportable.
- If the biological hazard level is higher, or suspected to be higher, than the level for which the laboratory is accredited, send the autopsy to a site capable of handling the biohazard.
- Determine the manner of transmission of the infection to determine what personal protective equipment is required.
- If the infectious organism is unknown but is believed to be within the hazard level for which the laboratory is accredited, and/or the method of transmission is unknown, use the most stringent personal protective equipment available.
- Perform the autopsy with adequate personal protective equipment. Designate 1 individual as the "clean" investigator to take notes. Another individual should perform the autopsy in order to reduce transmission of infective materials and contamination.

Case Scenario

A 41-year-old female has a perforated appendix with a mass in the right lower quadrant. The slide shows a tumor with neuroendocrine and mucinous features.

181. What is the differential diagnosis?

- Goblet cell adenocarcinoma.
- Mucinous adenocarcinoma.
- Low grade and high grade mucinous neoplasm.
- Signet-ring cell carcinoma.
- Mixed neuroendocrine-nonneuroendocrine neoplasm.
- Neuroendocrine carcinoma.
- Metastatic mucinous adenocarcinoma.

182. Outline the steps of gross examination of an appendix containing a mucinous lesion.

- Measure the length and diameter range of the appendix, and the width of the mesoappendix.
- Describe the color and appearance of the serosa. Inspect the serosa for perforation and mucinous implants.
- Ink the appendiceal margin and the serosa.
- Make a longitudinal section of the tip and serially section the remainder of the appendix at 3 mm intervals.
- Measure and describe the location, color, and appearance of the lesion(s).
- Measure the wall thickness and describe the mucosa and luminal content.
- Submit the entire specimen, with the resection margin en face in a separate cassette.

183. What morphologic features are diagnostic of goblet cell adenocarcinoma?

Presence of goblet-like mucinous cells in tubules or clusters, intermixed with endocrine and Paneth-like cells.

184. Compare low grade and high grade histologic features in goblet cell adenocarcinoma.

- Low grade features: tubules or clusters of goblet-like mucinous cells, endocrine cells, Paneth-like cells.
- High grade features: mucinous or nonmucinous cells invading in single cell pattern or forming complex anastomosing tubules, cribriforming structures, and sheets; large aggregates of goblet-like cells or signet ring–like cells with high grade cytology, numerous mitoses with atypical mitotic figures and necrosis.

185. How do you grade this type of tumor histologically?

Based on proportion of low and high grade components.

GRADE	TUBULAR/CLUSTERED PATTERN	LOSS OF TUBULAR/CLUSTERED PATTERN
1	> 75%	< 25%
2	50–75%	25–50%
3	< 50%	> 50%

186. What histologic finding allows you to distinguish high grade goblet cell adenocarcinoma from signet-ring cell adenocarcinoma of appendix?

Presence of low grade goblet cell adenocarcinoma component.

187. How do you stage appendiceal carcinoma based on the AJCC staging manual?

pTX: tumor cannot be assessed.

pT0: no evidence of primary tumor.

pTis: carcinoma in situ or LAMN confined to muscularis propria.

pT1: tumor invades submucosa (not applicable to LAMN).

pT2: tumor invades muscularis propria (not applicable to LAMN).

pT3: tumor invades through muscularis propria into subserosa or mesoappendix (including acellular mucin or mucinous epithelium for LAMN).

pT4a: tumor invades through visceral peritoneum (including acellular mucin or mucinous epithelium in LAMN).

pT4b: tumor invades adjacent organs/structures.

pNX: regional lymph nodes cannot be assessed.

pN0: no regional lymph node metastasis.

pN1: 1–3 regional lymph node metastases or presence of tumor deposits in absence of positive lymph nodes.

pN1a: 1 regional lymph node metastasis.

pN1b: 2–3 regional lymph node metastases.

pN1c: tumor deposits in subserosa/mesentery in absence of positive lymph nodes.

pN2: ≥ 4 regional lymph node metastases.

pM0: no distant metastasis.

pM1: distant metastasis.

  pM1a: intraperitoneal acellular mucin.

  pM1b: intraperitoneal metastasis, including mucinous deposits with tumor cells.

  pM1c: metastasis to sites other than peritoneum.

188. What is the prognosis for this patient?
- The prognosis depends on tumor stage and grade.
- Low grade goblet cell adenocarcinomas are mostly present in early stages (I–II), with an overall survival of 84–204 months.
- High grade goblet cell adenocarcinomas are mostly present with stage IV disease, with an overall survival of 29–45 months.

Case Scenario

The slide of an anal resection for a 60-year-old male shows a small blue cell tumor.

189. List the primary anal tumors that can show this morphology.
- Squamous cell carcinoma, poorly differentiated.
- Basaloid squamous cell carcinoma (previously cloacogenic carcinoma).
- Neuroendocrine tumor.
- Basal cell carcinoma.
- Lymphoma.
- Melanoma.

190. What is the differential diagnosis of anal squamous cell carcinoma?
- Adenocarcinoma.
- Small cell carcinoma.
- Perianal tumor extending into the anal canal.
- Urothelial carcinoma.
- Melanoma.
- Adenosquamous carcinoma.
- Mucoepidermoid carcinoma.
- In situ neoplasm.

191. What immunostains do you use to sort out the small blue tumor differential?
- Cytokeratin.
- CD45.
- CD56.
- Synaptophysin.
- p63.
- p40.
- S100.
- SOX10.

Case Scenario

A slide shows a poorly differentiated carcinoma of the cecum.

192. List 3 possible entities to consider in your differential diagnosis.
- Colorectal adenocarcinoma.
- Gastrointestinal stromal tumor.
- Melanoma.

193. What ancillary tests would you order?

Immunohistochemistry stains for pancytokeratin, CD117, DOG-1, S100, SOX10.

194. What is microsatellite instability (MSI)? How is it detected?

- MSI: results from dysfunction of DNA mismatch repair genes including *MLH1*, *MSH2*, *MSH6*, and *PMS2*.
- Detection:
  - Testing by 4-antibody immunohistochemistry against *MLH1*, *MSH2*, *MSH6*, and *PMS2*.
- PCR based genotyping at these sites (depending on the clinical context).
- Testing for direct microsatellites by looking at 2 mononucleotide repeats (*BAT25*, *BAT26*) and 3 dinucleotide repeats (*D5S346*, *D2123*, *D17S250*).

195. Outline an algorithmic approach for colorectal cancer tumor testing for MSI/Lynch syndrome.

- Mismatch repair (MMR) protein IHC:
  - If MLH1 loss: BRAFV600E IHC or MLH1 hypermethylation testing.
    › If negative: germline testing.
  - If MSH2, MSH6 or PMS2 loss: germline testing.

196. Define Lynch syndrome.

Lynch syndrome: a hereditary disorder caused by germline mutation in a mismatch repair gene in which affected individuals have a higher-than-normal chance of developing colorectal cancer, endometrial cancer, and various other types of aggressive cancers, often at a young age.

College of American Pathologists (CAP) Protocols for Examining and Reporting Primary Carcinoma of the Colon and Rectum

197. What are the recommended reporting elements for polypectomy?

- Tumor site.
- Specimen integrity.
- Polyp size.
- Polyp configuration.
- Size of invasive carcinoma.
- Histologic type.
- Histologic grade.
- Microscopic tumor extension.
- Margins.
- Lymphovascular invasion.
- Tumor budding.
- Type of polyp in which the invasive carcinoma arose.
- Additional pathologic findings.
- Ancillary studies.

198. What are the recommended reporting elements for colon cancer resections?

- Procedure.
- Tumor site.
- Tumor location.
- Tumor size.
- Macroscopic tumor perforation.
- Macroscopic intactness of the mesorectum.
- Histologic type.
- Histologic grade.
- Microscopic tumor extension.
- Margins.
- Treatment effect (neoadjuvant therapy).
- Lymphovascular invasion.
- Perineural invasion.
- Tumor budding.
- Tumor deposits (discontinuous extramural extension).
- Type of polyp in which the invasive carcinoma arose.
- Regional lymph nodes.
- Pathologic staging (pTNM).
- Additional pathologic findings.
- Ancillary studies.

199. What do you do if 2 subsites of the colon are affected by a tumor?

- Tumors located at the border between 2 subsites of the colon (e.g., cecum and ascending colon) are registered as tumors of the subsite that is more involved.
- If 2 subsites are involved to the same extent, the tumor is classified as an "overlapping" lesion.

200. How can you say that you have transitioned from the sigmoid to the rectum? Describe the anatomic landmarks of the rectum.

- The tenia coli of the sigmoid fuse to form a circumferential longitudinal muscle of the rectal wall 12–15 cm from the dentate line.
- Clinically, the rectum commences opposite the sacral promontory and ends at the anorectal ring, which corresponds to the proximal border of the puborectalis muscle (palpable on digital rectal exam).

201. How do you classify a rectal tumor or a rectosigmoid tumor?

- A tumor is classified as rectal if:
  - Its inferior margin lies < 16 cm from the anal verge.
  - – or –
  - If any part of the tumor is located at least partly within the supply of the superior rectal artery.
- A tumor is classified as rectosigmoid when differentiation between the rectum and sigmoid according to the previously mentioned guidelines is not possible.

202. What are the histologic types of colorectal malignant epithelial tumors according to the WHO classification?

- Adenocarcinoma, NOS.
- Serrated adenocarcinoma.
- Adenoma-like adenocarcinoma.
- Micropapillary adenocarcinoma.
- Mucinous adenocarcinoma.
- Poorly cohesive carcinoma.
- Signet-ring cell carcinoma.
- Medullary adenocarcinoma.
- Adenosquamous carcinoma.
- Carcinomam undifferentiated, NOS.

- Carcinoma with sarcomatoid component.
- Neuroendocrine tumor (NET), NOS.
- NET grade 1.
- NET grade 2.
- NET grade 3.
- Neuroendocrine carcinoma (NEC), NOS:
  · Large cell NEC.
  · Small cell NEC.
- Mixed neuroendocrine-nonneuroendocrine neoplasm (MiNEN).

203. Which histologic types of carcinomas have been shown to have adverse prognostic significance independent of stage?

- Signet-ring cell carcinoma.

- Poorly differentiated neuroendocrine carcinomas (large and small cell).

204. What is the genetic abnormality associated with medullary carcinoma?

- Medullary carcinoma is a distinctive histologic type frequently associated with microsatellite instability (MSI-H), often with *BRAF* mutations.

- Medullary carcinoma may occur either sporadically or in association with Lynch syndrome.

205. What are the histologic characteristics of medullary carcinoma?

- Solid growth of malignant cells with ample eosinophilic cytoplasm, vesicular nuclei, prominent nucleoli.
- Numerous tumor-infiltrating lymphocytes and neutrophilic granulocytes.

- No immunohistochemical evidence of neuroendocrine differentiation.
- Aberrant loss of caudal-type homeobox 2 (CDX2) and cytokeratin 20 (CK20).

206. How are colorectal cancers graded?

- There is no single accepted standard.
- Most systems grade as follows:
  · Grade 1: well differentiated (> 95% gland formation).
  · Grade 2: moderately differentiated (50–95% gland formation).
  · Grade 3: poorly differentiated (< 50% gland formation).
  · Grade 4: undifferentiated (no gland formation or mucin; no squamous or neuroendocrine differentiation).

- The majority of studies on grading and the WHO classification use 2-tiered stratification:
  · Low grade: well-differentiated and moderately differentiated (≥ 50% gland formation).
  · High grade: poorly differentiated and undifferentiated (< 50% gland formation).
- By convention, signet-ring cell carcinomas, small cell carcinomas, and undifferentiated carcinomas are high grade.

207. In patients with lymphovascular invasion (LVI) and perineural invasion (PNI), what are independent indicators of unfavorable outcome?

- Venous, lymphatic, and perineural invasion are all independent indicators of poor prognosis.
- Invasion of extramural veins, in particular, has been shown to be an independent indicator of unfavorable outcome

and increased risk of the occurrence of hepatic metastasis. However, the significance of intramural venous invasion is less clear.

208. How is the quality of a mesorectal resection grossly assessed?

- Evaluate the distance between the tumor and closest margins (distal, proximal, and circumferential).
- Circumferentially examine the nonperitonealized surface of the fresh specimen to score the completeness of mesorectum according to the worst area.

- Assess specimen's bulk, the integrity of the surface, and the presence or absence of coning of the distal end of the mesorectum resection.

209. What does "incomplete mesorectal excision" mean?

- The mesorectum has little bulk.
- Defects in the mesorectum extend to the muscularis propria.

- After transverse sectioning, the circumferential margin appears very irregular.

210. What does "nearly complete mesorectal excision" mean?
- Moderate bulk to the mesorectum.
- Irregularity of the mesorectal surface with defects > 5 mm, but none extending to the muscularis propria.
- No areas of visibility of the muscularis propria except at the insertion site of the levator ani.

211. What does "complete mesorectal excision" mean?
- The mesorectum is intact and bulky with a smooth surface.
- The mesorectal surface has only minor irregularities.
- There are no surface defects > 5 mm in depth.
- There is no coning toward the distal margin of the specimen.
- After transverse sectioning, the circumferential margin appears smooth.

212. Why is it important to identify MSI-H tumors?
- They are a prognostic marker of patient outcome.
- They are a predictive marker of response to chemotherapy and immunotherapy.
- They are a screening tool for Lynch syndrome.

213. What are Lynch-associated tumors?
- Cancers of the stomach, small and large bowel, pancreas and hepatobiliary tract, endometrium and ovary, kidney, renal pelvis, ureter, bladder, and prostate.
- Brain tumors.
- Sebaceous skin tumors.

214. What is the Crohn disease–like peritumoral infiltrate?
- Lymphoid aggregates or follicles at the tumor's edge.
- Not associated with preexisting lymph nodes.

215. What types of tumor-infiltrating lymphocytes are of significance?
- Peritumoral infiltrates that resemble Crohn disease.
- 3 or more tumor-infiltrating lymphocytes per HPF using H&E stained sections.

216. What are MSI-H histologic features?
- Tumor-infiltrating lymphocytes.
- Crohn disease–like lymphocytic reaction.
- Mucinous/signet ring cell differentiation.
- Medullary growth pattern.
- Right-sided location.
- Intratumoral heterogeneity (mixed conventional, mucinous, and poorly differentiated).
- High grade histology.
- Lack of dirty necrosis.

217. What margins require assessment in colorectal specimens? How is the radial margin defined?
- Proximal.
- Distal.
- Circumferential (radial margin) — the adventitial soft tissue margin closest to the deepest penetration of the tumor and the margin created surgically by blunt or sharp dissection of the retroperitoneal or subperitoneal aspect, respectively.
- Mesenteric margin — only pertinent in segments completely encased by peritoneum.

218. What is usually inked in colorectal specimens?
- All margins.
- Any area of puckering on the serosal surface to facilitate the microscopic assessment of tumor perforation or serosa involvement.

219. Why is it important to assess the radial margin, especially in cases of rectal cancer?
- Multivariate analysis has suggested that tumor involvement of the circumferential (radial) margin is the most critical factor in predicting local recurrence in rectal cancer.
- A positive circumferential (radial) margin in rectal cancer increases the risk of recurrence by 3.5 times and doubles the risk of death from disease.

220. What is considered a negative versus a positive radial margin?
- Negative: tumor is > 1 mm from the inked nonperitonealized surface.
- Positive: tumor is located ≤ 1 mm from the nonperitonealized surface, because local recurrence rates are similar with clearances of 0–1 mm.
- This assessment includes tumors within a lymph node as well as direct tumor extension, but if circumferential margin positivity is based solely on an intranodal tumor, this should be stated.

221. What are considered adequate distal margins?
- Distal resection margin of 2 cm is considered adequate.
- For T1 and T2 tumors, 1 cm may be sufficient.
- Anastomotic recurrences are rare when the distance is ≥ 5 cm.

222. If there is carcinoma arising in inflammatory bowel disease, how should the resection margins be assessed?

- In addition to the same evaluation as for non-IBD associated colorectal carcinoma, the proximal and distal resection margins evaluated for:
  - · Dysplasia.
  - · Active inflammation.

223. How is treatment effect measured according to the modified Ryan scheme?

TUMOR REGRESSION GRADE	NUMBER OF VIABLE TUMOR CELLS
0: complete response	• No viable tumor cells.
1: moderate response	• Single or small groups of viable tumor cells.
2: partial response	• Residual cancer with evidence of tumor regression (more than single or small groups of viable tumor cells).
3: poor response	• Extensive residual cancer with no evidence of tumor regression.

224. How should you handle acellular pools of mucin? Should they be used for TNM staging?

- Acellular pools of mucin in specimens from patients receiving neoadjuvant therapy represent completely eradicated tumors.
- They are not used to assign pT stage or counted as positive lymph nodes.

225. What is considered a tumor deposit?

- A discrete tumor deposit separates from the leading edge of the tumor, located in pericolic or perirectal fat or in adjacent mesentery, within the territory of lymphatic drainage of the primary tumor.
  - · There is no evidence of residual lymph node tissue.
  - · There is no identifiable vascular or neural structure.

226. What is the significance of tumor deposits? How should they be reported?

- They are associated with reduced disease-free survival and overall survival.
- The number of tumor deposits should be recorded in the surgical pathology report.
- They should be classified as pN1c in the absence of unequivocal lymph node metastases.
- pN1c is usually an indication for adjuvant therapy irrespective of pT staging.
- They do not influence the pT staging.

227. What are the T categories in colorectal cancer?

pTX: tumor cannot be assessed.
pT0: no evidence of primary tumor.
pTis: carcinoma in situ.
pT1: tumor invades submucosa.
pT2: tumor invades muscularis propria.

pT3: tumor invades through the muscularis propria into pericolorectal tissues.
pT4: tumor invades visceral peritoneum or invades/adheres to adjacent organs/structures.
  pT4a: tumor penetrates the visceral peritoneum.
  pT4b: tumor directly invades or is adherent to other organs or structures.

228. What does "pTis" mean in colorectal carcinomas?

Cancer cells have crossed the basement membrane and invaded the lamina propria but not through the muscularis mucosae (intramucosal carcinoma).

229. How is pT4 evaluated?

- Direct invasion of other organs or structures including invasion of other segments of the colorectum by way of the serosa or mesocolon (e.g., invasion of the sigmoid colon by carcinoma of the cecum) is classified as pT4b.
- A tumor that is adherent to other organs or structures macroscopically is classified clinically as cT4. However, if no tumor is found within the adhesion microscopically, the tumor should be classified as T3.
- For rectal tumors, invasion of the external sphincter and/or the levator ani is classified as T4b.

230. When is the peritoneum considered involved?

- When tumors that are present at the serosal surface with an inflammatory reaction, mesothelial hyperplasia, and/or erosion/ulceration.
- When free tumor cells are present on the serosal surface (in the peritoneum) with underlying ulceration of the visceral peritoneum.
- When tumor cells directly extend through a perforation to reach the serosal surface.

231. Why is it important to report penetration of the peritoneum?

Although both visceral peritoneal involvement (T4a) and invasion of adjacent structures (T4b) are associated with decreased survival, invasion limited to the visceral peritoneum has a 10–20% better 5-year survival than locally invasive carcinomas.

232. How are lymph nodes staged in colorectal carcinomas?

pNX: cannot be assessed.

pN0: no regional lymph node metastasis.

pN1: 1–3 regional lymph node metastases or presence of tumor deposit(s).

  pN1a: 1 regional lymph node metastasis.

  pN1b: 2–3 regional lymph node metastases.

pN1c: tumor deposit(s) in the subserosa, mesentery or nonperitonealized pericolic or perirectal tissues in absence of regional lymph node metastasis.

pN2: ≥ 4 regional lymph node metastases.

  pN2a: 4–6 regional lymph node metastases.

  pN2b: ≥ 7 regional lymph node metastases.

233. What are the regional lymph nodes for the anatomic subsites?

- Cecum: pericolic, ileocolic, right colic.
- Ascending colon: pericolic, ileocolic, right colic, right branch of middle colic.
- Hepatic flexure: pericolic, ileocolic, middle colic, right colic.
- Transverse colon: pericolic, middle colic.
- Splenic flexure: pericolic, middle colic, left colic.

- Descending colon: pericolic, left colic, inferior mesenteric, sigmoid.
- Sigmoid colon: pericolic, sigmoid, inferior mesenteric, superior rectal.
- Rectosigmoid: pericolic, sigmoid, superior rectal.
- Rectum: mesorectal, superior rectal, inferior mesenteric, internal iliac, inferior rectal.

234. What is the pM staging?

pM1a: metastasis to single organ/site (e.g., liver, lung, ovary, nonregional lymph node) without peritoneal metastasis.

pM1b: metastasis to ≥ 2 organs/sites without peritoneal metastasis.

pM1c: metastasis to the peritoneal surface is identified alone or with metastasis from other organ/site.

235. For rectal cancers, which lymph nodes are considered distant metastases?

Metastases in the external iliac or common iliac lymph nodes are classified as a distant metastasis.

236. What is the suggested minimum number of lymph nodes that should be submitted for microscopic examination in colorectal carcinomas? How are the nodes submitted?

- The recommended minimum target is 12 lymph nodes.
- The greater the number of nodes examined, the greater the likelihood that metastasis will be found, suggesting that if fewer than 12 lymph nodes are found, re-examining the specimen for additional lymph nodes, with or without visual enhancement techniques, should be considered.

- All grossly negative or equivocal lymph nodes are to be submitted entirely: colorectal cancer is often found in small lymph nodes (< 5 mm in diameter).
- Grossly positive lymph nodes may be partially submitted for microscopic confirmation of metastasis.

237. What factors affect the number of nodes recovered?

- Surgical technique.
- Surgery volume.

- Patient factors (e.g., age and anatomic variation, obesity, neoadjuvant therapy).
- Diligence and skill of the pathologist in identifying and harvesting lymph nodes in the resection specimen.

238. How are micrometastasis and isolated tumor cells defined? How are they staged?

- A micrometastasis is defined as a nodal metastatic deposit measuring > 0.2 mm and ≤ 2.0 mm in its greatest dimension. A lymph node containing a micrometastasis is considered positive and is classified as pN1. A designation of pN1mi can be used but is not mandatory.

- Isolated tumor cells (ITCs) are defined as single tumor cells or small clusters of tumor cells measuring ≤ 0.2 mm, usually found by special techniques such as immunohistochemical staining. A lymph node containing ITCs is considered negative and is classified as N0. The number of lymph nodes involved by ITCs should be reported.

CAP Protocol for Reporting Biomarker Results of Colorectal Carcinoma

239. What is the staining pattern for DNA MMR expression?
- Intact nuclear staining is the normal pattern for MMR protein expression.
- Complete loss of nuclear staining is required to interpret the test as abnormal.
- Nuclear staining in background nonneoplastic tissue, such as in lymphocytes, is used as an internal control to make sure the IHC is satisfactory.

240. What are the possible IHC results for MMR and their risk for MSI?
- No loss of nuclear expression of MMR proteins; low probability MSI-H.
- Loss of nuclear expression of *MLH1* and *PMS2* (testing for *MLH1* promoter methylation and/or *BRAF* mutation should follow: presence of *BRAF* V600E and/or *MLH1* methylation favors sporadic tumor; absence of *BRAF* V600E and *MLH1* methylation suggests possible Lynch syndrome).
- Loss of nuclear expression of *MSH2* and *MSH6*; high probability of Lynch syndrome.
- Loss of nuclear expression of *MSH6* only; high probability of Lynch syndrome.
- Loss of nuclear expression of *PMS2* only; high probability of Lynch syndrome.

241. What is the recommended next step if loss of nuclear expression of *MLH1* and *PMS2* is found?
- Testing for methylation of the *MLH1* promoter and/or *BRAF* mutation.
- Genetic testing of the *MLH1* gene (this can be considered in at-risk patients — e.g., < 50 years old, 1 first-degree relative with colorectal or endometrial cancer).

242. What does the *BRAF* V600E mutation or *MLH1* methylation imply in MMR testing?
- The presence of a *BRAF* V600E mutation and/or *MLH1* methylation suggests that the tumor is sporadic and germline evaluation is probably not indicated.
- Absence of both *MLH1* methylation and *BRAF* V600E mutation suggests Lynch syndrome; sequencing and/or large deletion/duplication testing of germ line *MLH1* may be indicated.

243. What is the recommended next step if MSH2 and MSH6 IHC shows negative nuclear staining?
Sequencing and/or large deletion/duplication testing of germline *MSH2*; if negative, sequencing and/or large deletion/duplication testing of germline *MSH6*.

244. What is the recommended next step if only MSH6 IHC shows negative nuclear staining?
Sequencing and/or large deletion/duplication testing of germ line *MSH6*.

245. What is the recommended next step if only PMS2 IHC shows negative nuclear staining?
Sequencing and/or large deletion/duplication testing of germline *PMS2*.

246. What are microsatellite islands? What happens when the MMR genes are defective?
- Microsatellite islands are short, repeated nucleotide sequences that are virtually unique for each individual.
- The repeated sequences are 4–5 nucleotides in length and the lengths (number of repeats) are also unique.
- Mistakes are usually made in these during DNA replication; mismatch repair enzymes can correct these mistakes.
- Defective MMR genes produce enzymes that cannot repair nucleotide mismatches during replication, which leads to microsatellite instability and changes in the numbers of repeated sequences.
- In addition to affecting the microsatellite islands, defects in MMR lead to the accelerated accumulation of mutations that can affect critical genes in malignant progression.

247. How is MSI assessment performed?
- The National Cancer Institute (NCI) recommends the assessment of 5 microsatellite markers:
  · These need to include 3 dinucleotide (which may have lower sensitivity and specificity) and 2 mononucleotide repeats.
  · Many labs use a commercial kit that includes 5 mononucleotide repeats.
  · Possible markers include BAT-25, BAT-26, NR-21, NR-24, Mono-27, D2S123, D5S346, and D17S250.
- PCR based methods using either isotopes or fluorescence primers are used to detect markers.
- Multiple peaks (multiple lengths of PCR products due to variable number of repeats) suggest microsatellite instability at that marker.
- False negatives can occur with contamination of noncancer cells (therefore you need at least 70% cancer cells).

248. How are the results of MSI interpreted?
- MSI–stable (MSS).
- MSI–low (MSI-L):
  · Instability exhibited in 1–29% of the NCI or mononucleotide markers.
  · Instability exhibited in 1 of the NCI or mononucleotide markers.
- MSI–high (MSI-H):
  · Instability exhibited in ≥ 30% of the NCI or mononucleotide markers.
  · Instability exhibited in ≥ 2 of the NCI or mononucleotide markers.
- MSI cannot be determined.

249. What does *MLH1* promoter methylation imply?

In contrast to loss of expression due to a germline mutation as seen in Lynch syndrome, loss of expression of *MLH1* in sporadic MSI-H colorectal carcinomas typically occurs due to methylation of the *MLH1* promoter region.

250. What are some of the methods used to obtain DNA for molecular pathology from slides/blocks?
- Laser capture microdissection.
- Manual under microscopic observation.
- Manual without microscopic observation.
- Cored from a block.
- Whole tissue section.

251. What are some of the methods that can be used for mutation analysis?
- IHC (BRAF and PTEN).
- Nucleotide based:
  · Direct (Sanger) sequencing.
  · Pyrosequencing.
  · High resolution melting analysis.
- PCR, allele specific hybridization.
- Real-time PCR.
- Duplication/deletion testing (via multiplex ligation-dependent probe assay [MLPA]).
- Whole exome/genome sequencing.

252. Why is it important to detect Lynch syndrome?
- It accounts for 2–3% of all colorectal carcinomas.
- It increases the risks of certain cancers:
  · Colorectal carcinoma (80%).
  · Endometrial carcinoma (60%).
  · Ovarian carcinoma (12%).
  · Stomach, pancreaticobiliary, urothelial carcinoma (inverted growth), kidney, small bowel, brain, skin (sebaceous adenomas and carcinomas and keratoacanthomas: Muir-Torre syndrome).
- It has clinical implications for treatment of the affected patient and family members.

253. What are the possible causes of an MSI-H result?
- Germline mutation in 1 of the MMR genes (Lynch syndrome):
  · MLH1.
  · MSH2.
  · MSH6.
  · PMS2.
- Germline mutation in genes adjacent to the MMR genes (Lynch syndrome):
  · *EPCAM* (affects *MSH2*).
  · *LRRFIP2* (affects *MLH1*).
- Hypermethylation of the *MLH1* promoter (15% of sporadic colorectal carcinomas).

254. How do you interpret discordant results between molecular and IHC (e.g., MSI-H PCR results with normal IHC; or abnormal IHC but MSS)?
- Normal IHC but MSI-H PCR:
  · Specimen mix-up.
  · Technical factors such as improper tissue fixation and inadequate antigen retrieval, which can affect immunohistochemical staining.
  · Missense mutation (especially in *MLH1*) that can lead to a nonfunctional protein but retained antigenicity (5% of families).
  · Defects in lesser-known MMR enzymes (rare).
- Abnormal IHC but MSS PCR:
  · Contamination with normal cells.
  · Specimen mix-up.
  · Suboptimal IHC (check the internal positive control).
  · Possible loss of MSH6 IHC staining in cases with prior chemotherapy or radiotherapy.
  · Possible absence of MSI-H in patients with germline *MSH6* mutations.

255. What is considered a positive IHC (normal) pattern of expression?
- Any positive reaction in the nuclei of tumor cells is considered as intact expression (normal).
- It is common for intact staining to be somewhat patchy.
- An interpretation of expression loss in tumor cells should be made only if a positive reaction is seen in internal control cells, such as the nuclei of stromal, inflammatory, or nonneoplastic epithelial cells.

256. What are the implications of *KRAS* mutations?
- *RAS* mutations have been shown to be associated with a lack of clinical response to targeted EGFR therapies (cetuximab and panitumumab).
- Current recommendations from the American Society of Clinical Oncology (ASCO) state that all patients considered for anti-EGFR therapy should be tested.
- Mutational analysis should include *KRAS* and *NRAS* codons 12, 13, 61, 117, and 146.

257. What are the implications of *BRAF* mutations?
- *MLH1* promoter hypermethylation is believed to cause defective mismatch repair in sporadic carcinomas.
- In tumors with *MLH1* promoter hypermethylation, 70% carry the *BRAF* V600E mutation, but not in Lynch associated cancers with *MLH1* or *MSH2* mutations.
- If there is MSI-H with loss of *MLH1*, it may be more cost effective to test for *MLH1* promoter hypermethylation and/
- or test for the *BRAF* V600E mutation rather than performing germ line genetic testing.
- They have been associated with *PMS2* mutations.
- The *BRAF* mutation has been associated with limited clinical response to EGFR-targeted therapies (cetuximab or panitumumab).

258. What are the implications of *PIK3CA* mutations?
- *PIK3CA* mutations activate the *PI3K-PTEN-AKT* pathway that is downstream from both the EGFR and the *RAS-RAF-MAPK* pathways.
- AKT activation plays an important role in carcinogenesis, *KRAS* mutation, and MSI.
- In *KRAS*-wild type colorectal carcinomas, *PIK3CA* mutations may be associated with worse clinical outcome and negatively predict response to anti-EGFR therapy.
- Mutation of exon 20 is associated with lack of cetuximab activity in *KRAS* wild type tumors and a shorter median progression-free survival and overall survival.
- Mutations in exon 9 are associated with *KRAS* mutations and do not have an independent effect on cetuximab efficacy.
- *PIK3CA* mutations may also positively predict response to acetylsalicylic acid.

259. What are the implications of *PTEN* mutations?
- *PTEN* loss occurs in 19–36% of colorectal cancer.
- The impact of *PTEN* loss in colorectal cancer prognosis and therapy is unclear.
- It has a possible effect on the response rate and survival or progression-free survival.
- Loss of *PTEN* expression may negatively predict response to cetuximab, although data remains inconclusive.
- There is no standard method for *PTEN* analysis.
- *PTEN* mutations occur with *KRAS*, *BRAF*, and *PIK3CA* mutations.

260. What are the implications of c-Met overexpression?
- c-Met is a receptor tyrosine kinase that is frequently overexpressed in colorectal carcinomas.
- *MET* copy-number gains or *MET* exon 14 skipping mutations may predict response to c-Met inhibitors.

CAP Protocols for Examining and Reporting Gastrointestinal Stromal Tumors (GISTs)

261. What elements should be included when reporting GIST?
- Procedure.
- Tumor site.
- Tumor size.
- Tumor focality.
- Histologic subtype.
- Mitotic rate.
- Necrosis.
- Histologic grade.
- Risk assessment.
- Margins.
- Pathologic staging (pTNM).
- Ancillary studies.
- Preresection treatment effect.

262. How are mitoses assessed in GIST?
- Count per 5 mm^2.
- With the use of older model microscopes, 50 HPF is equivalent to 5 mm^2. Most modern microscopes with wider x40 lenses/fields require only 20 HPF to embrace 5 mm^2.

263. At which location of the gastrointestinal tract does GIST have the best prognosis?
Stomach.

264. How is the grade determined in GIST?
- It is based solely on mitotic count:
  - GX: grade cannot be assessed.
- G1: low grade; mitotic rate ≤ 5/5 mm^2.
- G2: high grade; mitotic rate > 5/5 mm^2.

265. Is lymphadenectomy required in staging GIST? Explain.

No, GISTs rarely metastasize to lymph nodes. Consequently, lymphadenectomy is unnecessary (with the rare exception of clinically suspicious lymph nodes).

266. What immunohistochemistry is usually performed in the context of GIST? For each marker, what is the likelihood of a positive result?
- c kit (positive in 95% of GISTs).
- DOG1 (positive in 99% of GISTs).
- CD34 (positive in 70% of GISTs).
- Smooth muscle actin (positive in 30–40%).
- SDHB (negative in 5–10% of GISTs).
- Less common:
  - S100 (5% are positive, usually focal).
  - Desmin (5% are positive, usually focal).
  - Keratin (1–2% are positive, weak/focal).

Note: loss of SDHB suggests a genetic defect in 1 of the SDH-related genes and is seen in SDH-deficient neoplasms.

267. List molecular genetic studies that should be carried out in the context of GIST and what is their clinical significance?
- *KIT* mutations are seen in 75% of GISTs.
  - Exons 9, 11, 13, and 17 are usually tested.
  - Exon 11 responds to imatinib.
  - Exon 9 has poor response to imatinib: may benefit from higher dose or an alternative tyrosine kinase inhibitor (e.g., sunitinib).
- Exon 13, 14, 17 (and 18) confer acquired resistance to imatinib.
- *PDGFRa* mutations are seen in 10% of GISTs.
  - Exons 12, 14, and 18 are usually tested.
  - Exon 18 confers primary resistance to imatinib.
- Other mutations that can be tested: *BRAF, SDHA/B/C/D, NF1*.

268. What molecular alterations are associated with best and worst clinical outcome in GISTs?
- Best clinical outcome: *PDGFRa* exon 12, *BRAF, KIT* exon 11 mutations.
- Worst clinical outcome: *KIT* exon 9, *KIT* exon 11, *PDGFRa* exon 18.

CAP Protocols for Examining and Reporting Carcinoma of the Ampulla of Vater

269. What elements need to be reported for carcinoma of ampulla of Vater?
- Procedure.
- Tumor site.
- Tumor size.
- Histologic type.
- Histologic grade.
- Microscopic tumor extension.
- Margin.
- Lymphovascular space invasion.
- Perineural invasion.
- Regional lymph nodes.
- Pathologic staging (pTNM).
- Additional pathologic findings.
- Ancillary studies.

270. What tumor sites need to be distinguished for ampullary adenocarcinoma and how are they defined?
- Intraampullary: within the duct lined by pancreaticobiliary-type epithelium.
- Periampullary: on the duodenal surface of the papilla.

271. What are the possible histologic types?
- Adenocarcinoma, NOS.
  - Intestinal-type adenocarcinoma.
  - Pancreatobiliary-type.
  - Tubular adenocarcinoma with mixed features.
- Mucinous adenocarcinoma.
- Signet-ring cell carcinoma or poorly cohesive cell carcinoma.
- Medullary carcinoma, NOS.
- Adenosquamous carcinoma.
- Neuroendocrine carcinoma, NOS.
  - Large cell neuroendocrine carcinoma.
  - Small cell neuroendocrine carcinoma.
- Mixed neuroendocrine-nonneuroendocrine neoplasm (MiNEN).
- Undifferentiated carcinoma.

272. What are the margins on a Whipple specimen?
- Proximal margin (stomach or duodenum).
- Distal margin (duodenum or jejunum).
- Common bile duct margin.
- Uncinate process (retroperitoneal) margin.
- Pancreatic parenchymal resection margin.

273. Define the pT staging for carcinoma of the ampulla of Vater.

pTX: tumor cannot be assessed.

pT0: no evidence of primary tumor.

pTis: carcinoma in situ.

pT1a: tumor limited to the ampulla of Vater or the sphincter of Oddi.

pT1b: tumor invades beyond the sphincter of Oddi (perisphincteric invasion) and/or into the duodenum submucosa.

pT2: tumor invades the muscularis propria of the duodenum.

pT3a: tumor directly invades the pancreas up to 0.5 cm.

pT3b: tumor invades the pancreas > 0.5 cm or extends into peripancreatic or periduodenal tissue or duodenal serosa, but without involvement of the celiac axis or superior mesenteric artery.

pT4: tumor with vascular involvement of the superior mesentery artery, celiac axis, and/or common hepatic artery.

274. Which nodes are considered regional and how are they broadly categorized?
- Superior: superior to the head, body, and tail of the pancreas.
- Inferior: inferior to the head, body, and tail of the pancreas.
- Anterior: anterior pancreaticoduodenal, pyloric, and proximal mesenteric.
- Posterior: posterior pancreaticoduodenal, common bile duct, pericholedochal and proximal mesenteric.
- Also: hepatic artery, infrapyloric, subpyloric, celiac, superior mesenteric, retroperitoneal, and lateral aortic.

275. What is the suggested minimum number of lymph nodes that should be submitted for microscopic examination in a Whipple specimen?

The recommended minimum target is 12 lymph nodes.

276. How do you define well, moderately and poorly-differentiated carcinoma of the ampulla of Vater?
- Well-differentiated: > 95% of tumor composed of glands.
- Moderately differentiated: 50–95% of tumor composed of glands.
- Poorly differentiated: < 49% of tumor composed of glands.

277. Where do most local recurrences occur within the region of the pancreatic head?

Most recur at the uncinate margin (retroperitoneal margin). Therefore, this is a critical margin and the closest tumor should be carefully submitted.

278. How is noninvasive ampullary carcinoma with papillary growth pattern classified in terms of T staging?

It is staged as pTis.

279. Should multiple levels or special stains be done for routine examination of lymph nodes?

Data are currently insufficient to recommend any special measures to detect micrometastases or isolated tumor cells in lymph nodes.

CAP Protocols for Examining and Reporting Carcinoma of the Anus

280. What elements are needed in the report?
- Procedure.
- Tumor site.
- Tumor size.
- Histologic type.
- Histologic grade.
- Microscopic tumor extension.
- Margins status.
- Treatment effect.
- Regional lymph nodes.
- Pathologic staging (pTNM).
- Additional pathologic findings.
- Ancillary studies.

281. Why is it important to properly document the tumor site?
- There is a difference in staging between cancers of the anal canal and the rectum or the perianal skin.
- The regional lymph nodes at risk for metastasis are different for different sites.

282. What is the most commonly used anatomic definition of the anal canal?
- The surgical definition is the most widely used and accepted.
- The anal canal begins at the point where the rectum enters the puborectalis sling at the apex of the anal sphincter complex. Termination of the anal canal is defined as the junction of the distal squamous mucosa of the anal canal with the perianal hair-bearing skin.

283. What are the 3 epithelial zones found in the anal canal?
- The narrow zone of rectal type glandular mucosa.
- The anal transition zone of variable length between the glandular and squamous mucosa (which may contain multilayered transitional mucosa resembling squamous metaplasia or urothelium at the dentate line; anal glands may be found in the submucosa).
- The squamous epithelial mucosa zone lacking skin appendages.

284. How do you distinguish tumors of the anal canal from tumors of the perianal region?
- Tumors are classified as anal canal tumors if they arise from the anal canal and cannot be visualized entirely by traction on buttocks.
- Tumors are classified as perianal if they 1) arise from skin at, or distal to, the squamous mucocutaneous junction; 2) can be visualized entirely by traction on buttocks; and 3) are located within 5 cm of the anus.

285. What is the WHO classification of malignant epithelial tumors of the anal canal?
- Squamous cell carcinoma, NOS.
  - Verrucous squamous cell carcinoma.
- Adenocarcinoma, NOS.
- Neuroendocrine tumor (NET), NOS.
  - NET, grade 1.
  - NET, grade 2.
- NET, grade 3.
- Neuroendocrine carcinoma (NEC), NOS.
  - Large cell NEC.
  - Small cell NEC.
- Mixed neuroendocrine-nonneuroendocrine neoplasm (MiNEN).

286. What is the histologic type of most tumors of the anal canal?
Squamous cell carcinoma.

287. Which histological features are related to high-risk human papillomavirus infection?
- Basaloid features.
- Small tumor cell size.

288. Name 2 variants of squamous cell carcinoma that have a different prognosis than typical squamous cell carcinoma (SCC).
- Verrucous carcinoma: better prognosis compared to SCC, NOS.
- Squamous cell carcinoma with mucinous microcysts (cystic spaces containing Alcian blue or PAS positive mucin): worse prognosis compared to SCC, NOS.

289. How does verrucous carcinoma compare to SCC, NOS with respect to HPV status?
- Verrucous carcinoma is mostly associated with low-risk HPVs (types 6, 11).
- SCC, NOS is mostly associated with high-risk HPVs (type 16).

290. Name 2 aggressive tumor types with poor prognosis (classified as grade 4) found in the anal canal.
- Small cell carcinoma.
- Anaplastic (undifferentiated) carcinoma.

291. What is the pT staging for carcinoma of the anal canal?
pTX: tumor cannot be assessed.
pT0: no evidence of primary tumor.
pTis: high grade squamous intraepithelial lesion.
pT1: tumor ≤ 2 cm.
pT2: tumor > 2 cm and ≤ 5 cm.
pT3: tumor > 5 cm.
pT4: tumor of any size that invades adjacent organs (vagina, urethra, bladder).

Note: invasion of the rectal wall, perianal skin, subcutaneous tissue or sphincter muscle are not classified as pT4.

292. What are the regional lymph nodes for anal carcinoma?
- Mesorectal.
- Superior rectal (hemorrhoidal).
- External iliac.
- Internal iliac (hypogastric).
- Inguinal (superficial and deep).

293. What is the pN classification for carcinoma of the anal canal?

pN0: no regional lymph node metastasis.

pN1: metastasis in inguinal, mesorectal, internal iliac or external iliac lymph nodes.

   pN1a: metastasis in inguinal, mesorectal, or internal iliac lymph nodes.

pN1b: metastasis in external iliac lymph nodes.

pN1c: metastasis in external iliac with any N1a lymph nodes.

294. What type of cancer has been reported in the setting of chronic anorectal fistulae in long-standing Crohn disease?

- Adenocarcinoma has been reported.
- A link between longstanding perianal Crohn disease and squamous cell carcinoma has also been reported, although not confirmed in large-scale studies.

295. Which IHC can be used to distinguish poorly differentiated squamous cell carcinoma of the anal canal and anal gland carcinoma, and what is the expected staining?

- Squamous cell carcinoma: positive for CK7, CK5/6, p53, and p63; negative for CK20.
- Anal gland carcinoma: positive for CK7, and MUC5AC; negative for CK5/6, p63, and CK20.

296. Which IHC can be used to differentiate primary anal Paget disease from secondary Paget disease of the perianal area associated with colorectal carcinoma?

- Primary anal Paget disease (intraepithelial carcinoma with perianal skin appendage differentiation): positive for gross cystic disease fluid protein 15 (GCDFP-15) and CK7; negative for CK20 and CDX2.
- Secondary anal Paget disease (underlying colorectal adenocarcinoma): positive for CK20, CDX2, often also CK7; negative for GCDFP-15.

CAP Protocols for Examining and Reporting Pancreaticoduodenectomy (Whipple) and Small Bowel Resection

297. Define the radial margin in small bowel resections and pancreaticoduodenectomy (Whipple procedure).

- For segmental small bowel resections, margins include the proximal, distal, and mesenteric margins of resection. For all small bowel segments, except the duodenum, the mesenteric resection margin is the only pertinent radial margin.
- For pancreaticoduodenectomy specimens of carcinomas of the duodenum, the nonperitonealized surface of the uncinate process constitutes a deep radial (nonperitonealized soft tissue) margin.
  - In such specimens, the proximal margin of stomach or duodenum (pylorus-sparing Whipple resection) and the distal resection margin of the duodenum are more biologically relevant than in pancreaticoduodenectomy procedures performed for pancreatic carcinoma and should always be sampled.

298. Describe pT3 and pT4 small bowel tumors.

- pT3: tumor invades through the muscularis propria into the subserosa or into the nonperitonealized perimuscular tissue (mesentery or retroperitoneum) without serosal penetration.
- pT4: tumor perforates the visceral peritoneum or directly invades other organs or structures (including other loops of small and/or large bowel, mesentery, abdominal wall by way of serosa; and for duodenum only — invasion of the pancreas or bile duct).

299. Name common tumor types in the small bowel.

- Adenocarcinomas (24–44%).
- Low grade neuroendocrine tumors (20–42%).
- Lymphoma (12%–27%).
- Gastrointestinal stromal tumors (7–9%).

300. What grades are assigned to signet-ring cell carcinoma and small cell carcinoma in the small bowel?

- By convention, signet-ring cell carcinoma is always assigned grade 3.
- By convention, small cell neuroendocrine carcinoma and undifferentiated carcinoma are assigned grade 4.

301. List the predisposing factors for small bowel adenocarcinoma.

- Crohn disease.
- Celiac disease.
- Ileal conduits and reservoirs.
- Inherited polyposis syndromes:
  - Familial adenomatous polyposis.
  - Peutz-Jeghers syndrome.
- Lynch syndrome.

CAP Protocols for Examining and Reporting Carcinoma of the Stomach

302. What are recommended reported elements for local resection?

- Procedure.
- Tumor site.
- Tumor size.
- Histologic type (Lauren classification or WHO).
- Histologic grade.
- Microscopic extent of tumor.
- Margins.
- Treatment effect.
- Lymphovascular invasion.
- Perineural invasion.
- Regional lymph nodes.
- Pathologic staging (pTNM).
- Additional pathologic findings.
- Ancillary studies.

303. What anatomical subsites do you use for reporting stomach cancer?

- Gastric region: cardia (including EGJ), fundus, body, antrum, pylorus.
- Greater curvature, lesser curvature.
- Anterior wall, posterior wall.

304. How is gastric carcinoma of proximal stomach distinguished from EGJ carcinoma?

- If the tumor involves the EGJ and its epicenter is located > 2 cm into the proximal stomach, it is defined as gastric carcinoma.
- If it does not involve the EGJ and its epicenter is located ≤ 2 cm into the proximal stomach, it is defined as gastric carcinoma.
- If it involves the EGJ and its epicenter is located ≤ 2 cm into the proximal stomach, it is defined as EGJ carcinoma.

305. What is the Siewert classification of adenocarcinomas of the EGJ?

- Type I: adenocarcinoma of the distal esophagus, with or without infiltration of the EGJ from above (tumor epicenter is 1–5 cm above the EGJ).
- Type II: true carcinoma of the gastric cardia arising from the cardiac epithelium or short segments with intestinal metaplasia at the EGJ (tumor epicenter is within 1 cm above and 2 cm below the EGJ).
- Type III: subcardial gastric carcinoma, which infiltrates the EGJ and distal esophagus from below (tumor epicenter is between 2–5 cm below EGJ).

306. What are histologic types of gastric neuroendocrine carcinoma based on the WHO classification?

- Large cell neuroendocrine carcinoma.
- Small cell neuroendocrine carcinoma.
- Mixed neuroendocrine-nonneuroendocrine neoplasm.

307. List the malignant epithelial tumors of stomach based on the WHO classification.

- Adenocarcinoma, NOS.
  - Tubular adenocarcinoma.
  - Parietal cell carcinoma.
  - Adenocarcinoma with mixed subtypes.
  - Papillary adenocarcinoma, NOS.
  - Micropapillary carcinoma, NOS.
  - Mucoepidermoid carcinoma.
  - Mucinous adenocarcinoma.
  - Signet-ring cell carcinoma.
  - Poorly cohesive carcinoma.
  - Medullary carcinoma with lymphoid stroma.
  - Hepatoid adenocarcinoma.
  - Paneth cell carcinoma.
- Squamous cell carcinoma, NOS.
- Adenosquamous carcinoma.
- Carcinoma, undifferentiated, NOS.
- Gastroblastoma.
- Neuroendocrine tumor (NET), NOS.
  - NET, grade 1.
  - NET, grade 2.
  - NET, grade 3.
- Neuroendocrine carcinoma (NEC), NOS.
  - Large cell NEC.
  - Small cell NEC.
- Mixed neuroendocrine-nonneuroendocrine neoplasm (MiNEN).

308. What is the Lauren classification?

- Intestinal type.
- Diffuse type (signet-ring cell carcinoma if > 50% signet ring cells).
- Mixed (approximately equal amounts of intestinal and diffuse).

309. Does differentiating tumor types have prognostic value?

- Small cell neuroendocrine carcinoma of the stomach has an unfavorable prognosis.
- Otherwise, most multivariate analyses show no effect of tumor type, independent of stage, on prognosis.

310. What are benign epithelial tumors and precursors of stomach carcinoma based on the WHO classification?
- Glandular intraepithelial neoplasia, low and high grade.
- Intestinal-type adenoma, low and high grade.
- Adenomatous polyp, low and high grade.

311. What is the histologic grading for adenocarcinomas?
- Grade X: cannot be assessed.
- Grade 1: well-differentiated (> 95% of the tumor is composed of glands).
- Grade 2: moderately differentiated (50–95% of the tumor is composed of glands).
- Grade 3: poorly differentiated (≤ 49% of the tumor is composed of glands).
  - Signet-ring cell carcinomas, undifferentiated carcinoma (grouped with poorly differentiated carcinomas), and small cell neuroendocrine carcinomas are classified as grade 3.

312. What is the impact of grade?
- Grade has been shown to have little impact on survival for patients undergoing complete tumor resection.
- Grade has a significant impact on margin-negative resectability, with higher grade tumors less likely to be resectable.

313. What are the margins in gastric resection specimens?
- Proximal resection margin.
- Distal resection margin.
- Radial margins: nonperitonealized soft tissue margins closest to the deepest penetration of tumor.
  - In the stomach, these are:
    › The lesser omental (hepatoduodenal and hepatogastric ligaments) margin.
    › The greater omental resection margin.
  - In endoscopic resections, these are:
    › Peripheral mucosal margins.
    › Deep margin of resection.

314. What are the implications of LVI and PNI?
- Both venous and lymphatic vessel invasion have been shown to be adverse prognostic factors and are predictive of lymph node metastases in early gastric cancers.
- Perineural invasion has been shown to be an adverse prognostic factor and has been associated with lymph node metastases in early gastric cancer in univariate but not multivariate analyses.
- These do not impact the T staging.

315. What is the pT staging for gastric cancer?
pTX: tumor cannot be assessed.
pT0: no evidence of primary tumor.
pTis: carcinoma in situ (high grade dysplasia, intraepithelial tumor without invasion of the lamina propria).
pT1: tumor invades lamina propria, muscularis mucosae, or submucosa.
  T1a: tumor invades lamina propria or muscularis mucosae.
  T1b: tumor invades submucosa.
pT2: tumor invades muscularis propria.
pT3: tumor penetrates subserosal connective tissue without invasion of visceral peritoneum or adjacent structures (includes extension into gastrocolic, gastrohepatic ligaments, and greater or lesser omentum).
pT4: tumor invades serosa (visceral peritoneum) or adjacent structures.
  pT4a: tumor invades serosa (visceral peritoneum).
  pT4b: tumor invades adjacent structures (spleen, transverse colon, liver, diaphragm, pancreas, abdominal wall, adrenal gland, kidney, small intestine, and retroperitoneum).

316. What is the pN staging for gastric cancer?
pNX: regional lymph nodes cannot be assessed.
pN0: no regional lymph node metastasis.
pN1: 1–2 regional lymph node metastases.
pN2: 3–6 regional lymph node metastases.
pN3: ≥ 7 regional lymph node metastases.
  pN3a: 7–15 regional lymph node metastases.
  pN3b: ≥ 16 regional lymph node metastases.
- Lymph nodes containing isolated tumor cells (single tumor cells or small clusters of cells ≤ 0.2 mm in diameter) are classified as pN0.
- Discontinuous tumor deposits without evidence of residual lymph node and located in the subserosal tissue adjacent to a gastric carcinoma are considered regional lymph node metastases.

317. What are the regional lymph nodes of the stomach?
- Greater curvature of stomach: left paracardial (cardioesophageal), perigastric along greater curvature (including greater curvature and greater omental), infrapyloric (including gastroepiploic).
- Lesser curvature of stomach: right paracardial (cardioesophageal), perigastric along lesser curvature (including lesser curvature and lesser omental), suprapyloric (including gastroduodenal), left gastric artery, common hepatic artery, celiac artery, and hepatoduodenal.
- Splenic area: splenic artery, splenic helium.

318. What is the suggested minimum number of lymph nodes that should be submitted for microscopic examination in a gastrectomy specimen?

The recommended minimum target is 16 lymph nodes.

319. What is the pM staging for gastric cancer?

M0: no distant metastasis

M1: distant metastasis

- Implants on the peritoneal surface are classified as distant metastasis.

- Involvement of other intraabdominal lymph nodes, such as retropancreatic, pancreaticoduodenal, peripancreatic, superior mesenteric, middle colic, retroperitoneal, and para-aortic, is classified as distant metastasis.

320. What are some other findings that are often reported in gastric resection specimens?

- Intestinal metaplasia.
- Dysplasia.
- Gastritis:
- *Helicobacter pylori.*
- Autoimmune atrophic chronic gastritis.
- Gastric polyp (most commonly large hyperplastic polyps in the setting of atrophic gastritis).

CAP Protocol for Reporting *HER2* Results in Adenocarcinoma of the Stomach or Esophagogastric Junction

321. What is *HER2* and where is it located in the genome?

- *HER2* is a protooncogene.
- It is a receptor belonging to the epidermal growth factor receptor (EGFR) family whose phosphorylation initiates signaling pathways that lead to cell division, proliferation, differentiation, and apoptosis.
- It is located on chromosome 17.
- The approved symbol designated by Human Genome Organization is *ERBB2* (*HER2* and *NEU* are designated as synonyms).

322. Where is *HER2* gene product normally expressed? Where is it abnormally expressed?

- It is expressed in normal epithelial cells.
- Amplification and/or overexpression of this gene has been reported in up to:
- 30% of breast cancers.
- 9–38% of gastric cancer (intestinal > diffuse; moderately differentiated > poorly differentiated).

323. Why is *HER2* testing important for gastric cancer?

Anti-*HER2* humanized monoclonal antibody trastuzumab (herceptin) is effective in prolonging survival compared with chemotherapy alone in patients with *HER2* positive adenocarcinoma of the stomach and the gastroesophageal junction.

324. Is *HER2* a predictive or prognostic factor for gastric cancer?

For gastric cancer, it predicts response to trastuzumab therapy but its prognostic value is uncertain at the time.

325. When is it recommended to analyze *HER2* expression in gastric cancers?

In patients with inoperable locally advanced, recurrent, or metastatic adenocarcinoma of the stomach or esophagogastric junction for whom trastuzumab is under consideration for therapy.

326. How is *HER2* expression/amplification interpreted in gastric cancer?

- *HER2* is assessed in either biopsies or surgical resection specimens.
- IHC evaluates membranous protein expression of cancer cells (intensity and percentage are assessed).
- In situ hybridization (ISH) is used to verify IHC-equivocal cases. Most assays use a *HER2* probe and chromosome enumeration probe (CEP17) to determine the ratio of *HER2* to copies of chromosome 17. ISH includes:
- Fluorescence in situ hybridization (FISH).
- Chromogenic in situ hybridization (CISH).
- Silver-enhanced in situ hybridization (SISH).
- Dual in situ hybridization (DISH).

327. How is IHC for *HER2* different between breast and gastric cancers?

- It is more heterogeneous in gastric cancer than in breast cancer.
- The completeness of membrane staining required for positivity in breast cancer is infrequent in gastric adenocarcinoma, which often has a basolateral staining pattern.
- Surgical specimens and biopsy specimens (cell clusters) use different methods of evaluation in gastric cancer.

328. What constitutes a positive HER2 expression in gastric cancer as defined by immunohistochemistry (IHC)?

- In surgical specimens, at least 10% of cancer cells should demonstrate strong, complete, basolateral or lateral membranous staining with HER2 IHC.
- In biopsy specimens, a cluster of at least 5 tumor cells should demonstrate strong, complete, basolateral or lateral membranous staining with HER2 IHC.

Note: overexpression of *HER2* is reported in 9–38% of gastric cancers.

329. How is *HER2* gene amplification by FISH scored?

- It is scored similarly to breast cancer recommendations.
- The minimum assessment area is ≥ 10% stained tumor cells for resection specimens and a small cluster of cells (≥ 5 neoplastic cells) for biopsy specimens.
- *HER2* amplification is defined as a *HER2*-to-CEP17 ratio ≥ 2.

330. When is *HER2* considered amplified? When is trastuzumab an option?

- *HER2* positive gastric cancer has been defined as:
  · US and Japan: IHC 3+ or ISH positive.
  · Europe: IHC 3+ or 2+ and ISH positive.
- In the US, the FDA has approved trastuzumab with chemotherapy limited to patients with metastatic gastric carcinoma with a score of IHC 3+ or 2+ with ISH positivity.
- No significant survival benefit demonstrated for patients with IHC 0 or 1+ with FISH positivity. Trastuzumab is not recommended if the IHC score is 0 or 1+.

CAP Protocols for Examining and Reporting Esophageal Carcinoma

331. What is the WHO classification of malignant epithelial tumors of esophagus? Which of these are not graded?

- Adenocarcinoma, NOS.
- Adenoid cystic carcinoma.*
- Mucoepidermoid carcinoma.*
- Adenosquamous carcinoma.
- Squamous cell carcinoma, NOS.
  · Verrucous squamous cell carcinoma.
  · Squamous cell carcinoma, spindle cell.
  · Basaloid squamous cell carcinoma.
- Carcinoma, undifferentiated, NOS.
  · Lymphoepithelioma-like carcinoma.
- Neuroendocrine tumor (NET), NOS.*
  · NET, grade 1.
  · NET, grade 2.
  · NET, grade 3.
- Neuroendocrine carcinoma (NEC), NOS.*
  · Large cell NEC.
  · Small cell NEC.
- Mixed neuroendocrine-nonneuroendocrine neoplasm (MiNEN).
  · Combined small cell adenocarcinoma.
  · Combined small cell-squamous cell carcinoma.

*Note: these types are not generally graded.

332. What should we record about the tumor size and location?

- To establish the exact site of origin of the tumor, the pathologist should record:
  · The maximum longitudinal dimension of the tumor mass.
- · The distance of the tumor midpoint from the EGJ.
- · The relative proportions of the tumor mass located in the esophagus and in the stomach.

333. How are esophageal squamous cell carcinomas and adenocarcinoma graded?

GRADING OF SQUAMOUS CELL CARCINOMA: BASED ON ATYPIA, MITOTIC ACTIVITY, AND EVIDENCE OF KERATINIZATION

GRADE	FEATURES
Grade 1: well differentiated	• Minimal cytologic atypia, low mitotic rate, keratin pearls.
Grade 2: moderately differentiated	• Evident cytologic atypia, easily found mitotic figures, infrequent keratin pearls.
Grade 3: poorly differentiated	• Basal-like cells, high mitotic rate, only occasional keratinizing cells.

(continued on next page)

(continued from previous page)

GRADING OF ADENOCARCINOMA: BASED ON GLAND FORMATION

GRADE	FEATURES
Grade 1: well-differentiated	• Glands compose > 95% of tumor.
Grade 2: moderately differentiated	• Glands compose 50–95% of tumor.
Grade 3: poorly differentiated	• Glands compose ≤ 49% of tumor.

334. How are undifferentiated carcinomas staged?

All undifferentiated carcinomas are staged as grade 3 squamous cell carcinomas.

335. What is a common artifact after chemoradiation and how does it affect tumor staging?

Sizable pools of acellular mucin may be present after chemoradiation, but should not be interpreted as representing a residual tumor and should not affect the staging.

CAP Protocols for Examining and Reporting Appendix Tumors

336. How do you distinguish tumors at the base of the appendix from cecal carcinoma extending into the appendix?

- Gross exam: determine the location of the bulk of the tumor.
- Microscopic exam: look for the presence of a precursor lesion whose location may indicate the primary site of origin.

337. What is important to report for intraabdominal mucin pools?

The presence or absence of neoplastic cells should be clearly noted in the surgical pathology report.

338. What is the morphological distinction between low grade and high grade mucinous neoplasms and mucinous adenocarcinoma of the appendix?

- The pattern of invasion is the morphological distinction:
  · Low grade and high grade appendiceal mucinous neoplasms penetrate into or through the appendiceal wall with a broad pushing front. Pools of acellular mucin may be present in the wall. Mucinous implants, acellular or containing a few neoplastic cells, may be found on the peritoneal surface.
  · Mucinous adenocarcinomas are composed of infiltrative glands and crowded, expansile mucin pools with detached strips/glands/clusters of atypical neoplastic cells.

339. How are appendiceal carcinomas graded?

GRADING OF NONMUCINOUS CARCINOMAS: BASED ON GLAND FORMATION

GRADE	FEATURES
Grade 1: well-differentiated	• Glands compose > 95% of tumor.
Grade 2: moderately differentiated	• Glands compose 50–95% of tumor.
Grade 3: poorly differentiated	• Glands compose ≤ 49% of tumor.

GRADING OF MUCINOUS CARCINOMAS: BASED ON CYTOLOGY AND ARCHITECTURE

GRADE	FEATURES
Grade 1: well-differentiated	• Low grade cytology; no signet ring cells; tumor involving peritoneum that shows acellular mucin or low cellularity; no infiltrative invasion of peritoneum.
Grade 2: moderately differentiated	• Mix of low and high grade cytology or diffuse high grade cytology; no signet ring cells.
Grade 3: poorly differentiated	• High grade cytology; signet ring cells.

340. What are the margins required for the appendix?

- Simple appendectomy specimens:
  - Proximal margin is taken en face to allow evaluation of the entire appendiceal mucosa and muscularis circumferentially.
  - Mesenteric resection margin represents the radial margin.
- For a retrocecal appendix that is retroperitoneal, measure the distance between the invasive carcinoma and the nonperitonealized resection margin.
- Right hemicolectomy specimens:
  - Report the distance between the tumor and the ileal (proximal) and colonic (distal) margins. These margins are considered to be grossly negative if they are > 5 cm from the tumor.

IMAGES: GASTROINTESTINAL PATHOLOGY

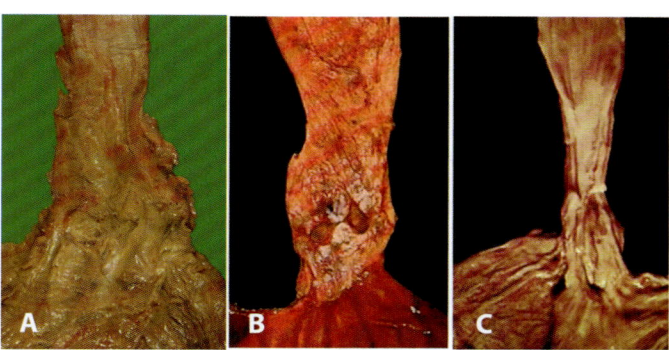

IMAGE 9.1 Image A: esophageal varices. Image B: reflux esophagitis with benign ulcer. Image C: esophagus with a benign stricture.

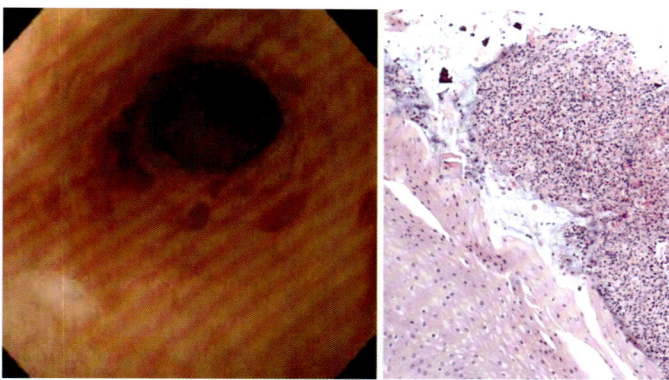

IMAGE 9.3 Pill esophagitis. Left: endoscopy shows scattered hemorrhagic ulcers. Right: mucosa ulceration with Kayexalate crystals admixed with inflammatory exudates.

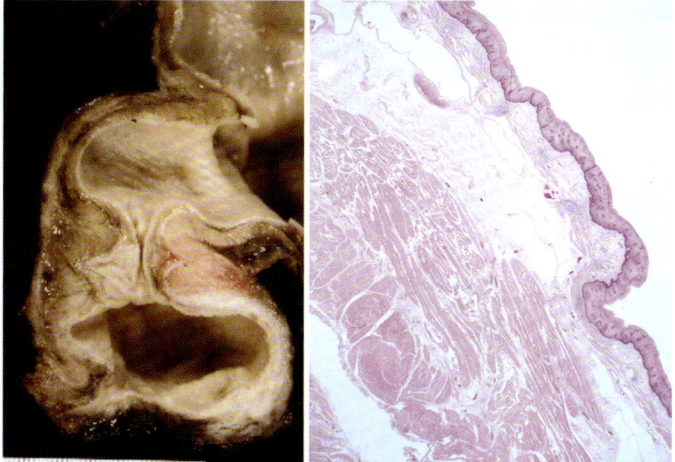

IMAGE 9.2 Achalasia. Left: the gross specimen shows a narrowing of the esophageal lumen due to muscle contraction. Right: full thickness tissue section shows complete absence of myenteric ganglion cells (H&E, x10).

Left: courtesy of Dr. Olga Aleynikova.

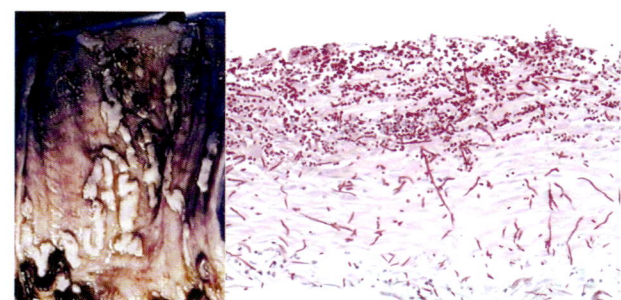

IMAGE 9.4 *Candida* esophagitis. Left: the gross specimen shows white plaques on the mucosa surface. Right: PAS stain demonstrates the characteristic budding yeast cells and pseudohyphae (x100).

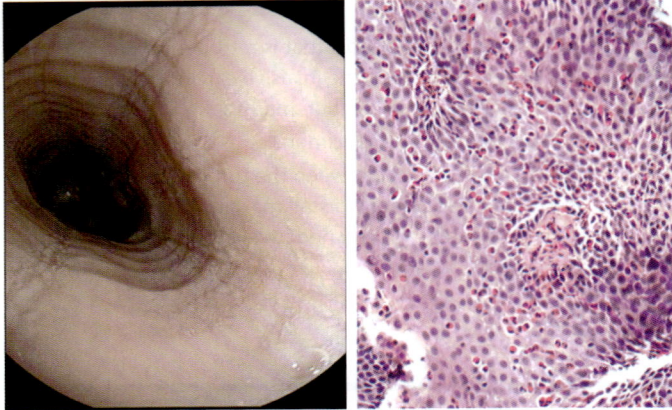

IMAGE 9.5 Eosinophilic esophagitis. Left: endoscopy shows feline esophagus with mucosal rings. Right: histology shows eosinophils infiltrating squamous mucosa (H&E, x200).

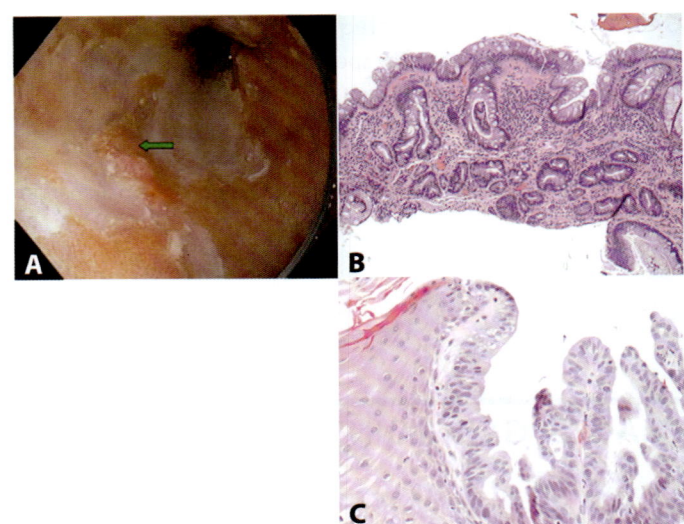

IMAGE 9.8 Barrett esophagus. Image A: endoscopy showing replacement of white squamous epithelium by pink glandular epithelium. Image B: intestinal metaplasia of the glandular epithelium (H&E, x100). Image C: dysplasia in the glandular epithelium (H&E, x100).

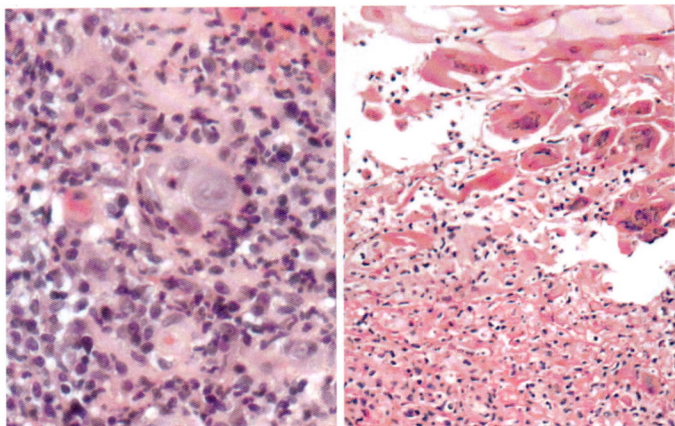

IMAGE 9.6 Left: cytomegalovirus esophagitis (H&E, x200). Note the pink intranuclear and intracytoplasmic viral inclusions. Right: herpes esophagitis (H&E, x100). Note the molding of nuclei, marginalization of chromatin, and intranuclear viral inclusions.

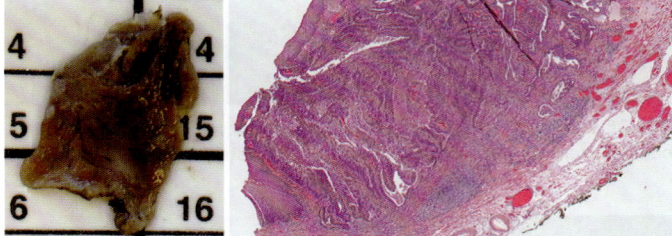

IMAGE 9.9 Esophageal mucosal resection. Left: gross. Right: microscopic section of esophageal adenocarcinoma invading into muscularis mucosae (H&E, x40).

Right: courtesy of Dr. Sophie Camilleri-Broët.

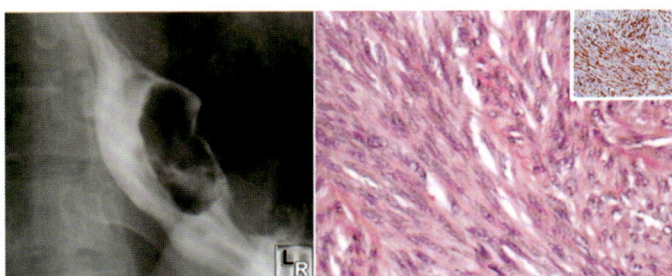

IMAGE 9.7 Esophageal leiomyoma. Left: radiology image. Right: H&E, x200, with inset showing the tumor stained positive for desmin.

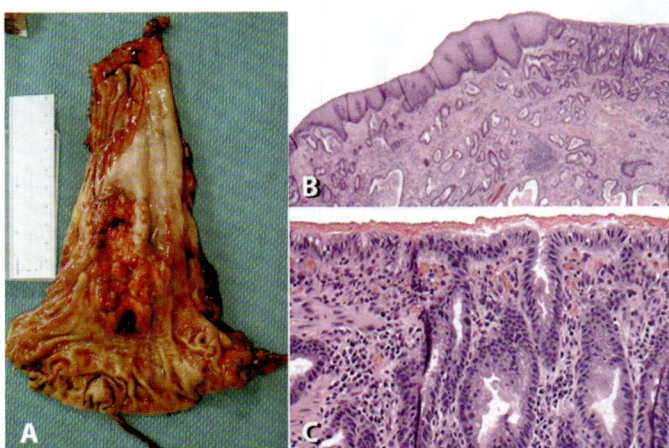

IMAGE 9.10 Esophageal adenocarcinoma. Image A: gross specimen showing an ulcerating tumor mass at the gastroesophageal junction. Image B: tumor glands infiltrating under the squamous mucosa (H&E, x20). Image C: high grade dysplasia of mucosa epithelium from which the invasive tumor arises (H&E, x100).

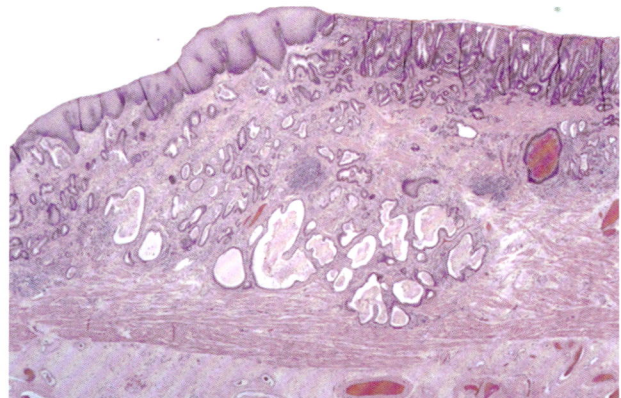

IMAGE 9.11 Recurrent esophageal carcinoma. Duplication of muscularis mucosae after mucosal resection (H&E, x20).

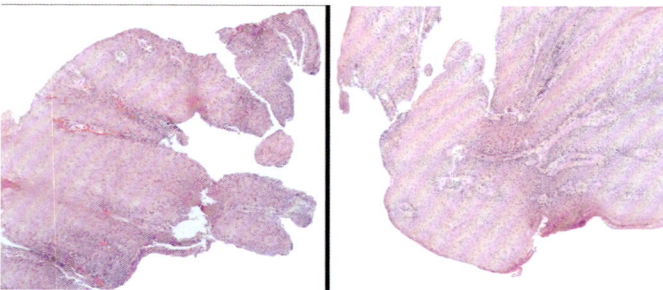

IMAGE 9.14 Esophageal verrucous carcinoma (both images: H&E, x20). The tumor is characterized by papillomatous proliferation of squamous cells with very mild cytological atypia. The basal aspect shows a broad-based pushing interface.

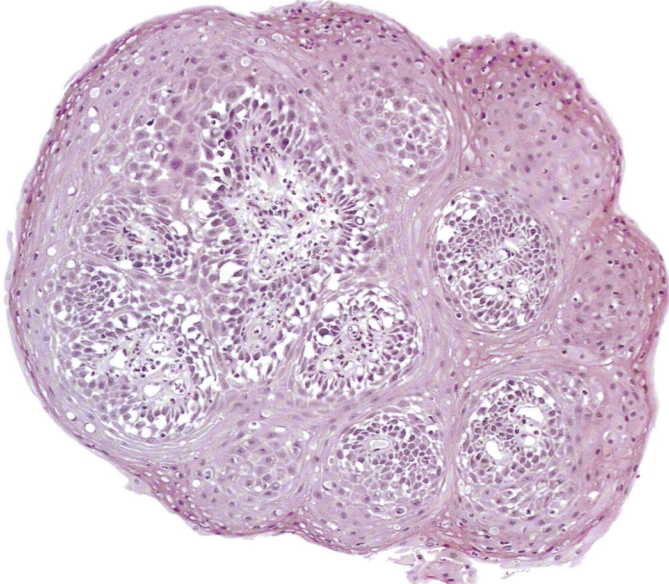

IMAGE 9.12 Esophageal squamous papilloma (H&E, x100).

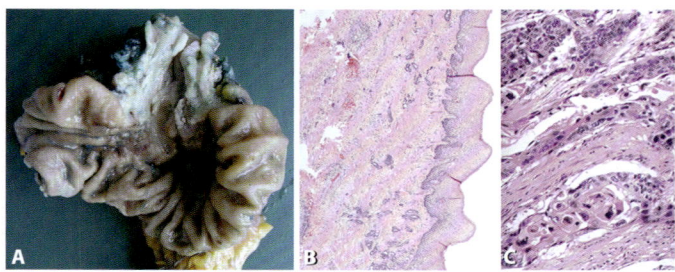

IMAGE 9.15 Esophagogastric junction carcinoma. Image A: gross. Image B: esophageal side showing the tumor infiltrating under the normal squamous mucosa (H&E, x10). Image C: gastric side (H&E, x40) showing the tumor glands infiltrating under the normal gastric mucosa.

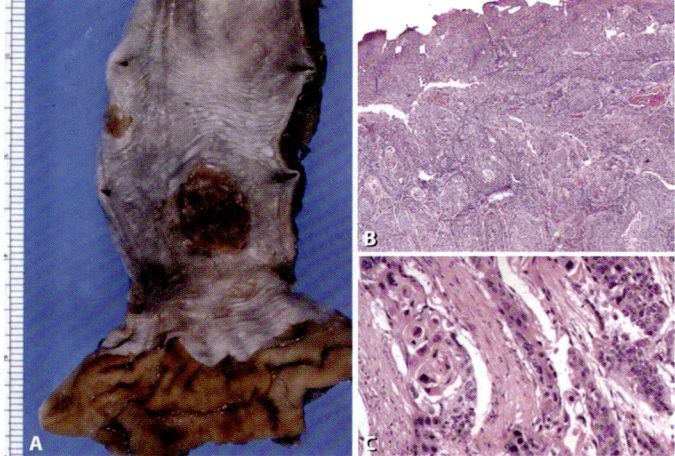

IMAGE 9.13 Esophageal squamous cell carcinoma. Image A: the gross specimen showing an ulcerating tumor located well above the gastroesophageal junction. Histologically, the tumor demonstrates typical squamous differentiation. Image B: H&E, x20. Image C: H&E, x200.

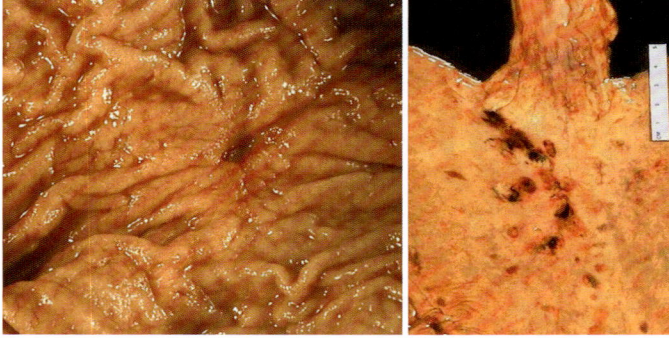

IMAGE 9.16 Stomach. Left: benign peptic ulcer. Right: mucosal erosion-stress ulcer.

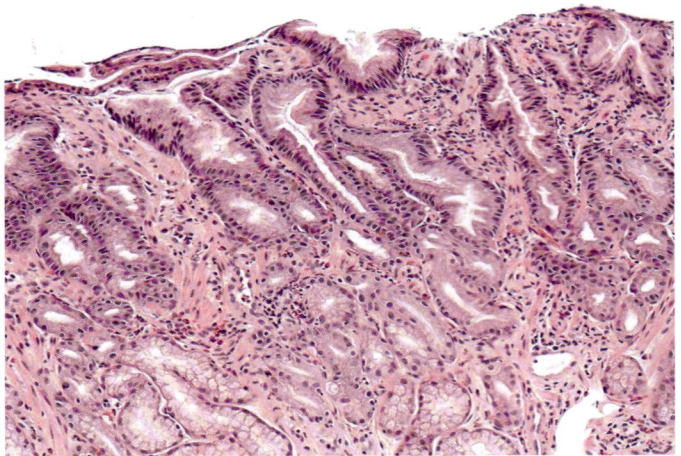

IMAGE 9.17 Chemical/reactive gastropathy (H&E, x100). The foveolar epithelium appears blue due to regeneration and mucin loss. The lamina propria shows smooth muscle proliferation. There is only minimal inflammation.

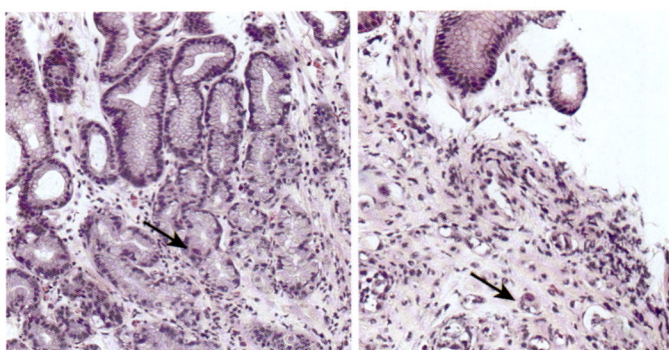

IMAGE 9.20 Cytomegalovirus gastritis (H&E, x200). Characteristic nuclear and cytoplasmic inclusions can be seen in glandular (left) and stromal (right) cells.

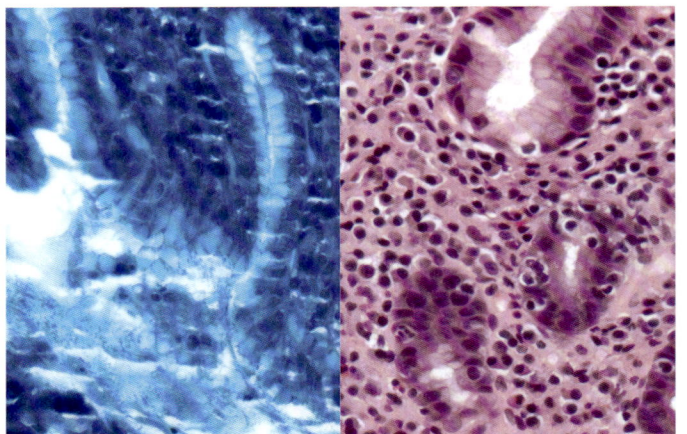

IMAGE 9.18 Left: *Helicobacter pylori* gastritis (Giemsa, x400). Right: lymphoepithelial lesion in mucosa associated lymphoid tissue (MALT) caused by *H. pylori* gastritis (H&E, x400).

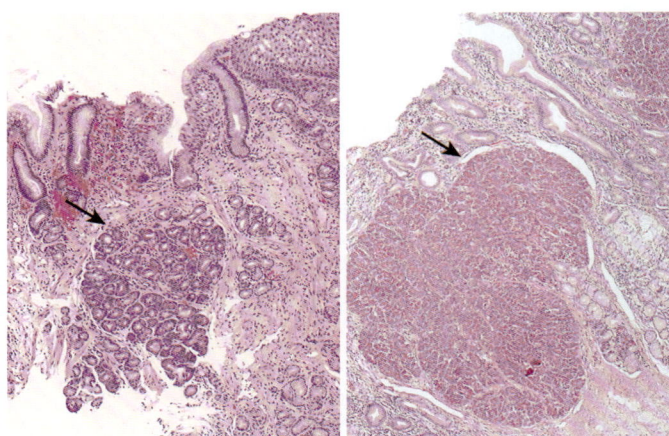

IMAGE 9.21 Ectopic pancreas tissue (arrows). Left: at esophagogastric junction (H&E, x100). Right: in duodenum (H&E, x20).

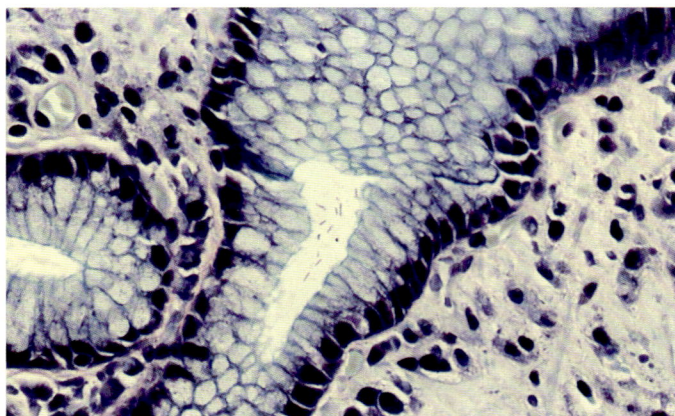

IMAGE 9.19 *Helicobacter heilmannii* gastritis (Giemsa, x600). In comparison to *H. pylori,* these organisms are larger, with a straight, tightly coiled corkscrew appearance, and lie freely within the lumen rather than attaching to the surface.

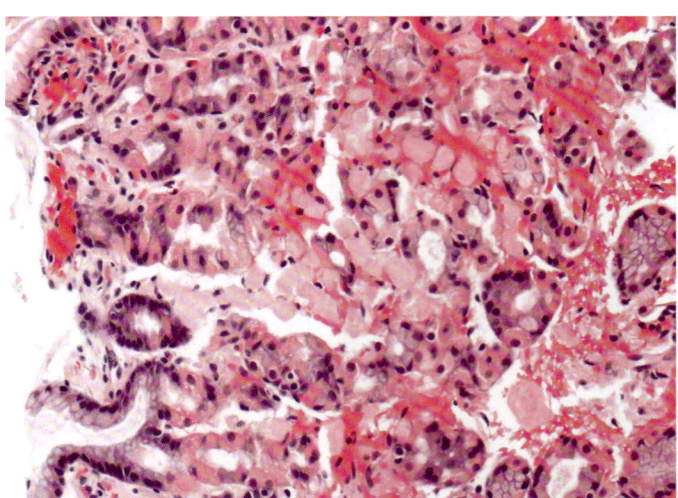

IMAGE 9.22 Amyloidosis involving the stomach (H&E, x200). Here the amyloid presents as globoid amorphous material in the lamina propria.

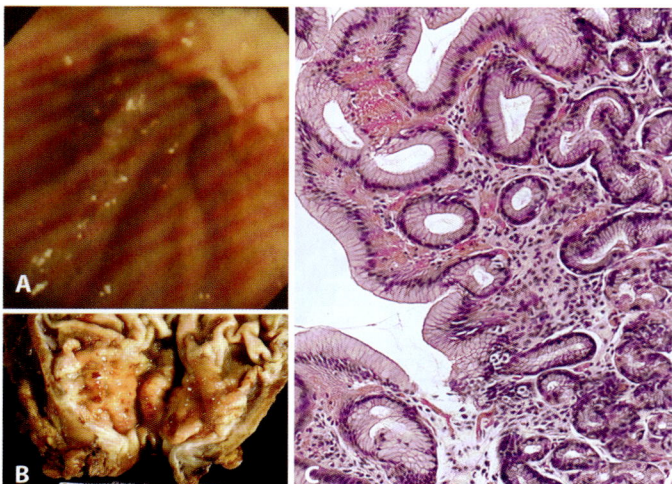

IMAGE 9.23 Gastric antral vascular ectasia. Image A (endoscopy) and Image B (gross): macroscopically, antral mucosal folds reveal tortuous ectatic vessels meriting the designation of "watermelon" stomach. Image C: microscopically, the mucosa shows dilated capillaries beneath the surface epithelium, intraluminal fibrin thrombi, and fibrohyalinosis of adjacent lamina propria (H&E, x200).

Left upper: courtesy of Dr. Olga Aleynikova.

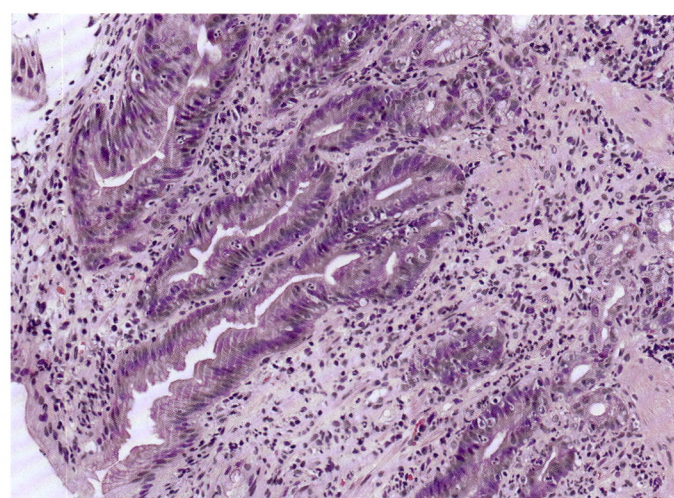

IMAGE 9.26 Graft versus host disease. The gastric mucosa glands contain many apoptotic cells (H&E, x100).

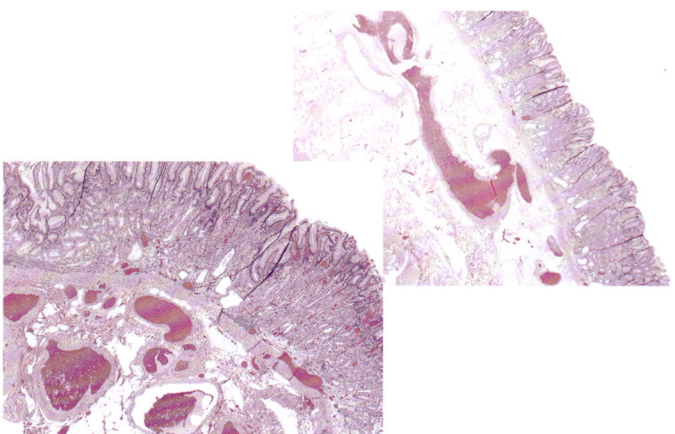

IMAGE 9.24 Stomach Dieulafoy lesion. Large dilated vessels in the submucosa penetrate through the muscularis mucosae. Left: H&E, x20. Right: H&E, x10.

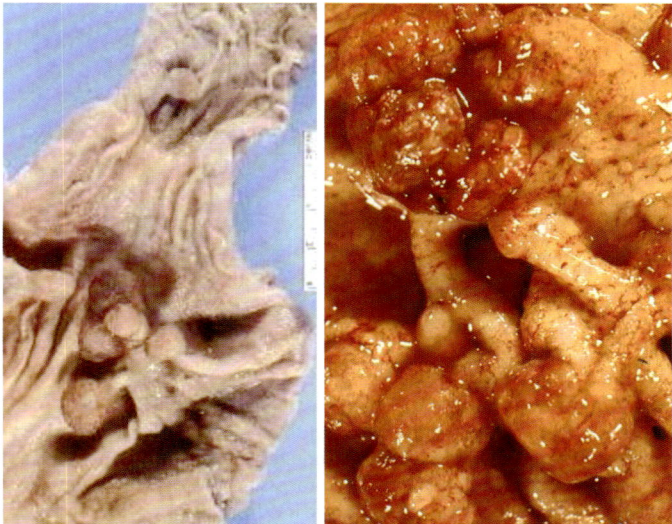

IMAGE 9.27 Gastric hyperplastic polyps. Gross specimens show pedunculated polyps protruding into gastric lumen.

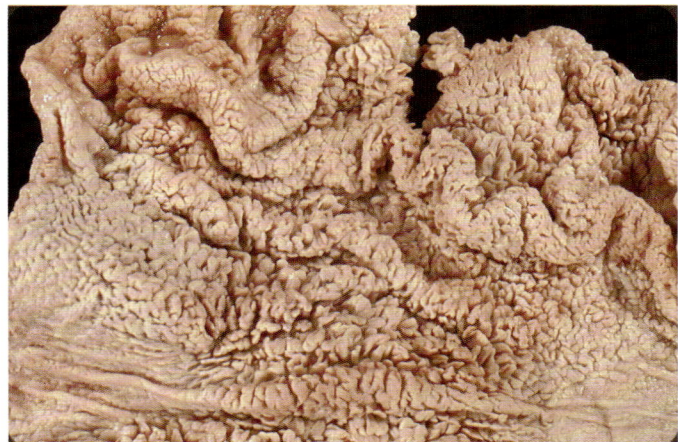

IMAGE 9.25 Ménétrier disease. Gross appearance is characterized by markedly hypertrophic rugal folds.

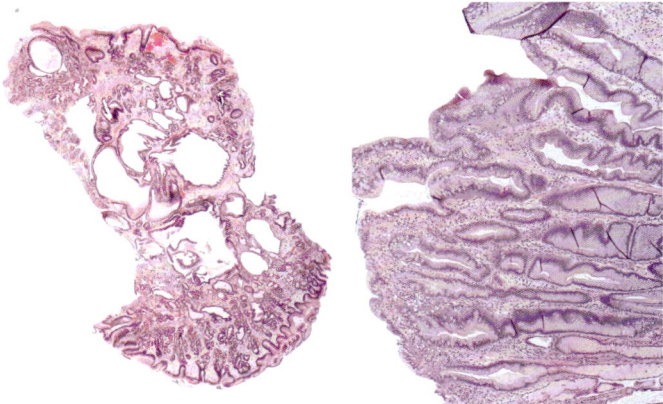

IMAGE 9.28 Left: fundic gland polyp in which the cystically dilated glands are lined by parietal and chief cells (H&E, x20). Right: gastric hyperplastic polyp with proliferation of foveolar epithelium (H&E, x40).

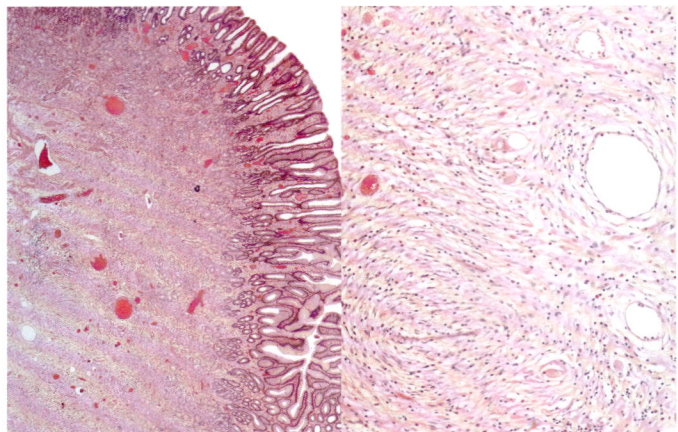

IMAGE 9.29 Inflammatory fibroid polyp of the gastric antrum. Left: H&E, x20. Right: H&E, x100. Histological features include edema, eosinophils infiltration, and perivascular "onionskin" arrangements of spindle cells.

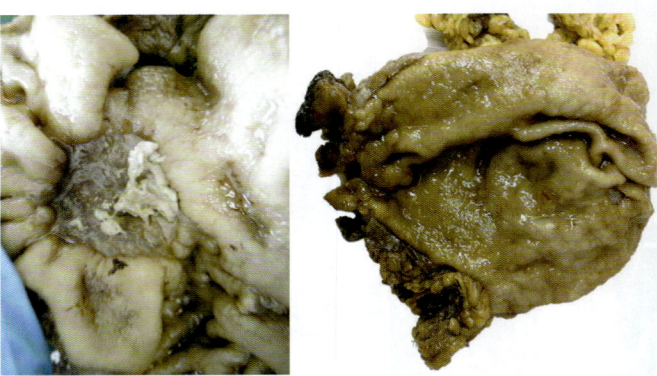

IMAGE 9.32 Gastric adenocarcinoma. Left: intestinal-type adenocarcinoma consisting of central ulcer with heaped-up borders. Right: infiltrative-type adenocarcinoma (linitis plastica).

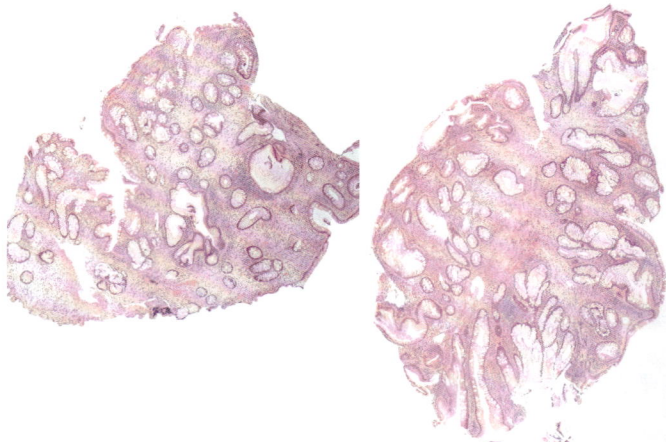

IMAGE 9.30 Stomach mucosa with Cronkhite-Canada syndrome (H&E, x20). It is morphologically similar to gastric hyperplastic polyp and Ménétrier disease. Definitive diagnosis requires knowledge of other clinical features and distribution of the disease process in the stomach: Ménétrier involves the body only, hyperplastic polyp involves the polypoid area only. Cronkhite-Canada syndrome diffusely involves the entire stomach mucosa.

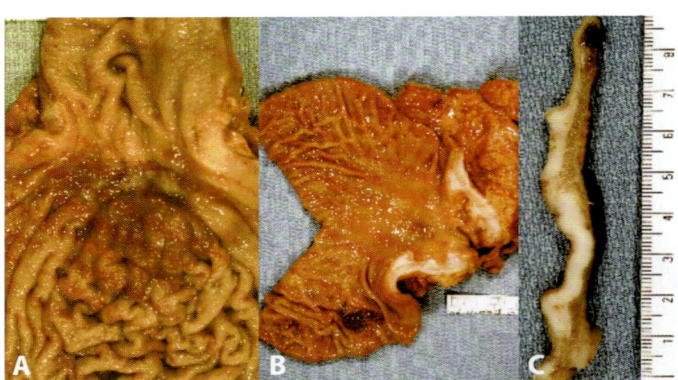

IMAGE 9.33 Gastric linitis plastica. Image A: diffuse gastric carcinoma can present as thick mucosa folds. Image B: it can also present as flattening of mucosa folds. Image C: the image shows diffuse invasion of stomach wall by the cancer.

Courtesy of Dr. Olga Aleynikova.

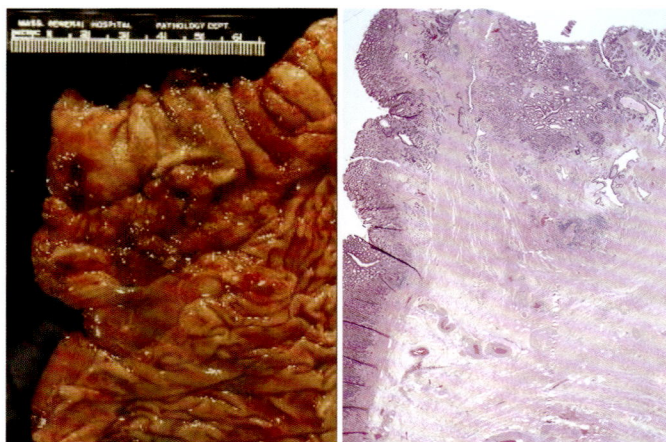

IMAGE 9.31 Gastritis cystica profunda. Left: the gross specimen shows irregular translucent polypoid mucosa protrusions. Right: the histological section shows lobulated benign mucosa glands located in the submucosa. Some glands are irregular and cystically dilated, which need to be differentiated from invasive carcinoma.

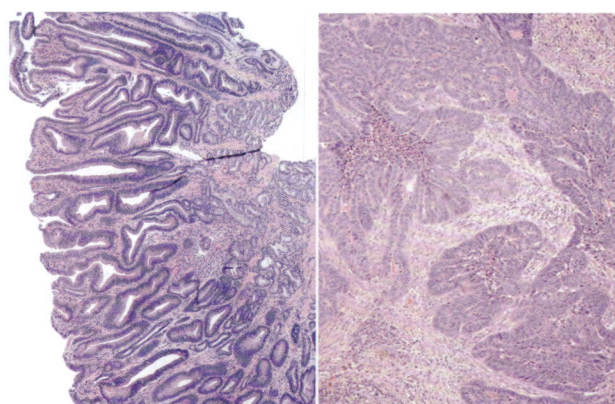

IMAGE 9.34 Left: gastric adenoma (H&E, x100). Right: gastric invasive adenocarcinoma (H&E, x40).

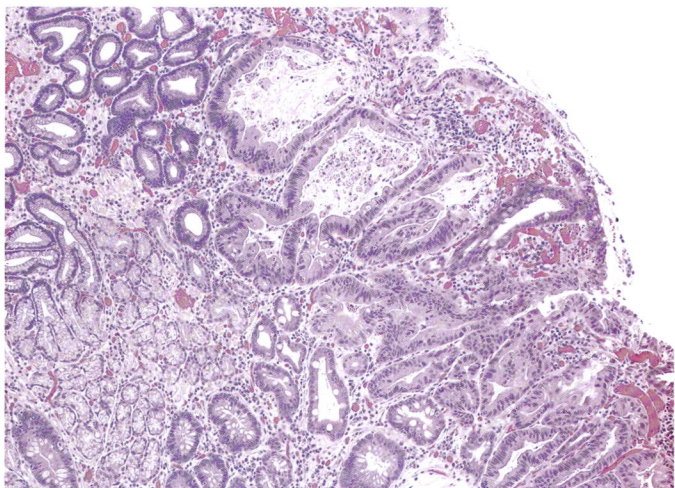

IMAGE 9.35 Early gastric carcinoma shows irregularly dilated dysplastic glands with intraluminal necrosis (H&E, x100).

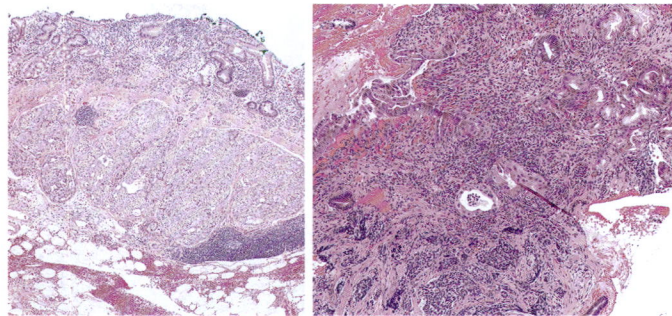

IMAGE 9.38 Gastric neuroendocrine tumor in background atrophic gastritis. Left: H&E, x40. Right: H&E, x100.

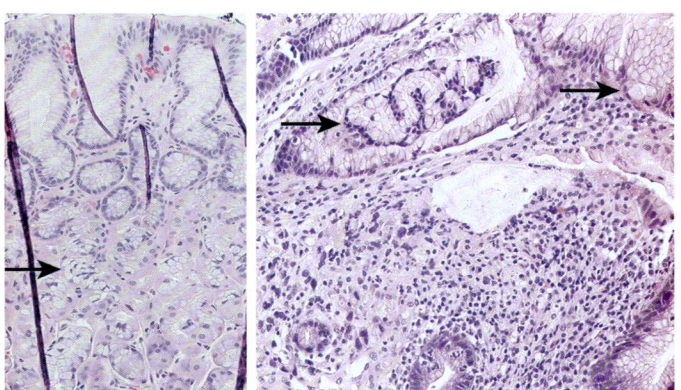

IMAGE 9.36 Globoid dysplasia (arrows), with adjacent invasive signet-ring cell carcinoma (right) (H&E, x200).

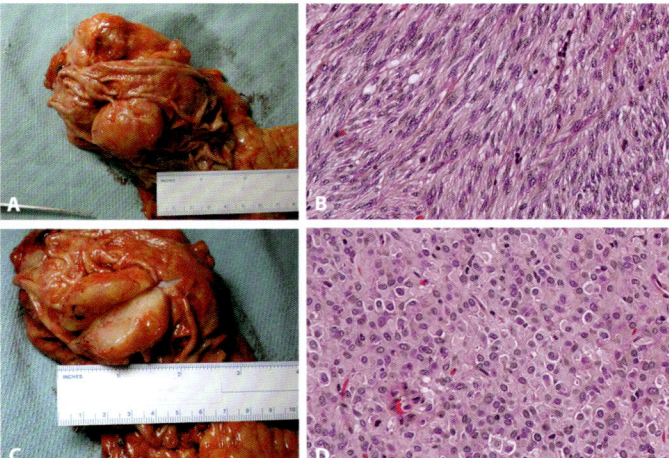

IMAGE 9.39 Stomach gastrointestinal stromal tumor (GIST). Left (images A, C): gross. Right: spindle cell (image B) and epithelioid (image D) morphology (H&E, x200).

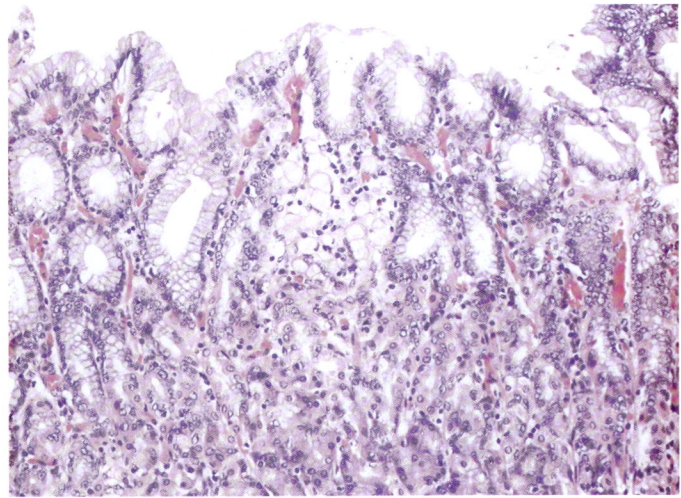

IMAGE 9.37 Signet-ring cell carcinoma found on preventive total gastrectomy (H&E, x200).

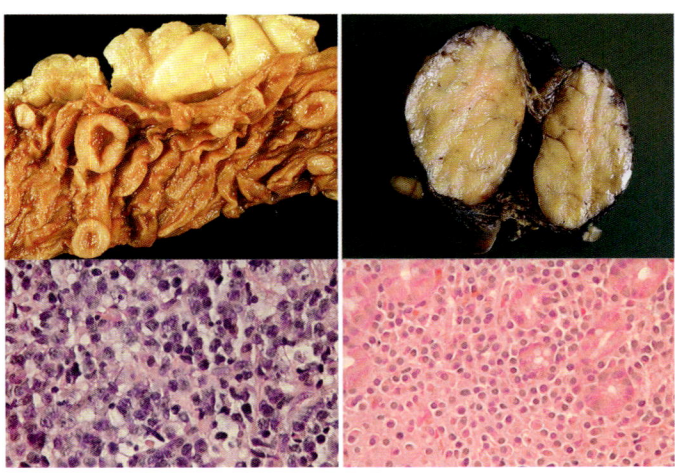

IMAGE 9.40 Left: diffuse large B-cell lymphoma. (Upper: gross. Lower: H&E, x400.) Right: MALT lymphoma. (Upper: gross. Lower: H&E, x200.)

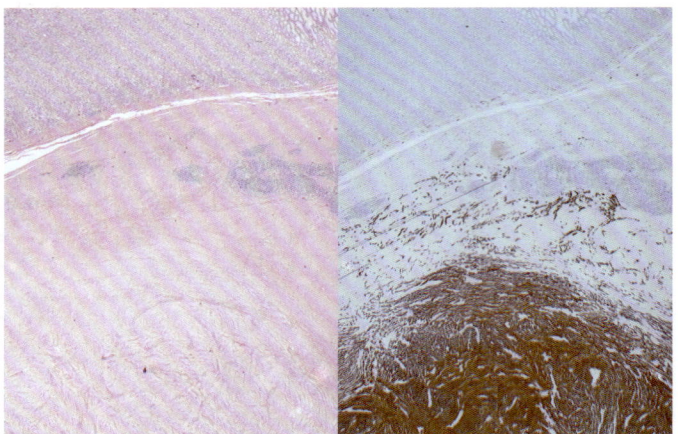

IMAGE 9.41 Gastric schwannoma. Left: H&E, x20. Right: S100, x20. Note the lymphoid aggregates at the periphery of the spindle cell tumor.

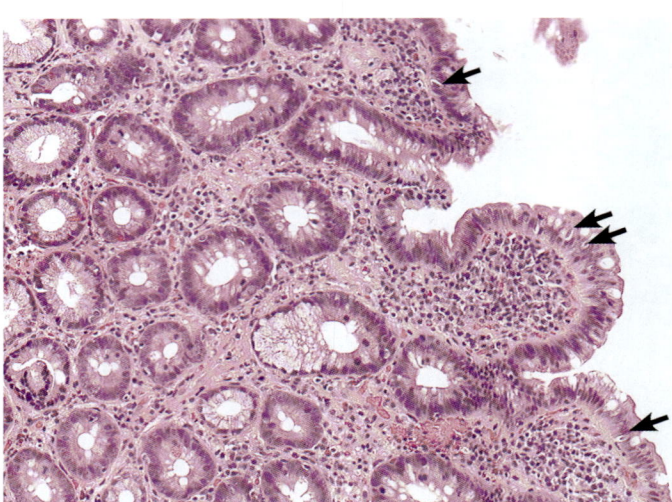

IMAGE 9.44 *Cystoisospora belli* infection shows ovoid developmental forms (arrows) inside the cytoplasm of enterocytes at the villus tip (H&E, x200).

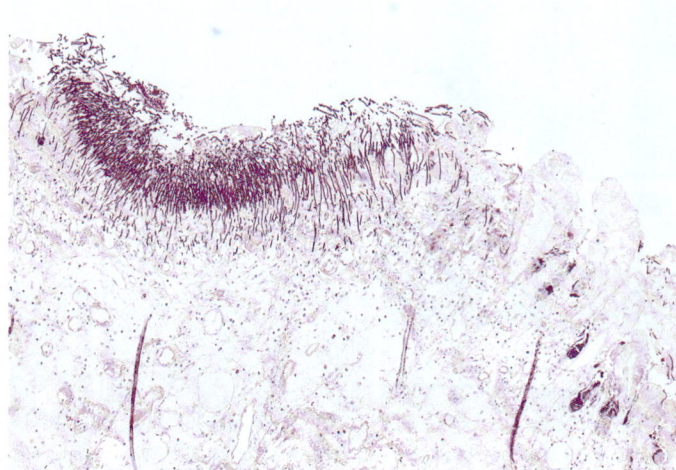

IMAGE 9.42 Small bowel *Candida* infection (PAS, x40).

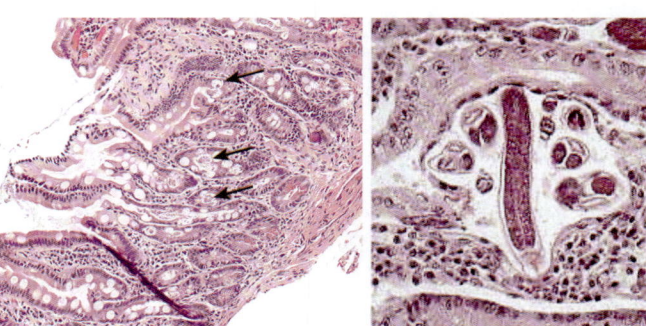

IMAGE 9.45 *Strongyloides stercoralis,* also called threadworm in the UK and Australia. The adult parasitic stage lives in tunnels in the mucosa of the small intestine. Left: H&E, x200 (arrows). Right: H&E, x400.

Right: courtesy of Dr. Jason Karamchandani.

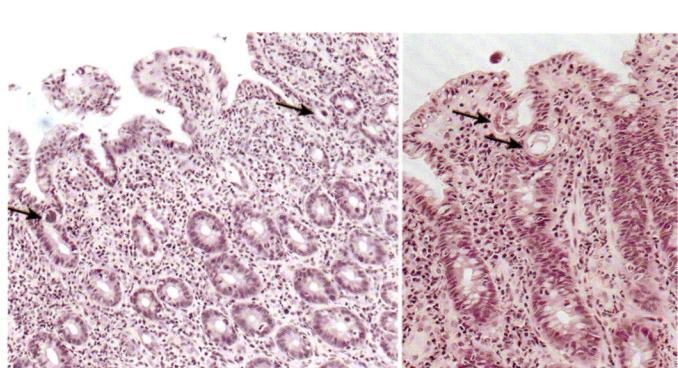

IMAGE 9.43 Nematodes *Capillaria philippinensis*. Large eggs (arrows) are deposited in the crypts. Left: H&E, x100. Right: H&E, x200.

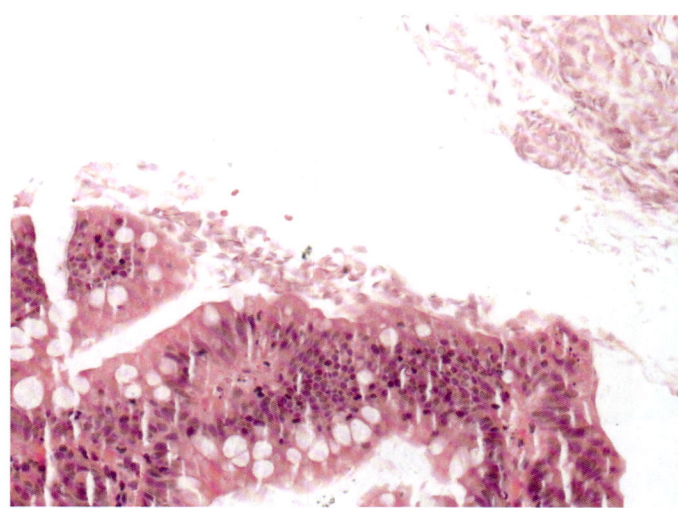

IMAGE 9.46 Giardia (H&E, x200). The parasite appears like "schools of fish" or "fallen leaves" on the mucosa surface.

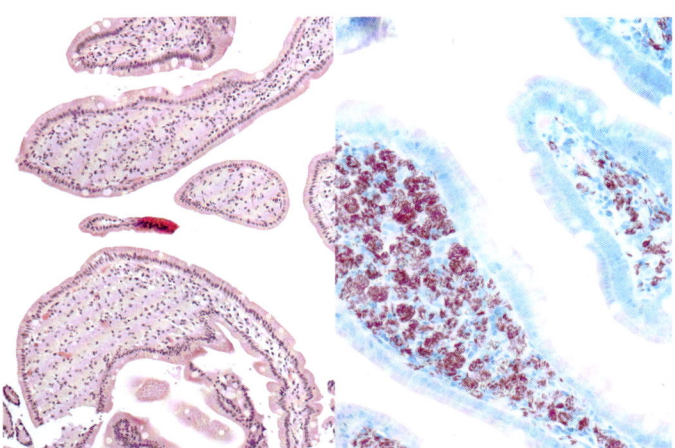

IMAGE 9.47 Duodenum with mycobacterial infection. Left: H&E, x100. Right: Ziehl–Neelsen, x400.

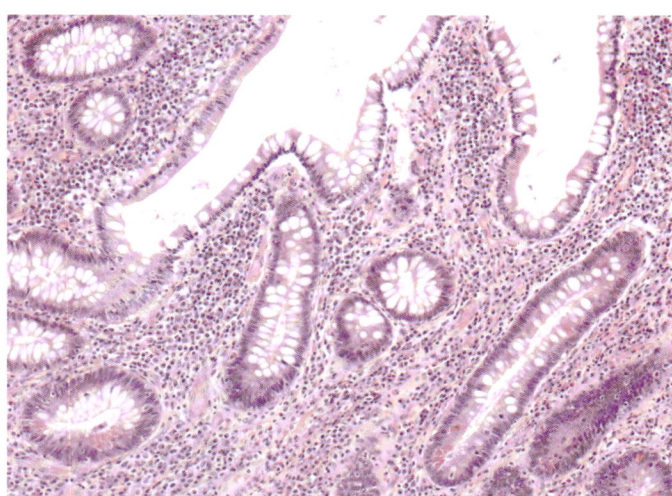

IMAGE 9.50 Small bowel mastocytosis (H&E, x100). There are sheets of mast cells in the lamina propria.

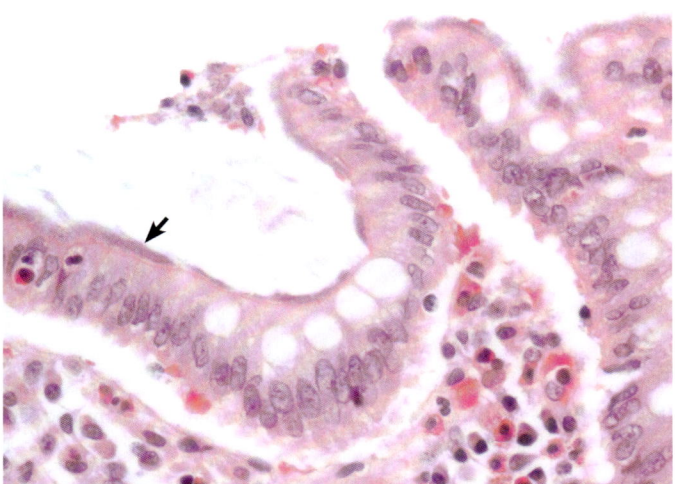

IMAGE 9.48 Intestinal spirochetosis (arrow) (H&E, x400). The brush border appears thickened and has a blue tinge.

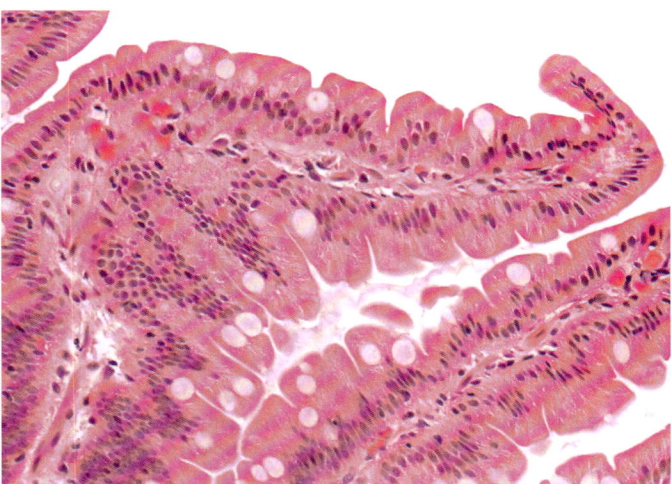

IMAGE 9.51 Duodenum biopsy specimen from a patient with hypogammaglobulinemia (H&E, x200). Note the lack of plasma cells in the lamina propria.

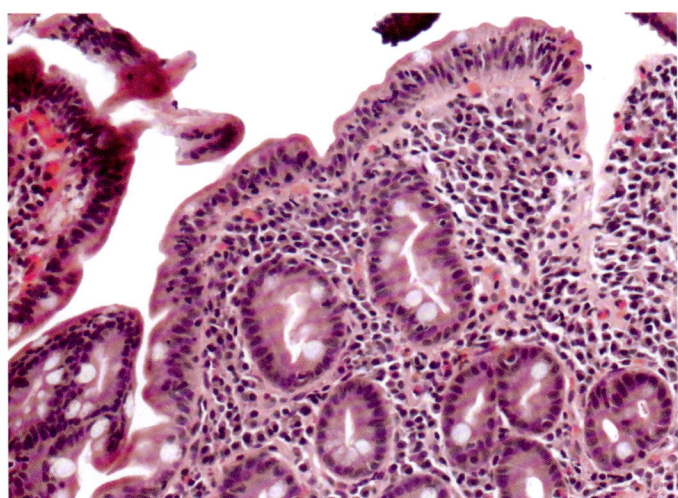

IMAGE 9.49 Celiac disease with partial villus atrophy and increased intraepithelial lymphocytes (H&E, x200).

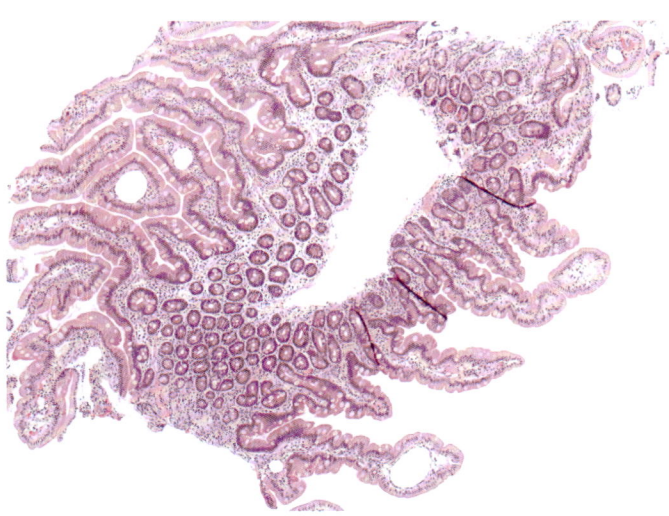

IMAGE 9.52 Duodenum with lymphangiectasia (H&E, x40).

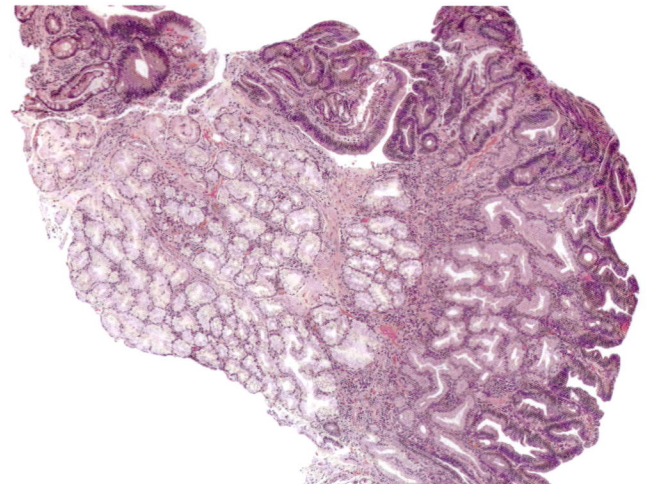

IMAGE 9.53 Duodenal adenoma (H&E, x40).

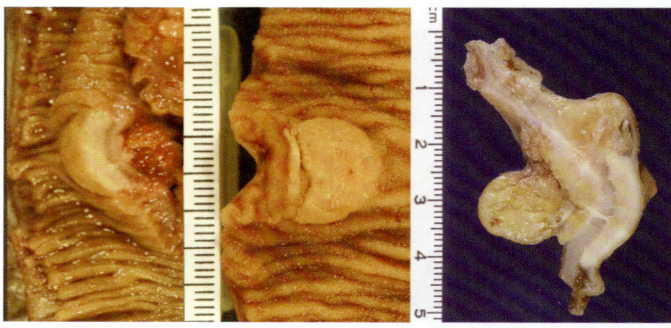

IMAGE 9.56 All images: neuroendocrine tumor of the small bowel showing glistening yellow cut surface.

Right: courtesy of Dr. Olga Aleynikova.

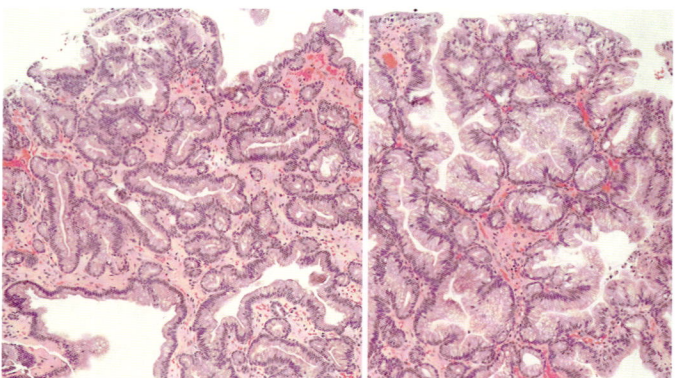

IMAGE 9.54 Duodenal pyloric gland adenoma (both images: H&E, x40). The polyp consists of tightly packed tubules of cuboidal or low-columnar cells with round uniform basal nuclei and foamy eosinophilic cytoplasm.

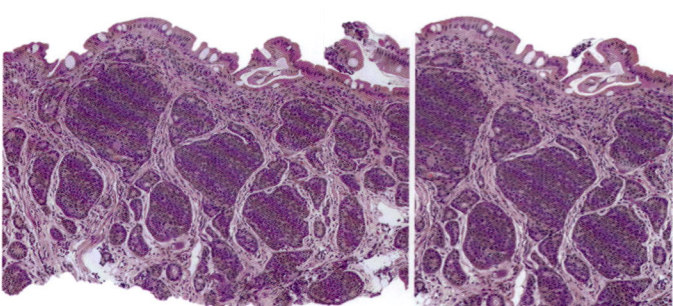

IMAGE 9.57 Well-differentiated neuroendocrine tumor of the small bowel. Left: H&E, x20. Right: H&E, x200.

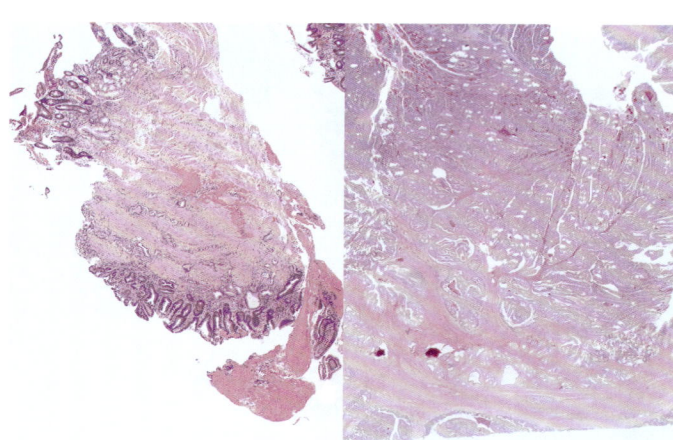

IMAGE 9.55 Left: ampulla adenoma shows benign glands and smooth muscle under the dysplastic epithelium in contrast to the Brunner glands of adjacent duodenum mucosa (H&E, x40). Right: ampulla carcinoma arising from an ampulla adenoma (H&E, x40).

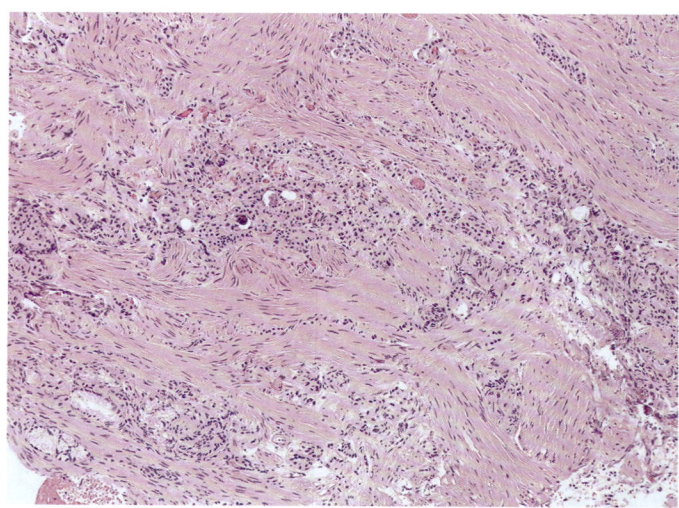

IMAGE 9.58 Psammomatous somatostinoma at the ampulla (H&E, x100).

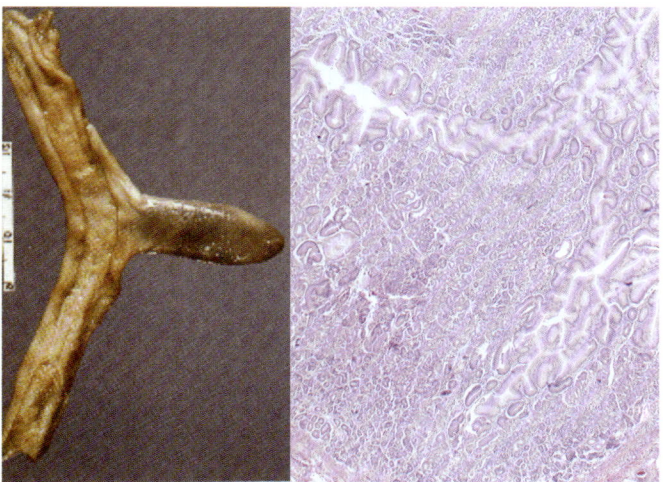

IMAGE 9.59 Meckel diverticulum. Left: a blind pouch protrudes at the side of the bowel wall. Right: ectopic gastric mucosa within the diverticulum (H&E, x40).

Left: courtesy of Dr. Olga Aleynikova.

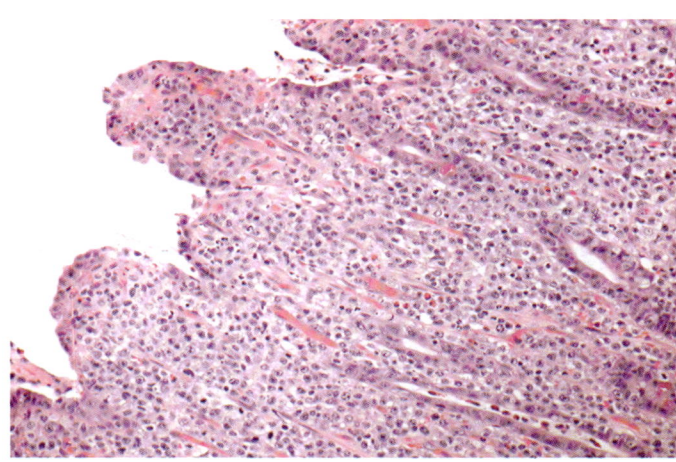

IMAGE 9.62 Mucosa-associated T-cell lymphoma in the small intestine in a patient with celiac disease (H&E, x100). T-cell lymphomas tend to have a clear halo around the neoplastic lymphocytes.

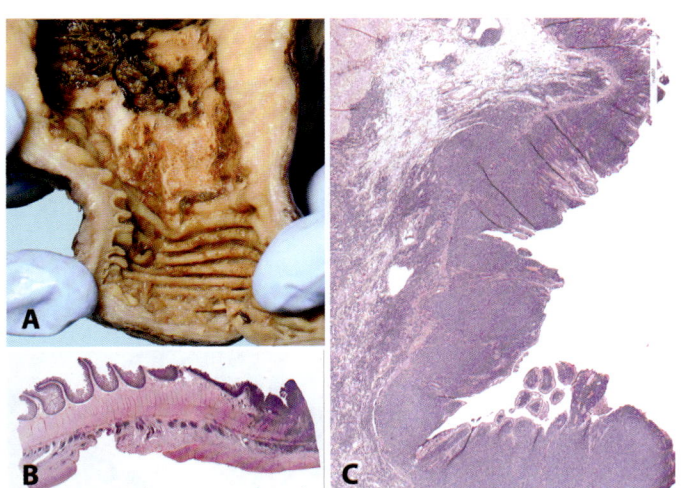

IMAGE 9.60 Small bowel follicular lymphoma. Image A: gross. Image B: H&E, x10. Image C: H&E, x20.

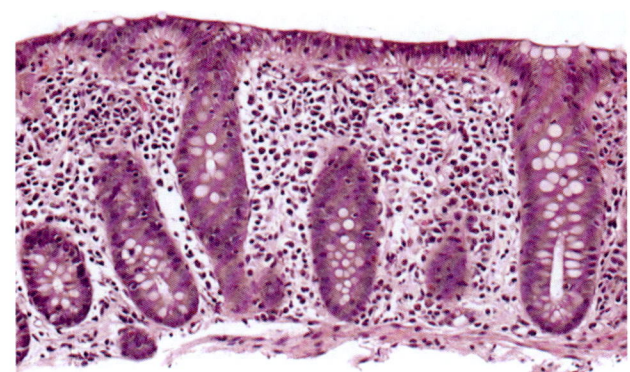

IMAGE 9.63 Lymphocytic colitis (H&E, x100). Note the increase of intraepithelial lymphocytes.

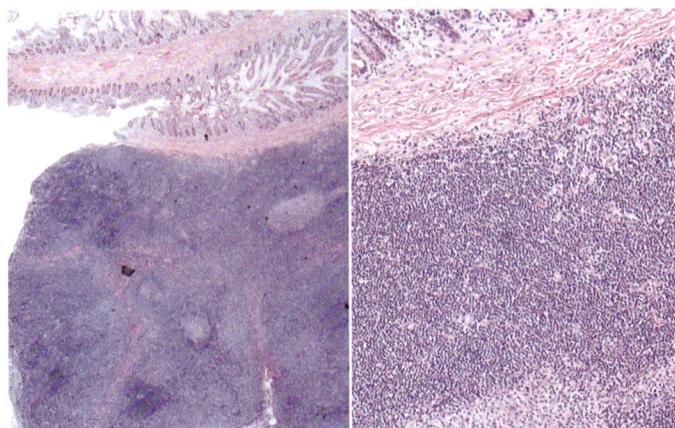

IMAGE 9.61 Marginal zone lymphoma (H&E, left x20, right x100). The marginal zone is expanded by sheets of lymphocytes.

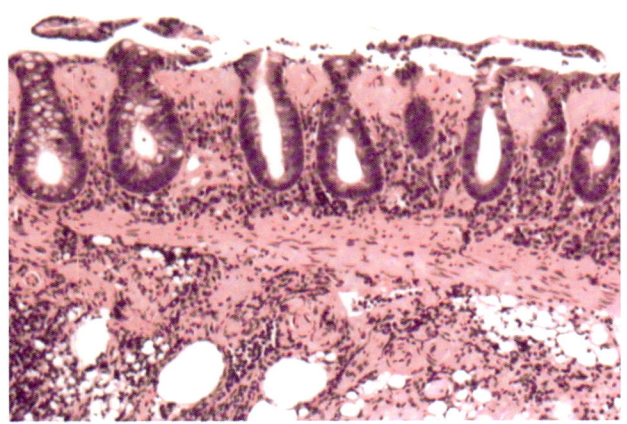

IMAGE 9.64 Collagenous colitis (H&E, x100). Note the thickening of subepithelial collagen and detachment of surface epithelium.

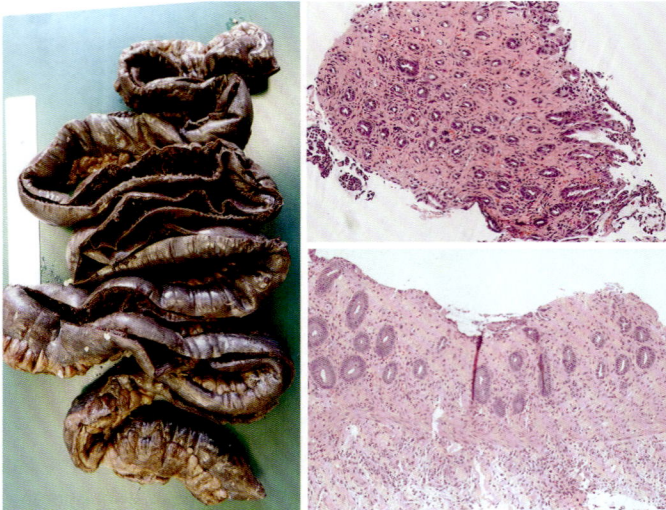

IMAGE 9.65 Left: ischemic necrotic bowel. Right (both images): ischemic colitis (H&E, x100). Note the surface erosion, stromal hyalinization, and the withering of the crypts.

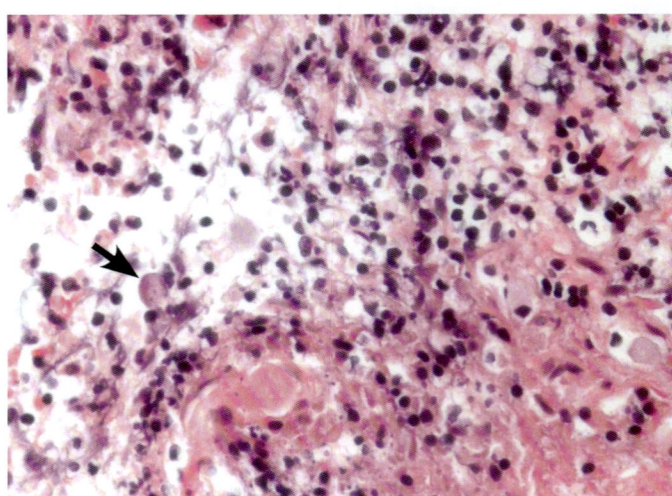

IMAGE 9.68 Amoebiasis (H&E, x400). Histology tends to show abundant necrotic debris. *Entamoeba histolytica* have small dot-like nuclei and foamy cytoplasm (arrow).

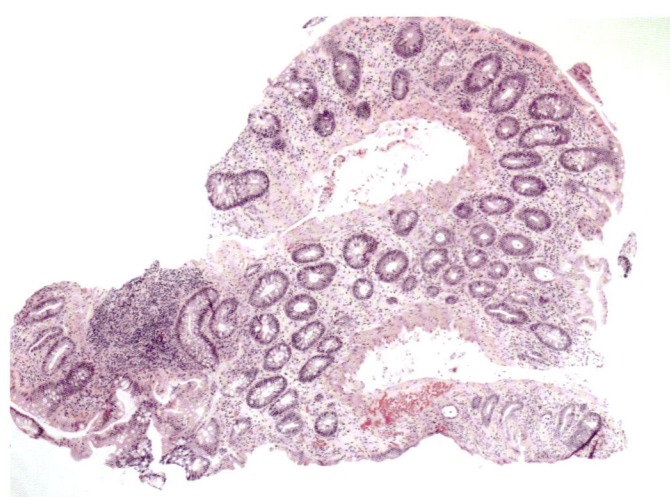

IMAGE 9.66 Mycophenolate mofetil-related colitis (H&E, x40). Colonic mucosa shows crypt architecture alteration, crypt apoptosis/atrophy, and reactive/reparative epithelial cytology.

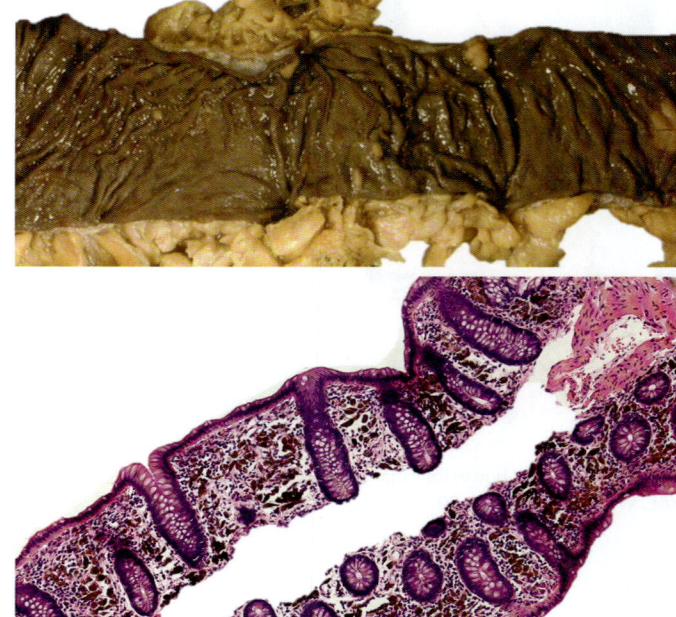

IMAGE 9.69 Melanosis coli. Upper: the gross image shows brown discoloration of colon. Lower: microscopy shows pigment-laden macrophages in the lamina propria (H&E, x100).

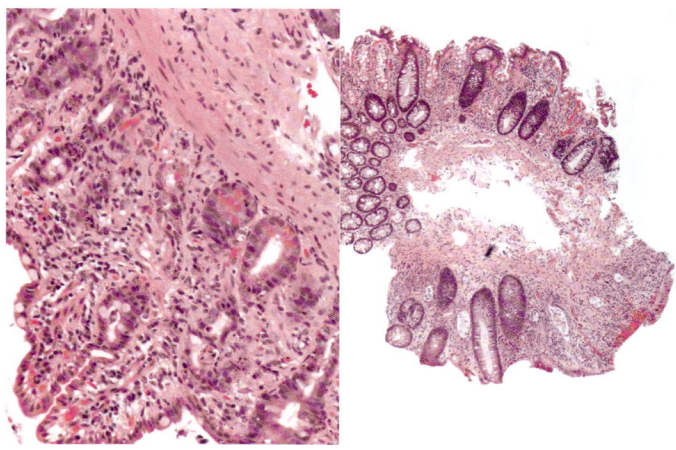

IMAGE 9.67 Graft versus host disease. Left: grade 2 with epithelial apoptosis (H&E, x200). Right: grade 3 with crypt loss (H&E, x40).

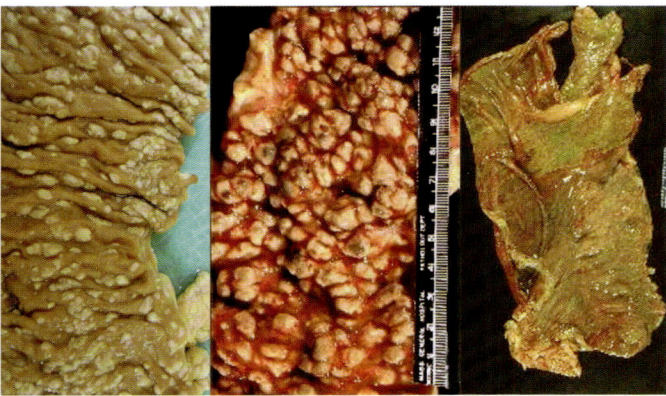

IMAGE 9.70 Pseudomembranous colitis. These gross images show different degrees of disease severity and extent of mucosa involvement.

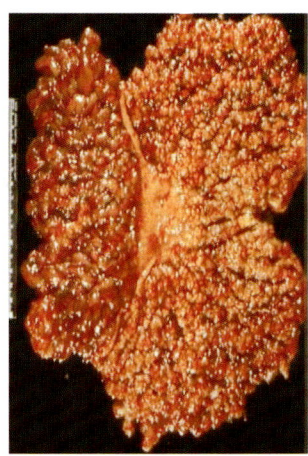

IMAGE 9.73 Cronkhite-Canada syndrome. The gross specimen shows the colonic mucosa carpeted by small polyps.

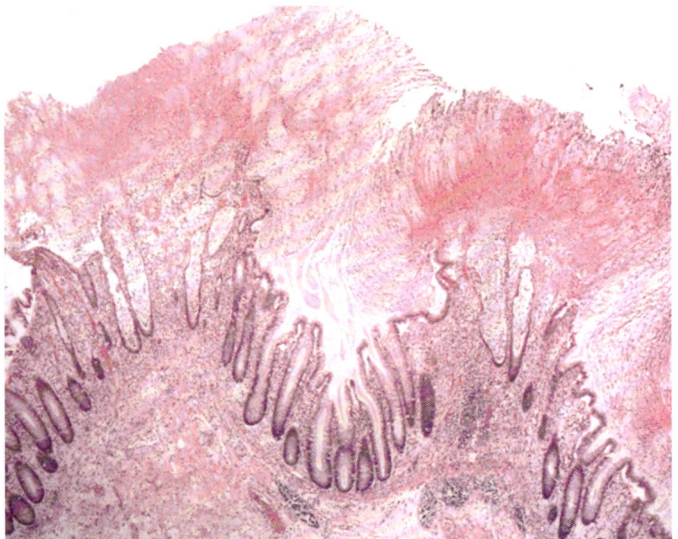

IMAGE 9.71 Pseudomembranous colitis (H&E, x40). Note the eruption of the top part of crypts and the characteristic appearance of the inflammatory exudate.

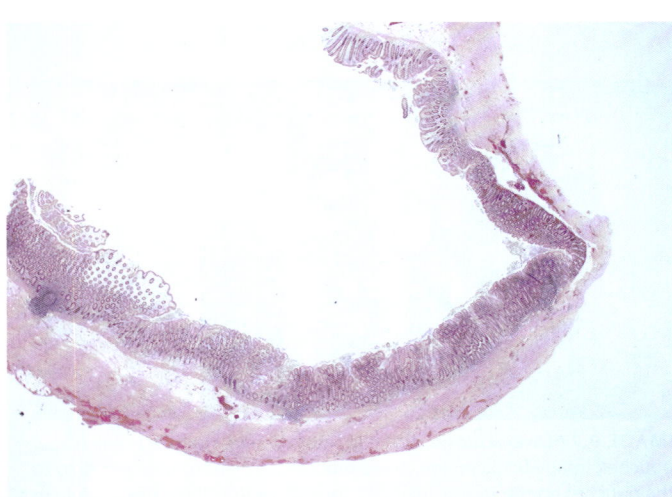

IMAGE 9.74 Ehlers-Danlos syndrome shows a severely attenuated muscle wall (H&E, x10).

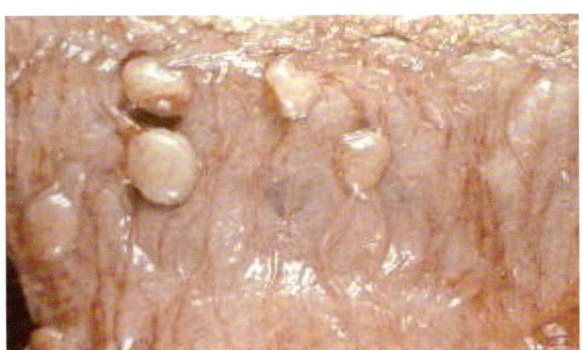

IMAGE 9.72 Cowden syndrome. The gross image shows multiple lipomas on colonic mucosa.

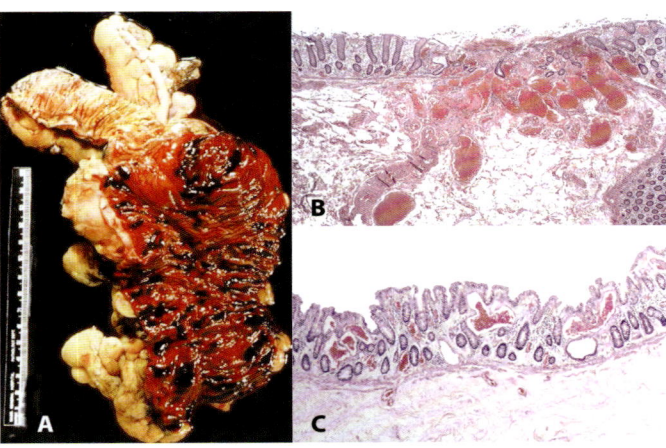

IMAGE 9.75 Angiodysplasia with hemorrhage. Left (image A): gross. Right (images B and C): many thick-walled vessels in the submucosa, which is the source of bleeding (image B: H&E, x100; image C: H&E, x40).

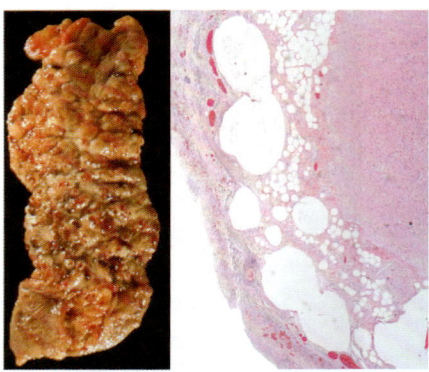

IMAGE 9.76 Pneumatosis coli. Left: the gross image shows translucent irregular mucosa with polypoid protrusions. Right: histology shows submucosal irregular air spaces without endothelial lining (H&E, x40).

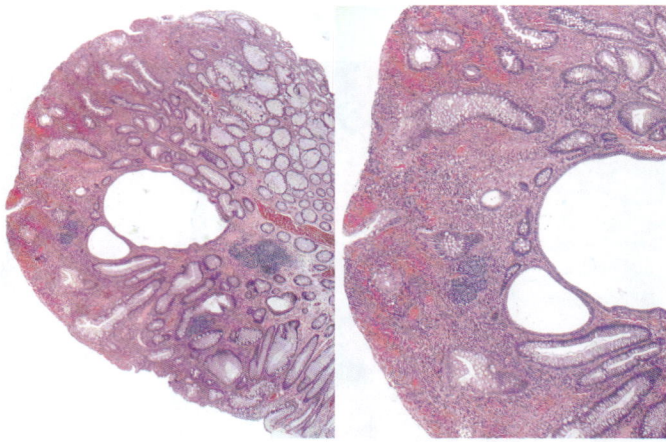

IMAGE 9.79 Solitary rectal ulcer. The mucosa can be polypoid with distortion of crypt architecture. Left: H&E, x20. Right: H&E, x100.

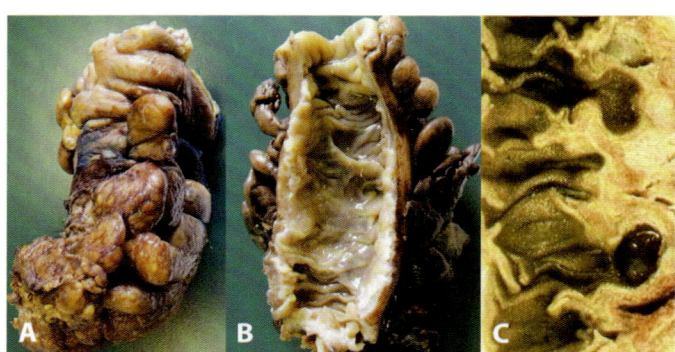

IMAGE 9.77 Diverticulosis. Image A: serosa shows multiple bulging pouches. Image B: the image shows mucosa herniation corresponding to the pouches on the serosa. Image C: coronal section illustrates the mucosa herniation.

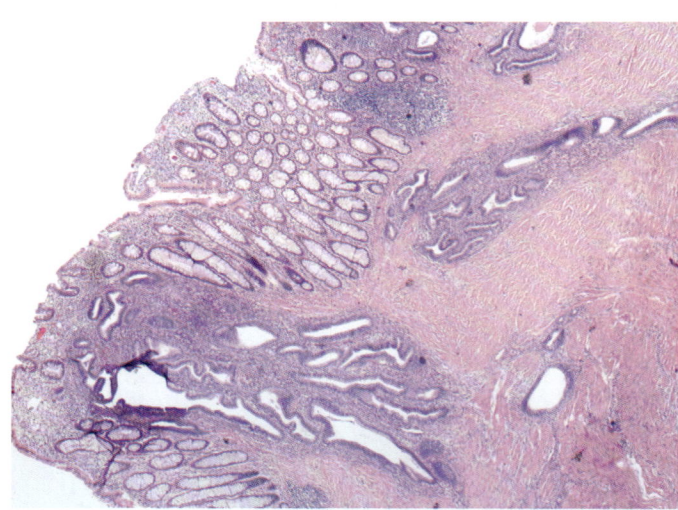

IMAGE 9.80 Endometriosis (H&E, x20). Endometrial glands typically are surrounded by endometrial stroma, which can help to differentiate them from carcinoma.

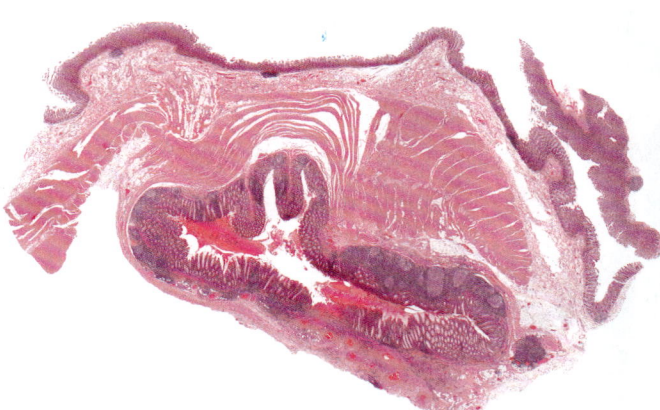

IMAGE 9.78 Diverticulum with hemorrhage (H&E, x1).

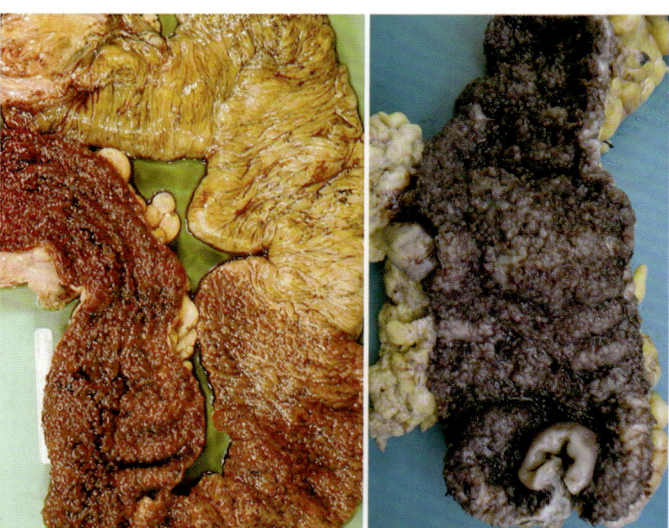

IMAGE 9.81 Ulcerative colitis gross features. Left: colorectum shows diffuse continuous involvement with a sharp demarcation from uninvolved bowel. Right: the affected mucosa is erythematous and granular, diffusely covered by small inflammatory pseudopolyps. The ileocecal valve is uninvolved.

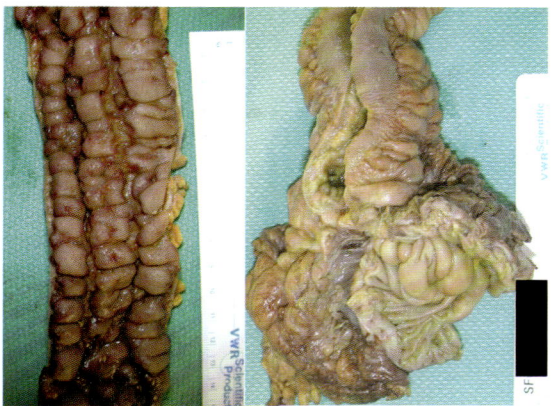

IMAGE 9.82 Crohn disease gross features. Left: "cobblestone" mucosa with linear ulcers. Right: creeping fat and adhesion.

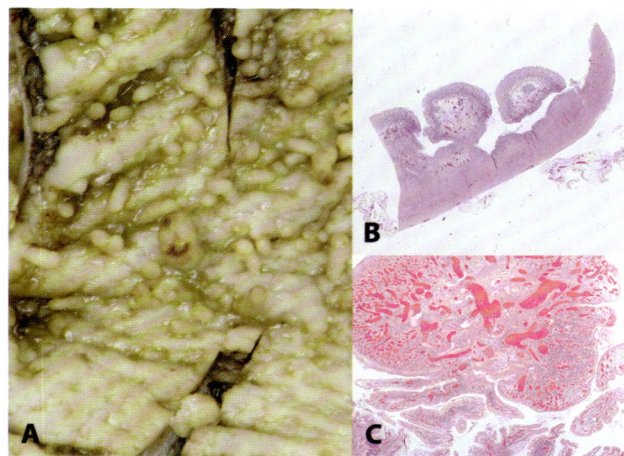

IMAGE 9.85 Ulcerative colitis with inflammatory pseudopolyps. Image A: gross. Image B: H&E, x1. Image C: H&E, x20.

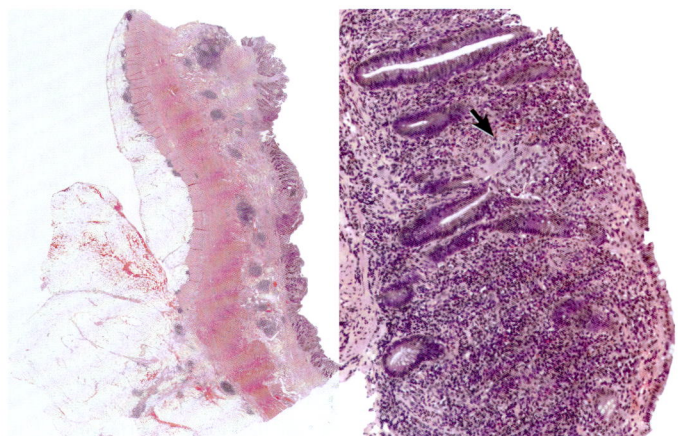

IMAGE 9.83 Crohn disease. Left: serosal and submucosal lymphoid aggregates (H&E, x1). Right: crypt architecture alteration and granuloma (arrow) in the lamina propria (H&E, x100).

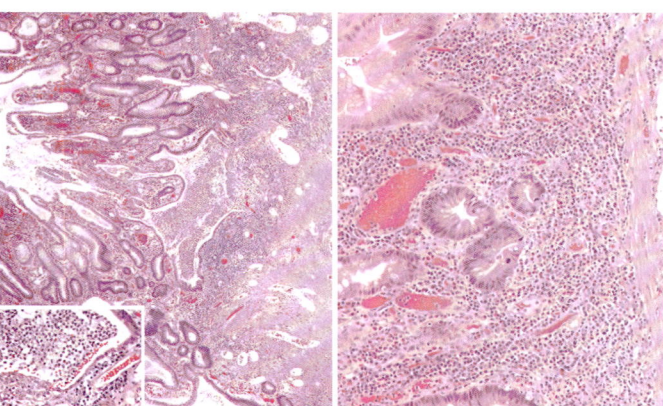

IMAGE 9.86 Ulcerative colitis. Left: crypt architecture alteration and crypt abscess (H&E, x20; inset: H&E, x100). Right: basal plasmacytosis (H&E, x100).

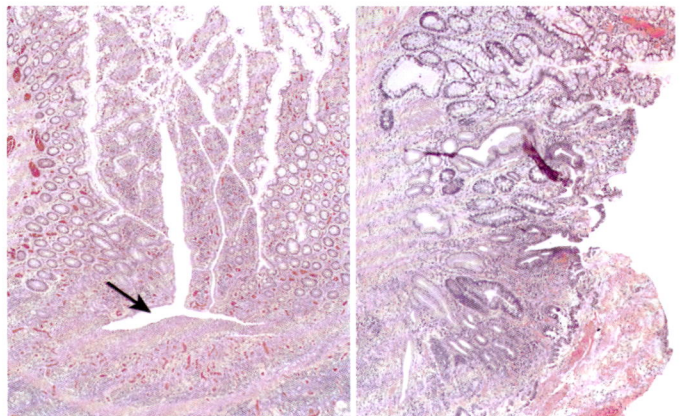

IMAGE 9.84 Crohn disease. Left: early stage with aphthous ulcer formation (H&E, x20). Right: late stage with focal low grade dysplasia (H&E, x100).

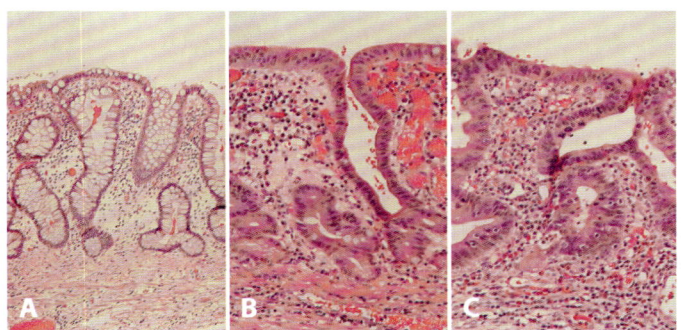

IMAGE 9.87 Ulcerative colitis with dysplasia (H&E, x100). Image A: no dysplasia. Image B: low grade dysplasia. Image C: high grade dysplasia.

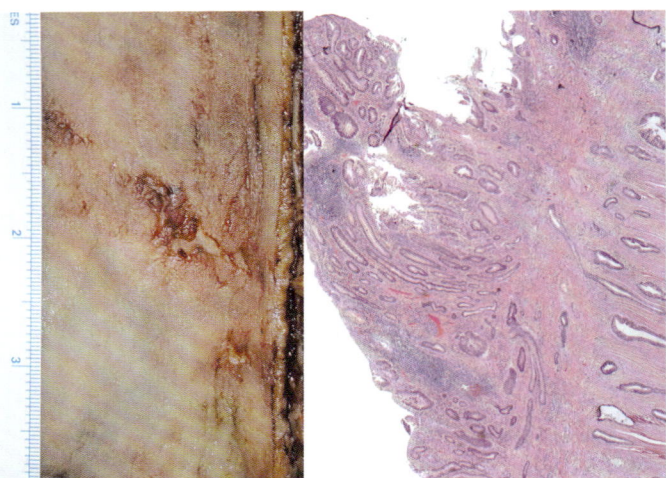

IMAGE 9.88 IBD-associated dysplasia and carcinoma. Left: the gross image shows a visible lesion in colorectal resection from a patient with ulcerative colitis. Right: note the invasive carcinoma under the mucosa with low grade dysplasia (H&E, x20).

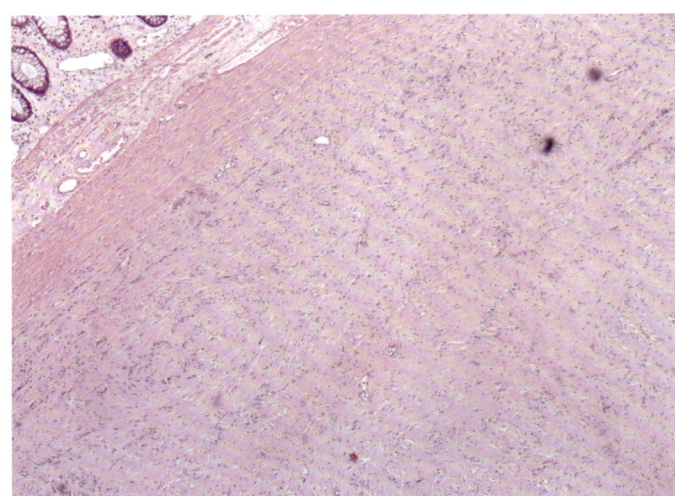

IMAGE 9.91 Colon schwannoma (H&E, x20). This lesion is in the submucosa. It can also present as a mucosal polyp.

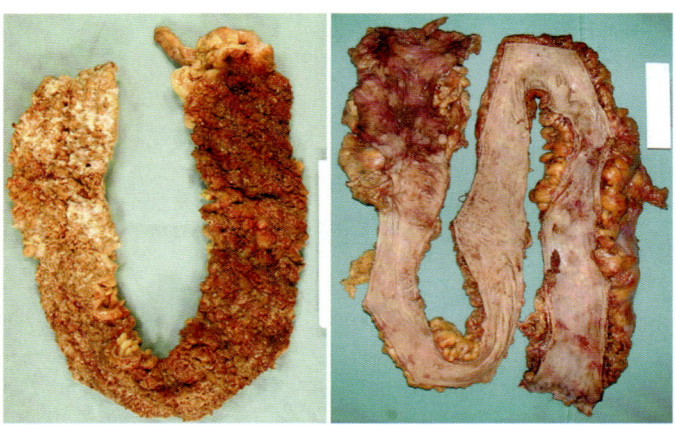

IMAGE 9.89 Left: fulminant colitis. Right: quiescent colitis.

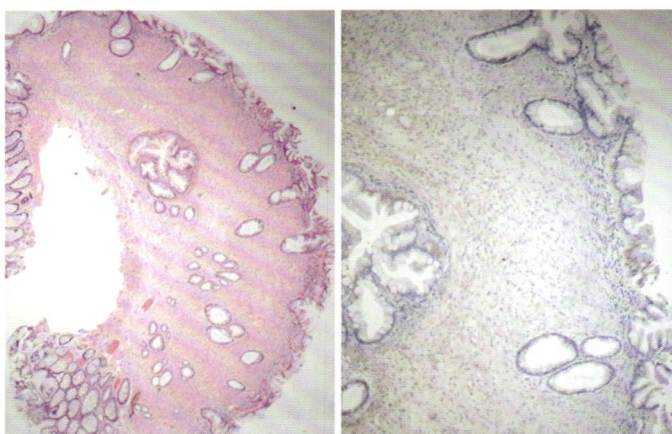

IMAGE 9.92 Perineurioma. Left: well-demarcated spindle cell lesion containing bland cells with tapering wavy nuclei infiltrating between hyperplastic-appearing crypts (H&E, x1). Right: the spindle cells stained positively for EMA (x100).

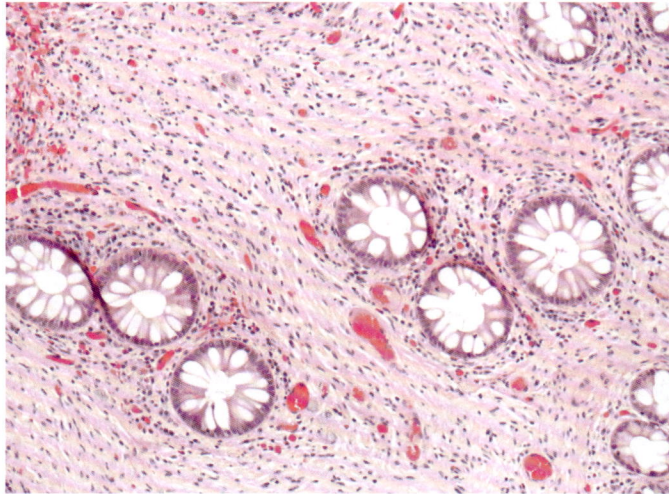

IMAGE 9.90 Ganglioneuroma (H&E, x100). The neoplastic ganglioneuroma cells push the normal crypts and glands apart.

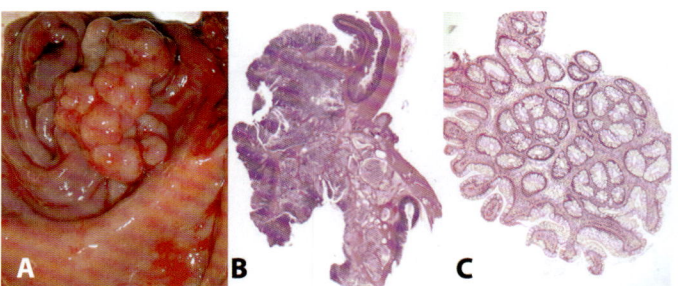

IMAGE 9.93 Hamartomatous polyps in a patient with Peutz-Jeghers syndrome. Image A: gross. Image B: polyp (H&E, x2). Image C: polyp (H&E, x40). The polyps have a typical branched (arborizing) architecture of overgrowth of mucosa and muscularis mucosa.

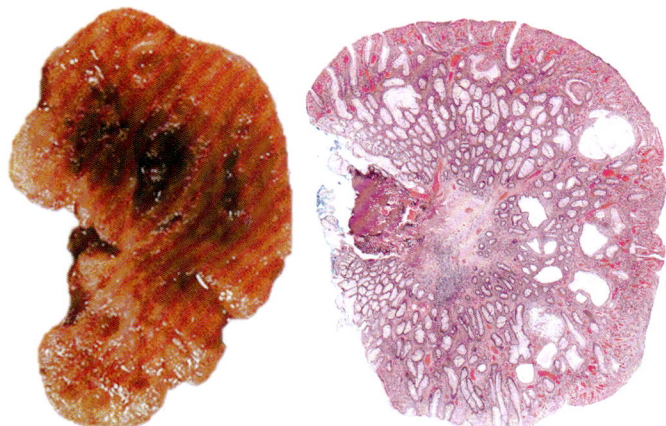

IMAGE 9.94 Juvenile (or retention) polyp. Left: gross. Right: characteristic juvenile polyp with a smooth contour and cystically dilated glands (H&E, x1).

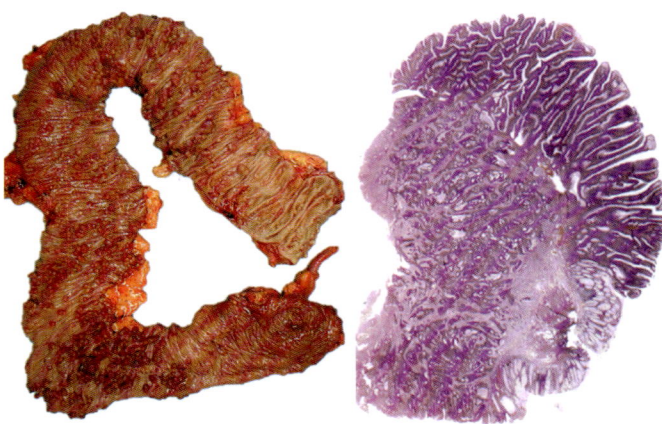

IMAGE 9.97 Familial adenomatous polyposis coli. Left: gross. Right: an adenocarcinoma arising from one of the polyps with positive margin.

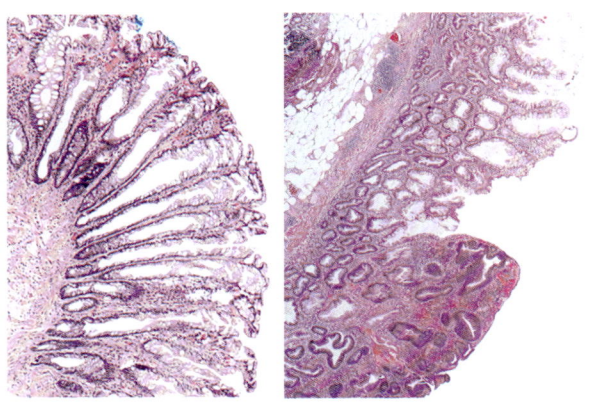

IMAGE 9.95 Colorectal hyperplastic polyps. Left: hyperplastic polyp (H&E, x40). Right: mixed hyperplastic-adenomatous polyp (H&E, x40).

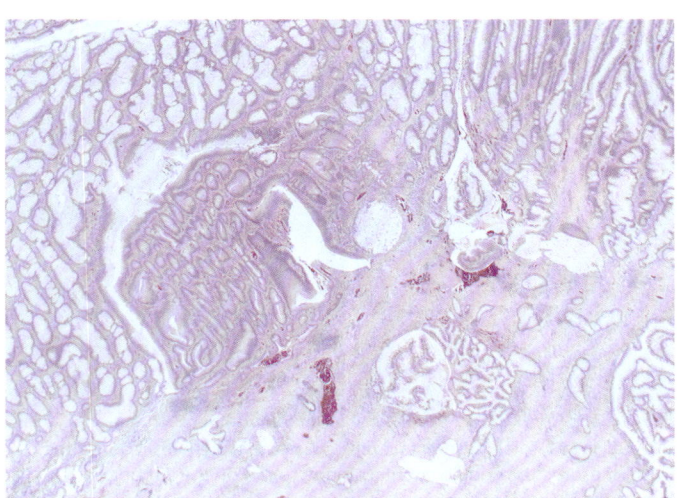

IMAGE 9.98 Tubular adenoma with pseudoinvasion. Note the lamina propria around the displaced glands with less dysplasia than the glands above, acellular mucin, and fresh hemorrhage on the surface of the polyp (H&E, x20).

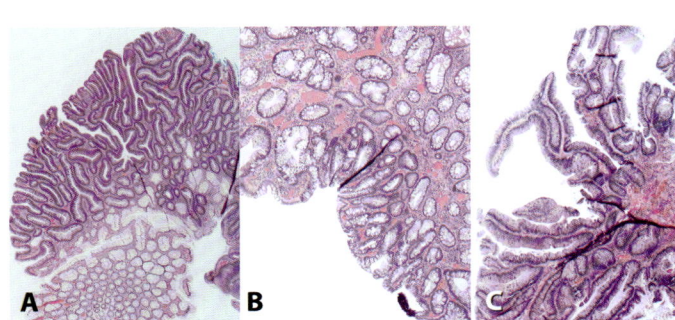

IMAGE 9.96 Colorectal adenomas (H&E, x40). Image A: pedunculated tubular adenoma. Image B: sessile flat tubular adenoma. Image C: large villous adenoma.

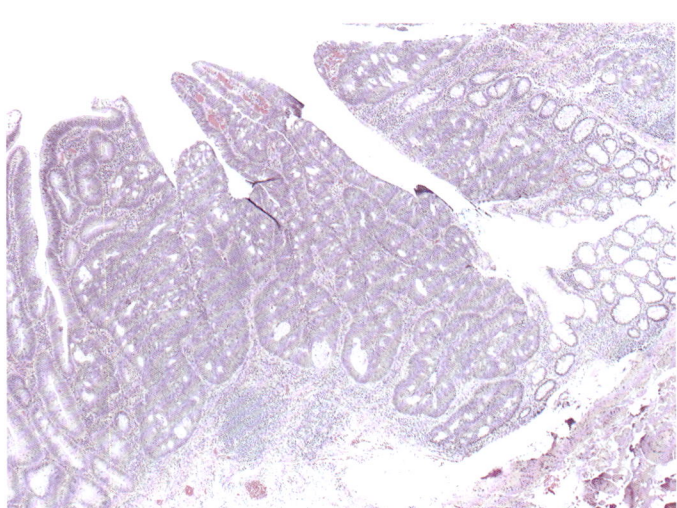

IMAGE 9.99 Intramucosal carcinoma showing cribriform high grade dysplastic glands (H&E, x40).

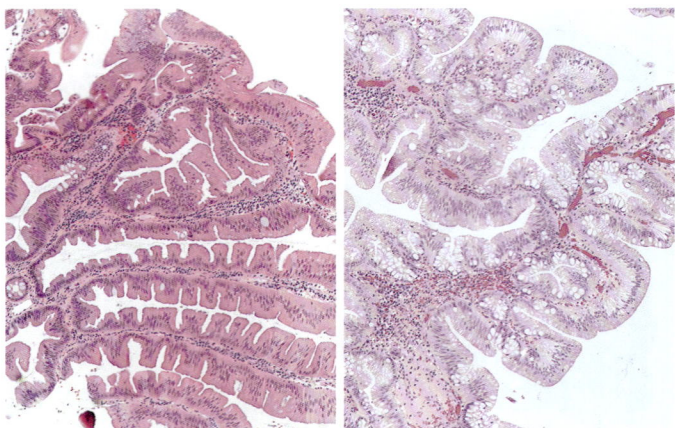

IMAGE 9.100 Traditional serrated adenoma shows eosinophilic cytoplasm and lesser degree of dysplasia on the surface (both images: H&E, x100).

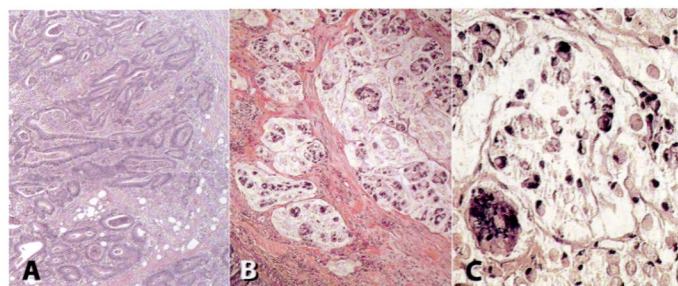

IMAGE 9.103 Colorectal adenocarcinoma. Image A: well-differentiated tumor glands (H&E, x40). Image B: mucinous differentiation (H&E, x200). Image C: poorly differentiated signet ring cell–type (H&E, x400).

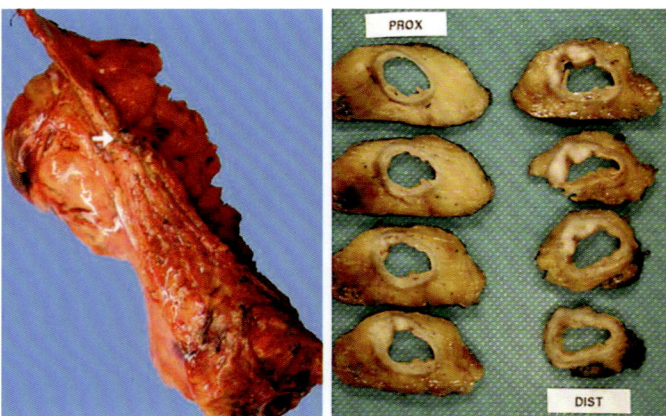

IMAGE 9.101 Total mesorectal excision. Left: complete resection with intact mesorectum and no conning. Right: tumor on the left upper quadrant and its depth of invasion.

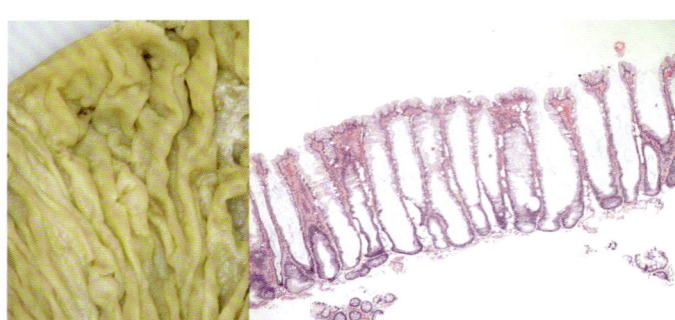

IMAGE 9.104 Sessile serrated lesion. Left: gross. Right: note the flask-shaped basal crypts (H&E, x40).

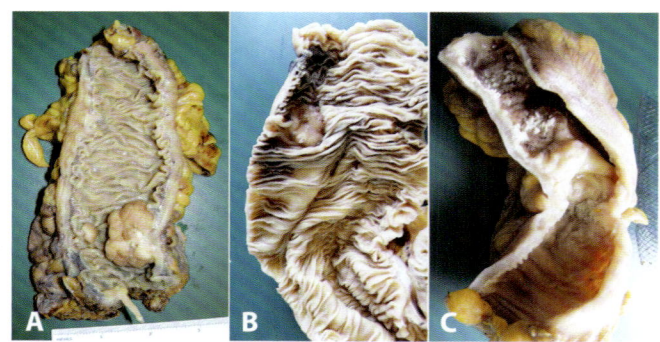

IMAGE 9.102 Colon cancer growth pattern. Image A: polypoid luminal protrusion. Image B: mucosa ulcer with raised edges. Image C: circumferential stricture.

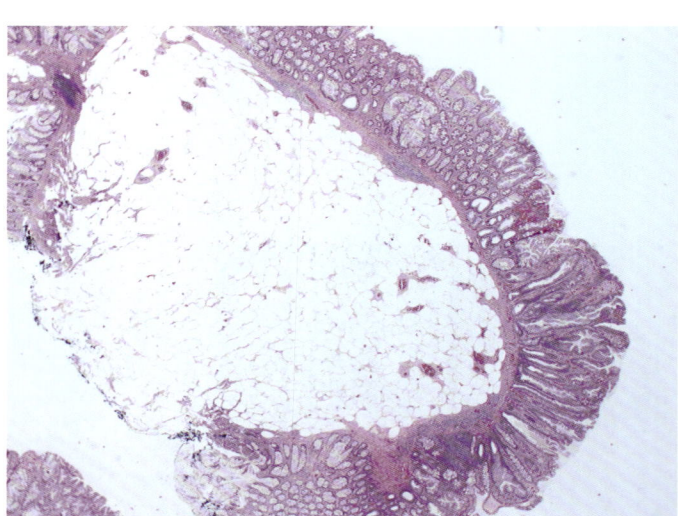

IMAGE 9.105 Fat in the submucosa of a sessile serrated lesion, which is a common phenomenon (H&E, x20).

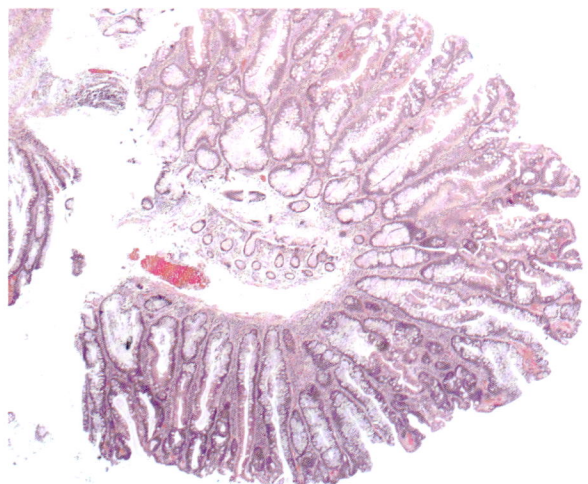

IMAGE 9.106 Sessile serrated lesion with dysplasia (H&E, x20). Cytological dysplasia is present in the lower part of the polyp.

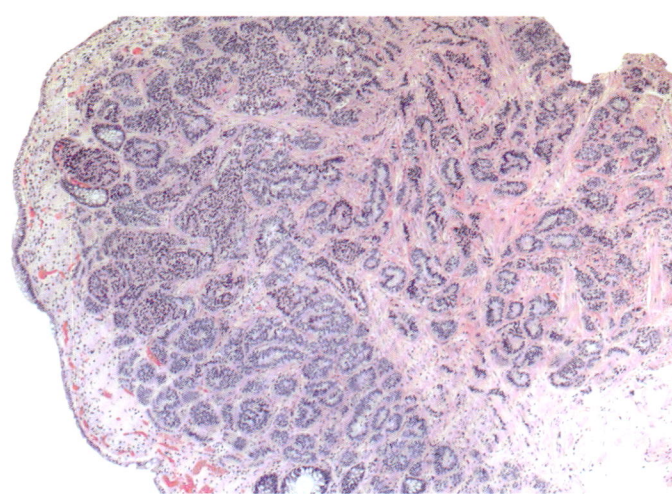

IMAGE 9.109 Rectal well-differentiated neuroendocrine tumor (H&E, x40).

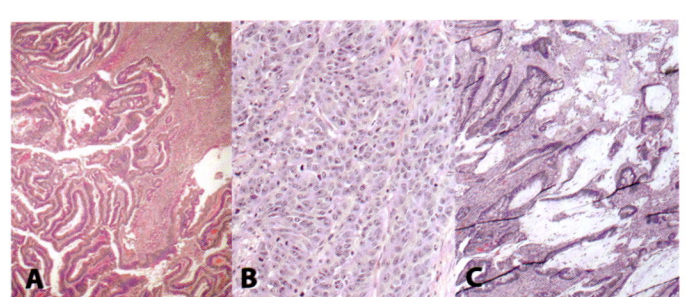

IMAGE 9.107 Proximally located colonic adenocarcinoma with histologic features suggestive of microsatellite instability (H&E, x100). Image A: pushing border, inflammatory cells, and serrated glands. Image B: poorly differentiated medullary carcinoma. Image C: mucinous adenocarcinoma with serrated glands.

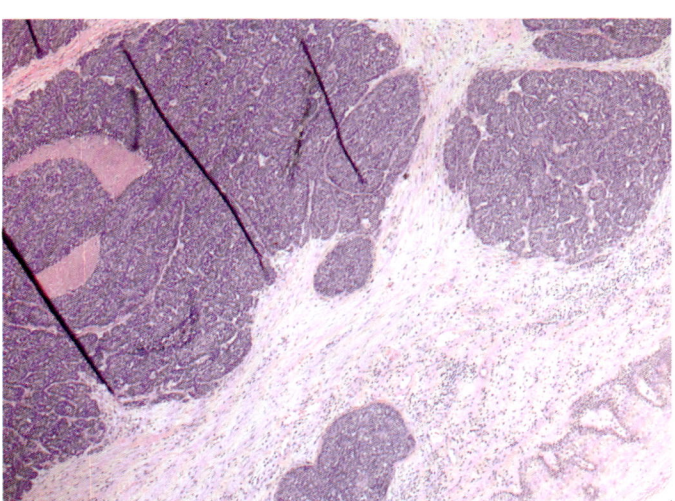

IMAGE 9.110 Anal basaloid squamous cell carcinoma (H&E, x40). Note the pronounced hyperchromasia, scant cytoplasm and peripheral palisading of the malignant glands.

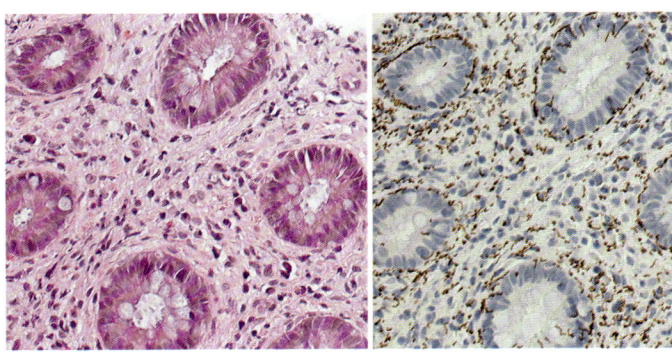

IMAGE 9.108 Syphilitic proctitis. Left: numerous plasma cells are conspicuous in the lamina propria (H&E, x400). Right: IHC highlights slender, helically coiled treponemal spirochetes (anti-*Treponema pallidum* IHC, x400).

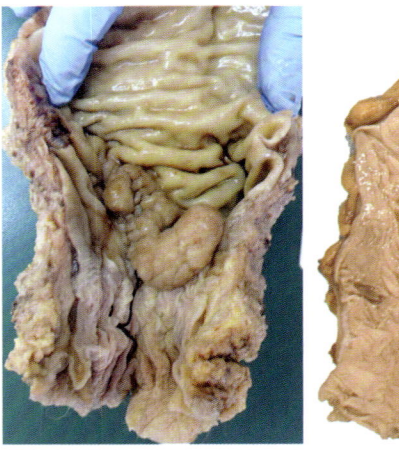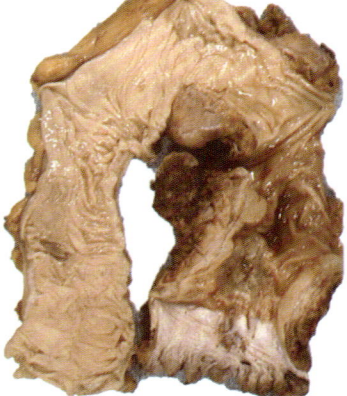

IMAGE 9.111 Left: low rectum adenocarcinoma. Right: anal squamous cell carcinoma.

Right: courtesy of Dr. Olga Aleynikova.

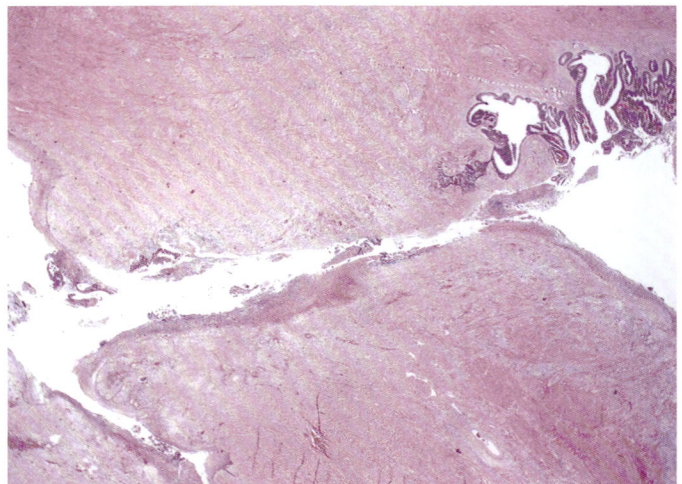

IMAGE 9.112 Adenocarcinoma with anal fistula (H&E, x20).

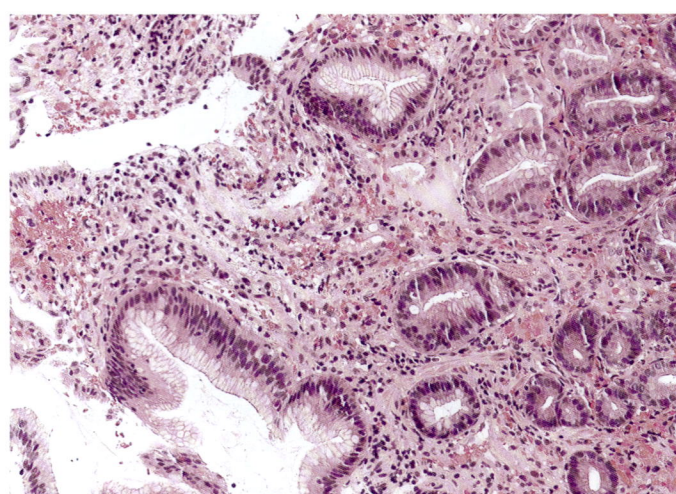

IMAGE 9.115 Kaposi sarcoma in colonic mucosa (H&E, x200). In the lamina propria, there are monomorphic spindle cells separated by slit-like spaces and associated with fresh hemorrhage.

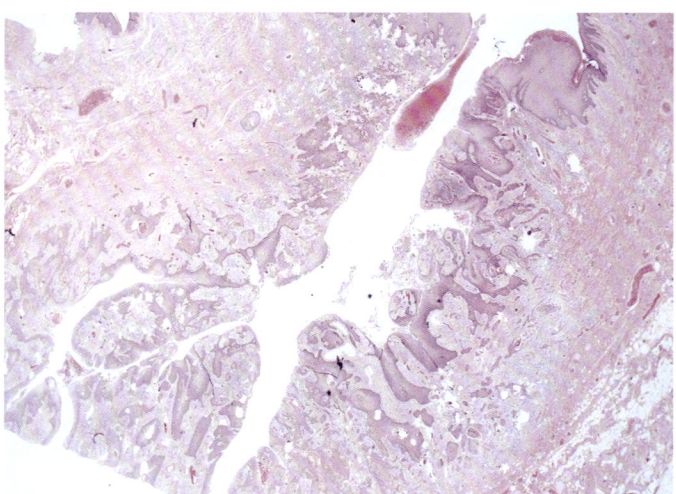

IMAGE 9.113 Squamous cell carcinoma with anal fistula (H&E, x20).

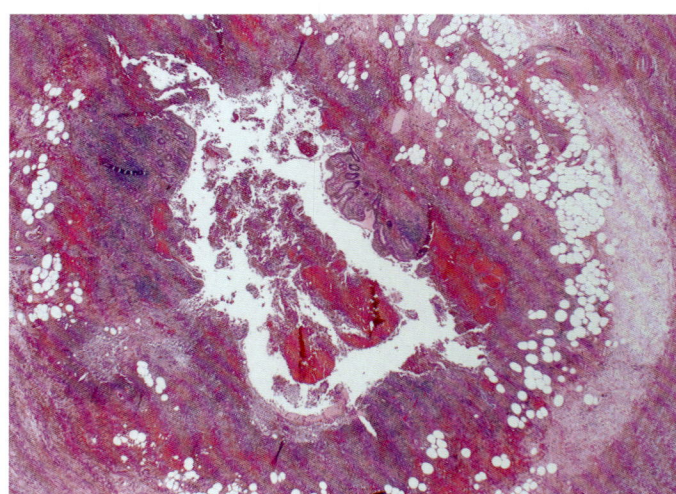

IMAGE 9.116 Acute appendicitis (H&E, x20).

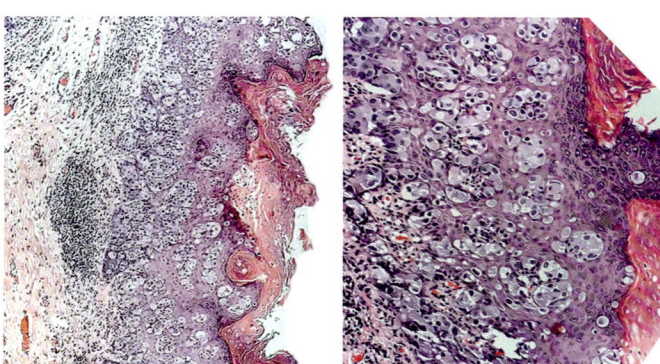

IMAGE 9.114 Extramammary Paget disease (both images: H&E, x10). Mucin-containing pagetoid cells infiltrating anal squamous mucosa.

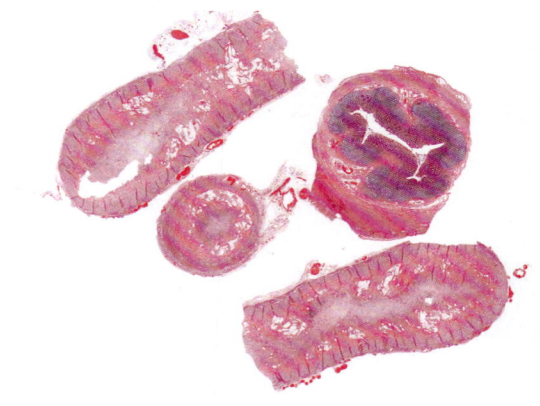

IMAGE 9.117 Fibrous obliteration of appendix (H&E, x1).

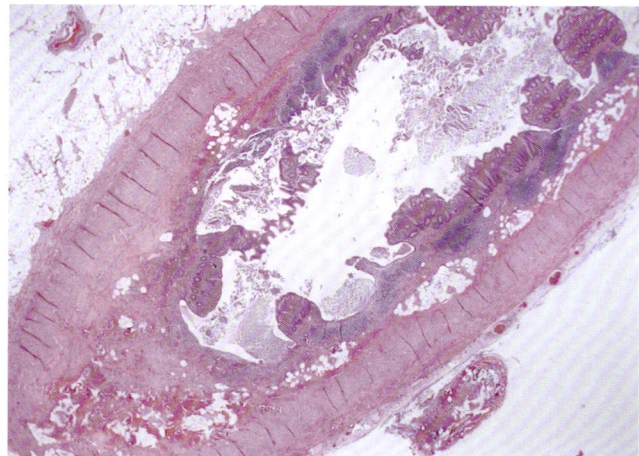

IMAGE 9.118 Crohn disease involving the appendix shows characteristic mucosa ulceration, pseudopolyps, and submucosa inflammatory aggregates (H&E, x20).

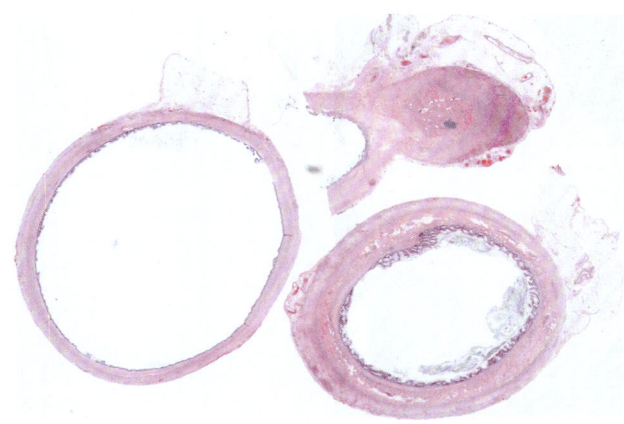

IMAGE 9.121 LAMN. The lumen is dilated and the epithelial lining is mostly flattened, with the characteristic effacement of lamina propria (H&E, x1).

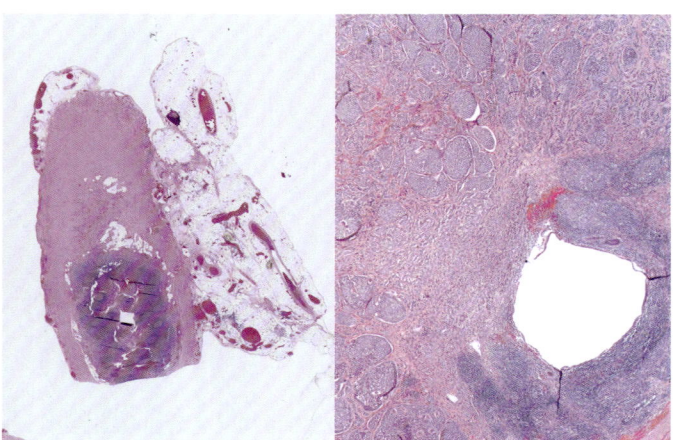

IMAGE 9.119 Appendiceal well-differentiated neuroendocrine tumor. Left: H&E, x1. Right: H&E, x40. The tip of the appendix is the most common site.

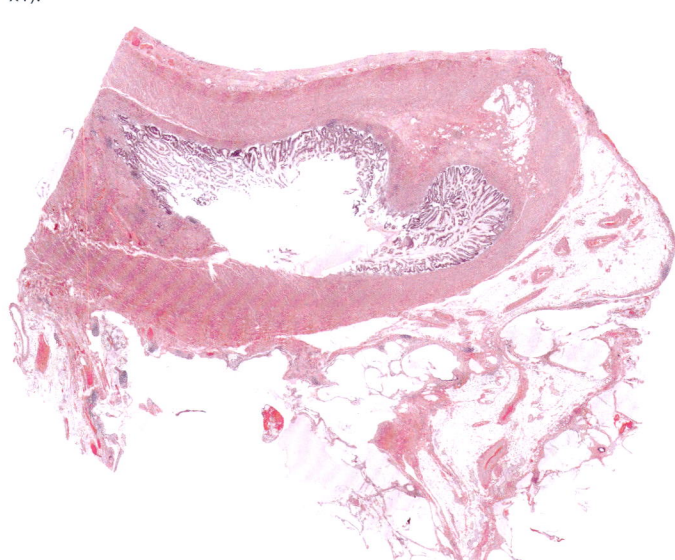

IMAGE 9.122 Appendiceal mucinous adenocarcinoma with pseudomyxoma peritonei (H&E, x1).

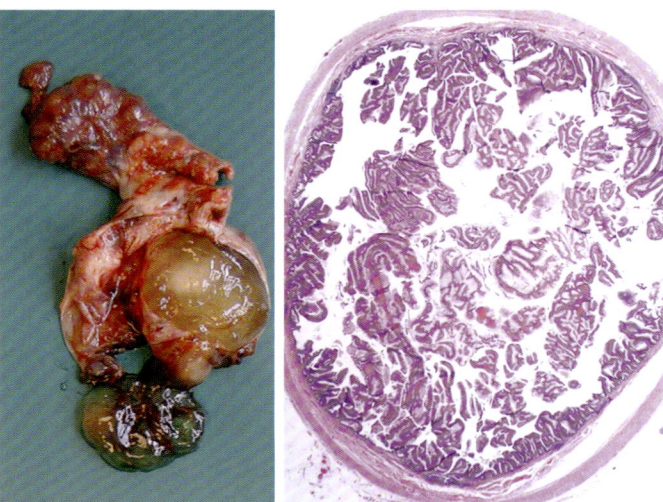

IMAGE 9.120 Low grade appendiceal mucinous neoplasm (LAMN). Left: gross. Right: the neoplastic epithelium showing low grade dysplasia with papillary projections into the appendiceal lumen (H&E, x40). There is no invasion to the appendiceal wall.

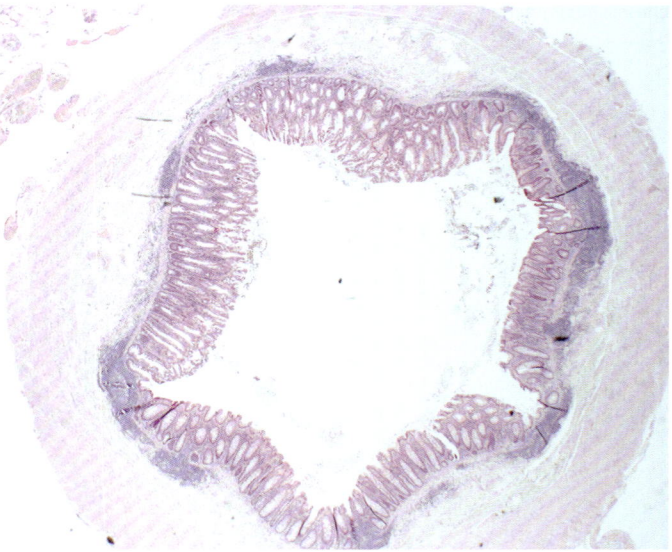

IMAGE 9.123 Appendiceal serrated lesion (H&E, x20). The lesion shows serrated and dilated crypts analogous to colonic sessile serrated lesion. Note that here lamina propria is mostly preserved unlike in LAMNs.

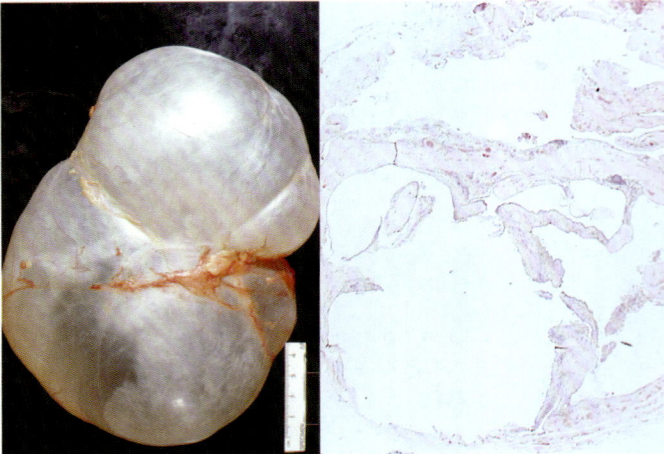

IMAGE 9.124 Benign peritoneal cyst. Left: gross. Right: the cysts are lined by a single layer of benign mesothelium (H&E, x10).

Left: courtesy of Dr. Olga Aleynikova.

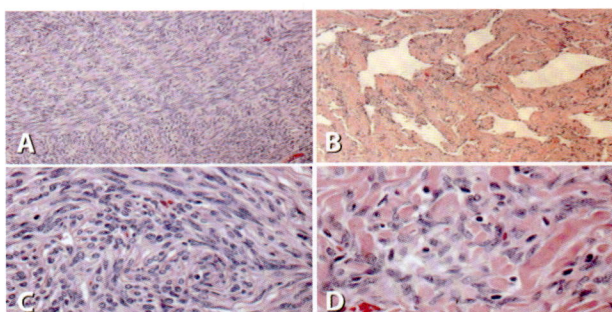

IMAGE 9.127 Solitary fibrous tumor. The 4 images show the characteristic alternating areas of hyper- and hypocellularity, branching staghorn vessels, patternless arrangement of bland oval-to-spindled cells, and prominent ropy keloidal collagen.

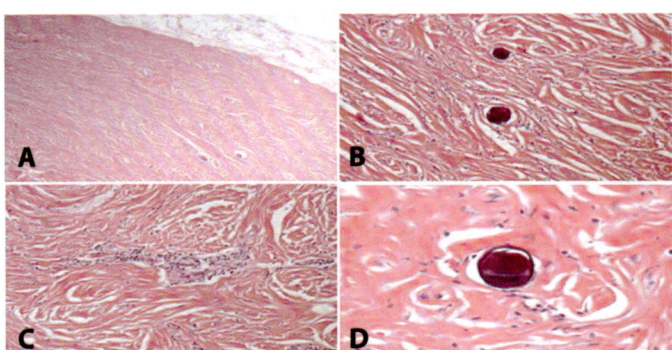

IMAGE 9.125 Calcifying fibrous tumor of the mesentery. The 4 images show the characteristic circumscribed border, low cellularity, hyalinized collagenous stroma, psammomatous calcifications and patchy, perivascular chronic inflammation.

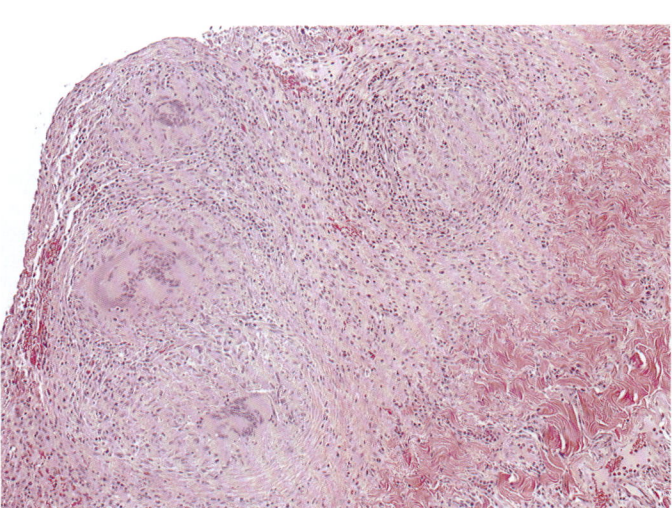

IMAGE 9.128 Peritoneum tuberculosis showing multiple granulomata (H&E, x40).

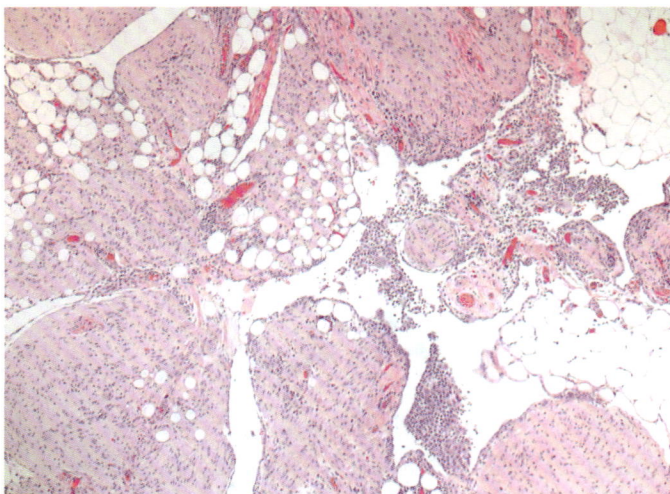

IMAGE 9.126 Mesenteric gliomatosis (H&E, x20). Nodules of mature glial tissue are embedded within the omentum.

Reference

1. Boudreaux JP, Klimstra DS, Hassan MM, et al. The NANETS consensus guideline for the diagnosis and management of neuroendocrine tumors: well-differentiated neuroendocrine tumors of the jejunum, ileum, appendix, and cecum. Pancreas. 2010;39(6):753-66. doi: 10.1097/MPA.0b013e318ebb2a5

Bibliography

Amin MB, Edge S, Greene F, et al, editors. AJCC cancer staging manual. 8th ed. New York: Springer; 2017.

Bartley AN, Christ J, Fitzgibbons P, et al; Cancer Biomarker Reporting Committee, College of American Pathologists. Template for reporting results of HER2 (ERBB2) biomarker testing of specimens from patients with adenocarcinoma of the stomach or gastroesophageal junction (Version: GastricHER2Biomarkers 1.0.0.1) [Internet]. College of American Pathologists; 2017. Available from www.cap.org.

Bartley AN, Hamilton SR, Alsabeh R, et al; Cancer Biomarker Reporting Committee, College of American Pathologists. Template for reporting results of biomarker testing of specimens from patients with carcinoma of the colon and rectum (Version: Colon and Rectum Biomarkers 1.2.0.1) [Internet]. College of American Pathologists; 2014. Available from www.cap.org.

Blair VR, McLeod M, Carneiro F, et al. Hereditary diffuse gastric cancer: updated clinical practice guidelines. Lancet Oncol. 2020; 21(8): e386-e397. doi: 10.1016/S1470-2045(20)30219-9

Boudreaux JP, Klimstra DS, Hassan MM, et al. The NANETS consensus guideline for the diagnosis and management of neuroendocrine tumors: well-differentiated neuroendocrine tumors of the jejunum, ileum, appendix, and cecum. Pancreas. 2010; 39:753. doi: 10.1097/MPA.0b013e3181ebb2a5

Burgart LJ, Kakar S, Shi C, et al; Cancer Committee, College of American Pathologists. Protocol for the examination of resection specimens from patients with primary carcinoma of the colon and rectum (Version: Colon and Rectum Resection 4.1.0.0) [Internet]. College of American Pathologists; 2020. Available from www.cap.org.

Burgart LJ, Shi C, Adsay V, et al; Cancer Committee, College of American Pathologists. Protocol for the examination of specimens from patients with carcinoma of the ampulla of Vater (Version: AmpullaVater 4.1.0.0) [Internet]. College of American Pathologists; 2020. Available from www.cap.org.

Burgart LJ, Shi C, Berho ME, et al; Cancer Committee, College of American Pathologists. Protocol for the examination of excisional biopsy specimens from patients with primary carcinoma of the colon and rectum (Version: Colon and Rectum Biopsy 4.1.0.0) [Internet]. College of American Pathologists; 2020. Available from www.cap.org.

Burgart LJ, Shi C, Driman DK, et al; Cancer Committee, College of American Pathologists. Protocol for the examination of specimens from patients with carcinoma of the anus (Version: Anus 4.1.0.0) [Internet]. College of American Pathologists; 2020. Available from www.cap.org.

Burgart LJ, Shi C, Driman DK, et al; Cancer Committee, College of American Pathologists. Protocol for the examination of specimens from patients with carcinoma of the appendix (Version: Appendix 4.1.0.0) [Internet]. College of American Pathologists; 2020. Available from www.cap.org.

Cancer Genome Atlas Research Network. Comprehensive molecular characterization of gastric adenocarcinoma. Nature. 2014;513(7517):202–09. doi: 10.1038/nature13480

Dellon ES, Liacouras CA, Molina-Infante J, et al. Updated international consensus diagnostic criteria for eosinophilic esophagitis: proceedings of the AGREE conference. Gastroenterology. 2018;155(4):1022–33.e10. doi: 10/1053.j.gastro.2018.07.009

Dixon MF, Genta RM, Yardley JH, et al. Classification and grading of gastritis. The updated Sydney System. International Workshop on the Histopathology of Gastritis, Houston 1994. Am J Surg Pathol. 1996;20(10):1161–81. Medline:8827022. doi: 10.1097/00000478-199610000-00001

Farraye FA, Odze RD, Eaden J, et al; AGA Institute Medical Position Panel on Diagnosis and Management of Colorectal Neoplasia in Inflammatory Bowel Disease. AGA medical position statement on the diagnosis and management of colorectal neoplasia in inflammatory bowel disease. Gastroenterology. 2010;138(2):738–45. Medline:20141808. doi 10.1053/j.gastro.2009.12.037

Gavioli M, Luppi G, Losi L, et al. Incidence and clinical impact of sterilized disease and minimal residual disease after preoperative radiochemotherapy for rectal cancer. Dis Colon Rectum. 2005;48(10):1851-57. doi:10.1007/s10350-005-0133-6

Goldblum J, Lamps L, McKenney J, et al. Rosai and Ackerman's surgical pathology. 11th ed. Philadelphia (PA): Elsevier; 2017.

Kumar V, Abbas AK, Aster JC. Robbins and Cotran pathologic basis of disease. 10th ed. North York (ON): Elsevier Canada; 2020.

Laine L, Kaltenbach T, Barkun A, et al. SCENIC international consensus statement on surveillance and management of dysplasia in inflammatory bowel disease. Gastroenterology. 2015; 148(3):639–51.e28. doi: 10.1053/j.gastro.2015.01.031

Laurini JA, Blanke CD, Cooper K, et al; Cancer Committee, College of American Pathologists. Protocol for the examination of resection specimens from patients with gastrointestinal stromal tumor (GIST) (Version: GIST Resection 4.1.0.0) [Internet]. College of American Pathologists; 2019. Available from www.cap.org.

Laurini JA, Hameed M, Corless CL, et al; Cancer Committee, College of American Pathologists. Template for reporting results of biomarker testing of specimens from patients with gastrointestinal stromal tumors (Version: GIST biomarkers 1.0.0.2) [Internet]. College of American Pathologists; Feb 2020 [revised 2020 Feb, accessed 2020 Dec]. 10 p. Available from www.cap.org.

Lester SC. Manual of surgical pathology. 3rd ed. Philadelphia (PA): Elsevier Saunders; 2010.

Longacre TA, editor. Mills and Sternberg's diagnostic surgical pathology. 7th ed. Philadelphia (PA): Wolters Kluwar; 2022.Odze RD, Goldblum JR, editors. Odze and Goldblum surgical pathology of the GI tract, liver, biliary tract, and pancreas. 3rd ed. Philadelphia (PA): Saunders/Elsevier; 2015.

Park JG, Vasen HF, Park KJ, et al. Suspected hereditary nonpolyposis colorectal cancer: International Collaborative Group on Hereditary Non-Polyposis Colorectal Cancer (ICG-HNPCC) criteria and results of genetic diagnosis. Dis Colon Rectum. 1999;42(6):710-716. doi:10.1007/BF02236922

Sepulveda AR, Hamilton SR, Allegra CJ, et al. Molecular biomarkers for the evaluation of colorectal cancer: Guideline From the American Society for Clinical Pathology, College of American Pathologists, Association for Molecular Pathology, and the American Society of Clinical Oncology. J Clin Oncol. 2017; 35(13): 1453–86. doi: 10.1200/JCO.2016.71.9807

Shaheen, NJ, Falk GW, et al. Diagnosis and management of Barrett's esophagus: an updated ACG guideline. Am J Gastroenterol. 2022;117(4):559-587. doi: 10.14309/ajg.0000000000001680

Shi C, Berlin J, Branton PA, et al; Cancer Committee, College of American Pathologists. Protocol for the examination of specimens from patients with carcinoma of the esophagus (Version: Esophagus 4.1.0.0) [Internet]. College of American Pathologists; 2020. Available from: www.cap.org.

Shi C, Berlin J, Branton PA, et al; Cancer Committee, College of American Pathologists. Protocol for the examination of specimens from patients with carcinoma of the small intestine (Version: Small Intestine 4.1.0.0) [Internet]. College of American Pathologists; 2020. Available at www.cap.org.

Shi C, Berlin J, Branton PA, et al; Cancer Committee, College of American Pathologists. Protocol for the examination of specimens from patients with carcinoma of the stomach (Version: Stomach 4.1.0.0) [Internet]. College of American Pathologists; 2020. Available from: www.cap.org.

Spechler SJ, Sharma P, Souza RF, et al; American Gastroenterological Association. American Gastroenterological Association medical position statement on the management of Barrett's esophagus. Gastroenterology. 2011;140(3):1084–91. Medline:21376940. doi: 10.1053/j.gastro.2011.01.031

Umar A, Boland CR, Terdiman JP, et al. Revised Bethesda guidelines for hereditary nonpolyposis colorectal cancer (Lynch syndrome) and microsatellite instability. J Natl Cancer Inst. 2004;96(4):261-68. doi:10.1093/jnci/djh034

Vasen HF, Mecklin JP, Khan PM, et al. The International Collaborative Group on Hereditary Non-Polyposis Colorectal Cancer (ICG-HNPCC). Dis Colon Rectum. 1991;34(5):424-25. doi:10.1007/BF02053699

WHO Classification of Tumours Editorial Board. WHO classification of tumours. 5th ed. Vol. 1, Digestive system tumours. Lyon (France): IARC; 2019.

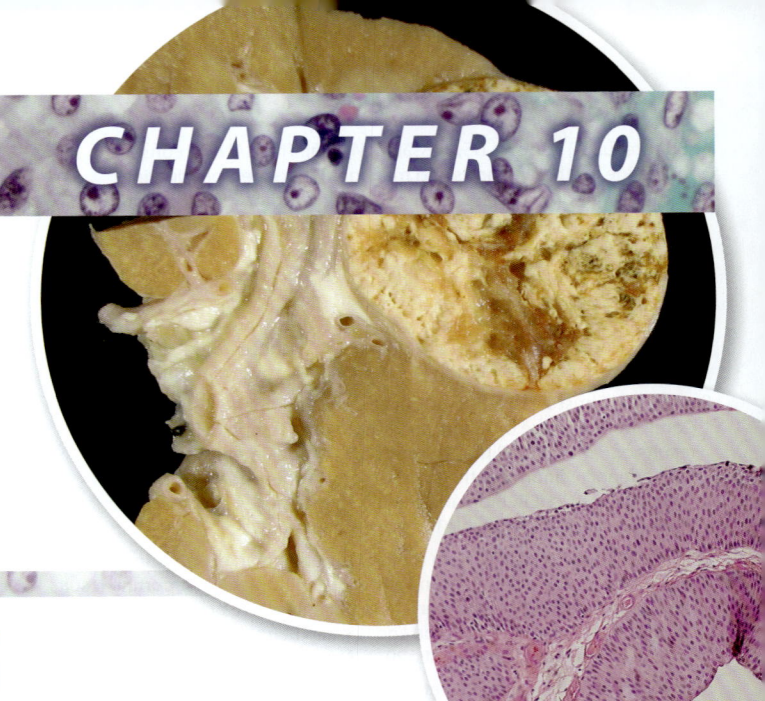

CHAPTER 10

Genitourinary & Renal Pathology

YUAN GAO, CHENG WANG, JENNIFER MERRIMEN

Genitourinary and Renal Pathology Exam Essentials

MUST KNOW

Nonneoplastic entities

You should be familiar with nonneoplastic entities in the genitourinary (GU) tract (e.g., amyloid, xanthogranulomatous pyelonephritis, cystic renal diseases, malakoplakia, cystitis, ectopic tissues, developmental anomalies, prostatic hyperplasia, granulomatous inflammation, torsion, testicular biopsy findings in infertility, penile inflammatory skin diseases, morphologic findings in sexually transmitted diseases).

World Health Organization (WHO) classifications

High-yield topics include:

- The WHO classification of tumors of the urinary system and male genital organs, including:
  - Kidney.
  - Urinary tract.
  - Prostate.
  - Testis and paratesticular tissue.
  - Penis.
- Renal cell carcinoma (RCC) and its various subtypes, genetic syndromes involving RCC, and clinical features including risk factors.
- An approach to the diagnosis of renal neoplasms of various morphologies (e.g., cystic renal neoplasms, eosinophilic renal neoplasms).

- Classification of, and relevant risk factors for, bladder carcinoma including: urothelial carcinoma and its clinically significant variants; adenocarcinoma; and squamous cell carcinoma.
- Diagnostic criteria of prostatic adenocarcinoma and Gleason grading, and important variants. Be familiar with mimics of adenocarcinoma and have an approach to differentiate these from carcinoma. Understand the differential diagnosis of cribriform glandular lesions, including intraductal carcinoma and its significance.
- Germ cell tumors, including: key morphologic and immunohistochemistry (IHC) features, the tumors associated with germ cell neoplasia in situ (GCNIS), molecular changes, relevant epidemiology, relevant serum markers, and issues around germ cell tumor regression.
- Sex cord stromal tumors of the testis.
- Tumors that can arise in the paratesticular region.
- Common skin diseases affecting the penis and foreskin, including squamous neoplasms, Paget disease, and inflammatory skin diseases.

AJCC and College of American Pathologists (CAP) protocols

High-yield topics include:

- Important staging and reporting features for renal cell carcinoma, including: International Society of

Urological Pathology (ISUP) grade; other prognostic features such as sarcomatoid differentiation and rhabdoid differentiation; and necrosis.
- Important staging features of tumors of the urinary bladder, ureter, and renal pelvis.
- Staging of prostatic adenocarcinoma and important features to report on biopsy and resection specimens.
- Key features of testicular tumor staging and relevant anatomy.

Medical renal diseases
- You should know commonly encountered medical kidney diseases, including their basic mechanism, clinical manifestations, morphologic features, and ancillary tests (e.g., immunofluorescence and electron microscopy findings).
- Basic knowledge of medical renal disease includes: nephritic versus nephrotic syndrome; common clinical presentations; and crescentic glomerulonephritis including main types.

Genetic and syndromic conditions
High-yield topics include:
- Common hereditary syndromes and genetic conditions that affect the GU tract: von Hippel-Lindau (VHL) syndrome; hereditary papillary RCC; Birt-Hogg-Dubé syndrome; tuberous sclerosis; hereditary leiomyomatosis and RCC; and succinate dehydrogenase-deficient-associated diseases, including Carney triad and Carney-Stratakis syndrome.
- Genetic syndromes that affect the testis, including Klinefelter syndrome and androgen insensitivity syndrome.

MUST SEE
High-yield slides include:
- Nonneoplastic renal entities such as:
  · Common glomerulopathies (morphology, and findings on electron microscopy [EM] and immunofluorescence [IF]):
    › Nephrotic diseases: minimal change disease, focal segmental glomerulosclerosis (FSGS), membranous nephropathy, diabetes, amyloid.
    › Mixed nephritic and nephrotic diseases: lupus, membranoproliferative glomerulonephritis, IgA nephropathy.
    › Nephritic diseases: Goodpasture syndrome and antiglomerular basement membrane (anti-GBM) glomerulonephritis; IgA nephritis (Berger disease) and Henoch-Schönlein purpura (HSP); postinfectious glomerulonephritis; antineutrophil cytoplasmic antibody (ANCA) associated vasculitis.
- Benign and malignant renal neoplasms such as:
  · Clear cell RCC.
  · Multilocular renal neoplasm of low malignant potential.

- Type 1 and 2 papillary RCC.
- Chromophobe RCC.
- Collecting duct RCC.
- Medullary RCC.
- Xp11 and microphthalmia (MiT) family translocation RCC.
- Tubulocystic RCC.
- Oncocytoma.
- Metanephric adenoma.
- Nephroblastoma.
- Pediatric cystic nephroma.
- Rhabdoid tumor.
- Angiomyolipoma.
- Mixed epithelial and stromal tumor (MEST).
- Paraganglioma.
- Renal papillary adenoma.
- Gross and morphologic findings of common renal pathologic entities:
  · Autosomal dominant and autosomal recessive polycystic kidney disease.
  · Papillary renal necrosis.
  · Hypertensive changes, diabetic changes, and renal infarct.
  · Pyelonephritis, including xanthogranulomatous pyelonephritis.
  · Nephrolithiasis.
  · Congenital anomalies of kidney and ureter.
- Common pathologic entities of the bladder and collecting system:
  · Hemorrhagic cystitis.
  · Schistosomiasis.
  · Cystitis cystica et glandularis.
  · Amyloid.
  · Malakoplakia.
  · Nephrogenic adenoma.
  · Urothelial neoplasms (papilloma, including inverted papilloma; papillary urothelial neoplasm of low malignant potential (PUNLMP); low grade papillary urothelial carcinoma; high grade papillary urothelial carcinoma; carcinoma in situ, including subtypes).
  · Variants of urothelial carcinoma with adverse prognosis.
  · Squamous cell carcinoma.
  · Adenocarcinoma, including those from urachal remnant.
  · Small cell carcinoma.
  · Inflammatory myofibroblastic tumor.
  · Paraganglioma.
  · Melanoma.
  · Postoperative spindle cell nodule.
- Common pathologic entities of the prostate:
  · Benign nodular hyperplasia.
  · Acinar prostatic adenocarcinoma and variants (e.g., atrophic, hyperplastic).

- Other carcinomas seen in prostate such as: ductal carcinoma, small cell carcinoma, urothelial carcinoma.
- Morphology and application of Gleason patterns.
- Cribriform lesions including: clear cell cribriform hyperplasia, ductal carcinoma, high grade prostatic intraepithelial neoplasia (HGPIN), and intraductal carcinoma.
- Mimics of prostate cancer, including atrophy, Cowper glands, and atypical adenomatous hyperplasia.
- Acute, chronic, and granulomatous prostatitis.
- Common entities in the testis and paratestis:
  - Infertility findings: Sertoli cells only, testicular atrophy, hypospermatogenesis, normal spermatogenesis, and germ cell maturation arrest.
  - Hydrocele and spermatocele.
  - Testicular infarct and testicular torsion.
  - Cryptorchid testis.
  - Germ cell neoplasms, including GCNIS, seminoma, embryonal carcinoma, yolk sac tumor, choriocarcinoma, teratoma, mixed germ cell tumor, regressed germ cell tumor, and spermatocytic tumor.
  - Sex cord stromal tumors, including Leydig cell tumor and Sertoli cell tumor.

- Lymphoma.
- Common paratesticular tumors, including adenomatoid tumor, mesothelioma, lipoma, and liposarcoma.
- Common penile lesions, including types related and unrelated to human papillomavirus and Paget disease: balanitis xerotica obliterans (penile lichen sclerosus), Zoon balanitis, penile intraepithelial neoplasia (PeIN), and small cell carcinoma (SCC).

MUST DO

- Practice generating differential diagnoses, and requesting additional relevant clinical information.
- List additional ancillary tests, histochemical stains, immunohistochemical stains, and molecular tests to narrow or confirm a diagnosis.
- List relevant risk factors and genetic syndromes for GU neoplasms.
- Describe the grossing protocol for biopsies and resections of GU organs and how they relate to determining the pathologic staging of tumors.
- Describe how to handle common fresh specimens in GU pathology (e.g., frozen section procedures and submitting tissue for EM and IF in medical kidney biopsies).

MULTIPLE CHOICE QUESTIONS

1. What is the cell of origin for adenomatoid tumors?

a. Renal tubular epithelial cell.
b. Interstitial cells of Cajal.
c. Mesothelial cell.
d. Hilar cell.
e. Undifferentiated mesenchymal cell.

Answer: c

2. Renal papillary necrosis is seen in the following situations **except**:

a. Diabetes mellitus.
b. Urinary tract obstruction.
c. Acute pyelonephritis.
d. Wegener granulomatosis.
e. Analgesic abuse.

Answer: d

3. A prostate needle biopsy specimen contains a conventional prostatic adenocarcinoma, with the following Gleason patterns: pattern 4 about 65%, pattern 3 about 30%, and pattern 5 about 5%. What is the Gleason score?

a. 8.
b. 7.
c. 7 with a tertiary pattern 5.
d. 9.
e. 12.

Answer: d

4. In the prostate, the basal layer of the epithelium stains for:

a. Prostate specific antigen (PSA).
b. p63.
c. Actin.
d. p53.
e. Prostatic acid phosphatase (PAP).

Answer: b

5. What is the most common malignancy of the spermatic cord of adult males?

a. Liposarcoma.
b. Leiomyosarcoma.
c. Embryonal rhabdomyosarcoma.
d. Undifferentiated sarcoma.
e. Angiosarcoma.

Answer: a

6. What condition is associated with granular IgA, IgG, IgM, and C3 within glomeruli?

a. Alport disease.
b. Lupus nephritis.
c. Antineutrophil cytoplasmic antibody (ANCA) associated vasculitis.
d. Postinfectious glomerulonephritis.
e. Membranous nephropathy.

Answer: b

7. Which is **not** a common histologic finding seen in cyclosporine and tacrolimus (FK506) nephrotoxicity?

a. Tubular isometric vacuolization.
b. Hyaline arteriopathy.
c. Acute thrombotic microangiopathy.
d. Crescentic glomerulonephritis.
e. Normal histology.

Answer: d

8. In myeloma cast nephropathy, what causes renal damage?

a. Hypercalcemia.
b. Tissue infiltration by neoplastic cells.
c. Immunoglobulin light chains.
d. Infection.
e. Secondary to chemotherapeutic agents.

Answer: c

9. In invasive urothelial carcinoma of the bladder, stage pT2 corresponds to:

a. Invasion of the lamina propria.
b. Invasion of the muscularis mucosae.
c. Invasion of the submucosa.
d. Invasion of the muscularis propria.
e. Invasion of the prostate.

Answer: d

10. Which is considered a premalignant lesion in the prostate?

a. High grade prostatic intraepithelial neoplasia (HPIN).
b. Postatrophic hyperplasia.
c. High grade preinvasive neoplasm.
d. Nephrogenic metaplasia.
e. Columnar cell change.

Answer: a

11. Which is **not** a typical morphological feature of balanitis xerotica obliterans (lichen sclerosis)?

a. Orthokeratotic hyperkeratosis.
b. Atrophy of the epidermis.
c. Homogenization of collagen in the upper dermis.
d. Interstitial hemorrhage and hemosiderin deposition.
e. Lymphoplasmacytic lichenoid inflammatory infiltrate.

Answer: d

12. Which stain is typically **negative** in classic seminoma?

a. Cytokeratin (AE1/AE3).
b. Placental alkaline phosphatase (PLAP).
c. OCT 4.
d. C-kit.
e. Periodic acid–Schiff (PAS).

Answer: a

13. What is the common genetic alteration seen in testicular germ cell tumors in adulthood?

a. t(11;22).
b. Loss of 3p.
c. Isochromosome 12p.
d. t(X;11).
e. Gain of 13q.

Answer: c

14. Which condition is **not** commonly associated with renal cell carcinoma?

a. Birt-Hogg-Dubé syndrome.
b. Autosomal dominant polycystic kidney disease.
c. Tuberous sclerosis.
d. Von Hippel-Lindau disease.
e. End stage renal disease.

Answer: b

15. What is the T stage of a renal cell carcinoma that shows direct growth into the ipsilateral adrenal gland?

a. pT2c.
b. pT3a.
c. pT3b.
d. pT3c.
e. pT4.

Answer: e

16. What is the characteristic morphological finding in malakoplakia?

a. Cytoplasmic lipid.
b. Weibel-Palade bodies.
c. Michaelis-Gutmann bodies.
d. Asteroid bodies.
e. Giant mitochondria.

Answer: c

17. Patients with which variant of urothelial carcinoma listed below have the best prognosis?

a. Sarcomatoid urothelial carcinoma.
b. Urothelial carcinoma with syncytiotrophoblasts.
c. Micropapillary urothelial carcinoma.
d. Nested urothelial carcinoma.
e. Mixed urothelial and small cell carcinoma.

Answer: b

18. What is the pT stage of a prostatic adenocarcinoma that invades the base of the seminal vesicle?

a. pT2c.
b. pT3a.
c. pT3b.
d. pT3c.
e. pT4.

Answer: c

19. Which of the following patterns is **not** a description of Gleason pattern 4?

a. Cribriform glands with central necrosis.
b. Carcinoma with ductal differentiation.
c. Glandular structures showing glomerulations.
d. Chains of fused glandular structures.
e. Poorly formed small glandular structures.

Answer: a

20. Which is **not** a mimic of invasive prostatic adenocarcinoma?

  a. Glandular atrophy.
  b. Atypical adenomatous hyperplasia.
  c. Cowper glands.
  d. Granulomatous prostatitis.
  e. Corpora amylacea.

Answer: e

21. Which entity is **not** associated with germ cell neoplasia in situ (GCNIS)?

  a. Cryptorchidism.
  b. Majority of post-pubertal mature teratoma.
  c. Embryonal carcinoma.
  d. Spermatocytic tumor.
  e. Mixed germ cell tumor.

Answer: d

22. On smear preparations received with male fertility biopsy specimens, which 2 patterns would you expect to show spermatozoa?

  a. Germ cell maturation arrest and hypospermatogenesis.
  b. Sertoli-cell-only syndrome and germ cell maturation arrest.
  c. Hypospermatogenesis and obstruction of sperm excretory ducts.
  d. Testicular atrophy and Sertoli-cell-only syndrome.
  e. Obstruction of sperm excretory ducts and Sertoli-cell-only syndrome with immature Sertoli cells.

Answer: c

23. Which is **not** a pattern seen in urothelial carcinoma in situ?

  a. Clinging/denuding pattern.
  b. Small cell pattern.
  c. Pagetoid pattern.
  d. Undermining pattern.
  e. Microcystic pattern.

Answer: e

24. Which is the most common genetic alteration in clear cell renal cell carcinoma?

  a. Loss of 3p.
  b. Isochromosome 12p.
  c. t(X;11).
  d. Gain of 13q.
  e. t(11;22).

Answer: a

25. Which of the following entities does **not** typically present with nephrotic syndrome?

  a. Minimal change disease.
  b. Focal segmental glomerulosclerosis.
  c. Membranous glomerulopathy.
  d. Thin basement membrane disease.
  e. Membrano-proliferative glomerulonephritis.

Answer: d

26. Which of the following is associated with fibrin and platelet thrombi within glomeruli?

  a. Alport syndrome.
  b. Hemolytic uremic syndrome.
  c. Immunotactoid glomerulopathy.
  d. Acute interstitial nephritis.
  e. Acute tubular necrosis.

Answer: b

27. Which of the following is true regarding immunostaining patterns in testicular neoplasms?

  a. Caudal-type homeobox 2 (CDX2) stains seminoma.
  b. Oct3/4 is positive in teratoma.
  c. Glypican 3 highlights yolk sac tumor.
  d. Epithelial membrane antigen (EMA) stains all types of germ cell tumors.
  e. Classic seminoma is positive for CD20.

Answer: c

28. In addition to clear cell renal cell carcinoma, von Hippel-Lindau (VHL) syndrome is also associated with which of the following?

  a. Renal cysts.
  b. Adrenal pheochromocytoma.
  c. Clear cell pancreatic neuroendocrine neoplasm (PEN).
  d. Papillary cystadenoma of epididymis or broad ligament.
  e. All of the above.

Answer: e

29. Which of the following is involved in von Hippel-Lindau syndrome?

  a. Hamartin.
  b. Hypoxia inducible factor.
  c. Folliculin.
  d. Merlin.
  e. Tuberin.

Answer: b

30. Inverted urothelial carcinoma of the renal pelvis is associated with which of the following?

  a. Lynch syndrome.
  b. Tuberous sclerosis.
  c. Birt-Hogg-Dubé syndrome.
  d. End stage of renal disease.
  e. None of the above.

Answer: a

31. Sickle cell trait is associated with which of the following?

  a. Wilms tumor.
  b. Oncocytoma.
  c. Clear cell tubulopapillary renal cell carcinoma.
  d. Renal medullary carcinoma.
  e. None of the above.

Answer: d

32. Which of the following statements about adenomatoid tumor is (are) correct?

a. Adenomatoid tumors are the most common tumor of the testicular adnexa and are usually asymptomatic.

b. By immunohisto-chemistry, adenomatoid tumor is positive for mesothelial markers including calretinin and Wilms tumor protein 1 (WT1). Adenomatoid tumor is negative for splicing factor 1 protein (SF1), which can be used in cases difficult to differentiate from Sertoli cell tumors.

c. Histologically, adenomatoid tumor is composed of cords or tubules of neoplastic cells with bland nuclei, open chromatin, and intracytoplasmic clear vacuoles.

d. The surrounding stroma of an adenomatoid tumor often shows prominent smooth muscle differentiation and acquires a more reactive appearance in cases with infarction.

e. All of the above.

Answer: e

33. Which of the following statements about testicular teratomas is correct?

a. All prepubertal testicular teratomas are malignant.

b. Testicular dermoid cysts are benign and may be amenable to conservative management.

c. The features of prepubertal-type teratoma include the presence of all of the following: cytological atypia, GCNIS, significant tubular atrophy/tubular sclerosis, scarred zones, impaired spermatogenesis, microlithiasis, and evidence of chromosome 12p amplification.

d. Postpubertal-type teratomas are subclassified further into immature and mature subtypes as they possess distinct biologic behaviors.

e. All of the above.

Answer: b

34. According to the World Health Organization (WHO) classification of genitourinary tumors,* the nonchoriocarcinomatous trophoblastic tumors include the following:

a. Epithelioid trophoblastic tumor (ETT).

b. Placental site trophoblastic tumor (PSTT).

c. Cystic trophoblastic tumor (CTT).

d. Answers a, b, and c.

e. None of the above.

Answer: d

*This chapter uses the fourth edition of the WHO classification of tumors of the urinary system and male genital organs.

35. What immunohistochemical markers are useful in differentiating epithelioid trophoblastic tumor (ETT) and placental site trophoblastic tumor (PSTT)?

a. p63.

b. Ki 67.

c. Human placental lactogen (hPL).

d. Answers a, b, and c.

e. None of the above.

Answer: d

36. Membranous nephropathy is a form of chronic immune complex glomerulonephritis induced by antibodies against glomerular antigens. An antigen frequently involved in membranous nephropathy is:

a. Podocyte antigen phospholipase A2 receptor (PLA2R).

b. Collagen type IV antigen.

c. HIV.

d. Hepatitis B virus (HBV).

e. All of the above.

Answer: a

Prostate
Prostate Adenocarcinoma

37. Describe the 5 Gleason patterns of prostatic adenocarcinomas.

PATTERN	DESCRIPTION
1*	• Circumscribed nodule of medium sized acini. • Acini: closely packed but separate, uniform, and round to oval in shape. • Larger glands than in pattern 3.
2*	• Like pattern 1: fairly circumscribed, but minimal infiltration at the edge of the nodule. • Glands more loosely arranged and not quite as uniform as in pattern 1.
3	• Discrete glandular units. • Typically smaller glands than in pattern 1 or 2. • Infiltrates in and among nonneoplastic prostate acini. • Variation in size and shape.
4	• Fused microacinar glands. • Poorly defined glands with poorly formed glandular lumina. • Large cribriform glands and cribriform glands with an irregular border. • Glomeruloid structures.
5	• Essentially no glandular differentiation — composed of solid sheets, cords, or single cells. • Comedocarcinoma with central necrosis surrounded by papillary, cribriform, or solid masses.

*Note: Gleason pattern 1 and 2 are no longer assigned on prostate biopsies based on current recommendations, and rarely assigned on other specimens.

38. What are the prostate prognostic grade groupings (GG) endorsed by the WHO and the International Society of Urological Pathology (ISUP)?
- Grade group 1: Gleason score 6/10 (3 + 3).
- Grade group 2: Gleason score 7/10 (3 + 4).
- Grade group 3: Gleason score 7/10 (4 + 3).
- Grade group 4: Gleason score 8/10 (4 + 4, 3 + 5, 5 + 3).
- Grade group 5: Gleason score 9–10/10 (4 + 5, 5 + 4, 5 + 5).

39. How is Gleason grading applied in prostate core biopsy specimens?
- The Gleason score is the sum of the primary Gleason grade (the predominant grade in terms of surface area of involvement) and the secondary) Gleason grade (the grade second in predominance).
  - For example, in a specimen with 60% Gleason pattern 3 and 40% Gleason pattern 4:
    › Prostate adenocarcinoma GG2, Gleason Score 3+4 = 7.
- When no secondary Gleason grade exists, the primary Gleason grade is doubled to arrive at a Gleason score.
  - For example, in a specimen with 100% Gleason pattern 4:
    › Prostate adenocarcinoma GG4, Gleason Score 4+4 = 8.
- In specimens where there is a minor secondary component (less than 5% of the tumor):
- If the minor pattern is of lower grade, it need not be included. For example, in a specimen with 95% Gleason pattern 4 and < 5% Gleason 3:
  › Prostate adenocarcinoma GG4, Gleason Score 4+4 = 8.
- If the minor pattern is of higher grade, it should be included. For example, in a specimen with 95% Gleason pattern 4 and < 5% Gleason 5:
  › Prostate adenocarcinoma GG4, Gleason Score 4+5 = 9.
- If 3 patterns are present, use the most predominant pattern and worst pattern of the remaining 2.
  - For example, in a specimen with 50% Gleason pattern 3, 35% Gleason pattern 4, and 15% Gleason pattern 5:
    › Prostate adenocarcinoma GG4, Gleason Score 3+5 = 8.

40. How is Gleason grading applied in transurethral resection specimens?
The rules of grading are the same as prostate biopsy specimens.

41. How is Gleason grading applied differently in radical prostatectomies?
- Similar to prostate biopsies, the Gleason score is the sum of the primary Gleason grade and the secondary Gleason grade.
- Tertiary Gleason patterns are common in radical prostatectomy specimens. When Gleason pattern 5 is present as a tertiary pattern, its presence should be specially recognized.

(continued on next page)

- When tertiary Gleason Pattern 5 is less than 5% of overall tumor volume, the report should document it as a tertiary pattern.
  - For example, in a specimen with 50% Gleason pattern 3, 45% Gleason pattern 4, and < 5% Gleason pattern 5:
    › Prostate adenocarcinoma GG3, Gleason Score 3+4 = 7, tertiary pattern 5 less than 5%.
- When Gleason Pattern 5 is more than 5% of overall tumor volume, it should be incorporated in the Gleason score.

- For example, in a specimen with 50% Gleason pattern 3, 35% Gleason pattern 4, and 15% Gleason pattern 5:
  › Prostate adenocarcinoma GG3, Gleason Score 3+5 = 8.
- For radical prostatectomy specimens, a Gleason score should be assigned to the dominant nodule(s), if present. Where more than 1 separate tumor is clearly identified, the Gleason scores of individual tumors can be recorded separately, or, at the very least, a Gleason score of the dominant or most significant lesion should be recorded.

Intraductal Carcinoma

42. What is intraductal carcinoma of the prostate?

Intraductal carcinoma of the prostate is defined as proliferation of malignant prostate epithelial cells within ducts and acini that have intact basal cell layers.

43. What are the typical histologic features of intraductal carcinoma?

- Large ducts or acini with solid, loose, or dense cribriforming growth, or micropapillary growth.
- Malignant epithelial cells that line the ducts and acini, and that feature nucleomegaly (6x usual size), nuclear pleomorphism, and prominent nucleoli.
- Nonfocal comedonecrosis.
- Intact basal cell layers.

44. What is intraductal carcinoma associated with?

- High volume, high grade prostate carcinoma.
- Metastatic disease and worse clinical prognosis.

Variants of Prostate Adenocarcinoma

45. What is ductal adenocarcinoma of the prostate?

- Ductal adenocarcinoma is an uncommon variant of invasive prostate carcinoma composed of glands lined by pseudostratified columnar cells.
- The morphology resembles intestinal and endometrioid carcinomas.
- It should not be confused with intraductal carcinoma of the prostate.

46. List 3 morphologic patterns of prostate ductal adenocarcinoma.

- Cribriform.
- Papillary.
- Solid.

47. What is mucinous adenocarcinoma of prostate?

It is prostate adenocarcinoma with at least 25% of the tumor having extracellular mucin pool. This diagnosis should be reserved for radical prostatectomies.

48. How are mucinous and ductal carcinomas of the prostate graded?

- Ductal carcinoma of the prostate: this is graded as patterns 4 and 5 (with necrosis).
- Mucinous carcinoma: the mucin is ignored; grading is based on the underlying architecture.

49. List special types of carcinoma that occur in the prostate and that are not Gleason graded.

- Prostate adenocarcinoma demonstrating treatment effects (usually in the setting of androgen withdrawal and radiation therapy).
- Small cell and other neuroendocrine carcinomas.
- Squamous cell and adenosquamous carcinomas.
- Basaloid and adenocystic carcinomas.
- Urothelial carcinomas.
- Undifferentiated carcinomas.

50. List variants of acinar prostate carcinoma mimicking benign conditions.

- Atrophic.
- Pseudohyperplastic.
- Foamy.
- Microcystic.

Challenging Issues in Prostate Adenocarcinoma

51. List benign histologic findings mimicking prostate adenocarcinoma.

- Normal structures: small benign prostate glands, ejaculatory duct or seminal vesicle glands, Cowper glands, mesonephric remnants, and paraganglia.
- Metaplastic lesions: mucinous metaplasia.
- Hyperplastic lesions: adenosis, sclerosing adenosis, nodular hyperplasia, basal cell hyperplasia, and verumontanum hyperplasia.
- Atrophic lesions: glandular atrophy, partial atrophy, and postatrophic hyperplasia.
- Other lesions: nephrogenic adenoma, radiation atypia, reactive atypia, granulomatous prostatitis, and xanthoma.

52. What workup would you recommend for small atypical glandular lesions seen on a prostate needle biopsy?

- Immunohistochemical tests for high molecular weight keratin (34βE12 or CK5/6 or others), or p63, or a combination of the 2, with AMACR/racemase (P504S) in a double or triple cocktail.
- Serial sections and/or deeper tissue levels.

53. When the overall diagnosis of a prostate biopsy is "atypical," what would you recommend to the clinician as a next step?

- Recommend repeat prostate needle biopsy in < 6 months.
- Many of these patients (40–50%) show prostatic adenocarcinoma on follow-up biopsy.

54. What is the significance of high grade prostatic intraepithelial neoplasia (HPIN)?

- HPIN is thought to be the precursor lesion for prostatic adenocarcinoma.
- The presence of an isolated HPIN should be reported in all biopsy specimens. The reporting of HPIN in biopsies with carcinoma is considered optional. Low grade PIN is not reported.
- The reporting of HPIN in prostatectomy specimens is optional.
- HPIN in a biopsy without evidence of carcinoma has in the past been a risk factor for the presence of carcinoma on subsequent biopsies, but the magnitude of the risk has diminished, and, in some studies, high grade PIN was not a risk factor at all, unless multiple cores were positive for HPIN.

55. List 4 histologic features used in pT staging of prostate carcinoma.

- Extraprostatic extension.
- Invasion of seminal vesicles.
- Microscopic invasion of the bladder neck.
- Tumor that is fixed or invades adjacent structures or organs.

56. What is the differential diagnosis of cribriform glandular lesions in the prostate?

- HPIN.
- Cribriform prostatic adenocarcinoma, Gleason pattern 4.
- Clear cell cribriform hyperplasia.
- Central zone prostatic glands.
- Ductal adenocarcinoma of the prostate.
- Intraductal carcinoma.

57. What features help differentiate cribriform glandular lesions in the prostate?

LESION	LOCATION	MORPHOLOGY	BASAL CELL LAYER
HPIN	• Peripheral lobes.	• Enlarged nuclei with prominent nucleoli. • Flat, micropapillary, cribriform and tufted patterns.	• Present, may be fragmented.
Invasive prostatic adenocarcinoma, Gleason pattern 4	• Peripheral lobes.	• Enlarged nuclei with prominent nucleoli.	• Absence of basal cells.
Clear cell cribriform hyperplasia	• Transition zone.	• No nuclear atypia.	• Polarized areas of prominent basal cells.
Central zone prostatic glands	• Central zone, near base.	• No nuclear atypia, Roman bridge configuration with nuclear streaming.	• Present.
Ductal adenocarcinoma of the prostate	• Transition zone.	• True papillary architecture; back to back glands and detached cribriform fragments. • +/– necrosis.	• Patchy basal cells or absent.
Intraductal carcinoma	• Peripheral lobes.	• Nucleomegaly, pleomorphism, prominent nucleoli.	• Present, usually continuous.

58. You receive a radical prostatectomy specimen and, after an initial review, you do not identify an obvious carcinoma. What are your next steps?

- Review the slides again and ask a colleague to review them.
- Submit all tissue if the prostate was not submitted in toto.
- Review the prostate needle biopsy that was diagnosed as carcinoma to confirm the diagnosis and note sextant location.
- Consult the imaging if it was done prior to the biopsy or procedure.
- Inquire whether the patient received therapy that may make carcinoma difficult to identify — e.g., antihormone treatment.
- Perform immunostaining and deeper sections on all slides with high grade prostatic intraepithelial neoplasia or atypical prostatic glands.
- Flip blocks from the sextant site with cancer on the biopsy and do 1 level. If atypical glands or HPIN are noted, perform stains and deeper levels as above.
- Pursue molecular testing to confirm that the prostate needle biopsy and the radical prostatectomy are from the same individual.
- Communicate with the clinician regarding your workup of the case and possible explanations for this phenomenon.

59. What are some possible explanations for failing to identify a carcinoma after a thorough review of the radical prostatectomy slides?

- The carcinoma is in tissue that was not submitted.
- The carcinoma is in the part of paraffin block that was not sectioned.
- The carcinoma was lost during block trimming.
- The carcinoma is obscured by treatment — e.g., antihormone treatment.
- The carcinoma is obscured by inflammation or infarction.
- The carcinoma was extremely focal and removed by biopsy procedure.
- In a radical prostatectomy, the prostatectomy was incomplete (capsular incision) and tissue with carcinoma remains in the surgical bed.
- The prostate needle biopsy tissue was misidentified.
- The prostate needle biopsy was misdiagnosed.

College of American Pathologists (CAP) Protocols for Examining and Reporting Prostate Carcinoma

60. How is adenocarcinoma quantified in a biopsy specimen?

- The number of positive cores involved out of the total number of cores should always be reported, except in situations where fragmentation precludes accurate counting.
- The estimated proportion (percent) of prostatic tissue involved by tumor and/or the linear millimeters of the tumor should also be reported.
- Reporting of the positive core with the greatest percentage of tumor is also an option.

61. What histological clues are useful to determine extraprostatic invasion in biopsy specimens?

- Extraprostatic invasion is present if periprostatic fat is present and involved by tumor.
- In needle biopsy specimens, it is difficult to distinguish between seminal vesicle and ejaculatory duct tissue. It

is important not to overinterpret the ejaculatory duct as seminal vesicle, since involvement of the ejaculatory duct by tumor does not constitute pT3b disease.

62. How is a transurethral resection specimen submitted?

- Transurethral resection specimens that weigh ≤ 12 g should be submitted in their entirety, usually in 6–8 cassettes.
- For specimens that weigh > 12 g, the initial 12 g are submitted (6–8 cassettes), and 1 cassette may be submitted for every additional 5 g.
- In general, random chips are submitted; however, if some chips are firmer or have a yellow or orange-yellow appearance, they should be submitted preferentially.
- If an unsuspected carcinoma is found in tissue submitted, and it involves ≥ 5% of the tissue examined, the remaining tissue may be submitted for microscopic examination, especially in younger patients.

63. Describe how to prepare a gross assessment of a radical prostatectomy specimen.

- Check the requisition and container identifiers.
- Weigh the specimen, ink resection margins (right and left require different colors), and determine the dimensions of the prostate and seminal vesicle. Note that, technically, weight should exclude seminal vesicles.
- Amputate the prostatic apex and base, section the remaining specimen, and submit.
- Section the remainder of the prostate in 3 mm slices and, if < 35 g, submit in toto. If > 35 g, submit at least 75% of the tissue, with preference given to the posterior. Trim transitional zone tissue. Other variations of partial submission of radical prostatectomy specimens can be used.
- Always include sections where seminal vesicles meet the base of the prostate.

64. How is adenocarcinoma quantified in a transurethral resection specimen and a radical prostatectomy?
- Provide an estimate of the percentage of prostatic tissue involved.
- When prostate cancer is discovered incidentally (i.e., discovered in specimens submitted for clinically benign disease, usually benign prostatic hyperplasia), the percentage involvement is used to determine the clinical T1 substage:
  - If ≤ 5% involvement: cT1a.
  - If > 5% involvement: cT1b.
- In radical prostatectomy specimens, it may be possible to measure a dominant tumor nodule in at least 2 dimensions.

65. How do you determine extraprostatic extension (EPE) on radical prostatectomy?
- Tumor is admixed with periprostatic fat.
- Tumor invades connective tissue in the plane or beyond the plane of fat.
- Tumor invades beyond the confines of normal prostate gland in the anterior prostate.
- Evaluation of EPE in the anterior apex of the prostate is controversial and should generally be avoided unless the margin is positive at this location.

66. How is EPE quantified and reported in radical prostatectomy?
- The specific location(s) and the number of sites (blocks) of EPE are useful to report.
- Descriptors of EPE (focal versus nonfocal) should be used.
  - Focal EPE equates with only a few neoplastic glands being outside the prostate or a tumor extending outside the prostate involving < 1 high power field in 1–2 sections.
  - Nonfocal (established) EPE is more extensively spread beyond the prostatic edge.

67. How is seminal vesicle invasion defined?
Seminal vesicle invasion is defined by involvement of the muscular wall.

68. How are negative and positive margins defined in radical prostatectomy?
- Surgical margins should be designated as "negative" if the tumor is not present at the inked margin and as "positive" if tumor cells touch the ink at the margin.
- When the tumor is located close to an inked surface but is not actually in contact with the ink, the margin is considered negative.
- Positive surgical margins should not be interpreted as extraprostatic extension.

69. How do you report a positive margin in a radical prostatectomy specimen?
- If the surgical margin finding is positive, the pathologist should state that explicitly, although this finding is not relied on for pathologic staging.
- The specific locations of the positive margins should be reported, and it should be specified whether EPE or intraprostatic incision is present at each site of margin positivity.
- The apex should be carefully examined because it is a common site of margin positivity.
- There should be some indication of the extent of margin positivity (it can be measured in mm).

70. What is the pathological T staging for prostate carcinoma (pT)?
Primary tumor (pT).
- pT2: organ confined.
- pT3: extraprostatic extension.
  - pT3a: extraprostatic extension (unilateral or bilateral) or microscopic invasion of bladder neck.
  - pT3b: tumor invades seminal vesicle(s).
- pT4: tumor is fixed or invades adjacent structures other than seminal vesicles (e.g., external sphincter, rectum, bladder, levator muscles, and/or pelvic wall).

Note: there is no pathologic T1 classification. Subdivision of pT2 disease is problematic and has not proven to be of prognostic significance.

71. If there is an intraprostatic incision, what is the pT?
- Prostrate carcinoma with positive intraprostatic margins in the setting of intraprostatic incision is classified as pT2+ disease.
- Surgical incision can create stage pT2+ from either pT2 or pT3 disease.

72. What is the pathological N staging (regional lymph node involvement) for prostate carcinoma?
pNX: regional lymph nodes cannot be assessed.
pN0: no regional lymph node metastasis.
pN1: metastasis in regional lymph node or nodes.

73. Which lymph nodes are considered regional?

- The regional lymph nodes are the nodes of the true pelvis, which essentially are the pelvic nodes below the bifurcation of the common iliac arteries. They include the following groups:
  - Pelvic, not otherwise specified (NOS).
- Hypogastric.
- Obturator.
- Iliac (internal, external, or NOS).
- Sacral (lateral, presacral, promontory [Gerota], or NOS).
- Laterality does not affect the N classification.

74. Which lymph nodes are considered distant and how are they considered in the staging system?

- Distant lymph nodes include:
  - Aortic (paraaortic lumbar).
  - Common iliac.
  - Inguinal, deep.
  - Superficial inguinal (femoral).
- Supraclavicular.
- Cervical.
- Scalene.
- Retroperitoneal, NOS.
- Involvement of distant lymph nodes is classified as M1a.

75. What is the pM?

- pM1: distant metastasis.
- pM1a: nonregional lymph nodes(s).
- pM1b: bone(s).
- pM1c: other site(s) with or without bone disease.

Note: when > 1 site of metastasis is present, the most advanced category is used. pM1c is most advanced.

Kidney (Nonmedical)
Cystic Diseases of the Kidney

76. What is the classification of cystic diseases of the kidney?

- The classification is:
  - Multicystic renal dysplasia.
  - Polycystic kidney disease.
    - › Autosomal dominant (adult) polycystic disease.
    - › Autosomal recessive (childhood) polycystic disease.
  - Medullary cystic disease.
    - › Medullary sponge kidney.
    - › Nephronophthisis.
  - Acquired (dialysis associated) cystic disease.
  - Localized (simple) renal cysts.
- Renal cysts in hereditary malformation syndromes (e.g., tuberous sclerosis).
- Glomerulocystic disease.
- Extraparenchymal renal cysts (pyelocalyceal cysts, hilar lymphangitic cysts).
- Cystic changes are also very common in renal tumors (e.g., in clear cell renal cell carcinoma [RCC], clear cell tubulopapillary RCC, tubulocystic RCC, mixed epithelial and stromal tumor).

77. What are the common extrarenal manifestations of autosomal dominant polycystic kidney disease?

- Cysts in the liver (polycystic liver disease).
- Cysts in the spleen, pancreas, and lungs (less frequent).
- Intracranial berry aneurysms in the circle of Willis.
- Mitral valve prolapse and other cardiac valvular anomalies.

78. What immunostaining is helpful in highlighting the classic ovarian-appearing stroma in mixed epithelial and stromal tumors (MEST).

Estrogen receptor (ER) and progesterone receptor (PR).

79. What are the causes and morphology of multicystic renal dysplasia?

- Causes:
  - Ureteropelvic obstruction.
  - Ureteral agenesis or atresia.
  - Other anomalies of the lower urinary tract.
- Morphology:
- Gross features: enlarged, irregular, and multicystic with cysts of variable size.
- Histology: presence of islands of undifferentiated mesenchyme, often with cartilage, and immature collecting ducts.

Renal Cell Carcinoma

80. List the risk factors that predispose patients to RCC and the syndromes associated with RCC.

- Risk factors:
  - Smoking.
  - Obesity.
  - Hypertension.
  - Unopposed estrogen therapy.
  - Exposure to asbestos, petroleum products, and heavy metals.
  - Chronic renal failure.
  - Acquired cystic disease.
- Associated syndromes:
  - Birt-Hogg-Dubé syndrome.
  - Tuberous sclerosis.
  - Von Hippel-Lindau (VHL) syndrome.
  - Hereditary (familial) clear cell carcinoma.
  - Hereditary papillary RCC.
  - Familial leiomyomatousis and renal cell carcinoma syndrome.

81. List at least 3 paraneoplastic syndromes associated with RCC.

- Polycythemia.
- Hypercalcemia.
- Hypertension.
- Hepatic dysfunction.
- Feminization or masculinization.
- Cushing syndrome.
- Eosinophilia.
- Leukemoid reactions.
- Amyloidosis.

82. What areas must be sampled when performing the gross assessment of a kidney tumor?

- Margins — renal vein, ureter, renal artery, and any soft tissue margins that are suspicious for tumor involvement.
- Sections of the tumor — typically 1 section per cm of largest tumor dimension, with care taken to show various areas, such as well-preserved tumor tissue for typing and grading, areas suspicious for sarcomatoid differentiation, areas of tumor-type necrosis.
- Extent of invasion — areas suspicious for large vessel invasion, perinephric fat invasion, and renal sinus fat invasion. In larger tumors (e.g., > 5 cm) that are centrally located, submit at least 5–7 sections of the tumor where it pushes into the renal sinus fat. The renal hilum lacks a capsule: when this area is undersampled, these tumors are often understaged.
- Normal tissue — background renal tissue and adrenal gland if present.

83. List the common types of renal cell tumors and their typical gross appearance.

- Clear cell RCC:
  - This is a solitary well-circumscribed cortical mass with a golden yellow color (usual).
  - Cystic change, hemorrhage, necrosis, calcification, and fibrous areas are common.
- Papillary:
  - This is a well-circumscribed cortical tumor with a fibrous pseudocapsule.
  - Necrosis and hemorrhage are common.
  - It is more likely to be bilateral or multifocal than other types of RCC.
- Chromophobe RCC:
  - This is a solitary, round, well-circumscribed unencapsulated mass, with a tan-to-light-brown color.
  - Central scar is sometimes present.
- Oncocytoma:
  - This is a well-circumscribed mass, with a mahogany-brown-to-tan or yellow color.
  - Central or eccentric scar is commonly present.
- Angiomyolipoma:
  - This is well-demarcated, but unencapsulated.
  - Gross appearance varies from yellow to red/pinkish tan, depending on the proportions of each of the 3 components that make up the tumor.
- Sarcomatoid areas of RCC:
  - This has a gray-white "fish flesh" appearance.

84. List features that should be included in a report for RCC.

- Histologic type.
- Invasion of renal vein or its muscle-containing branches.
- Invasion of renal sinus and perinephric adipose tissue.
- WHO/ISUP nuclear grade.
- Vascular invasion.
- Sarcomatoid morphology (and quantity).
- Geographic necrosis.
- Invasion of collecting system.
- Resection margin status.
- Any other tissues involved — e.g., adrenal gland involvement.
- Assessment of background kidney parenchyma.

85. Outline the WHO/ISUP grading system for renal cell carcinomas.

- Applicable for clear cell RCC and papillary RCC only.
- Assesses nuclear features visible with a x10 and x20 objective lens.
- Grades tumors according to the highest-grade features present.

(continued on next page)

- Incorporates nucleolar prominence, pleomorphism, and sarcomatoid and/or rhabdoid morphology:
  - Grade 1: these tumors have nucleoli that are inconspicuous and basophilic at x400 magnification.
  - Grade 2: these tumors have nucleoli that are clearly visible at x400 magnification and eosinophilic.
- Grade 3: these tumors have clearly visible nucleoli at x100 magnification.
- Grade 4: these tumors have extreme pleomorphism or rhabdoid and/or sarcomatoid morphology.

Clear Cell Renal Cell Carcinoma

86. List the histologic features of clear cell RCC.
- Alveolar nests or sheets of clear cells interspersed by a delicate vascular network.
- Various other growth patterns: cystic, pseudopapillary, trabecular, tubular, etc.
- Sarcomatoid and rhaboid differentiations (not uncommon).

87. What is the typical immunoprofile of clear cell RCC?
- Positive: carbonic anhydrase IX (CAIX), CD10, vimentin.
- Negative: CK7 (can be focally positive), α-methylacyl-CoA racemase (AMCAR), CD117.

88. What syndrome is most commonly associated with clear cell RCC?
- Von Hippel-Lindau syndrome is most commonly associated (the VHL gene is located on chromosome 3).
- Sporadic clear cell RCC also shows chromosome 3p deletion in the majority cases.

89. What is the prognosis of clear cell RCC?
Approximately a third of patients with clinically localized disease develop local and distant recurrence after surgery. Approximately half of patients die of the disease.

Papillary Renal Cell Carcinoma

90. List the histologic features of papillary RCC.
- It is circumscribed and pseudoencapsulated.
- It exhibits papillary growth with delicate fibrovascular cores that often contain foamy macrophages.
- It frequently has associated necrosis and hemorrhage.
- Psammoma bodies may be present.

91. What histologic features distinguishe papillary adenoma from papillary RCC?
- Unencapsulated tumors with papillary, tubular, or tubulopapillary growth.
- Diameter < 1.5 cm.
- Low nuclear grade: WHO/ISUP grade 1 or 2.

92. What genetic abnormalities are commonly associated with papillary RCC?
- Sporadic tumors may be associated with trisomy 7 or 17, and loss of Y chromosome.
- A small percentage is associated with *MET* mutation.

Chromophobe Renal Cell Carcinoma and Oncocytoma

93. List the histologic features of chromophobe RCC.
- Cells are arranged in solid sheets, with occasional tubulocystic architecture.
- The mass is randomly intersected by broad fibrous septa with medium-sized blood vessels.
- Cell nuclei are irregular and hyperchromatic, with wrinkled contours and occasional multinucleation.
- Two types of tumor cell are present:
  - Chromophobe cell — a large polygonal cell with thick "plantlike" cell borders and finely vesicular cytoplasm; it is usually found adjacent to the blood vessels.
  - Eosinophilic cell — a smaller cell with less abundant granular eosinophilic cytoplasm, and perinuclear clearing or "halo."

94. List the histologic features of oncocytoma.
- This is a well-circumscribed tumor typically demonstrating compacted nested growth.
- It is composed of eosinophilic cells with indistinct membrane, granular cytoplasm, and round-to-ovoid nuclei.
- Small and conspicuous nucleoli may be present.
- Bizarre degenerative nuclei may be present.

95. What features help distinguish chromophobe RCC from oncocytoma?

FEATURE	CHROMOPHOBE RCC	ONCOCYTOMA
Nuclear	• Binucleation. • Wrinkled nuclei with perinuclear halos.	• Round with prominent nucleoli. • Occasionally degenerative nuclear atypia.
Colloidal iron stain	• Diffuse staining.	• Usually negative.
Electron microscopy	• Cytoplasm with many microvesicles 150–300 nm.	• Cytoplasm with dilated mitochondria.
CD117	• Positive.	• Positive.
CK7	• Diffuse positivity.	• Mostly negative, with scattered positivity.

96. What features help distinguish eosinophilic variant chromophobe RCC from eosinophilic variant clear cell RCC?

FEATURE	CHROMOPHOBE RCC	CLEAR CELL RCC
Vascular pattern	• Randomly arranged broad fibrous septa with predominantly medium-caliber blood vessels.	• Small, delicate sinusoidal blood vessels.
CAIX	–	+
CK7	+	–
CD10	–	+
Vimentin	–	+
CD117	+	–

97. What is the prognosis for patients with chromophobe RCC compared to clear cell RCC?

The prognosis for chromophobe RCC is much better for than clear cell RCC: mortality is < 10% and 5-year disease survival is > 90%.

98. What are the genetic changes in chromophobe RCC?

Multiple losses of whole chromosomes, usually Y, 1, 2, 6, 10, 13, 17, and 21.

99. What genetic syndrome is associated with multiple chromophobe RCCs and oncocytomas?

• Birt-Hogg-Dubé syndrome — characterized by cutaneous fibrofolliculomas, pulmonary cysts, and multifocal renal tumors consisting of chromophobe RCCs, oncocytomas, clear cell RCCs, and hybrid tumors with features of both chromophobe RCC and oncocytoma.

• These tumors are called hybrid oncocytic/chromophobe tumors (HOCTs), which can also occur sporadically. They are associated with a mutation in the *FLCN* gene, which codes for the protein folliculin.

Angiomyolipoma

100. List the 3 histologic components of angiomyolipoma.

• Smooth muscle cells that typically form a collar around the blood vessels and may be oriented perpendicular to the vessel.

• Adipocytes.
• Dysmorphic blood vessels: thick walled artery-like blood vessels that lack elastic.

101. What clinical syndrome is associated with angiomyolipoma?

Tuberous sclerosis: an autosomal dominant tumor suppressor gene syndrome associated with cerebral cortical tubers, cardiac rhabdomyoma, facial angiofibroma, renal angiomyolipoma, and lymphangioleiomyoma.

102. What is the cell of origin of angiomyolipoma?

The perivascular epithelioid cell.

103. What is the immunoprofile of angiomyolipoma?

• Coexpression of smooth muscle markers (muscle specific actin, smooth muscle actin) and melanocytic markers (human melanoma black 45 [HMB45], Melan-A).

• Angiomyolipoma is also positive for cathepsin K.

Rhabdoid Tumor of the Kidney

104. What are the clinical features of rhabdoid tumor of the kidney, and what is the prognosis for patients?

- Clinical features: infants (< 24 months) with hematuria, often with advanced disease at presentation.
- Prognosis: extremely poor, with < 25% survival at 1 year.
- Approximately 10–15% of patients develop atypical teratoid or rhabdoid tumors of the central nervous system, often resembling primitive neuroectodermal tumor (PNET) morphologically.

105. What are the histologic features of rhabdoid tumor of the kidney?

Sheets of large cells with vesicular nuclei, eosinophilic cytoplasmic inclusions, and very infiltrative tumor borders.

106. What are the immunohistochemical and ultrastructural features of rhabdoid tumor of the kidney?

- Immunohistochemical: vimentin positive (strong and diffuse), focal EMA and cytokeratin positivity.
- Ultrastructural: inclusions are made up of intermediate filaments tightly whorled together.

107. What is the differential diagnosis of rhabdoid tumor of the kidney?

- Nephroblastoma.
- Neuroblastoma.
- Mesoblastic nephroma.
- Medullary renal carcinoma.
- Clear cell sarcoma of the kidney — however, if rhabdoid morphology is seen in these tumors, it is focal.

108. How do you report sarcomatoid features in nephrectomy specimens?

- Give the percentage of sarcomatoid element.
- The lesion should be reported as unclassified RCC if either of the following is found:
  · Pure sarcomatoid carcinoma.
  · Sarcomatoid carcinoma associated with epithelial elements that do not conform to usual types of renal carcinoma.

109. Where would you find lymph nodes in a radical nephrectomy specimen?

In the renal hilum around major vessels (only a few may be present).

110. How do you assess microscopic tumor extension? What sections need to be taken to carefully assess it?

- Extension into perinephric soft tissues (section of tumor in relation to renal capsule).
- Extension into renal sinus (generous sampling of renal sinus fat).
- Extension beyond Gerota fascia (gross inspection).
- Extension into major vein (section of tumor in relation to renal vein or its segmental branches).
- Extension into pelvicalyceal system (section of tumor in relation to calyces).
- Extension into adrenal glands (section of tumor and adrenal gland, including soft tissue in between, to assess for direct versus indirect invasion).
- Extension into other organs.

111. Where is extrarenal extension most underrecognized and associated with a more aggressive outcome?

- Extension in the renal sinus fat, which is rich in small vessels and lymphatics, is underrecognized and associated with aggressive tumors.
- The renal sinus should be very carefully assessed; every nodule in the area should be sampled.

112. How do you classify adrenal gland involvement?

pT4: contiguous involvement/direct invasion.

pM1: noncontiguous involvement.

113. What are the margins to assess in a partial nephrectomy and radical nephrectomy?

- Partial:
  · Renal parenchymal margin.
  · Perinephric fat overlying the tumor, if present.
- Radical:
  · Ureteric margin.
  · Major vascular margins (vein and artery).
  · Soft tissue margins (Gerota fascia, renal sinus).

114. How should a nonneoplastic kidney be assessed?

- Medical kidney diseases should be looked for in each case, with special stains as needed.
- Consultation with a nephropathologist should be requested if needed.

115. What findings in a nonneoplastic kidney point to significant decline in renal function 6 months after radical nephrectomy?

A finding of > 20% global glomerulosclerosis or a finding of advanced diffuse diabetic glomerulosclerosis.

116. What is the pT classification of renal cell carcinoma?

pT0: no evidence of primary tumor.

pT1: tumor ≤ 7 cm in greatest dimension, limited to the kidney.

pT1a: tumor ≤ 4 cm in greatest dimension, limited to the kidney.

pT1b: tumor > 4 cm but not > 7 cm in greatest dimension, limited to the kidney.

pT2: tumor > 7 cm in greatest dimension, limited to the kidney.

pT2a: tumor > 7 cm but ≤ 10 cm in greatest dimension, limited to the kidney.

pT2b: tumor > 10 cm, limited to the kidney.

pT3: tumor extends into major veins or perinephric tissues but not into the ipsilateral adrenal gland and not beyond Gerota fascia.

pT3a: Tumor grossly extends into the renal vein or its segmental (muscle containing) branches, or tumor invades perirenal and/or renal sinus fat but not beyond Gerota fascia.

pT3b: tumor grossly extends into the vena cava below the diaphragm.

pT3c: tumor grossly extends into vena cava above diaphragm or invades the wall of the vena cava.

pT4: tumor invades beyond Gerota fascia (including contiguous extension into the ipsilateral adrenal gland).

Kidney (Medical)
Acute Tubular Necrosis

117. List the common causes of acute tubular necrosis (ATN).
- Ischemia due to shock or inadequate blood flow.
- Neophrotoxicity due to drugs/medications (e.g., gentamicin, radiographic contrast, heavy metal, organic solvents) or endogenous elements (e.g., myoglobin, hemoglobin, monoclonal light chains, bile/bilirubin).
- Combined causes (e.g., hemolytic crises with hemoglobinuria or skeletal muscle injury with myoglobinuria).

118. Describe characteristic histology of renal toxicity caused by mercuric chloride, carbon tetrachloride, and ethylene glycol.
- Mercuric chloride: severely injured tubular cells containing large acidophilic inclusions.
- Carbon tetrachloride: accumulation of neutral lipids in injured tubular cells.
- Ethylene glycol: hydropic degeneration of proximal convoluted tubular epithelium; presence of calcium oxalate crystals.

Rapidly Progressive Glomerulonephritis

119. What is the typical clinical presentation of rapidly progressive glomerulonephritis?

Rapid and progressive loss of renal function associated with severe oliguria and nephritic syndrome.

120. What is the morphological finding that corresponds to a diagnosis of rapidly progressive glomerulonephritis?

Glomerular crescents affecting > 50% of glomeruli.

121. What are the major immunopathological categories of crescentic glomerulonephritis?
- Type I: antiglomerular basement membrane (anti-GBM) antibody mediated.
- Type II: immune complex mediated.
- Type III: pauci-immune.

122. What are the findings of each category on direct immunofluorescence? List a few examples of diseases in each category.

IMMUNOPATHOLOGIC CATEGORY	CLASSIC DIRECT IMMUNOFLUORESCENCE FINDINGS	EXAMPLES
Anti-GBM antibody mediated	• Linear staining along glomerular basement membrane with IgG. • +/− interrupted granular C3.	• Anti-GBM antibody disease. • Goodpasture syndrome.
Immune complex mediated	• Granular deposits of Ig and C3 along GBM, in mesangium, or in both locations.	• Postinfectious glomerulonephritis. • Lupus nephritis. • IgA nephropathy. • Henoch-Schönlein purpura.
Pauci-immune	• Absent or very low Ig staining.	• ANCA associated vasculitis. • Granulomatosis with polyangiitis. • Microscopic polyangiitis.

Primary Membranous Nephropathy

123. Describe the typical clinical presentation of primary membranous nephropathy.
- Nephrotic syndrome characterized by:
  · Heavy proteinuria (> 3.5 g/day).
  · Hypoalbuminemia.
  · Severe edema.
  · Hyperlipidemia.
  · Lipiduria.

124. List the findings for membranous nephropathy seen on light microscopy.
- Usually all glomeruli are affected to a similar extent.
- Glomerular capillary walls are diffusely thickened. Silver stains show "spikes" as the glomerular basement membrane expands around immune deposits; later "bicycle chain" morphology is seen.
- Tubular epithelial cells often show reabsorption droplets.
- Foam cells may be in the interstitium or between tubular epithelial cells due to reabsorption of filtered lipoproteins.

125. Describe the characteristic findings of primary membranous nephropathy on electron microscopy and direct immunofluorescence.
- Direct immunofluorescence findings: finely to coarsely granular IgG deposits along the glomerular basement membrane; presence of C3 (often).
- Ultrastructural findings: subepithelial electron-dense deposits; intramembranous electron-dense deposits in later disease (possible).

Immunoglobulin A (IgA) Nephropathy

126. What are the findings of IgA nephropathy on light microscopy, direct immunofluorescence, and electron microscopy?
- Light microscopy:
  · The range of findings includes normal morphology, mesangial proliferative glomerulonephritis, proliferative glomerulonephritis, crescent formation.
  · Later, lesions may become sclerotic.
- Direct immunofluorescence:
  · Dominant or codominant IgA deposition in the mesangium is present.
  · Lesser staining with other Igs may be present.
  · Mesangial staining with C3 is strong.
- Electron microscopy:
  · Mesangial and paramesangial electron-dense deposits are present.

127. What are the important differential diagnostic considerations for IgA nephropathy?
- Lupus nephritis:
  · This can show predominant IgA deposition, but also can show strong C1q on direct immunofluorescence (this should be absent in IgA nephropathy).
  · It is important to assess for subendothelial electron-dense deposits and perform serologic testing to rule out this differential.
- Henoch-Schönlein purpura:
  · This has identical kidney findings to lupus nephritis, but the nephritis is accompanied by arthralgia, purpura caused by leukocytoclastic vasculitis of dermal vessels, and abdominal pain caused by involvement of small vessels in the gastrointestinal tract.

128. What factors determine prognosis for patients with IgA nephropathy?
- More severe renal insufficiency at presentation.
- Greater proteinuria.
- Extensive crescent formation.
- More extensive glomerular or tubulointerstitial scarring.

129. What is the clinical presentation of IgA nephropathy?
- Asymptomatic microscopic hematuria or intermittent gross hematuria.
- Less commonly: nephritic syndrome or renal failure.

Renal Manifestations of Systematic Lupus Erythematosus

130. What is the classification of lupus nephritis and how does it relate to prognosis?

CLASSIFICATION	PROGNOSIS
Class I: minimal mesangial lupus nephritis	• Excellent.
Class II: mesangial proliferative lupus nephritis	• Good.
Class III: focal lupus nephritis	• Moderate.
Class IV: diffuse segmental or global lupus nephritis	• Moderate to poor.
Class V: membranous lupus nephritis	• Moderate.
Class VI: advanced sclerosing lupus nephritis	• Poor.

131. What are some examples of active and chronic glomerular lesions?
- Active glomerular lesions:
  - Endocapillary hypercellularity.
  - Karyorrhexis.
  - Fibrinoid necrosis.
  - Rupture of glomerular basement membrane.
  - Crescents, cellular or fibrocellular.
  - Subendothelial deposits identified by light microscopy (wire loops).
  - Intraluminal immune aggregates (hyaline thrombi).
- Chronic glomerular lesions:
  - Glomerular sclerosis (segmental, global).
  - Fibrous adhesions.
  - Fibrous crescents.

Diabetic Nephropathy

132. List 4 glomerular lesions seen in diabetic nephropathy.
- Capillary basement membrane thickening — widespread thickening of the glomerular basement membrane.
- Diffuse mesangial sclerosis — prominent PAS positive material in the mesangial area, possible mild cellular proliferation.
- Nodular glomerular sclerosis — also known as Kimmelstiel-Wilson nodules, which are PAS positive laminated nodules of matrix in the periphery of the glomerulus that are surrounded by patent capillaries.
- Accumulation of hyaline material — called "fibrin caps" when material accumulates on capillary loops, and "capsular drops" when material is adherent to Bowman capsule.

133. List 2 nonglomerular renal findings in diabetes mellitus.
- Renal vascular lesions — these include renal atherosclerosis and arteriolosclerosis, which show similar findings to atherosclerosis at other sites.
- Pyelonephritis — acute and chronic pyelonephritis are more common in diabetics than the general population. Specifically, necrotizing papillitis or papillary necrosis is more common in diabetic patients.

134. List 2 findings of diabetic nephropathy on electron microscopy.
- Thickened glomerular basement membrane due to protein insudation which appears as electron-dense material.
- Mesangial matrix expansion.

135. List differential diagnoses for the glomerular changes of diabetic nephropathy.
- Mesangial proliferative glomerulonephritis.
- Monoclonal immunoglobulin deposition disease.
- IgA nephropathy.
- Lupus nephritis.
- Focal segmental glomerular sclerosis (FSGS).
- Membranous glomerulopathy.
- Minimal change disease.

Medication-Associated Changes to the Kidney

136. Name medications associated with changes to the renal and urinary tracts and describe the changes in each case.

- Cyclosporine:
  - Acute nephrotoxicity: possible absence of morphologic abnormality, acute tubular injury, and/or tubular cell vacuolization (isometric).
  - Arteriolopathy: individual smooth muscle cell degeneration, vacuolization, necrosis, and loss with myocytes replaced by hyaline deposits in a beaded pattern in the media.
  - Thrombotic microangiopathy.
  - Chronic nephrotoxicity with patchy tubular atrophy and interstitial fibrosis.
- Nonsteroidal antiinflammatory drugs:
  - Hemodynamically induced acute renal failure, due to the decreased synthesis of vasodilatory prostaglandins.
  - Acute hypersensitivity interstitial nephritis.
  - Acute interstitial nephritis and minimal change disease.
  - Membranous nephropathy.
- Phenacetin:
  - Chronic tubulointerstitial nephritis and renal papillary necrosis.

Renal Lesions Associated With Plasma Cell Dyscrasia

137. List at least 3 renal lesions associated with plasma cell dyscrasia and describe their features on light microscopy, direct immunofluorescence, and electron microscopy.

LESION	LIGHT MICROSCOPY	DIRECT IMMUNOFLUORESCENCE	ELECTRON MICROSCOPY
Myeloma cast nephropathy	• Large, brittle casts with fracture lines or fragments surrounded by tubular epithelium, neutrophils, and multinucleate giant cells. • PAS negative, brightly eosinophilic or fuchsinophilic on Masson trichrome. • Sometimes Congo red positive.	• Monoclonal light chain.	• Cast: composed of a mass of deeply electron-dense material.
Monoclonal Ig deposition disease	• Nodular glomerulopathy, but possible normal appearance and mesangial expansion. • Widened tubular basement membranes.	• Monoclonal Ig bound to all basement membranes.	• Clustered, punctate, dense deposits external to tubular basement membranes and within vascular and glomerular basement membranes.
Amyloidosis	• Amorphous, pale eosinophilic material in mesangium +/− capillary wall and arteriole involvement. • Congo red positive, with apple green birefringence.	• AL amyloid: possible positive for light chain Ig.	• Randomly arranged fibrils, 10–12 nm in arterioles, arteries, mesangium, +/− interstitium.
Fibrillary glomerulonephritis	• Increase in mesangial cellularity and irregularly thickened capillary walls. • Congo red negative.	• Coarse linear/confluent granular IgG, C3, and 1 or both light chains.	• Fibrils, 10–20 nm in diameter throughout mesangial matrix and basement membrane.
Immunotactoid glomerulopathy	•Membranoproliferative glomerulonephritis type 1 pattern.	• Granular capillary IgG, complement, and 1 or both light chains.	• Coarse, hollow cored fibrils 20–80 nm thick.

138. Define Bence-Jones protein.

Bence-Jones protein: monoclonal light chain found in blood or urine.

139. What are the 2 mechanisms by which Bence-Jones proteins cause renal toxicity?

- Light chains are directly toxic to epithelial cells.
- Bence-Jones proteins combine with the urinary glycoprotein (Tamm-Horsfall protein) to form tubular casts that obstruct the tubular lumens and induce an inflammatory reaction around the casts (light chain cast nephropathy).

Renal Transplant Biopsies

140. What are the adequacy criteria for renal transplant biopsy specimens?
- At least 10 glomeruli and 2 muscular-walled small arteries on tissue for light microscopy.
- At least 1 glomerulus on tissue for direct immunofluorescence and electron microscopy.

141. How do you classify transplant rejection?
- Temporally: hyperacute, acute, and chronic.
- By mechanism: cellular and humoral.

142. Briefly outline the Banff classification scheme for reporting renal transplant biopsies.
- Class I: normal.
- Class II: antibody mediated rejection.
- Class III: borderline changes suspicious for acute cellular rejection.
- Class IV: T-cell mediated rejection.
- Class V: interstitial fibrosis and tubular atrophy.
- Class VI: other changes not related to rejection (e.g., ATN, drug toxicity).

143. What are the histologic features of acute cellular rejection?
- Interstitial mononuclear inflammatory infiltrate.
- Tubulitis.
- Intimal arteritis.
- Vasculitis with fibrinoid necrosis.
- Glomerulitis.

144. What are the features of acute antibody-mediated rejection?
- Light microscopy: ATN-like with minimal inflammation; capillaritis; and vasculitis.
- Direct immunofluorescence: C4d staining in peritubular capillaries.
- Presence of circulating antidonor antibodies.

Testes
Testicular Biopsy for Infertility

145. What are the indications for testicular biopsy for infertility?
- Patients with either azoospermia or severe oligospermia: to differentiate between obstructive azoospermia (obstruction) and primary seminiferous tubule failure.
- Patients with nonobstructive azoospermia: to assess fertility potential.

146. List the major histologic patterns seen in testicular biopsies performed to investigate male infertility.
- Normal spermatogenesis.
- Sertoli-cell-only syndrome.
- Germ cell maturation arrest.
- Hypospermatogenesis.
- Tubular hyalinization.

147. List the causes of infertility associated with normal histology.
- Excurrent duct obstruction.
- Abnormalities of sperm head or tail.
- Spermatozoa transport problems.
- Young syndrome and ciliary dyskinesia.

148. List 4 causes of Sertoli-cell-only syndrome.
- Chemotherapy.
- Radiation.
- Exposure to toxin.
- Cryptorchidism.

Testicular Germ Cell Tumors

149. List risk factors for testicular germ cell tumors.
- Caucasian.
- Previous germ cell tumor in contralateral testis.
- Testicular dysgenesis syndromes.
- Cryptorchidism.
- Testicular microlithiasis.
- Family history of testicular germ cell tumors.

150. What is the most common cytogenetic abnormality in germ cell tumors?
Isochromosome p12.

151. What is the classification of germ cell tumors in the testes?
- Seminomatous tumors.
  · Seminoma.
- Nonseminomatous tumors.
  · Embryonal carcinoma.
  · Yolk sac (endodermal sinus) tumor.
- Choriocarcinoma.
- Teratoma.
- Spermatocytic tumor.
- Mixed germ cell tumors.

152. List the 3 hormones that can be used as biomarkers for germ cell tumors of the testes.
- Lactate dehydrogenase (LDH).
- α fetoprotein (AFP).
- β-HCG.

153. List the precursor lesions of germ cell tumors.
- Germ cell neoplasia in situ (GCNIS).
- Intratubular seminoma.
- Intratubular nonseminoma.

154. What immunohistochemical stains are positive for GCNIS?
- PLAP.
- OCT 3/4.
- C-kit.
- D2-40.

155. List at least 3 germ cell tumors that are not associated with GCNIS.
- Prepubertal type yolk sac tumor.
- Prepubertal type teratoma, including dermoid cyst, epidermoid cyst and well-differentiated neuroendocrine tumor.
- Prepubertal type mixed teratoma and yolk sac tumor.
- Spermatocytic tumor.

156. How do immunohistochemical stains differentiate between the major germ cell tumor types?

TUMOR	CYTOKERATIN	PLAP	OCT3/4	CD30	AFP	β-HCG
Classic seminoma	Variable.	+	+	−	−	Focal.
Embryonal carcinoma	+	+	+	+	Variable.	−
Teratoma	+	−	−	−	Focal.	−
Yolk sac tumor	+	Variable.	−	Variable.	+	−
Choriocarcinoma	+	+	−	−	−	+
Spermatocytic Tumor	−	Variable.	−	−	−	−

157. What are the recommendations for sampling a testicular tumor?
- Sample the entire tumor if it fits in ≤ 10 blocks. If > 10 blocks; 1 block/cm.
- Tissues sampled include:
  · Tumor, including interface with surrounding testis and tunica albuginea (best areas to see lymphatic invasion).
  · All of the grossly different appearing areas in the tumor.
  · Testicular hilum/mediastinum testis.
  · Uninvolved testis, including tunica albuginea.
  · Epididymis.
  · Spermatic cord, including cord margin.
  · Other lesion(s).
  · All identifiable lymph nodes.
  · Other tissue(s) submitted with specimen.

158. List the features to report for germ cell tumors of the testes.
- Tumor types and quantities of each.
- Tumor size.
- Structures that the tumor is or is not invading (e.g., rete testis, tunicae, epididymis, hilar soft tissue, spermatic cord).
- Lymphovascular invasion.
- Resection margin status.
- Background parenchyma, including presence of GCNIS and spermatogenesis.

159. What is the significance of a testicular scar? What features are seen?
- In patients with metastatic disease with clinically apparent primaries, a testicular scar may represent regressed, "burnt-out" testicular germ cell tumors.
- If there is residual disease, a partial regression may signify 1 of the components is regressed.
- Established criteria for diagnosing testicular scar includes:
  · Scar associated with GCNIS.
  · Scar with associated intratubular calcification.
- Other histologic features include:
  · Lymphoplasmacytic infiltrate.
  · Hemosiderin-containing macrophages.
  · Testicular atrophy.

160. What is the clinical behavior of Sertoli cell tumors and Leydig cell tumors?
Most Sertoli cell tumors and Leydig cell tumors are benign, but approximately 10% of each can be malignant.

Seminoma

161. What are the histologic features of classic seminoma?
- Sheets and lobules of loosely cohesive cells divided by fibrous septa containing lymphocytes and plasma cells.
- Round or polygonal cells with sharp cell membranes, clear-to-eosinophilic cytoplasm.
- Large and vesicular nuclei with prominent nucleoli.
- Possible areas of necrosis, syncytiotrophoblasts.

162. What is the typical presentation of pure classic seminoma?
- Incidence peaks between the fourth and fifth decade.
- In 75% of patients, disease is confined to testis at presentation.
- In 20% of patients, disease has retroperitoneal involvement.
- In 5% of patients, disease has involvement above the diaphragm or visceral metastases.
- In 1–2% of patients, disease is bilateral; it may be synchronous or asynchronous.

163. What variant of seminoma is associated with elevated serum β-HCG levels?
- Seminoma with syncytiotrophoblasts.
  - This is a variant of classic seminoma and does not represent a form of mixed germ cell tumor.
- The prognosis is similar to classic seminoma without syncytiotrophoblasts.

164. What is the prognosis for patients with classic seminoma?
Excellent, and classic seminoma is very responsive to radiotherapy.

Spermatocytic Tumor

165. What are the histologic features of spermatocytic tumor (formerly spermatocytic seminoma)?
- Cells arranged in sheets in an edematous stroma.
- 3 cell types:
  - Small cells: 6–8 μm, smudged chromatin, and scant cytoplasm.
  - Intermediate cells: 15–20 μm, scant cytoplasm, and round nuclei with granular or filamentous chromatin.
  - Giant cells: 50–100 μm, uninucleate or multinucleate, and possible filamentous chromatin.
- Little or no intervening stroma, and no or scant lymphocytic infiltration.
- Absence of GCNIS.

166. What is the prognosis for patients with spermatocytic tumor?
Patients with pure spermatocytic tumor have an excellent prognosis and are treated with resection alone.

167. What is the immunohistochemical staining pattern of spermatocytic tumor?
- PLAP: variable, rarely positive.
- C-kit: 40–50% positive.
- Other germ cell tumor markers and keratin: negative (OCT3/4, AE1/3, CD30).
- Cam5.2: 40% positive.

Teratoma

168. How do adult testicular teratoma and childhood testicular teratoma behave differently?
- In children, mature teratoma is considered benign. Immature teratoma requires close follow-up.
- In postpubertal males, the majority of teratomas are regarded as malignant and capable of metastasis, irrespective of the maturity of tumor elements.

169. What are the most common sites of teratoma in adults and children?
- In adults: the testes and ovaries.
- In children: sacrococcygeal sites.

Testicular Lymphoma

170. List the most common types of testicular lymphoma in **decreasing** order of frequency.
- Diffuse large B-cell lymphoma.
- Burkitt lymphoma.
- Epstein-Barr-virus-positive extranodal NK/T-cell lymphoma.

171. How do testicular lymphomas behave differently from lymphomas arising at other sites?

Testicular lymphomas have a higher propensity for central nervous system involvement than similar lymphomas arising in other sites.

Paratesticular Tumor

172. List the most common spermatic cord and paratesticular benign tumors.
- Lipoma is the most common tumor involving the spermatic cord.
- Adenomatoid tumor is the most common benign paratesticular tumor.

173. What are the most common malignant paratesticular tumors in children and adults?
- In children: rhabdomyosarcoma.
- In adults: liposarcoma.

CAP Protocols for Examining and Reporting Malignant Germ Cell and Sex Cord–Stromal Tumors of the Testis

174. What are margins in a testicular resection?
- Spermatic cord margin.
- Scrotal skin.
- Parietal layer of tunica vaginalis.

175. What are the major types of tumors from the modified Armed Forces Institute of Pathology (AFIP) and WHO histologic classification of testicular tumors?
- Germ cell tumors.
- Mixed germ cell sex cord–stromal tumors.
- Sex cord–stromal tumors.
- Miscellaneous.

176. List the types of sex cord–stromal tumors and their variants.
- Leydig cell tumor.
- Sertoli cell tumor:
  · Variant: large cell calcifying Sertoli cell tumor.
  · Variant: sclerosing Sertoli cell tumor.
- Granulosa cell tumor:
  · Adult type.
  · Juvenile type.
- Mixed and indeterminate (unclassified) sex cord–stromal tumor.

177. How are tumors invading the rete testis, epididymis, testicular hilar soft tissue, or tunica vaginalis staged by the American Joint Committee on Cancer (AJCC)?*
- Rete testis invasion:
  · Does not upstage tumor if limited to testis and there is no vascular invasion (pT1).
  · Some reports suggest higher risk of relapse for seminomas if the rete is involved.
- Epididymis invasion, hilar soft tissue invasion, and/or penetration of visceral mesothelial layer covering the external surface of tunica albuginea (tunica vaginalis):
  · Classified as pT2.

*This chapter uses the eighth edition of the AJCC cancer staging manual.

178. How is venous or lymphatic vessel invasion handled clinically?
- The presence of vascular space invasion (usually lymphatic but possibly also capillary or venous invasion) has been correlated with a significantly elevated risk for distant metastasis.
- Patients who have clinical stage I disease (no evidence of spread beyond the testis by clinical examination and radiographic and serum marker studies) require close follow-up only.

179. How is invasion of the vessels of the spermatic cord handled?
- AJCC staging does not address this specific issue.
- CAP recommends:
  · Invasion of the spermatic cord is pT3.
- Vascular invasion in the cord is pT2 unless the tumor penetrates into the cord.
- Clinical outcomes in the above situations are similar.

180. What else should be reported if the lymph nodes are involved?
- Size of the largest lymph node involved.
- Size of the largest metastatic deposit.
- Extranodal extension.
- Histologic subtype.

181. What is the Royal Marsden system and how should it be used?
- These are additional criteria for staging seminomas.
- Studies show that staging with the TNM system for local tumors does not provide useful prognostic information.
- CAP recommends the use of the TNM system with optional use of the modified Royal Marsden staging system for patients with seminoma.

182. How do you stage with the modified Royal Marsden staging system?

Stage I: tumor confined to the testis.
Stage II: infradiaphragmatic nodal involvement.
  Stage IIA: greatest dimension of involved nodes < 2 cm.
  Stage IIB: greatest dimension of involved nodes ≥ 2 cm and < 5 cm.
  Stage IIC: greatest dimension of involved nodes ≥ 5 cm and < 10 cm.
  Stage IID: greatest dimension of involved nodes ≥ 10 cm.
Stage III: supraclavicular or mediastinal involvement.
Stage IV: extranodal metastases.

183. How is any residual tumor staged after therapy?

RX: presence of residual tumor cannot be assessed.
R0: no residual tumor.
R1: microscopic residual tumor.
R2: macroscopic residual tumor.

184. What is the use of serum markers in evaluating testicular tumors?
- Serum marker studies play a key role in the clinical management of patients with testicular germ cell tumors.
- Elevated serum levels of AFP or β-HCG may indicate the need for additional sections of certain specimens if the initial findings do not account for such elevations.
- Preorchiectomy serum markers are also important in clinical staging.

185. What are some common additional pathologic findings reported in testicular neoplasms?
- Leydig cell hyperplasia, which may be correlated with β-HCG elevation.
- Features that may indicate regression of a tumor, such as scarring and presence of hemosiderin-laden macrophages.
- Intratubular calcification.
- Testicular atrophy.
- Abnormal testicular development (e.g., dysgenesis or androgen insensitivity syndrome).

186. Why is it important in residual metastatic disease following chemotherapy to differentiate metastatic residual teratoma from nonteratomatous types of germ cell tumors?
- Pure teratomatous metastasis is generally treated by surgical excision alone.
- Other residual germ cell tumor components are usually treated with additional chemotherapy.

187. What is the AJCC pT staging for testicular neoplasms?

pTX: cannot be assessed.
pT0: no evidence of primary tumor.
pTis: germ cell neoplasia in situ.
pT1: tumor limited to the testis (including rete testis invasion) without lymphovascular invasion; tumor may invade tunica albuginea but not tunica vaginalis.
  pT1a*: tumor < 3 cm.
  pT1b*: tumor ≥ 3 cm.
pT2: tumor limited to the testis (including rete testis invasion) with lymphovascular invasion, **or** tumor invading hilar soft tissue or epididymis or penetrating visceral mesothelial layer covering the external surface of tunica albuginea with or without lymphovascular invasion.
pT3: tumor invades the spermatic cord with or without lymphovascular invasion.
pT4: tumor invades the scrotum with or without lymphovascular invasion.

*Note: subclassification of pT1 applies only to pure seminoma.

188. What is the AJCC N staging for testicular neoplasms?

pNX: cannot be assessed.
pN0: no regional lymph node metastasis.
pN1: metastasis with a lymph node mass ≤ 2 cm in greatest dimension and ≤ 5 nodes positive, none > 2 cm in greatest dimension.
pN2: metastasis with a lymph node mass > 2 cm and ≤ 5 cm in greatest dimension; or > 5 nodes positive, none > 5 cm; or evidence of extranodal extension of tumor.
pN3: metastasis with a lymph node mass > 5 cm in greatest dimension.

189. What is the AJCC M staging for testicular neoplasms?

pM1: distant metastasis present.

pM1a: nonretroperitoneal nodal or pulmonary metastases.

pM1b: nonpulmonary visceral metastases.

Urothelial Tract
Metaplastic Lesions of the Urothelium

190. List 3 types of metaplasia seen in the urinary bladder and describe their significance.
- Intestinal metaplasia in cystitis glandularis and cystitis cystica:
  - Intestinal metaplasia without dysplasia has no risk of adenocarcinoma.
  - Intestinal metaplasia with dysplasia has increased risk of concurrent or subsequent adenocarcinoma.
- Squamous metaplasia:
  - Nonkeratinizing squamous metaplasia is usually not associated with increased risk of squamous cell carcinoma. It is commonly seen in the female trigon region.
  - Keratinizing squamous metaplasia is a risk factor for squamous cell carcinoma.
- Nephrogenic metaplasia/adenoma:
  - This is a benign lesion. When the tubular component of nephrogenic adenoma involves the superficial muscularis propria, it could be misinterpreted as a malignant process.

191. Discuss the pathogenesis of nephrogenic adenoma (nephrogenic metaplasia).
- Recent evidence from renal transplant patients suggests that this lesion is derived from renal tubular epithelial cells and is not a metaplastic lesion.
- It is associated with:
  - Calculi.
  - Instrumentation of, or trauma to, the genitourinary tract.
  - Cystitis.

192. List the histopathological features of nephrogenic adenoma.
- Tubular (most common), cystic, polypoid, papillary, and polypoid patterns.
- Cuboidal to low columnar epithelium with scant cytoplasm (occasionally clear cytoplasm); hobnail cells (common).
- Hyalin around tubules in basement membrane (possible).

193. Name the anatomic sites where nephrogenic adenoma may be found.
- Urinary bladder.
- Ureter.
- Urethra.
- Renal pelvis.

194. List stains that help differentiate nephrogenic adenoma from prostatic adenocarcinoma.

STAIN	NEPHROGENIC ADENOMA	PROSTATIC ADENOCARCINOMA
P504S (racemase/AMACR)	+	+
HMW keratin	−	−
P63	−	−
PSA, PAP, NKX3.1	−	+
CK7	+	− (usually)
PAX8	+	−

Neoplastic Urothelial Lesions

195. List the risk factors for urothelial carcinoma.
- Cigarette smoking.
- Industrial exposure to arylamines.
- Long-term use of analgesics.
- Heavy long-term exposure to cyclophosphamide.
- Irradiation.

196. What is the classification scheme for urothelial lesions according to the WHO and ISUP?

MORPHOLOGY	CLASSIFICATION	CLINICAL NOTES AND BEHAVIOR
Flat	Urothelial proliferation of uncertain malignant potential (formerly flat hyperplasia).	• If not associated with other papillary lesions, no follow-up needed.
	Atypia of unknown significance.	• Predominantly good outcomes.
	Urothelial dysplasia, low grade.	• Can be marker of urothelial instability denoting progression and recurrence.
	Urothelial carcinoma in situ.	• Mortality of 7–15% if not associated with invasion.
Papillary	Urothelial proliferation of uncertain malignant potential (formerly papillary hyperplasia).	• Continued monitoring required, due to association with papillary neoplasia.
	Urothelial papilloma.	• Favorable clinical course.
	Papillary urothelial lesion of low malignant potential.	• Excellent prognosis. • Lower recurrence rate than low grade papillary carcinoma.
	Papillary urothelial carcinoma (noninvasive), low grade.	• Recurrence in 48–71% of cases. • Progression and death in < 5% of cases.
	Papillary urothelial carcinoma (noninvasive), high grade.	• Progression to invasion in 15–40% of cases.
Invasive	Invasive urothelial carcinoma.	• 5-year survival ~70% in pT1. • Variable survival rates in pT2–T4.

197. List the common variants of urothelial carcinoma that are known to behave more aggressively than the usual variant.
- Nested variant.
- Micropapillary variant.
- Sarcomatoid variant.
- Plasmacytoid/signet ring variant.
- Undifferentiated variant.

198. List 2 common genetic alterations associated with urothelial carcinoma.
- Gain-of-function mutations in *FGFR3*, found predominantly in noninvasive low grade papillary carcinomas.
- Loss-of-function mutations in the *TP53* and *RB* tumor suppressor genes, almost always seen in high grade tumors and frequently seen in muscle invasive tumors.

199. List 5 prognostic factors in reporting urothelial carcinoma in radical cystectomy specimens.
- Tumor grade.
- Tumor extension and depth of invasion.
- Associated flat carcinoma in situ in the nearby mucosa.
- Resection margins.
- Lymphovascular invasion and lymph node metastasis.

200. List the morphologic features that suggest invasion in urothelial carcinoma.
- Irregularly shaped nests and single cell infiltration.
- Absent basement membrane.
- Fingerlike projections into lamina propria.
- "Paradoxical differentiation."
- Desmoplastic stromal response.
- Myxoid stroma.
- Pseudosarcomatous stroma.
- Retraction artifact.
- Inflammation.

201. Which stains help differentiate urothelial carcinoma from prostatic carcinoma?

STAIN	UROTHELIAL CARCINOMA	PROSTATIC ADENOCARCINOMA
NKX3.1, PSA, and PAP	−	+
CK7	+	− (usually)
CK20	+	− (usually)
HMW keratin	+	−
P63	+	−
P504S racemase	+	+

202. List 2 nonurothelial carcinoma of the bladder and risk factors for each.

- Squamous cell carcinoma:
  - *Schistosoma hematobium* infection.
  - Bladder diverticula.
  - Nonfunctioning bladder.
  - Transplant patients.
- Adenocarcinoma:
  - Nonfunctioning bladder.
  - Exstrophy.
  - Intestinal metaplasia.
  - Urachal remnant.

203. Name 1 common localized therapy to the urinary bladder, and the morphological changes seen after treatment.

- Therapy: bladder instillation of bacillus Calmette-Guérin (BCG).
- Morphological changes: dense chronic inflammatory infiltrate in the lamina propria with interspersed small granulomas composed of epithelioid histiocytes and multinucleate giant cells.

Urachal Adenocarcinoma

204. Where is urachal adenocarcinoma typically located?

Usually centered in the muscular wall of the bladder dome.

205. What are the subtypes of urachal adenocarcinoma?

- Mucinous.
- Enteric.
- Signet ring cell.
- Not otherwise specified (NOS).
- Mixed types.

206. What are the specific criteria used to classify a tumor as urachal in origin?

- Tumor at the dome of the bladder.
- Sharp demarcation between the tumor and the normal surface epithelium.
- Exclusion of primary adenocarcinoma elsewhere that has spread secondarily to the bladder (especially colonic adenocarcinoma).

207. What is the importance of distinguishing between urachal and nonurachal adenocarcinoma in the urinary bladder and why?

- Resection of urachal adenocarcinoma must include removal of the entire urachal remnant.
- Because the urachus is usually found along the free surface of the bladder, urachal carcinomas are frequently amenable to partial cystectomy. The entire length of the median umbilical ligament may harbor urachal remnants that may develop carcinoma synchronously or metachronously. For this reason, the surgery of choice should include en bloc resection of the entire length of the ligament, including the umbilicus.

208. Which immunohistochemical stains reliably distinguish between colonic adenocarcinoma and urachal adenocarcinoma?

- There is no reliable Immunohistochemical stain.
- ß-catenin has some utility. It typically shows nuclear positivity in colonic adenocarcinoma, and shows only cytoplasmic and/or membranous staining in urachal adenocarcinoma.

Postoperative Spindle Cell Nodules in the Urinary Bladder

209. State the common clinical setting of postoperative spindle cell nodules in the bladder.

- Usually occurs within 3 months of a previous resection procedure.
- Develops as a nodule at the same site.

210. List the histologic features of postoperative spindle cell nodules in the bladder.

- Interlacing fascicles of mitotically active spindle cells with uniform nuclei and little pleomorphism.
- Delicate vasculature, scattered inflammatory cells, small foci of hemorrhage, edema, and focal myxoid change.

211. What lesion has a similar morphological appearance but lacks the clinical setting described in the previous question? List a key immunohistochemical stain for this lesion.

- Lesion: inflammatory pseudotumor.
- Stain: anaplastic lymphoma kinase protein (ALK 1).

212. List important differential diagnoses of postoperative spindle cell nodules in the bladder.

- Sarcomatoid carcinoma.
- Leiomyosarcoma.

213. List other histologic changes in the urinary bladder often seen postinstrumentation.
- Postsurgical necrobiotic granulomas.
- Nephrogenic adenoma.
- Eosinophilic inflammation/cystitis.

CAP Protocols for Examining and Reporting Bladder Cancer

214. List required elements for reporting transurethral resection of bladder tumor (TURBT) and biopsy.
- Procedure (required only for TURBT).
- Tumor type.
- Histologic type.
- Associated epithelial lesions.
- Histologic grade.
- Adequacy of material for determining muscularis propria invasion.
- Lymphovascular invasion.
- Microscopic tumor extension.

215. What is meant by relevant patient history in the setting of bladder cancer?
- Relevant patient history includes:
  · Cystoscopy findings.
  · History of renal stones, recent urinary tract procedures, infections, or obstruction.
- · History of neoplasia.
- · Prior therapy (systemic or intravesical chemotherapy, immunotherapy, radiation, etc.).
- The method of collection and date should be specified in urine cytology specimens.

216. What is the most common histologic type of bladder cancer?
- Most bladder cancers are urothelial cell carcinomas (95%).
- Pure squamous or pure glandular histology is required for diagnosing squamous cell carcinoma or adenocarcinoma.
- No urothelial carcinoma in situ or associated papillary urothelial neoplasms can be present; if they are present, this favors invasive urothelial carcinoma with squamous or glandular differentiation.

217. How should invasion be reported in urothelial carcinoma?
- Pathologists are encouraged to provide some assessment of the extent of lamina propria invasion — i.e., focal versus extensive, or depth in millimeters, or by level (above, at, or below muscularis mucosae).
- Designation of a tumor as merely muscle invasive is inappropriate, but the type of muscle invasion — i.e., muscularis mucosae (pT1 tumors) versus muscularis propria (pT2 tumors) — needs to be clearly stated.
- Fat can be found in the lamina propria and submucosa, and thus extravesical involvement can be identified only on resection.

218. List the margins that need to be assessed and reported in radical cystectomy.
- Ureteral margin.
- Distal urethra margin.
- Deep soft tissue margin.

219. What is the AJCC T staging for carcinoma of the urinary bladder?

pTX: primary tumor cannot be assessed.
pT0: no evidence of primary tumor.
pTa: noninvasive papillary carcinoma.
pTis: urothelial carcinoma in situ.
pT1: tumor invades subepithelial connective tissue (lamina propria).
pT2a: tumor invades superficial muscularis propria (inner half).

pT2b: tumor invades deep muscularis propria (outer half).
pT3a: tumor invades perivesical tissue (microscopically).
pT3b: tumor invades perivesical tissue (macroscopically/extravesical mass).
pT4a: extravesical tumor invades directly into prostatic stroma, uterus, or vagina.
pT4b: extravesical tumor invades pelvic or abdominal wall.

CAP Protocols for Examining and Reporting Carcinoma of the Ureter and Renal Pelvis

220. What history is important for the interpretation of carcinoma of the upper urinary tract?
- A history of renal stones or recent urinary tract procedures, infections, or obstruction can influence the interpretation of random biopsies obtained from patients with hematuria.
- Any neoplasms previously diagnosed should be specified, especially as part of Lynch syndrome.
- Analgesic abusers have nephropathy, papillary necrosis, and an increase in renal pelvic tumors.

(continued on next page)

- Previous therapy (intravesicular or systemic chemotherapy, immunotherapy, radiation) may affect interpretation.

- Site of collection of urine cytology specimens may affect interpretation (ureter or renal pelvis may be overinterpreted).

221. How are primary squamous cell carcinoma or adenocarcinoma distinguished from urothelial carcinoma with aberrant squamous or glandular differentiation?

- The primary classification requires pure histology of squamous cell carcinoma or adenocarcinoma.
- If the histology shows recognizable papillary, invasive, or flat carcinoma in situ (CIS) and, in addition, there is

a urothelial component present, the recommended classification is urothelial carcinoma with squamous or glandular differentiation.

222. What are important considerations when assessing the extent of invasion in neoplasms of the upper urinary tract?

- Depth of invasion and pathologic stage are the most important prognostic indicators.
- For renal pelvis carcinoma, the type of tumor involvement of the kidney, when present, impacts stage (pT3) or perinephric fat (pT4).
- In situ extension of carcinoma into renal collecting ducts and renal tubules does not affect stage.

- The lamina propria is absent beneath the urothelium that lines the renal papillae in the pelvis, and is thin along the minor calyces. There is no accepted approach for assessing depth of lamina propria invasion, but you can provide an assessment of extent — e.g., focal versus extensive, or depth in millimeters, or by level (above, at, or below muscularis mucosae).

223. What are the regional lymph nodes for the renal pelvis and for the ureter?

- Renal pelvis: renal hilar, paracaval, aortic, and retroperitoneal.

- Ureter: renal hilar, iliac (common, internal [hypogastric], external), paracaval, periureteral, and pelvic.
- Other lymph nodes: considered distant metastasis.

224. How is a residual tumor described?

- A tumor remaining in a patient after therapy with curative intent (e.g., surgical resection for cure) is categorized by a system known as R classification:
  - RX: presence of residual tumor cannot be assessed.

R0: no residual tumor.
R1: microscopic residual tumor.
R2: macroscopic residual tumor.

225. How are sections submitted for biopsies and segmental ureterectomy?

- Ureteroscopic biopsies: submit entire specimen (can be submitted for cytology cell block preparation).
- Needle core biopsies (renal masses): submit entire specimen.
- Segmental ureterectomy (proximal and midureter tumors):
  - Record the length and diameter of the intact ureter.
  - Search for a mass by palpation and inspection.

- Ink the outer aspect of ureter.
- Take proximal and distal cross-section margins.
- Open the ureter longitudinally to assess mucosal abnormalities.
- Take sections to demonstrate deepest level of invasion.
- Take 1 section of uninvolved ureter.

226. Describe how to submit sections for radical nephroureterectomy with bladder cuff.

- Gross examination and sampling should document the relationship of the tumor to adjacent renal parenchyma, peripelvic fat, nearest soft tissue margin, and ureter.
- Ink the outer aspect of ureter.

- Open the ureter longitudinally to assess mucosal abnormalities.
- Take sections to demonstrate deepest level of invasion.
- Submit the bladder cuff margin as a shave.
- Obtain sections of unremarkable kidney, pelvis, and ureter.

227. What are the margins in renal pelvis, ureter, and nephroureterectomy specimens?

- Radial hilar soft tissue margin.
- Bladder cuff margin.
- Ureteric margin.

- Renal parenchymal margin.
- Gerota fascia margins.

228. How is lymphovascular invasion assessed? What diagnostic difficulties can be encountered?

- This is an important prognostic factor in upper urinary tract urothelial carcinoma.
- Pitfalls include:
  - Artifactual space formation by tumor cells (especially when urothelial cells invade into the lamina propria);

however, blood vessels can be highlighted by immunohistochemical staining for factor VIII–related antigen, CD31, or CD34.
  - Artifactual space around clusters of micropapillary variant.

229. What is the T staging for ureter and renal pelvis tumors?

pTX: cannot be assessed.

pT0: no evidence of primary tumor.

pTa: papillary noninvasive carcinoma.

pTis: flat carcinoma in situ.

pT1: tumor invades subepithelial connective tissue (lamina propria).

pT2: tumor invades muscularis propria.

pT3: for renal pelvis only: tumor invades beyond muscularis into peripelvic fat or into the renal parenchyma. For ureter only: tumor invades beyond muscularis into periureteric fat.

pT4: tumor invades adjacent organs, or through the kidney into the perinephric fat.

230. What is the N staging for renal pelvis and ureter tumors?

pNX: cannot be assessed.

pN0: no regional lymph node metastasis.

pN1: metastasis in a single regional lymph node ≤ 2 cm in greatest dimension.

pN2: metastasis in a single regional lymph node > 2 cm; or multiple lymph nodes.

CAP Protocols for Examining and Reporting Urethra Tumor Resection Specimens

231. What is the pertinent history in evaluation of urethral biopsies?

- Renal stones, recent urinary tract procedures, infections, obstruction, or prior therapy (intravesical or systemic chemotherapy, local radiation) — these can lead to reactive epithelial changes potentially mimicking malignancy.

- History of neoplasms, including histologic type, primary site, and histologic grade.

232. How does the anatomic location influence tumor type in urethral tumors?

- Carcinomas of the urethra vary in histologic type, depending on the type of epithelium lining the urethra in a given anatomic location.

- In women, squamous cell carcinoma is the most common histologic subtype (approximately 75%) and is most common in the anterior urethra (distal third). Urothelial (transitional cell) carcinoma is next in frequency, followed by adenocarcinoma (approximately 10–15% each), including clear cell adenocarcinomas (rare in men).

- In men, most tumors involve the bulbomembranous urethra, followed by penile urethra and prostatic urethra. Most carcinomas of the male urethra (80%) are squamous cell carcinoma, followed by urothelial (transitional cell) origin. Urothelial carcinomas are typically more proximal. Primary urethral adenocarcinomas are rare in men.

233. How is depth of invasion reported in urethral tumors?

- The surrounding anatomic structures vary by location within the urethra but include the subepithelial connective tissue, corpus spongiosum, corpus cavernosum, prostate, periurethral muscle, extraprostatic soft tissue, anterior vagina, bladder neck, or other adjacent organs.

- In the prostatic urethra, invasion may arise from a tumor lining the urethral lumen or from carcinoma in situ colonizing the prostatic ducts.

- Invasion arising from the prostatic ducts is designated as at least pT2.

- In papillary urothelial tumors, invasion occurs most often at the base of the tumor and less frequently in the stalk.

234. What sections need to be taken for microscopic evaluation in urethral samples?

- In transurethral specimens, submit 1 section per centimeter of tumor diameter (up to 10 cassettes).

- If the tumor is noninvasive by the initial sampling, additional submission of tissue (including possibly submitting all tissue) is necessary to diagnose or rule out the presence of invasion.

- In urethrectomy specimens, submit 1 section per centimeter of tumor, including the macroscopically deepest penetration.

- Documentation of the tumor in relation to surrounding anatomic structures (such as corpus spongiosum, corpus cavernosum, prostate, periurethral muscle, vagina, and bladder) is critical to proper staging.

- The distal and proximal urethral margins should be submitted (or distal urethra and bilateral ureteral margins if bladder is included). Submit en face or perpendicular sections if the tumor is close to the margin.

- The surrounding radial soft tissue margins should also be submitted, guided by the closest approximation of the tumor to ink by gross evaluation.

- Other tissues:
  · Submit 1 or more sections of other organs included in the resection.
  · Demonstrate microscopically any invasion of neighboring organs, if present.

(*continued on next page*)

- Submit several sections of the urinary bladder mucosa remote from the carcinoma, especially if abnormal, including the lateral wall(s), dome, and trigone, because urothelial neoplasia is frequently multifocal.
- Submit 1 section from each ureteral margin if not evaluated by frozen section. Representative sections

of the peripheral zone, central zone, and seminal vesicles should be included because concomitant prostatic adenocarcinoma is not uncommon. The gross examination may help target sampling of selective abnormal-appearing areas.

235. Describe the pathologic T stages in urethral carcinoma.

- Primary tumor (pT) (male penile urethra and female urethra):
    - pTX: cannot be assessed.
    - pT0: no evidence of primary tumor.
    - pTa: noninvasive papillary carcinoma.
    - pTis: carcinoma in situ.
    - pT1: tumor invades subepithelial connective tissue.
    - pT2: tumor invades any of the following: corpus spongiosum, periurethral muscle.
    - pT3: tumor invades any of the following: corpus cavernosum, anterior vagina.
    - pT4: tumor invades other adjacent organs (invasion of the bladder wall).

- Primary tumor (pT) (prostatic urethra):
    - pTX: cannot be assessed.
    - pT0: no evidence of primary tumor.
    - pTa: noninvasive papillary, polypoid, or verrucous carcinoma.
    - pTis: carcinoma in situ, involving the prostatic urethra or periurethral or prostatic ducts without stromal invasion.
    - pT1: tumor invades urethral subepithelial connective tissue immediately underlying the urothelium.
    - pT2: tumor invades the prostatic stroma surrounding ducts either by direct extension from the urothelial surface or by invasion from the prostatic ducts.
    - pT3: tumor invades the periprostatic fat.
    - pT4: tumor invades other adjacent organs (e.g., extraprostatic invasion of the bladder wall, rectal wall).

Penis
Penile Squamous Cell Carcinoma

236. What subtypes of squamous cell carcinoma have a better prognosis for patients?
- Verrucous carcinoma.
- Warty carcinoma.
- Papillary carcinoma.
- Pseudohyperplastic carcinoma.

237. What subtypes of squamous cell carcinoma have a poorer prognosis for patients?
- Basaloid carcinoma.
- Sarcomatoid carcinoma.

238. What are the risk factors for penile squamous cell carcinoma?
- Phimosis.
- Chronic inflammatory conditions (e.g., balanitis xerotica obliterans [BXO]).
- Smoking.
- Ultraviolet irradiation.
- Human papilloma virus (HPV) infection.

239. What conditions are associated with squamous cell carcinoma?
- HPV infection.
- Penile intraepithelial neoplasia/squamous cell carcinoma in situ.
- BXO — particularly in patients without HPV infection.

240. How do you classify penile intraepithelial neoplasia (PeIN)?
- Undifferentiated PeIN (uPeIN) — HPV associated; p16 positive.
- Differentiated PeIN (dPeIN) — non-HPV associated; p16 negative; aberrant expression of p53 (usually).

241. What are the important features to include when reporting penile squamous cell carcinoma?
- Histologic type.
- Histologic grade.
- Extent of invasion (e.g., subepithelial tissue, corpora cavernosa and spongiosum, urethra, prostate, adjacent structures).
- Maximum depth measurement.
- Lymphovascular invasion.
- Perineural invasion.
- Resection margin status.
- Associated lesions — e.g., carcinoma in situ, dysplasia, BXO.

242. What are the clinical features of bowenoid papulosis, and how does its behavior differ from Bowen disease and erythroplasia de Queyrat?

- It usually occurs in younger patients (20–40 years old) who present with papules on the shaft that can undergo spontaneous regression.
- Histology is similar among all 3 lesions.

CAP Protocols for Examining and Reporting Carcinoma of the Penis

243. How are circumcision specimens grossed?

- Take measurements, describe the specimen, and identify and describe the tumor.
- Identify and ink the mucosal and cutaneous margins with different colors.
- Most squamous cell carcinomas arise from the mucosal surface of the foreskin; therefore, the coronal sulcus (mucosal) margin is especially important.
- Lightly stretch and pin the specimen. Fix for several hours in formalin. Cut vertically through the urethra in the 12-to-6 o'clock plane to divide the penile glans, foreskin, and shaft into right and left portions.

244. How are penectomy specimens grossed?

- Take measurements, describe the specimen, and identify and describe the tumor.
- If present, classify the foreskin as short, medium, long, and/ or phimotic.
- Cut the proximal margin of resection en face making sure to include the entire circumference of the urethra (this may be retracted, so find it!).
- The urethra and periurethral cylinder can be placed in 1 cassette.
- The skin of the shaft with dartos and fascia can be included together with the corpora cavernosa (you may need more than 1 cassette).
- Fix the rest of the specimen overnight.
- Using the meatus and proximal urethra as reference points, cut longitudinally and centrally (do not probe the urethra) and separate the specimen into halves.
- Cut 2–6 serial sections of each half.
- If the tumor is small and asymmetric, the central portion of the tumor may be used as the axis of sectioning.
- If the tumor is large, do not remove the foreskin.
- If there is a small carcinoma in the glans without foreskin involvement, you may remove the foreskin leaving 3 mm of redundant edge around the sulcus (gross as per circumcision protocol).

245. What part of the penis do squamous cell carcinomas usually arise from?

Most arise from the epithelium of the distal portion of the organ (glans, coronal sulcus, and mucosal surface of the prepuce); the tumor may involve 1 or more of these anatomical compartments.

246. What are the different types of foreskin?

- Short foreskin: the preputial orifice is located behind the glans corona.
- Medium foreskin: the orifice is between the corona and the meatal orifice.
- Long foreskin: the entire glans is covered and the meatus is not identified without retracting the foreskin.
- Phimotic foreskin: the foreskin is unretractable and long (phimotic foreskin is present in half of patients with penile cancer and considered a risk factor).

247. What is the significance of the number of lymph nodes involved in penile carcinoma and what impact does it have surgically?

- The number and percentage of positive nodes involved has an impact on survival.
- More than 2 positive lymph nodes in 1 inguinal basin increases the likelihood of contralateral inguinal and ipsilateral pelvic nodal involvement.
- Prophylactic contralateral inguinal and ipsilateral pelvic lymphadenectomy is advised in these cases.

248. What are the types of tumor base infiltration and what is their significance?

- Infiltrating:
  - Invasion in blocks of small solid strands of cell tumors broadly infiltrating the stroma.
- Pushing:
  - Tumor cells invading in large cell blocks with well-defined tumor-stroma interface.
- Significance: the infiltrating pattern of invasion is associated with a higher risk for nodal involvement.

249. What are the recognized histologic types of penis cancers?

- Squamous cell carcinoma.
- Usual (keratinizing).
- Basaloid.
- Warty (condylomatous) (optional).

(continued on next page)

- Verrucous.
- Cuniculatum (optional).
- Papillary, not otherwise specified (NOS) (optional).
- Sarcomatoid.
- Pseudohyperplastic (optional).
- Acantholytic (pseudoglandular) (optional).
- Mixed squamous cell carcinomas (optional).

- Adenosquamous.
- Primary neuroendocrine carcinoma.
- Paget disease.
- Adnexal carcinoma (specify type).
- Clear cell carcinoma.
- Carcinoma, type cannot be determined.
- Other (specify).

250. Divide the histologic subtypes of penile squamous cell carcinoma into prognostic risk groups.

- There are 3 main prognostic groups that have correlation with regional/nodal and systemic dissemination:
  · Low-risk (verruciform tumors):
    › Verrucous, papillary, and warty/condylomatous carcinomas.
    › Pseudohyperplastic and carcinoma cuniculatum.
  · Intermediate risk:

  › Usual type squamous cell carcinomas.
  › Mixed neoplasm (such as hybrid verrucous carcinomas).
  › High grade variants of warty/condylomatous carcinomas.
  · High risk:
    › Basaloid, sarcomatoid, adenosquamous, and poorly differentiated squamous cell carcinoma of the usual type.

251. How are penile squamous cell carcinomas graded?

- Grade 1 is an extremely well-differentiated carcinoma, with a minimal deviation from the morphology of normal/hyperplastic squamous epithelium.
- Grade 2 tumors show a more disorganized growth as compared to grade 1 lesions, higher nuclear-cytoplasmic ratio, evident mitoses, and, although present, less prominent keratinization.
- Grade 3 are tumors showing any proportion of anaplastic cells, identified as solid sheets or irregular small aggregates,

cords or nests of cells with little or no keratinization, high nuclear-cytoplasmic ratio, thick nuclear membranes, nuclear pleomorphism, clumped chromatin, prominent nucleoli, and numerous mitosis.
- A tumor should be graded according to the least differentiated component.
- Any proportion of grade 3 should be noted in the report.

252. How should the specimen or tumor be sectioned?

- The tumor depth in small lesions is best obtained by perpendicularly sectioning along the tumor central axis.

- For large glans tumors, section the specimen longitudinally in half, with additional parallel sections of each half, using as an axis the central and ventral penile urethra.

253. How is tumor depth or thickness measured?

- Depth of invasion of squamous cell carcinoma is defined as a measurement in millimeters from the epithelial-stromal junction of the adjacent nonneoplastic epithelium to the deepest point of invasion.

- For large tumors, especially verruciform ones, the tumor is measured from the surface (minus the keratin layer).

254. How is depth or thickness correlated with prognosis?

- Minimal risk for metastasis has been reported for tumors measuring < 5 mm in thickness.
- Tumors invading deeper into penile anatomical levels are usually associated with a higher risk for nodal involvement.

- Depth is usually correlated with grade (some exceptions occur).
- Tumors invading into corpus cavernosum are at higher risk than those invading into corpus spongiosum.

255. Name 4 key penile resection margins.

- Proximal urethra and surrounding periurethral cylinder consisting of epithelium, subepithelial connective tissue (lamina propria), corpus spongiosum, and penile fascia.
- Proximal shaft with corresponding corpora cavernosa separated and surrounded by the tunica albuginea and Buck fascia.

- Skin of shaft with underlying dartos and penile fascia.
- In circumcisions: coronal sulcus margin and cutaneous margin.

256. What are the most important predictive factors of mortality in penile tumors that are 5–10 mm thick?

- Histologic grade.

- Perineural invasion.

257. What factors best predict nodal metastases and survival in penile squamous cell carcinoma, and form the basis of the prognostic index for this entity?

- Histologic grade.
- Deepest anatomical level of infiltration.

- Presence of perineural invasion.

258. What are the subtypes of penile intraepithelial neoplasia (PeIN)? What are their associations with HPV?

- Differentiated (simplex) PeIN: parakeratosis, epithelial thickening, elongation of rete ridges, prominent bridges, basal cell atypia, enlarged nuclei, and prominent nucleoli.
  - This subtype is HPV independent; it is associated with lichen sclerosus (p16 negative).
- Penile intraepithelial neoplasia, HPV associated.
  - This subtype has high association with HPV.
  - It includes:

> Warty PeIN, basaloid PeIN and warty/basaloid PeIN: warty (spiky surface with parakeratosis). The normal epithelium is replaced by markedly pleomorphic cells showing prominent koilocytosis.
> Basaloid: replacement of the normal epithelium by small, uniform cells with round nuclei and scant cytoplasm.
> Warty/basaloid: variable mixture of warty and basaloid cells.

Note: the Lower Anogenital Squamous Terminology (LAST) Project recommends a 2-tiered nomenclature system for HPV-related anogenital lesions: 1) low grade squamous intraepithelial lesion (LGSIL); and 2) high grade squamous intraepithelial lesion (HGSIL). Warty, basaloid, and warty basaloid PeIN are classified as HGSIL (usually p16 positive).

259. What are common optional additional pathologic findings reported?

- HPV-related PeIN.
- Non-HPV-related PeIN (Differentiated (simplex) PeIN).
- Lichen sclerosus.
- Squamous hyperplasia.
- Condyloma acuminatum.

260. What is the AJCC T staging for penile cancers?

pTX: primary tumor cannot be assessed.

pT0: no evidence of primary tumor.

pTis: carcinoma in situ (PeIN).

pTa: noninvasive localized squamous cell carcinoma.

pT1: **glans**: tumor invades lamina propria; **foreskin**: tumor invades dermis, lamina propria, or dartos fascia; **shaft**: tumor invades connective tissue between epidermis and corpora regardless of location.

> pT1a: tumor is without lymphovascular invasion or perineural invasion and is not high grade (i.e., grade 3 or sarcomatoid).

pT1b: tumor exhibits lymphovascular invasion and/or perineural invasion or is high grade (i.e., grade 3 or sarcomatoid).

pT2: tumor invades into corpus spongiosum (either glans or ventral shaft) with or without urethral invasion.

pT3: tumor invades into corpora cavernosum (including tunica albuginea) with or without urethral invasion.

pT4: tumor invades into adjacent structures (i.e., scrotum, prostate, pubic bone).

261. What is the AJCC N staging for penile cancers?

pNX: regional lymph nodes cannot be assessed.

pN0: no lymph node metastasis.

pN1: ≤ 2 unilateral inguinal metastases, no extranodal extension.

pN2: ≥ 3 unilateral inguinal metastases or bilateral metastases.

pN3: extranodal extension of lymph node metastases or pelvic lymph node metastases.

262. What is the AJCC M staging for penile cancers?

- The M staging refers to distant metastasis (pM) and has 2 categories: not applicable; and pM1: distant metastasis present.
- Distant metastasis also involves lymph node metastasis outside of the true pelvis in addition to visceral or bone sites.

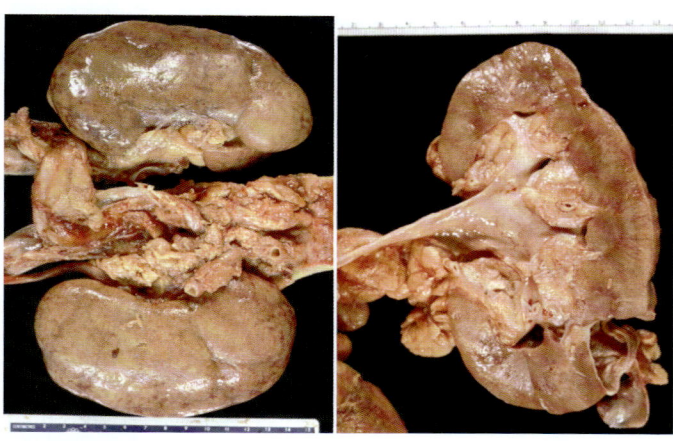

IMAGE 10.1 Kidney with amyloidosis. Both kidneys are enlarged with a pale, firm, and waxy appearance (right cross-section).

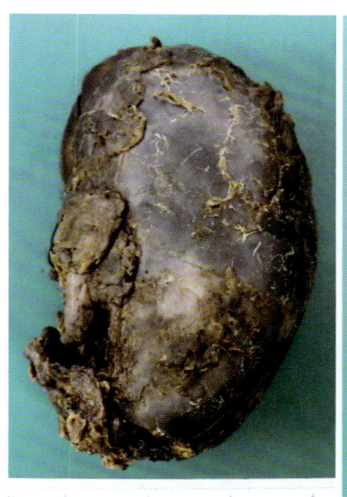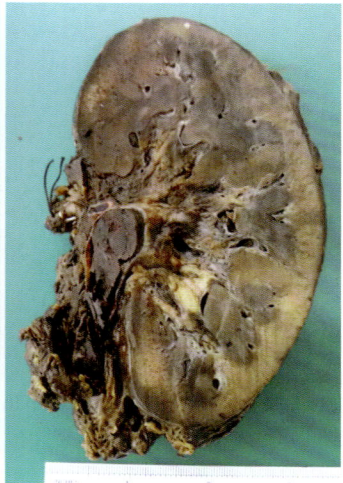

IMAGE 10.4 Necrotic kidney allograft due to renal vein thrombosis.

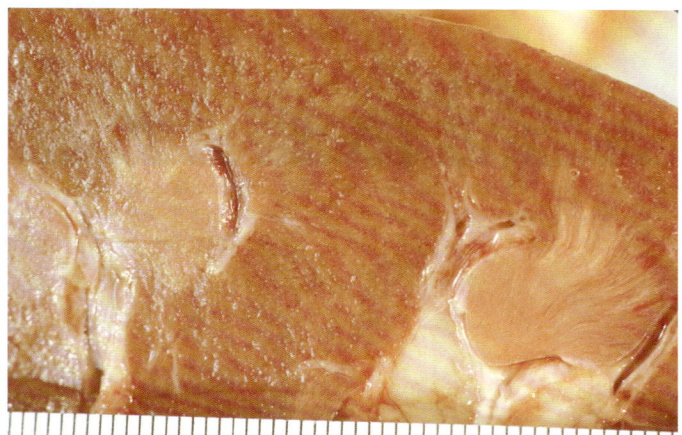

IMAGE 10.2 Diabetic kidney. The kidney shows hypertrophy of cortex and papillae.

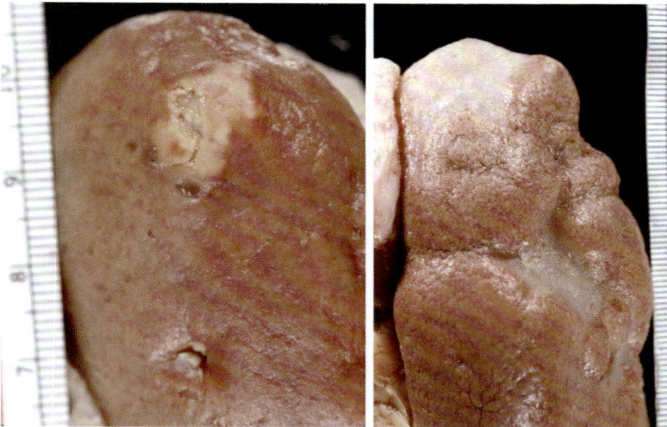

IMAGE 10.5 Kidney infarct. Left: recent infarct. Right: remote infarct.

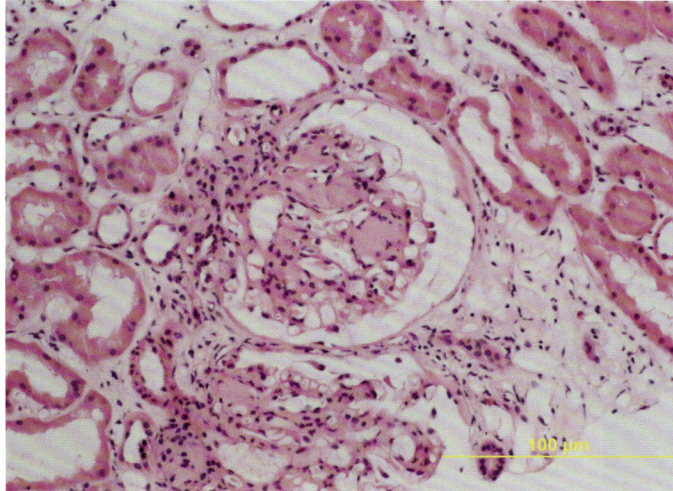

IMAGE 10.3 Diabetic nephropathy with Kimmelstiel-Wilson nodules (H&E, x200).

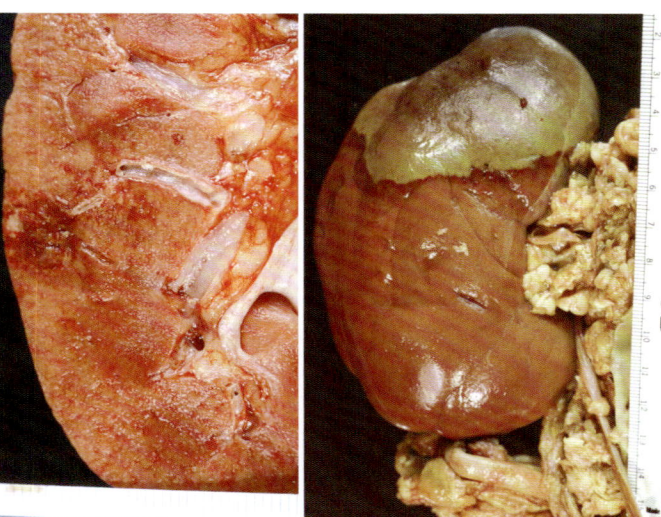

IMAGE 10.6 Left: kidney septal infarct due to bacterial endocarditis. Right: kidney infarct due to mucormycosis emboli.

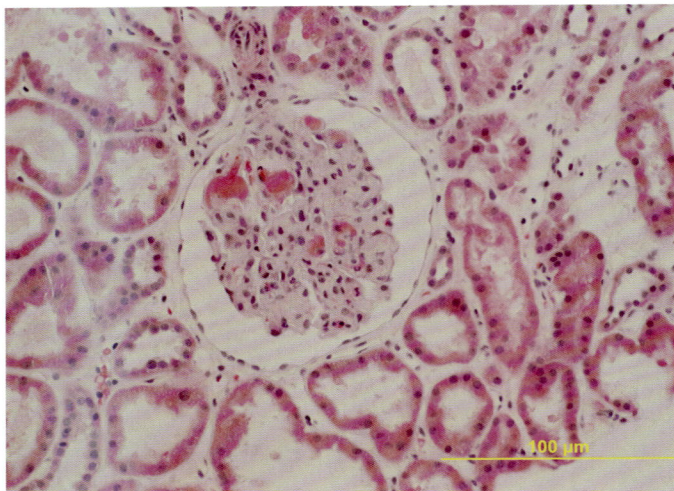

IMAGE 10.7 Glomerulus with fibrin thrombi, typically seen in thrombotic microangiopathy (H&E, x200).

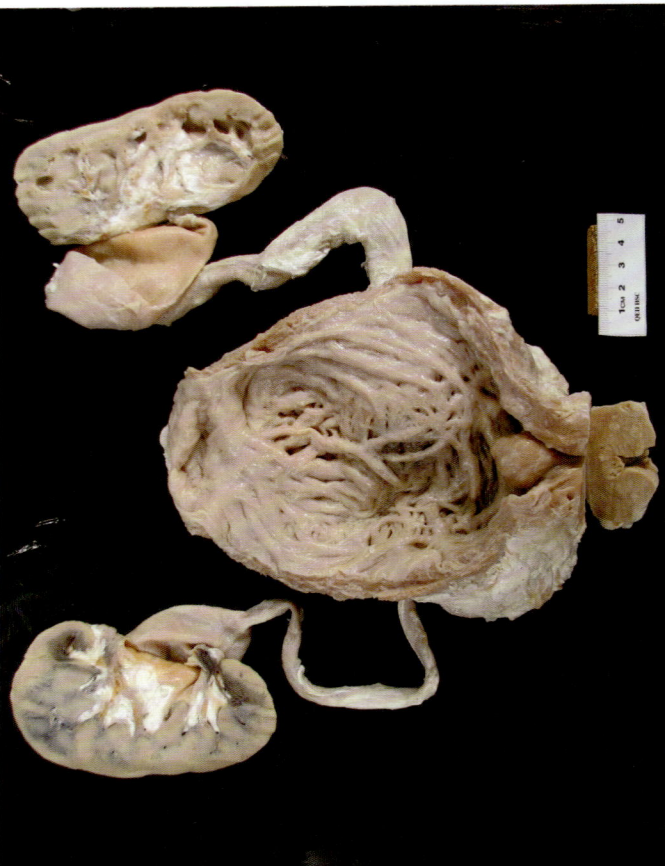

IMAGE 10.9 Hydronephrosis secondary to benign prostatic hyperplasia. Note trabeculation of bladder wall and dilatation of ureters and renal pelvis.

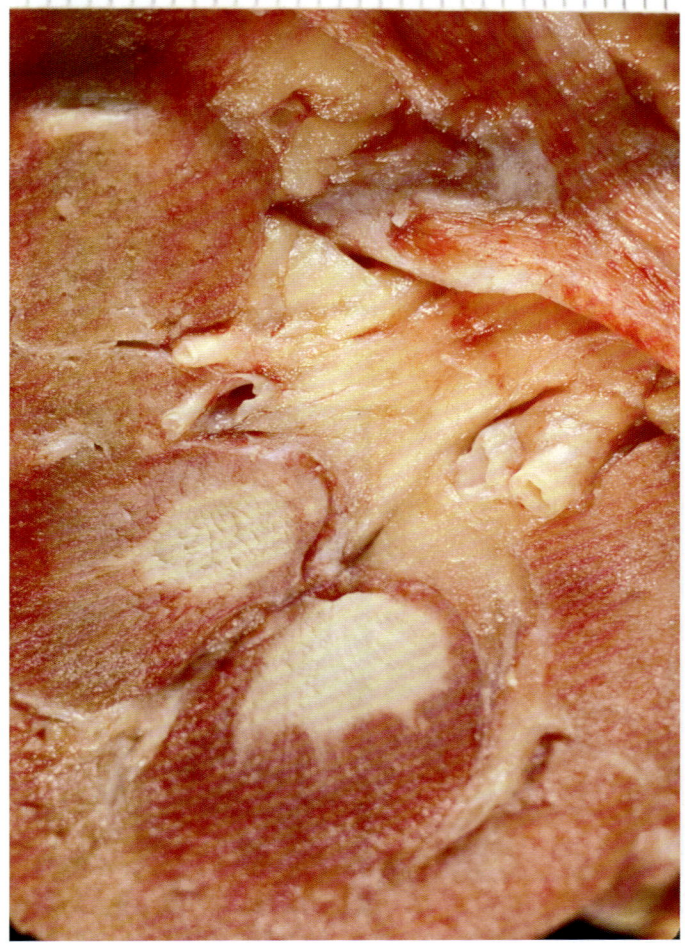

IMAGE 10.8 Kidney papillary necrosis due to acute pyelonephritis.

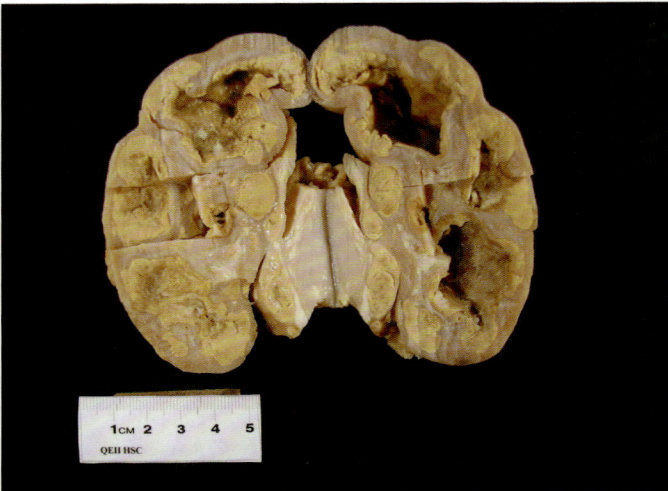

IMAGE 10.10 Xanthogranulomatous pyelonephritis. The image shows dilated renal pelvis and calyces filled with yellow-brown material.

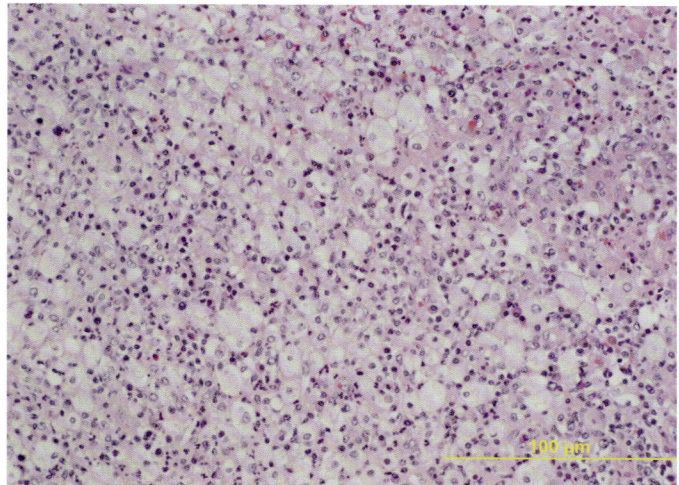

IMAGE 10.11 Xanthogranulomatous pyelonephritis with large collections of mixed inflammatory cells including foamy histiocytes, lymphocytes, plasma cells, and neutrophils (H&E, x200).

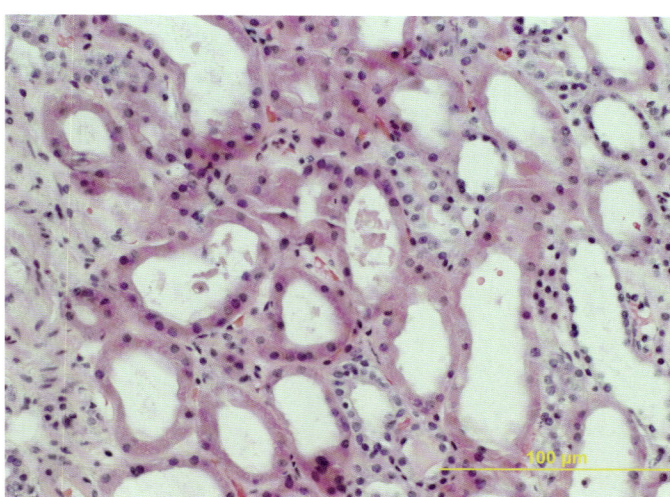

IMAGE 10.14 Acute tubular necrosis. Note dilated tubules and sloughed epithelial cells within lumens (H&E, x200).

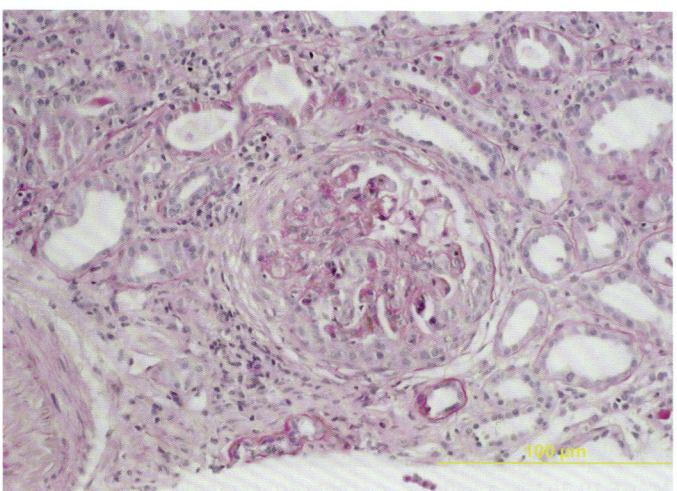

IMAGE 10.12 Glomerulus with cellular crescent (PAS, x200).

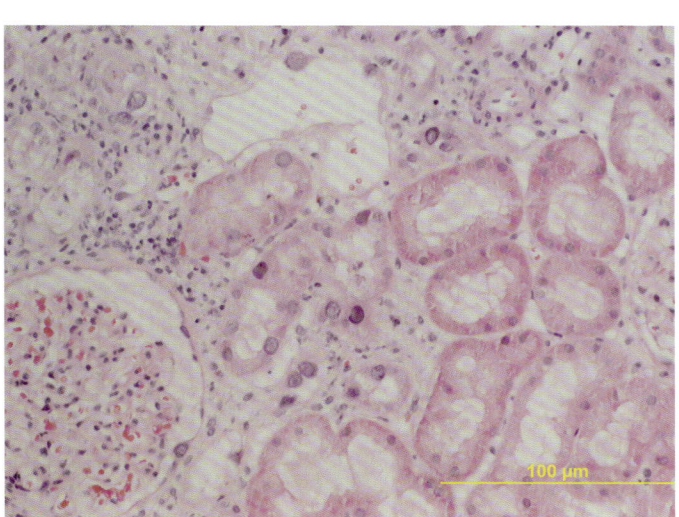

IMAGE 10.13 Polyoma virus infection in transplant kidney. Note enlarged nuclei in tubular epithelium with smudged nuclear inclusions (H&E, x200).

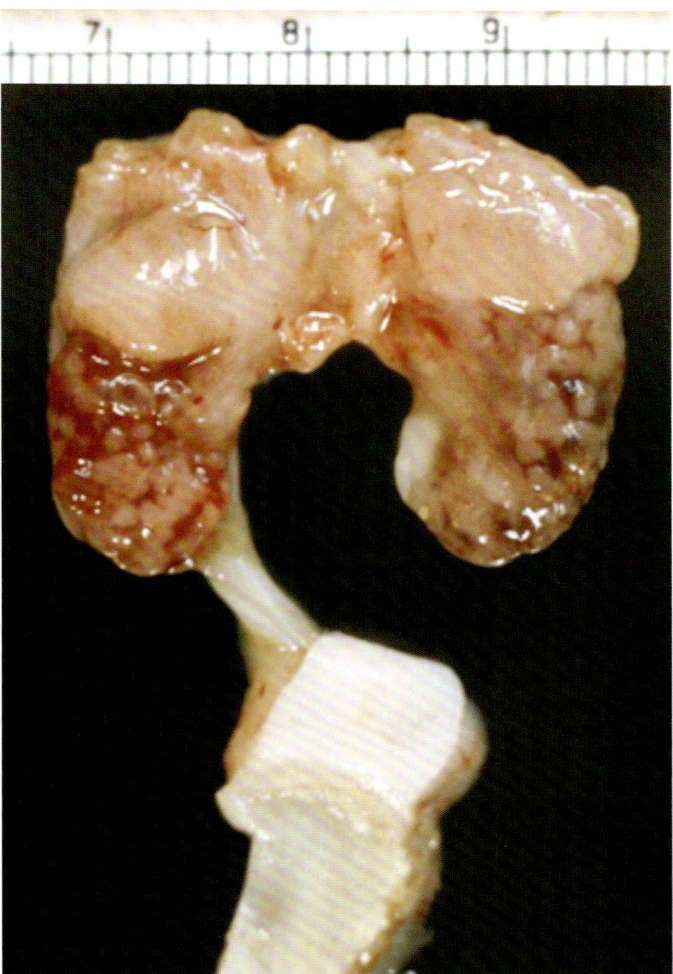

IMAGE 10.15 Horseshoe kidney with a single ureter draining into a dystrophic bladder.

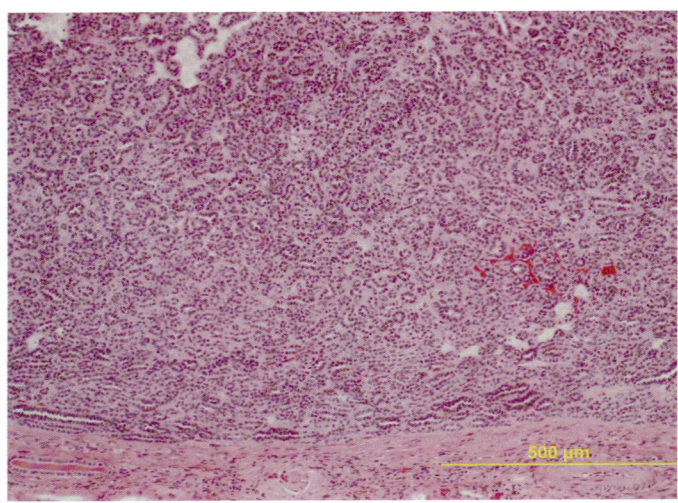

IMAGE 10.16 Metanephric adenoma composed of small tubules with small cells with bland nuclei. Note lack of pseudocapsule (H&E, x40).

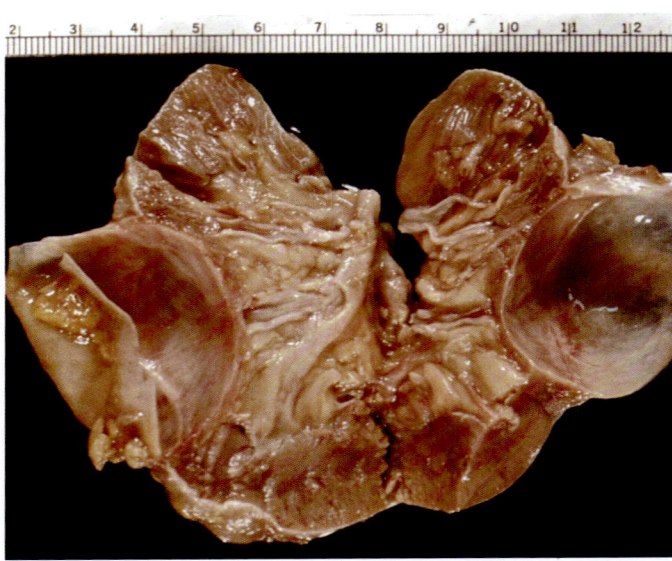

IMAGE 10.19 Kidney simple cyst. The cyst has smooth lining and contains clear fluid.

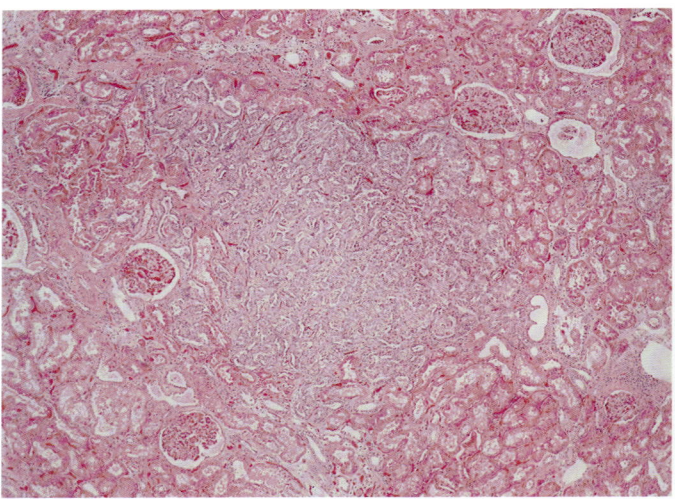

IMAGE 10.17 Renal papillary adenoma (H&E, x40). This is a benign lesion composed of glands forming tubulopapillary architecture.

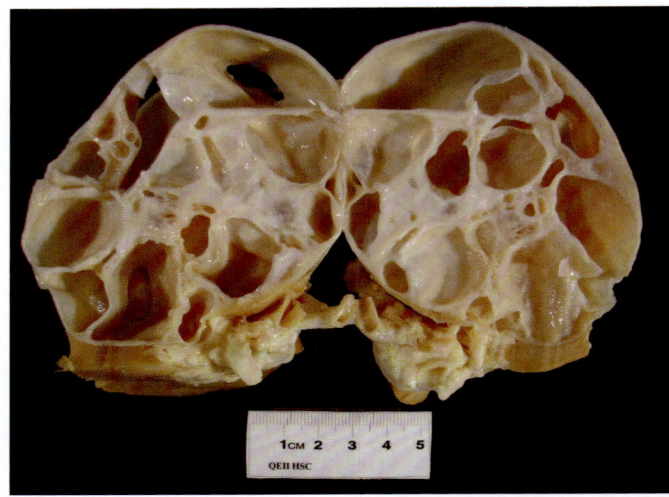

IMAGE 10.20 Mixed epithelial and stromal tumor The lesion shows a well-circumscribed, multilocular cystic mass.

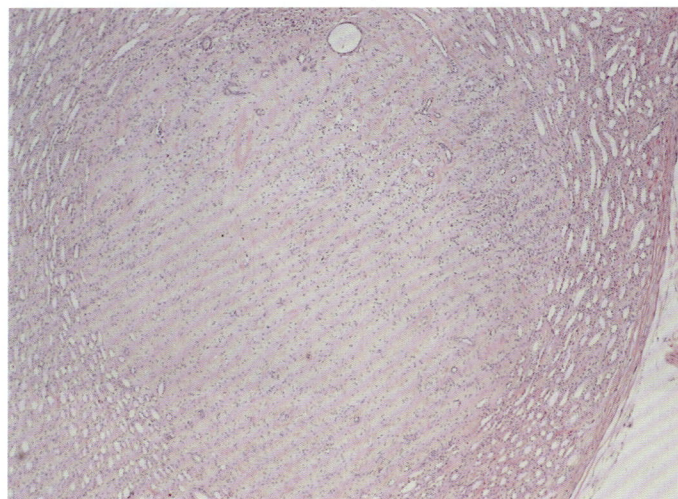

IMAGE 10.18 Renal medullary interstitial cell tumor (H&E, x40). The tumor has spindle and stellate cells in a fibrotic stroma, and contains entrapped tubules.

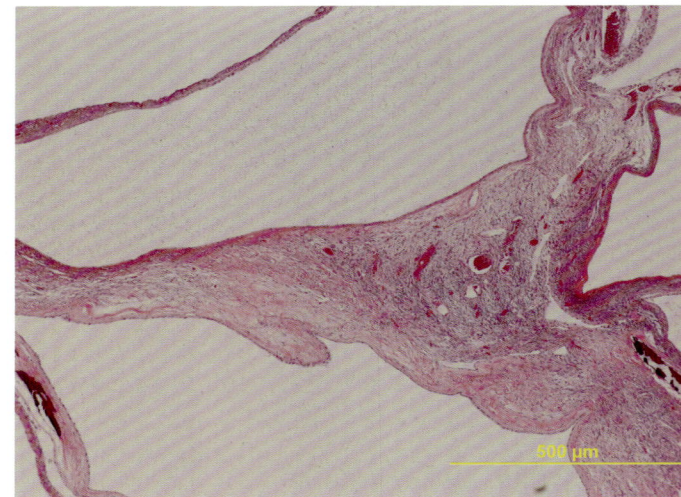

IMAGE 10.21 Mixed epithelial and stromal tumor of kidney with cysts lined by cuboidal cells. Note the "ovarian-type" stroma within the septae (H&E, x40).

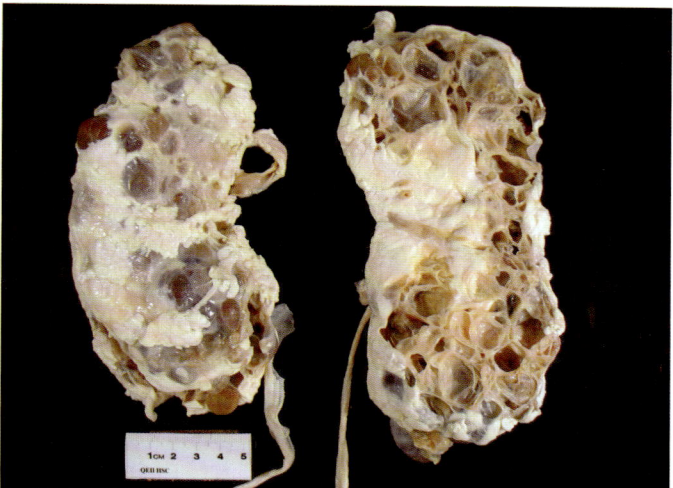

IMAGE 10.22 Autosomal dominant polycystic kidney disease with enlarged kidneys due to cysts of variable size replacing the entire parenchyma.

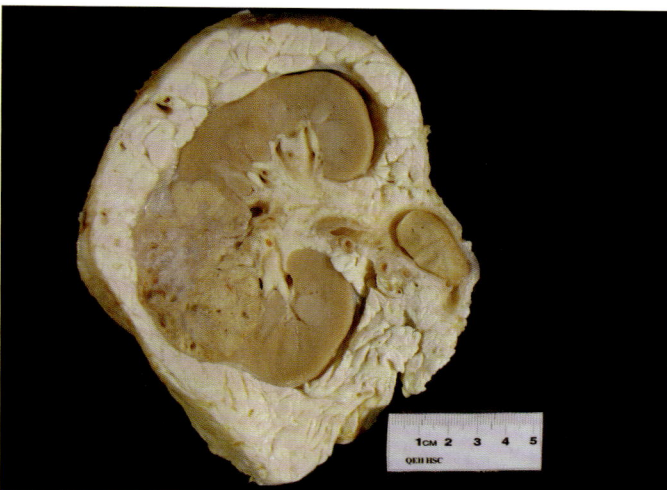

IMAGE 10.25 Clear cell renal cell carcinoma invading renal vein.

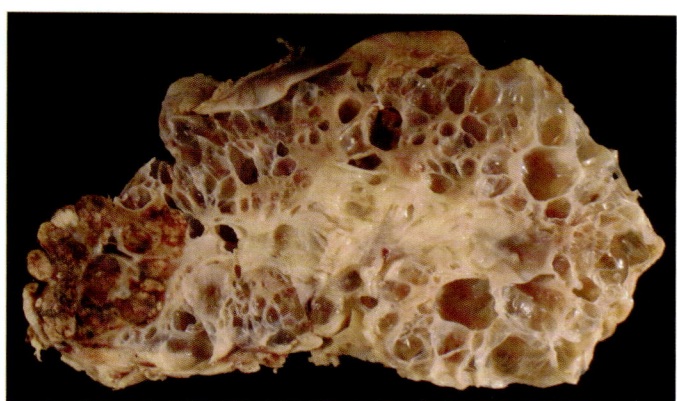

IMAGE 10.23 Polycystic kidney with renal cell carcinoma. The renal cell carcinoma on the left side of the image shows a solid, yellowish cut surface.

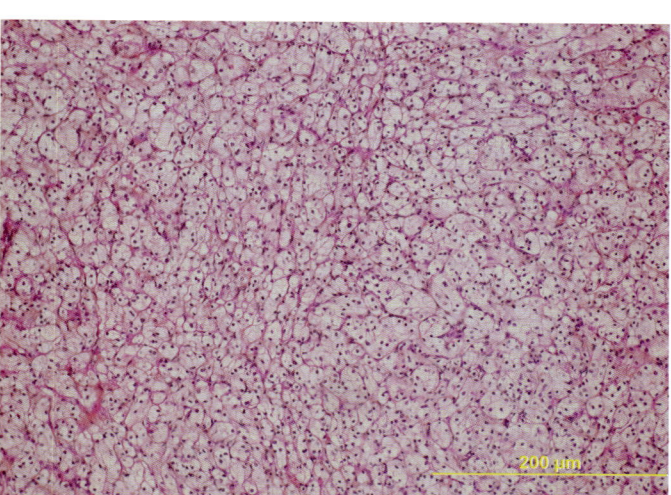

IMAGE 10.26 Clear cell renal cell carcinoma grade 1 with tumor cells having thin, distinct cell membranes, clear cytoplasm, and a delicate capillary vascular network (H&E, x100).

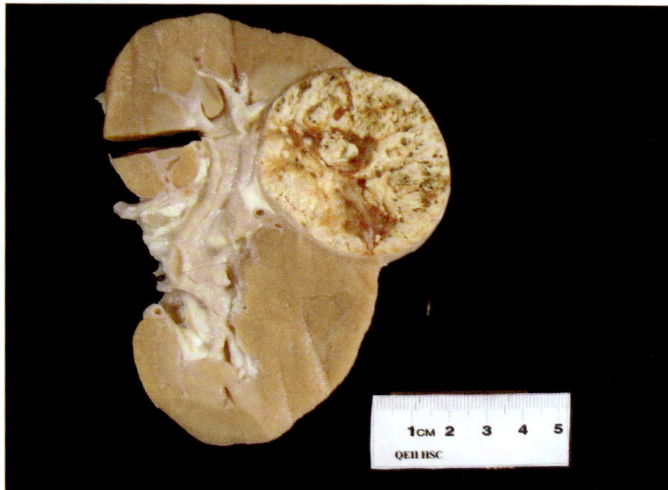

IMAGE 10.24 Clear cell renal cell carcinoma. The tumor is confined to the kidney with a typical yellow cut surface.

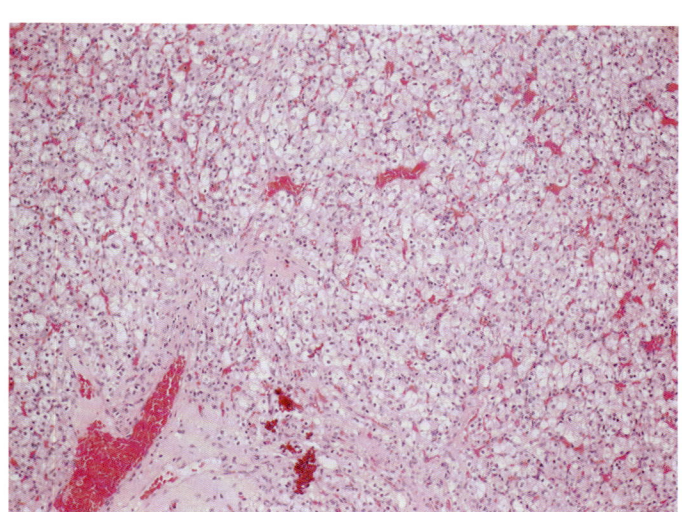

IMAGE 10.27 Clear cell renal cell carcinoma, grade 2 (H&E, x100).

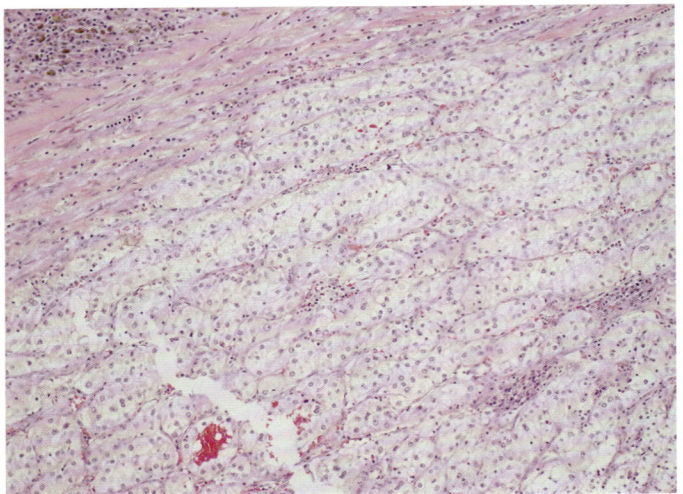

IMAGE 10.28 Clear cell renal cell carcinoma, grade 3 (H&E, x100).

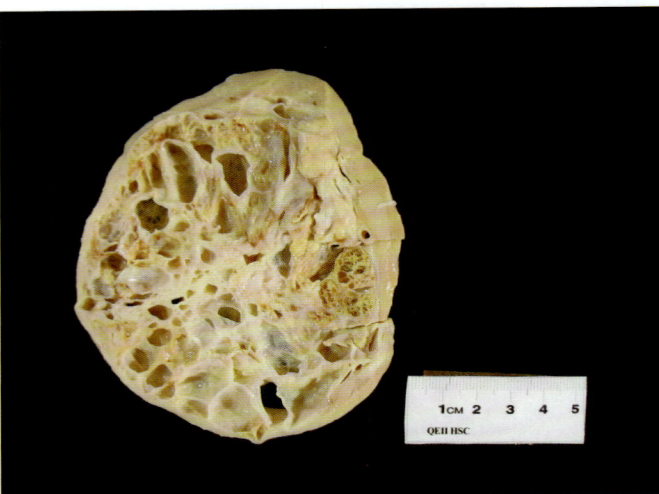

IMAGE 10.31 Renal cell carcinoma with prominent cystic architecture. The solid yellow nodules of tumor exclude the diagnosis of multilocular cystic renal cell carcinoma.

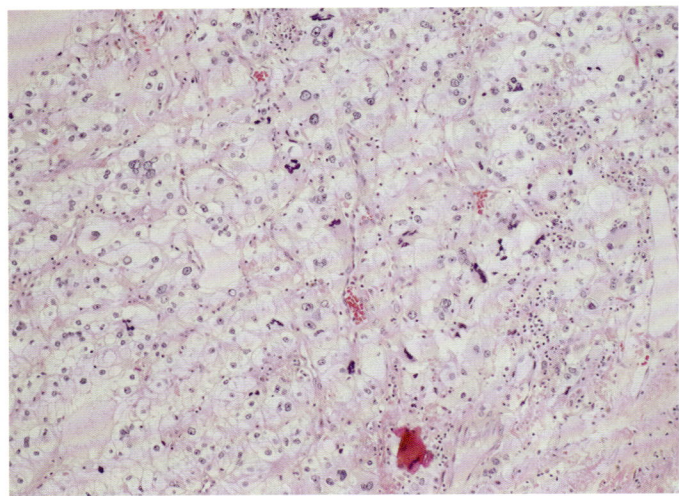

IMAGE 10.29 Clear cell renal cell carcinoma, grade 4 (H&E, x100).

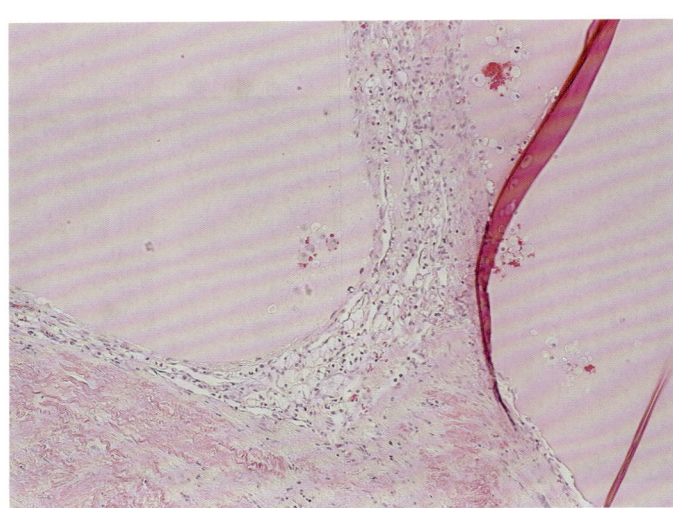

IMAGE 10.32 Multilocular cystic renal cell carcinoma with collections of clear cells within septae (H&E, x100).

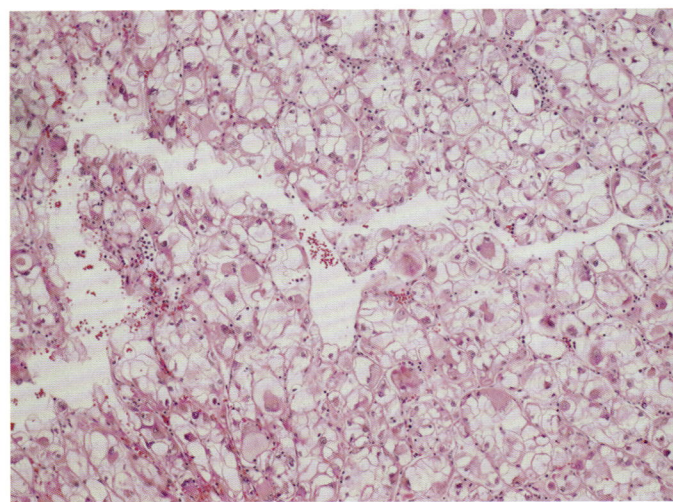

IMAGE 10.30 Clear cell renal cell carcinoma, grade 4 with rhabdoid morphology (H&E, x100).

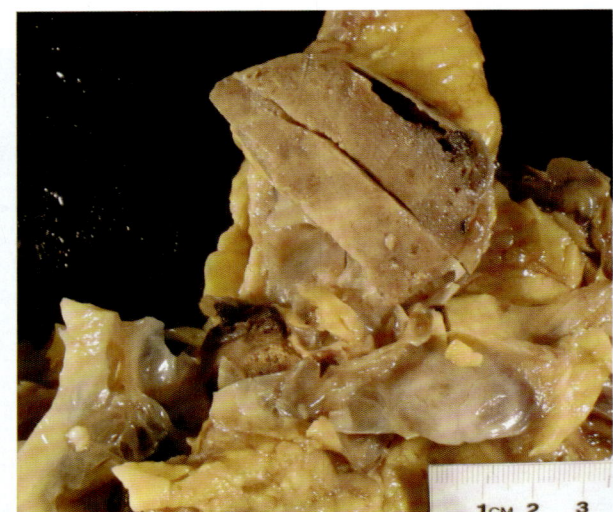

IMAGE 10.33 Acquired cystic disease–associated renal cell carcinoma. The cyst shows a smooth lining. The renal cell carcinoma above the cyst shows a yellowish, homogenous cut surface.

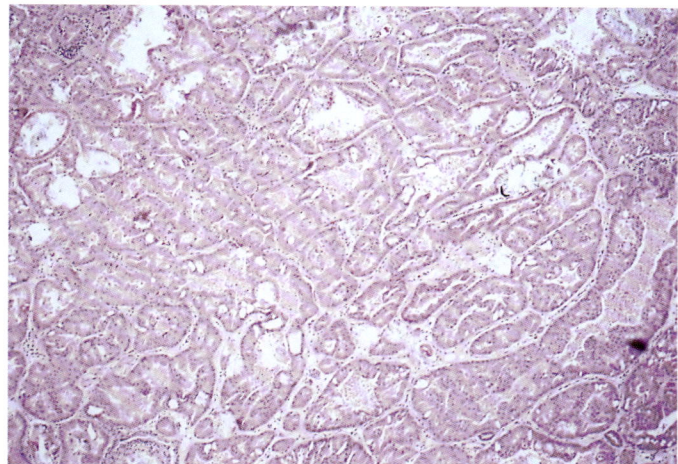

IMAGE 10.34 Acquired cystic disease–associated renal cell carcinoma. The tumor is composed of eosinophilic neoplastic cells forming tubular, alveolar, or cribriform architectures. Intracytoplasmic and intercellular lumina are present. There are also intratumoral oxalate crystals (H&E, x40).

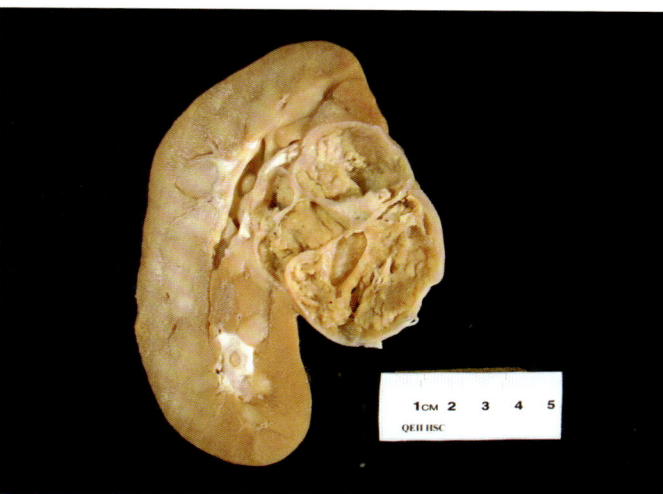

IMAGE 10.37 Papillary renal cell carcinoma. The tumor appears friable and yellowish, and has a pseudocapsule.

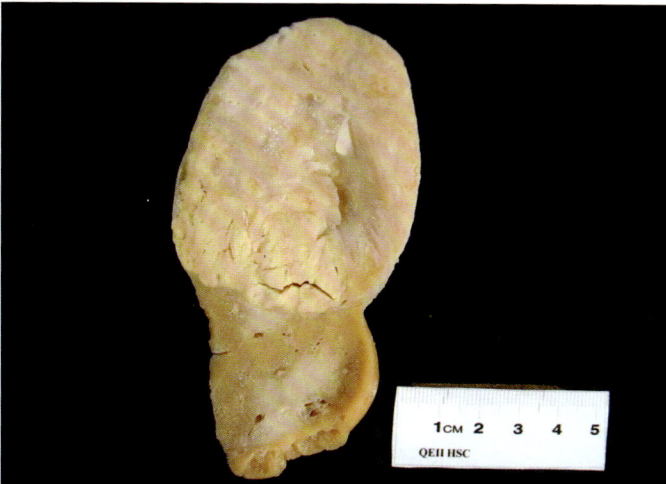

IMAGE 10.35 Clear cell renal cell carcinoma with sarcomatoid differentiation in the superior aspect of renal mass. Note the white, fleshy cut surface in the sarcomatoid area compared to the yellow of the remaining area of classic renal cell carcinoma in the lower part of the specimen.

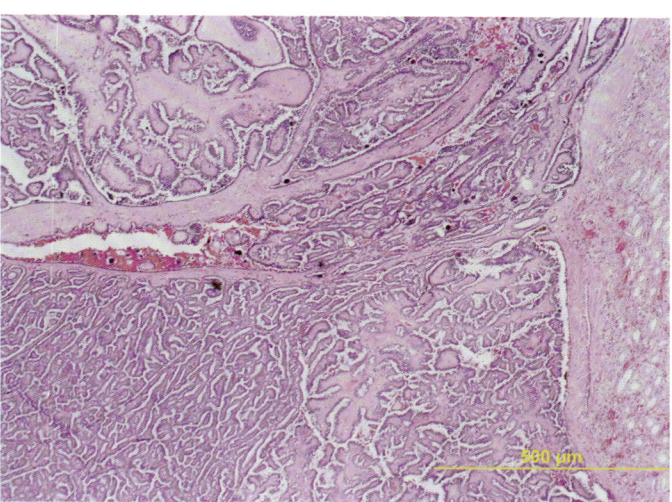

IMAGE 10.38 Papillary renal cell carcinoma, type 1, showing papillary architecture with psammomatous calcifications and occasional foam cells. Small cells with scanty cytoplasm line the papillae (H&E, x40).

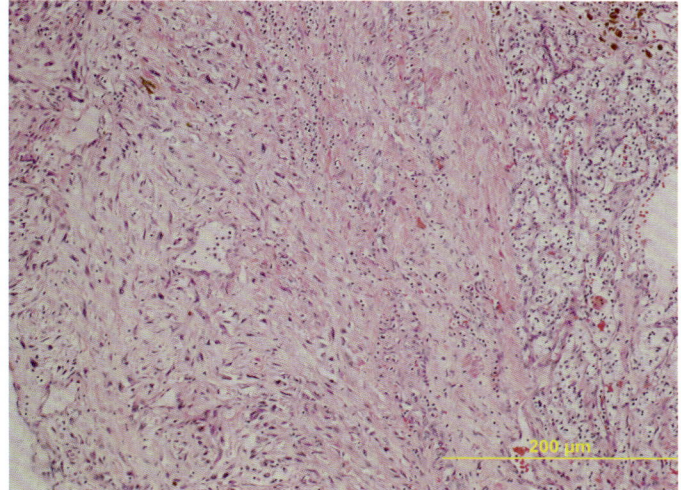

IMAGE 10.36 Clear cell renal cell carcinoma (right) with sarcomatoid differentiation (left) (H&E, x100).

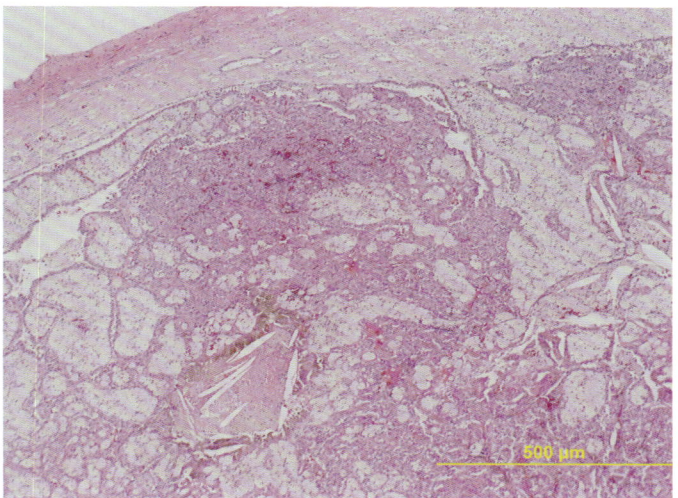

IMAGE 10.39 Papillary renal cell carcinoma, type 2, showing papillary architecture with prominent foam cells within the papillae. Papillae are lined by large cells with abundant eosinophilic cytoplasm (H&E, x40).

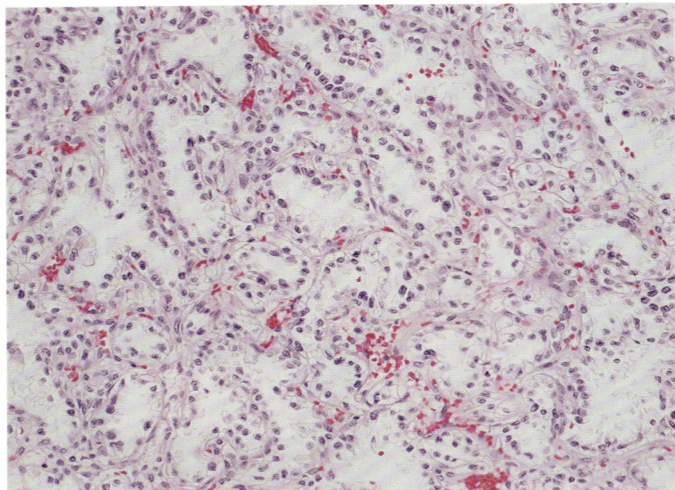

IMAGE 10.40 Clear cell tubulopapillary renal cell carcinoma. Note the reverse polarization of the nucleus with the cell (H&E, x200).

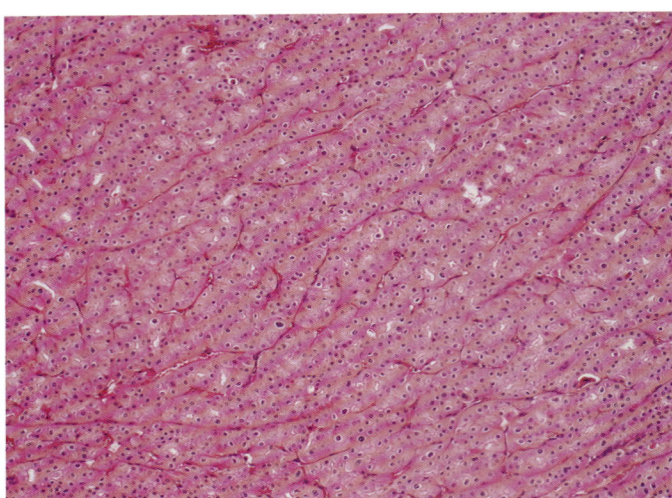

IMAGE 10.43 Chromophobe renal cell carcinoma, eosinophilic type (H&E, x100).

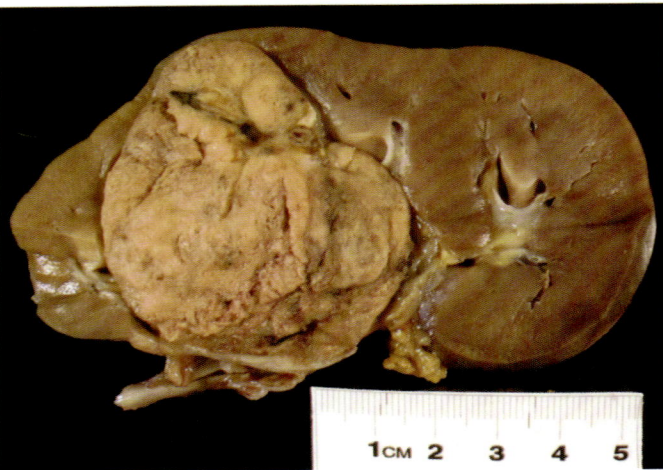

IMAGE 10.41 Chromophobe renal cell carcinoma. The tumor is large but relatively well circumscribed with a homogenously brown-tan cut surface.

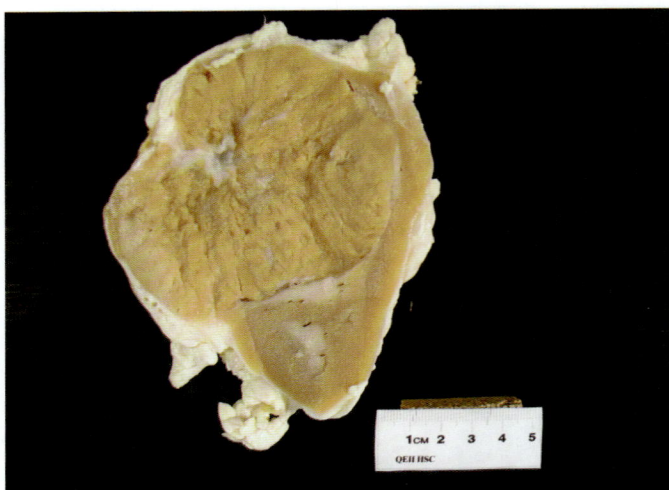

IMAGE 10.44 Oncocytoma showing a tan-colored tumor with central scar.

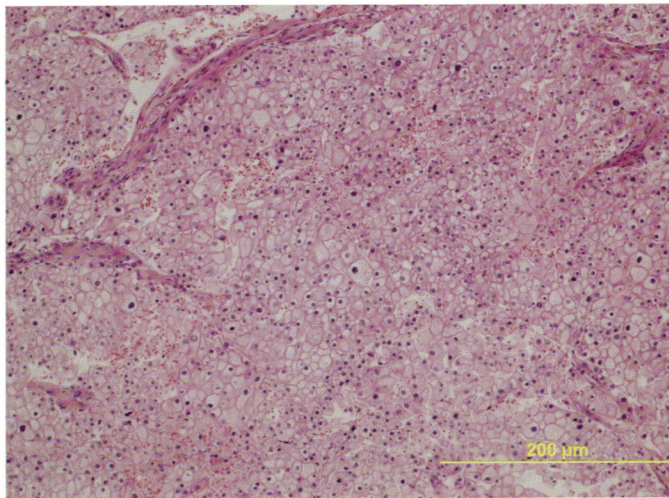

IMAGE 10.42 Chromophobe renal cell carcinoma with tumor cells with thick plantlike cell borders intersected by fibrous bands containing medium-sized blood vessels (H&E, x100).

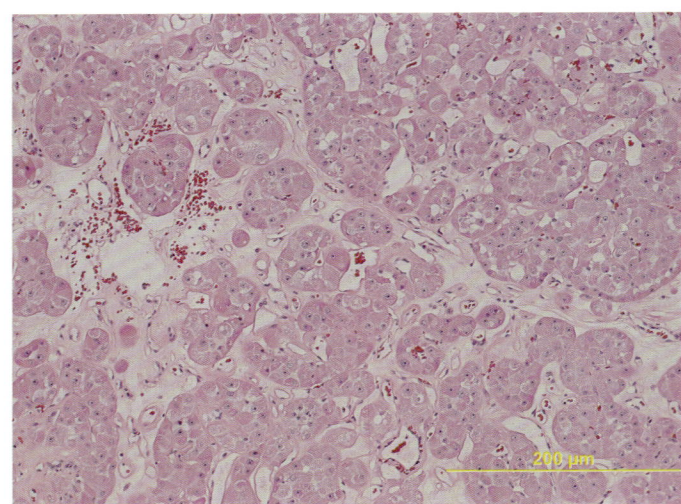

IMAGE 10.45 Renal oncocytoma with nests of cells with abundant granular eosinophilic cytoplasm within an edematous stroma (H&E, x100).

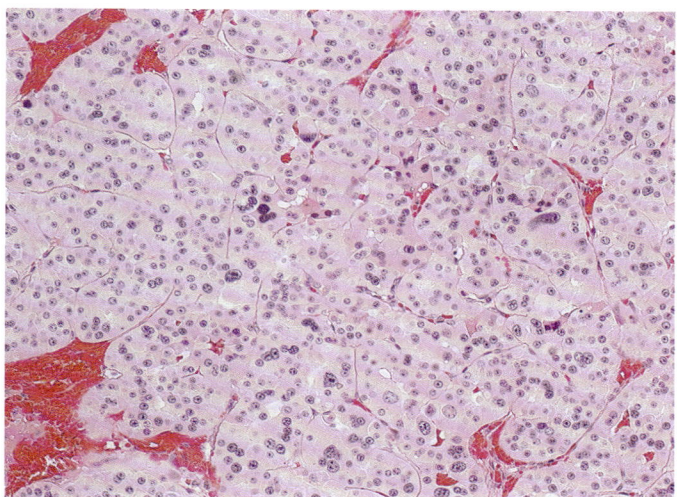

IMAGE 10.46 Oncocytoma with zones of degenerative atypia (H&E, x200).

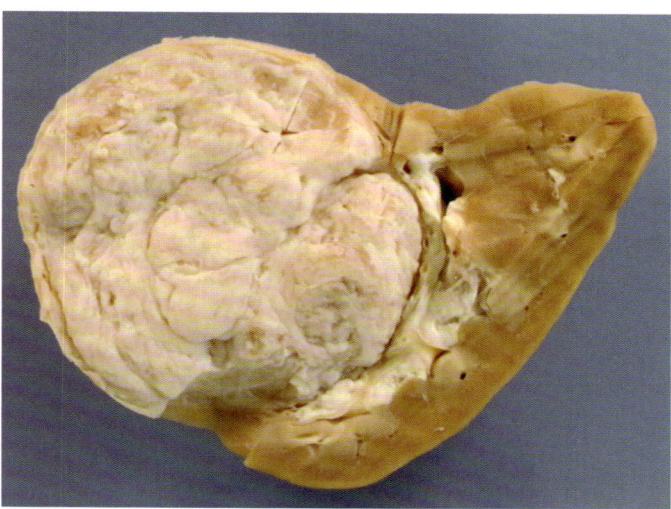

IMAGE 10.49 Angiomyolipoma, muscle predominant. The cut surface of the tumor has a lobulated, slightly whorled appearance.

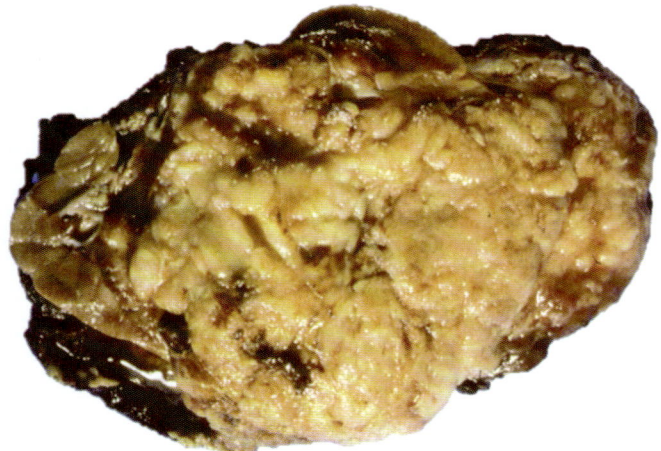

IMAGE 10.47 Wilms tumor. The kidney contains a large, solitary, well-circumscribed renal mass of yellow-tan color, with lobular pattern and some areas of hemorrhage and necrosis.

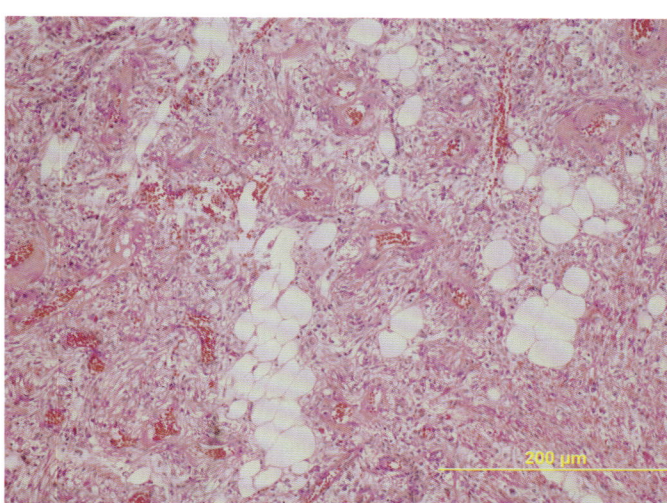

IMAGE 10.50 Renal angiomyolipoma showing adipocytes, dystrophic blood vessels, and spindle cells (H&E, x100).

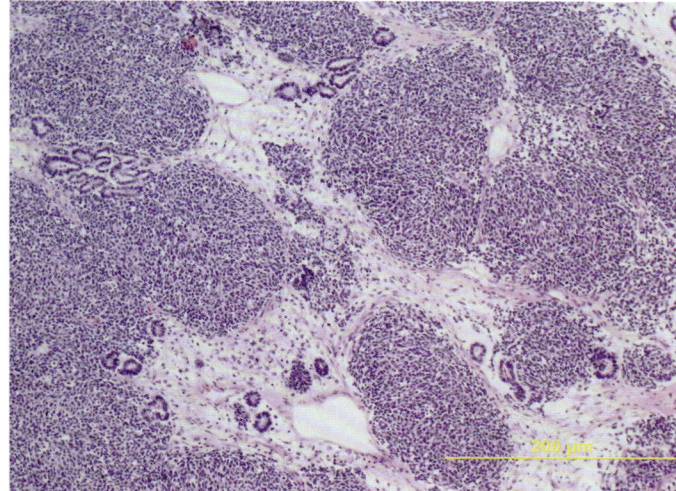

IMAGE 10.48 Wilms tumor. Note triphasic appearance with blastemal, stromal, and primitive epithelial components (H&E, x100).

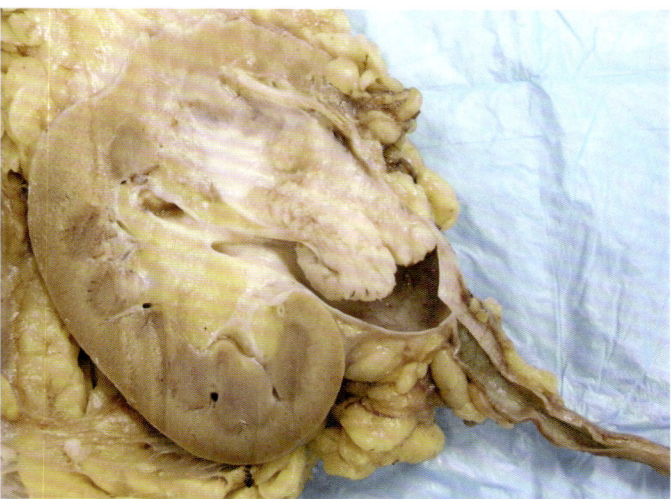

IMAGE 10.51 High grade papillary urothelial carcinoma arising from the renal pelvis.

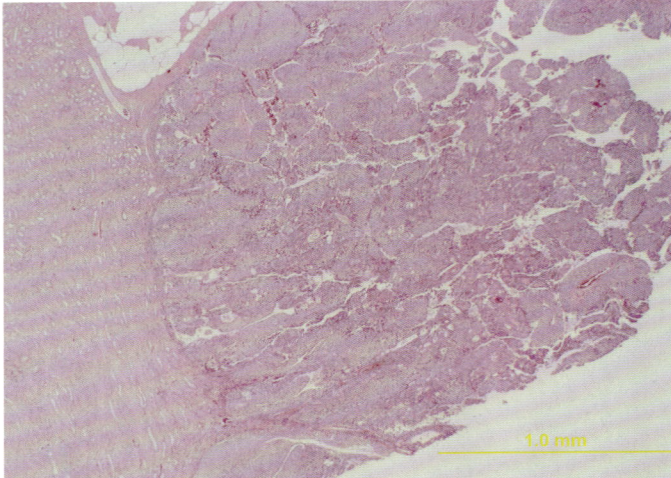

IMAGE 10.52 Papillary urothelial carcinoma, high grade, arising in the renal pelvis (H&E, x20).

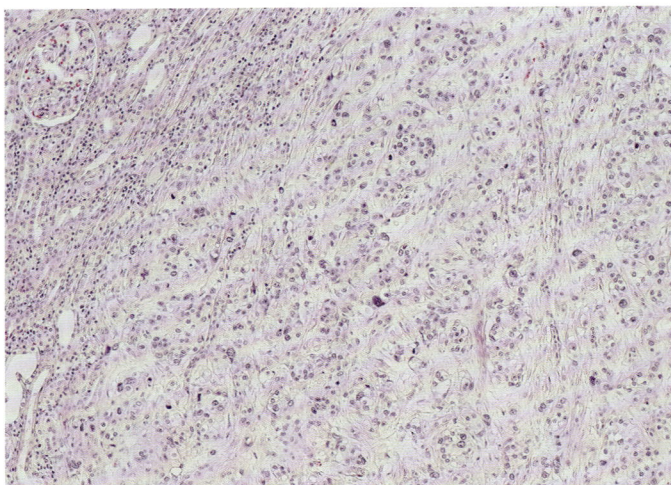

IMAGE 10.53 Invasive urothelial carcinoma within kidney (H&E, x100).

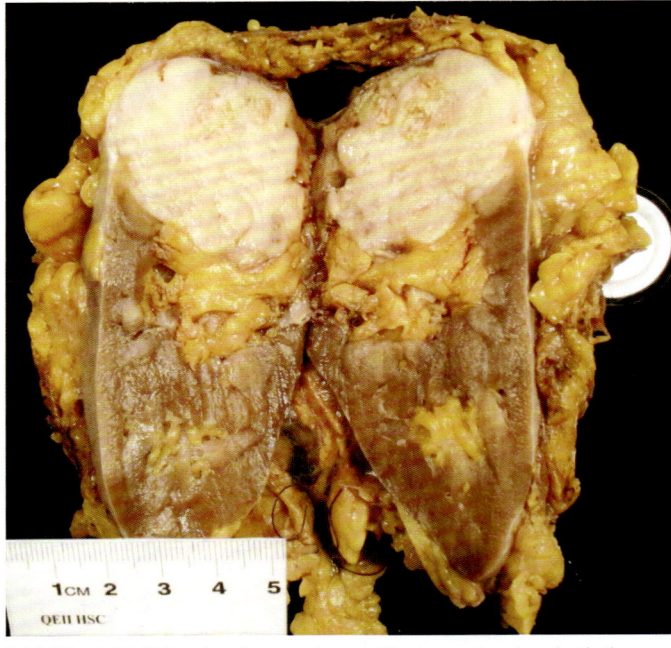

IMAGE 10.54 Collecting duct carcinoma. The tumor involves both the renal cortex and medulla, and has invaded renal sinus fat. The tumor shows a tan-white cut surface with focal yellow areas of tumor necrosis.

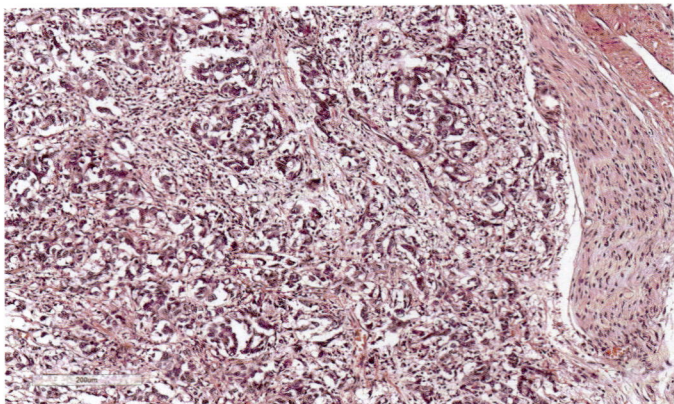

IMAGE 10.55 Collecting duct carcinoma (x1, x4, and x10). This high grade adenocarcinoma consists of markedly atypical neoplastic cells forming variable architectures, including tubular, cribriform, acinar, cord, and solid patterns. Desmoplastic stromal reaction, intratumoral inflammatory infiltrate, and perineural invasion are present (H&E, x100).

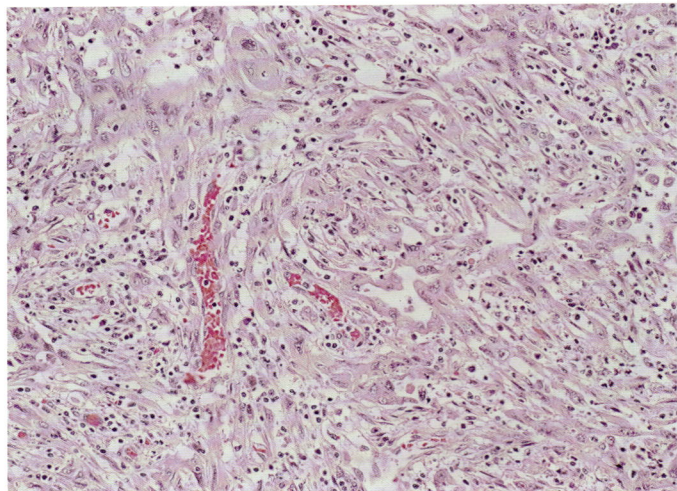

IMAGE 10.56 Medullary carcinoma. Note the sickled red blood cells (H&E, x200).

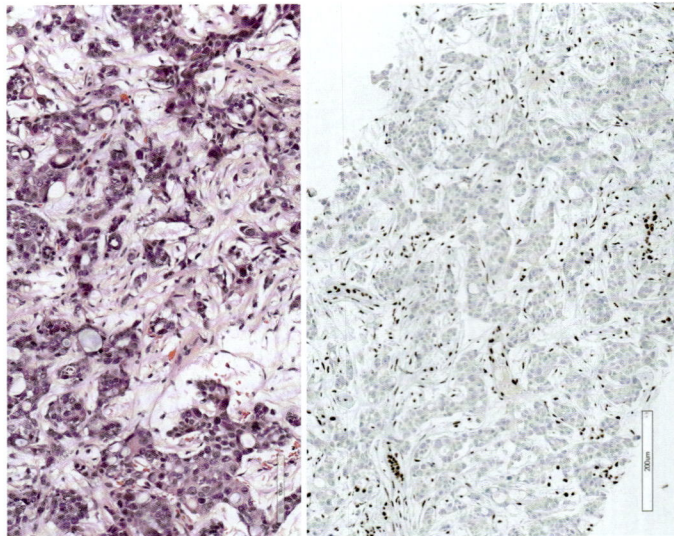

IMAGE 10.57 Medullary carcinoma. Left: H&E, x100. Right: INI1 immunohistochemistry showing negative epithelial and positive endothelial staining (immune peroxidase, x100).

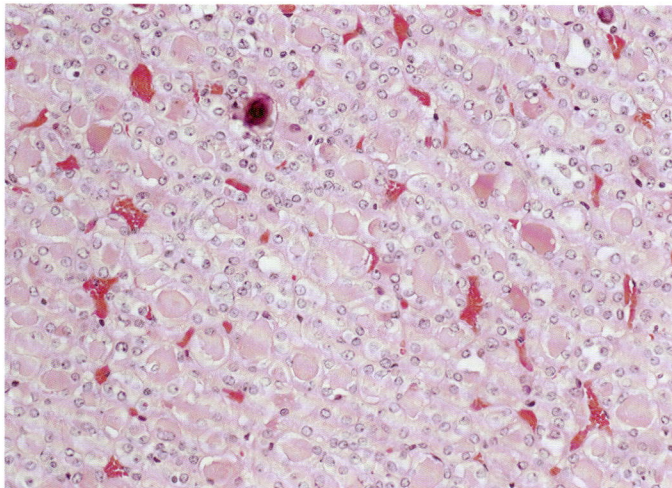

IMAGE 10.58 Primary thyroid-like follicular carcinoma of the kidney (H&E, x200).

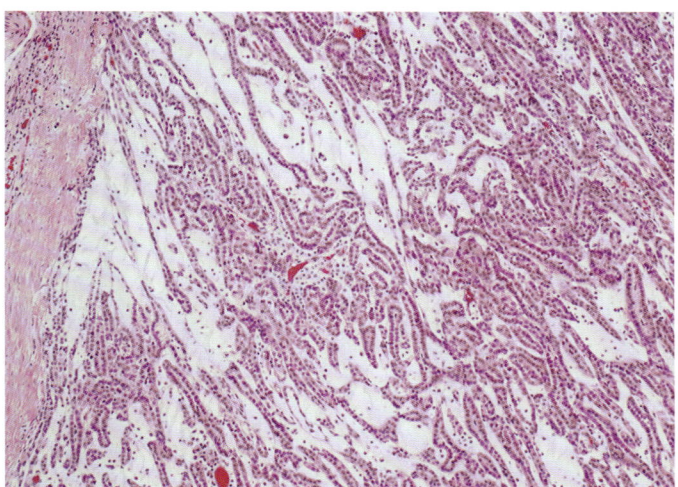

IMAGE 10.59 Mucinous tubular and spindled carcinoma of the kidney (H&E, x100).

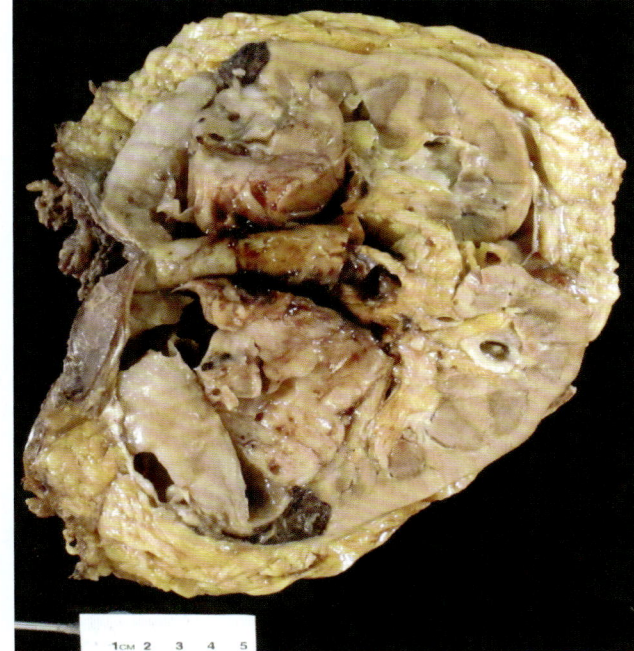

IMAGE 10.60 Renal synovial sarcoma. The tumor involves the renal collecting duct system in the mid and lower pole with extensive venous invasion.

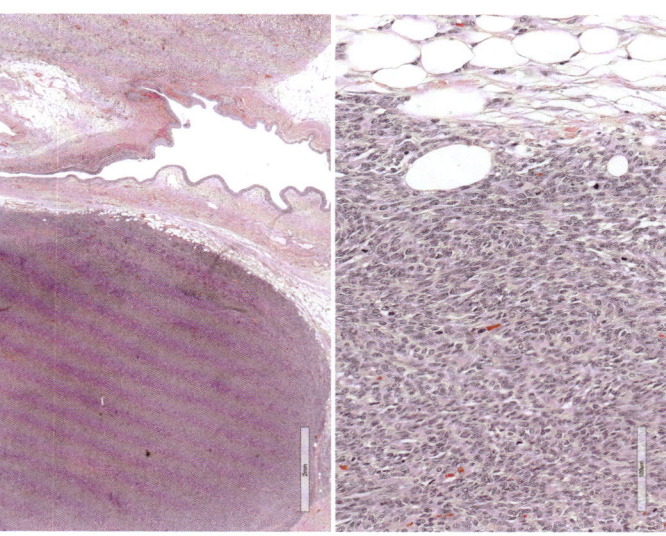

IMAGE 10.61 Renal synovial sarcoma. Left (H&E, x10): low power shows lobulated architecture and infiltrative borders. Right (H&E, x200): high power shows interlacing fascicles of spindle neoplastic cells with frequent mitosis.

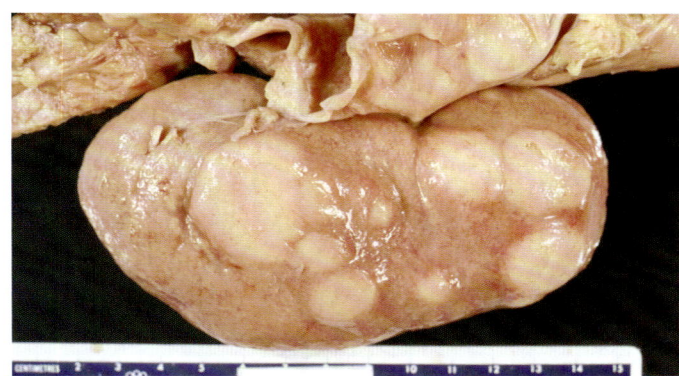

IMAGE 10.62 Kidney involved by diffuse large B-cell lymphoma. Multiple variable sized white tumor nodules protrude to the surface of the kidney.

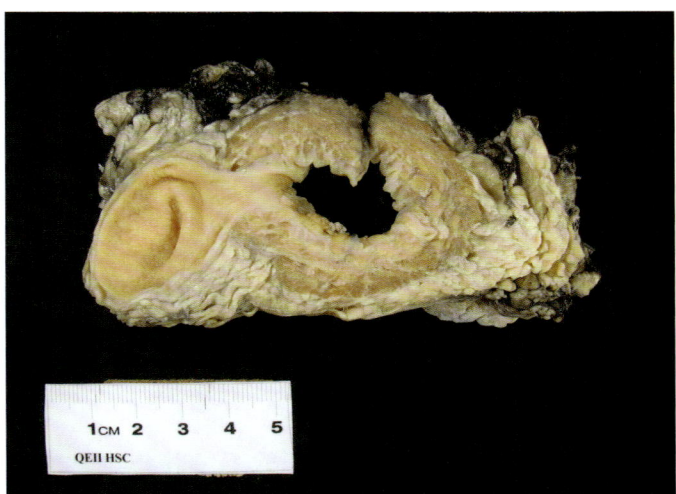

IMAGE 10.63 Urinary bladder with acquired diverticulum.

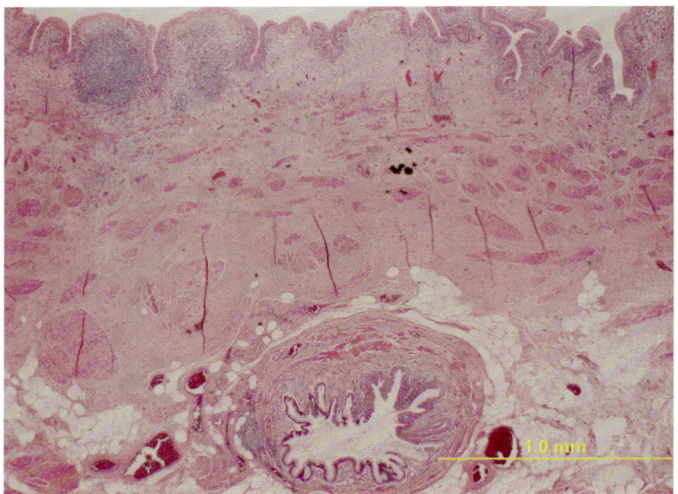

IMAGE 10.64 Urachal remnant located at bladder dome (H&E, x20).

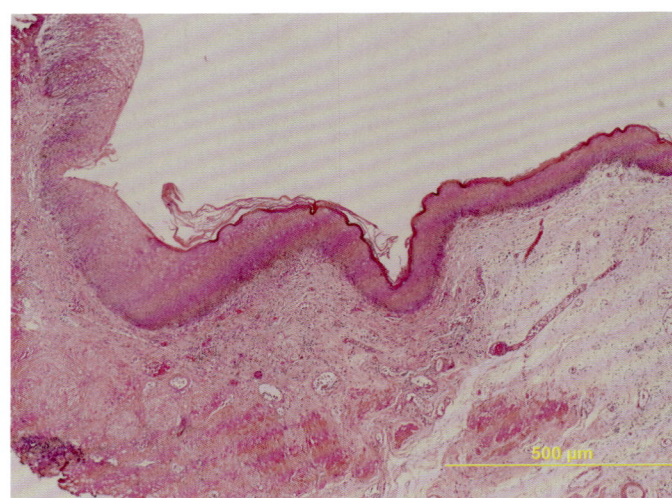

IMAGE 10.67 Keratinizing squamous metaplasia of the urinary bladder (H&E, x40).

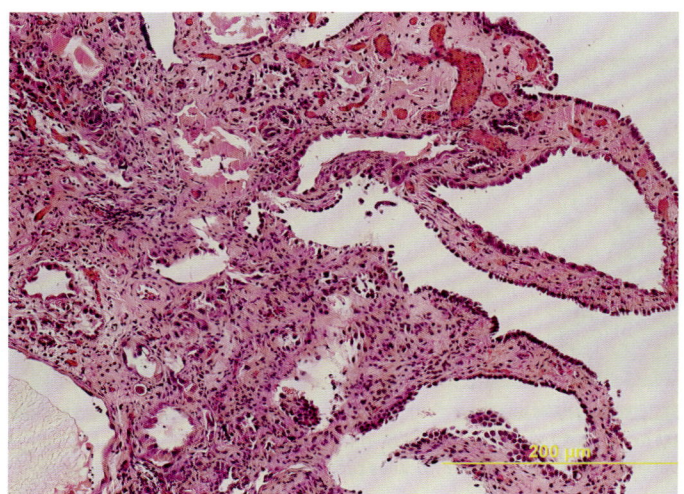

IMAGE 10.65 Nephrogenic metaplasia of the urinary bladder. Note papillary and tubular architecture with hobnail cells (H&E, x100).

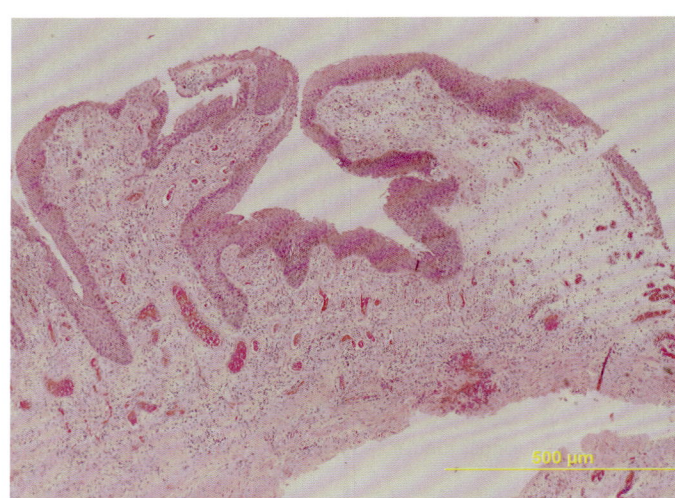

IMAGE 10.68 Polypoid cystitis (H&E, x40).

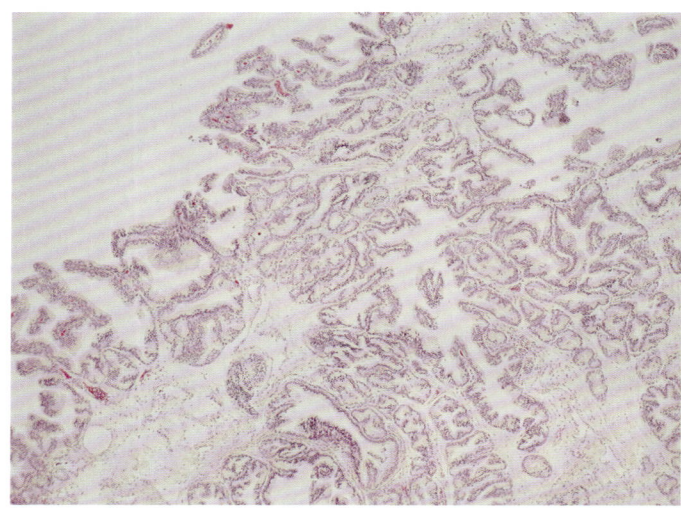

IMAGE 10.66 Bladder with ectopic prostatic tissue (H&E, x40).

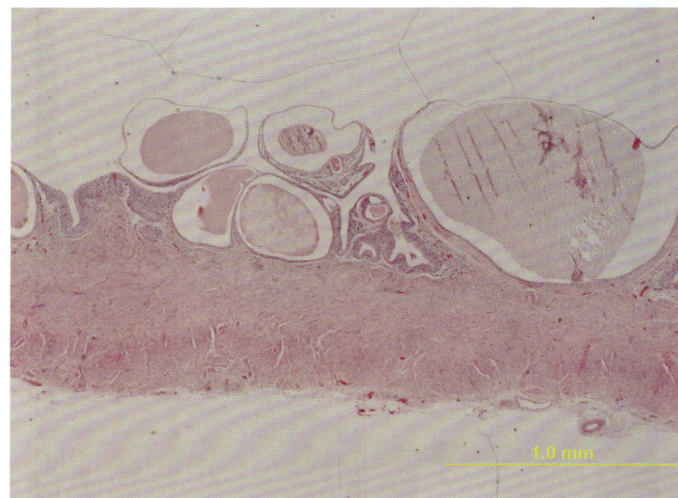

IMAGE 10.69 Cystitis cystica (H&E, x20). Variable-sized cystic cavities filled with eosinophilic fluid are present.

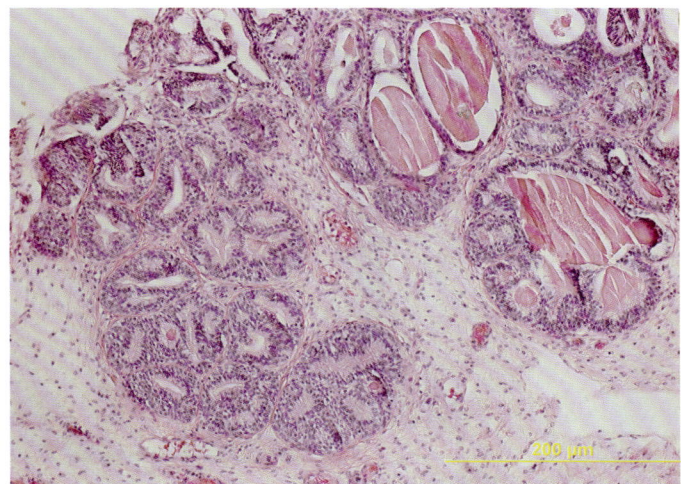

IMAGE 10.70 Cystitis cystica et glandularis, usual type (H&E, x100).

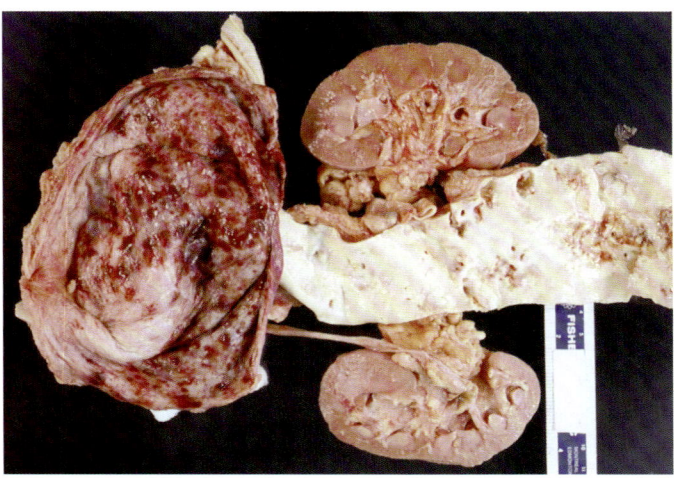

IMAGE 10.73 Bladder with hemorrhagic cystitis.

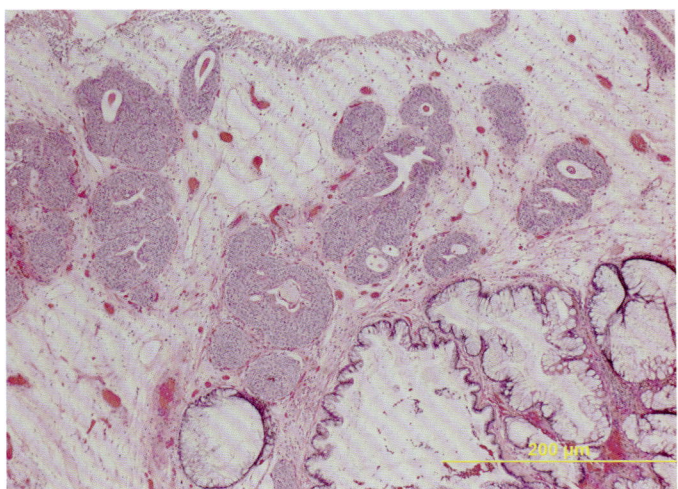

IMAGE 10.71 Cystitis cystica et glandularis, enteric type (H&E, x100).

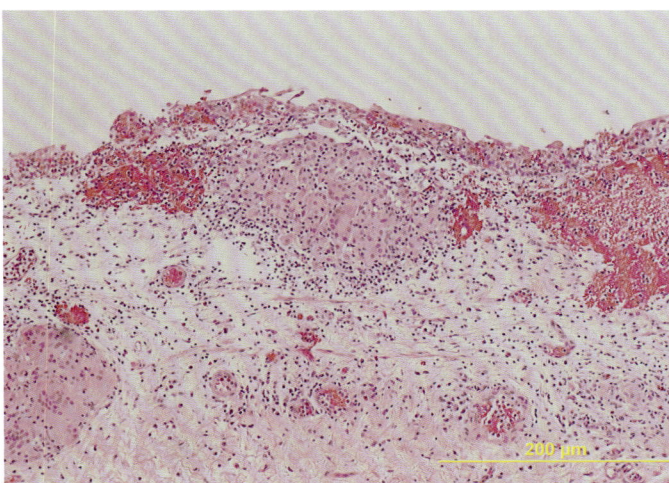

IMAGE 10.74 Bacillus Calmette-Guérin–related hemorrhage and granulomatous inflammation in the urinary bladder (H&E, x100).

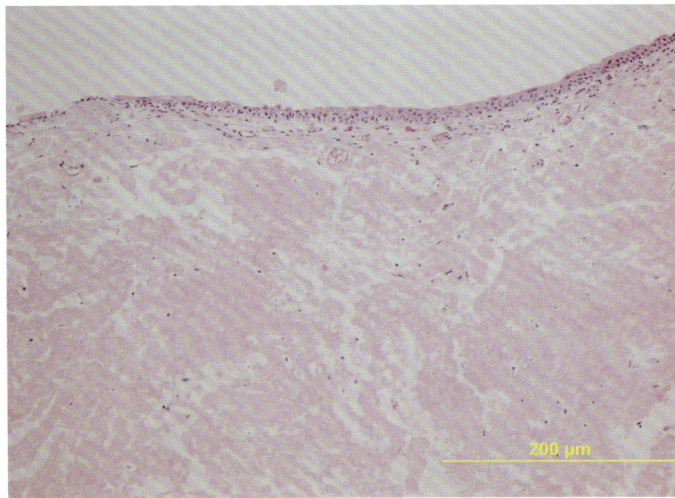

IMAGE 10.72 Localized amyloidosis of the urinary bladder (H&E, x100).

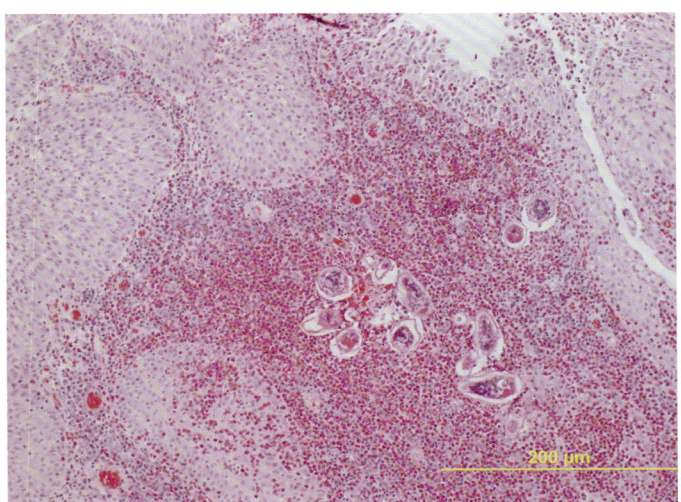

IMAGE 10.75 Schistosomiasis eggs and a marked mixed inflammatory reaction with abundant eosinophils (H&E, x100).

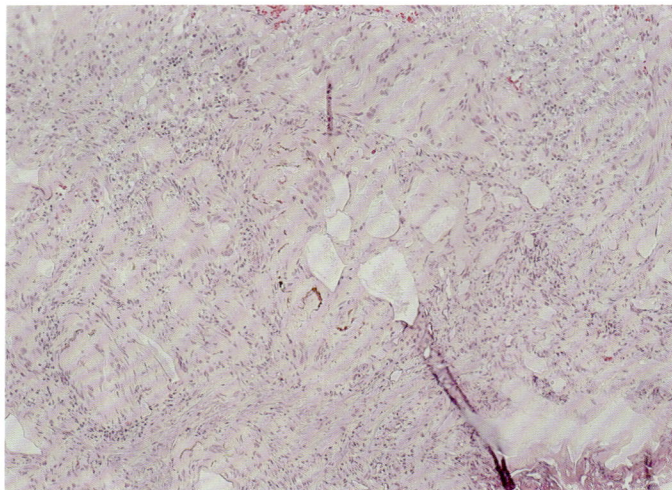

IMAGE 10.76 Bladder with postprocedural granulomas (H&E, x100).

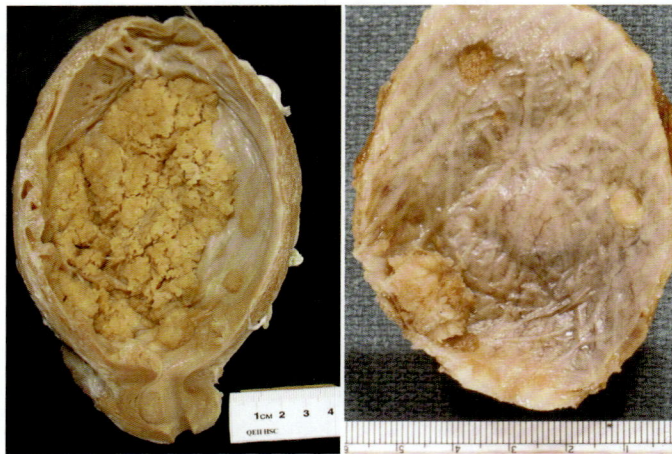

IMAGE 10.79 Papillary urothelial carcinoma of bladder. Note multifocal tumors with papillary appearance.

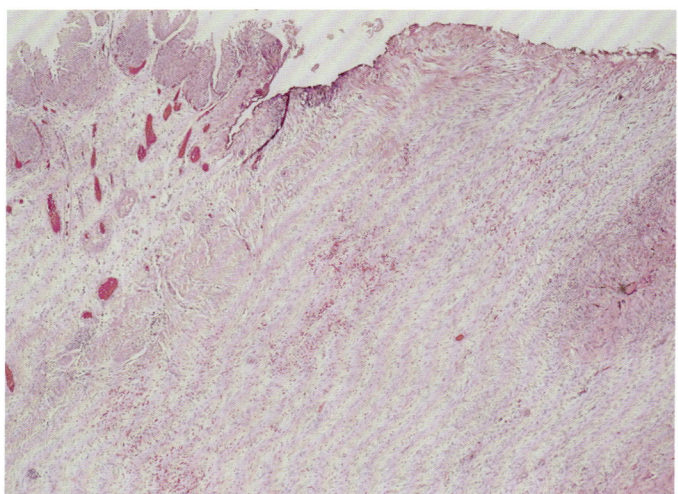

IMAGE 10.77 Bladder with postoperative spindle cell nodule and postprocedural granuloma (H&E, x40).

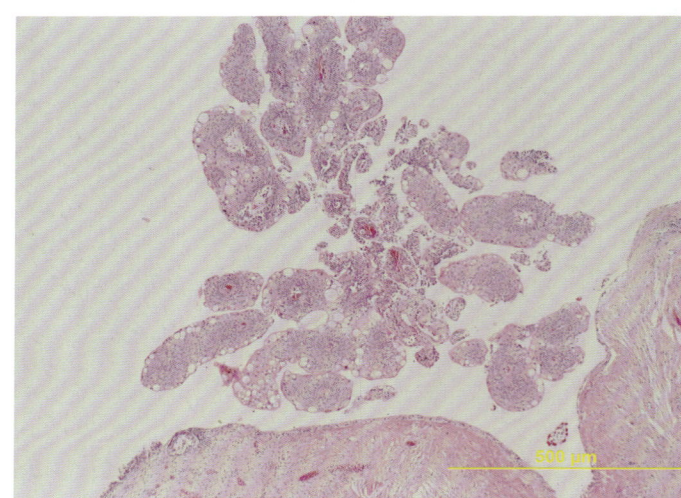

IMAGE 10.80 Urothelial papilloma showing delicate papillae lined by normal urothelium. (H&E, x40).

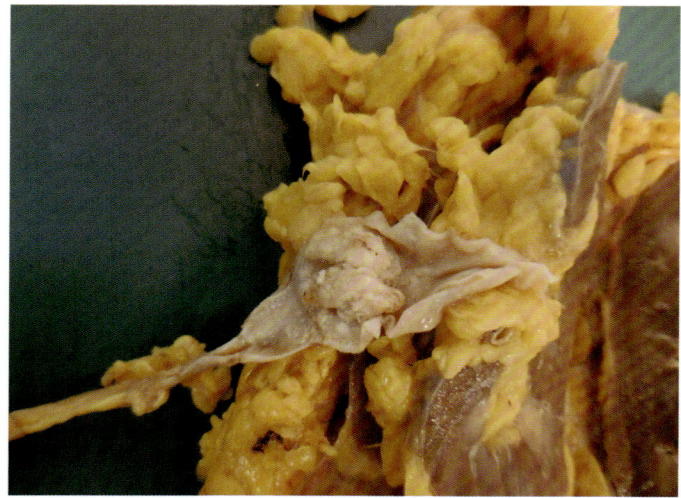

IMAGE 10.78 Ureter with papillary noninvasive urothelial carcinoma.

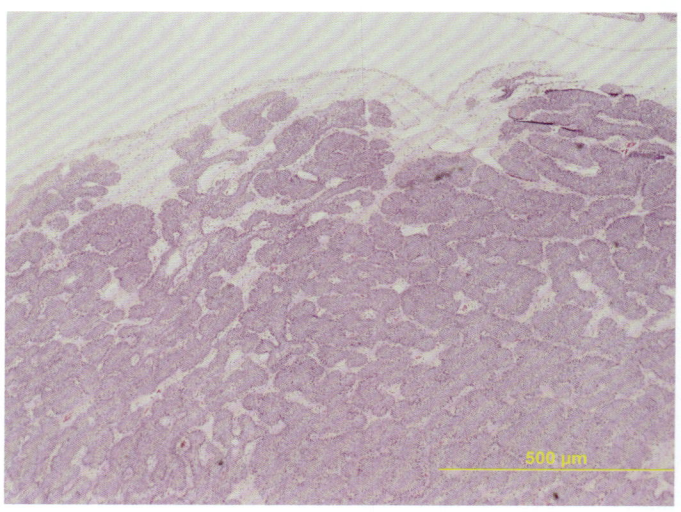

IMAGE 10.81 Urothelial inverted papilloma (H&E, x40).

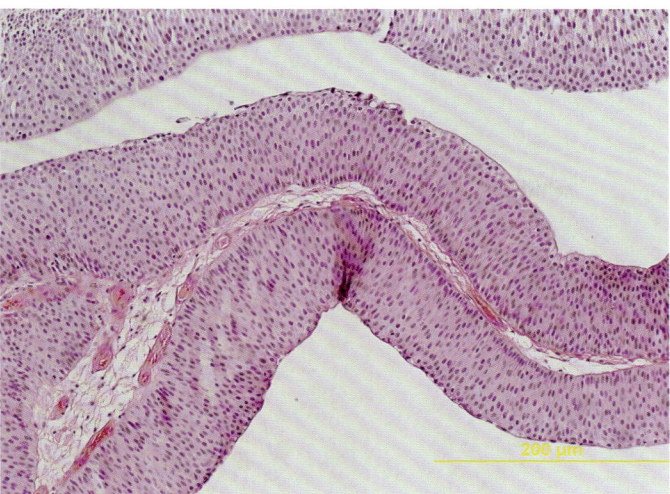

IMAGE 10.82 Papillary urothelial neoplasm of low malignant potential showing papillae lined by thickened urothelium with bland nuclear features (H&E, x100).

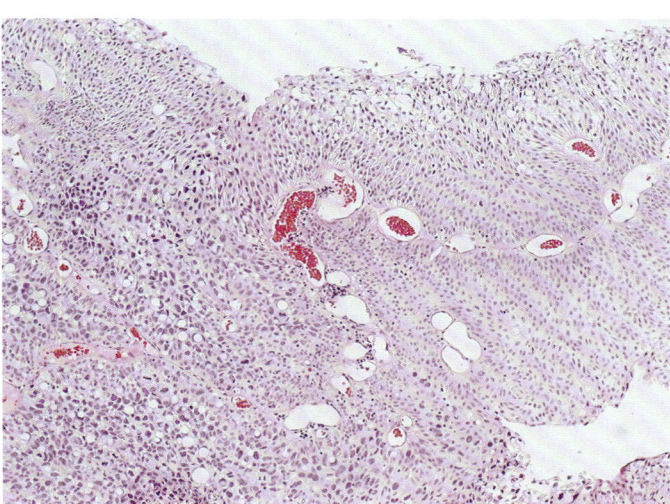

IMAGE 10.85 Papillary urothelial carcinoma with mixed low grade and high grade areas (H&E, x100).

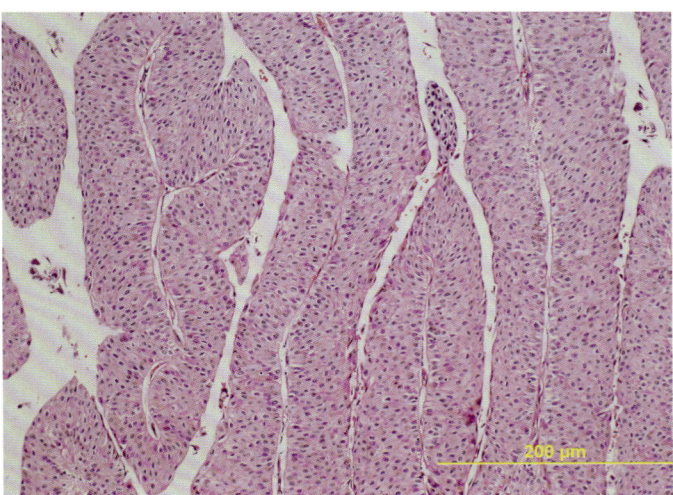

IMAGE 10.83 Papillary urothelial carcinoma, low grade. Papillae are lined by urothelial cells with low grade atypia and preserved cell polarity (H&E, x100).

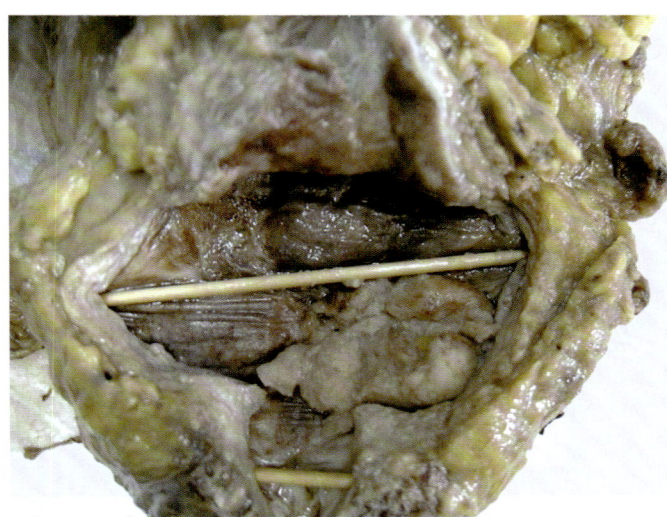

IMAGE 10.86 Invasive papillary urothelial carcinoma showing a fungating mass at the left posterior wall of the bladder.

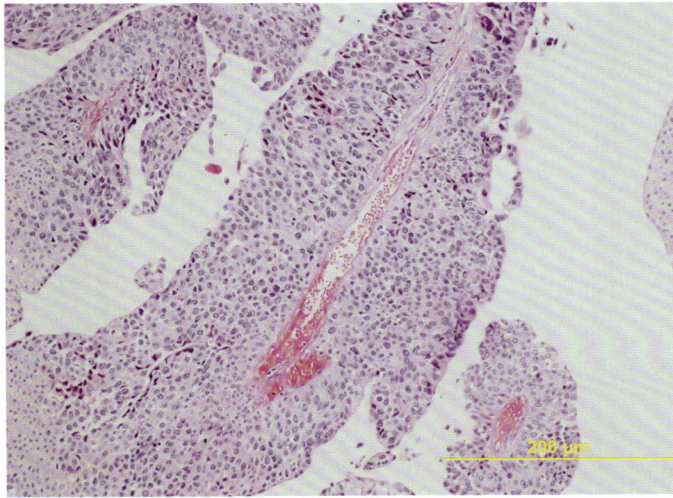

IMAGE 10.84 Papillary urothelial carcinoma, high grade. Papillae are lined by urothelial cells with high grade atypia and disordered cell polarity (H&E, x100).

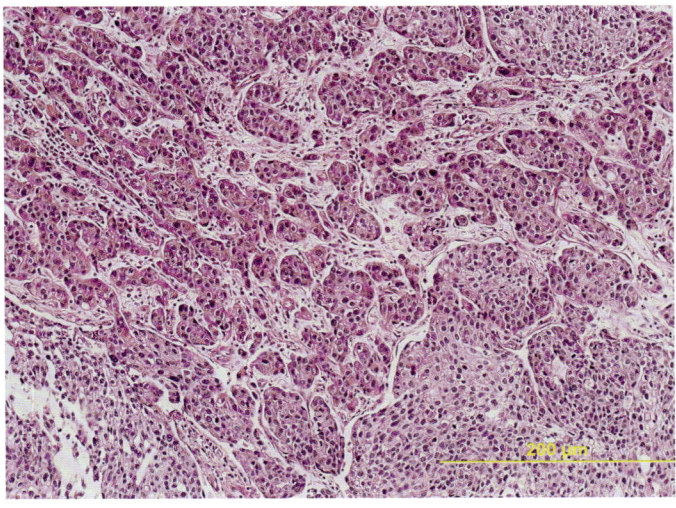

IMAGE 10.87 Papillary urothelial carcinoma, high grade, with invasion of the lamina propria (H&E, x100).

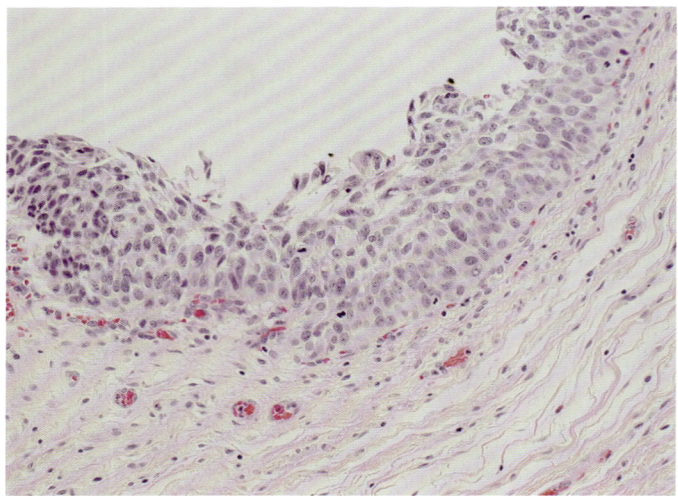

IMAGE 10.88 Flat urothelial carcinoma in situ (H&E, x200).

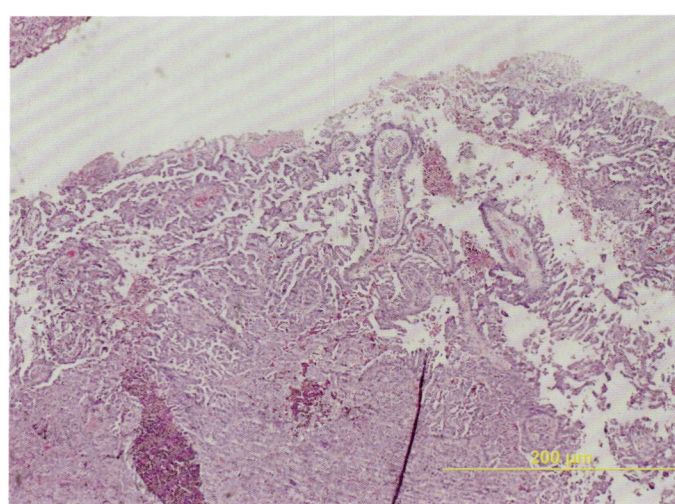

IMAGE 10.91 Urothelial carcinoma, micropapillary variant (H&E, x100).

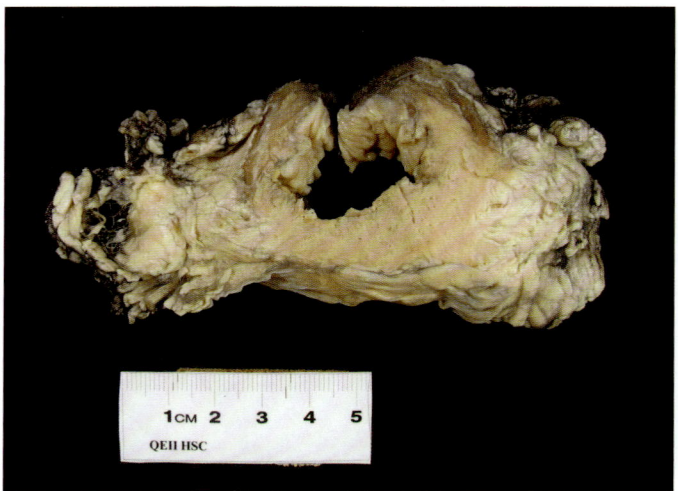

IMAGE 10.89 Invasive urothelial carcinoma of bladder showing invasion through muscularis propria into adipose tissue on right side.

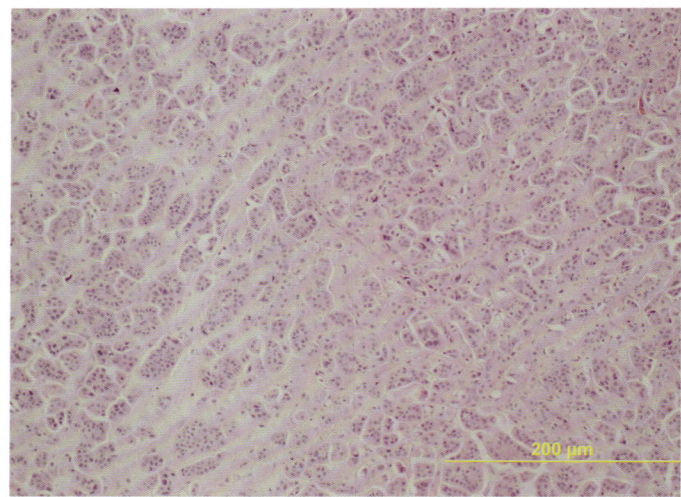

IMAGE 10.92 Invasive urothelial carcinoma, micropapillary variant (H&E, x100).

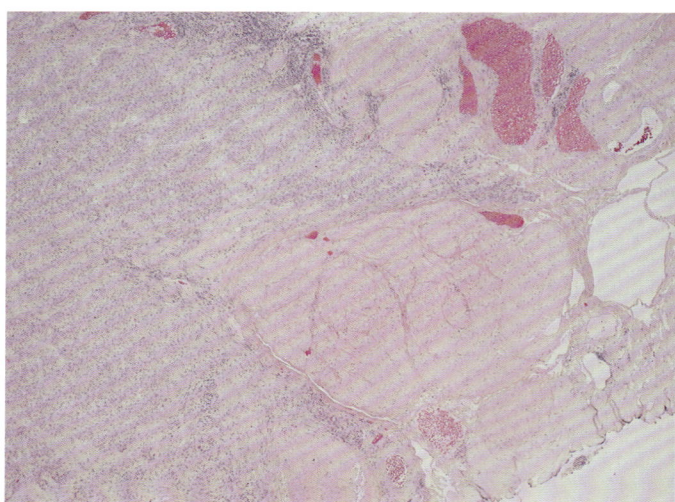

IMAGE 10.90 Urothelial carcinoma invading muscularis propria (H&E, x40).

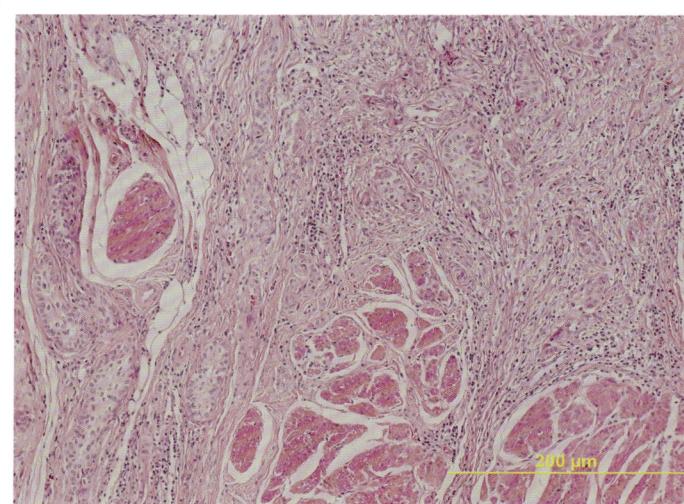

IMAGE 10.93 Invasive urothelial carcinoma, nested variant, showing deeply infiltrative nests of urothelial cells with deceptively bland nuclear features (H&E, x100).

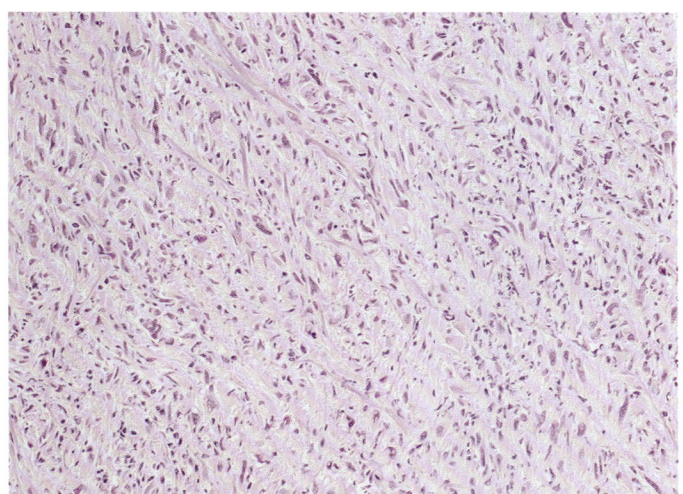

IMAGE 10.94 Sarcomatoid urothelial carcinoma (H&E, x200).

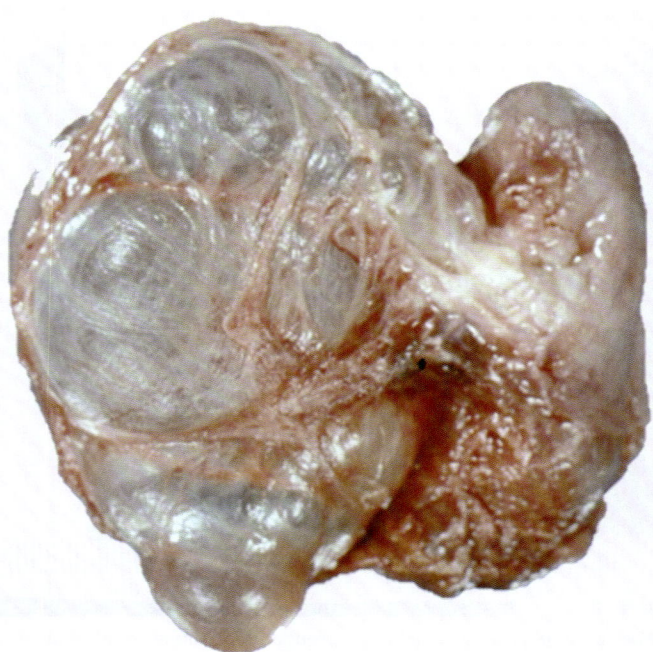

IMAGE 10.96 Epididymal cyst. These are cystic dilatations of the rete testis or the head of the epididymis. These cysts are filled with sperm. If an epithelial lining is identified histologically, these lesions are called spermatocele.

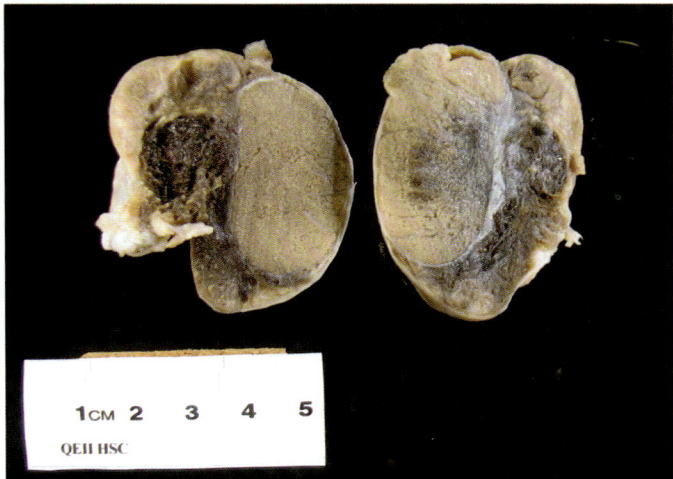

IMAGE 10.95 Testicular torsion showing hemorrhagic infarction of the testicle and epididymis.

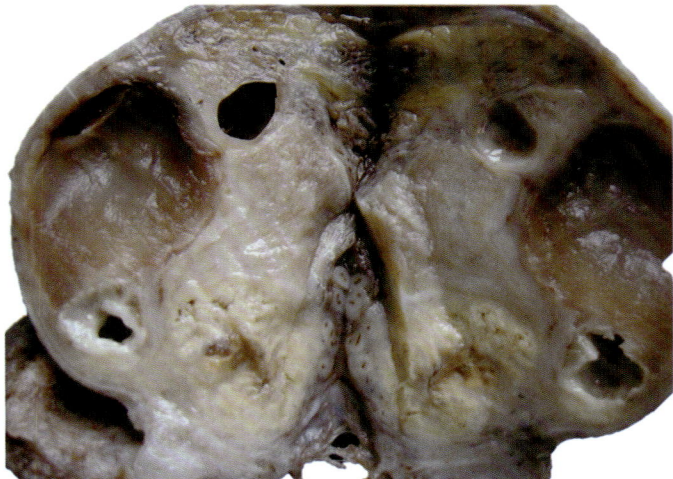

IMAGE 10.97 Infectious epididymoorchitis. The epididymis and adjacent testis contains an irregular, white, necrotic mass with areas of hemorrhage, necrosis, and cystic degeneration.

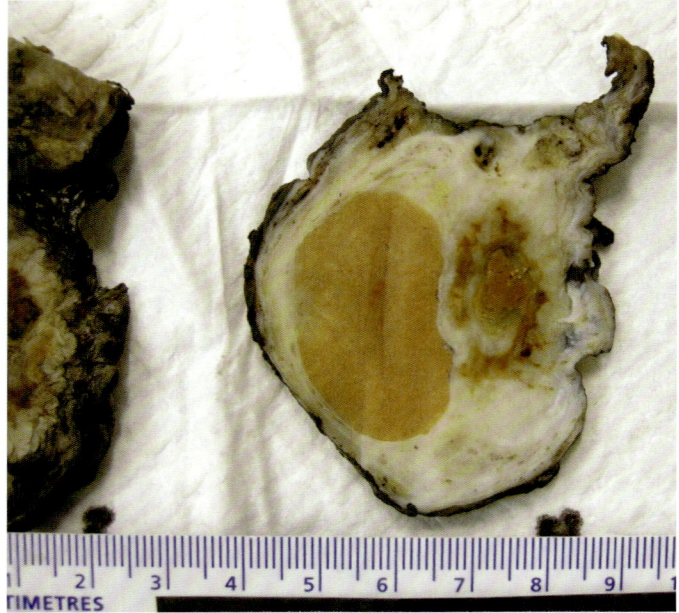

IMAGE 10.98 Paratesticular fibrous pseudotumor. This is a rare benign mass-forming spindle cell lesion in the paratesticular region. These lesions typically do not involve the testicular parenchyma.

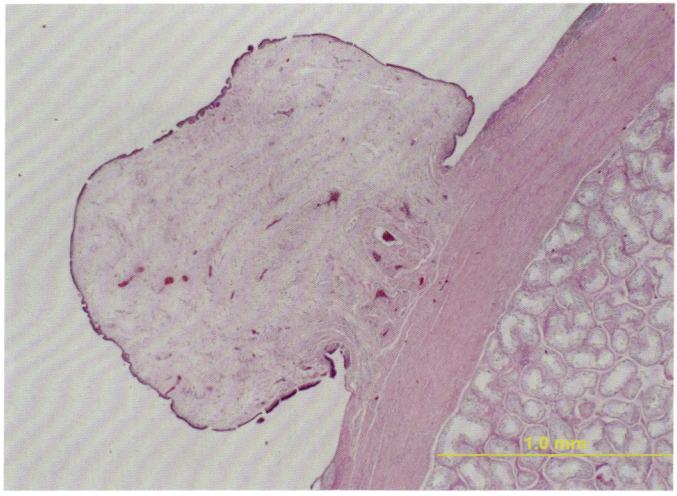

IMAGE 10.99 Appendix of testis (H&E, x20). This structure has fibrovascular tissue lined by a layer of benign columnar epithelium that can show variable degrees of surface invagination.

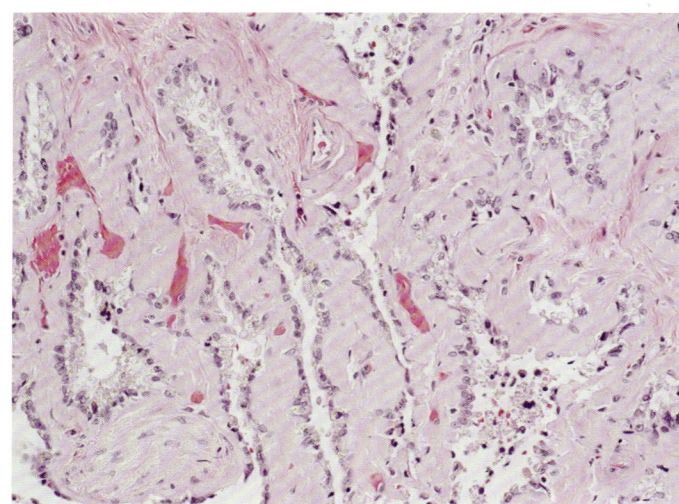

IMAGE 10.100 Senile amyloidosis of seminal vesicle (H&E, x200).

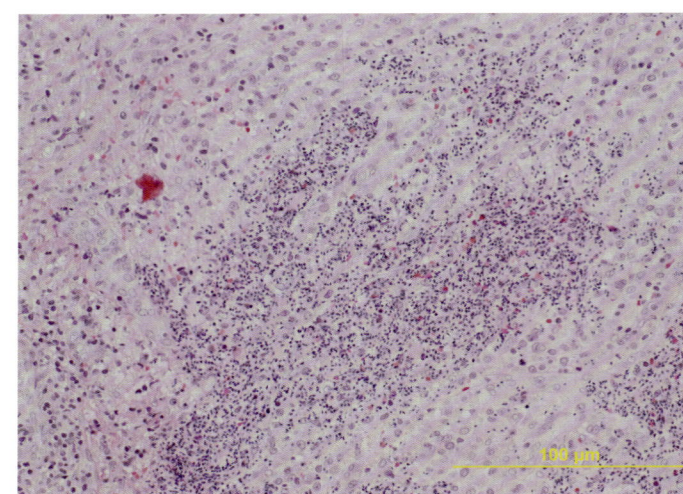

IMAGE 10.101 Sperm granuloma in testis (H&E, x200).

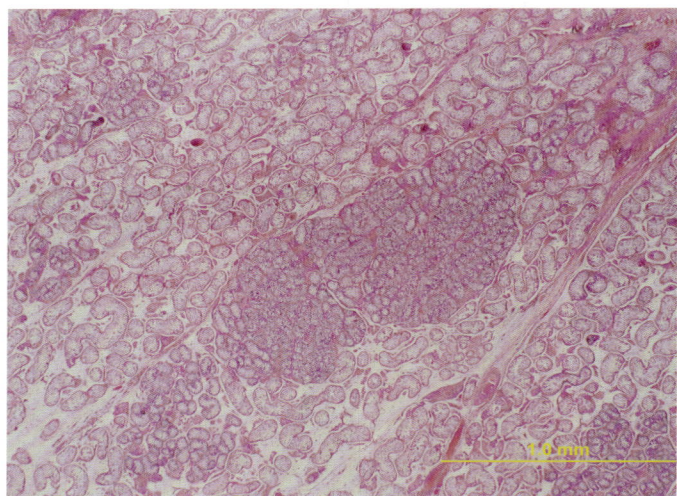

IMAGE 10.102 Sertoli cell hyperplasia ("Pick adenoma") of testis (H&E, x20).

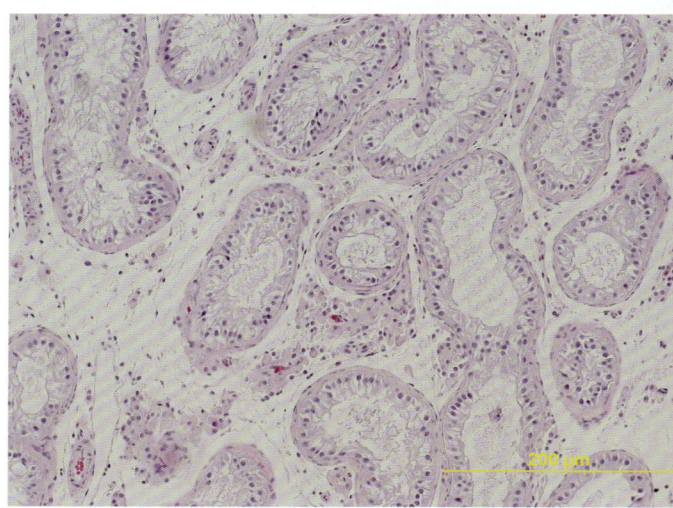

IMAGE 10.103 Male fertility biopsy showing Sertoli-cell-only pattern (H&E, x100).

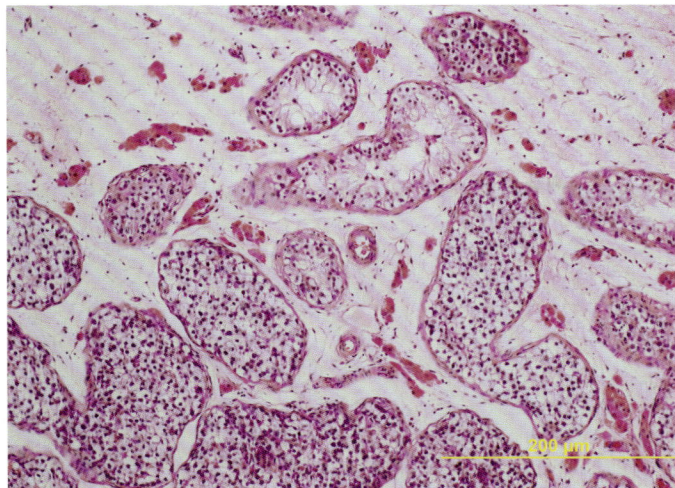

IMAGE 10.104 Germ cell neoplasia in situ of testis. Tubules at the bottom of the field show intratubular seminoma (H&E, x100).

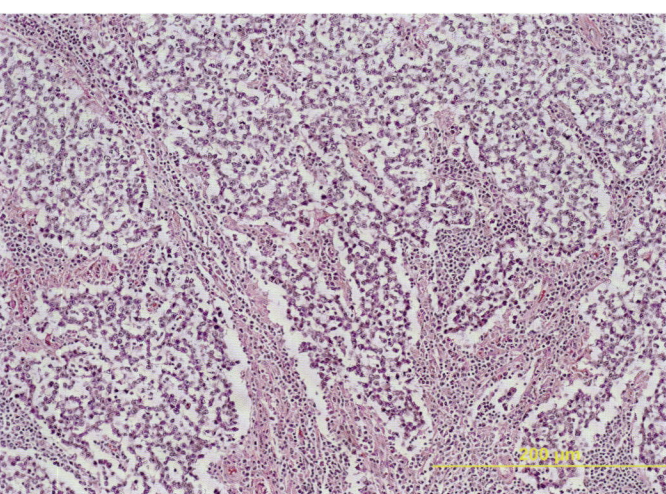

IMAGE 10.107 Classic seminoma. Islands of discohesive cells with clear-to-eosinophilic cytoplasm, large nuclei, prominent nucleoli, and intervening fibrous septae containing abundant chronic inflammatory cells (H&E, x100).

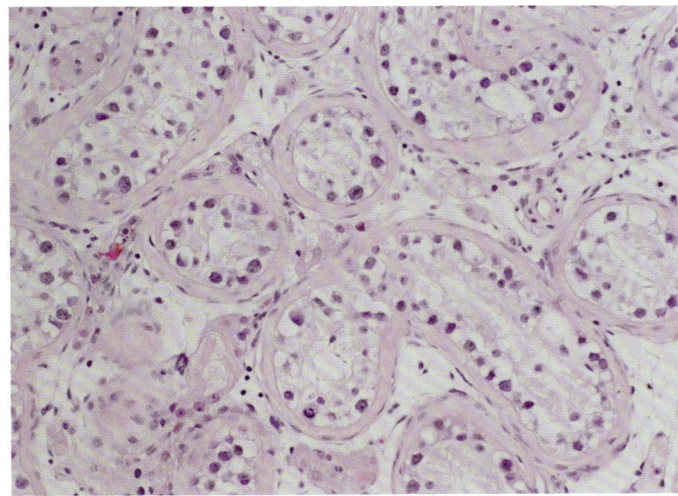

IMAGE 10.105 Germ cell neoplasia in situ arising in a cryptorchid testis (H&E, x200).

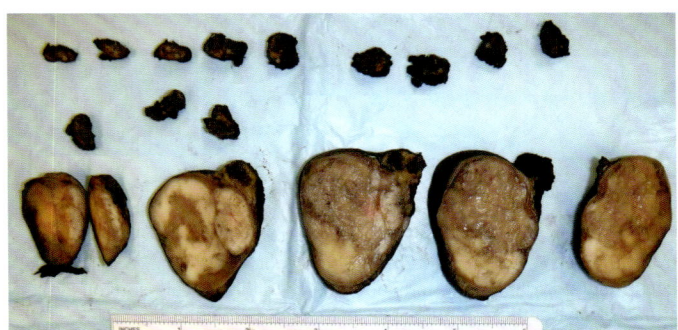

IMAGE 10.108 Testicle seminoma with syncytiotrophoblasts. The upper part of the tumor appears more hemorrhagic and irregular.

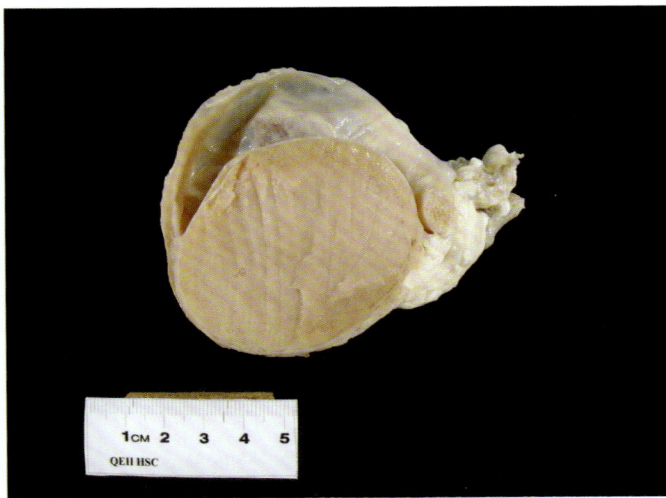

IMAGE 10.106 Classic seminoma showing uniform tan tumor replacing most of the testicle. Hydrocele is also present.

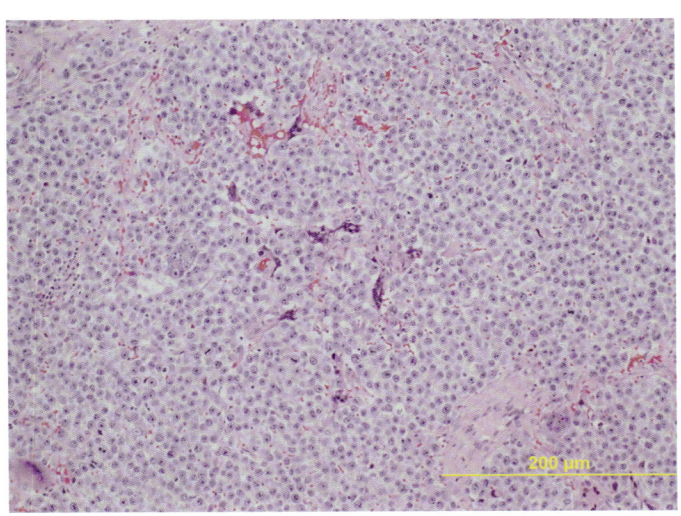

IMAGE 10.109 Seminoma with syncytiotrophoblasts (H&E, x100).

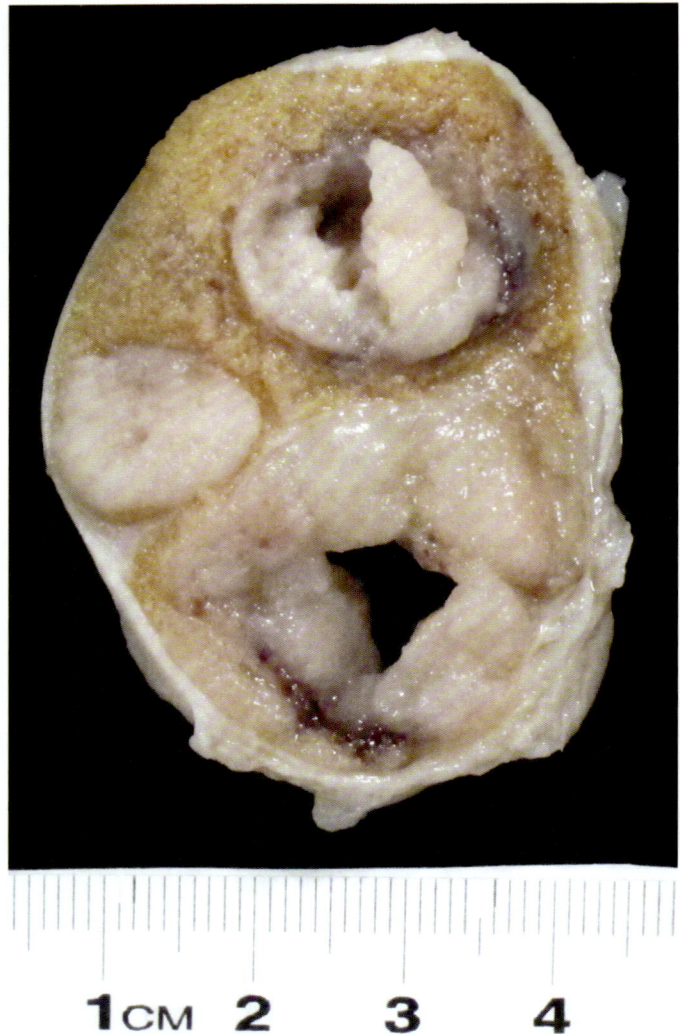

IMAGE 10.110 Testicular spermatocytic tumor. The testicle contains 3 well-circumscribed, friable, pale-tan nodules with mildly mucoid and bulging cut surface. None of the lesions grossly involves the tunica albuginea.

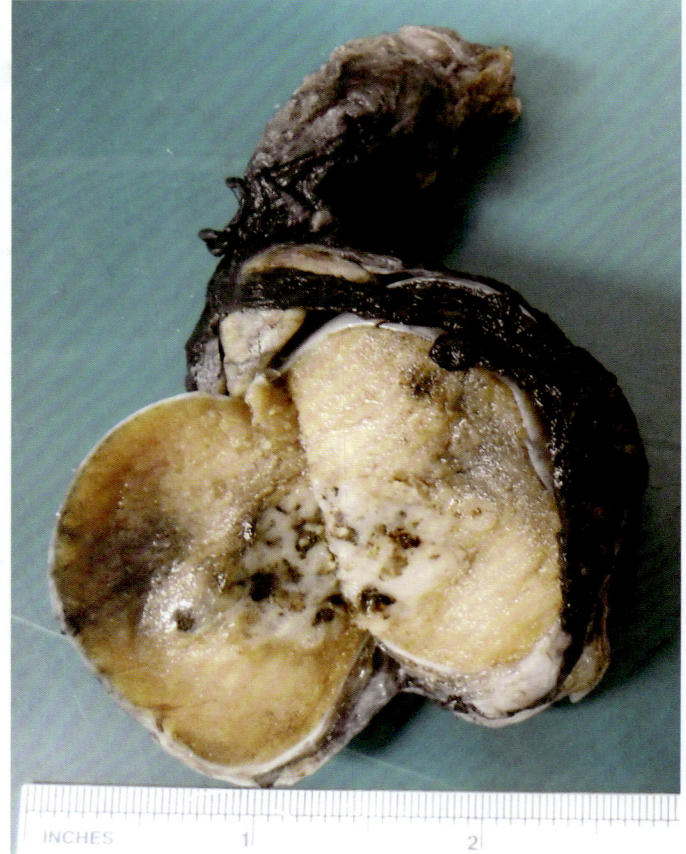

IMAGE 10.112 Left testicle embryonal carcinoma. The tumor shows a variegated appearance with areas of hemorrhage and necrosis.

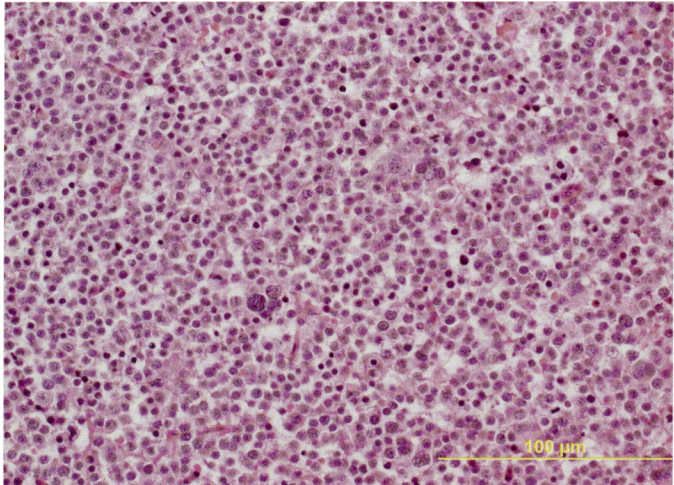

IMAGE 10.111 Spermatocytic tumor of testis. Note the intermediate, small, and large cells (H&E, x200).

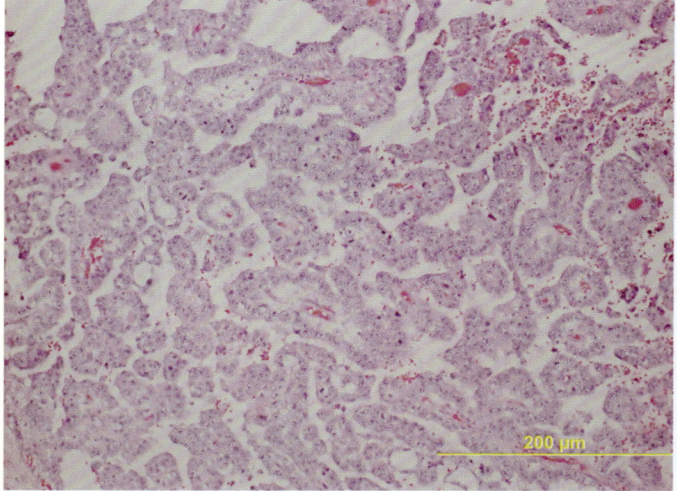

IMAGE 10.113 Embryonal carcinoma of testis showing papillary growth pattern (H&E, x100).

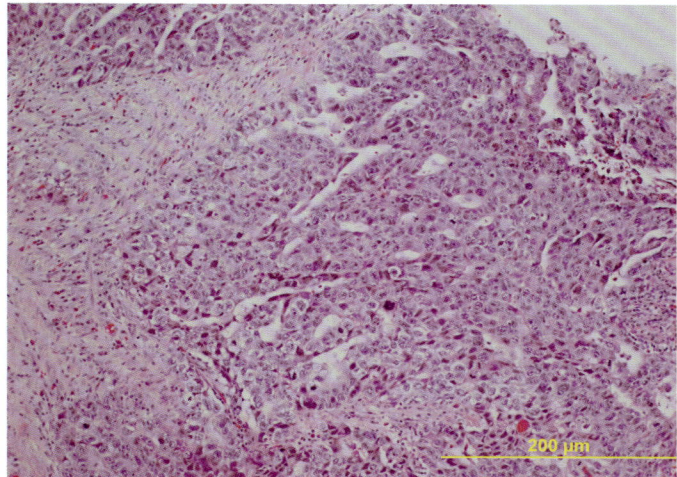

IMAGE 10.114 Embryonal carcinoma of testis showing cribriform glandular growth pattern (H&E, x100).

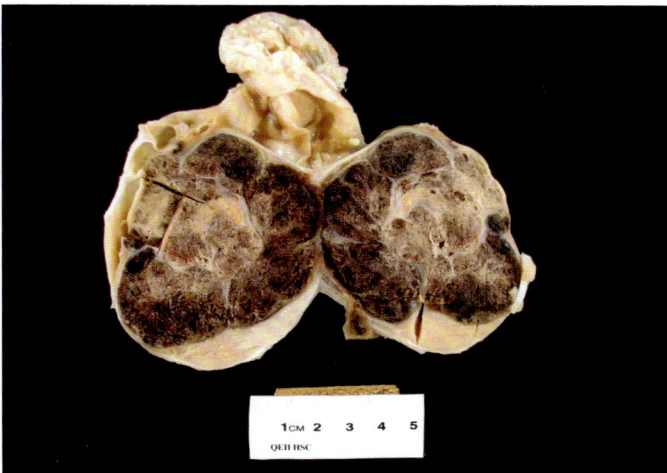

IMAGE 10.115 Mixed germ cell tumor of testis with prominent choriocarcinoma component. Note the extensive areas of hemorrhage within the tumor.

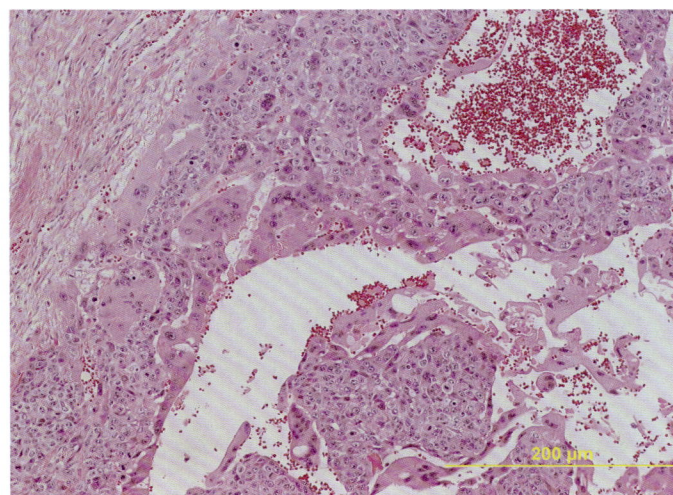

IMAGE 10.116 Choriocarcinoma of testis showing syncytiotrophoblasts, cytotrophoblasts and areas of hemorrhage (H&E, x100).

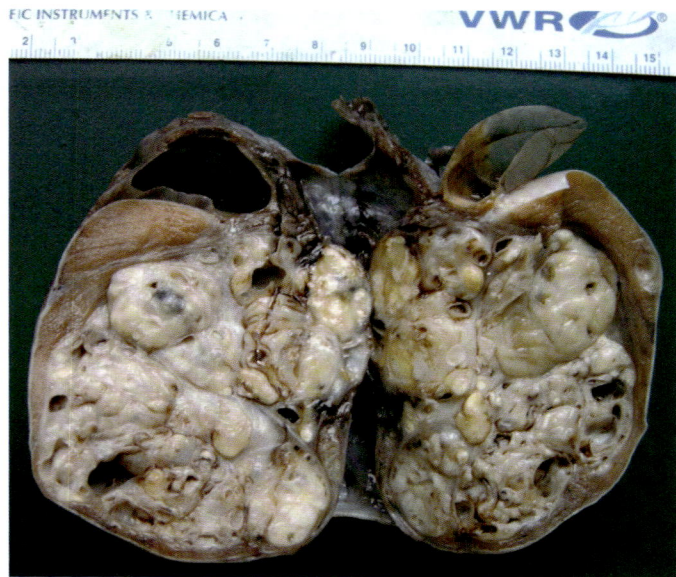

IMAGE 10.117 Testicle teratoma. The tumor appears heterogeneous, with solid and cystic features due to the presence of different tissue components. Fleshy or hemorrhagic areas likely represent more primitive elements.

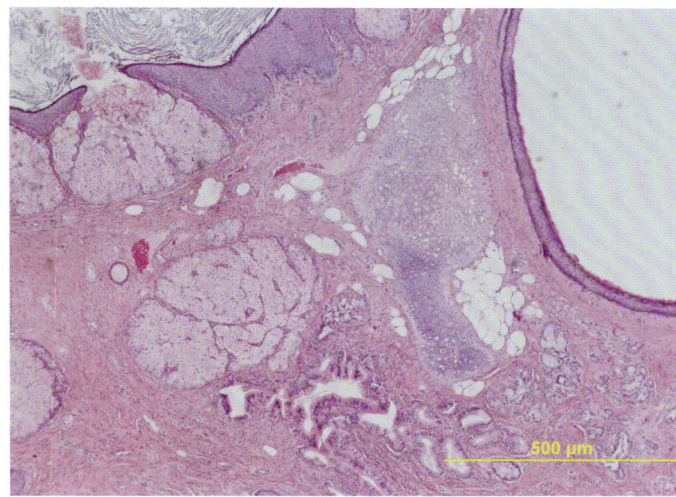

IMAGE 10.118 Teratoma of testis with mature ectodermal, mesenchymal, and endodermal derived tissue (H&E, x40).

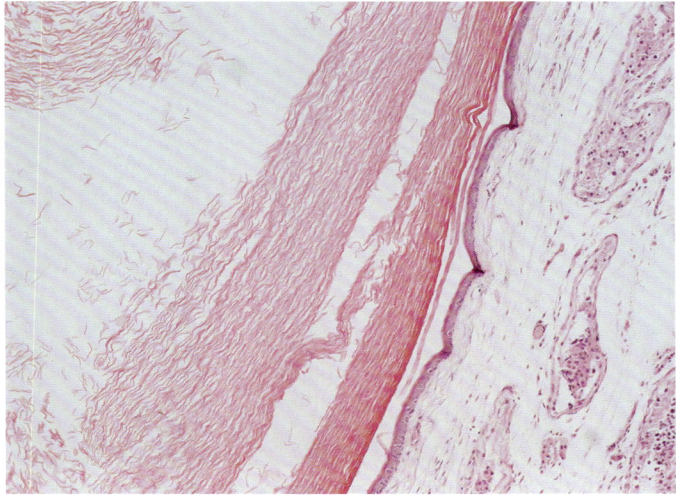

IMAGE 10.119 Epidermoid cyst of testis (H&E, x100).

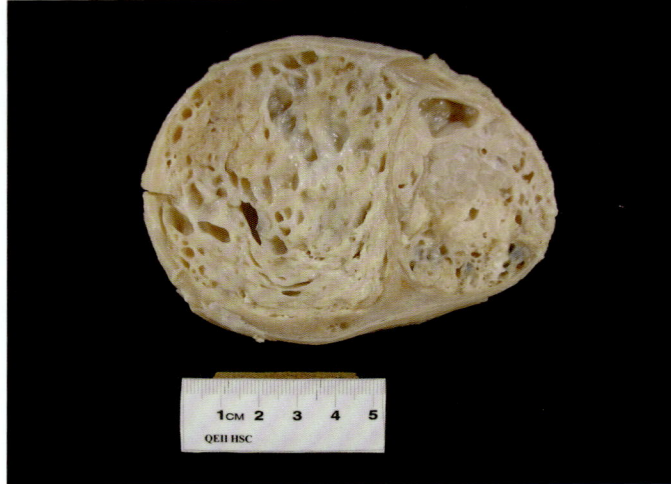

IMAGE 10.120 Mixed germ cell tumor of testis with prominent teratoma component. Note cyst formation and cartilage (right).

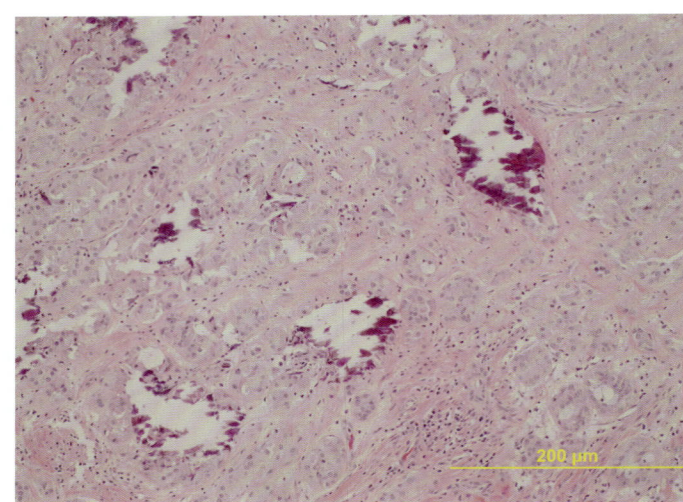

IMAGE 10.123 Large cell calcifying Sertoli cell tumor of testis (H&E, x100).

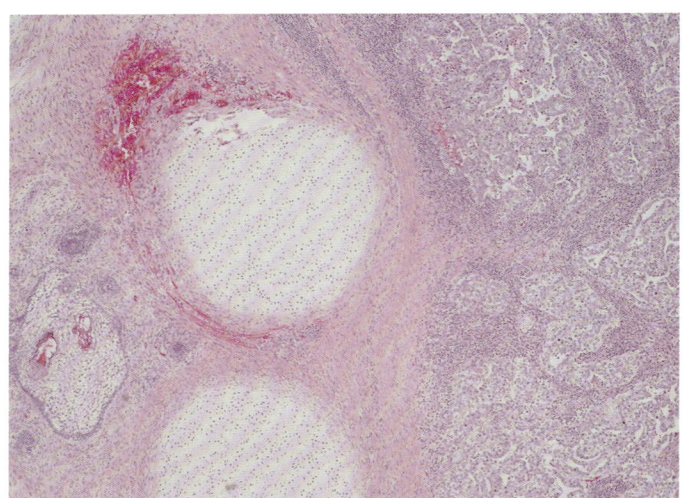

IMAGE 10.121 Mixed germ cell tumor with embryonal carcinoma and teratoma (H&E, x40).

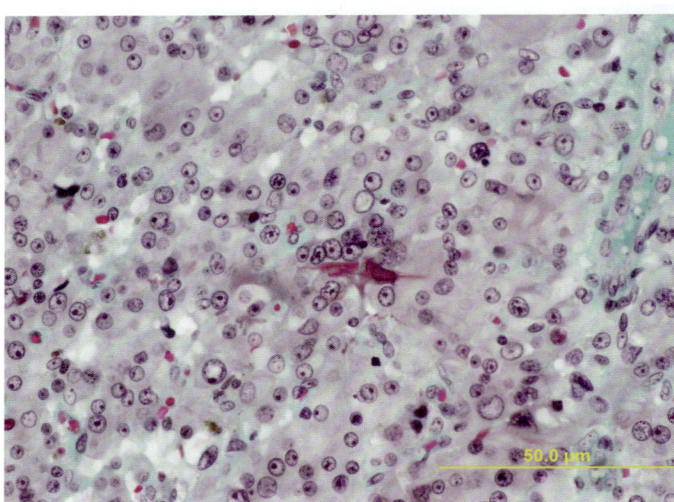

IMAGE 10.124 Leydig cell tumor with Reinke crystalloid (Masson, x400).

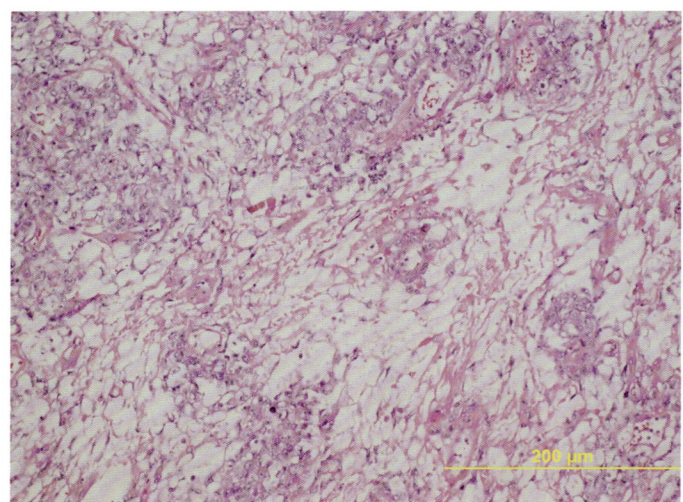

IMAGE 10.122 Yolk sac tumor of testis showing reticular or microcystic growth pattern and hyaline globules (H&E, x100).

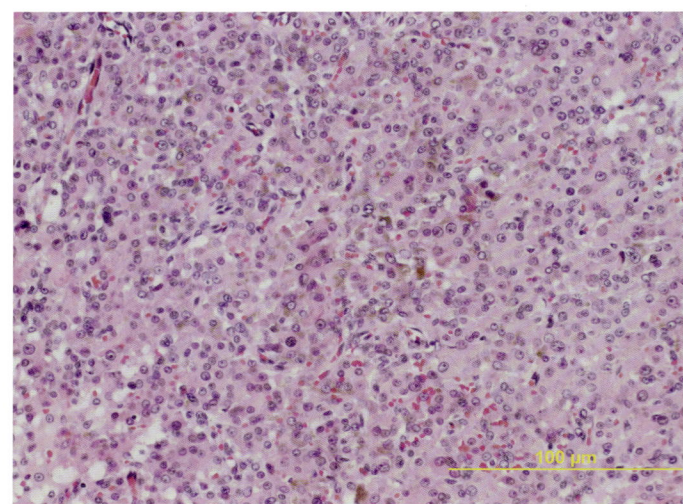

IMAGE 10.125 Leydig cell tumor of testis with lipochrome pigment (H&E, x200).

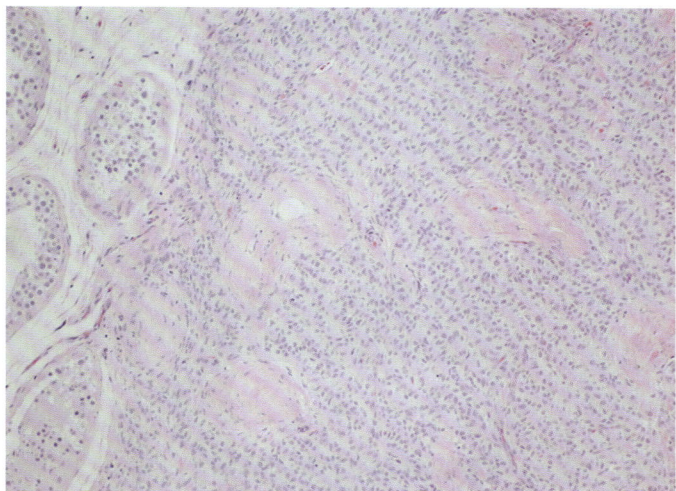

IMAGE 10.126 Granulosa cell tumor of testis (H&E, x100). The tumor is composed of small, bland, cuboidal-to-polygonal cells with angulated nuclei, some of which show nuclear grooves (better appreciated with higher power).

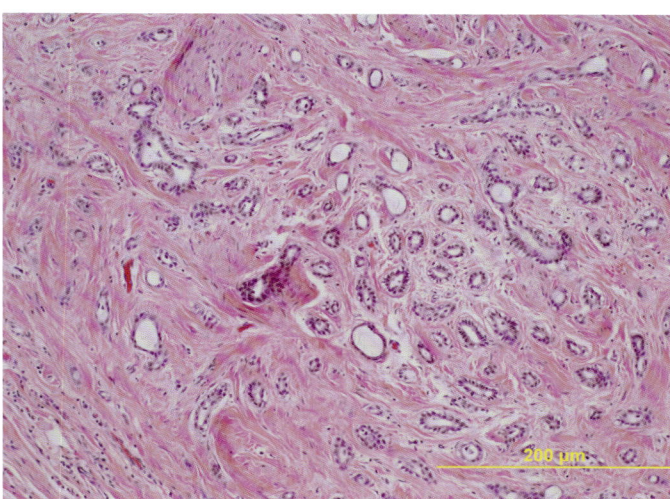

IMAGE 10.128 Adenomatoid tumor in the paratestis (H&E, x100). Tumor cells are arranged in gland-like, tubule-like, and cyst-like structures.

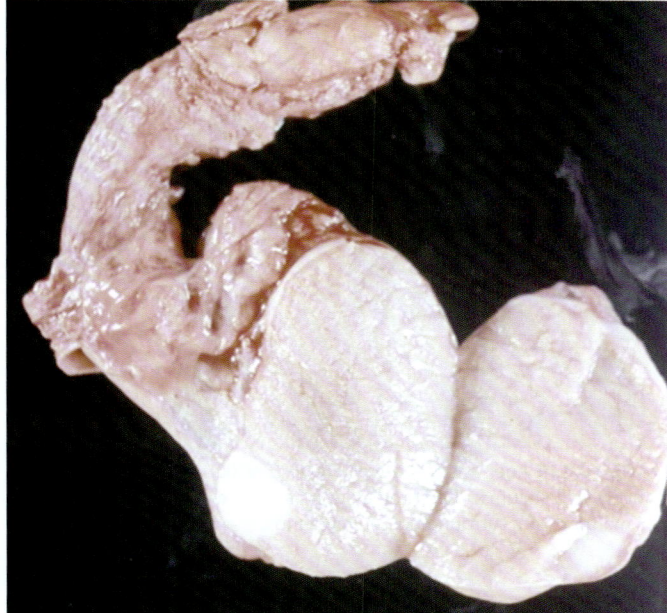

IMAGE 10.127 Adenomatoid tumor. It is usually < 2 cm in size, and is a solitary, white, fibrous nodule attached to the head or tail of the epididymis or the tunica albuginea.

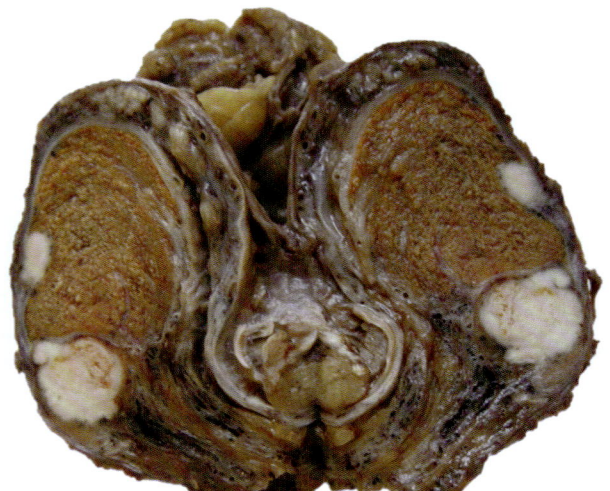

IMAGE 10.129 Paratesticle malignant mesothelioma. The lesion shows 2 white, solid tumor nodules at the tunica albuginea, and invades into the testicular parenchyma and the paratesticular adipose tissue.

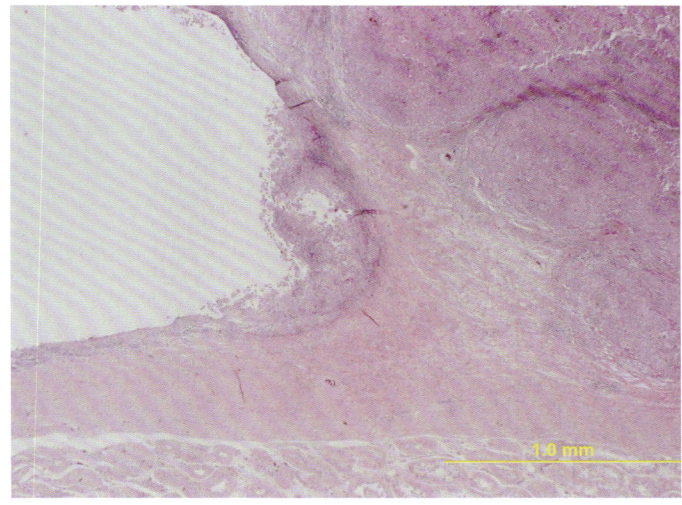

IMAGE 10.130 Mesothelioma arising from the tunica vaginalis (H&E, x20).

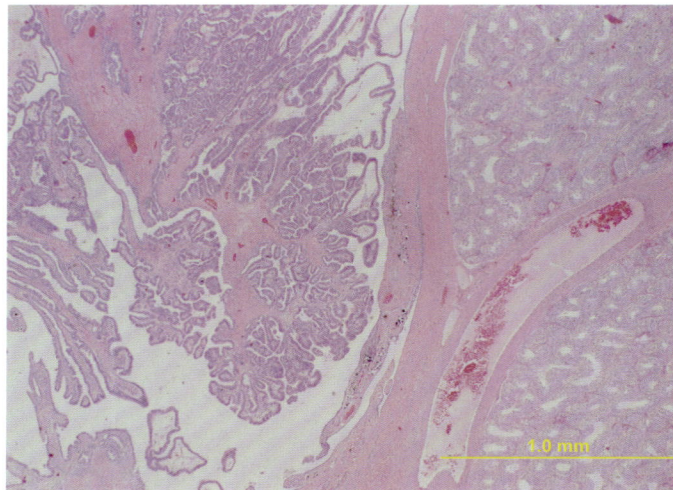

IMAGE 10.131 Borderline serous tumor of the tunica vaginalis (H&E, x20).

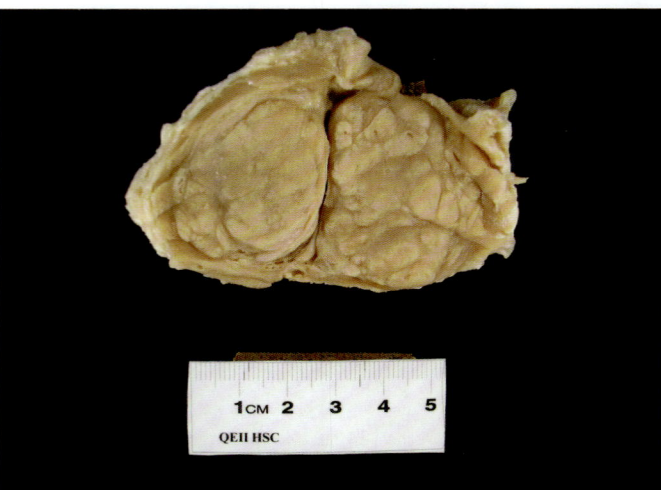

IMAGE 10.134 Benign nodular hyperplasia of prostate with prominent periurethral nodules.

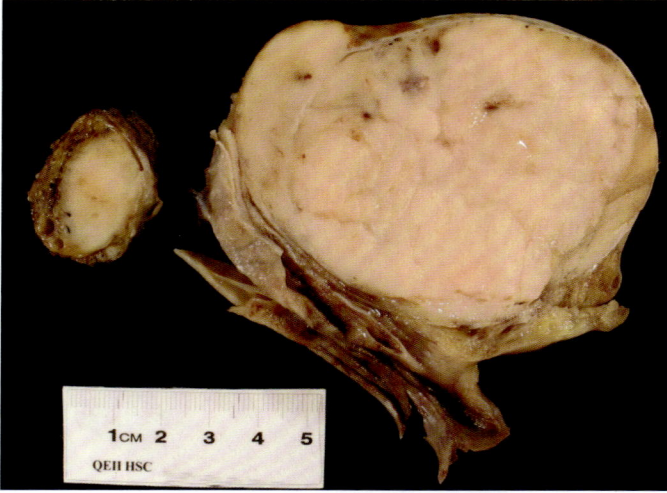

IMAGE 10.132 Testicle diffuse large B-cell lymphoma. The testicle is diffusely enlarged with a homogenous, white, fleshy cut surface.

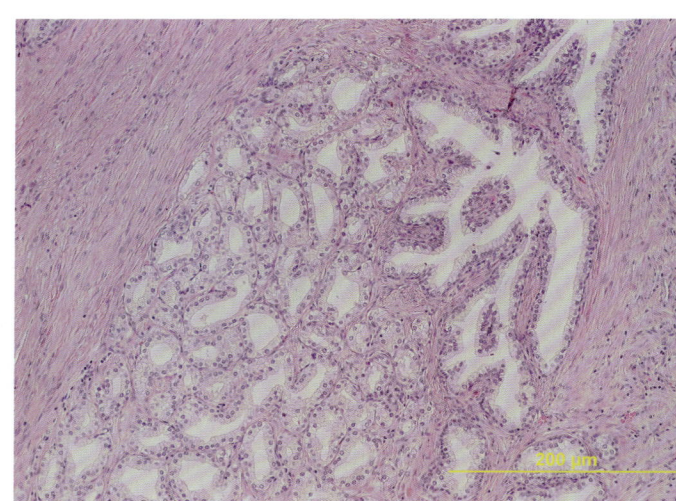

IMAGE 10.135 Adenosis of the prostate (H&E, x100). The lesion shows a relatively well-circumscribed proliferation of small, crowded, closely spaced acini merging with surrounding benign glands.

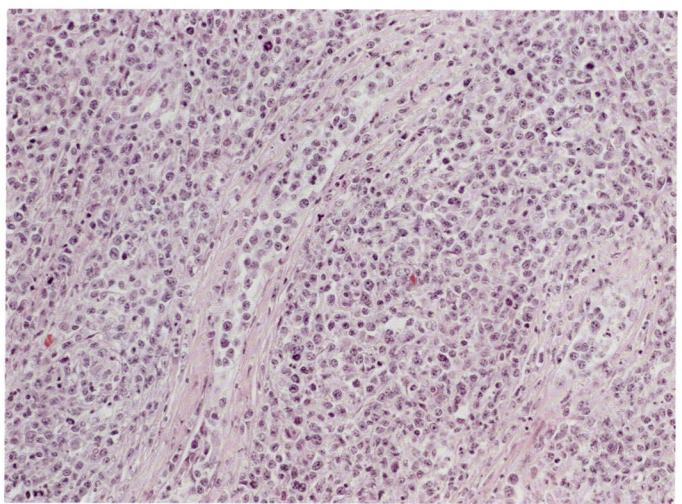

IMAGE 10.133 Diffuse large B-cell lymphoma presenting as a testicular mass.

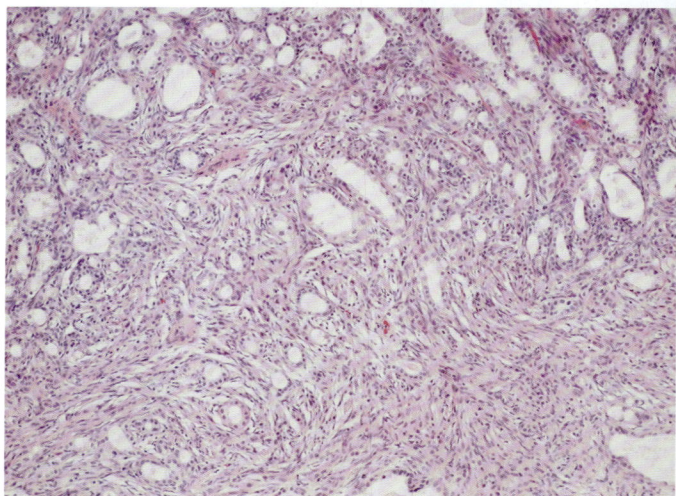

IMAGE 10.136 Sclerosing adenosis in the prostate (H&E, x100). The lesion shows a circumscribed proliferation of small acini in a background of cellular spindle cell stroma.

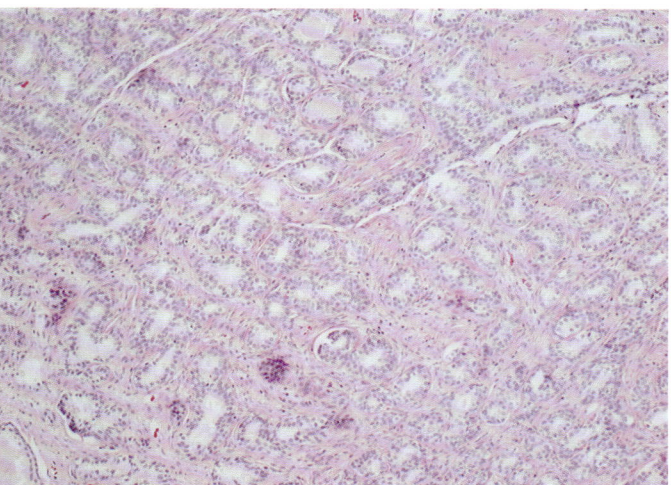

IMAGE 10.137 Basal cell hyperplasia in the prostate (H&E, x100).

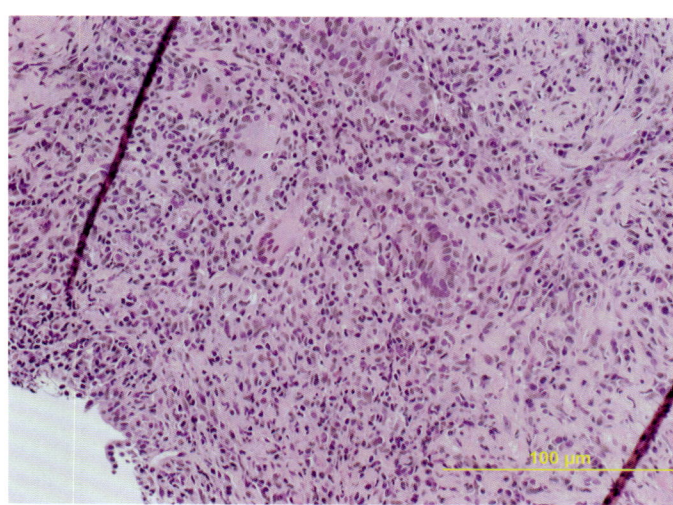

IMAGE 10.140 Granulomatous prostatitis (H&E, x200).

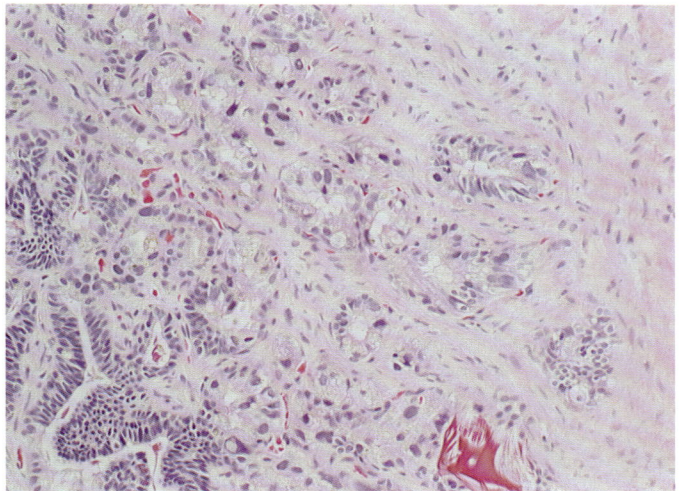

IMAGE 10.138 Prostate needle biopsy with ejaculatory duct/seminal vesicle glands (H&E, x200).

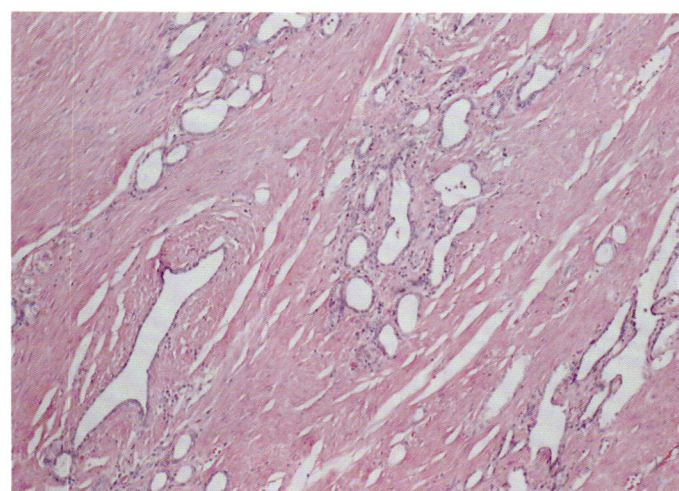

IMAGE 10.141 Glandular atrophy in the prostate (H&E, x100).

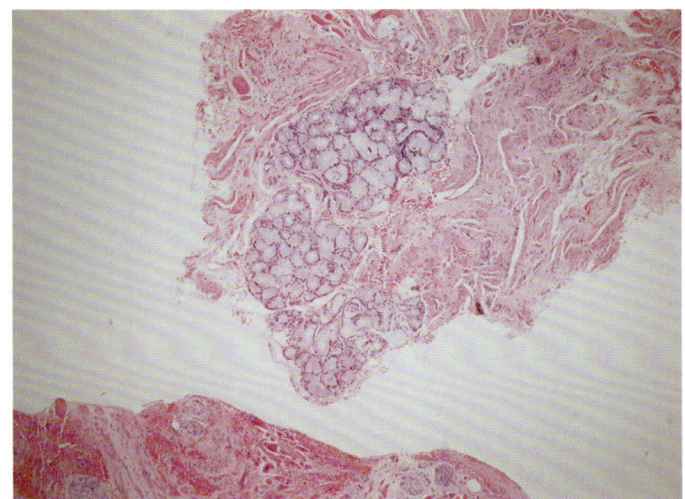

IMAGE 10.139 Prostate needle biopsy with Cowper glands (H&E, x200).

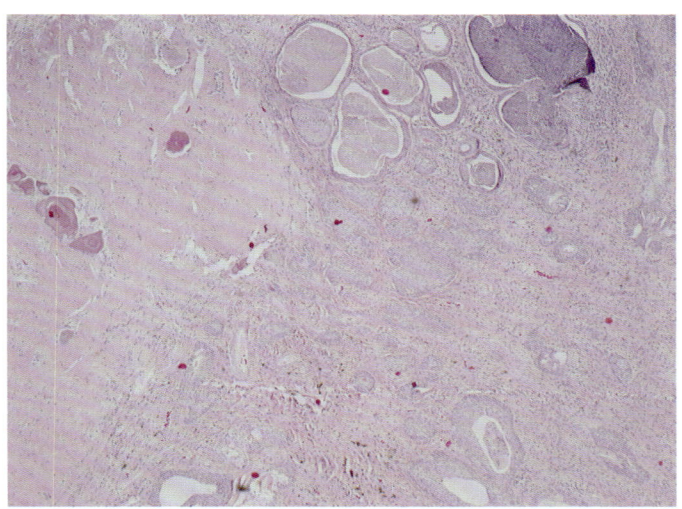

IMAGE 10.142 Prostatic infarct with adjacent squamous metaplasia (H&E, x40).

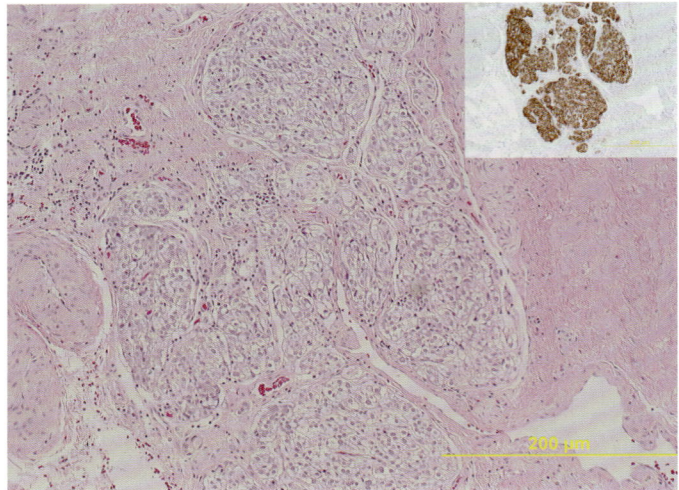

IMAGE 10.143 Paraganglion in periprostatic tissue. (H&E, x100) Inset shows synaptophysin stain.

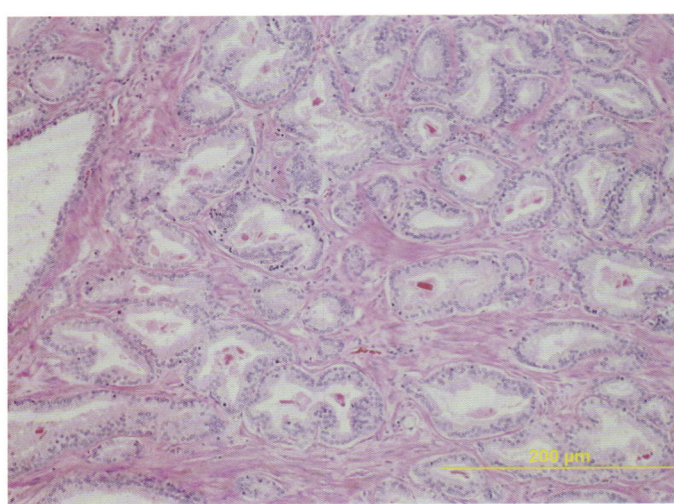

IMAGE 10.146 Invasive prostatic adenocarcinoma, Gleason pattern 3, showing prominent eosinophilic luminal crystalloids (H&E, x100).

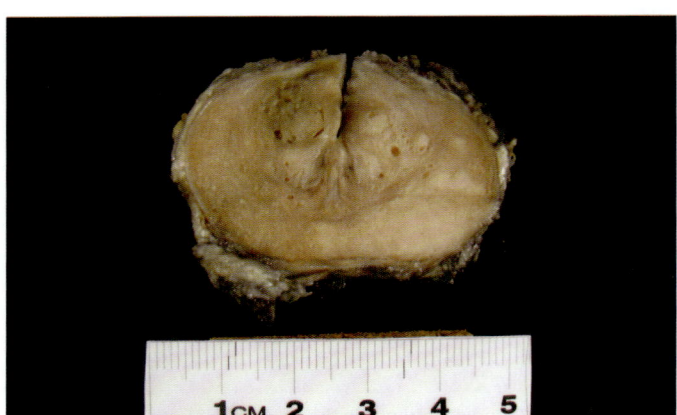

IMAGE 10.144 Prostatic adenocarcinoma. Note the yellow-tan tumor in the posterior aspect of the right lobe.

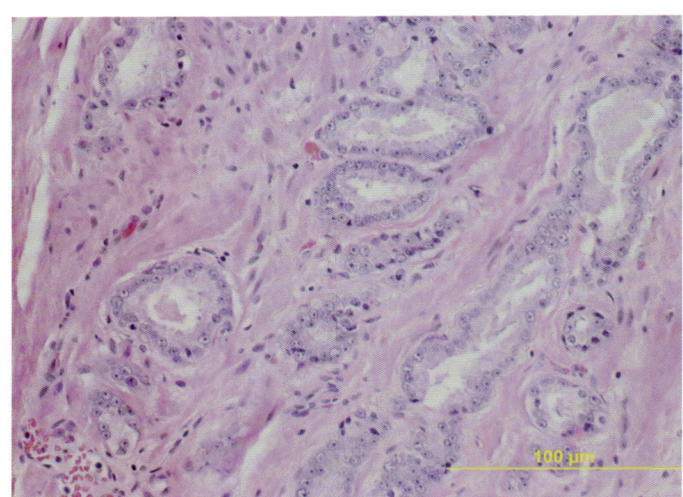

IMAGE 10.147 Prostatic adenocarcinoma, acinar type showing Gleason pattern 3 well-formed gland morphology (H&E, x200).

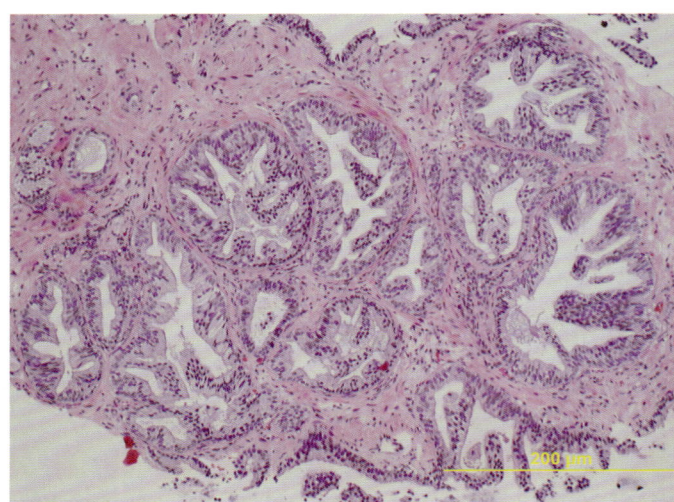

IMAGE 10.145 High grade prostatic intraepithelial neoplasia (H&E, x100).

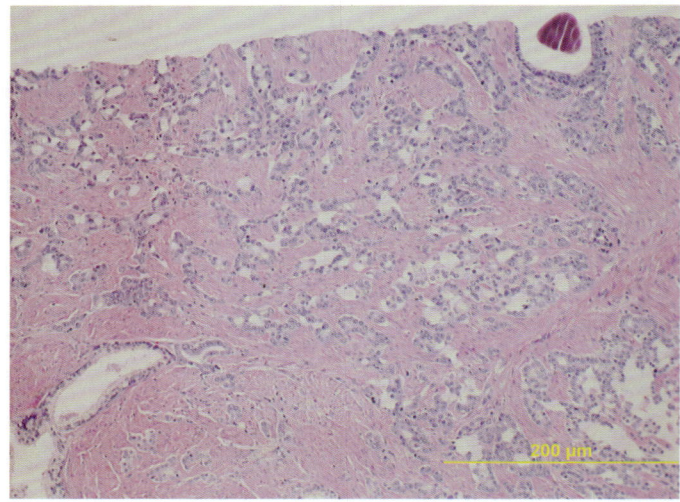

IMAGE 10.148 Prostatic adenocarcinoma, acinar type showing Gleason pattern 4 fused gland growth pattern (H&E, x100).

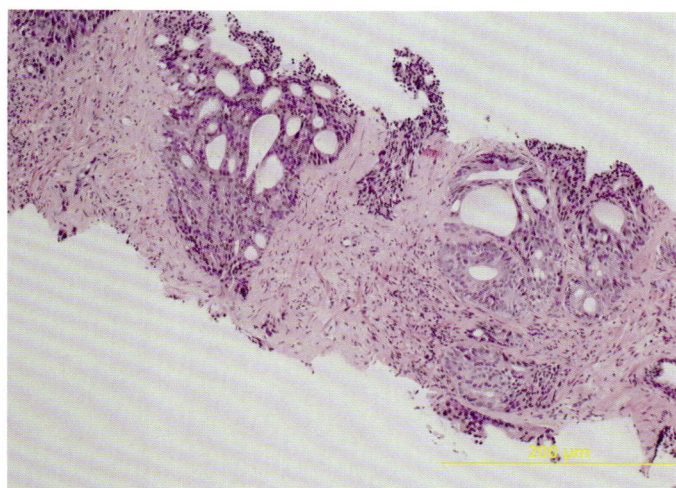

IMAGE 10.149 Prostatic adenocarcinoma, acinar type showing Gleason pattern 4 cribriform growth pattern (H&E, x100).

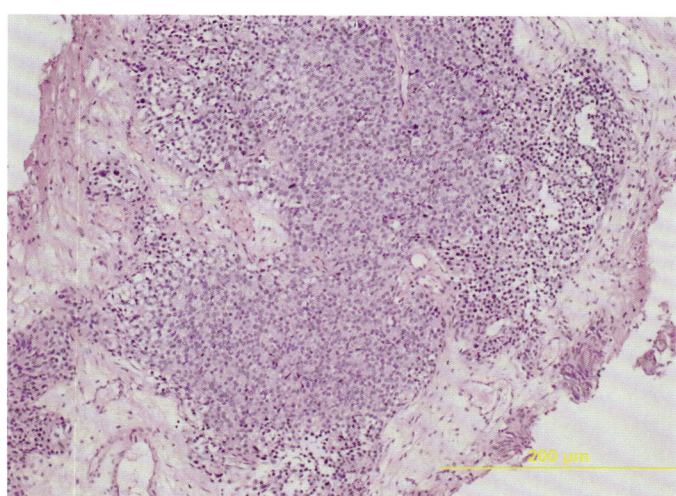

IMAGE 10.152 Prostatic adenocarcinoma, acinar type, showing Gleason pattern 5 solid growth pattern (H&E, x100).

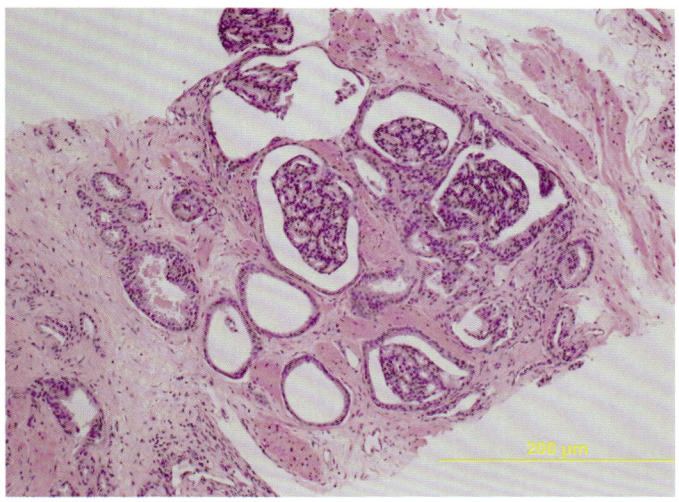

IMAGE 10.150 Prostatic adenocarcinoma, acinar type, showing Gleason pattern 4 glomeruloid growth pattern (H&E, x100).

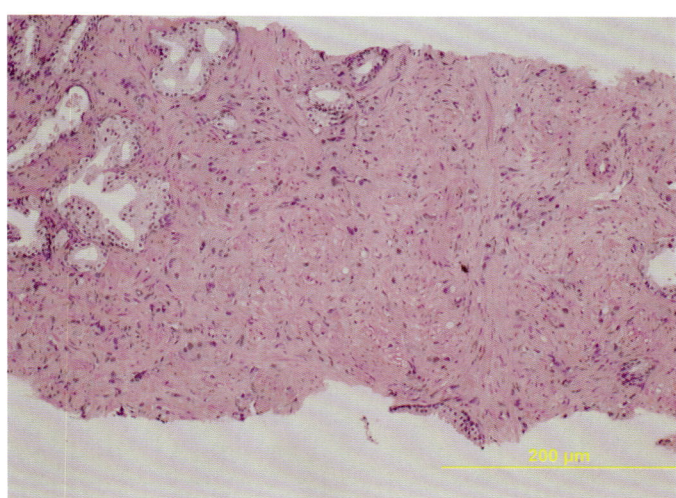

IMAGE 10.153 Prostatic adenocarcinoma, acinar type, showing Gleason pattern 5 single infiltrating neoplastic cells (H&E, x100).

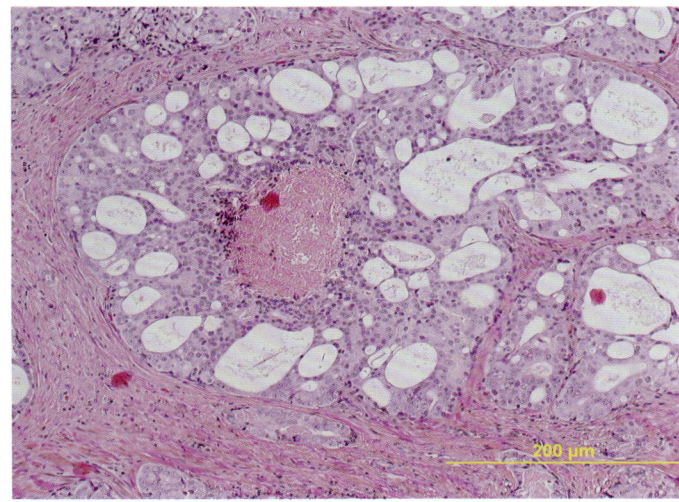

IMAGE 10.151 Prostatic adenocarcinoma, acinar type, showing Gleason pattern 5 cribriform glands with necrosis morphology (H&E, x100).

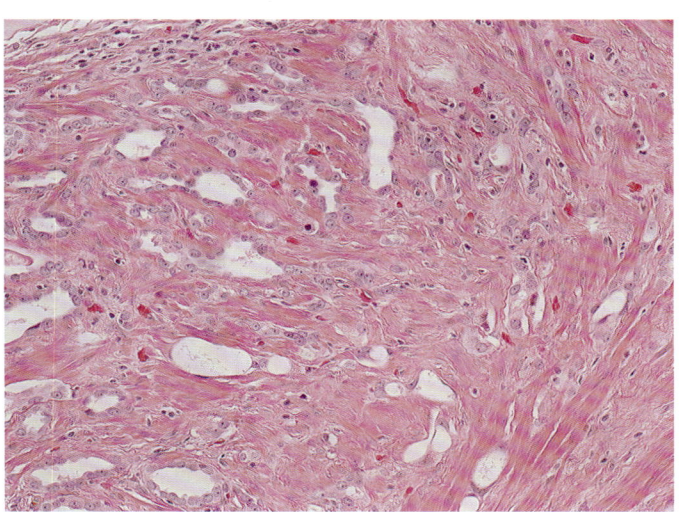

IMAGE 10.154 Prostatic carcinoma with atrophic pattern (H&E, x200).

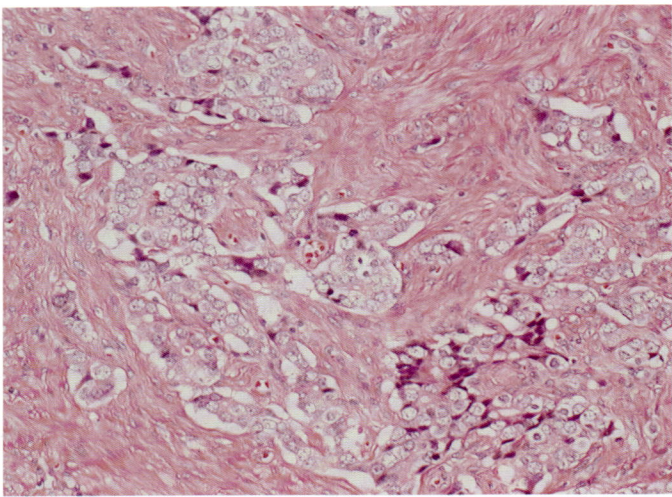

IMAGE 10.155 Prostatic carcinoma treated with antiandrogens (H&E, x200).

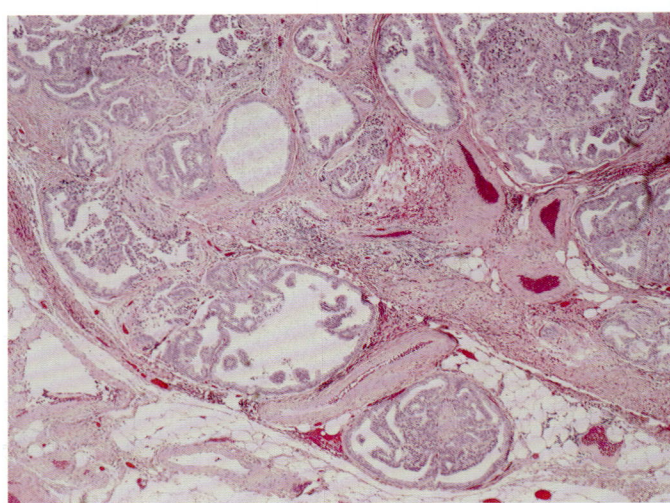

IMAGE 10.158 Prostatic carcinoma with extraprostatic extension (H&E, x40).

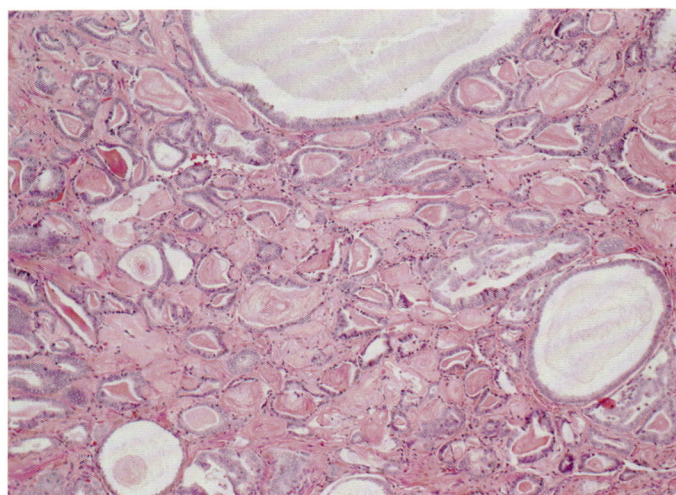

IMAGE 10.156 Prostatic carcinoma with collagenous micronodules (H&E, x100).

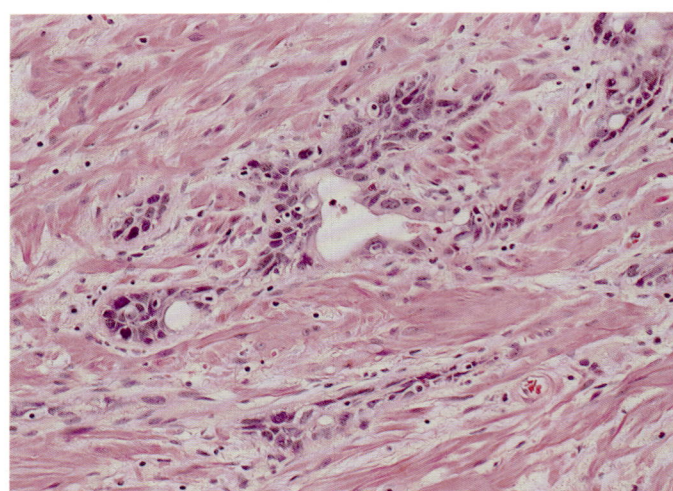

IMAGE 10.159 Prostatic tissue with radiation effects (H&E, x200). The striking change is nuclear enlargement and hyperchromasia of basal cells, but glands should still retain their lobular architecture.

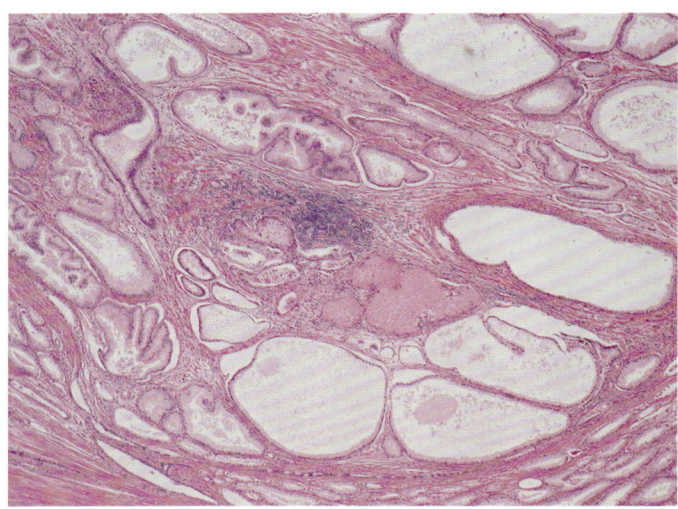

IMAGE 10.157 Prostatic carcinoma with pseudohyperplastic pattern (H&E, x40).

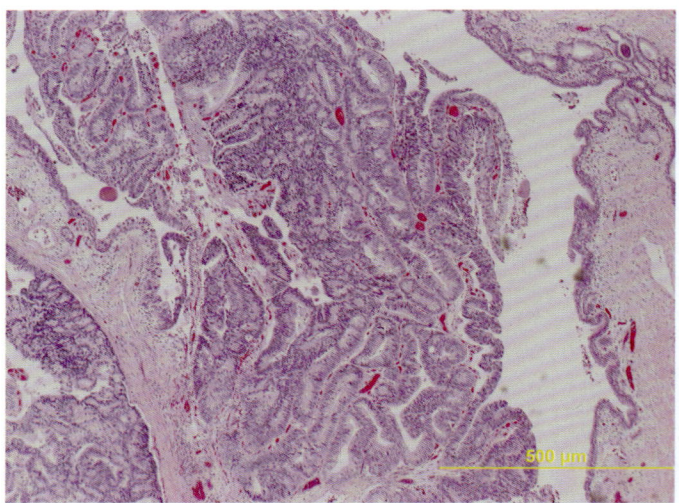

IMAGE 10.160 Ductal carcinoma of the prostate (H&E, x40).

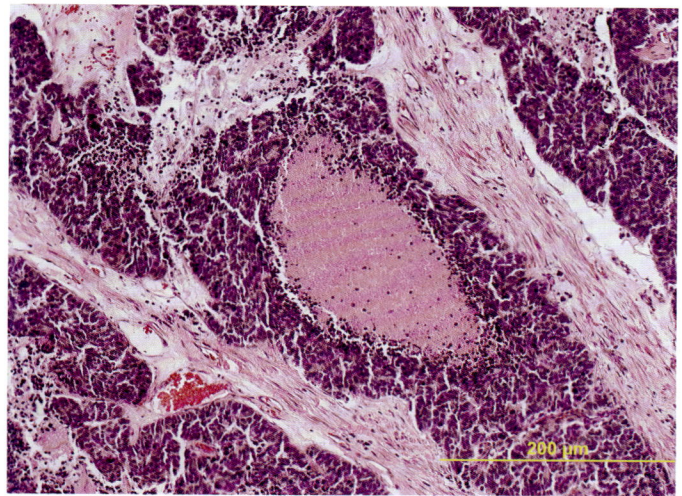

IMAGE 10.161 Small cell carcinoma of the prostate (H&E, x100).

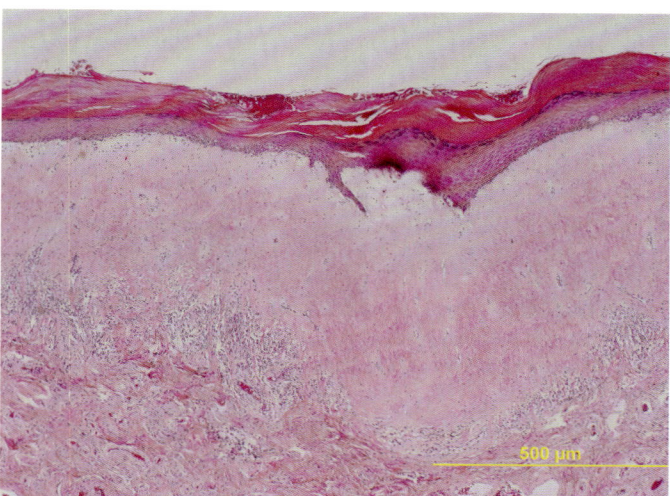

IMAGE 10.163 Balanitis xerotica obliterans showing an atrophic and hyperkeratotic epidermis, homogenization of the superficial dermis, and a lichenoid chronic inflammatory infiltrate (H&E, x40).

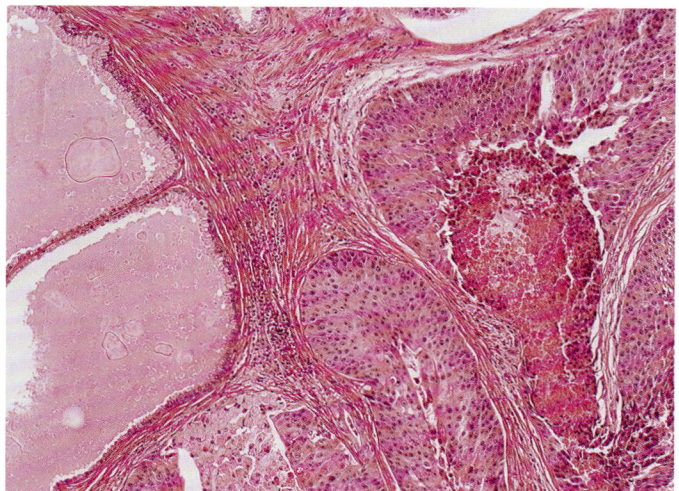

IMAGE 10.162 Prostatic tissue with urothelial carcinoma in situ colonizing glands (H&E, x100).

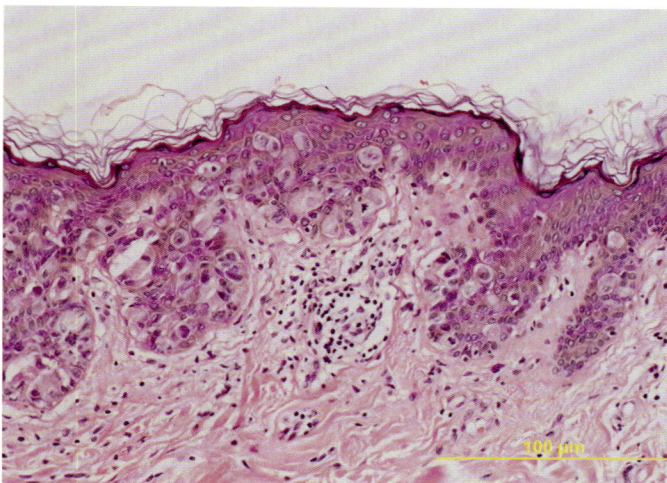

IMAGE 10.164 Paget disease of the scrotum. Note the large, atypical cells spreading through the epithelium in a pagetoid pattern (H&E, x200).

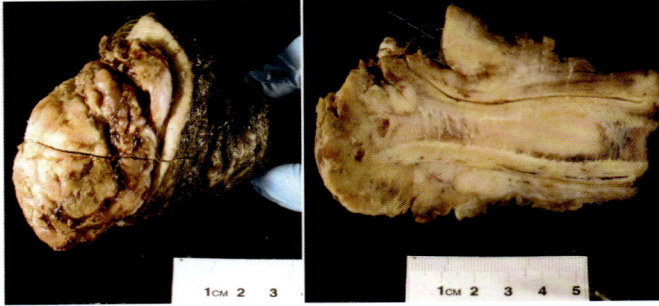

IMAGE 10.165 Penile squamous cell carcinoma. The tumor involves the mucosal surface of foreskin, entire glans, and part of the shaft, with a white cut surface.

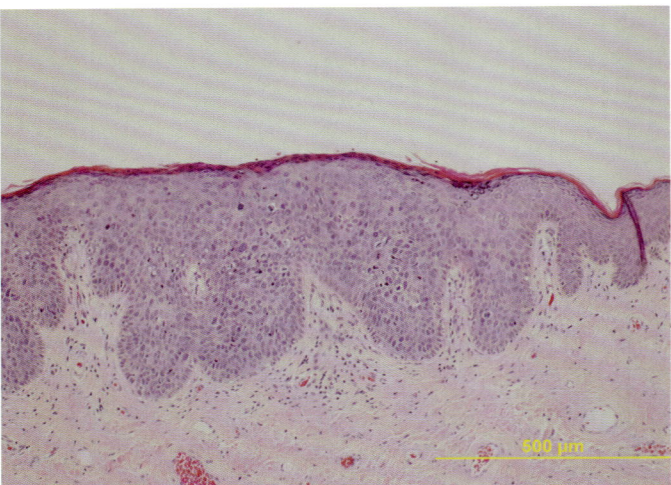

IMAGE 10.166 Squamous cell carcinoma in situ of the penis (H&E, x40).

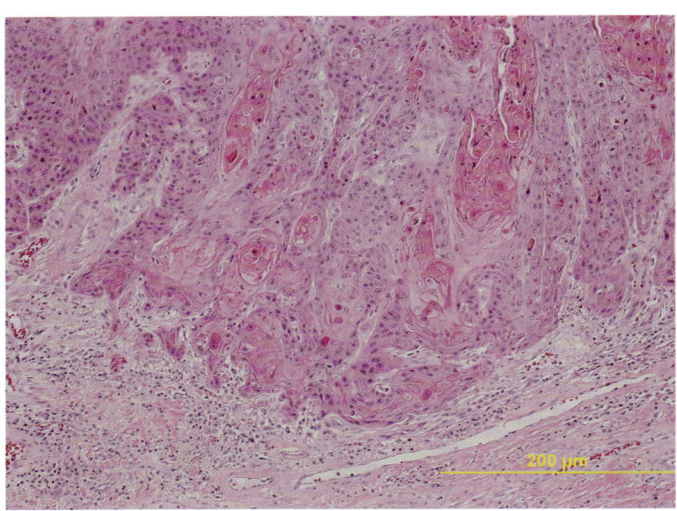

IMAGE 10.167 Invasive squamous cell carcinoma of the penis (H&E, x100).

Bibliography

Amin MB, Delahunt B, Bochner BH, et al; Cancer Committee, College of American Pathologists. Protocol for the examination of specimens from patients with carcinoma of the urinary bladder (Version: UrinaryBladder 4.0.2.0) [Internet]. College of American Pathologists; 2020. Available from www.cap.org.

Amin MB, Edge S, Greene F, et al, editors. AJCC cancer staging manual. 8th ed. New York: Springer; 2017.

Amin MB, Grigon DJ, Humphrey PA, et al. Gleason grading of prostate cancer, a contemporary approach. Philadelphia (PA): Lippincott Williams & Wilkins; 2010.

Bishop M, Hicks MJ; Cancer Committee, College of American Pathologists. Protocol for the examination of specimens from pediatric and adult patients with extragonadal germ cell tumors (Version: GermCell 3.1.0.0) [Internet]. College of American Pathologists; 2016. Available from www.cap.org.

Cheng L, Maclennan GT, Bostwick DG. Urologic surgical pathology. 4th ed. North York (ON): Elsevier Canada; 2019.

Epstein JI, Reuter VE, Amin MB. Biopsy interpretation of the bladder. 3rd ed. Philadelphia (PA): Wolters Kluwar; 2016.

Epstein JI, Yang XJ. Biopsy interpretation of the prostate. 6th ed. Philadelphia (PA): Wolters Kluwar; 2020.

Fogo AB, Alpers CE, Cohen AH, et al. Fundamentals of renal pathology. 2nd ed. New York: Springer; 2014.

Humphrey PA, Amin MB, Chang A, et al; Cancer Committee, College of American Pathologists. Protocol for the examination of specimens from patients with carcinoma of the prostate gland (Version: Prostate 4.1.0.1) [Internet]. College of American Pathologists; 2020. Available from www.cap.org.

Humphrey PA, Amin MB, Chang A, et al; Cancer Committee, College of American Pathologists. Protocol for the examination of specimens from patients with carcinoma of the ureter and renal pelvis (Version: UreterRenalPelvis 2.1.0.0) [Internet]. College of American Pathologists; 2019. Available from www.cap.org.

Kumar V, Abbas AK, Aster JC. Robbins and Cotran pathologic basis of disease. 10th ed. North York (ON): Elsevier Canada; 2020.

McKenney JK, Amin MB, Epstein JI, et al; Cancer Committee, College of American Pathologists. Protocol for the examination of specimens from patients with carcinoma of the urethra (Version: Urethra 4.0.3.0) [Internet]. College of American Pathologists; 2020. Available from www.cap.org.

Morgado M, Costa-Silva A, Monteiro CP. Adenomatoid paratesticular tumour: rare presentation in a child. Urol Case Rep. 2018;21:34-35. doi: 10.1016/j.eucr.2018.08.008

Petersen RO, Sesterhenn IA, Davis CJ. Urologic pathology. 3rd ed. Philadelphia (PA): Lippincott Williams & Wilkins; 2009.

Reddy VB, David O, Spitz DJ, et al. Gattuso's differential diagnosis in surgical pathology. 4th ed. Philadelphia (PA): Elsevier; 2021.

Sheng B, Zhang Y-P, Wei H-H, et al. Primary adenomatoid tumor of the testis: report of a case and review of literature. Int J Clin Exp Pathol. 2015;8(5):5914-8. PMID: 26191318

Srigley JR, Amin MB, Campbell SC, et al; Cancer Committee, College of American Pathologists. Protocol for the examination of specimens from patients with invasive carcinoma of renal tubular origin (Version: Kidney 4.0.2.0) [Internet]. College of American Pathologists; 2020. Available from www.cap.org.

Tickoo SK, Reuter VE, Amin MB, et al; Cancer Committee, College of American Pathologists. Protocol for the examination of specimens from patients with malignant germ cell and sex cord–stromal tumors of the testis (Version: Testis 4.0.1.2) [Internet]. College of American Pathologists; 2019. Available from www.cap.org.

Velazquez EF, Amin MB, Epstein JI, et al; Cancer Committee, College of American Pathologists. Protocol for the examination of specimens from patients with carcinoma of the penis (Version: Penis 4.1.0.1) [Internet]. College of American Pathologists; 2017. Available from www.cap.org.

WHO Classification of Tumours Editorial Board. WHO classification of tumours. 5th ed. Vol. 8, Urinary and male genital tumours, Lyon (France): IARC Press; 2016.

Zhang C, Berney DM, Hirsch MS, et al. Evidence supporting the existence of benign teratomas of the postpubertal testis. Am J Surg Pathol. 2013;37(6):827-35. doi: 10.1097/PAS.0b013e31827dcc4c

Zhou M, Magi-Galluzzi C. Genitourinary pathology. In: Foundations in diagnostic pathology. Goldblum JR, editor. Philadelphia (PA): Saunders; 2015.

Zhou M, Netto G, Epstein J. Uropathology. High-yield pathology [series]. 2nd ed. Philadelphia (PA): Elsevier; 2022.

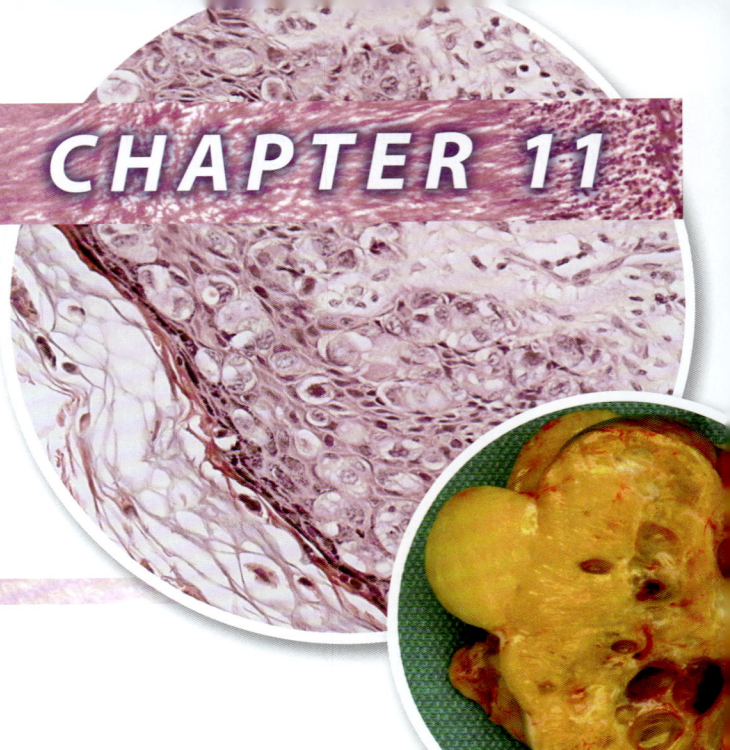

CHAPTER 11

Gynecologic Pathology

TUYET NHUNG TON NU, GUANGMING HAN

Gynecologic Pathology Exam Essentials

MUST KNOW

World Health Organization (WHO) classification

- You should be familiar with the organs and anatomic sites that fall under the WHO classification of tumors of the female reproductive tract, fifth edition, including:
  - Ovary and fallopian tube.
  - Peritoneum, broad and other uterine ligaments (although these are seldom tested).
  - Uterine corpus.
  - Gestational trophoblastic disease (GTD).
  - Cervix.
  - Vagina and vulva.
- Ovarian tumors are classically divided into epithelial tumors, sex cord and stromal tumors, and germ cell tumors. All 3 categories are high yield, either in the written component of the exam or the practical component. High-yield topics include:
  - Epithelial tumors:
    › Classification and associated biological behavior.
    › Grading and histologic criteria.
    › Molecular changes, especially p53.
    › Syndromes associated with ovarian tumor, such as *BRCA1*.
    › Peritoneal implants versus metastasis.

- Sex cord and stromal tumors:
  › Separation of tumors into pure sex cord or stromal categories.
  › Possible hormonal effect of these tumors.
  › Genetic changes, such as *FOXL1* in granulosa cell tumor.
- Germ cell tumors: the approach is identical to that of testicular germ cell tumors (see chapter 10).
- High-yield topics in fallopian tube pathology include:
  - Precursor lesions to serous carcinoma, including serous tubal intraepithelial lesions (STILs) and serous tubal intraepithelial carcinoma (STIC).
  - Molecular changes responsible for serous tumors.
  - How to use morphology, p53, and Ki 67 to differentiate them.
  - Modern theory on pathogenesis of ovarian serous tumors.
- For the peritoneum and uterine ligament, the exam mainly focuses on serous carcinoma and metastasis, and implants from other gynecologic sites.
- The uterine corpus is divided into epithelial tumors and mesenchymal tumors (especially smooth muscle tumors and endometrial stromal tumors), both of which are frequently examined. Some important points include:
  - Types of hyperplasia.
  - Classification and grading of carcinomas.

- Mimics of carcinomas.
- Benign mesenchymal tumors, including subtypes of leiomyoma.
- Differential diagnosis and workup of leiomyosarcoma.
- Uterine stromal tumors, including how to differentiate endometrial stromal nodule (ESN) from low grade and high grade endometrial stroma sarcoma (ESS), and their molecular changes.
- Mixed epithelial-mesenchymal tumors.
- Molecular changes in carcinomas and sarcomas, especially ESS.
- GTD is a popular topic and worth spending effort on. Some important topics include:
  - Classification of trophoblastic tumors: choriocarcinoma, placental site trophoblastic tumor (PSTT), epithelioid trophoblastic tumor (ETT).
  - How to differentiate trophoblastic tumors with immunohistochemistry (IHC).
  - Nonneoplastic counterparts: exaggerated placental site reaction, and placental site nodule and plaque.
  - Molar pregnancy classification: complete, partial, and invasive.
  - Differences among molar pregnancies in clinical presentation, serum findings, radiology findings, genetics, gross findings, microscopic findings, IHC workup, and treatment ramifications, and in comparison to hydropic abortus and dysmorphic villi in genetic disease.
- For the uterine cervix, the tumors are mainly squamous cell carcinoma and adenocarcinoma. High-yield topics include:
  - Risk factors for various types of cervical cancer.
  - Tumors related and unrelated to human papillomavirus (HPV).
  - Grading of cervical dysplasia.
  - How to detect HPV and HPV types, and the molecular mechanism of oncogenesis.
  - How to differentiate cervical from endometrial adenocarcinoma.
  - Syndromes with increased risk of cervical cancer, such as Peutz-Jeghers syndrome.
  - Benign mimics of cervical cancer.
  - Correlation of cervical Pap smear with histology.
- For the vagina and vulva, the exam mostly focuses on squamous lesions and human papillomavirus (HPV), as with the cervix. Some additional considerations include:
  - Vulvar melanoma.
  - Extramammary Paget disease.

AJCC and College of American Pathologists (CAP) protocols

- The ovary, fallopian tube, and peritoneum share the same CAP and AJCC protocol. Some topics worth studying include:

- How to determine site of origin for high grade serous carcinomas involving multiple gynecologic organs.
- How to differentiate (noninvasive) implants from invasive carcinoma (formerly invasive implants) (serous borderline tumor [or seromucinous borderline tumor] versus low grade serous carcinoma or seromucinous carcinoma).
- Some important factors that affect tumor (pT) staging for ovaries. Note both the TNM and the International Federation of Gynecology and Obstetrics (FIGO) staging protocols are complex, so don't try to memorize them verbatim.
- The uterine corpus is divided into CAP and AJCC protocols for endometrium sarcomas (including endometrium biomarkers) and uterine sarcomas, both of which have important information that can be examined.
  - The endometrium protocol has the following important points:
    › Histologic typing, especially in cases with mixed types.
    › How to distinguish atypical hyperplasia (or endometrial intraepithelial neoplasia [EIN]) from low grade endometrioid adenocarcinoma.
    › FIGO grading.
    › How to measure myometrial invasion.
    › The various structures involved in pT staging.
    › Definition of micrometastasis and macrometastasis for lymph node (pN) staging.
    › Biomarker testing by IHC, such as mismatch repair proteins (MMRs), estrogen receptor (ER), progesterone receptor (PR), and HER2 (for serous endometrial cancer).
  - The sarcoma protocol has the following important points:
    › Classification of definition of various sarcomas.
    › Affect of tumor size on pT staging of some sarcomas.
    › Margins.
- The GTD protocol is limited and the exam is likely to focus on basic pathophysiology. Nonetheless some important points include:
  - Classification of GTD.
  - Tumor that is confined to the uterus versus extending into to other genital structures.
  - Important IHC to differentiate various trophoblastic tumors.
  - The WHO scoring system.
- The cervix protocol is relatively complex. Focus on:
  - Tumor classification, such as HPV-associated versus HPV-independent tumors (p16 IHC is mandatory).
  - pT staging factors, with special attention to depth of invasion and effect on adjacent structures as staging factors.
  - How to measure tumor size and depth of stromal invasion.

- Various margins.
- Definition of isolated tumor cells, micrometastasis, and macrometastasis for pN staging.
- Using IHC to separate endocervical from endometrial adenocarcinoma.

- The vagina protocol is not frequently tested, and there are only few topics:
  - Diethylstilbestrol (DES) exposure as related to vaginal (and cervical) lesions.
  - Squamous lesions, squamous tumors, and precursors.

- The vulva protocol focuses on squamous and glandular lesions, and contains some important points, including:
  - WHO classification of squamous lesions, and HPV-associated versus HPV-independent tumors (p16 IHC is mandatory).
  - How to measure tumor size and depth of stromal invasion.
  - Margins.
  - Different pathogenesis pathways of invasive vulvar squamous carcinoma, and its epidemiology, histologic features, IHC, and prognosis.

Nonneoplastic diseases

In the gynecologic tract, these conditions can be mainly divided into infectious and congenital lesions, including:
- Ovary:
  - Benign cysts.
  - Endometriosis.
- Fallopian tube:
  - Salpingitis and pelvic inflammatory disease (PID).
  - Ectopic pregnancy.
- Uterus:
  - Complications of intrauterine device (IUD).
  - Causes of abnormal uterine bleeding.
  - Benign lesions such as polyps and metaplasia.
  - Congenital malformations of the uterus.
- Cervix:
  - Cervicitis.
- Vagina and vulva:
  - Inflammatory dermatoses that can involve the vulva.
  - Sexually transmitted infections, HPV-related lesions such as warts.

Genetic and syndromic conditions

High-yield topics include:
- *BRCA1*- and *BRCA2*-associated hereditary breast and ovarian cancer syndrome.
- Lynch syndrome.
- Cowden syndrome.
- Li-Fraumeni syndrome.
- Peutz-Jeghers syndrome.
- Ataxia-telangiectasia.
- Carney complex.
- *DICER1* syndrome.
- Ovarian dysgenesis.

- Von Hippel-Lindau syndrome.
- Hereditary leiomyomatosis and renal cell carcinoma.
- Other genetic tumor syndromes.

MUST SEE

High-yield gross and microscopic images include:
- Ovary:
  - Benign cysts, corpus luteum cysts.
  - Endometriosis.
  - Epithelial tumors: benign, borderline, and malignant.
  - Endometrioid, mucinous, seromucinous, clear cell, Brenner, carcinosarcoma.
  - Peritoneal implants of serous lesions.
  - Krukenberg tumors.
  - Sex cord stromal tumors: fibroma, thecoma, granulosa cell tumor (adult and juvenile), Sertoli-Leydig cell tumor, steroid cell tumor.
  - Germ cell neoplasm (GCN): teratoma, monodermal teratomas, dysgerminoma, yolk sac tumor (YST).
- Fallopian tube:
  - Ectopic pregnancy.
  - Salpingitis and salpingitis isthmica nodosa.
  - p53 signature, STIC, STIL.
  - Serous adenocarcinoma.
- Uterus:
  - IUD changes, complications such as actinomyces, endometritis.
  - Phases of menstrual cycle: proliferative, secretory, menstrual.
  - Atrophy.
  - Pregnancy, Arias-Stella reaction.
  - Leiomyoma, including various types.
  - Adenomatoid tumor.
  - Hyperplasia with and without atypia.
  - Carcinoma and subtypes.
  - Carcinosarcoma, adenosarcoma.
  - Endometrial stromal nodule and sarcoma.
  - Leiomyosarcoma, undifferentiated uterine sarcoma.
  - Perivascular epithelioid cell tumor (PEComa).
- GTD:
  - Complete versus partial mole.
  - Choriocarcinoma.
  - PSTT, ETT.
- Cervix:
  - Microglandular hyperplasia.
  - Squamous intraepithelial lesions and glandular in situ lesions.
  - Squamous cell carcinoma and adenocarcinoma, including variants.
- Vagina and vulva:
  - Hidradenoma papilliferum.
  - Squamous intraepithelial lesions (vaginal intraepithelial neoplasm [VaIN], vulval intraepithelial neoplasm [VIN]).

- Squamous cell carcinoma, and variants.
- Melanoma.
- Extramammary Paget disease.
- Inflammatory lesions, such as lichen simplex chronicus and lichen sclerosus.
- Syphilis.
- Zoon vulvitis.

MUST DO

- For each of the entities in the Must See section, you should be comfortable generating a differential diagnosis, and listing relevant additional studies such as histochemical or IHC stains.
- When studying in groups, practice:
  - Listing tumors associated with endometriosis.
  - Distinguishing primary versus metastatic tumors to the ovary, including gross and microscopic clues, and workup.
- You should be able to describe the grossing protocols for, and independently gross, key specimens, including:

- Oophorectomy +/– salpingectomy for benign reasons such as ectopic pregnancy, endometrioma, or simple cysts.
- Prophylactic salpingectomy in *BRCA*, using the SEE-FIM (**S**ectioning and **E**xtensively **E**xamining the **F**imbriated **E**nd) protocol
- Salpingo-oophorectomy for ovarian and/or fallopian tube malignancy.
- Hysterectomy for benign reasons such as leiomyoma.
- Hysterectomy +/– salpingo-oophorectomy for malignancy, which may involve multiple organs.
- Pelvic exenteration for extensive tumors involving multiple organs.
- Products of conception for GTD.
- Cervical cone biopsies and loop electrosurgical excision procedure (LEEP).
- Hysterectomy +/– vaginectomy for cervical or vaginal carcinoma.
- Small vaginal and vulvar biopsies.
- Vulvectomy for malignancy.
- You should be able to describe and handle fresh specimens and frozen sections of ovarian tumors sent for tumor classification and assessment of malignancy.

MULTIPLE CHOICE QUESTIONS

1. Which of the following statements is **not** true about adult granulosa cell tumors of the ovary?

a. The majority of the tumors are unilateral, with only a small number of cases presenting as bilateral ovarian masses.

b. The *FOXL2* mutation occurs in nearly all adult granulosa cell tumors of the ovary.

c. Positive *FOXL2* immunohistochemistry

(IHC) can be used to distinguish adult granulosa cell tumor from other ovarian sex cord–stromal tumors.

d. Reticulin is useful in distinguishing between granulosa cell tumors and thecomas.

Answer: c

2. Ovarian low grade serous carcinoma (LGSC) and high grade serous carcinoma (HGSC) differ in which of the following?

a. HGSC has more solid areas within the tumor than LGSC.

b. Mitotic rate is typically higher in HGSC than in LGSC.

c. Total absence of P53 IHC is usually seen with HGSC but not LGSC.

d. Both b and c.

Answer: d

3. A 36-year-old woman has recently had her intrauterine device (IUD) removed. The endometrial biopsy specimen shows lymphoid follicles with increased numbers of plasma cells. Which of the following statements is true?

a. The likely diagnosis is acute endometritis.

b. Acute salpingitis is often associated with this condition.

c. The etiology for this condition is usually noninfectious.

d. Plasma cells are not seen in normal menstrual endometrium.

Answer: b

4. When examining a hysterectomy specimen labeled "fibroid uterus," a single lesion in the myometrium is identified. A diagnosis of uterine perivascular epithelioid cell tumor (PEComa) is made. Which of the following statements is **not** true?

a. PEComa is similar in morphology and IHC to epithelioid angiomyolipoma, lymphangioleiomyoma, and clear cell "sugar" tumors.

b. Patchy HMB-45 positivity is usually seen in PEComa.

c. PEComa can be positive for muscle markers such as smooth muscle actin and desmin.

d. All PEComas are considered malignant neoplasms.

Answer: d

5. Which of the following IHC markers is **not** useful to distinguish serous carcinoma from peritoneal mesothelioma?

a. WT1.

b. PAX8.

c. Estrogen receptor (ER).

d. Calretinin.

Answer: a and b

6. The following diagnoses can be reliably made on endometrial curettage **except**:

a. Endometrial carcinosarcoma.

b. Atypical endometrial hyperplasia.

c. Adenosarcoma.

d. Endometrial stromal nodule.

Answer: d

7. Some gynecological tumors are known to be associated with specific mutations. The following tumor associated mutations can be seen as germ line mutations with the exception of:

a. *FOXL2* and adult granulosa cell tumor.

b. *BRCA1* and high grade ovarian serous carcinoma.

c. *SMARCA4* and ovarian small cell carcinoma, hypercalcemic type.

d. *DICER1* and Sertoli-Leydig cell tumor.

Answer: a

8. A patient with which of the following conditions may present with an elevated serum human chorionic gonadotropin (β-hCG)?

a. Choriocarcinoma.

b. Molar pregnancy.

c. Germ cell tumor.

d. All of the above.

Answer: d

9. Which of the following gynecological tumors are **not** known to be associated with Peutz-Jeghers syndrome?

a. Endocervical gastric type adenocarcinoma.

b. Bilateral ovarian fibromas.

c. Adnexal mucinous neoplasms.

d. Sex cord tumor with annular tubules.

Answer: b

10. Which of these features are **not** seen with uterine adenosarcoma?

a. Leaflike architecture.

b. Sarcomatous overgrowth.

c. Rhabdomyoblastic differentiation.

d. Malignant glandular epithelium.

Answer: d

11. Which of the following statements is true regarding uterine adenosarcoma?

a. Its clinical behavior is similar to carcinosarcoma.

b. Deep myometrial invasion is an adverse prognostic factor.

c. It is staged in the same way as endometrial stromal sarcoma.

d. The presence of sex cord–like elements is an adverse prognostic factor.

Answer: b

12. An 18-year-old woman has been diagnosed with a low grade squamous intraepithelial lesion. Which of the following statements is **not** true?

a. Human papillomavirus (HPV) types 6 or 11 may be responsible for the lesion.

b. HPV types 16 or 18 may be responsible for the lesion.

c. As this is a precursor lesion to squamous cell carcinoma, the patient requires cone biopsy as the next step of management.

d. The presence of koilocytic change is often seen with this diagnosis.

Answer: c

13. Which feature is useful in distinguishing low grade endometrial stromal sarcoma from endometrial stromal nodule?

a. Presence of smooth muscle differentiation.

b. Mitotic rate.

c. Infiltrative border.

d. Positive for estrogen receptor IHC.

Answer: c

14. Which of the following statements regarding differentiated vulvar intraepithelial neoplasm (differentiated VIN) is **not** true?

a. It is associated with high-risk HPV infection.

b. P53 expression is believed to be abnormal in differentiated VIN; however, it is difficult to interpret as a diagnostic IHC marker.

c. Differentiated VIN usually occurs in older patients compared to the usual VIN.

d. Differentiated VIN is more likely than the usual VIN to progress to invasive carcinoma.

Answer: a

15. For uterine smooth muscle tumors, which of the following statements is true?

a. Infiltrative border is a required diagnostic criterion for leiomyosarcoma.

b. Increased mitotic rate > 10/10 high power field is, on its own, sufficient to diagnose smooth muscle tumor with uncertain malignant potential.

c. Benign leiomyoma should not have tumor cell necrosis.

d. A combination of CD10 and desmin can reliably distinguish smooth muscle tumor from endometrial stromal neoplasm.

Answer: c

16. Which gynecologic tumor is associated with *SMARCA4* mutation?

  a. Large cell neuroen-docrine carcinoma.

  b. Signet-ring stro-mal tumor.

  c. Gonadoblastoma.

  d. Small cell carcinoma of the ovary of hypercalcaemic type.

Answer: d

17. What IHC tests for *SMARCA4* mutation and what is the staining pattern?

  a. BRG1 with positive nuclear staining.

  b. BRG1 with positive nuclear and cyto-plasmic staining.

  c. INI1 with loss of nuclear staining.

  d. BRG1 with loss of nuclear staining.

  e. BRG1 and INI1 with loss of nuclear staining.

Answer: d

SHORT ANSWER QUESTIONS

Ovary: Nonneoplastic
Ovarian Cysts

18. What are the gross and microscopic characteristics of ovarian polycystic disease?

- Gross:
  - Rounded and slightly enlarged ovaries; bilateral disease (usual).
  - Multiple small subcortical follicles, typically similar in size.
- Microscopic:
  - Fibrous and thick ovarian capsule.
  - Hyperplastic ovarian stroma (+/− luteinized).
  - No stigmata of prior ovulation (often).

19. List the nonneoplastic cysts found in the ovary, and briefly describe the histology of each.

- Epithelial inclusion cyst.
  - Usually a single layer with flat to cuboidal to columnar lining (+/− ciliated).
  - < 1.0 cm (if > 1.0 cm, considered a serous cystadenoma).
- Follicular cyst.
  - 2.5–10 cm.
  - Uniloculated with an inner layer composed of granulosa cells and an outer layer composed of theca cells.
  - Note: large solitary luteinized follicle cyst of pregnancy and puerperium may show nuclear pleomorphism and hyperchromasia.
- Corpus luteum cyst.
  - Lined by luteinized granulosa cells with an outer layer of luteinized theca cells.
- Endometriotic cyst.
  - Endometrial glandular epithelium lining the cyst, often denuded in areas.
  - Underlying endometrial stroma and/or hemosiderin laden macrophages.
- Polycystic ovarian disease.
  - Fibrous and thick ovarian capsule.
  - Hyperplastic ovarian stroma (+/− luteinized).
  - Stigmata of prior ovulation often absent.
- Hyperreactio luteinalis.
  - Multiple follicular cysts with luteinized theca and granulosa layers.
  - Edema within the stroma and theca layer.
  - Luteinized stroma.

Ovary: Neoplastic
Epithelial Neoplasms of the Ovary

20. List the histologic types of epithelial neoplasms of the ovary.

- Serous — benign, borderline, malignant (including low grade and high grade serous carcinomas).
- Endometrioid — benign, borderline, malignant.
- Clear cell — benign, borderline, malignant.
- Mucinous — benign, borderline, malignant.
- Seromucinous — benign, borderline, malignant.
- Brenner tumor — benign, borderline, malignant.
- Other carcinomas — mesonephric-like adenocarcinoma; undifferentiated and dedifferentiated carcinomas; carcinosarcoma; mixed carcinoma.

21. When should the term *mixed carcinoma* be used?

- Essential diagnostic criteria: presence of at least 2 ovarian carcinoma histological types with the components showing distinct and unequivocal differences by histomorphology.
- Desirable diagnostic criteria: differences between the 2 components based on ancillary testing.

22. Why is it important to classify epithelial tumors of the ovary based on histology?
- Tend to present at different stages.
- Require different treatment/adjuvant treatment.
- May have different responses to chemotherapy.
- Are different in prognosis and survival rate.
- Are associated with different genetic abnormalities.

23. What are the College of American Pathologists (CAP) protocols* for reporting resection specimens of ovarian and fallopian tube tumors?
- Clinical history.
- Procedure.
- Hysterectomy type.
- Specimen integrity.
- Tumor site.
- Tumor size.
- Histologic type.
- Histologic grade (required for: serous, endometrioid, mucinous, and seromucinous carcinomas; immature teratomas; and Sertoli-Leydig cell tumors).
- Ovarian surface involvement.
- Fallopian tube surface involvement.
- Implants (required for advanced stage serous/seromucinous borderline tumors only).
- Other tissue and organ involvement.
- Largest extrapelvic peritoneal focus.
- Peritoneal/ascitic fluid involvement.
- Chemotherapy response score (CRS).
- Regional lymph node status.
- Distant site(s) involved.

*This chapter uses the CAP protocols updated in March 2022.

24. Why should the ovarian surface be examined carefully? Why is it important to know the integrity of the ovary and whether there is a rupture?
- The surface of the ovary should be handled as gently as possible; avoid rubbing and scraping it, and do not allow it to dry.
- It is important to stage tumors limited to the ovary; surface involvement may influence treatment.
- Patients with a family history of ovarian and/or breast cancer may have small carcinomas centered at the ovarian surface that are potentially lethal.
- If the tumor has ruptured, malignant cells may have spilled into the abdominal cavity.
- In tumors that have an admixture of benign, borderline, and/or malignant areas, it may also be important to know which area is ruptured.

25. How is the omentum grossed?
- If the tumor is grossly identifiable, representative sections are enough.
- For borderline tumors or immature teratoma with grossly apparent implants, multiple sections of the implants should be taken.
- Take 5–10 sections of grossly normal omentum.

26. What is the importance of lymphovascular invasion in ovarian epithelial carcinomas?
- The presence or absence of lymphovascular invasion does not impact tumor staging.
- Prognostic significance has not been demonstrated.
- In some cases, such as otherwise well-differentiated mucinous carcinoma, the presence of lymphovascular invasion should raise suspicion for metastatic disease to the ovary.

27. Describe the TNM staging system for reporting ovary, fallopian tube, and primary peritoneal cancer, as described by the AJCC and the Union for International Cancer Control (UICC).*

pT category
  pT not assigned (cannot be determined based on available pathological information).
  pT0: No evidence of primary tumor.
  pT1: Tumor limited to ovaries (1 or both) or fallopian tube(s).
    pT1a: Tumor limited to 1 ovary (capsule intact) or fallopian tube, no tumor on ovarian or fallopian tube surface; no malignant cells in ascites or peritoneal washings.
    pT1b: Tumor limited to both ovaries (capsules intact) or fallopian tubes; no tumor on ovarian or fallopian tube surface; no malignant cells in ascites or peritoneal washings.

pT1c: Tumor limited to one or both ovaries or fallopian tubes, with any of the following:
    pT1c1: Surgical spill.
    pT1c2: Capsule ruptured before surgery or tumor on ovarian or fallopian tube surface.
    pT1c3: Malignant cells in ascites or peritoneal washings.
  pT1 (subcategory cannot be determined).
pT2: Tumor involves 1 or both ovaries or fallopian tubes with pelvic extension below pelvic brim or primary peritoneal cancer.
    pT2a: Extension and/or implants on the uterus and/or fallopian tube(s) and/or ovaries.
    pT2b: Extension to and/or implants on other pelvic tissues.
  pT2 (subcategory cannot be determined).

(continued on next page)

pT3: Tumor involves 1 or both ovaries or fallopian tubes, or primary peritoneal cancer, with microscopically confirmed peritoneal metastasis outside the pelvis and/or metastasis to the retroperitoneal (pelvic and/or paraaortic) lymph nodes.

  pT3a: Microscopic extrapelvic (above the pelvic brim) peritoneal involvement +/- positive retroperitoneal lymph nodes.

  pT3b: Macroscopic peritoneal metastasis beyond pelvis ≤ 2 cm in greatest dimension +/- metastasis to the retroperitoneal lymph nodes.

  pT3c: Macroscopic peritoneal metastasis beyond pelvis > 2 cm in greatest dimension +/- metastasis to the retroperitoneal lymph nodes (includes extension to capsule of liver and spleen without parenchymal involvement of either organ).

  pT3 (subcategory cannot be determined).

pN category

  pN not assigned (no nodes submitted or found.

pN not assigned (cannot be determined based on available pathological information).

pN0: No regional lymph node metastasis.

pN0 (i+): Isolated tumor cells in regional lymph node(s) ≤ 0.2 mm.

pN1: Positive retroperitoneal lymph nodes only (histologically confirmed).

  pN1a: Metastasis up to 10 mm in greatest dimension.

  pN1b: Metastasis > 10 mm in greatest dimension.

pN1 (subcategory cannot be determined).

pM category (required only if confirmed pathologically)

  Not applicable - pM cannot be determined from the submitted specimen(s).

  pM1a: Pleural effusion with positive cytology.

  pM1b: Liver or splenic parenchymal metastases; metastases to extraabdominal organs (including inguinal lymph nodes and lymph nodes outside the abdominal cavity); transmural involvement of intestine.

  pM1 (subcategory cannot be determined).

*This chapter uses the eighth edition of the AJCC-UICC classification and the 2018 Cancer Report of the International Federation of Gynecology and Obstetrics (FIGO).

Familial Ovarian Carcinoma

28. What is the most common histologic type of familial ovarian carcinoma, and what are the common mutations associated with it?

- High grade serous carcinoma.
- *BRCA1/2*.

29. How should the ovary and fallopian tubes be submitted in patients with *BRCA* mutations or with suspected increased risk of hereditary breast or ovarian cancer?

- All ovarian and tubal tissue should be serially sectioned and submitted in toto.
  · Ovaries are sectioned at 2–3 mm.
- Protocol for sectioning and extensively examining the fimbriated end (SEE-FIM) of the fallopian tube:

· Amputate the distal fimbriated ends and section parallel to the long axis of the fallopian tube to maximize the amount of tubal epithelium available for histological examination.

· The remainder of the fallopian tube is submitted as serial cross-sections at 2–3 mm intervals.

Serous Neoplasms of the Ovary

30. List the types of serous neoplasm of the ovary and their histologic characteristics.

- Serous cystadenoma, cystadenofibroma, adenofibroma, surface papilloma.
  · Cystic or papillary with broad papillae and/or small glands and cysts in a prominent fibromatous stroma or as small simple papillae on the surface.
  · Single layer of ciliated cuboidal to columnar lining cells similar to fallopian tube epithelium.
- Serous borderline tumors (SBTs).
  · Hierarchical branching papillae with variable amounts of stroma in the cores.
  · Stratified epithelial lining with tufting and cell detachment.
  · Mild to moderate cytological atypia.
  · Implant: extraovarian disease, noninvasive.

· Autoimplant: desmoplastic implant on the ovarian surface.

· SBT with microinvasion: < 5 mm based on WHO definition.

- SBT, micropapillary/cribiform subtypes.
  · Area of pure micropapillary/cribiform growth ≥ 5 mm.
  · Elongated micropapillae without stromal cores (at least 5 times longer than wide) directly emanating from large papillae (Medusa head appearance).
  · Small punched-out cribriform spaces.
- Low grade serous carcinoma.
  · SBT with extraovarian invasion (invasive implant).
  · Variety of patterns: small nests, glands, papillae, micropapillae, or inverted macropapillae.
  · Frequently free-floating within unlined clear spaces.

(*continued on next page*)

- Psammoma bodies (often present).
- Mild-moderate nuclear atypia.
- Rare necrosis.
- Coexisting SBT.
- High grade serous carcinoma.
  - Heterogeneous patterns: papillary, labyrinthine (with slit-like spaces), glandular, cribriform, or SET (**s**olid, **e**ndometrial-like, **t**ransitional).

- Significant cytological atypia, sometimes with bizarre nuclei.
- Markedly increased mitotic rate, atypical mitoses.
- Necrosis and multinucleated cells.

31. Describe differences in the management of the various types of serous neoplasm.
- Benign: requires no further treatment after unilateral oophorectomy.
- Borderline: removal of all visible disease with peritoneal and omental sampling (recommended), no retroperitoneal lymph node sampling.
- Low grade serous carcinoma:
  - Surgery: hysterectomy, bilateral salpingo-oophorectomy, omentectomy, lymph node dissection, and resection of all visible disease.
  - Postoperative therapy (if required and depending on stage): chemotherapy, hormone therapy.
- High grade serous carcinoma: neoadjuvant therapy as required, surgery, and chemotherapy.

32. What is the prognosis associated with each type of serous neoplasm?
- Benign: good prognosis with 100% survival.
- Borderline: depends on stage.
  - Stage I: good prognosis.
  - Advanced stage: 4 to 7% of women with SBT develop LGSC, rarely HGSC.
  - Poor prognostic factors include micropapillary or cribriform subtype; advanced stage; bilaterality; ovarian surface involvement; and residual disease after surgery.
- LGSC: depends on stage.
  - Early stage: good prognosis.
  - Advanced stage: poor prognosis (median progression-free: 28 months; overall survival time: 100 months).
- HGSC: generally poor prognosis.

33. What is the significance of finding SBT in lymph nodes?
- It occurs in up to a third of patients with SBT who have undergone lymphadenectomy.
- It requires exclusion of the following: endosalpingiosis involving lymph nodes; psammomatous calcifications without epithelial cells; nodal mesothelial hyperplasia; and metastatic low grade serous carcinoma involving lymph nodes.
- It is more common in subcapsular sinuses than parenchyma.
- Definitive SBT in a lymph node is not considered an adverse prognostic factor.

Endometrioid Neoplasms of the Ovary

34. How do you classify endometrioid tumors of the ovary?
- Benign: endometrioid cystadenoma or cystadenofibroma.
- Borderline: endometrioid borderline tumor.
- Malignant: endometrioid carcinoma.

35. Name 1 benign finding associated with endometrioid neoplasms.
Endometriosis.

36. Describe the morphological features of each type of endometrioid neoplasm.
- Cystadenomas:
  - Cysts lined by endometrial epithelium.
  - No endometrial stroma.
  - Often associated with endometriosis, mucinous metaplasia.
- Cystadenofibroma:
  - Cystic spaces lined by endometrial epithelium within fibromatous stroma.
  - Often associated with endometriosis, mucinous metaplasia.
- Borderline tumor:
  - Two growth patterns: adenofibromatous (more common) and intracystic:
    › Adenofibromatous: background of endometrioid adenofibroma; crowded glands (resembling endometrial atypical hyperplasia); mild-moderate atypia; squamous metaplasia/morule; mucinous metaplasia.
    › Intracystic: simple papillary architecture protruding into an endometriotic cyst.
  - Areas of microinvasion (< 5 mm).
- Carcinoma:
  - Morphological resemblance to endometrioid carcinoma of the endometrium.
  - Confluent back-to-back glands (common), destructive pattern of invasion, solid pattern.
  - Association with squamous, mucinous differentiation, endometriosis.
  - Rare morphology: oxyphilic, ciliated, and corded and hyalinized.

37. How do you grade endometrioid adenocarcinoma of the ovary?
- There is more than 1 system currently used in practice:
  - Silverberg grading system based on architecture patterns, nuclear grade, and mitotic activity.
- FIGO grading system like the one used for endometrial endometrioid carcinoma.
- Binary nuclear grading system.

38. List the molecular alterations found in endometrioid adenocarcinoma.
- *ARID1A*: 30%.
- *PTEN*: 17%.
- *PIK3CA*: 40%.
- Mismatch repair protein genes.
- *CTNNB1* — low grade tumor, often with squamous differentiation: 53%.
- *TP53* — high grade tumors.
- *KRAS*: 33%.

39. Discuss the prognosis associated with each type of endometrioid neoplasm classified by the WHO.
- Benign: excellent.
- Borderline: excellent.
- Malignant: better prognosis compared to serous carcinoma in general.
- A high proportion of endometrioid adenocarcinoma presents as stage I disease.
- The higher the FIGO stage, the worse the prognosis. The 5-year survival rate for patients with stage I tumors is > 75%, compared to < 10% for patients with stage IV tumors.

40. How do you distinguish metastatic endometrial endometrioid adenocarcinoma of the ovary from synchronous ovarian and endometrial primary adenocarcinomas?

FINDING	SYNCHRONOUS	METASTATIC
Myometrial invasion	• Superficial or no myometrial invasion.	• Deep.
Lymphovascular invasion	• Absent.	• Present.
Endometriosis	• Present (+/− atypia).	• Absent.
Ovarian involvement	• Parenchymal location, solitary, unilateral.	• Surface, small tumor, multinodular, bilateral.
Spread of tumor to other locations	• Absent.	• Present.

41. What is the clinical significance of metastatic disease versus synchronous primary tumors?
Synchronous primary tumors are associated with excellent prognosis when the tumor is limited to the endometrium and ovary.

Clear Cell Neoplasms of the Ovary

42. List the different types of clear cell neoplasms of the ovary.
- Benign: clear cell cystadenoma or cystadenofibroma.
- Borderline: borderline clear cell tumor (rare).
- Malignant: clear cell carcinoma.

43. Name 1 associated benign finding for clear cell neoplasm of the ovary.
Endometriosis.

44. Describe the morphology of clear cell carcinoma of the ovary.
- Varied patterns: solid, papillary, tubulocystic, or mixed.
- Hobnailed cells with relatively uniform hyperchromatic nuclei, prominent nucleoli.
- Clear or eosinophilic cytoplasm, with relatively low mitotic activity.
- Presence of hyaline globules or psammoma bodies (possible).
- Hyalinized stroma.

45. Describe the differential diagnosis of clear cell carcinoma.
- Serous carcinoma.
- Endometrioid carcinoma with clear cell changes.
- Yolk sac tumor.
- Dysgerminoma.
- Metastatic clear cell carcinoma from an extraovarian site.
- Steroid cell tumors.

Mucinous Neoplasms of the Ovary

46. How should you handle a cystic, mucinous ovarian mass at the time of frozen section and grossing?

- Frozen section:
  - Weigh and measure the specimen.
  - Inspect capsule for intactness, and record any surface lesions or rupture.
  - Ink the outer surface.
  - Cut and open as many cystic components as possible, if multiloculated.
  - Examine for solid/papillary areas and submit more than 1 block for frozen section, if needed.
- Grossing:
  - Start with sampling 1 block per centimeter of the tumor's greatest dimension, and any suspicious areas (solid, papillary, necrosis). More sections may be required.
  - Sample the fallopian tubes.
  - Assess any other tissue sent with ovarian mass and sample appropriately, including:
    › Omentum.
    › Uterus/cervix: sample endometrium/myometrium with/ serosa.
    › Opposite ovary +/− fallopian tube.
    › Appendix and/or other tissue.

47. What does the frozen section diagnosis of a mucinous ovarian neoplasm mean to the surgeon?

- The type of surgery to proceed with.
- Whether an additional staging procedure is needed.
- Whether assessment of the appendix and intestines is required.

48. Describe the morphological features of ovarian mucinous borderline tumor, and list the differential diagnosis.

- Morphology:
  - Cysts lined by gastrointestinal type mucinous epithelium: stratification, tufting, villous or slender filiform papillae.
  - Mild to moderate cytological atypia.
  - Epithelial proliferation: >10% of the tumor volume.
  - Associated with mucinous cystadenoma, Brenner tumor, or mature cystic teratoma.
  - Mural nodules.
- Differential diagnosis:
  - Adenocarcinoma (primary or secondary).

49. How do seromucinous borderline tumors differ from mucinous borderline tumors?

MUCINOUS BORDERLINE TUMORS	SEROMUCINOUS BORDERLINE TUMORS
• Most common subtype in Asia. • Second most common subtype of borderline tumor in North America and Europe.	• Rare.
• Mean age: 45 years.	• Mean age: 34–39 years.
• Association with Brenner tumor or mature cystic teratoma.	• Association with endometriosis.
• *KRAS* mutation, p53 mutation (rare).	• *ARID1A* mutations.
• Mean tumor size: 20 cm. • Unilateral. • Smooth external surface. • Multiloculated.	• Mean tumor size: 9 cm. • 30% bilateral. • Smooth external surface. • Uniloculated.
• Gastrointestinal type epithelium.	• Papillae, hierarchical branching. • Admixture of Mullerian cell types: endometrioid, endocervical-type mucinous, ciliated, hobnail. • Clear and eosinophilic cells.
• CK7: positive. • CK20, CDX2: usually positive. • PAX8: focally positive or negative. • ER, PR: negative.	• PAX8, ER, PR, CK7: usually positive. • CK20, CDX2: negative.

Case Scenario

A patient presents with bilateral ovarian mucinous tumors.

50. What are the differential diagnoses?

- Primary — ovarian mucinous borderline tumor, ovarian mucinous carcinoma.
- Secondary — metastasis (e.g., from gastrointestinal tract, breast).

51. What are the sources of common metastases to the ovary?

- Gastrointestinal tract (GI) — stomach, appendix, pancreas, and colon.
- Breast.
- Other female genitourinary sites — endometrium, cervix.

52. How do you differentiate a primary ovarian tumor from a metastasis?

- Features favoring primary ovarian tumor:
  - Unilateral.
  - 1 large mass.
  - Mainly parenchymal involvement.
  - No history of extraovarian lesions.
  - IHC patterns compatible with ovarian primary.
- Features favoring metastasis:
  - Bilateral.
  - Multiple small foci or single cells infiltrating through the parenchyma.
  - Surface and parenchymal involvement.
  - Extensive lymphovascular spread.
  - Pools of mucin (rare exception includes an appendiceal/GI-type mucinous tumor arising from a mature teratoma).
  - History of extraovarian malignancy.
  - Histologic features such as dirty necrosis.
  - IHC patterns of an extraovarian origin such as GI, breast, lung.

Ovarian sex cord–stromal tumors
OVARIAN ADULT GRANULOSA CELL TUMORS (AGCTS)

53. What are the clinical features of AGCTs?

- Patients are most often middle-aged and postmenopausal females.
- Patients have amenorrhea, abnormal uterine bleeding.
- The tumors are more frequently estrogen secreting — increased association with endometrial hyperplasia and carcinoma.
- Androgenic changes are rare.
- Hemoperitoneum.
- May have elevated serum levels of B-inhibin.
- Patients with early stage disease have a good prognosis in general: 90% 10-year survival with stage I tumors.

54. Describe the gross and microscopic findings of AGCTs. What is the characteristic mutation?

- Gross:
  - Unilateral (majority); average size: 10 cm.
  - Solid and cystic component.
  - Soft, yellow/tan, +/– hemorrhagic.
- Microscopic:
  - Varied patterns: cords, trabecular, insular, diffuse, solid-tubular, microfollicular, macrofollicular, watered silk, gyriform, pseudopapillary.
  - Granulosa cells: ovoid cells with grooves (coffee bean nuclei) +/– Call-Exner bodies.
  - Low mitotic activity.
  - Rare: increased mitotic activity, bizarre nuclei, mucinous epithelium and hepatic differentiation.
- Molecular abnormality:
  - *FOXL2* mutation.

55. List the differential diagnosis of AGCTs.

- Poorly differentiated or undifferentiated carcinoma.
- Endometrioid adenocarcinoma.
- Small cell carcinoma.
- Endometrioid stromal sarcoma.
- Thecoma and cellular fibroma.
- Stromal tumors with minor sex cord elements.
- Large solitary luteinized follicle cyst of pregnancy.
- Yolk sac tumor.

56. Discuss how to differentiate AGCTs from poorly differentiated carcinomas, based on clinicopathological findings.

AGCTS	POORLY DIFFERENTIATED CARCINOMAS
• Rarely bilateral.	• Bilateral tumor more frequent.
• Indolent course even when clinically malignant; patients have a good prognosis.	• Rapid course; patients have a poor prognosis.
• Typically low stage.	• Typically high stage.
• Cell nuclei uniform, pale, some with grooves.	• Cell nuclei hyperchromatic, unequal size and shape.
• Low mitotic count.	• High mitotic count with atypical mitosis.
• IHC: inhibin+, calretinin+, WT1+, CD10+, FOXL2+, PAX8–, CK7–, EMA–.	• IHC: WT1+/–, inhibin–, calretinin–, CD10–, FOXL2c PAX8+, CK7+, EMA+.

57. List the clinicopathologic features that differentiate AGCTs from juvenile granulosa cell tumors (JGCTs).

AGCTS	JGCTS
• Perimenopausal women.	• Mean patient age: 13 years. • Rarely associated with Maffucci syndrome, Ollier disease, or DICER1 syndrome.
• Somatic *FOXL2* missense mutation.	• *AKT1*, *GNAS* mutation. • *IDH1*, *IDH2* mutations (associated with Maffucci syndrome or Ollier disease). • Association with tuberous sclerosis, p53, *PTEN* mutations. • *DICER1* mutations.
• Unilateral. • Average size: 10 cm. • Solid and cystic. • Hemorrhage.	• Unilateral. • Average size: 12 cm. • Solid (common) or solid and cystic. • Hemorrhage.

• Many patterns:
  · Ovoid cells with grooves (coffee bean nuclei) +/− Call-Exner bodies.
  · Nuclei that are uniform, pale, more often with a groove.
  · Bizarre nuclei, mucinous epithelium, hepatic differentiation.
  · No immature follicles.
  · Low mitotic rate.
	• Nodular or diffuse architecture.
	• Wide variation in nuclear atypia, hyperchromatic, rarely grooved.
	• Presence of immature follicles; Call-Exner bodies rare.
	• Vary in mitotic rate, higher than AGCTs.

• SF1+, WT1+, CD99+, CD56+, inhibin=, calretinin+, FOXL2+, SMA, desmin, CD10+. • EMA−.	• SF1+, WT1+, EMA+, CD99+, CD56+, inhibin=, calretinin+, FOXL2+/−.

58. A spindle cell neoplasm found in an ovary was thought to be a primary ovarian neoplasm within the fibroma/thecoma group. List 3 possible diagnoses within this group, and briefly describe their clinical features and microscopic findings.

TYPE OF NEOPLASM	CLINICAL FINDINGS	MICROSCOPIC FINDINGS
Fibroma	• Most common ovarian stromal tumor. • Patients: any age, commonly middle-aged. • Occasionally hormonal symptoms. • Symptoms related to adnexal mass. • Associated with Meig syndrome (pleural effusion, ascites), and nevoid basal cell carcinoma syndrome (Gorlin syndrome).	• Spindle cells arranged in intersecting bundles within a variably collagenous stroma, calcification, rare mitosis. • Cellular fibroma: may have increased mitotic activity, hyper and hypocellular areas. • No cytologic atypia.
Fibrosarcoma	• Very rare.	• Uniform hypercellularity with significant cytological atypia and conspicuous mitotic activity. • Occasionally hemorrhage and necrosis.
Thecoma	• Patients: older age group. • Often unilateral. • Hormonal symptoms. • Symptoms related to adnexal mass.	• Sheets of cells with fibrous bands and hyaline. • Cells often oval or rounded with ill-defined borders and abundant cytoplasm. • Keloid-like sclerosis. • Steroid-type cells with eosinophilic or clear cytoplasm.
OTHER RARE TUMORS		
Sclerosing stromal tumor	• Patients: second and third decades, mean age of 29 years. • Abnormal uterine bleeding. • Rare hormonal symptoms. • Symptoms related to adnexal mass. • Rarely associated with Meigs syndrome.	• Pseudolobular pattern. • Cellular and fibrous areas, sometimes myxoid, hypocellular edematous, collagenous stroma. • Bland epithelioid (clear or eosinophilic vacuolated cytoplasm, signet ring cells) and spindle cells. • Low mitosis.
Signet-ring stromal tumor	• Patients: adults. • Nonfunctioning, benign. • No hormonal symptoms. • Symptoms related to adnexal mass.	• Spindled cells and signet ring–like cells in the background of stroma.
Microcystic stromal tumor	• Patients: adults, mean age 45 years. • No hormonal symptoms. • Symptoms related to adnexal mass. • Uncertain behavior. • Possible association with familial adenomatous polyposis.	• Classic triad: microcysts, solid cellular zone and fibrous stroma with hyaline plaques. • Intracytoplasmic vacuoles. • Low mitosis.

Ovarian Germ Cell Tumors

TYPES OF OVARIAN GERM CELL TUMORS

59. List the types of ovarian germ cell tumors, including classification, clinical features, gross and microscopic findings, and prognosis.

TYPE OF TUMOR	CLINICAL	GROSS	MICROSCOPIC	PROGNOSIS
Mature teratoma	• Cystic variant: most common ovarian germ cell neoplasm. • Most common in reproductive years, but wide age distribution. • Abdominal pain or mass. • Rarely associated with anti-NMDAR encephalitis.	• Rare solid variant. • Sebaceous material, hair, teeth or cartilage. • Typically, presence of a solid nodule lined by hair-bearing skin (Rokitansky protuberance) along the cyst lining.	• Ectoderm: squamous epithelium and cutaneous adnexal structures. • Neuroectoderm: glia, ependyma, and cerebellum. • Mesoderm: adipose, bone, cartilage, and smooth muscle. • Endoderm: gastrointestinal, respiratory/bronchial. • Epithelium, thyroid, salivary glands, etc. • Can see all 3 layers.	• Complications (torsion, infection, rupture), malignancy arising in the tumor. • Patients have good prognosis after tumor excision.
Immature teratoma	• Uncommon. • Often occurs in first 2 decades.	• Large, unilateral. • Fleshy, greyish-tan, and solid-cystic areas. • Hemorrhage and necrosis.	• Immature tissues: mostly neuroectodermal tubules and rosettes with ectoderm and endoderm. • May be in combination with other germ cell tumors.	• Malignant with rapid growth.
Dysgerminoma	• Children and young women. • Women with gonadal dysgenesis. • Most common malignant germ cell tumor. • Rare after menopause. • Elevated serum LDH.	• Large tumor, about 15 cm. • Bilateral 20%. • Fleshy, yellow, cream-colored, solid, and lobulated. • Cystic degeneration, hemorrhage, and necrosis.	• Uniform cell population arranged in sheets or groups separated by thin fibrous septa with infiltrating lymphocytes. • Sometimes syncytiotrophoblast may be seen (β-hCG). • Polygonal cells, well-defined cell borders, abundant clear or eosinophilic cytoplasm. • One central nucleus with 1 or 2 prominent nucleoli. • Mitoses frequent.	• Depends on stage. • Mets and local spread. • Less aggressive than other germ cell tumors. • 10-year progression-free survival rate is > 90%.
Yolk sac tumor	• Second most common malignant ovarian germ cell neoplasm. • Occurs in second and third decades, rare after menopause. • AFP: elevated.	• Almost always unilateral. • Usually solid with cystic areas. • Friable, hemorrhagic, necrotic.	• Many patterns: reticular/microcystic (the most common), endodermal sinus (Schiller-Duval bodies), papillary pattern, solid, festoon, glandular, etc. · Hyaline droplets (PAS+, AFP+).	• Malignant. • Early metastasis. • Good response to chemotherapy.
Embryonal	• Occurs in children and young adults. • Precocious puberty. • Menstrual abnormalities. • Serum β-hCG and/or AFP may be elevated.	• Solid gray mass with necrosis and hemorrhage. • Unilateral, 16 cm.	• Solid, nested, glandular, and papillary. • Patterns: monomorphic to pleomorphic cells: polygonal, abundant amphophilic or clear cytoplasm. • Mitotically active. • Often admixed with other malignant germ cell tumor.	• Malignant. • Aggressive locally.
Nongestational choriocarcinoma	• Children and young adults. • Pelvic mass, and vaginal bleeding. • Elevated β-hCG.	• Unilateral, solid gray mass. • Hemorrhage and necrosis.	• Population of cytotrophoblasts, intermediate trophoblasts, and syncytiotrophoblasts. • Extensive hemorrhage and necrosis. • Can be admixed with other malignant germ cell tumor.	• Malignant. • Frequent lymphatic and intraperitoneal spread. • Good response with chemotherapy.
Mixed	• Various presentations (see above). • Dysgerminoma and yolk sac. • Tumor (most common).	• Various presentations (see above).	• More than 1 germ cell tumor component. • Usually classified per predominant type.	• Various presentations (see above).

Abbreviations: AFP: α_1-fetoprotein; β-hCG: human chorionic gonadotropin; PAS: periodic acid–Schiff stain.

A 24-year-old female has an ovarian mass. The frozen section slide shows an immature teratoma.

60. What do you tell the surgeon at the time of frozen section?
- Indicate that an immature component is seen, and provide a grade if possible.
- Indicate if any other germ cell tumor component is present.
- Discuss further management, since an immature component is considered malignant.

61. What is most likely the immature component in an immature teratoma?
Immature neuroepithelium.

62. How do you grade an immature teratoma according to the WHO?
- Immature teratomas are graded based on the amount of immature neuroepithelium they contain.
  - Grade 1 (low grade): rare immature neuroepithelium ≤ 1 low power field (x40) on any slide.
- Grade 2 (high grade): immature neuroepithelium > 1 but ≤ 3 low power fields.
- Grade 3 (high grade): immature neuroepithelium > 3 low power fields.

63. What prognosis do patients with immature teratomas have?
- It depends on the stage and grade of the primary tumor.
- It depends on grade of the metastatic tumor.
- The 5-year overall survival rate is > 90%.
- Increased immaturity with poor differentiation equates with poor prognosis.

64. What do you include in the final surgical report on an immature teratoma?
- Procedure.
- Specimen integrity.
- Primary tumor site.
- Ovarian surface involvement.
- Tumor size.
- Presence of other germ cell components.
- Presence of other malignancy arising from teratoma.
- Histologic grade.
- Implants (if applicable).
- Extent of involvement of other tissues/organs.
- Peritoneal ascitic fluid.
- Pleural fluid.
- Regional lymph nodes.
- Pathologic stage classification.
- Optional:
  - Additional pathologic findings.

65. List the types of malignancy arising from teratomas.
- Any type of malignancy can arise from the different cell lineages.
  - Most common: squamous cell carcinoma.
- Others reported: colonic type adenocarcinoma, mucinous carcinoma, papillary thyroid carcinoma, carcinoid tumor, malignant melanoma, basal cell carcinoma, chondrosarcoma, leiomyosarcoma, angiosarcoma.

66. What other tumors in the genital tract can have heterologous elements?
- Carcinosarcomas — i.e., malignant mullerian mixed tumors (MMMT).
- Endometrioid adenocarcinoma.
- Adenosarcoma.
- Sertoli-Leydig cell tumor.
- Gynandroblastoma.

YOLK SAC TUMORS

67. List the histologic patterns of yolk sac tumors.
- Microcystic or reticular.
- Endodermal sinus.
- Solid.
- Alveolar-glandular.
- Polyvesicular vitelline.
- Myxomatous.
- Papillary.
- Macrocystic.
- Hepatoid.
- Parietal.
- Sarcomatoid.

68. List the IHC of ovarian germ cell tumor.
- Yolk sac tumor:
  - Positive: AFP, CAM5.2, SALL4, GLYPICAN-3.
  - Negative: OCT4, CD117–/+, D2–40, SOX2.
- Dysgerminoma:
  - Positive: OCT4, CD117, D2–40, SALL4.
  - Negative: AFP, often negative or weak cytokeratin, SOX2.
- Embryonal carcinoma:
  - Positive: OCT4, CAM5.2, SOX2, CD30, SALL4.
  - Negative: CD117, D2–40.
- Choriocarcinoma:
  - Positive: SALL4, β-hCG.

69. How do you distinguish yolk sac tumors from clear cell carcinoma of the ovary by histopathology?

YOLK SAC TUMOR	CLEAR CELL CARCINOMA
• Similarity: both can have tubulocystic , papillary, solid patterns, clear cytoplasm, hyaline globules.	
• No association with endometriosis.	• Background endometriosis possible.
• Various patterns: reticular, endodermal sinus, alveolar-glandular, etc.	• More regular tubular patterns, +/− solid, papillary areas. • Hobnail cells, cuboidal cells. • Stromal hyalinization, myxoid stromal. • Can have eosinophilic cytoplasm.
• Schiller-Duval bodies possible.	• No Schiller-Duval bodies.
• AFP+, SALL4+, glypican + CK7−, EMA−. • CDX2+ (intestinal pattern), HepPar1+ (hepatoid pattern), TTF1+ (respiratory pattern).	• AFP− (rare exceptions), CK7+, EMA+, HNF1-β+, NapsinA+, SALL4−.

Abbreviations: AFP: α$_1$-fetoprotein; EMA: antiendomysial antibody; HNF1-β: hepatocyte nuclear factor-1β; SALL4: sal-like protein 4.

SALPINGITIS

70. List the **common** types of salpingitis, and their etiology and complications.

TYPE OF SALPINGITIS	ETIOLOGY	COMPLICATIONS
Acute salpingitis	• Young females. • Ascending infections from *Chlamydia* and gonorrhea. • Polymicrobial infection (PID).	• Infertility. • Ectopic pregnancy.
Chronic salpingitis	• Resolving acute salpingitis.	• Hydrosalpinx.
Granulomatous salpingitis	• Tuberculosis. • Fungal. • Crohn disease. • Sarcoid.	• Infertility. • Ectopic pregnancy.
Salpingitis isthmica nodosum	• Young females. • Etiology unclear.	• Infertility. • Ectopic pregnancy.

FALLOPIAN TUBE TUMORS AND PRECURSOR LESIONS

71. What is the significance of fallopian tubes in the origin of ovarian cancers?
- Recent data suggest that the fallopian tube may be the primary source for at least a significant number of high grade serous carcinomas involving the ovary, fallopian tube and peritoneum.
- Literature has shown that 50% of cases with pelvic serous carcinoma have serous tubal intraepithelial carcinomas (STIC).
- Prophylactic salpingo-oophorectomy specimens in *BRCA+* patients have shown most early carcinomas are in the tubal fimbria or in the form of STICs.

72. Describe the morphological and IHC features of STIC.
- Discretely different population of epithelial cells replacing the normal tubal mucosa.
- Epithelial stratification.
- Increased nuclear to cytoplasmic ratio with rounded hyperchromatic nuclei, loss of cell polarity, and prominent nucleoli.
- Absence of ciliated cells.
- Increased mitotic activity, possibly with abnormal mitosis.
- Cells that exhibit abnormal staining for p53 and markedly increased Ki 67 (40–100%).

73. Describe p53 signature lesion versus tubal intraepithelial lesion. What is the clinical significance of these lesions?
- p53 signature lesion has foci of at least 12 consecutive morphologically benign but abnormal p53 IHC with low Ki 67.
- Tubal intraepithelial lesion in transition (TILT) has abnormal p53 IHC foci with features intermediate between p53 signature and STIC.

Uterus
Endometrium Nonneoplastic
COMPLICATIONS ASSOCIATED WITH IUDS

74. List 4 pathological changes or complications associated with IUDs.
- Actinomyces infection.
- Endometritis.
- Squamous metaplasia.
- Uterine perforation or laceration (rare).

ENDOMETRIAL METAPLASIA

75. List the types of endometrial metaplasia.
- Tubal.
- Squamous.
- Eosinophilic.
- Mucinous.
- Papillary syncytial (glandular change associated with endometrial breakdown; it is not a true metaplasia).
- Papillary.
- Hobnail.
- Secretory.

DYSFUNCTIONAL UTERINE BLEEDING

76. List 4 nonmalignant causes of uterine bleeding.
- Pregnancy.
- Atrophy.
- Anovulatory cycles.
- Exogenous hormone use.
- Other medications.

77. List 4 causes of a hyperestrogenic state.
- Exogenous estrogens such as estrogen replacement therapy.
- Endogenous hyperestrogenism such as polycystic ovarian syndrome.
- Obesity (peripheral conversion of androgens to estrogens).
- Estrogen secreting tumor, such as ovarian functional granulosa cell tumor.

Uterine Epithelial Neoplasms
ENDOMETRIAL HYPERPLASIA AND OTHER PRECURSOR LESIONS

78. Describe the WHO classification for endometrial hyperplasia and give the risk of developing carcinoma for each type.
- Hyperplasia without atypia: threefold to fourfold increased risk.
- Atypical hyperplasia (AH) and endometrioid intraepithelial neoplasia (EIN): 14-fold increased risk in early 4-class hyperplasia studies; 45-fold increased risk in 2-class EIN studies.

79. What is the differential diagnosis of endometrial hyperplasia, and how do you distinguish hyperplasia from well-differentiated carcinoma?
- Differential diagnosis:
  · Well-differentiated adenocarcinoma.
  · Secretory endometrium.
  · Endometrial polyp.
  · Metaplasia.
- Endometrial gland and stromal breakdown.
- Hyperplasia versus carcinoma:
  · Architecture — well-differentiated carcinoma often has higher complexity with solid area, fused glands, cribriform glands, desmoplastic stroma.
  · Cytology — not as helpful.

80. What is currently considered the precursor lesion for endometrial serous carcinoma (EIC)? List its histologic and IHC features.
- Serous endometrial intraepithelial carcinoma:
  · Often on surface of a polyp, or lining preexisting endometrial glands in background atrophic endometrium.
  · Composed of cells with marked cytologic atypia, including high nuclear-cytoplasmic ratio, atypical mitotic figures, hyperchromasia, and prominent nucleoli.
- IHC: p53 overexpression or complete absence or diffuse cytoplasmic staining, increased Ki 67 (50–75% of cells), usually p16 diffusely positive or, rarely, completely negative.

Note: SEIC shows cytological and IHC features that are identical to serous carcinoma.

Case Scenario

A 38-year-old female presented clinically with an endometrial polyp. Pathology reported atypical polypoid adenomyoma.

81. What are the differential diagnoses of a polypoid lesion of the endometrial cavity?

- Benign endometrial polyp.
- Secretory endometrium.
- Atypical polypoid adenomyoma.
- Polyp with atypical hyperplasia or EIN.
- Adenosarcoma.
- Polyp with area of carcinoma (endometrioid carcinoma, serous carcinoma or SEIC).
- Carcinosarcoma (MMMT).

82. How does atypical polypoid adenomyoma behave clinically? What are the clinical implications of the diagnosis?

- It occurs in premenopausal and nulliparous females, and may be associated with infertility.
- It has a high recurrence rate if incompletely excised.
- Patients have a risk of developing endometrioid adenocarcinoma (similar to atypical endometrial hyperplasia).

ENDOMETRIAL ADENOCARCINOMA

83. List the hereditary syndromes that can cause familial endometrial carcinoma.

- Lynch syndrome.
  - It is autosomal dominant.
  - It involves mutation in 1 of 4 DNA mismatch repair genes: *MSH2* (2p21), *MLH1* (3p22.2), *MSH6* (2p16.3), and PMS2 (7p22.1) or EPCAM.
  - It can be associated with any tumor types: endometrioid, clear cell, mixed endometroid and clear cell, undifferentiated, and dedifferentiated carcinomas.
  - Muir-Torre syndrome (sebaceous skin tumor with visceral cancer) is a subtype.
- Cowden syndrome (*PTEN* hamartoma tumor syndrome).
  - It is caused primarily by *PTEN* mutation.
  - It is autosomal dominant, causing endometrial carcinomas (low grade endometrioid type, rarely serous endometrial carcinomas) and uterine leiomyomas.
- Li-Fraumeni syndrome.
  - It is autosomal dominant and involves p53 germline mutation.
  - It is most frequently associated with ovarian neoplasm, followed by the uterine corpus, the cervix and the vagina.

84. Why is it important to screen for Lynch syndrome in patients with endometrial cancer? What can be done?

- The lifetime risk for endometrial carcinoma in women with Lynch syndrome may be as high as 60%. Endometrial cancer may be the sentinel cancer that develops in these women before the onset of colorectal cancer.
- Family history alone has poor predictive value.
- Gynecologic cancers associated with Lynch syndrome can develop at any age.
- Patients should be considered for genetic counselling.
- IHC is the preferred test (MLH1, MLH2, MSH6, and PMS2).
- Lynch syndrome–related endometrial carcinoma is predominantly associated with *MLH2* mutations and *MSH6* mutations in particular.
- The majority of *MLH1* IHC loss is due to hypermethylation.
- *PMS2* IHC loss is often associated with loss of *MLH1* and is only independently meaningful if *MLH1* is intact.
- Non-IHC based testings include *MLH1* hypermethylation testing, polymerase chain reaction (PCR) assays to detect microsatellite instability (MSI), and DNA sequencing to determine mutations.

85. Give the WHO histologic classification of endometrial carcinoma.

- Endometrioid adenocarcinoma, NOS.
  - Pole-ultra mutated.
  - Mismatch repair-deficient.
  - p53 mutated.
  - Nonspecific molecular profile.
- Mucinous carcinoma, intestinal type.
- Serous carcinoma.
- Clear cell adenocarcinoma.
- Mixed cell carcinoma.
- Mesonephric-like adenocarcinoma.
- Squamous cell carcinoma.
- Undifferentiated carcinoma.
- Carcinosarcoma.

86. When should the term *mixed carcinoma* be used?

- The term applies when 2 or more distinct subtypes of endometrial carcinoma are identified, in which at least 1 component is either serous or clear cell; dedifferentiated carcinoma and carcinosarcoma are excluded.
- The term can also apply to any percentage of high grade carcinoma.
- Major and minor types should be specified.

87. When should tumors be classified as "carcinoma, subtype cannot be determined"?
- Classify high grade tumor with ambiguous features (histology and IHC) this way.
- This is an infrequent situation: every effort should be made to subclassify such tumors.

88. What are the CAP protocols* for reporting resection specimens for endometrial cancer?
- Clinical history.
- Procedure.
- Hysterectomy type.
- Specimen integrity.
- Tumor site.
- Tumor size.
- Histologic type.
- Histologic grade.
- Myometrial invasion.
- Adenomyosis.
- Uterine serosa involvement.
- Lower uterine segment involvement.
- Cervical stroma involvement.
- Other tissue/organ involvement.
- Peritoneal/ascitic fluid.
- Lymphovascular invasion.
- Margin status.
- Regional lymph node status.
- Distant site(s) involved.

*This chapter uses the CAP protocols updated in June 2021.

89. Why are procedure and specimen integrity important to report?
- Occasionally certain laparoscopic procedures may result in venous tumor emboli that are likely iatrogenic.
- In unsuspected uterine cancer cases where the uterus was received morcellated, there is a risk of spreading tumor cells to the pelvis and peritoneal cavity.
- Different hysterectomy procedures, such as subtotal hysterectomy, total hysterectomy, and radical hysterectomy, require that different margins be reported.

90. Describe grading methods for 3 common types of endometrial tumors.
- Endometrioid carcinoma:
  · FIGO grading system: grade on percentage of solid component.
    › Grade 1: ≤ 5% solid.
    › Grade 2: 6–50% solid.
    › Grade 3: > 50% solid.
  · Note: if severe nuclear atypia, upgrade by 1.
  · Note: squamous areas are not considered solid areas.
- Mucinous carcinoma: grade on the same criteria as endometrioid carcinoma.
- Serous, clear cell, small cell, large cell neuroendocrine carcinoma, undifferentiated carcinomas, dedifferentiated carcinoma and carcinosarcoma:
  · High grade based on tumor type.
- Mixed carcinoma: the highest grade should be assigned.

91. List at least 3 types of endometrial carcinoma associated with poor prognoses.
- Serous carcinoma.
- Clear cell carcinoma.
- Undifferentiated carcinoma.
- Dedifferentiated carcinoma.
- Carcinosarcoma.
- Small cell and large cell neuroendocrine carcinoma.

92. List 4 pathological prognostic factors in endometrial carcinoma limited to the uterine corpus.
- Tumor type.
- Tumor grade.
- Lymphovascular invasion.
- Depth of myometrial invasion.

93. List 5 factors used as staging criteria for endometrial carcinoma.
- Uterine serosa involvement.
- Depth of myometrial invasion.
- Presence of cervical stromal involvement.
- Presence of extrauterine tumor involvement.
- Lymph node involvement.

94. How does staging guide management for endometrial carcinoma?

Higher stage tumors may need postoperative adjuvant therapy including radiation/chemotherapy.

95. Describe the TNM staging systems for reporting endometrial carcinomas, as described by the AJCC, UICC, and FIGO.

pT category

pT not assigned (cannot be determined based on available pathological information).

pT0: No evidence of primary tumor.

pT1: Tumor confined to the corpus uteri, including endocervical glandular involvement.

pT1a: Tumor limited to endometrium or invading less than half the myometrium.

pT1b: Tumor invading one half or more of the myometrium.

pT1 (subcategory cannot be determined).

(continued on next page)

pT2: Tumor invading the stromal connective tissue of the cervix but not extending beyond the uterus. Does not include only endocervical glandular involvement.

pT3: Tumor involving serosa, adnexa, vagina, or parametrium.

  pT3a: Tumor involving serosa and/or adnexa (direct extension or metastasis).

  pT3b: Vaginal involvement (direct extension or metastasis) or parametrial involvement.

  pT3 (subcategory cannot be determined).

pT4: Tumor invading bladder mucosa and/or bowel mucosa (bullous edema is not sufficient to classify a tumor as T4).

pN category

pN not assigned (no nodes submitted or found).

pN not assigned (cannot be determined based on available pathological information).

pN0: No regional lymph node metastasis.

pN0(i+): Isolated tumor cells in regional lymph node(s) ≤ 0.2 mm.

pN1: Regional lymph node metastasis to pelvic lymph nodes.

pN1mi: Regional lymph node metastasis (> 0.2 mm but ≤ 2.0 mm in diameter) to pelvic lymph nodes.

pN1a: Regional lymph node metastasis (> 2.0 mm in diameter) to pelvic lymph nodes.

pN1 (subcategory cannot be determined).

pN2: Regional lymph node metastasis to paraaortic lymph nodes, +/- positive pelvic lymph nodes.

  pN2mi: Regional lymph node metastasis (> 0.2 mm but ≤ 2.0 mm in diameter) to paraaortic lymph nodes, +/- positive pelvic lymph nodes.

  pN2a: Regional lymph node metastasis (> 2.0 mm in diameter) to paraaortic lymph nodes +/- positive pelvic lymph nodes.

  pN2 (subcategory cannot be determined).

pM category

Not applicable — pM cannot be determined from the submitted specimen(s).

pM1: Distant metastasis (includes metastasis to inguinal lymph nodes, intraperitoneal disease, lung, liver, or bone; excludes metastasis to pelvic or paraaortic lymph nodes, vagina, uterine serosa, or adnexa).

Uterine Mesenchymal Neoplasms
UTERINE SMOOTH MUSCLE TUMORS

96. List the different histologic subtypes of leiomyoma.

- Cellular leiomyoma.
- Mitotically active leiomyoma.
- Epithelioid leiomyoma.
- Myxoid leiomyoma.
- Leiomyoma with bizarre nuclei.
- Lipoleiomyoma.
- Fumarate hydratase-deficient leiomyoma.
- Hydropic leiomyoma.
- Apoplectic leiomyoma.
- Dissecting leiomyoma.
- Diffuse leiomyomatosis.

97. List the gross and microscopic features used to distinguish between benign and malignant smooth muscle tumors.

- Leiomyoma (LM), classical type, gross features:
  · Range widely in size.
  · Usually multiple.
  · Sharply circumscribed, uncapsulated.
  · Typically firm, white whorled cut surface.
  · With or withoug degeneration (yellow-brown to red softening).
- Leiomyosarcoma (LMS) gross features:
  · Larger tumor size.
  · Usually single tumor mass.
  · Poorly circumscribed/poorly demarcated from surrounding normal myometrium.
  · Hemorrhagic, soft/necrotic, "fish flesh" texture on cut surface.
  · Locally invasive growth.
- Histologic criteria for LMS:
  · Depends on the histologic type: spindle cell type, epithelioid cell type, or myxoid type.

· Spindle cell type: the presence of 2 of the following 3 features indicates LMS.
  › Diffuse moderate to severe cytologic atypia.
  › True tumor cell necrosis (coagulative necrosis).
  › Increased mitotic activity (≥ 10 mitoses /10 high power field).
· Epithelioid cell type: similar to spindle cell type, but the criterion for mitotic activity is lower: ≥ 4 mitoses/10 high power field.
· Myxoid type: predominantly myxoid smooth muscle tumors with significant cytologic atypia, or tumor cell necrosis, and > 1 mitosis/ 10 high power field.
· IHC markers suggestive of malignant tumor:
  › p16+ overexpression (high percentage of cells showing positive nuclear/cytoplasmic staining).
  › p53+ overexpression.
  › High Ki 67.

98. Define STUMP.

- STUMP: **s**mooth **m**uscle **t**umor of **u**ncertain **m**alignant **p**otential. The term is used when there is:
  - Uncertainty of the type of smooth muscle differentiation.
  - Uncertainty of benign behavior for a certain group of tumors due to a lack of adequate clinicopathologic information.
- Uncertainty of the mitotic index — sometimes marked atypia with uncertain mitotic count or borderline mitotic count, or associated with uncertain type of necrosis.
- Uncertainty of the presence or type of tumor necrosis.

ENDOMETRIAL STROMAL NEOPLASMS AND RELATED TUMORS

99. List the gross and histologic features of each type of endometrial stromal tumor and related tumors.

- Gross:
  - Endometrial stromal nodule (ESN): well-circumscribed, yellow/soft, usually solitary.
  - Low grade endometrial stromal sarcoma: poorly circumscribed/demarcated, diffuse permeative growth, yellow/soft cut surface, intravascular tumor plugs.
  - High grade endometrial stromal sarcoma: bulky, intracavitary or intramural, tan-yellow, fleshy masses, often with hemorrhage and necrosis.
  - Undifferentiated uterine sarcoma (UUS): similar to leiomyosarcoma; large intracavitary or intramural, tan-yellow, fleshy masses with hemorrhage and necrosis.
- Histologic:
  - ESN: circumscribed, or at most may have 3 finger-like projections < 3 mm from the margin; bland round to oval small cells with scant cytoplasm; round to oval nuclei;
  inconspicuous nucleoli, sometimes arranged around hyalinized arterioles.
  - Low grade endometrial stroma sarcoma (ESS): similar cytological features to ESN, but more than 3 finger-like projections > 3 mm from the margin; permeative growth with lymphovascular invasion; sometimes necrosis; low mitotic activity.
  - High grade ESS: permeative, infiltrative growth; lymphovascular invasion; high mitosis; necrosis; nests of round cells with eosinophilic cytoplasm; high grade nuclei; scant or moderate amounts of cytoplasm; associated with low grade ESS.
  - UUS: destructive pattern of invasion; sheets of uniform or pleomorphic epithelioid and/or spindled cells; associated with brisk mitotic activities; easily identified necrosis, lymphovascular invasion.

100. List the IHC markers used to distinguish low grade ESS and high grade ESS.

- Low grade ESS:
  - It tends to be diffusely positive for estrogen receptors (ER), progesterone receptor (PR), CD10, and SMA.
  - Cyclin D1 is often negative.
- High grade ESS:
- IHC markers in *YWHAE-NUTM2A/B* fusion are: positive cyclin D1, SCOR, c-KIT, CD56, and CD99; and negative CD10, ER, PR, and SMA.
- In *ZC3H7B-BCOR* fusion, they are: positive CD10 and cyclin D1; ER, PR, SMA, and SCOR are often negative.

Note: high grade ESS can have areas that resemble low grade ESS in morphology and IHC.

101. List the IHC markers used to distinguish uterine smooth muscle tumors from endometrial stromal neoplasms.

- CD10.
  - CD10+ favors endometrial stromal neoplasm.
- Desmin/caldesmon.
  - Desmin/caldesmon+ favors smooth muscle tumor.
- This is **not** absolute.
- Note that molecular genetics may be helpful. The most common translocations are:
  - Low grade ESS: t(7;17) *JAZF1-JJAZ1(SUZ12)*.
  - High grade ESS: t(10;17) *YWHAE-FAM22*.

102. Describe morphological characteristics of UUS.

- This is a high grade sarcoma that lacks specific differentiation.
- It has marked uniform or cellular pleomorphism and abundant mitotic activity with atypical forms; it lacks the typical growth pattern and vascularity of ESS.
- It often resembles the homogenous sarcomatous component of a carcinosarcoma.
- It is usually negative for ER and PR.
- UUS should be a diagnosis of exclusion (leiomyosarcomas and other high grade tumors such as rhabdomyosarcoma and malignant PEComa, should be excluded).

103. What should be included in the report of a uterine sarcoma according to CAP cancer protocols?

- Procedure.
- Hysterectomy type.
- Specimen integrity.
- Tumor site.
- Tumor size.
- Histologic type.
- Histologic grade (only for adenocarcinoma).
- Myometrial invasion (only for adenocarcinoma).

(continued on next page)

- Other tissue/organ involvement.
- Lymphovascular invasion.
- Peritoneal/ascitic fluid.
- Margin status.
- Regional lymph node status.
- Distant site(s) involved.

104. Describe the TNM staging system for reporting LMS, ESS, and UUS, as described and approved by CAP.

pT category

  pT not assigned (cannot be determined based on available pathological information).

  pT0: No evidence of primary tumor.

  pT1: Tumor limited to the uterus.
    pT1a: Tumor ≤ 5 cm in greatest dimension.
    pT1b: Tumor > 5 cm.
    pT1 (subcategory cannot be determined).

  pT2: Tumor extends beyond the uterus, within the pelvis.
    pT2a: Tumor involves adnexa.
    pT2b: Tumor involves other pelvic tissues.
    pT2 (subcategory cannot be determined).

  pT3: Tumor infiltrates abdominal tissues.
    pT3a: Tumor infiltrates abdominal tissues in one site.
    pT3b: Tumor infiltrates abdominal tissues in more than one site.

  pT3 (subcategory cannot be determined).

  pT4: Tumor invades bladder or rectum.

pN category

  pN not assigned (no nodes submitted or found).

  pN not assigned (cannot be determined based on available pathological information).

  pN0: No regional lymph node metastasis.

  pN0(i+): Isolated tumor cells in regional lymph node(s) ≤ 0.2 mm.

  pN1: Regional lymph node metastasis.

pM category

  Not applicable — pM cannot be determined from the submitted specimen(s).

  pM1: Distant metastasis (excluding adnexa, pelvic, abdominal tissues, and regional lymph nodes).

Combined Epithelial-Mesenchymal Neoplasms
CLASSIFICATION AND CLINICAL PROGNOSIS

105. Briefly discuss the classification of, and clinical prognosis associated with, combined epithelial-mesenchymal neoplasms in the uterus.

- Carcinosarcoma (staged and reported in the same way as endometrial carcinoma).
  - Patients have a poor prognosis.
- Adenosarcoma.
  - It has low malignant potential (generally).
  - If it recurs, patients may have a poor prognosis.
- Carcinofibroma.
  - Patients have an uncertain prognosis — it is an uncommon entity.
- Possible factors in prognosis include stage, depth of myometrial invasion, and histology.
- Adenofibroma.
  - It is benign.
  - It may recur if not completely removed.
- Adenomyoma.
  - It is benign.
  - It may recur if not completely removed.

106. How is sarcomatous overgrowth defined in uterine adenosarcoma?

By the presence of pure sarcoma, usually high grade and without an epithelial component, occupying at least 25% of the tumor.

107. Describe the TNM staging system for reporting uterine adenosarcoma, as described and approved by CAP.

pT category

  pT not assigned (cannot be determined based on available pathological information).

  pT0: No evidence of primary tumor.

  pT1: Tumor limited to the uterus.
    pT1a: Tumor limited to the endometrium/endocervix.
    pT1b: Tumor invades to less than half of the myometrium.
    pT1c: Tumor invades one half or more of the myometrium.
    pT1 (subcategory cannot be determined).

  pT2: Tumor extends beyond the uterus, within the pelvis.

    pT2a: Tumor involves adnexa.
    pT2b: Tumor involves other pelvic tissues.
    pT2 (subcategory cannot be determined).

  pT3: Tumor infiltrates abdominal tissues.
    pT3a: Tumor infiltrates abdominal tissues in 1 site.
    pT3b: Tumor infiltrates abdominal tissues in > 1 site.
    pT3 (subcategory cannot be determined).

  pT4: Tumor invades bladder or rectum.

pN category

  pN not assigned (no nodes submitted or found).

  pN not assigned (cannot be determined based on available pathological information).

(continued on next page)

pN0: No regional lymph node metastasis.

pN0(i+): Isolated tumor cells in regional lymph node(s) ≤ 0.2 mm.

pN1: Regional lymph node metastasis.

pM category

Not applicable — pM cannot be determined from the submitted specimen(s).

pM1: Distant metastasis (excluding adnexa, pelvic, abdominal tissues, and regional lymph nodes.

Gestational Trophoblastic Disease (GTD)

TYPES OF GTD

108. List the types of gestational trophoblastic diseases.
- Hydatidiform mole:
  · Complete hydatidiform mole.
  · Partial hydatidiform mole.
  · Invasive hydatidiform mole.
- Nonmolar lesions:
  · Placental site trophoblastic tumor.
- Epithelioid trophoblastic tumor.
- Gestational Choriocarcinoma.
- Benign trophoblastic lesions:
  › Exaggerated implantation site reaction.
  › Placental site nodule/atypical placental site nodule.
  › Mixed trophoblastic tumors.

109. Compare complete hydatidiform moles with partial moles.

COMPLETE MOLE	PARTIAL MOLE
• Empty ovum.	• Normal ovum.
• Diploid, 46, XX or 46, XY.	• Triploid, 69, XXY, or 69, XXX.
• Markedly increased β-hCG.	• Normal to moderately increased β-hCG.
• "Snow storm" sign on ultrasound.	• Uterus small for dates.
• Large edematous villi with circumferential trophoblastic proliferations.	• 2 populations of villi, scalloping, some degree of trophoblastic proliferation.
• Trophoblastic atypia often present.	• Trophoblastic atypia usually absent.
• No fetal parts.	• Fetal parts can be identified.
• p57− (absent or very low nuclear staining in villous cytotrophoblast and villous stromal cells).	• p57+.

110. What is the cause of a complete mole?

Fertilization of an empty ovum by 2 sperms or by 1 sperm with duplication — therefore paternally derived.

111. What is the cause of a partial mole?

Fertilization of a normal haploid ovum by 2 sperms with a haploid set of chromosomes **or** by a sperm with a diploid set (diandric).

112. Describe the treatment and prognosis for molar pregnancy.
- After evacuation of a molar pregnancy, the patient is followed with serial serum β-hCG levels to monitor for development of persistent GTD.
  · Risk of persistent GTD:
    › Complete mole: 15–20%.
    › Partial mole: 0.5–5%.
- Patients who have had complete moles are at greater risk of choriocarcinoma.
- Risk of choriocarcinoma:
  › Complete mole: 2–3%.
  › Partial mole: < 0.5%.
- Invasive moles are the most common type of persistent GTD. They may develop following either complete or partial moles.
- In general, patients who have had a molar pregnancy can anticipate a normal

Case Scenario

A uterine curettage specimen from a 37-year-old female showed edematous villi and a single piece of tissue suggestive of squamous cell carcinoma.

113. How do you differentiate hydatidiform moles from hydropic abortus?

- Clinical presentation, β-hCG levels, radiological findings.
- Morphological features:
  - Complete and partial moles: see question 110.
  - Hydropic abortus: no gross abnormality, smooth villi contour with mild hydrops, no significant trophoblastic proliferation (may have mild proliferation in a polarized distribution); no trophoblastic atypia, no trophoblastic inclusions.
- p57 IHC staining:
  - Absent in complete moles; present in partial moles and hydropic abortus.
- Flow cytometry/ploidy analysis:
  - Partial moles: triploid.
  - Complete moles and hydropic abortus: diploid.
- DNA microsatellite marker analysis.

114. Your colleague signed out this case as a molar pregnancy, but you believe it is a nonmolar hydropic change. How would you resolve the discrepancy?

- Discuss the case with your colleague: suggest the ancillary tests listed above.
- If there is no agreement, suggest obtaining another opinion (either intra- or extradepartmental consultation).
- If a final agreement is reached resulting in a change of diagnosis, a revised report should be issued by the original pathologist, and the clinician should be informed.

115. List 4 differential diagnoses for the single fragment of tissue suggestive of squamous cell carcinoma.

- Endometrioid adenocarcinoma of the endometrium, with squamous cell differentiation/morule.
- Squamous cell carcinoma of the cervix or elsewhere in the lower female genital tract.
- Gestational trophoblastic neoplasms including choriocarcinoma, epithelioid trophoblastic tumor (rare).
- Contamination from a different case (floater).

116. How do you prove that the fragment is a contaminant?

- Check levels and deeper slides.
- Cut additional histology sections.
- Check the paraffin block to see whether the tissue fragment is embedded in the block.
- Perform DNA testing.

NONMOLAR TROPHOBLASTIC DISEASES

117. Describe the characteristic histologic and IHC features of placental site trophoblastic tumor (PSTT).

- Histology:
  - Large, pleomorphic implantation-site intermediate trophoblastic cells (mononucleated, amphophilic cells) forming confluent sheets or single cells, with infiltrative growth.
  - Scattered multinucleated cells.
  - Low mitosis.
  - Often vascular invasion.
  - Fibrinoid deposits and dissection of smooth muscle.
- IHC:
  - hPL+++, CD10+, MUC4+, p63–, Ki 67 (10–30%).

118. List the differential diagnosis of PSTT.

- Exaggerated placental site.
- Choriocarcinoma.
- Squamous cell carcinoma, undifferentiated carcinoma.
- Epithelioid trophoblastic tumors.
- Epithelioid smooth muscle tumors.
- Placental site nodule and plaque.

119. Give the prognosis for a patient with PSTT and list some poor prognostic features.

- Some patients (25–30%) may develop recurrent disease or metastasis and about a half of those may die of the disease.
- Poor prognostic features of PSTT include:
  - Clear cytoplasm.
  - Deep myometrial invasion.
  - Large tumor size.
  - Necrosis.
  - High mitotic count (> 5 mitoses/10 high power field).
  - Advanced stage.
  - At least 48 months since antecedent pregnancy.
  - Age more than 40 years.

120. List 2 differences and 2 similarities between PSTT and epithelioid trophoblastic tumors (ETT).

- Differences:
  - Cell of origin.
    - › PSTT: implantation-site intermediate trophoblasts, similar to exaggerated placental site (EPS).
    - › ETT: chorionic type intermediate trophoblasts, similar to placental site nodule (PSN).
  - IHC profile — e.g., PSTT is hPL+++ and p63–; ETT is hPL+/– and p63+ (also see table in answer to question 123).
- Similarities:
  - Clinical presentation.
  - Patient prognosis.

121. What IHC markers does CAP recommend to differentiate trophoblastic lesions?

	PLACENTAL SITE NODULE	PLACENTAL SITE TROPHOBLASTIC TUMOR	EPITHELIOID TROPHOBLASTIC TUMOR	CHORIOCARCINOMA
Mel-Cam (CD146) (membranous)	0–2%	75–100%	0–2%	6–75%
HPL	0–2%	25–75%	0–2%	Positive in IT and ST
ß-hCG	0–25%	0–25%	0–25%	Positive in ST
P63	> 50–75%	Negative	< 25 up to 75%	< 25%
Ki 67 (MIB-1)	3–10%	> 10%	> 10%	69 +/– 20%
Cyclin E	Focal		> 50%	

Abbreviations: HPL: human placental lactogen; IT: intermediate trophoblast; ST: syncytiotrophoblast.

122. What are the most useful IHC stains to differentiate ETT and squamous cell carcinoma (SCC)?

	ETT	SQUAMOUS CELL CARCINOMA
P63	+	+
CK5/6	– or focal	+
P16	–	+ (in HPV associated SCC)
Inhibin	+	20%
CD10	+	20%
HPL	+/–	–
Mel-CAM	+/–	–

123. What is the TNM staging system for reporting gestational trophoblastic tumors, as described and approved by CAP?

Primary tumor (T):

pTX: primary tumor cannot be assessed.

pT0: no evidence of primary tumor.

pT1: tumor confined to uterus.

pT2: tumor extends to other genital structures (vagina, ovary, broad ligament, fallopian tube) by metastasis or direct extension.

Regional lymph nodes (N): this classification does not apply to gestational trophoblastic tumors. Nodal involvement in these tumors is rare but has an extremely poor prognosis. Nodal metastases should be classified as metastatic M1b disease.

Distant metastasis (M):

pM0: no distant metastasis.

pM1: distant metastasis:

pM1a: lung metastasis.

pM1b: all other distant metastasis.

124. What is the FIGO staging system for gestational trophoblastic tumors?

Stage I: disease confined to the uterus.

Stage II: tumor extends outside of the uterus, but is limited to the genital structures (adnexa, vagina, broad ligament).

Stage III: tumor extends to the lungs, +/– known genital tract involvement.

Stage IV: all other metastasis.

Note: stages I to IV are subdivided into low risk and high risk based on prognostic scores.

Cervix
Tumors of the Uterine Cervix

125. Provide the classification for neoplastic squamous tumors.

- Condyloma acuminatum.
- Low grade squamous intraepithelial lesion.
- High grade squamous intraepithelial lesion.
- Squamous cell carcinoma, HPV-associated.
- Squamous cell carcinoma, HPV-independent.
- Squamous cell carcinoma, NOS.

126. What is the appearance of a cervix with low grade squamous intraepithelial lesions on colposcopic examination?

Acetic acid accentuates white changes, iodine negativity, mosaicism, and punctuation which may indicate productive lesions.

127. List methods to diagnose HPV infection.
- Pap smear cytology or H&E morphology.
- IHC p16 as a surrogate marker.
- In situ hybridization.
- DNA HPV testing.

128. Name at least 2 noncervical carcinomas associated with HPV.
- Oropharyngeal squamous cell carcinoma.
- Anal squamous cell carcinoma.
- Vulvar and vaginal squamous cell carcinoma.
- Penile squamous cell carcinoma.

129. List 3 high-risk HPV types and 2 low-risk HPV types.
- High-risk HPV: 16, 18, and 31.
- Low-risk HPV: 6 and 11.

130. Briefly describe the molecular mechanisms by which high-risk HPV causes cancer.
- Two HPV viral proteins, E6 and E7, act to overcome the activity of cell cycle inhibitors.
- E6 binds to p53, inactivating p53 by enhancing its degradation through ubiquitin dependent proteolysis.
- E7 binds to RB, disrupting the E3F/RB complex and promoting the degradation of RB.
- The inhibition of p53 and RB, 2 important tumor suppressor proteins, leads to dysregulation of apoptosis and growth restriction.

Precursor Lesions and Invasive Carcinoma of the Cervix

131. List risk factors for developing cervical cancer.
- HPV infection.
- Smoking.
- Oral contraceptives.
- Immunosuppression.
- Multiparity.

132. What is the prognosis for squamous cell carcinoma (SCC), HPV-independent?
- Frequently presents with advanced stage.
- Higher rate of lymph node metastasis means reduced disease-free and survival rate.

133. Provide the classification of adenocarcinoma of endocervix.
- Adenocarcinoma in situ, NOS.
- Adenocarcinoma in situ. HPV-associated.
- Adenocarcinoma in situ, HPV-independent.
- Adenocarcinoma, NOS.
- Adenocarcinoma, HPV-associated.
- Adenocarcinoma, HPV-independent (NOS, gastric, clear cell, mesonephric type).
- Endometrioid adenocarcinoma, NOS.
- Carcinosarcoma, NOS.
- Adenosquamous carcinoma.
- Mucoepidermoid carcinoma.
- Adenoid basal carcinoma.
- Carcinoma, undifferentiated, NOS.

134. Name the precursor lesion for adenocarcinoma of the uterine cervix.
- Adenocarcinoma in situ, NOS.
- Adenocarcinoma in situ, HPV-associated.
- Adenocarcinoma in situ, HPV-independent.

135. What are the histologic features of adenocarcinoma in situ, HPV-associated?
- Confined to existing glandular architecture.
- Cell crowding.
- Decrease of cytoplasmic mucin.
- Pseudostratification, hyperchromasia.
- Nuclear enlargement/elongation and atypia.
- Increased apical mitoses (floating mitoses) and basal karyorrhexis, apoptotic debris.
- Presence or absence of goblet cells.
- p16 overexpression.

136. Discuss the role of early screening for adenocarcinoma of the uterine cervix.
- Adenocarcinoma is less common than squamous cell carcinoma.
- If atypical glandular cells are present, proceed to colposcopy.
- Sometimes a patient with a squamous intraepithelial lesion (SIL) on screening may have adenocarcinoma/AIS on cone or hysterectomy.

137. List 3 types of invasive cervical carcinoma that are not HPV related.

- Gastric type endocervical adenocarcinoma.
  - The extremely well-differentiated forms are also known as minimal deviation adenocarcinoma/adenoma malignum (not recommended terminology).
  - Association with Peutz-Jeghers syndrome has been noted (*STK11* mutation).
- Clear cell carcinoma.
  - This is associated with diethylstilbestrol (DES) exposure.
- Mesonephric carcinoma.
  - This is associated with mesonephric remnants.

138. Describe how to gross a cone specimen and a radical hysterectomy specimen.

- Cone specimen:
  - Orient the specimen if possible, and ink the margins.
  - Open and measure.
  - Serially section into wedge shaped sections along the axis of cervical canal.
  - Submit 1 section per cassette; respect the order.
  - Submit in toto.
- Radical hysterectomy specimen:
  - Orient; ink resection margins; identify and examine parametrial tissue; assess vaginal extension and margins.
  - Amputate the cervix with vaginal cuff; open at 12 o'clock position.
  - If the tumor is grossly identified, measure the size of the tumor; take representative blocks to demonstrate the maximum depth of invasion. Sample the vaginal tissue (submit entire vaginal cuff if tumor is at or close to vaginal margin). Carefully assess the parametrium for lymph nodes. Sample parametrium. Sample the rest of the uterus and adnexa accordingly.
  - If the tumor is not grossly identified, submit the entire cervix in a fashion similar to a cone biopsy.

139. What mandatory information does CAP recommend in reporting cervical cancer for a resection specimen?

- Procedure.
- Hysterectomy type.
- Tumor site.
- Tumor size.
- Histologic type.
- Histologic grade.
- Stromal invasion.
- Other tissue/organ involvement.
- Lymphovascular invasion.
- Margin status for invasive carcinoma.
- Margin status for HSIL or AIS.
- Regional lymph node status.
- Distant site(s) involved.

140. In the CAP protocol, which margins should be reported? How should you report the margin status?

- Margins to report in 1 specimen include:
  - Endocervical/lower uterine segment margin.
  - Ectocervical margin.
  - Radial/circumferential margin.
  - Vaginal margin (if applicable).
- For margin status:
  - Report margin status for invasive carcinoma as:
    › Margins involved by invasive carcinoma: specify the involved margin.
    › All margins negative for invasive carcinoma: measure the distance of invasive carcinoma to the closest margin in mm; specify the closest margin.
  - Report margin status for HSIL/AIS as:
    › HSIL/AIS present at margin: specify the involved margin.
    › All margins negative for HSIL/AIS.

141. How is the depth of invasion measured in cervical cancer? Does presence of lymphovascular invasion alter the staging?

- The depth of invasion is measured from its HSIL origin, that is, from the base of the epithelium, whether epithelial surface or an endocervical gland that is involved by HSIL to the deepest point of invasion.
- If there is no obvious epithelial origin, the depth is measured from the deepest focus of tumor invasion to the base of the nearest surface epithelium, regardless of whether it is dysplastic or not.
- In situations where carcinomas are exclusively or predominantly exophytic, there may be little or no invasion of the underlying stroma. The tumor thickness (from the surface of the tumor to the deepest point of invasion) should be measured. The depth of invasion should not be provided in these cases.
- Vascular space involvement, either venous or lymphatic, does not alter the staging.
  - The presence of lymphovascular invasion in biopsy or cone specimens may change the extent of subsequent surgical treatment.
  - The presence of lymphovascular invasion may be an independent risk factor for recurrence.

142. How do you define superficial invasive squamous cell carcinoma (SISCCA)?

- The diagnosis of SISCCA must meet the following 3 criteria:
  - The carcinoma is strictly confined to the cervix.
  - The carcinoma can be diagnosed only by microscopy.
  - The depth of the carcinoma is ≤ 3 mm of stromal invasion.

A slide shows a well-differentiated adenocarcinoma from uterine curettings.

143. What is the major differential diagnosis?
- Endometrioid adenocarcinoma of the endometrium.
- Endocervical adenocarcinoma.

144. What morphological features establish the diagnosis?
- Endometrioid adenocarcinoma:
  - Background endometrial atypical hyperplasia/EIN.
  - Squamous metaplasia.
  - Foamy macrophages in the stroma.
  - Lack of squamous intraepithelial lesion.
- Endocervical adenocarcinoma:
  - Markedly increased apical mitotic rate and apoptotic bodies.
  - Elongated "pencil shape" nuclei.
  - Background AIS and/or SIL.
  - No evidence of endometrial hyperplasia.

145. List IHC markers to differentiate endometrial from endocervical carcinoma.

IHC MARKER	ENDOCERVICAL ADENOCARCINOMA, HPV ASSOCIATED	ENDOMETRIAL (ENDOMETRIOID)
p16	+++ (block staining)	+/− ("skip pattern")
CEA, monoclonal	+++	+/−
ER	+/−	+++
PR	+/−	+++
Vimentin	+/−	+++

- Additional ancillary test: HPV in situ hybridization.

146. Describe the TNM staging system for reporting cervical cancer, as described and approved by CAP.

pT category

pT not assigned (cannot be determined based on available pathological information).

pT0: No evidence of primary tumor.

pT1: Carcinoma is strictly confined to the cervix (extension to the corpus should be disregarded).

  pT1a: Invasive carcinoma that can be diagnosed only by microscopy with maximum depth of invasion ≤ 5 mm.

  pT1a1: Measured stromal invasion ≤ 3 mm in depth.

  pT1a2: Measured stromal invasion > 3 mm and ≤ 5 mm in depth.

  pT1a (subcategory cannot be determined).

  pT1b: Invasive carcinoma with measured deepest invasion greater than 5 mm (greater than stage IA); lesion limited to the cervix uteri with size measured by maximum tumor diameter.

  pT1b1: Invasive carcinoma > 5 mm depth of stromal invasion and ≤ 2 cm in greatest dimension.

  pT1b2: Invasive carcinoma > 2 cm and ≤ 4 cm in greatest dimension.

  pT1b3: Invasive carcinoma > 4 cm in greatest dimension.

  pT1b (subcategory cannot be determined).

  pT1 (subcategory cannot be determined).

pT2: Carcinoma invades beyond the uterus, but has not extended onto the lower third of the vagina or to the pelvic wall.

  pT2a: Involvement limited to the upper two-thirds of the vagina without parametrial invasion.

  pT2a1: Invasive carcinoma ≤ 4 cm in greatest dimension.

  pT2a2: Invasive carcinoma > 4 cm in greatest dimension.

  pT2a (subcategory cannot be determined).

  pT2b: With parametrial invasion but not up to the pelvic wall.

  pT2 (subcategory cannot be determined).

pT3: Carcinoma involves the lower third of the vagina and/or extends to the pelvic wall and/or causes hydronephrosis or nonfunctioning kidney.

  pT3a: Carcinoma involves lower third of the vagina, with no extension to the pelvic wall.

  pT3b: Extension to the pelvic wall and/or hydronephrosis or nonfunctioning kidney (unless known to be due to another cause).

  pT3 (subcategory cannot be determined).

pT4: Carcinoma has involved (biopsy-proven) the mucosa of the bladder or rectum, or has spread to adjacent organs. (Bullous edema, as such, does not permit a case to be assigned to stage 4.)

pN category

pN not assigned (no nodes submitted or found).

pN not assigned (cannot be determined based on available pathological information).

pN0: No regional lymph node metastasis.

pN0(i+): Isolated tumor cells in regional lymph node(s) ≤ 0.2 mm, or single cells or clusters of cells ≤ 200 cells in a single lymph node cross-section.

(continued on next page)

pN1mi: Regional lymph node metastasis (> 0.2 mm but ≤ 2.0 mm) to pelvic lymph nodes.

pN1a: Regional lymph node metastasis (> 2.0 mm diameter) to pelvic lymph nodes.

pN1 (subcategory cannot be determined).

pN2mi: Regional lymph node metastasis to paraaortic lymph nodes (> 0.2 mm but ≤ 2.0 mm +/- positive pelvic lymph nodes.

pN2a: Regional lymph node metastasis to paraaortic lymph nodes (> 2.0 mm in diameter) +/- positive pelvic lymph nodes.

pN2 (subcategory cannot be determined).

pM category (required only if confirmed pathologically)

Not applicable - pM cannot be determined from the submitted specimen(s).

pM1: Distant metastasis (includes metastasis to inguinal lymph nodes, intraperitoneal disease, lung, liver, or bone; excludes metastasis to pelvic or paraaortic lymph nodes, or vagina). Uterine serosa and adnexa involvement are considered M1 disease.

Vagina
Primary Vaginal Malignancy

147. Why are clinical history and pathological history important in diagnosing primary vaginal malignancy? Give examples of relevant history.

- Many tumors extend to the vagina and are thus not vaginal primary, including:
  - Squamous cell carcinomas that also involve vulva or cervix.
  - Adenocarcinoma involving the vagina either by direct extension or metastases, commonly from the endometrium, colorectal, ovary, vulva, urethra, or urinary bladder.
- Helpful clinical and pathological history includes:
  - A history of dysplasia, carcinoma in situ, or invasive carcinoma of the cervix, as well as details of microscopic features.
  - A history of a carcinoma higher in the female genital tract.
  - Prior pathology slides and reports (should be reviewed if needed).
  - A history of DES exposure.

148. Provide the classification for neoplastic squamous tumors of the vagina.

- Condyloma acuminatum.
- Low grade squamous intraepithelial lesion.
- High grade squamous intraepithelial lesion.
- Squamous cell carcinoma, HPV-associated.
- Squamous cell carcinoma, HPV-independent.
- Squamous cell carcinoma, NOS.

149. Provide the classification for neoplastic glandular tumors of the vagina.

- Adenocarcinoma, NOS.
- Adenocarcinoma, HPV-associated.
- Endometrioid adenocarcinoma, NOS.
- Clear cell carcinoma, NOS.
- Mucinous carcinoma, gastric type.
- Mucinous adenocarcinoma.
- Mesonephric adenocarcinoma.
- Carcinosarcoma, NOS.
- Mixed tumors, NOS.
- Carcinoma of Skene (Cowper and Littré) glands.
- Adenosquamous carcinoma.
- Adenoid basal carcinoma.

150. List reporting elements recommended by CAP for vaginal resection specimens.

- Procedure.
- Tumor site.
- Tumor size (in cm).
- Histologic type.
- Histologic grade.
- Site(s) involved by direct tumor extension.
- Margins.
- Lymphovascular invasion.
- Regional lymph nodes.
- Pathological stage.

151. Describe the TNM staging system for reporting vaginal carcinoma, as described in the AJCC and UICC.

Primary tumor (T)

pTX: Primary tumor cannot be assessed.

pT0: No evidence of primary tumor.

pT1: Tumor confined to vaginal wall.
  pT1a: Tumor confined to vaginal wall, ≤ 2 cm.
  pT1b: Tumor confined to vaginal wall, > 2 cm.

pT2: Tumor invades paravaginal tissues but no the pelvic wall.
  pT2a: Tumor invades paravaginal tissues but not the pelvic wall, ≤ 2 cm.
  pT2b: Tumor invades paravaginal tissues but not the pelvic wall, > 2 cm.

(continued on next page)

pT3: Tumor extends to pelvic wall and/or causing hydronephrosis or nonfunctioning kidney.

pT4: Tumor invades mucosa of bladder or rectum and/or extends beyond the true pelvis (Bullous edema is not sufficient to classify a tumor as T4).

Regional lymph nodes (N)

pNX: Regional lymph nodes cannot be assessed.

pN0: No regional lymph node metastasis.

pN0(i+): Isolated tumor cells in regional lymph node(s) ≤ 0.2 mm.

pN1: Pelvic or inguinal lymph node metastasis.

Distant metastasis (M)

pM0: No distant metastasis.

pM1: Distant metastasis.

Vulva
Nonsquamous Neoplasms of the Vulva

152. List examples of primary glandular carcinoma of the vulva.
- Paget disease.
- Adenocarcinoma of the mammary gland type.
- Bartholin gland carcinomas.
- Sweat gland type carcinomas.
- Phyllodes tumors, malignant.
- Adenocarcinoma of anogenital mammary-like glands.
- Adenoid cystic carcinoma.
- Neuroendocrine tumor, NOS.
- Adenocarcinoma, intestinal type.

Extramammary Paget Disease

153. List the possible sites for extramammary Paget disease.
- Vulva.
- Perineum.
- Anus.
- Scrotum.
- Axilla.

154. Describe the morphological features and IHC profile for primary vulvar Paget disease.
- Cells lying singly or in small clusters within the epidermis (basal layers) and its appendages.
- Large round cells with pale cytoplasm, a large nucleus, and prominent nucleolus.
- "Halo" around cells — each cell has a clear separation from the surrounding epithelial cells.
- Finely granular cytoplasm containing mucin.
- Inflammatory response in the superficial dermis.
- Positive for CK7, EMA, CEA, GATA3, HER2/neu (ERBB2), androgen receptor, GCDFP-15; negative for S100, HMB45, CK20, ER, PR, uroplakin-3, CDX2.

155. List the differential diagnoses of primary vulvar Paget disease.
- Primary squamous intraepithelial lesion, HPV-associated.
- Vulvar intraepithelial neoplasia, HPV-independent.
- Melanoma.
- Merkel cell carcinoma intraepithelial component.
- Secondary Paget disease: colorectal, bladder, cervical carcinoma.

Squamous Vulvar Lesions

156. List 4 types of lesions in the vulva that can have a verruciform appearance.
- Condyloma.
- Seborrheic keratosis.
- Verrucous carcinoma.
- Verruciform squamous cell carcinoma.

157. Provide the classification for vulvar squamous precursors.
- Squamous intraepithelial lesions, HPV-associated:
  · Low grade squamous intraepithelial lesion (VIN 1).
  · High grade squamous intraepithelial lesion (VIN 2, 3).
- Squamous intraepithelial neoplasia, HPV-independent/ differentiated vulvar intraepithelial neoplasia (VIN):
  · Differentiated exophytic vulvar intraepithelial lesion.
  · Vulvar acanthosis with altered differentiation.

158. Compare the 2 types of vulvar squamous precursors.

SQUAMOUS INTRAEPITHELIAL LESIONS, HPV-ASSOCIATED	DIFFERENTIATED VIN
• Associated with high-risk HPV (most commonly HPV 16), cigarette smoking, immunocompromise. • Younger females. • Often asymptomatic, pruritus and irritation. • Multifocal and multicentric lesions. • White, erythematous, or pigmented macules, papules, or verrucous plaques. • Loss of maturation, nuclear hyperchromasia, high nuclear-cytoplasmic ratios and mitoses. • Basaloid and/or warty patterns. • Precursor lesion for squamous cell carcinoma variants: basaloid, warty (condylomatous), mixed, keratinizing (rare). • p16: diffuse, block staining, p53 wild type. • Relatively low risk of progression into an invasive squamous cell carcinoma.	• Associated with preexisting inflammatory disorder (lichen sclerosus or lichen planus). • Postmenopausal women. • Long history of itching and burning, pruritus, irritation, pain. • Often unifocal and unicentric lesions. • Thick keratinized plaques; erosive erythematous macules or plaques. • Often normal maturation, basal hyperchromasia, basal atypical mitoses, atypical keratinocytes, parakeratosis, dyskeratosis. • Can have basaloid, warty exophytic growth, acanthotic or verruciform architecture. • Background of vulvar dystrophy. • Precursor lesion for keratinizing squamous cell carcinoma, usually well differentiated, verrucous carcinoma. • p53 abnormal in basal layer; p16 normal or negative. • High risk and short time of progression into an invasive squamous cell carcinoma.

159. Provide the classification for squamous cell carcinoma of the vulva.
- Squamous cell carcinoma (SCC), HPV-associated.
- Squamous cell carcinoma (SCC), HPV-independent.
- Squamous cell carcinoma (SCC), NOS.

160. List 3 differential diagnoses of invasive vulvar squamous cell carcinoma.
- Pseudoepitheliomatous hyperplasia.
- Keratoacanthoma.
- Tangential sectioning, or adnexal involvement by squamous intraepithelial lesions.

161. How do you measure depth of invasion and tumor thickness in vulvar carcinoma?
- Depth of invasion: in millimeters, measured from the dermal-epidermal junction of the adjacent most superficial dermal papilla to the deepest point of invasion.
- Tumor thickness: in millimeters, measured from the surface of the tumor or, if there is surface keratinization, from the bottom of the granular layer to the deepest point of invasion.

162. Describe the management implications of VIN and invasive carcinoma in the vulva.
- Squamous intraepithelial lesions, HPV-associated: topical imiquimod, local excision, cidofovir, and photodynamic or laser therapy.
- Squamous intraepithelial neoplasia, HPV-independent/differentiated VIN: complete excision.
- Squamous cell carcinoma, stage IA (size ≤ 2 cm, depth of invasion ≤ 1 mm): wide local excision without vulvectomy or node sampling.
- Higher stage squamous cell carcinoma: more extensive surgery including partial or total vulvectomy, with groin lymph node assessment.

163. List recommended CAP reporting elements for vulvar cancer.
- Procedure.
- Specimen size.
- Tumor site.
- Tumor size.
- Tumor focality.
- Histologic type.
- Histologic grade.
- Depth of invasion.
- Other tissue/organ involvement.
- Margins.
- Lymphovascular invasion.
- Lymph nodes.
- Distant site(s) involved.
- Pathologic stage.

164. What is the significance of vascular space invasion in vulvar squamous cell carcinoma?
Vascular space invasion by squamous cell carcinoma has been associated with a poorer prognosis, including a risk factor for regional lymph node metastasis.

165. Why does extranodal extension matter?
Extranodal extension and the size of lymph node metastasis have been shown to reflect a poor prognosis.

166. Describe the TNM staging system for reporting vulvar carcinoma, as described and approved by CAP.

Primary tumor (T):

pTX: primary tumor cannot be assessed.

pT0: no evidence of primary tumor.

pT1a: lesions ≤ 2 cm in size, confined to the vulva or perineum and with stromal invasion ≤ 1.0 mm.

pT1b: lesions > 2 cm in size or any size with stromal invasion > 1.0 mm, confined to the vulva or perineum.

pT2: tumor of any size with extension to adjacent perineal structures (lower/distal third of urethra, lower/distal third of vagina, anal involvement).

pT3: tumor of any size with extension to any of the following: upper/proximal two-thirds of urethra, upper/proximal two thirds of vagina, bladder mucosa, rectal mucosa, or fixed to pelvic bone.

Regional lymph nodes (N):

pNX: regional lymph nodes cannot be assessed.

pN0: no regional lymph node metastasis.

pN0(i+): isolated tumor cells in regional lymph node(s) ≤ 0.2 mm.

pN1: 1–2 regional lymph nodes with the following features:

pN1a: 1–2 lymph node metastasis each < 5 mm.

pN1b: 1 lymph node metastasis ≥ 5 mm.

pN2: regional lymph nodes metastasis with the following features:

pN2a: 3 or more lymph node metastasis each < 5 mm.

pN2b: 2 or more lymph node metastasis ≥ 5 mm.

pN2c: lymph node metastasis with extranodal spread.

pN3: fixed or ulcerated regional lymph node metastasis.

Distant metastasis (M):

pM0: no distant metastasis.

pM1: distant metastasis, including pelvic lymph node metastasis.

Miscellaneous Lesions
Endometriosis

167. List common sites of involvement by endometriosis.
- Ovaries.
- Uterine ligaments.
- Fallopian tubes.
- Rectovaginal septum.
- Pelvic peritoneum.
- Laparotomy scars.
- Umbilicus.
- Vagina.
- Vulva.
- Appendix.

168. Outline 3 theories of pathogenesis for endometriosis.
- Regurgitation/implantation theory: retrograde menstruation through the fallopian tube out into the peritoneum, cervical mucosa.
- Metaplastic theory: arises from coelomic epithelium, from which mullerian ducts and endometrium originate.
- Vascular or lymphatic dissemination theory: pelvic veins and lymphatics spread to lungs and lymph nodes.

169. Name tumors associated with endometriosis.
- Endometrioid carcinoma.
- Clear cell carcinoma.
- Seromucinous borderline tumor.
- Rare: endometrial stromal sarcoma, carcinosarcoma, adenosarcoma.

170. List the fibroblastic and myofibroblastic tumors of the lower genital tract.
- Postoperative spindle cell nodule: location: vagina, vulva, cervix, endometrium.
- Fibroepithelial stromal polyp: location: vagina ++, rare in vulva, cervix.
- Prepubertal fibroma: location: vulva.
- Superficial myofibroblastoma: location: vagina ++, rare in vulva, cervix.
- Myofibroblastoma: location: vagina/vulva, peritoneum.
- Cellular angiofibroma: location: vagina/vulva.
- Angiomyofibroblastoma: location: vulva.
- Solitary fibrous tumor: location: vagina, vulva, rarely cervix.
- Dermatofibrosarcoma protuberans: location: labia majora > mons pubis > clitorus.
- NTRK-rearranged spindle cell neoplasm (emerging): location: cervix and/or lower uterine segment.

IMAGES: GYNECOLOGIC PATHOLOGY

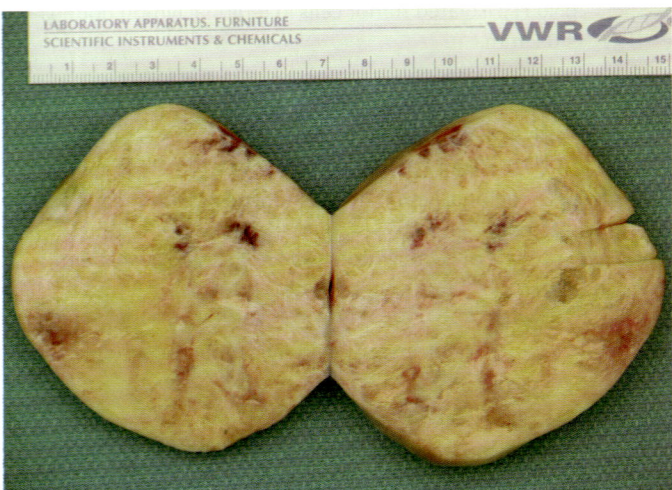

IMAGE 11.1 Ovarian fibroma. Ovarian fibromas are solid firm masses with white lobulated cut surfaces. Myxoid changes may be present.

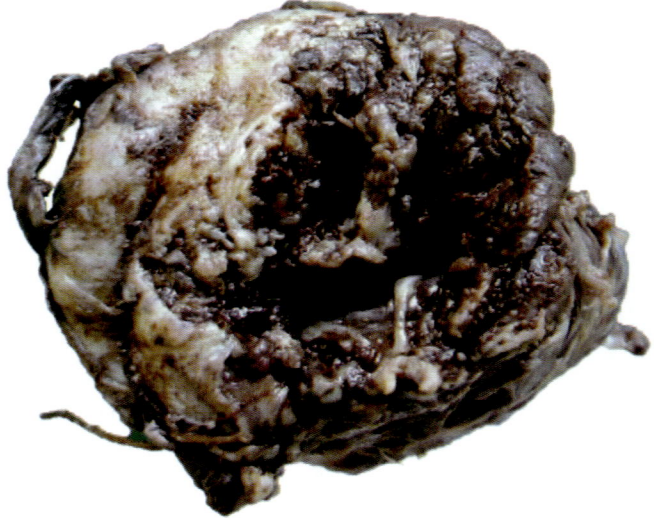

IMAGE 11.2 Cystic ovarian lesion (endometriosis). This dark brown cystic lesion of the ovary is consistent with endometriosis microscopically.

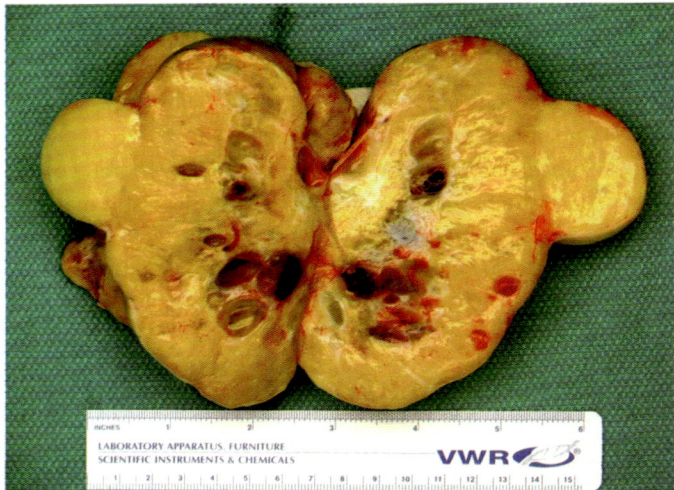

IMAGE 11.3 Ovarian thecoma. Ovarian thecomas are solid masses with cystic changes. Cut surface is yellow.

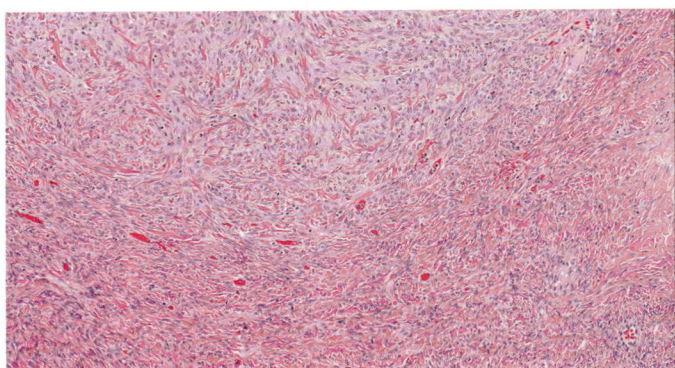

IMAGE 11.4 Ovarian thecoma. The image shows diffuse growth of uniform tumor cells with oval to round nuclei, pale-grey cytoplam, indistinct cell membranes. Reticulin stain will surround individual cells.

IMAGE 11.5 Ovarian cellular fibroma. The image shows dense, bland fibromatous spindle cells. There is no severe nuclear atypia, necrosis, or high mitosis.

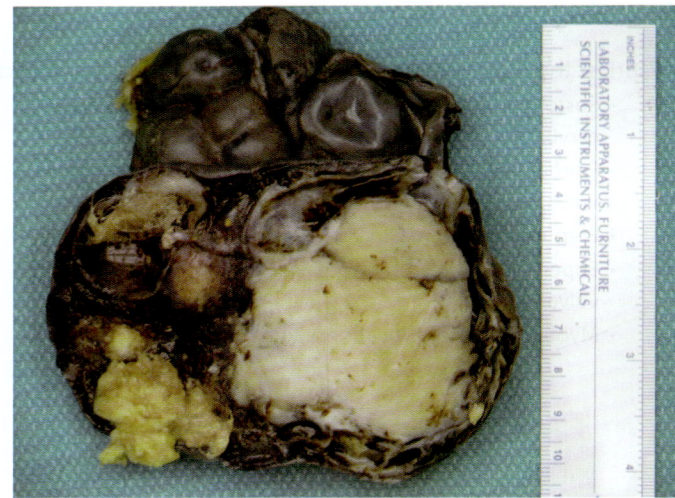

IMAGE 11.6 Ovarian mature teratoma. These are often cystic with keratinaceous debris, hair, and occasionally areas of cartilage and pigmentation.

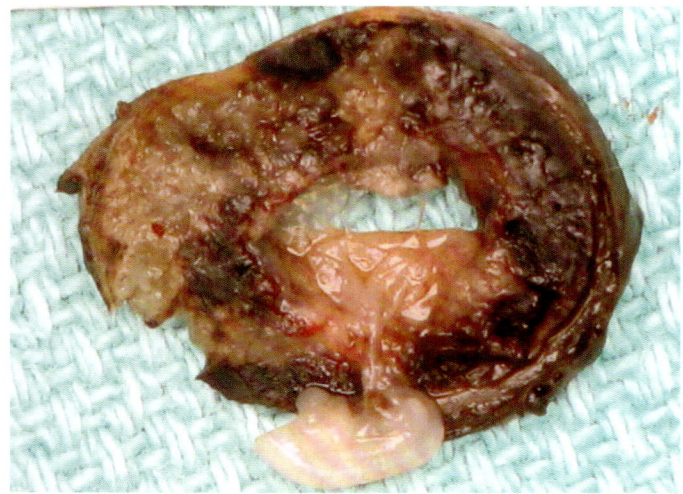

IMAGE 11.7 Tubal pregnancy. The image shows an edematous fallopian tube with areas of hemorrhage. A small embryo is present at the bottom of the image.

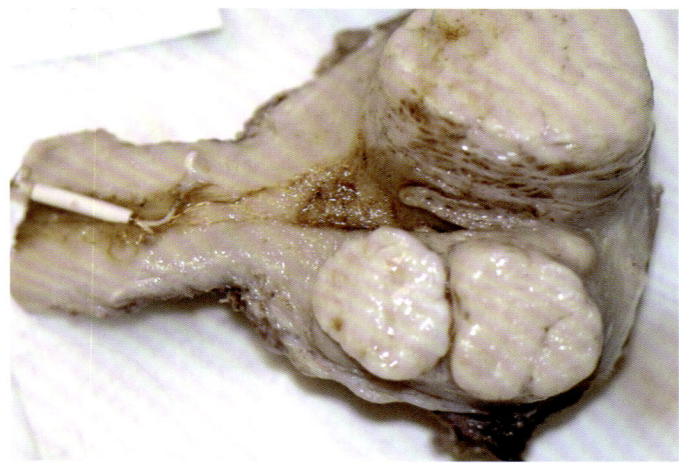

IMAGE 11.10 IUD and leiomyomata. An IUD is seen in the endocervical canal. The cut surfaces of the leiomyomata are white and whorled.

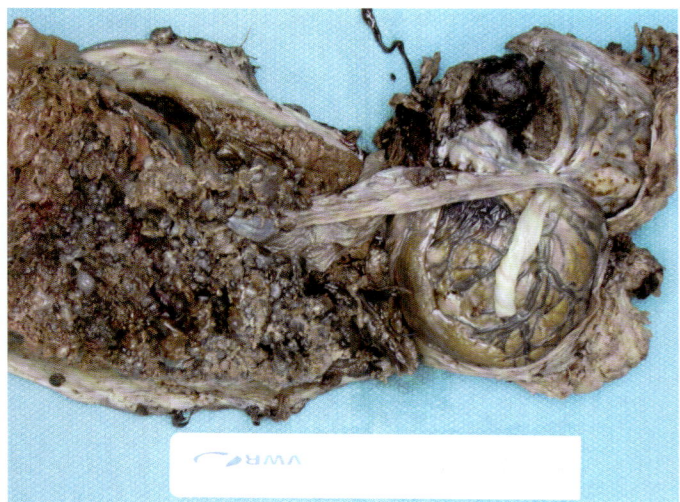

IMAGE 11.8 Twin with molar pregnancy. On the right, there is a normal placenta with an umbilical cord identified along with membranes. On the left, there is a molar pregnancy.

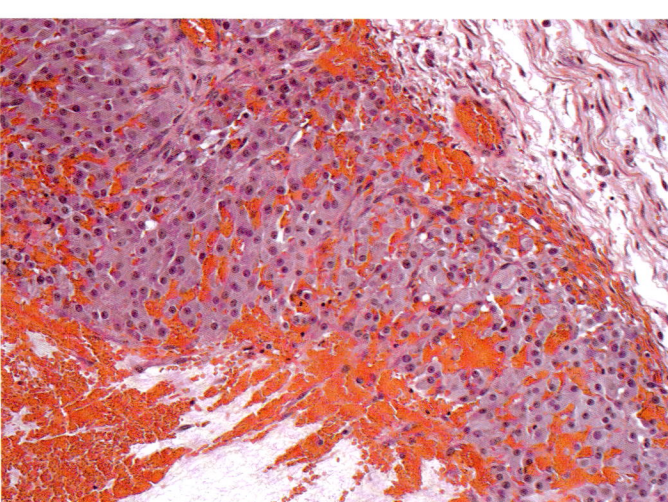

IMAGE 11.11 Ovary corpus luteal cyst. The cyst wall is composed of a luteinized inner granulosa cell layer and an outer theca cell layer.

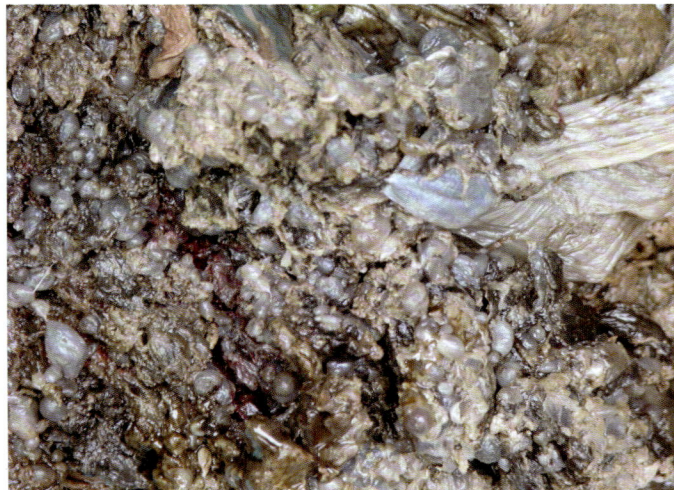

IMAGE 11.9 Twin with molar pregnancy. The image shows a close-up of the hydropic villi in the molar pregnancy.

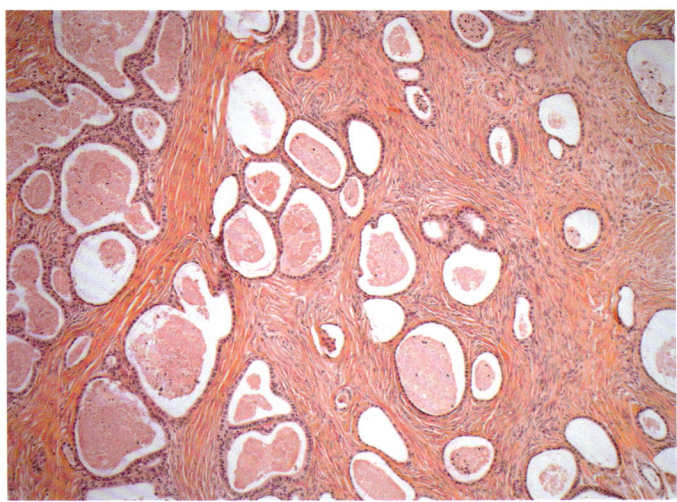

IMAGE 11.12 Ovarian serous cystadenofibroma. This lesion has a glandular pattern with a dense fibrous stroma.

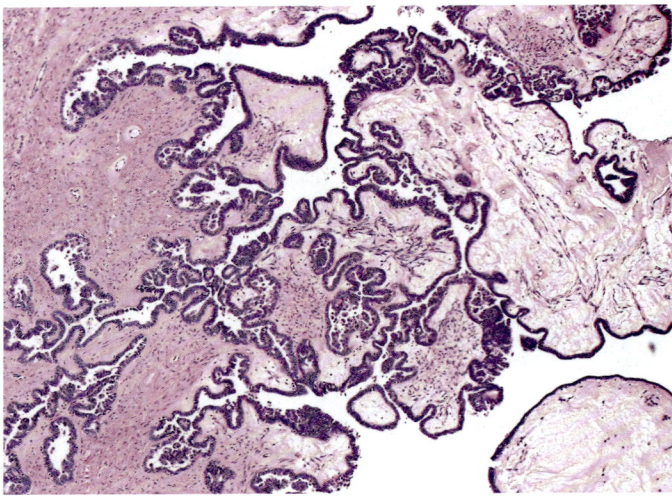

IMAGE 11.13 Ovarian SBT (serous borderline tumor). This lesion has papillary architecture with smaller tufts and epithelial hyerplasia. Note that there are no areas of invasion or solid and cribriform architecture.

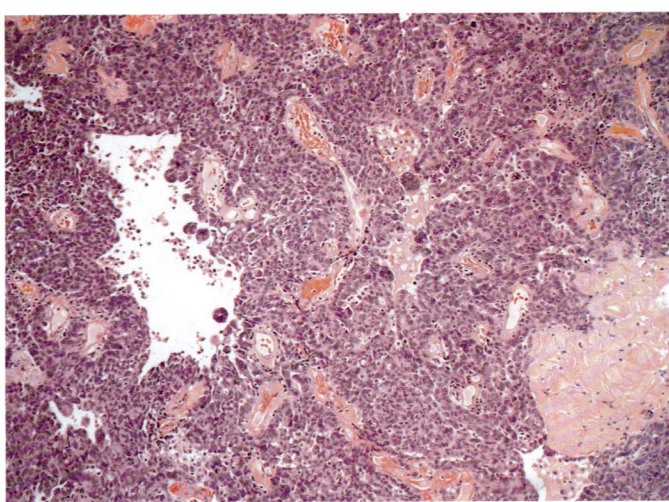

IMAGE 11.16 Ovarian HGSC (high grade serous carcinoma). The image shows solid and papillary growth with marked cytologic atypia.

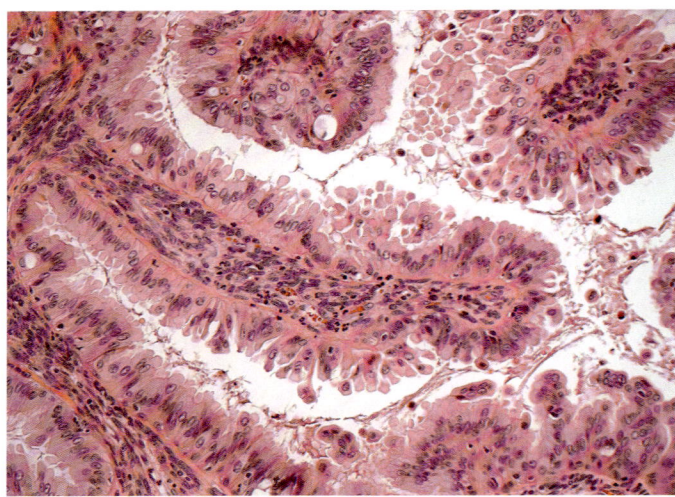

IMAGE 11.14 Ovarian seromucinous borderline tumor (endocervical type mucinous borderline tumor). This lesion has papillary architecture with columnar cells that have bland basal nuclei and apical mucin.

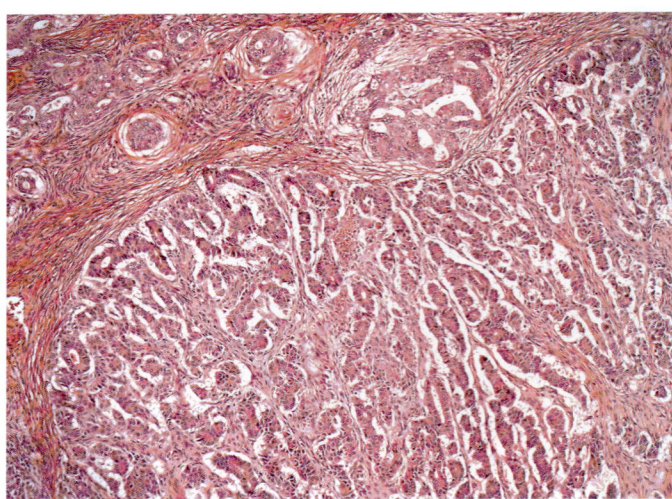

IMAGE 11.17 Ovarian endometrioid adenocarcinoma. The image shows glandular growth with glands that resemble endometrial epithelium.

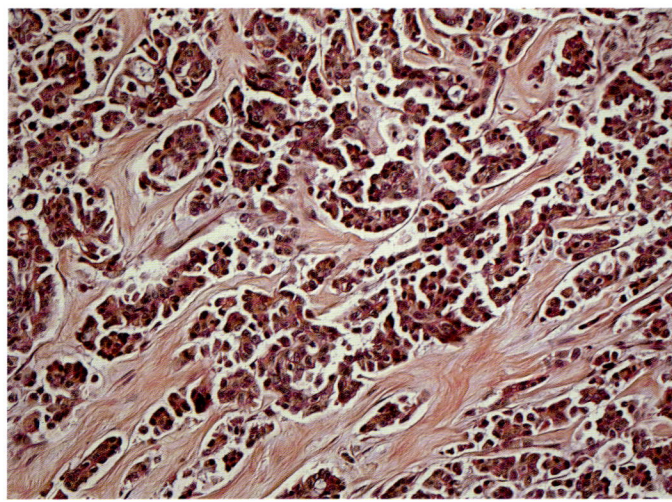

IMAGE 11.15 Ovarian LGSC (low grade serous carcinoma). The tumor infiltrates stroma with micropapillary growth pattern.

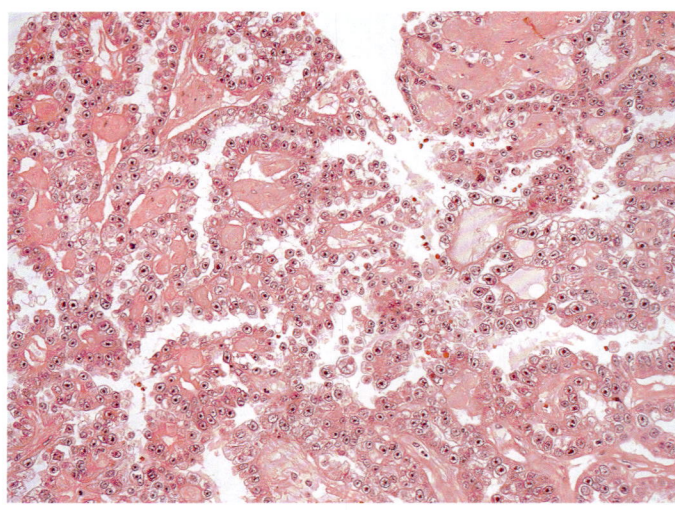

IMAGE 11.18 Ovarian clear cell carcinoma. This carcinoma has papillary architecture with hobnail cells and clearing of the cytoplasm. Note the prominent nucleoli and stromal hyalinization.

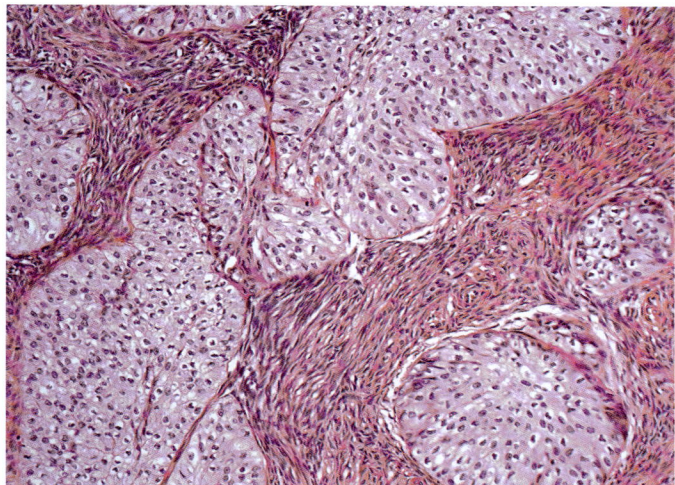

IMAGE 11.19 Ovarian benign Brenner tumor. The image shows nests of cells that resemble the urothelial epithelium.

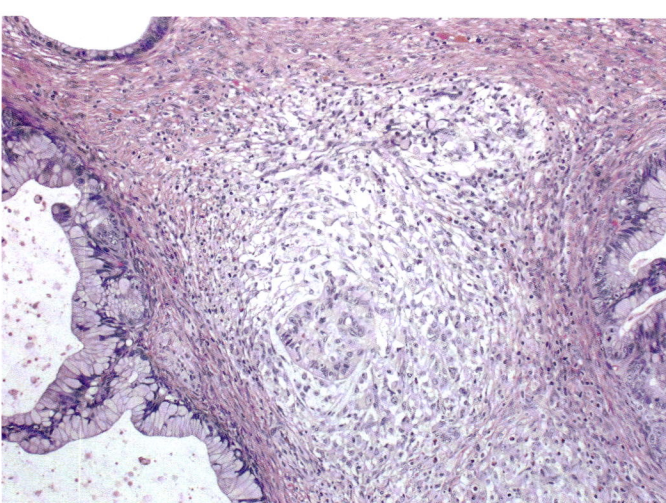

IMAGE 11.22 Ovarian mucinous borderline tumor with microinvasion.

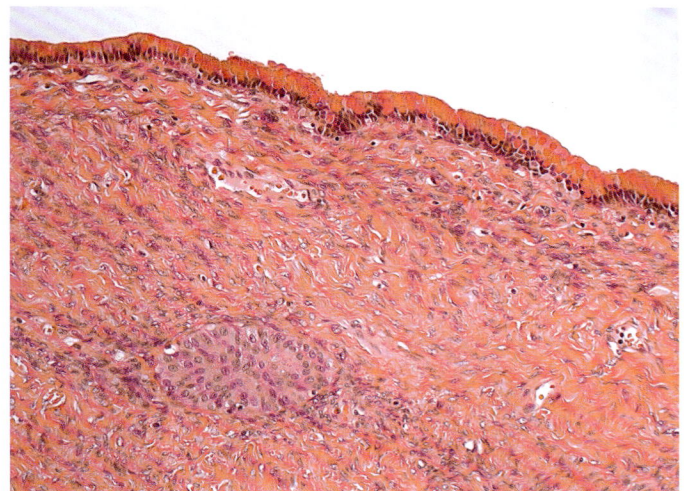

IMAGE 11.20 Ovarian mucinous cystadenoma with Brenner tumor. The top part of the image demonstrates a mucinous epithelial lining; in the stroma, there is a nest of cells resembling urothelial epithelium.

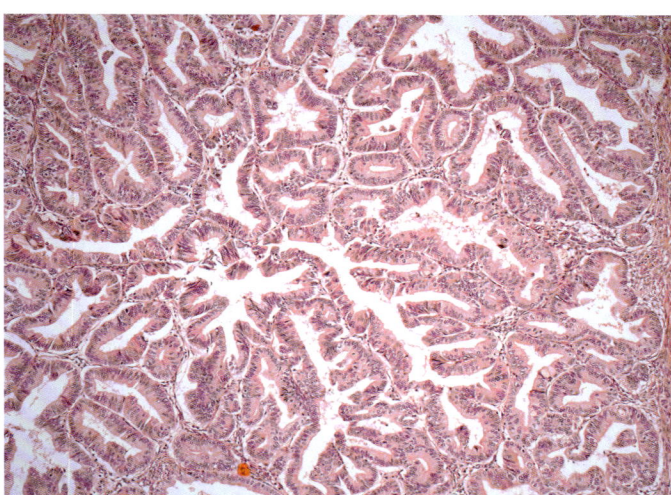

IMAGE 11.23 Ovarian mucinous adenocarcinoma. The image shows a complex pattern of glands with expansile type of invasion.

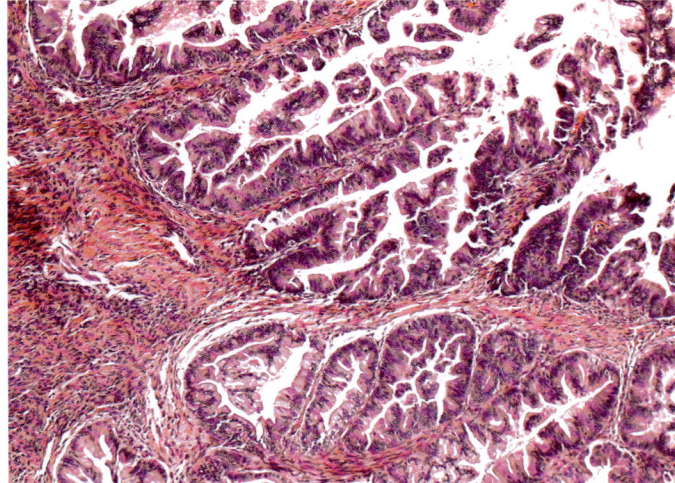

IMAGE 11.21 Ovarian mucinous borderline tumor. The image shows stratified epithelium with tufting present.

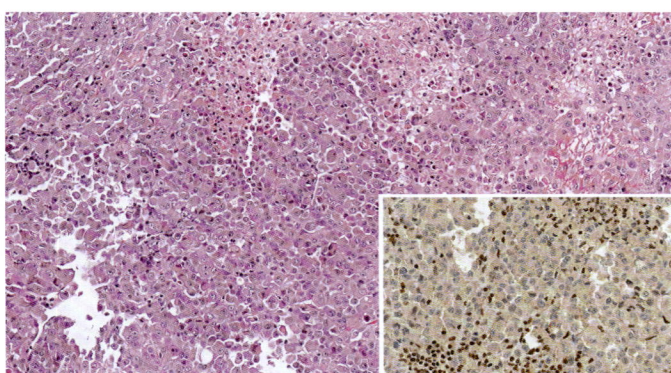

IMAGE 11.24 Ovarian small cell carcinoma, hypercalcemic type. The image shows round and oval cells with nucleoli and focal rhabdoid appearance; tumor necrosis and high mitosis; and loss of BRG1 nuclear staining (internal control-lymphocytes: normal-intact nuclear staining).

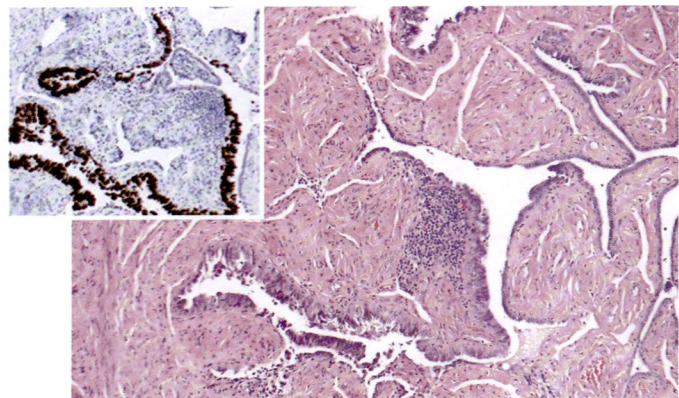

IMAGE 11.25 Serous tubal intraepithelial carcinoma (STIC). The image shows epithelial tufting, loss of polarity, nuclear enlargement, hyperchromasia, nucleolar prominence, and presence of mitosis and apoptosis. The finding for p53 is abnormal, overexpression.

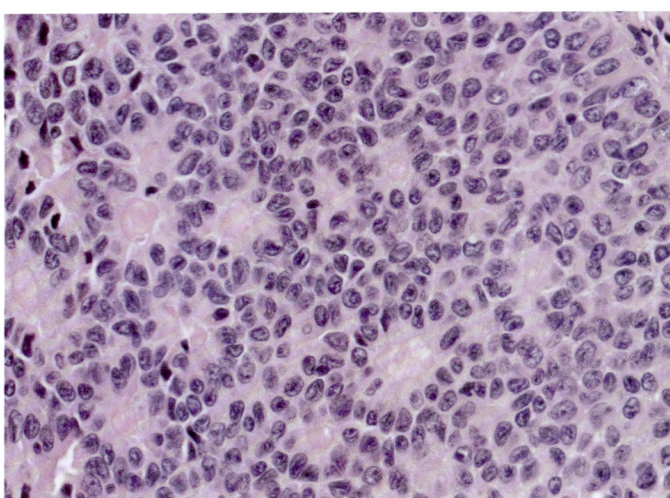

IMAGE 11.28 Ovarian AGCT. This is a high power view of the Call-Exner bodies. Grooves can be seen in some of the nuclei.

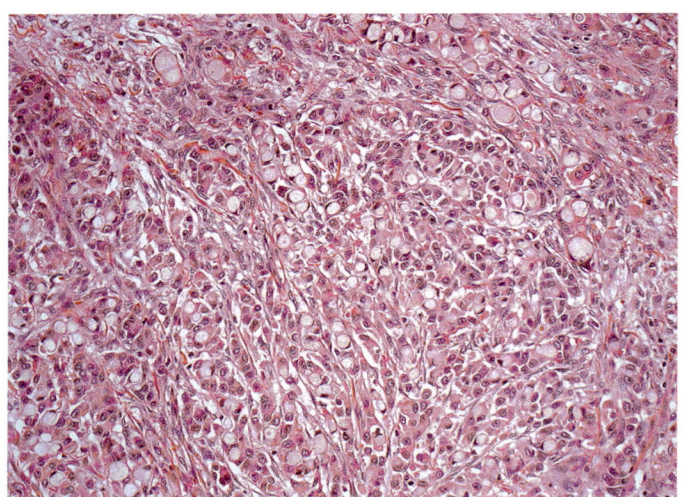

IMAGE 11.26 Metastatic signet-ring cell carcinoma to the ovary. The image shows solid proliferation replacing the parenchyma with cords and single cells with signet ring appearance.

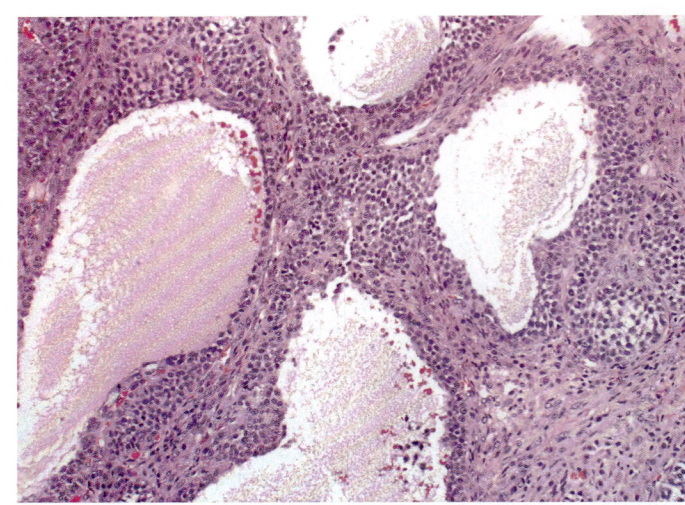

IMAGE 11.29 Ovarian JGCT (juvenile granulosa cell tumor). The image shows solid areas with immature follicles.

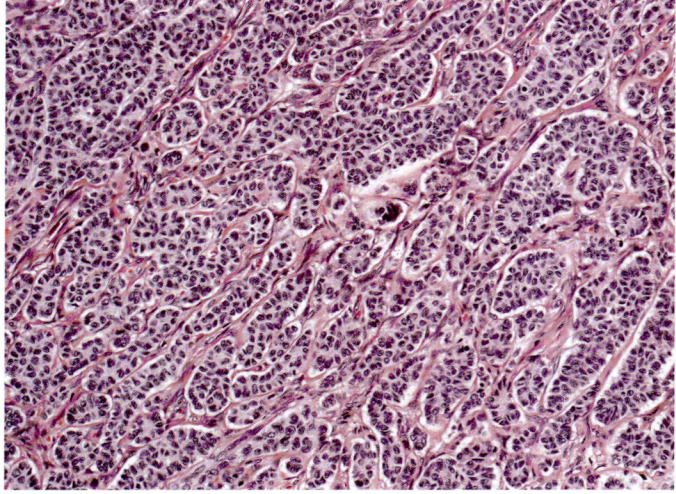

IMAGE 11.27 Ovarian AGCT (adult granulosa cell tumor). This is a low power view showing calcification.

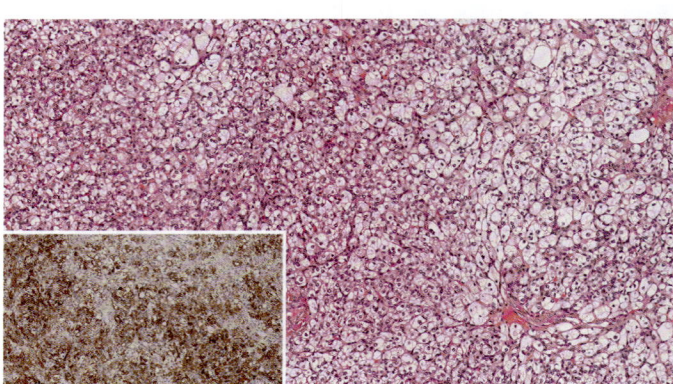

IMAGE 11.30 Ovarian steroid cell tumor. The image shows diffuse growth of large polygonal cells with abundant vacuolated (lipid-rich) cytoplasm; and scant fibrous bands in the stroma. Ovarian steroid cell tumor is diffusely positive with inhibin.

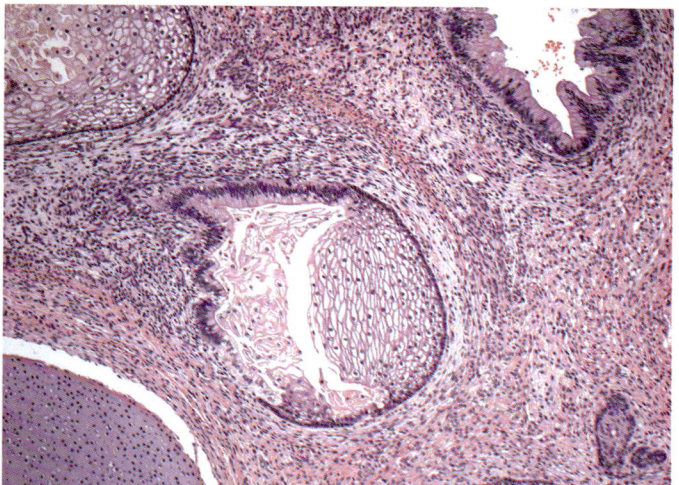

IMAGE 11.31 Ovarian mature teratoma. The image shows mucinous, squamous, and cartilaginous differentiation.

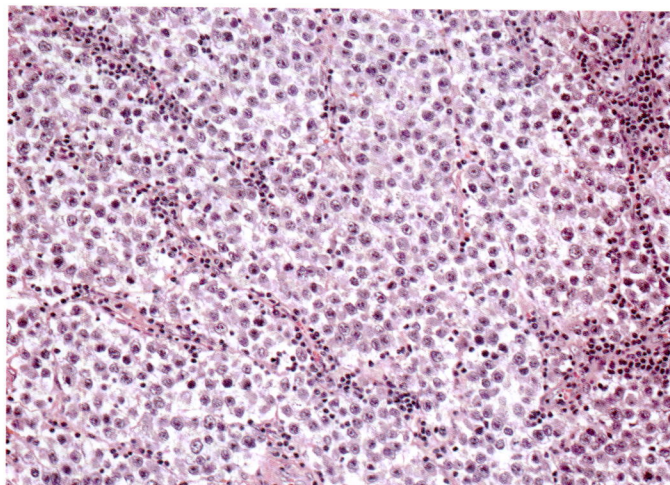

IMAGE 11.34 Ovarian dysgerminoma. The image shows a solid sheet of primitive germ cells with interspersed lymphocytes. This lesion resembles a testicular seminoma.

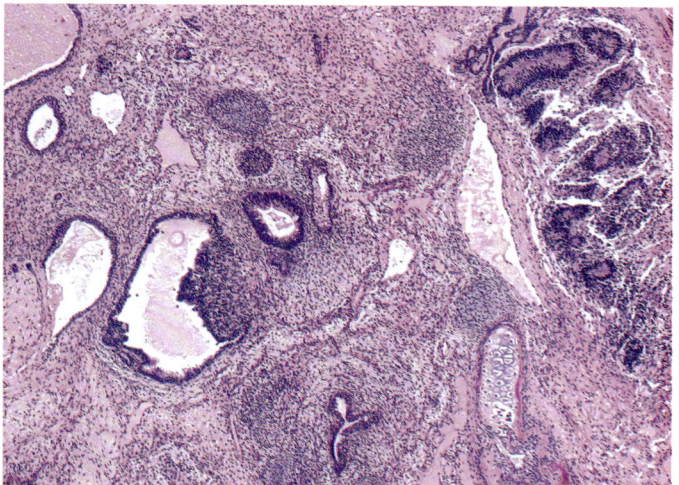

IMAGE 11.32 Ovary immature teratoma with mature areas. Immature teratomas often have a mixture of mature and immature areas from the 3 germ lines.

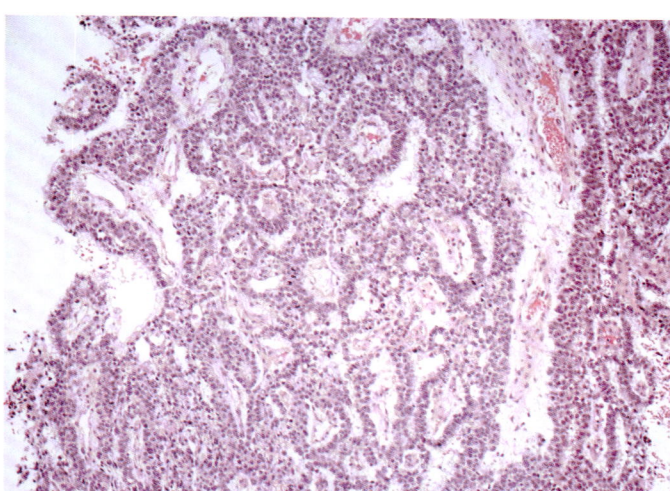

IMAGE 11.35 Ovarian yolk sac tumor. This is a low power view of a microcystic pattern with occasional Schiller-Duval bodies composed of fibrovascular projections surrounded by epithelium.

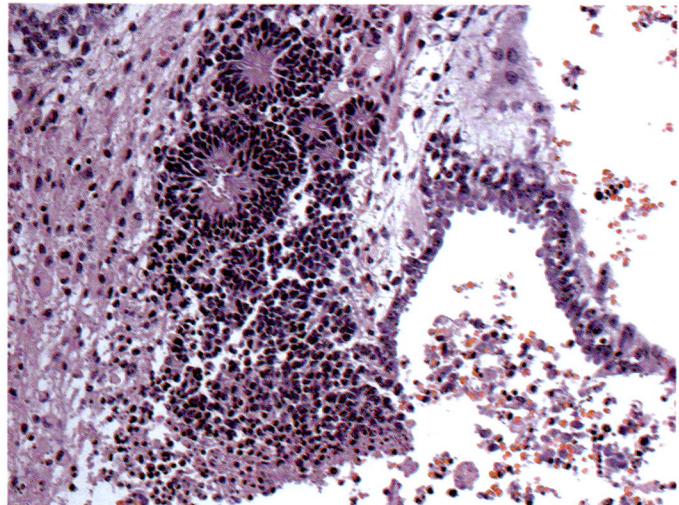

IMAGE 11.33 Ovarian immature teratoma. This is a high power view of primitive neuroepithelium with rosette formation.

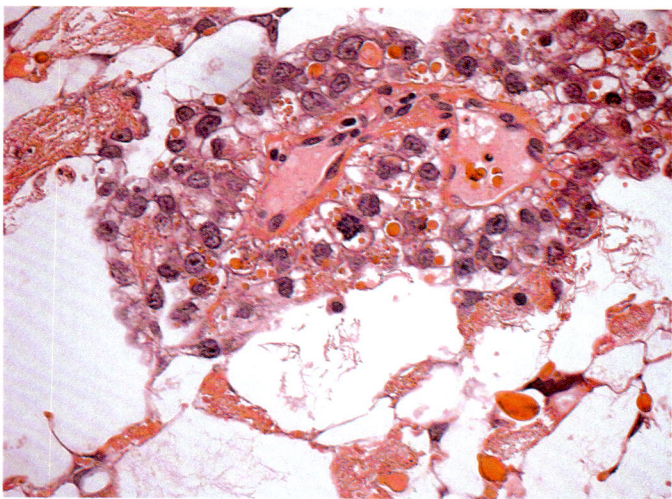

IMAGE 11.36 Ovarian yolk sac tumor. This is a high power view of hyaline globules.

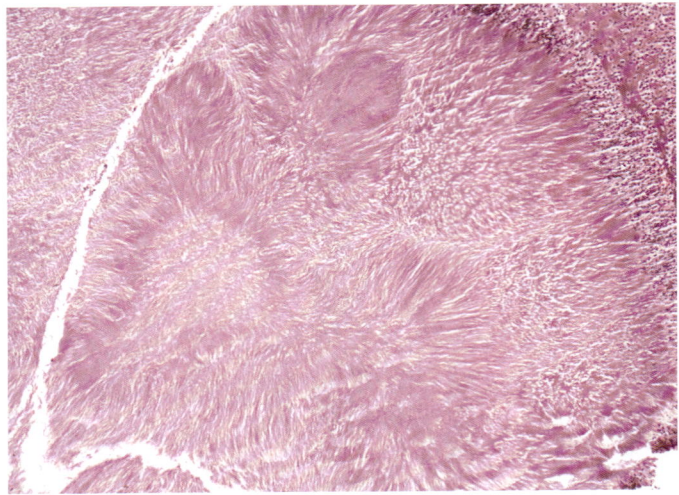

IMAGE 11.37 Uterus with actinomyces. This condition is often seen with an IUD.

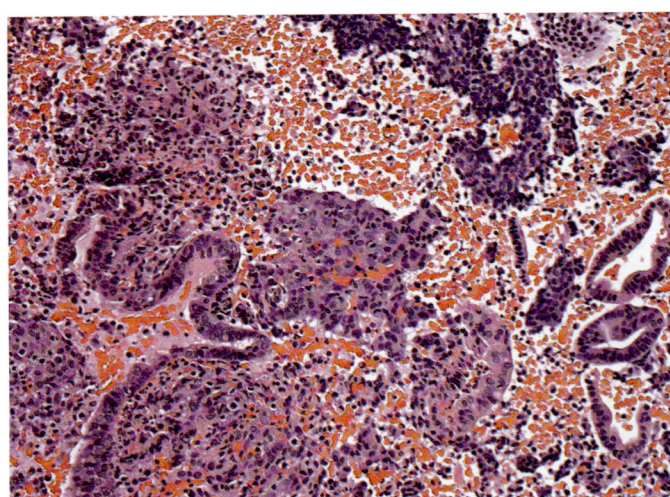

IMAGE 11.40 Menstrual endometrium. The aggregation of stromal cells in the top right corner can form "blue balls" on cytology. Note the collapsed endometrial glands with neutrophils and hemorrhage.

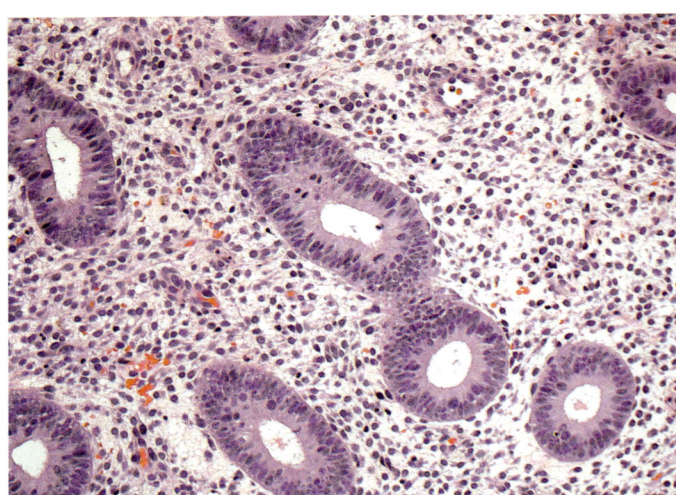

IMAGE 11.38 Proliferative endometrium. The image shows tubular endometrial glands with mitoses identified.

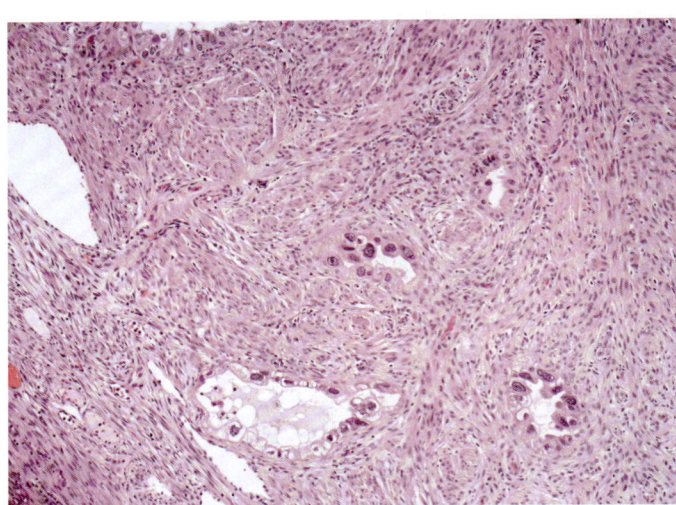

IMAGE 11.41 Arias-Stella reaction. Glands demonstrate clearing and vacuolization of the cytoplasm, and nuclear enlargement with a hobnail appearance.

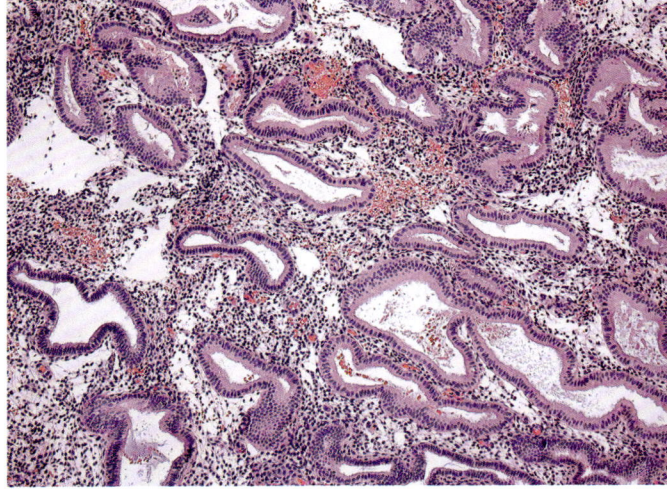

IMAGE 11.39 Secretory endometrium, day 20. The image shows midsecretory phase glands with luminal secretions.

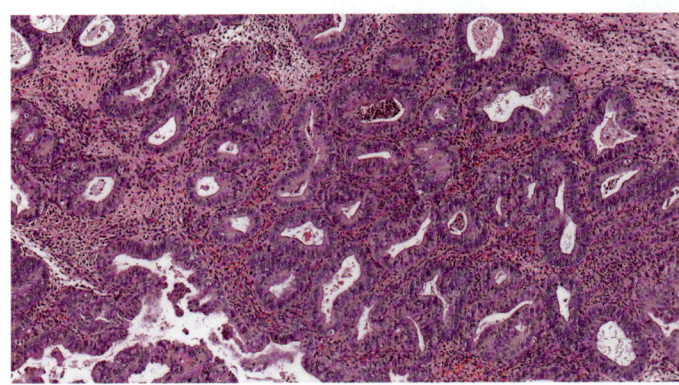

IMAGE 11.42 Endometrial biopsy in a 70-year-old woman. This shows atypical hyperplasia/endometrioid intraepithelial neoplasia.

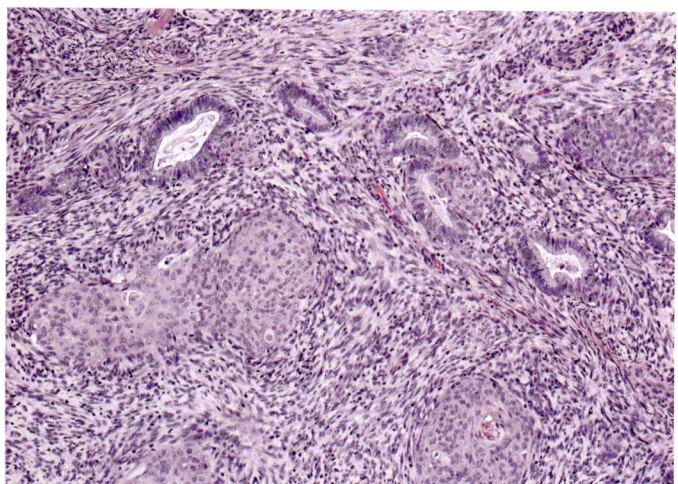

IMAGE 11.43 Atypical polypoid adenomyoma. The image shows endometrial glands with architectural and cytologic atypia, extensive squamous morules, and a background of smooth muscles in the stroma.

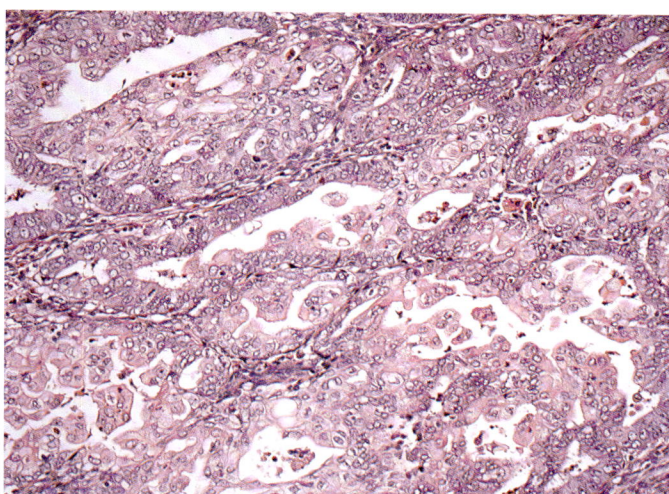

IMAGE 11.46 Endometrioid adenocarcinoma with small, nonvillous papillae.

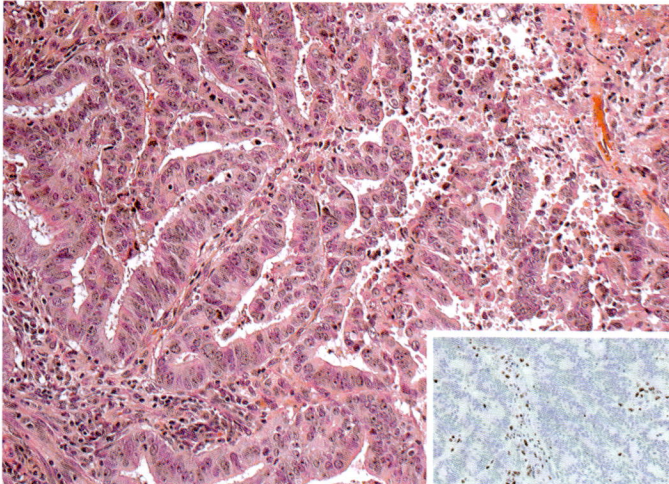

IMAGE 11.44 Endometrioid adenocarcinoma of the endometrium. This specimen has a predominantly glandular appearance with loss of stroma between glands. The glands demonstrate cellular crowding and moderate nuclear atypia. There is loss of nuclear staining of *MLH1*.

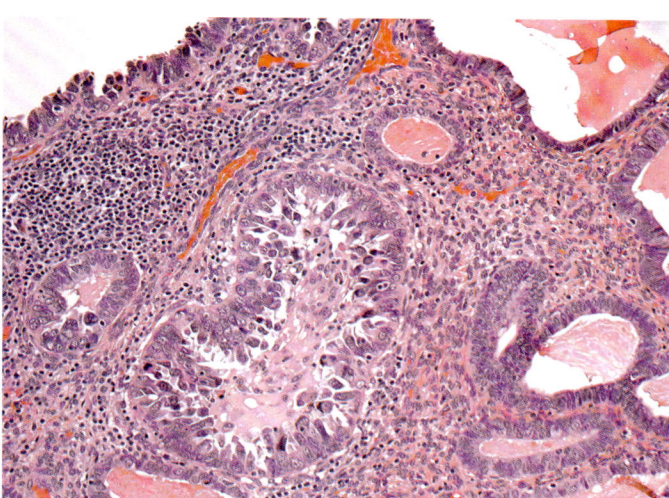

IMAGE 11.47 Endometrium with serous carcinoma. The image shows sloughing of cells into the lumen with severe nuclear atypia.

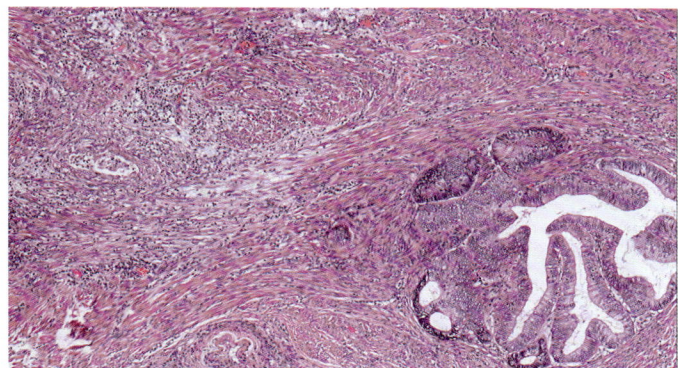

IMAGE 11.45 Endometrioid adenocarcinoma, low grade, with MELF (microcystic elongated and fragmented) pattern of invasion.

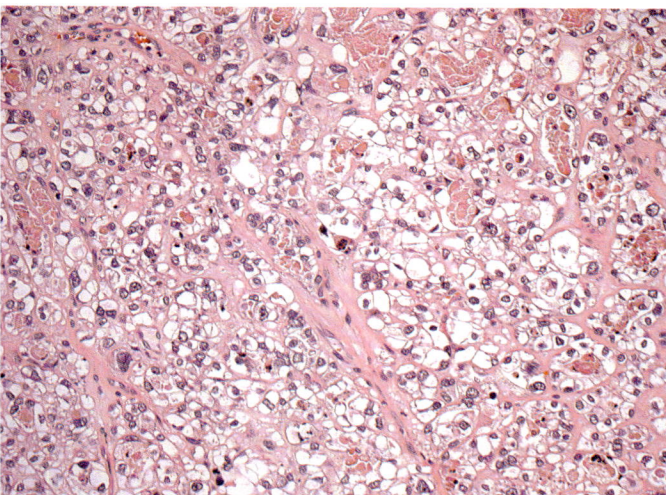

IMAGE 11.48 Endometrium with clear cell adenocarcinoma. The image shows solid growth of clear cells with hyalinized areas in the stroma. The morphology of this lesion resembles ovarian clear cell carcinoma.

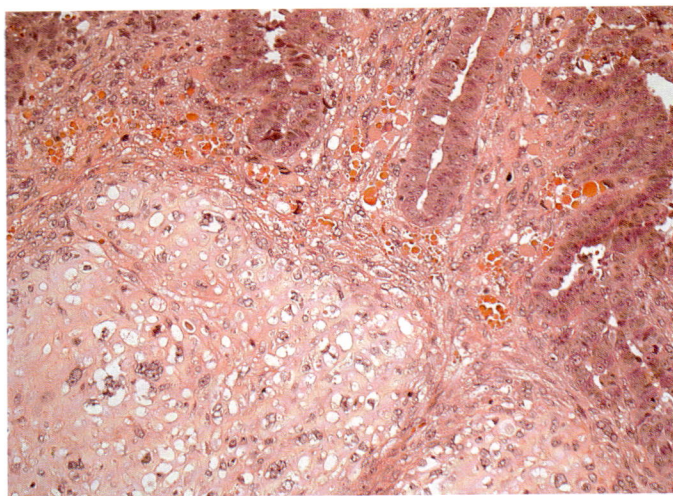

IMAGE 11.49 Endometrial carcinosarcoma with heterologous elements and a chondrosarcoma element at the bottom of the image. Both the glandular and stromal components are malignant.

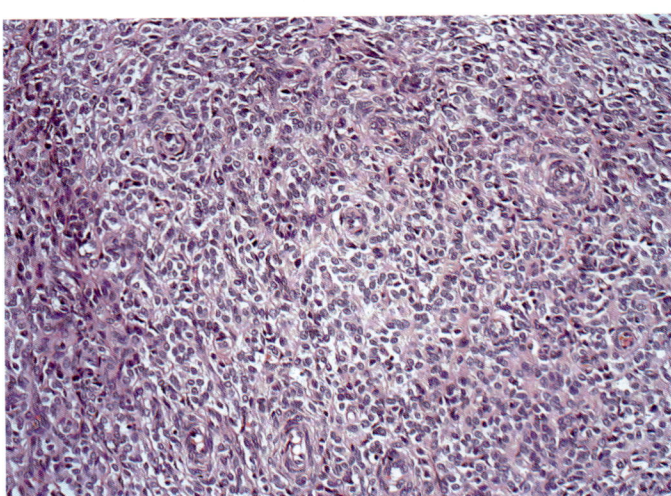

IMAGE 11.52 Low grade endometrial stromal sarcoma. This is a cellular, spindled tumor with minimal mitotic activity and vessels that resemble spiral arteries.

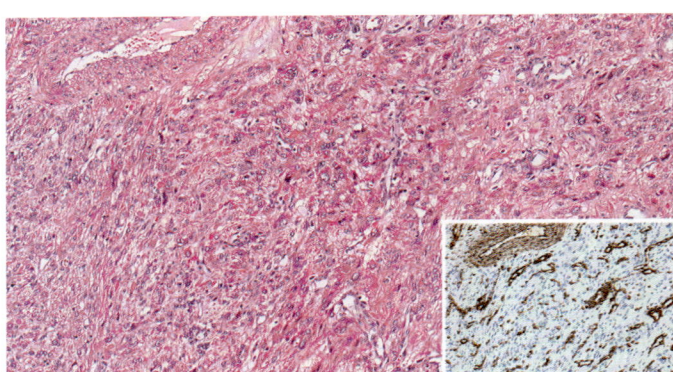

IMAGE 11.50 Hereditary leiomyomatosis and renal cell carcinoma. Uterine leiomyomas show scattered bizarre nuclei, eosinophilic cytoplasmic inclusions, prominent eosinophilic nucleoli surrounded by perinucleolar haloes, and abnormal fumarase staining or loss of fumarase staining.

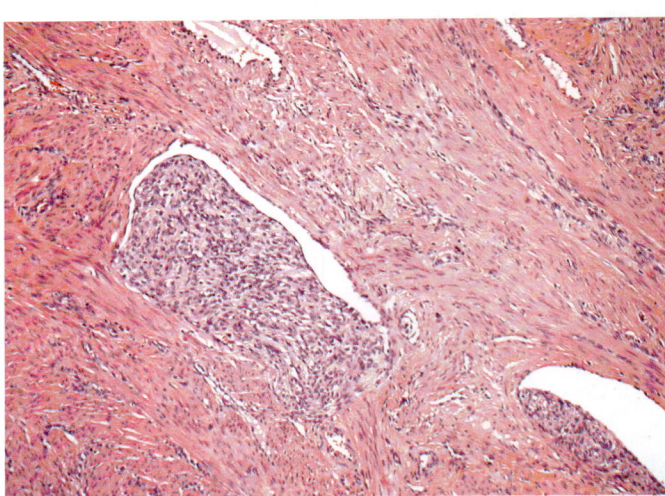

IMAGE 11.53 Low grade endometrial stromal sarcoma. The image shows the characteristic invasion of the lymphatic and vascular channels.

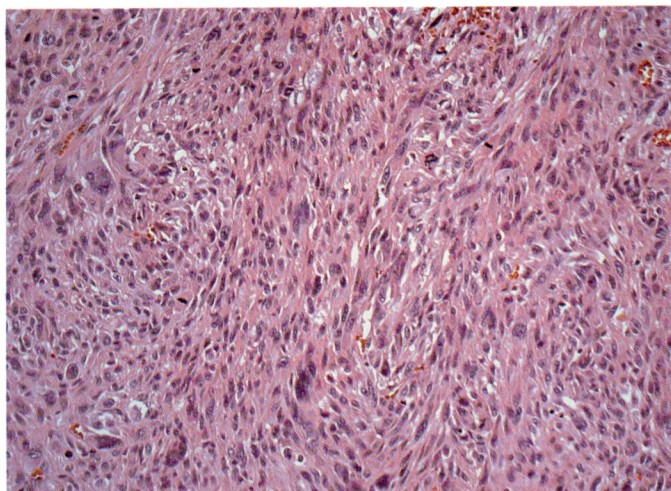

IMAGE 11.51 Uterine LMS (leiomyosarcoma). This is a cellular, smooth muscle tumor with diffuse severe nuclear atypia, increased mitotic rate, and atypical mitosis.

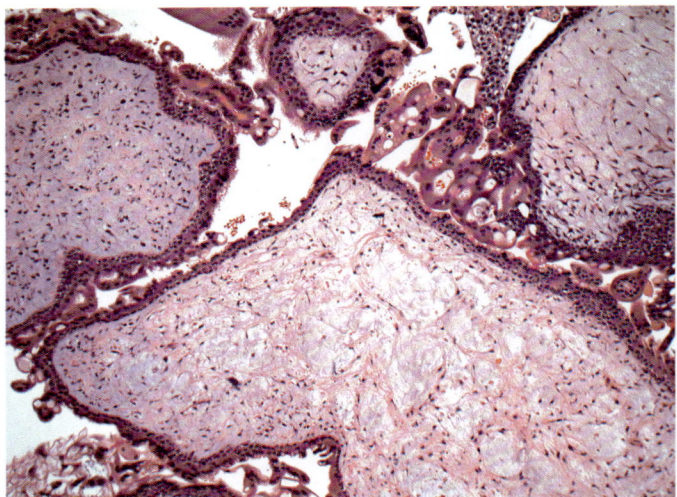

IMAGE 11.54 Complete hydatidiform mole. The image shows hydropic villi with prominent trophoblastic proliferation. Villi usually lack fetal vessels and nucleated red blood cells. Villous stroma often appears myxoid in early complete mole.

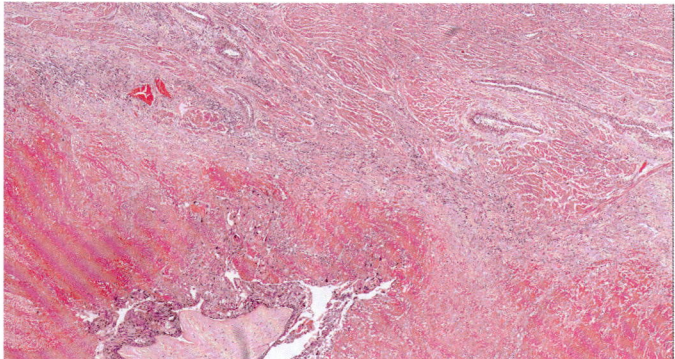

IMAGE 11.55 Invasive hydatidiform mole. Complete hydatidiform mole invades the myometrium.

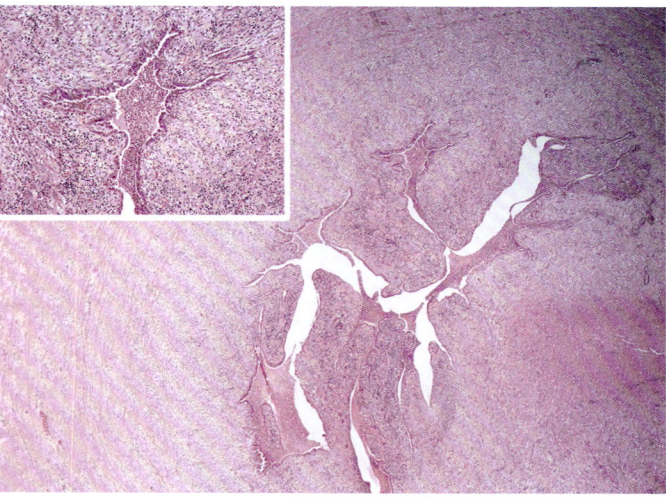

IMAGE 11.58 Acute salpingitis. The image shows the edematous wall of the fallopian tube with marked neutrophilic transmural infiltration.

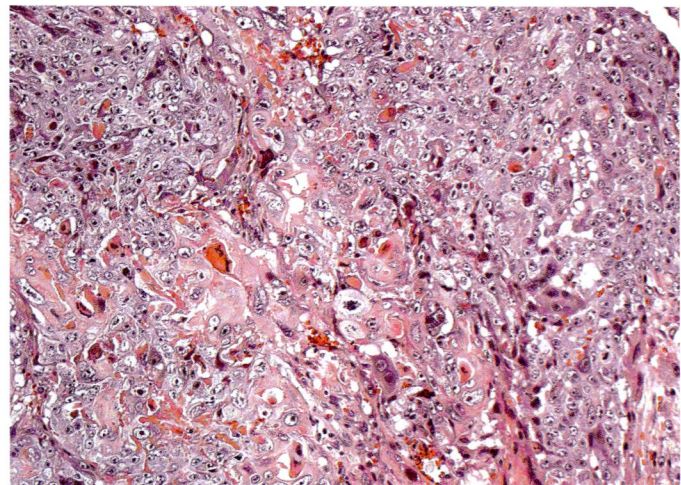

IMAGE 11.56 Choriocarcinoma. The image shows groups of cytotrophoblasts with surrounding syncytiotrophoblasts. Atypical mitotic figures and necrotic cells are seen.

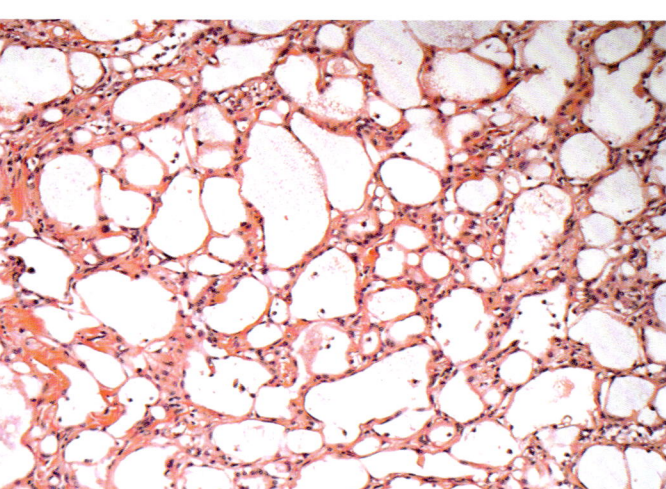

IMAGE 11.59 Adenomatoid tumor. The image shows small interconnecting spaces with flat to cuboidal lining. This tumor is mesothelial in origin.

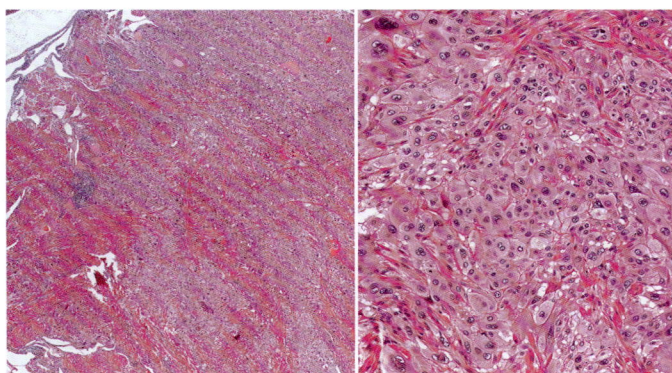

IMAGE 11.57 Placental site trophoblastic tumor. This tumor has large, polyhedral-to-round, mainly mononucleated cells (rarely multinucleated cells). Tumor cells infiltrate the myometrium. The cells have abundant amphophilic cytoplasm.

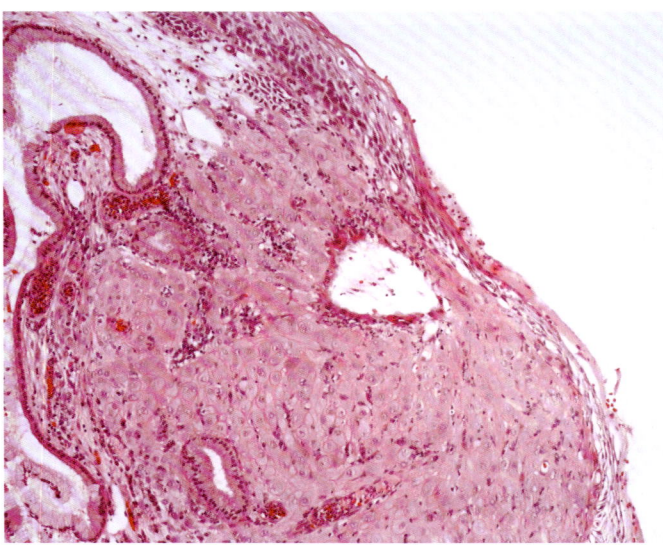

IMAGE 11.60 Cervix with decidual changes. Within the cervical stroma, the cells become more eosinophilic and plump, and resemble decidua.

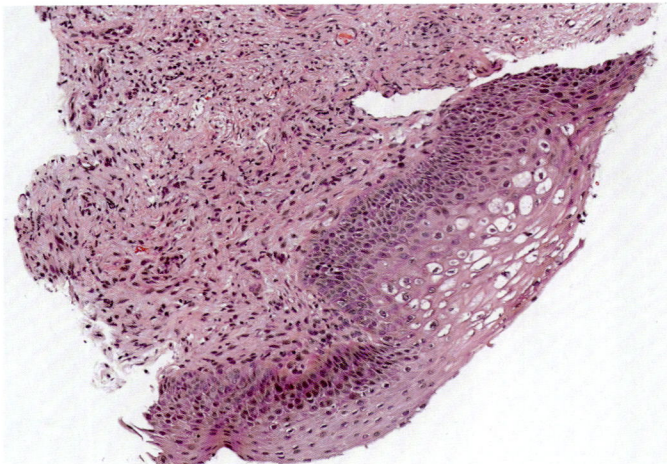

IMAGE 11.61 Cervix with low grade squamous intraepithelial lesion. The image shows evidence of koilocytosis.

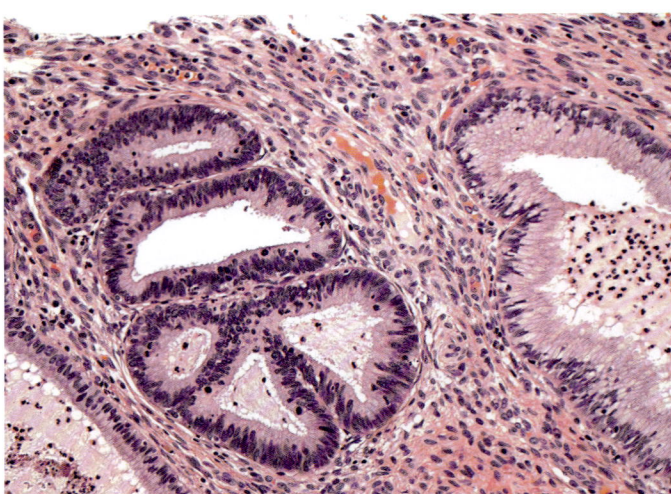

IMAGE 11.64 AIS (adenocarcinoma in situ) of the cervix showing crowded, atypical columnar cells with elongated nuclei, increased mitotic figures, and apoptotic bodies. Note the adjacent benign endocervical glands.

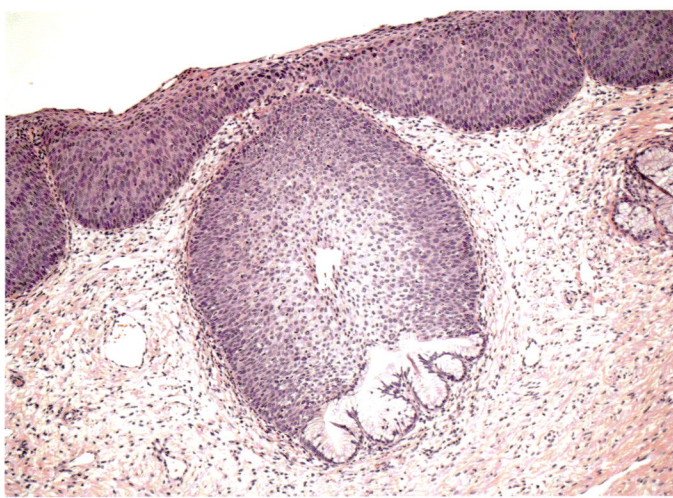

IMAGE 11.62 HSIL (high grade squamous intraepithelial lesion) involving an endocervical gland.

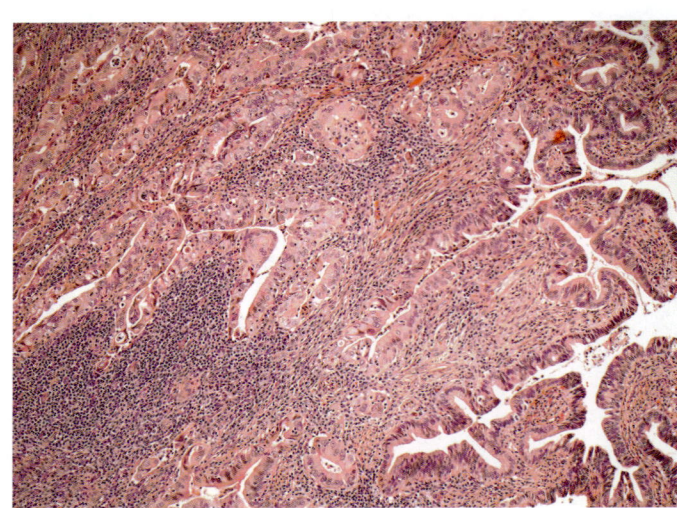

IMAGE 11.65 Cervical adenocarcinoma. The image shows invasive glands that have pale cytoplasm and a prominent lymphocytic infiltrate that surrounds the invasive component.

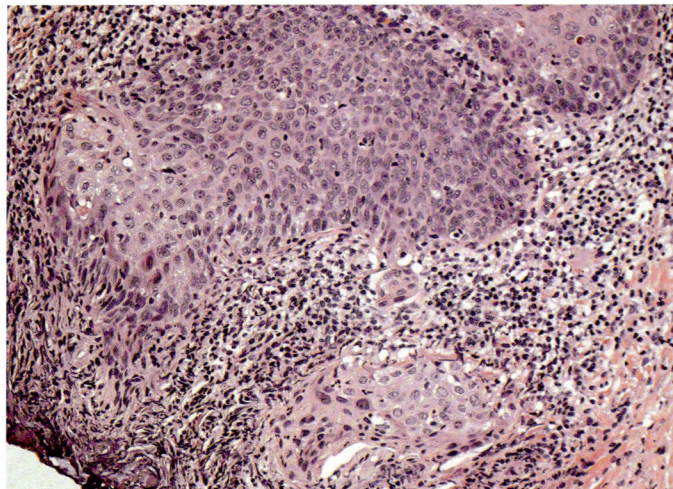

IMAGE 11.63 Cervix with focally invasive squamous cell carcinoma. The image shows pseudomaturation of the invasive component. The basement membrane is no longer visualized and there is a dense surrounding inflammatory component.

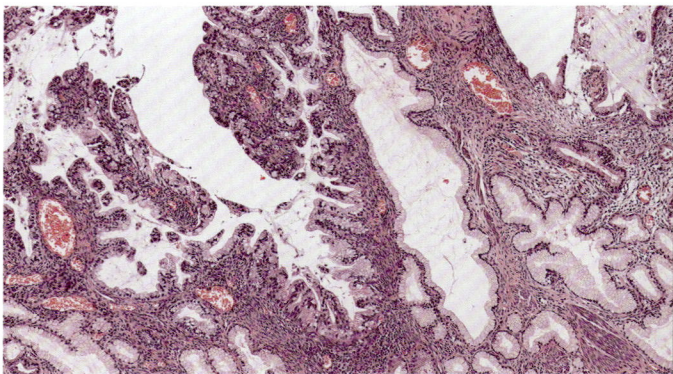

IMAGE 11.66 Endocervical adenocarcinoma, HPV-independent, gastric type. This tumor is defined by abundant clear-to-pale eosinophilic cytoplasm, distinct cell borders, rare apical mitoses, and rare apotosis.

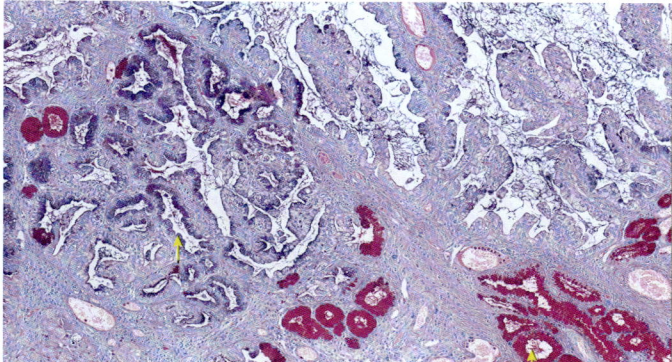

IMAGE 11.67 Endocervical adenocarcinoma, HPV-independent, gastric type with alcian blue/PAS stain.

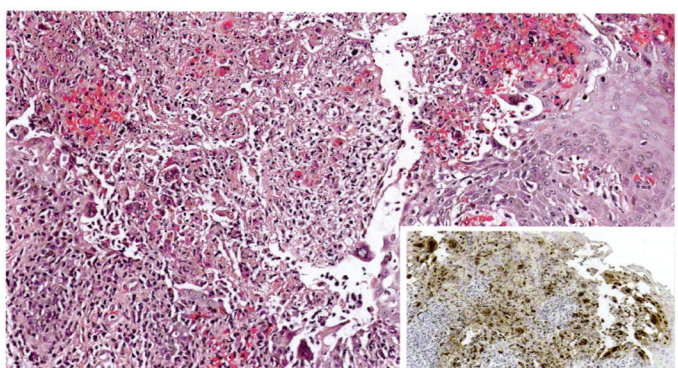

IMAGE 11.70 Herpes simplex vulvitis. The image shows ulcerated squamous mucosa with viral cytopathic effects, including multinucleation, molding, and nuclear margination. The diagnosis is confirmed by HSV IHC.

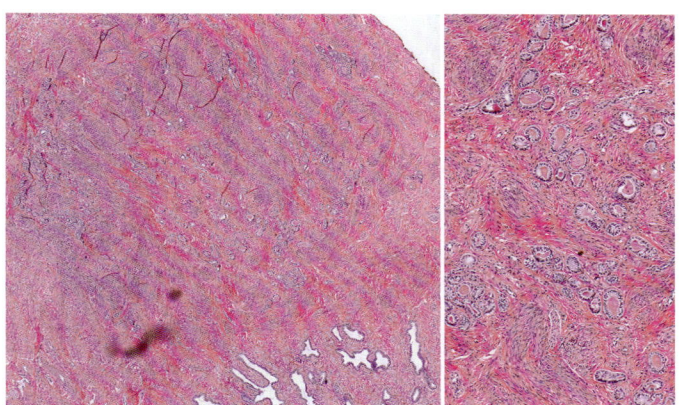

IMAGE 11.68 Endocervix with mesonephric hyperplasia: proliferation of mesonephric tubules. The image shows tubules lined by cuboidal bland cells with intraluminal eosinophilic secretions.

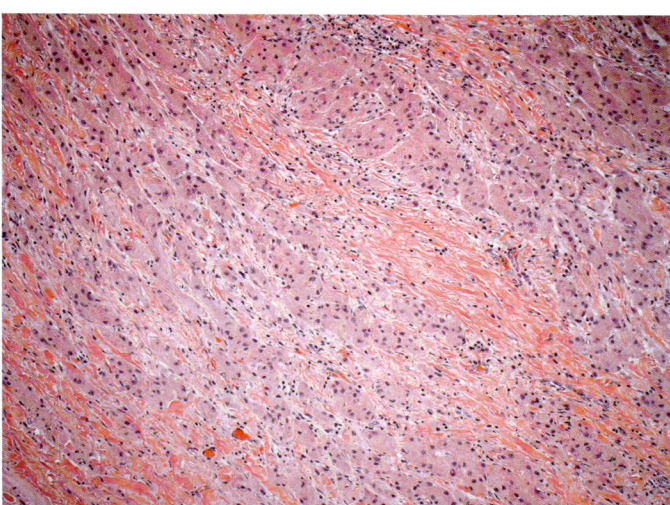

IMAGE 11.71 Granular cell tumor of the vulva. The image shows cords and nests of large, eosinophilic cells with granular cytoplasm and bland nuclei.

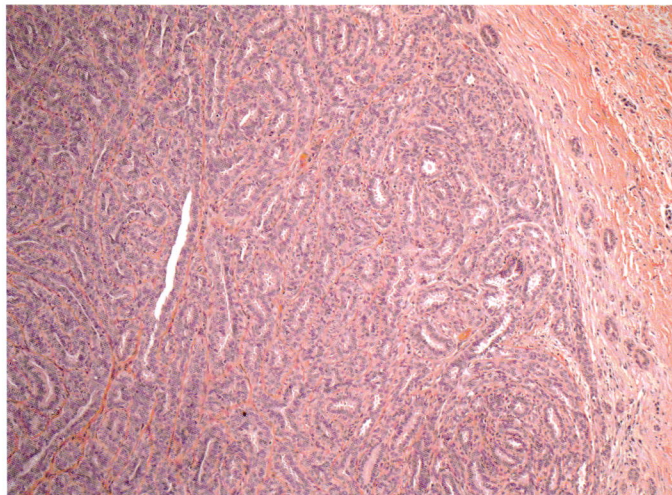

IMAGE 11.69 Hidradenoma papilliferum of the vulva. This is a well-demarcated lesion consisting of papillae and tubules with an apocrine appearance.

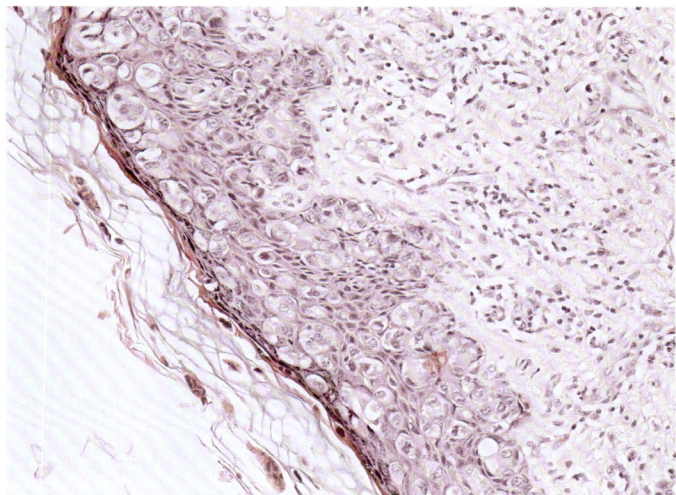

IMAGE 11.72 Extramammary Paget disease of the vulva. The image shows large single cells and clusters are scattered throughout the epidermis. Cells have an amphophilic cytoplasm and prominent nucleoli.

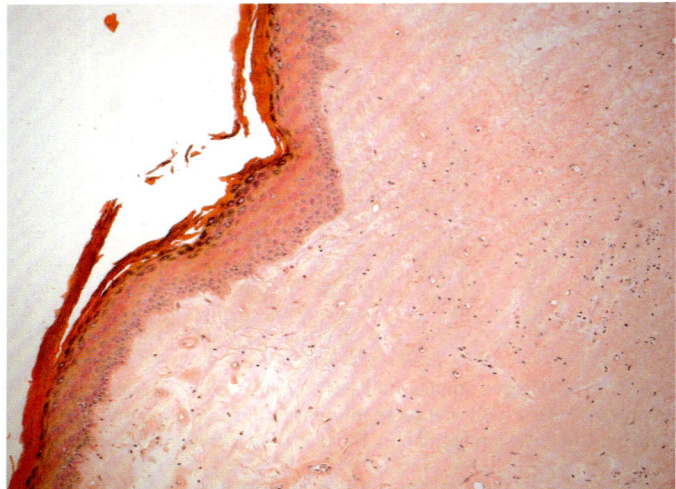

IMAGE 11.73 Lichen sclerosus of the vulva. The image shows epidermis with loss of rete ridges, and a subepithelial band of hyalinization and edema.

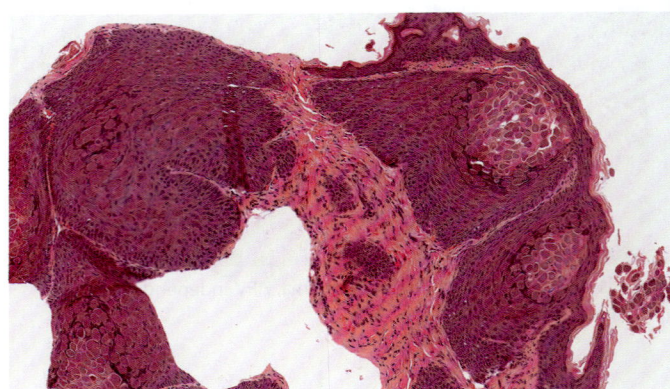

IMAGE 11.76 Vulva: molluscum contagiosum. This is a cup-shaped lesion with Henderson-Paterson or molluscum bodies, which are large intracytoplasmic eosinophilic inclusion bodies.

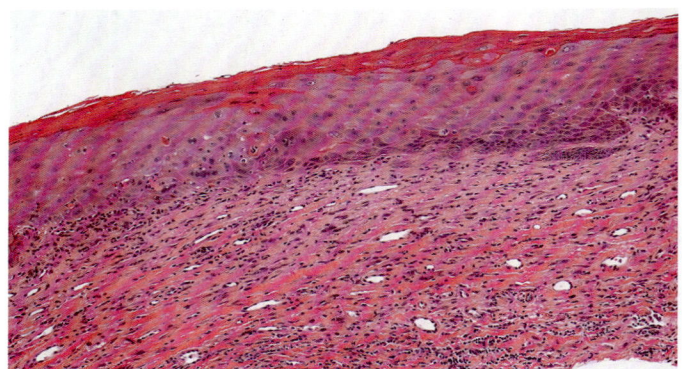

IMAGE 11.74 Vulvar intraepithelial neoplasia, HPV-independent/differentiated vulvar intraepithelial neoplasia. The image shows dyskeratosis and atypical keratinocytes confined to the basal and parabasal layers with hyperchromasia and atypical mitoses.

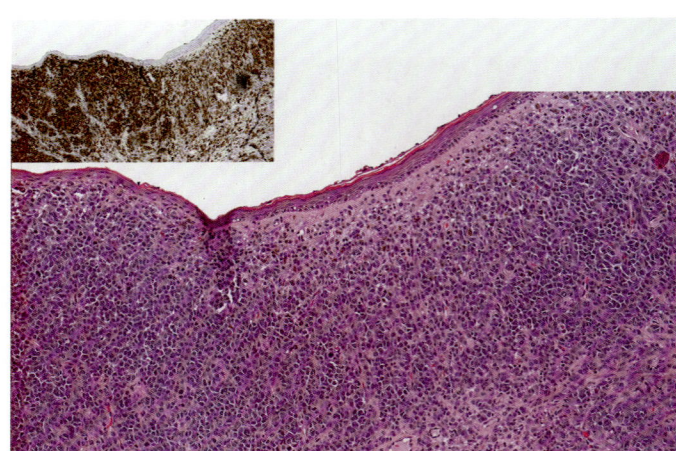

IMAGE 11.77 Vulvar melanoma. This is defined by large pleomorphic epithelioid malignant melanocytes, prominent nucleoli, abundant mitosis, and the presence of melanin. MART is positive.

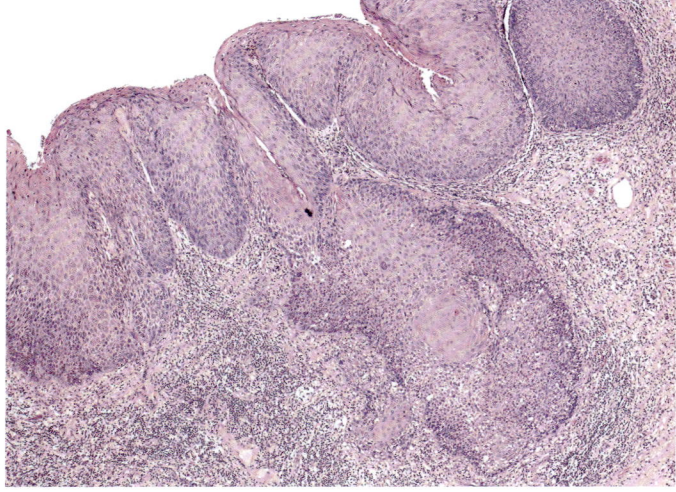

IMAGE 11.75 Squamous cell carcinoma arising in the vulva. The image shows dense subepithelial lymphocytic infiltrate with an invasive finger-like extension into the stroma by nests of pseudomature, invasive squamous cells.

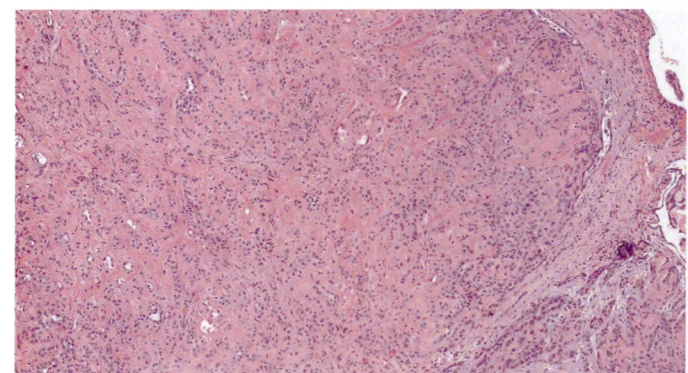

IMAGE 11.78 Malignant peritoneal mesothelioma. This is an epithelioid tumor in tubular and solid architecture. It has mild to moderate nuclear atypia and rare mitosis. Fifty percent of tumors show loss of nuclear BAP1 expression.

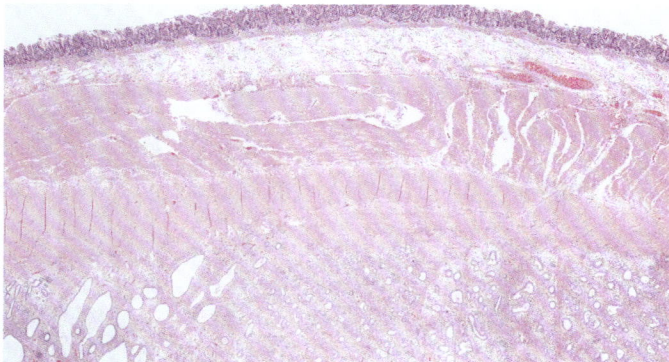

IMAGE 11.79 Colon with adenosarcoma arising from endometriosis.

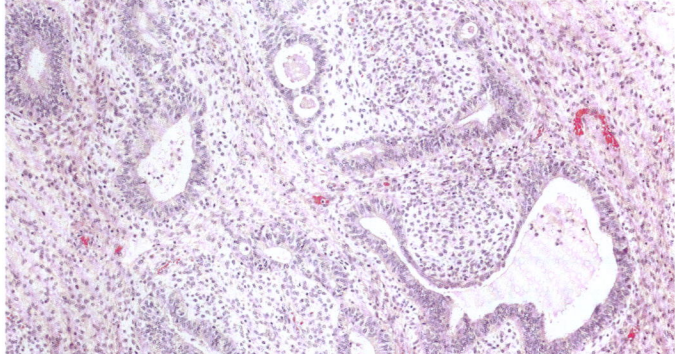

IMAGE 11.80 Adenosarcoma. The image shows cleft-like, dilated glands lined by benign endometrium and a distinct cuff of neoplastic stroma (atypia, increased mitosis, atypical mitosis).

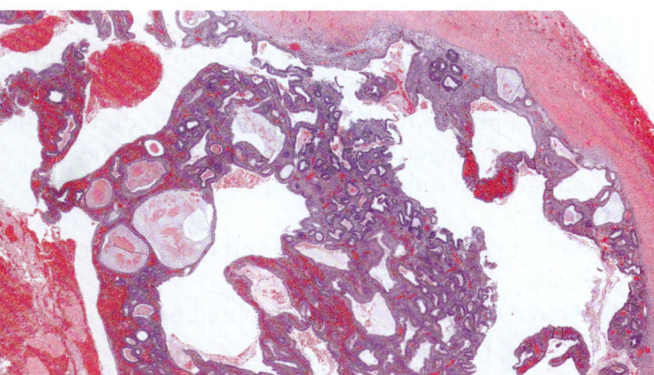

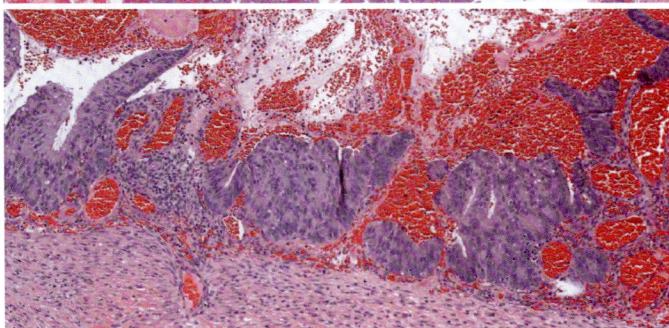

IMAGE 11.81 Diaphragm with endometrioid carcinoma arising from endometriosis. The images show glandular cribriform and nuclear atypia in a background of extensive endometriosis.

Bibliography

Amin MB, Edge S, Greene F, et al, editors. AJCC cancer staging manual. 8th ed. New York: Springer; 2017.

Clement PB, Stall J, Young R. Atlas of gynecologic surgical pathology. 4th ed. Philadelphia (PA): Elsevier; 2019.

FIGO Committee on Gynecologic Oncology. Current FIGO staging for cancer of the vagina, fallopian tube, ovary, and gestational trophoblastic neoplasia. Int J Gynaecol Obstet. 2009;105(1):3-4. Medline:19322933. doi: 10.1016/j.ijgo.2008.12.015

FIGO Committee on Gynecologic Oncology. FIGO staging for carcinoma of the vulva, cervix, and corpus uteri. Int J Gynaecol Obstet. 2014;125(2):97-8. Medline:24630859. doi: 10.1016/j.ijgo.2014.02.003

Fitzgibbons PL, Bartley AN, Longacre TA, et al; Cancer Biomarker Reporting Committee, College of American Pathologists. Template for reporting results of biomarker testing of specimens from patients with carcinoma of the endometrium (Version: Endometrium Biomarkers 1.2.0.0) [Internet]. College of American Pathologists; 2019. Available from www.cap.org.

Goldblum JR, Lamps LW, McKenny J, et al. Rosai and Ackerman's surgical pathology. 11th ed., vol. 2. Philadelphia (PA): Elsevier; 2017.

Klatt EC. Robbins and Cotran atlas of pathology. 3rd ed. North York (ON): Elsevier Canada; 2020.

Krishnamurti U, Movahedi-Lankarani S, Bell DA, et al; Cancer Committee, College of American Pathologists. Protocol for the examination of specimens from patients with primary gestational trophoblastic malignancy (Version: Trophoblast 4.0.0.0) [Internet]. College of American Pathologists; 2017. Available from www.cap.org.

Krishnamurti U, Movahedi-Lankarani S, Bell DA, et al; Cancer Committee, College of American Pathologists. Protocol for the examination of specimens from patients with primary carcinoma of the uterine cervix (Version: Uterine Cervix 4.3.0.0) [Internet]. College of American Pathologists; 2020. Available from www.cap.org.

Krishnamurti U, Movahedi-Lankarani S, Bell DA, et al; Cancer Committee, College of American Pathologists. Protocol for the examination of resection specimens from patients with primary carcinoma of the vagina (Version: Vagina 4.2.0.1) [Internet]. College of American Pathologists; 2020. Available from www.cap.org.

Krishnamurti U, Movahedi-Lankarani S, Bell DA, et al; Protocol for the examination of specimens from patients with sarcoma of the uterus (Version: Uterine Sarcoma 4.1.0.0) [Internet]. College of American Pathologists; 2018. Available from www.cap.org.

Krishnamurti U, Crothers BA; Cancer Committee, College of American Pathologists. Protocol for the examination of specimens from patients with carcinoma and carcinosarcoma of the endometrium (Version: Uterus 4.2.0.0) [Internet]. College of American Pathologists; 2021. Available from www.cap.org.

Kumar V, Abbas AK, Aster J. Robbins and Cotran pathologic basis of disease. 10th ed. North York (ON): Elsevier Canada; 2020.

Kurman RJ, Carcangiu ML, Harrington CS, et al, editors. World Health Organization classification of tumours. 4th ed. Vol. 6, WHO classification of tumours of the female reproductive organs. Lyon (France): IARC; 2014.

Kurman RJ, Ellenson LH, Ronnett BM, editors. Blaustein's pathology of the female genital tract. 7th ed. New York: Springer; 2019.

Lacey JV Jr, Sherman ME, Rush BB, et al. Absolute risk of endometrial carcinoma during 20-year follow-up among women with endometrial hyperplasia. J Clin Oncol. 2010;28(5):788-92. Medline:20065186. doi: 10.1200/JCO.2009.24.1315

Longacre TA, editor. Mills and Sternberg's diagnostic surgical pathology. 7th ed. Philadelphia (PA): Wolters Kluwar; 2022.

Movahedi-Lankarani S, Krishnamurti U, Bell DA, et al; Cancer Committee, College of American Pathologists. Protocol for the examination of specimens from patients with primary tumors of the ovary or fallopian tube (Version: Ovary Fallopian 1.1.1.0) [Internet]. College of American Pathologists; 2020. Available from www.cap.org.

Movahedi-Lankarani S, Krishnamurti U, Bell DA, et al; Cancer Committee, College of American Pathologists. Protocol for the examination of specimens from patients with carcinoma of the vulva (Version: Vulva 4.1.0.1) [Internet]. College of American Pathologists; 2020. Available from www.cap.org.

Mutch DG, Prat J. 2014 FIGO staging for ovarian, fallopian tube and peritoneal cancer. Gynecol Oncol. 2014;133(3):401-4. Medline:24878391. doi: 10.1016/j.ygyno.2014.04.013

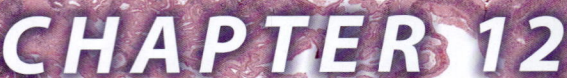

CHAPTER 12

Head & Neck Pathology

MARTIN BULLOCK

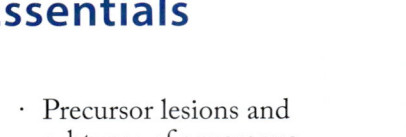

Head and Neck Pathology Exam Essentials

MUST KNOW

High-yield topics include:

- The clinical and pathological features of a wide variety of diseases of the head and neck, including those of soft tissue, bone, skin, and hematologic origin.
- Normal histology and basic embryology of the head and neck region.
- The major types of surgery performed for head and neck cancers (and what structures they typically include), such as segmental versus rim mandibulectomy, total versus infrastructure maxillectomy, orbital exenteration, total laryngectomy, superficial versus radical parotidectomy, and the categories of neck dissection.
- Major entities in each chapter of the World Health Organization (WHO) classification of head and neck tumors (nasal cavity and paranasal sinuses; nasopharynx; hypopharynx, larynx, and trachea; oral cavity and oropharynx; salivary glands; odontogenic tumors; ear; paraganglionic system). Of particular relevance are:
  - Salivary gland tumor classification, with its multiple entities with overlapping features, evolving terminology, and associated molecular alterations.
  - The large and expanding classification of sinonasal tumors, including at least a cursory knowledge of uncommon but often distinctive tumors with specific molecular alterations, such as nuclear protein of the testis (NUT) midline carcinoma, and *SMARCB1*-mutated and *INI1*-mutated tumors.

- Precursor lesions and subtypes of squamous cell carcinoma, and how these differ depending on site (e.g., human papillomavirus–mediated (HPV-mediated) carcinomas in oropharynx, nonkeratinizing carcinoma in nasal cavity, basaloid carcinoma in hypopharynx).
- A basic approach to the classification of odontogenic tumors (odontogenic epithelium, mesenchyme/ odontogenic ectomesenchyme, or both), with a few examples.
- The most common soft tissue and bone tumors of each site.
- The most common hematolymphoid neoplasms in each site.
- The major features of the College of American Pathologists (CAP) synoptic reporting protocols and the TNM staging for each site, with particular relevance to:
  - The determination and reporting of margin status for high grade dysplasia and invasive squamous cell carcinoma.
  - The importance of tumor size versus anatomical site involvement for tumor (pT) categorization (e.g., tumor size is not required for categorization of laryngeal carcinoma, but is relevant in the oral cavity).

- The measurement and importance of depth of invasion in oral cavity cancers.
- Factors that increase carcinomas in each site to the pT4 categories.
- The lymph node (pN) categories, including the importance of extranodal extension in most sites.
- The importance of the distinction between HPV-related and HPV-unrelated oropharyngeal squamous cell carcinoma.
- The unique staging systems for some tumors such as nasopharyngeal carcinoma and mucosal melanoma.
- The key elements of the CAP biomarker protocol, including when to order and how to interpret p16.

MUST SEE

Study cases that illustrate common and/or challenging problems in head and neck pathology, including:
- Small blue cell tumors of the nasal cavity.
- Destructive nasal lesions that raise the broad differential diagnosis of infectious, inflammatory, and neoplastic conditions.
- Glandular lesions of the nasal cavity: benign versus malignant, salivary versus nonsalivary type.
- Nasal polyps that raise the differential diagnosis of inflammatory polyp, papilloma, hamartoma, and polypoid neoplasms.
- The subclassification of squamous cell carcinoma, with further investigation as appropriate, such as p16 or HPV-specific testing.
- Spindle cell tumors of any site in the head and neck.
- Lymphoid infiltrates that raise the differential diagnosis of reactive conditions versus hematopoietic neoplasia.
- Atypia in mucosal biopsies, including the correct interpretation of dysplasia versus reactive atypia (or conveying uncertainty when appropriate).
- Grading dysplasia in various mucosal sites.
- In situ versus invasive squamous cell carcinoma: features that allow a confident diagnosis of invasion.
- Small biopsies of any site with inconclusive findings. How much immunohistochemistry (IHC) is reasonable? When should you ask for additional tissue? When should you consult a colleague?
- Biopsies of low grade salivary neoplasms, particularly in the oral cavity. Which IHC panel will be most useful? How conclusive should you be?
- Jaw cysts: how diagnose the most common.
- Fibroosseous and giant cell lesions of the oral cavity and jaws: correlation with clinical impression and imaging.
- Lichenoid and blistering oral lesions: correlation with immunofluorescence.
- Salivary gland tumors, including difficult ones requiring IHC and potentially molecular workup.
- Cystic neck masses.

- Tumors and lesions of unusual sites, such as the parapharyngeal space, skull base, and temporal bone.
- Presumed metastatic tumors to head and neck sites, including the salivary glands, jaws, and lymph nodes.
- Large head and neck resections illustrating common problems that arise in tumor staging (e.g., depth of invasion measurement in oral cancer, determination of bone invasion).

MUST DO

- Practice grossing a wide variety of head and neck specimens and develop an approach to dealing with these anatomically complex specimens. This includes:
  - Being familiar with the regional anatomy of the head and neck, including the orbit, nasal cavity and sinuses, larynx, pharynx and oral cavity.
  - Accurately describing the structures included in a resection specimen, their involvement by tumor and the margin status.
  - Correctly measuring a tumor, including its thickness and estimated depth of invasion.
  - Applying ink(s) to specimen margins judiciously.
  - Decalcifying tissues appropriately, with pre- and postdecalcification sampling.
  - Sampling tumors and margins correctly, using the reporting protocols and TNM staging system as a guide.
  - Describing, inking (as necessary) and sampling neck dissection specimens, using anatomical landmarks to guide the designation of levels, as necessary.
  - Dealing with challenging specimens, such as tumors resected in multiple parts.
  - Knowing when to involve the surgeon in the orientation of difficult specimens.
- Practice reporting a wide variety of head and neck specimens, including:
  - Ordering special stains and immunohistochemistry appropriately.
  - Writing relevant comments that permit clinicopathological correlation by the recipient.
  - Knowing which reporting components result in changes to the pT or pN categories and/or significant treatment alteration (such as the addition of radiation and/or chemotherapy).
  - Knowing how to further investigate and interpret potentially subjective areas of specimen reporting, such as margin status and extranodal extension.
  - Writing clear reports that convey your final interpretation of margin status, tumor size, and other parameters, in cases with multiple specimens.
  - Knowing when to apply the term *cannot be determined* to reporting parameters.
- Independently perform evaluations of head and neck frozen sections, including:
  - Orienting and describing tumor resection specimens.

- Specimen inking, using multiple inks as necessary.
- Appropriate specimen sampling.
- Preservation of the specimen for final grossing, postfixation.
- Orientation and correct submission of tumor bed margins.
- Communicating with the surgeon, with an appropriate level of certainty and confidence.
- Knowing when a second opinion is advisable.
- Using your time wisely: balancing time constraints with the additional value of information that may be provided by extra workup.

- Working with technologists collegially to obtain the best result, including requesting extra technical assistance in cases with multiple specimens.
- Dealing with special circumstances, such as the need for additional tissue, fresh tissue, or culture.
- Attend head and neck oncology rounds: present the pathological findings, when possible, to master the relevance of pathological findings and treatment.
- Correlate findings from fine-needle aspiration with results of surgical specimens and review together when possible.

MULTIPLE CHOICE QUESTIONS

1. Pleomorphic adenomas may show any of the following **except**:

a. Foci of mucinous and squamoid differentiation mimicking mucoepidermoid carcinoma.

b. Recurrence in the form of multiple nodules within fibrous and adipose tissue.

c. Frequent perineural invasion.

d. Rounded "buds" protruding through the tumor capsule.

e. Adenoid cystic-like pattern.

Answer: c

2. Which of the following is **not** true of mucoepidermoid carcinoma?

a. Keratin pearls are seen frequently in the epidermoid component.

b. Goblet cells are common in low grade tumors.

c. The translocation *MECT1-MALM2* may have diagnostic utility.

d. High grade tumors are most often purely or predominantly solid.

e. A clear cell component may be seen that is distinct from the mucinous component.

Answer: a

3. Which of the following is true of carcinoma arising in pleomorphic adenoma?

a. Adenoid cystic carcinoma is commonly the malignant component.

b. Carcinoma confined to the capsule of the pleomorphic adenoma is associated with a poor prognosis.

c. A history of a long-standing mass with recent sudden growth is rare.

d. Minimally invasive carcinoma, defined as extension < 1.5 mm beyond the capsule of the pleomorphic adenoma, is associated with an excellent prognosis.

e. Salivary duct carcinoma is rarely the malignant component.

Answer: d

4. Which of the following is **not** true of Warthin tumors?

a. Solid nodules composed of oncocytic cells that may mimic oncocytoma are occasionally seen.

b. Squamous metaplasia with atypia when infected may mimic squamous cell carcinoma, particularly with specimens from fine-needle aspiration (FNA) biopsy.

c. Malignancy may develop in either the epithelial or lymphoid component.

d. Occasional goblet cells may be present within the epithelium, raising the differential diagnosis of oncocytic mucoepidermoid carcinoma.

e. Stroma poor variants (epithelial component ≥ 70–80%) have a higher recurrence rate than typical cases.

Answer: e

5. A 44-year-old man presents with a hard palate mass that he has had for 6 months. He thinks it has gradually enlarged during that period. A specimen from an incisional biopsy shows a solid proliferation of cells with eosinophilic cytoplasm and eccentrically located mildly atypical nuclei, consistent with hyaline or plasmacytoid myoepithelial cells. Which of the following statements is true?

a. It is important to notify the clinician that low grade myoepithelial carcinoma cannot be ruled out until the tumor is removed and assessed for invasive growth.

b. Myoepithelial cells of this type are seen in myoepithelioma, myoepithelial carcinoma, pleomorphic adenoma,

and adenoid cystic carcinoma.

c. Myoepitheliomas will almost always stain positively for pan-keratin, smooth muscle myosin heavy chain, smooth muscle actin, and desmin.

d. S100 rarely stains tumor cells in myoepithelioma.

e. Chondroid differentiation is common.

Answer: a

6. All of the following statements are true about acinic cell carcinoma of the salivary gland **except**:

a. It may occur in minor and major salivary glands.

b. It is among the most common salivary gland malignancies in children.

c. Occasional tumors are composed of a single cyst with minimal solid component.

d. Acinic cell carcinoma is graded based on nuclear and architectural features.

e. High grade transformation (dedifferentiation) is rare and associated with poor prognosis.

Answer: d

7. Basal cell adenoma shows all of the following features **except**:

a. The membranous variant is sometimes associated with cutaneous neoplasms that have an identical morphologic appearance.

b. Basal cell adenoma may be grossly cystic.

c. Cells with a myoepithelial phenotype

are not present in basal cell adenoma.

d. The membranous variant has also been termed "dermal analogue tumor."

e. Infiltrative growth into adjacent salivary gland tissue indicates basal cell adenocarcinoma.

Answer: c

8. The differential diagnosis of adenoid cystic carcinoma includes a number of other tumors. Which of the following is **not** typically considered in the differential diagnosis?

a. Membranous variant of basal cell adenoma.

b. Basaloid squamous cell carcinoma.

c. Polymorphous adenocarcinoma.

d. Salivary duct carcinoma.

e. Epithelial-myoepithelial carcinoma.

Answer: d

9. All of the following are true for nasopharyngeal angiofibroma **except**:

a. It may grow into the middle cranial fossa.

b. It occurs most commonly in young women.

c. It typically presents with epistaxis and nasal obstruction.

d. It contains thin walled vessels lacking

elastic fibers and with incomplete smooth muscle coats.

e. Characteristic site of origin is the posterolateral roof of the nasopharynx in the area of the sphenopalatine foramen.

Answer: b

10. Which of the following statements is true regarding sinonasal papillomas?

a. Inverted papillomas have a low rate of recurrence with simple excision.

b. Exophytic (fungiform) papillomas typically occur on the lateral wall of the nasal cavity and paranasal sinuses.

c. The risk of malignant transformation is higher with exophytic papillomas than with oncocytic

schneiderian (cylindrical cell) papillomas.

d. Bilateral inverted papillomas are common.

e. While the malignant tumor that arises most frequently with inverted papilloma is squamous cell carcinoma, other tumor types such as mucoepidermoid carcinoma, clear cell carcinoma, and verrucous carcinoma also occur.

Answer: e

11. Which of the following is least likely to be seen on microscopic examination of an olfactory neuroblastoma?

a. Neurofibrillary stroma.

b. Homer-Wright pseudorosettes.

c. S100 positive staining of sustentacular

cells at the periphery of cell nests.

d. Nests of squamous cells surrounded by neuroblasts.

e. Strong staining with synaptophysin.

Answer: d

12. A 51-year-old man presents with a cystic mass just anterior to the sternocleidomastoid muscle in the upper neck. Clinically and radiologically, this is felt to be consistent with a branchial cleft cyst. Excision shows variable morphology of the cyst lining, with some areas lined by a multilayered maturing squamous epithelium with mild atypia and some regions of frank squamous cell carcinoma. Which of the following statements is **not** true with respect to this situation?

a. Branchial cleft cysts are less common than metastatic squamous cell carcinoma in this age group.
b. Malignant transformation of a branchial cleft cyst is an uncommon but well-recognized complication.
c. Staining for p16 would be supportive evidence of origin from the oropharynx.
d. Cystic metastases of squamous cell carcinoma in this location are most often of palatine or lingual tonsillar origin.
e. Human papilloma virus–related (HPV-related) squamous cell carcinoma of the head and neck shows greater response to radiotherapy than non-HPV-related cancers.

Answer: b

13. Which of the following is least likely to be a cystic lesion of the neck?

a. Metastatic papillary thyroid carcinoma.
b. Parathyroid adenoma.
c. Metastatic squamous cell carcinoma.
d. Parathyroid cyst.
e. Thyroglossal duct cyst.

Answer: b

14. Jugulotympanic paraganglioma (glomus tympanicum, glomus jugulare) is the most common tumor of the middle ear. Which of the following statements is true regarding these tumors?

a. The rate of malignant behavior is approximately 30%.
b. They are closely related to glomus tumor of the skin.
c. The chief cells would be expected to stain positively with chromogranin, S100, and synaptophysin.
d. Predicting malignant behavior from the histologic appearance is impossible.
e. The tumors are typically readily recognized at the time of surgery as nonvascular whitish masses.

Answer: d

15. With respect to cholesteatoma, which of the following is true?

a. It is a neoplasm and is in essence a well-differentiated squamous cell carcinoma.
b. The histologic appearance typically consists of a proliferation of squamous cells in solid nests and trabecular patterns.
c. It may show clinical evidence of extensive bone destruction.
d. It is most often seen in the external auditory canal.
e. It rarely metastasizes.

Answer: c

16. A 78-year-old man who has a long history of smoking and alcohol use presents with hoarseness of 3 month's duration. Examination of the vocal cords shows an exophytic mass on the right vocal cord. Biopsy shows invasive moderately differentiated squamous cell carcinoma. Which of the following statements is true?

a. The primary treatment in this situation should be radical laryngectomy.
b. Squamous cell carcinomas at this site are more often related to human papilloma virus than to tobacco and alcohol use.
c. Tumors confined to the vocal cord are associated with a better prognosis
d. Laryngeal squamous cell carcinoma involving a tracheostomy site is associated with a good prognosis.
e. Most squamous cell carcinomas at this site are preceded by a recognized prolonged period of squamous dysplasia/carcinoma in situ.

Answer: c

17. Which of the following statements is true regarding otologic tumors?

a. Tumors of the ceruminous glands are typically malignant.
b. Tumors of the ceruminous glands may be of salivary gland type.
c. The majority of schwannomas arising in the temporal bone ("acoustic neuroma") are associated with neurofibromatosis type 2.
d. Squamous cell carcinoma of the external auditory canal has a better prognosis than that of the external ear.
e. Most meningiomas of the ear/temporal bone region are not associated with an intracranial meningioma.

Answer: b

18. You receive a specimen labeled "sinus contents" from a 42-year-old man. The sections show inflamed mucosa with many eosinophils, and thick, laminated mucin containing Charcot-Leyden crystals and degenerating granulocytes. You suspect allergic/eosinophilic fungal rhinosinusitis. Which of the following statements is incorrect about this disease?

a. Fungi may be difficult to identify within the mucin, even with special stains.

b. This condition may cause an expansile mass, leading to bone erosion or proptosis.

c. Cultures are invariably positive for *Aspergillus* species.

d. Patients often have allergic symptoms, with peripheral eosinophilia and elevated IgE.

e. Slides should be carefully examined to rule out invasive fungal sinusitis.

Answer: c

19. Which of the following tumors may present as an exophytic or polypoid mass in the supraglottic larynx?

a. Granular cell tumor.

b. Adult type rhabdomyoma.

c. Spindle cell/sarcomatoid variant

of squamous cell carcinoma.

d. Neuroendocrine carcinoma.

e. All of the above.

Answer: e

20. In the context of evaluating a clinically designated squamous papilloma of the larynx, which of the following statements is true?

a. A single representative section is sufficient for adequate histological evaluation.

b. Squamous cell carcinomas with papillary architecture are extremely rare in this location.

c. HPV-related squamous papillomas

are typically heavily keratinized.

d. In situ hybridization for HPV should be performed routinely.

e. Occasional suprabasal mitoses, ciliated or columnar cells, and koilocytes are common findings in benign papillomas.

Answer: e

21. Which of the following statements about hematopoietic neoplasms of the upper aerodigestive tract mucosa is correct?

a. Diffuse large B-cell lymphoma is more commonly found on the nasal septum than in the oropharynx.

b. Extramedullary plasmacytoma is not associated with systemic plasma cell neoplasms.

c. Nasal natural killer/T-cell lymphoma is typically negative on in situ hybridization for Epstein-Barr

virus–encoded RNA (EBER).

d. Nasal natural killer/T-cell lymphoma should be considered in the differential diagnosis of destructive, inflammatory conditions of the nasal and oral cavities.

e. Hodgkin lymphoma is more common than non-Hodgkin lymphoma among older adults.

Answer: d

22. You receive a biopsy specimen from the lining of a cyst surrounding the crown of a mandibular third molar tooth that contains inflamed, nondysplastic squamous epithelium. Which of the following entities can be excluded?

a. Radicular cyst.

b. Conventional type ameloblastoma.

c. Dentigerous cyst.

d. Unicystic ameloblastoma.

e. Odontogenic keratocyst/keratocystic odontogenic tumor.

Answer: a

23. Which of the following statements is untrue regarding ossifying fibroma of the jaw?

a. Clinical and radiographic correlation are crucial when attempting to distinguish this entity from other fibro-osseous conditions.

b. It is considered a neoplasm.

c. Aggressive/active variants are more

common in adults than children.

d. Lesions are typically well-demarcated from the surrounding native bone and "shell out" easily.

e. They may contain giant cells.

Answer: c

24. Which of the following statements is correct regarding fibromas of the oral cavity?

a. The most common site is the floor of the mouth.

b. They are always traumatic in origin.

c. Atrophy and hyperkeratosis of the surface epithelium are distinctly unusual

and should raise the possibility of low grade fibrosarcoma.

d. Stellate, multinucleated cells may occur in some cases.

e. They are considered a premalignant condition.

Answer: d

25. Which of the following statements about secretory carcinoma of salivary glands is **not** true?

a. Distant metastases are common at presentation.

b. It typically stains positively for S100, mammaglobin, vimentin, and *GATA3*.

c. The differential diagnosis can include acinic cell carcinoma; adenocarcinoma, not otherwise specified

(NOS); and mucoepidermoid carcinoma.

d. It shares its most common translocation with secretory carcinoma of the breast, congenital fibrosarcoma, and congenital mesoblastic nephroma.

e. It can occur over a wide age range.

Answer: a

26. Which of the following statements regarding genetic alterations in salivary gland tumors is **not** true?

a. Most clear cell carcinomas have an *EWSR1-ATF1* translocation.

b. Membranous expression of HER2 by immunohistochemistry can be a useful feature in the diagnosis of salivary duct carcinoma.

c. The majority of adenoid cystic carcinomas will have

either a *MYB-NFIB* or *MYBL1-NFIB* gene rearrangement.

d. The commonest gene rearrangement in secretory carcinoma is *ETV6-RET*.

e. Tumors categorized as polymorphous carcinoma may have either point mutations or rearrangements of the *PRKD1* gene.

Answer: d

27. Which of the following statements is true about nasopharyngeal carcinoma (NPC)?

a. It is never keratinizing type.

b. It rarely stains positively with p63.

c. Basaloid squamous cell carcinoma was added as a category in the last World Health Organization (WHO) classification.

d. It includes categories with glandular differentiation.

e. Identifying the growth patterns Regaud and Schminke are relevant to the prognosis and treatment of undifferentiated type NPC.

Answer: c

28. All of the following entities typically enter the differential diagnosis of a sinonasal "small round cell" tumor, **except**:

a. Sinonasal undifferentiated carcinoma.

b. Intestinal-type adenocarcinoma.

c. Olfactory neuroblastoma.

d. Ewing sarcoma.

e. Nuclear protein of the testis (*NUT*) midline carcinoma.

Answer: b

29. Which of the following statements about spindle cell tumors of the sinonasal tract is **not** true?

a. The differential diagnosis is broad and can include tumors of salivary type.

b. Tumors with a "herringbone" growth pattern can include malignant peripheral nerve sheath tumor, low grade sinonasal sarcoma with neural and myogenic differentiation, synovial sarcoma, and fibrosarcoma.

c. Skeletal muscle differentiation can

occur in teratocarcinosarcoma, low grade sinonasal sarcoma with neural and myogenic differentiation, and sarcomatoid carcinoma.

d. Virtually all sarcomas can occur in this location.

e. Sinonasal glomangiopericytoma is typically positive for CD34 and negative for smooth muscle actin.

Answer: e

30. Which of the following statements is true about reporting oral cancer resection specimens

a. *Depth of invasion* and *tumor thickness* are synonymous terms.

b. Depth of invasion can be measured from the base of an ulcerated tumor.

c. *Worst pattern of invasion* is a core data element in the College of American

Pathologists (CAP) reporting protocol.

d. Superficial erosion of cortical bone alone is insufficient to increase the tumor (pT) category.

e. Extranodal extension from lymph nodes is an optional data element in the CAP reporting protocol.

Answer: d

31. Which of the following statements is **incorrect** about the gross examination and submission of total laryngectomy specimens?

a. The cricothyroid membrane should be examined as a site of potential extralaryngeal extension in tumors with subglottic extension.

b. Subglottic extension, involvement of a tracheostomy site, and the arytenoid cartilage are all adverse prognostic findings.

c. The greatest dimension of the tumor is not required to determine the pT category.

d. Prior therapeutic radiation can cause chondronecrosis of the laryngeal cartilages.

e. All statements are correct.

Answer: e

32. Which of the following statements is correct about tumors of the hypopharynx?

a. It is the most common site for paragangliomas of the upper aerodigestive tract.
b. Squamous cell carcinoma is more common in the pyriform sinus than in the posterior wall or postcricoid areas.
c. The postcricoid area includes the upper third of the esophagus.
d. Squamous cell carcinomas are typically HPV-mediated.
e. They commonly present at an early stage.

Answer: b

33. Which of the following immunohistochemical (IHC) stains is most frequently **negative** in Langerhans cell histiocytosis of the jaw?

a. CD1a.
b. S100.
c. CD30.
d. *BRAF* V600E.
e. Langerin.

Answer: c

34. Which of the following statements is **incorrect** about oral mucosal pigmented lesions?

a. Melanotic macules and amalgam tattoo are common benign causes.
b. The *BRAF* V600E mutation is uncommon in melanoma of the oral mucosa.
c. Melanoma is more common in sites with underlying bone (e.g., gingiva, palate) than in those without (e.g., floor of mouth, tongue).
d. Black hairy tongue is a predisposing condition to oral melanoma.
e. Most melanomas arise de novo, rather than from a pre-existing nevus.

Answer: d

35. Which of the following is the **least** common cause of a gingival nodule in an adult?

a. Pyogenic granuloma.
b. Peripheral ossifying fibroma.
c. Irritation fibroma.
d. Peripheral giant cell lesion/granuloma.
e. Granular cell tumor.

Answer: e

36. All of the following entities are typically associated with pseudoepitheliomatous hyperplasia **except**:

a. Pleomorphic adenoma.
b. Granular cell tumor.
c. Osteoradionecrosis.
d. Fungal infections.
e. Necrotizing sialometaplasia.

Answer: a

37. Which statement is **incorrect** about salivary gland mucocele of the oral cavity?

a. The most common site is the lower lip.
b. Retention type mucocele (mucus retention cyst) is more common than extravasation type mucocele.
c. It can present as a floor of mouth or neck mass.
d. The histological differential diagnosis can include mucoepidermoid carcinoma.
e. It may occur secondary to trauma.

Answer: b

38. Which of the following statements is correct about lymphoepithelial sialadenitis?

a. Quantification of lymphoepithelial lesions is required for evaluating minor salivary gland biopsies for Sjögren syndrome.
b. It is considered an IgG4-mediated disorder.
c. It is a risk factor for development of salivary gland lymphoma.
d. It never results in the formation of cysts.
e. The majority of cases are not associated with Sjögren syndrome.

Answer: c

39. Which of the following is the **least** likely histologic finding in a nasal biopsy from a patient with granulomatosis with polyangiitis?

a. Ulceration.
b. Geographic-type necrosis.
c. Vasculitis.
d. Mixed inflammation with microabscesses.
e. Well-formed, sarcoid-type granulomas.

Answer: e

40. Which of the following statements is **incorrect** about squamous cell carcinoma (SCC) and precursors in the oral cavity?

a. The majority of biopsies from lesions labelled "leukoplakia" are not dysplastic or malignant.
b. Proliferative verrucous leukoplakia is most common in older women.
c. Multiple primary malignancies may occur due to the field cancerization phenomenon.
d. Oral lichen planus is a common precursor of squamous cell carcinoma.
e. Accurate assessment of depth of invasion of SCC is aided by both gross and microscopic examination of a resection specimen.

Answer: d

Salivary Gland Tumors

41. List the benign and malignant epithelial tumors in the 2017 WHO Classification. (List as many as you can!)

BENIGN	MALIGNANT
• Pleomorphic adenoma.	• Mucoepidermoid carcinoma.
• Basal cell adenoma.	• Adenoid cystic carcinoma.
• Warthin tumor.	• Acinic cell carcinoma.
• Oncocytoma.	• Carcinoma ex pleomorphic adenoma.
• Myoepithelioma.	• Adenocarcinoma, not otherwise specified (NOS).
• Canalicular adenoma.	• Polymorphous adenocarcinoma.
• Cystadenoma.	• Basal cell adenocarcinoma.
• Sebaceous adenoma.	• Intraductal carcinoma.
• Lymphadenoma.	• Salivary duct carcinoma.
• Sialadenoma papilliferum.	• Epithelial-myoepithelial carcinoma.
• Ductal papilloma.	• Secretory carcinoma.
	• Squamous cell carcinoma.
	• Myoepithelial carcinoma.
	• Poorly differentiated carcinoma (3 subtypes).
	• Lymphoepithelial carcinoma.
	• Clear cell carcinoma.
	• Oncocytic carcinoma.
	• Carcinosarcoma.
	• Sebaceous adenocarcinoma.
	• Sialoblastoma.

42. List the common morphologic features of pleomorphic adenoma.
- It is a circumscribed, typically encapsulated tumor (encapsulation may be absent, particularly in minor salivary glands).
- Often, there is rounded "budding" through the capsule.
- A mixture of stromal and epithelial components is present in varying proportion.
- The stromal component is myxoid or myxochondroid. It may be hyalinized or contain bone or adipose tissue.
- Myoepithelial cells can have varying cytomorphologies, often spindled or plasmacytoid.
- The epithelial component is usually small ducts or glands, surrounded by proliferating "abluminal" cells.
- Squamous, oncocytic and mucinous metaplasia may occur.

43. List the common morphologic features of basal cell adenoma.
- It is a circumscribed, typically encapsulated tumor composed of uniform basaloid cells, with few or no mitoses and no necrosis.
- It is biphasic (luminal and abluminal cells are present).
- Four patterns occur: tubular, trabecular, solid, and membranous.
- The tubular pattern is composed of glands with 1 to several layers of basaloid cells surrounding luminal cells.
- The trabecular pattern is composed of anastomosing ribbons of basaloid cells in myxoid to collagenous stroma.
- The solid pattern is composed of variably sized and shaped nests of basaloid cells, often with peripheral palisading. Areas of cribriform growth may create confusion with adenoid cystic carcinoma.
- The membranous pattern is composed of nests of basaloid cells in "jigsaw puzzle" arrangement surrounded by basement membrane material.
- The stroma may be more cellular and contain S100-positive spindle cells.

44. List the common morphologic features of Warthin tumor.
- It is a circumscribed tumor with 2 components: epithelial and lymphoid and varying degrees of cyst formation.
- The epithelial component is classically composed of bilayered oncocytic epithelium arranged in papillary structures.
- The lymphoid component is composed of small lymphocytes, frequently with germinal centers.
- Oncocytes may proliferate to form solid areas.

(continued on next page)

- Cysts contain degenerated columnar cells, inflammatory cells and debris (often recognizable on an FNA).

- Squamous metaplasia, infarction may occur, particularly following FNA, sometimes with worrisome atypia.

45. List the common morphologic features of myoepithelioma.

- It is a circumscribed, often encapsulated tumor composed of myoepithelial cells with variable cytomorphology (spindle, plasmacytoid, epithelioid, clear) and architecture.
- The cells have uniform oval nuclei without mitoses and necrosis.
- Spindle shaped cells are typically arranged in fascicles.
- Plasmacytoid cells are often arranged in sheets and nests; most commonly seen in minor salivary gland (e.g., palatal) tumors.

- Epithelioid cells are often arranged in trabecular, reticular, solid, or nested patterns.
- Tumor cells are usually keratin (including CK7) and S100 positive, variably positive for actins or calponin.
- Only rare, focal ductal differentiation is permitted.
- Stroma is variable in quantity, and is myxoid or hyalinized.

46. List the common morphologic features of mucoepidermoid carcinoma.

- The features are highly variable, depending on the grade and combination of cell types; it may be circumscribed or infiltrative.
- It is composed of a mixture of mucin-producing, intermediate, and squamoid cells.
- Mucinous cells most commonly have goblet cell morphology (usually key to their recognition).
- Squamoid cells are polygonal, with moderate to abundant eosinophilic cytoplasm, organized in a "paving stone" arrangement. Cell bridges may be seen, but keratinization is extremely uncommon (suggests an alternative diagnosis).
- Intermediate cells are small, cuboidal, nondescript cells that lack cytoplasmic mucin or squamoid differentiation. They typically proliferate around mucin-producing cells in low and intermediate grade tumors.

- Clear cells are also common; oncocytes may be present (dominant in the uncommon oncocytic variant).
- Low grade tumors are predominantly cystic, with numerous mucinous cells and minor components of intermediate and squamoid cells. The have bland nuclear features and minimal/no mitotic activity.
- Intermediate grade tumors are usually predominantly solid, with a large component of intermediate cells; they have minor nuclear atypia and little mitotic activity.
- High grade tumors often infiltrate in small nests, are solid, with a high proportion of squamoid cells and minor mucinous and intermediate components. All show significant nuclear atypia and mitotic activity +/− necrosis.
- See also the question on grading below.

47. List the common morphologic features of adenoid cystic carcinoma.

- It is a circumscribed (unenecapsulated) or infiltrative, firm, gray-white mass on gross examination.
- Three patterns can occur: tubular, cribriform, and solid.
- The cribriform pattern is classic, and consists of variably sized groups of cells with pseudocystic spaces filled with acid mucin and/or basement membrane material, as well as less frequent and inconspicuous small true duct lumina containing neutral mucin.
  › Pseudocystic spaces are lined by cells showing myoepithelial differentiation with nuclei arranged tangentially to the space.

  › True duct lumina are lined by cells showing glandular differentiation with nuclei arranged radially around the space.
- The tubular pattern consists of bilayered tubules with an inner epithelial layer and outer myoepithelial layer, the latter with dark angular nuclei and clear cytoplasm.
- The solid pattern is composed of sheets or islands of cells, sometimes with central (comedo-like) necrosis; cells in these regions often have slightly larger nuclei with more open chromatin and increased mitotic activity.
- Adenoid cystic carcinoma is highly infiltrative and perineural invasion is present in the majority of cases.

48. List the common morphologic features of acinic cell carcinoma.

- Most are grossly circumscribed and may be mistaken for benign neoplasms.
- They are composed of several cell types arranged in a variety of architectural patterns.
- All cell types typically show bland uniform nuclei with rare mitoses and no significant pleomorphism (except following high grade transformation).
- The most characteristic is serous acinar cell with abundant cytoplasm containing basophilic granules. These should be present in all cases, though some tumors may have few and require PAS stain to identify the granules.

- Other cell types are vacuolated (1 to several large vacuoles), intercalated duct (small cuboidal cells with scant cytoplasm), clear cells (infrequent), and nonspecific glandular cells.
- Patterns are solid, microcystic, papillary cystic, and follicular.
  · The solid pattern is common and composed of sheets of cells. These regions often are composed predominantly of serous acinar cells.
  · The microcystic pattern is distinctive and seen in a high percentage of cases, often with a mixture of acinar cells, intercalated duct cells, and vacuolated cells with numerous microcystic spaces, either empty or containing eosinophilic material.

(continued on next page)

- The papillary cystic pattern has cystic spaces with papillary epithelial proliferations projecting into them. Cells lining the papillae often have a hobnail or tombstone appearance. Rare tumor and secretory carcinoma must be excluded.
- The follicular pattern has structures resembling thyroid follicles lined by intercalated duct type cells.

- A tumor-associated lymphoid proliferation (TALP) is common.
- Dedifferentiation or high grade transformation occurs rarely, typically to undifferentiated carcinoma or poorly differentiated adenocarcinoma.
- Key point: immediate recognition from low power is possible with a blue/purple hue, and a combined microcystic and solid pattern with TALP.

49. List the common morphologic features of carcinoma ex pleomorphic adenoma.

- This is a malignant epithelial tumor arising from a preexisting pleomorphic adenoma, or in a site from which a pleomorphic adenoma has been previously removed.
- The pleomorphic adenoma component may be small and inconspicuous, or may represent the majority of the tumor. In many instances, the tumor shows stromal hyalinization, and there may only be a well-circumscribed hyalinized nodule identified. The latter can be identified as a pleomorphic adenoma with greater certainty if:
  - S100-positive (myoepithelial) spindle cells are present in the stroma or surrounding nests of malignant cells.
  - – or –
  - Abundant elastic tissue is present within the nodule.

- The carcinoma component is usually a high grade adenocarcinoma: adenocarcinoma, NOS, and salivary duct carcinoma are common. Other tumor types include undifferentiated carcinoma, myoepithelial carcinoma, and squamous cell carcinoma. Sarcomatous differentiation can occur. The extent of the malignant component must be further characterized as:
  - Noninvasive: carcinoma confined within the capsule of the preexisting pleomorphic adenoma (excellent prognosis).
  - Minimally invasive: carcinoma extends < 1.5 mm beyond the capsule (excellent prognosis).
  - Invasive: carcinoma extends > 1.5 mm beyond the capsule (poor prognosis).

50. List the morphologic features of adenocarcinoma, NOS.

- This is a very uncommon tumor type, especially with proper classification and adjunctive molecular techniques.
- It is a malignant tumor with ductal or glandular differentiation that lacks the distinctive histologic features of the specific adenocarcinomas of salivary glands (e.g., acinic, adenoid cystic, polymorphous low grade).
- It may be low, intermediate, or high grade.

51. Discuss the treatment, prognosis, and behavior of adenoid cystic carcinoma.

- Treatment involves wide local excision +/− radiotherapy. Complete excision is often not possible or assumed.
- Prognosis depends on location, is generally worsening: parotid is better than submandibular; sublingual and minor salivary glands better than nasal.
- Its behavior is characterized by indolent but persistent growth, with frequent distant metastases late in the course of the disease. Lymph nodes metastases are less common.

- Most tumors tend to metastasize to lung and, to a lesser extent, bone, liver, brain.
- The overall 10-year survival is 50–70%.
- Prognosis has been correlated with tumor stage, site, margin status, invasion of large nerves, and patient age.
- It can be graded (I–III) according to architecture and extent of solid pattern. Generally, solid architecture > 30% confers worse prognosis.

52. List reactive lesions and tumors to be considered in the differential diagnosis of mucoepidermoid carcinoma (MEC).

- There is a broad differential diagnosis depending on the grade, location, and variant of MEC.
  - Nonneoplastic entities: necrotizing sialometaplasia, cysts of salivary duct origin, odontogenic cysts (if intraosseous in jaws).
  - Benign neoplasms: pleomorphic adenoma, Warthin tumor with squamous and mucinous metaplasia, cystadenoma, oncocytoma, sclerosing polycystic adenoma (adenosis).

- Malignant neoplasms: squamous cell carcinoma, adenosquamous carcinoma, salivary duct carcinoma, secretory carcinoma, acinic cell carcinoma, oncocytic carcinoma, clear cell carcinoma, metastatic renal cell carcinoma.
- Some examples are listed in the following table.

REACTIVE LESION/TUMOR	FEATURES THAT MAY OVERLAP	DIFFERENTIATION FROM MUCOEPIDERMOID CARCINOMA
Necrotizing sialometaplasia	• It presents as an ulcer or swelling, most commonly involving the palate. • Salivary glands show squamous metaplasia of ducts +/− acini. • It resembles low grade MEC because of residual benign mucinous cells admixed with metaplastic squamous epithelium.	• Lobular architecture of the preexisting salivary gland is maintained. • It lacks an intermediate cell component. • Pseudoepitheliomatous hyperplasia of the surface is present. • Necrosis of deep salivary acini is present (if obtained in biopsy). • Classic history and location apply.
Acinic cell carcinoma	• It has vacuolated cells that may resemble goblet cells. • Clear cells may be present.	• Serous acinar cells are invariably present. • It lacks a squamous component. • Microcystic and follicular patterns not typical of MEC are present.
Pleomorphic adenoma	• It occasionally has foci of mucinous and squamous differentiation.	• Myxochondroid stroma, and plasmacytoid myoepithelial cells are present. • There is no infiltrative growth.
Adenosquamous carcinoma	• Both are found in mucosal sites. • It overlaps with high grade MEC. • It contains mucin-producing and squamous cells.	• There is usually a greater degree of cytologic atypia. • It may keratinize. • It may have overlying dysplasia. • It lacks an obvious intermediate cell component. • Zonation is common (deep glandular component).

53. Describe the histologic features that are used to grade mucoepidermoid carcinoma.

- There is no universally accepted or recommended grading scheme. The most common are: traditional morphological (modified Healey), Armed Forces Institute of Pathology, Brandwein and Memorial Sloan-Kettering.
- The traditional grading scheme relies on proportion of cell type (mucinous, intermediate, squamoid), solid/cystic architecture, nuclear atypia/mitoses, and infiltrative growth.
  - Low grade: typically cystic; high proportion of mucinous cells; absent nuclear atypia and mitoses; and no infiltrative growth.
  - Intermediate grade: predominance of intermediate cells; lesser cystic component; occasional mitoses and mild nuclear atypia; often a minor infiltrative component.
  - High grade: predominantly or purely solid; marked predominance of squamoid cells; mitotic activity and moderate nuclear atypia; significant component of infiltrative growth.
- The AFIP and related Brandwein systems assign a numerical value to various findings that are added to produce a score, which is then converted to a grade. In the Brandwein system, if none of the following adverse findings is present, the tumor is considered low grade. If only 1 is present, the tumor is considered intermediate grade. If 2 or more are present, it is considered high grade:
  - Intracystic component < 25%.
  - Tumor front that invades in small nests and islands.
  - Pronounced nuclear atypia.
  - Lymphatic and or vascular invasion.
  - Bony invasion.
  - > 4 mitoses/10 high power fields (HPF).
  - Perineural spread.
  - Necrosis.

54. List the features of Warthin tumor on FNA.

- Oncocytes: cells with abundant granular eosinophilic cytoplasm and vesicular nuclei with prominent central nucleoli. Typically present in clusters with minimal overlapping nuclei (versus acinic cell carcinoma).
- Lymphocytes: predominantly small mature lymphocytes with occasional large cells; possible presence of tangible body macrophages. The features are consistent with a reactive lymphoid population.
- Macrophages (foamy or hemosiderin laden): consistent with cystic component.
- Other features: squamous cells +/− atypia, particularly with inflamed/infected tumors, degenerated columnar oncocytes, and amorphous debris.

55. List salivary gland tumors with their most common gene rearrangements.

- Pleomorphic adenoma — *PLAG1* and *HMGA2* translocations.
- Mucoepidermoid carcinoma — t(11;19) and t(11;15) translocations with *CRTC1-MAML2* and *CRTC3-MAML2*, respectively.
- Adenoid cystic carcinoma — t(6;9) and t(8;9) translocations with *MYB-NFIB* and *MYBL1-NFIB*, respectively.
- Secretory carcinoma — t(12;15) translocation with *ETV6-NTRK3*.
- Clear cell carcinoma — t(12;22) translocation with *EWSR1-ATF1*.

Nasopharyngeal Carcinoma (NPC)

56. What is the etiology of nasopharyngeal carcinoma? Describe the predisposing factors.

- Etiology: infection by Epstein-Barr virus (EBV). Individuals with NPC are more likely than people with other forms of cancer to have IgA antibodies to EBV and those with greater tumor burdens have higher titers of IgA antibody. EBV DNA is present in almost all tumor cells and is present in a clonal form, indicating integration of EBV DNA prior to clonal expansion.
- Predisposing factors: genetic susceptibility (the major factor). There is a markedly higher incidence of nasopharyngeal carcinoma in individuals from China (both native and foreign born) and other regions in Southeast Asia (Thailand, Philippines and Vietnam), and in Indigenous people of Alaska and northern Canada. This increased incidence decreases when they emigrate to low incidence regions, but it still is higher than in the non-Chinese population.
- Other factors of less significance: diet (high in nitrosamines), poor hygiene, and exposure to agents such as tobacco smoke, wood, grass, and incense.

57. Describe the WHO classification and histologic features of each type of nasopharyngeal carcinoma.

- Current classification:
  - Nonkeratinizing carcinoma (differentiated and undifferentiated).
  - Keratinizing squamous cell carcinoma.
  - Basaloid squamous cell carcinoma.
- Histology: see the table that follows.

TYPE	HISTOLOGIC FEATURES

Nonkeratinizing carcinoma	• It is subdivided into differentiated and undifferentiated subtypes.
	  · Differentiated subtype: typically grows in multilayered and plexiform patterns. Not infrequently, the tumor resembles a transitional cell carcinoma of the urinary bladder. Tumor cells have well-developed cell borders and euchromatic nuclei.
	  · Undifferentiated subtype (also known as lymphoepithelioma): more often grows in sheets and nests with a syncytial pattern. The individual cells have pale, vesicular nuclei with prominent nucleoli. Some examples show prominent spindling of the tumor cells. Lymphocytes surrounding and infiltrating the nests of tumor cells are common, though are not invariably present.

Keratinizing squamous cell carcinoma	• It resembles squamous cell carcinoma arising in other sites within the head and neck. • Tumors infiltrate either in broad tongues, small irregular shaped nests, or single cells. • Tumor cells show prominent intercellular bridges and individual cell keratinization. • Keratin pearls may be found.

Basaloid squamous cell carcinoma	• There are 2 components present:
	  · First component: a population of basaloid cells, which is typically the dominant component. The cells have scant cytoplasm and hyperchromatic nuclei. They have a high mitotic rate and necrosis is frequent, often with a comedo necrosis-like pattern. Common accompaniments of this component are small mucin pools and stromal hyalinization.
	  · Second component: differentiated squamous cells (typically minor). This may consist only of squamous cell carcinoma in situ, or may include a keratinizing, invasive component.

58. Describe the typical patterns of spread of nasopharyngeal carcinoma.

- Local spread into the cranial vault, paranasal sinuses, infratemporal fossa, and orbit.
- High rate of spread via lymphatics to regional lymph nodes. The most commonly involved lymph node is jugulodigastric (level IIa). Posterior triangle lymph nodes are also frequently involved. Presentation as a neck mass in NPC is seen in up to 42% of patients.
- Distant metastases to lungs, liver, and bone (notably ribs and spine) in a disproportionately high percentage of cases, particularly with nonkeratinizing, undifferentiated carcinomas.

59. Describe the treatment and prognosis for patients with nasopharyngeal carcinoma.

- Standard treatment:
  - External beam radiotherapy.
- Prognosis:
  - Tumor stage (most important): the stage I disease-free 5-year survival is 98%. This falls to 73% for stage IV.
  - Tumor type: nonkeratinizing carcinomas are associated with a better prognosis than keratinizing squamous cell carcinomas.

60. List immunostains or ancillary tests useful in the workup of nasopharyngeal carcinoma.

- Pancytokeratin (AE1/AE3) — establishes the diagnosis of carcinoma.
- P63, P40 or CK5/6 — confirms squamous differentiation.
- EBER in situ or PCR for EBV — establishes EBV infection.

(continued on next page)

- S100, HMB45, Melan-A — rules out melanoma.
- LCA — rules out lymphoma.
- P16 — may help rule out exclude oropharyngeal carcinoma (if direct spread suspected or in a metastatic tumor).

61. List tumors that should be considered in the differential diagnosis of a cervical lymph node containing metastatic nasopharyngeal carcinoma.
- Malignant melanoma.
- Large cell lymphoma.
- Hodgkin lymphoma.
- Rhabdomyosarcoma.
- Lymphoepithelioma-like/undifferentiated carcinoma of other sites in upper aerodigestive tract.
- Sinonasal undifferentiated carcinoma.

Fungal Infections of the Sinonasal Tract

62. Classify fungal infections of the sinonasal tract and briefly describe the clinical and pathological features of each.
- Noninvasive fungal infections:
  - Fungus ball, also known as mycetoma.
    - Is a noninvasive collection of fungus not causing an allergic response.
    - Is typically found unilaterally in the maxillary sinus.
    - Microscopically, consists of dense laminated masses of fungal hyphae, usually *Aspergillus*.
  - Allergic fungal sinusitis.
    - Is associated with an allergic response, peripheral eosinophilia, and elevated IgE.
    - May be locally destructive.
    - Has dense "allergic type" mucin with Charcot-Leyden crystals.
    - Requires fungal stains to confirm, but organisms may be scant and culture is required for speciation.
- Invasive fungal infections:
  - Acute.
    - Is typically associated with diabetes and immunosuppression.
    - May exhibit vascular invasion and rapid spread with central nervous system invasion.
    - Has high rate of mortality.
    - Shows necrosis and vascular invasion by fungi in tissue sections.
  - Chronic.
    - Is usually seen in immunocompetent patients, commonly diabetics.
    - Is a slowly progressive, low grade invasive infection, typically caused by *Aspergillus fumigatus*.

Papillomas and Hamartomas of the Nasal Cavity and Paranasal Sinuses

63. List the histologic subtypes of Schneiderian papilloma of the nasal cavity and paranasal sinuses.
- Three histologic subtypes of papilloma arise from the ectodermally derived specialized mucosa of the sinonasal tract (Schneiderian mucosa):
- Inverted papilloma.
- Exophytic (fungiform, septal) papilloma.
- Oncocytic (cylindrical cell) papilloma.

64. List the subtypes of Schneiderian papilloma in order of frequency.
- Inverted.
- Exophytic.
- Oncocytic.

65. Describe the etiology of papilloma of the nasal cavity and paranasal sinuses.
- The most consistent etiologic agent is HPV. The strongest association is with exophytic papillomas, where approximately 50% of cases evaluated by various methods, such as PCR or in situ hybridization, can be shown to be HPV positive. The most common types of HPV identified are 6 and 11. Inverted papillomas evaluated in the same manner show HPV positivity in 38% of cases, again with 6 and 11 most common. Occasionally, HPV types 16 and 18 are found.
- Limited studies have demonstrated Epstein Barr virus in a high percentage of inverted papillomas, but these results have not been reproduced.
- No etiologic agent has been identified in oncocytic schneiderian papilloma.

66. Describe the natural history of papilloma of the nasal cavity and paranasal sinuses.
- All 3 types of sinonasal papilloma have high local recurrence rates. Some studies report a recurrence rate as high as 74%.
- Inverted papilloma and oncocytic schneiderian papilloma have a propensity to undergo malignant transformation.
  - Rate for inverted papilloma: 11%, reported in a large collective review.

(continued on next page)

- Rate for oncocytic schneiderian papilloma: reported as 4–17%.
- Exophytic papillomas: no, or negligible, propensity to undergo malignant transformation.
- The majority of tumors that arise from both inverted and oncocytic types of schneiderian papilloma are squamous

cell carcinomas. Other tumor types encountered less frequently include mucoepidermoid carcinoma, clear cell carcinoma, small cell carcinoma, sinonasal undifferentiated carcinoma, verrucous carcinoma, and spindle cell carcinoma.

67. List 3 types of nasal hamartoma, with major pathological features.
- Respiratory epithelial adenomatoid hamartoma (REAH).
  - Has elongated, large glands lined by ciliated epithelium; prominent periglandular hyalinization; variable quantities of stroma.
- Seromucinous hamartoma.
  - Has small glands, often budding from larger REAH-type glands; is S100 positive; lacks a basal/myoepithelial layer.
- Chondroosseous and respiratory epithelial adenomatoid hamartoma (COREAH).
  - Is basically a REAH with a central chondroid and/or osseous component.
- Combinations of REAH and seromucinous hamartoma are common. REAH and seromucinous glandular collections may be found in association with chronic rhinosinusitis.

Olfactory Neuroblastoma (ONB, Esthesioneuroblastoma)

68. Name 4 entities in the differential diagnosis of olfactory neuroblastoma.
- Most important entities:
  - Lymphoma.
  - Sinonasal undifferentiated carcinoma.
  - Neuroendocrine carcinoma (carcinoid, atypical carcinoid, small cell carcinoma).
  - Sinonasal malignant melanoma.
  - Nonkeratinizing squamous cell carcinoma.
- Other less common entities:
  - Rhabdomyosarcoma.
  - Ewing sarcoma/primitive neuroectodermal tumor (PNET).
  - Pituitary adenoma.
  - NUT midline carcinoma.

69. List IHC stains that are important in the diagnosis of olfactory neuroblastoma.
- Most useful stains:
  - Synaptophysin — most ONBs show strong cytoplasmic positivity in a diffuse pattern.
  - Chromogranin — less often positive in ONB, but is more specific and in some tumors shows strong positivity when synaptophysin is negative or weak.
  - S100 — stains cells that surround the nests of tumor cells (sustentacular cells) in the majority of cases (highly specific staining pattern). Occasionally S100 stains the majority of tumor cells, making it difficult to evaluate. Sometimes S100 positive dendritic cells are present also within cell nests.
  - Cytokeratin — broad spectrum keratin stains are useful to rule out carcinoma. A minority of ONBs may show focal weak positivity; they rarely show strong diffuse positivity.

  When they show strong diffuse positivity, S100 staining of sustentacular cells and evidence of neuroendocrine differentiation together with the morphology on routine stains assumes greater importance.
- Other IHC stains of importance, particularly in selected cases (to rule out alternative diagnoses):
  - CD45 — rules out lymphoma.
  - CD99 — rules out Ewing/PNET.
  - Myogenin/Myo D1 — rule out rhabdomyosarcoma.
  - Pituitary hormone markers, including follicle-stimulating hormone (FSH), luteinizing hormone (LH), growth hormone (GH), prolactin — rule out pituitary adenoma.
  - Calretinin — has high sensitivity for ONB; is helpful in small biopsies.

70. What is the most common location for ONB?
ONB arises from the superior portion of the nasal cavity, in particular the region of the cribriform plate.

Other Sinonasal Pathology

71. Give a broad classification of sinonasal adenocarcinoma.
- Salivary type carcinomas (most commonly adenoid cystic).
- Nonsalivary adenocarcinoma.
  - Intestinal type adenocarcinoma (5 subtypes).
  - Nonintestinal type adenocarcinoma (low or high grade).

72. List the major pathological findings in granulomatosis with polyangiitis (GPA).
- Vasculitis (small- to medium-sized vessels, polymorphous).
- Granulomatous inflammation (poorly formed, usually loose aggregates of giant cells).
- Necrosis (so-called "geographic" necrosis, with granular blue hue and sometimes palisaded histiocytes).

(continued on next page)

Note: all 3 findings are uncommon in small biopsies, but may be present in more substantial specimens. Always consider destructive nasal processes in the diagnosis.

73. List entities in the differential diagnosis of granulomatosis with polyangiitis in a nasal biopsy.
- Infectious (particularly invasive fungal disease).
- Drug abuse (e.g., intranasal cocaine or other drug abuse).
- Lymphoma (nasal type NK/T cell; less commonly others).
- Other inflammatory processes (e.g., Churg-Strauss syndrome, chronic rhinosinusitis).

74. List the most common sites of involvement of GPA in the head and neck.
- Most common: nasal cavity, paranasal sinuses.
- Less common: oral cavity, nasopharynx, ear.
- Rare: salivary glands, skin.

Case Scenario

A 55-year-old man presents with a cystic neck lesion. An FNA biopsy specimen reveals atypical and anucleate squamous cells and debris.

75. List the major entities in the differential diagnosis and describe the histologic features of each.
- Squamous cell carcinoma, metastatic (top entity for consideration).
  · This clinical scenario signifies metastasis to a cervical lymph node in most cases. Histologic findings would include partial or total replacement of the lymph node by a squamous proliferation of variable differentiation.
  · When the metastatic tumor is the presenting feature, a common location of the primary tumor is tonsil (palatine/lingual). Tumors from this site are commonly HPV driven and have basaloid morphology. Clusters of basaloid malignant cells should be sought in the FNA specimen, but are not always present.
- Branchial cleft cyst (second branchial cleft anomaly).
  · This shows a cystic lesion lined by multilayered squamous epithelium with surrounding lymphoid tissue.
  · The epithelium is bland, and the lymphoid tissue may be organized as a lymph node (capsule, subcapsular sinus). On FNA, the squamous atypia is generally mild and necrotic debris is usually absent.
  · If infected, the epithelium may be partially or completely lost, and lymphoid tissue is replaced by fibrous tissue.
- Epidermal inclusion cyst.
  · This is lined by bland squamous epithelium with granular layer and filled with keratin. Evidence of rupture may be present. On FNA, the squamous atypia is generally mild.
- Warthin tumor.
  · This may be considered a neck mass when located in the tail of the parotid gland.
  · Typically, it is partially cystic with papillary fronds covered by oncocytic bilayered epithelium with reactive lymphoid tissue cores.
  · When infected, the oncocytic epithelium frequently shows squamous metaplasia and may be atypical. Aspiration biopsies containing atypical squamous epithelium and lymphocytes may lead to a diagnosis of squamous cell carcinoma, unless the alternative diagnosis is considered.
- Other entities: thyroglossal duct cyst with squamous metaplasia, pilomatricoma, and dermoid cyst, depending on the clinical history and location of the lesion.
  · Pilomatricoma is a particular pitfall on FNA because it contains basaloid cells that may be mitotically active. Ghost cells and superficial location are a clue to the correct diagnosis.

76. What additional tests could be done?
- IHC stain for p16 — possibly useful if there is a cell block available, but a firm diagnosis of malignancy should be based on cytomorphology, not IHC.
  · Strong nuclear and cytoplasmic positivity in the squamous cells would support of a diagnosis of metastatic squamous cell carcinoma, and would also be evidence in support of a tonsil/base of tongue primary tumor.
  · A negative stain is less helpful, as some squamous cell carcinomas, particularly keratinizing tumors, are negative and the stain works best on clusters of preserved cells rather than isolated, desquamated cells.
  · A branchial cleft cyst may be p16 positive, so a malignant diagnosis should be based on the degree of atypia rather than this finding alone.
- Additional investigation of the patient to determine the location of the cystic mass and whether there are other enlarged lymph nodes or lesions in the upper aerodigestive tract.
  · Positron emission tomography (PET scan) may be ordered to search for a primary site. Head and neck surgeons try to avoid "diagnostic" lymph node resections for squamous cell carcinoma, as it disturbs the surgical site of a subsequent neck dissection.

Laryngeal Carcinoma

77. Classify laryngeal carcinoma according to location.

- Supraglottic squamous cell carcinoma involves the supraglottic larynx (superior to the apex of the ventricle), including the epiglottis, aryepiglottic folds, arytenoids, and false vocal cords.
- Glottic squamous cell carcinoma involves the true vocal cords, and the anterior and posterior commissures.
- Subglottic squamous cell carcinoma involves the subglottis, defined as beginning 1 cm below the apex of the ventricle to its lower border represented by the rim of the cricoid cartilage.
- Transglottic carcinoma crosses the ventricles in a vertical direction; it may arise in glottic or supraglottic larynx.

78. List the primary site of laryngeal cancers in order of frequency.

- Glottic (60–65%).
- Supraglottic (30–35%).
- Subglottic (< 5%).

79. What is the prognostic implication of this classification?

- Glottic squamous cell carcinomas indicate a better prognosis than either subglottic or supraglottic.
- Transglottic tumors are typically advanced stage tumors and indicate a worse prognosis.

80. Describe how you would perform gross examination, sectioning, and sampling of a laryngectomy specimen.

- Examine, measure, and describe the external aspect of the specimen.
- Open the specimen along the posterior aspect and examine, measure, and describe the internal aspect of the larynx as well as any tumor that is present (size, sites of involvement).
- Fix the specimen overnight, and then sample the tumor prior to decalcification.
- Decalcify the specimen. Note: the laryngeal cartilage is ossified in most adults and requires a short period of decalcification.
- Following decalcification, section the larynx in either the sagittal plane (preferable) or in the transverse plane. Take sections in order to document the following:

- Tumor and relation to ventricle/cords (establish site of tumor).
- Tumor and relation to laryngeal cartilages (establish invasion of cartilage or extralaryngeal tumor spread).
- Resection margins — epiglottic/tongue base, tracheal ring, soft tissue, pyriform sinuses, postcricoid.
- Thyroid (and relation to tumor if closely approached or invaded).
- Tracheal stoma site (if present).
- Search for and submit any lymph nodes and parathyroid glands.

Note: pay particular attention to tumor spread into the preepiglottic space, and extension through the cricothyroid membrane and around the trachea.

Verrucous Carcinoma

81. What are the common sites of occurrence of verrucous carcinoma in the head and neck region?

- In head and neck region: oral cavity (about 70%) and larynx.
- Within oral cavity: buccal mucosa and gingiva.
- Within larynx: vocal cords.
- Other sites (uncommon): nose and nasopharynx.

82. Describe the typical gross and microscopic features of verrucous carcinoma.

- Gross features:
  - This is a white, or white and red, broadly based exophytic lesion with a rough, papillary surface.
- Microscopic features:
  - It is characterized by a lack of squamous dysplasia and by infiltrative growth in broad pushing invaginations.
- The surface often shows pronounced hyperkeratosis ("church spire" pattern).
- A chronic inflammatory cell infiltrate is frequently present within the stroma adjoining the tumor.
- Adjacent epithelium is typically hyperplastic and hyperkeratotic, but not obviously dysplastic.

83. What entities are typically considered in the differential diagnosis of verrucous carcinoma? Describe the features that allow differentiation of these entities.

- Differential diagnosis is largely with 3 lesions:
  - Reactive squamous hyperplasia — typically, the proliferating squamous epithelium is composed of slender rete pegs with sharp ends, which contrasts with broad pegs with blunt ends in verrucous carcinoma. It does not form an expansile mass extending into the stroma below the adjacent mucosa (it may be difficult to determine in small or superficial biopsies).

(continued on next page)

 566 Head & Neck Pathology

- Squamous papilloma — this shows more complex exophytic growth with lack of keratin production, which contrasts with the markedly keratotic surface of verrucous carcinoma.

- Conventional squamous cell carcinoma — this has the nuclear atypia of malignancy, which precludes a diagnosis of verrucous carcinoma. It usually invades as smaller, infiltrative nests.

84. What is the prognosis for patients with verrucous carcinoma?
- Generally good — with extensive surgery, disease-free 5-year survival rates are 80–90% for oral tumors, and 85–95% for laryngeal tumors.
- Verrucous carcinoma does not metastasize. Surgical excision (in the larynx, laser may be employed) is the

mainstay of treatment, though radiotherapy may be employed where surgery is not practical or for salvage. Neck dissection is not required. However, it should be remembered that approximately 20% of verrucous carcinomas harbor a conventional squamous cell carcinoma ("hybrid" tumors) and these have a risk of nodal metastases.

Tumors and Cysts of the Jaw

85. Name the typical site of origin and list the major pathological features of a dentigerous cyst.
- Site of origin: surrounding the crown of an unerupted tooth, typically a third molar.
- Pathology: a flat epithelium composed of several layers of cuboidal to squamoid cells, with or without mucous

or ciliated cells. Inflammation may cause epithelial hyperplasia, spongiosis, and a frankly squamous appearance.

86. List the 4 major entities in the clinical and radiographic differential diagnosis of a dentigerous cyst.
- Odontogenic keratocyst.
- Unicystic ameloblastoma.
- Hyperplastic dental follicle.
- Odontogenic myxoma.

87. List the major clinical and pathological features of a periapical or radicular cyst.
- Clinical:
  - Is associated with carious, nonvital teeth, due to pulp necrosis and inflammation.
  - Occurs at the apex of the tooth root, less commonly lateral to it.
  - May arise at any age or be associated with any tooth.
  - May result in tooth pain (e.g., while eating) and tooth sensitivity to percussion.
- Pathological features:
  - Is preceded by a periapical granuloma (heavily inflamed granulation tissue with large numbers of plasma cells, foamy macrophages, and cholesterol clefts).
  - Is lined by nonkeratinizing squamous epithelium, with or without mucous cells.
  - Occasionally contains respiratory type epithelium (especially maxillary). Sometimes contains Rushton bodies (variably shaped eosinophilic, lamellated structures).

88. List 3 major entities considered in the broad category of fibroosseous lesions of the jaw.
- Fibrous dysplasia.
- Ossifying fibroma.
- Cementoosseous dysplasia.

89. List common entities in the clinical differential diagnosis of a gingival nodule.
- Pyogenic granuloma.
- Fibroma/fibrous hyperplasia.
- Peripheral ossifying fibroma (or other peripheral variants of odontogenic neoplasms).
- Peripheral giant cell lesion (rule out extraosseous extension of central giant cell lesion).

Note: there are innumerable less common causes, including reactive, neoplastic, benign, and malignant causes (including occasional metastases!).

IgG4-Related Diseases of the Head and Neck

90. List 3 IgG4-related entities of the head and neck.
- Mikulicz disease (IgG4-related dacryoadenitis and sialadenitis).
- Sclerosing sialadenitis (Küttner tumor: IgG4-related submandibular gland disease).
- Inflammatory orbital pseudotumor (IgG4-related orbital inflammation or orbital inflammatory pseudotumor).
- Chronic sclerosing dacryoadenitis (lacrimal gland enlargement, IgG4-related dacryoadenitis).
- Riedel thyroiditis (IgG4-related thyroid disease).

91. List at least 3 IgG4-related diseases in other parts of the body.
- Type 1 autoimmune pancreatitis (IgG4-related pancreatitis).
- IgG4-related sclerosing cholangitis.
- "Idiopathic" retroperitoneal fibrosis (Ormond disease) and related disorders (retroperitoneal fibrosis, and mesenteritis) in a subset of patients where the disease process is IgG4 related.
- Chronic sclerosing aortitis and periaortitis (IgG4-related aortitis or periaortitis).
- IgG4-related interstitial pneumonitis and pulmonary inflammatory pseudotumors (IgG4-related lung disease).
- IgG4-related kidney disease (including tubulointerstitial nephritis and membranous glomerulonephritis secondary to IgG4-RD).
- IgG4-related hypophysitis.
- IgG4-related pachymeningitis.

92. List the histologic features of IgG4-related disease in salivary glands.
- Storiform fibrosis.
- Dense lymphoplasmacytic infiltrate.
- Obliterative phlebitis.
- IHC: elevated absolute IgG4 count > 100/HPF, or IgG4/IgG ratio > 40%.

93. List 3 clinical/radiological differential diagnoses of IgG4-related salivary disease.
- Obstructive sialadenitis.
- Lymphoma (sclerosing variant of follicular lymphoma).
- Inflammatory pseudotumor.
- Radiation-induced sialadenitis.

CAP Protocols for Examining and Reporting Specimens From Head and Neck Sites (Larynx, Pharynx, Lip and Oral Cavity, Major Salivary Glands, Nose and Paranasal Sinuses)

94. True or false: the CAP protocol for the nose and paranasal sinuses applies to mucosal melanomas of this site.

True.

95. What is considered a "close margin" in head and neck cancer?
- It varies depending on the site.
- Generally, a close margin is ≤ 5 mm.
- For glottic tumors it is 2 mm.
- Note: margins should be reported for both invasive cancer and dysplasia of moderate degree or above.

96. What is the most common location of sinus tumors?

Maxillary sinus.

97. What are the subdivisions of the maxillary sinus? What is their importance?
- The maxillary sinus (or antrum) is divided approximately into halves by the Ohngren line, which extends from the medial canthus of the eye to the angle of the mandible. It divides the sinus into an anteroinferior portion (infrastructure) and superoposterior portion (suprastructure).
- Carcinomas of the suprastructure are associated with a worse prognosis than those of the infrastructure because of their closer proximity to the base of the skull and the eye.

98. Why is reporting of perineural invasion important in head and neck cancers?
- It is associated with poor local control and regional control.
- It has increased incidence of regional lymph node involvement.
- It indicates a decrease in disease specific survival and overall survival.
- It has a possible association with distant metastasis (conflicting data).
- It may be an indication for adjuvant chemoradiation.

99. What parameters are included when reporting lymph node involvement by head and neck cancers?
- Note: the status of the cervical lymph nodes is the most important prognostic factor in head and neck cancers.
- Mandatory elements to report:
  · Number of lymph nodes examined.
  · Number of lymph nodes involved.
- Extranodal extension (present, not identified or indeterminate).
- Optional elements to report, but reporting is suggested:
  · Greatest dimension of metastatic focus in a lymph node.
  · Extent of extracapsular extension (distance in millimeters of tumor from lymph node capsule).

100. What is the significance of extranodal extension?

It is a predictor of locoregional recurrence and distant metastasis and is an indication for postoperative radiotherapy (+/− chemotherapy) in patients with non-HPV related squamous cell carcinomas. This is not necessarily the case for HPV-related oropharyngeal carcinomas.

101. Describe the 3 anatomical subsites of the pharynx.

- Oropharynx: portion of the pharynx extending from the plane of the superior surface of the soft palate to the superior surface of the hyoid bone or floor of the vallecula. It includes:
  · Soft palate.
  · Palatine tonsils.
  · Anterior and posterior tonsillar pillars.
  · Tonsillar fossa and pillars.
  · Uvula.
  · Base of tongue, including the lingual tonsils.
  · Vallecula.
  · Posterior oropharyngeal wall.

- Nasopharynx: situated behind the nasal cavity and above the soft palate. It begins anteriorly at the posterior choana and extends along the plane of the airway to the level of the free border of the soft palate. It includes:
  · Nasopharyngeal tonsils (adenoids).
  · Orifice of eustachian tubes.
  · Fossa of Rosenmüller.
- Hypopharynx: extends from the plane of the superior border of the hyoid bone (or floor of vallecula) to the plane corresponding to the lower border of the cricoid cartilage. It includes:
  · Piriform sinuses (right and left).
  · Lateral and posterior hypopharyngeal walls.
  · Postcricoid region.

102. What is Waldeyer ring?

- A group of extranodal lymphoid tissues surrounding the upper end of the pharynx. It consists of the:
  · Palatine tonsils.

  · Pharyngeal tonsils (adenoids).
  · Base of tongue/lingual tonsils.
  · Adjacent submucosal lymphatics.

103. Classify the histologic types of neuroendocrine carcinoma of the upper aerodigestive tract, based on the 2017 WHO classification.

- Well-differentiated neuroendocrine carcinoma (carcinoid, neuroendocrine carcinoma, grade 1).
- Moderately differentiated neuroendocrine carcinoma (atypical carcinoid, neuroendocrine carcinoma, grade 2).

- Poorly differentiated neuroendocrine carcinoma (neuroendocrine carcinoma grade 3; includes large cell and small cell neuroendocrine carcinoma).

104. What ancillary study is required for squamous cell carcinoma of oropharynx (OPSCC) and how is it reported?

- Some form of high hisk HPV testing is required.
- IHC for p16 is a very good surrogate marker of active HPV infection in oropharyngeal squamous cell carcinoma, and should be reported as follows:
  · Positive (> 70% diffuse and strong nuclear and cytoplasmic staining).

  · Equivocal (< 70% but > 50% diffuse and strong nuclear and cytoplasmic staining).
  · Negative (< 50% diffuse and strong nuclear and cytoplasmic staining).
  · Indeterminate (explain).

105. List other HPV testing methods for OPSCC.

- HPV DNA by in situ hybridization.
- HPV E6/E7 mRNA by in situ hybridization.

- HPV DNA by polymerase chain reaction.
- HPV E6/E7 mRNA by polymerase chain reaction.

Note: these methods can be used as a substitute for p16 or for equivocal or indeterminate p16 results.

106. What are the recommendations for confirmatory HPV testing in oropharyngeal squamous cell carcinoma based on morphology and p16 staining profile?

MORPHOLOGY	P16	REQUIRES HPV-SPECIFIC TESTING CONFIRMATION
Nonkeratinizing or predominantly nonkeratinizing.	Strong and diffuse (cytoplasmic and nuclear, i.e., > 70%).	No.
Nonkeratinizing or predominantly nonkeratinizing.	Negative or only focally positive.	Yes.
Keratinizing.	Strong and diffuse (cytoplasmic and nuclear, i.e., > 70%).	Yes.
Keratinizing.	Negative or only focally positive.	No.

107. Is there any indication to test nasopharyngeal, oral cavity, or laryngeal cancers for HPV?

- Rare nonkeratinizing (differentiated or undifferentiated) nasopharyngeal carcinomas are HPV related, so testing is indicated if they are EBV negative.
- There is no established role for routine HPV testing of the oral cavity or laryngeal carcinomas.

108. Describe the AJCC staging* for occult primary squamous cell carcinoma of the neck.

pT category: T0.

pN category: assigned as per nasopharynx if EBV related; as per HPV-mediated oropharynx if HPV/p16 positive; as per the generic N categorization for head and neck squamous cell carcinoma (HNSCC) if both EBV and HPV are negative.

Note: EBV and HPV/p16 testing is suggested for nonkeratinizing and/or basaloid neck tumors with an occult primary tumor, although as oropharyngeal carcinomas are much more common, upfront p16 is the most practical approach.

*This chapter uses the eighth edition of the AJCC staging manual.

109. True or false: superficial erosion alone of the bone/tooth socket by gingival primary tumor is not sufficient to classify a tumor as T4.

True.

Note: superficial erosion can be difficult to distinguish from true bone invasion in circumscribed (pushing) tumors and in patients with alveolar bone recession. A general staging guideline is to choose the lower staging parameter when there is uncertainty.

110. Explain the difference between tumor thickness and depth of invasion in oral cancers.

- Tumor thickness (TT): from mucosal surface to deepest point of tissue invasion.
- Depth of invasion (DOI): from basement membrane of adjacent normal mucosa to deepest point of invasion.
  - Note: TT and DPI are not interchangeable terms. TT can exceed DOI in exophytic tumors; TT can be less than DOI in ulcerated tumors.
- DOI is measured from a vertical "plumb" line intersecting with a horizontal line extending across the tumor surface from intact adjacent surface.
- DOI measurement can be difficult because of tumor and site irregularity. Should be correlated with proper gross description.

111. Discuss how DOI affects the pT category.

- The important cutoffs are 5 mm and 10 mm, and DOI can increase the pT category independent of the greatest dimension of the tumor.
- Tumors ≤ 2 cm but DOI > 5 mm are pT2.
- Tumors > 2 cm and ≤ 4 cm but DOI > 10 mm are pT3.
- Tumors > 4 cm can be pT3 or pT4 if DOI ≤ 10 mm or > 10 mm, respectively.

112. What is meant by *worst pattern of invasion type 5* when reporting oral cavity cancers?

It means dispersion of ≥ 1 mm between tumor satellites. These dispersions are found around the leading edge of a tumor, and may be due to direct infiltration of tumor, perineural or lymphovascular spread. The intervening tissue should be normal.

113. Is WPOI-5 (versus WPOI 1-4) an optional or mandatory element in the CAP oral cavity reporting protocol?

Optional: however, it is an adverse prognostic factor for oral cavity cancers.

114. Is histologic grade a good prognostic factor in squamous cell carcinoma? Do all squamous cell carcinoma require grading?

- For conventional squamous cell carcinoma, histologic grading does not perform well as a prognosticator, but is required.
- Variants of squamous cell carcinoma (e.g., verrucous, sarcomatoid, basaloid) have an intrinsic biologic potential and do not require grading.
- HPV-mediated OPSCC does not require grading and the behavior is independent of morphology (e.g., papillary, nonkeratinizing, adenosquamous).

115. What is important about the assessment of extraparenchymal extension as it pertains to the pT3 classification of major salivary gland tumors?

Microscopic evidence of extraparenchymal extension is not sufficient for a pT3 designation. A classification of pT3 requires clinical or macroscopic evidence of invasion of soft tissues or nerves. (Note: involvement of the facial nerve is considered pT4a disease.)

116. How is carcinoma ex pleomorphic adenoma graded and evaluated?

- Histologic grade:
  - Low grade.
  - High grade (typically adenocarcinoma, NOS or salivary duct carcinoma).
- Extent of invasion:
  - Noninvasive (intracapsular) cancers: completely confined within the capsule of the preexisting pleomorphic

adenoma without penetration into extracapsular tissue. The entire lesion must be submitted in order to exclude invasion.
  - Minimally invasive cancers: ≤ 1.5 mm of extracapsular extension.
  - Invasive carcinomas: > 1.5 mm of invasion.

117. What types of intraepithelial dysplasia exist and how are they graded?

- Nonkeratinizing ("classic") dysplasia.
- Keratinizing dysplasia.
- For both types, grading includes mild, moderate, and severe categories. Severe keratinizing dysplasia is synonymous

with carcinoma in situ as it has a similar propensity for progression.
- In the larynx only, the WHO recommends a 2-tiered system with low grade dysplasia (keratosis, hyperplasia, mild dysplasia) and high grade dysplasia (moderate, severe, CIS).

118. What are important features of dysplasia of the upper aerodigestive tract?

- Full thickness dysplasia (carcinoma in situ) is uncommon, but may occur, for instance in the floor of mouth and ventral tongue.
- Invasive carcinoma can develop from non-full-thickness keratinizing dysplasia, even when atypia is limited to the lower third (basal zone) of the surface epithelium.
- The grading is problematic and lacks reproducibility among pathologists.

- Keratinizing severe dysplasia is often multifocal (field effect) and frequently occurs adjacent to or near synchronous foci of invasive carcinoma. The entire upper aerodigestive tract should be evaluated.
- Keratinizing severe dysplasia has a rate of progression to invasive carcinoma that is greater than that of "classic" carcinoma in situ and requires therapeutic intervention.

119. How do you report mucosal margins in the setting of keratinizing dysplasia?

- The presence of keratinizing mild dysplasia at (or near) a surgical margin should not be viewed/reported as a positive margin.
- The presence of keratinizing moderate or severe dysplasia at (or near) a surgical margin should be viewed/reported as a positive margin.

- The distance in millimeters of moderate or greater dysplasia from the margin should be reported, as should the site of this margin, if known.

120. Where do mucosal melanomas most frequently occur? What is their minimal T stage?

- Incidence:
  - Two-thirds arise in the sinonasal tract.
  - One-quarter arise in the oral cavity.
  - The rest arise sporadically in other mucosal sites of the head and neck.

- To reflect aggressive behavior:
  - Primary cancers limited to the mucosa are considered T3 lesions.
  - Advanced mucosal melanomas are classified as T4a and T4b.

121. What is leukoplakia? What are the risks for malignant transformation in a patient with white mucosal lesions (leukoplakia)?

- Leukoplakia refers to white mucosal lesions that cannot be removed by rubbing and which cannot be characterized as any other clinically definable lesion. Leukoplakias can be divided into homogenous (smooth appearance) and nonhomogenous (irregular appearing surface).
- It is a clinical term that correlates to keratosis, but does not necessarily imply a histological diagnosis of dysplasia or malignancy.

- The following features increase the risk for dysplasia:
  - Location at the floor of the mouth, tongue (lateral and ventral), and vermilion border of the lip.
  - Nonhomogeneous appearance: the incidence of malignant transformation for homogeneous leukoplakia is 3% and for nonhomogeneous leukoplakia is 15%.

122. What is erythroplakia? What is its risk for malignant transformation?

- Erythroplakia are so-called red mucosal lesions.
- In erythroplakic lesions, invasive carcinoma is present in 50% of cases, carcinoma in situ in 40%, and mild to moderate dysplasia in 10%.

- Carcinomas developing from erythroplakia are usually the nonkeratinizing type.

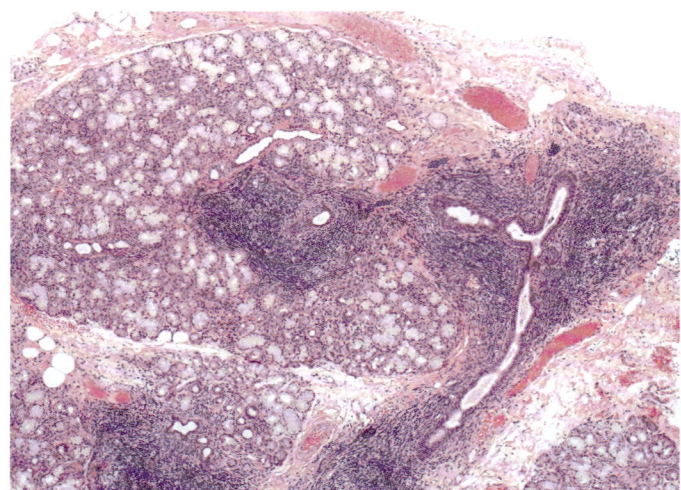

IMAGE 12.1 Sjögren syndrome. A minor salivary gland shows dense lymphocytic infiltration surrounding, and adjacent to, salivary ducts (H&E, x40).

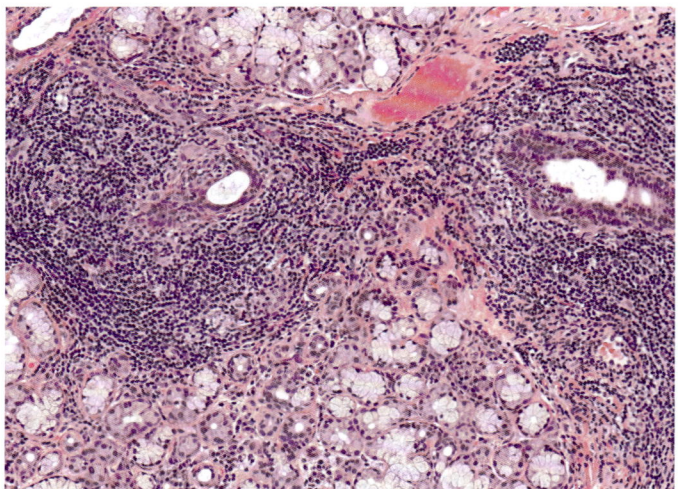

IMAGE 12.2 Sjögren syndrome. A lymphoepithelial lesion is shown, with proliferating ductal epithelium infiltrated by lymphocytes, and a dense lymphoid infiltrate in the surrounding tissues (H&E, x100).

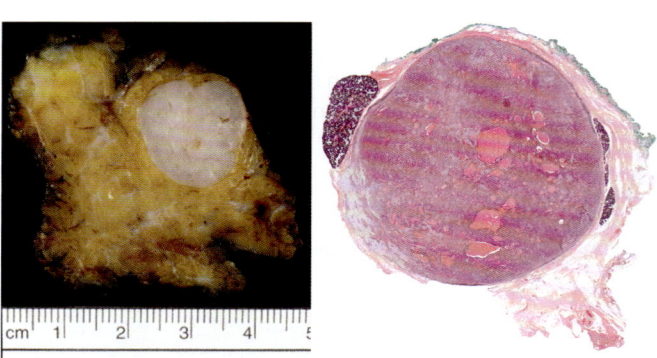

IMAGE 12.3 Pleomorphic adenoma. Left: gross shows a circumscribed nodule with glistening and somewhat translucent cut surface surrounded by normal parotid gland tissue. Right: scanning magnification shows another pleomorphic adenoma with adjacent minor salivary gland tissue.

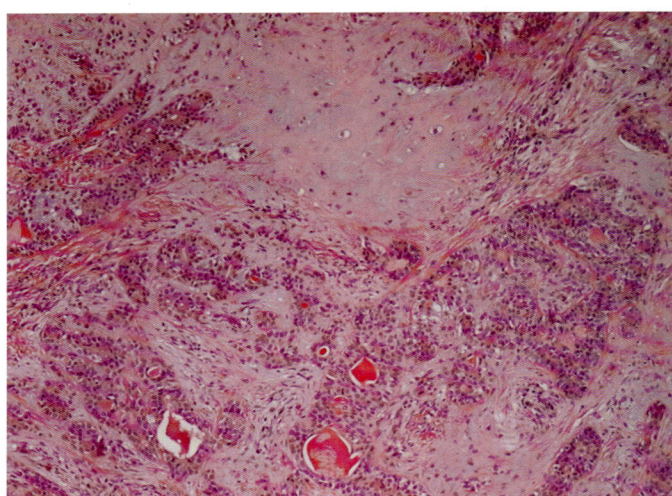

IMAGE 12.4 Pleomorphic adenoma with bilayer tubules containing eosinophilic secretion in the lower field and chondroid stroma in upper central region (H&E, x100).

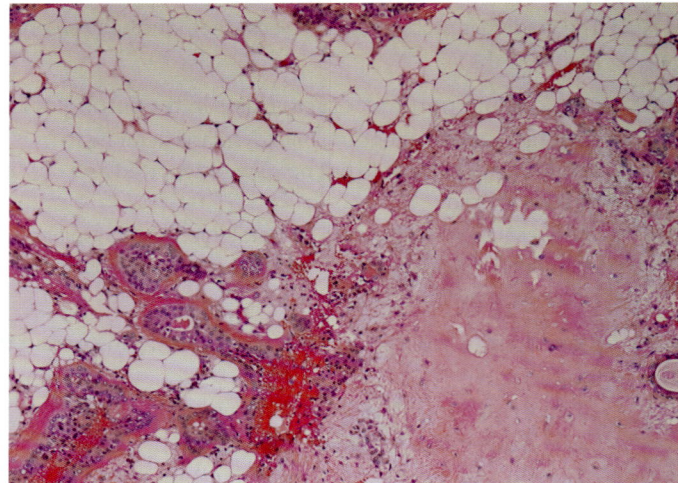

IMAGE 12.5 Pleomorphic adenoma. The image shows chondroid stroma in the lower right field with upper and left portions containing adipose stroma (H&E, x100).

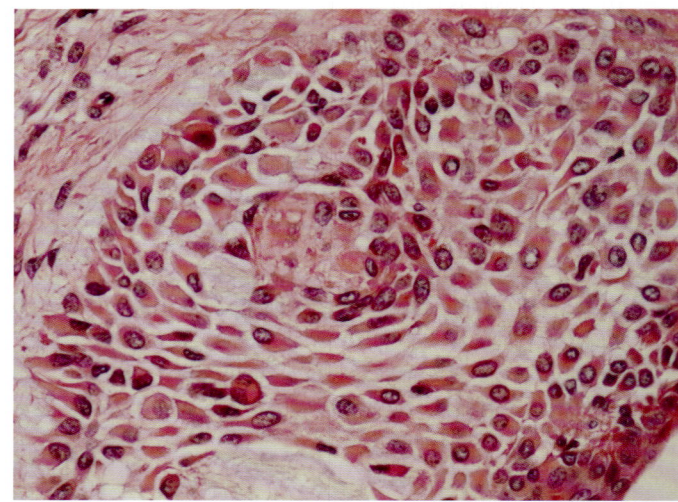

IMAGE 12.6 Pleomorphic adenoma. This field contains a predominance of hyaline (plasmacytoid) myoepithelial cells (H&E, x200).

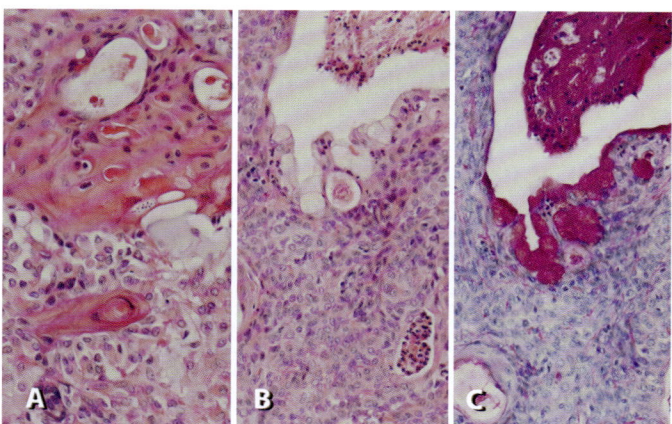

IMAGE 12.7 Pleomorphic adenoma with mucoepidermoid differentiation. Image A: squamous differentiation with keratinization (H&E, x200). Keratinization would be unusual in low grade mucoepidermoid carcinoma. Image B: numerous goblet cells (H&E, x200). Image C: goblet cells highlighted by PAS plus diastase stain (PAS plus diastase, x200).

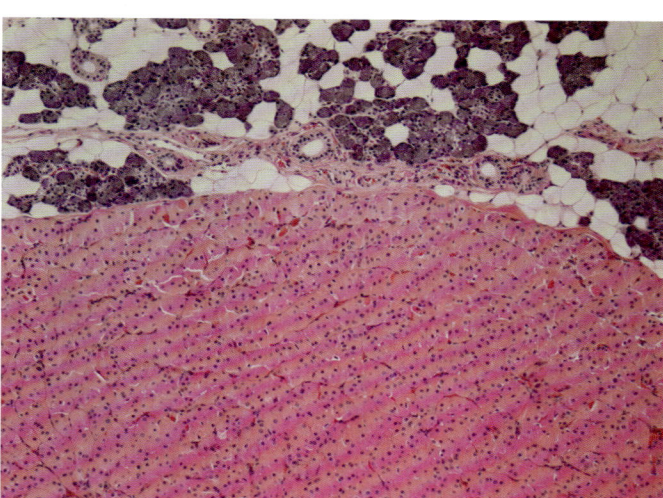

IMAGE 12.10 Oncocytoma, parotid gland. The image shows a circumscribed nodule with normal parotid gland tissue above (H&E, x100).

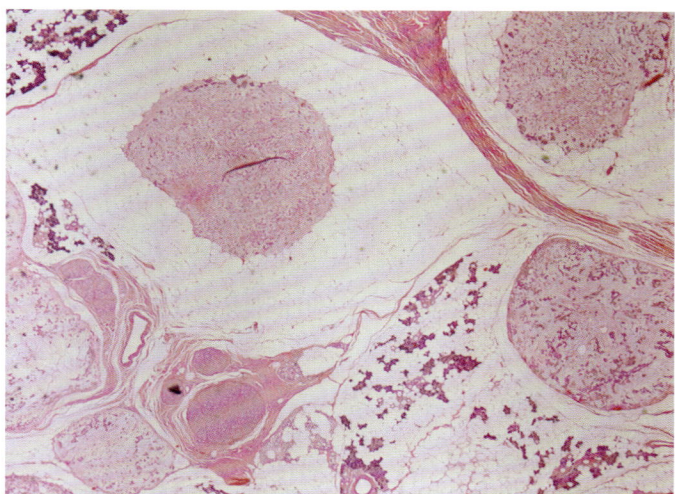

IMAGE 12.8 Pleomorphic adenoma. Multiple nodules as seen here indicate recurrent pleomorphic adenoma in every instance (H&E, x40).

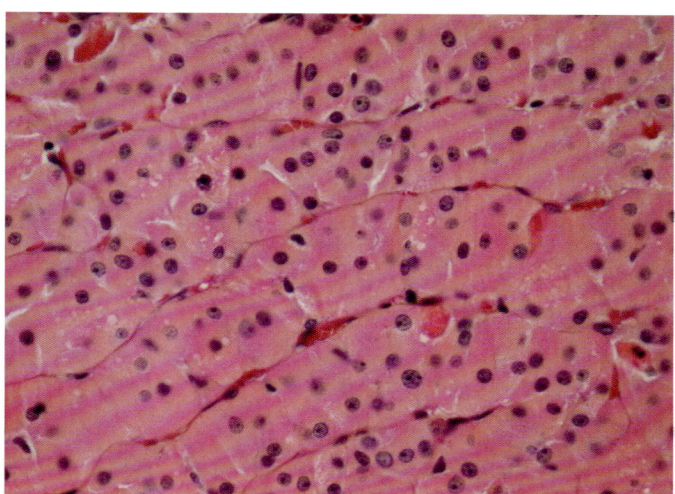

IMAGE 12.11 Oncocytoma, parotid gland. The image shows cells with abundant granular eosinophilic cytoplasm and vesicular nuclei with conspicuous nucleoli (H&E, x400).

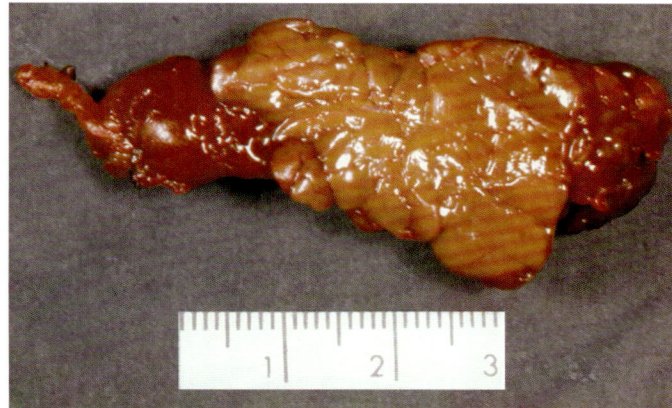

IMAGE 12.9 Oncocytoma, parotid gland. This is a circumscribed, homogeneous brown tumor.

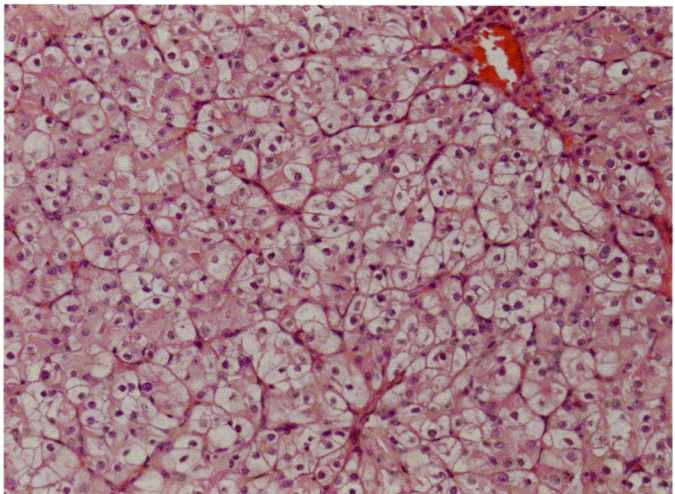

IMAGE 12.12 Oncocytoma, parotid gland. Some oncocytomas are composed predominantly or purely of cells with clear cytoplasm, requiring differentiation from metastatic renal cell carcinoma (H&E, x200).

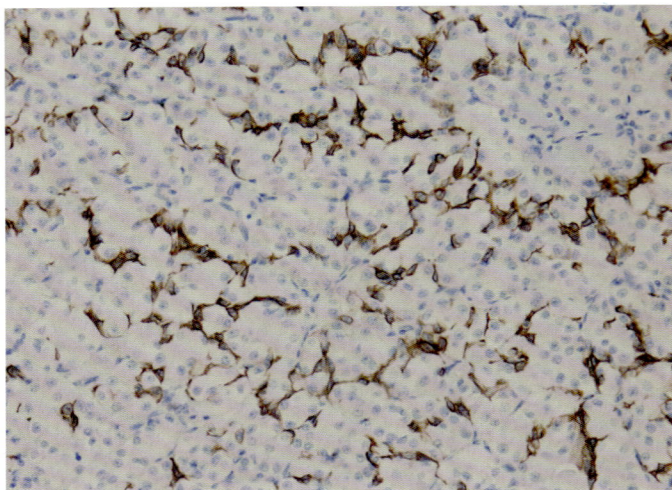

IMAGE 12.13 Oncocytoma, parotid gland. Basal cells stain positive with high molecular weight cytokeratins in oncocytoma; basal cells are not present in metastatic renal cell carcinoma (cytokeratin 5, x200).

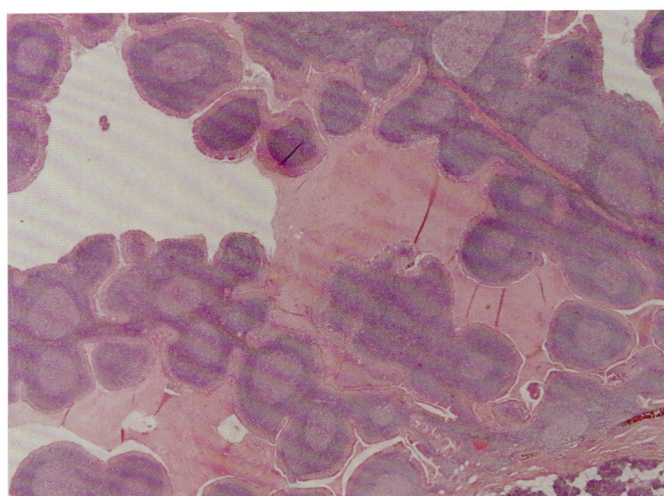

IMAGE 12.16 Warthin tumor. Low magnification shows lymphoid follicles covered by eosinophilic epithelium (H&E, x20).

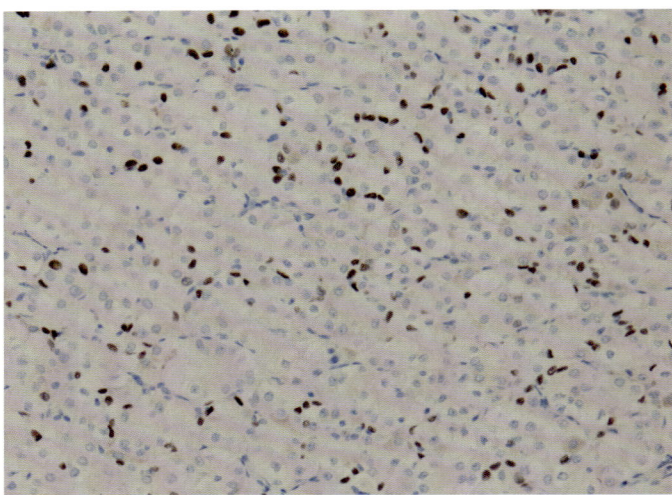

IMAGE 12.14 Oncocytoma, parotid gland. Basal cells are also positive for p63 in oncocytoma (p63, x200).

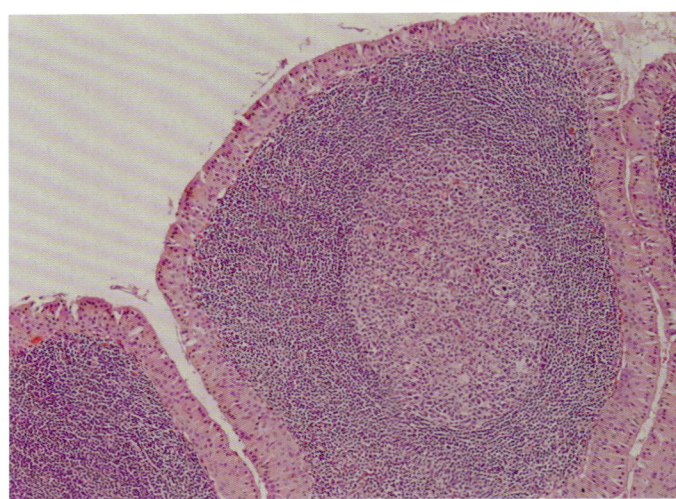

IMAGE 12.17 Warthin tumor. High magnification shows lymphoid follicles covered by a double layer of oncocytic cells (H&E, x200).

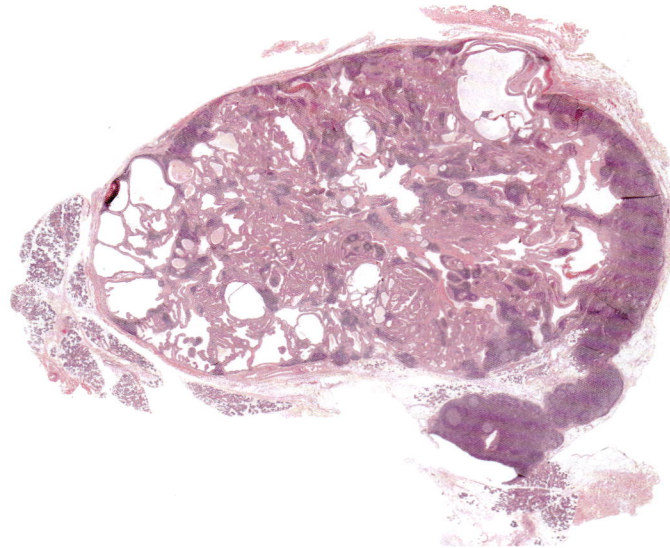

IMAGE 12.15 Warthin tumor. Scanning magnification shows a well-demarcated cystic tumor.

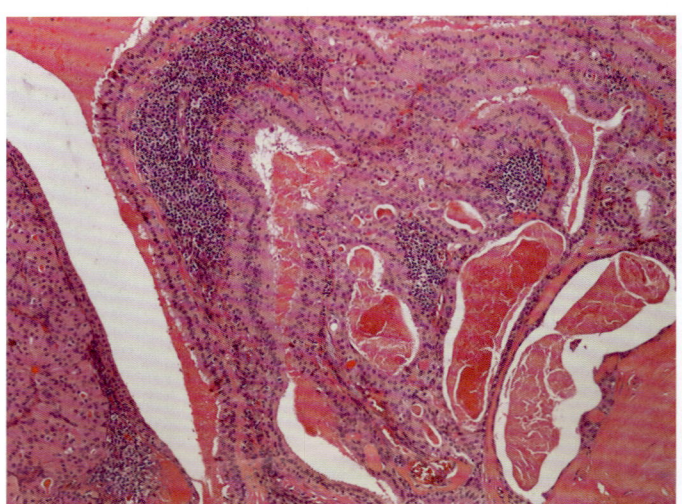

IMAGE 12.18 Warthin tumor, parotid gland. Glands and papillary structures have a surface of bilayer oncocytic epithelium with reactive lymphoid stroma (H&E, x100).

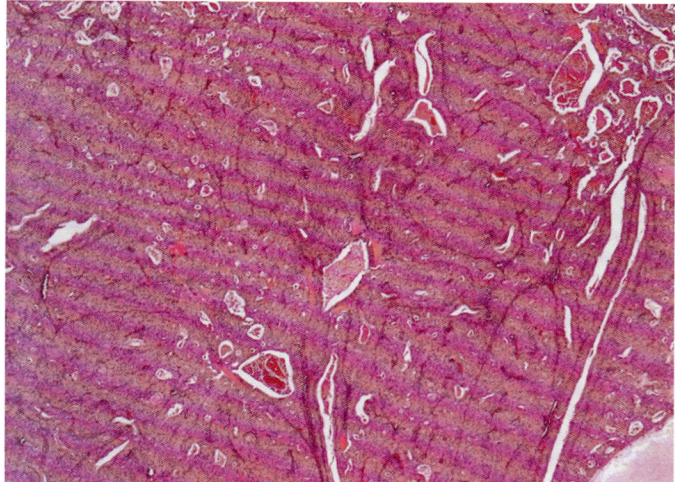

IMAGE 12.19 Warthin tumor, parotid gland. The image shows a lymphocyte poor region with oncocytic hyperplasia, resembling oncocytoma (H&E, x40).

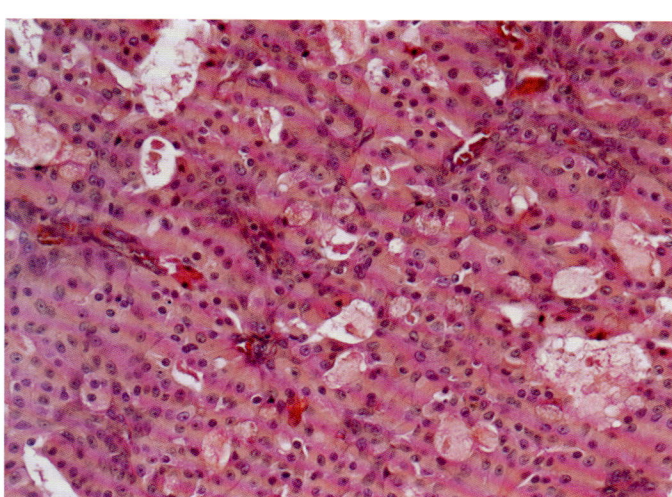

IMAGE 12.20 Warthin tumor, parotid gland. Foci containing mucinous (goblet) cells may lead to confusion with mucoepidermoid carcinoma, a tumor that may show prominent mucinous differentiation (H&E, x200).

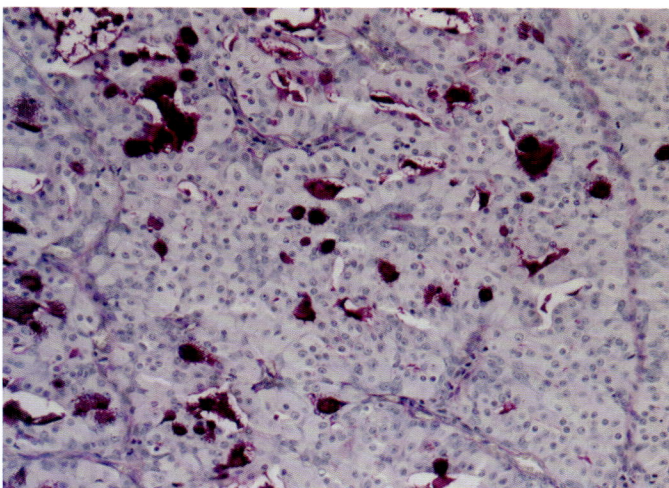

IMAGE 12.21 Warthin tumor, parotid gland. Presence of mucinous cells is confirmed with PAS plus diastase stain (PAS plus diastase, x200).

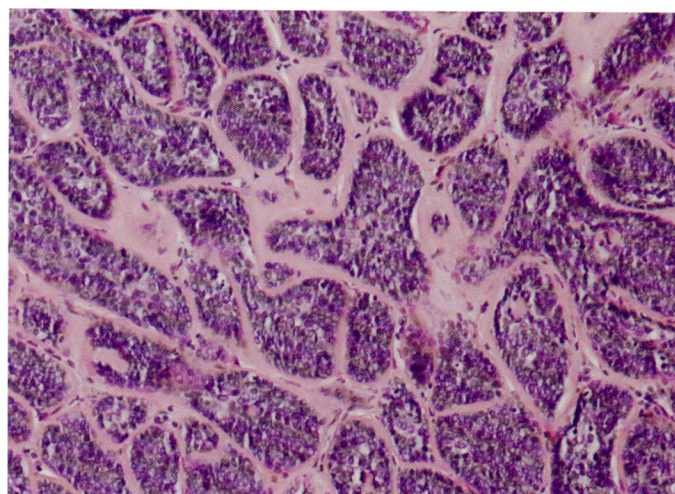

IMAGE 12.22 Basal cell adenoma, membranous variant. The image shows nests of small basaloid cells with scant cytoplasm surrounded by a cuff of eosinophilic hyaline material and scattered droplets of hyaline material within nests (H&E, x100).

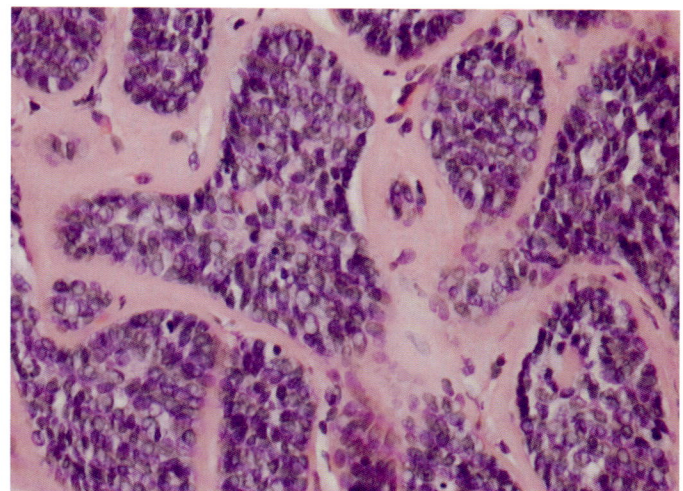

IMAGE 12.23 Basal cell adenoma, membranous variant (H&E, x400).

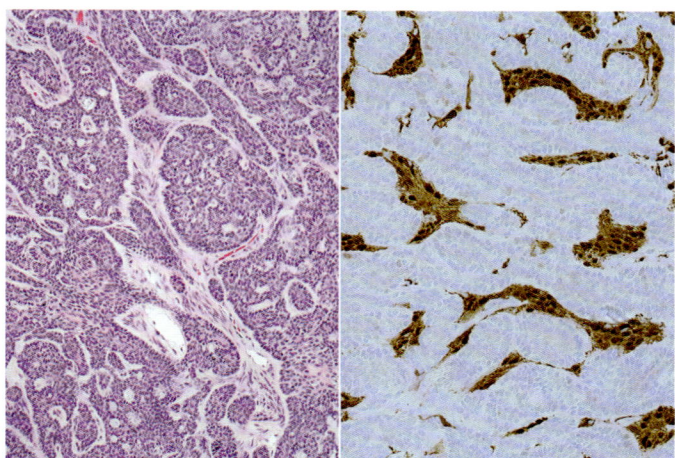

IMAGE 12.24 Basal cell adenoma. Left: the image shows a basal cell adenoma with combined solid and trabecular patterns and a cellular spindle stroma (H&E, x100). Right: the image shows S100 stain, with strong positivity of the spindle cell stroma.

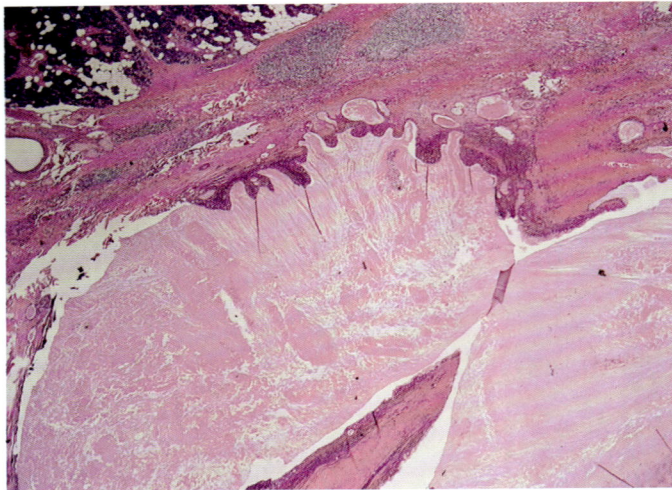

IMAGE 12.25 Mucoepidermoid carcinoma, parotid gland. This tumor consists of an irregular unilocular cyst. Note the lymphoid aggregates adjacent to the tumor, common in mucoepidermoid carcinoma (H&E, x20).

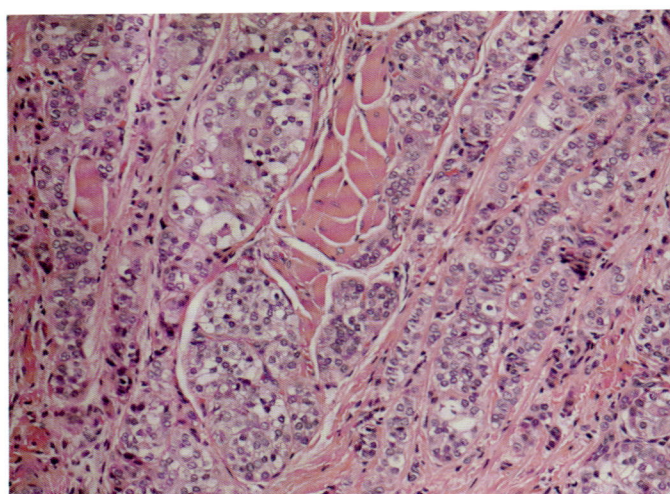

IMAGE 12.28 Mucoepidermoid carcinoma, high grade, parotid gland. This tumor grows in small nests and cords that invade skeletal muscle (H&E, x200).

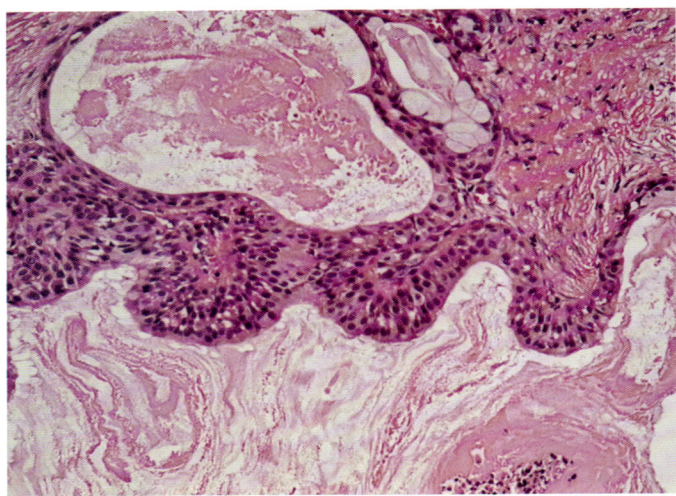

IMAGE 12.26 Mucoepidermoid carcinoma, parotid gland. This is a low grade carcinoma composed of mucinous cells and intermediate cells lining the cystic space (H&E, x100).

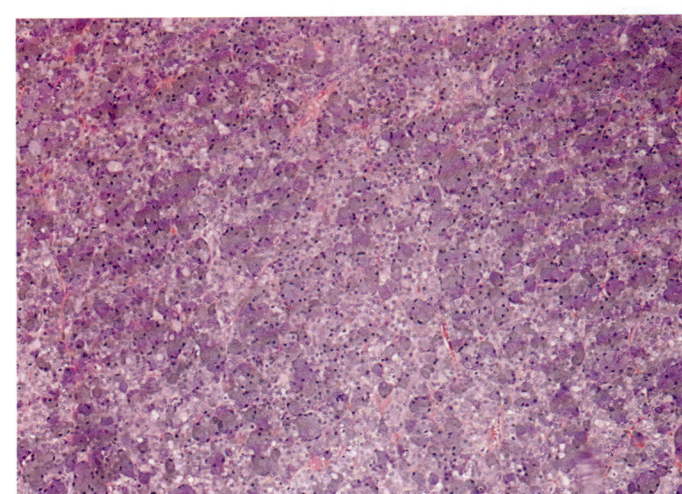

IMAGE 12.29 Acinic cell carcinoma. The image shows a solid growth pattern composed of serous acinar cells and intercalated duct cells (H&E, x100).

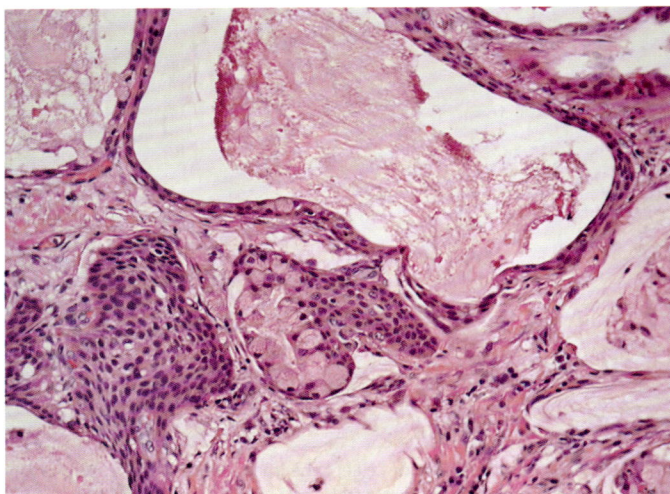

IMAGE 12.27 Mucoepidermoid carcinoma, palate. This is a low grade carcinoma composed of mucinous and squamoid cells (H&E, x200).

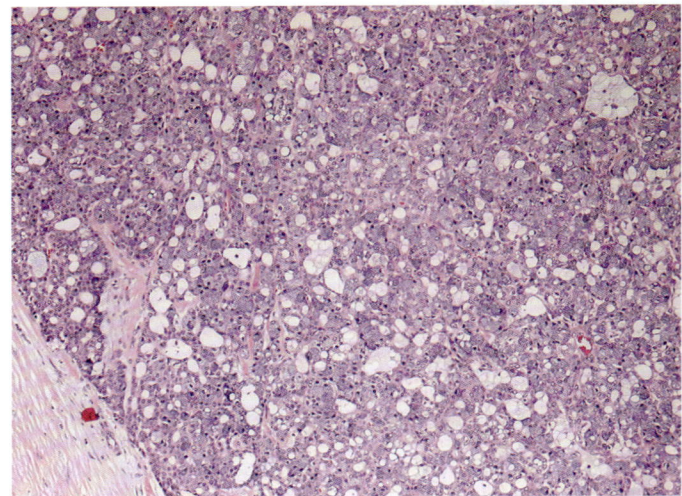

IMAGE 12.30 Acinic cell carcinoma, microcystic pattern (H&E, x100).

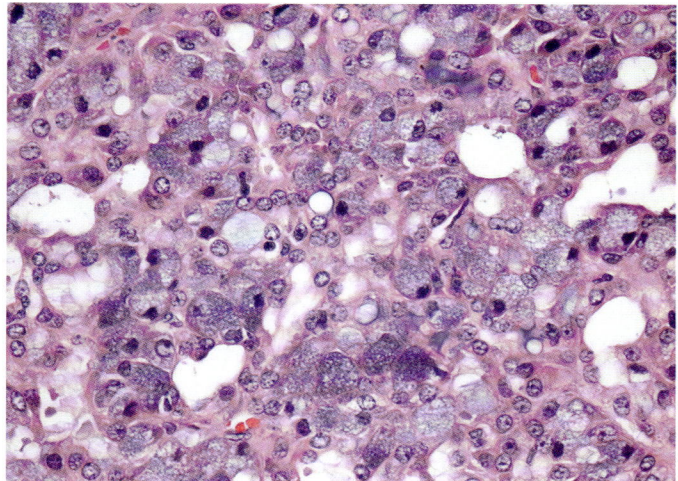

IMAGE 12.31 Acinic cell carcinoma. The image shows serous acinar cells with abundant granular basophilic cytoplasm and small regular hyperchromatic nuclei (H&E, x400).

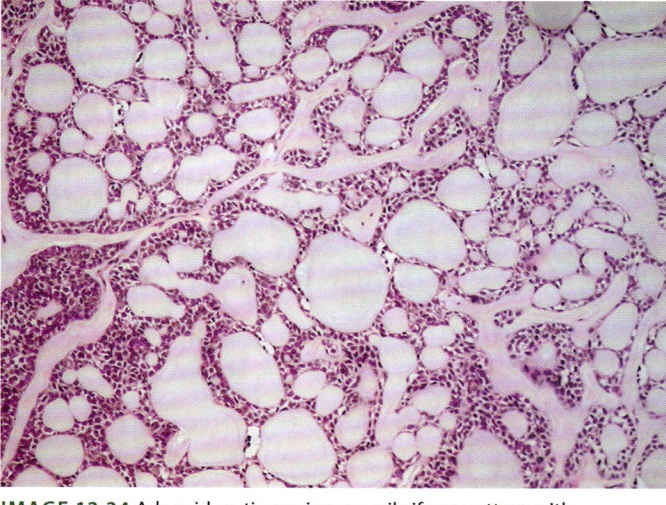

IMAGE 12.34 Adenoid cystic carcinoma, cribriform pattern with predominance of pseudocystic spaces filled with acid mucin (pale blue-gray) and eosinophilic fibrillar material (H&E, x100).

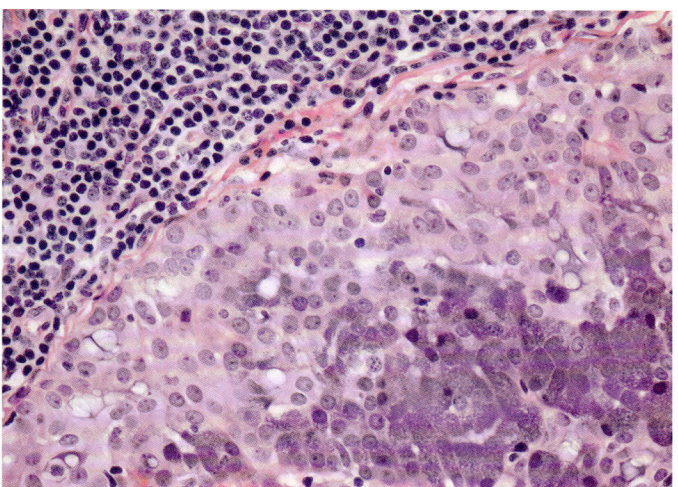

IMAGE 12.32 Acinic cell carcinoma. Note the serous acinar cells with abundant granular basophilic cytoplasm in the lower right, and the intercalated duct cells with moderate amounts of pale eosinophilic cytoplasm and vesicular nuclei with conspicuous nucleoli to the left and above. Lymphoid tissue, in the upper left, is a common finding in acinic cell carcinoma (H&E, x400).

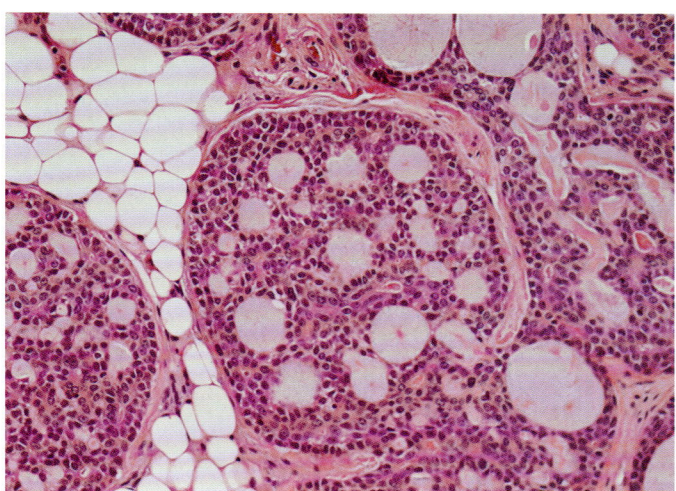

IMAGE 12.35 Adenoid cystic carcinoma, cribriform pattern with predominance of pseudocystic spaces filled with acid mucin (pale blue-gray). True ductal lumina are inconspicuous and contain eosinophilic secretion (H&E, x200).

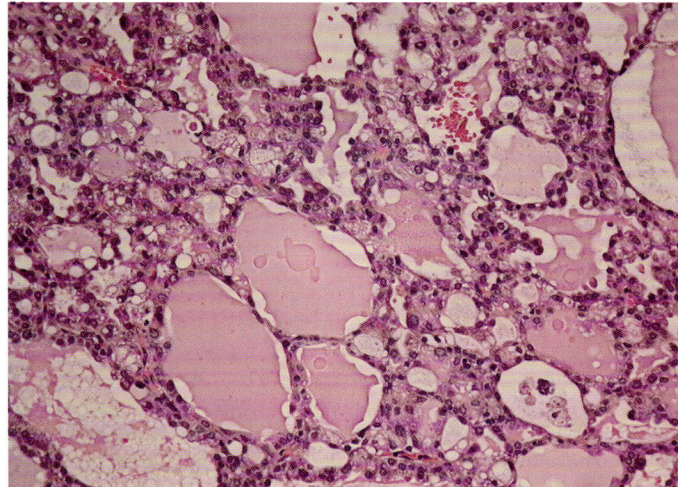

IMAGE 12.33 Acinic cell carcinoma, follicular pattern (H&E, x200).

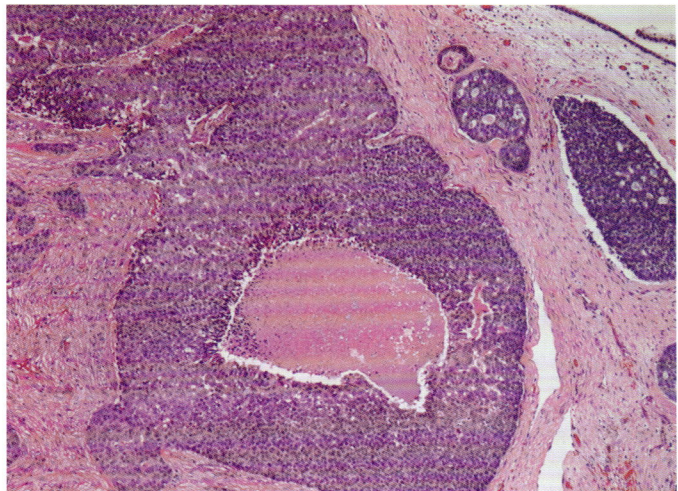

IMAGE 12.36 Adenoid cystic carcinoma, solid pattern with comedo-like necrosis (H&E, x40).

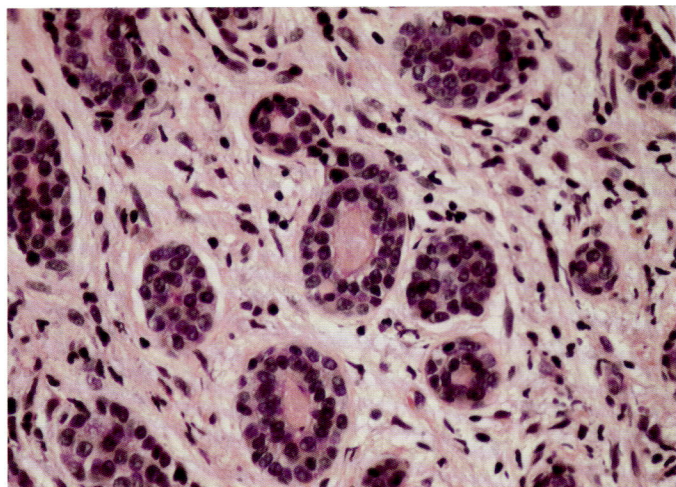

IMAGE 12.37 Adenoid cystic carcinoma, tubular pattern with bilayer tubules (H&E, x400).

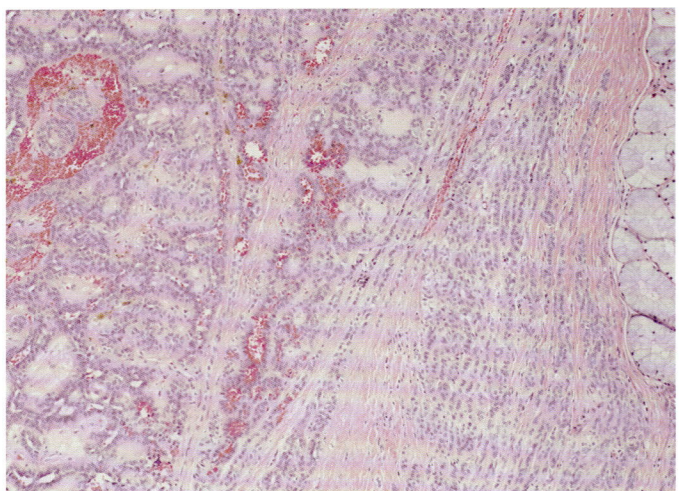

IMAGE 12.38 Polymorphous low grade adenocarcinoma. This palatal tumor shows several architectural patterns, including strands of cells in a single file pattern (right). The tumor cells are monomorphous. Note residual mucinous acini on the far right (H&E, x200).

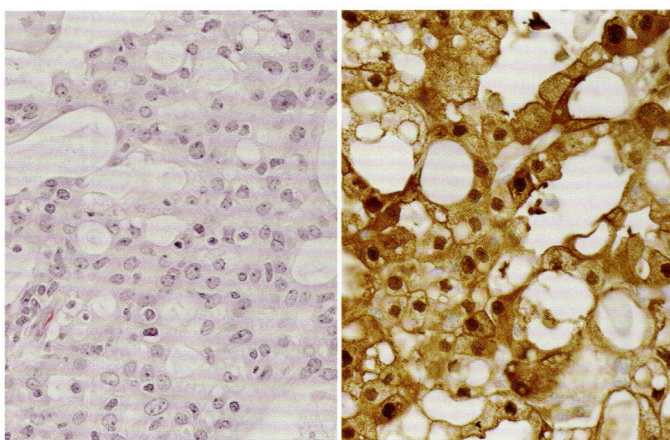

IMAGE 12.39 Secretory carcinoma (formerly mammary analog secretory carcinoma). Right: the tumor forms glands containing bubbly secretions and is composed of cells with eosinophilic, vacuolated cytoplasm. The nuclei have easily visible, often central nucleoli, with occasional nuclear grooves (H&E, x400). Left: S100 stain showing moderate to strong nuclear and cytoplasmic positivity (x400).

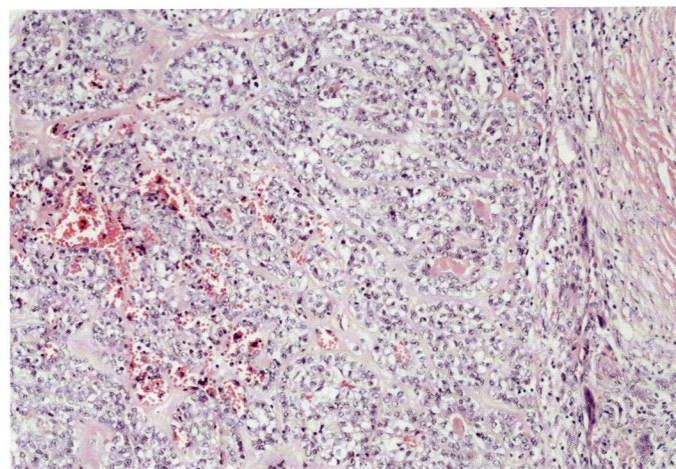

IMAGE 12.40 Epithelial-myoepithelial carcinoma. There is a predominance of clear myoepithelial cells in nests with less conspicuous epithelial cells forming lumens with central eosinophilic mucin (H&E, x100).

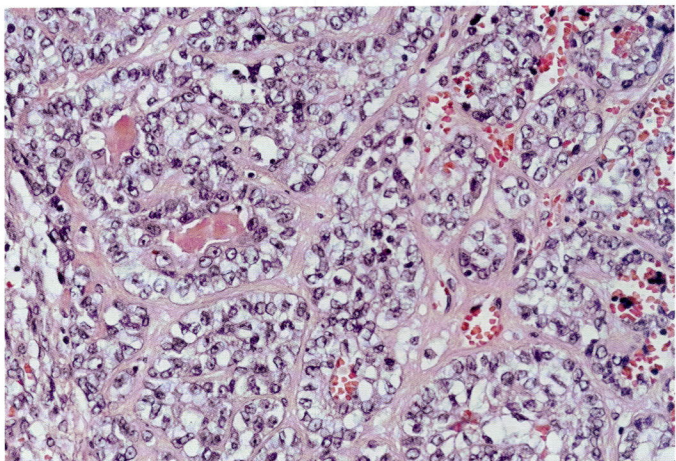

IMAGE 12.41 Epithelial-myoepithelial carcinoma. Nuclear atypia is present in both elements, somewhat more than is typical for these low grade tumors (H&E, x200).

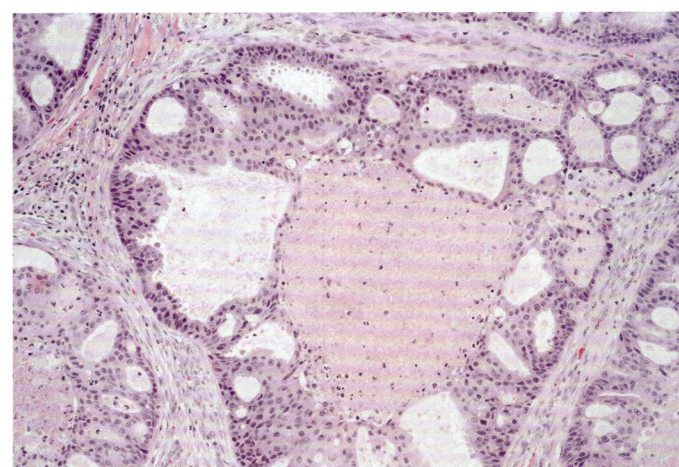

IMAGE 12.42 Salivary duct carcinoma. This resembles high grade comedo type ductal carcinoma in situ of the breast. The tumor cells exhibit apocrine differentiation. They are typically androgen receptor positive, and may exhibit membranous HER2 positivity (H&E, x40).

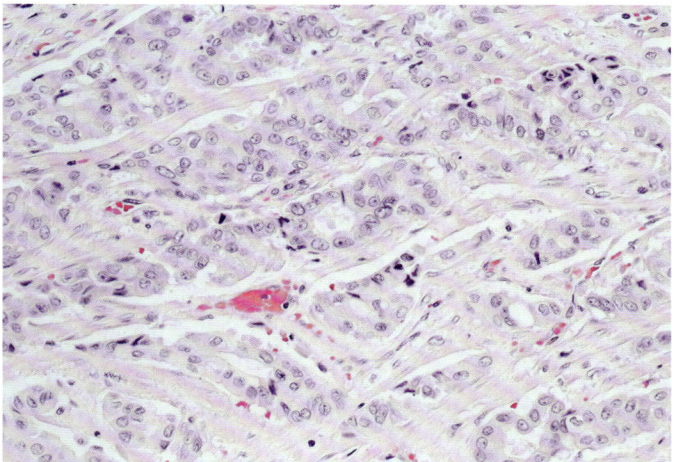

IMAGE 12.43 Salivary duct carcinoma, with an obvious invasive component (H&E, x200).

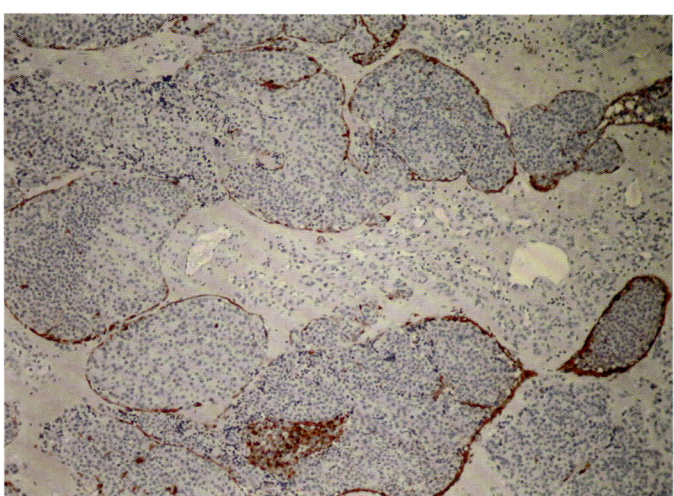

IMAGE 12.46 Olfactory neuroblastoma. The image shows sustentacular cells at the periphery of nests highlighted by S100 stain (S100, x100).

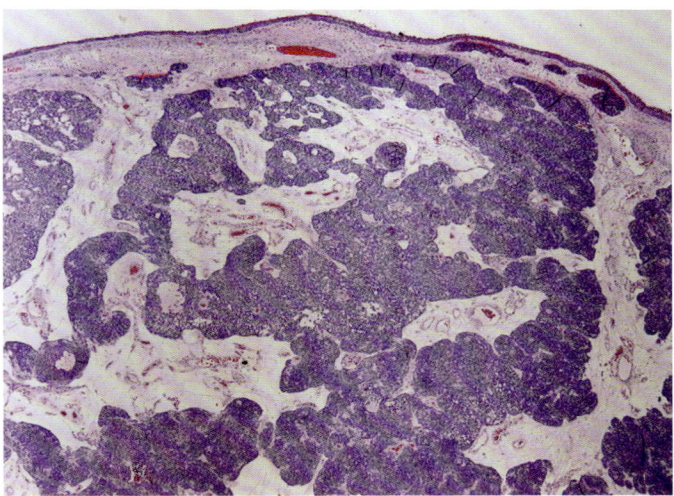

IMAGE 12.44 Olfactory neuroblastoma. The image shows a small cell neoplasm organized into broad trabeculae with intervening loose, vessel-rich stroma (H&E, x40).

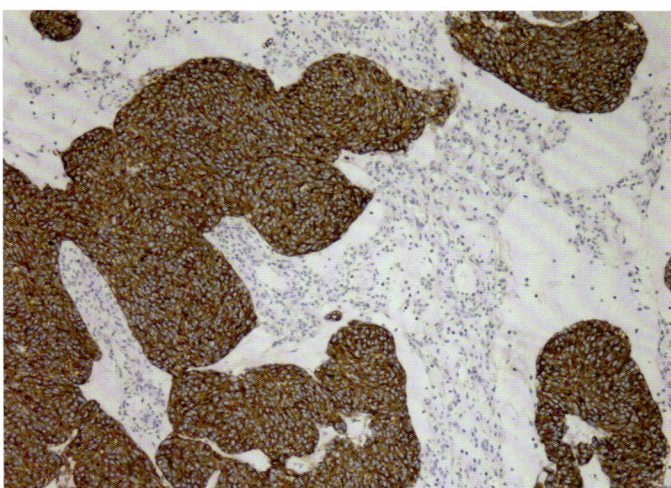

IMAGE 12.47 Olfactory neuroblastoma. The image shows a strong positive staining for synaptophysin (synaptophysin, x100).

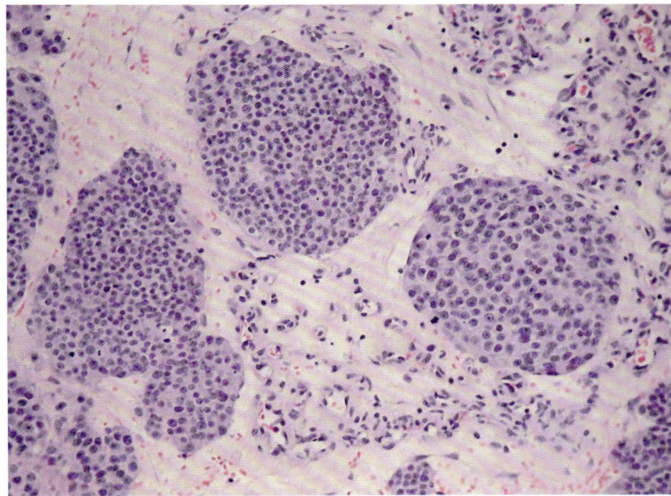

IMAGE 12.45 Olfactory neuroblastoma. The image shows large nests of relatively uniform cells with moderate cytoplasm and scattered ill-defined rosettes. The stroma is richly vascular (H&E, x200).

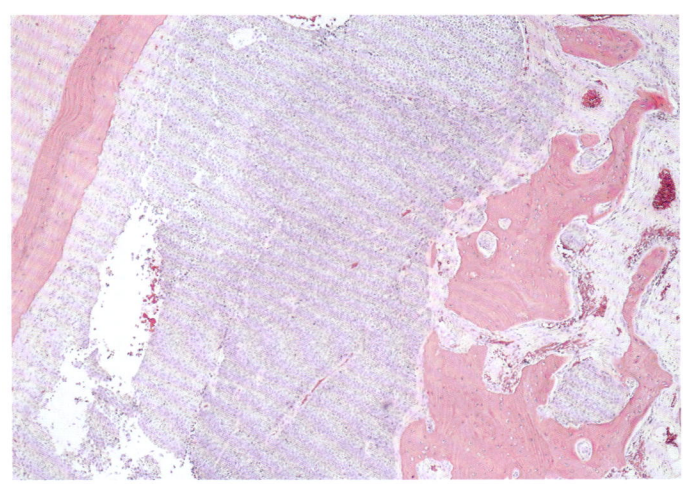

IMAGE 12.48 Nonkeratinizing squamous cell carcinoma of the nasal cavity, with bone invasion (H&E, x40).

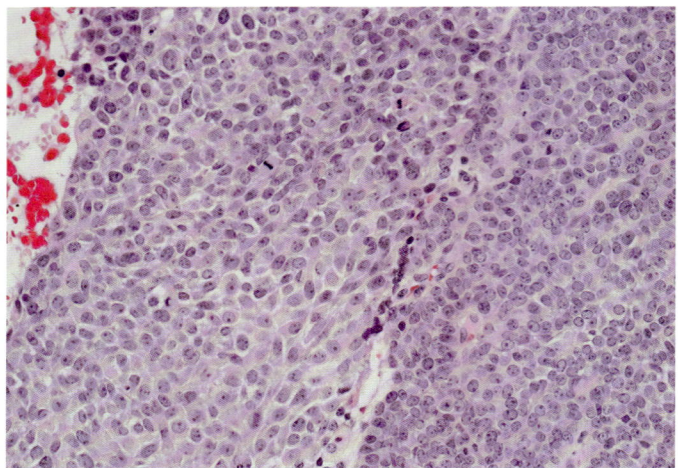

IMAGE 12.49 Nonkeratinizing squamous cell carcinoma of the nasal cavity. Most of the tumor is basaloid; areas on the left are more polygonal and squamoid. Glandular differentiation may be found in some cases (H&E, x200).

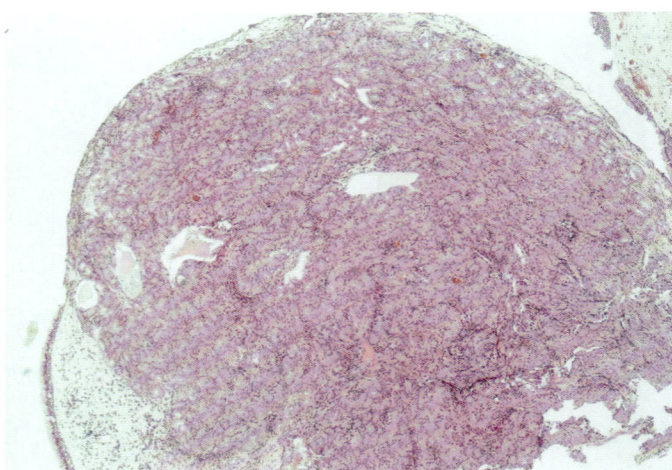

IMAGE 12.52 Low grade sinonasal nonintestinal type adenocarcinoma. The image shows a mass of closely packed glands (H&E, x40).

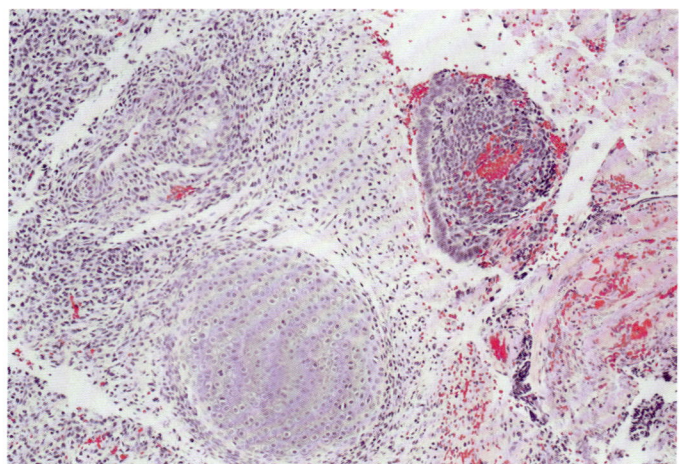

IMAGE 12.50 Sinonasal teratocarcinosarcoma. This image shows a mixture of nondescript spindle areas, chondroid, epithelial, and small blue (blastema-like) components (H&E, x100).

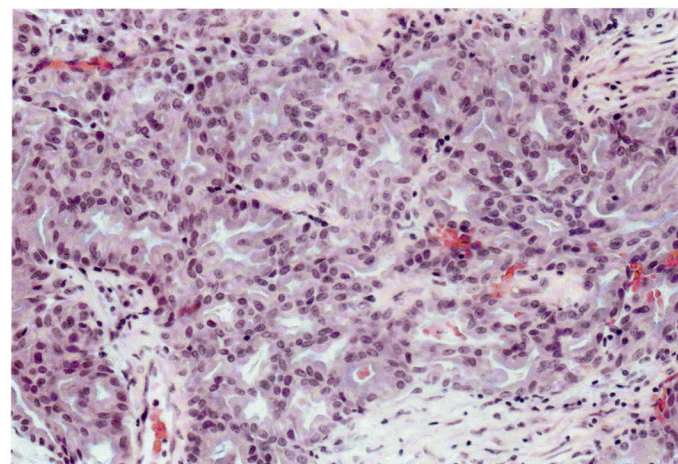

IMAGE 12.53 Low grade sinonasal nonintestinal type adenocarcinoma. The image shows closely packed, fused glands with minimal atypia (H&E, x200).

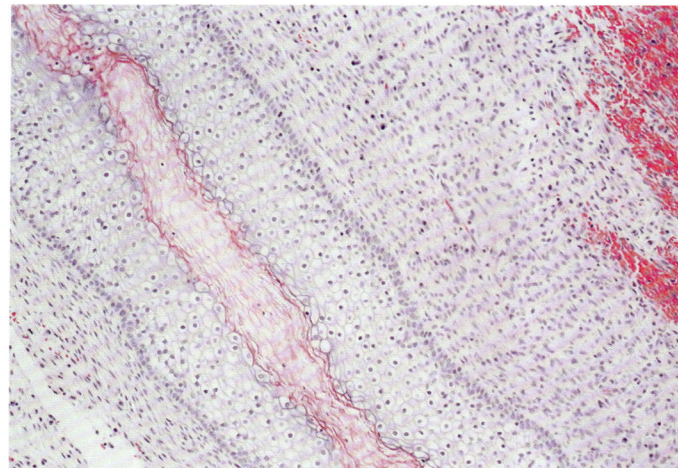

IMAGE 12.51 Sinonasal teratocarcinosarcoma. The image shows a portion of squamous epithelium with clear cells (fetal-appearing). This is a common feature of the squamous elements (H&E, x100).

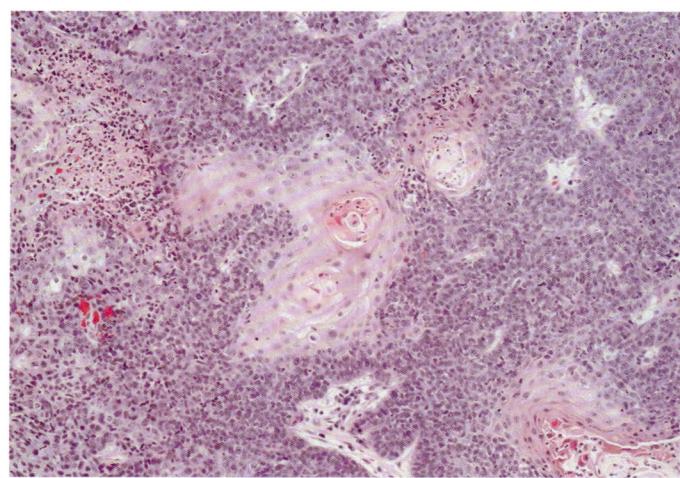

IMAGE 12.54 NUT midline carcinoma. An undifferentiated high grade component surrounds an abrupt area of squamous differentiation. An infiltrate of neutrophils is common (H&E, x200).

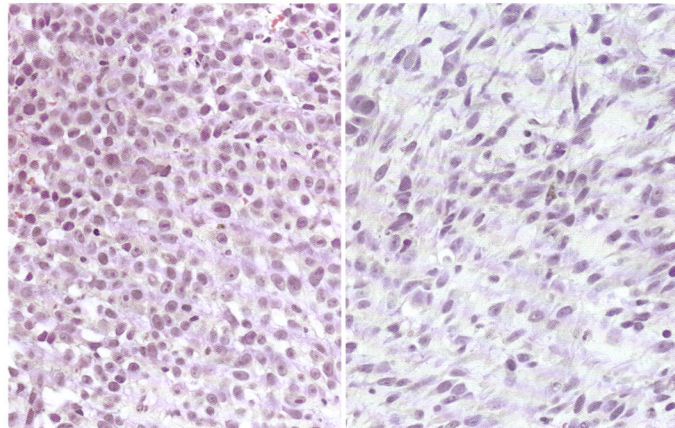

IMAGE 12.55 Nasal melanoma. Left: nasal melanomas are often amelanotic. They demonstrate the spectrum of histological findings found in melanomas of other locations. This area shows an epithelioid pattern of growth (H&E, x400). Right: part of the same tumor showing a spindle pattern of growth with a myxoid background. Note the focal melanin deposition (H&E, x400).

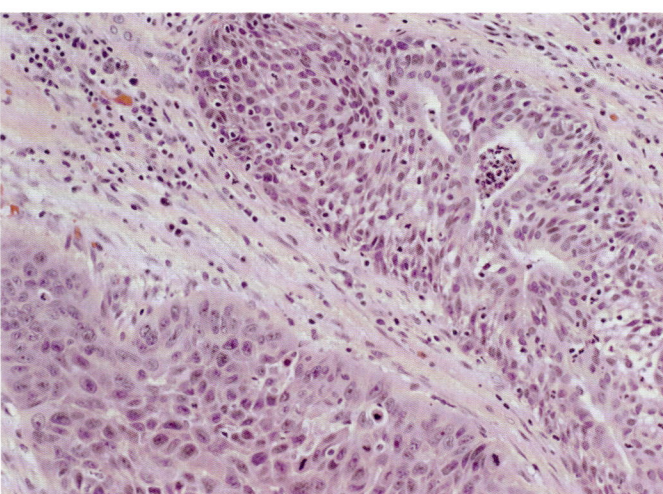

IMAGE 12.58 Squamous cell carcinoma arising in an inverted papilloma. Note the abrupt transition between squamous cell carcinoma in the lower left and the residual inverted papilloma in the upper right (H&E, x100).

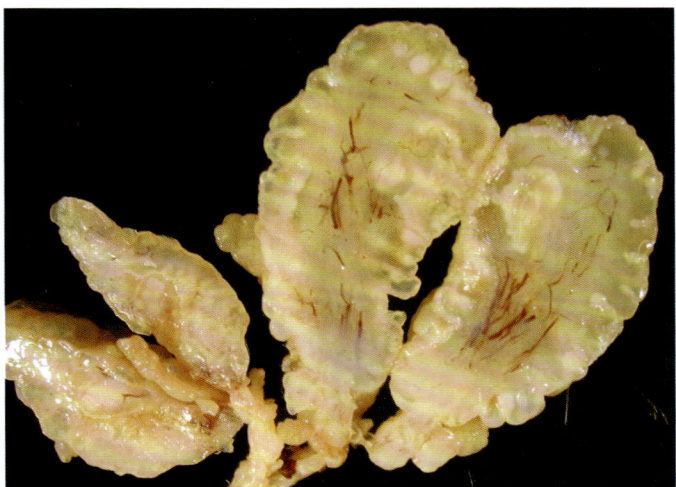

IMAGE 12.56 Inverted schneiderian papilloma. This image shows a polypoid mass with a cerebriform surface, vascular stroma, and pale tan ribbons of invaginating epithelium extending into the stroma.

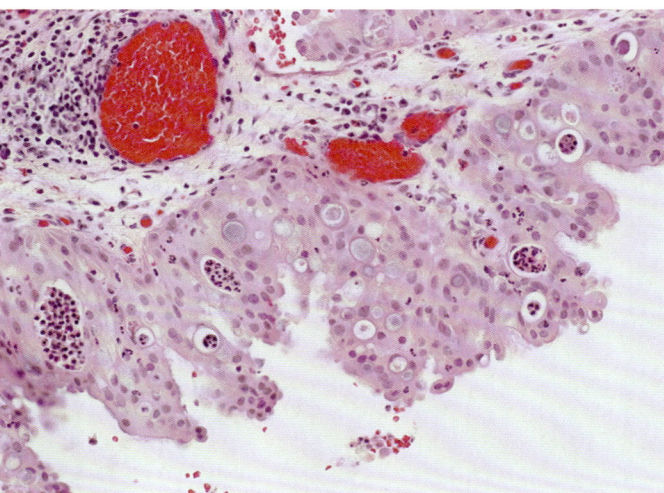

IMAGE 12.59 Oncocytic schneiderian papilloma. The irregular surface epithelium is composed of cells with abundant pink cytoplasm, interspersed microabscesses, and mucous cysts (H&E, x200).

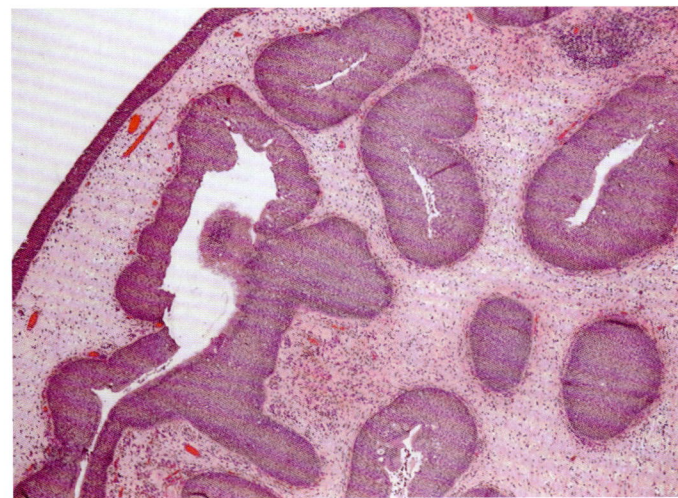

IMAGE12.57 Inverted papilloma. The image shows broad downgrowths with rounded contours embedded in a nasal-polyp-like stroma (H&E, x40).

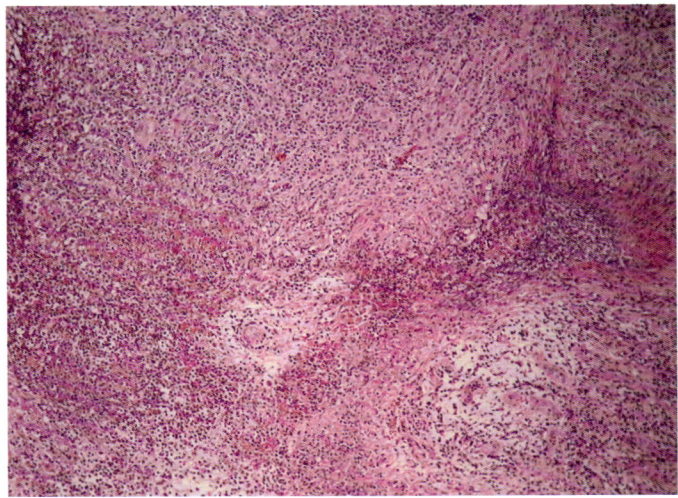

IMAGE 12.60 Granulomatosis with polyangiitis (Wegener granulomatosis). The image shows geographic necrosis (H&E, x100).

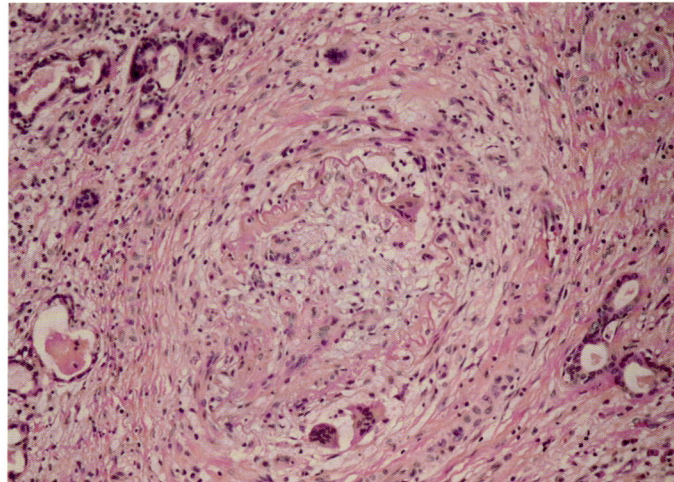

IMAGE 12.61 Granulomatosis with polyangiitis. The image shows healing granulomatous vasculitis (H&E, x200).

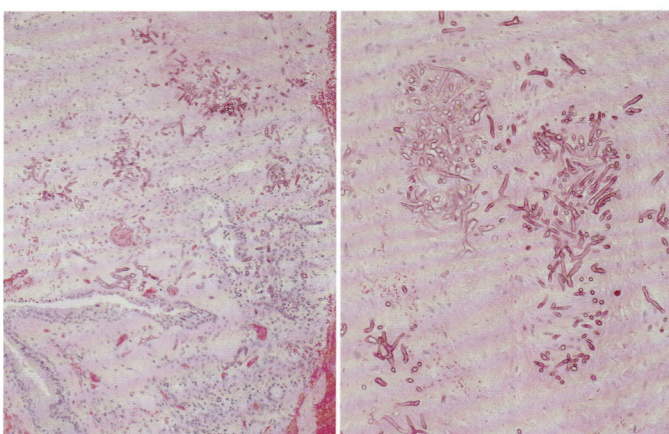

IMAGE 12.64 Invasive fungal rhinosinusitis. Left: this patient was immunosuppressed following a bone marrow transplant for lymphoma. Note the numerous irregular fungal hyphae throughout the necrotic nasal mucosa (H&E, 100x). Right: necrotic blood vessels invaded by fungi, confirmed by culture to be *Rhizomucor* species. Note the lack of inflammation (H&E, 200).

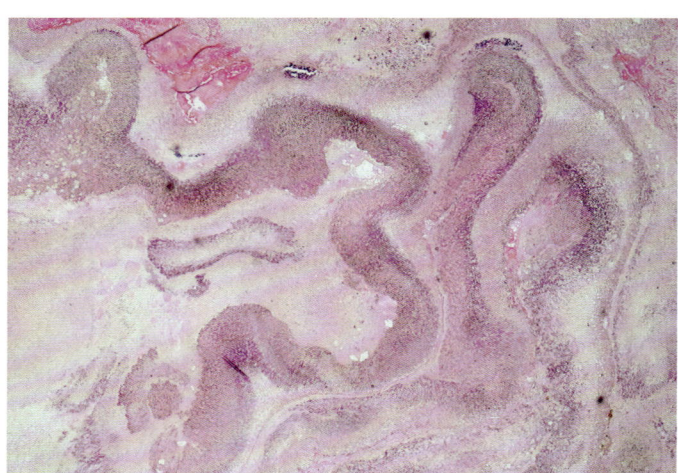

IMAGE 12.62 Sinus fungal ball (mycetoma). Note the laminated pattern from low power (H&E, x40).

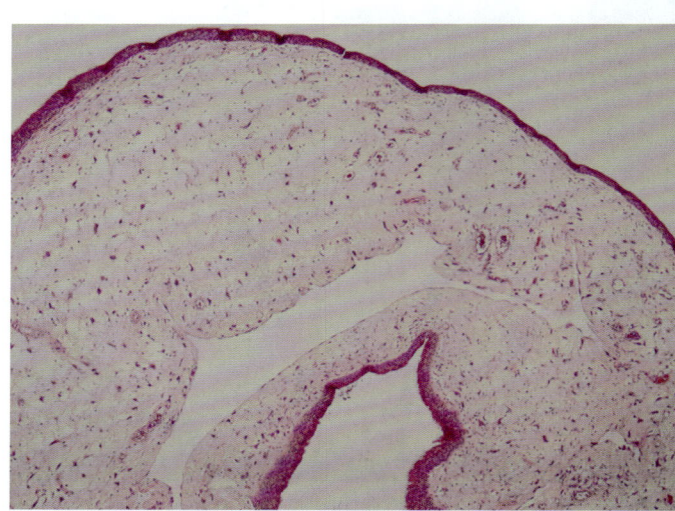

IMAGE 12.65 Sinonasal inflammatory polyp with stromal atypia (H&E, x40).

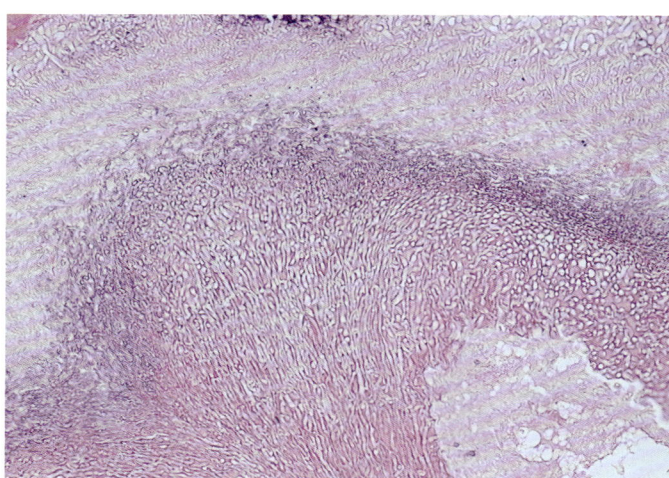

IMAGE 12.63 Sinus fungal ball. The image shows a complex mass of hyphae. Occasional "fruiting bodies" may be noted in some cases (H&E, x200).

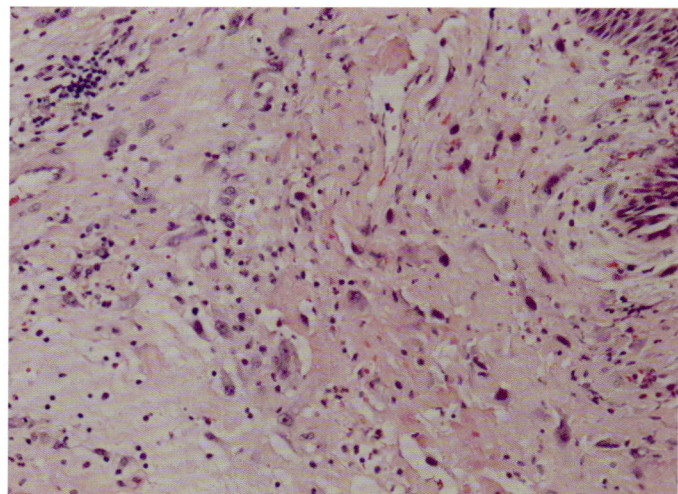

IMAGE 12.66 Sinonasal inflammatory polyp with stromal atypia. The image shows scattered cells with enlarged nuclei and prominent nucleoli. Absence of mitoses and lack of hypercellularity distinguishes this lesion from sarcoma (H&E, x200).

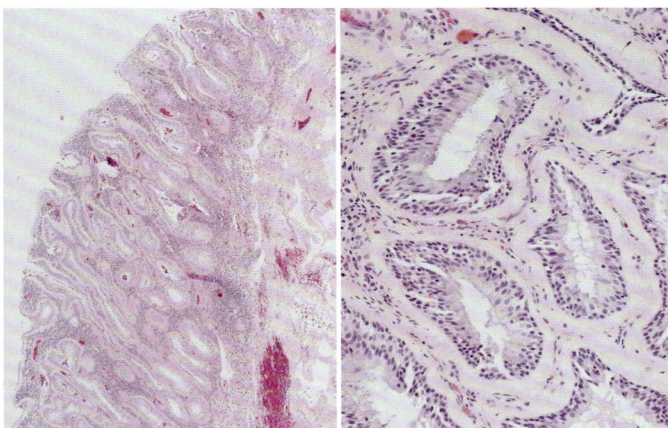

IMAGE 12.67 Respiratory epithelial adenomatoid hamartoma. Left: elongated glands with prominent periglandular hyalinization and interspersed inflammatory infiltrate (H&E, x40). Right: large glands lined by ciliated respiratory type epithelium with surrounding periglandular hyalinization (H&E, x200).

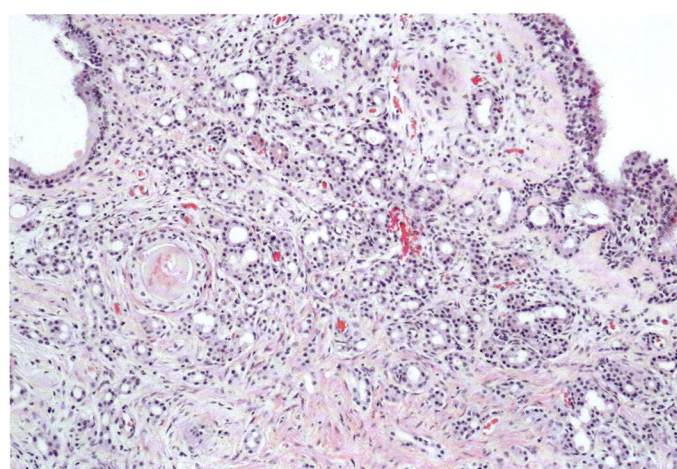

IMAGE 12.68 Seromucinous hamartoma. The image shows a polypoid mass containing numerous small uniform glands. Some larger glands (resembling those in REAH) are also present (upper left), from which the small glands may arise (H&E, x40).

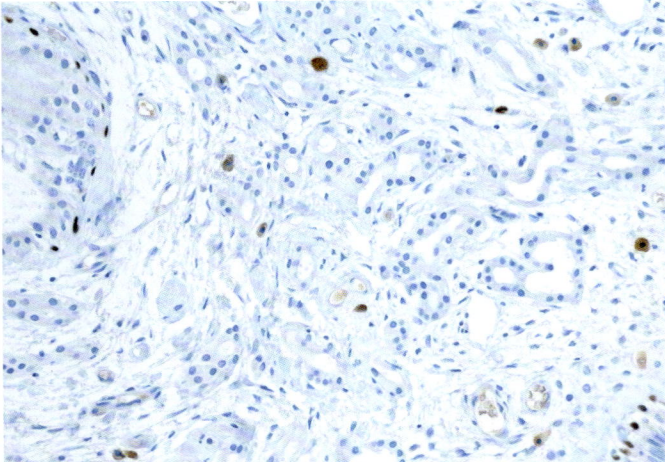

IMAGE 12.69 Seromucinous hamartoma. The lack of p63 positive basal cells around the proliferating glands is typical, and not an indication of malignancy. The cytoplasm of these small glands is often slightly eosinophilic and they stain with S100 (not shown) (p63, x200).

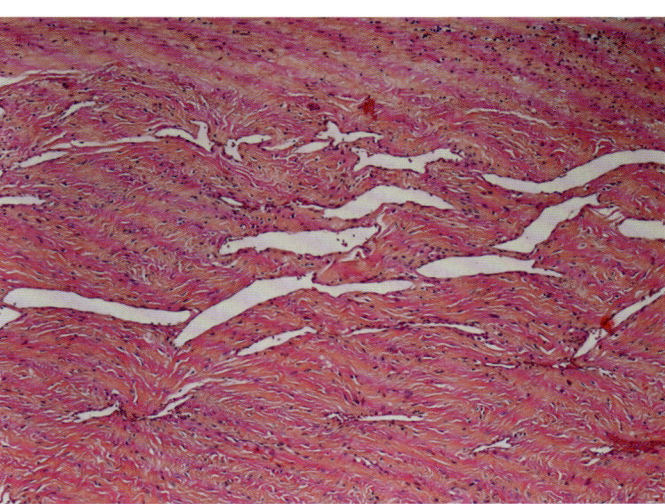

IMAGE 12.70 Nasopharyngeal angiofibroma. The image shows thin-walled vessels embedded in densely fibrous stroma (H&E, x100).

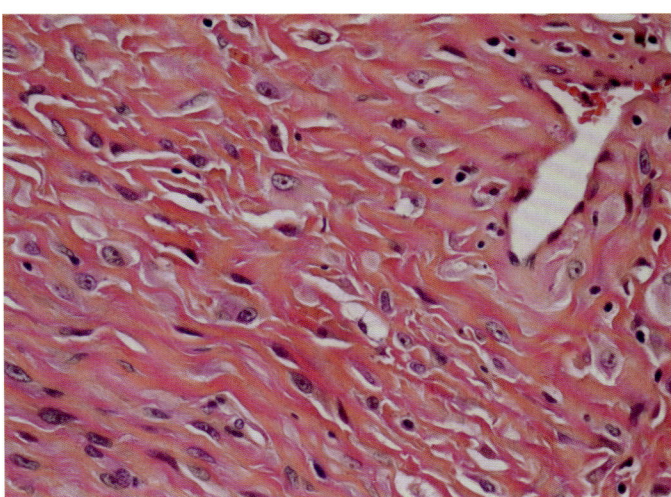

IMAGE 12.71 Nasopharyngeal angiofibroma. The image shows characteristic epithelioid fibroblasts with vesicular nuclei and conspicuous nucleoli (H&E, x400).

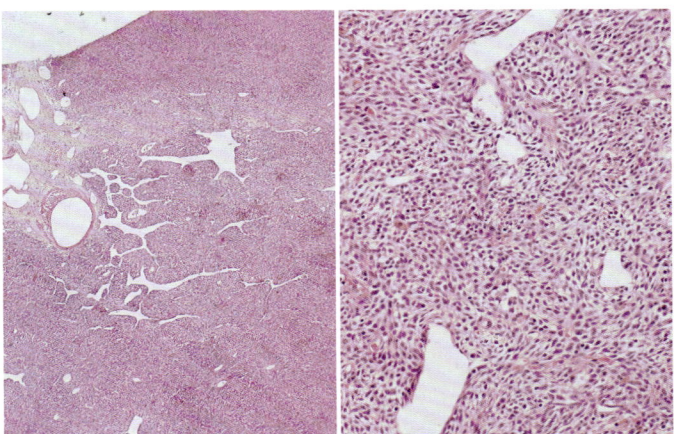

IMAGE 12.72 Glomangiopericytoma (nasal type hemangiopericytoma). Left: branching, thin-walled staghorn-type blood vessels are visible at low power (H&E, x20). Right: bland spindle cells in short intersecting fascicles. Note the lack of significant cytological atypia (H&E, x200).

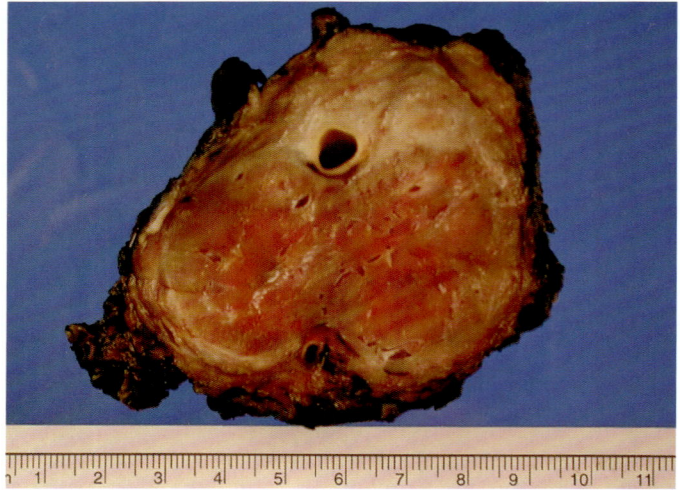

IMAGE 12.73 Carotid body tumor. This tumor partially envelops the branches of the carotid artery.

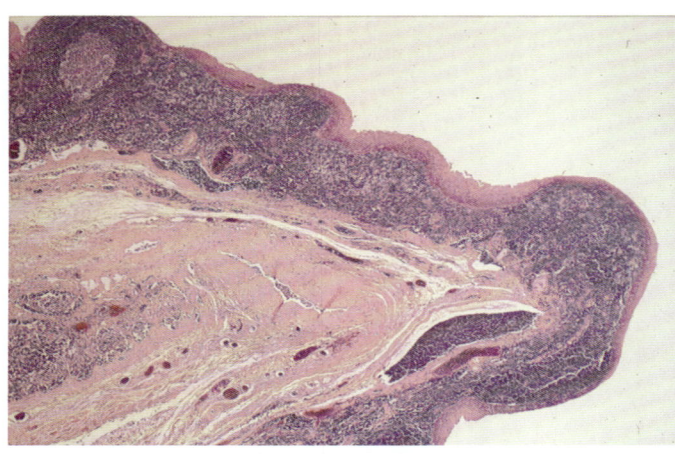

IMAGE 12.76 Branchial cleft cyst. The image shows a squamous epithelium lined cyst surrounded by reactive lymphoid tissue. (H&E, x40).

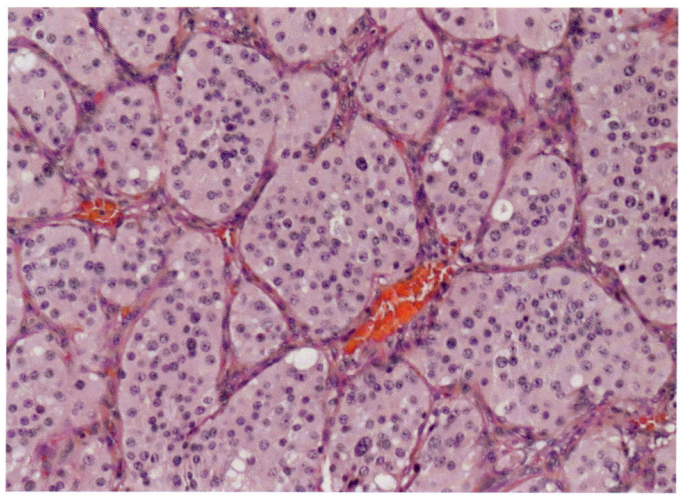

IMAGE 12.74 Carotid body tumor with nests (Zellballen) composed of cells with moderate eosinophilic cytoplasm and surrounded by vascular stroma (H&E, x200).

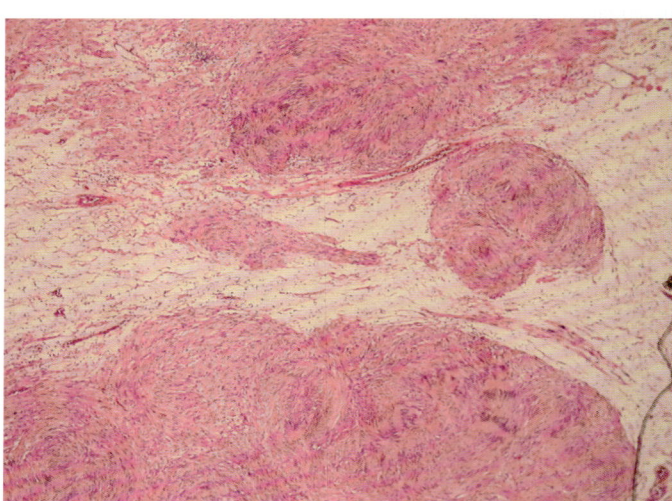

IMAGE 12.77 Cervical mass: schwannoma. The image shows Antoni A tissue above and below intervening Antoni B tissue (H&E, x40).

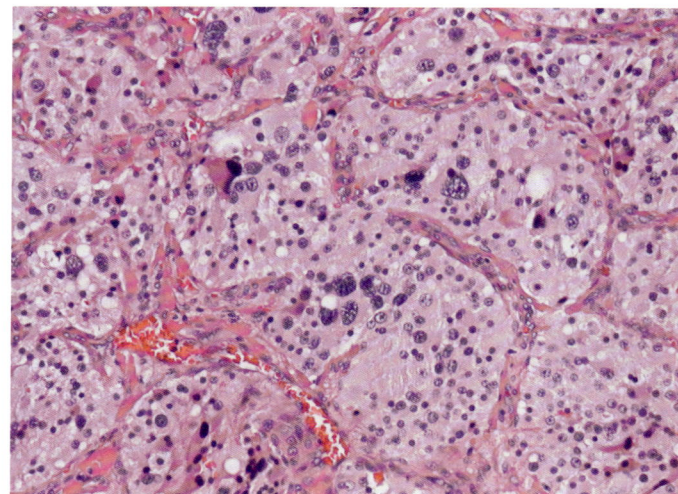

IMAGE 12.75 Carotid body tumor with scattered pleomorphic nuclei ("endocrine atypia"). This is a common finding in carotid body tumors and does not signify more aggressive behavior (H&E, x200).

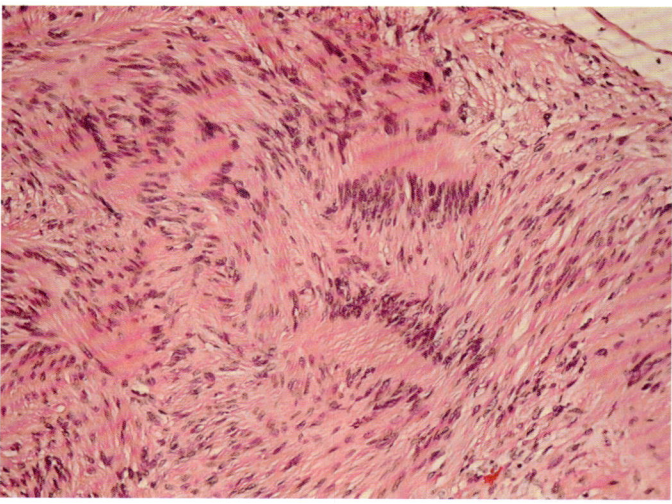

IMAGE 12.78 Schwannoma. The image shows palisading nuclei with Verocay body formation (H&E, x200).

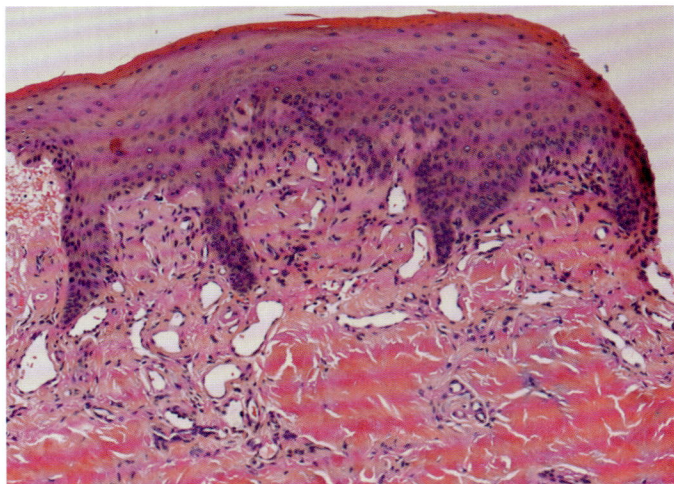

IMAGE 12.79 Laryngeal amyloidosis (bilateral supraglottic nodular swelling). The image shows deposits of amorphous eosinophilic material underlying the epithelium (H&E, x100).

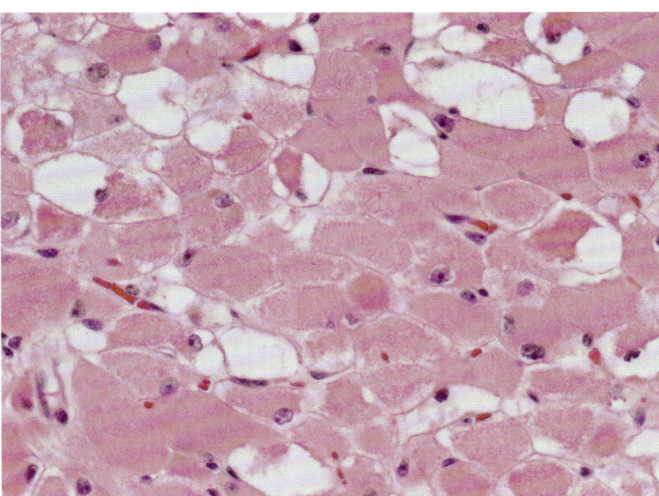

IMAGE 12.82 Adult rhabdomyoma of the larynx. Note the large polygonal rhabdomyoblasts with eosinophilic cytoplasm and easily visible cross-striations in some cells (H&E, x400).

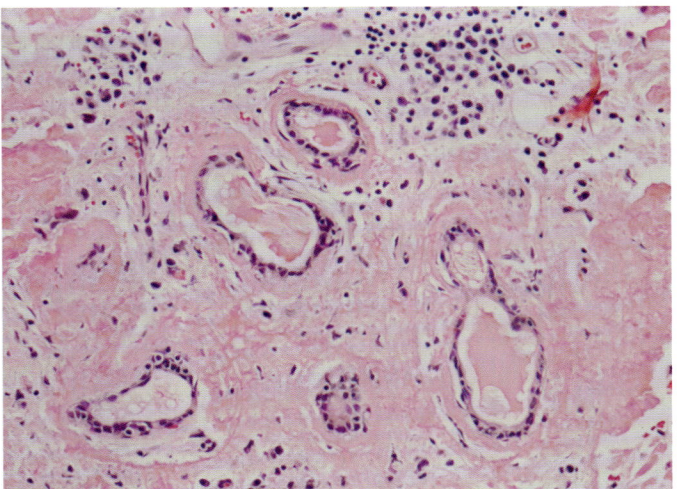

IMAGE 12.80 Laryngeal amyloidosis. The image shows atrophic mucoserous glands surrounded by amorphous eosinophilic deposits of amyloid (H&E, x200).

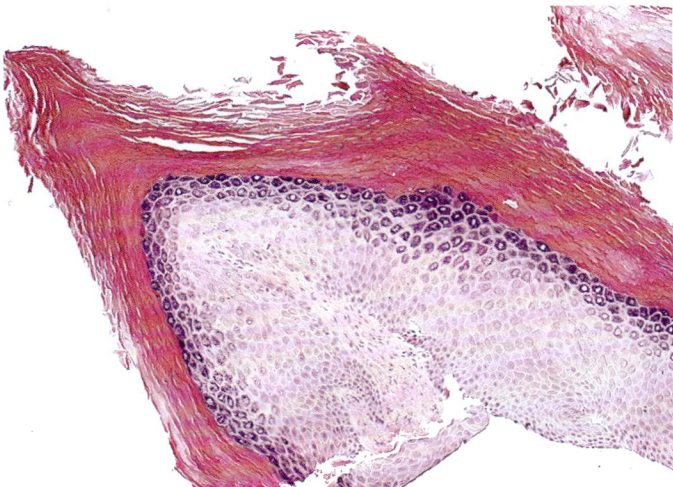

IMAGE 12.83 Papillary keratosis of larynx with heavy surface keratinization and lack of dysplasia. These lesions are common in smokers and are usually heavily keratinized and solitary, unlike HPV-related papillomas of the larynx (H&E, x100).

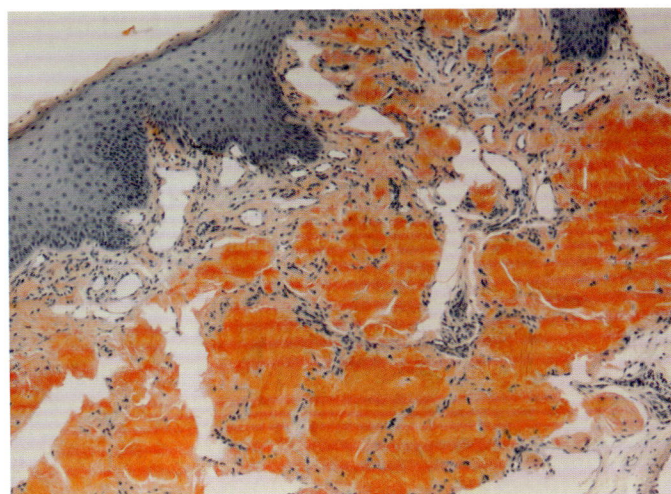

IMAGE 12.81 Laryngeal amyloidosis. The image shows strong Congo red positivity (Congo red, x100).

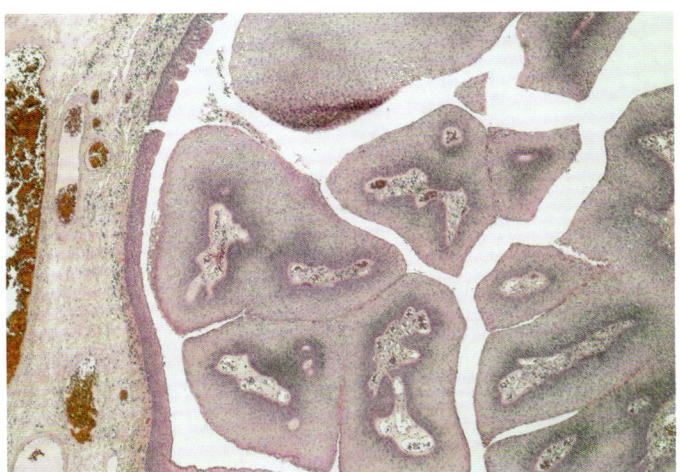

IMAGE 12.84 Laryngeal nonkeratinizing papilloma. These complex, branching papillomas are typical or recurrent respiratory papillomatosis. They may keratinize if they become inflamed or traumatized (H&E, x40).

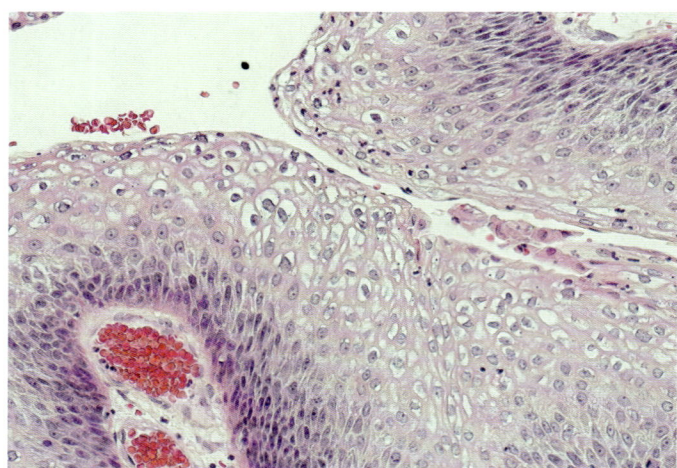

IMAGE 12.85 Laryngeal nonkeratinizing papilloma. The image shows bland squamous epithelium with viral effects. Mild atypia is common, but overt dysplasia is less common and is rarely high grade (H&E, x200).

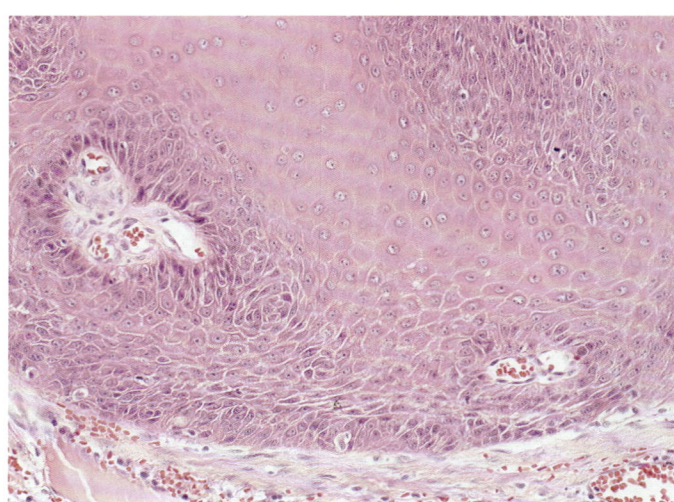

IMAGE 12.88 Verrucous carcinoma. The leading edge of the tumor shows a lack of atypia or appreciable mitotic activity (H&E, x200).

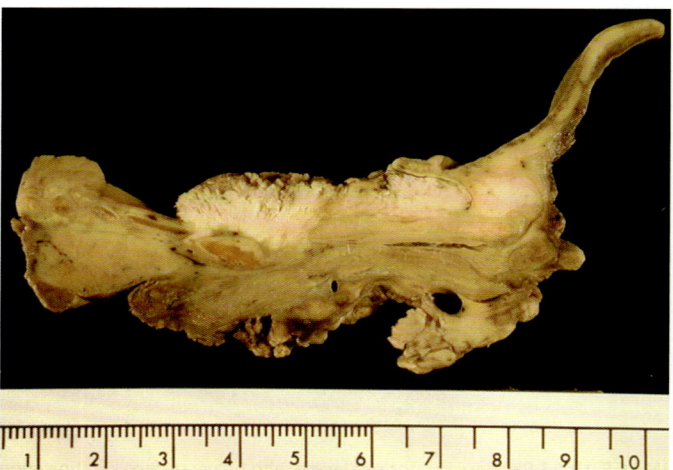

IMAGE 12.86 Verrucous carcinoma, larynx. Note the erosion of the thyroid/cricoid cartilage.

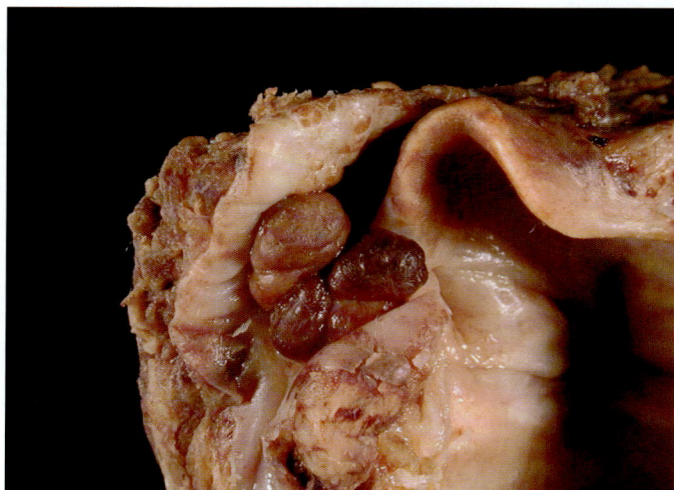

IMAGE 12.89 Spindle cell carcinoma, left aryepiglottic fold/pyriform sinus. The image shows characteristic polypoid growth.

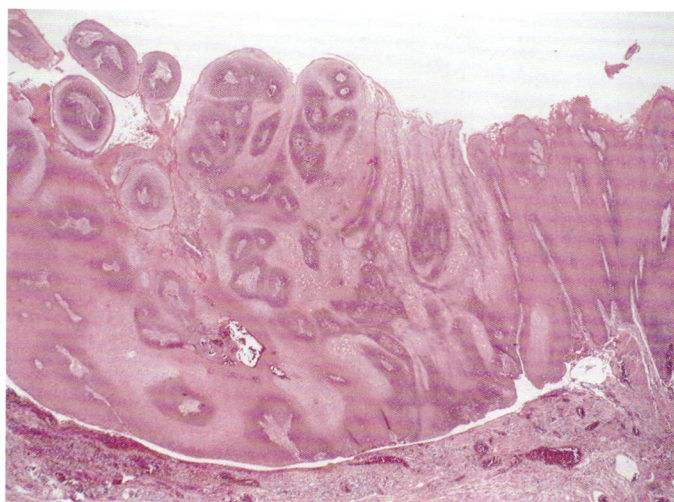

IMAGE 12.87 Verrucous carcinoma. The image shows papillomatous and verruciform surface architecture with a broad pushing invasive front. Note the artifactual cleft between the tumor and underlying stroma (H&E, x20).

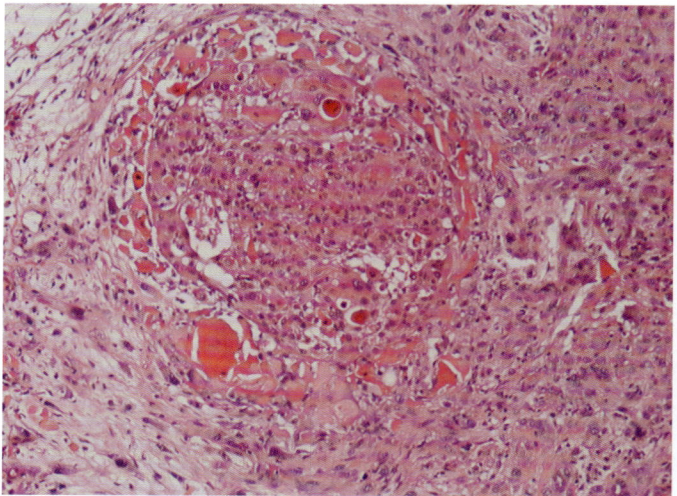

IMAGE 12.90 Spindle cell carcinoma, larynx. The image shows a nest of keratinizing squamous epithelial cells surrounded by atypical spindle cells (notably in the lower left) (H&E, x200).

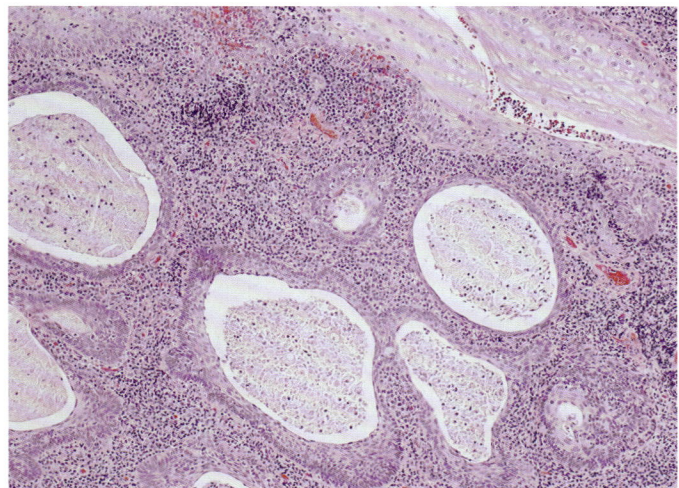

IMAGE 12.91 HPV-associated nonkeratinizing squamous cell carcinoma of the tonsil. These tumors often invade as circumscribed nests with minimal desmoplasia and central necrosis or cyst formation (H&E, x40).

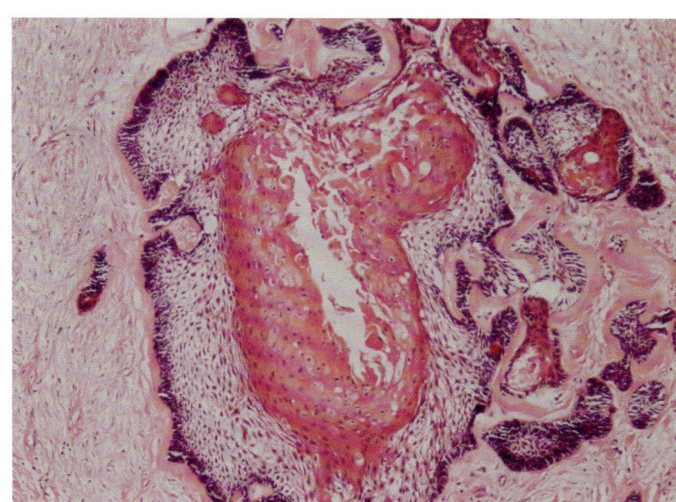

IMAGE 12.94 Ameloblastoma, mandible, acanthomatous variant. Squamous differentiation is present within the stellate reticulum zone (H&E, x100).

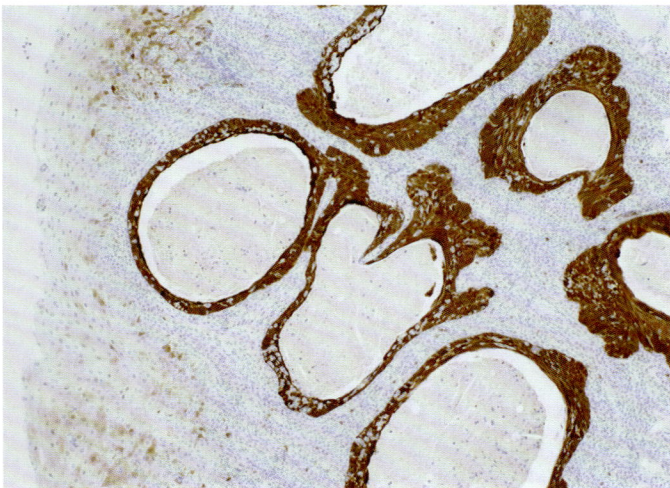

IMAGE 12.92 HPV-associated nonkeratinizing squamous cell carcinoma of the tonsil. The p16 immunostain shows strong, diffuse nuclear and cytoplasmic positivity. The surface of the epithelium shows patchy, weak "mosaic type" pattern (H&E, x40).

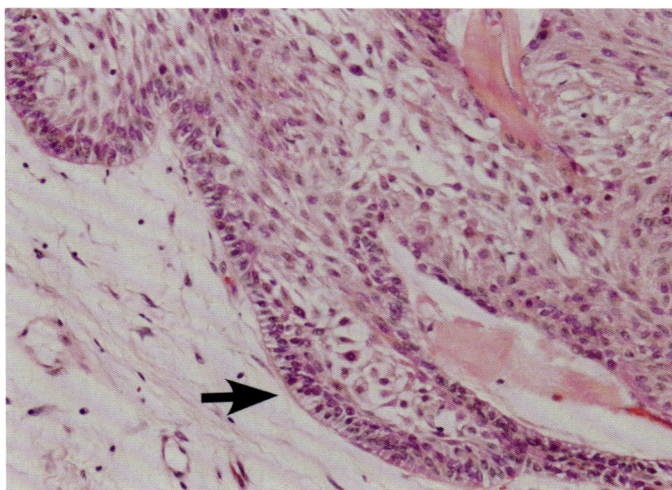

IMAGE 12.95 Ameloblastoma, mandible. Note the peripheral cells with reverse polarity (arrow) surrounding loose stellate reticulum (H&E, x200).

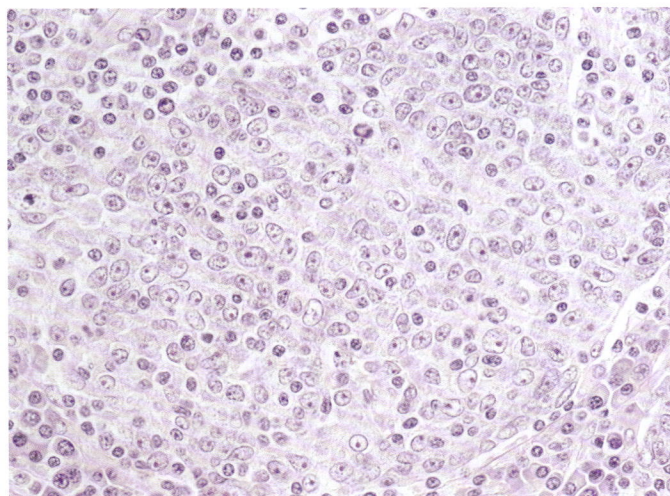

IMAGE 12.93 Nasopharyngeal carcinoma, undifferentiated type. Note the syncytial mass of malignant cells interspersed with and surrounded by benign lymphocytes and plasma cells (H&E, x400).

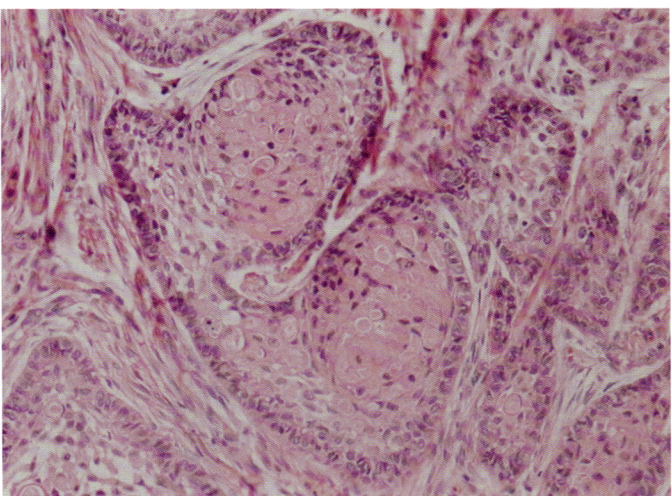

IMAGE 12.96 Ameloblastoma, maxilla, granular cell variant. Cells with granular cytoplasm are noted centrally within the stellate reticulum (H&E, x200).

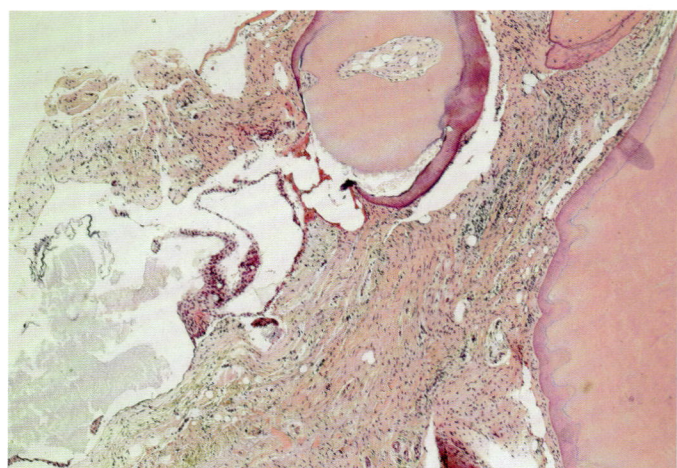

IMAGE 12.97 Compound odontoma. This image shows aggregates of dentin and cementum on the left and immature enamel matrix surrounded by enamel epithelium on the lower right. The designation of compound or complex type is often not possible except with clinical and imaging correlation (H&E, x40).

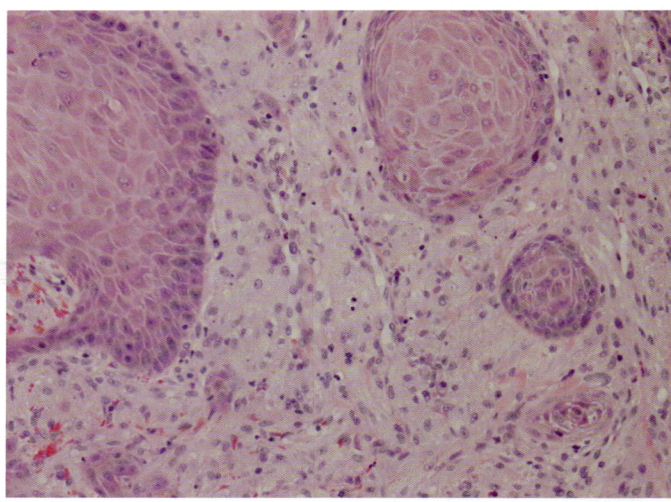

IMAGE 12.100 Granular cell tumor, tongue. Cells with abundant granular cytoplasm with ill-defined cell borders fill the stroma (H&E, x200).

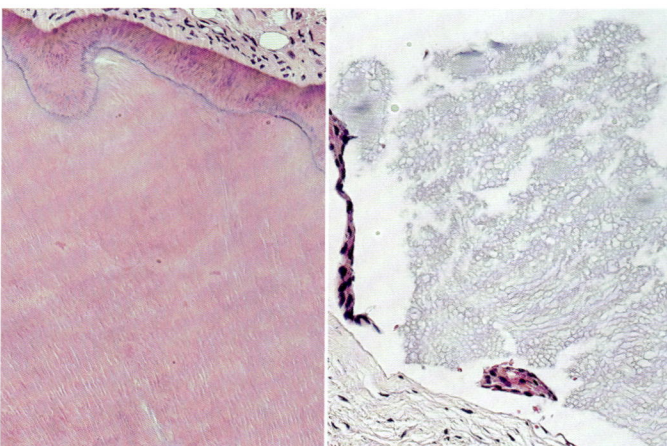

IMAGE 12.98 Odontoma. On the left there is immature dentin with a rim of cementum. Note the dentinal tubules. On the right is pale, laminated immature enamel matrix, which is typically absent in mature teeth (H&E, x200).

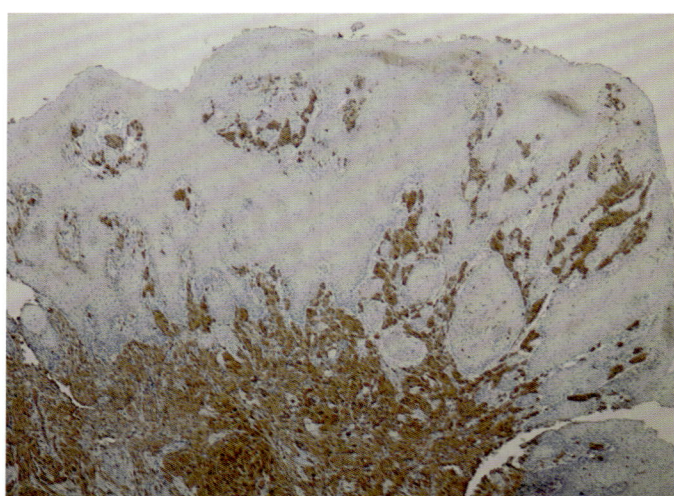

IMAGE 12.101 Granular cell tumor. S100 highlights the tumor cells, which are of Schwann cell origin (S100, x40).

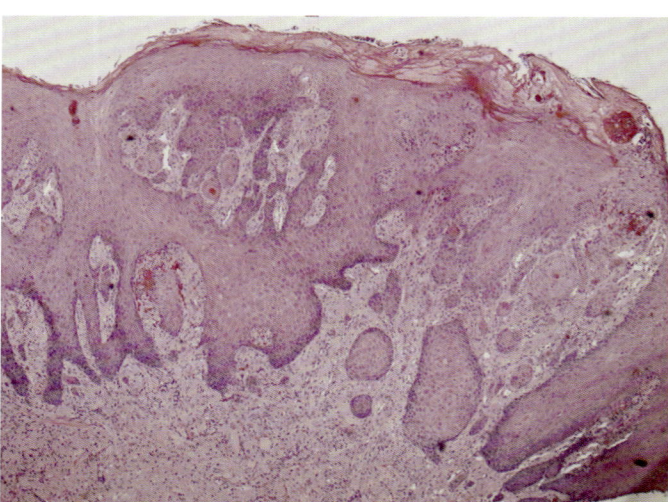

IMAGE 12.99 Granular cell tumor, tongue. The image shows pseudocarcinomatous (pseudoepitheliomatous) hyperplasia of the overlying epithelium with indistinct infiltrate of granular cells (H&E, x40).

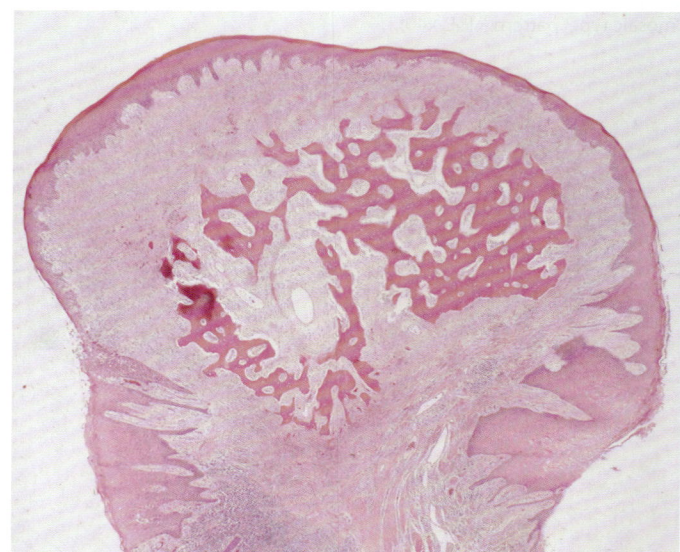

IMAGE 12.102 Peripheral ossifying fibroma. The nodular gingival lesion is covered by attenuated surface epithelium and contains an irregular mass of woven bone within a cellular fibrous stroma (H&E, x20).

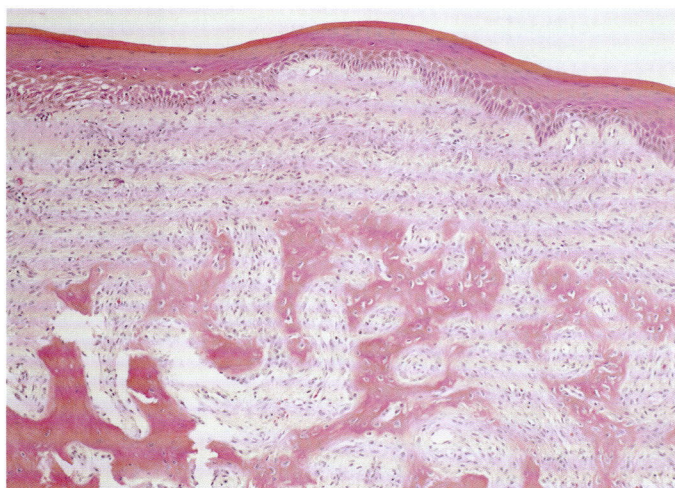

IMAGE 12.103 Peripheral ossifying fibroma. Note the anastomosing trabeculae of woven bone with a surrounding stroma of bland, spindled fibroblasts (H&E, x20).

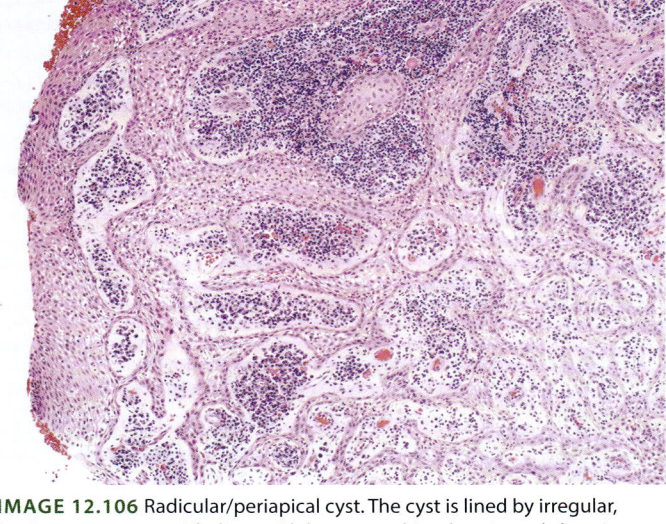

IMAGE 12.106 Radicular/periapical cyst. The cyst is lined by irregular, benign squamous epithelium with heavy combined acute and chronic inflammation. (H&E, x40).

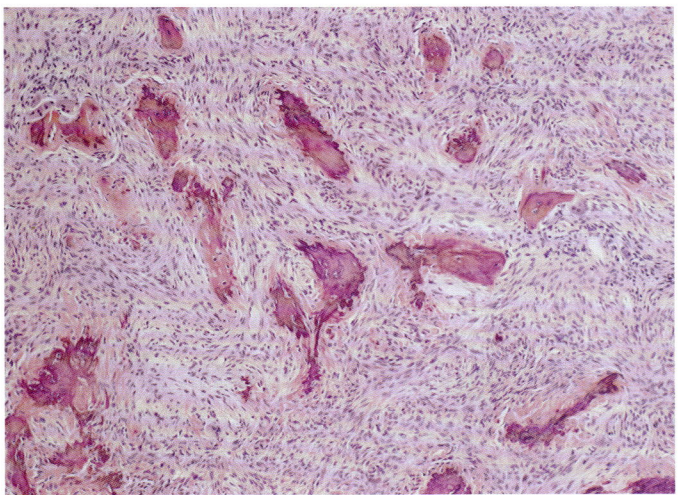

IMAGE 12.104 Central ossifying fibroma. Note the irregular deposits of calcified matrix, some resembling woven bone, set in a moderately cellular, bland, spindle cell stroma (H&E, x100).

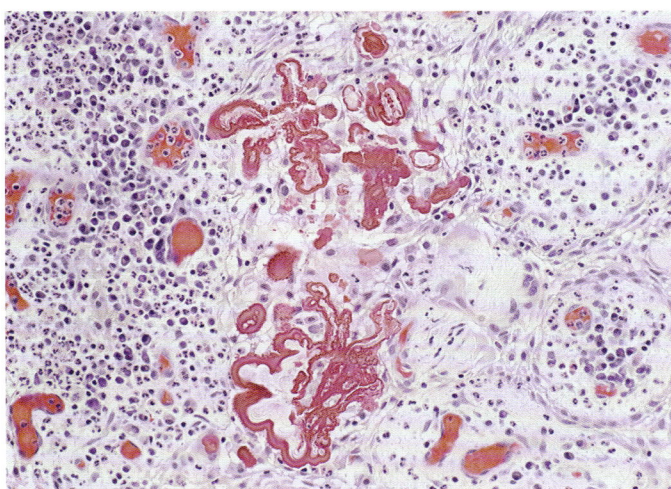

IMAGE 12.107 Radicular/periapical cyst. Note the Rushton bodies in the wall of the cyst. These irregular, eosinophilic, laminated structures are commonly found in the wall of these cysts, but are not pathognomonic for this entity (H&E, x200).

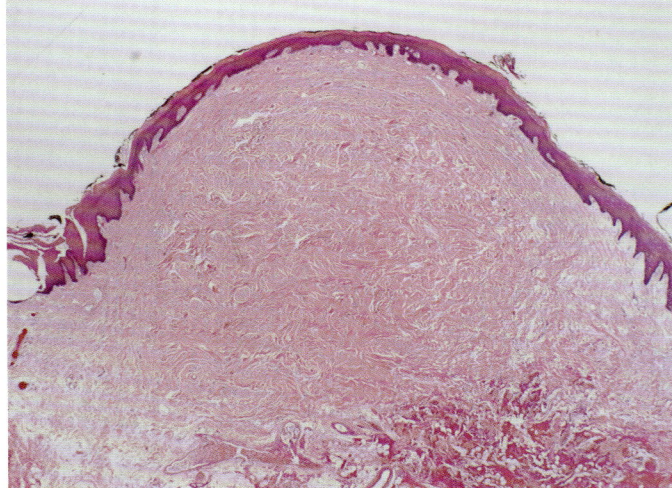

IMAGE 12.105 Irritation/traumatic fibroma. A nodular mass of dense fibrous tissue protrudes above the surrounding mucosa, with attenuated, slightly keratinized surface epithelium (H&E, x20).

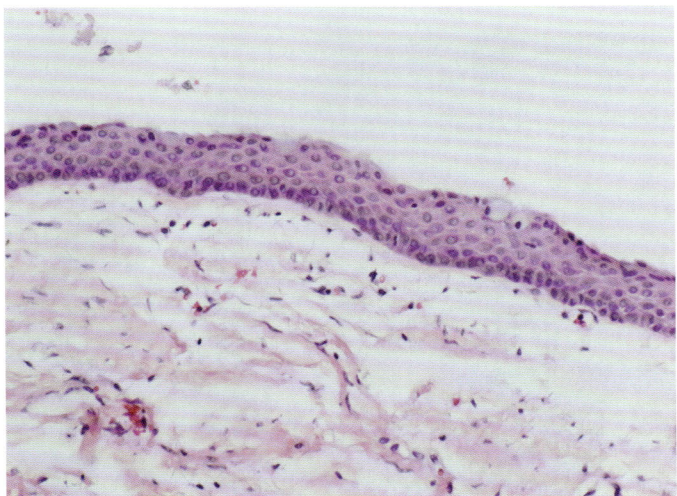

IMAGE 12.108 Dentigerous cyst. This cyst surrounded the root of an unerupted third molar. Note the thin, flat, cuboidal lining with scattered interspersed mucous cells (H&E, x200).

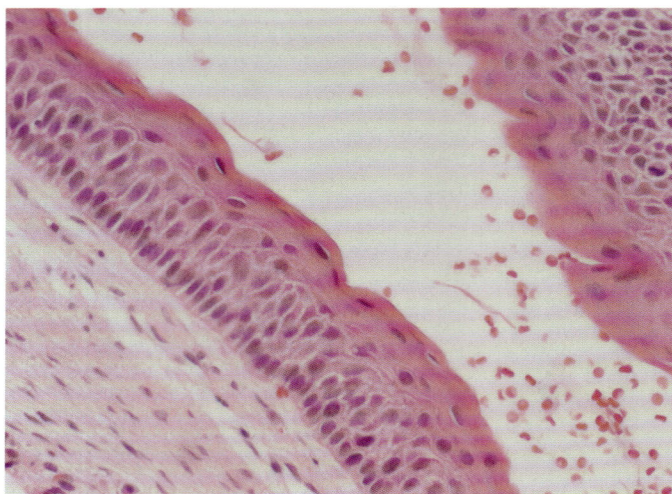

IMAGE 12.109 Odontogenic keratocyst. The characteristic lining has wavy or corrugated surface parakeratin with a palisaded basal layer (H&E, x400).

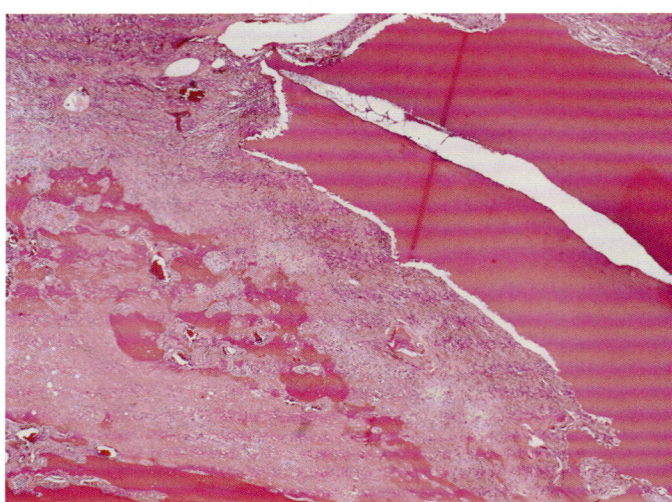

IMAGE 12.112 Osteosarcoma of the mandible. This bone-forming tumor shows an irregular mass of woven bone in the lower left that is destroying a tooth (upper right). The residual tooth tissue consists of cementum (H&E, x20).

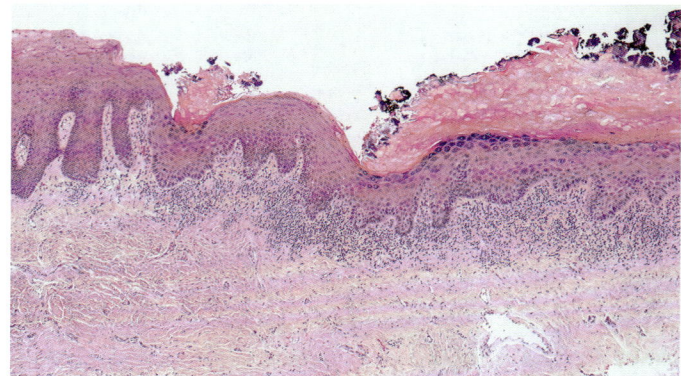

IMAGE 12.110 Mild keratinizing dysplasia of the oral cavity. Note the abrupt switch from nonkeratinized to keratinized epithelium, which is common for dysplasia. There is a mild lichenoid infiltrate (H&E, x40).

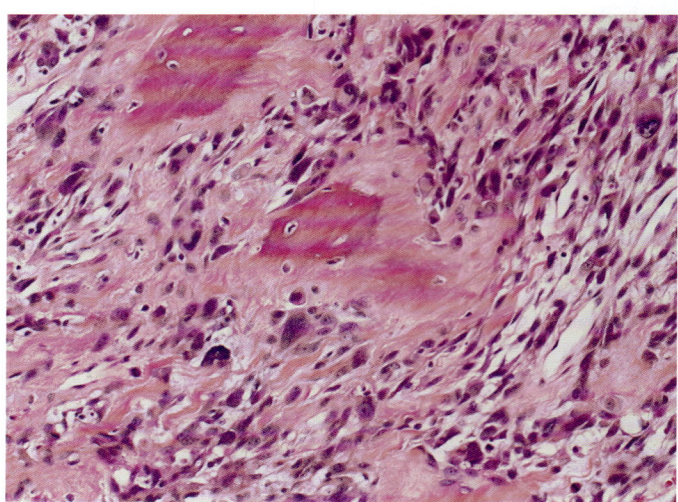

IMAGE 12.113 Osteosarcoma of the mandible. The image shows high grade malignant spindle cells surrounding irregular portions of osteoid and immature bone (H&E, x400).

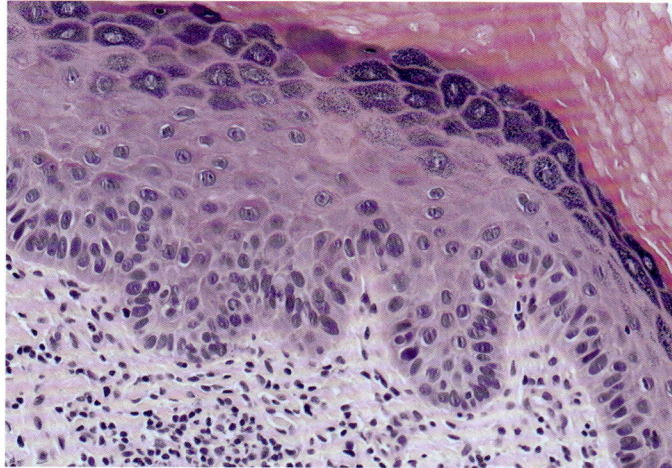

IMAGE 12.111 Mild keratinizing dysplasia. There is rounded budding of the basal epithelium, with crowding, hyperchromasia, and some enlargement of the basal cells (H&E, x200).

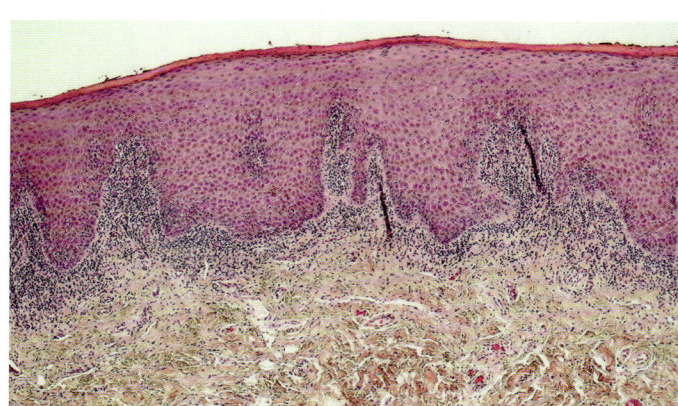

IMAGE 12.114 Lichen planus of oral cavity. The epithelium is hyperplastic and hyperkeratotic, with a dense infiltrate of lymphocytes confined to the upper aspect of the lamina propria (H&E, x100).

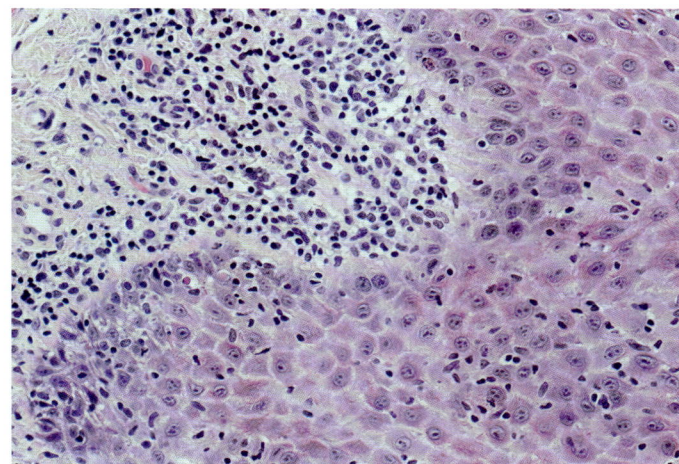

IMAGE 12.115 Lichen planus of oral cavity. The lymphoid infiltrate extends into the basal epithelium with occasional dyskeratotic keratinocytes (colloid bodies). There is slight vacuolization of the basal zone and minimal reactive atypia (H&E, x200).

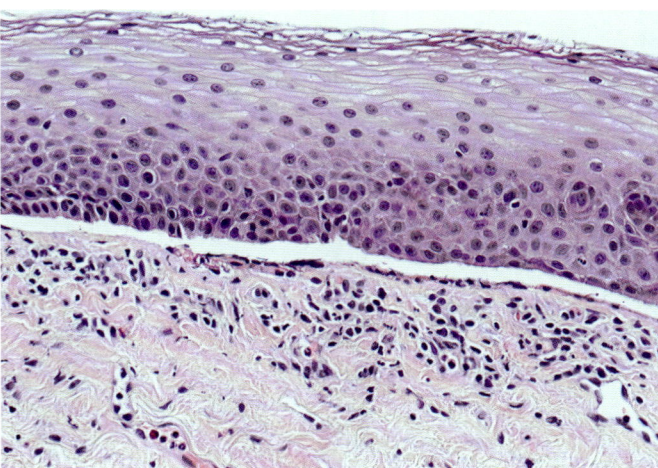

IMAGE 12.117 Mucous membrane pemphigoid. Only mild inflammation is present, with rare eosinophils. The basal epithelial cells are slightly rounded or flattened. Direct immunofluorescence (IF) showed a continuous linear band of IgG (H&E, x200).

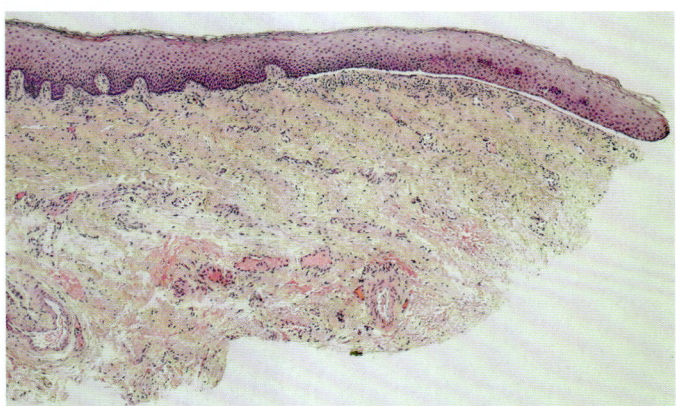

IMAGE 12.116 Mucous membrane pemphigoid. There is a subepithelial blister. The affected epithelium is slightly attenuated, which helps to distinguish this from artifactual separation (H&E, x40).

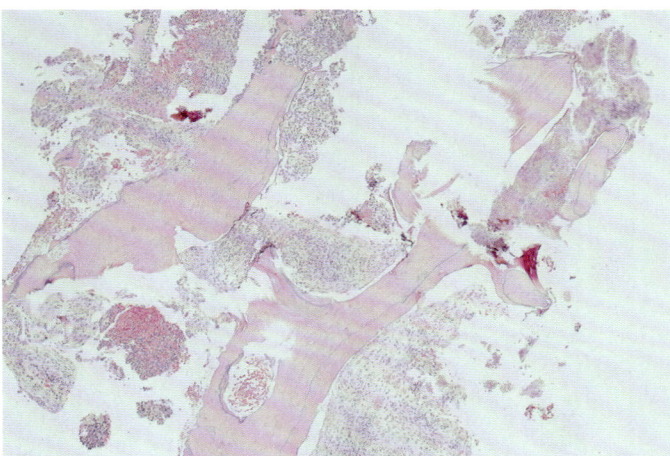

IMAGE 12.118 Medication-related osteonecrosis of the jaw. The image shows irregular fragments of necrotic bone embedded within inflamed granulation and organizing fibrous tissue (H&E, x40).

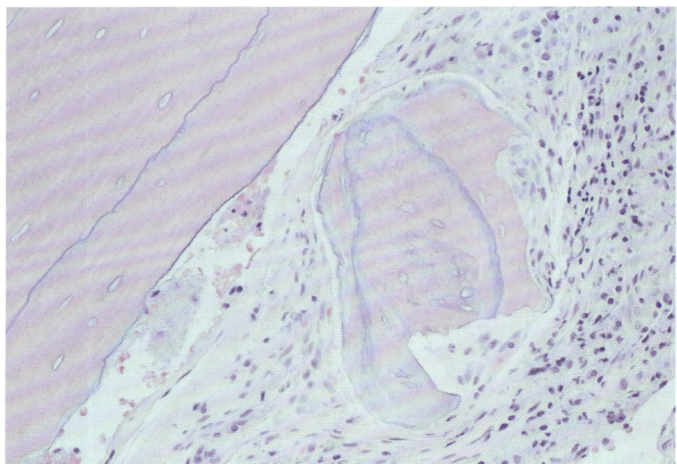

IMAGE 12.119 Medication-related osteonecrosis of the jaw. An entrapped bone fragment with a "moth-eaten" periphery. Sometimes the necrotic bone is engulfed by surface epithelium (not shown) (H&E, x200).

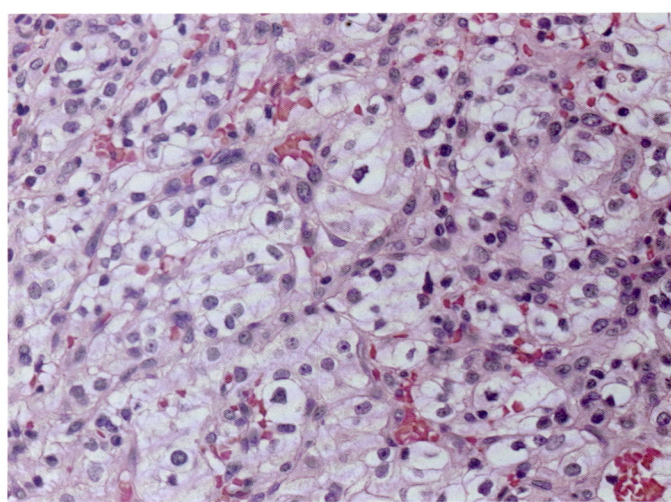

IMAGE 12.121 Metastatic renal cell carcinoma to the palate. Note the nests of cells with abundant, clear cytoplasm and prominent background vascularity, typical of renal cell carcinoma (H&E, x400).

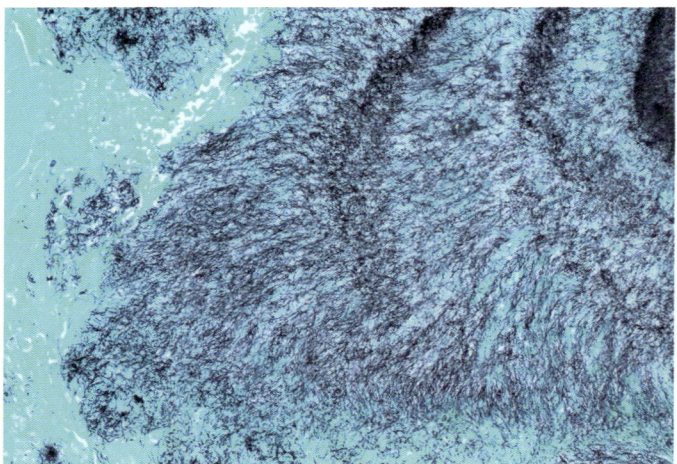

IMAGE 12.120 Medication-related osteonecrosis of the jaw. Bacterial aggregates are frequent, including filamentous actinomyces colonies, which can be highlighted with gram and GMS stains (GMS, x200).

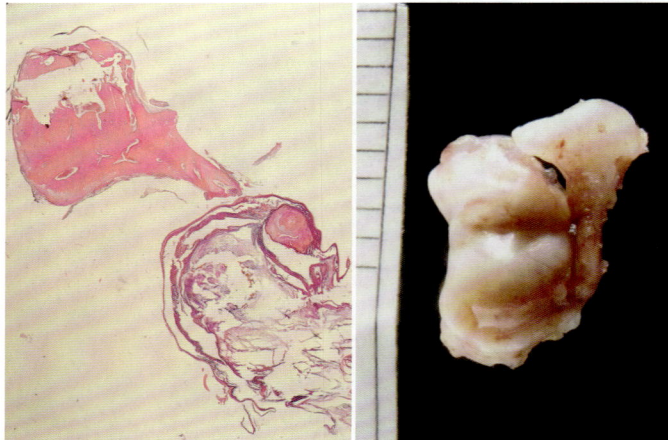

IMAGE 12.122 Cholesteatoma. Right: the gross photograph shows a smooth, "pearly" cyst attached to the incus (above). Left: incus on lower left has attached cholesteatoma containing abundant laminated keratin (H&E, x10).

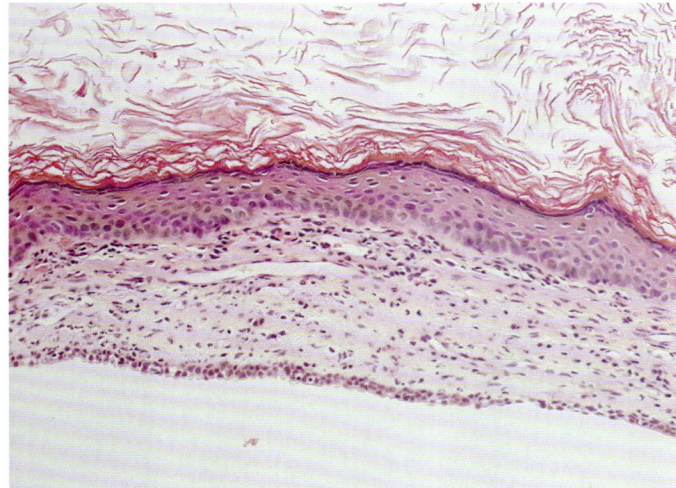

IMAGE 12.123 Cholesteatoma showing the thin, flat, keratinizing squamous lining that is typical of cholesteatoma. Note the residual cuboidal epithelium of the middle ear in the lower portion of the field that is covering the external aspect of the cyst.

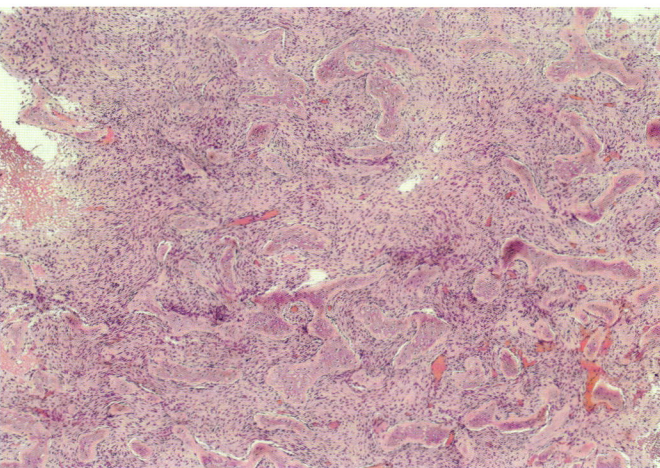

IMAGE 12.125 Fibrous dysplasia of the temporal bone. The image shows complex anatomosing trabeculae of woven bone (resembling ginger roots) in a fibrous stroma (H&E, x100).

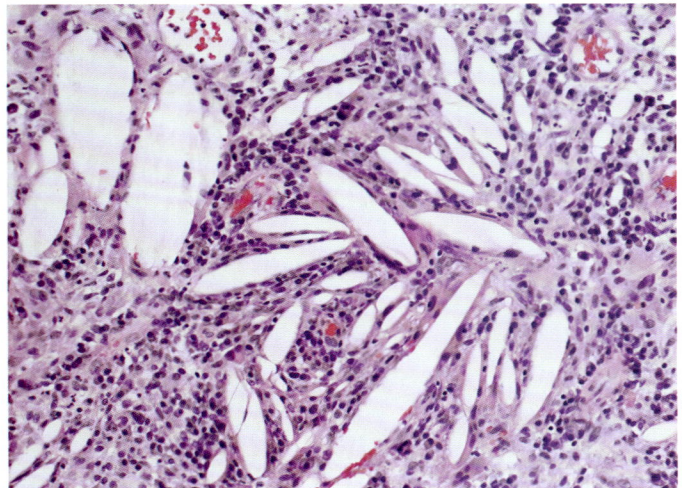

IMAGE 12.124 Cholesterol granuloma. On this background of inflammatory cells, including numerous plasma cells, note the elongated, oval, and pointed cholesterol clefts, some surrounded by multinucleated giant cells (H&E, x400).

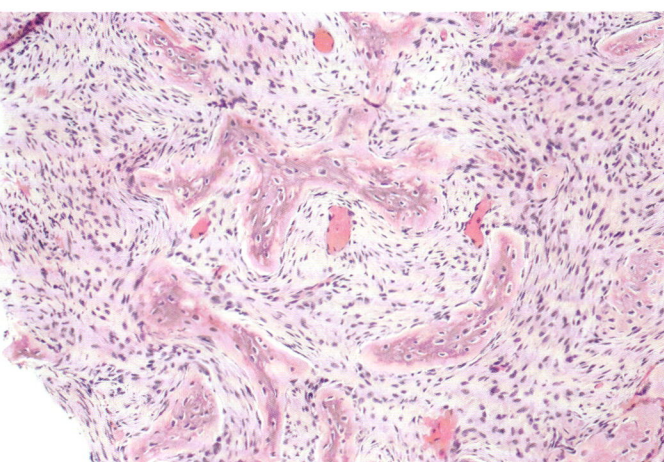

IMAGE 12.126 Fibrous dysplasia. The woven bone shows no atypia and there is no osteoblastic rimming in this image (although it may be found focally). The stroma is bland, and in this case is rather cellular (H&E, x200).

Bibliography

Amin MB, Edge S, Greene F, et al. editors. AJCC cancer staging manual. 8th ed. New York: Springer; 2017.

Carlson DL, Weinreb I, McHugh JB, et al; Cancer Committee, College of American Pathologists. Protocol for the examination of specimens from patients with carcinomas of the salivary glands (Version: SalivaryGland 4.1.0.0) [Internet]. College of American Pathologists; 2021. Available from www.cap.org.

El-Nagar AK, Chan JKC, Grandis JR, et al, editors. WHO classification of tumors. 4th ed. Vol. 9, WHO classification of head and neck tumours. Lyon (France): IARC Press; 2017.

Kumar V, Abbas AK, Aster J. Robbins and Cotran pathologic basis of disease. 10th ed. North York (ON): Elsevier Canada; 2020.

Lester SC. Manual of surgical pathology. 3rd ed. Philadelphia (PA): Elsevier Saunders; 2010.

Longacre TA, editor. Mills and Sternberg's diagnostic surgical pathology. 7th ed. Philadelphia (PA): Wolters Kluwar; 2022.

Seethala RR, Carlson DL, Weinreb I, et al; Cancer Committee, College of American Pathologists. Protocol for the examination of specimens from patients with carcinomas of the pharynx (Version: Pharynx 4.0.0.2) [Internet]. College of American Pathologists; 2019. Available from www.cap.org.

Seethala RR, Weinreb I, Bullock M, et al; Cancer Committee, College of American Pathologists. Protocol for the examination of specimens from patients with carcinomas of the larynx (Version: Larynx 4.1.0.0) [Internet]. College of American Pathologists; 2021. Available from www.cap.org.

Seethala RR, Weinreb I, Bullock M, et al; Cancer Committee, College of American Pathologists. Protocol for the examination of specimens from patients with carcinomas of the lip and oral cavity (Version: LipOralCavity 4.0.0.1) [Internet]. College of American Pathologists; 2017. Available from www.cap.org.

Wenig BM. Atlas of head and neck pathology. 5th ed. Philadelphia (PA): Elsevier; 2016.

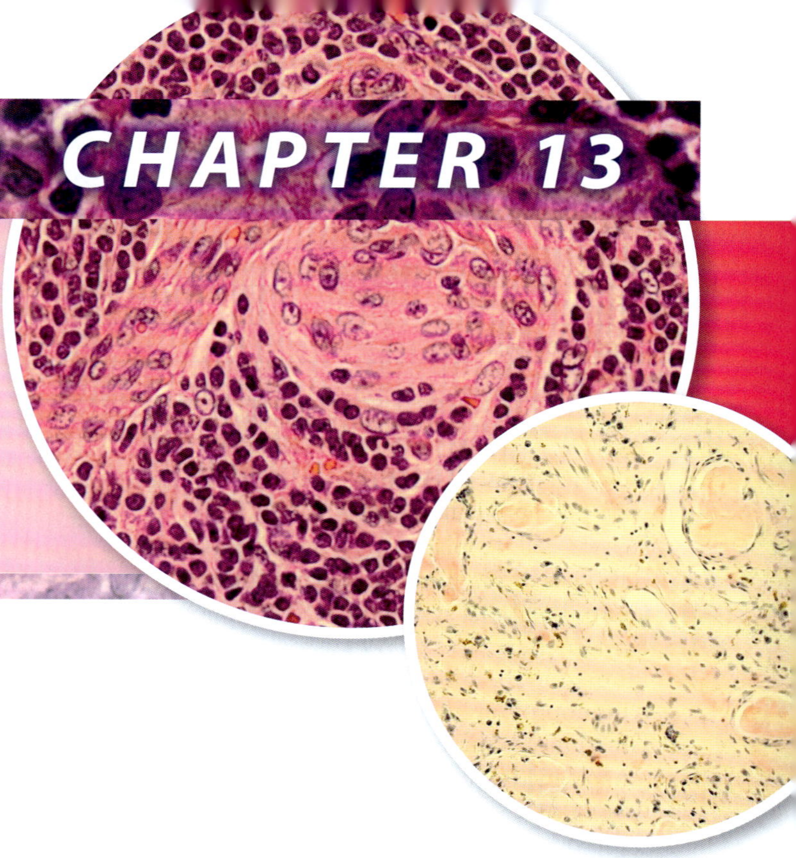

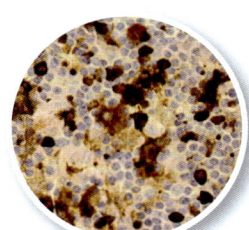

CHAPTER 13

Hematological Pathology

MEER-TAHER SHABANI-RAD

Hematological Pathology Exam Essentials

MUST KNOW

World Health Organization (WHO) classification

- The hematologic system is a complex and daunting area in pathology, as reflected in the voluminous nature of the WHO classification. The focus of your pathology specialty (hematologic pathology, general pathology, or anatomic pathology) determines your focus within this classification. This chapter is oriented to anatomic pathology (AP).
- Within hematopathology, the AP exam mostly focuses on mature B-cell lymphomas. High-yield AP categories within the WHO classification are indicated with an asterisk, below, and include:
  - Myeloproliferative neoplasms.*
  - Myelodysplastic syndrome.
  - Acute myeloid leukemia (AML).
  - Precursor lymphoid neoplasms.
  - Mature B-cell neoplasms.*
  - Mature T- and NK-cell neoplasms.
  - Hodgkin lymphomas.*
  - Immunodeficiency-associated lymphoproliferative disorders.
  - Histiocytic disorders.
- Within myeloproliferative neoplasms, you should be able to name at least 5 examples and their common mutations. Some of the more commonly examined

myeloproliferative neoplasms include:
  - Chronic myeloid leukemia (CML).
  - Polycythemia vera.
  - Primary myelofibrosis.
  - Essential thrombocythemia.
  - Mastocytosis (although the WHO lists this separately).
- Within myelodysplastic syndrome (MDS), you should be able to list some subtypes. Although each subtype contains many details, these details appear to be low yield.
- As with MDS, AML and precursor lymphoid neoplasms have numerous subtypes and genetic changes, but the details are less relevant. You should have some basic knowledge about AML and acute lymphoblastic leukemia (ALL).
- Mature B-cell neoplasm is an important category for the AP exam. Although the WHO lists innumerable entities within this category, some categories stand out. These can be categorized as either stand-alone B-cell lymphoma, where location is irrelevant (e.g., chronic lymphocytic leukemia/small lymphocytic lymphoma [CLL/SLL], follicular lymphoma), or lymphoma associated with a location (e.g., breast effusion lymphoma, MALT lymphoma). An alternate categorization is based on general patterns of CD5 and CD10 stains, which a table makes easier to memorize.

	CD5	CD10
CLL/SLL	+	–
Mantle cell	+	–
Follicular	–	+
Diffuse large B-cell lymphoma (DLBCL)	–	+
Burkitt	–	+
Lymphoplasmacytic	–	–
Marginal zone	–	–
Hairy cell	–	–

- A few other special entities in addition to those mentioned above include:
  · Plasma cell neoplasms.
  · Subtypes of marginal zone lymphoma.
  · Central nervous system (CNS) lymphoma.
  · Epstein-Barr virus (EBV) associated lymphomas.
  · Human herpesvirus 8 (HHV-8) associated lymphoproliferative disease.
  · Effusion-associated lymphoma.
  · Anaplastic lymphoma kinase (ALK) associated lymphoma.
  · Subtypes of Burkitt lymphoma.
  · Castleman disease.
  · Splenic tumors, which include lymphomas, leukemias, littoral cell angiomas, and metastasis.
- The NK/T cell category is unfamiliar to most AP examinees, but surprisingly contains several entities of interest within specific anatomic locations:
  · EBV-positive NK/T-cell lymphoma, especially in the head and neck region.
  · Intestinal T-cell lymphoma, especially in the context of celiac disease.
  · Mycosis fungoides/Sezary syndrome.
  · Anaplastic large cell lymphoma, especially those with *ALK* translocations.
- You should be well versed in Hodgkin lymphoma (HL) and all its variants. This includes clinical symptoms, pathogenesis, morphologic findings, and ancillary studies for:
  · Classic HL.
  · Nodular lymphocyte predominant HL.
- For immunodeficiency related lymphoproliferative disorders, the context will likely be HIV.
- For histiocytic disorders, the key focus will be on Langerhans cell histiocytosis and variants.
- Thymus pathology is included here, and there are a few small topics worth knowing:
  · Types of thymoma.
  · Other anterior mediastinal lesions.

AJCC and College of American Pathologists (CAP) protocols

The CAP/AJCC has only 4 protocols for bone marrow, Hodgkin lymphoma, plasma cell neoplasms, and an assortment of non-Hodgkin lymphomas. Because of the

unique nature of hematologic neoplasms compared to solid organ neoplasms, you should focus on the following aspects:
- Any specific or unique clinical presentations (e.g., Burkitt lymphoma presenting as jaw mass).
- Findings on peripheral smear.
- Any particular flow cytometry finding.
- Any bone marrow biopsy finding (especially myeloproliferative neoplasms and myelodysplastic syndromes).
- Lymph node findings.
- Findings in other involved locations, such as skin, spleen, gastrointestinal system, or other organs.
- Immunophenotype of the entities already mentioned. For B-cell lymphomas, use the CD5/CD10 categorization approach.
- Any additional study used for diagnosis (e.g., *TCR* rearrangement studies, cytogenetics, sequencing, fluorescence in situ hybridization [FISH], Epstein-Barr encoding region in situ hybridization [EBER ISH]).
- Don't forget about metastasis to bone and lymph nodes, especially on the practical portion of the exam. Just because the specimen seems hematological doesn't mean the tumor is of hematopoietic origin.
- Don't forget that lymphomas can mimic other small round blue cell tumors in various organs.

Nonneoplastic diseases

Overall, the major focus in hematopathology is on neoplastic conditions (especially B cell related). Nonetheless, there are some high-yield, nonneoplastic conditions worth considering, especially within the lymph node (for a more comprehensive list, see the Must See section):
- Differential diagnoses for benign conditions that mimic lymphoma in various organs (e.g., skin dermatoses that mimic mycosis fungoides).
- The multitude of causes of follicular hyperplasia.
- Lymph node infections.
- Infectious and vascular changes in the spleen.
- Causes of splenomegaly.
- Red and white pulp expansion of the spleen, especially causes.
- Extramedullary hematopoiesis.

Genetic and syndromic conditions

There aren't many syndromes in this chapter that are of great relevance to the AP exam. Review:
- Histiocytosis and related syndromes.
- Neurofibromatosis (NF1) with juvenile myelomonocytic leukemia.

MUST SEE
- Gross pathology is a very minor area in hematopathology.

- Although the number of entities in the WHO classification is daunting, filter out those related to specific genetic changes and instead focus on that category's "big picture."
- Many entities within hematopathology cannot be diagnosed on H&E alone, and require correlation with clinical impression, blood smear, flow cytometry, bone marrow aspirate, or other ancillary studies such as FISH. Hence it is uncommon to encounter hematopathology questions on the quick slide portion of the exam. They are ideal, however, for oral questions.
- Other than H&E images, you should find images of the immunostain results to correlate with entities' H&E impression. Knowing the pattern of staining and intensity of staining is especially important in hematopathology, and sometimes the result is beyond simply categorizing it as "positive" or "negative." In some cases, other ancillary studies might be important too, such as reticulin stains in myelofibrosis.
- The focus will be on lymph nodes and bone marrow specimens. Although peripheral smear and bone marrow aspirate examination is a critical component in many cases, these are more within the realm of GP and are rarely asked on the AP exam.
- The myeloid lesions of interest include:
  - CML.
  - Polycythemia vera.
  - Primary myelofibrosis.
  - Essential thrombocythemia.
  - Cutaneous mastocytosis (urticaria pigmentosa).
  - MDS with single and multilineage dysplasia.
  - AML.
- The B-cell lymphomas of interest include:
  - CLL/SLL.
  - Marginal zone lymphoma, including splenic and nodal types.
  - Hairy cell leukemia.
  - Lymphoplasmacytic lymphoma.
  - Plasma cell myeloma and plasmacytoma.
  - Amyloidoma.
  - MALT lymphoma.
  - Follicular lymphoma.
  - Mantle cell lymphoma.
  - DLBCL, including CNS DLBCL, thymic large B-cell lymphoma.
  - Effusion related lymphoma.
  - Burkitt lymphoma.
- The other miscellaneous lesions of interest include:
  - Hodgkin lymphoma, both classic and nodular lymphocyte predominant types.
  - NK/T-cell lymphoma, nasal type.
  - Intestinal T-cell lymphoma.
  - Mycosis fungoides/Sezary syndrome.
  - Anaplastic large cell lymphoma (ALCL).
  - Langerhans cell histiocytosis (LCH).
- Thymoma and thymic carcinoma.
- Metastases (don't forget about these).
- Nonneoplastic conditions of interest include:
  - Reactive follicular hyperplasia.
  - Progressive transformation of germinal centers.
  - Toxoplasma.
  - Kikuchi disease.
  - Catscratch disease.
  - Dermatopathic lymphadenopathy.
  - Kimura disease.
  - Rosai Dorfman disease.
  - Systemic lupus erythematosus adenopathy.
  - HIV adenopathy.
  - Castleman disease, and variants.
  - Granulomatous lymphadenitis.
  - Sarcoidosis.
- The spleen also contains a few interesting lesions:
  - Littoral cell angioma.
  - Red and white pulp expansion.
  - Splenic marginal zone lymphoma.
  - Angiosarcoma.
  - Amyloidosis (Sago and Lardaceous spleen).
  - Infarction.

MUST DO

- For each of the entities outlined in the Must See section, you should be comfortable generating a differential diagnosis and listing additional studies (e.g., histochemical or immunohistochemical stains).
- When studying in groups, practice:
  - The molecular changes in myeloproliferative neoplasm (MPN).
  - Using immunohistochemistry (IHC) and other studies to differentiate various B-cell lymphomas.
  - The various stages of mycosis and Sezary syndrome.
  - The various patterns of reactive lymphadenopathy and differential diagnosis.
  - The differential diagnosis for granulomatous lymphadenopathy.
  - The symptoms and complications of multiple myeloma in various organs.
- Grossing of hematologic specimens is relatively simple. Focus less on this area compared to solid organs. High-yield topics include:
  - Core biopsies of lymph node.
  - Excision of lymph node.
  - Submission of specimen for flow cytometry.
  - Touch prep.
  - Making peripheral smear.
  - How to perform bone marrow biopsy (consider watching a video).
- You should be able to describe and handle fresh tissue for lymphoma protocol.

MULTIPLE CHOICE QUESTIONS

1. Which of the following is not classified as a microcytic anemia?

a. Iron deficiency.

b. Thalassemia.

c. Anemia of chronic disease.

d. Aplastic anemia.

e. Sideroblastic anemia.

Answer: d

2. Which of the following anemias will **not** show an increased reticulocyte count?

a. Fanconi anemia.

b. Hemolytic anemia.

c. Hemorrhagic anemia.

d. Partially treated folic acid deficiency.

e. Glucose-6-phosphate dehydrogenase (G6PD) deficiency.

Answer: a

3. Which of the following does not demonstrate Burr cells in a blood smear?

a. Acute renal failure.

b. Bleeding ulcer.

c. Myelofibrosis.

d. Gastric carcinoma.

e. Pyruvate kinase deficiency.

Answer: c

4. Spherocytes may appear with all of the following **except**:

a. Hemoglobin C disease.

b. Transfusion.

c. Autoimmune hemolytic anemia.

d. Burns.

e. ABO incompatibility.

Answer: a

5. Which condition is **not** usually associated with the presence of schistocytes?

a. Thrombotic thrombo-cytopenic purpura.

b. Hemolytic ure-mic syndrome.

c. Severe burns.

d. Disseminated intra-vascular coagulation.

e. Hereditary elliptocytosis.

Answer: e

6. Rouleaux formation is seen in all of the following **except**:

a. Paraproteinemia.

b. Multiple myeloma.

c. Hereditary spherocytosis.

d. Diabetes mellitus.

e. Acute and chronic inflammation.

Answer: c

7. Which condition does **not** show target cells in a peripheral blood smear?

a. Thalassemia.

b. Iron deficiency anemia.

c. Liver disease.

d. Megaloblas-tic anemia.

e. Hemoglobin C disease.

Answer: d

8. Ovalocytes are seen in all of the following conditions **except**:

a. Thalassemia.

b. Iron deficiency anemia.

c. Folate deficiency.

d. Hereditary elliptocytosis.

e. Sideroblastic anemia.

Answer: e

9. Which of the following is **not** associated with stomatocytes in a peripheral blood smear?

a. Myelofibrosis.

b. Immune hemo-lytic anemia.

c. Rh null syndrome.

d. Chronic liver disease.

e. Erythrocyto-toxic agents.

Answer: a

10. Which of the following conditions is **not** usually associated with teardrop cells?

a. Splenectomy.

b. Aplastic anemia.

c. Myelofibrosis.

d. Thalassemia.

e. Metastatic bone marrow.

Answer: b

11. Acanthocytes are typically seen in all of the following conditions **except**:

a. Abetalipoproteinemia.

b. Chronic alcoholism.

c. Sickle cell anemia.

d. Severe liver disease.

e. Splenectomy.

Answer: c

12. Which of the following conditions does **not** show t(9;22)?

a. Acute myeloid leukemia.

b. Chronic myelog-enous leukemia.

c. Acute B-lympho-blastic leukemia/lymphoma.

d. Acute T-lympho-blastic leukemia/lymphoma.

e. All of the above.

Answer: d

13. Which of the following statements about chronic myeloid leukemia (CML) is **not** correct?

a. *BCR-ABL1* fusion is the most important factor in pathogenesis of CML.

b. Tyrosine kinase inhibitors are the main treatment modality in treatment of CML.

c. Increased blast percentage > 10% but < 20% is the only diagnostic criteria for progression of CML into accelerated phase.

d. CML cases with normal cytogenetic studies may show *BCR-ABL1* fusion gene by reverse transcription polymerase chain reaction (RT-PCR).

e. Transformed CMLs associated with altered *TP53, RB1, MYC, CDKN2A, NRAS, KRAS, RUNX1, MECOM (EVI1), TET2, CBL, ASXL1, IDH1,* and *IDH2* genes.

Answer: c

14. Which of the following statements about polycythemia vera (PV) is **not** correct?

a. The annual incidence of PV in western countries is higher than in Japan and East Asia.

b. Most PV patients (> 95%) demonstrate subnormal erythropoietin (EPO), endogenous erythroid colony (EEC), or *JAK2* mutations.

c. Most PV cases demonstrate sufficient morphological

features, even in the early prepolycythemic stage.

d. Most PV cases (> 95%) show no evidence of stainable iron in bone marrow aspirate and biopsy.

e. Later myelofibrotic stages of PV are defined by progressive erythropoiesis and decreased megakaryocytic proliferation.

Answer: e

15. Which of the following statements is **not** applicable to primary myelofibrosis (PMF)?

a. The prefibrotic stage of PMF is characterized by hypercellular marrow with atypical megakaryocytic proliferation.

b. The fibrotic stage of PMF is defined by leukoerythroblastic reaction and organomegaly.

c. The prefibrotic stage of PMF is associated with the presence of frequent

teardrop red cells in peripheral blood.

d. Marked increase in bone marrow reticulin fibrosis and intravascular hematopoiesis are characteristic morphological findings seen in PMF.

e. Atypical megakaryocytes with cloud-like nuclei and extramedullary hematopoiesis are common features of PMF.

Answer: c

16. Which of the following statements is **not** applicable to essential thrombocythemia (ET)?

a. Persistent marked thrombocytosis > 450 x 10E9/L is a diagnostic feature of ET, especially when it is supported by the presence of *JAK2* mutation.

b. Some ET cases with marked thrombocytosis are associated with chromosome 3 abnormalities.

c. Bone marrow biopsy may be helpful to exclude other myeloid neoplasms presenting with thrombocytosis (e.g., myelodysplastic syndrome [MDS]

with chromosome 5q deletion, and myelodysplastic/myeloproliferative neoplasm with ring sideroblasts and thrombocytosis [MDS/MPN-RS-T]).

d. Proliferation of giant megakaryocytic forms displaying staghorn lobulated nuclei is a characteristic feature of ET.

e. ET cases demonstrate *JAK2* mutation (50–60%) and/or *CALR* mutation (30%), or *MPL* mutation (3%), and 12% are triple negative.

Answer: b

17. Which of the following statements are not applicable to chronic myelomonocytic leukemia (CMML)?

a. The presence of persistent monocytosis (> 1 x 10^9/L), accounting for ≥ 10% of leukocytes, for at least 3 months is the first precondition for the diagnosis of CMML.

b. CMML cases may demonstrate mild to moderate bone marrow dysplasia.

c. CMML cases with eosinophilia associated with t(5;12) do not require

further molecular or genetic testing for subclassification.

d. Extramedullary involvement of splenic red pulp, skin, hepatic sinusoids and lymph nodes may be seen with CMML.

e. Nodular proliferation of plasmacytoid dendritic cells (plasmacytoid monocytes) is a morphological feature seen in CMML cases.

Answer: c

18. Which of the following statements about myelodysplastic syndrome (MDS) is **not** correct?

a. Dysplastic megakary-ocytes and dyseryth-ropoiesis may be seen with exposure to chemo agents, viral infections, toxins, and congenital disorders.

b. In the presence of *SF3B1* mutation, the diagnosis of myelo-dysplastic syndrome with ring sideroblasts (MDS-RS) does not require correlation with the percentage of ringed sideroblasts.

c. The presence of Auer rods in MDS cases with < 5% blasts has been associated with poor prognosis and should be classified as MDS with excess blasts-2 (MDS-EB2).

d. Pelger-Huet neutro-phils may be seen in MDS as well as non-neoplastic conditions.

e. Approximately 10% of MDS cases may demonstrate hypo-plastic marrow or bone marrow fibrosis.

Answer: b

19. Which of the following statements about acute myeloid leukemia (AML) with recurrent genetic abnormalities is **not** correct?

a. All myeloid neo-plasms with t(8;21)(q22;q22), inv(16)(p13.1;q22), and t(15;17)(q22;q12), regardless of blast count, are clas-sified as AML.

b. Blasts in AML with t(8;21)(q22;q22) usually demonstrate abundant granular cytoplasm with prom-inent perinuclear halo and increased eosino-philic precursors.

c. All myeloid neo-plasms with t(9;11)(p23;q34), inv(3)(q21;q26.2), and t(3;3)(q21;q26.2), regardless of blast

count, are also diagnosed as AML.

d. AML cases with inv(16)(p13.1;q22) usually demonstrate myelomonocytic features with variable number of eosino-philic precursors with large eosino-philic granules.

e. Acute promyelocytic leukemia (APL) cases with t(15;17) *PML-RARA* are sensitive to treatment with all-trans retinoic acid (ATRA) and expres-sion of CD56 is associated with less favorable prognosis.

Answer: c

20. Which of the following statements is **not** applicable to variants of AML?

a. Most AML cases with multilineage dysplasia are not correlated to previous cytotoxic therapy.

b. In the 2016 WHO revised classification, most of previously diagnosed acute erythroleukemia cases (erythroid/myeloid subtype) will be categorized as MDS-RAEB2.

c. Therapy related myeloid neoplasms, including t-AML/t-MDS or t-AML/t-MDS/t-MPN, account for 10–20% of AML cases and are usually correlated to a previ-ous treatment with

alkylating agents/radiation therapy.

d. Cases of AML with minimal differen-tiation presenting with medium size agranular blasts may require immuno-phenotypic studies to be distinguished from acute lympho-blastic leukemia (ALL) or megakaryo-blastic leukemia.

e. AML with maturation cases account for 10% of AML cases and fre-quently display Auer rods. Promyelocytes, myelocytes, and neutrophils account for at least 10% of bone marrow cells.

Answer: a

21. Which immunophenotypic marker is not usually present on immature stem cells or early progenitor/precursor lymphoid blasts?

a. Terminal deoxy-nucleotidyl trans-ferase (TdT).

b. CD34.

c. CD1a.

d. CD10.

e. Cytoplasmic IgM heavy chain (μ).

f. CD68.

Answer: f

22. B-lymphoblastic leukemia/lymphoma is the most common type of acute leukemia in children. What clinical and cytogenetic/molecular factors adversely affect the prognosis for children with this disease?

a. Age: < 2 years and > 10 years.

b. White blood cell (WBC) count at pre-sentation > 100 000.

c. *KMT2A* (also called *MLL*) fusions (*KMT2A*-rearranged

B-lymphoblastic leukemia/lymphoma).

d. Presence of t(9;22).

e. Minimal residual dis-ease (MRD) detection following induction chemotherapy.

f. None of the above.

g. All of the above.

Answer: g

23. Which of the following statements is **not** applicable to B-lymphoblastic leukemia/lymphoma (B-ALL)?

a. Many treatment protocols consider 25% blast count in bone marrow as a cutoff for defining this neoplasm as acute lymphoblastic leukemia.

b. B-ALL is most common in children and 75% of cases occur in children under 6 years of age.

c. The most common form of extramedullary involvement is mediastinal mass.

d. Patients with B-lymphoblastic lymphoma without leukemia are usually asymptomatic and most have a limited stage disease.

e. B-ALL has a good prognosis and > 95% of children with ALL show complete remission.

Answer: c

24. Which of the following statements about T-lymphoblastic leukemia/lymphoma (T-ALL) is **not** correct?

a. T-ALL cases account for 15% of childhood ALL and are more common in adolescent males.

b. T-ALL cases usually present with high leukocyte counts; however, the diagnosis should be avoided when blasts are < 20%. Compared to B-ALL trilineage, hematopoiesis is relatively spared.

c. T-ALL cases with hyperdiploid chromosomes are commonly seen among older children and are associated with a very favorable prognosis.

d. T-ALL cases are usually TdT positive and express cytoplasmic CD3 with frequent coexpression of CD4 and CD8 (thymocyte T cell immunophenotype).

e. T-ALL in childhood is a high-risk disease and no favorable subtypes with recurrent genetic abnormalities have been recognized for this entity.

Answer: c

25. Which of the following immunophenotypic features are **not** seen with neoplastic plasma cells?

a. Expression of CD138, CD38, eosine-5-maleimide (EMA), MUM1.

b. Expression of cyclin D1/D3.

c. Monotypic immunoglobulin light chain restriction.

d. Aberrant expression of CD56 and CD117.

e. Absence of CD45/CD20/CD43.

Answer: e

SHORT ANSWER QUESTIONS

Red Cell Disorders
Anemia

26. List the laboratory tests used in the diagnosis of iron deficiency anemia.

- Serum iron.
- Total iron binding capacity (TIBC).
- Free erythrocyte protoporphyrin.
- Serum soluble transferrin receptor.
- Complete blood count.
- Serum ferritin.

27. Compare the underlying cause, symptoms, significant laboratory test findings, and treatments of iron deficiency anemia and sideroblastic anemia.

ANEMIA	UNDERLYING CAUSE	SYMPTOMS	LABORATORY FINDINGS	TREATMENT
Iron deficiency anemia	• Intake inadequacy; poor iron absorption; blood loss.	• Pallor, fatigue nail spooning, cheilitis, glossitis.	• Decreased serum iron and ferritin, increased TIBC, decreased bone marrow storage iron, target cells.	• Oral iron therapy or parenteral iron dextran.
Sideroblastic anemia	• Inherited; alcoholism; lead poisoning; congenital sideroblastic anemia.	• Weakness, pallor, palpitations.	• Increased serum iron, decreased TIBC, increased bone marrow storage iron, ringed sideroblasts in bone marrow aspirate, Pappenheimer bodies.	• Pyridoxine or removal of the causative toxic substance (i.e., drugs, alcohol, lead).

28. How are iron deficiency anemia and anemia of chronic disease differentiated?

- Serum iron levels is approximately the same in both conditions.
- The percentage of transferrin saturation is decreased in both, but is > 10% in chronic disease and < 10% in iron deficiency.
- The main difference is in serum ferritin levels, which are increased in chronic disease and decreased in iron deficiency.
- TIBC is decreased with chronic disease, but increased with iron deficiency.

29. What are the main pathophysiologic mechanisms for anemia of chronic disease (ACD), including chronic renal disease?

- The primary mechanism in ACD is an immunologic cytokine reaction to either infection or other entities (e.g., neoplasms), leading to iron blockade within macrophages and decreased erythropoiesis in bone marrow.
- The primary mechanism at work in anemia of chronic renal disease is decreased erythropoiesis due to lower production of erythropoietin by the kidneys.

30. What are some of the disease states and conditions frequently correlated with ACD?

- Inflammatory conditions (i.e., lupus, rheumatoid arthritis, and ulcerative colitis).
- Infections (i.e., HIV, tuberculosis, pyelonephritis).
- Malignancy (i.e., lymphoma, leukemia, carcinoma).

31. List the underlying causes and mechanisms of megaloblastic anemia.

- Megaloblastic anemia is caused by deficiency in the coenzymes folate and vitamin B_{12}.
- This deficiency causes flawed DNA synthesis: specifically, multiplying cells are not able to produce enough DNA to permit mitosis to occur. With more cells in the DNA synthesis phase, and RNA synthesis not being dependent on folate or vitamin B_{12}, there is a discrepancy between the maturation of the nucleus and cytoplasm.
- This discrepancy causes giant, immature-appearing nuclei coupled with outwardly appearing more mature cytoplasm.

32. What are the main laboratory tests that aid in the diagnosis of megaloblastic anemia?

- Serum vitamin B_{12}.
- Serum and red blood cell folate.
- Intrinsic factor antibodies.
- Lactate dehydrogenase (LDH).
- Homocysteine.
- Serum iron.
- Methylmalonic acid.

33. What are the red cell protein defects associated with hereditary spherocytosis and hereditary elliptocytosis?

- Hereditary spherocytosis is most commonly associated with a protein defect correlated to the ankyrin gene (*ANK1*).
- Flow cytometric assessment of EMA binding provides high sensitivity and specificity in the diagnosis of hereditary spherocytosis.
- Hereditary elliptocytosis is most commonly associated with protein defects in spectrin α chains, spectrin β chains, and protein 4.1 genes.

34. What are the main laboratory tests employed in the diagnosis of hereditary spherocytosis? What are the associated findings?

TEST	FINDING
Peripheral blood smear	• Spherocytes are present; increased reticulocytes.
Osmotic fragility test	• Osmotic fragility is increased.
Flow cytometric EMA staining	• Fluorescence from EMA is reduced.

35. Compare and contrast the peripheral blood smear morphology of pyruvate kinase (PK) deficiency and glucose-6-phosphate dehydrogenase (G6PD) deficiency.

DISORDER	MORPHOLOGY
PK deficiency	• Spicular red cells, marked anisopoikilocytosis, polychromasia (reticulocytosis).
G6PD deficiency	• Heinz bodies, bite cells, polychromasia (reticulocytosis).

36. What are the most commonly used tests for detecting G6PD deficiency?

- Quantitative G6PD assay.
- Fluorescent spot test.
- Methemoglobin reduction test.
- Blood smear analysis for bite cells.
- Heinz body screening (supravital staining).

37. What is the most common clinically significant hemoglobinopathy? What is its etiology? What are its clinical consequences?

- Most common: hemoglobin S (HbS).
- Etiology: HbS results from replacement of glutamic acid by valine in beta chains causing alterations in hemoglobin solubility.
- Consequences:

· The homozygous condition results in sickle cell anemia.
· Sickle cell anemia is characterized by moderate to severe hemolysis.
· This results in painful sickle cell crises due to the irregularly shaped red cells blocking the blood vessels, causing ischemic and microthrombotic events.

38. What laboratory tests are used in the diagnosis of hemoglobin disorders?

- Complete blood count (CBC) and peripheral blood smear (PBS).
- Hemoglobin S solubility test (SICKLEDEX).
- Liquid chromatography (high-performance liquid chromatography).

- Hemoglobin acid/alkaline gel electrophoresis.
- Molecular studies (polymerase chain reaction and DNA/amino acid sequencing).
- Isopropanol stability test.

39. Compare and contrast hemoglobin C disease, hemoglobin E disease, and hemoglobin H disease in terms of red cell morphology.

DISEASE	RED CELL MORPHOLOGY
Hemoglobin C disease	• Numerous target cells, hemoglobin C crystals and folded red cells.
Hemoglobin E disease	• Hypochromic microcytes.
Hemoglobin H disease	• Brilliant cresyl blue stain shows hemoglobin H precipitates.

40. List the cause of thalassemia and 2 main categories of thalassemia.

- Cause: thalassemia is characterized by hemoglobin gene defects causing impairment in globin chain synthesis and consequent imbalance in the number of paired chains (α and β chains).
- Categories: the 2 main categories of thalassemia are α thalassemia and β thalassemia:

· α thalassemia is associated with variants of gene deletion (3.7, 4.2, *SEA*, and *FIL*).
· β thalassemia is caused by gene mutation/posttranscriptional defects (globin mRNA defects).

41. Describe the variant hemoglobin M and its genetic associations.

- Hemoglobin M (HbM) is characterized by a single amino acid substitution favoring the formation of methemoglobin, and by its inability to bind oxygen or sustaining reduced heme iron.

- HbM is seen with inherited autosomal dominant methemoglobinemia.
- Heterozygote individuals who inherit HbM display cyanosis; however, since the homozygous HbM is lethal, the status of these genes is not well known.

42. Tabulate the main clinical and laboratory features of autoimmune hemolytic anemias (AIHA).

CLINICAL FINDINGS	WARM AIHA	COLD AIHA
Onset	• Sudden.	• Gradual.
Jaundice	• Present.	• Usually absent.
Splenomegaly	• Present.	• Absent.
Immunoglobulin type	• IgG mediated.	• IgM mediated.
Red cell morphology	• Spherocytes.	• Agglutinated red cells.
Clinical association	• Usually autoimmune.	• Usually infections.
DAT (Direct antiglobulin test)	• Positive (monospecific anti-IgG).	• Positive (monospecific C3d).
Mechanism of hemolysis	• Extravascular (mononuclear phagocyte system).	• Intravascular (complement).

43. What are the main causes of microangiopathic hemolytic anemia (MAHA) and which drugs are associated with it?

- Causes: MAHA results from red cell fragmentation (schistocytes) due to endothelial injury of arterioles due to blockade by platelet microthrombi and ischemic consequences.

- This group includes thrombotic thrombocytopenic purpura (TTP), hemolytic uremic syndrome (HUS), and disseminated intravascular coagulation (DIC).
- Associated drugs: mitomycin, cyclosporine, and tacrolimus have been known to cause secondary TTP.

44. Compare and contrast the 3 causes of MAHA.

ANEMIA	CAUSE	SYMPTOMS	TREATMENT
TTP	• Idiopathic; autoimmune disorders.	• Thrombocytopenia, fever, renal failure, neurological signs.	• Plasmapheresis and immunosuppressants.
HUS	• Hemorrhagic colitis.	• Bloody diarrhea, bleeding, pain.	• Supportive care is usually sufficient.
DIC	• Sepsis; cancer; trauma; obstetrical complications and snakebites.	• Hemorrhage.	• Coagulation factor replacement with cryoprecipitate.

45. Compare and contrast malarial infection, babesiosis infection, and bartonellosis (catscratch disease).

INFECTION	CAUSE	LOCATION	SYMPTOMS	LABORATORY FINDINGS
Malaria	• *Plasmodium* species.	• Africa, Asia, (Tropical regions).	• Cyclic fevers, anemia, and splenomegaly.	• Intracellular red cell inclusions +/– gametocytes +/– Schuffner dots.
Babesiosis	• *Babesia microti.*	• Northeast United States.	• Noncyclic fevers, headache.	• Intra- and extracellular ring-shaped inclusions with tetrad formation.
Bartonellosis or catscratch disease	• *Bartonella henselae.*	• Worldwide.	• Fever, fatigue, lymphadenopathy (necrotizing lymphadenitis).	• Bacilli detected by Warthin-Starry stain.

46. What are the tests commonly used in detection of paroxysmal nocturnal hemoglobinuria (PNH), and what is its association with myeloid neoplasm?
- Tests:
  · Flow cytometry for CD55 and CD59.
  · Acidified serum test.
  · Associated with myelodysplastic syndromes.

47. What are the causes of primary and secondary aplastic anemia?
- Primary aplastic anemia is usually idiopathic and may be associated with an autoimmune process.
- Secondary aplastic anemia is often caused by infections, such as HIV, Epstein-Barr virus, hepatitis, or influenza.
- Secondary aplastic anemia is also commonly linked with various drugs and toxins, such as benzene, chloramphenicol, nonsteroidal antiinflammatory drugs (NSAIDs), chemotherapy drugs, and insecticides.

48. Describe the peripheral blood and bone marrow findings in aplastic anemia.
- The peripheral blood shows marked pancytopenia.
- Red cells are often found to be macrocytic.
- The bone marrow is hypocellular, often with < 10% cellularity.
- Bone marrow plasma cells and reactive small lymphoid cells are usually increased in number.

Bone Marrow Pathology
Ancillary Studies in Bone Marrow Pathology

49. List common aspiration/biopsy sites.
- Posterior iliac crest.
- Alternative site: sternum.

50. Immunophenotypic studies are essential for the accurate subclassification of hematolymphoid disorders, as required by the WHO classification of tumors of hematopoietic and lymphoid tissues. Name and briefly describe the 2 laboratory methods that result in immunophenotypic characterization of the cells of interest.
- Flow cytometric immunophenotyping:
  · Viable and unfixed cell suspensions (i.e., peripheral blood, bone marrow/tissue aspirates, bodily fluids, cell suspensions of tissue from biopsies) are stained with antibodies against various CDs (clusters of differentiation) conjugated to fluorochromes, then washed and subsequently laser/computer analyzed for specific staining patterns.
  · The cell bearing the antigen specifically binds the fluorochrome conjugated antibody.
  · Once attached to the specific cellular antigen, the fluorochrome emits light of a particular wavelength, which is measured by cytometer detectors.
  · The light is converted into electrical signals, depicted as cell plots/histograms.
  · The histograms are evaluated by trained pathologists, who construct the cell immunophenotype and interpret the results in conjunction with clinical/morphological findings.

(continued on next page)

- Immunohistochemistry methodology:
  - This uses formalin fixed and paraffin embedded tissue and heat induced antigen retrieval to enhance the detection of the specific antibody-antigen reaction. It requires:
    - A cellular antigen of interest.
    - A primary antibody targeting that antigen.
    - A detection system to visualize the antigen-antibody complex.
    - A trained pathologist to interpret the results in the context of morphological findings.

51. List common cytochemical/special stains used in bone marrow assessment.
- Iron stain (Prussian blue stain).
- Reticulin stain.
- Cytochemical stains (no longer required for the diagnosis of most disorders):
- Peroxidase special stain.
- Leukocyte alkaline phosphatase.
- Naphthol-ASD chloroacetate esterase.

52. Name 3 ancillary studies, other than immunohistochemistry (IHC) and flow cytometry, commonly used in the diagnosis and subclassification of hematolymphoid neoplasms. Give 1 or 2 examples of specific tests performed in these studies.
- Molecular cytogenetics: fluorescence in situ hybridization (FISH) for *c-MYC* and *BCR-ABL1*.
- Molecular studies:
- Polymerase chain reaction (PCR): *IgH/TCR/BCL-2/BCL-1/JAK2/FLT-3*.
- In situ hybridization (ISH): Epstein-Barr encoding region (EBER), cytomegalovirus (CMV).

53. What kind of information do you need to appropriately interpret bone marrow biopsy specimens?
- Clinical and medication history.
- Routine and molecular laboratory tests.
- Flow cytometric analysis and IHC.
- Imaging studies and skeletal X-ray survey.
- Information from peripheral blood smear, bone marrow aspirate specimen, aspirate clot section (cell block), and previous bone marrow core biopsy.

54. How do you handle a bone marrow biopsy specimen?
- Record the number of stained and unstained peripheral blood, bone marrow aspirate, and bone marrow core biopsy touch preparation smears.
- Record the length of the bone marrow core biopsy specimen.
- Submit for cytogenetic studies in a sodium heparin tube (method of choice) or in saline or RPMI transport medium.
- Submit bone marrow aspirate specimen for immunophenotyping by flow cytometry (ACD tube; yellow top tube) or EDTA tube (lavender top tube).
- Care must be taken not to under- or overdecalcify the bone marrow biopsy specimen.

55. What are recommended reported elements for biopsy/resection?
- Specimen type.
- Diagnostic line.
- Status of trilineage hematopoiesis and percentage of abnormal elements.
- Presence or absence of excess blats/residual disease.
- Abnormal findings in peripheral blood.
- Result of ancillary studies:
  - Ancillary studies (flow cytometry and IHC).
  - Cytogenetic and fluorescence in situ hybridization (FISH) studies.
  - Routine molecular tests (*BCR-ABL1* and *JAK2* p.V617F mutation).
  - Next-generation sequencing.

56. What is the first step for molecular evaluation of myeloproliferative neoplasm (MPN)?
- *BCR-ABL1* fusion/t(9;22) and *JAK2* test for MPNs.
- FISH for *PDGFRA/B* and *FGFR1* fusions when myeloid neoplasms accompanied by eosinophilia.
- Cytogenetics (karyotyping) and FISH.
- Next-generation sequencing.
- Additional molecular genetic tests are done when cytogenetics and/or FISH results are nonspecific or negative (e.g., trisomies +8 and/or +9 are often identified).
- Additional molecular genetic tests are done when cytogenetics and/or FISH results are nonspecific or negative (e.g., trisomies +8 and/or +9 are often identified).

57. What diseases are often associated with *JAK2* p.V617F (c.1849G>T)?
- This mutation is a characteristic finding with chronic myeloproliferative neoplasms.
- Almost all patients with polycythemia vera (95%) are positive for *JAK2* p.V617F mutation (others have insertions/deletions in exon 12).
- Many patients (40–50%) with primary myelofibrosis or essential thrombocythemia are positive for *JAK2* p.V617F mutation.

58. What are methods to evaluate for *JAK2* p.V617F (c.1849G>T) mutation testing?
- Allele-specific PCR.
- Sanger sequencing.
- Pyrosequencing.
- Next-generation sequencing.

59. For what diseases—which are treated with tyrosine kinase inhibitors (TKIs)—is *c-KIT* mutation clinically important?
- Mastocytosis (*c-KIT* mutation; D816V).
- Soft tissue neoplasm; gastrointestinal stromal tumor.
- Acute myeloid leukemia (*c-KIT* D816V).
- Melanoma.

60. List the lymphoid cell associated markers used in flow cytometry.
- B cell–associated markers: CD19, CD20, CD22, CD79a, CD10, kappa, lambda.
- T cell–associated markers: sCD3/cyCD3, CD2, CD5, CD7, CD4, CD8, and TdT.
- T/NK cell–associated markers: CD1a, CD3, CD2, CD5, CD7, CD4, CD8.

Myeloid Neoplasms and Acute Myeloid Leukemias

61. Briefly describe important clinical and diagnostic features of CML.
- CML is defined by marked peripheral leukocytosis with neutrophilic and myelocytic peaks.
- Phases of CML include chronic phase, accelerated phase, and blastic phase.

62. List findings that can establish the diagnosis of the accelerated phase of CML.
- Persistent leukocytosis > 10 x 10⁹/L.
- Persistent thrombocytosis with eosinophil counts > 1000 x 10⁹/L.
- Persistent thrombocytopenia with eosinophil counts < 100 x 10⁹/L.
- Basophilia of ≥ 20% in peripheral blood.
- Increased blasts (10–19%) in peripheral blood or bone marrow.
- Clonal cytogenetic evolution.
- Persistent/progressive splenomegaly.
- Hematological resistance to first TKI.
- Hematological and/or genetic evidence of resistance to 2 sequential TKIs.
- During therapy, > 1 mutation in *BCR-ABL1* fusion gene.

63. What is the most important cytogenetic abnormality associated with CML? Describe the tests used to detect this abnormality.
- Cytogenetic abnormality: t(9;22)(q34;q11.2), known as the Philadelphia chromosome, resulting in *BCR-ABL1* fusion.
- Tests:
  - Conventional karyotyping, FISH, or quantitative reverse transcription polymerase chain reaction (qRT-PCR).
- Application of FISH for *BCR-ABL1* fusions increases the sensitivity of the technique by detection of rare cryptic variants.
- FISH is also important for detecting genomic duplication or amplification of the *BCR-ABL1* locus, which may contribute to TKI resistance in a subset of CML patients.

64. What is the most sensitive method used for detecting *BCR-ABL1* fusion and monitoring CML patient response, resistance, or progression?
- Serial testing of patients for *BCR-ABL1* by qRT-PCR during TKI therapy.
- Reporting the result of PCR with the standardized reporting scale, known as the International Scale (IS).
- Major molecular response (MMR) is defined as *BCR-ABL1* qRT-PCR values ≤ 0.1% IS and a 3-log reduction from the standardized baseline.
- Defining a complete molecular response (CMR) as undetectable *BCR-ABL1* levels using a test with 4.5-log sensitivity.

65. How do CML patients on TKI manifest signs of therapeutic resistance?
- Progression to accelerated or blast phase.
- Failure to achieve timely cytogenetic or molecular milestones.
- Signs of loss of previously achieved response.

66. Briefly describe the diagnostic and prognostic markers in PV patients.
- No abnormal immunophenotypic features have been reported for PV.
- Recurring chromosomal abnormalities are seen in 20% of PV cases. These abnormalities, especially +8 and +9, are associated with disease progression to post-PV myelofibrosis in 80–90% of cases.

(continued on next page)

- Most PV patients die from thrombosis or hemorrhage and up to 20% may transform to MDS or AML.
- Although *JAK2* V617F and exon 12 mutation are found in > 95% of PV patients, so far no PV specific genetic defect has been discovered.

67. Briefly describe the clinical and diagnostic bone marrow features applicable to PMF patients.

- Varying degrees of splenomegaly may be seen in up to 90% of PMF patients.
- Patients may show vascular proliferation with perivascular localization of atypical megakaryocytes with hyperchromatic smeared nuclear features.
- Varying degrees of reticulin fibrosis (none to mild in pre-PMF) and/or collagen fibrosis (moderate to severe in overt fibrotic stage) are seen.
- Elevated lactate dehydrogenase (LDH), leukoerythroblastosis, and tear drop cells are present.
- Patients with PMF demonstrate mutations in *JAK2* V617F (50–60%), *CALR* (24%), and *MPL* (8%), and are triple negative in the rest of cases.
- Presence of del(13)(q12–22) or der(6)t(1;6) are strongly supportive of transformation of PMF to AML (30% of cases).

68. Briefly describe the clinical and diagnostic features applicable to ET patients.

- Slightly more than 50% of ET cases are asymptomatic at the time of presentation with marked thrombocytosis with an ongoing rate of 1–2% thrombotic events per year afterward.
- Basophilia, leukoerythroblastosis, and teardrop red cells are usually not seen in ET.
- Since some CML patients may initially present with thrombocytosis without leukocytosis, the exclusion of *BCR-ABL1* fusion genes is recommended at the time of diagnosis.
- The criteria for CML, PV, PMF are not met.
- Transformation of ET to AML, MDS, or post-ET myelofibrosis occurs in < 5% of patients.

69. Briefly describe the common features of specific subtypes of MDS/MPN.

- Chronic myelomonocytic leukemia (CMML) is defined by persistent peripheral monocytosis (> 1 10⁹/L), and hypercellular marrow with dysplastic changes and increased monocytic/mature myeloid cells. Based on the expansion of blasts, it may be subclassified to CMML-0 (< 5% blast), CMML-1 (5–9% blasts), or CMML-2 (10–19% blasts) in bone marrow.
- *BCR-ABL1* negative atypical chronic myeloid neoplasm falls into the category of MDS/MPN and is characterized by the lack of absolute monocytosis (monocytes < 10%), peripheral neutrophilia with dysgranulopoiesis, and negative genetic testing.
- Juvenile myelomonocytic leukemia (JMML) occurs among children < 3 years (75% of JMML cases), and it is more common among boys. In some cases, it is associated with neurofibromatosis (NF1). Germline mutation of *PTPN11* (coding SHP2) is commonly seen among these patients.
- JMML cases may show significantly elevated hemoglobin F, marked hypersensitivity to granulocyte-macrophage colony-stimulating factor (GM-CSF), and marked hepatosplenomegaly. Clinical presentation may mimic severe viral disease. There are 5 canonical RAS pathway mutations (in *PTPN11, NRAS, KRAS, NF1, and CBL*).
- MDS/MPN with ring sideroblasts (MDS/MPN-RS-T) is characterized by thrombocytosis, ≥ 15% ringed sideroblasts, erythroid dyplasia +/– multilineage dysplasia, without increased blasts.
- MDS/MPN unclassifiable (MDS/MPN-U) is characterized by thrombosis/leukocytosis and myelodysplasia while not meeting criteria for other myeloid neoplasms (60% are *JAK2* positive).

70. Briefly describe the morphological features seen among specific subtypes of MDS.

- MDS-EB-1 (excess blasts-1) cases have 2–4% blasts in peripheral blood (PB) or 5–9% blasts in bone marrow (BM).
- MDS-EB-2 (excess blasts-2) category includes cases displaying Auer rods regardless of blast count, or have 5–19% blasts in PB or 10–19% blasts in BM. A third of patients progress to AML.
- MDS with isolated del(5q) cases may have 1 additional abnormality — except loss of chromosome 7 or del(7q) — and hypolobated and/or monolobated megakaryocytes, without pancytopenia. Clonal suppression is possible with lenalidomide.
- MDS-MLD-RS (multilineage dysplasia with ringed sideroblasts) cases account for approximately 13% of MDS and have 2–3 lineages with > 10% dysplasia and ≥ 15% ringed sideroblasts (5% if *SF3B1* mutated).
- MDS-MLD cases account for 30% of MDS and have ≥ cytopenias and 2–3 dysplastic lineages.
- MDS-SLD-RS (single lineage dysplasia with ringed sideroblasts) cases account for up to 11% of MDS and are not associated with pancytopenia. Patients usually present with macrocytic anemia and dyserythropoiesis.
- MDS-SLD cases account for up to 20% of MDS and are not associated with pancytopenia.
- MDS-U (unclassified) cases: 1) have 1% blasts in PB (with < 5% blasts in BM) on ≥ 2 occasions, 2) represent MDS-SLD/MDS-del(5q) with pancytopenia, or 3) have a MDS-defining chromosomal abnormality in the absence of dysplasia.

Note: the prognosis of MDS is defined by the Revised International Prognostic Scoring System (IPSS-R). There are 5 risk groups: very low (score ≤ 1.5), low (2–3), intermediate (3.5–4.5), high (5–6), and very high (> 6).

Acute Myeloid Leukemia (AML) and Related Precursor Neoplasms

71. Describe the common features of specific subtypes of acute myeloid leukemia (AML).

- Acute promyelocytic leukemia (APL) is defined by presence of abnormal promyelocytes showing characteristic immunophenotypic features: lack of expression of HLA-DR and CD34, bright CD33/CD13 with aberrant coexpression of CD56.
- Abnormal erythroblasts of pure erythroid leukemia are often negative for HLA-DR and CD34, but express CD117 and CD36 in absence of myeloid markers such as CD13 and CD33.
- Acute megakaryoblastic leukemia is an uncommon type of AML with expression of CD41/CD42 (platelet markers) that are associated with hepatosplenomegaly, dysplastic changes, and marked marrow fibrosis.
- Myeloid sarcoma is an entity defined by extramedullary tumor mass consistent with myeloid blasts and, in a significant number of cases, demonstrates myelomonocytic/monoblastic features.

72. Describe the common features of blastoid plasmacytoid dendritic cell neoplasm (BPDCN).

- BPDCN is a clinically aggressive disease, which presents with skin, BM, PB, and lymph node involvement.
- The tumor cells express CD4, CD43, CD56, and CD123 (plasmacytoid dendritic associated marker) and are negative for myeloperoxidase.
- Two-thirds of patients with BPDCN have an abnormal karyotype involving 5q21, 5q34 (seen in 72% of cases), 12p13 (in 64%), 13q13-21 (in 64%), 6q23-qter (in 50%), 15q (in 43%), and loss of chromosome 9 (in 28%).
- Next-generation sequencing has revealed mutations in *NRAS* (present in 27.3% of cases); *ATM* (in 21.2%); *MET, KRAS, IDH2*, and *KIT* (in 9.1% each); *APC* and *RB1* (in 6.1% each); and *VHL, BRAF, MLH1, TP53*, and *RET* (in 3% each).

73. Tabulate prognostic classification of AML subtypes with and without recurrent genetic abnormalities.[1]

CLASS	PROGNOSIS	MORPHOLOGY/COMMENTS
I. AML WITH RECURRENT GENETIC ABNORMALITIES		
AML with t(8;21)(q22;q22.1); *RUNX1-RUNX1T1*	• Favorable.	• This features granulocytic maturation (predominantly neutrophilic); and blasts with abundant basophilic cytoplasm, azurophilic granules, frequent Auer rods and prominent Golgi.
AML with inv(16)(p13.1;q22) or t(16;16)(p13.1;q22); *CBFB-MYH11*	• Favorable.	• This features monocytic and granulocytic differentiation; and abnormal eosinophilic precursors with basophilic granules.
Acute promyelocytic leukemia with *PML-RARA*; (15;17) (q22;q11-22)	• Favorable.	• The hypergranular variant has multiple primary granules and Auer rods (often in bundles), and the hypogranular variant has inconspicuous granules. Both variants have bilobed nuclei, and a high incidence of disseminated intravascular coagulation.
AML with t(9;11)(p21.3;q23.3); *KMT2A-MLLT3*	• Intermediate (poor with *MECOM* overexpression).	• This has monocytic/monoblastic morphology, and this category is reserved for this specific translocation. Other rearrangements of *KMT2A* should be classified as "appropriate."
AML with t(6;9)(p23;q34.1); *DEK-NUP214*	• Poor.	• Monocytic features may be present. It is often associated with multilineage dysplasia (MLD) and basophilia. *FLT3*-ITD mutations are common.
AML with inv(3)(q21.3;q26.2) or t(3;3)(q21.3;q26.2); *GATA2, MECOM*	• Poor.	• Megakaryocytic dysplasia is frequently present and MLD is common.
AML (megakaryoblastic) with t(1;22)(p13.3;q13.1); *RBM15-MKL1*	• Poor.	• This is a rare entity. Megakaryocytic maturation and dysplasia are present; it occurs in infants and young children (≤ 3 years) without trisomy 21. Patients have marked organomegaly.
AML with *BCR-ABL1* (provisional)	• Poor.	• This is de novo AML; treatment is TKI and HSCT.
AML with mutated *NPM1*	• Favorable.	• This has myelomonocytic or monocytic features; IHC for NPM1 shows abnormal cytoplasmic staining; > 85% have normal karyotype.
AML with biallelic mutation of CEBPA	• Favorable.	• Good prognosis is related only to biallelic mutations; > 70% have normal karyotype.
AML with mutated *RUNX1* (provisional)	• Unclear (possibly poor).	• This is de novo AML; it lacks the genetic alterations of the above categories.

CLASS	PROGNOSIS	MORPHOLOGY/COMMENTS
II. AML WITH MYELODYSPLASIA-RELATED CHANGES (3 CRITERIA; 24–35% OF AML)		
With prior history of MDS or MDS/MPN	• Poor.	• Diagnosis is based on clinical history.
Multilineage dysplasia	• Poor.	• Diagnosis requires ≥ 2 cell lines with ≥ 50% dysplastic cells; cases of de novo AML with mutated *NPM1* or biallelic mutated *CEBPA* are excluded.
With MDS-related cytogenetic abnormality	• Poor.	• This is most commonly associated with del(5q), t(5q), del(7q), or complex karyotype.
III. THERAPY-RELATED MYELOID NEOPLASMS (10–20% OF AML)		
AML, therapy-related	• Very poor.	• Patients have a history of chemotherapy with alkylating agents, topoisomerase II inhibitor (e.g., etoposide), or radiation therapy; MDS-like cytogenetic aberrations (e.g., 5q–, 7q– [the majority]) or balanced translocations (e.g., *KMT2A*; minority) are present.
IV. AML, NOS (NOT OTHERWISE SPECIFIED) (FRENCH-AMERICAN-BRITISH [FAB] CLASSIFICATION INCLUDED)		
AML with minimal differentiation (M0)	• Intermediate.	• No morphocytochemical evidence of maturation is present; diagnosis requires flow cytometry to identify myeloblasts (+CD117/CD13/CD33) lacking markers of myelomonocytic maturation.
AML without maturation (M1)	• Intermediate.	• At least 3% of blasts are positive for myeloperoxidase; < 10% granulocytes are mature.
AML with maturation (M2)	• Intermediate.	• Morphology includes myelocytic maturation (> 10% of nucleated cells) with < 20% of monocyte lineage.
Acute myelomonocytic leukemia (M4)	• Intermediate.	• Myelocytic and monocytic differentiation are present (> 20% nucleated cells each).
Acute monoblastic and monocytic leukaemia (M5)	• Intermediate.	• Monocytic lineage is present (≥ 80% of nucleated cells); ≥ 80% of monocytic cells are monoblasts in acute monoblastic leukemia.
Pure erythroid leukemia (M6)	• Very poor.	• This has near exclusive commitment to erythroid lineage (> 80% of nucleated cells) with ≥ 30% proerythroblasts and no significant myeloblastic component.
Acute megakaryoblastic leukemia (M7)	• Poor.	• Blasts or megakaryocytic lineage predominate (≥ 50% of blasts); flow cytometry is positive for platelet glycoproteins (CD41/CD61/CD42a); patients with trisomy 21 are excluded (classified as myeloid leukemia associated with Down syndrome, despite being morphologically identical).
Acute basophilic leukemia	• Poor.	• This is very rare; morphology primarily involves differentiation to basophils.
Acute panmyelosis with myelofibrosis	• Very poor.	• This is very rare; it features de novo, acute panmyeloid proliferation with > 20% blasts and fibrosis.

Precursor Lymphoid Neoplasms: B-ALL and T-ALL

74. Describe the common features of specific subtypes of B-ALL with recurrent genetic abnormalities.[1]

SUBTYPE	PROGNOSIS	COMMENTS
B-ALL/LBL with t(9;22) (q34.1;q11.2); *BCR-ABL1*	• Poor.	• This is more common in adults (25% of adult ALL); it is usually +CD10/CD19/TdT and frequently shows myeloid associated CD13/CD33 expression; a minor breakpoint occurs in children (m-bcr) versus both major and minor breakpoints in adults (M-bcr & m-bcr); the treatment is TKI therapy.
B-ALL/LBL with t(v;11q23.3); *KMT2A*-rearranged	• Poor.	• This has bimodal peaks: it is the most common leukemia in infants and has a second peak in adulthood; CNS involvement is frequent; it has > 100 fusion partners.
B-ALL/LBL with t(12;21) (p13.2;q22.1); *ETV6-RUNX1*	• Very favorable.	• Common in childhood (25% of childhood ALL); excellent prognosis: > 90% cure rate in children with favorable risk factors.
B-ALL/LBL with hyperdiploidy	• Very favorable.	• This is common in childhood (25% of childhood ALL); it is defined by > 50 chromosomes; it has excellent prognosis with a > 90% cure rate in children; trisomies of chromosomes 4 and 10 carry the best prognosis.
B-ALL/LBL with hypodiploidy	• Poor.	• This is defined by < 46 chromosomes; worse prognosis is associated with near-haploid ALL (23–29 chromosomes).
B-ALL/LBL with t(5;14) (q31.1;q32.1); *IGH-IL3*	• Intermediate.	• This is rare; it is associated with peripheral eosinophilia (reactive, nonleukemic population).
B-ALL/LBL with t(1;19) (q23;p13.3); *TCF3-PBX1*	• Intermediate.	• This is relatively common in children (6%); it is characterized by blasts with pre-B phenotype (+CD19/CD10/cytoplasmic μ heavy chain and lack CD34 expression).
B-ALL/LBL, *BCR-ABL1*-like (provisional entity)	• Poor.	• This has a gene-expression profile similar to ALL with *BCR-ABL1*; it requires complex lab analysis to identify; several translocations are implicated (e.g., *CRLF2*); it features increased incidence with age (10–25% of ALL).
B-ALL/LBL with *iAMP21*	• Poor.	• This occurs in older children (2% of ALL); it involves amplification of a portion of chromosome 21; increased treatment intensity may improve outcome.

75. T-lymphoblastic leukemia/lymphoma often presents as a mediastinal mass. What is the differential diagnosis of this entity when it presents as a mediastinal mass?

- Thymic lesions (hyperplastic thymus, thymoma, or thymic carcinoma).
- Hodgkin lymphoma.
- Germ cell tumor.
- Metastases.
- Primary mediastinal large B-cell lymphoma.

Plasma Cell Neoplasms and Amyloidosis

76. List the types of plasma cell neoplasms.

- Plasma cell myeloma (PCM), known as multiple myeloma and its variants:
  · Smouldering (asymptomatic) PCM.
  · Nonsecretory myeloma.
  · Plasma cell leukemia.
- Plasmacytoma and its variants:
  · Solitary plasmacytoma of bone.
  · Extraosseous (extramedullary) plasmacytoma.
- Monoclonal immunoglobulin depositions diseases:
  · Primary amyloidosis.
  · Systemic light and heavy chain deposition diseases.
- Plasma cell neoplasms with associated paraneoplastic syndromes:
  · POEMS syndrome (**p**olyneuropathy, **o**rganomegaly, **e**ndocrinopathy, **m**onoclonal gammopathy, **s**kin changes).
  · TEMPI syndrome (provisional) (**t**elangiectasias, **e**levated erythropoietin and erythrocytosis, **m**onoclonal gammopathy, **p**erinephric fluid collection, **i**ntrapulmonary shunting).
- Non-IgM (plasma cell) monoclonal gammopathy of undetermined significance (MGUS).

77. What are the diagnostic criteria for plasma cell myeloma (PCM)?

- M protein in serum/urine (most cases > 30g/L IgG, or > 25g/L of IgA or > 1g/24 hours of urine light chain; some patients have less).
- Bone marrow clonal plasmacytosis (≥ 10%) OR biopsy-proven plasmacytoma.
- Also requires ≥ 1 myeloma defining event: end-organ damage OR ≥ 1 biomarker of malignancy.
- End organ damage (CRAB): hyper**c**alcemia, **r**enal insufficiency, **a**nemia, **b**one lesions (≥ 1 osteolytic lesions on X-ray or CT scan).
- Biomarkers of malignancy: BM clonal plasmacytosis (≥ 60%), serum free light chain ratio ≥ 100, or > 1 focal lesion on MRI.

78. List the factors causing kidney dysfunction in symptomatic PCM.

- Renal tubular reabsorption of nephrotoxic Bence Jones protein.
- Hypercalcemia.
- Hyperuricemia.
- Hyperviscosity.
- Recurrent bacterial infections and pyelonephritis.
- Extramedullary plasma cell infiltrates.
- Amyloid light chains.
- NSAIDs/cytotoxic medications.
- Contrast/radiographic studies.
- Myeloma cast nephropathy.

79. How is PCM staged?

STAGE	DURIE-SALMON SYSTEM[2]	REVISED INTERNATIONAL STAGING SYSTEM[3]
I	• All of the following:* · Hemoglobin: > 10g/dL. · Serum Ca: normal or < 10.5 mg/dL. · Bone x-ray: normal or solitary plasmacytoma. · M-component production rate: low (IgG < 5 g/dL; IgA < 3 g/dL). · Urine light chain M-component: < 4 g/24hrs.	• Serum albumin: > 3.5 g/dL. • Serum β_2-microglobulin: < 3.5 mg/L. • Cytogenetics: no high-risk features. • Serum LDH: normal.
II	• No fit with stage I or III.*	• No fit with stage I or III.
III	• At least 1 of:* · Hemoglobin: < 8.5 g/dL. · Serum Ca: > 12 mg/dL. · Advanced lytic bone lesions. · M-component production rate: high (IgG > 7 g/dL; IgA > 5 g/dL). · Urine light chain M-component: > 12 g/24hrs.	• Serum β_2-microglobulin: > 5.5 mg/L. • **And** 1 of the following: · High-risk cytogenetics: t(4;14), t(14;16), del(17p). · Elevated serum LDH.

Abbreviations: LDH: lactate dehydrogenase; M-component: monoclonal component.
*Subclassifications include: A: normal renal function (serum creatinine < 2.0 mg/dL; B: abnormal renal function (serum creatinine > 2.0 mg/dL).

80. According to the International Myeloma Working Group, what are recommended baseline genetic tests for PCM?[4]

CATEGORY	STANDARD RISK (60%)	INTERMEDIATE RISK (20%)	HIGH RISK (20%)
Cytogenetics	• t(11;14). • t(6;14). • Hyperdiploid. • All others.	• t(4;14). • Del 13. • Hypodiploid.	• Del 17p. • t(14;16). • t(14;20). • GEP — high risk.

81. What are the cytogenetic risk groups of PCM?

Unfavorable	• Aneuploid or hypodiploid karyotype. • −13 or del(13q). • t(4;14)(p16;q32). • t(14;16)(q32;q23). • del(17p13).
Favorable	• Hyperdiploid karyotype. • t(11;14)(q13;q32).

82. What is the definition of amyloid? Name 2 major subgroups and subtypes of amyloidosis.[5]

- Amyloid: a β-pleated sheet deposited in vivo and appearing as amorphous eosinophilic material (H&E stain) and fibrillar material (electron microscopy).

- Systemic amyloidosis is categorized into 2 major subgroups: primary systemic amyloidosis (AL type; amyloid light chain) and secondary system amyloidosis (non-AL types; other amyloid associated proteins).

TYPE (HUMAN AMYLOIDOSIS)	TYPE OF AMYLOID PROTEIN	MAIN CLINICAL SETTINGS
Systemic	• Immunoglobulin light chains.	• Plasma cell disorders.
	• Transthyretin.	• Familial amyloidosis, senile cardiac amyloidosis.
	• A amyloidosis.	• Inflammation associated amyloidosis, familial Mediterranean fever.
	• β_2-microglobulin.	• Dialysis-associated amyloidosis.
	• Immunoglobulin heavy chains.	• Systemic amyloidosis.
Hereditary	• Fibrinogen alpha chain.	• Familial systemic amyloidosis.
	• Apolipoprotein AI.	• Familial systemic amyloidosis.
	• Apolipoprotein AII.	• Familial systemic amyloidosis.
	• Lysozyme.	• Familial systemic amyloidosis.
Central nervous system	• Beta protein precursor.	• Alzheimer disease, Down syndrome, hereditary cerebral hemorrhage with amyloidosis (Dutch).
	• Prion protein.	• Creutzfeldt-Jakob disease, Gerstmann-Sträussler-Scheinker disease, fatal familial insomnia, kuru.
	• Cystatin C.	• Hereditary cerebral hemorrhage with amyloidosis (Icelandic).
	• ABri precursor protein.	• Familial dementia (British).
	• ADan precursor protein.	• Familial dementia (Danish).
Ocular	• Gelsolin.	• Familial amyloidosis (Finnish).
	• Lactoferrin.	• Familial corneal amyloidosis.
	• Keratoepithelin.	• Familial corneal dystrophies.
Localized	• Calcitonin.	• Medullary thyroid carcinoma.
	• Amylin (islet amyloid polypeptide amyloidosis).	• Insulinoma, type 2 diabetes.
	• Atrial natriuretic factor amyloidosis.	• Isolated atrial amyloidosis.
	• Prolactin.	• Pituitary amyloid.
	• Keratin.	• Cutaneous amyloidosis.
	• Medin.	• Aortic amyloidosis in elderly people.

Mature B-Cell Neoplasms

Also see lymph node pathology.

83. Describe the clinicopathological features of chronic lymphocytic leukemia/small lymphocytic lymphoma (CLL/SLL).

- CLL is the most common mature B-cell lymphoma, presenting with leukemic phase.
- Affected patients are often middle-aged or elderly men.
- Almost all patients have blood and bone marrow involvement.
- Patients are often asymptomatic and detected incidentally on complete blood counts (lymphocytosis of $\geq 5.0 \times 10^9$/L).

- Flow cytometry shows monotypic CD5+ B cells with dim surface immunoglobulin (IgM/IgD), negative for CD10 and FMC7.
- SLL is the extramedullary variant of CLL, which is less common and may present with lymphadenopathy and splenomegaly.

84. Describe the clinicopathological features of hairy cell leukemia (HCL).

- HCL is a red pulp disease that presents with massive splenomegaly.

- Most patients are men (20–80 years old).

(continued on next page)

- Patients have excellent prognosis with appropriate treatment.
- The most common presentation is pancytopenia (50%) and dry tap due to marrow fibrosis (30–50%).
- Features of HCL include:
  · Medium-size lymphoid cells with hairy cytoplasmic projections in peripheral blood.

- Atypical lymphoid cells of HCL with diffuse marrow involvement displaying honeycomb pattern.
- CD20 positive B cells, coexpressing CD103 and CD25 by flow cytometry.
- Nearly all classic HCL cases have *BRAF* V600E mutation.

85. Describe the clinicopathological features of HCL-variant.

- Patients present with lymphocytosis composed of medium size cells displaying prominent nucleoli and blastic/convoluted nuclei.
- By flow cytometry, cells are positive for CD103 but negative for CD25.
- Tartrate resistant acid phosphatase (TRAP) special stain and annexin A1 by IHC are negative.

- Patients are resistant to conventional chemo and interferon.
- Patients are often men with massive splenomegaly and marked lymphocytosis.
- At onset, the disease features a lack of neutropenia and monocytopenia.

86. Describe the clinicopathological features of lymphoplasmacytic lymphoma (LPL).

- LPL is a low grade B-cell lymphoma with primary involvement of bone marrow (80% of cases).
- Most patients present with monoclonal serum IgM gammopathy and Waldenstrom macroglobulinemia with hyperviscosity, coagulopathy, or cryoglobulinemia.
- LPL features bone-marrow-infiltrated small lymphoid cells showing plasmacytoid or plasma cell differentiation.
- Flow cytometry reveals monotypic B cells with concurrent monotypic plasma cells (CD5/CD10 negative).

- Some patients (30%) have leukemia composed of lymphocytes and lymphoplasmacytoid cells.
- Neoplastic lymphoid/lymphoplasmacytoid B cells may display cytoplasmic Russell and nuclear Dutcher bodies.
- More than 90% of LPL cases have the *MYD88 L265P* mutation.
- LPL may have poorer prognosis than other small B-cell lymphomas.

Lymph Node Pathology
Lymphoma Protocol and Ancillary Studies

87. What types of fixatives are used in handling lymphoma specimens and what are their advantages and disadvantages?

- Zinc formalin or B5 produces superior cytologic detail but is not suitable for DNA extraction and may impair some immunostains (e.g., CD30). B5 requires hazardous materials disposal.
- Formalin fixation is preferable when the tissue sample is limited, as it is most suitable for IHC and many other ancillary tests, such as molecular/genetic studies and in situ hybridization.
- Overfixation (≥ 24 hours in formalin and ≥ 4 hours in zinc formalin or B5) affects immunophenotypic reactivity, and recovery of RNA and phosphoproteins from fixed tissues. Record fixation time.

88. How should you section a lymph node for lymphoma protocol?

Serial sectioning at 2 mm intervals perpendicular to the long axis of the lymph node.

89. How should you handle a specimen for lymphoma protocol?

- Make sure tissue is received fresh.
- Record size, color, consistency, nodularity.
- Consider making touch imprints for cytogenetics.
- Consider snap freezing a portion of tissue for DNA or RNA extraction.

- Submit a portion of tissue in RPMI for flow cytometry.
- Snap freeze a portion of tissue for DNA or RNA extraction.
- Put the remainder of the tissue in fixative such as zinc formalin, B5, or formalin; specify which fixative is used.
- Consider a fresh portion of tissue for culture if needed.

90. Compare the advantages and disadvantages of the 2 methods of immunophenotyping: flow cytometry and IHC.

- Flow cytometry:
  · Is rapid (hours).
  · Is quantitative.

  · Allows multiple antigens to be evaluated on the same cell simultaneously.
  · Detects minimal residual disease.
  · Cannot correlate antigen reactivity with architecture or cytological features.

(continued on next page)

- IHC:
  - Requires hours/days to perform.
  - Provides only subjective quantitation.
- Allows correlation of antigen expression with architecture and cytology.
- Provides targeted therapy-related biomarkers: CD20 (rituximab) and CD30 (brentuximab).

91. What are recommended as elements to report for biopsy/resection specimens?
- Specimen type.
- Procedure type.
- Specimen/tumor site.
- Synoptic reports recommended by professional working groups (e.g., CAP).
- Cytogenetic (karyotyping and FISH) and molecular studies (PCR and next-generation sequencing).
- Clinical, histological, and immunophenotypic prognostic factors and indices.

92. What are some of the uses of molecular studies in hematopoietic neoplasms?
- Establishing clonality.
- Determining lineage.
- Establishing the diagnosis of specific disease entities.
- Monitoring minimal residual disease.
- Providing prognostication markers.
- Identifying predictive markers.
- Identifying actionable targeted therapies.

93. List cytogenetic aberrations that are detectable on FISH and that may assist in B-cell lymphoma subclassification and/or prognosis.
- Follicular lymphoma:
  - t(14;18)(q32;q21).
  - 17p (p53 gene)—associated with transformation to diffuse large B-cell lymphoma (DLBCL).
  - Additional BCL6 and c-MYC gene aberrations resulting in poor prognosis ("double/triple hit" disease).
- MALT associated marginal zone lymphoma:
  - Trisomy of chromosome 3.
  - t(11;18)(q21;q21) or API2 gene/MALT gene rearrangements associated with resistance to Helicobacter pylori eradication therapy, but not associated with gastric MALT progression to diffuse large B-cell lymphoma.
- Splenic marginal zone lymphoma:
  - Loss of 7q21–32 (dysregulation of the CDK6 gene).
- Diffuse large B-cell lymphoma:
  - t(14;18)/BCL2 rearrangement (present in 20–30%).
  - Rearrangement of BCL6 gene (locus on 3q27).
  - Additional c-MYC aberrations resulting in poor prognosis ("double/triple hit" disease).
- Primary mediastinal (thymic) large B-cell lymphoma:
  - Hyperdiploidy.
  - Mutations of BCL6 gene.
- Gain of chromosome 9q, 12q and Xq.
- REL protooncogene amplification.
- Burkitt lymphoma:
  - Rearrangements of c-MYC with t(8;14) or variant translocations involving loci on chromosome 2p12 or 22q11.2.
  - 17p mutations (TP53).
  - Clonal Epstein-Barr virus (EBV) genome in tumor cells.
- Chronic lymphocytic leukemia/small lymphocytic lymphoma:
  - TP53 and IGHV somatic hypermutation.
- Lymphoplasmacytic lymphoma (LPL)/Waldenstrom macroglobulinemia (WM):
  - MYD88 L265P mutation (90% of cases).
  - CXCR4 mutations (30%).
- Mantle cell lymphoma:
  - t(11;14)(q13;q32) with IGH-CCND1 leading to cyclin D1 overexpression (>95% cases).
  - Tetraploidy (in 80% of pleomorphic and 36% of blastoid variants).
  - Cyclin D1-negative mantle cell lymphoma (MCL): SOX11 expression, may have CCND2 translocation.
  - Mutations of ATM gene (ataxia telangiectasia gene).

Note: many of the aberrations listed above are not specific to 1 lymphoma type.

Reactive Lymphadenitis

94. What are the 4 basic architectural patterns of chronic nonspecific lymphadenitis/lymphadenopathy? List distinct clinicopathological conditions associated with each pattern.
- Follicular hyperplasia.
  - Rheumatoid arthritis.
  - Systemic lupus erythematosus.
  - Toxoplasmosis.
  - Early HIV infection.
- Sinus pattern.
  - Sinus histiocytosis with massive lymphadenopathy (Rosai-Dorfman disease).
- Local drainage of areas affected by cancer.
- Paracortical hyperplasia.
  - Dermatopathic lymphadenopathy.
  - Infectious mononucleosis.
- Mixed pattern.
  - Chronic/late HIV infection.

95. Dermatopathic lymphadenitis is a common nodal reaction pattern. What are the morphological and IHC features of this specific lymph node reaction pattern?

- It is common in lymph nodes draining areas affected by cutaneous irritation or underlying skin disease (i.e., exfoliative dermatitis).
- The macronodules in the paracortical T-zone are best observed on low power.
- It has a mottled appearance.

- It has a pleomorphic infiltrate, which is composed of:
  - S100+ interdigitating dendritic cells.
  - CD1a+ Langerhans cells.
  - CD68+ macrophages laden with pigment (melanin or hemosiderin).

96. Sinus histiocytosis with massive lymphadenopathy (SHML), known as Rosai-Dorfman disease, is a spontaneously remitting condition of unknown etiology. What are the morphological features of this entity?

- Nodal enlargement (common) or extranodal mass (rare).
- Exuberant expansion of sinuses.
- Sinuses filled with S100/CD68/CD4 positive histiocytes lacking CD1a.

- Emperipolesis.
- Polyclonal plasmacytosis in the medulla and association with IgG4.

97. What is the definition of emperipolesis?

Emperipolesis: a process of engulfment of viable/intact cells into the intracytoplasmic vacuoles, which protect the engulfed cells from enzymatic degradation (usually lymphocytes taken by histiocytes).

98. Toxoplasmosis lymphadenitis affects predominantly a solitary cervical lymph node and is caused by protozoan *Toxoplasma gondii* infection of the immunocompetent host. What is the characteristic histologic triad associated with toxoplasmosis lymphadenopathy?

- Background of florid follicular hyperplasia.
- Monocytoid B-cell hyperplasia in subcapsular/trabecular sinuses.

- Presence of clusters of epithelioid histiocytes (microgranuloma) at margins and within reactive germinal centers.
- "Moth eaten" borders at periphery of germinal centers that contain many tingible body macrophages.

99. *Bartonella henselae* is the causative bacillus of catscratch disease. What are the morphological features of this nodal infection?

- Background of follicular hyperplasia and monocytoid B cell reaction.
- Stellate microabscesses/granulomas surrounded by palisading macrophages, forming suppurative/caseous granulomatous lesions.

- Areas of necrosis with neutrophils, which may appear caseous.

Note: *Bartonella henselae* may be present in the vessel walls and/or areas of necrosis and can be detected with Warthin-Starry silver stain.

100. Define Kikuchi lymphadenitis.

Kikuchi lymphadenitis: a self-limited and spontaneously regressing granulomatous/histiocytic necrotizing lymphadenitis commonly affecting young adults, particularly young women from East Asia.

101. What are the morphological features of the necrotizing type of Kikuchi lymphadenitis?

- Morphological changes similar to the pattern of lupus lymphadenitis.
- Patchy areas of paracortical necrosis with karyorrhectic debris devoid of neutrophils.
- Aggregates of MPO+/CD68+/lysozyme+ histiocytes with characteristic crescentic nuclei.

- Paracortical expansion by CD8 positive T lymphocytes and immunoblasts.
- Paucity of CD20+ lymphocytes.
- Increased numbers of CD68/CD4/CD123/CD4/CD43 plasmacytoid dendritic cells.

102. What are the salient diagnostic features that may indicate the presence of syphilis related (luetic) lymphadenitis?

- Extensive follicular hyperplasia.
- Lymphoplasmacytic periarteritis and arteritis obliterans.
- Epithelioid granulomas and rare giant cells.
- Thickened capsule.
- Prominent vessels in interfollicular areas.

- Extensive plasmacytosis in interfollicular areas.
- Spirochetes (*T. pallidum*): observable with silver impregnation stain (Warthin-Starry stain) or dark field/immunofluorescence techniques.

103. What are the morphological and immunophenotypic features of acute lymphadenitis caused by EBV?

- Expanded lymph node paracortex by a heterogenous population of immunoblasts, centroblasts, and plasma cells.
- Immunoblastic reaction that may be florid, creating a "moth eaten" pattern.
- Numerous immunoblasts highlighted by CD30 immunostain.
- Abundance of background CD3/CD8+ cytotoxic T cells.

104. In the context of congenital or acquired immunodeficiency, what human viruses of the Herpesviridae family, other than EBV, may cause distinctive lymph node reaction patterns?

- Human herpesvirus type 1(HHV-1) and type 2 (HHV-2), resulting in herpes simplex virus lymphadenitis.
- Cytomegalovirus (HHV-5), resulting in CMV lymphadenitis.
- Kaposi sarcoma virus (HHV-8), resulting in Castleman lymphadenopathy, plasma cell variant.
- Varicella herpes zoster (HHV-3), resulting in varicella-herpes zoster lymphadenitis.

105. Lymphadenopathy may be part of the clinical presentation of HIV/AIDS. What are the 3 distinct patterns of HIV lymphadenitis that also correspond to clinical stages of HIV infection/immunosuppression?

- The type 1 pattern features follicular and paracortical hyperplasia, and is associated with chronic lymphadenopathy.
- The type 2 pattern, which shows diffuse lymphoid hyperplasia but loss of germinal centers, signifies evolution of chronic lymphadenopathy to AIDS.
- The type 3 pattern shows marked lymphocytic depletion and represents the end-stage lymph node seen in fatal AIDS.

106. What are the morphological features that may suggest the presence of the acute phase of HIV related lymphadenopathy?

- Florid follicular hyperplasia.
- Expanded, large, and irregularly shaped germinal centers.
- Attenuated mantle zones resulting in "naked germinal centers" and folliculolysis.
- Aggregates of plasma cells, macrophages, monocytoid B cells, and immunoblasts in interfollicular areas with occasional:
  · Warthin-Finkeldey–type multinucleate giant cells.
  · Neutrophil infiltration in sinuses.

107. What are the morphological features diagnostic of progressive transformation of germinal centers (PTGC)?

- Retained nodal architecture with a background of follicular hyperplasia.
- Well-demarcated macronodular structures with regressed germinal centers.
- Intact interfollicular areas.
- Poorly defined but expanded mantle zones, infiltrating into germinal centers by IgM/IgD positive naive mantle B cells.
- Possible collections of epithelioid histiocytes surrounding the PTGC macronodules.
- Absence of lymphocyte predominant cells (LP cells, previously called L&H cells) cells of nodular lymphocyte predominant Hodgkin lymphoma.

108. What are the clinicopathological variants of Castleman lymphadenopathy?

- Hyaline vascular variant.
  · Unicentric/localized.
- Plasma-cell variant.
- · Unicentric/localized.
- · Multicentric.

109. What are the salient features of the hyaline vascular type of Castleman lymphadenopathy?

- Atrophic appearing and lymphocyte depleted germinal centers often with hyaline deposits.
- Mantle zone hyperplasia featuring concentric layers forming "onionskin/target" lesions.
- Prominent interfollicular vascularity.
- Vessels penetrating into germinal centers forming "lollipop" lesions.
- Lymphocyte depleted germinal centers containing mostly CD21/CD23/CD35 positive follicular dendritic cells.
- Collections of CD123 positive plasmacytoid dendritic cells in the interfollicular areas.

110. Describe genetic abnormalities and the pathogenesis of autoimmune lymphoproliferative syndrome (ALPS).

- ALPS is an autosomal dominant immune regulation immunodeficiency disorder, with variable genotype/penetrance, resulting in variable onset (birth to late teens), and variable clinical presentation and severity.
- There are 5 genetic types, which are most often autosomal dominant:
- · ALPS-FAS (*FAS* gene; 65% cases).
- · ALPS-sFAS (somatic *FAS* mutations).
- · ALPS-FASLG (germline mutations of *FASL*).
- · ALPS-CASP10 (germline mutations of *CASP10* gene).
- · ALPS-U (unknown defects; 25% cases).

111. What are the clinical and morphologic/phenotypic features of ALPS?

- Clinical features:
  - Generalized lymphadenopathy.
  - Splenomegaly.
  - Hypergammaglobulinemia.
  - Autoimmune cytopenias.
  - Preponderance of bacterial infections.
  - Increased risk for lymphoma development, as in any case of congenital or acquired immunodeficiency.
- Morphologic/phenotypic features:
  - Paracortical hyperplasia.
  - Florid follicular hyperplasia.
- Presence of PTGC.
- Polyclonal plasmacytosis.
- Massive sinus histiocytosis resembling Rosai-Dorfman disease.
- Increased fraction of circulating naive and polytypic CD5+ B cells.
- Expansion of circulating naive CD45RA/HLA-DR+CD3/TCR α/β T cells lacking CD45RO/CD4/D8 expression ("double negative T cells") and exhibiting expression of cytotoxic antigens (i.e., perforin, TIA/CD57).
- Defective apoptotic in vitro assays.

112. Lymphoproliferative disorders are more common in immunocompromised individuals. Name at least 3 clinical conditions that may result in impaired immune function.

- Congenital immunodeficiency disorders:
  - Cellular type.
  - Humoral type.
  - Combined type.
- Chronic viral infections, including HIV, HHV-8, and human T-cell lymphotrophic virus.
- Iatrogenic and immunosuppressive therapy:
  - Post bone marrow transplant.
  - Post solid organ transplant.
  - Treatment of autoimmune conditions—rheumatoid arthritis, systemic lupus erythematosus.
- Autoimmune disorders—Sjögren syndrome, Hashimoto thyroiditis, ulcerative colitis, Crohn disease.

Mature Non-Hodgkin B-Cell Lymphoma

113. The notion that a majority of lymphoid neoplasms result from autonomous expansion of a clone, which represents a putative stage of B cell or T/NK cell differentiation, is the basis of the WHO classification of hematopoietic and lymphoid tissues. What are the 5 broad categories of lymphoid neoplasms in that classification?

- Precursor B-cell neoplasms; neoplasms of B lymphoblasts (B-ALL).
- Precursor T-cell neoplasms; neoplasms of T lymphoblasts (T-ALL).
- Mature B-cell lymphomas; neoplasms of mature B cells and plasma cells.
- Mature T-cell and NK-cell neoplasms; neoplasms of mature T/NK cells.
- Hodgkin lymphoma; B-cell neoplasms of altered germinal center B cells, which are incapable of immunoglobulin transcription and show markedly suppressed B cell programming.

114. In some clinical scenarios, fine needle aspiration (FNA) may be used in the diagnosis of malignant lymphoma. What are the cytomorphological features that suggest the presence of neoplastic lymphoid cells in FNA material?

- Abundant monomorphic lymphoid cells (large or small).
- Scanty cytoplasm.
- Coarsely clumped chromatin with conspicuous nucleoli (small cells).
- Distinct nuclear membrane.

115. In general, CLL/SLL has a slow progressive clinical course. However, some patients may undergo an abrupt clinical deterioration known as Richter transformation. What are the clinical features associated with this abrupt change?

- Marked increase in LDH.
- Sudden increase in lymphadenopathy or splenomegaly.
- Markedly worsening cytopenias and/or transfusion requirements.
- New and rapidly enlarging lymph node/splenic or extranodal mass.

116. Why do we perform molecular studies on CLL/SLL?

- For predicting the prognosis.
  - Patients with *IgVH* unmutated genes have a more aggressive disease and are more resistant to therapy than those with mutated *IgVH* genes.
  - Determining *IgVH* mutations requires specific equipment and is laborious, expensive, and time consuming.
  - Detection of immunoglobulin VH3–21 usage by sequencing of *IgH* rearrangements has been associated with poor outcomes in CLL and should be reported when detected by IgH sequencing.

117. List FISH testing of markers of CLL and their prognostic value.

MARKER POSITIVE BY FISH	APPROXIMATE FREQUENCY	PROGNOSIS	NOTES
Del 13q14	• 35–45%.	• Low risk.	
Trisomy 12	• 11–16%.	• Intermediate to high risk.	
Del 11q22–23 (*ATM: BIRC3*)	•	• Intermediate to high risk.	• Bulk disease, aggressive clinical course, shorter survival.
Del 17p (*TP53*)	• 3–7%.	• High risk.	• Frequently no response to therapy or relapse after therapy.
No abnormality		• Low to intermediate risk.	

118. Mantle cell lymphoma (MCL) is a clinically aggressive mature B-cell neoplasm commonly involving the gut (lymphomatous polyposis), spleen, Waldeyer ring, lymph nodes, and bone marrow. What are the morphological and immunohistochemical features that indicate a worse prognosis for patients with mantle cell lymphoma?

- Pleomorphic and blastoid morphological variants.
- Enhanced proliferation index (Ki 67 > 30%).

119. The presence of cyclin D1 and/or t(11;14) is not pathognomonic for MCL. List other B-cell neoplasms that rarely may be associated with this cytogenetic abnormality/cyclin D1 expression.

- Plasma cell neoplasm.
- Splenic marginal zone lymphoma (SMZL).
- HCL.
- B-cell prolymphocytic leukemia.

120. In a tabulated form, compare and contrast clinical, morphological, IHC, and genetic features of mature B-cell neoplasms that may present with splenomegaly: CLL/SLL, MCL, and HCL.

FEATURES	CLL/SLL	MCL	HCL
Clinical course	• Indolent disease.	• Aggressive.	• Indolent/curable.
Associated entities	• Persistent lymphocytosis.	• Rare lymphocytosis.	• Leukopenia/monocytopenia.
BM involvement	• Common.	• Sometimes present.	• Always present.
Lymphadenopathy	• Present.	• Present.	• Sometimes present (28%).
Histological	• Small lymphoid cells. • Proliferation centers. • Paraimmunoblasts.	• Notched lymphoid cells. • Patchy sclerosis. • Pink histiocytes.	• Bean shaped nuclei. • Cytoplasmic projections. • "Fried egg" appearance.
IHC	• Positive: CD20/CD5/bcl-2. • Variable: CD23/CD43. • Negative: Bcl-6/CD10. • Negative: cyclin D1. • Positive: LEF1 (92% specific, 70% sensitivity).	• Positive: CD20/CD5/bcl-2. • Variable: CD23/CD43. • Negative: Bcl-6/CD10. • Positive: cyclin D1 (95%). • Positive: SOX11 (90%).	• Positive: CD20/11C/CD103. • Positive: CD25/DBA.44/TRAP. • Negative: CD5/BCL6/CD10. • Positive: cyclinD1 (variable). • Positive: annexin A1.
Genetic	• t(11;14): negative. • del 13q(50%), trisomy 12 (20%).	• t(11;14): positive.	• t(11;14): negative. • *BRAF* V600E: mutated.

121. What differentiates SMZL from mucosa associated lymphoid tissue (MALT) lymphoma and nodal marginal zone lymphoma?

- Almost exclusive involvement of spleen, peripheral blood, and bone marrow.
- Characteristic intrasinusoidal bone marrow infiltrates.
- Association with hepatitis C infection.
- Presence of small serum monoclonal paraprotein—up to 28% of cases.
- Chromosome 7q21 deletion—reported to be present in up to 40% of cases and associated with a more aggressive course.
- Greater frequency of transformation to high grade lymphoma—13% of cases.
- Presence of villous lymphocytes in peripheral blood smear.
- Possibility of cure by splenectomy (some cases).

122. Other than SMZL, what hematolymphoid neoplasms may preferentially involve the spleen?

- HCL, classic and variant types.
- MCL.
- Splenic diffuse red pulp small B-cell lymphoma.
- Chronic myeloproliferative neoplasms—particularly chronic myelogenous leukemia.
- Hepatosplenic T-cell lymphoma.

123. MALT (specialized mucosa associated lymphoid tissue) protects permeable mucosal surfaces from external pathogens. What are the anatomic site-specific physiologic/native MALT formations?

- Gut associated Peyer patches.
- Waldeyer ring, including tonsils.
- Salivary and lacrimal glands.
- Thyroid.
- Respiratory tract.
- Genitourinary tract.
- Vermiform appendix.

124. T cell–mediated chronic antigenic stimulation of various infectious agents has been implicated in the development of extranodal marginal zone lymphoma of MALT, a finding that warrants antibiotic therapy in initial stages of the disease. Link commonly accepted associations of pathogens with distinct anatomic sites of MALT lymphomas.

- Skin associated MALT lymphoma: *Borrelia burgdorferi*.
- Gastric MALT lymphoma: *Helicobacter pylori*.
- Ocular adnexa MALT lymphoma: *Chlamydia psittaci*.
- Immunoproliferative small intestinal disease (IPSID): *Campylobacter jejuni*.

125. What are the clinical and morphological features of IPSID?

- Clinical:
  · It occurs in the Middle East and the cape region of South Africa.
  · It affects young adults.
  · It results in severe malabsorption.
  · *Campylobacter* species as *C. jejuni* or *C. coli* have been recently identified as a causative agents in some cases.
- It may respond to antibiotics: *Campylobacter* species have been identified as a causative agent in a subset of cases.
- Morphological:
  · It is a form of MALT associated neoplasm with prominent plasmacytoid differentiation.
  · It is associated with the production of truncated alpha heavy chains without light chains.

126. Describe the cytomorphological features of centrocytes (the predominant neoplastic cells of follicular lymphoma [FL]) and centroblasts (the neoplastic cells of DLBCL).

- A centrocyte is a small sized lymphoid cell also known as "small cleaved cell." It features:
  · Elongated and convoluted/irregular nuclear contours.
  · Indiscernible nucleoli.
  · Scanty cytoplasm.
- A centroblast is a large sized cell with a nucleus at least twice the size of the nucleus of a reactive lymphocyte/ histiocyte or an endothelial cell. It is also known as a "transformed cell" or "large noncleaved cell" ("blast" in European lymphoma nomenclature). It features:
  · Vesicular nuclear chromatin pattern.
  · Few inconspicuous and nuclear membrane bound nucleoli.
  · A rim of basophilic cytoplasm.

127. FL grading remains controversial and subjective. Currently, only 2 principal FL grades are recognized: FL grade 1–2/3 and FL grade 3/3. Describe guiding criteria for FL grading based on the WHO classification of hematopoietic and lymphoid tissues.

- FL grade 1–2/3 is defined as 1–15 centroblasts per unselected high power field (HPF).
- FL grade 3/3 is defined as > 15 centroblasts per unselected HPF.
- Subcategories of FL grade 3/3 include:
- Grade 3a/3: pleomorphic mix of small centrocytes accompanied by centroblasts > 15/HPF.
- Grade 3b/3: solid sheets of centroblasts within neoplastic follicles. This FL subtype is important to recognize, as it is regarded as a high grade B-cell lymphoma and treated similarly to DLBCL.

128. What are the morphological negative prognosticators in FL?

- Presence of diffuse areas with sheets of centroblasts (i.e., FL grade 3b/3).
- Blastic cytomorphology with high proliferative index.
- In addition to t(14;18), cytogenetic "hits," including:
  · Inactivation of *TP53*.
- Dysregulation of P38/MAPK on 3q27.
- Activation of *c-MYC/BCL6* genes (chromosome 3q27).
- Loss of BCL-2 protein and acquisition of MUM-1 expression (IHC).

129. FL is the most common form of indolent adult B-cell lymphoma in North America and Europe. What is the molecular hallmark of this entity and the pathogenesis underlying its progression to DLBCL?

- Molecular hallmark:
  · t(14;18)(q32;q21)—detectable in up to 90% of FL cases.
- Pathogenesis:
  · t(14;18) juxtaposes *IGH* gene with locus on chromosome 14 next to *BCL2* gene with locus on chromosome 18.
  · This fusion leads to overexpression of BCL-2 protein.
- BCL-2 protein disrupts the apoptosis pathway and leads to neoplastic transformation of the affected cell.
- Ongoing somatic mutations (e.g., inactivation of *TP53/CDKN2A*, activation of *MYC/BCL6*) have been associated with transformation to DLBCL.

130. What is the Follicular Lymphoma International Prognostic Index (FLIPI)?

- FLIPI: evaluates 5 adverse prognostic risk factors, including:
  · Age (> 60 years versus ≤ 60 years).
  · Ann Arbor stage (III–IV versus I–II).
  · Hemoglobin level (< 120 g/L versus ≥ 120 g/L).
  · Number of nodal areas (> 4 versus ≤ 4).
  · Serum LDH level (above normal level versus normal or below).
- Patients are stratified into 3 risk groups:
  · Low risk (0–1 adverse factors), intermediate risk (2 adverse factors), and poor risk (≥ 3 adverse factors).

131. List the IHC stains that have a prognostic value in DLBCL and explain why.

- CD5: a small subset (5–10%) of DLBCL cases with coexpression of CD5 show more aggressive clinical course.
- c-MYC and BCL-2: in addition to patients with double/triple hit lymphoma, DLBCL cases with coexpression of c-MYC and BCL-2 immunostains (double expressors) show poor prognosis and a higher frequency of central nervous system involvement.

132. Why is it important to perform CD20 in DLBCL?

- The standard therapy for DLBCL patients is R-CHOP (rituximab, cyclophosphamide, doxorubicin, vincristine, and prednisone).
- Knowledge of CD20 expression provides justification for using rituximab.

133. Is there a difference between a germinal center derived DLBCL and a nongerminal center derived DLBCL?

In general, DLBCL of germinal center subtype is associated with a better prognosis. However, the majority of double hit, high grade B-cell lymphomas (HGBCL [85%]) demonstrate germinal center B-cell immunophenotype (GCB) (see Han's algorithm).

HAN'S ALGORITHM

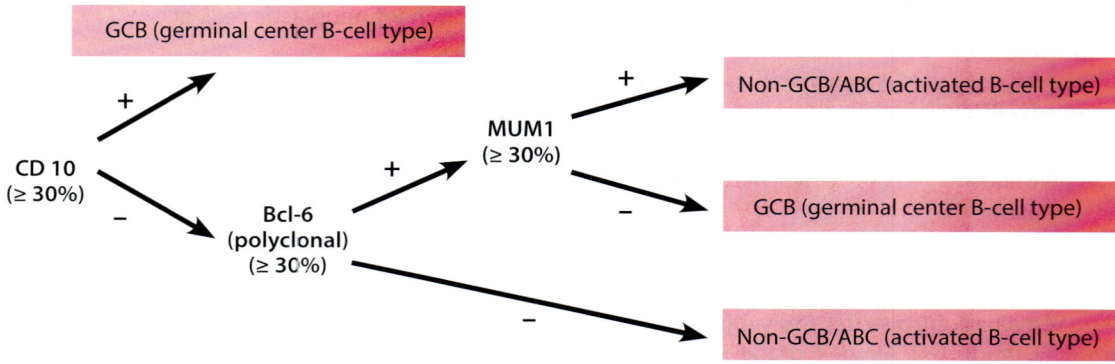

Adapted from Hans CP et al. Confirmation of the molecular classification of diffuse large B-cell lymphoma by immunohistochemistry using a tissue microarray. Blood. 2004;103(1):275–282.

134. DLBCL may present with some distinct features resulting in a unique clinical behavior. List at least 5 distinct clinicopathology subtypes of DLBCL as recognized by the WHO classification:

- Primary mediastinal (thymic) large B-cell lymphoma.
- Primary effusion lymphoma.
- Primary cutaneous large B-cell lymphoma.
- Intravascular large B-cell lymphoma.
- T cell/histiocyte rich large B-cell lymphoma.
- Primary DLBCL of the central nervous system (CNS).
- Cutaneous diffuse large B-cell lymphoma, leg type.
- EBV positive DLBCL, not otherwise specified (NOS).
- Lymphomatoid granulomatosis (LyG).
- DLBCL associated with chronic inflammation.
- ALK positive large B-cell lymphoma.
- Plasmablastic lymphoma.
- HHV-8+ DLBCL, NOS.

135. Why is it important to perform CD30 in DLBCL?

- CD30 assessment is recommended because of the potential utility of the anti-CD30 antibody drug conjugate brentuximab vedotin.
- Approximately 10–15% of DLBCL cases express CD30, and these patients may be eligible for this agent if they fail standard therapy.
- Expression of CD30 is commonly associated with EBV positive lymphomas.

136. Describe the unique clinical and genotypic/viral characteristics of the endemic (African) variant of Burkitt lymphoma.

- Clinical characteristics:
  - Affects children in sub-Saharan Africa.
  - Presents as rapidly enlarging mass with predilection for mandible, kidneys, ovaries, and adrenal glands.
  - Rarely involves peripheral blood and bone marrow.
- Genotypic/EBER characteristics:
  - The molecular characteristic of this tumor is a sole reciprocal translocation: t(8;14), t(8;22), or t(2;8).
  - Any of these translocations reposition the *c-MYC* gene from its locus on chromosome 8 next to the Ig promoter/enhancer sequences, resulting in *c-MYC* overexpression leading to tumorigenesis.
  - The break in the *IgH* locus is usually within the class switch regions.
  - The presence of *c-MYC* rearrangement/overexpression results in cells autonomously dividing and being in perpetual cell cycle.
  - Nearly all endemic Burkitt lymphomas show evidence of individually unique and clonal presence of EBV DNA.

137. Since the clinical approach to high grade lymphoma differs depending on tumor subclassification, compare the salient clinical, morphological, IHC, and molecular features associated with the following: DLBCL, HGBCL, and Burkitt lymphoma (BL).

FEATURES	DLBCL	HGBCL	BL
Clinical	• Any age. • Nodal mass. • IPI index. • De novo or secondary. • EBV < 10%.	• Any age. • Nodal/extranodal. • Aggressive. • De novo or secondary. • Variable.	• Children/young. • Often extranodal. • Limited stage. • Rarely leukemic involvement. • Endemic (100% EBV)/Sporadic (< 30% EBV).
Morphological	• Centroblastic/immunoblastic.	• Intermediate size. • Starry sky.	• Intermediate size. • Starry sky.
IHC			
CD20/cCD79a	• Positive.	• Positive.	• Positive.
CD10	• Variable.	• Positive.	• Positive.
BCL-2	• Variable.	• Variable.	• Negative.
Bcl-6	• Variable.	• Positive.	• Positive.
Ki 67	• Variable.	• High.	• Near 100%.
MOLECULAR/GENETIC			
c-MYC	• 5–8%.	• 35–50%.	• > 95%; (8;22), t(2;8) or t(14;22).
BCL-2 [t(14;18)]	• 20–30%.	• 15%.	• Absent.
Bcl-6	• Up to 70%.	• 10%.	• Absent.
Complex	• Possible.	• Double/triple hit.	• Absent.

Staging and Prognostic Indicators of Non-Hodgkin B-Cell Lymphoma

138. What factors are used to determine treatment in adult patients with lymphoma?

- Histologic type.
- Stage of the disease.
- The International Prognostic Index score (IPI score).

139. What is the IPI score for DLBCL?

- The score represents the 5 pretreatment characteristics that have been shown to be independently statistically significant:
  - Age in years (≤ 60 versus > 60).
  - Tumor stage I or II (localized) versus III or IV (advanced).
  - Number of extranodal sites of involvement (0 or 1 versus > 1).
  - Patient's performance status (0 or 1 versus 2–4).
  - Serum LDH (normal versus abnormal).
- Based on the number of risk factors, patients can be assigned to 1 of 4 risks groups: low (0 or 1), low intermediate (2), high intermediate (3), or high (4 or 5).
- A revised IPI (R-IPI) has been proposed for patients with diffuse large B-cell lymphoma who are treated with rituximab plus CHOP chemotherapy.

140. What are the clinical findings that have prognostic value in Hodgkin and non-Hodgkin lymphoma?

- B symptoms, which include:
  - Fever (> 38°C).
  - Unexplained weight loss (> 10% body weight) in the 6 months before diagnosis.
- Drenching night sweats.
- Note that the stage and bulk of disease does not correlate with prognosis, but has treatment implications.

141. What are other factors that have prognostic value for lymphoma?

- HIV status.
- BCL-2 expression.
- Serum interleukin-10 (IL-10) levels before treatment.
- DLBCL-specific factors:
  - Tumor bulk (masses ≥ 10 cm).
- Male sex.
- Vitamin D deficiency.
- Concordant bone marrow involvement.
- Low absolute lymphocyte/monocyte count.

Hodgkin Lymphoma

142. Group and name 5 distinct subtypes of Hodgkin lymphoma, according to the 2017 WHO classification of hematopoietic and lymphoid tissues.

- Nodular lymphocyte predominant Hodgkin lymphoma (NLPHL).
- Classic Hodgkin lymphoma (CHL):
  - Nodular sclerosis Hodgkin lymphoma (NS).
- Lymphocyte rich classical Hodgkin lymphoma (LR).
- Mixed cellularity Hodgkin lymphoma (MC).
- Lymphocyte depleted Hodgkin lymphoma (LD).

143. What is the immunophenotype of Reed-Sternberg (RS) cells in CHL?

- RS cells in all subtypes of CHL (NS, LR, MC, and LD) show similar classical immunophenotype:
  - Positive for CD30.
- Negative for CD45, EMA.
- +/−: CD15+/−, PAX5+/−, CD20−/+, CD79a−/+, EBER−/+.

144. Describe the characteristic disease distribution in different types of Hodgkin lymphoma.

- NLPHL: usually presents with isolated lymphadenopathy of long duration; involves cervical and axillary nodes; commonly involves liver and spleen in high stage disease.
- NS type: occurs above the diaphragm in the lower cervical, supraclavicular and mediastinal nodes; develops into bulky mediastinal disease in 50% of cases.
- MC type: usually occurs below or on both sides of the diaphragm; involves the spleen in 30% of cases and bone marrow in 10%.
- LRCHL: is similar to NLPHL; presents as stage I and II in 70% of cases; does not usually develop into bulky disease.
- LD type: is not well described; usually presents in elderly patients with higher stage disease; involves abdominal organs and bone marrow.

145. What are common sites for Hodgkin lymphoma?

- Hodgkin lymphoma is nearly always nodal based with cervical lymph nodes more commonly involved.
- Other sites include mediastinal, axillary, and para-aortic lymph nodes.
- Extranodal Hodgkin lymphoma is rare.
- Anatomic distribution varies on type.

146. What is the immunophenotype of lymphocyte predominant cells (LP cells; previously called L&H cells) in nodular lymphocyte predominant Hodgkin lymphoma?

- Positive for CD20, CD79a, PAX5, CD45, Bcl-6.
- OCT-2+ and BOB-1+ (only 1 of 2 is positive in RS cells of classical Hodgkin lymphoma).
- Negative for CD15, CD30, CD43, EBER.
- CD3/CD57/PD1-positive T cells surround LP cells (T cell "rosettes").
- EMA +/−.

147. Compare morphological, IHC, and molecular features that distinguish CHL from NLPHL.

FEATURES	CHL	NLPHL
Morphologic	• Macronodules. • Fibrotic bands. • Pleomorphic background: lymphocytes, eosinophils, epithelioid histiocytes. • Mononucleate or binucleate Reed-Sternberg cells with conspicuous nucleoli.	• Macronodules. • No fibrosis. • Monotonous background of small lymphocytes. • Polylobated LP cells with inconspicuous nucleoli.
IHC (neoplastic cells)	• Positive: CD30/CD15/PAX5/MUM-1. • Variably positive: CD20/EBER. • Mostly negative: OCT1/OCT2/BOB1. • Negative: CD45/CD3.	• Positive: CD45/CD20/PAX5/MUM-1. • Variably positive: EMA. • Positive: OCT1/OCT2/BOB1. • Negative: CD15/CD30/CD3.
Molecular	• EBER: variably positive. • *IgH/TCR*: negative.	• EBER: negative (> 95%). • *IgH*: may be positive.

148. What is the International Prognostic Score and what are the factors used to predict outcome?

- The International Prognostic Score (IPS) was developed for Hodgkin lymphoma to predict outcome based on the following adverse factors:
  · Serum albumin < 4g/dL.
  · Hemoglobin concentration < 10.5 g/dL.
  · Male sex.
  · Age ≥ 45 years.
- · Stage IV disease.
- · WBC count ≥ 15,000/mm^3.
- · Lymphopenia < 600/mm^3 or < 8%.
- The rate of freedom from progression by risk category is 0 factors 84%, 1 factor 77%, 2 factors 67%, 3 factors 60%, 4 factors 51%, and ≥ 5 factors 42%.

149. Describe the Cotswold revision of the Ann Arbor staging classification of Hodgkin lymphomas.

- Stage I: involvement of a single lymph node region (I), or lymphoid structure (e.g., spleen, thymus, Waldeyer ring).
- Stage II: involvement of 2 or more lymph node regions on the same side of the diaphragm (II) (the mediastinum is considered a single site).
- Stage III: involvement of lymph node regions on both sides of the diaphragm (III), which may be accompanied by extralymphatic extension in association with lymph node involvement (IIIE) or splenic involvement (IIIS).
- Stage IV: involvement of extranodal site(s) beyond those designated E.

Mature T-Cell and NK-Cell Neoplasms

150. The putative cell of origin of angioimmunoblastic T-cell lymphoma (AITL) is a follicular helper type T cell (T FH). What are the clinical and morphological/molecular features of this T-cell neoplasm?

- Clinical features:
  · Fever.
  · Weight loss.
  · Skin rash.
  · Polyclonal hypergammaglobulinemia.
  · Autoimmune hemolytic anemia/circulating immune complexes.
  · Increased susceptibility to infections.
  · Diffuse lymphadenopathy.
  · Hepatosplenomegaly.
  · Profound immunodeficiency.
- Morphological/molecular features:
- · Effaced nodal architecture with pleomorphic background of lymphocytes, plasma cells, eosinophils, and immunoblasts.
- · Characteristic sparing of subcapsular sinuses.
- · Prominent vascularity with arborizing vessels.
- · Extrafollicular proliferation of CD21/CD23 positive follicular dendritic cells.
- · Scattered neoplastic T cells with clear cytoplasm expressing T FH phenotype CD3/CD4/Bcl-6/PD1/CXCL 13.
- · Coexistent proliferation of CD20 positive B immunoblasts.
- · EBER expression in majority of cases.
- · Cytogenetics: trisomy of chromosomes +3, +5, +X.
- · Clonal rearrangements of *TCR* (75–90% of cases) and *IgH* (25–30% of cases).

151. What are the clinical, morphological, immunohistochemical, and cytogenetic features of systemic/nodal anaplastic large cell lymphoma (ALCL)?

- Clinical features:
  - More commonly occurs in young adults.
  - Presents at nodal and extranodal sites (skin, bone, lung, liver) with advanced stage disease.
  - Is clinically aggressive, but responds well to multiagent chemotherapy.
- Morphological features:
  - Cohesive and sinusoidal type proliferation of neoplastic T/null cells.
  - Subcapsular and sinusoidal involvement.
  - Presence of "hallmark" cells: poly obated wreath-like or doughnut shaped, large sized neoplastic cells with multiple conspicuous nucleoli.

- Note: morphological variants exist (classic/common, small cell, Hodgkin-like, lymphohistiocytic, sarcomatous).
- Immunohistochemical/cytogenetic features:
  - CD30/EMA positive "hallmark" cells with variable expression of CD45/CD3/CD2/CD4/CD43/ALK-1/TIA-1; neoplastic cells are usually positive for granzyme B and perforin, and negative for EBV-EBER.
  - Constitutive activation of a chimeric tyrosine kinase from reciprocal t(2;5)9p23;q35) involving *ALK/NPM* gene.
  - Other variant translocations: t(1;2)(q25;p23), t(2;3) (p23;q35), inv(2)(p23;q35), t(2;17)(p23;q11).
  - Note: ALK-1 expression may be cytoplasmic, nuclear, or nucleolar depending on type of reciprocal translocation.

152. List the clinically significant extranodal T-cell lymphoma subtypes with characteristic immunophenotypic markers.

- Extranodal NK/T-cell lymphoma (sCD3–/cCD3+/CD56+/EBV+).
- Enteropathy-associated T-cell lymphoma (CD3+/CD4–/CD8–/CD5–/CD56+).
- Nodal peripheral T-cell lymphoma with TFH phenotype (PTCL-TFH) defined by the expression of at least 2 or 3 TFH markers (CD10, BCL6, PD-1, CXCL13, and ICOS).
- Hepatosplenic T-cell lymphoma (CD3+/CD56+/–/TIA1+).
- Cutaneous T-cell lymphomas:

- Mycosis fungoides (CD4+ T cells with loss of CD5/7).
- Subcutaneous panniculitis-like T-cell lymphoma (CD8+/granzymeB+/perforin+/CD56–).
- Primary cutaneous CD4 positive small/medium T-cell lymphoproliferative disorder.
- Primary cutaneous CD30 positive T-cell lymphoproliferative disorder (CD30+/EMA+ but ALK–).
- Lymphomatoid papulosis.
- Primary cutaneous anaplastic large cell lymphoma.

Immune Deficiency Associated Lymphoproliferative Disorder (PTLD)

153. Describe the clinicopathological features of posttransplant lymphoproliferative disorder (PTLD).

- PTLD is a lymphoproliferative disorder arising in the background of transplant procedures (solid organ, stem cell, and bone marrow transplant) that is usually EBV-driven.
- PTLD cases are classified into major categories of nondestructive PTLD, polymorphic PTLD, monomorphic PTLD and CHL PTLD.
- Treatment of polymorphic PTLD is withdrawal or reduction of immunosuppression.

- Monomorphic PTLD and CHL PTLD are classified as lymphomas of immunocompetent individuals.
- Indolent B-cell lymphomas (follicular and EBV-negative MALT) in allograft recipients are not considered PTLD and should be classified as primary lymphomas similar to lymphomas in immunocompetent individuals.
- The most important risk factor for EBV driven PTLD is EBV seronegativity at the time of transplantation.

Histiocytic and Dendritic Cell Neoplasms

154. Describe the clinical and cytomorphological features of Langerhans cell histiocytosis (LCH) and how it differs from other histiocytic disorders.

- Clinical features:
  - May be part of other syndromes:
    - › Hand-Schuller-Christian disease: indolent disease of children and young adults.
    - › Hashimoto-Pritzker disease: congenital but self-limited form of LCH.
    - › Letterer-Siwe disease: systemic variant of LCH in infants.
- Cytomorphological features:
  - LCH is a clonal neoplastic proliferation of immature dendritic cells.

- It is composed of epithelioid cells with horseshoe shaped nuclei displaying vesicular chromatin and linear grooves or folds.
- Electron microscopy reveals Birbeck granules that are pentalaminar tubules, often with a dilated terminal end producing a tennis racket–like appearance.
- Lung, bone, and lymph node are common sites of involvement.

(continued on next page)

- LCH cells are positive for HLA-DR, S100, CD1a, CD68, and Langerin by IHC.
- About half harbor *BRAF* V600E mutation and a quarter have *MAP2K1* mutation.

HISTIOCYTIC AND DENDRITIC CELL NEOPLASMS (CELL OF ORIGIN AND IMMUNOPHENOTYPE)[1]

NEOPLASM	CELL TYPE	PHENOTYPE
Histiocytic sarcoma	• Macrophage.	• Positive: CD45/CD68/CD163/CD4/lysozyme. • Negative: FDC markers/S100/CD1a/Langerin.
Langerhans cell histiocytosis/sarcoma	• Langerhans cell (LC).	• Positive: CD45(weak)/CD68/CD163/CD4/lysozyme(weak)/S100/CD1a/Langerin. • Negative: FDC markers.
Interdigitating dendritic cell sarcoma	• Interdigitating dendritic cell (IDC).	• Positive: CD45(weak)/S100/fascin. • Negative: FDC markers (except fascin)/CD1a/Langerin. • Variable (+/−): CD68/CD163/CD4/lysosome.
Follicular dendritic cell sarcoma	• Follicular dendritic cell (FDC).	• Positive: FDC markers (CD21/CD23/CD35/fascin/clusterin/CXCL13). • Negative: generally all others. • Variable (+/−): S100.
Inflammatory EBV+ follicular dendritic cell sarcoma	• FDC.	• Positive: FDC markers, EBV-EBER. • Negative: generally all others. • Variable: SMA (in FDC marker negative cases).
Disseminated juvenile xanthogranuloma	• Uncertain.	• Positive: vimentin/sCD14/CD68/CD163/fascin/FXIIIa. • Negative: CD1a/Langerin/FDC markers (except fascin). • Variable(+/−): S100.
Erdheim-Chester disease	• Non-Langherans histiocytes.	• Positive: CD14/CD68/CD163/fascin/FXIIIa. • Negative: CD1a/Langerin/FDC markers (except fascin). • Variable (+/−): S100.
Blastic plasmacytoid dendritic cell neoplasm (BPDCN)*	• Plasmacytoid dendritic cell (PDC) precursor.	• Positive: CD56/CD123/CD4/CD68. • Negative: CD45/CD163/lysozyme/S100/CD1a/Langerin. • Variable (+/−): TdT.

*Note: BPDCN is a clinically aggressive tumor derived from the precursors of PDCs that has a dedicated chapter the WHO classification.

HISTIOCYTIC DISORDERS: IMMUNOPHENOTYPIC FEATURES AND CELL OF ORIGIN[7]

MARKER/DIAGNOSIS	LCH	HLH	SHML
Cell of origin	LC	M/M	Histiocyte
CD1a	++	−	−
CD14	−	++	++
CD68 (KP-1, PGM-1)	+/−	++	++
CD163	−	++	++
Langerin	++	−	−
Fascin	−	+/−	+
S100	+	+/−	+
Lysozyme	−	++	++

Thymus Pathology

155. What is the WHO classification of thymomas?

- Type A thymoma.
- Type AB thymoma.
- Type B1 thymoma.
- Type B2 thymoma.
- Type B3 thymoma.

- Other:
  - Micronodular thymoma.
  - Metaplastic thymoma.
  - Microscopic thymoma.
  - Sclerosing thymoma.
  - Lipofibroadenoma.

156. What is the WHO classification of thymic carcinomas?

- Squamous cell carcinoma.
- Basaloid carcinoma.
- Mucoepidermoid carcinoma.
- Lymphoepithelioma-like carcinoma.
- Clear cell carcinoma.
- Sarcomatoid carcinoma.
- Papillary adenocarcinoma.
- Thymic carcinoma with adenoid cystic carcinoma-like features.
- Mucinous adenocarcinoma.
- Adenocarcinoma, NOS.
- NUT carcinoma (also known as t(15;19) carcinoma).
- Undifferentiated carcinoma.
- Large cell neuroendocrine carcinoma.
- Small cell carcinoma.
- Combined thymic carcinomas.

157. What items should be included in the report of a thymic tumor?

- Specimen.
- Procedure.
- Specimen integrity.
- Specimen weight.
- Tumor size.
- Histologic type.
- Tumor extension.
- Margins.
- Treatment effect.
- Lymphovascular invasion.
- Regional lymph nodes.
- Pathologic staging for thymomas (modified Masaoka stage).
- Implants/distant metastasis.
- Pathologic staging for thymic carcinomas (pTNM).
- Additional pathologic findings (select all that apply):
  - Age appropriate involution changes.
  - Fibrosis.
  - Cortical hyperplasia.
  - Cystic changes in tumor.
  - Cystic changes in adjacent thymus.
  - Other (specify).
- Ancillary studies.
  - Immunohistochemical staining.

158. How are thymomas staged?

- Modified Masaoka staging system:
  - Stage I: grossly and microscopically encapsulated (includes microscopic invasion into, but not through, the capsule).
  - Stage IIa: microscopic transcapsular invasion.
  - Stage IIb: macroscopic capsular invasion.
  - Stage III: macroscopic invasion of neighboring organs.
  - Stage IVa: pleural or pericardial dissemination.
  - Stage IVb: hematogenous or lymphatic dissemination.
  - Cannot be determined.

159. What are the important prognostic parameters for a thymus tumor?

- Tumor stage.
- Histologic type.
- Completeness of resection.

160. Where do thymic tumors metastasize most frequently?

- Lung.
- Liver.
- Skeletal system.
- Pleura and pericardium.

161. What immunostains are useful to help distinguish a thymoma from other mediastinal tumors?

- Cytokeratins are helpful in distinguishing between thymomas and lymphoid lesions.
- CD1a and TdT may be helpful in defining the cortical thymocyte phenotype of thymoma, as distinguished from the typical peripheral T cell phenotype of tumor infiltrating lymphocytes associated with other tumors.
- CD5/CD117 immunostains may be helpful in distinguishing thymic carcinoma from thymoma and other mediastinal tumors, however keep in mind that B3 thymomas may express CD5/CD117.
- Immunostains for human chorionic gonadotropin (hCG), placental alkaline phosphatase (PLAP), carcinoembryonic antigen (CEA), α-fetoprotein, SALL4, OCT4, and CD30 can be used to differentiate among thymic carcinomas and mediastinal germ cell tumors.

Red Cell Disorders

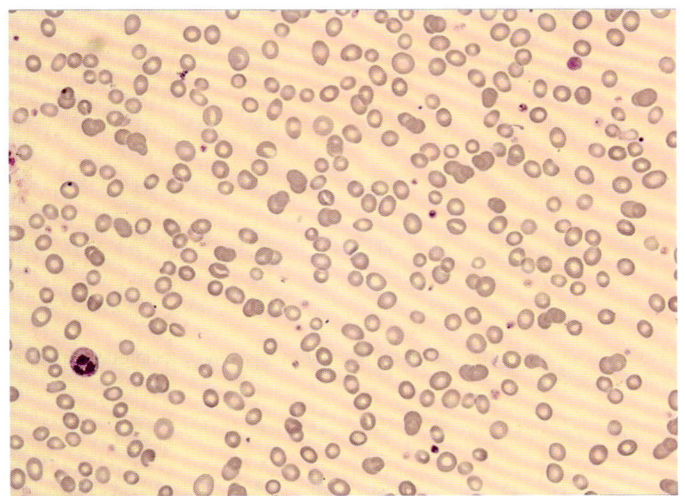

IMAGE 13.1 Microcytic red cells. This finding may be associated with iron deficiency, anemia of chronic disease, or thalassemia trait.

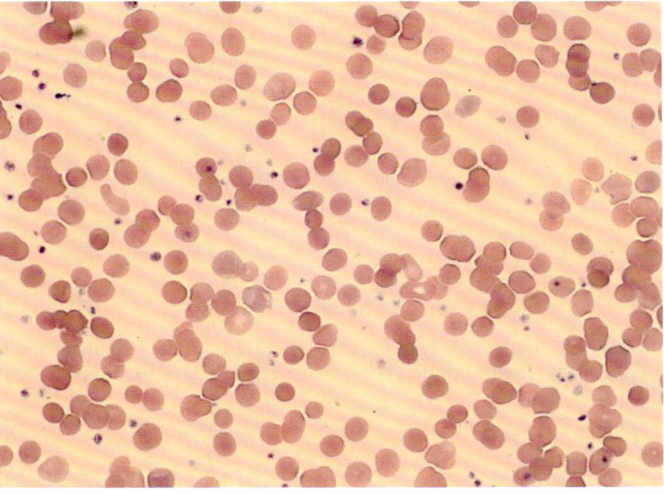

IMAGE 13.4 Spherocytosis is usually associated with hemolytic anemia or ABO incompatibility causing HDN (hemolytic disease of newborn).

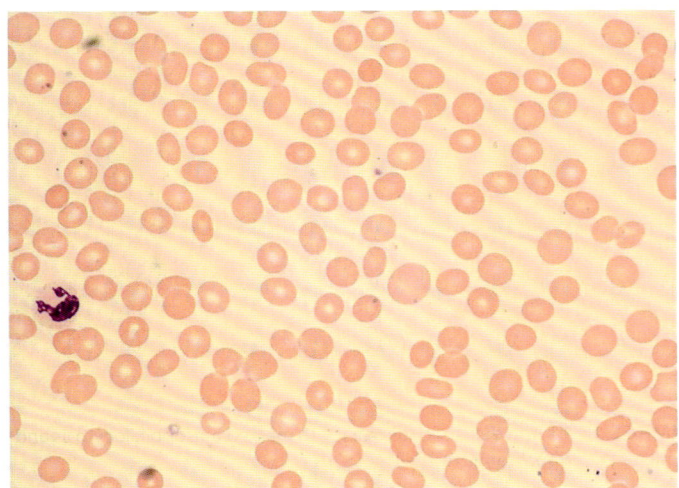

IMAGE 13.2 Macrocytic red cells.

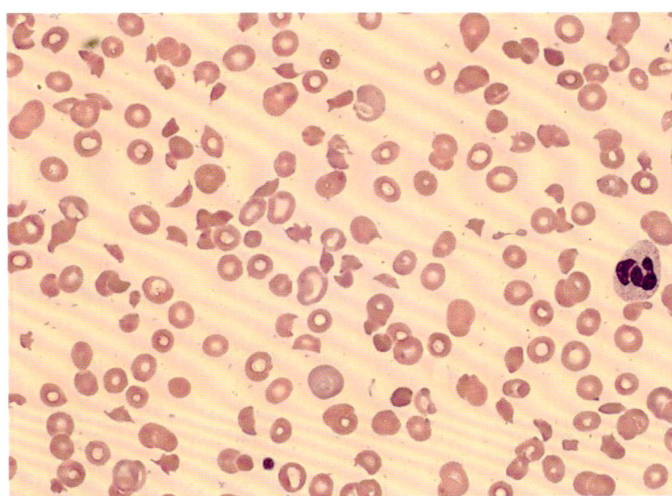

IMAGE 13.5 Schistocytes are fragmented or dysmorphic red cells associated with acute DIC (disseminated intravascular coagulopathy).

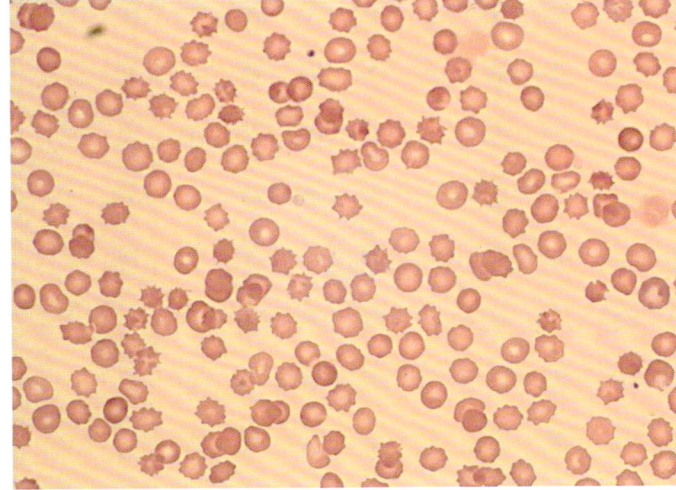

IMAGE 13.3 Burr cells display irregular peripheral spikes and are usually associated with acute renal failure or hyperammonemia.

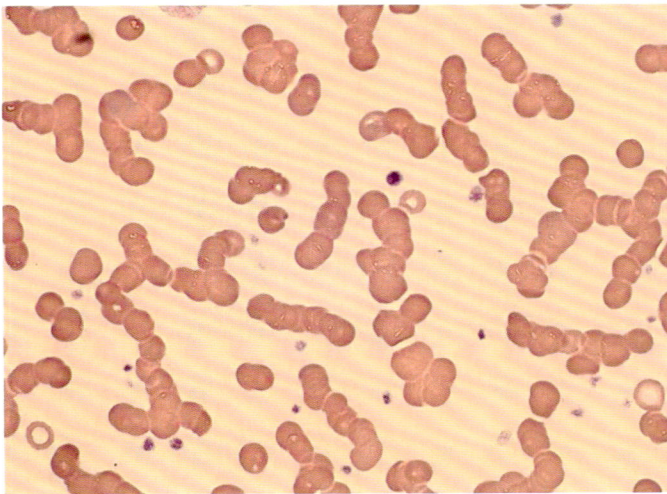

IMAGE 13.6 Rouleaux formation showing linear stacks of red cells that are seen with acute inflammation or increased monoclonal proteins.

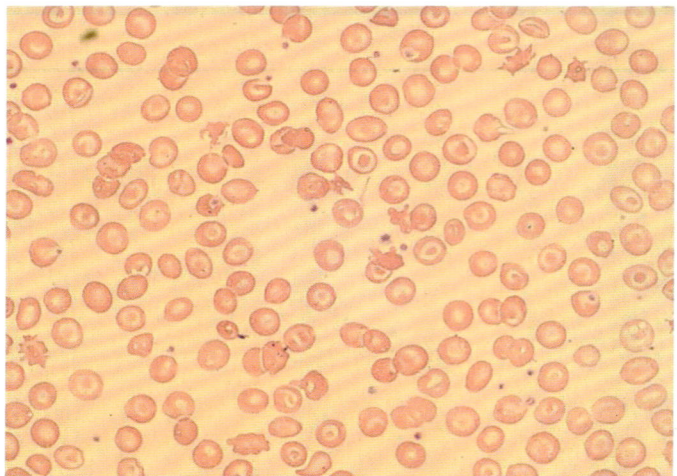

IMAGE 13.7 Target cells: red cells with bulls eye appearance that are commonly seen with chronic liver disease or hemoglobinopathies.

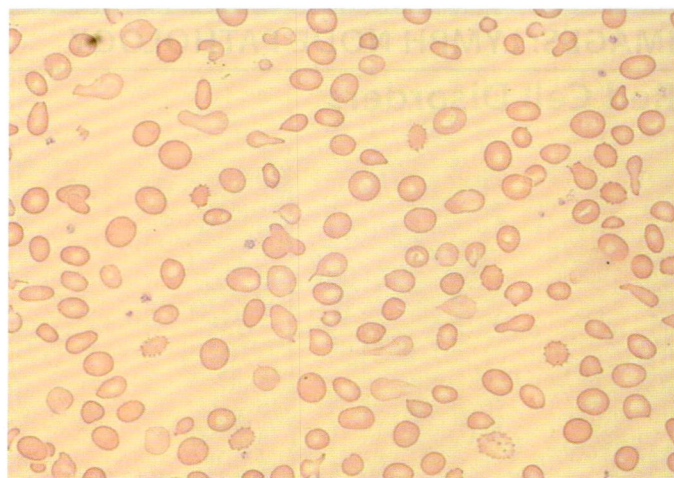

IMAGE 13.10 Teardrop red cells (dacrocytes): usually associated with bone marrow fibrosis.

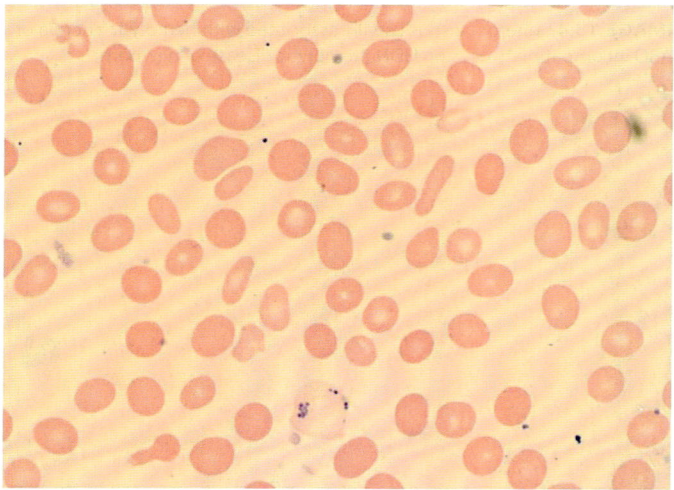

IMAGE 13.8 Elliptocytes/ovalocytes: oval shaped red cells that are usually seen with chronic anemia or anemia of iron deficiency.

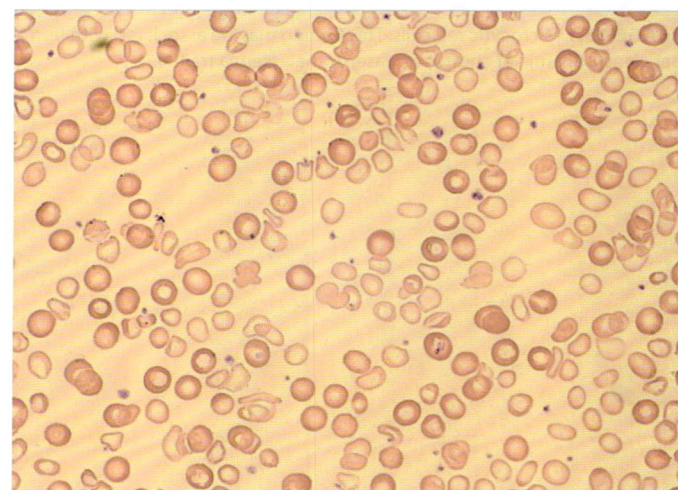

IMAGE 13.11 Iron deficiency anemia with marked anisopoikilocytosis and microcytic hypochromic red cells.

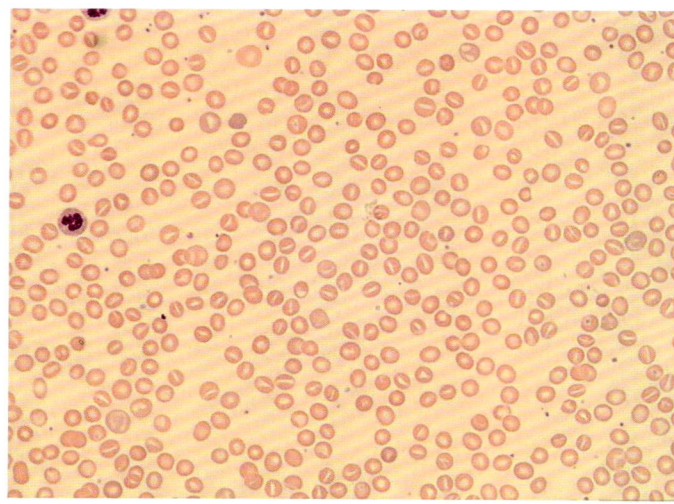

IMAGE 13.9 Stomatocytes: red cells with a central pallor that resembles a fish mouth.

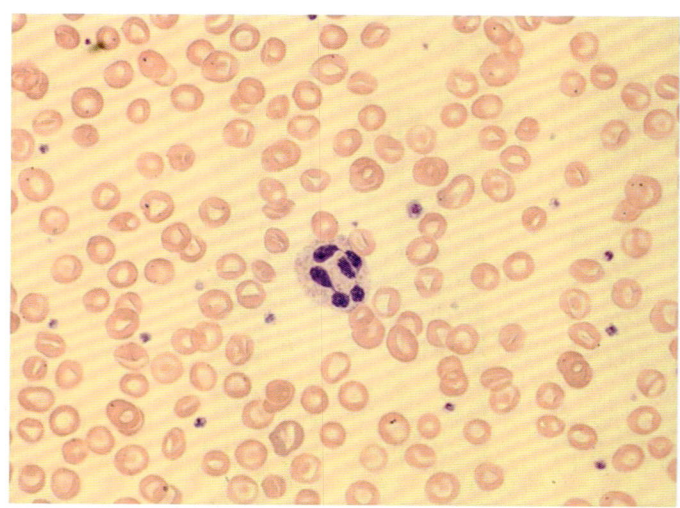

IMAGE 13.12 Hypersegmented neutrophil (nucleus with 5 or more segments): usually seen with macrocytic anemia or cytotoxic drugs.

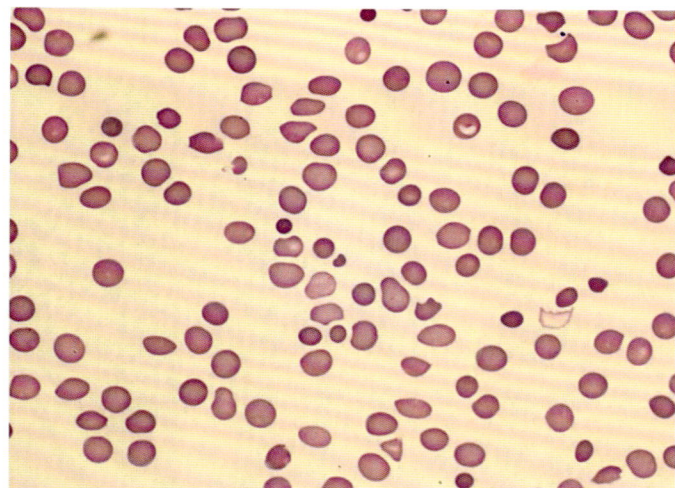

IMAGE 13.13 Autoimmune hemolytic anemia showing frequent spherocytes and few characteristic microspherocytes at the center.

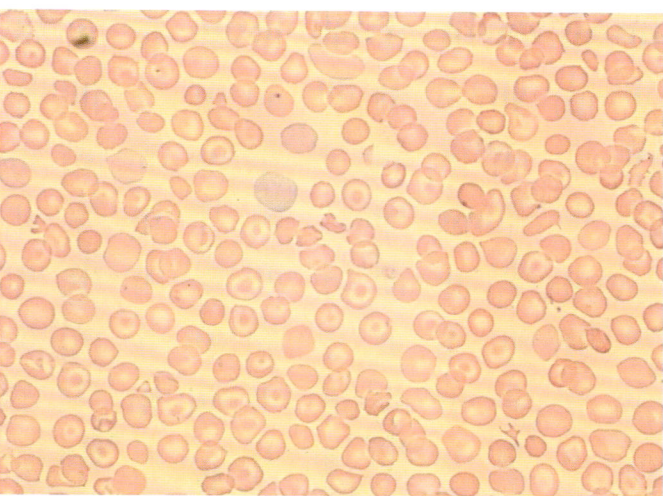

IMAGE 13.16 Hemoglobin C disease. The image shows numerous target cells with occasional folded or cigarette shaped abnormal erythrocytes.

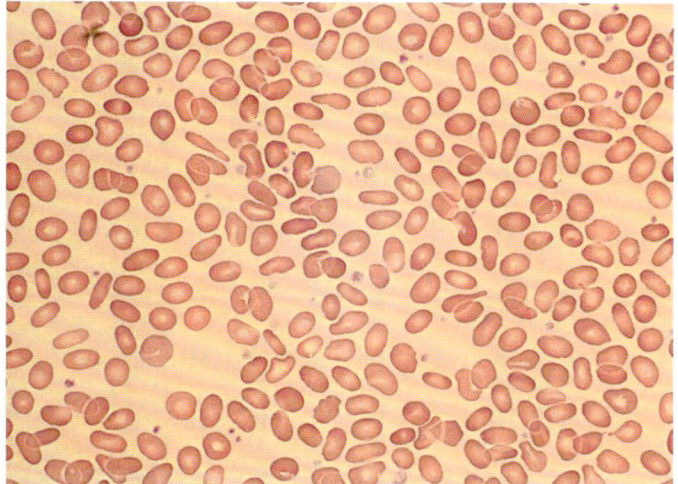

IMAGE 13.14 Hereditary elliptocytosis. Elliptocytes/ovalocytes account for > 25% of red cells in this hereditary condition.

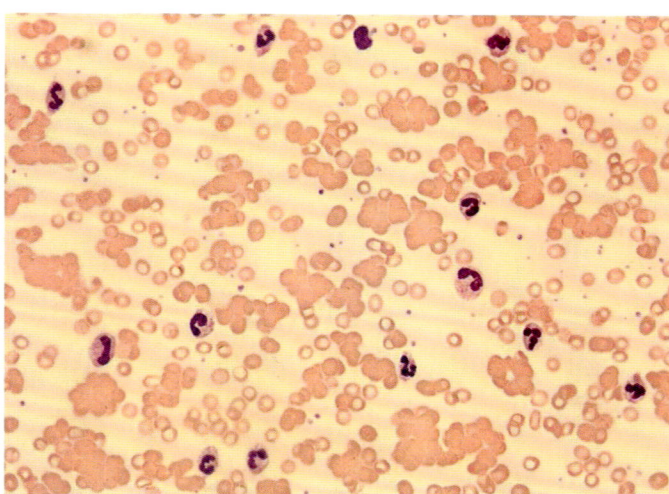

IMAGE 13.17 Cold agglutinin disease, characterized by the presence of 3-dimensional aggregates of red cells.

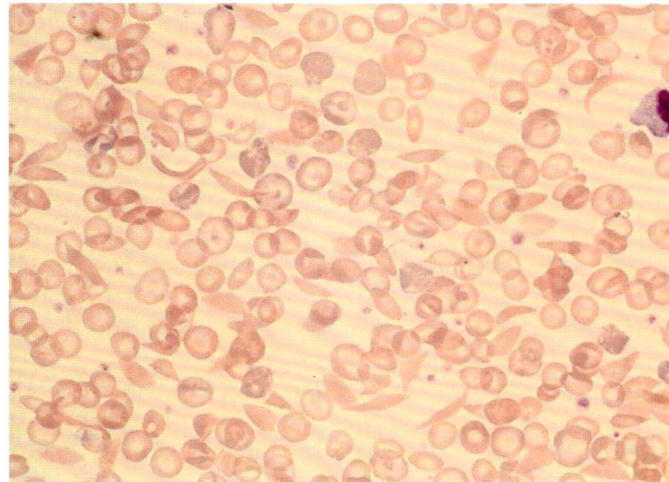

IMAGE 13.15 Hemoglobin S disease. Frequent sickle cells are indicative of sickle cell hemolytic crisis.

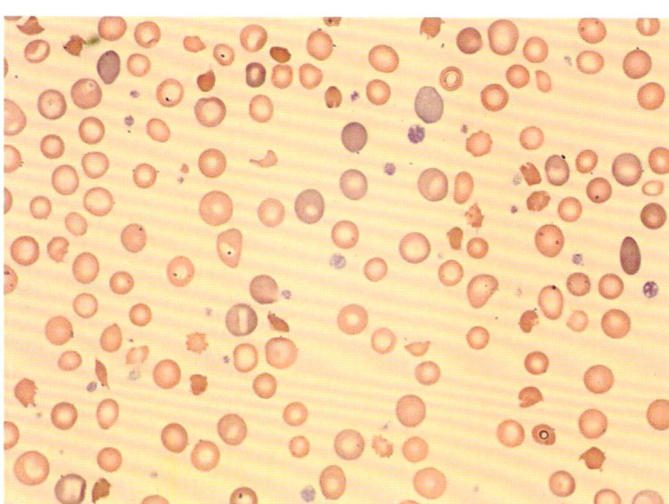

IMAGE 13.18 DIC, characterized by an increased number of schistocytes and helmet cells.

Bone Marrow Pathology

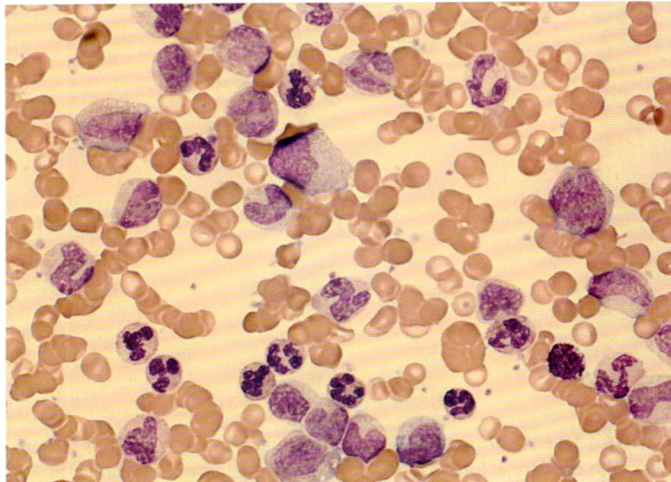

IMAGE 13.19 CML (chronic myeloid leukemia). Neutrophilic and myelocytic/metamyelocytic peaks are characteristic findings in blood.

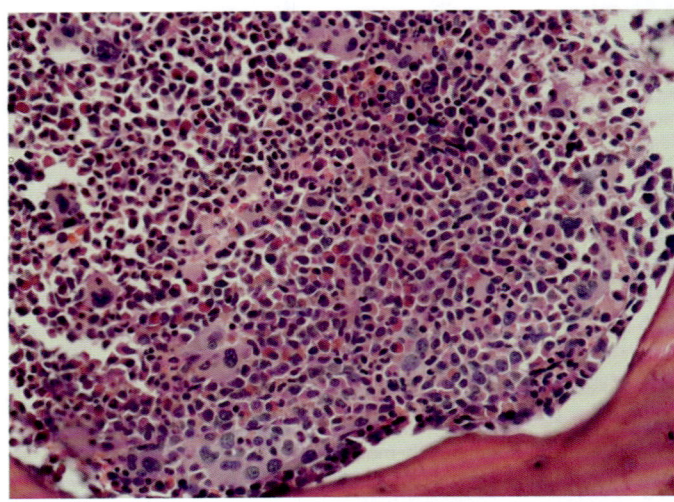

IMAGE 13.22 CML is characterized by myeloid preponderance and proliferation of micromegakaryocytes (small megakaryocytes).

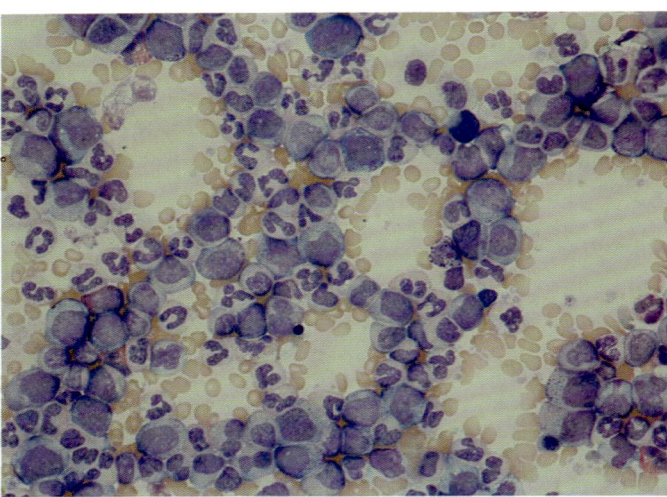

IMAGE 13.20 CML usually presents with marked leukocytosis, which may cause leukostasis syndrome.

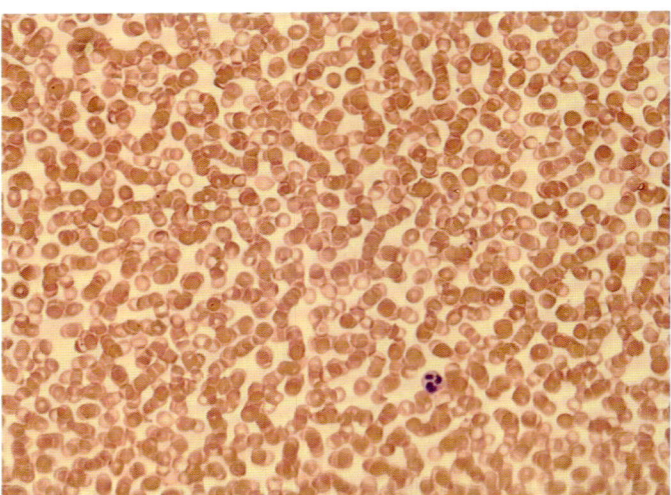

IMAGE 13.23 PV (polycythemia vera). An increase in hemoglobin and red cell mass and positive *JAK2* V617F mutation are characteristic findings.

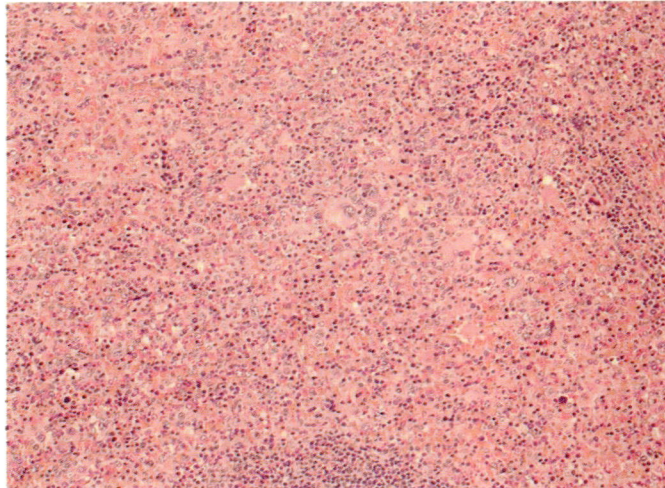

IMAGE 13.21 With CML, the bone marrow is always hypercellular and reveals marked proliferation of myeloid and megakaryocytic lineages.

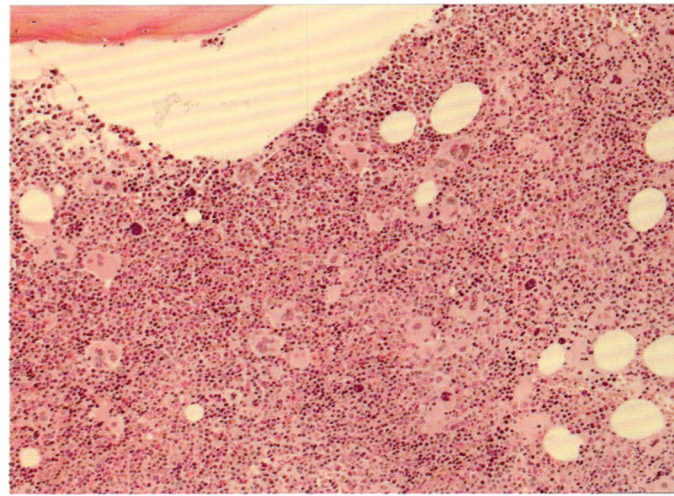

IMAGE 13.24 PV, characterized by hypercellular marrow with increased erythroids and loose clusters of megakaryocytes.

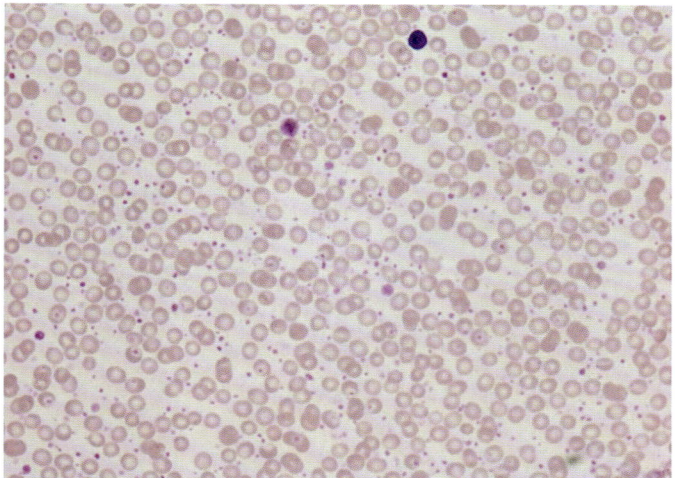

IMAGE 13.25 ET (essential thrombocythemia). Markedly increased platelets with hypogranular morphology are characteristic findings.

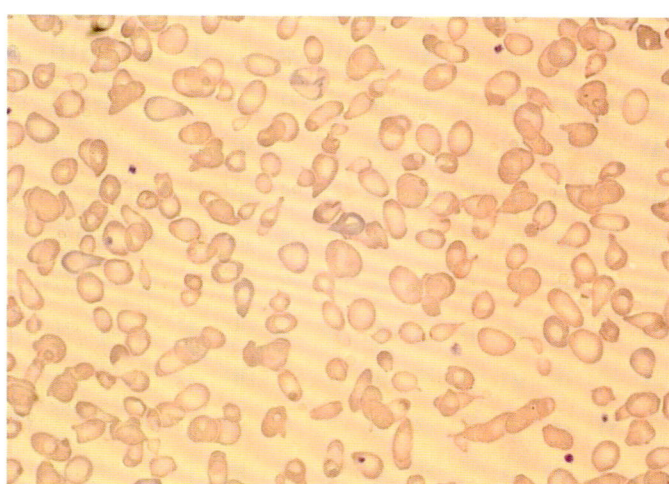

IMAGE 13.28 PMF (primary myelofibrosis). Teardrop red cells and leukoerythroblastic reaction are typical findings seen in PMF patients.

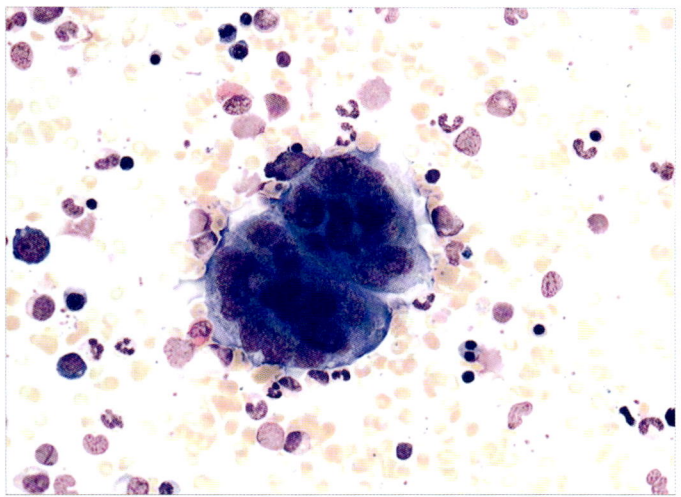

IMAGE 13.26 ET. Megakaryocytic proliferation with giant variants are typical findings.

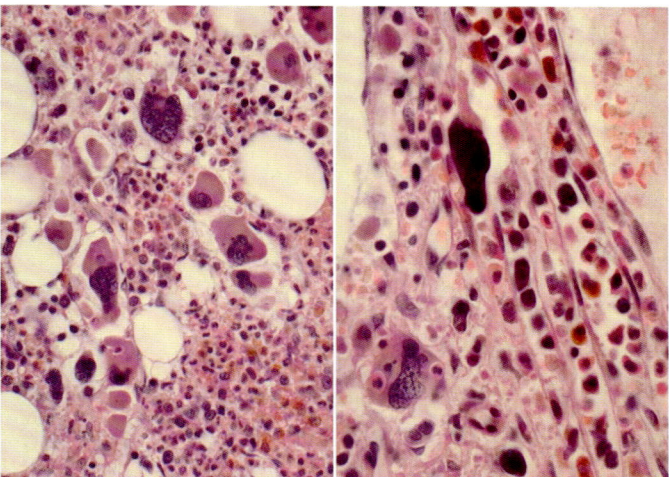

IMAGE 13.29 PMF. Bone marrow fibrosis, atypical megakaryocytosis, and intravascular hematopoiesis are characteristic features of PMF.

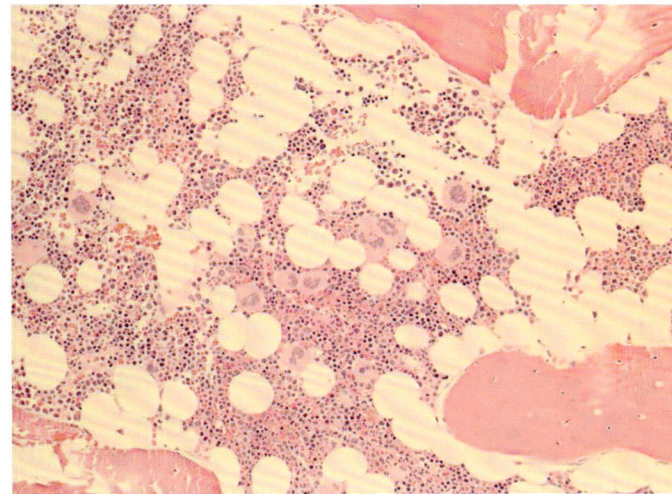

IMAGE 13.27 ET, characterized by atypical megakaryocytosis, which includes giant forms with staghorn nuclear features.

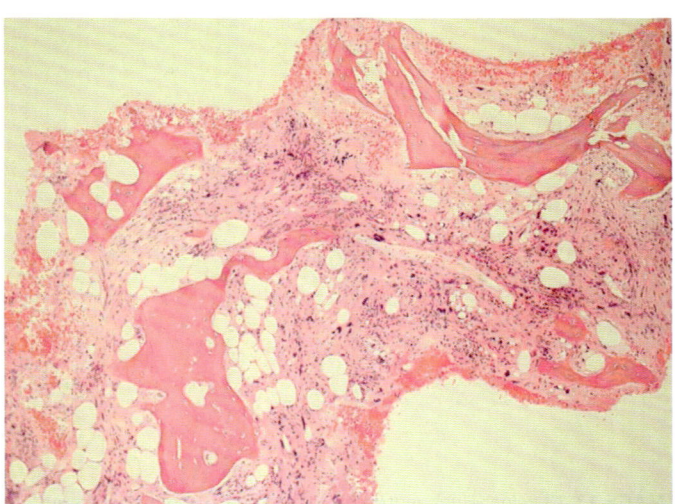

IMAGE 13.30 PMF. Bone marrow fibrosis and atypical megakaryocytes with cloudy and smeared nuclear features are characteristic findings.

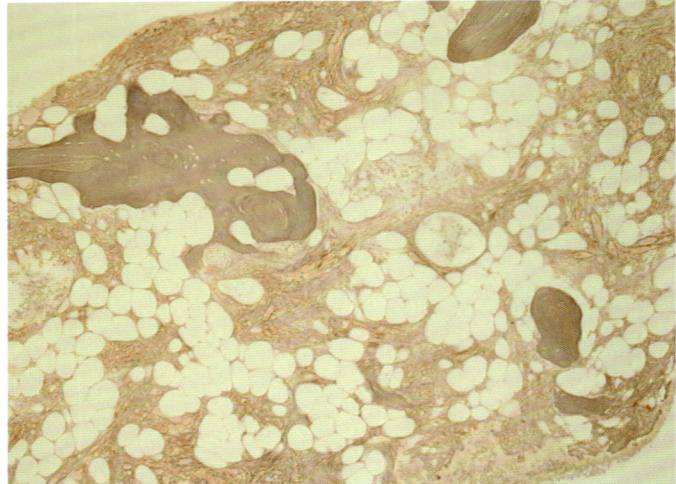

IMAGE 13.31 PMF. Bone marrow fibrosis can be highlighted by special reticulin stain, which is required for proper grading.

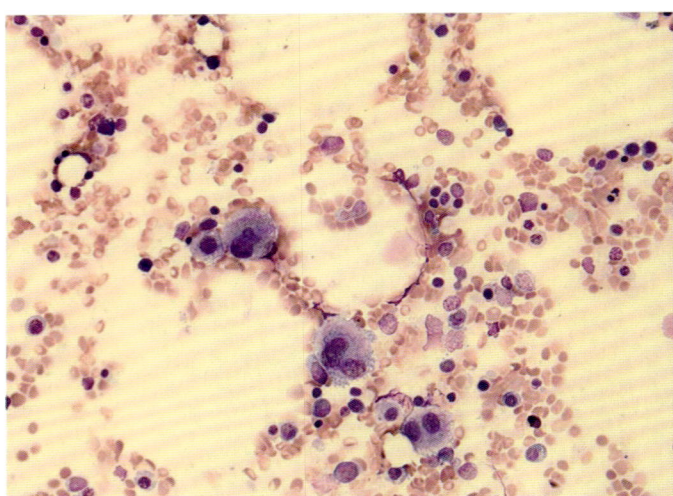

IMAGE 13.34 MDS (myelodysplastic syndrome). The presence of dysplastic megakaryocytes is the most characteristic finding in MDS.

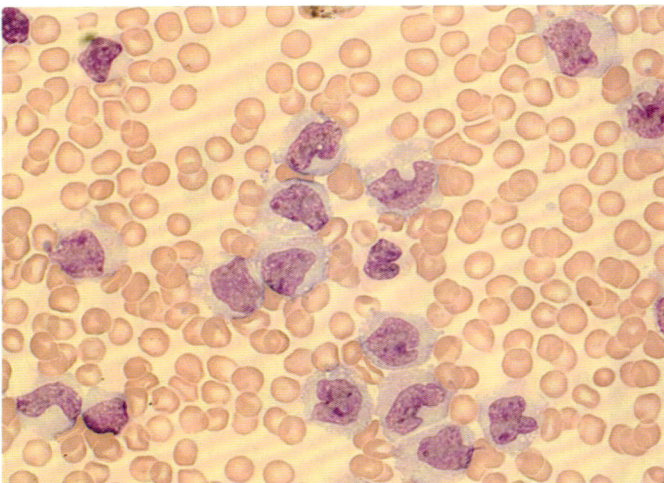

IMAGE 13.32 CMML (chronic myelomonocytic leukemia) is characterized by persistent monocytosis (> 3 month) without known etiology.

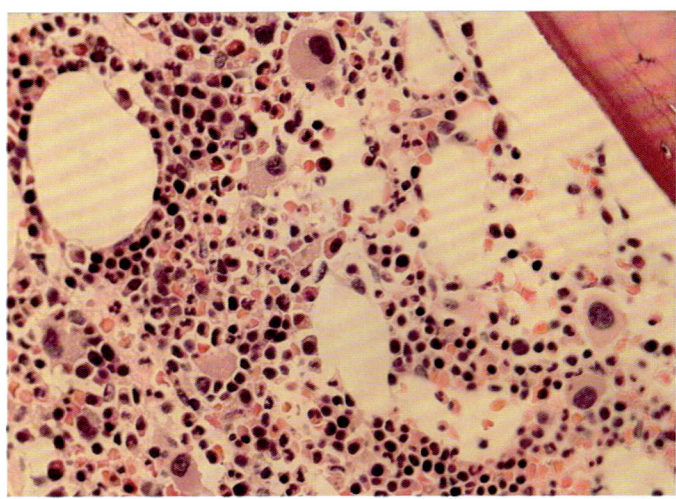

IMAGE 13.35 MDS. Erythroid preponderance with dyserythropoiesis and dysplastic megakaryocytes are common findings in RCMD.

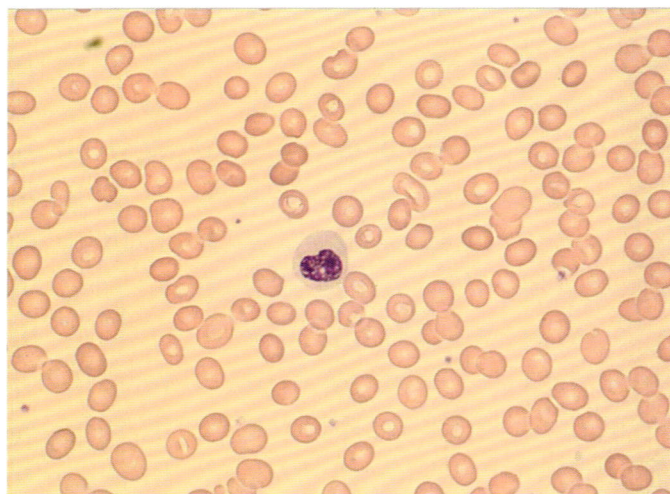

IMAGE 13.33 Pelger-Huet neutrophil. Hypogranular and monolobated neutrophils are common features of myelodysplasia.

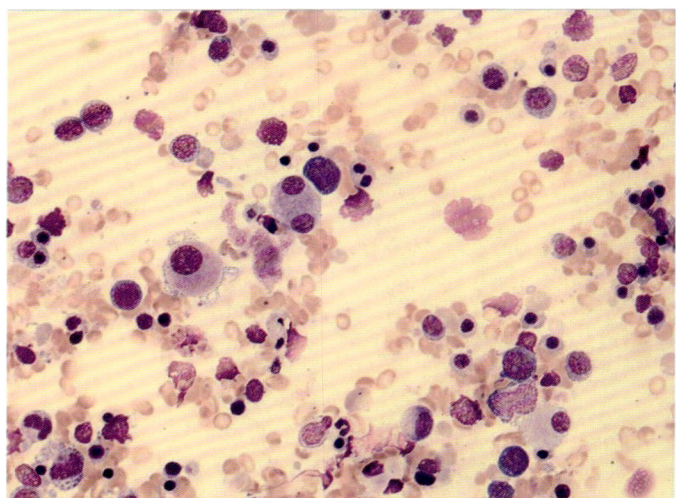

IMAGE 13.36 MDS (−5q syndrome): characterized by peripheral thrombocytosis and/or macrocytosis, as well as frequent bone marrow small megakaryocytes.

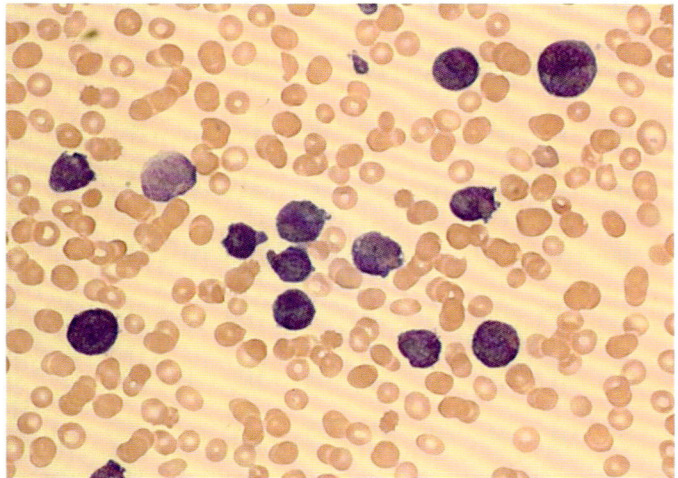

IMAGE 13.37 AML-M0 (acute myeloid leukemia with minimal differentiation, FAB classification).

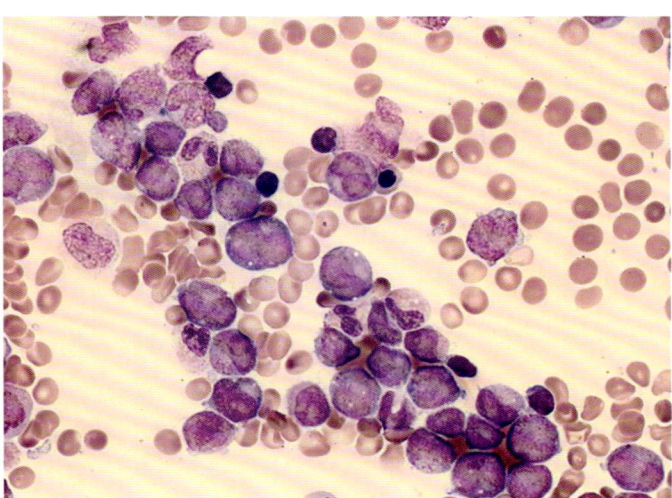

IMAGE 13.40 AML-M3 (APL: acute promyelocytic leukemia, FAB classification).

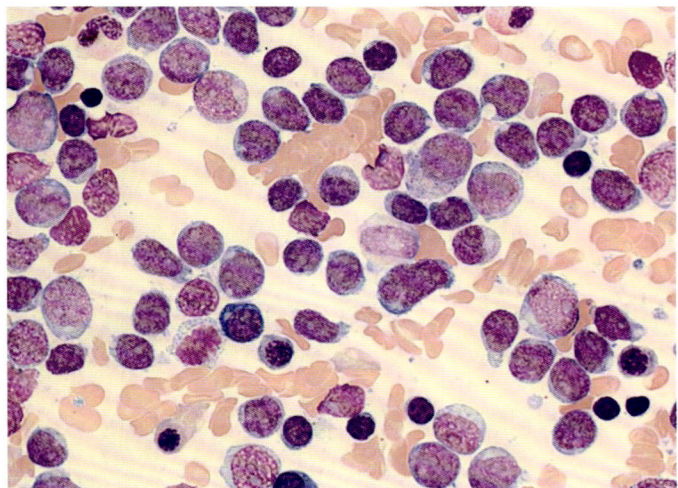

IMAGE 13.38 AML-M1 (acute myeloid leukemia without maturation, FAB classification).

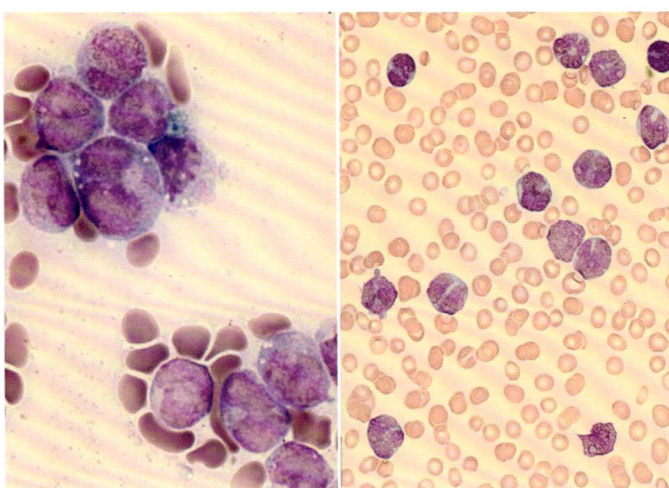

IMAGE 13.41 APL-M3 (acute promyelocytic leukemia). Bilobed butterfly cells (right image) and Auer rod (left image) are characteristic findings.

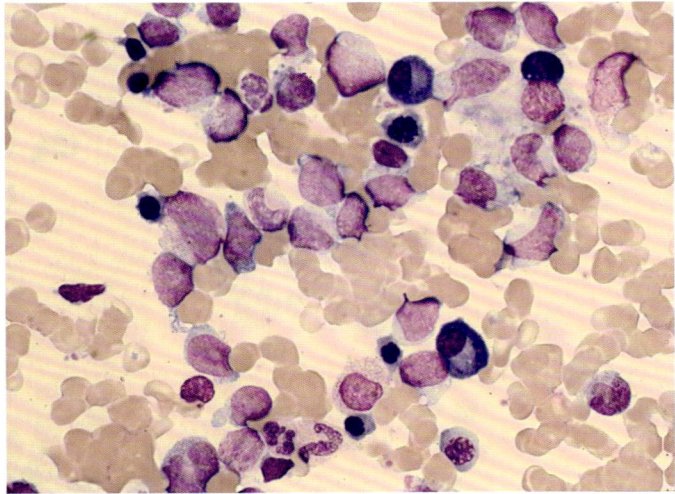

IMAGE 13.39 AML-M2 (acute myeloid leukemia with maturation, FAB classification).

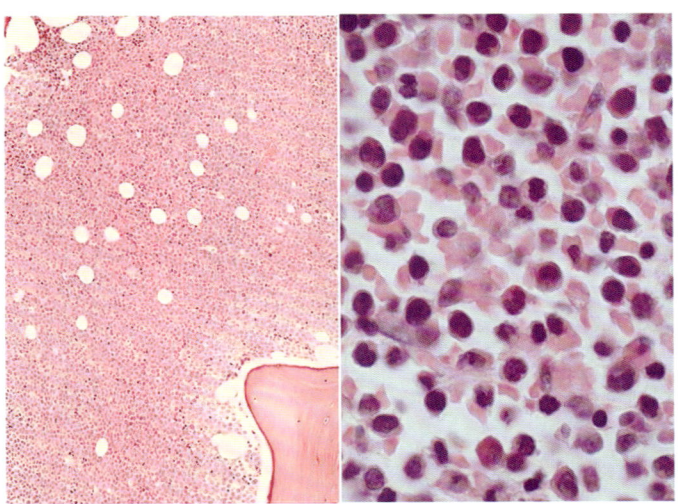

IMAGE 13.42 APL-M3 (acute promyelocytic leukemia). Bone marrow biopsy reveals sheets of atypical promyelocytes with pink cytoplasm.

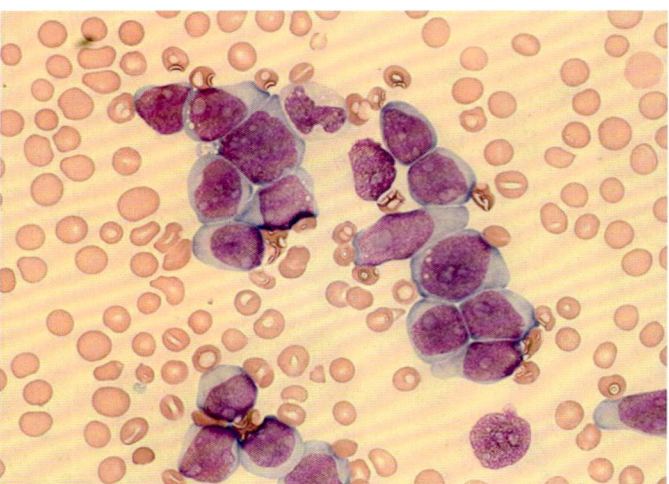

IMAGE 13.43 AML-M4 (acute myeloid leukemia with myelomonocytic differentiation, FAB classification).

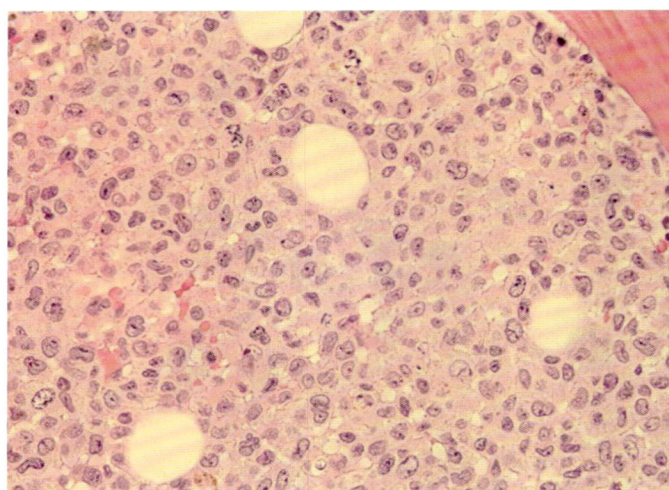

IMAGE 13.46 AML with monoblastic/monocytic differentiation (M5). Bone marrow biopsy reveals sheets of blasts with lobulated nuclei.

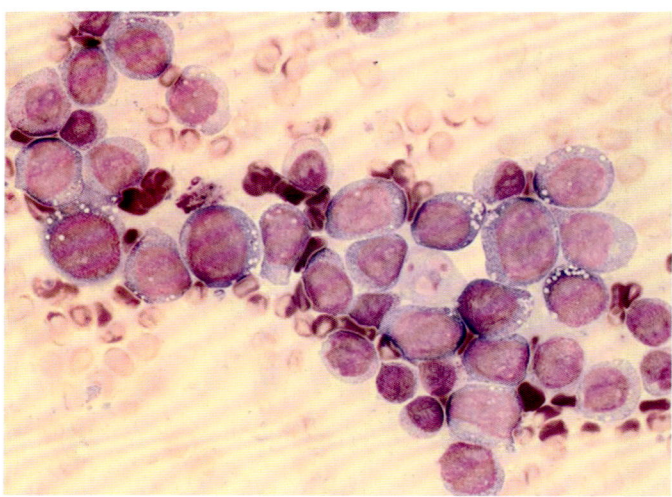

IMAGE 13.44 AML-M5A (acute myeloid leukemia with monoblastic differentiation, FAB classification).

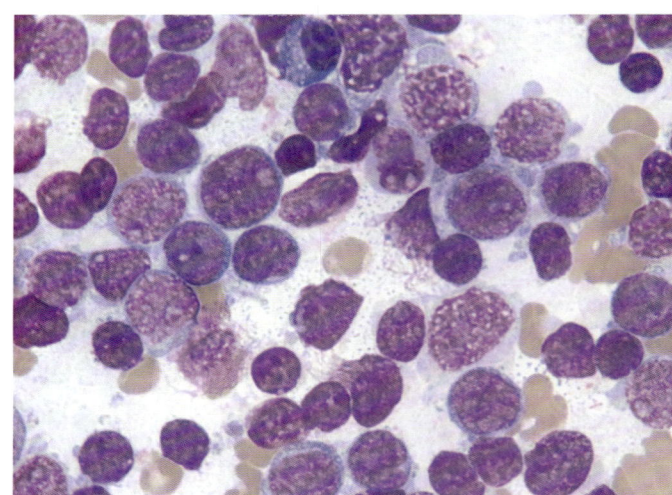

IMAGE 13.47 AML-M6 (AEL: acute erythroid leukemia, FAB classification). Blasts were positive for GPA and CD36 by flow cytometry.

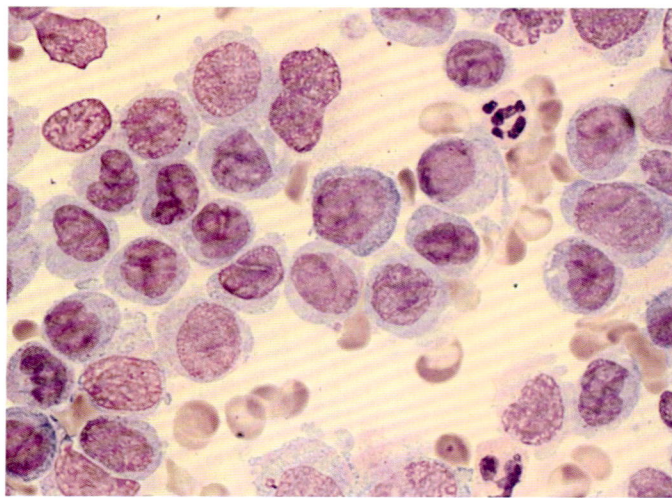

IMAGE 13.45 AML-M5B (acute myeloid leukemia with monocytic differentiation, FAB classification).

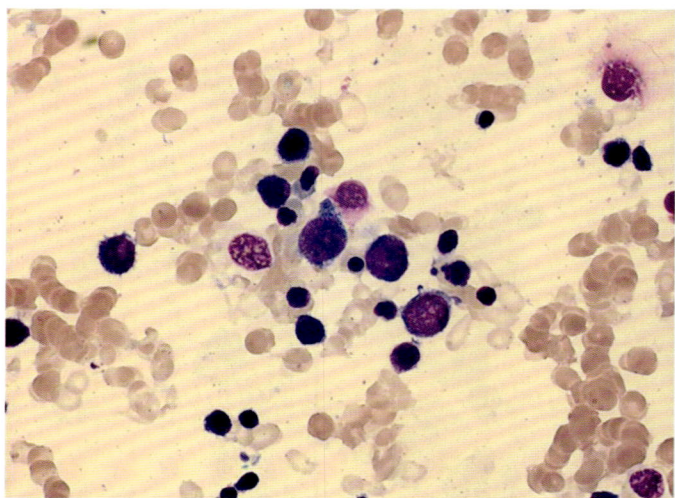

IMAGE 13.48 AML-M7 (AMKL: acute megakaryoblastic leukemia, FAB classification). Blasts were positive for CD41 and CD61 by flow cytometry.

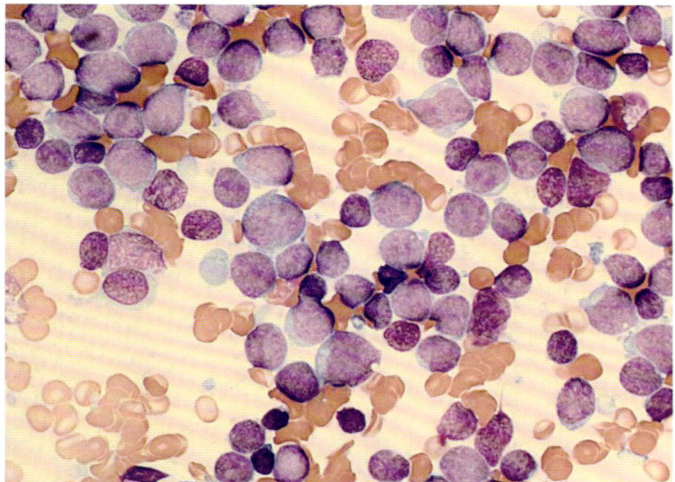

IMAGE 13.49 B-ALL (B lymphoblastic leukemia/lymphoma).

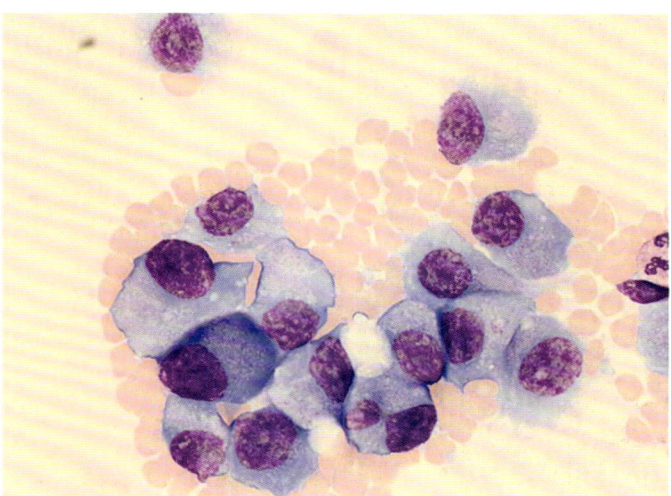

IMAGE 13.52 PCM (plasma cell myeloma), characterized by markedly increased plasma cells. Clinical correlation is required for final diagnosis.

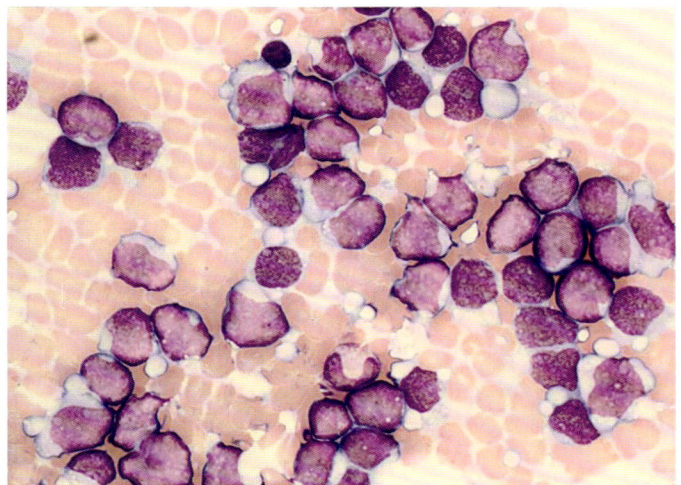

IMAGE 13.50 T-ALL (T lymphoblastic leukemia/lymphoma).

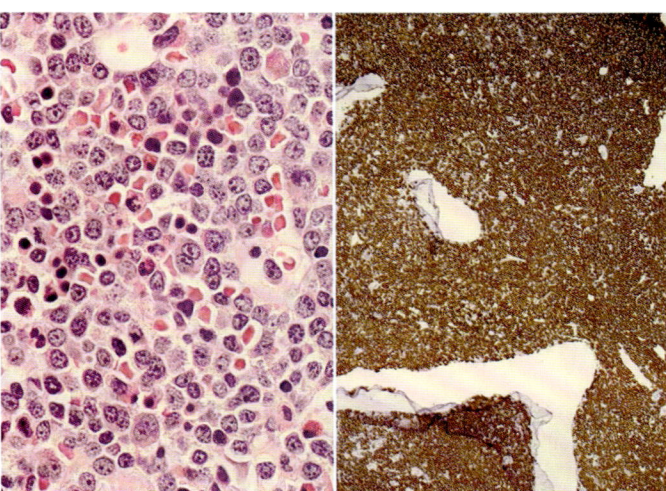

IMAGE 13.53 PCM. Bone marrow biopsy reveals sheets of plasma cells which are positive for CD138 by immunohistochemistry.

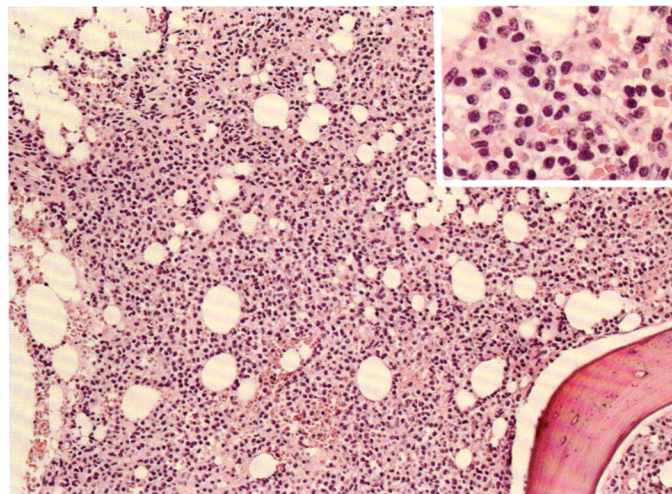

IMAGE 13.51 HCL (hairy cell leukemia) showing small neoplastic lymphoid cells with interstitial distribution and fried egg appearance.

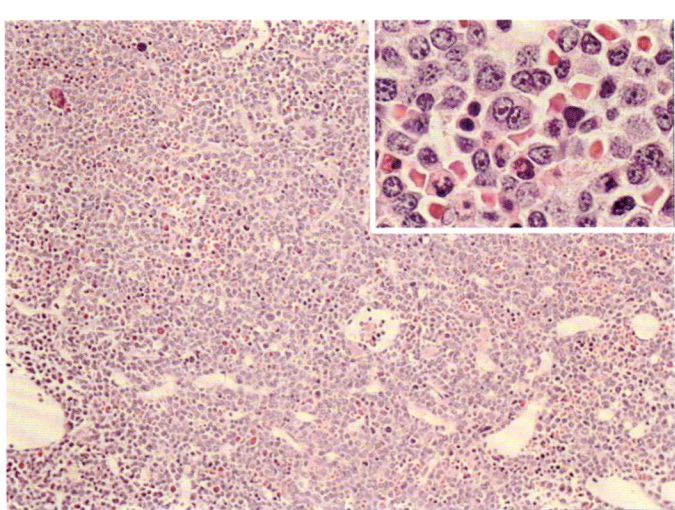

IMAGE 13.54 PCM with plasmablastic features.

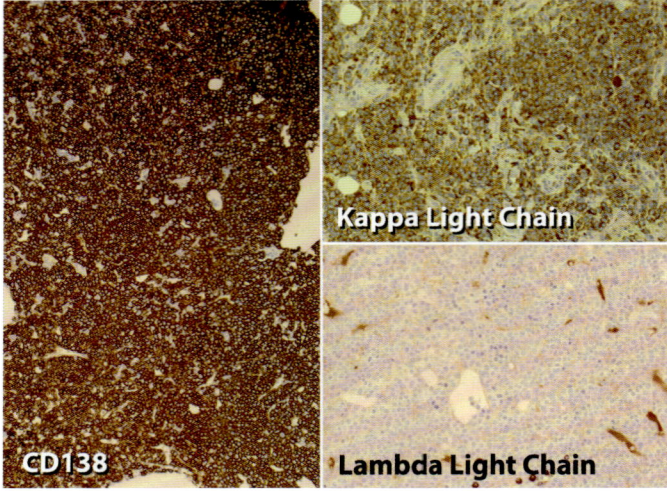

IMAGE 13.55 PCM (CD138 positive) with kappa light chain restriction.

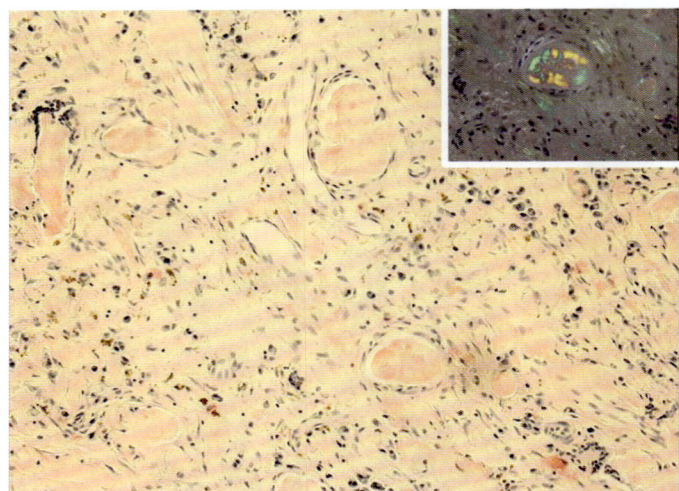

IMAGE 13.56 Extensive soft tissue involvement by amyloidosis, Congo red special stain under polarized light (apple green birefringence).

Lymph Node Pathology

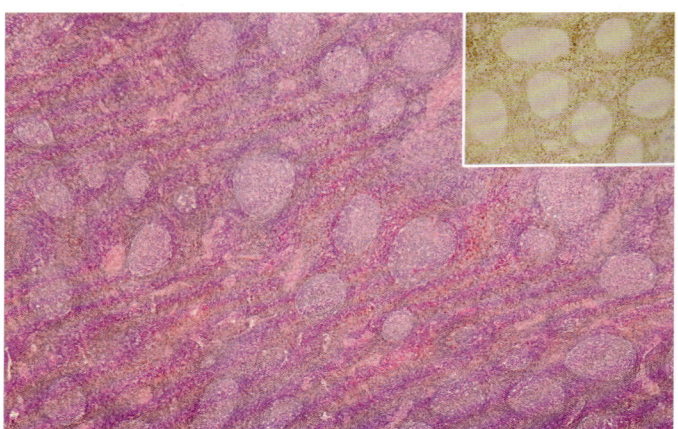

IMAGE 13.57 Reactive follicular hyperplasia. Germinal centers are BCL-2 negative by IHC.

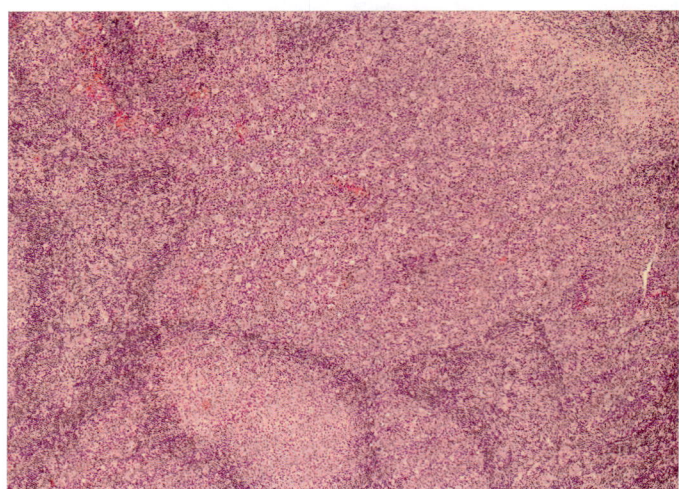

IMAGE 13.59 Reactive hyperplastic follicles with geographic pattern. This pattern may be seen in early phase of HIV associated lymphadenopathy.

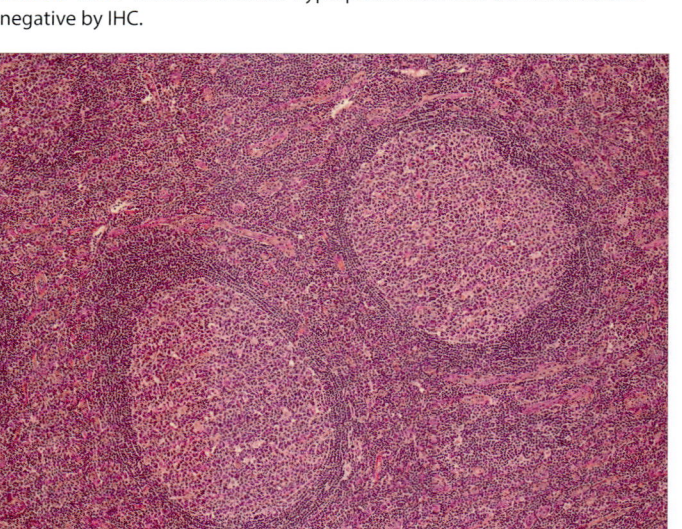

IMAGE 13.58 Reactive hyperplastic follicles. Preserved mantle zones, polarization, and tingible body macrophages are characteristic findings.

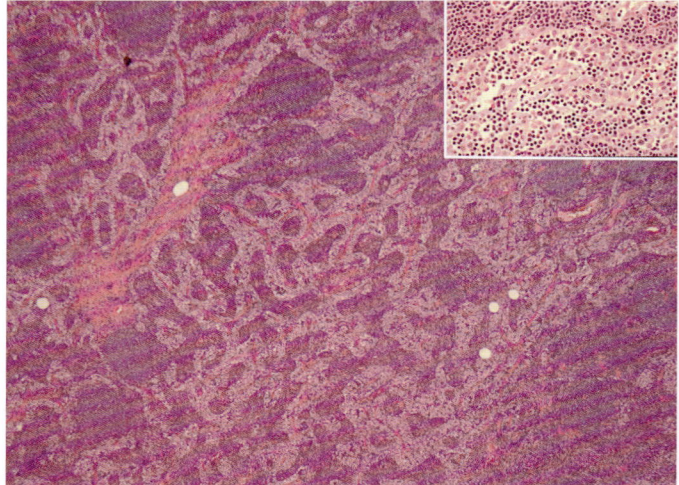

IMAGE 13.60 Sinusoidal hyperplasia. Reactive histiocytes display pale pink cytoplasm.

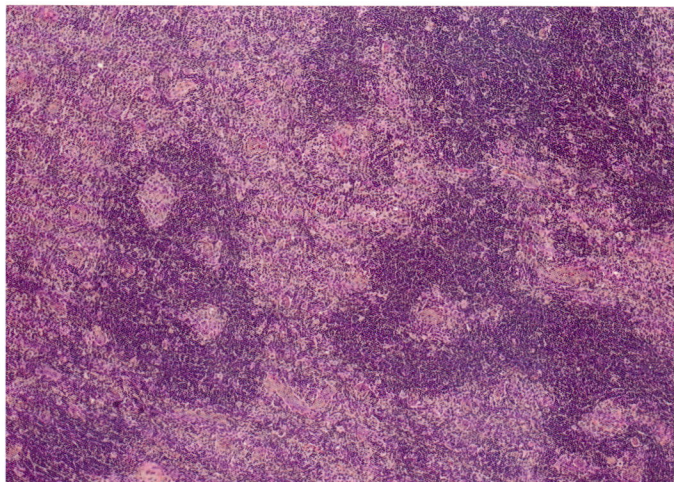

IMAGE 13.61 Lymph node with mixed hyperplasia: interfollicular and mantle cell hyperplasia.

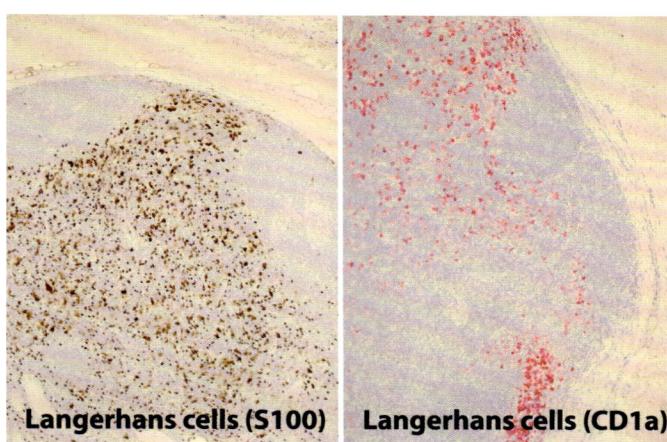

Langerhans cells (S100)   Langerhans cells (CD1a)

IMAGE 13.64 Dermatopathic lymphadenitis. Note the interfollicular nodular hyperplasia with proliferation of histiocytes and Langerhans cells.

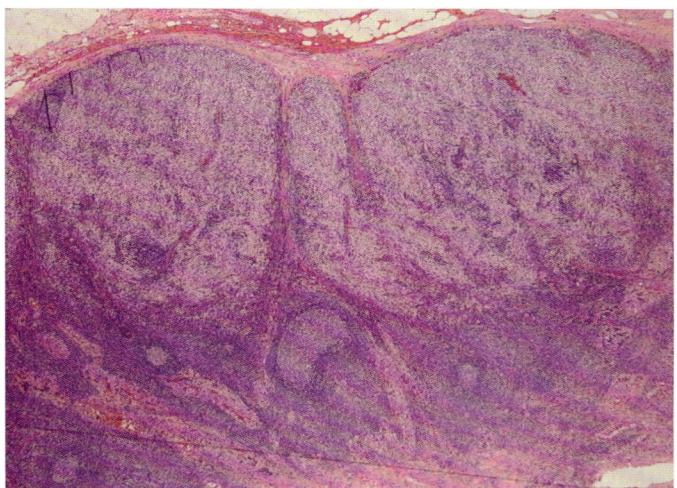

IMAGE 13.62 Dermatopathic lymphadenitis. Note the wedge shaped lymphohistiocytic proliferation with base of lesion at the periphery.

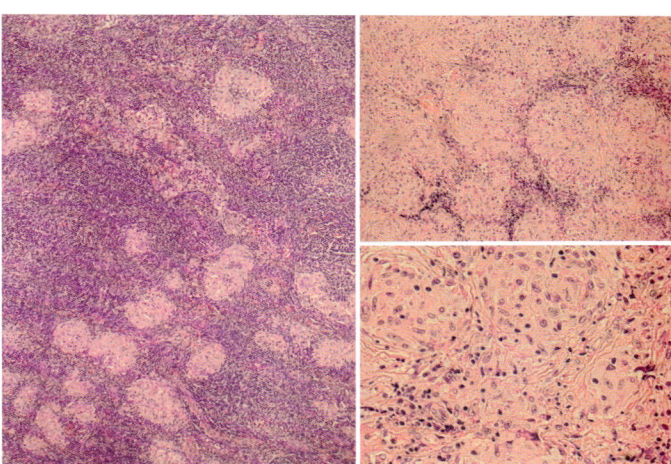

IMAGE 13.65 Granulomatous lymphadenitis with epithelioid histiocytes (sarcoidosis).

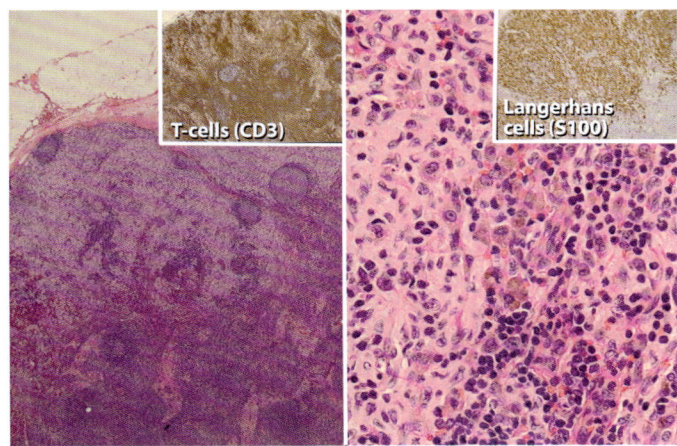

T-cells (CD3)   Langerhans cells (S100)

IMAGE 13.63 Dermatopathic lymphadenitis. The images show interfollicular nodular hyperplasia associated with pigments and increased Langerhans cells.

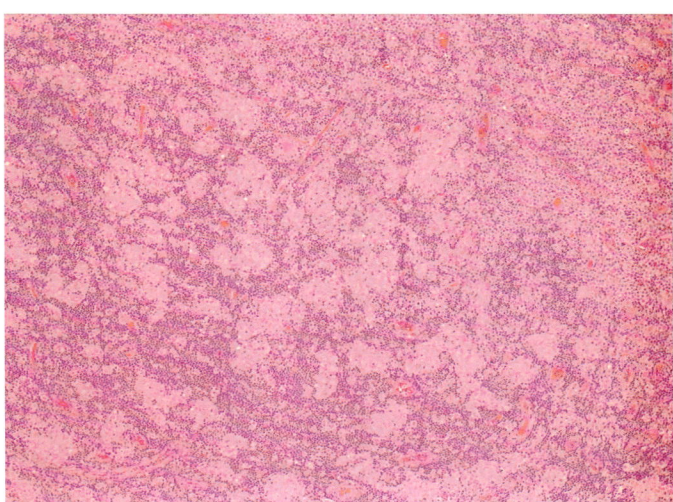

IMAGE 13.66 Granulomatous lymphadenitis with frequent microgranulomata and intrafollicular granulomata.

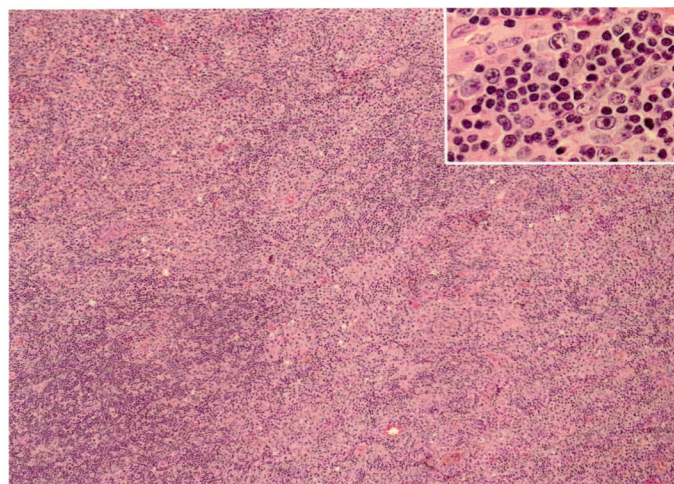

IMAGE 13.67 EBV associated lymphadenitis showing mixed lymphoid proliferation with occasional large reactive immunoblasts.

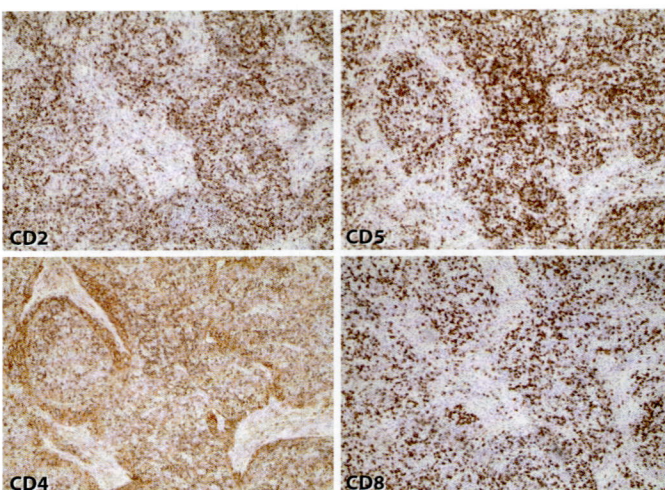

IMAGE 13.70 CAEBV is usually associated with loss of normal lymph node structure by a dense T cell infiltrate.

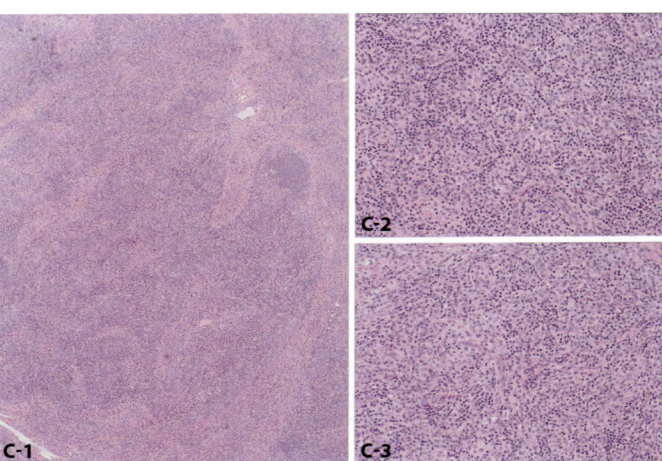

IMAGE 13.68 Chronic active Epstein-Barr virus infection (CAEBV) is a rare complication of EBV infection, which can lead to immune system failure with life-threatening complications, and it is commonly mistaken with T-cell lymphoma, namely angioimmunoblastic T-cell lymphoma.

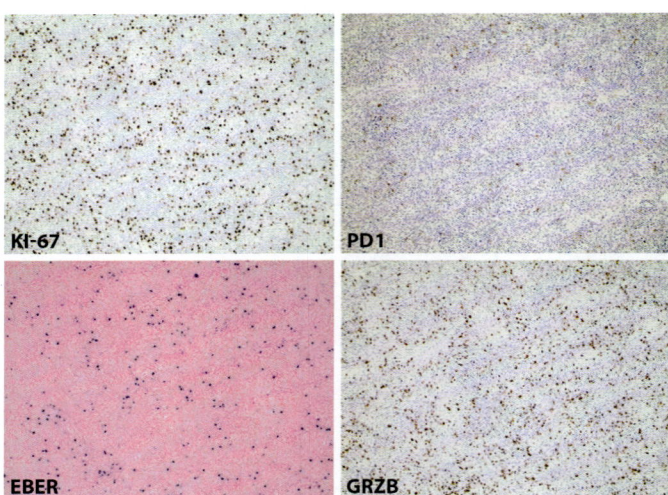

IMAGE 13.71 CAEBV is usually associated with the EBV infection of T cells in lymph node tissue, however the diagnosis is based on the clinical symptoms, organomegaly and high EBV DNA titer by qPCR test in blood.

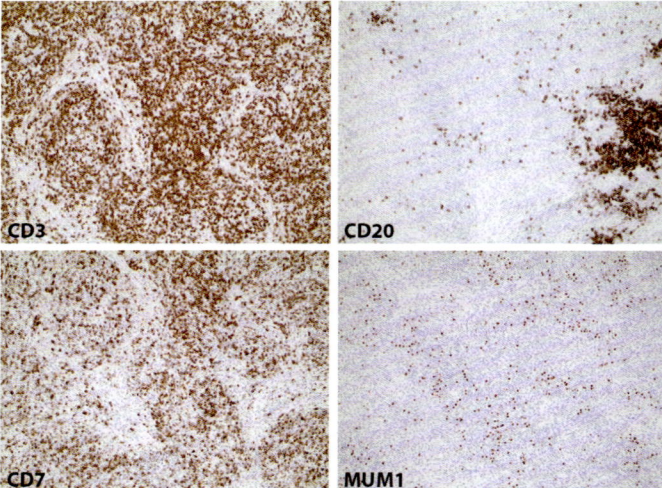

IMAGE 13.69 CAEBV is usually associated with loss of normal lymph node structure and replacement of B cells by a dense T cell infiltrate.

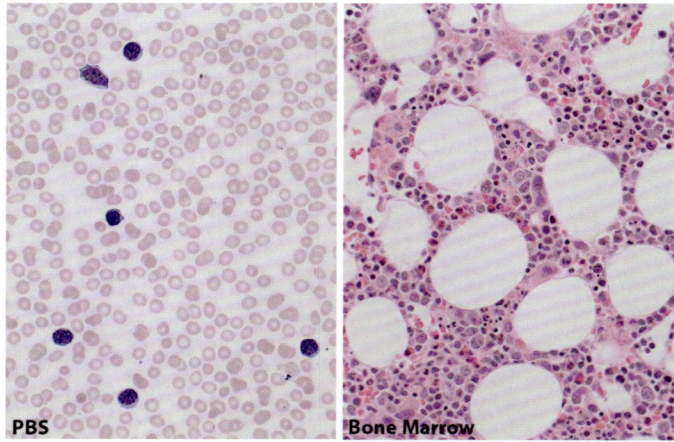

IMAGE 13.72 CAEBV may involve peripheral blood and bone marrow. Atypical lymphoid cells with variable morphology may be seen in peripheral blood. The bone marrow biopsy shows evidence of hemophagocytois (HLH) and extensive infiltration by EBV positive T cells (see next image).

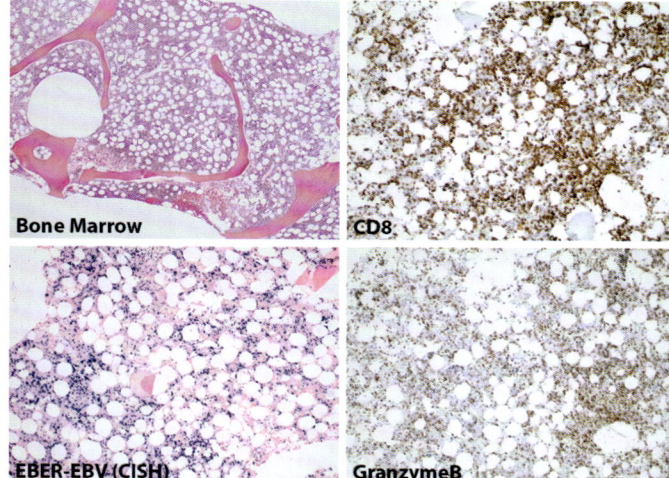

IMAGE 13.73 CAEBV is a systemic disease and may also involve bone marrow. This bone marrow biopsy shows a dense infiltrate of CD8 positive cytotoxic T cells and extensive infiltration by EBV positive T cells.

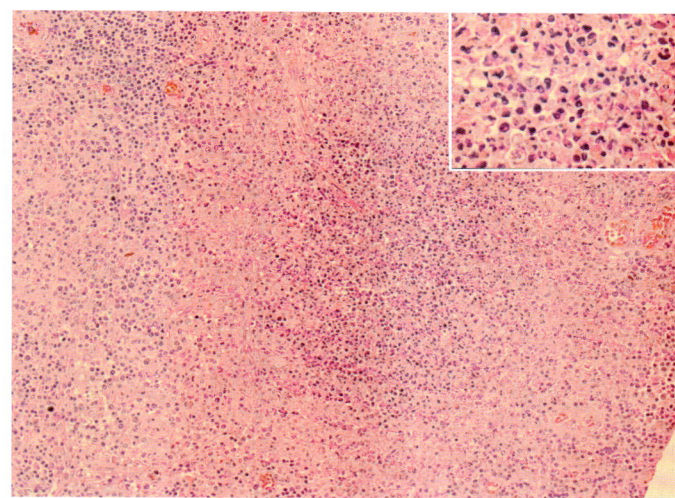

IMAGE 13.76 Neutrophilic necrotizing lymphadenitis: cat scratch disease.

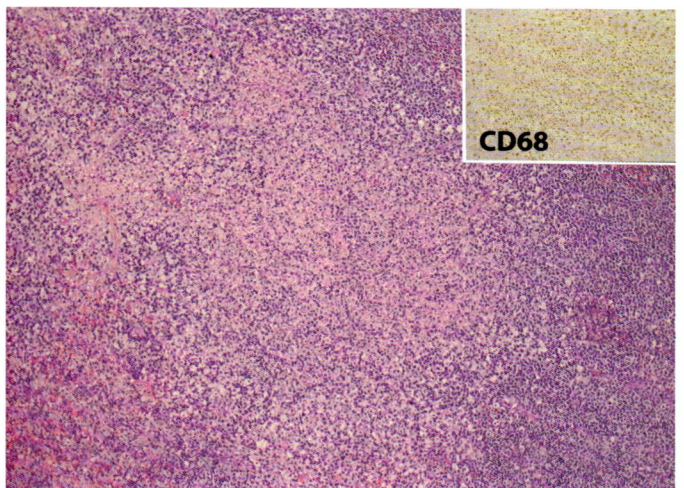

IMAGE 13.74 Necrotizing lymphadenitis. The image shows aneutrophilic inflammation and abundant karyorrhectic debris (Fujimata-Kikuchi disease).

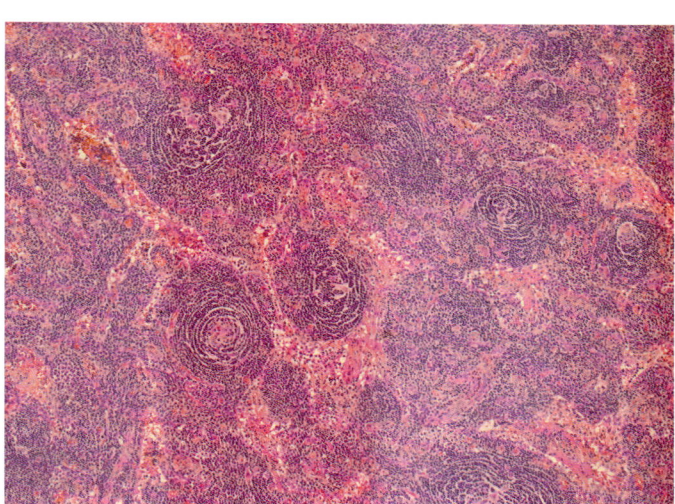

IMAGE 13.77 Castleman disease: hyaline vascular type (angiofollicular hyperplasia).

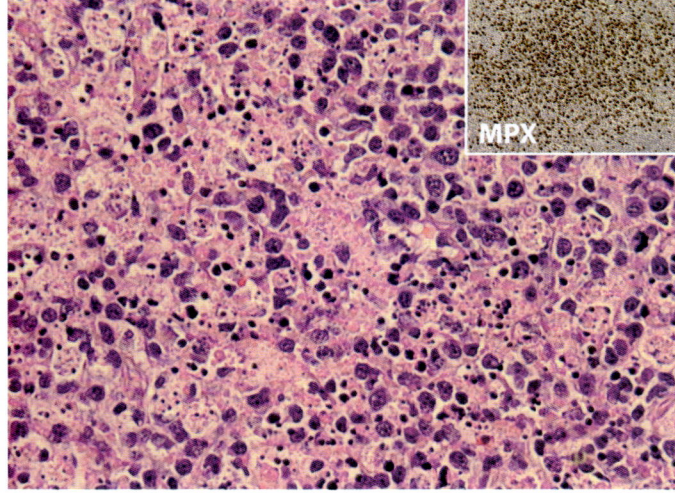

IMAGE 13.75 Histiocytic necrotizing lymphadenitis: Kikuchi-Fujimoto disease, the expression of myeloperoxidase by histiocytes.

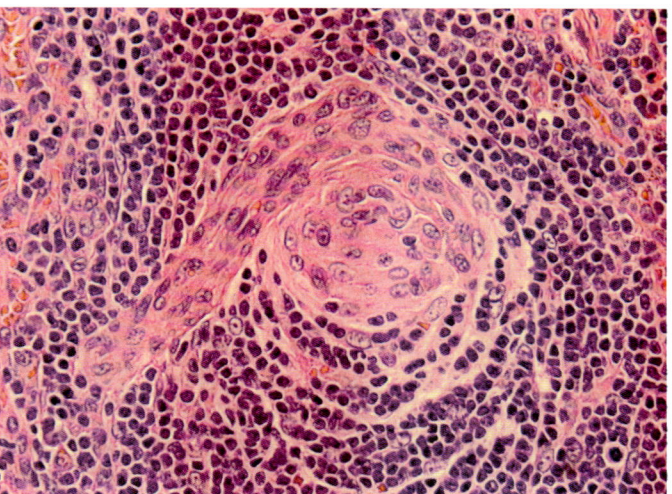

IMAGE 13.78 Castleman disease. The image displays germinal centers with vascular hyalinization, which shows "lollipop" pattern, and an expanded mantle zone with "onionskin" pattern.

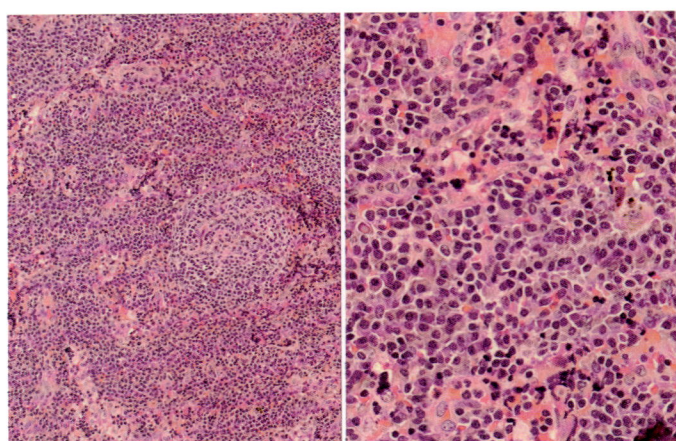

IMAGE 13.79 Castleman disease, plasmacytic variant: characterized by expanded sheets of plasma cells within interfollicular areas.

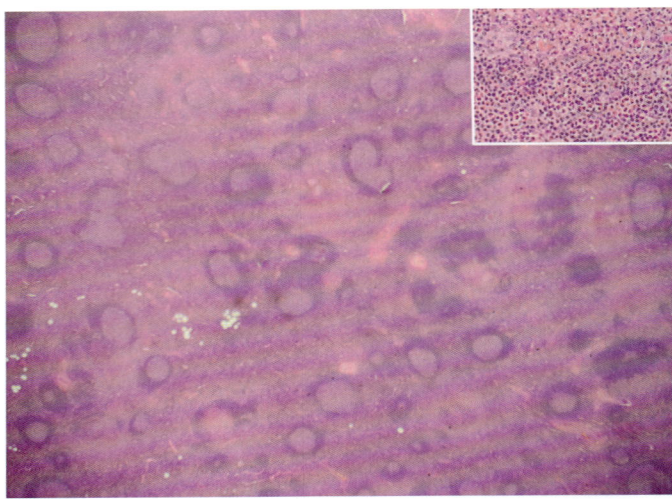

IMAGE 13.82 Kimura disease. The image shows follicular hyperplasia and expanded interfollicular areas with abundant eosinophils.

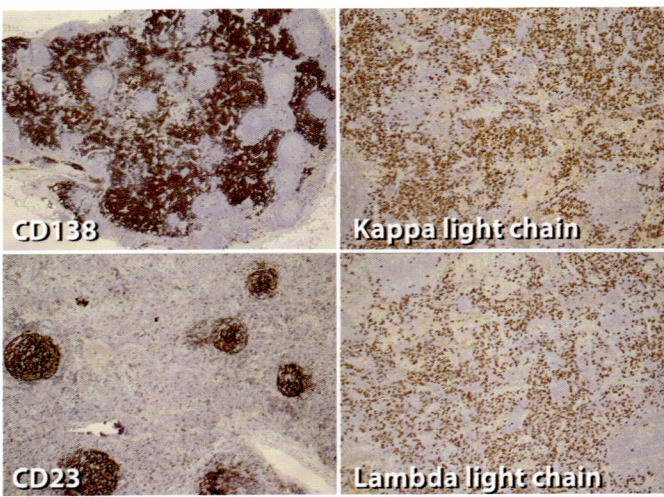

IMAGE 13.80 Castleman disease, plasmacytic variant: interfollicular polytypic plasma cells (CD138) and dense dendr tic meshwork (CD23).

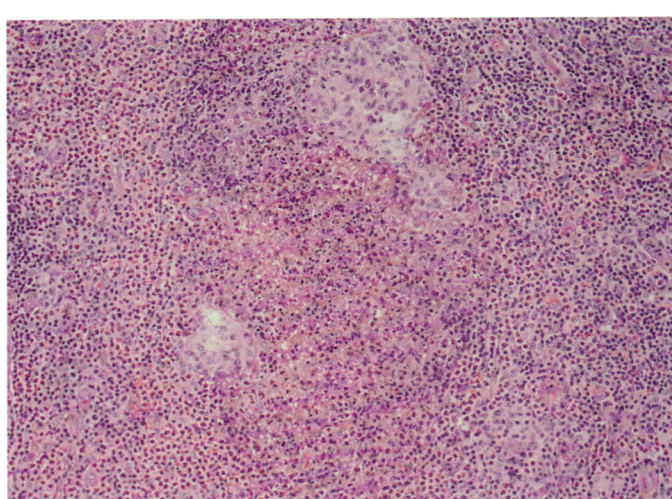

IMAGE 13.83 Kimura disease. Note the eosinophil rich granulomatous inflammation with epithelioid histiocytes and necrosis.

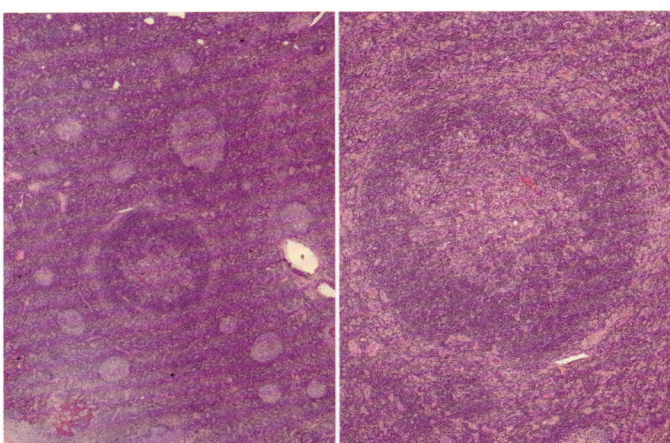

IMAGE 13.81 PTGC (progressive transformation of germinal centers). Note the expansion and extension of mantle cells into hyperplastic macrofollicles.

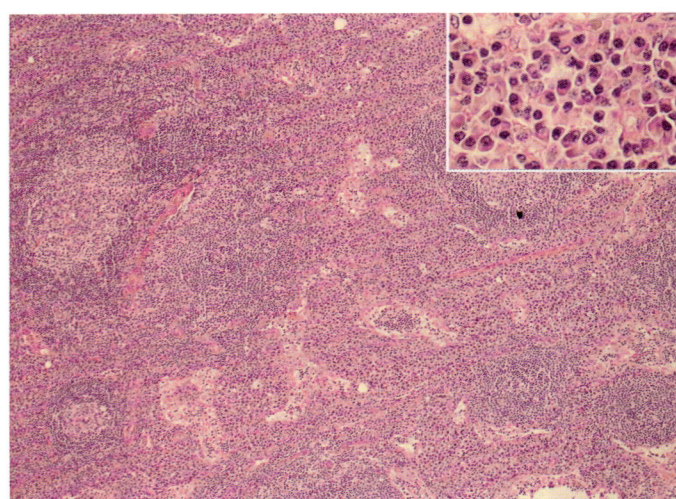

IMAGE 13.84 Reactive lymph node with plasmacytic proliferation. This may be seen with autoimmune disease, syphilis, or Castleman disease.

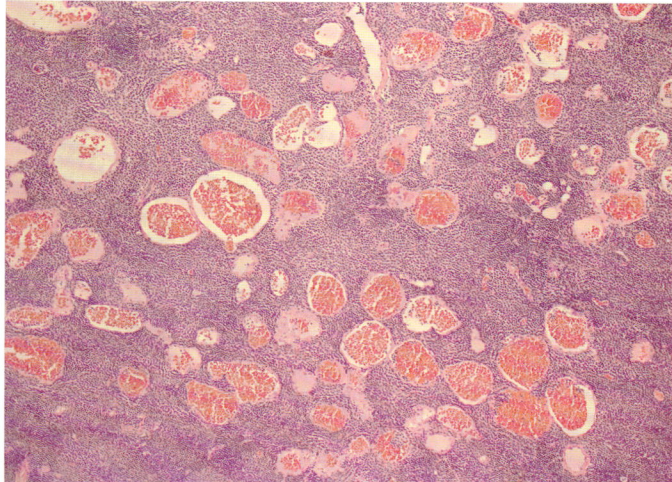

IMAGE 13.85 Lymph node involved by cavernous hemangioma. Background small lymphoid cells show monocytoid hyperplasia.

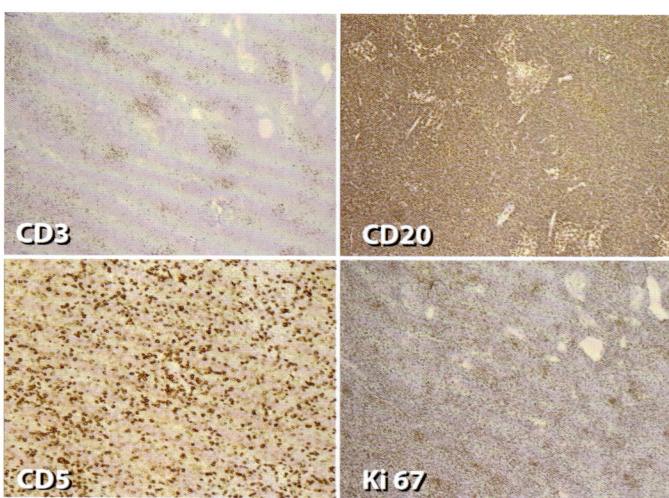

IMAGE 13.88 CLL/SLL. The proliferation centers are highlighted by dense T cell infiltration (CD3), higher proliferation index (Ki 67), and dim CD5.

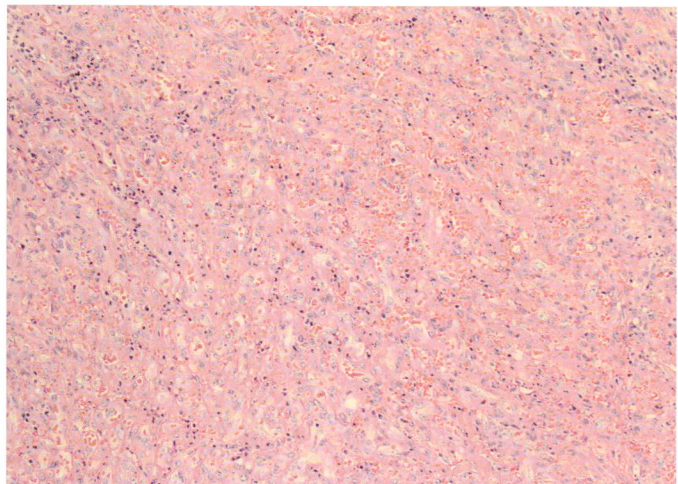

IMAGE 13.86 Lymph node with extensive involvement by Kaposi sarcoma, HIV associated (haphazard proliferation of arborizing vessels).

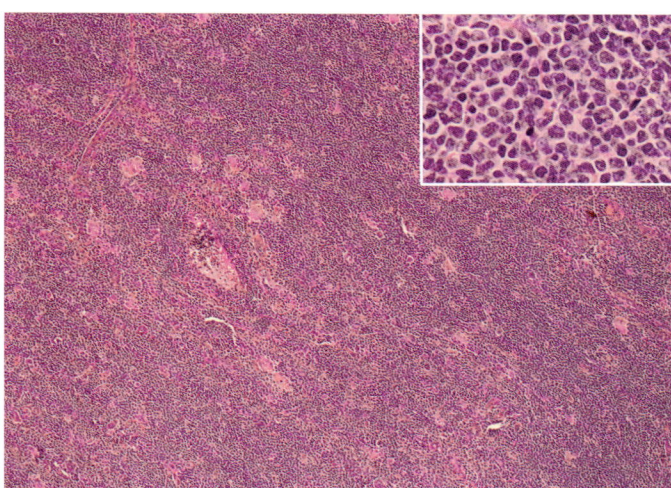

IMAGE 13.89 MCL (mantle cell lymphoma). The image shows small lymphoid cells with irregular nuclear features (notched cells), pink histiocytes, and patchy sclerosis.

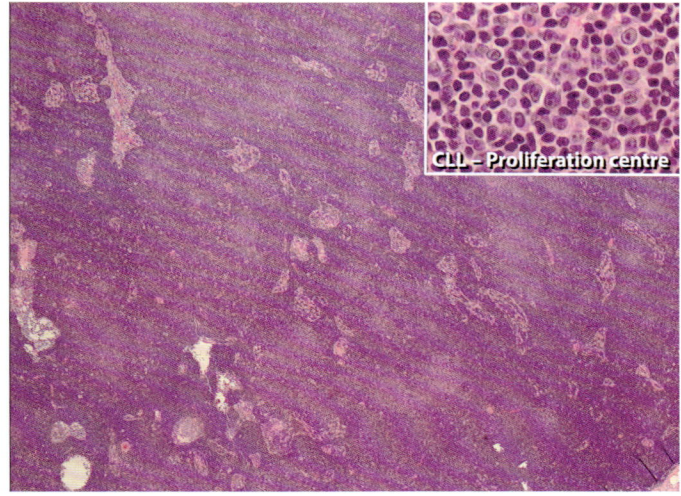

IMAGE 13.87 CLL/SLL (chronic lymphocytic leukemia/small lymphocytic lymphoma). Note the pale proliferation centers with paraimmunoblasts.

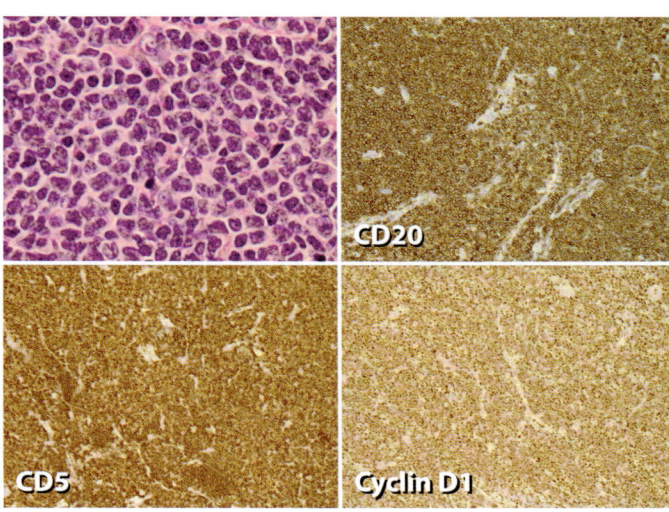

IMAGE 13.90 MCL. The neoplastic B cells are positive for CD20 and CD5 and show nuclear expression of CyclinD1.

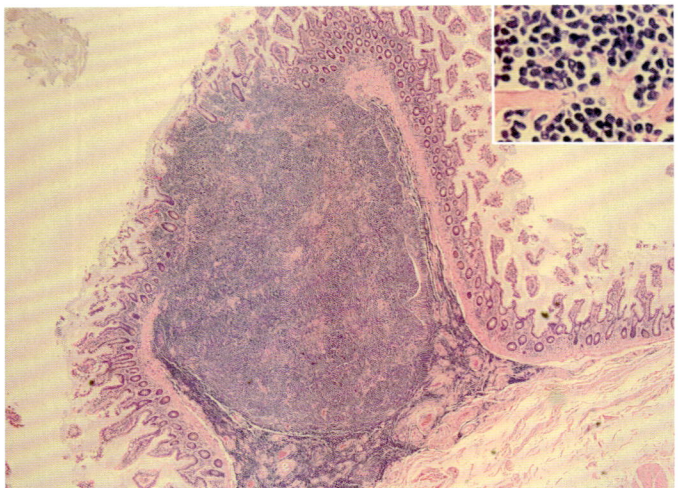

IMAGE 13.91 MCL involving small intestinal wall (lymphomatoid polyposis).

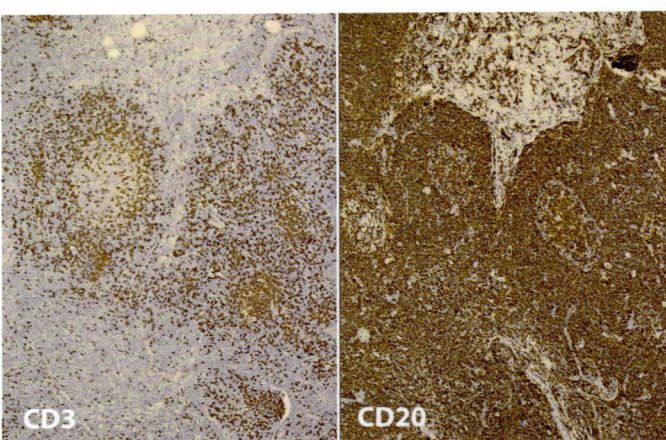

IMAGE 13.94 Nodal marginal zone lymphoma showing abnormal follicles with expanded marginal zones positive for CD20+ B cells.

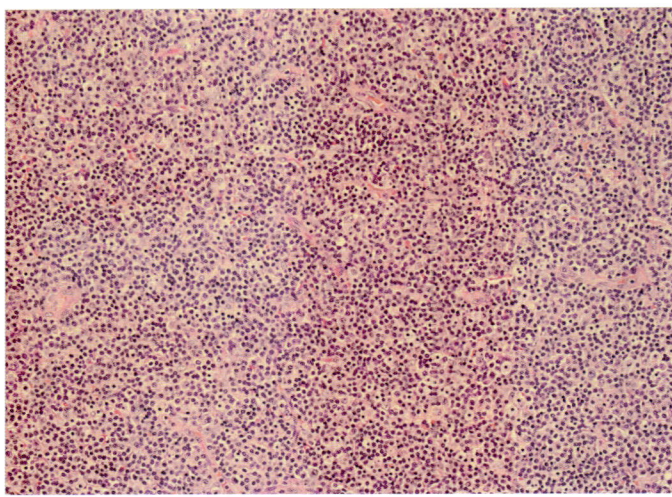

IMAGE 13.92 Nodal marginal zone lymphoma. Note the lack of normal nodal architecture and diffuse lymphoid infiltrate of small lymphoid cells.

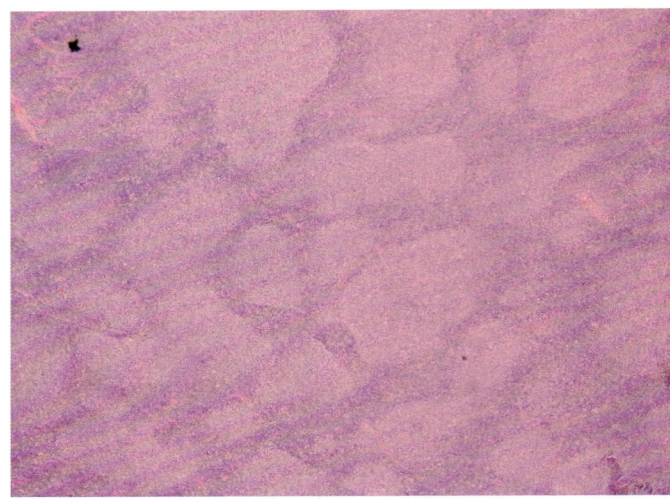

IMAGE 13.95 Follicular lymphoma. Note the atypical follicular proliferation with expanded germinal centers and loss of mantle zones.

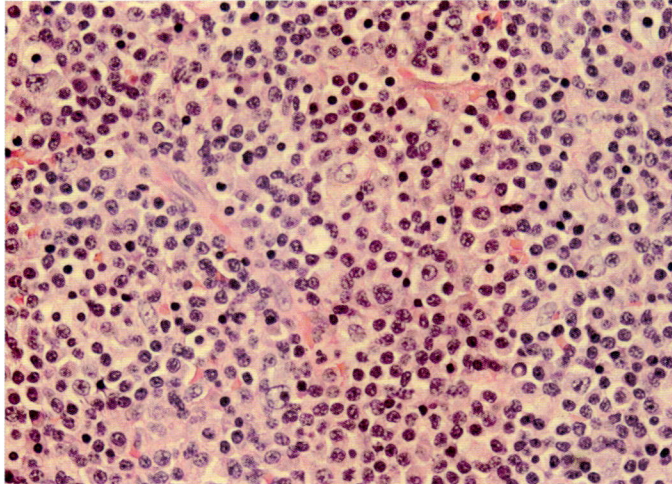

IMAGE 13.93 Nodal marginal zone lymphoma. The image shows small lymphoid cells with pink cytoplasm, monocytoid features, and plasmacytic differentiation.

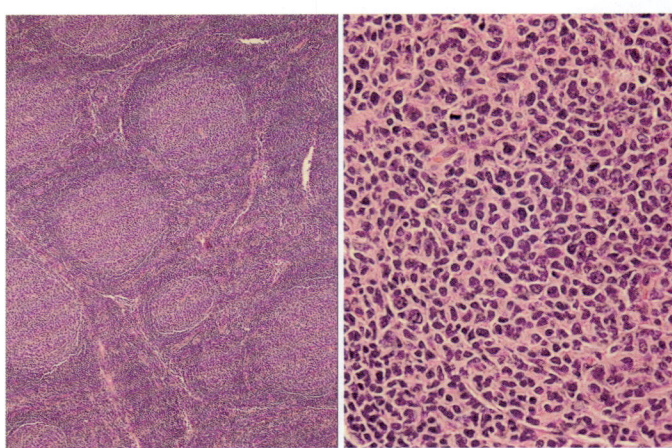

IMAGE 13.96 Follicular lymphoma. Note the atypical follicles with expanded germinal centers that are predominantly composed of centrocytes.

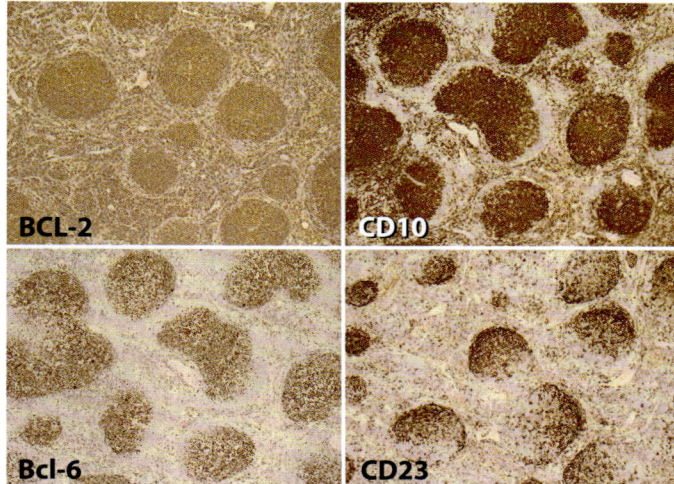

IMAGE 13.97 Follicular lymphoma with expanded germinal centers, which are Bcl-6+/CD10+/CD23+ and aberrantly express BCL-2.

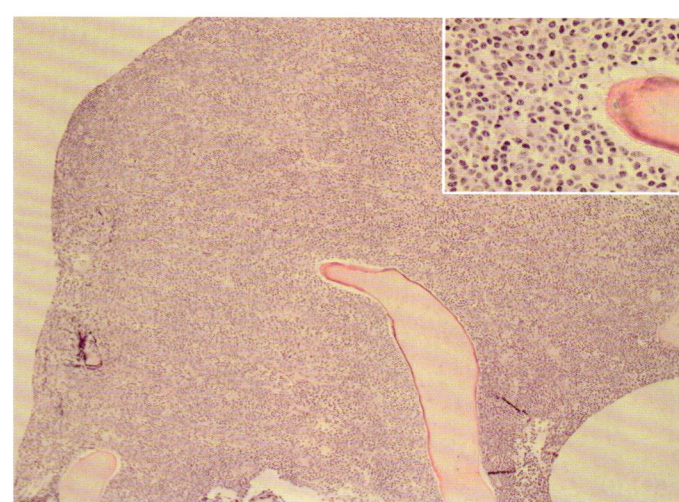

IMAGE 13.100 Lymphoplasmacytic lymphoma. The lymphoid infiltrate is composed of small lymphoid, lymphoplasmacytoid, and plasma cells.

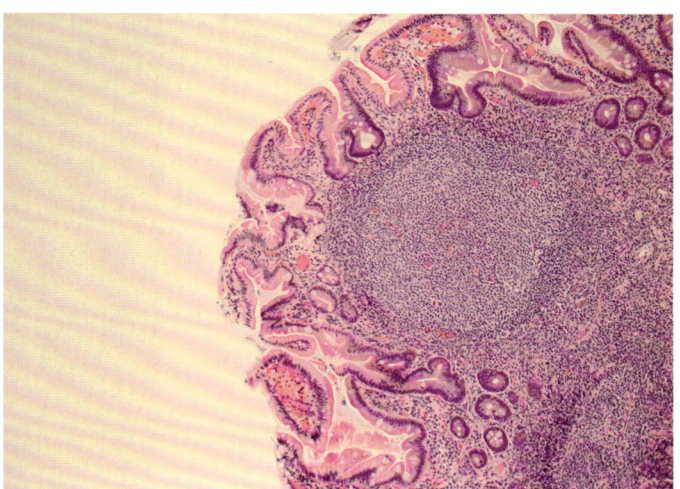

IMAGE 13.98 Intestinal follicular lymphoma.

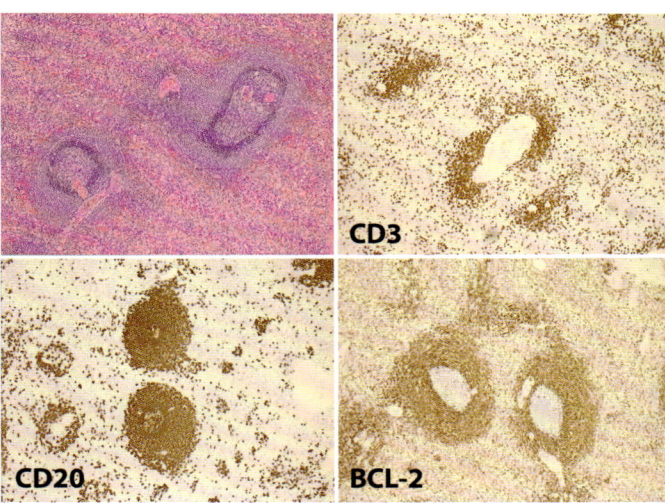

IMAGE 13.101 Splenic marginal zone lymphoma with prominent white pulps highlighted by CD20 and BCL-2. No red pulp involvement is noted.

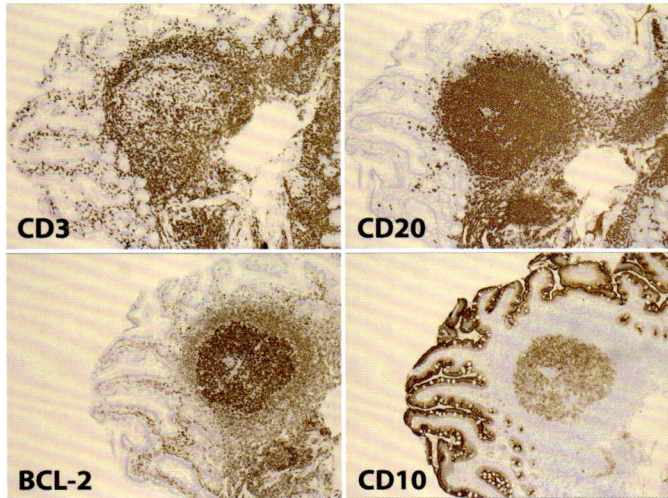

IMAGE 13.99 Intestinal follicular lymphoma showing neoplastic germinal centers (CD20+) with expression of CD10 and BCL-2.

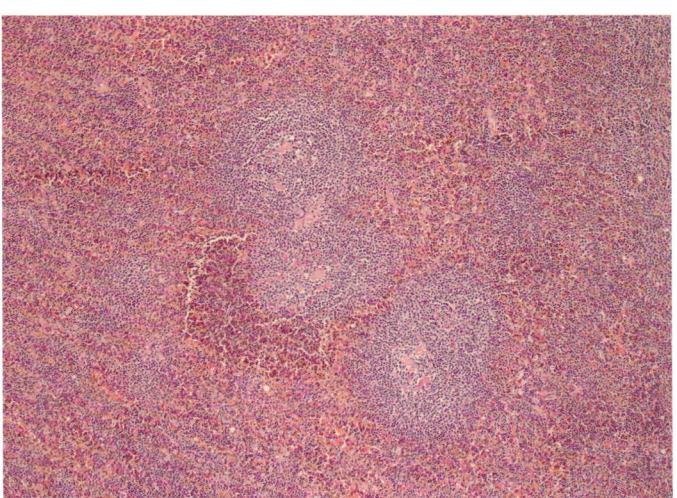

IMAGE 13.102 Splenic diffuse red pulp small B-cell lymphoma. The image shows red pulp infiltration by small lymphoid cells and mildly prominent white pulps.

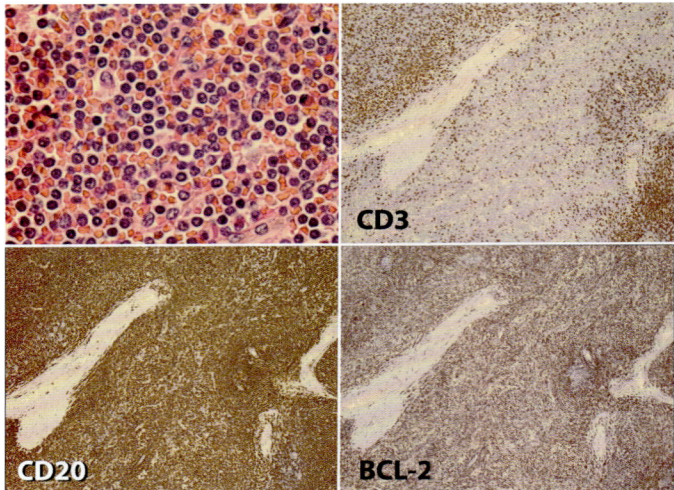

IMAGE 13.103 Splenic diffuse red pulp small B-cell lymphoma; red pulp infiltrated by BCL-2 positive B cells (CD20+).

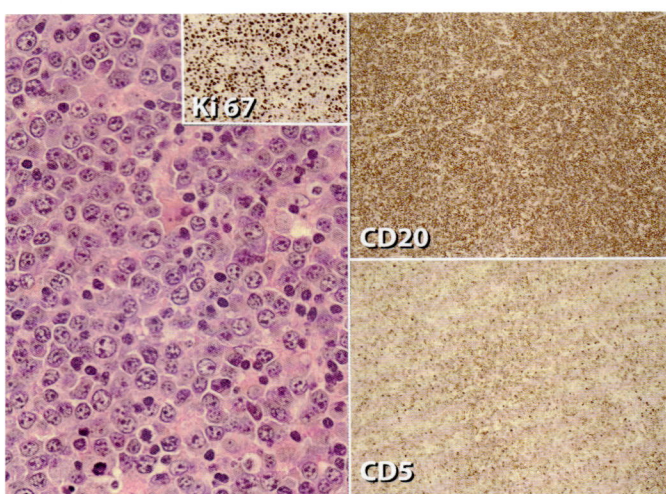

IMAGE 13.106 DLBCL, CD5 positive (variable and dim).

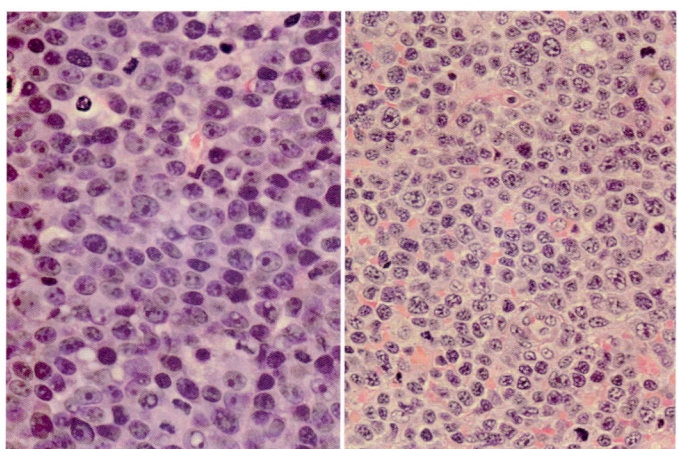

IMAGE 13.104 DLBCL (diffuse large B-cell lymphoma), NOS, cytomorphological variants; immunoblastic (left) and centroblastic (right) variants.

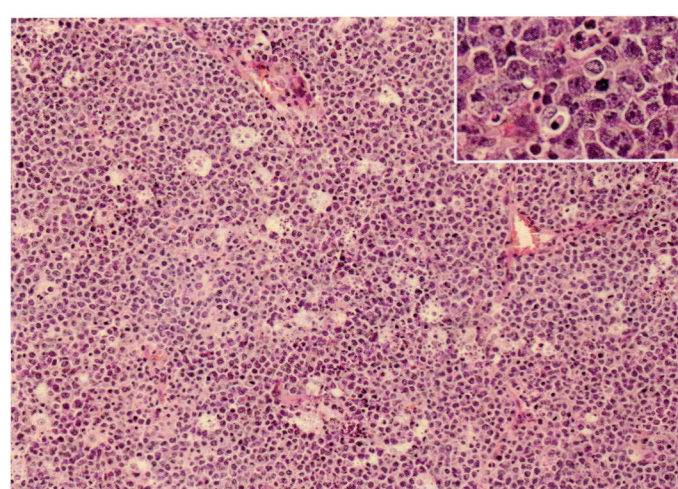

IMAGE 13.107 High grade B-cell lymphoma, NOS.

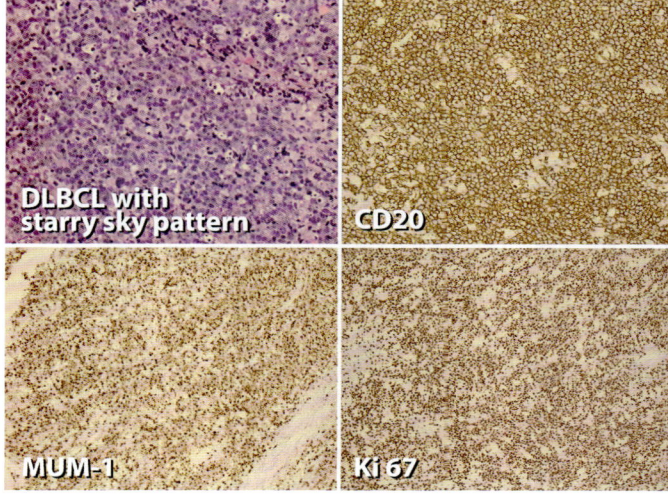

IMAGE 13.105 DLBCL with starry sky pattern anc ABC subtype (MUM1+) and 80% Ki 67 proliferation index.

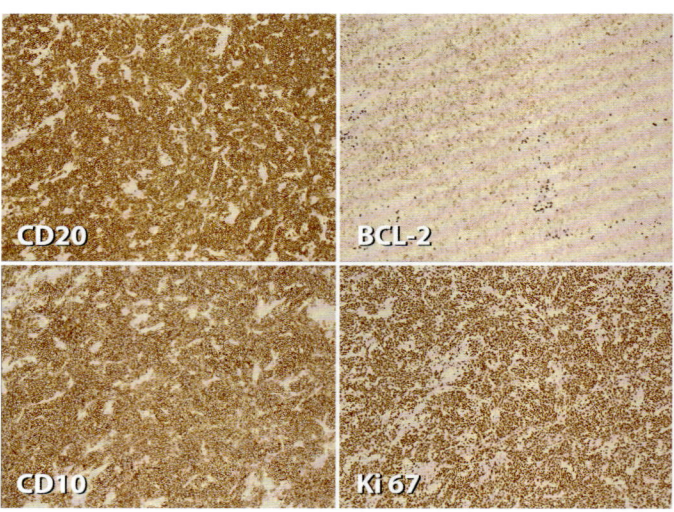

IMAGE 13.108 High grade B-cell lymphoma, NOS (Burkitt-like immunophenotype).

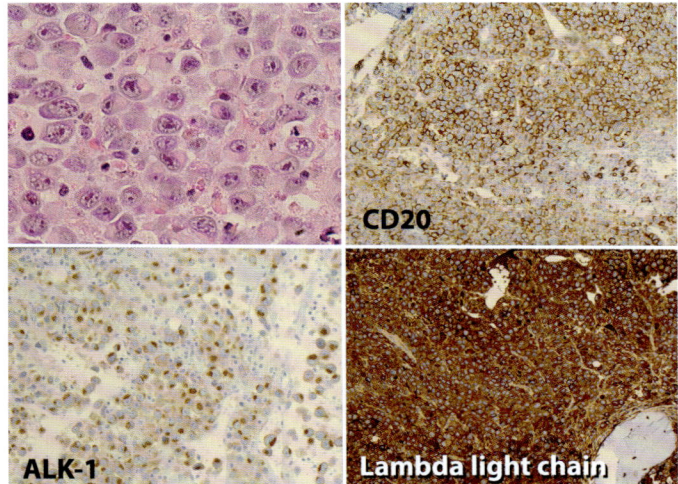

IMAGE 13.109 ALK-positive DLBCL.

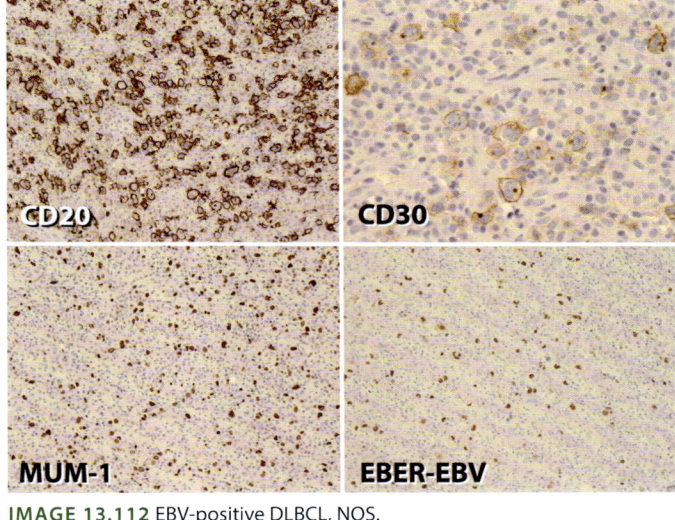

IMAGE 13.112 EBV-positive DLBCL, NOS.

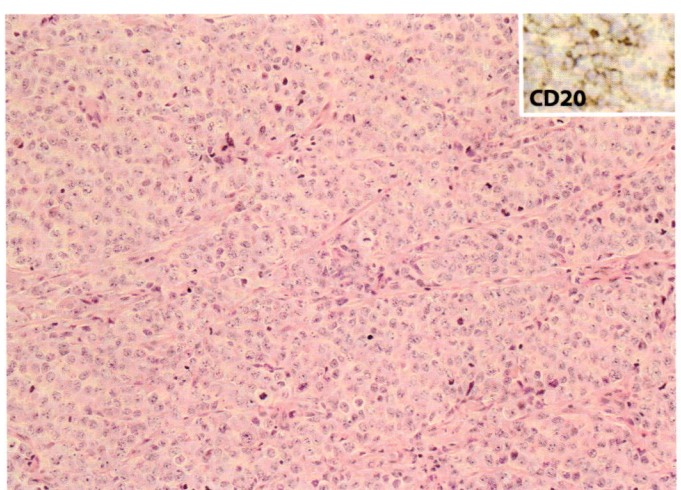

IMAGE 13.110 Primary mediastinal large B-cell lymphoma.

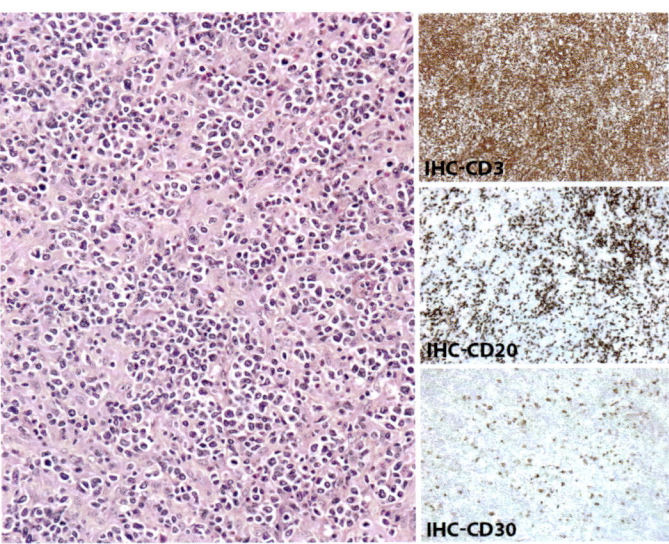

IMAGE 13.113 T cell/histiocyte-rich large B-cell lymphoma is a specific subtype of DLBCL with numerous T cells in background. Some cases of TCHRB-CL arising in the background of NLP-HL may express CD30 (30%).

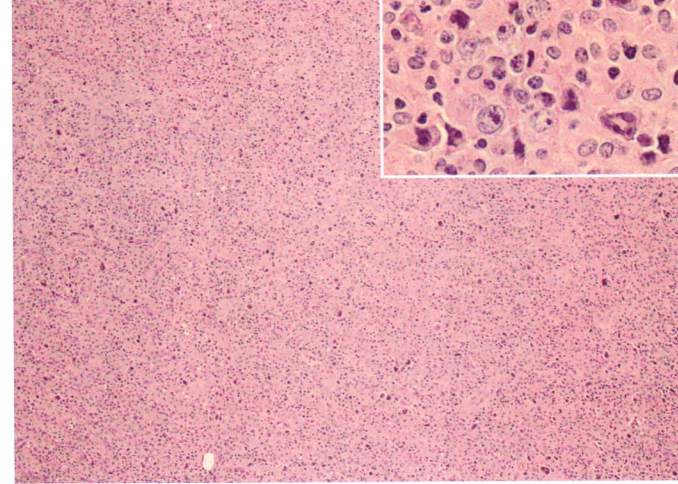

IMAGE 13.111 EBV-positive DLBCL, NOS.

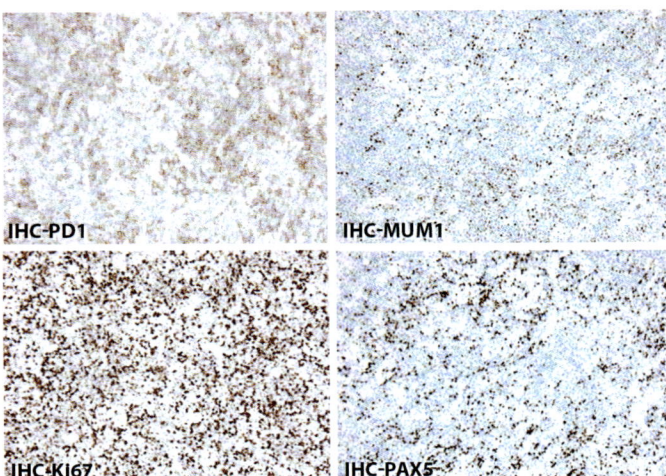

IMAGE 13.114 TCHRB-CL cases are defined by the presence of < 10% large B cells in a T cell/histiocyte rich background. T follicular helper cells with the expression of PD1 may be also seen.

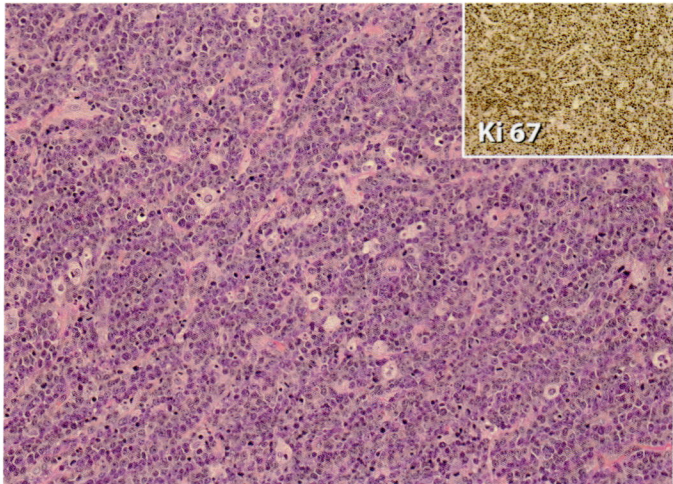

IMAGE 13.115 Classical Burkitt lymphoma, starry sky pattern with monotonous population of intermediate size cells.

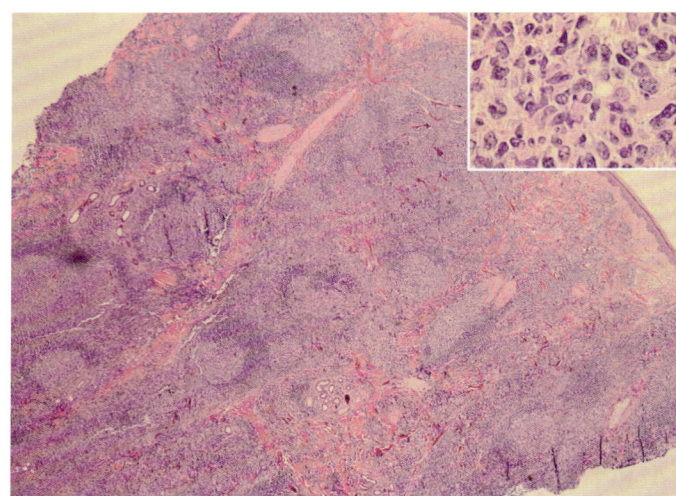

IMAGE 13.118 Primary cutaneous follicular center lymphoma. Germinal centers are composed of intermediate size centrocytes.

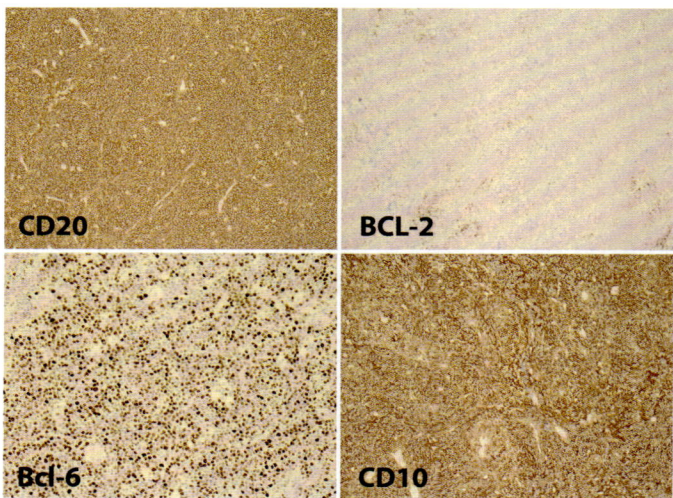

IMAGE 13.116 Burkitt lymphoma with classical immunophenotype.

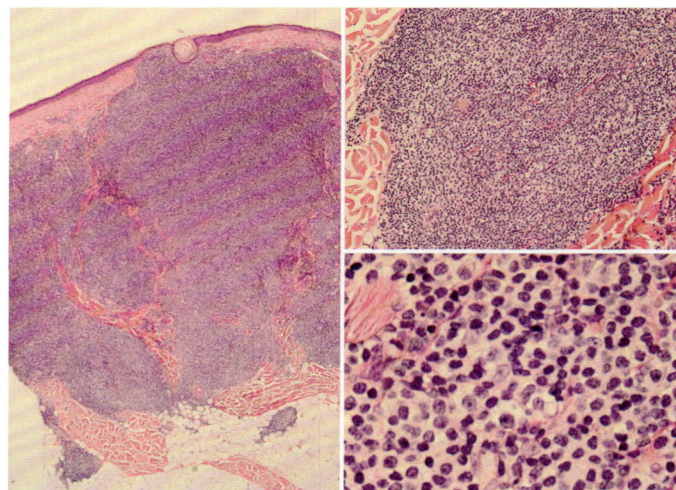

IMAGE 13.119 Primary cutaneous marginal zone lymphoma. Neoplastic B cells demonstrate monocytoid features.

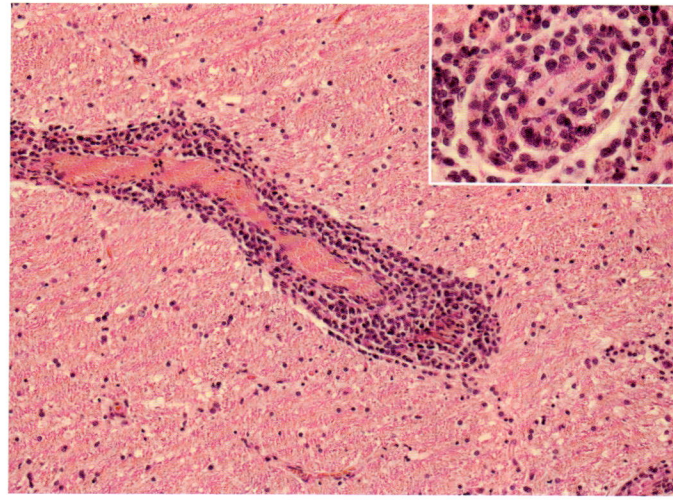

IMAGE 13.117 Primary central nervous system DLBCL with characteristic perivascular pattern.

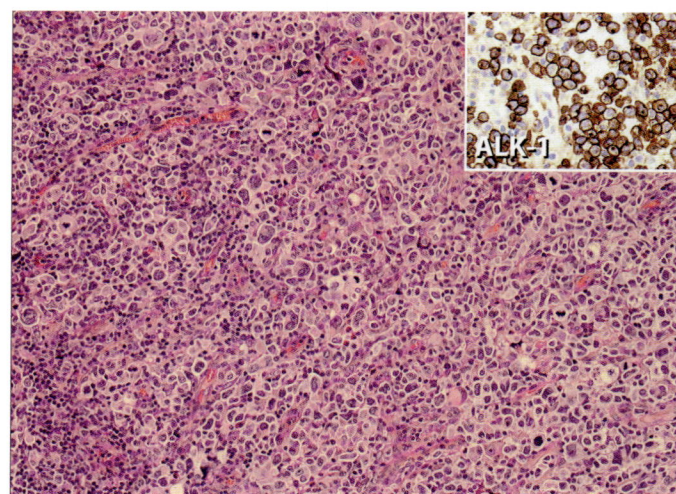

IMAGE 13.120 Anaplastic large cell lymphoma-ALK-1 positive. The image shows large hallmark cells with frequent perinuclear eosinophilic region/inclusion.

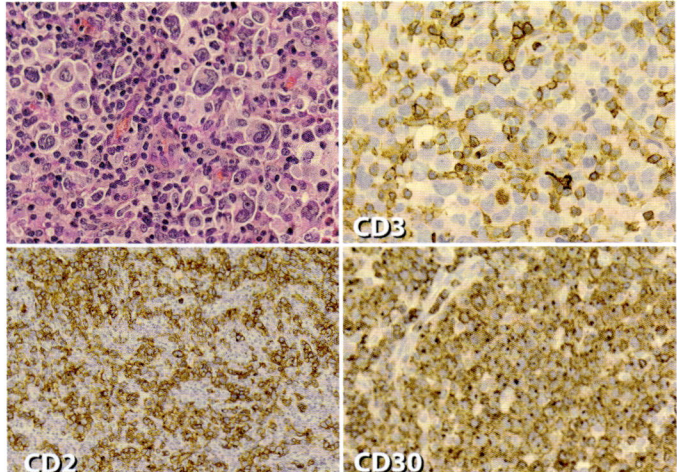

IMAGE 13.121 Anaplastic large cell lymphoma-ALK-1 positive. The neoplastic cells are negative for CD3, but positive for CD2 and CD30.

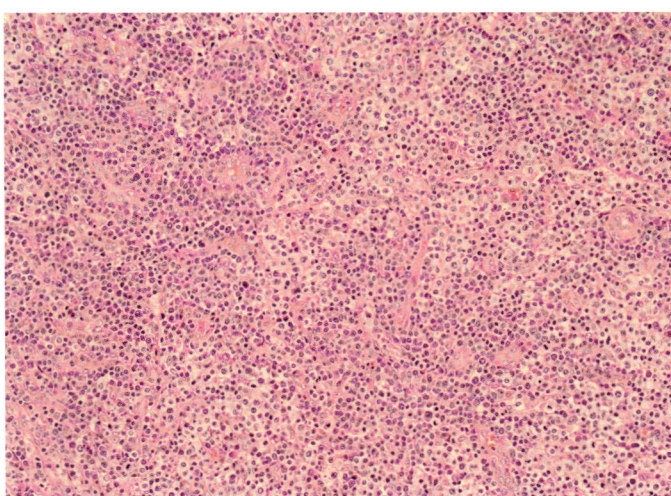

IMAGE 13.124 Peripheral T-cell lymphoma (PTCL) displaying neoplastic T cells with clear cytoplasm.

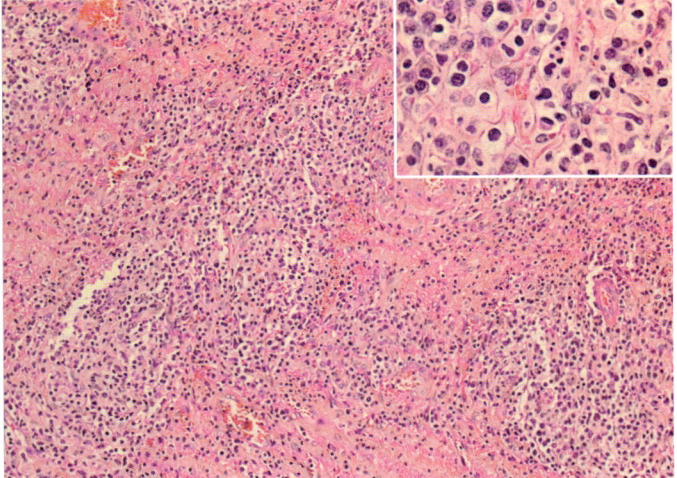

IMAGE 13.122 AITL (angioimmunoblastic T-cell lymphoma). The image shows neoplastic T cells with clear cytoplasm and prominent vascular proliferation of HEVs.

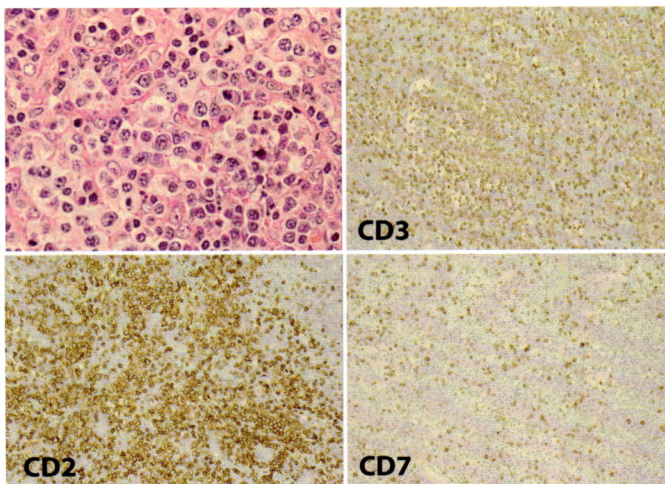

IMAGE 13.125 Peripheral T-cell lymphoma. Note the neoplastic T cells with clear cytoplasm and aberrant loss of CD2 (partial) and CD7.

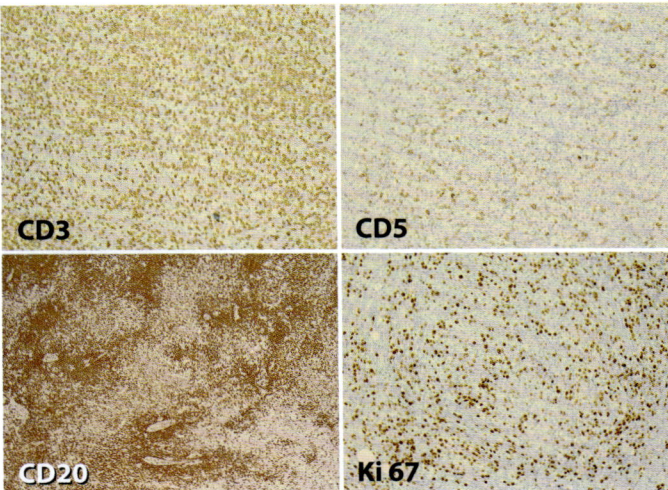

IMAGE 13.123 AITL with loss of CD5 and perivascular arrangements of B cells (CD20 positive).

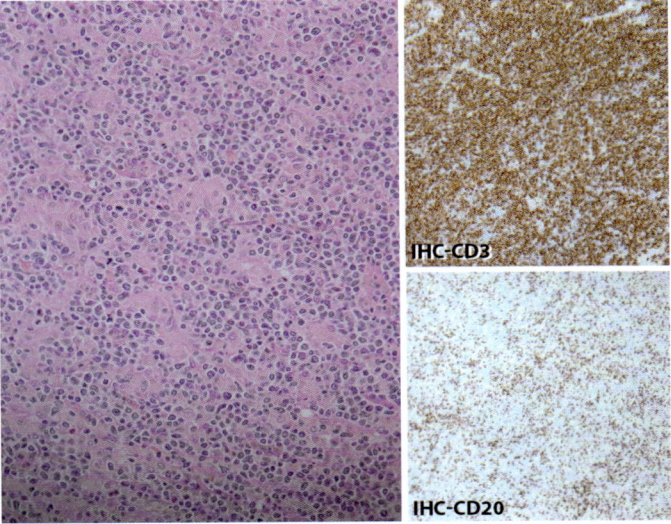

IMAGE 13.126 PTCL with TFH phenotype is a subset of the peripheral T-cell lymphomas, NOS which show a T follicular helper (TFH) cell phenotype.

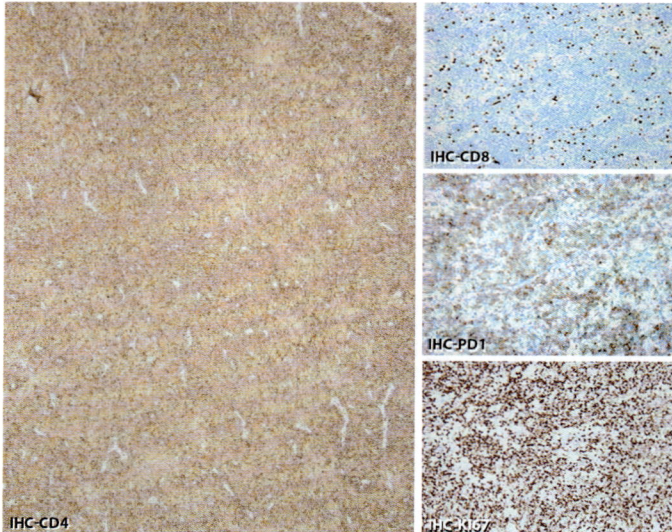

IMAGE 13.127 PTCL with TFH phenotype. Neoplastic T cells are mainly composed of CD4 positive cells with expression of PD1 (T follicular helper cell marker).

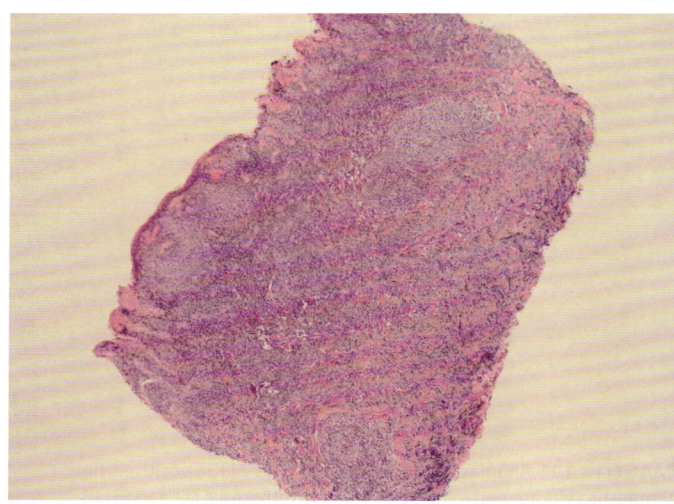

IMAGE 13.130 Lymphomatoid papulosis, characterized by scattered large neoplastic cells that appear in a background of small lymphoid cells.

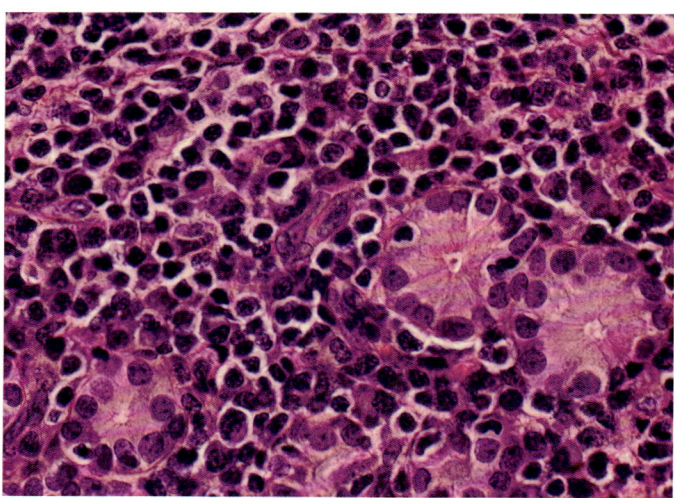

IMAGE 13.128 NK/T-cell lymphoma, nasal type. The image shows neoplastic T cells with dense chromatin and irregular nuclear outlines.

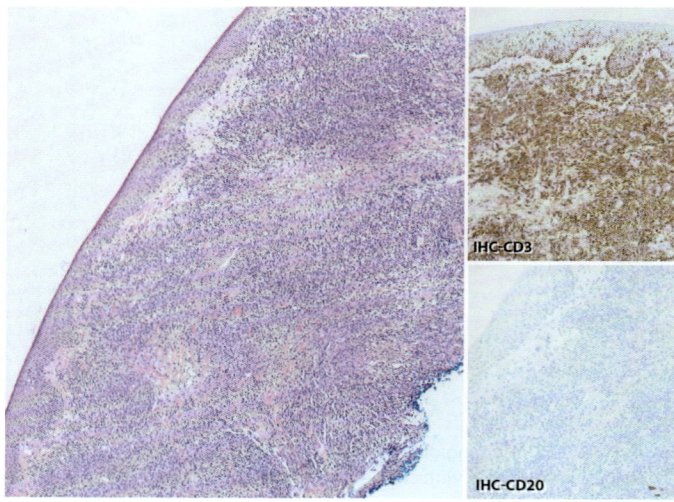

IMAGE 13.131 Lymphomatoid papulosis with DUSP22-IRF4 rearrangement. CD3 immunostain highlights both dermal and intraepidermal infiltrate of atypical lymphoid cells (CD4/CD8 negative).

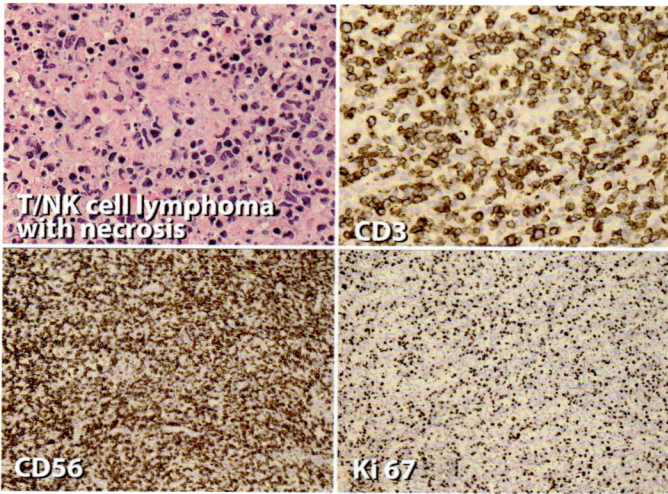

IMAGE 13.129 NK/T-cell lymphoma, nasal type. The neoplastic T cells demonstrate tumor cell necrosis and are positive for CD3 and CD56.

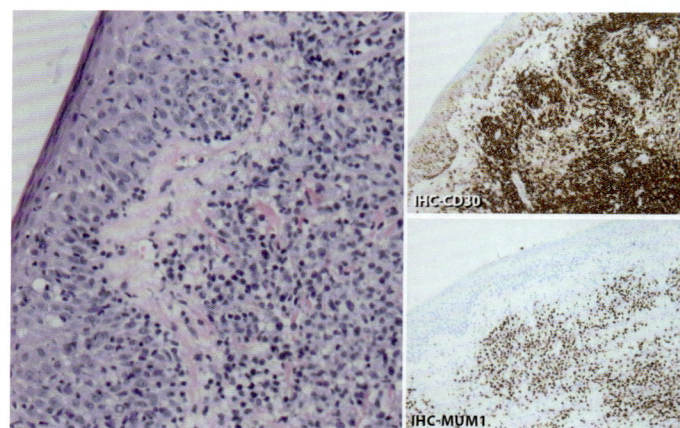

IMAGE 13.132 Lymphomatoid papulosis with DUSP22-IRF4 rearrangement. Both dermal and intraepidermal components are CD30 positive. Dermal component demonstrate nuclear expression of MUM1.

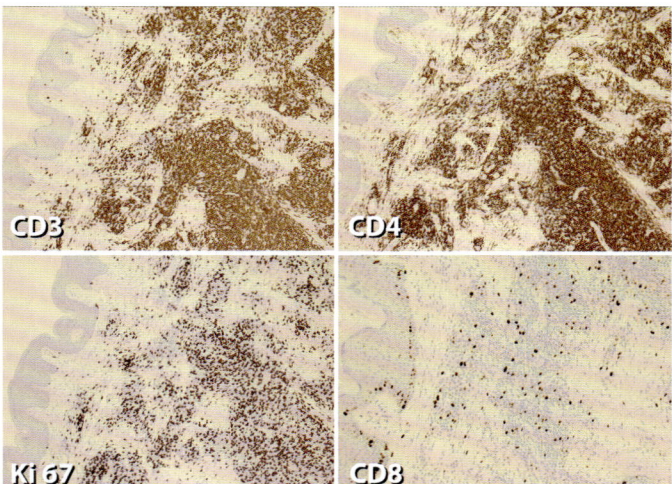

IMAGE 13.133 Primary cutaneous CD4+ small/medium T-cell lymphoproliferative disorder, showing low Ki 67 proliferation index.

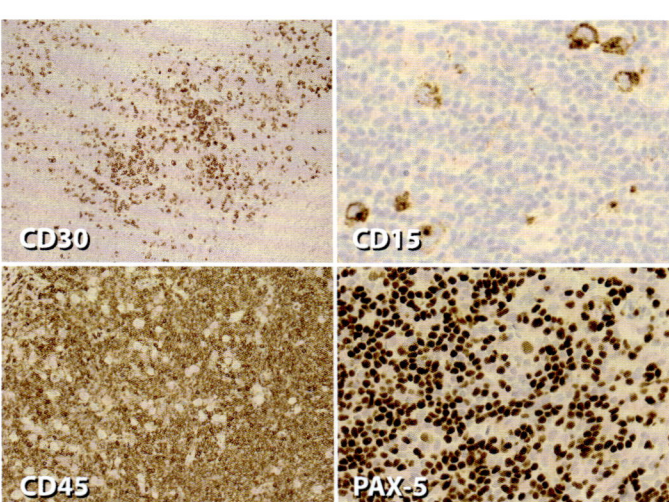

IMAGE 13.136 Classical Hodgkin lymphoma. The Reed-Sternberg cells express CD30, CD15, and PAX5 (dim) but are negative for CD45 and CD20.

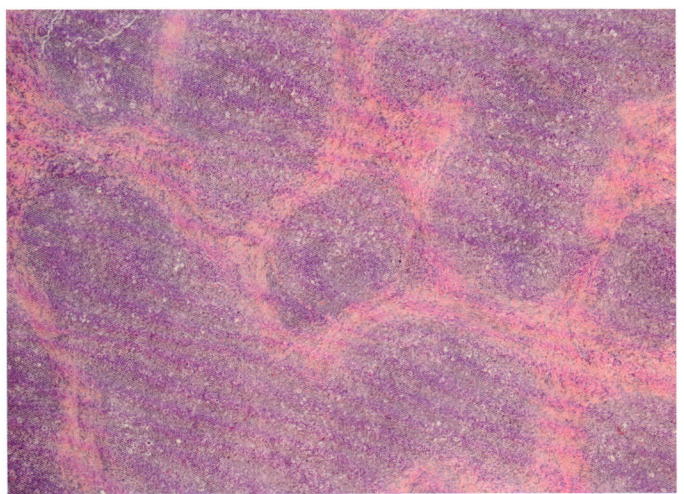

IMAGE 13.134 Nodular sclerosis classical Hodgkin lymphoma. Note the nodular proliferation with thick fibrous tissue extended into lymph node.

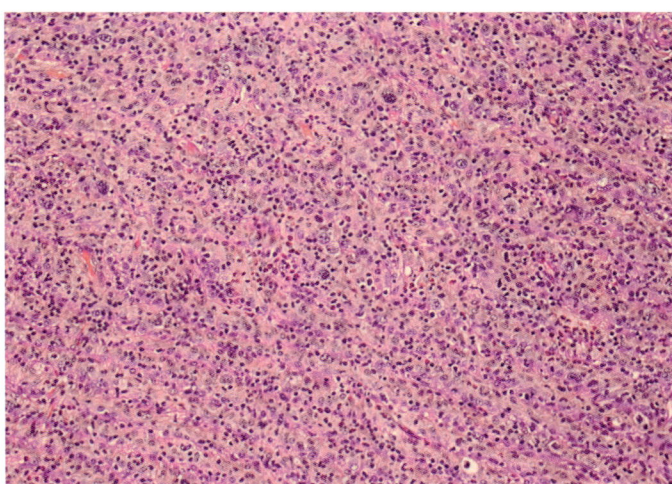

IMAGE 13.137 Mixed cellularity classical Hodgkin lymphoma. Note the abundant Reed-Sternberg cells in an inflammatory/eosinophilic background.

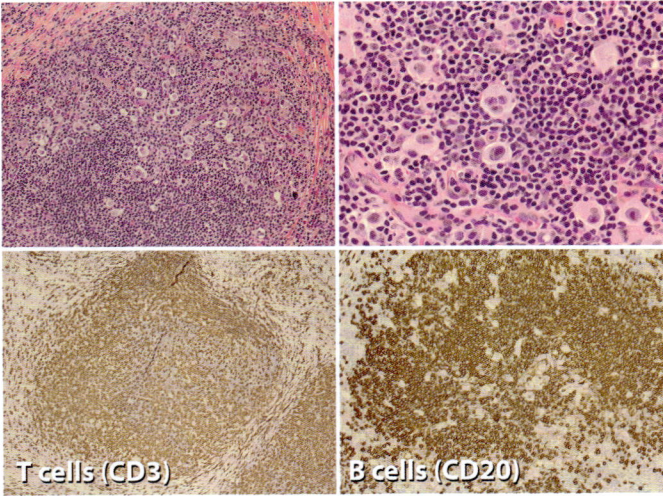

IMAGE 13.135 Nodular sclerosis classical Hodgkin lymphoma. The image shows Reed-Sternberg cells (CD20 negative) in the background of reactive T and B cells.

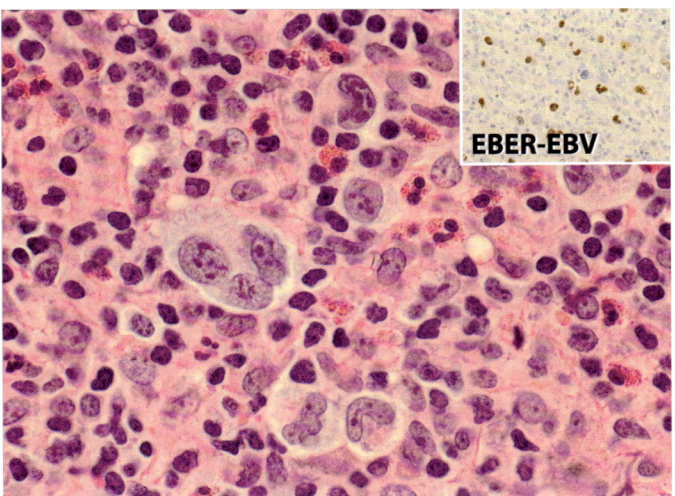

IMAGE 13.138 Mixed cellularity classical Hodgkin lymphoma. Reed-Sternberg cells are frequently positive for EBER-EBV by in situ hybridization.

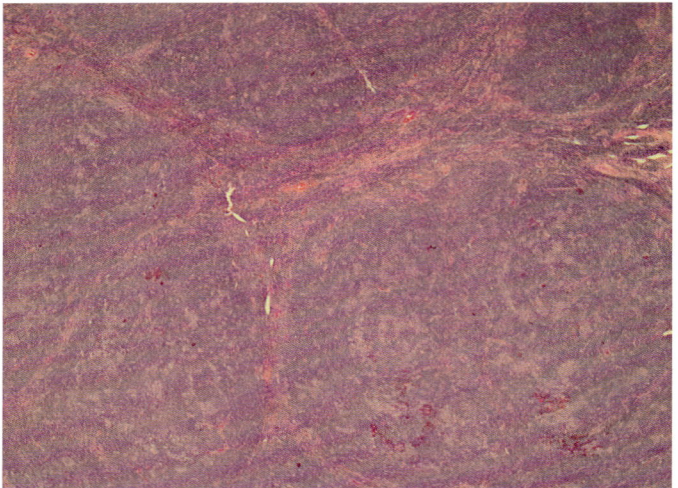

IMAGE 13.139 Nodular lymphocyte predominant Hodgkin lymphoma (NLP-HL). Note the lymph node with a macronodular pattern.

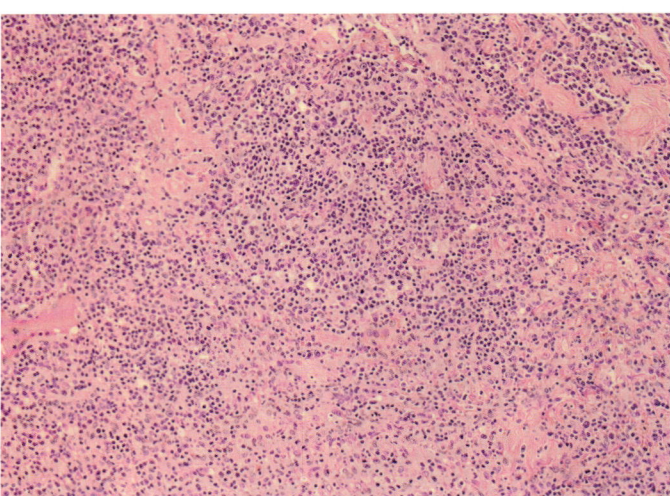

IMAGE 13.142 PTLD (posttransplant lymphoproliferative disorder), polymorphic type, defined by mixed lymphoid/plasmacytic proliferation.

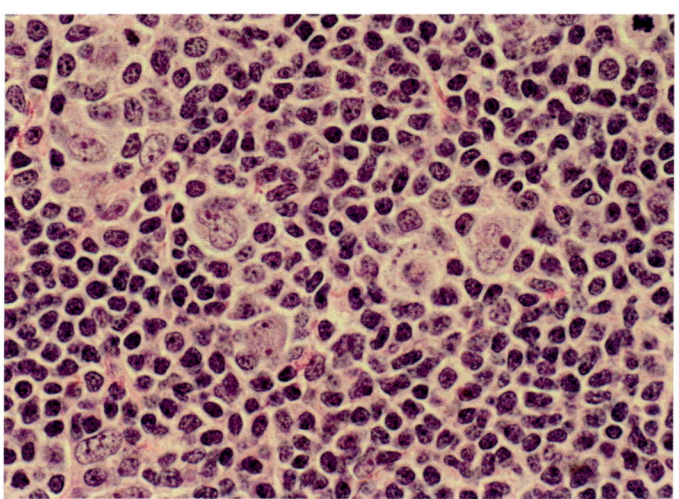

IMAGE 13.140 NLP-HL showing characteristic L&H cells surrounded by standby T lymphocytes.

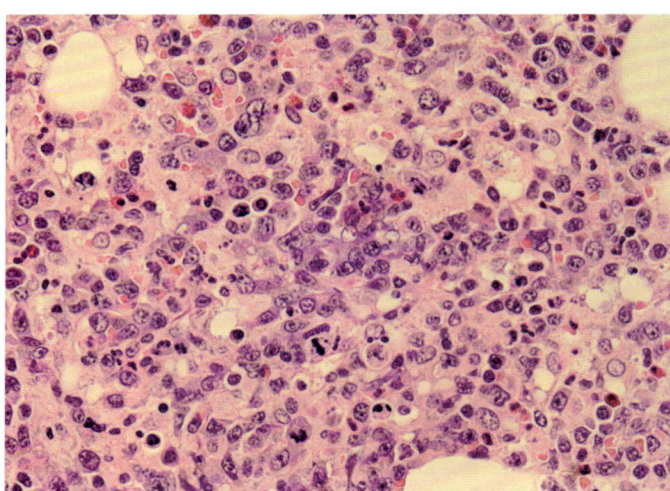

IMAGE 13.143 PTLD, polymorphic type, showing mixed lymphoid and plasmacytic infiltrate.

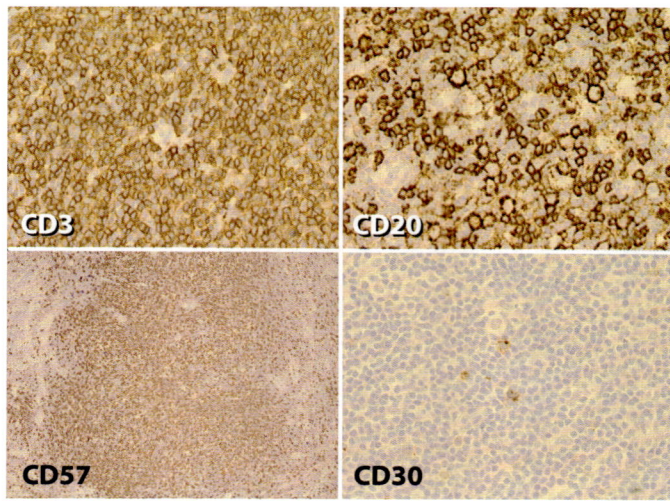

IMAGE 13.141 NLP-HL. The image shows CD20 positive L&H cells in a background of standby T cells (CD57+ and PD1+).

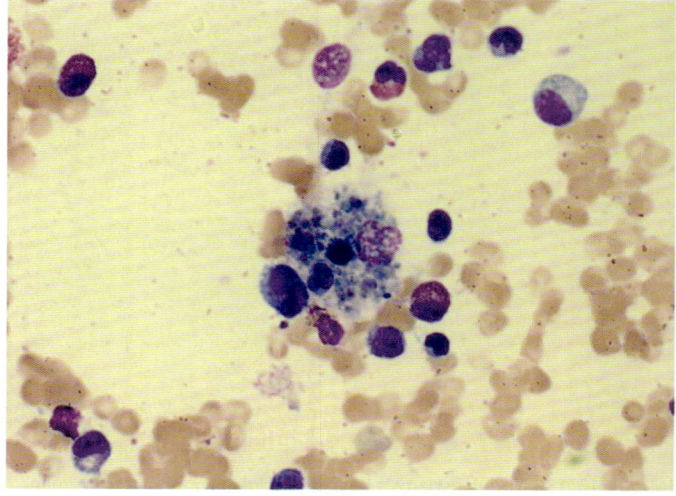

IMAGE 13.144 Hemophagocytic syndrome. Marrow aspirate reveals a histiocyte with ingested intracytoplasmic hematopoietic elements.

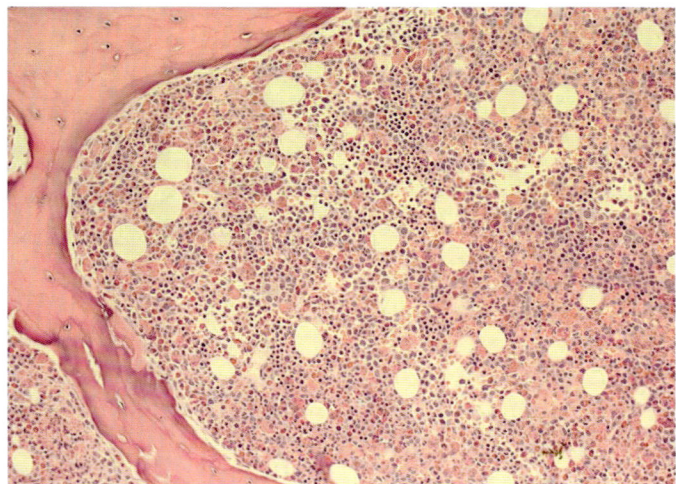

IMAGE 13.145 Hemophagocytic syndrome. Marrow biopsy reveals histiocytes with intracytoplasmic hematopoietic elements.

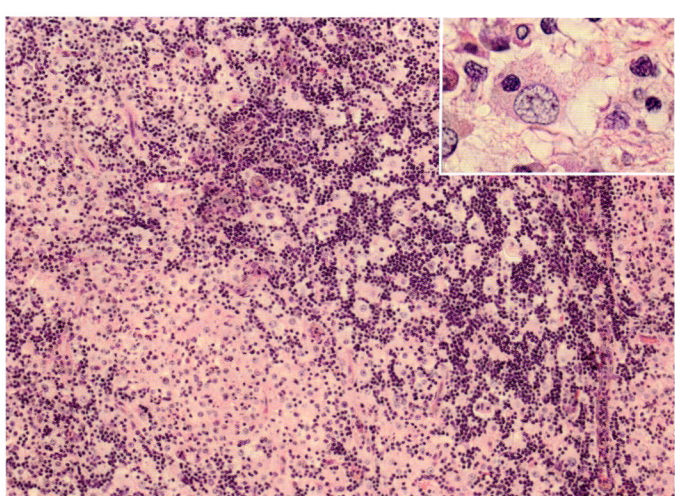

IMAGE 13.148 Rosai-Dorfman disease. The image shows a lymph node with histiocytic proliferation and lymphophagocytosis (emperipolesis).

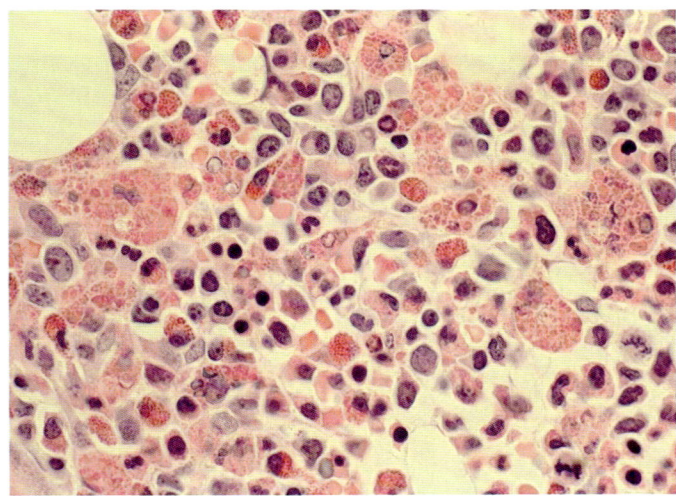

IMAGE 13.146 Hemophagocytic syndrome. Marrow biopsy reveals frequent histiocytes with intracytoplasmic hematopoietic elements.

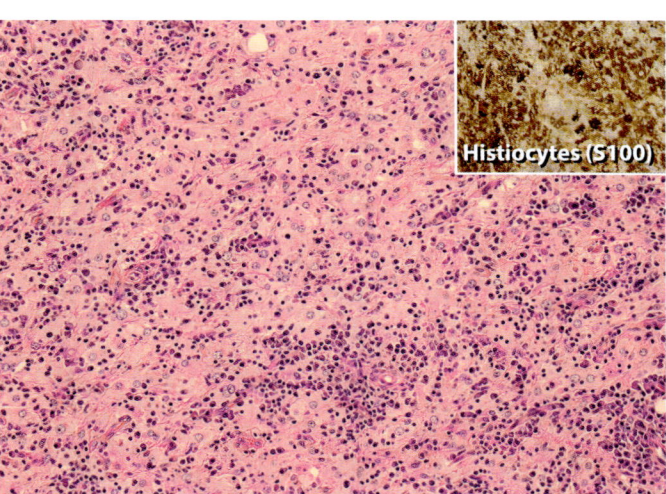

IMAGE 13.149 Rosai-Dorfman disease. The image shows a lymph node with histiocytic proliferation and lymphophagocytosis (emperipolesis).

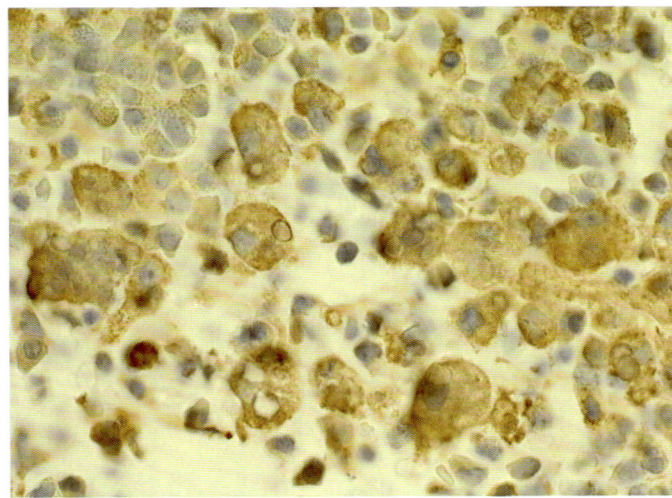

IMAGE 13.147 Hemophagocytic syndrome. Marrow biopsy reveals frequent hemophagocytic histiocytes highlighted by CD68 immunostain.

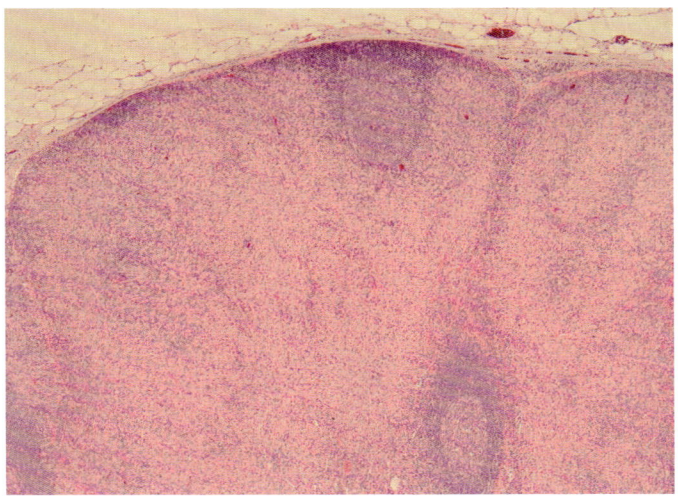

IMAGE 13.150 LCH (Langerhans cell histiocytosis), characterized by histiocytic proliferation and increased eosinophils in the background.

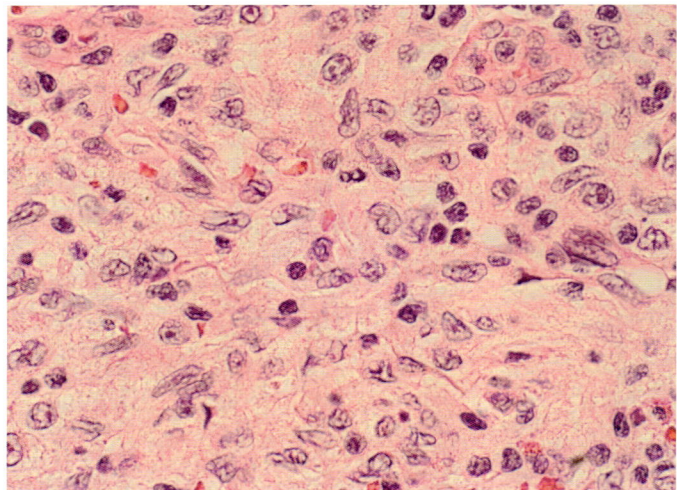

IMAGE 13.151 LCH showing neoplastic histiocytes with pink cytoplasm and horseshoe shaped, grooved nuclei.

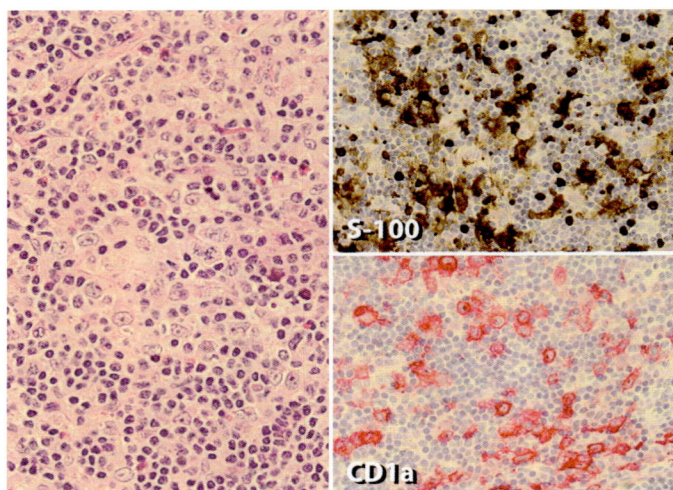

IMAGE 13.152 LCH. The neoplastic histiocytes demonstrate coexpression of S-100 and CD1a by IHC.

Thymus Pathology

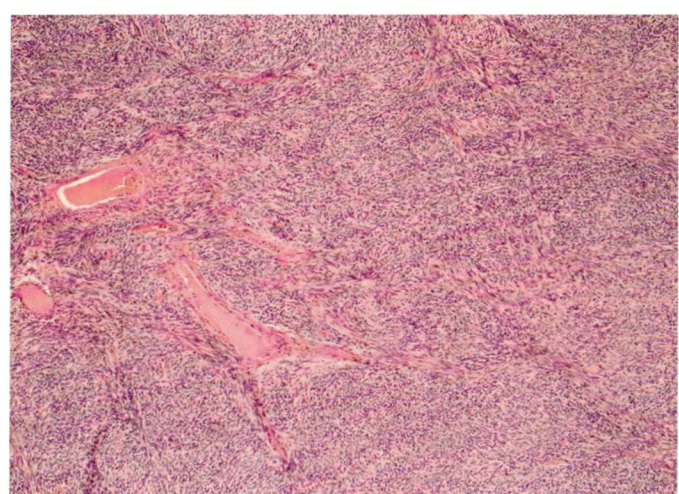

IMAGE 13.153 Spindle cell/medullary thymoma (type A), characterized by spindle/oval shaped epithelial cells and lack of nuclear atypia.

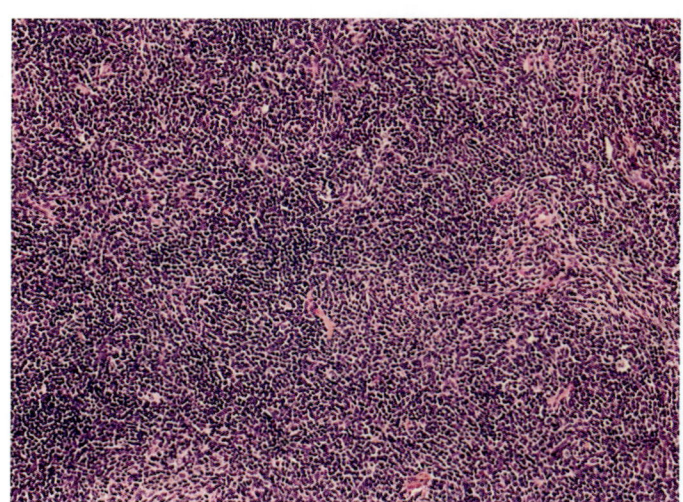

IMAGE 13.155 Lymphocyte rich thymoma (type B1), characterized by dense thymic T cell component and normal looking thymic cortical areas.

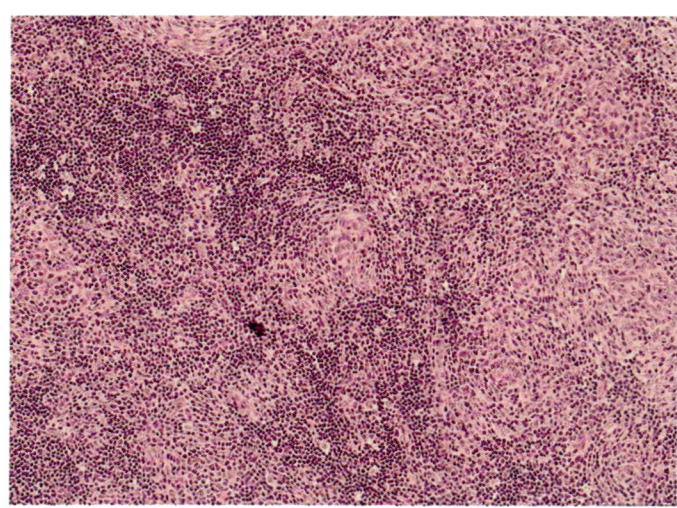

IMAGE 13.154 Mixed thymoma (type AB), characterized by mixed spindle cell and lymphocytic rich cortical type areas.

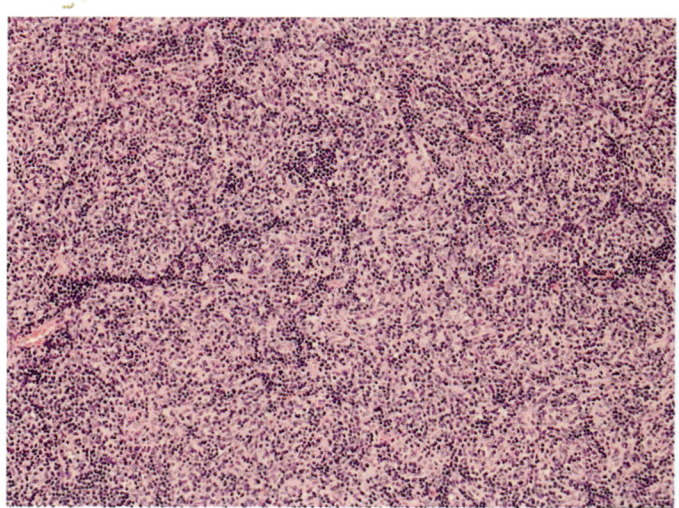

IMAGE 13.156 Lymphocytic cortical type thymoma (type B2), highlighted by epithelioid cells and significant lymphocytic component.

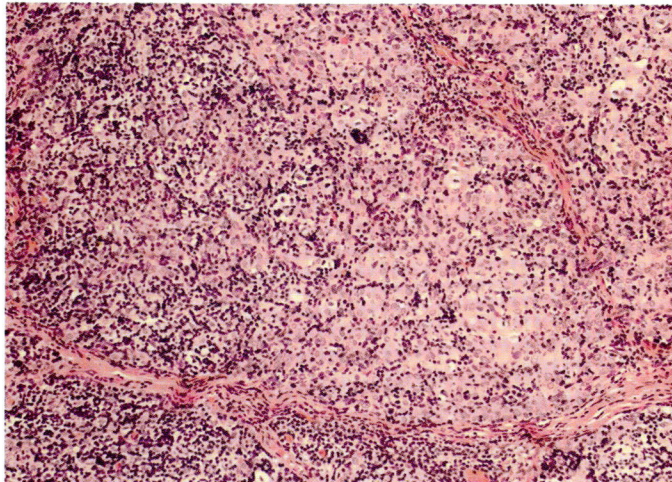

IMAGE 13.157 Thymoma type B3. The epithelial cells are round or polygonal and show mild atypia, squamous metaplasia, and few lymphocytes.

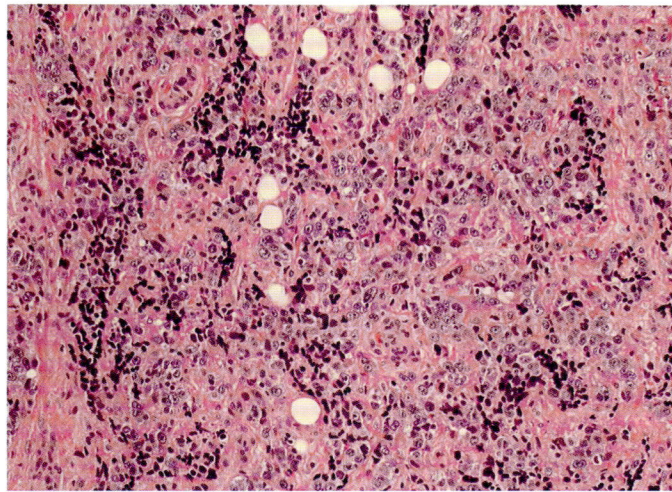

IMAGE 13.158 Thymic carcinoma (type C), defined by sheets of neoplastic cells that may show squamous or sarcomatoid features.

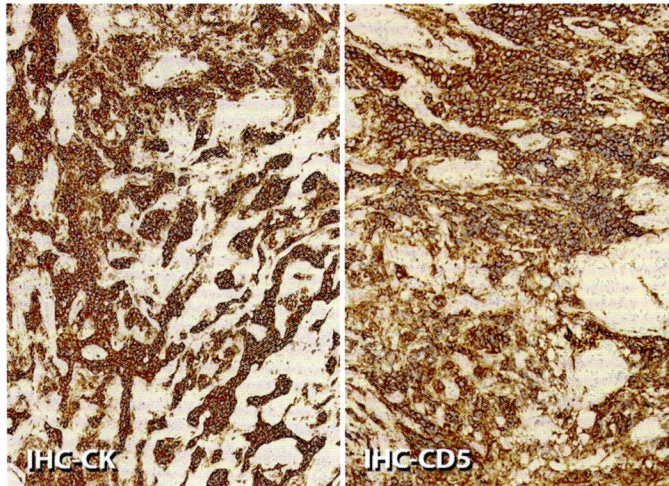

IMAGE 13.159 Thymic carcinoma (type C). The tumor cells are positive for cytokeratin and aberrantly express CD5.

References

1. Swerdlow S, Campo E, Harris N, et al. WHO classification of tumours of haematopoietic and lymphoid tissues. Revised 4th ed. Lyon (France): IARC; 2017.

2. International Myeloma Foundation [Internet]. Los Angeles: International Myeloma Foundation; c1990-2022. Durie-Salmon staging system; [updated 2021 Jul 20; cited 2022 Aug 31]. Available from myeloma.org/durie-salmon-staging.

3. Leukemia and Lymphoma Society [Internet]. Rye Brook (NY): Leukemia and Lymphoma Society: n.d. Myeloma staging; [cited 2022 Aug 31]. Available from lls.org/myeloma/diagnosis/myeloma-staging.

4. Chesi M, Bergsagel PL. Molecular pathogenesis of multiple myeloma: basic and clinical updates. Int J Hematol. 2013:97(3):313-23. doi: 10.1007/s12185-013-1291-2

5. Holmes RO, Jacobson DR, Baethge BA, et al. Amyloidosis [Internet]. Medscape [updated 2014 Nov 26; cited 2016 Jul 30]. Available from emedicine.medscape.com/article/335414-overview#a2.

6. Hans CP, Weisenburger DD, Greiner TC, et al. Confirmation of the molecular classification of diffuse large B-cell lymphoma by immunohistochemistry using a tissue microarray. Blood. 2004;103(1):275-82. doi: 10.1182/blood-2003-05-1545

7. Weitzman S, Egeler RM, editors. Histiocytic disorders of children and adults: basic science, clinical features, and therapy. Cambridge (UK): Cambridge University Press; 2011.

Bibliography

Bradley KT, Arber DA, Brown MS, et al; Cancer Committee, College of American Pathologists. Protocol for the examination of specimens from patients with hematopoietic neoplasms of the ocular adnexa (Version: OcularAdnexa 3.0.0.0) [Internet]. College of American Pathologists; 2010. Available from www.cap.org.

Chesi M, Bergsagel PL. Molecular pathogenesis of multiple myeloma: basic and clinical updates. Int J Hematol. 2013:97(3):313-23. doi: 10.1007/s12185-013-1291-2

Dacic S, Beasley MB, Berman M, et al; Cancer Committee, College of American Pathologists. Protocol for the examination of specimens from patients with thymic tumors (Version: Thymus 4.0.0.1) [Internet]. College of American Pathologists; 2017. Available from www.cap.org.

Duncavage E, Advani RH, Agosti S, et al; Cancer Biomarker Reporting Committee, College of American Pathologists. Template for reporting results of biomarker testing of specimens from patients with chronic lymphocytic leukemia/small lymphocytic lymphoma (Version: CLLBiomarkers 1.0.0.2) [Internet]. College of American Pathologists; 2017. Available from www.cap.org.

Duncavage E, Advani RH, Agosti S, et al; Cancer Biomarker Reporting Committee, College of American Pathologists. Template for reporting results of biomarker testing of specimens from patients with diffuse large B-cell lymphoma, not otherwise specified (NOS) (Version: DLBCL Biomarkers 1.0.0.2) [Internet]. College of American Pathologists; 2017. Available from www.cap.org.

Hans CP, Weisenburger DD, Greiner TC, et al. Confirmation of the molecular classification of diffuse large B-cell lymphoma by immunohistochemistry using a tissue microarray. Blood. 2004;103(1):275-82. doi: 10.1182/blood-2003-05-1545

Holmes RO, Jacobson DR, Baethge BA, et al. Amyloidosis [Internet]. Medscape [updated 2014 Nov 26]. Available from http://emedicine.medscape.com/article/335414-overview#a2.

Hussong JW, Arber DA, Bradley KT, et al; Cancer Committee, College of American Pathologists. Protocol for the examination of specimens from patients with non-Hodgkin lymphoma/lymphoid neoplasms (Version: NonHodgkin 3.2.0.1) [Internet]. College of American Pathologists; 2013. Available from www.cap.org.

International Myeloma Foundation [Internet]. Los Angeles: International Myeloma Foundation; c1990-2022. Durie-Salmon staging system; [updated 2021 Jul 20]. Available from myeloma.org/durie-salmon-staging.

Jaffe E, Arber DA, Campo E, et al. Hematopathology. 2nd ed. Philadelphia (PA): Elsevier; 2016.

Kelley TW, Alsabeh R, Arber DA, et al; Cancer Biomarker Reporting Committee, College of American Pathologists. Template for reporting results of biomarker testing for myeloproliferative neoplasms (Version: MPNBiomarkers 1.0.0.2) [Internet]. College of American Pathologists; 2017. Available from www.cap.org.

Kelley TW, Alsabeh R, Arber DA, et al; Cancer Biomarker Reporting Committee, College of American Pathologists. Template for reporting results of monitoring tests for patients with chronic myelogenous leukemia (*BCR-ABL1+*) (Version: CML Biomarkers 1.0.0.1) [Internet]. College of American Pathologists; 2015. Available from www.cap.org.

Khoury JD, Dogan A, Foucar K, et al; Cancer Committee, College of American Pathologists. Protocol for the examination of specimens from patients with plasma cell neoplasms (Version: Plasma Cell Neoplasms 1.0.0.2) [Internet]. College of American Pathologists; 2015. Available from www.cap.org.

Khoury JD, Hussong JW, Arber DA, et al; Cancer Committee, College of American Pathologists. Protocol for the examination of specimens from patients with hematopoietic neoplasms involving the bone marrow (Version: Bone Marrow 3.1.0.0) [Internet]. College of American Pathologists; 2018. Available from www.cap.org.

Kumar V, Abbas AK, Aster J. Robbins and Cotran pathologic basis of disease. 10th ed. North York (ON): Elsevier Canada; 2020.

Leukemia and Lymphoma Society [Internet]. Rye Brook (NY): Leukemia and Lymphoma Society: n.d. Myeloma staging; [cited 2022 Aug 31]. Available from www.lls.org/myeloma/diagnosis/myeloma-staging.

Medereiros J. Ioachim's lymph node pathology. 5th ed. Philadelphia (PA): Wolters Kluwar; 2021.

Swerdlow S, Campo E, Harris N, et al. WHO classification of tumours of haematopoetic and lymphoid tissues. Revised 4th ed. Lyon (France): IARC; 2017.

Weitzman S, Egeler RM, editors. Histiocytic disorders of children and adults: basic science, clinical features, and therapy. Cambridge: Cambridge University Press; 2011.

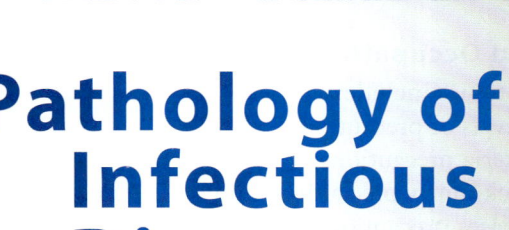

CHAPTER 14

Pathology of Infectious Disease

**LIK HANG LEE,
ANN MARIE NELSON**

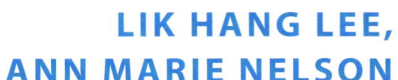

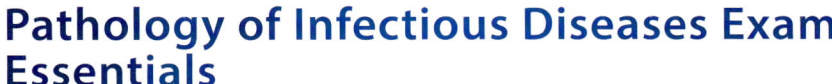

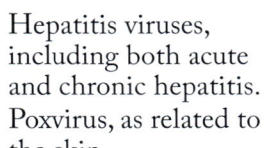

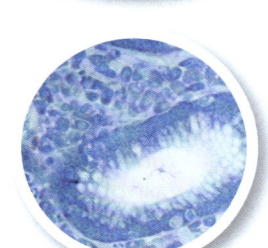

Pathology of Infectious Diseases Exam Essentials

MUST KNOW

Key information about infectious diseases

This section presents a noncomprehensive list of infectious diseases classified according to their taxonomy. For each taxonomic group, you should focus on which body system each infectious agent primarily affects, how to detect the infectious agent, and complications from infection. You should also understand the general characteristics and basic biology of each taxonomic group. Finally, you should know, in general, methods for identifying infectious agents, including histochemical stains, cultures, and molecular techniques.

Viruses and prions:
  Viral pneumonia and influenza.
  Viral gastroenteritis.
  HIV, including associated opportunistic infections.
  Cytomegalovirus (CMV).
  Epstein Barr virus (EBV).
  BK virus.
  Herpes simplex virus (HSV), as related to the skin, esophagus, and gynecologic tract.
  Parvovirus, as related to placental and fetal anomalies.
  Human papillomavirus (HPV), as related to the head and neck, skin, genitourinary and reproductive systems.
  Hepatitis viruses, including both acute and chronic hepatitis.
  Poxvirus, as related to the skin.
  Oncogenic viruses: human herpes virus 8 (HHV-8), EBV, hepatitis B virus (HBV), hepatitis C virus (HCV), Merkel cell polyomavirus (MCV), HPV.
  Prion diseases including Creutzfeldt-Jakob disease (CJD), vCJD (variant CJD), fatal familial insomnia, kuru.

Bacteria:
  Bacterial pneumonia, including unusual organisms such as *Legionella* spp.
  Bacterial colitis, including *Clostridium difficile* colitis.
  Septic joint.
  Helicobacter pylori and *Helicobacter heilmannii*.
  Poststreptococcal glomerulonephritis.
  Tropheryma whippeli, as related to the gastrointestinal tract.
  Bartonella henselae, as related to the lymph nodes.
  Yersinia pestis, as related to the lymph nodes.
  Pseudomonas aeruginosa, as related to cystic fibrosis.
  Treponema pallidum, as related to the reproductive organs.
  Gardnerella vaginalis, as related to the cervix.
  Lyme disease (*Borrelia burgdorferi*), as related to the skin and lymph nodes.

Staphylococcus aureus, as related to the skin.

Tuberculosis (*Mycobacterium tuberculosis*).

Atypical mycobacterial infections, including *Mycobacterium avium-intracellulare*, and *Mycobacterium leprae*.

Coxiella burnetti, as related to the bone marrow.

Fungi:

Candida spp, as related to the skin, esophagus, gynecologic tract, placenta, and other organs.

Pulmonary fungal infections, including *Histoplasma* spp., *Blastomyces* spp., and *Coccidioides* spp.

Cryptococcus neoformans, as related to the cerebrospinal fluid and the lung.

Actinomyces spp. infections, as related to the endometrium.

Pneumocystis jiroveci, as related to the lung.

Aspergillus spp. and *Zygomycetes* (including *Mucor* spp.) infectious, as related to the lung and sinonasal tract.

Parasites:

Protozoa:

Entamoeba histolytica, as related to the gastrointestinal tract.

Toxoplasma gondii, as related to the brain and placenta.

Malaria (*Plasmodium* spp.).

Helminths (cestodes, trematodes, and nematodes):

Taenia spp. tapeworm, as related to the brain and gastrointestinal tract.

Echinococcus spp., as related to the lung and hepatobiliary system.

Schistosoma spp., as related to the skin, bladder, and gastrointestinal tract.

Filariasis, as related to lymphedema.

Strongyloides spp., as related to the gastrointestinal tract.

Ascaris lumbricoides, as related to the gastrointestinal tract and lungs.

Arthropods:

Demodex spp., as related to skin.

Scabies.

Ticks, including those related to Lyme disease.

Detection methods

High-yield topics include:
- Bacterial stains, including:
  · Gram stains: Brown-Brenn, Brown-Hopps.
  · Acid-fast stains: Ziehl-Neelson, Kinyoun, Fite, auramine-rhodamine.
  · Silver stains: Warthin-Starry, Dieterle.
  · Other stains: Giemsa, Wright-Giemsa.
- Fungal stains: Grocott methenamine silver (GMS), periodic acid-Schiff (PAS), PAS with diastase (PASD).
- Stain for bacterial or fungal capsules: India ink, mucicarmine, Fontana-Masson.
- Immunohistochemistry (IHC).

- Immunofluorescence.
- Electron microscopy.
- Culture.
- Polymerase chain reaction (PCR).

Safety and Occupational Health

High-yield topics include:
- Various levels of precautions.
- Mycobacteria precautions.
- Needlestick injury precautions and procedures.
- Prion diseases precautions.

MUST SEE

- For each of the infectious agents outlined in the Must Know section, focus on organ systems that are most likely affected, and the gross and microscopic findings seen.
- The exam may include images of gross infectious lesions (e.g., pneumonia, hydatid cyst), but these are less common than microscopy images. Infectious diseases often make good oral examination questions, including questions about occupational safety.
- High-yield images include:
  · Viruses and prions:
    › Viral pneumonias.
    › Viral gastroenteritis, nonspecific changes.
    › HIV and complications, such as colitis, encephalitis, opportunistic infections, and associated malignancies.
    › CMV changes in esophagus, gastrointestinal tract, placenta, gynecologic tract.
    › EBV, especially the related lymphoproliferative disease.
    › Polyomavirus on urine cytology (decoy cells).
    › HSV skin bulla, esophagitis, Pap smear findings.
    › MCV and Merkel cell carcinoma.
    › Acute and chronic viral hepatitis, cirrhosis.
    › Low- and high-risk HPV lesions: condyloma; verruca; squamous dysplasia and carcinoma of head and neck, skin, anogenital region, and gynecologic tract.
    › Kaposi sarcoma of the skin due to HHV-8.
    › Parvovirus infection of the placenta.
    › Molluscum contagiosum (poxvirus) of the skin.
    › Orf of the skin.
    › Changes in the central nervous system due to prion disease.
  · Bacteria:
    › Lobar pneumonia versus bronchopneumonia, red versus grey hepatization.
    › Pseudomembranous colitis.
    › Septic joint hardware.
    › Peptic ulcer disease.
    › Poststreptococcal glomerulonephritis, including immunofluorescence and electron microscopy findings.

- › Lymphadenitis and necrotizing lymphadenitis due to various organisms.
- › Pneumonia related to cystic fibrosis.
- › Syphilis, including chancre, and also secondary (skin) and neurosyphilis.
- › Gynecologic cytology findings, such as bacterial vaginosis and actinomycosis.
- › Erythema migrans.
- › Infection of the skin causing impetigo and bullae.
- › Granulomatous pneumonia due to mycobacterial infections.
- › *Mycobacterium avium–intracellulare* complex findings in the lymph node and gastrointestinal tract.
- › Q fever in the bone marrow.
- · Fungi:
  - › *Candida* dermatitis, esophagitis, vulvitis, etc.
  - › Granulomatous fungal pneumonias (histoplasmosis, blastomycosis, coccidioidomycosis, cryptococcosis, aspergillosis, and pneumocystosis.)
  - › Mycetoma, including invasive fungal infections of the sinonasal tract.
- · Parasites:
  - › Amoebiasis.
  - › Toxoplasmosis abscess in the brain.
  - › Hydatid cyst in the lung and liver.
  - › Malaria, including blood smears.
  - › Schistosomiasis in the skin, bladder, and gastrointestinal tract.
  - › Elephantiasis (lymphatic filariasis).
  - › Gastrointestinal flatworms and roundworms, including their pathologic effect on other body organs.
  - › Arthropod bite skin reaction.
  - › Arthropod body and mouth parts.

MUST DO

- For each of the entities outlined in the Must See section, you should be comfortable generating a

differential diagnosis for the relevant histologic finding. The exam may give you only a pattern of finding rather than pathognomonic changes (such as granulomas, or acute necrotizing process). In these cases, you should think of both infectious and noninfectious causes (e.g., drugs, vasculitis, autoimmune disease), and be prepared to offer ancillary studies such as histochemical or immunohistochemical stains to elucidate the diagnosis.

- When studying in groups, example topics to practice include:
  - · Differential diagnosis of granulomatous disease in various organs (skin, lung, lymph node, etc.).
  - · Necrotizing lymphadenitis.
  - · Critical values related to infectious causes.
  - · Safety, occupational health, and public health issues related to infectious diseases.
  - · Using ancillary studies to confirm infectious organisms.
  - · Oncogenic viruses, the neoplasms they cause, and their mechanism of pathology.
  - · Acute and chronic changes in viral hepatitis.
  - · Causes of abundant macrophages in the lamina propria in the gastrointestinal tract.
- There is no specific grossing protocol for most infectious diseases. However, the issue of safety may be of particular concern if previous infection is known. You should be familiar with:
  - · Specimen fixation.
  - · Handling of prion disease tissue.
  - · Knife and needlestick injuries.
  - · Tissue transport and disposal.
  - · Public health and reportable diseases.
- You should be able to describe and handle fresh specimens and frozen sections. Key topics include:
  - · Taking fresh tissue for culture.
  - · Analyzing frozen section of lung nodules of unknown etiology.
  - · Conducting autopsies on patients with infectious diseases, especially HIV, HCV, and tuberculosis.

MULTIPLE CHOICE QUESTIONS

1. Which of the following is **not** a cause of diffuse alveolar damage?

- a. Tinea versicolor.
- b. Coronavirus disease 2019 (COVID-19).
- c. Herpes simplex virus.
- d. *Pneumocystis jiroveci.*
- e. *Mycobacterium tuberculosis.*

Answer: a

2. Which organism is a commensal organism on human skin?

- a. *Trichophyton interdigitale.*
- b. *Hortaea werneckii.*
- c. *Malassezia furfur.*
- d. *Microsporum gypseum.*
- e. *Neisseria meningitidis.*

Answer: c

3. Which of the following is **not** a method of vertical transmission of infectious agents?

a. Transmission through sperm during fertilization.

b. Transplacental transmission.

c. Transmission during birth by direct contact with birth canal.

d. Transmission through maternal breast milk.

e. Break in maternal fetal barrier during amniocentesis.

Answer: a

4. Which of the following tissue reactions is **not** commonly associated with the listed infection?

a. Cytopathic or cytoproliferative reaction due to Epstein-Barr virus (EBV).

b. Suppurative reaction due to human papillomavirus (HPV).

c. Granulomatous reaction due to tuberculosis.

d. Tissue necrosis due to *Clostridium perfringens*.

e. Scarring due to hepatitis C virus (HCV).

Answer: b

5. Which of the following is **not** a category A disease/agent of bioterrorism, as categorized by the Centers for Disease Control and Prevention (CDC)?

a. Bacillus anthracis.

b. Yersinia pestis.

c. Clostridium botulinum toxin.

d. Variola major virus.

e. Rickettsia prowazekii.

Answer: e

6. Which statement about organisms that live in or on other organisms is correct?

a. Mutualistic symbiotic organisms and their hosts have a mutually advantageous arrangement.

b. Parasitic organisms do the host no good and no harm.

c. Commensal organisms thrive while harming the host.

d. Saprophytic organisms live off internal organs of the host.

e. Vectors are the infectious microorganisms that have been transmitted into a host by an insect.

Answer: a

7. A patient with rheumatoid arthritis receiving treatment of antitumor necrosis factor (anti-TNF) agents complains of cough and night sweats. Chest X-ray shows a left lung apical nodule. Biopsy of the nodule reveals a granulomatous lesion, which is negative for microorganisms on Ziehl–Neelsen stain. What is the most appropriate next step you should recommend?

a. Culture.

b. Start treatment with isoniazid and rifampin.

c. Sputum acid-fast smear.

d. DNA probes.

e. Gas-liquid chromatography.

Answer: b

8. Brain tissue from an HIV patient with a CD4 count of 50 and a ring enhancing lesion would most commonly be positive for:

a. *Pneumocystis jiroveci*.

b. Primary central nervous system (CNS) lymphoma.

c. *Toxoplasma gondii*.

d. Cytomegalovirus (CMV).

e. HSV.

Answer: c

9. Which viral infection below is the **least** likely cause of interstitial nephritis?

a. HSV.

b. CMV.

c. EBV.

d. BK virus.

e. Hantavirus.

Answer: a

10. Which disease has **no** proven association with human herpesvirus 8 (HHV-8)?

a. Acute myelogenous leukemia.

b. Kaposi sarcoma.

c. Multicentric Castleman disease.

d. Primary effusion lymphoma.

Answer: a

11. Which virus does **not** cause hemorrhagic fevers?

a. Lassa virus.

b. Ebola virus.

c. Corona virus.

d. Marburg virus.

e. Machupo virus.

Answer: c

12. Negri bodies are seen in:

a. HIV encephalitis.

b. CMV encephalitis.

c. HSV encephalitis.

d. West Nile encephalitis.

e. Rabies encephalitis.

Answer: e

13. A young man presents with fever, sore throat, and cervical adenopathy. Monospot test was positive. If a cervical lymph node is submitted for biopsy, which type of immune cell would most likely appear atypical on histologic section?

a. CD21+ B cell.

b. Follicular dendritic cell.

c. T cell.

d. Langerhans cell.

e. Mantle zone B cell.

Answer: c

14. A resident grossing a partially resected liver hemangioma specimen accidentally cuts his finger. The specimen is from a patient with negative serology for hepatitis B virus (HBV) and hepatitis C virus (HCV). What should the resident do after reporting the incident to his supervisor?

a. Obtain the patient's consent to do an HIV screening test.
b. Watch and wait to see if the resident develops flu-like symptoms.
c. Test the resident for HIV using enzyme-linked immunosorbent assay (ELISA).
d. Prophylactically give the resident antiviral drugs.
e. Test the resident for HIV with a Western blot assay.

Answer: a

15. Which of the following pairings of polyoma viruses and clinical diseases is **incorrectly** matched?

a. Merkel cell polyomavirus and Merkel cell carcinoma.
b. BK polyoma virus and polyomavirus-associated nephropathy.
c. JC polyomavirus and progressive multifocal leukoencephalopathy.
d. Trichodysplasia spinulosa polyomavirus and trichodysplasia spinulosa.
e. Simian vacuolating virus 40 (SV40) and simian human immunodeficiency.

Answer: e

16. Postmortem lung samples from a patient who died of acute community acquired pneumonia reveal acute necrotizing bronchopneumonia. Gram stains are negative for organisms, but silver staining shows coccobacilli. The most likely etiologic agent is:

a. Panton-Valentine toxin positive *S. aureus* infection.
b. *Streptococcus pneumoniae.*
c. *Legionella pneumophila* serogroup 1.
d. *Hemophilus influenzae* serotype B 2a.
e. *Bartonella henselae.*

Answer: c

17. Poststreptococcal kidney failure usually shows which pattern of injury in a kidney biopsy specimen?

a. Acute tubular necrosis.
b. Diffuse proliferative glomerulonephritis.
c. Membrano-proliferative glomerulonephritis.
d. Focal segmental glomerulosclerosis.
e. Gram-positive cocci in chains.

Answer: b

18. Which of the following organisms does **not** stain positive with a modified acid-fast stain?

a. *Nocardia asteroides.*
b. *Mycobacterium marinum.*
c. *Actinomyces israelii.*
d. *Legionella micdadei.*
e. *Rhodococcus equi.*

Answer: c

19. Catscratch associated lymphadenitis is caused by:

a. *Streptococcus pyogenes.*
b. *Rickettsia cattii.*
c. *Tropheryma whippeli.*
d. *Bartonella henselae.*
e. *Toxoplasma gondii.*

Answer: d

20. Which of the following is a finding in colon biopsy specimens from patients infected by *Shigella* organisms?

a. Extensive eosinophilia of the lamina propria.
b. Multiple cytoplasmic inclusions in the colonic enterocytes.
c. Granulomas throughout the mucosa of the colon.
d. Cryptitis, crypt abscess, and pseudomembranes.
e. Crypt distortion, branching, and hypertrophy.

Answer: d

21. What is a finding in pseudomonas infections?

a. Laryngotracheo-bronchitis.
b. Necrotizing pneumonia.
c. Chronic renal disease.
d. Multiple hemorrhagic foci in the mediastinum.
e. Extensive rash on trunk of the body.

Answer: b

22. Which is **not** a feature of syphilis infections?

a. Chancre on the penis/scrotum/vulva/cervix.
b. Argyll Robertson pupils.
c. Endarteritis of proximal aorta.
d. Gummas of the skin, bone, and liver.
e. Closed angle glaucoma.

Answer: e

23. Which statement about Whipple disease is **false**?

a. It is caused by the gram-positive actinomycete *Tropheryma whippeli.*
b. Clinical symptoms are caused by accumulation of organism laden macrophages in the bile ducts.
c. A histologic feature is dense accumulation of distended, foamy macrophages in the small intestinal lamina propria.
d. Small intestinal histologic findings of Whipple disease can be mistaken for intestinal tuberculosis.
e. The foamy macrophages contain PAS-positive, diastase-resistant granules, but do not stain positively with acid-fast stain.

Answer: b

24. A young woman presents with genital itch and a foul, fishy smell from the genital area. Her Pap smear shows *Trichomonas vaginalis* and epithelial cells covered by numerous coccobacilli. Which organism is associated with vaginal pH elevation?

a. *Lactobacillus.*

b. Group B *Streptococci* spp.

c. *Gardnerella vaginalis.*

d. *Peptostreptococcus anaerobius.*

e. *Atopobium vaginae.*

Answer: c

25. Which of the following histochemical stains do **not** detect acid-fast bacilli?

a. Ziehl-Neelsen.

b. Kinyoun.

c. Fite.

d. Rhodanine.

e. Auramine-rhodamine.

Answer: d

26. Which of the following bacteria are **not** frequently intracellular?

a. *Shigella* spp.

b. Invasive *Escherichia coli.*

c. *Mycobacterium tuberculosis.*

d. *Vibrio cholerae.*

e. *Listeria monocytogenes.*

Answer: d

27. Which of the following statements regarding *Histoplasma capsulatum* is true?

a. Grocott-Gomori methenamine-silver stain (GMS stain) is positive for yeast organisms 5–10 μm in diameter.

b. Yeasts exhibit broad based budding.

c. Mucicarmine staining shows large capsules.

d. The organism is positive with Romanowsky/Giemsa stain.

e. Granulomatous inflammation is uncommon.

Answer: d

28. Dimorphic fungi in histology samples appear as:

a. Yeast structures only.

b. Yeast with occasional pseudohyphae.

c. Yeast and hyphal elements.

d. Hyphae with conidia formation.

e. Periodic acid-Schiff (PAS) positive intracellular inclusions.

Answer: b

29. Which statement about fungi is correct?

a. Fungi are prokaryotes with cell walls that give them their shape.

b. Fungi can grow as multicellular filaments called yeasts, and single cells or chains of cells called molds.

c. *Candida* species infections are the most frequent cause of human fungal infections.

d. *Cryptococcus* most commonly presents as meningoencephalitis in otherwise healthy individuals.

e. Aspergillosis is an opportunistic infection caused by "bread mold fungi."

Answer: c

30. Which of the following statements is true regarding cysticercosis in humans?

a. Sheep are the host of the tapeworm stage of the life cycle.

b. Lesions are most commonly seen in the liver.

c. Stool examination is usually positive for tapeworm eggs.

d. Cysts are typically 10–15 cm in size.

e. It is uncommon in the Middle East.

Answer: e

31. What is a cause of elephantiasis?

a. Bacterial infection of the cardiac valves, causing heart failure.

b. Viral infection of the veins, breaking down the venous valves.

c. Lymphoma destroying the lymph nodes of the lower limbs and inguinal region.

d. Worms in the lymphatic system causing damage to the lymphatic system.

Answer: d

32. A 38-year-old male returns from bear hunting and has eaten undercooked bear meat. He presents with myalgia, fever, and periorbital edema. Which of the following organisms is most likely responsible for his illness?

a. *Trichinella spiralis.*

b. *Echinococcus granulosus.*

c. *Taenia solium.*

d. *Borrelia burgdorferi.*

e. *Echinococcus multilocularis.*

Answer: a

33. Which of the following statements regarding *Taenia solium* is **false**?

a. The 2 known reservoirs of *T. solium* are pigs and humans.

b. Pigs are the definitive host and humans are the primary intermediate host.

c. *T. solium* can be transmitted through the consumption

of undercooked pork products.

d. Taeniasis is the infection of the intestines by adult tapeworms.

e. Neurocysticercosis occurs when *T. solium* larvae invade tissue of the brain and form cysts.

Answer: b

34. Which of the following statements regarding filariasis is **false**?

a. Adult filaria mate and release microfilaria into the blood.

b. Filariasis is endemic in central Africa and southeast Asia.

c. *Brugia malayi* and *Brugia timori* are the most common cause of filarial infections worldwide.

d. Humans are the only hosts for *Wuchereria bancrofti* filariasis.

e. Intact adult worms develop within lymphatics and can cause lymphatic obstruction leading to lymphedema and peau d'orange skin.

Answer: c

35. Which statement about schistosomiasis is **incorrect**?

a. *S. haematobium* eggs are oval with a terminal spine; *S. japonicum* eggs are round to oval with a very small subterminal spine or no spine; *S. mansoni* eggs are oval with a well-defined lateral spine.

b. Adult schistosomes inhabit the blood capillaries of the mesentery or plexus of the bladder.

c. In tissues, schistosomiasis eggs are often calcified with granulomatous reaction or fibrosis.

d. Schistosomiasis infection in the bladder is associated with carcinomas of the bladder.

e. Schistosomes are simultaneous hermaphrodites.

Answer: e

SHORT ANSWER QUESTIONS

Prions
Prion Disease

36. Name at least 4 human prion diseases.
- Creutzfeldt-Jakob disease (CJD).
- Gerstmann-Sträussler-Scheinker syndrome.
- Fatal familial insomnia.
- Kuru.
- Variant CJD.

37. What is another name for prion diseases?
Transmissible spongiform encephalopathies.

38. What are prions, and how do they differ from all other known infectious agents?
- Prions are infectious agents composed of misfolded proteins that cause transmissible neurodegenerative disorders.
- Prions do not contain nucleic acids, unlike all other infectious agents.

39. Describe the pathogenesis of prion disease.
- Normal prion protein (PrP), which is normally present in neurons, undergoes a conformational change to an abnormal form, making it resistant to digestion with proteases.
- Infectious (misfolded) prion protein (PrP^{Sc}) binds to normal prion protein (PrP^c), catalyzing a conformational change into PrP^{Sc}.
- The new PrP^{Sc} further catalyzes the transformation of more PrP^c to PrP^{Sc}.
- This abnormal prion protein accumulates in neural tissues, causing pathology in the tissue.

40. What are 3 methods by which prion diseases arise in humans?
- Acquired.
- Familial.
- Sporadic.

41. What are the clinical presentations of prion disease?
- Personality changes.
- Psychiatric problems such as depression.
- Lack of coordination.
- Ataxia.
- Myoclonus.
- Sensory changes.
- Insomnia.
- Confusion.
- Memory problems.
- Dementia.
- Paralysis.

Creutzfeldt-Jakob Disease

42. Name key pathologic differences between classic and variant CJD.
- "Florid plaques" are absent in classic CJD and present in variant CJD.
- Protease resistance prion proteins (PrP-res) show variable accumulation in classic CJD, and significant accumulation in variant CJD. This can be seen on immunohistochemistry against PrP-res or by the presence of increased glycoform ratio on immunoblot analysis of PrP-res.
- The infective agent is often seen in lymphoid tissue in variant CJD, but not in classic CJD.

43. How is CJD classified?
- Classic Creutzfeldt-Jakob disease (CJD).
- Sporadic Creutzfeldt-Jakob disease (sCJD).
- Iatrogenic Creutzfeldt-Jakob disease (iCJD).
- Familial Creutzfeldt-Jakob disease (fCJD).
- Variant Creutzfeldt-Jakob disease (vCJD).

44. Describe the microscopic features of CJD.
- Spongiform transformation of cerebral cortex and, frequently, the caudate and putamen.
- Uneven distribution of variably sized small microscopic vacuoles within the neuropil and, sometimes, the perikaryon of neurons. These may expand into cyst-like spaces (status spongiosus).
- Severe neuronal loss and reactive gliosis in advanced cases.
- Kuru plaques (aggregates of PrP^{Sc}), frequently in the cerebellum.
  - Also in the cerebral cortex in vCJD.
  - Congo red and PAS positive.

45. What immunohistochemistry stain is seen in all prion diseases?
Proteinase K-resistant PrP^{Sc}.

46. Which prion disease does not show spongiform change? What are its characteristic histologic findings?
- Disease: fatal familial insomnia.
- Histologic findings:
  - Neuronal loss in anterior ventral and dorsomedial nuclei of thalamus, and in inferior olivary nuclei.
  - Reactive gliosis in anterior ventral and dorsomedial nuclei of thalamus.

Viruses
Viruses: General

47. What 4 factors affect viral tropism?
- Host cell receptors for the virus.
- Cellular transcription factors that respond to viral enhancers and promoter sequences.
- Anatomic barriers.
- Local environment, including temperature, pH, and host defenses.

48. Through what 3 mechanisms do viruses cause damage to human hosts?
- Direct cytopathic effects.
- Eliciting an immune response that damages tissues.
- Transforming infected cells into neoplastic cells.

49. What are the 3 components of the virus particle?
- Envelope.
- Capsid.
- Core.

50. List the Baltimore classification of viruses and give an example of each.

- I: dsDNA viruses — herpesvirus.
- II: ssDNA viruses — parvovirus B19.
- III: dsRNA viruses — reovirus.
- IV: (+)ssRNA viruses — West Nile virus.
- V: (–)ssRNA viruses — rabies virus.
- VI: ssRNA-RT viruses — HIV.
- VII: dsDNA-RT viruses — hepatitis B.

51. List at least 6 oncogenic viruses and 1 malignancy associated with each.

VIRUS	ASSOCIATED MALIGNANCY
HBV	• Hepatocellular carcinoma.
HVC	• Hepatocellular carcinoma.
Human T-lymphotrophic virus	• Adult T-cell leukemia.
Merkel cell polyomavirus	• Merkel cell carcinoma.
EBV	• Burkitt lymphoma. • Hodgkin lymphoma. • Posttransplant lymphoproliferative disorder. • Nasopharyngeal carcinoma. • Gastric carcinoma.
HHV-8	• Kaposi sarcoma. • Multicentric Castleman disease. • Primary effusion lymphoma.
HPV	• Cervical carcinoma. • Anal carcinoma. • Penile carcinoma. • Vulvar and vaginal carcinomas. • Oropharyngeal carcinoma.

Human Papilloma Virus (HPV)

52. List 3 lesions caused by HPV.

- Condyloma.
- Verruca vulgaris planus.
- Squamous papilloma.
- Cervical/anal/oropharynx squamous intraepithelial or invasive neoplasm.
- Cervical adenocarcinoma/adenosquamous carcinoma.
- Acquired epidermodysplasia verruciformis (in immunocompromised hosts).

53. List 2 genotypes of high-risk HPV and 2 genotypes of low-risk HPV.

- High-risk HPV:
  - In the cervix, types 16 and 18 cause up to 70% of cervical cancer cases.
- Others include types 31, 33, 39, 45, 51, 52, 56, 58, 59, 66, 68, and 73, which are covered by FDA approved diagnostic DNA tests.
- Low-risk HPV:
  - In the cervix, types 6 and 11 cause condyloma acuminata.

54. Describe 2 HPV proteins/genes in HPV carcinogenesis.

- E6 protein binds p53, thereby stimulating the degradation of p53 and preventing its function.
  - Functions of p53 include cell cycle arrest and apoptosis.
- E7 protein binds Rb protein, thereby preventing normal Rb function.
  - Rb protein binds E2F-family transcription factors, which prevents E2F from stimulating cellular proliferation. Therefore, E7 allows E2F to function, which promotes cell proliferation.
- As a feedback mechanism, p16 is overexpressed, allowing p16 to serve as a surrogate marker for HPV infection.

Viral Hepatitis

55. What is the classification of viral hepatitis?
- By clinical syndrome:
  - Acute asymptomatic infection with recovery (serologic evidence only).
  - Acute symptomatic hepatitis with recovery, with or without icterus.
  - Chronic hepatitis, without or with progression to cirrhosis.
  - Fulminant hepatitis with massive to submassive hepatic necrosis.
- By type of virus:
  - Hepatotropic viruses: hepatitis A, B, C, D, E.
  - Nonhepatotropic viruses including CMV, EBV, herpesvirus, adenovirus, HIV.

56. What is the definition of chronic hepatitis?
Chronic hepatitis: symptomatic, biochemical, or serologic evidence of continuing or relapsing hepatic disease for > 6 months.

57. While all hepatotropic viruses can cause acute asymptomatic or symptomatic infections, not all lead to chronic infections. What is the frequency of chronic liver disease for each hepatotropic virus?
- Hepatitis A virus (HAV): does not cause chronic hepatitis.
- Hepatitis B virus (HBV): 10% of infected adults.
- Hepatitis C virus (HCV): 80% of infected adults.
- Hepatitis D virus (HDV): 5% in coinfections with HBV, and up to 80% in superinfections with HBV.
- Hepatitis E virus (HEV): does not cause chronic hepatitis.

58. Which genotypes of HCV have the best response to treatment?
Genotypes 2 and 3.

59. What is the "carrier" state of HBV?
- The state of an infected individual who can transmit the virus, but is asymptomatic with either no liver disease or with nonprogressive liver damage.
  - Serologically, these patients have anti-HBe, normal aminotransferases, and low serum HBV DNA.
  - They do not have HBeAg, but have HBsAg.
  - Liver biopsy would show a lack of significant inflammation and a lack of significant necrosis.

60. What are the laboratory and histologic findings in a healthy carrier of HBV?
- HBsAg+.
- HBeAg−
- Anti-HBe+.
- Alanine aminotransferase (ALT) and aspartate aminotransferase (AST): normal.
- HBV DNA: low or undetectable.
- Liver biopsy: lack of significant inflammation and lack of significant necrosis.

61. What are the histologic findings in acute viral hepatitis?
- Hepatocyte ballooning degeneration (diffuse hepatocyte swelling).
- Cholestasis.
- Lymphocytic infiltrate, most prominent in zone 3.
- Apoptotic hepatocytes with fragmented nuclei and intensely eosinophilic cytoplasm.
- Focal dropout of hepatocytes with scavenger macrophage aggregates.
- Kupffer cell hypertrophy and hyperplasia with lipofuscin pigment.
- Portal tract infiltration with mixed inflammatory cells.

62. What are some specific histologic features of acute HAV and HBV?
- HAV:
  - Lobular predominant, spotty necrosis, abundant apoptotic bodies.
  - Plasma cell predominant inflammatory infiltrate involving portal, periportal, and lobular areas.
  - Perivenular cholestasis.
  - Extensive microvesicular steatosis.
- HBV:
  - No specific histologic pattern suggests HBV.
  - Ground-glass hepatocytes, classic of chronic HBV, may not be seen.

63. What are the histologic findings of chronic hepatitis?
- Predominantly lymphocytic portal inflammatory infiltrate, with or without interface hepatitis.
- Varying degrees of necrosis or bridging necrosis.
- Varying degrees of fibrosis, ranging from periportal to bridging fibrosis.

64. What are some specific histologic features of chronic HBV and HCV?

- HBV:
  - Ground-glass hepatocytes.
- HCV:

· Lymphoid aggregates with or without germinal centers and bile duct reactive changes in portal tracts.
· Focal macrovesicular steatosis — more prevalent in HCV genotype 3.

65. What are the histologic findings of cirrhosis?

Hepatocytes divided into irregularly sized nodules separated by thick bands of fibrosis.

66. What are several common grading and staging systems for viral hepatitis?

- Hepatic activity index.
- Ishak modification of the hepatic activity index.
- Scheuer classification for grading and staging of chronic hepatitis.

- METAVIR classification for staging HCV liver disease.
- Batts-Ludwig system.

67. What is reported in a grading and staging system for viral hepatitis?

- Grade: degree of inflammation and necrosis.

- Stage: degree of fibrosis.

68. What is fulminant hepatic failure?

Hepatic insufficiency that progresses from the onset of symptoms to hepatic encephalopathy within 2–3 weeks in an individual who does not have chronic liver disease.

69. What are the morphological findings of fulminant hepatitis?

- Massive loss of liver mass.
- Limp, red colored tissue.
- Wrinkled capsule.

- Necrotic red interior with hemorrhage.
- Complete destruction of hepatocytes leaving a collapsed reticulin and preserved portal tracts.

70. Describe the route of transmission, incubation period, and diagnostic investigations for each hepatotropic virus.

VIRUS	TRANSMISSION	INCUBATION	DIAGNOSIS
Hepatitis A	• Fecal-oral.	• 2–6 weeks.	• Anti-HAV (IgM).
Hepatitis B	• Parenteral or equivalent. • Vertical.	• 6 weeks–6 months.	• HBsAg or HBcAg antibody.
Hepatitis C	• Parenteral.	• 5–10 weeks.	• HCV RNA (by PCR) or anti-HCV (IgG/IgM).
Hepatitis D	• Nonparenteral (close contact in endemic areas). • Parenteral.	• 6 weeks–6 months.	• Anti-HDV (IgG/IgM), HDV RNA in serum, or HDAg in liver.
Hepatitis E	• Fecal-oral.	• 2–6 weeks.	• Anti-HEV (IgG/IgM) or HEV RNA (by PCR).

Abbreviations: HBcAg: hepatitis B core antigen; HBsAg: hepatitis B surface antigen; HDAg: hepatitis D antigen; PCR: polymerase chain reaction.

71. Which immunohistochemical stains are useful in HBV, and how are they used?

- HBV core antigen (HBcAg) and HBV surface antigen (HBsAg).
  - These markers are not uncommonly negative in acute hepatitis B.
  - They may be positive in chronic hepatitis B with positivity usually decreasing with increasing degree of inflammation.

· HBsAg is a cytoplasmic staining.
· HBcAg is a nuclear staining, representing active viral replication.
· If HBsAg is also membranous, and HBcAg is also cytoplasmic, this indicates unopposed viral replication, likely in immunocompromised individuals.

72. Describe the serological and polymerase chain reaction (PCR) findings of hepatitis B in various clinical scenarios.

CLINICAL STATE	HBSAG	ANTI-HBS	HBEAG	ANTI-HBE	ANTI-HBC	HBV DNA
Acute HBV	+	−	+	−	IgM	+
Chronic HBV (high infectivity)	+	−	+	−	IgG	+
Chronic HBV (low infectivity)	+	−	−	+	IgG	+/−
Recovered	−	+	−	+/−	IgG	−
Immunized	−	+	−	−	−	−

73. What are risk factors for HCV infection?

- Intravenous drug use.
- Multiple sex partners.
- Recent surgery (last 6 months).
- Needle stick injury.
- Multiple contacts with HCV infected people.
- Employment in medical or dental fields.
- Remote blood transfusions (prior to the early 1990s).
- Dialysis.
- Body piercings and tattoos.

74. What is the natural history of HCV infections?

- Persistent infection and chronic hepatitis occurs in 80% of cases.
- Cirrhosis develops over 5–20 years after acute infection in 20–30% of patients with persistent infections.

75. Describe the morphology and immunohistochemistry of HDV.

- Histology: same features as for HBV.
- Immunohistochemistry: HDAg.

76. Describe HDV acute coinfection, superinfection, and helper independent latent infection.

- Acute coinfection: occurs on exposure to serum containing both HDV and HBV.
  - HBV is established first, providing HBsAg necessary for HDV virions.
  - Hepatitis ranges from mild to fulminant, but chronicity rarely develops.
- Superinfection: occurs when chronic HBV carriers are exposed to new HDV.
  - Acute hepatitis develops 30–50 days later.
- It frequently develops into to chronic disease and cirrhosis.
- Helper independent latent infection: occurs in liver transplants.
  - HDV is detected in nuclei of transplant without evidence of HDV infection or HBV reinfection.
  - It occurs due to infection of graft by HDV alone. HBV is prevented by administering hepatitis B immunoglobulins.

77. Define hepatitis G virus (HGV). How is it transmitted, and what disease does it cause?

- HGV: a flavivirus related to HCV; also known as GB virus C (GBV-C).
- It is transmitted by blood and sexual contact.
- It replicates primarily in lymphocytes.
- Although it was initially thought to be associated with chronic hepatitis, extensive investigation has failed to identify any association between this virus and clinical illness. It is not hepatotropic and does not cause elevations in ALT or AST.

78. What is the relationship between HGV and HIV?

- HGV commonly coinfects HIV patients.
- This dual infection appears to be somewhat protective against HIV disease.

79. What should you do if you cut your finger while doing an autopsy?

- Follow your facility's policies.
- Wash the wound with warm water and soap.
- Hold the affected limb down to get it to bleed.
- Do not squeeze the wound or soak it in bleach.
- Apply an antiseptic if necessary (e.g., povidone-iodine 10%).
- Contact the occupational health or hospital emergency department as soon as possible.

Epstein-Barr Virus (EBV)

80. What is the usual clinical presentation of infectious mononucleosis?

- Fever.
- Fatigue.
- Generalized lymphadenopathy.
- Splenomegaly.
- Sore throat.
- Maculopapular rash.

81. What are uncommon complications of acute EBV infection?

- Splenic rupture.
- Upper airway obstruction.
- Hepatitis.
- Encephalitis.
- Pneumonitis.
- Hemophagocytic lymphohistiocytosis.

82. What is the epidemiology of infectious mononucleosis?

- In developed nations: late adolescents or young adults in upper socioeconomic classes.
- In developing world: childhood; asymptomatic.

83. What is seen in the blood of patients with infectious mononucleosis?

- Lymphocytosis.
  - Between 5 and 80% of lymphocytes are atypical: large; abundant cytoplasm with multiple clear vacuolations; oval, indented, or folded nucleus; scattered cytoplasmic azurophilic granules.
  - Most express CD8.

84. What are the pathological changes in the spleen of a patient with infectious mononucleosis?

- The spleen is enlarged, weighing 300–500 g.
- It is soft and fleshy with hyperemic cut surface.
- It has red pulp congestion and hyperplastic white pulp.
- There is a blurred border between the red pulp and white pulp.
- There is variable follicular hyperplasia in the white pulp, and polymorphic cellular population in the red pulp and sinusoids, causing their expansion.

Human Immunodeficiency Virus (HIV)

85. What lymph node abnormalities are seen in HIV patients?

- The features of HIV-associated lymphadenopathy depend on the stage of HIV infection:
  - Early stage:
    › Reactive lymphoid hyperplasia.
    › Absent or indistinct mantle zones.
    › Enlarged, hyperplastic germinal centers with irregular shapes.
    › Germinal centers with disruption from hemorrhage, increased T lymphocytes, and follicular dendritic cell meshwork destruction.
    › Sinuses expanded by monocytoid B lymphocyte hyperplasia.
    › Atrophic interfollicular zones filled with increased plasma cells and large multinucleate giant cells.
  - Intermediate/late stage:
    › Follicular involution.
    › Paracortex lymphocyte depletion.
    › Vascular proliferation.
    › Immunostaining with p24 of the follicular dendritic network, CD4 T cells, and/or macrophages (more common in early and intermediate stages).

86. List at least 3 malignancies suggestive of underlying HIV infection.

- Kaposi sarcoma.
- Immunoblastic lymphoma.
- Burkitt lymphoma.
- Primary CNS lymphoma.

87. What are the components of the HIV virion?

- Envelope — lipid bilayer from the host cell containing the gp41 transmembrane and gp120 surface glycoproteins.
- Matrix — composed of p17 protein.
- Core — capsid of core protein p24 surrounding 2 single strands of HIV RNA, each of which has a complete copy of the virus's genome, and enzymes including reverse transcriptase, integrase, and protease.

88. What are the modes of transmission of HIV?

- Unprotected anal, vaginal, and — rarely — oral intercourse.
- Sharing of HIV contaminated needles or injection equipment.
- Transfusion of contaminated blood products.
- Needle stick injury or other parenteral health care exposure — 0.3%.
- Vertical transmission from mother to child in utero, at delivery, or during breastfeeding.

89. List the methods of laboratory diagnosis for HIV.

- ELISA to detect serum antibodies to HIV — antibodies usually detectable within 3 months (seroconversion takes 2–8 weeks); confirmed by follow-up Western blot to detect antibodies to at least 2 HIV protein bands (p24, gp41, gp120/160).
- Rapid test, then confirmation with Western blot.
- PCR to detect HIV DNA in plasma.
- ELISA to detect p24 antigen.

90. What is the sensitivity and specificity of the rapid test and the Western blot in testing for HIV antibodies?

- Rapid test: 96% sensitivity, > 99.9% specificity.
- Western blot: > 99% sensitivity, > 99.99% specificity.

91. What are several complications and symptoms of HIV at the following CD4 counts?

- < 500 cells/mm^3:
  - Constitutional symptoms.
  - Mucocutaneous lesions — seborrheic dermatitis, oral hairy leukoplakia (EBV), Kaposi sarcoma, shingles (varicella zoster virus), HSV.
  - Lymphoma.
  - Oral, esophageal, and vaginal candidiasis.
  - Pulmonary and extrapulmonary tuberculosis.
- < 200 cells/mm^3:
  - *Pneumocystis jiroveci* pneumonia.

(*continued on next page*)

- Toxoplasmosis.
- *Bartonella* infection.
- Visceral Kaposi sarcoma.
- Local or disseminated fungal infections, including *Cryptococcus*, *Coccidioides*, and *Histoplasma*.
- < 100 cells/mm³:
  - Progressive multifocal leukoencephalopathy (PML) due to JC virus.

- CNS toxoplasmosis.
- < 50 cells/mm³:
  - *Mycobacterium avium* complex (MAC).
  - CMV infection causing retinitis, colitis, cholangiopathy, and CNS disease.
  - Invasive aspergillosis.
  - Bacillary angiomatosis (disseminated *Bartonella*).
  - CNS lymphoma.

Bacteria
Bacteria: General

92. What are 3 helpful features to distinguish *Helicobacter heilmannii* from *Helicobacter pylori*?

- *Helicobacter heilmannii* is acquired from domestic animals and pets.
- *H. heilmannii* are larger than *Helicobacter pylori* and have a corkscrew morphology.

- *H. heilmannii* often lie freely in gastric foveolar lumen or surface while *H. pylori* are more often adherent to the epithelium.
- *H. heilmannii* is usually associated with less inflammation and activity than *H. pylori*.

93. What are the pathogens and relevant stains for bacillary angiomatosis, erythema chronicum migrans, leprosy, chancre syphilis, and impetigo?

DISEASE	PATHOGEN	STAINS
Bacillary angiomatosis	*Bartonella* family bacilli	• Gram stain negative. • Warthin Starry.
Erythema chronicum migrans	*Borrelia burgdorferi* spirochete	• Gram stain negative. • Steiner, Warthin-Starry. • Dieterle stain.
Leprosy	*Mycobacterium leprae*	• Modified acid-fast stain (FITE)
Chancre syphilis	*Treponema pallidum* spirochete	• Gram stain negative. • Steiner, Warthin-Starry. • Dieterle stain. • Dark field examination. • Immunohistochemistry/immunofluorescence for *Treponema pallidum*.
Impetigo	*Staphylococcus aureus* cocci	• Gram stain positive. • Silver stain.

94. Photochromogens, scotochromogens, and nonchromogens are 3 groups of slowly growing nontuberculous mycobacteria that take > 7 days to form colonies clearly visible to the naked eye. List at least 1 representative example of each. Also list at least 1 representative example of a rapid-growing nontuberculous mycobacteria.

- Photochromogens (develop yellow pigment when exposed to light): *Mycobacterium kansasii, Mycobacterium marinum*.
- Scotochromogens (develop yellow pigment in the dark or in the light): *Mycobacterium gordonae, Mycobacterium scrofulaceum*.

- Nonchromogens (do not produce pigment): *Mycobacterium avium* and *Mycobacterium intracellulare* (known together as MAI); *Mycobacterium ulcerans*.
- Rapid growers (colonies form in < 5 days and do not produce pigment): *Mycobacterium fortuitum, Mycobacterium peregrinum, Mycobacterium abscessus, Mycobacterium chelonae*.

Yersinia Enterocolitis

95. List the common clinical features of *Yersinia* enterocolitis infection.

- Fever, diarrhea, nausea, vomiting, abdominal tenderness.

- Peyer patch invasion and involvement of regional lymphatics, mimicking acute appendicitis.

96. What are the common extraintestinal features of *Yersinia* enterocolitis infection?
- Pharyngitis.
- Arthralgia.
- Erythema nodosum.

97. How is *Yersinia* enterocolitis infection detected?
- Stool cultures on *Yersinia* selective agar.
- Cultures of lymph nodes or blood (if extraintestinal).

98. What are the common postinfectious complications of *Yersinia* enterocolitis infection?
- Sterile arthritis.
- Reiter syndrome.
- Myocarditis.
- Glomerulonephritis.
- Thyroiditis.

99. How is gastrointestinal *Yersinia* contracted most commonly?
- Ingestion of:
  - Pork.
  - Raw milk.
  - Contaminated water.

100. What are the gross features of *Yersinia* enterocolitis infection?
- Involvement of ileum, appendix, and right colon.
- Bowel wall thickening.
- Hyperplastic lymphoid follicles.
- Hemorrhagic mucosa over lymphoid tissue.
- Aphthous ulcers.

101. What are the microscopic features of *Yersinia* enterocolitis infection?
- Lymph node and Peyer patch hypertrophy.
- Acute cryptitis.
- Granulomas, neutrophilic or stellate.
- Lamina propria densely infiltrated with plasma cells, lymphocytes, and neutrophils.

Legionnaires' Disease

102. What is the agent of Legionnaires' disease and what are its characteristics?
- Agent:
  - *Legionella pneumophila*.
- Characteristics:
  - Aerobic gram-negative bacteria.
  - Facultative intracellular bacterium that can invade and replicate inside amoebae.

103. What environment does *Legionella pneumophila* live in?
Artificial aquatic environments, particularly warm ones, such as hot tubs, cooling towers, hot water tanks, large plumbing systems, air conditioning systems, and indoor ornamental fountains.

104. How is *Legionella pneumophila* transmitted?
- Inhalation of aerosolized organisms.
- Aspiration of contaminated water.

105. What is the epidemiology of Legionnaires' disease?
- Middle-aged and older individuals, particularly those who smoke, have chronic lung diseases, or are immunocompromised.
- Organ transplant patients (particularly susceptible).

106. What are the signs and symptoms of Legionnaires' disease?
- High fever and pneumonia, chills, and cough with or without sputum.
- Potential derangement of renal and liver function tests, and electrolytes, including hyponatremia.
- Fever with bradycardia (Faget sign, also known as sphygmothermic dissociation).
- Bibasilar consolidation on chest X-ray.
- Headache and confusion.
- Development of symptoms: 2–10 days after exposure to bacteria.

107. What is Pontiac fever?
- Mild disease caused by *L. pneumophila*, featuring fever and muscle aches without pneumonia.
- Development of symptoms: within hours to days of infection.
- Recovery: generally spontaneous within 2–5 days without treatment.

108. How is Legionnaires' disease diagnosed?
- *Legionella* antigens in urine.
- Positive fluorescent antibody test on bronchoalveolar lavage samples.
- Legionnaire antibody levels in 2 blood samples taken 3–6 weeks apart.
- Culture or detection by nucleic acid amplification.

109. How do *Legionella* organisms survive in the host?
- *L. pneumophila* invade and replicate in macrophages.
- Inside the macrophage, the bacteria enter/live in a membrane bound vacuole.
- They have several methods, including effector proteins, of interfering with the fusion of the vacuole with lysosomes and endosomes.

Lyme Disease

110. List 4 infectious diseases caused by spirochetes.
- Intestinal spirochetosis (*Brachyspira pilosicoli* and *Brachyspira aalborgi*).
- Leptospirosis (*Leptospira* species).
- Lyme disease (*Borrelia burgdorferi*, *Borrelia garinii*, and *Borrelia afzelii*).
- Relapsing fever (*Borrelia recurrentis*).
- Syphilis (*Treponema pallidum*).
- Yaws (*Treponema pallidum pertenue*).

111. How is Lyme disease transmitted? What is the most common vector?
- Arthropod-borne illness.
- Spread by the bite of infected tick, most commonly several ticks of the *Ixodes* genus.

112. Describe the 3 stages of Lyme disease.

STAGE	INCUBATION PERIOD	SIGNS/SYMPTOMS
1 (early localized)	3–32 days	• Erythema migrans skin rash. • Fever. • Lymphadenopathy.
2 (early disseminated)	Weeks to months	• Multisystem involvement due to dissemination of spirochetes. • Multiple secondary erythema migrans lesions. • Neurologic presentations (aseptic meningitis, cranial nerve palsies, neuropathies, radiculopathy, intracranial hypertension). • Cardiac presentations (carditis, heart block). • Lymphadenopathy.
3 (late persistent)	Months to years	• Chronic monoarthritis or oligoarthritis. • Skin and soft tissue presentations (chronic atrophic acrodermatitis, borrelial lymphocytoma). • Neurologic presentations (polyneuropathies, radiculopathies, encephalomyelitis).

113. Describe the macroscopic and microscopic findings of the hallmark dermatologic lesion of Lyme disease.
- Erythema migrans.
- Macroscopic:
  › It begins as a small macule or papule that enlarges over days.
  › It is initially uniformly red.
  › Later, a central clearing may develop around the initial tick bite that remains red (bull's-eye lesion).
  › Annular skin rash, 5–20 cm in diameter, is present.
  › Multiple lesions may develop.
- Microscopic:
  › Superficial and deep perivascular and interstitial lymphocytic infiltrate is present.
  › Plasma cells and eosinophils may be present (eosinophils more likely present at the site of the bite).
  › Vascular proliferation and dermal necrosis may be present at site of the bite.
  › Warthin-Starry silver stain or immunohistochemical staining with monoclonal antibodies against *Borrelia* species may identify spirochetes.

114. What is the differential diagnosis for erythema migrans?
- Other arthropod bites (especially southern tick-associated rash illness [STARI]).
- Bacterial cellulitis.
- Contact dermatitis.
- Infections with herpes simplex or varicella.
- Tinea.
- Urticaria.
- Fixed drug eruption.

115. How is Lyme disease diagnosed?

- It is often a difficult diagnosis.
- History of tick exposure in endemic areas is extremely helpful; however, documentation of a tick bite is not necessary.
- Clinical presentation of the classic erythema migrans rash, acquired in an endemic area, may be sufficient for diagnosis.
- Laboratory testing includes:
  - Serology: 2-tier testing with ELISA and Western blot assay or enzyme immunoassay.
  - Microbiological culture.
  - Tissue: immunohistochemistry or immunofluorescent identification.
  - Molecular: PCR.

116. Describe common histologic findings in the skin from an arthropod bite.

- Wedge shaped superficial and deep mixed inflammatory infiltrate with lymphocytes, histiocytes, eosinophils, and sometime neutrophils.
- Scattered eosinophils away from vessels.
- Dermal edema.
- Possible lymphoid reaction with germinal centers and secondary vasculitis.
- Variable epidermal changes, including spongiosis, acanthosis, and parakeratosis; possible excoriation.

117. List 2 diseases that can coinfect with Lyme disease.

Lyme disease, ehrlichiosis, and babesiosis can be transmitted by a "deer tick": *Ixodes scapularis*.

Other Bacteria and Related Diseases

118. What organisms cause the following diseases?

- Syphilis: *Treponema pallidum*.
- Bacillary angiomatosis: *Bartonella henselae* and *Bartonella quintana*.
- Impetigo: primarily *Staphylococcus aureus*, occasionally *Streptococcus pyogenes*.
- Erythema chronicum migrans: *Borrelia burgdorferi sensu lato* — i.e., the cause of Lyme disease.
- Leprosy: *Mycobacterium leprae*.
- Typhus fever: *Rickettsia prowazekii*.
- Cholera: *Vibrio cholera*.
- Whooping cough: *Bordetella pertussis*.
- Typhoid fever: *Salmonella typhi*.
- Bubonic plague: *Yersinia pestis*.
- Catscratch disease: *Bartonella henselae*.
- Molluscum contagiosum: molluscum contagiosum virus.
- Chagas disease: *Trypanosoma cruzi*.
- Sleeping sickness: *Trypanosoma brucei gambiense* (95% of cases) and *Trypanosoma brucei rhodesiense* (5% of cases).
- Filariasis: *Wuchereria bancrofti*, *Brugia malayi*, and *Brugia timori*.

Case Scenario

A young man presents with an MAI mycobacterial pseudotumor in a mesenteric node.

119. What is MAI?

- MAI includes 2 species of bacteria: *Mycobacterium avium* and *Mycobacterium intracellulare* that cause similar infections.
- The bacteria are referred to together as *M. avium-intracellulare* complex (MAI).

120. In what environment is MAI normally found, and how does it gain access to hosts?

- Environment: soil, water, dust, domestic animals.
- Access to hosts: inhalation or ingestion.

121. In what patient population is MAI common?

- AIDS patients.
- Cystic fibrosis patients.
- Other people with low numbers of CD4+ lymphocytes (< 60 cells/mm³).
- Elderly men and women with chronic lung disease (pulmonary MAI infection).

122. What are the clinical findings of MAI in HIV patients?

- Fever, night sweats, weight loss, cough if respiratory infection.
- Diarrhea and abdominal pain if gastrointestinal involvement.
- Anemia and neutropenia if bone marrow involvement.
- Bacteria in blood, sputum, and bone marrow cultures (possible).

123. What are the gross findings of MAI infection?
- Infection is widely disseminated, including the lungs and gastrointestinal system.
- The most common sites in the gastrointestinal system include the large bowel, small bowel, liver, esophagus, and the associated intraabdominal lymph nodes. Yellow plaques often present on intestinal surfaces.
- Infection may be localized to the lungs (pulmonary MAI infection).

124. What are the microscopic findings of MAI infection?
- Hallmark finding: abundant foamy macrophages/histiocytes stuffed with acid-fast bacilli.
  - These can be disseminated throughout the body, including lymph nodes, liver, and spleen.
    - Nodes have extensive infiltration of the paracortical regions by infected histiocytes.
  - In the gastrointestinal system, they are found in lamina propria (Whipple-like expansion and flattening of villi in the small intestine).
  - They can be localized to the lungs.
- Organisms are slender, curvilinear, and sometimes beaded, measuring 4–6 μm in length.
- Affected organs may have yellow pigmentation, due to the large number of bacteria.
- Granulomas, lymphocytes, and tissue destruction are possible — granulomas are more likely in immunocompetent patients.
- Granulomas may have macrophages of spindled morphology, especially in the lymph nodes, lung, and bone marrow.

125. Describe the overall diagnostic approach for MAI, including the use of special stains.
- Acid-fast stain: identifies significant numbers of acid-fast bacilli within the foamy macrophages, frequently in parallel arrays.
- Silver stains: highlight the bacteria.
- Other stains: PAS+ and PAS-diastase resistant. Gram+ but usually not seen unless in large numbers.
- Cultures to rule out tuberculosis and to determine antibiotic sensitivities.

126. What is the differential diagnosis of MAI? Include storage diseases presenting with foamy macrophages.
- Whipple disease.
- Gaucher disease.
- Niemann-Pick disease.
- Cholesteryl ester storage disease.
- Mucopolysaccharidoses.
- Glycogen storage diseases.

127. List causes of immunosuppression associated with MAI, other than AIDS.
- Hairy cell leukemia.
- Severe combined immunodeficiency disorder.
- IFN gamma and IL-12 pathway disorders.
- Immunosuppressive chemotherapy.

128. How do you reduce the risk of transmission of infection from cryostats?
- Consider cryostats contaminated each time specimens are processed, and decontaminate them frequently with 70% alcohol.
- Wear stainless steel mesh gloves when handling blades in cryostats.
- Consider tissue that collects around the edges of cryostats infectious and remove it during decontamination.
- Treat cryostats with glutaraldehyde or another tuberculocidal agent at least weekly and after any known case of tuberculosis.

Case Scenario

A 32-year-old female has granulomatous lymphadenitis in a cervical lymph node.

129. Name 6 morphologic features of granulomas (they may overlap).
- Nonnecrotizing.
- Necrotizing.
- Palisading.
- Suppurative.
- Necrobiotic.
- Fibrin ring.

130. List at least 4 differential diagnoses of nonnecrotizing granulomas.
- Sarcoidosis.
- Beryllium disease.
- Hypersensitivity pneumonitis.
- Drug reactions.
- Tuberculoid leprosy.
- Crohn disease.

131. List at least 4 differential diagnoses of necrotizing granulomas.
- Tuberculosis.
- Fungal infections.
- Rheumatoid nodules.
- Wegener granulomatosis.
- Necrobiotic postsurgical granulomas.

132. List at least 1 differential diagnosis associated with palisading granulomas.
- Rheumatoid nodules.
- Postsurgical necrobiotic granuloma.

133. List at least 2 differential diagnoses of suppurative granulomas.
- Catscratch disease (*Bartonella henselae*).
- Lymphogranuloma venereum (*Chlamydia trachomatis*).
- Tularemia.
- *Yersinia*.

134. List at least 3 differential diagnoses of necrobiotic granulomas.
- Granuloma annulare.
- Rheumatoid nodule.
- Necrobiosis lipoidica diabeticorum.
- Wegener granulomatosis.
- Postsurgical necrobiotic granulomas.

135. List 1 differential diagnosis associated with fibrin ring granulomas.
Q fever (found in liver and bone marrow).

136. How do you proceed if, clinically, a node appears to indicate tuberculosis but the acid-fast stain is negative?
- Ensure the acid-fast stain has been examined carefully at high power (100x/oil immersion objective may be required to see rare acid-fast bacilli).
- Suggest sending samples for culture, with tuberculosis in the differential diagnosis of the granulomatous inflammation.
- Consider trying to visualize the acid-fast bacilli by fluorescent microscopy using the auramine-rhodamine stain, which makes the bacilli appear golden in color.
- Consult with microbiologist/infectious disease on requesting PCR on tissue for *M. tuberculosis*.

137. What are risk factors for acquiring tuberculosis?
- Drinking unpasteurized milk.
- Living in or emigrating from a country with high endemic rate of tuberculosis.
- Incarceration in prisons.
- Homelessness.
- Poverty.
- Crowding.
- Alcoholism.
- Immunosuppression (e.g., HIV, drugs).

138. What conditions increase the risk of developing active tuberculosis, once a patient is infected?
- Age — young and old.
- Malnutrition.
- Diabetes.
- Immunosuppression.
- Alcoholism.
- Chronic lung disease.
- Chronic renal failure.

139. What precautions prevent the transmission of airborne infections during the processing of frozen sections?
- Ensure there is adequate air exchange in the frozen section room/cabinet, with HEPA filtration or external venting of air.
- Follow universal precautions, including gloving at all times and handwashing.
- Wear N95 mask protection and goggles.
- Section and manipulate specimens in a biosafety cabinet whenever possible.
- Clean surfaces appropriately.

Case Scenario

A 45-year-old man presents with a year-long history of an unintentional gradual weight loss of 15 kg, diarrhea, and abdominal pain. He also has of migratory joint pain. An occult stool blood test is negative. A CT scan identifies mesenteric and retroperitoneal lymphadenopathy, and prominent duodenal and jejunal folds. An upper endoscopy is performed and duodenal biopsies taken. The duodenum shows a dense accumulation of foamy cells within the lamina propria causing villous expansion.

140. List at least 6 pathologic differential diagnoses of abundant foamy cells in the lamina propria of the small intestine.
- Microorganisms:
  - *Mycobacterium avium-intracellulare* infection.
  - Whipple disease.
  - Histoplasmosis.
  - Leishmaniasis.
  - *Pneumocystis jiroveci*.

(continued on next page)

- Neoplastic entities:
  - Signet-ring cell carcinoma.
  - Metastatic carcinomas.
  - Mastocytosis.
  - Langerhans cell histiocytosis.
  - Rosai-Dorfman disease.
  - Waldenström macroglobulinemia.
- Metabolic storage diseases.

- Other entities:
  - Crushed Brunner glands.
  - Xanthoma/xanthelasma.
  - Mineral oil ingestion.
  - Crystal storing histiocytosis.
  - *Pseudomelanosis coli*.
  - Various pigment accumulations.

141. Histology suggests the foamy cell infiltrate is composed of macrophages. What ancillary tests would you perform?
- CD68 immunohistochemistry.
- PAS or PAS-diastase histochemical staining.
- Acid-fast bacilli stain (Ziehl-Neelsen stain or auramine rhodamine stain).

142. You find that the foamy cells are positive for CD68, PAS, and PAS-diastase, and negative for acid-fast bacilli. What is the most likely diagnosis?
Whipple disease.

143. Briefly describe Whipple disease.
- It is a chronic systemic infection caused by *Tropheryma whippeli*, a gram positive intracellular actinomycete.
- It most often affects the small intestine, but can also affect other organs including the joints, central nervous system, lungs, and heart.

144. List at least 1 method to confirm a diagnosis of Whipple disease.
- Anti-*T. whippeli* immunohistochemical staining.
- PCR study.
- Electron microscopy.

145. What is the primary mechanism for the diarrhea of Whipple disease?
Bacteria-laden macrophages accumulate within the small intestinal lamina propria and mesenteric lymph nodes, causing lymphatic obstruction. The impaired lymph drainage causes malabsorptive diarrhea.

Fungi
Blastomycosis

146. What organism causes blastomycosis?
Blastomyces dermatitidis.

147. What environment does the blastomycosis fungus live in, and where is the fungus found in North America?
- Environment: soil.
- Location: Mississippi, Ohio, St. Lawrence, and Tennessee river basins.

148. List 4 key clinical forms of blastomycosis infection.
- Primary cutaneous blastomycosis.
- Pulmonary blastomycosis.
- Osseous blastomycosis.
- Disseminated blastomycosis.

149. Describe the clinical presentation of pulmonary blastomycosis.
- It presents as an abrupt illness with a productive cough, headache, chest pain, weight loss, fever, abdominal pain, night sweats, chills, and anorexia.
- Chest X-rays reveal lobar consolidation, multilobar infiltrates, perihilar infiltrates, multiple nodules, or miliary infiltrates.
- The upper lobes are most frequently involved.
- The natural progression is either spontaneous resolution, persistent infection, or progression to chronic lesion.

150. Describe the histology of pulmonary blastomycosis.
- Suppurative granulomas in the lung, which form because macrophages have limited ability to ingest and kill the organism, leading to recruitment of neutrophils.
- Yeast in tissue: 5–15 µm yeast cells, which divide with broad based budding and have thick double contoured cell walls and multiple nuclei.

151. Describe the gross appearance of cutaneous blastomycosis lesions.

Typical cutaneous lesions show central healing with microabscesses at the periphery.

152. Describe the histology of blastomycosis involving the epithelium.

Marked epithelial hyperplasia (pseudoepitheliomatous hyperplasia), possibly mistaken for squamous cell carcinoma.

Histoplasmosis

153. Which organs/tissues are usually involved in histoplasmosis?
- Lungs.
- Bone marrow.
- Liver.
- Spleen.

154. In what region of North America is histoplasmosis common, and in what ecologic niches are the organisms most commonly found?
- Region in North America: most common in the midwestern United States, within the Ohio and Mississippi river valleys; in Canada within the St. Lawrence River valleys.
- There is also global distribution, including southern and east Africa, and in Southeast Asia.
- Ecologic niche: blackbird roosts, chicken houses, and bat guano.

155. What are 3 common symptomatic clinical presentations of histoplasmosis?
- Acute pulmonary (flu-like illness).
- Chronic pulmonary.
- Disseminated.

156. Describe the symptoms of histoplasmosis.
- Asymptomatic (most common).
- Dyspnea.
- Productive cough with possibly purulent or bloody sputum.
- Anorexia.
- Weight loss.
- Night sweats.

157. What is the classic appearance of histoplasmosis on chest X-ray?
- Bilateral interstitial infiltrates.
- Hilar and mediastinal adenopathy are common in acute infection.
- Coin lesions (healed granuloma) may be seen in remote infection.

158. What is the histology of pulmonary histoplasmosis?
- It is a narrow based, budding, small yeast with a blunt and a pointed/tapered end that stains with silver and Giemsa stains.
- It is often intracellular and in clusters.
- It may form a necrotizing granulomatous inflammation, with a thick fibrous capsule, possibly with calcification, and with organisms in the central necrotic areas.
- Organisms may occur within foamy macrophages — especially in immunocompromised patients.

Hyphal Fungi

159. Name the 4 most common fungi seen as hyphae in tissues.
- *Aspergillus*.
- *Zygomycetes*.
- *Fusarium*.
- *Pseudallescheria*.

160. Compare and contrast the hyphae of *Aspergillus* and *Zygomycetes* (mucormycosis) in terms of septation, outline appearance, branching pattern, and width.
- *Aspergillus* is septate, while *Zygomycetes* is aseptate or pauciseptate.
- The outline of *Aspergillus* appears as parallel lines, while *Zygomycetes* appears as irregular, nonparallel lines.
- *Aspergillus* shows a dichotomous branching pattern (i.e., the daughter branch has the same width as the parent branch) and branches at acute angles; *Zygomycetes* has a haphazard branching pattern and frequently branches at 90 degrees or greater.
- *Aspergillus* hyphae are 3–6 μm wide, while *Zygomycetes* hyphae are 6–50 μm wide.

Yeast-Like Fungi

161. List 3 dimorphic fungi, their associated endemic areas, and the diseases they cause.
- *Histoplasma capsulatum*: Ohio and Mississippi river valleys; lung infection similar to tuberculosis.
- *Blastomyces dermatitis*: eastern North America; skin and lung infections.
- *Coccidioides immitis*: southwestern United States; lung infection.

162. Name 5 fungi frequently seen as yeasts.
- *Histoplasma capsulatum*.
- *Blastomyces dermatitidis*.
- *Cryptococcus neoformans*.
- *Coccidioides immitis*.
- *Candida* species.

163. Name a key feature that distinguishes each of the following entities: *Histoplasma capsulatum*, *Blastomyces dermatitidis*, *Cryptococcus neoformans*, *Coccidioides immitis*, and *Candida* species.
- *Histoplasma capsulatum*, and *Candida* species are 2-6 μm in size; *Cryptococcus neoformans* is 5–20 μm; *Blastomyces dermatitidis* is 15-30 μm; *Coccidioides immitis* spherules are 20–100 μm, with endospores of 2-5 μm.
- All are round-to-oval in shape, but *Histoplasma capsulatum* may also be pear or teardrop shaped.
- *Blastomyces dermatitidis* demonstrates single broad-based budding, while *Histoplasma capsulatum*, *Cryptococcus neoformans*, and *Candida* species have narrow-neck budding.
- *Coccidioides immitis* demonstrates endosporulation.
- *Candida* species demonstrate pseudohyphae (rarely true hyphae); the others rarely demonstrate hyphae or pseudohyphae.
- *Blastomyces dermatitidis* has multiple nuclei; the others have single nuclei.
- *Histoplasma capsulatum* is positive on Giemsa stain; the others are negative.
- *Cryptococcus neoformans* is positive on mucicarmine stain: the others are negative.

Parasites
Echinococcus Granulosus

164. Describe the life cycle of *E. granulosus* and how humans are infected.
- Adult tapeworms live in canids and produce eggs that are passed with dog feces.
- Intermediate hosts such as sheep are infected by food contaminated with eggs shed by dogs.
- Eggs hatch into oncosphere larvae and penetrate intestinal walls, entering the blood and traveling to tissues such as the liver, lungs, bones, and brain.
- Larvae form hydatid cysts in host tissue.
- Larval worms are then eaten by dogs who prey on the usual herbivore intermediate hosts such as sheep.
- Humans are accidental intermediate hosts.

165. Describe the gross and microscopic appearance of *E. granulosus* infestation in humans.
- *E. granulosus* forms cysts.
  - Two-thirds are found in the liver, 5–15% in the lung, and the rest in bone, the brain, and other organs.
  - Cysts range in size from microscopic to > 10 cm in diameter.
  - Cysts consist of an outer, opaque, nonnucleated layer with a laminated appearance. There is an inner, nucleated, germinative layer, and opalescent fluid in the middle that contains a fine, sand-like sediment representing degenerating scolices.
- Around cysts, a host inflammatory reaction forms, consisting of a zone of fibroblasts, giant cells, mononuclear cells, and eosinophils.
- Smaller daughter cysts may form within larger cysts and contain protoscolices and hooklets.
- Larvae of *E. granulosus* may lodge in capillaries and create an inflammatory reaction composed of mononuclear leukocytes and eosinophils.

Malaria

166. What is the genus of the malarial parasite?

Plasmodium.

167. List at least 4 species of parasites that cause malaria. Which is the most common?

- *P. falciparum* — most common, most virulent.
- *P. vivax.*
- *P. ovale.*
- *P. malariae.*
- *P. knowlesi.*

168. Which genus of mosquitos transmits malaria?

Anopheles.

169. Describe the life cycle of malarial parasites.

- Malaria is infectious as sporozoites, which are found in the salivary glands of female mosquitoes.
- The mosquitoes infect people with sporozoites when they feed on human blood.
- The sporozoites attach to and invade liver cells.
- Sporozoites mature into schizonts and multiply rapidly in the liver into thousands of merozoites (asexual haploid form).
- Infected hepatocytes rupture releasing thousands of merozoites.
- The merozoites bind to and invade red blood cells.
- Within each red blood cell, the parasite develops into a trophozoite, defined by the presence of a single chromatin mass, then into a schizont, which has multiple chromatin masses.
- Each chromatin mass develops into a new merozoite.
- When an infected red blood cell bursts, the new merozoites infect other red blood cells.
- Some trophozoites within red blood cells develop into gametocytes — the sexual form of the parasite — which infect new mosquitoes when mosquitoes feed on human blood.

170. What are the clinical features of a malarial infection?

- Flu-like prodrome.
- Paroxysms of high fever and shaking chills, which are caused by synchronous systemic lysis of red blood cells at set time intervals (*P. vivax* and *P. ovale* cause chills and fever every 48 hours; *P. malariae* every 72 hours; *P. falciparum* at variable intervals).
- Abdominal pain, myalgias, headache, cough.
- Hepatosplenomegaly.

171. What are some specific complications caused by *P. falciparum*?

- *P. falciparum* causes tissue damage and is the form seen in tissue.
- CNS involvement causes seizures and coma (malignant cerebral malaria).
- Severe anemia.
- Acute renal failure.
- Acute respiratory distress syndrome.
- Of note, schizonts of *P. falciparum* do not circulate because they adhere to endothelial cells (and are therefore seldom seen in peripheral blood).

172. What are some gross morphological findings of malarial infection?

- Splenomegaly.
- Hyperplastic white pulp.
- Acute:
  · Congestion and enlargement of the spleen (can be > 1000 g).
  · Dark red parenchyma due to congestion and malarial pigment deposition.
- Splenic rupture.
- Chronic:
  · Fibrotic and brittle spleen.
  · Grey/black parenchyma.
  · Hepatomegaly with pigmentation.
  · Enlarged kidneys.

173. What are the microscopic features of malaria?

- Spleen/acute:
  · Parasitized red blood cells in venous sinuses.
  · Increased numbers of macrophages containing hemosiderin, red cell debris, and malarial pigment.
  · Desquamation of sinus lining cells containing phagocytosed erythrocytes.
  · Increased small lymphocytes in red pulp.
- Spleen/chronic:
  · Fibrosis and scarring.
  · Phagocytic cells containing more granular, brown-black, faintly birefringent hemozoin pigment concentrated around periarteriolar lymphoid sheaths.
- Liver:
  · Kupffer cell hyperplasia heavily laden with malarial pigment, parasites, and cellular debris from ruptured erythrocytes.
  · Some pigment in hepatocytes.
- Pigmented phagocytic cells dispersed throughout bone marrow, lymph nodes, subcutaneous tissues, and lungs.
- Kidney congestion and dusting of pigment in glomeruli and hemoglobin casts in tubules.

174. What are the histologic findings of malignant cerebral malaria?
- Brain vessels plugged with parasitized red cells.
- Ring hemorrhages around vessels, related to local hypoxia due to vascular stasis.
- Small focal inflammatory reactions (malarial or Dürck granuloma).
- If severe hypoxia:
  · Degeneration of neurons.
  · Focal ischemic softening.
  · Inflammatory infiltrates in meninges.

175. How can you determine if pigment is malarial pigment?
Malarial pigment is refractile, birefringent, and negative for melanin and iron stains.

Other Parasites

176. List 3 infections caused by larval cysts that can involve skeletal muscle.
- Cysticercosis from pork tapeworm.
- Echinococcosis from dog tapeworm.
- Trichinellosis from a roundworm transmitted from domestic or wild animals.

177. List 3 parasite larvae that can cause diseases by penetrating skin.
- *Strongyloides stercoralis* and *Necator americanus* are roundworms capable of penetrating bare skin (usually the foot). This is known as "ground itch."
- Schistosomes (flukes) can penetrate skin in snail-infested water. This is known as "swimmer's itch."

General Knowledge

178. List 4 organ systems that are common routes of entry for infectious diseases into the body.
- Skin.
- Gastrointestinal tract.
- Respiratory tract.
- Urogenital tract.

179. For each system, provide 1 major local defense system, and 1 potential method for the failure of this defense.

SITE	MAJOR LOCAL DEFENSE	POTENTIAL DEFENSE FAILURE
Skin	• Epidermal barrier.	• Mechanical defects (punctures, burns, ulcers, animal/insect bites).
	• Normal microbiota.	• Antibiotic use.
Gastrointestinal tract	• Epithelial barrier.	• Mechanical defects. • Attachment and local proliferation or invasion of microbes. • Uptake through M cells.
	• Acidic secretions.	• Acid-resistant cysts and eggs.
	• Peristalsis.	• Obstruction, ileus, postsurgical adhesions.
	• Bile and pancreatic enzymes.	• Resistant microbial external coats.
	• Normal protective microbiota.	• Antibiotic use.
Respiratory tract	• Epithelial barrier.	• Attachment and local proliferation or invasion of microbes.
	• Mucociliary clearance.	• Ciliary paralysis by toxins.
	• Resident alveolar macrophages.	• Resistance to killing by phagocytes.
Urogenital tract	• Epidermal/epithelial barrier.	• Mechanical defects. • Attachment and local proliferation or invasion of microbes.
	• Urination.	• Obstruction, microbial attachment.
	• Normal vaginal microbiota.	• Antibiotic use.

180. Define vertical transmission of infectious disease.

Vertical transmission is the transmission of infectious agents from mother to fetus or newborn child.

181. List 3 routes of vertical transmission of infectious agents and provide at least 1 example of each.

- Placental-fetal transmission: rubella infection.
- Transmission during birth: gonococcal and chlamydial conjunctivitis.
- Postnatal transmission in maternal milk: CMV, HIV, HBV.

182. List at least 5 strategies infectious microorganisms use to evade the immune system.

- Antigenic variation to avoid being recognized by the host.
- Resistance to antimicrobial peptides.
- Inactivation of antibodies or complement.
- Mechanisms to resist phagocytosis.
- Evasion of apoptosis and manipulation of replicate within a host cell.
- Suppression of the host adaptive immune response.
- Evasion of recognition by T cells through alteration of MHC antigen presentation.
- Downregulation of T cell response through immune checkpoint interference (e.g., PD-1).
- Establishing latency.
- Infecting and disabling or destroying immune cells.

183. List at least 5 major histologic tissue reactions or inflammatory responses to infections.

- Suppurative infection.
- Mononuclear and granulomatous inflammation.
- Cytopathic-cytoproliferative reaction.
- Tissue necrosis.
- Chronic inflammation/scarring.
- No reaction.

IMAGES: PATHOLOGY OF INFECTIOUS DISEASE

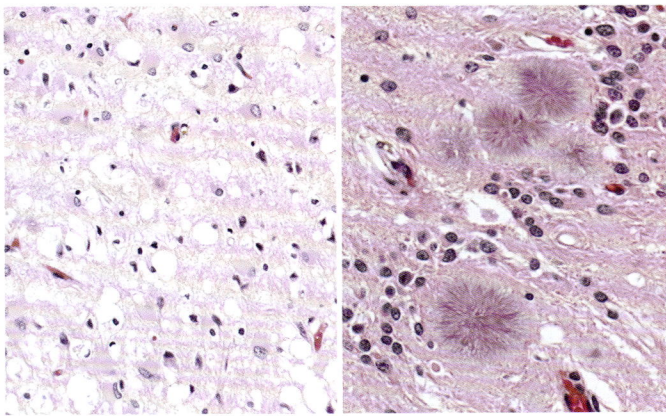

IMAGE 14.1 Variant Creutzfeldt-Jakob disease (vCJD). Left: the cerebral cortical neuropil shows prominent spongiotic change, termed spongiform encephalopathy (H&E, x100). Right: prion protein may precipitate as amyloid plaques that consist of a core with radiating fibrils and a surrounding pale halo (H&E, x200).

Source: CDC Public Health Image Library

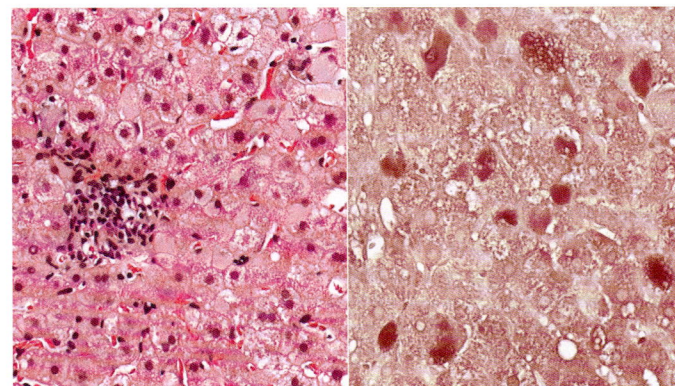

IMAGE 14.2 Chronic active hepatitis B (HBV) infection. Left: the liver shows hepatocellular ballooning, lobular inflammation, and many ground-glass hepatocytes with finely granular eosinophilic cytoplasm (H&E, x100). Right: ground-glass materials are positive for anti-HBsAg (immunoperoxidase, x100).

Source: Joint Pathology Center, Infectious Disease Archives

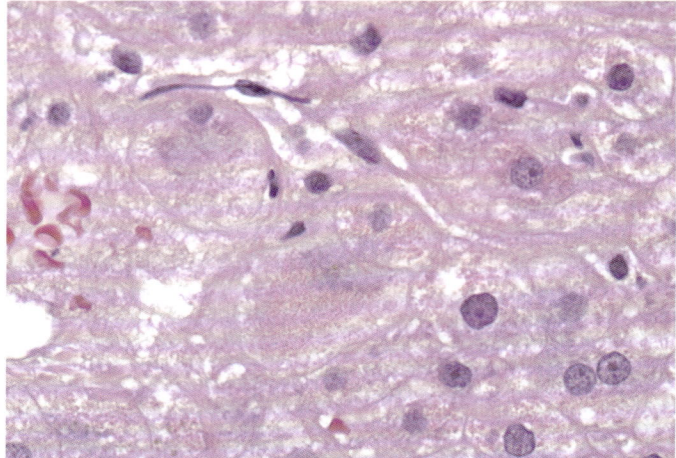

IMAGE 14.3 HBV infection. The liver shows many ground-glass hepatocytes with finely granular eosinophilic cytoplasm with a clear halo (H&E, x1000).

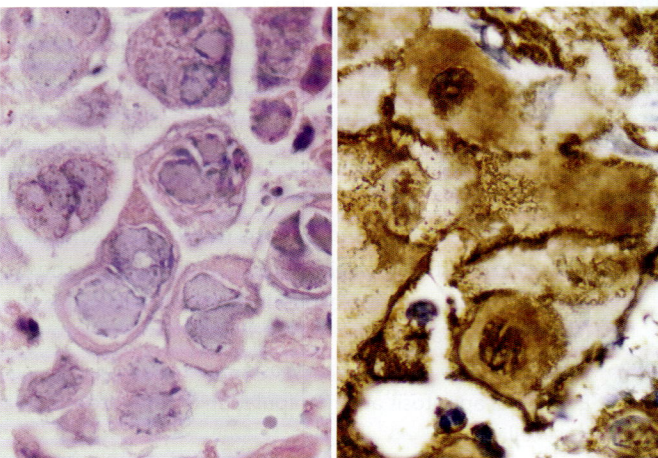

IMAGE 14.6 HSV infecting squamous cells. Left: H&E, x1000. Right: anti-HSV-1 and -2 immunoperoxidase, x1000.

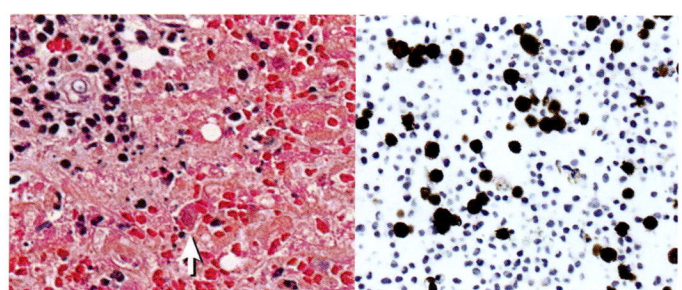

IMAGE 14.4 Herpes simplex virus (HSV) hepatitis. Left: the image shows coagulative necrosis with infected cells containing Cowdry type A intranuclear eosinophilic inclusion (arrow, H&E, x200). Right: infected cells are positive for anti-HSV-1 and anti-HSV-2 antibodies (immunoperoxidase, x200).

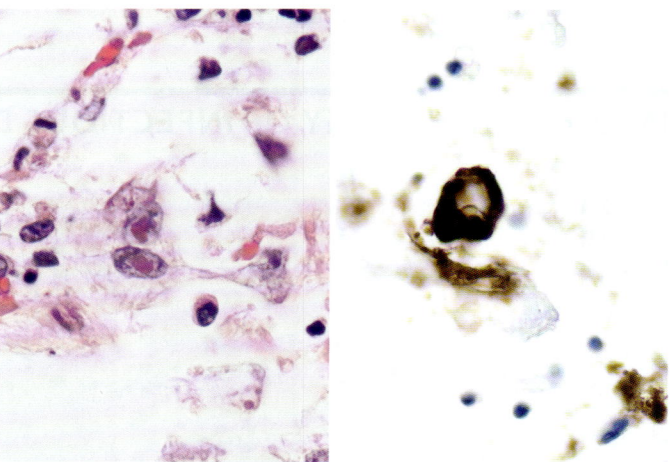

IMAGE 14.7 Varicella zoster virus. Left: histologic nuclear changes are similar to that seen in other herpes viruses. This virus shows a distinct nuclear inclusion (H&E, x1000). Right: infected cells are positive for anti-varicella zoster virus antibody (immunoperoxidase, x1000).

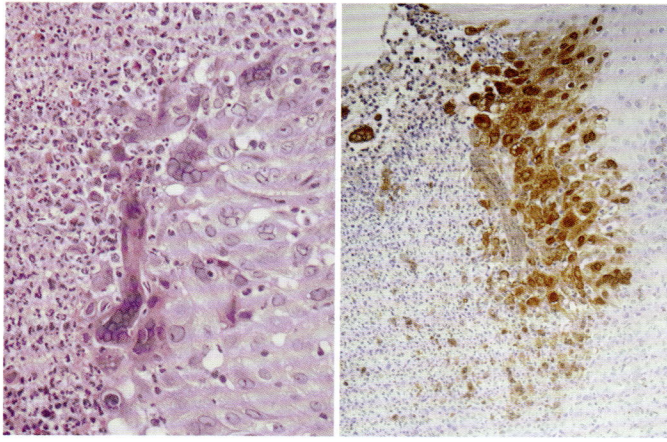

IMAGE 14.5 HSV genital ulcer. Left: this is an epithelial ulcer with classic herpes changes: multinucleation, nuclear molding, and margination of nuclear chromatin. There is a mixed inflammatory infiltrate in the submucosa (H&E, x400). Right: infected cells are positive for anti-HSV-1 and -2 antibodies (immunoperoxidase, x200).

Source: Joint Pathology Center, Infectious Disease Archives

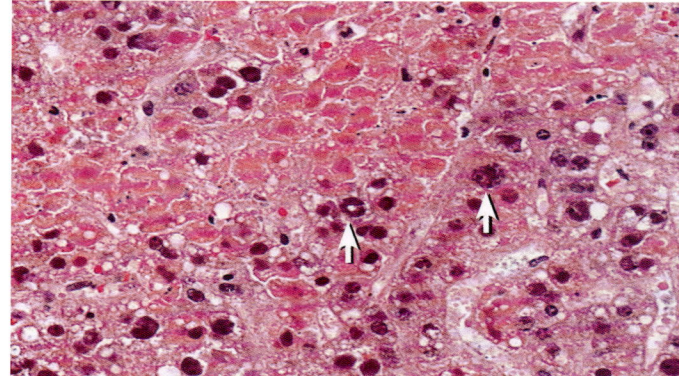

IMAGE 14.8 Adenovirus hepatitis. Hepatocellular coagulative necrosis with nuclear "blueberry muffin" inclusions (arrows) containing multiple basophilic particles (H&E, x200).

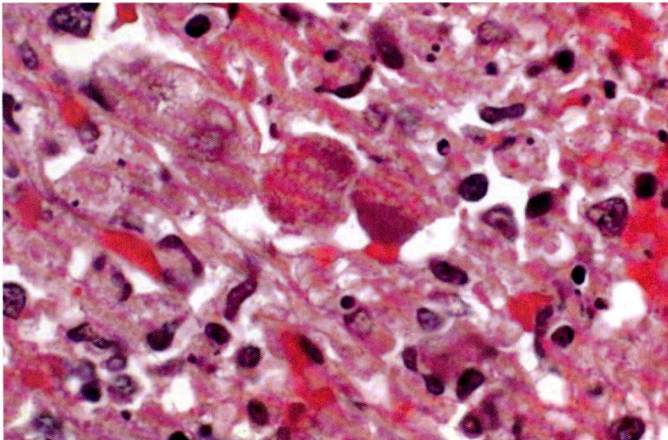

IMAGE 14.9 Adenovirus pneumonia (HIV-infected patient). Necrotizing pneumonia, enlarged cells with inclusions, and smudged nuclei are present (arrows, H&E, x500).

Source: Joint Pathology Center, Infectious Disease Archives

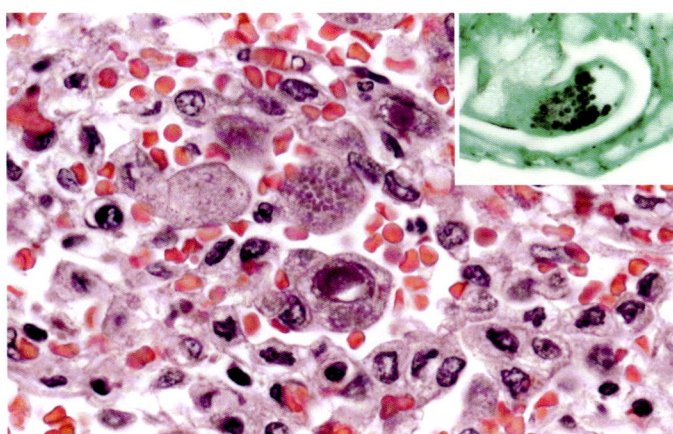

IMAGE 14.12 CMV pneumonia, hemorrhagic. The image depicts enlarged cells showing a spectrum of changes: classic eosinophilic "owl eye" intranuclear inclusion, amphophilic intracytoplasmic inclusions (inset, GMS+, x400), and other atypical CMV cells (H&E, x400).

Source: Joint Pathology Center, Infectious Disease Archives

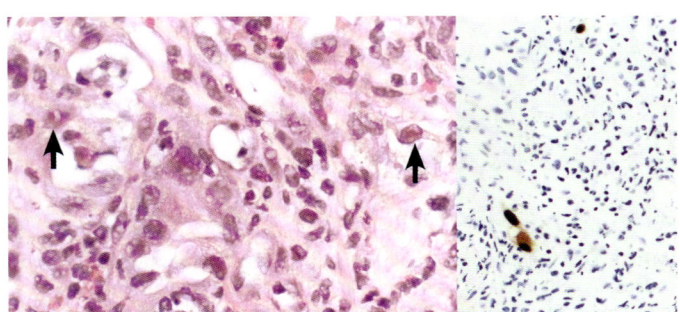

IMAGE 14.10 Gastric cytomegalovirus (CMV) infection. Left: the arrows point to the infected cells with characteristic intranuclear eosinophilic inclusion (H&E, x400). Right: the infected cells are positive for anti-CMV immunostaining (immunoperoxidase, x100).

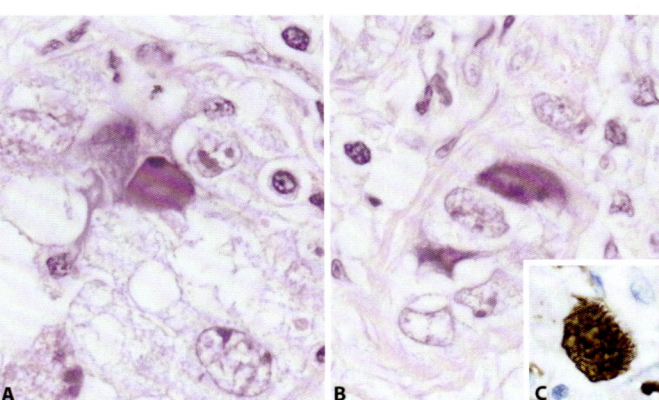

IMAGE 14.13 BK polyoma virus in transplant kidney. Images A and B: infected cells have a nucleus with a large, homogenous, purple intranuclear inclusion, often affecting the tubular epithelium (H&E, x1000). Image C (inset): the infected cells are cross-reactive for anti-simian virus 40 (anti-SV40) antibody (immunoperoxidase, x1000).

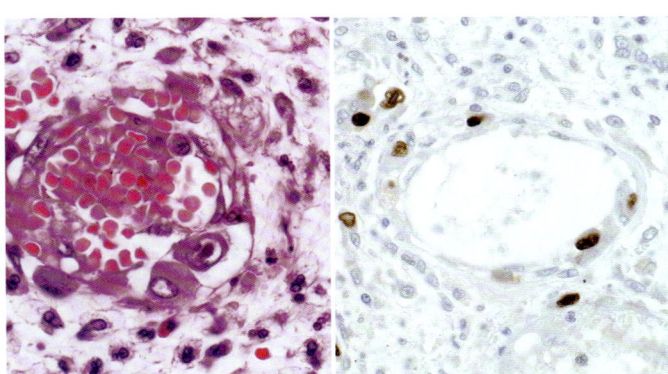

IMAGE 14.11 CMV infecting endothelial cells. Left: intranuclear eosinophilic "owl eye" inclusion and amphophilic intracytoplasmic inclusion are seen (arrow, H&E, x400). Right: the infected cells are positive for anti-CMV antibody (immunoperoxidase, x400).

Source: Joint Pathology Center, Infectious Disease Archives

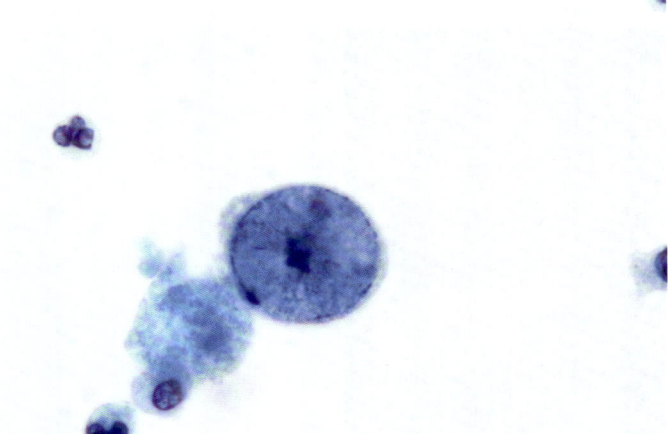

IMAGE 14.14 BK polyoma virus affecting a urothelial cell as seen on urine cytology. The so-called "decoy cell" is an enlarged cell with a large, homogenous, amorphous ground-glass-like intranuclear inclusion with a condensed rim of chromatin. There is often an incomplete rim of cytoplasm (ThinPrep Papanicolaou stain, x1000).

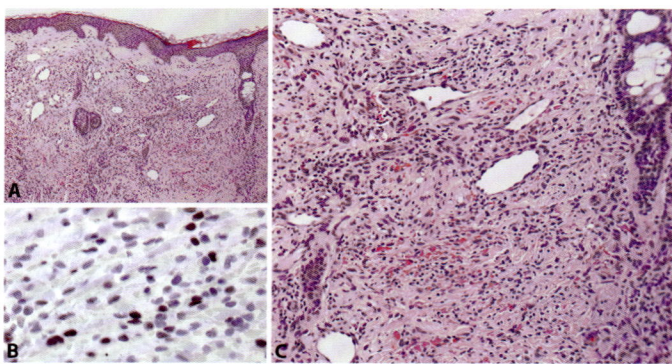

IMAGE 14.15 Kaposi sarcoma in the skin. Images A and B: this subcutaneous patch lesion shows angulated blood vessels, extravasated erythrocytes in dermis, and periadnexal vascular slits (H&E; A. x20; B. x200). Image C: the spindle cells are positive for latent nuclear antigen-1 of human herpes virus-8 (HHV-8) (immunoperoxidase, x400).

Source: Joint Pathology Center, Infectious Disease Archives

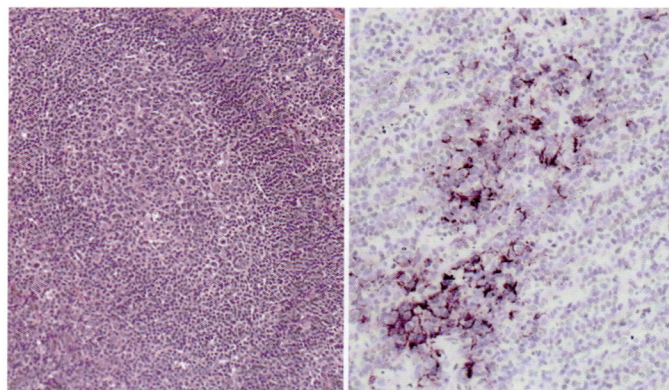

IMAGE 14.18 Lymph nodes, HIV infection. Left: follicular hyperplasia with loss of mantle zone (H&E, x40). Right: HIVp24 immunostain of viral particles on the follicular dendritic network with scattered individually infected T cells and macrophages (immunoperoxidase, x40).

Source: Joint Pathology Center, Infectious Disease Archives

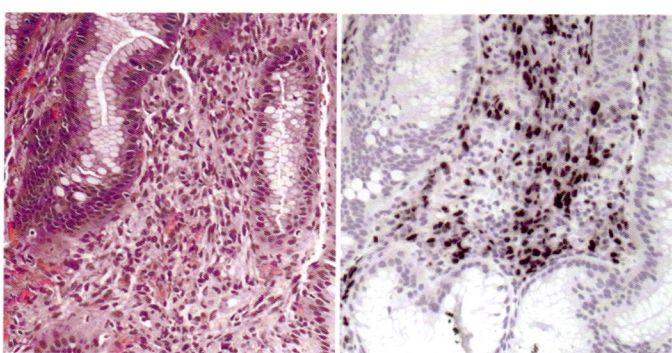

IMAGE 14.16 Kaposi sarcoma in the stomach. Left: vascular slits and extravasated erythrocytes in the submucosa are seen (H&E, x200). Right: the cells are positive for latent nuclear antigen-1 of HHV-8 (immunoperoxidase, x200).

Source: Joint Pathology Center, Infectious Disease Archives

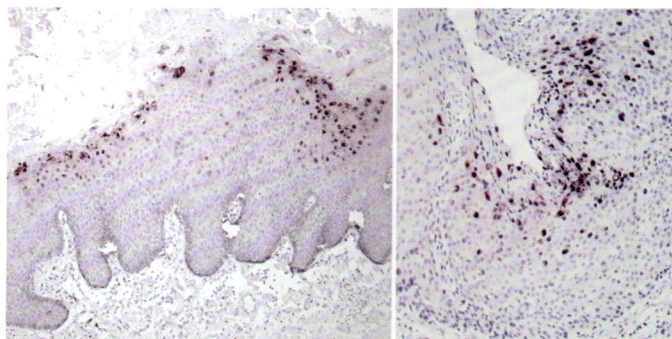

IMAGE 14.19 Human papilloma virus (HPV). Left: anal condyloma showing squamous cells infected with "low-risk" HPV-6 and/or -11 (chromogenic in situ hybridization, x100). Right: cervix high grade intraepithelial neoplasia with squamous cells infected with "high-risk" HPV-16 and/or -18 (chromogenic in situ hybridization, x200).

Source: Joint Pathology Center, Infectious Disease Archives

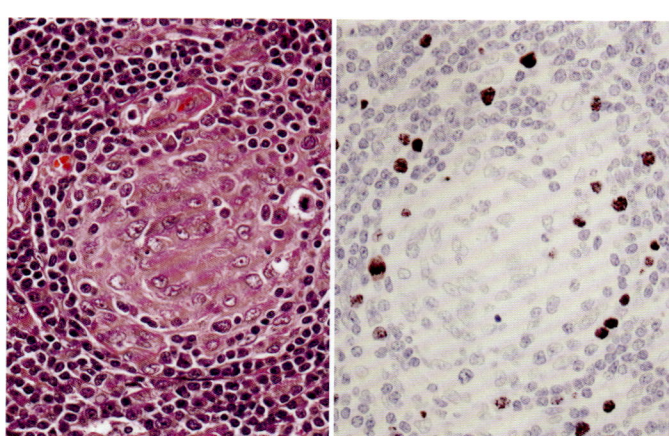

IMAGE 14.17 Castleman lymphadenopathy. Left: hyaline changes in the follicle and plasma cell expansion of the interfollicular areas (H&E, x400). Right: HHV-8 latent nuclear antigen positive lymphocytes (immunoperoxidase, x400).

Source: Joint Pathology Center, Infectious Disease Archives

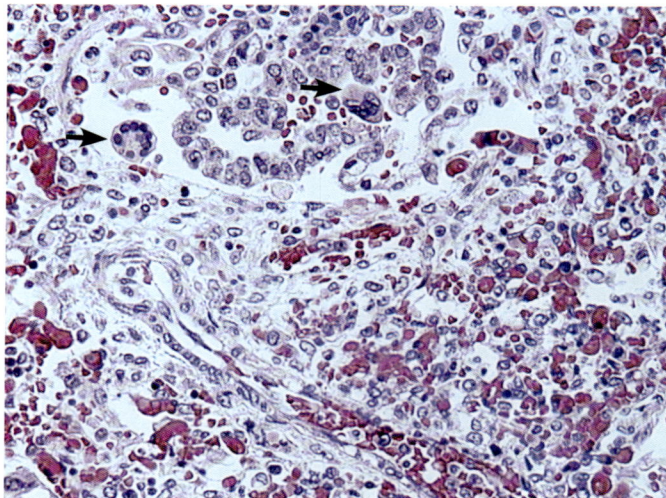

IMAGE 14.20 Lung with respiratory syncytial virus infection demonstrates characteristic giant multinucleated respiratory cells (arrows) in a mixed inflammatory background (H&E, x200).

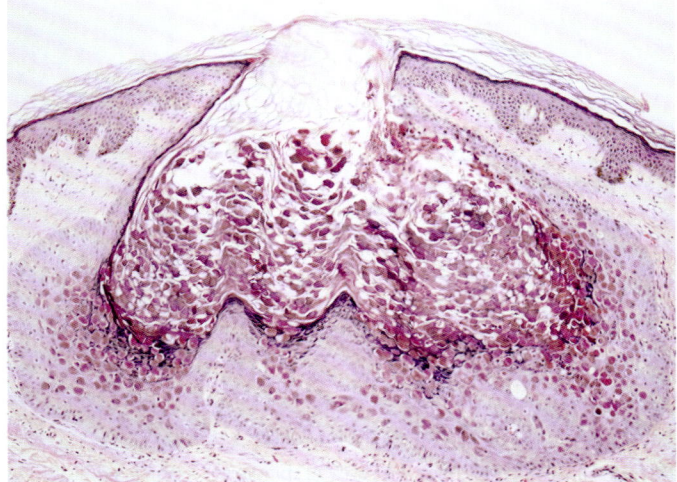

IMAGE 14.21 Skin, molluscum contagiosum. Lobular proliferation of basal cells with a central area containing molluscum bodies (H&E, x20).

Source: Joint Pathology Center, Infectious Disease Archives

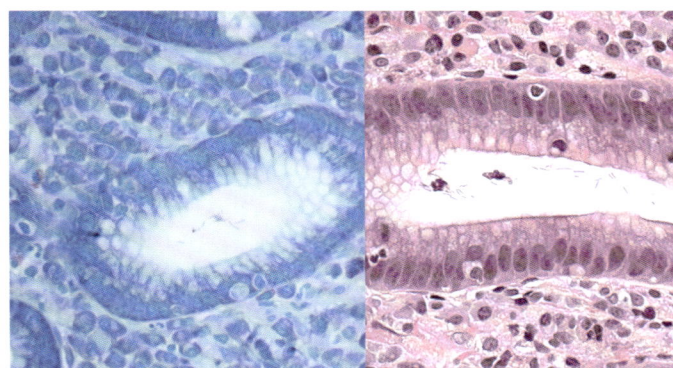

IMAGE 14.24 Stomach biopsy showing *Helicobacter heilmannii* infection. The bacteria have a characteristically thick, elongated, corkscrew appearance. Left: Giemsa stain, x400. Right: H&E, x400.

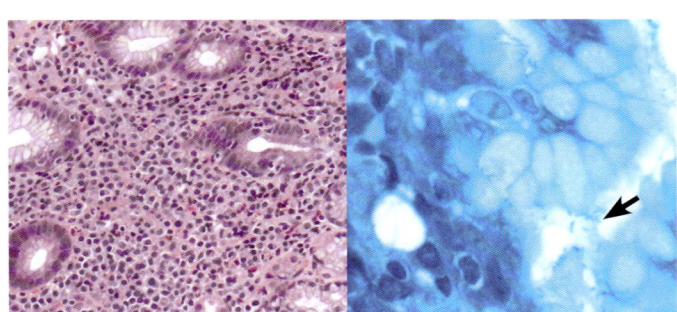

IMAGE 14.22 *Helicobacter pylori* gastritis. Left: H&E staining shows chronic active gastritis (x200). Right: Giemsa stain highlights the *Helicobacter pylori* bacteria (arrow, x400).

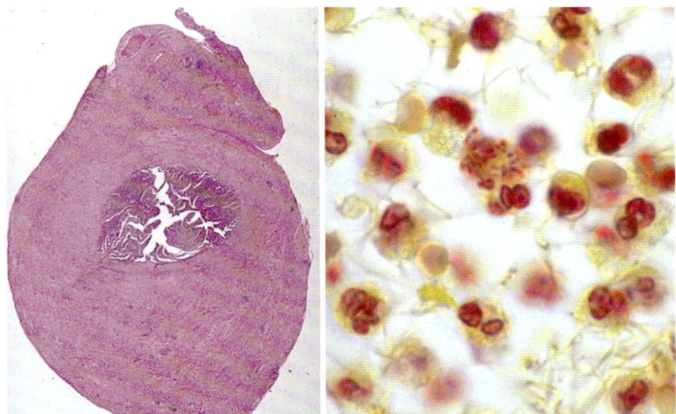

IMAGE 14.25 *Neisseria gonorrhea* salpingitis. Left: H&E shows a cross-section of a fallopian tube with a thickened wall and neutrophils in the lumen (H&E, x20). Right: Brown-Hopps Gram stain shows small gram-negative coccobacilli in the cytoplasm of a neutrophil (x1000).

Source: Joint Pathology Center, Infectious Disease Archives

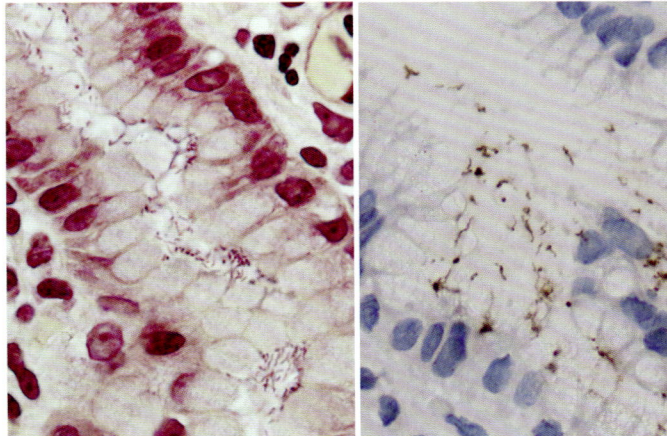

IMAGE 14.23 *Helicobacter pylori* gastritis. Left: *H. pylori* organisms are gram negative (Gram stain, x1000). Right: They are also positive for anti-*H. pylori* antibody (immunoperoxidase, x1000).

Source: Joint Pathology Center, Infectious Disease Archives

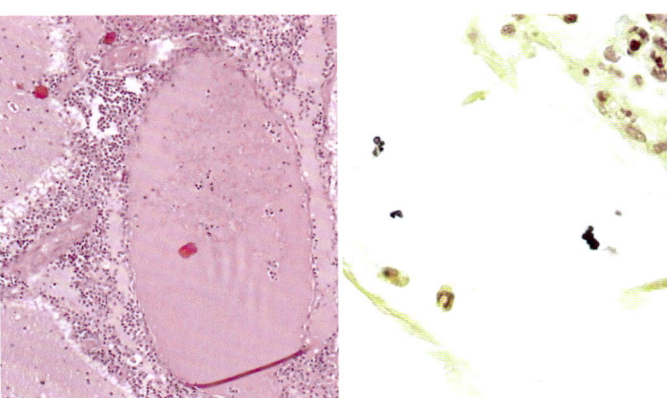

IMAGE 14.26 Brain, autopsy, streptococcal meningitis. Left: meninges are expanded by neutrophils (H&E, x40). Right: Brown-Hopps Gram stain reveals gram-positive cocci (x400).

Source: Joint Pathology Center, Infectious Disease Archives

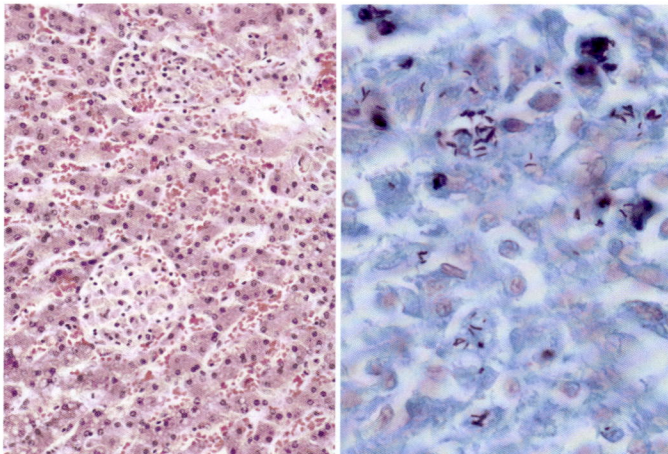

IMAGE 14.27 Liver with *Mycobacterium tuberculosis*. Left: multiple granulomata are seen (H&E, x200). Right: abundant acid-fast *Mycobacterium tuberculosis* bacteria are identified within the histiocytes of the granuloma (Ziehl-Neelsen stain, x600).

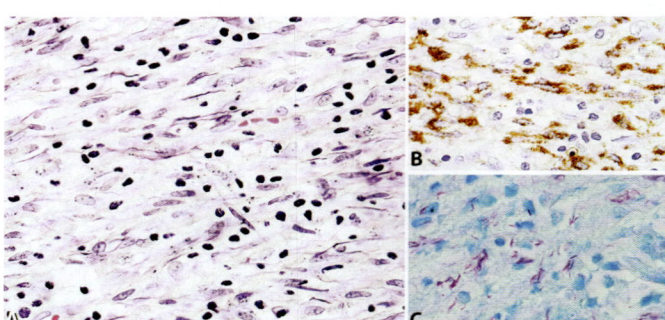

IMAGE 14.30 A lymph node with an MAI spindle cell lesion in an AIDS patient. Image A: the nodular lesion shows a spindled lesion (H&E/Silver, x200). Image B: the spindled cells are positive for CD68 (immunoperoxidase, x400). Image C: Ziehl-Neelsen stain identifies numerous fine acid-fast bacilli within the spindled cells (x600).

Source: Joint Pathology Center, Infectious Disease Archives

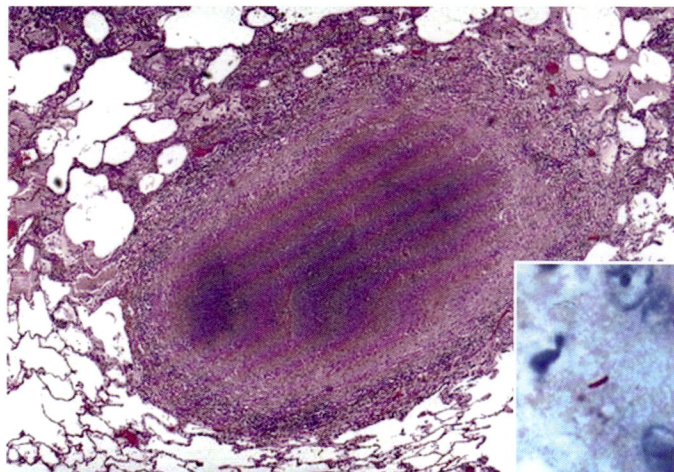

IMAGE 14.28 Lung with tuberculosis. Caseating granuloma are seen (H&E, x20). Inset: Ziehl-Neelsen stain identifies acid-fast mycobacteria in a giant cell (x600).

Source: Joint Pathology Center, Infectious Disease Archives

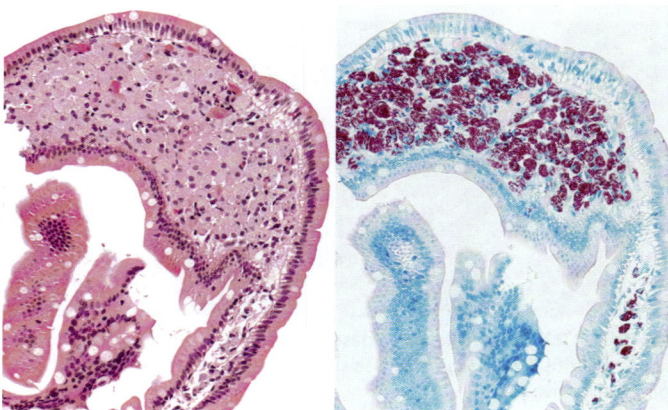

IMAGE 14.31 Small bowel with MAI infection. Left: the lamina propria is filled with foamy macrophages (H&E, x100). Right: MAI are identified by Ziehl–Neelsen stain as fine eosinophilic bacilli (x100).

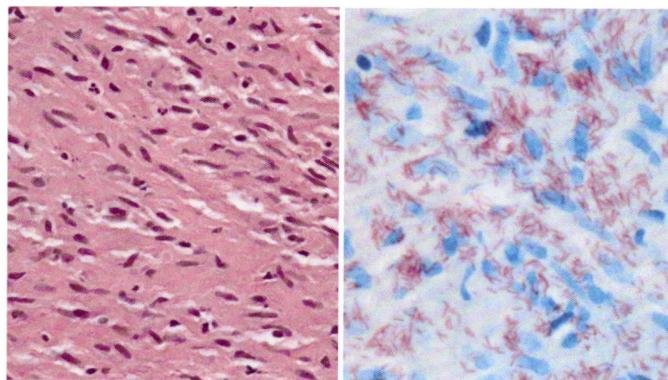

IMAGE 14.29 A retroperitoneal nodule with *Mycobacterium avium-intracellulare* complex (MAI) infection in an AIDS patient. Left: the nodular lesion shows an epithelioid granuloma (H&E, x100). Right: Ziehl-Neelsen stain identifies numerous fine acid-fast bacilli (x600).

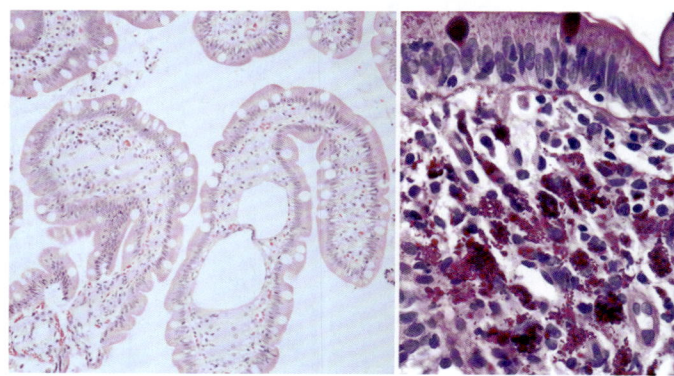

IMAGE 14.32 Whipple disease. Left: *Tropheryma whippeli* infection of the small bowel demonstrates characteristic foamy macrophages and dilated lacteals in the lamina propria of intestinal villi (H&E, x100). Right: PAS stain reveals masses of cytoplasmic granules (x400).

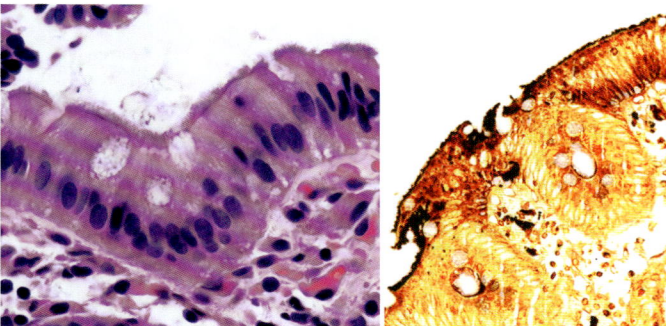

IMAGE 14.33 Intestinal spirochetosis. Note the characteristic "purple haze" of microorganisms on the surface of colonic epithelium (Left: H&E, x400; Right: Steiner silver stain, x200). The most common bacteria involved are *Brachyspira pilosicoli* and *Brachyspira aalborgi*.

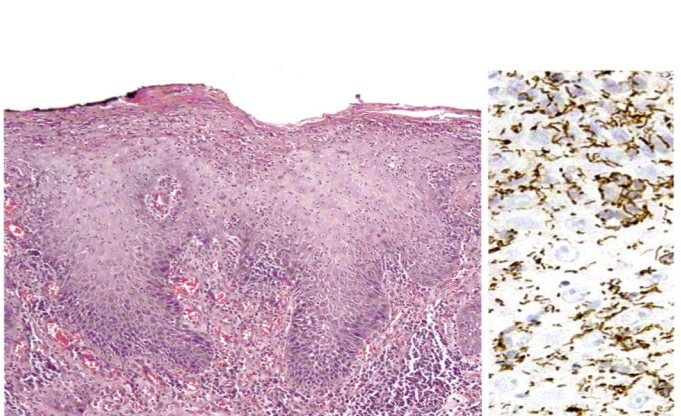

IMAGE 14.34 Anal syphilis. Left: this anal lesion has psoriasiform hyperplasia, exocytosis of neutrophils, and deep plasma cell infiltrate, characteristic of syphilis (H&E, x100). Right: immunohistochemistry highlights *Treponema pallidum* organisms (immunoperoxidase, x400).

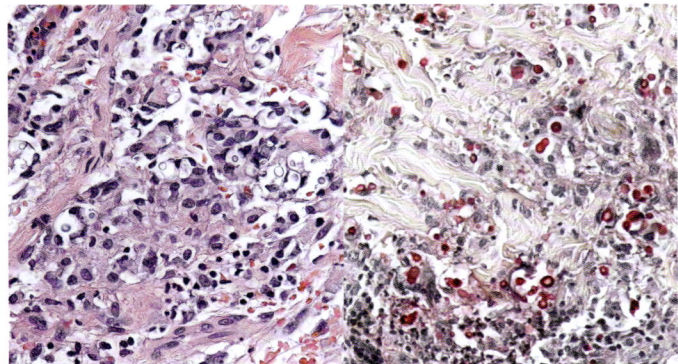

IMAGE 14.35 Skin *Cryptococcus neoformans* infection. Left: H&E shows pleomorphic, 4–10 µm yeasts with thick refractile capsules (x200). Right: mucicarmine stain shows bright red capsules with narrow-necked budding yeasts (x200).

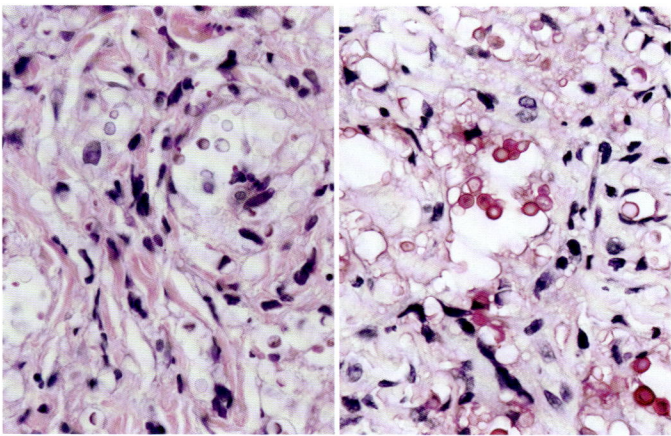

IMAGE 14.36 Lung *Cryptococcus neoformans* infection. Left: H&E shows pleomorphic, 4–10 µm yeasts that appear waxy on H&E (x400). Right: mucicarmine stain identifies bright red capsules with narrow-necked budding yeasts (x400).

Source: Joint Pathology Center, Infectious Disease Archives

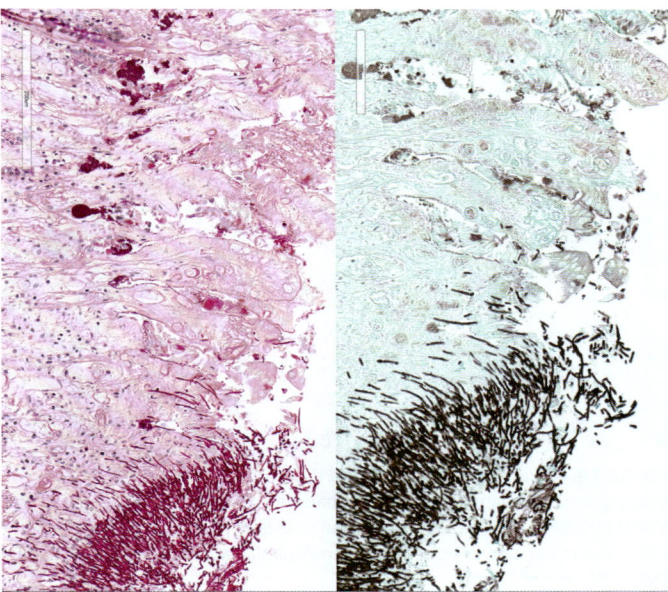

IMAGE 14.37 Small bowel *Candida albicans* infection in an immunocompromised patient. The images show densely matted pseudohyphae and spores in sections of necrotic villi. Left: H&E, x40. Right: Grocott, x40.

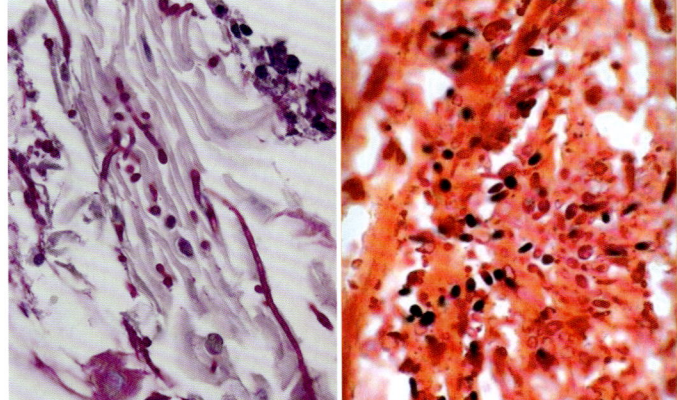

IMAGE 14.38 Esophageal *Candida albicans* infection in an immunocompromised patient. Left: pseudohyphae and spores are both visible on PAS stain (x400). Right: Brown-Hopps Gram variable yeast are seen (x400).

Source: Joint Pathology Center, Infectious Disease Archives

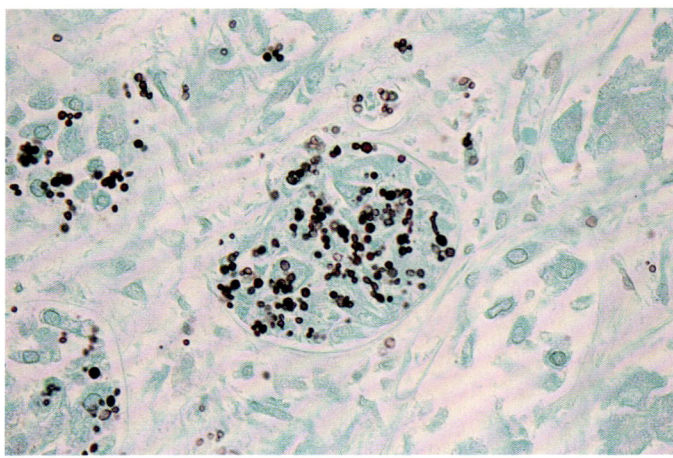

IMAGE 14.39 Kidney *Candida albicans* infection. The image shows yeasts 5–10 microns in size and a few pseudohyphae (Grocott, x200).

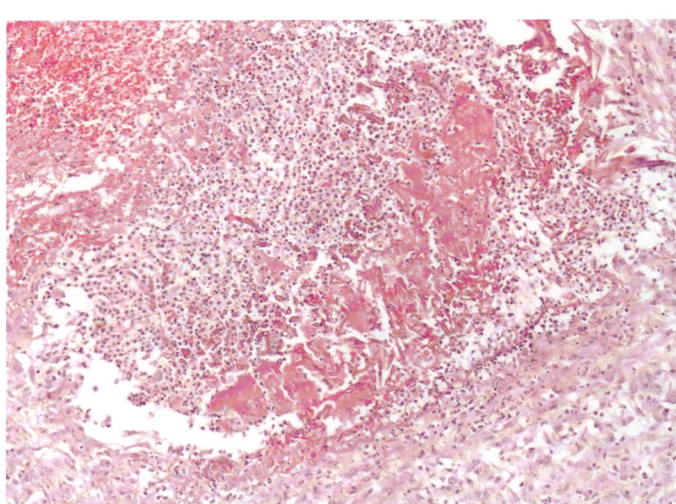

IMAGE 14.42 Fungal vasculitis. The image shows *Mucor* in the wall of a destroyed artery (H&E, x40).

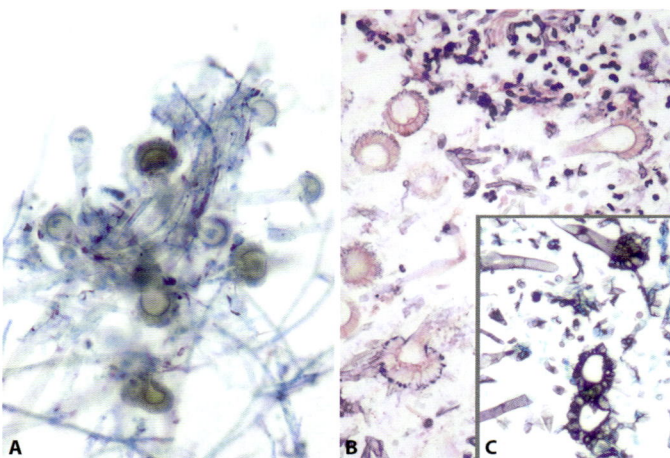

IMAGE 14.40 Pulmonary aspergillosis. A pulmonary cavity was seen on imaging and abundant *Aspergillus* hyphae were identified on bronchoscopy. Fruiting bodies (conidia) are uncommon to see on histology, but are more often seen in cavities. Image A: ThinPrep Papanicolaou stain, x400. Image B: H&E, x400. Image C (inset): GMS, x400.

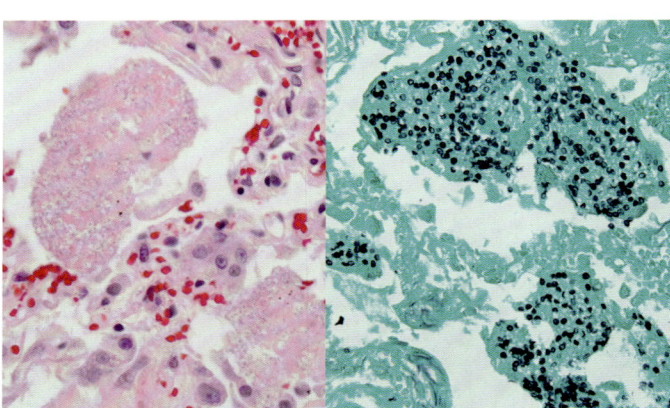

IMAGE 14.43 *Pneumocystis jiroveci* pneumonia. Left: alveolar spaces filled with pink, foamy amorphous material (H&E, x200). Right: yeasts with "dented table tennis ball" appearance (GMS, x200).

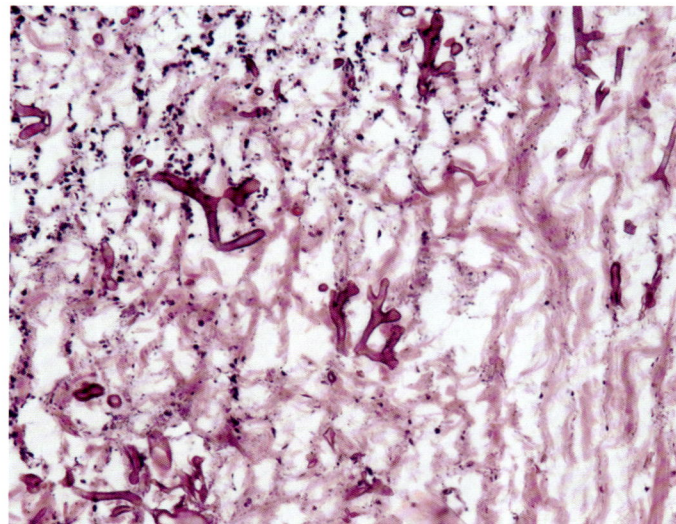

IMAGE 14.41 Sinonasal zygomycosis. The image shows *Mucor* infection characterized by broad, nonseptate, thin-walled hyphae in necrotic tissue (PAS, x100).

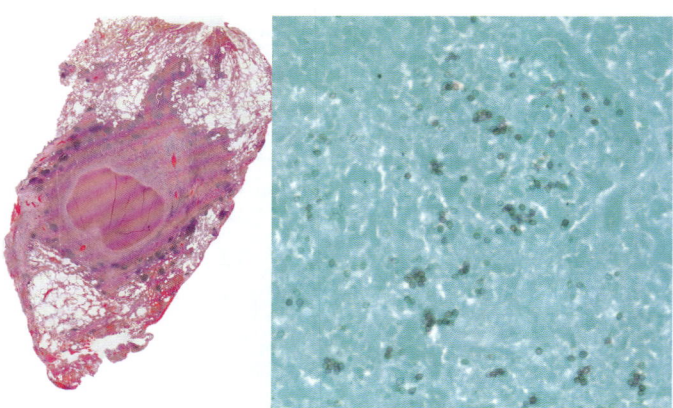

IMAGE 14.44 Lung *Histoplasma capsulatum*. Left: the image shows a necrotizing granulomatous inflammation with 3 zones: outer capsule, mummefactive necrosis, and caseating necrosis in the center (H&E, x1). Right: the necrotic area (right) shows 2–4 μm yeasts (GMS, x200).

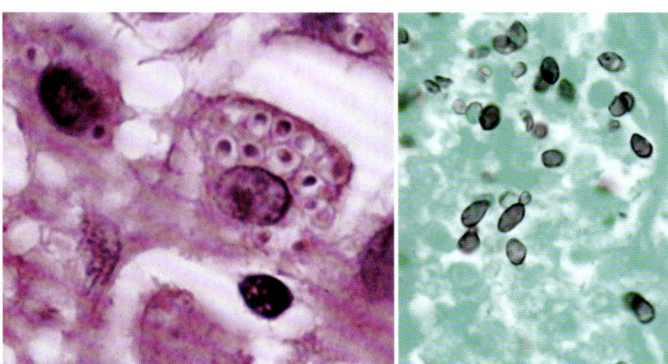

IMAGE 14.45 Pulmonary *Histoplasma capsulatum* infection. Left: H&E shows yeast in the cytoplasm of a macrophage. Note the halo (retraction artefact) (x1000). Right: GMS stain shows 2–4 μm yeasts (x1000).

Source: Joint Pathology Center, Infectious Disease Archives

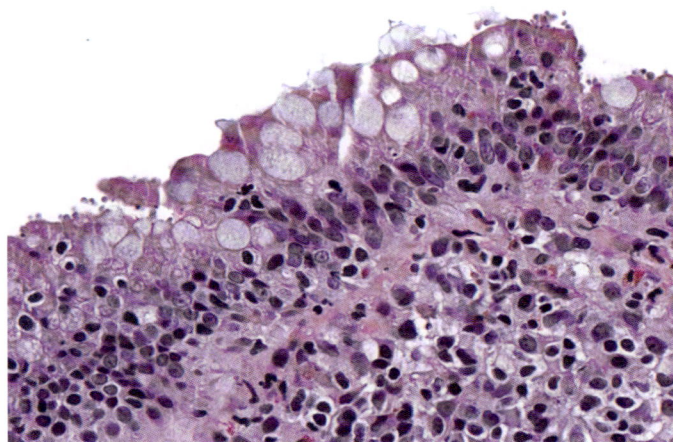

IMAGE 14.48 Cryptosporidiosis. H&E shows 2–5 μm *Cryptosporidium* on the surface of colonic epithelium (x400).

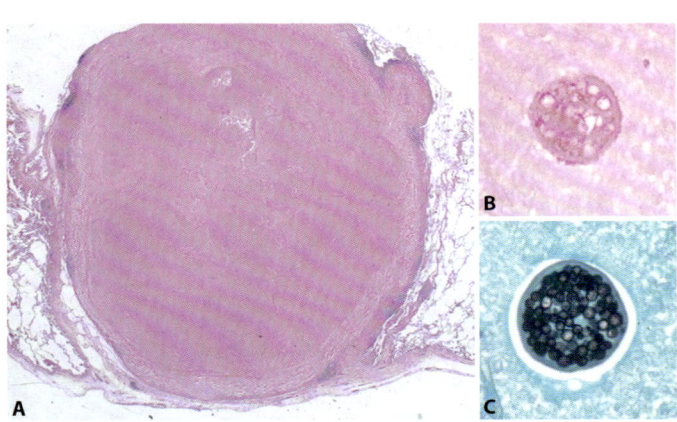

IMAGE 14.46 Pulmonary *Coccidioides immitis* infection. Image A: H&E shows a fibrocaseous granuloma (H&E, x20). Image B: a large mature spherule packed with endospores is seen (PAS, x600). Image C: GMS only stains the endospores, not the spherule (x600).

Source: Joint Pathology Center, Infectious Disease Archives

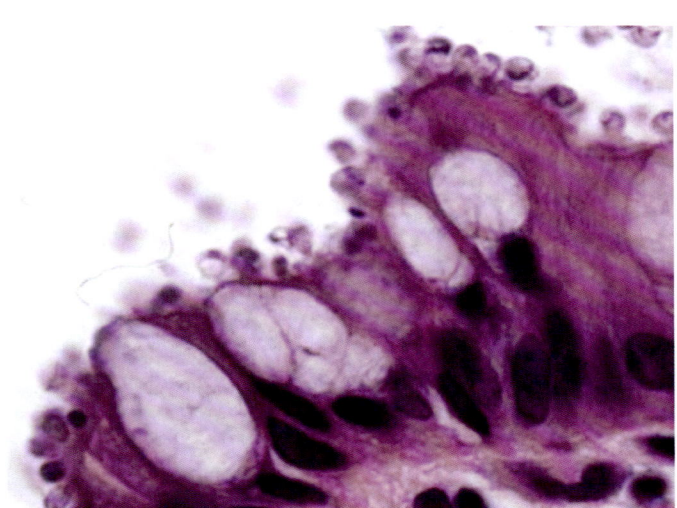

IMAGE 14.49 Cryptosporidiosis. H&E shows 2–5 μm *Cryptosporidium* on the surface of colonic epithelium (x1000).

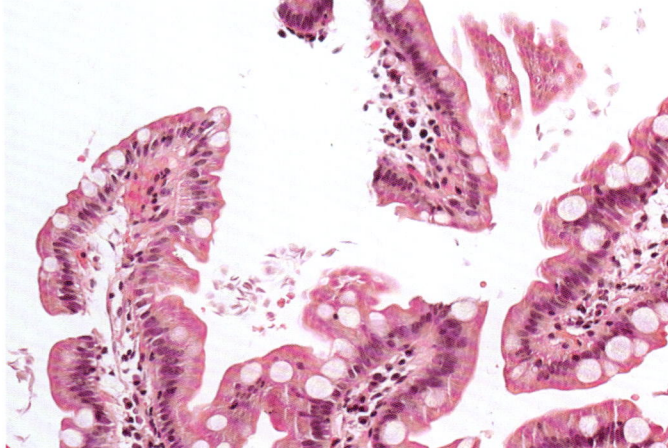

IMAGE 14.47 Small bowel giardiasis protozoan (*Giardia lamblia*). Organisms are teardrop (pear) shaped (like trichomonas) with paired nuclei in the lumen between almost intact villi. Note the lack of inflammation (H&E, x400).

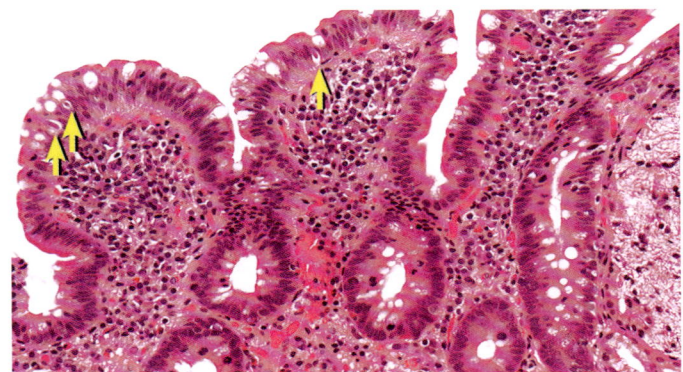

IMAGE 14.50 Small bowel *Cystoisospora (Isospora) belli* infection shows crescent- or banana-shaped asexual forms (unsporulated sporocyst) interposed between adjacent enterocytes (arrows, H&E, x200).

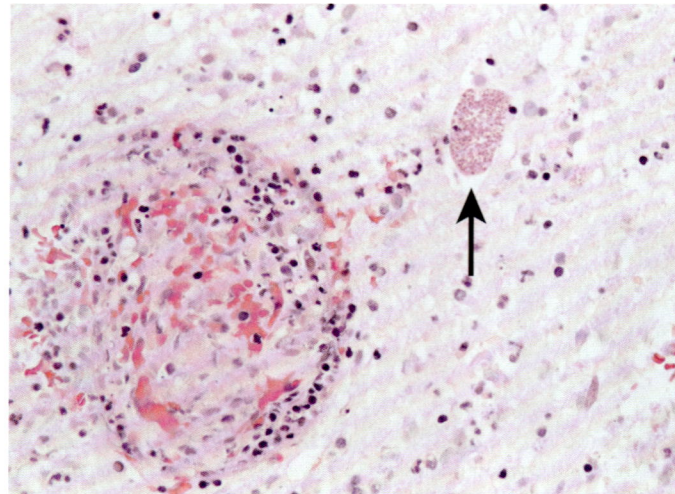

IMAGE 14.51 Central nervous system toxoplasmosis. There is a granuloma and a cyst filled with bradyzoites (arrow) of *Toxoplasma gondii* in brain tissue (H&E, x100).

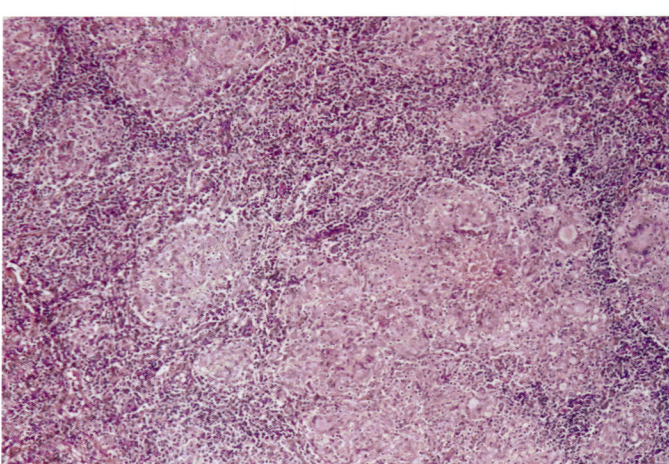

IMAGE 14.53 Toxoplasmosis. Lymph node *Toxoplasma gondii* infection is characterized by florid reactive follicular hyperplasia, germinal center granulomas, and sinusoidal distention by monocytoid B cells (H&E, x40).

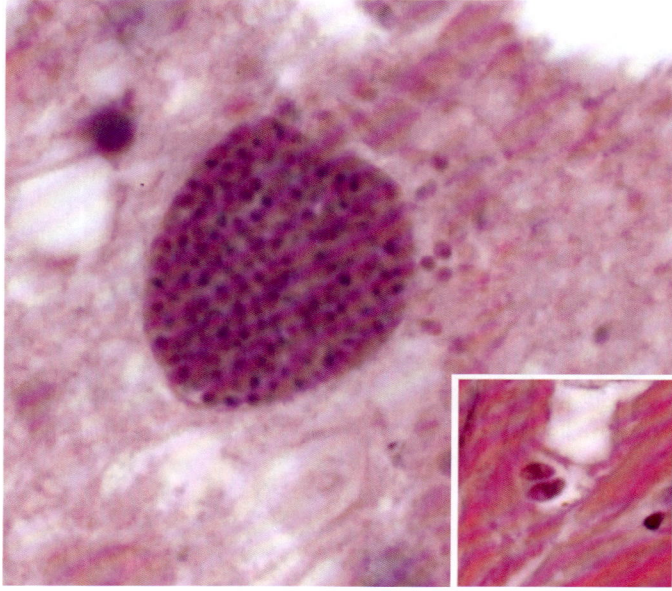

IMAGE 14.52 Central nervous system toxoplasmosis. There is a cyst filled with bradyzoites and scattered tachyzoites of *Toxoplasma gondii* in brain tissue (H&E, x400). Inset: crescent-shaped tachyzoites are present (H&E, x1000).

Source: Joint Pathology Center, Infectious Disease Archives

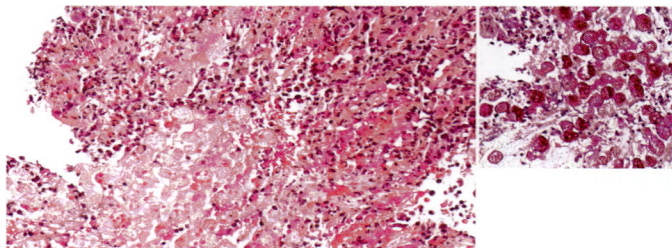

IMAGE 14.54 Colon amebiasis. The trophozoites of *Entamoeba histolytica* resemble macrophages admixed in ulcer debris. Left: H&E, x40. Right: PAS, x400.

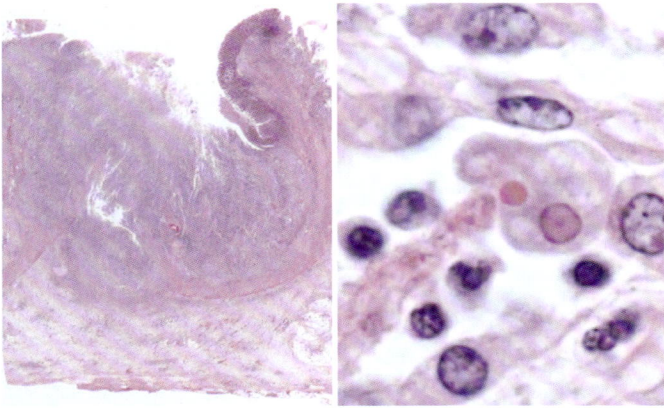

IMAGE 14.55 Colon amebiasis. Left: a deep ulcer extends into the submucosa (H&E, x20). Right: the trophozoites of *Entamoeba histolytica* resemble macrophages with abundant cytoplasm and vacuoles, and may contain ingested red blood cells. The nuclei are small and round with prominent nuclear membranes and a central karyosome (chromocenter) (PAS, x400).

Source: Joint Pathology Center, Infectious Disease Archives

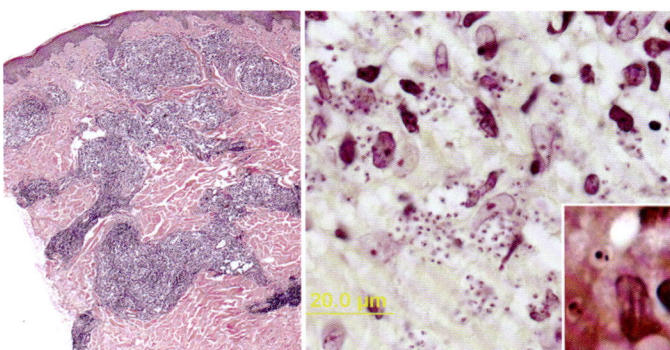

IMAGE 14.57 Skin, leishmaniasis. Left: multiple nodules of lymphocytes are present in the dermis (H&E, x20). Right: Brown-Hopps Gram stain shows clusters of amastigotes in the cytoplasm of macrophages (x400). Right inset: higher power clearly shows the amastigote nucleus and kinetoplast (x1000).

Source: Joint Pathology Center, Infectious Disease Archives

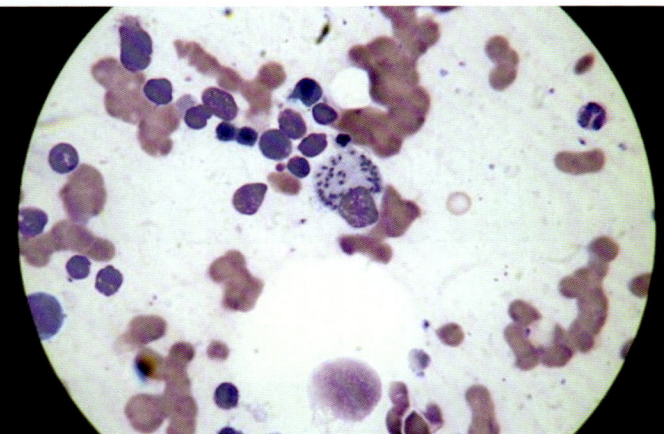

IMAGE 14.56 Bone marrow aspirate smear from an HIV+ Sudanese man showing *Leishmania* amastigotes within histiocytes (Wright-Giemsa stain, x600).

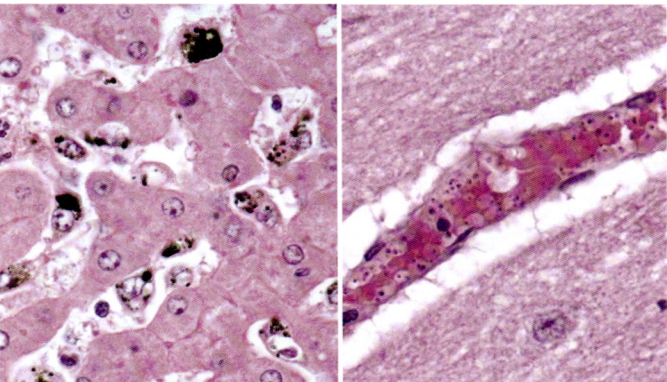

IMAGE 14.58 Malaria infections. Left: liver showing malarial pigment in Kuppfer cells and sinusoids (H&E, x200). Right: brain showing small vessels containing multiple schizonts of *Plasmodium falciparum* malaria (H&E, x1000).

Source: Joint Pathology Center, Infectious Disease Archives

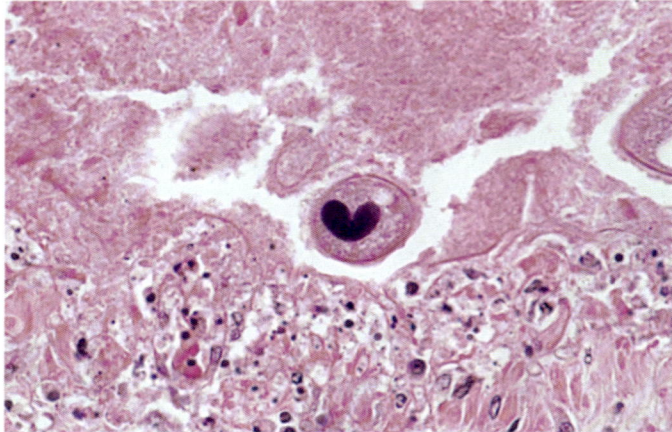

IMAGE 14.59 *Balantidium coli* in the intestine. The image shows a large ciliated trophozoite (H&E, x100).

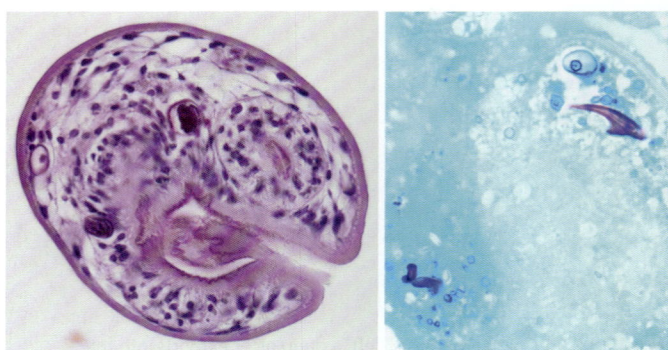

IMAGE 14.62 *Echinococcosis granulosus*. Left: scolex (H&E, x400). Right: hooklets revealed by acid-fast stain (x400).

Source: Joint Pathology Center, Infectious Disease Archives

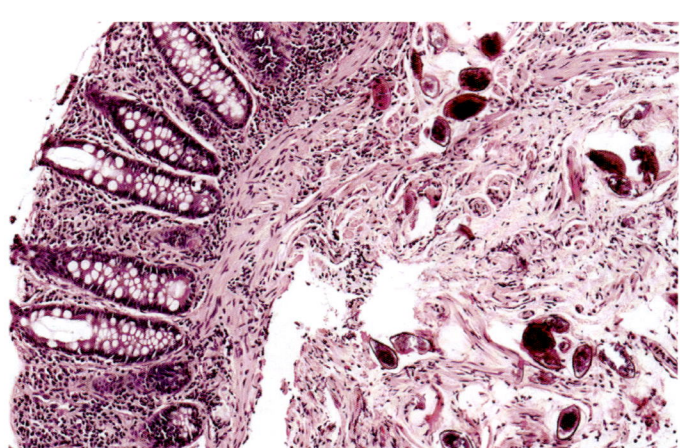

IMAGE 14.60 Schistosomiasis. Calcified eggs of *Schistosoma japonicum* with characteristic oval/round, minute, knob-like spines in the colonic submucosa and surrounded by a fibrogranulomatous reaction (H&E, x100).

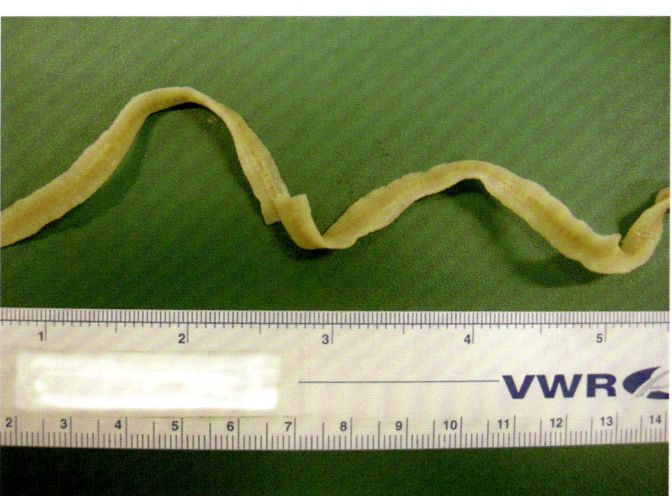

IMAGE 14.63 Tapeworms showing a flat, segmented appearance. Eating undercooked meat from infected animals is the main cause of tapeworm infection in humans.

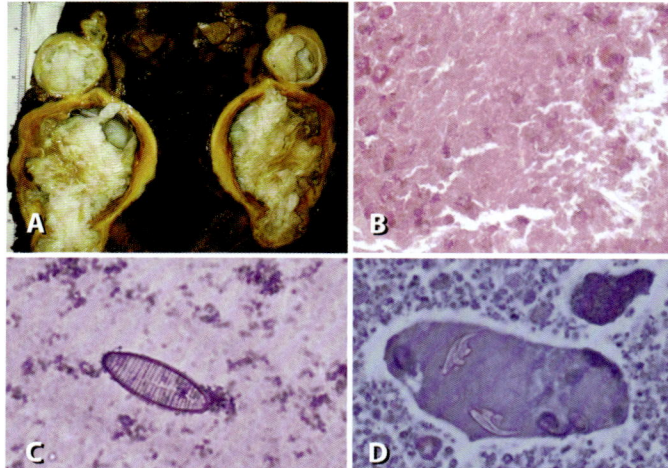

IMAGE 14.61 Echinococcosis. Image A: bladder showing a hydatid cyst (gross). Image B: cyst contents containing necrotic tissue and daughter cysts (H&E, x100). Image C: an *Echinococcus* egg (H&E, x200). Image D: Protoscolices with 2 hooklets (H&E, x400).

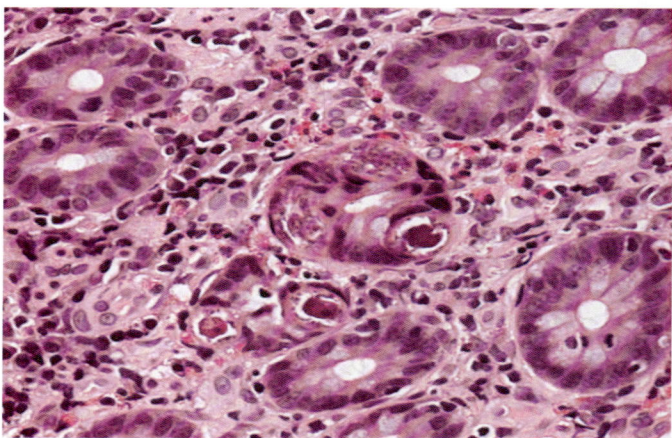

IMAGE 14.64 Colon *Capillaria philippinensis*. The image shows the round, basophilic granular appearance of the small nematodes in cross-section (H&E, x400).

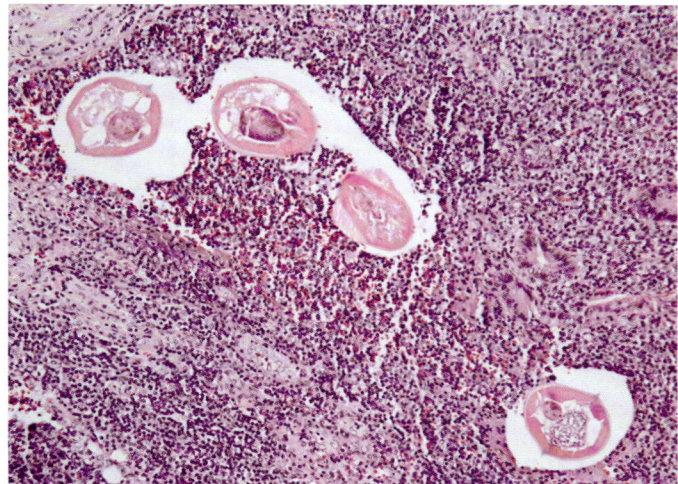

IMAGE 14.65 Enterobiasis (pin worm) in an appendectomy specimen. Cross-section of *Enterobius vermicularis* showing characteristic lateral spikes (H&E, x20).

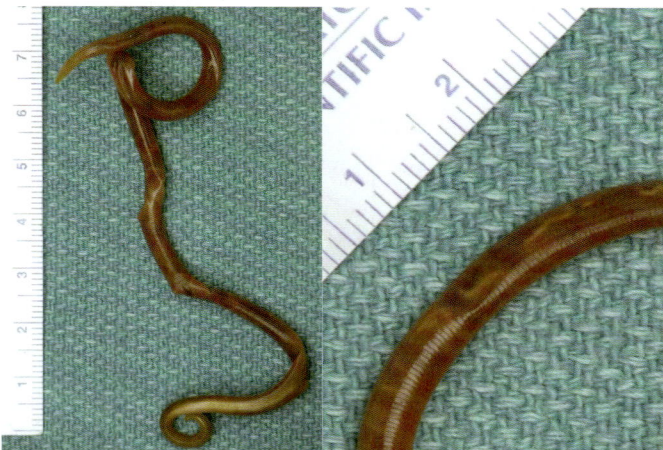

IMAGE 14.67 *Ascaris lumbricoides*. Images A and B: this parasite is 2–6 mm in diameter and can grow up to 50 cm long.

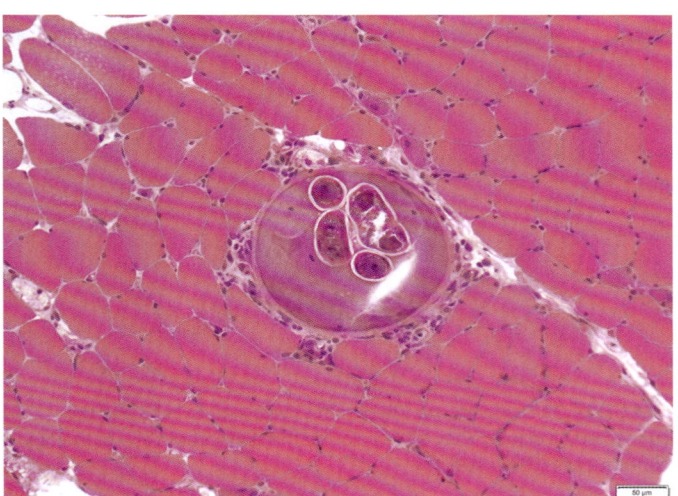

IMAGE 14.66 Trichinosis. Cross-section of *Trichinella spiralis* larval cyst in skeletal muscle tissue with surrounding inflammation (H&E, x40).

Courtesy of Dr. Jason Karamchandani.

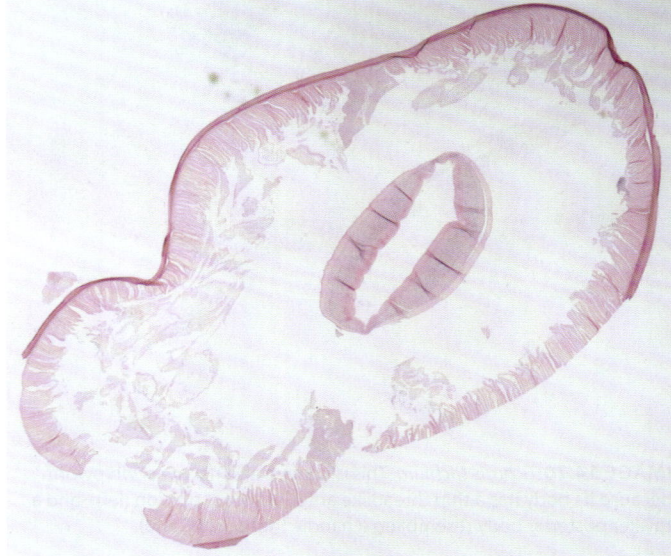

IMAGE 14.68 *Ascaris lumbricoides*. Histologic cross-section of an *Ascaris lumbricoides* adult (H&E, x10).

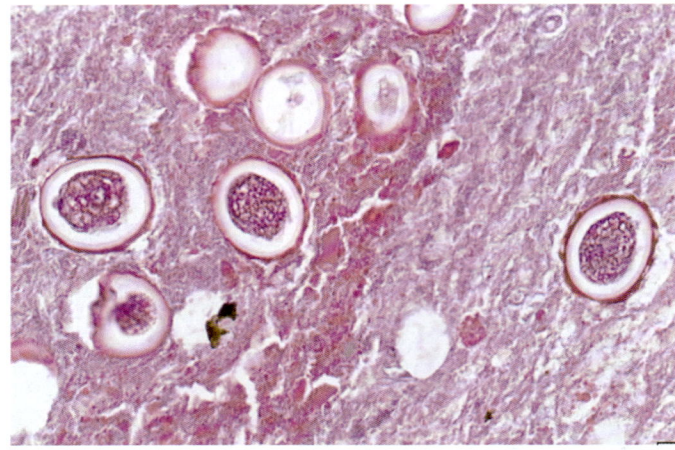

IMAGE 14.69 *Ascaris lumbricoides*. The image shows histologic sections of eggs (H&E, x200).

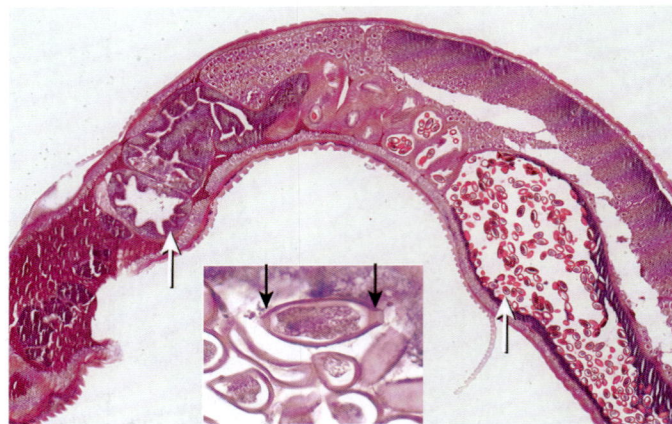

IMAGE 14.71 *Tichuris trichiura*. The image shows a longitudinal section of the posterior end of a gravid female demonstrating the intestine and eggs (white arrow) (H&E, x40). Inset: high magnification of the eggs demonstrates the characteristic "bipolar" plugs at both ends (black arrows, x400).

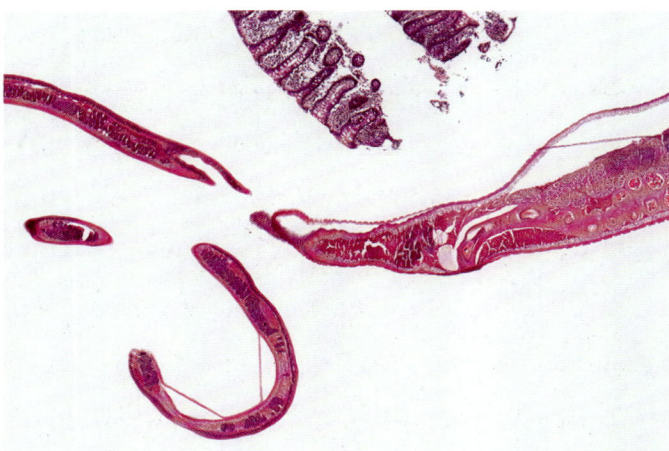

IMAGE 14.70 *Tichuris trichiura*. This is commonly known as "whipworm" because its body has a thin threadlike anterior "head" portion (left), and a thicker posterior body resembling a handle (right) (H&E, x40).

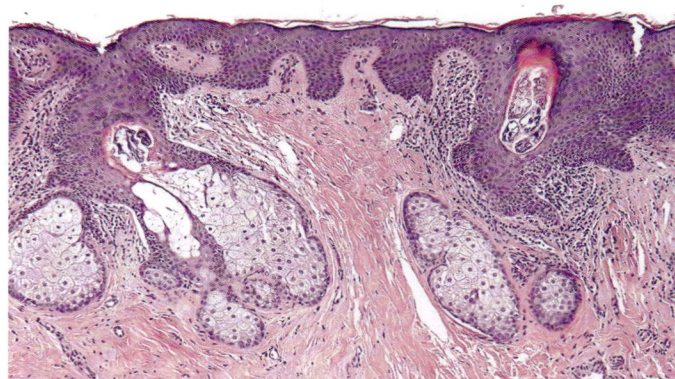

IMAGE 14.72 *Demodex* spp. These mites live in hair follicles and the connected oil glands. They often colonize the skin without any pathologic consequence (H&E, x100).

Acknowledgments

We wish to acknowledge the excellent contributions by one of the original authors of this chapter, Dr. Daniel Gregson, and one of the second edition authors, Dr. Yu Shi.

Bibliography

Belay ED, Schonberger LB. Variant Creutzfeldt-Jakob disease and bovine spongiform encephalopathy. Clin Lab Med. 2002;22(4):849–62, v–vi. doi: 10.1016/s0272-2712(02)00024-0

Centers for Disease Control and Prevention. Bovine spongiform encephalopathy (BSE), or mad cow disease [Internet]. Atlanta: Centers for Disease Control and Prevention, National Center for Emerging and Zoonotic Infectious Diseases, Division of High-Consequence Pathogens and Pathology; [updated 2018 Oct 9]. Available from http://www.cdc.gov/prions/bse/index.html.

Centers for Disease Control and Prevention. Creutzfeldt-Jakob disease, classic (CJD) [Internet]. Atlanta: Centers for Disease Control and Prevention, National Center for Emerging and Zoonotic Infectious Diseases, Division of High-Consequence Pathogens and Pathology; [updated 2018 Oct 9]. Available from http://www.cdc.gov/prions/cjd/index.html.

Centers for Disease Control and Prevention. Malaria [Internet]. Atlanta: Centers for Disease Control and Prevention, National Center for Emerging and Zoonotic Infectious Diseases, Division of High-Consequence Pathogens and Pathology; [updated 2020 Oct 6]. Available from https://www.cdc.gov/dpdx/malaria/index.html.

Cheng L, Bostwick DG, editors. Essentials of anatomic pathology. 4th ed. New York: Springer; 2016.

Connor DH, Schwartz DA, Lack EE, et al, editors. Pathology of infectious diseases. New York: McGraw-Hill; 1997.

Goldblum JR, Lamps LW, McKenney JK, et al, editors. Rosai and Ackerman's surgical pathology. 11th ed., vol. 2. Philadelphia (PA): Elsevier; 2017.

Jameson JL, Fauci A, Kasper D, et al, editors. Harrison's principles of internal medicine. 20th ed. New York: McGraw-Hill; 2018.

Kradin RL. Diagnostic pathology of infectious disease. 2nd ed. Philadelphia (PA): Elsevier; 2017.

Kumar V, Abbas AK, Aster J. Robbins and Cotran pathologic basis of disease. 10th ed. North York (ON): Elsevier Canada; 2020.

Longacre TA. Mills and Sternberg's diagnostic surgical pathology. 7th ed. Philadelphia (PA): Wolters Kluwer; 2022.

Milner D, editor. Diagnostic pathology: infectious diseases. 2nd ed. Philadelphia (PA): Elsevier; 2015.

Reddy VB, David O, Spitz DJ, et al. Gattuso's differential diagnosis in surgical pathology. 4th ed. Philadelphia (PA): Elsevier; 2021.

U.S. Public Health Service. Updated U.S. public health service guidelines for the management of occupational exposures to HBV, HCV, and HIV and recommendations for postexposure prophylaxis. MMWR Recomm Rep. 2001;50(RR-11):1-52.

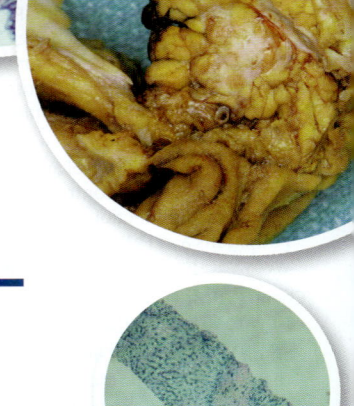

CHAPTER 15

Liver & Pancreas Pathology

ELIZAVETA CHERNETSOVA, ZU-HUA GAO

Liver and Pancreas Pathology Exam Essentials

MUST KNOW

World Health Organization (WHO) classification

Tumors of the liver and pancreas are contained within the WHO classification for the entire digestive system. However, the complexity of liver, pancreas, and bile ducts makes a separate discussion of these tumors worthwhile.

- You should know the basic anatomy of the liver (lobes, segments, vascular supply and drainage, biliary structure), be familiar with the normal histology of the liver, and understand the main functions of the liver.
- You should be familiar with which organs and anatomic sites fall under the WHO classification of liver, pancreas, and bile duct tumors, which specifically includes:
  · Liver and intrahepatic bile ducts.
  · Gallbladder and extrahepatic bile ducts.
  · Pancreas.
- For the liver and intrahepatic bile ducts, most of the focus is on tumors of hepatocellular origin:
  · Benign and malignant tumors of hepatocellular origin.
  · Subtyping of hepatocellular adenomas.
  · Differentiating massive regenerative nodule, nodular regenerative hyperplasia, focal nodular hyperplasia, and hepatocellular adenoma.
  · Biliary intraepithelial neoplasia and malignancy.
  · Combined tumors.

  · Liver metastasis (don't forget about this).
- For the gallbladder, the number of tumors is relatively low and the focus is on glandular lesions:
  · Adenomas.
  · Cystic neoplasms.
  · Biliary intraepithelial neoplasia.
  · Carcinomas.
- The pancreas contains a number of important tumors, including neuroendocrine tumors (note that the CAP/AJCC protocol separates neuroendocrine tumors [NET] from exocrine pancreas tumors):
  · Serous neoplasms.
  · Glandular intraepithelial neoplasia (pancreatic intraepithelial neoplasia [PanIN]), low and high grade
  · Pancreatic intraductal papillary mucinous neoplasm (IPMN).
  · Pancreatic intraductal oncocytic papillary neoplasm (IOPN).
  · Pancreatic mucinous cystic neoplasm (MCN).
  · Solid pseudopapillary tumor (SPPN).
  · Ductal adenocarcinoma.
  · Acinar cell carcinoma.
  · Functioning and nonfunctioning neuroendocrine tumors, neuroendocrine carcinomas, and mixed

neuroendocrine-nonneuroendocrine neoplasm (MiNEN).

AJCC and College of American Pathologists (CAP) protocols

- Note that the CAP/AJCC protocols classify hepatobiliary and pancreatic tumors differently than the WHO classification. Because of slight differences in staging, the CAP/AJCC protocol uses smaller anatomical areas, as follows (asterisks indicate high-yield areas):
  - Ampulla of Vater.
  - Distal extrahepatic bile ducts.
  - Gallbladder.
  - Hepatocellular carcinoma.*
  - Intrahepatic bile ducts.
  - Pancreas (exocrine).*
  - Perihilar bile ducts.
- The CAP/AJCC protocols for ampulla of Vater, bile ducts, and the gallbladder, which are very complex with subtle differences in tumor staging (pT staging) parameters, are generally low yield for this exam. You should glance over them at least once, but reserve in-depth review until after you have studied other areas thoroughly.
- The hepatocellular carcinoma (HCC) protocol has the following important details:
  - Subtypes of HCC.
  - Grading.
  - pT staging parameters.
  - What to do if there are multiple tumors.
- The exocrine pancreas protocol has the following important details:
  - Different types of pancreas resection.
  - The separation of tumors into ductal versus acinar cell tumors.
  - The complex nature of margins that need to be reported, and the importance of good grossing, especially for Whipple procedure specimens.
  - pT staging parameters.

Nonneoplastic diseases

This is an extremely important area, because the exam often covers hepatitis and pancreatitis. Liver transplantation is an esoteric subject not included in every training program, so not covered here. High-yield topics include:
- Liver:
  - Viral hepatitis.
  - Alcoholic steatohepatitis (ASH) and nonalcoholic steatohepatitis (NASH).
  - Acute versus chronic hepatitis; histologic changes; how to grade activity; causes such as drugs, autoimmune, vascular.
  - Cirrhosis, clinical findings, pathologic findings, staging, and sequelae/complications.

- Vascular diseases, such as Budd-Chiari syndrome and portal vein thrombosis.
- Metabolic diseases, including α_1-antitrypsin deficiency, hemochromatosis, and Wilson disease.
- Storage disorders, such as Gaucher disease.
- Traumatic liver injury, in the context of forensic topics such as motor vehicle collisions.
- Bile ducts:
  - Primary biliary cholangitis (PBC) and primary sclerosing cholangitis (PSC), including their associations, histologic findings.
  - Other causes of cholangitis.
- Gallbladder:
  - Cholelithiasis.
  - Other causes of cholecystitis.
  - Cholesterolosis.
- Pancreas:
  - Acute pancreatitis, including clinical findings, causes, sequelae, and complications.
  - Features of chronic pancreatitis.
  - Nonneoplastic cystic conditions, including pseudocysts.
  - Exocrine deficiencies, including diabetes.

Genetic and systemic conditions

High-yield topics include:
- Liver:
  - Hemochromatosis.
  - α_1-antitrypsin deficiency.
  - Wilson disease.
- Pancreas:
  - Syndromes that increase risk of pancreatic cancer, such as familial adenomatous polyposis (FAP), Lynch syndrome, familial atypical multiple mole melanoma syndrome (FAMMM), BRCA-associated hereditary breast and ovarian cancer syndromes (HBOC/BRCA), Peutz-Jeghers syndrome.
  - Cystic fibrosis.
- Bile ducts:
  - PSC with ulcerative colitis (UC).

MUST SEE

Because of the complex anatomy and unique appearance of some tumors, lesions in the liver and pancreas are frequently tested as gross and microscopic images. High-yield images include:
- Liver:
  - Hepatocellular adenoma.
  - Focal nodular hyperplasia.
  - HCC and variants.
  - Fibrolamellar HCC.
  - Hepatoblastoma.
  - PBC.
  - PSC.

- Biliary intraepithelial neoplasia, low and high grade:
  · Intrahepatic cholangiocarcinoma.
  · Neuroendocrine tumor.
  · Angiosarcoma.
  · Metastases.
  · Acute hepatitis.
  · ASH and NASH.
  · Viral hepatitis.
  · Cholestasis.
  · Vascular congestion.
  · Hydatid cyst.
- Gallbladder and extrahepatic bile ducts:
  · Biliary intraepithelial neoplasia, low and high grade.
  · Cholangiocarcinoma, including Klatskin tumors.
  · Acute cholangitis.
  · Gallbladder adenocarcinoma.
  · Cholelithiasis and chronic cholecystitis.
  · Cholesterolosis.
  · Adenomyomatous changes.
- Pancreas:
  · Serous cystadenoma.
  · Glandular intraepithelial neoplasia (PanIN), low and high grade.
  · IPMN and IOPN.
  · MCN.
  · Ductal adenocarcinoma.
  · Acinar cell carcinoma.
  · Pancreatoblastoma.
  · SPPN.
  · Pancreatic NET.
  · Neuroendocrine carcinoma.
  · Acute pancreatitis.
  · Chronic pancreatitis (including findings at frozen section).

· Pseudocyst.
· Fat necrosis.
· Amyloidosis.

MUST DO
- For each of the entities in the Must See section, you should be comfortable generating a differential diagnosis, and listing relevant additional studies such as histochemical or immunohistochemical stains.
- When studying in groups, practice listing:
  · Causes of hepatitis and pancreatitis.
  · Clinical findings and complications of hepatitis and pancreatitis.
- You should be able to describe the grossing protocol and independently gross the following specimens:
  · Liver core biopsy done for medical liver disease, as well as tumors.
  · Partial hepatectomy.
  · Total hepatectomy for liver transplant.
  · Resection of bile ducts for tumors, such as Klatskin tumors.
  · Cholecystectomy for benign and malignant lesions.
  · Whipple procedure.
  · Distal pancreatectomy +/– splenectomy.
- You should be able to describe and handle fresh specimens and frozen sections of the following specimens:
  · Whipple procedure margins.
  · Liver nodules to assess for benign versus malignant diseases.
  · Incidental peritoneal nodules found during hepatobiliary surgery and submitted to rule out metastasis.

MULTIPLE CHOICE QUESTIONS

1. Which cell type in the liver is mostly responsible for the development of hepatic fibrosis?

   a. Stem cell.
   b. Hepatocyte.
   c. Kupffer cell.
   d. Fibroblast.
   e. Stellate cell.

Answer: e

2. A patient with aplastic anemia has required repeated blood transfusions for several years. She has developed chronic viral hepatitis. Which virus type is most likely the cause?

   a. Hepatitis A virus (HAV).
   b. Hepatitis B virus (HBV).
   c. Hepatitis C virus (HCV).
   d. Hepatitis D virus (HDV).
   e. Hepatitis E virus (HEV).

Answer: c

3. Which of the following is the most common clinical indication for liver biopsy in HBV?

a. To grade the severity of inflammation.

b. To stage the degree of fibrosis.

c. To confirm HBV infection by HBsAg staining and confirm viral replication by HBcAg staining.

d. To rule out super-imposed diseases such as nonalcoholic fatty liver diseases.

e. To determine if there is active hepatitis in patients whose serological or bio-chemical data do not paint a clear picture of disease status.

Answer: e

4. A 3-year-old girl was treated with aspirin at home for flu-like symptoms. After a few days, she became irritable. Shortly afterwards, she became lethargic and died in the hospital. What histologic features are you most likely to find in the autopsy liver?

a. Microvesicular ste-atosis with panaci-nar distribution.

b. Acute hepatitis with many acido-phil bodies.

c. Cholestasis.

d. Giant mitochondria and Mallory bodies.

e. Portal and interface inflammation with many plasmacytes.

Answer: a

5. A liver biopsy specimen showed distinct eosinophilic globules accumulate in periportal hepatocytes on periodic acid-Schiff stain (PAS) with diastase stain. All of the following about the patient are true **except**:

a. The spectrum of liver abnormalities in adult patients includes chronic hepatitis, cir-rhosis, and hepato-cellular carcinoma.

b. Neonates and infants can present with giant cell hepatitis and a paucity of intra-hepatic bile ducts.

c. The patient can have emphysema and pul-monary dysfunction.

d. The intracel-lular inclusions stain positively for α1-antitrypsin antibody.

e. The patient's α1-antitrypsin phenotype is most likely *PiMM*.

Answer: e

6. An 18-year-old male with elevated liver enzymes, increased copper in the urine, and Kayser-Fleisher rings on slit lamp eye exam will most likely have:

a. A high serum level of antinuclear antibody and anti-smooth muscle antibody (anti-SMA).

b. Glucose intolerance.

c. Degeneration of the putamen in the brain.

d. High serum ceru-loplasmin level.

e. Low serum cop-per level.

Answer: c

7. A 30-year-old male presented with progressive jaundice and elevated liver enzymes. Endoscopic retrograde cholangiopancreatography (ERCP) showed alternating segments of stenosis and dilatation. A liver biopsy showed an onionskin pattern of fibrosis around interlobular bile ducts. He also had developed chronic diarrhea. What do you expect a colonic biopsy to show?

a. Crohn disease.

b. Microscopic colitis.

c. Bowel ischemia.

d. Pseudomembra-nous colitis.

e. Ulcerative colitis.

Answer: e

8. When evaluating a biopsy of suspected primary biliary cholangitis, which of the following findings would indicate probable overlap with autoimmune hepatitis?

a. The patient is a middle-aged female with a history of lupus nephritis.

b. The patient's serum antinuclear antibody level is elevated.

c. The biopsy shows significant balloon-ing degeneration and numerous

acidophil bodies associated with high transaminases.

d. The portal tract contains many plasmacytes.

e. Lymphocytes fill the sinusoids in the periportal region of the lobule.

Answer: c

9. Zone 3 necrosis associated with lymphocytic infiltration should raise concern for all the following entities **except**:

a. Autoimmune hepatitis.

b. Drugs.

c. Transplant rejection.

d. Alcohol.

e. Chronic hepatitis.

Answer: e

10. The single most important histologic feature on liver biopsy for establishing the diagnosis of extrahepatic biliary atresia in a neonate is:

a. Cholestasis.

b. Giant cell hepatitis.

c. Portal inflammation.

d. Ductular proliferation.

e. Paucity of inter-lobular bile ducts.

Answer: d

11. Which of the following statements about Mallory-Denk bodies is **incorrect**?

a. Mallory-Denk bod-ies can be seen in both alcoholic and nonalcoholic steatohepatitis.

b. Mallory-Denk bodies can be seen in patients with cholestasis.

c. Mallory-Denk bodies in Wilson disease are associated with copper overload.

d. Mallory-Denk bodies contain degener-ated mitochondria.

e. Mallory-Denk bod-ies contain cyto-keratin 8 and 18.

Answer: d

12. A 36-year-old woman with a history of long-term oral contraceptive use had a subcapsular mass resected from the right lobe of the liver. Histologically, the mass was composed of sheets and cords of cells resembling normal hepatocytes with abundant glycogen content. Thick-walled vessels were scattered throughout the lesion, but no portal tracts or central veins were found. This tumor can be associated with which of the following?

a. *KRAS* activation.

b. *p53* mutation.

c. *Jagged-1* mutations.

d. Hepatocyte nuclear factor-1a mutations.

e. *C-myc* mutations.

Answer: d

13. Which of the following special stains is most helpful in the diagnosis of hepatocellular carcinoma?

a. Reticulin.

b. Trichrome.

c. Iron.

d. PAS plus diastase (PAS-D).

e. Copper.

Answer: a

14. All of the following statements about hepatocellular carcinoma are correct **except**:

a. It can develop in noncirrhotic liver.

b. A single tumor can have different histologic patterns and grades in different areas.

c. The fibrolamellar variant is typically seen in young adults who have viral hepatitis or other well-defined risk factors.

d. Primary tumors resembling hepatocellular carcinoma (even with bile formation) can be found outside the liver such as in the stomach, ovary, and other sites.

e. Tumor cells can stain positive for CK7 and CK19.

Answer: c

15. Carcinoma of the gallbladder is most commonly associated with:

a. Chronic cholecystitis.

b. Cholelithiasis.

c. Cholesterolosis.

d. Porcelain gall bladder.

e. Sclerosing cholangitis.

Answer: b

16. Which of the following statements regarding gallbladder carcinoma is **incorrect**?

a. Elective cholecystectomy can be a preventive measure for gallbladder adenocarcinoma in some patients with gallstones and chronic cholecystitis.

b. Hyalinizing cholecystitis without calcifications is not associated with carcinoma.

c. The histological grading of gallbladder adenocarcinoma in the American Joint Committee on Cancer (AJCC) TNM classification system is based on the degree of glandular differentiation.

d. If high grade dysplasia is identified in the gallbladder, extensive sampling is warranted.

e. The gallbladder has ill-defined layers; therefore, the current staging protocols are problematic for early-stage tumors.

Answer: b

17. Cholangiocarcinoma is most commonly associated with:

a. Primary biliary cirrhosis.

b. Primary sclerosing cholangitis.

c. Schistosomiasis.

d. Cholelithiasis.

e. Viral hepatitis.

Answer: b

18. Graft versus host disease affecting the liver typically damages:

a. Hepatocytes.

b. Portal veins.

c. Central veins.

d. Arterials.

e. Interlobular bile ducts.

Answer: e

19. A patient underwent a Whipple resection of a pancreatic carcinoma. During the operation, several whitish capsular nodules were found in the liver incidentally. On biopsy, a nodule showed collections of irregular dilated glands in fibrous stroma, with some of the glands containing inspissated bile. The most likely diagnosis is:

a. Metastatic adenocarcinoma.

b. Von Meyenburg complex (bile duct malformation).

c. Bile duct adenoma.

d. Cholangiocarcinoma.

e. Biliary cystadenofibroma.

Answer: b

20. In North America, the most important cause of chronic pancreatitis is:

a. Alcohol.

b. Cholelithiasis.

c. Hereditary disease.

d. Malnutrition.

e. Hyperparathyroidism.

Answer: a

21. A patient with obstructive jaundice underwent a Whipple resection. The resected pancreas showed extensive ductal centric plasmacyte infiltration. These plasmacytes most likely stain positively with:

a. IgM.

b. IgG1.

c. IgG2.

d. IgG3.

e. IgG4.

Answer: e

22. A 60-year-old man presented with weight loss, jaundice, back pain, and elevated serum CA 19–9. Radiology and exploratory laparotomy showed a large mass located in the head of the pancreas and multiple omental nodules. A biopsy of the tumor showed invasive glands in a desmoplastic stroma. All the following statements are correct **except**:

a. The tumor glands stain positively for CK7 and CK19.

b. > 85% of the tumor will have *KRAS* mutation.

c. The back pain is likely caused by perineural invasion.

d. This tumor is more common in developing countries and is caused by chronic pancreatitis.

e. The 5-year survival rate for patients with this type of tumor is < 5%.

Answer: d

23. Which islet cell tumors are the most common and the least malignant?

a. Insulinoma.

b. Gastrinoma.

c. Somatostatinoma.

d. Glucagonoma.

e. VIPoma.

Answer: a

24. Which of the following histologic features is the most important in grading a pancreatic neuroendocrine tumor and predicting its metastatic potential?

a. Nuclear pleomorphism and cytological atypia.

b. Vascular invasion and capsular invasion.

c. Tumor size and type of hormone secreted.

d. Mitosis and Ki 67 proliferation index.

e. Genetic abnormality and aneuploidy.

Answer: d

25. Which of the following statements about intraductal papillary mucinous neoplasms of the pancreas (IPMN) is **not** true?

a. *KRAS* mutations and alterations of tumor suppressor genes (*p53, p16, SMAD4 [DPC4]*) play a role in the carcinogenesis.

b. They occur more frequently in males than females.

c. The survival rate is worse than for ductal carcinoma.

d. A large amount of mucous at the opening of ampulla of Vater can be observed endoscopically.

e. Biological behavior ranges from benign to borderline to malignant.

Answer: c

26. Which of the following statements about mucinous cystic neoplasms of the pancreas is true?

a. These tumors are all associated with a poor prognosis.

b. Genetic alterations of *KRAS, p53,* and *SMAD4/DPC4* play a role in their pathogenesis.

c. They occur more frequently in males than females.

d. Obstructive jaundice is usually the first clinical presentation.

e. They are associated with von Hippel-Lindau syndrome.

Answer: b

27. A 33-year-old female was found to have a cystic mass in the pancreas during a routine gynecological examination without obvious symptoms. The lesion was resected, and, histologically, it showed solid nests of tumor cells with abundant small blood vessels. Cells located distant to the vessels were more degenerative with more viable tumor cells cuffing each blood vessel. Hyaline globules and nuclear groves were found in some tumor cells. Which of the following statements regarding this lesion is **incorrect**?

a. This tumor is more common in women than men.

b. This is a biologically low grade tumor, and it will never metastasize.

c. The tumor cells stain positive for α1-antitrypsin.

d. The tumor cells often demonstrate abnormal nuclear β-catenin immunoexpression.

e. Occasionally, the tumor cells can stain positive for CD56 and synaptophysin.

Answer: b

Liver
Viral Hepatitis

28. What is the appropriate length of a liver biopsy specimen?
- It depends on what you are looking for:
  - For a mass lesion, the specimen is considered sufficient as long as tumor tissue is present no matter how small the specimen is.
- For most chronic diseases, a minimum of 1.5 cm in length and 6 portal tracts is usually sufficient.

29. What is the risk of becoming infected with hepatitis B (HBV) or hepatitis C (HCV) from a needle stick?
- HBV is 6–30% and HCV is 1.8%.
- HIV (for comparison): 0.3%.

30. What is the risk that chronic hepatitis will develop from HBV and from HCV?
- HBV: 5–10%.
- HCV: 80–90%.

31. List the viruses that can cause fulminant liver failure.
- Hepatitis A, B, C, D, and E virus.
- Herpes simplex virus (HSV) (even in immunocompetent patients).
- Epstein-Barr virus (EBV).
- Cytomegalovirus (CMV).
- Varicella-zoster virus.
- Parvovirus B19 in children.

32. What is a carrier in the setting of viral hepatitis?
- A carrier is an individual who harbors and can transmit an organism, but who has not manifested symptoms.
- In the case of HBV infection, a healthy carrier is often defined as an individual with positive HBsAg for > 6 months, without HBeAg, but with the presence of anti-HBe antibody, normal aminotransferases, low or undetectable serum HBV DNA, and liver biopsy showing a lack of significant inflammation and necrosis.

33. What is chronic hepatitis in the setting of viral hepatitis?
Symptomatic, biochemical, or serologic evidence of continuing or relapsing hepatic disease for > 6 months.

34. What is the role of pathologists in the diagnosis of viral hepatitis from liver biopsies?
- Confirm the diagnosis.
- Ascertain the etiology.
- Grade the activity.
- Stage the fibrosis.
- Rule out other superimposed disease processes.

35. Describe the positive serology that can aid in the diagnosis of hepatitis A, B, and C.
- Hepatitis A:
  - Acute infection: anti-HAV IgM.
  - Immunity: anti-HAV IgG.
- Hepatitis B:
  - Acute infection: HBsAg, anti-HBsAg, anti-HBc IgM, anti-HBc IgG.
  - Chronic infection (no replication): HBsAg, anti-HBc IgG.
  - Chronic replicating: HBsAg, anti-HBc IgG, HBV DNA.
  - Reactivation: HBsAg, HBV DNA, anti-HBc IgM, anti-HBc IgG.
  - Past exposure immunity: anti-HBsAg, anti-HBc IgG.
  - Vaccination immunity: anti-HBsAg.
- Hepatitis C:
  - Acute and chronic: HCV-RNA, anti-HCV IgG (not protective).

36. List the histologic clues that can aid in the differential diagnosis of the common types of viral infection of the liver.
- In immunocompetent patients:
  - Abundant plasma cells and cholestasis: HAV.
  - Predominant ballooning degeneration, ground-glass cytoplasmic inclusions: HBV.
  - Dense lymphoid aggregates, bile duct damage, sinusoidal lymphocytes, steatosis: HCV.
  - Portal and sinusoidal small lymphocytes, and granulomas with minimal hepatocyte damage: EBV/ CMV.
  - Confluent necrosis and cholangitis: hepatitis E (HEV).
- In immunocompromised patients:
  - Nuclear/cytoplasmic inclusions and microabscesses with neutrophils: CMV.
  - Portal infiltration of large lymphocytes (polymorphic B cell hyperplasia or lymphoma): EBV.
  - Randomly distributed coagulative necrosis and nuclear inclusions: herpes virus or adenovirus.
  - Extensive hepatocyte necrosis, prominent cholestasis, and pericellular fibrosis: fibrosing cholestatic HBV or HCV.

37. You see steatosis or steatohepatitis in a patient with HCV. What does that mean to the patient?
- Mild steatosis is probably HCV genotype 3.
- Steatosis favors viral replication since fat droplets provide a scaffold for viral assembly.
- Severe steatosis may represent superimposed disease processes (e.g., diabetes, alcohol, obesity).
- It is usually associated with more inflammatory activity and faster fibrosis.

38. List the conditions that morphologically simulate lymphoma/leukemia in the liver.
- HCV.
- EBV/CMV mononucleosis.
- Toxoplasmosis.
- Hemophagocytic syndrome.
- Small cell carcinoma.

39. Classify viral hepatitis based on mode of transmission.
- Fecal-oral: hepatitis A, hepatitis E.
- Parenteral, sexual: hepatitis B, C, D.
- Parenteral: hepatitis G.

40. List liver function test results and their corresponding histology.
- Liver cell necrosis: elevation of aspartate aminotransferase (AST), alanine aminotransferase (ALT).
- Cholestasis: elevation of Υ-glutamyltransferase (GGT), alkaline phosphatase (ALP), bilirubin.
- Hepatocyte dysfunction: low albumin and blood urea nitrogen (BUN); high prothrombin time/international normalized ratio (PT/INR), and ammonia.
- Autoimmune hepatitis: antinuclear antibodies (ANA), anti-smooth muscle antibody (anti-SMA), elevated IgG levels.
- Primary biliary cholangitis: antimitochondrial antibodies (AMA), elevated IgM.
- Primary sclerosing cholangitis: perinuclear antineutrophil cytoplasmic antibodies (pANCA).
- Hepatocellular carcinoma: AFP, decarboxy-prothrombin (DCP).

41. Give the differential diagnosis of ground-glass hepatocytes in a nonneoplastic setting.
- HBV.
- Drug induced hypertrophy of smooth endoplasmic reticulum (e.g., phenobarbital): centrilobular, PAS diastase negative, orcein negative.
- Fibrinogen storage disease: random location, PAS diastase positive.
- Alcohol aversion drug (cyanamide): secondary lysosome accumulation, periportal, PAS positive, PAS diastase negative.
- Glycogen storage disease type 4 or abnormal glycogen metabolism due to multidrug intake: mostly periportal, PAS positive, PAS diastase negative.
- Lafora disease (myoclonic epilepsy): periportal; positive for PAS, and for colloidal iron and polyglucosan immunostains. Composed of smooth endoplasmic reticulum and glycogen.

42. What are the main patterns of hepatocyte injury?
- Direct: characterized by fatty change, mitochondrial damage, central (zone 3) necrosis.
  - Common etiologies include alcohol, metabolic disorders, drugs, and metabolites toxicity.
- Immunological: characterized by damage to cell membranes with piecemeal necrosis of periportal (zone 1) hepatocytes and mononuclear-cell infiltration.
  - Common etiologies include chronic viral hepatitis, autoimmune hepatitis, primary biliary cholangitis, drug-induced (e.g., halothane).
- Cholestatic: characterized by portal edema, feathery degeneration of periportal hepatocytes, ductular proliferation, bile plugs in canalicular spaces, etc.
  - Etiologies are intrahepatic (such as sex-hormone induced cholestasis) and extrahepatic (such as biliary obstruction due to stones or malignancy).

43. What are the common causes of acute liver failure?
- Infections (hepatitis A, B, C, D).
- Drugs/toxins (paracetamol, aspirin, valproate, tetracycline, idiosyncratic reactions to medications, herbal supplements).
- Pregnancy complications (acute fatty liver of pregnancy, HELLP syndrome).
- Vascular causes (Budd-Chiari syndrome, hepatic arterial thrombosis).

44. Define acute liver failure and its gross and histological correlate.
- Acute liver failure is condition resulted from severe liver injury that occurs within 26 weeks of the initial insult in the absence of cirrhosis or preexisting liver disease and associated with encephalopathy and coagulopathy.
- Gross appearance: liver is small and shrunken.
- Microscopically there are 3 main patterns:
  - Massive hepatic necrosis alternating with islands of regenerating hepatocytes.
  - Diffuse microvesicular steatosis.
  - Histologic features specific to nonhepatotropic virus infection (CMV, HSV, adenovirus).

Autoimmune Hepatitis

45. Name 3 subtypes of autoimmune hepatitis and their characteristic autoimmune markers.
- Type 1. ANA, ASMA.
- Type 2. anti-liver-kidney microsomal antibody (anti-LKM).
- Type 3. antisoluble liver antigen or liver pancreas antigen.

46. Name the top 4 differentials for central zone necrosis with inflammation.
- Drug toxicity.
- Autoimmune hepatitis.
- Transplant rejection.
- Alcohol.

Liver Cirrhosis

47. What is cirrhosis?
- To diagnose cirrhosis, all the following criteria should be met:
  · Bridging fibrous septa.
- Parenchymal nodules.
- Disruption of the architecture of the entire liver.

48. What is the point of performing a biopsy on a cirrhotic liver?
- Confirm the diagnosis.
- Identify clues to the etiology.
- Rule out carcinoma.

49. What stains do we routinely use to analyze liver biopsy specimens? What is the use of each stain?
- Perls Prussian blue: iron.
- PAS: glycogen.
- PAS diastase: ceroid macrophages, a_1-antitrypsin, basement membrane of interlobular bile ducts, fungi.
- Orcein: elastic fibers for differentiating old fibrosis from new fibrosis, HBsAg, copper binding protein.
- Rhodanine: copper.
- Trichrome: collagen — for recognizing fibrosis.
- Reticulin: liver architecture, thickness of liver cell plates.
- CK7/CK19: ducts, ductules, and duct derived tumors.

50. What serology data are useful for liver biopsy interpretation in addition to liver function tests?
- Serology for viral hepatitides.
- Serology for ANA, AMA, and anti-SMA.
- Serology for IgG and IgM.
- Serum levels of ceruloplasmin and a_1-antitrypsin.
- Serum iron, ferritin levels.

51. List the 4 most common causes of liver cirrhosis.
- Alcohol abuse.
- Viral hepatitis.
- Nonalcoholic steatohepatitis (NASH).
- Biliary disease.

52. Describe the characteristic histology of 3 common causes of liver cirrhosis.
- Cirrhosis due to viral hepatitis: portal-to-portal bridging predominant, regenerative nodules, ongoing portal-based inflammation.
- Cirrhosis due to cardiac failure: central-to-central bridging, lack of inflammation, central venular congestion, and sinusoidal dilatation.
- Cirrhosis due to biliary disease: cholestasis, cholate stasis with periseptal clear halo, coarse fibrous septa subdividing the liver in a jigsaw-like pattern with no obvious regeneration.

53. List 4 clinical consequences of liver cirrhosis.
- Portal hypertension: ascites; formation of portosystemic venous shunts leading to upper gastrointestinal bleeding; splenomegaly.
- Hepatic dysfunction: coagulation defects, hypoalbuminemia, hepatic encephalopathy, hyperestrinism in males.
- Other important organ dysfunction: hepatorenal syndrome, hepatopulmonary syndrome.
- Increased incidence of hepatocellular carcinoma.

54. How do you differentiate cirrhosis from massive hepatic necrosis?
- Necrosis shows a collapsed reticulin network with no regenerative nodules.
- Cirrhosis shows collagen deposition with regenerative nodules.

55. How do you differentiate cirrhosis from nodular regenerative hyperplasia?

Nodular regenerative hyperplasia should not have fibrous septa.

56. When there is no well-formed nodule, what are the histologic clues to cirrhosis in a core biopsy specimen?

- Fragmentation of the biopsy specimen.
- Thin layers of connective tissue adhering to the rounded edges of a nodular fragment.
- Abnormal orientation of reticulin fibers.

- Abnormal spacing of portal tracts and central veins, more central veins than the number of portal tracts, tiny portal tracts.
- Liver cell regeneration (2-cell thick plates), or dysplasia (small or large cell change).

57. Define progressive cirrhosis and regressive cirrhosis.

- Progressive: broad fibrous septa with loosely aggregated collagen fibers (pale blue on trichrome stain), containing inflammatory cells and ductular reactions.

- Regressive: thin, dense and acellular stroma (dark blue on trichrome stain), perforated delicate septa, remnant portal tracts, and isolated collagen fibers.

α₁-Antitrypsin Deficiency

58. What is the function of α₁-antitrypsin?

Inhibition of proteases, particularly neutrophil elastase, cathepsin G, and proteinase 3, which are normally released from neutrophils at sites of inflammation.

59. What is the mechanism of α₁-antitrypsin deficiency (pathogenesis)?

- It is an autosome recessive disorder with a selective defect in the migration of α₁-antitrypsin from the endoplasmic reticulum to the Golgi apparatus; α₁-antitrypsin polymerizes in the endoplasmic reticulum, causing endoplasmic reticulum stress and leading to apoptosis.
- Alleles are inherited codominantly. The normal genotype is *PiMM*. The most common abnormal allele is Z.

- In *PiZZ* genotype, the polypeptide is abnormally folded and cannot be secreted into the blood, which leads to a low serum α₁-antitrypsin level.
- α₁-Antitrypsin accumulates in hepatocytes causing liver damage.

60. List 3 clinical consequences of α₁-antitrypsin deficiency.

- Liver damage in the form of neonatal hepatitis, liver cirrhosis, and increased risk of hepatocellular carcinoma.

- Pulmonary emphysema.
- Cutaneous panniculitis.

61. How do you confirm that cytoplasmic deposits are α₁-antitrypsin?

- Characteristic morphology.
- Periportal distribution.

- PAS diastase staining pattern.
- Positive immunohistochemical staining using α₁-antitrypsin antibody (if necessary).

Hemochromatosis

62. Define hemochromatosis and differentiate it from hemosiderosis.

- Hemochromatosis: an autosomal recessive inherited disorder caused by excessive iron absorption (also known as primary or hereditary hemochromatosis).

- Hemosiderosis: the accumulation of iron in tissues as a consequence of parenteral administration of iron, usually in the form of transfusions, or from other causes (also known as acquired hemochromatosis).

63. List 2 genetic abnormalities that can cause primary adult form hemochromatosis.

- Almost always caused by mutations of hemochromatosis gene (*HFE*), a gene located on the short arm of chromosome 6 at 6p21.3.

- Most common mutation: *C282Y* — a cystine to tyrosine substitution at amino acid position 282.
- Second common mutation: *H63D* — histidine to aspartate at amino acid position 63.

Note: mutations in transferrin receptor 2 (*TFR2*), and ferroportin can also cause adult hemochromatosis. Mutations of the hepcidin gene (*HAMP*) and hemojuvelin (*HJV*) cause severe juvenile hemochromatosis.

64. Briefly describe the pathogenesis of primary hemochromatosis.
- Unrestricted intestinal absorption of iron develops due to mutations of *HFE*.
- Iron stimulates the production of hydroxyl free radicals.
- Free radicals damage tissue and stimulate hepatic stellate cells to promote fibrosis.
- Free radical interactions with DNA predispose patients to hepatocellular carcinoma.
- Iron deposits in multiple organs cause damage: pancreas, heart, joints, skin.

65. List 3 secondary causes of hemochromatosis.
- Blood transfusions.
- Long term hemodialysis.
- Hemoglobinopathies (e.g., sickle cell disease, thalassemia, sideroblastic anemias).

66. List 5 organs involved in hemochromatosis and the resulting complications.
- Liver: cirrhosis, hepatocellular carcinoma.
- Pancreas: diabetes mellitus.
- Skin: pigmentation.
- Myocardium: dilated cardiomyopathy, arrhythmias.
- Joint synovial linings: synovitis, arthritis.

67. List 3 causes of death from hemochromatosis.
- Liver cirrhosis.
- Cardiac failure.
- Hepatocellular carcinoma.

68. List 3 types of pigments in the liver and the stains that can differentiate them.
- Iron: Perls stain, blue color.
- Copper: rhodamine stain (reddish orange color), orcein.
- Bilirubin: Hall stain, green color.

69. How do you handle liver biopsy specimens if hemochromatosis is suspected clinically?
- Biopsy specimens usually come as 2 separate cores:
  · Describe both cores in the usual fashion (e.g., color, length, diameter, fragmented or not).
- Put 1 core in formalin for routine histology.
- Wrap 1 core in lens paper and submit it for measurement of dry weight iron or molecular testing.

70. How do you calculate the hepatic iron index?
- HI = hepatic iron in µmol/g dry weight ÷ age.
- HI < 1: normal.
- HI > 2: diagnostic of hemochromatosis only when it is in a noncirrhotic liver and in livers with no other reason for excess iron accumulation.

71. List other primary liver diseases that can have hepatic siderosis.
- HCV.
- Fatty liver due to alcohol or nonalcoholic fatty liver disease (NAFLD).
- Hepatocellular carcinoma.
- Porphyria cutanea tarda.

Wilson Disease

72. What is Wilson disease?
- An autosomal recessive disorder caused by mutation of the *ATP7B* gene, which encodes a copper transport protein on the hepatocyte canalicular membrane.
- Pathogenesis:
  · It is due to defective hepatocyte transport of copper into bile for excretion, **not** due to increased absorption.
- It leads to failure to incorporate copper into ceruloplasmin and **low** serum ceruloplasmin due to decreased synthesis.
- Unbound copper accumulates in blood and deposits in other tissues, causing toxic effects.

73. List 4 characteristic histologic features of Wilson disease.
- Fatty change.
- Glycogenated nuclei.
- Mallory bodies.
- Copper pigment deposition especially in periportal hepatocytes.

Note: histomorphological changes are nonspecific. Hepatic copper content per dry weight of liver (> 250 µg/gram dry liver is essentially diagnostic) is the single most sensitive and accurate biochemical test for Wilson disease. Mutation analysis of *ATP7B* by direct sequencing should be performed if the diagnosis is difficult.

74. List 3 organs primarily affected by Wilson disease and the consequences.

- Liver: steatosis, acute/chronic hepatitis, cirrhosis.
- Eye: Kayser-Fleischer rings, green to brown deposits of copper in Descemet membrane in the limbus of the cornea.
- Brain: basal ganglia (particularly the putamen) atrophy and even cavitation; behavioral changes in patient, or psychosis, or tremor.

75. List 4 conditions that can be associated with increased hepatic copper.

- Cholestasis of any cause.
- α_1-Antitrypsin deficiency (neonatal).
- Wilson disease.
- Exposure to sprays containing copper sulfate (e.g., vineyard workers).

Amyloidosis

76. What are the patterns of amyloid deposition in the liver?

- Amorphous extracellular eosinophilic deposits in the sinusoid space of Disse, portal tract connective tissue, and vessel wall.
- They are mostly linear, but can be globular.

77. Name the 2 most common types of amyloid in the liver and their associated conditions.

- Amyloid light chain: plasma cell dyscrasia.
- Amyloid associated protein: chronic inflammatory disorders.

Alcoholic Steatohepatitis

78. List 5 histologic features of alcoholic steatohepatitis.

- Macrovesicular steatosis, especially in perivenular zone.
- Mallory-Denk bodies.
- Perivenular sinusoidal fibrosis ("chicken wire fence" pattern) and sclerosing hyaline necrosis.
- Lobular focal necroinflammatory change with neutrophils.
- Hepatocyte ballooning and necrosis.

79. List 5 clinical complications of chronic ethanol consumption.

- Liver: steatosis, steatohepatitis, cirrhosis, hepatocellular carcinoma.
- Central nervous system: Wernicke-Korsakoff syndrome.
- Gastrointestinal system: pancreatitis, gastritis.
- Malnutrition and deficiency of vitamins: anemia, dilated cardiomyopathy due to thiamine deficiency.
- Pregnancy: fetal alcohol syndrome.

80. Describe how alcohol causes steatosis in the liver.

- Shunting of normal substrates away from catabolism and toward lipid biosynthesis, as a result of excessive alcohol dehydrogenase and acetaldehyde dehydrogenase.
- Impaired assembly and secretion of lipoproteins.
- Increased peripheral catabolism of fat.

81. List 4 clinicopathological clues that help differentiate alcoholic steatohepatitis (ASH) from nonalcoholic steatohepatitis (NASH).

ASH	NASH
• History of alcohol intake.	• Obesity, diabetes, bypass surgery, hyperlipidemia, metabolic disease, and others.
• AST/ALT > 2.	• AST/ALT < 1.
• Central venular distribution of steatosis and fibrosis, more macrovesicular steatosis.	• More diffuse distribution, more microvesicular steatosis, more frequent portal fibrosis.
• Mallory-Denk bodies frequent.	• Mallory-Denk bodies less frequent.

82. Give the differential diagnosis of lobular neutrophilic infiltration.

- Alcoholic steatohepatitis.
- Liver infection or sepsis.
- Medication reaction.
- Surgical hepatitis.
- Virus in immunocompromised host — CMV, herpes.

83. What is the role of liver biopsy in the diagnosis of fatty liver disease?
- Confirm or exclude the diagnosis.
- Differentiate simple steatosis from steatohepatitis.
- Assess the extent of necroinflammatory activity and fibrosis.

84. What information needs to be provided in a pathology report for nonalcoholic fatty liver diseases?[1]

REPORT	ASSESSMENT
NAFLD activity score (NAS) — total score > 5 = NASH	• Percentage of steatosis: · < 5%: score 0. · 5–33%: score 1. · 34–66%: score 2. · 67–100%: score 3. • Lobular inflammation: · < 2 foci/20x field: score 1. · 2–4 foci/20x field: score 2. · > 4 foci/20x field: score 3. • Hepatocyte ballooning: · Mild: score 1. · Moderate to marked: score 2.
Degree of fibrosis	• 1a: mild centrilobular sinusoidal fibrosis. • 1b: moderate centrilobular sinusoidal fibrosis. • 1c: portal fibrosis only. • 2: centrilobular sinusoidal and periportal fibrosis. • 3: bridging fibrosis. • 4: cirrhosis.

Mallory Hyaline (Mallory-Denk bodies)

85. Describe the morphology of Mallory hyaline.
Eosinophilic cytoplasmic clumps in hepatocytes.

86. What is the molecular composition of Mallory hyaline?
Tangled skeins of cytokeratin intermediate filaments, such as cytokeratin 8 and 18, complexed with other proteins such as ubiquitin.

87. List 3 pathological conditions associated with Mallory hyaline.
- Alcoholic liver disease and nonalcoholic fatty liver diseases.
- Primary biliary cholangitis and other chronic cholestatic entities.
- Wilson disease.

88. List the histologic clues that differentiate Mallory hyaline due to alcohol from Mallory hyaline due to cholestasis.

HISTOLOGIC FEATURE	MALLORY HYALINE DUE TO CHOLESTASIS	MALLORY HYALINE DUE TO ALCOHOL
Location	• Periportal.	• Central venular.
Attraction for neutrophils	• Absent.	• Present.
Ductal damage, ductular proliferation	• Present.	• Absent.
Cholestasis	• Present.	• Absent.
Steatosis	• Usually absent, but can be present (Wilson).	• Present.
Giant mitochondria	• Absent.	• Present.

Drug-Induced Liver Injury

89. Describe Reye syndrome.

- A rare and potentially fatal syndrome of mitochondrial dysfunction in the liver, brain, and elsewhere that occurs predominantly in children.

- Associated with the administration of acetylsalicylic acid (aspirin) for the relief of fever.
- Histologically, characterized by extensive microvesicular steatosis in the liver.

90. Describe patterns of primary liver damage and drugs related to the patterns.

PATTERN OF INJURY	REPRESENTATIVE DRUGS
Lobular necrosis without inflammation	• Halothane, CCL4, acetaminophen, mushrooms.
Lobular necrosis with inflammation	• Phenytoin, isoniazid, rifampin, alpha-methyldopa.
Chronic hepatitis	• Nitrofurantoin, propylthiouracil.
Fibrosis	• Vitamin A, vinyl chloride, methotrexate.
Fatty change	• Corticosteroids, ethanol, tetracycline, methotrexate.
Granulomas	• Allopurinol (fibrin ring granuloma), diazepam, sulphonamides, methyldopa, phenylbutazone.
Cholestasis	• Oral contraceptives, cyclosporine A, tamoxifen, indomethacin, carbamazepine, anabolic steroids.
Vascular injury	• Arsenic, oral contraceptives, alkaloids.
Liver cell adenoma	• Oral contraceptives, anabolic steroids.
Hepatocellular carcinoma	• Aflatoxin, thorotrast.
Angiosarcoma	• Thorotrast, vinyl chloride, arsenic.
Cholangiocarcinoma	• Thorotrast.

91. Describe the characteristic liver changes in patients on long-term total parenteral nutrition.

- Intrahepatic cholestasis: perivenular bilirubin stasis, cholelithiasis.

- Macrovesicular steatosis, periportal.
- Portal and periportal fibrosis.

92. List 4 disease processes in the liver that are unique to pregnancy and their characteristic histologic features.

- Acute fatty liver of pregnancy: microvesicular steatosis.
- Intrahepatic cholestasis of pregnancy: perivenular canalicular and hepatocellular bilirubin stasis.
- Preeclampsia and eclampsia:
  · Macro: hemorrhages over the capsule and on the cut surface.

- · Micro: fibrin thrombi in portal vessels and sinusoids, periportal necrosis.
- HELLP syndrome (syndrome involving hemolysis, elevated liver function, and low platelets): periportal hemorrhage, fibrin and necrosis, glycogenated nuclei.

93. List the most common entities that typically present with granulomas in the portal tract.

- Sarcoidosis.
- Infection, especially mycobacteria.

- Drug hepatotoxicity.
- Primary biliary cholangitis.

94. List entities that cause macrovesicular steatosis and entities that cause microvesicular steatosis.

- Macrovesicular:
  · Alcohol.
  · Diabetes.
  · Drugs.
  · Total parenteral nutrition.

- Microvesicular:
  · Pregnancy.
  · Reye syndrome.
  · Drugs/toxins: valproic acid, mushrooms, tetracycline.
  · Adult-onset diabetes.

95. What are the histologic clues to drug-induced liver damage?

- Eosinophil infiltration.
- Centrilobular necrosis.
- Nonnecrotizing granulomas.

- Parenchymal giant cell hepatitis in adult patients.
- Cholestasis without obvious inflammation.

96. Describe the spectrum of liver changes in patients with diabetes.

- Steatosis, nonalcoholic fatty liver disease (NAFLD).
- Hepatocyte glycogenosis (glycogenic hepatopathy).
- Glycogenated hepatocyte nuclei.

- Hepatosclerosis — diffuse perisinusoidal fibrosis.
- Vascular disorders.

97. List 3 disease processes that can cause "nutmeg" liver.
- Congestive heart failure and/or left heart failure.
- Budd-Chiari syndrome.
- Constrictive pericarditis.

98. List 4 disease processes that can affect sinusoidal blood flow.
- Cirrhosis.
- Sickle cell disease.
- Metastatic carcinoma.
- Chemotherapy or cytotoxic preparation for bone marrow transplantation.

99. List 3 classic clinical features of Budd-Chiari syndrome.
- Marked enlargement of hepatic caudate lobe by imaging.
- Visible dilatation of lumbar veins posteriorly.
- Improvement after mesocaval shunt.

100. List 5 causes of hepatic venous thrombosis.
- Primary myeloproliferative disorders (e.g., polycythemia vera).
- Inherited disorders of coagulation (e.g., antithrombin deficiency; protein S or protein C deficiency; or mutations of factor V).
- Antiphospholipid syndrome.
- Paroxysmal nocturnal hemoglobinuria.
- Intraabdominal cancers, particularly hepatocellular carcinoma.

101. What is the most common cause of venoocclusive disease?
Bone marrow transplantation.

102. List 3 noninfectious causes of portal vein thrombosis.
- Vascular injury: trauma, catheterization.
- Stasis: cirrhosis, hepatocellular carcinoma.
- Hypercoagulable state: polycythemia vera, protein C or S deficiency, factor V Leiden.

103. List 5 autopsy findings of portal hypertension other than cirrhosis.
- Portal vein thrombosis.
- Hepatoportal sclerosis.
- Nodular regenerative hyperplasia.
- Splenomegaly.
- Esophageal varices.

104. List 4 drugs that can cause angiosarcoma.
- Thorotrast.
- Vinyl chloride.
- Arsenic.
- Androgens.

105. List the characteristic immunohistochemical markers for Kaposi sarcoma that allow differentiation from angiosarcoma.
- Human herpesvirus-8 (HHV-8).
- Bcl-2.

Liver Allograft Biopsy

106. In the context of liver steatosis, how do you define the adequacy of the liver graft?
- The assessment and decision are made based on the percentage of macrovesicular steatosis. The presence of microvesicular steatosis is generally acceptable for transplantation.
  - Mild steatosis (5–33%): favorable outcome.
- Moderate steatosis (34–66%): borderline; it may be acceptable depending on other factors.
- Severe steatosis (> 66%): it generally leads to an unfavorable outcome (primary nonfunction), and it is not usually transplanted.

107. List 3 types of allograft rejection and their characteristic histology.
- Hyperacute rejection.
  - Ischemic necrosis and predominantly neutrophilic infiltrates.
  - The diagnosis is strengthened if:
    › Neutrophilic or necrotizing arteritis is present.
    › Immunoglobulin deposits can be demonstrated.
    › Preformed antidonor antibodies are found.
- Acute cellular rejection.
  - Mixed, but predominantly mononuclear, portal inflammation, containing blastic or activated lymphocytes, neutrophils, and eosinophils (i.e., rejection type infiltrate).

(continued on next page)

- Subendothelial inflammation of portal and/or terminal hepatic veins.
  - Bile duct inflammation and damage.
- Chronic rejection.

- Early bile duct atrophy/pyknosis, later bile duct loss.
- Early zone 3 necroinflammatory lesions, later perivenular fibrosis with bridging, and/or fibrous luminal obliteration of the central vein.
- Foam cell obliterative arteriopathy.

108. Describe the Banff scoring system for acute cellular rejection.
- Pathologists first grade rejections descriptively (indeterminate, mild, moderate, severe).

- Pathologists then use the criteria given in the rejection activity index (RAI) to subjectively score from 0 to 3 each of the following: portal inflammation, bile duct damage, and venous endothelial inflammation.

109. How commonly does primary liver disease recur in the liver allograft after liver transplantation?
- HCV: > 90%; eventually they all recur.
- Primary sclerosing cholangitis (PSC), primary biliary cholangitis (PBC), autoimmune hepatitis (AIH), alcoholic hepatitis, NASH: 20–30%.

- Hepatocellular carcinoma: 15–20%.
- Cholangiocarcinoma: 90%.

110. What is fibrosing cholestatic hepatitis B? Histologically, what characterizes it?
- Fibrosing cholestatic hepatitis B is a form of rapidly progressive, recurrent hepatitis B after transplantation.
- Histologically, it is characterized by:
  - Extensive periportal fibrosis progressing to septal fibrosis.

- Marked hepatocellular swelling and lobular disarray.
- Occasional ground-glass cells.
- Immunohistochemistry (IHC) showing large amounts of HbcAg and/or HbsAg.

111. Give the differential diagnosis of portal eosinophil infiltration.
- Drugs.
- Parasite infestation.
- Acute allograft rejection.

- AIH, PBC, PSC.
- Extramedullary hematopoiesis.

Graft Versus Host Disease (GVHD)

112. What is GVHD?

GVHD occurs when immune competent cells or their precursors are transplanted into immunologically compromised recipients, and the transferred cells recognize alloantigens (HLA antigen) in the host as foreign and react against them.

113. In what clinical settings does GVHD occur?
- Hematopoietic stem cell transplantation.
- Bone marrow transplantation.

- Transplantation of solid organs rich in lymphoid cells (e.g., the liver).
- Transfusion of unirradiated blood.

114. List 3 organs commonly involved by acute GVHD.
- Skin: generalized rash, desquamation if severe.
- Liver: destruction of small bile ducts, causing jaundice; destruction of sinusoidal endothelium and central venous endothelium, resulting in venoocclusive disease.

- Intestine: mucosal apoptosis, crypt loss, ulceration, bloody diarrhea.

115. Describe the characteristic liver histology of acute and chronic GVHD.
- Acute GVHD: lobular and mild portal hepatitis, ductulitis.

- Chronic GVHD: portal tract inflammation, bile duct destruction (or complete loss), and portal fibrosis.

116. List the 2 most common liver complications after bone marrow transplantation.
- GVHD.

- Venoocclusive disease.

Benign Liver Nodules

117. List 3 benign nodules that enter the differential of hepatocellular carcinoma (HCC).
- Massive regenerative nodule.
- Focal nodular hyperplasia.
- Hepatocellular adenoma.

118. List 3 risk factors for HCC other than viral hepatitis.
- Fatty liver disease: alcohol, NASH, NAFLD.
- Food contaminants such as aflatoxin.
- Metabolic disease: hemochromatosis, α_1-antitrysin deficiency, glycogen storage disease, tyrosinemia.

119. Classify benign liver nodules.
- Tumor-like conditions: hydatid cyst (*E. Multilocularis*), macroregenerative nodule, dysplastic nodule, nodular regenerative hyperplasia, focal nodular hyperplasia.
- Benign liver cell tumor: hepatocellular adenoma.
- Benign bile duct tumors: bile duct hamartoma, bile duct adenoma.
- Benign vascular tumors: hemangioma.

120. List 3 stains that distinguish well-differentiated HCC from regenerative nodules.
- CD34.
- Glypican-3.
- Reticulin.

121. List 2 reasons why biopsy diagnosis of hepatocellular adenoma is clinically important.
- To differentiate from hepatocellular carcinoma.
  - Note: rarely, adenoma may transform into carcinoma, particularly when it arises in individuals with glycogen storage disease, or with β-catenin gene mutations.
- To diagnose subcapsular adenomas, which have a tendency to rupture, particularly during pregnancy, causing life threatening intraperitoneal hemorrhage.

122. Compare the pathogenesis of focal nodular hyperplasia and nodular regenerative hyperplasia. What do they have in common?

They both have either focal or diffuse alterations in hepatic blood supply, arising from obliteration of portal vein radicles, and compensatory augmentation of arterial blood supply.

123. List 3 gross features of focal nodular hyperplasia.
- Well-demarcated but unencapsulated nodule in noncirrhotic liver.
- Central gray-white, depressed stellate scar radiating to the periphery.
- No bile stain — differentiates from fibrolamellar hepatocellular carcinoma.

124. List 3 histologic features of focal nodular hyperplasia (FNH).
- Central scar contains large arteries with fibromuscular hyperplasia and eccentric or concentric narrowing of the lumen.
- Radiating septa contain lymphocytic infiltrates and exuberant bile duct proliferation along septal margins.
- Parenchyma between the septa lacks normal portal tracts or normal sinusoidal plate architecture, and contains normal hepatocytes forming thick plates characteristic of regeneration.

Note: multiple FNH syndrome is defined as multiple FNH **plus** 1 or more other lesions such as hepatic hemangioma, systematic arterial structural defects (berry aneurysm, brain telangiectasia), or brain tumors (astrocytoma, meningioma).

125. List 4 histologic features that differentiate hepatocellular adenoma (HCA) from carcinoma.

HISTOLOGIC FEATURE	HEPATOCELLULAR ADENOMA	HEPATOCELLULAR CARCINOMA
Background liver	• Mostly normal.	• Mostly cirrhotic.
Thickening of liver cell plate	• Absent (≤ 2 hepatocytes).	• Present (> 2 hepatocytes).
Cytological atypia	• No.	• Yes.
Invasion into surrounding liver or lymph vascular spaces	• No.	• Yes.

126. Classify HCA. List the molecular abnormalities, and IHC and histomorphology characteristics, of each subtype.

SUBTYPE	MOLECULAR ABNORMALITY	IHC	HISTOLOGY
Hepatocyte nuclear factor 1 α (HNF-1α) inactivated	• HNF-1α mutation.	• Loss of liver fatty acid binding protein (LFABP)	• Steatosis.
Inflammatory	• *JAK/STAT* pathway activation.	• Serum amyloid A (SAA) and/ or C-reactive protein (CRP) overexpression.	• Inflammation, ductular reaction, sinusoidal dilatation, dystrophic vessels.
Beta-catenin mutated	• Mutation or deletion of CTNNB1 (encoding β-catenin).	• Nuclear β-catenin staining; homogenous glutamine synthetase (GS) staining.	• Cytological atypia, small cell change, pseudoacini.
Sonic Hedgehog	• *GLI1* activation.	• Prostaglandin D synthase (PGTDS) and argininosuccinate synthase 1 (ASS1) overexpression.	• Hemorrhage, abnormal vessels.
Unclassified	• Unknown.	• No specific features.	• No specific features.

127. What are the top 3 common subtypes of HCA?
- Hepatocyte nuclear factor 1 α (HNF-1α) inactivated subtype.
- Inflammatory subtype.
- β-catenin subtype.

128. What subtype of HCA has the highest risk of malignant progression?

The β-catenin muted subtype: it has up to 40% risk of progressing to hepatocellular carcinoma.

Note: recent studies have shown that the exact mutation site (exon) determines the risk of malignant progression. See: Beaufrère A, Paradis V. Hepatocellular adenomas: review of pathological and molecular features. Hum Pathol. 2021;112:128-37.

129. List 5 lesions that commonly enter the differential diagnosis of subcapsular nodules in a frozen section during resection of a gastrointestinal malignancy.
- Metastatic carcinoma.
- Bile duct hamartoma (Meyenburg complex).
- Bile duct adenoma.
- Fibrous scar.
- Hemangioma.

130. Differentiate focal nodular hyperplasia from hepatocellular adenoma.

FEATURE	FOCAL NODULAR HYPERPLASIA	HEPATOCELLULAR ADENOMA
Demographic	• Female, all ages. • No clear association with oral contraceptives.	• Female, 20–40 years old. • Clear association with oral contraceptives.
Clinical	• Asymptomatic mass. • No risk of hemorrhage. • No risk of malignant transformation.	• Mass. • Risk of hemorrhage. • Small risk of malignant transformation.
Gross	• No capsule. • Nodular, stellate scar.	• Partial or complete capsule. • Homogeneous, no scar.
Hemorrhage, necrosis	• Uncommon.	• Common.
Bile ductules and bile stasis	• Bile ductules present, bile stasis absent.	• Bile ductules absent, bile stasis present.
Management	• No excision is needed.	• Excision is necessary in many cases.

Hepatocellular Carcinoma

131. List at least 4 noninfectious etiologies for the development of HCC.
- Aflatoxin exposure — causes mutation at the third nucleotide of codon 249 of *TP53*.
- Steatohepatitis due to alcohol or nonalcoholic causes.
- Metabolic diseases: hemochromatosis, tyrosinemia, α1-antitrypsin deficiency.
- Drugs: thorotrast, androgens/anabolic steroids, oral contraceptives.

132. List the specific etiologies highly associated with HCC carcinogenesis (> 15%).

- HBV, HCV.
- Hereditary hemochromatosis.
- Hereditary tyrosinemia.
- Porphyria cutanea tarda.
- Hypercitrullinemia.
- Membranous obstruction of inferior vena cava.

133. What are the carcinogenetic mechanisms of HBV infection?

- Integration of viral DNA into host genome, leading to chromosomal instability.
- Insertional mutations at specific sites, leading to activation of genes involve in cell proliferation.
- Expression of HBX viral protein to modulate cell proliferation and inactivate *p53* activities.

134. List the stains that can help differentiate primary hepatocellular carcinoma from metastatic adenocarcinoma. List their patterns of staining.

- Confirm hepatocellular origin:
  · Hep Par-1 (cytoplasmic, granular).
  · AFP (cytoplasmic).
  · Arginase 1 (cytoplasmic and nuclear).
  · CK8/18 (cytoplasmic).
  · TTF-1 (cytoplasmic).
  · Fluorescence in situ hybridization (FISH) for albumin mRNA.
- Confirm metastasis:
  · Monoclonal carcinoembryonic antigen (CEA) (cytoplasmic with membrane enhancement in adenocarcinoma; negative in hepatocellular carcinoma).
  · MOC-31 (membranous).
  · Mucin stains (highlight intra- and extracellular mucin in adenocarcinoma).

135. List special and immunohistochemical stains that help confirm malignancy in well-differentiated hepatocellular lesions. List their patterns of staining.

- Reticulin (loss).
- Glypican-3 (cytoplasmic and membranous).
- CD34 diffuse sinusoidal endothelium staining
- Polyclonal CEA, and CD10 (canalicular pattern of staining).

136. What are the common mutations in hepatocellular carcinoma?

- *TP53*.
- *CTNNB1* (β-catenin activation).
- *TERT* promoter mutations.
- *ARID1A*.

137. List 5 conditions that can have elevated serum α-fetoprotein (AFP) levels.

- Hepatocellular carcinoma.
- Hepatoblastoma.
- Pregnancy.
- Yolk sac tumor.
- Massive liver necrosis with regeneration.

138. What is the cutoff size for defining early hepatocellular carcinoma?

2 cm.

139. Both early hepatocellular carcinoma (eHCC) and small progressed hepatocellular carcinoma (spHCC) are < 2 cm in size. How do you differentiate them histologically?

	EHCC	SPHCC
Atypia	• Increased cell density and mild cytological atypia.	• More cytological atypia
Gross margin	• Indistinct.	• Distinct.
Tumor capsule	• Absent.	• Present.
Invasion	• Focal stromal invasion.	• Expansive/infiltrative growth
CD34 stain	• Scattered/low-density.	• Diffuse/high density.
"Nodule in nodule" pattern	• Absent.	• Present.

140. What is the cutoff size for defining a dysplastic nodule?

It is ≥ 1 mm.

Note: a dysplastic focus is < 1 mm.

141. How do you distinguish a low grade dysplastic nodule and a large regenerative nodule (e.g., macroregenerative nodule)?

The presence of unpaired arteries or cytological atypia greater than the background liver favors a dysplastic nodule.

142. List 3 cytological variants of hepatocellular carcinoma in addition to the fibrolamellar variant.
- Pleomorphic (giant cell).
- Clear cell.
- Sarcomatoid.

143. What are the histological subtypes of hepatocellular carcinoma according to the WHO classification of digestive tumors?*
- Steatohepatitic.
- Clear cell.
- Macrotrabecular (massive).
- Scirrhous (> 50% of tumor shows dense intratumoral fibrosis).
- Chromophobe.
- Fibrolamellar carcinoma.
- Neutrophil rich.
- Lymphocyte rich.

*This chapter uses the fifth edition of the WHO classification of digestive system tumors.

144. What are the main histological patterns of growth of HCC?
- Trabecular.
- Solid (compact).
- Pseudoglandular (pseudoacinar).
- Macrotrabecular (composed mostly of trabeculae [≥ 10 cells thick], which is associated with worse prognosis).
- Mixed pattern.

145. What are the main macroscopic patterns of growth of HCC?
- Single distinct nodule.
- Large dominant nodule with multiple smaller satellite nodules (usually present within 2 cm of the dominant nodule).
- Diffuse (cirrhotomimetic): dozens to hundreds HCC nodules that are approximately of the same size and shape as cirrhotic nodules.
- Multiple distinct nodules (represent independent primaries).
- Pedunculated HCC (protrudes from the surface of the liver).

146. What are the main parameters of the College of American Pathologists (CAP) protocols for reporting resection of HCC?
- Specimen.
- Procedure.
- Tumor size.
- Tumor focality.
- Satellitosis.
- Histologic type.
- Histologic grade.
- Tumor extension.
- Treatment effect.
- Margins.
- Lymphovascular invasion.
- Perineural invasion.
- Lymph node examination.
- Pathologic staging.
- Additional pathologic findings.
- Ancillary studies.

147. According to the Couinaud classification, how many segments are in the liver? What factors divide the segments from each other?
- There are 8 functionally independent segments.
- The hepatic veins are at the periphery of each segment.
- The center of each segment has branches of the portal veins, hepatic arteries, and bile ducts.
- Each segment can be resected without damaging the remaining tissue if the resection is made along the vessels that define the periphery of the segment.

148. What is another name for segment 1 of the liver? What are the characteristics of blood circulation to this segment?
- The caudate lobe, which:
  · May receive blood from both the right and left branches of the portal vein.
- Contains hepatic veins that drain directly into the inferior vena cava.

149. What is Cantlie line?
- It is an imaginary line that passes to the left of the vena cava all the way forward and sections the gallbladder into halves.
- The Cantlie line follows the middle hepatic vein, which divides the liver into left and right functional lobes.

150. What segments are in the right liver? What are in the left liver?
- The middle hepatic vein divides the liver into left and right lobes. The segments of the liver are numbered clockwise.
  - Left liver:
    › Lateral segments 2 and 3.
    › Medial segments 4a and 4b.
- Right liver:
  › Anterior segments 5 and 8.
  › Posterior segments 6 and 7.
  › The caudate lobe (segment 1) drains directly into the inferior vena cava, but based on the Cantlie line, most of the caudate lobe lies on the left side.

151. What are the CAP protocols for sampling a liver tumor?
- Sections should be taken from each major tumor nodule.
- Representative sampling of smaller nodules (macroscopically different) should be performed.
- Cirrhotic nodules that are larger than the surrounding background liver should be included.

152. For the purposes of staging, how does CAP approach satellite nodules, multifocal primary hepatocellular carcinomas, and intrahepatic metastases?
These are not distinguished and are considered simply as multiple tumors.

153. What is the WHO classification of malignant tumors of the liver and intrahepatic bile ducts?
- Hepatocellular carcinoma.
- Hepatoblastoma.
- Cholangiocarcinoma:
  - Large duct intrahepatic cholangiocarcinoma.
  - Small duct intrahepatic cholangiocarcinoma.
- Combined hepatocellular and cholangiocarcinoma.
- Carcinoma undifferentiated, not otherwise specified (NOS).
- Neuroendocrine tumours, NOS.
- Neuroendocrine tumors grades 1, 2, and 3.
- Neuroendocrine carcinoma, NOS:
  - Large cell neuroendocrine carcinoma.
  - Small cell neuroendocrine carcinoma.
- Mixed neuroendocrine-nonneuroendocrine neoplasm (MiNEN).
- Carcinoma, undifferentiated, NOS.

154. How do you classify a tumor displaying typical HCC, but which also has areas of fibrolamellar carcinoma?
It should be classified as hepatocellular carcinoma not fibrolamellar carcinoma.

155. List the AJCC grades* and WHO grades for hepatocellular carcinomas.

AJCC	WHO
• GX: grade cannot be assessed. • G1: well-differentiated. • G2: moderately differentiated. • G3: poorly differentiated. • G4: undifferentiated.	• G1: well-differentiated. • G2: moderately differentiated. • G3: poorly differentiated.

*This chapter uses the eighth edition of the AJCC cancer staging manual.

156. What does CAP recommend for the evaluation of margins?
- Consult the surgeon to determine the critical foci within the margins that require microscopic evaluation.
- Report the closest distance from margin.
  - If multiple tumors are present, the distance of the nearest tumor to the margin is reported.
- To evaluate wide transection margins:
  - If grossly positive, confirm the margins microscopically.
  - If grossly free, sample the region closest to the nearest identified tumor nodule.
  - Random sampling of the cut surface may be sufficient.

157. How often are macroscopic and microscopic invasion seen?
- Macroscopic invasion: 15%.
- Microscopic invasion: 43%.
- Both are associated with lower postresection survival.

158. When should vascular invasion be suspected?
- Larger tumors (> 5 cm).
- Multiple tumors.

159. What is the AJCC T staging for hepatocellular carcinoma?
TX: primary tumor cannot be assessed.
T0: no evidence of primary tumor.
T1: solitary tumor ≤ 2 cm or > 2 cm without vascular invasion.
T1a: solitary tumor ≤ 2 cm.

(continued on next page)

T1b: solitary tumor > 2 cm without vascular invasion.

T2: solitary tumor ≥ 2 cm with vascular invasion; or multiple tumors, none > 5 cm in greatest dimension.

T3: multiple tumors, at least 1 of which > 5 cm in greatest dimension.

T4: single tumor or multiple tumors of any size involving a major branch of the portal vein or hepatic vein, or tumor(s) with direct invasion of adjacent organs other than the gallbladder, or with perforation of visceral peritoneum.

160. What is the CAP protocol for the number of lymph nodes to examine? What are the regional nodes in the hepatic region?

- Histologic examination usually involves examination of 3 or more lymph nodes.

- The regional lymph nodes of the hepatic region include the hilar, hepatoduodenal ligament, inferior phrenic, caval, common hepatic artery and portal vein lymph nodes.

Fibrolamellar Hepatocellular Carcinoma

161. List 3 characteristic clinical features of fibrolamellar hepatocellular carcinoma.

- Patients are young (20–40 years old), male or female.
- They have no underlying chronic liver diseases.

- The outcome is similar to classical HCC in noncirrhotic liver.

162. What is the characteristic mutation and immunohistochemical pattern of fibrolamellar hepatocellular carcinoma?

- Mutation: a ~400 base pair deletion on chromosome 19 leads to fusion of *DNAJB1* and *PRKACA* genes, and a novel *DNAJB1-PRKACA* fusion transcript.

- Immunohistochemical pattern: CK7 and CD68 positive.

163. List 3 characteristic gross features of fibrolamellar hepatocellular carcinoma.

- Single, large, hard scirrhous tumor with fibrous bands running through it.

- Background liver shows no cirrhosis.
- Bile stains on cut surface.

164. List 2 characteristic microscopic features of fibrolamellar hepatocellular carcinoma.

- Well-differentiated polygonal cells with abundant eosinophilic cytoplasm and prominent nucleoli.

- Nests or cords of tumor cells separated by parallel lamellae of dense collagen bundles.

165. Differentiate usual fibrolamellar hepatocellular carcinoma (FL-HCC) from hepatocellular carcinoma (usual HCC).

FEATURE	FL-HCC	USUAL HCC
Demographic	• Peak third decade. • M = F.	• Six to seventh decade. • M:F = 3–6:1.
% of HCC	• 1–5%.	• 95–99%.
DCP, neurotensin, unsaturated B12 binding capacity	• Often increased.	• Rare.
Live enzyme abnormality	• Uncommon.	• Common.
Imaging: calcification, scar	• Common.	• Uncommon.
MACRO		
Multifocality	• Solitary, left lobe.	• Both lobes, can be multifocal.
Necrosis/hemorrhage	• Uncommon.	• Common.
Fibrous septa/scar	• Common.	• Uncommon.
Associated cirrhosis	• No.	• Yes.
MICRO		
Large cell/granular cytoplasm	• Common.	• Uncommon.
Pale bodies/hyaline globules	• Common.	• Uncommon.
Lamellar stroma bands.	• Present.	• Absent.
EM mitochondria	• Numerous.	• Less common.
OUTCOME AND RESECTABILITY		
5-year survival	• 30%.	• 7%.
Resectability	• 60%.	• 25%.

166. Describe the criteria for selecting HCC patients for liver transplantation.

- The Milan criteria for selecting patients with cirrhosis and early HCC:
  · Single lesion: < 5 cm.
- Multiple lesions: no more than 3 lesions with the largest measuring ≤ 3 cm.

Hepatoblastoma

167. What is the most frequent malignant liver tumor in children?
Hepatoblastoma.

168. List the histologic patterns of hepatoblastoma.

- Epithelial type:
  · Fetal pattern.
  · Embryonal pattern.
  · Macrotrabecular.
- Small cell undifferentiated.
- Mixed epithelial-mesenchymal type:
  · Teratoid.
  · Nonteratoid.

169. What syndromes are associated with hepatoblastoma? What are additional risk factors?

- Syndromic associations:
  · Familial adenomatous polyposis.
  · Beckwith-Wiedemann syndrome.
  · Trisomy 18 (Edwards syndrome).
- Additional risk factors:
  · Low birth weight.
  · Maternal smoking.

170. What are the genetic abnormalities in hepatoblastoma?

- Abnormalities in WNT/β-catenin signaling pathway due to:
  · Mutations in *CTNNB1*.
  · Mutations in *AXIN*.
- Mutations in *APC*.
- Mutations in *TP53*.
- Overexpression of cyclin D1, *MYC*, and *TERT*.

171. Differentiate hepatoblastoma from childhood hepatocellular carcinoma.

FEATURE	HEPATOBLASTOMA	CHILDHOOD HEPATOCELLULAR CARCINOMA
DEMOGRAPHIC		
Age	• < 5 years.	• > 5 years.
Sex	• M:F = 2:1.	• M:F = 10:1.
MACROSCOPIC		
Pseudocapsule	• Present.	• Absent.
Single lesion	• Approximately 75%.	• Approximately 30%.
Cirrhosis	• Absent.	• Approximately 15%.
MICROSCOPIC		
Light and dark pattern	• Present.	• Absent.
Trabeculae	• 2–3 cells thick.	• > 2–3 cells thick.
Cell size	• Smaller than normal hepatocyte.	• Larger than normal hepatocyte.
Pleomorphism	• Absent.	• Present.
Tumor giant cells	• Uncommon.	• Common.
Intranuclear inclusions	• Absent.	• Common.
Cytoplasmic hyaline globules	• Absent.	• Common.
Extramedullary hematopoiesis	• Present.	• Absent.

Intrahepatic Biliary Disease

172. Classify jaundice based on etiology.

- Predominantly **unconjugated** hyperbilirubinemia.
  - Excessive extrahepatic production of bilirubin (e.g., hemolytic anemia).
  - Reduced hepatocyte uptake (e.g., drug interference with membrane carrier systems).
  - Impaired bilirubin conjugation (e.g., viral hepatitis).

- Predominantly **conjugated** hyperbilirubinemia.
  - Decreased hepatocellular excretion (e.g., deficiency of canalicular membrane transporters: Dubin-Johnson syndrome).
  - Impaired bile flow (e.g., choledocholithiasis, PSC, PBC).

173. What clinicopathological clues differentiate mechanical duct obstruction, primary biliary cholangitis (PBC), and primary sclerosing cholangitis (PSC)?

FEATURES	MECHANICAL DUCT OBSTRUCTION	PRIMARY BILIARY CHOLANGITIS	PRIMARY SCLEROSING CHOLANGITIS
Associated disorders	• Biliary atresia. • Cholelithiasis. • Stricture. • Carcinoma of pancreatic head.	• 30% associated with inflammatory arthropathy, other autoimmune diseases.	• 70% associated with inflammatory bowel disease (chronic ulcerative colitis).
Sex predilection	• No.	• F:M = 9:1. • Middle age.	• F:M = 2:1. • 70% < 45 years old.
Cancer risk	• Not established.	• Mostly hepatocellular carcinoma.	• Mostly cholangiocarcinoma.
Laboratory findings	• Conjugated hyperbilirubinemia.	• Elevated serum IgM, M2 form of antimitochondrial antibody highly specific.	• Elevated serum IgM, hypergammaglobulinemia, atypical p-ANCA.
Cholangiogram	• Based on etiology, proximal dilatation.	• Normal.	• Beading.
Characteristic histology	• Acute cholangitis, cholestasis (canalicular or ductal), bile lakes, ductular proliferation with surrounding neutrophils, portal tract edema.	• Intrahepatic small duct. • Florid duct lesion. • Granulomas adjacent to bile duct.	• Extrahepatic and intrahepatic small and large bile ducts, periductal portal tract fibrosis, segmental stenosis.

174. List 4 liver conditions that can be associated with polycystic kidney disease.

- Polycystic liver disease.
- Congenital hepatic fibrosis.
- Caroli disease.
- Von Meyenburg complexes.

Note: these are all due to ductal plate malformation.

175. What is pathogenesis of congenital hepatic fibrosis? List the main histologic features and associated conditions.

- Autosomal-recessive congenital disorder of the liver due to mutations in *PKHD1* gene (encodes the protein fibrocystin/polyductin) result in defective remodeling of the ductal plate, abnormal development of the intrahepatic portal veins, and progressive periportal fibrosis.

- It is associated with fibropolycystic diseases (e.g., Caroli disease, polycystic kidney disease, nephronophthisis).
- Histology:
  - Bile ductular proliferation in fibrotic portal areas.
  - Portal-portal bridging fibrosis with no inflammation.
  - Normal hepatocellular plates and central veins.

176. What is the mode of inheritance and significance of Caroli disease?

- Caroli disease: autosomal-recessive disorder that usually presents in childhood and early adulthood.

- Significance: commonly associated with polycystic kidney disease and increased risks of cholangiocarcinoma.

177. What are the main pathologic features of Caroli disease?

Characterized by saccular dilatation of the intrahepatic bile ducts, with dilated segments alternate with segments of normal caliber.

178. What is Caroli syndrome?

Caroli syndrome: Caroli disease together with congenital hepatic fibrosis.

179. List the entities that typically show ductular proliferation at the portal-lobular interface.
- Extrahepatic biliary obstruction.
- Massive hepatocyte necrosis.
- PSC.
- PBC.

180. What are the histologic features of cholestasis?
- Parenchymal changes:
  - Bilirubin stasis (presence of bilirubin pigment in hepatocytes, bile canaliculi and bile ducts).
  - Cholestatic liver cell rosettes, canalicular cholestasis.
  - Feathery degeneration.
  - Xanthomatous cells.
  - Bile infarcts.
  - Copper accumulation, Mallory hyaline.
- Periportal and architectural changes:
  - Portal edema.
  - Cholate stasis (periportal hepatocyte swelling/feathery degeneration, with or without Mallory hyaline).
  - Ductular reaction.
  - Periductular fibrosis.
  - Biliary fibrosis and cirrhosis (jigsaw pattern).

181. What is the role of an extrahepatic duct biopsy in primary sclerosing cholangitis?
To rule out malignancy— not for the diagnosis of PSC.

182. What is the differential diagnosis of portal neutrophilic infiltrate?
- Ascending cholangitis.
- Total parenteral nutrition.
- Drugs.
- Extrahepatic biliary obstruction.
- Treated autoimmune hepatitis.

183. What is the differential diagnosis of granulomatous inflammation in liver parenchyma?
- Sarcoidosis.
- Drugs.
- Infection (*M. avium-intracellulare*, fungal, bacterial, parasitic, viral).
- Primary biliary cirrhosis.
- Foreign material.
- Lipogranuloma.
- Chronic granulomatous disease of childhood.
- Neonatal age.

184. List 7 key entities that can cause absence of bile ducts in the portal tract.
- Extrahepatic bile duct atresia or biliary atresia (BA), Alagille syndrome.
- Primary biliary disease processes: PBC, PSC.
- Overlap of autoimmune hepatitis with either PBC or PSC.
- Chronic liver allograft rejection.
- Graft versus host disease.
- Drugs.
- Idiopathic.

Cholangiocarcinoma

INTRAHEPATIC CHOLANGIOCARCINOMA AND RELATED TUMORS

185. What are histological subtypes of intrahepatic cholangiocarcinoma?
- Small duct type.
- Large duct type.

186. List the histologic characteristics of cholangiocarcinoma that allow differentiation from hepatocellular carcinoma.
- Gland formation.
- Mucin production.
- Stroma desmoplasia.
- No trabeculae.
- No bile.
- No cirrhosis.
- CK7+, CK19+, claudin-4+.

187. List 3 cytokeratin stains that help differentiate cholangiocarcinoma from metastatic colonic carcinoma.
- Cholangiocarcinoma: CK7+, CK19+, CK20−.
- Metastatic colon carcinoma: CK20+, CK7−, CK19−.

188. What is combined hepatocellular cholangiocarcinoma?
A malignant epithelial neoplasm characterized by the presence of both hepatocytic and cholangiocytic differentiation within the same tumor on H&E and confirmed by immunohistochemical markers.

189. List the features that differentiate bile duct hamartoma from bile duct adenoma.

FEATURE	BILE DUCT HAMARTOMA (VON MEYENBURG COMPLEX)	BILE DUCT ADENOMA (PERIBILIARY GLAND HAMARTOMA)
Multiple nodules	• Common.	• Uncommon.
Portal tracts	• Typical location.	• Often trapped in nodule.
Ducts with ectatic lumen	• Typical.	• Rare.
Ducts with bile	• Common.	• Absent.
Ducts with small or absent lumen	• Uncommon.	• Typical.
Ducts with mucin	• Absent.	• Common.
Prominent lymphocytes	• Absent.	• Common.

190. How do you report liver wedge resections?
- Specimen type: indicate they are wedge resections.
- Tumor type, size, grade.
- Extent of invasion: capsule, lymphovascular space, perineural.
- Tumor necrosis, if present.
- Resection margin.
- Nonlesional liver pathology, if appropriate (e.g., cirrhosis, inflammation, steatosis).

191. How do you address multifocal tumors?
- Sample each nodule.
- Intrahepatic cholangiocarcinoma, metastases, and satellite nodules are all considered as multiple tumors.

192. How does the AJCC grade cholangiocarcinoma?
- GX: grade cannot be assessed.
- G1: well-differentiated.
- G2: moderately differentiated.
- G3: poorly differentiated.

193. What are the 3 growth patterns observed in intrahepatic cholangiocarcinoma?
- Mass-forming type (60% of cases).
- Periductal infiltrating type (20% of cases) — it spreads in a diffuse longitudinal pattern along the bile duct, and it is associated with poor prognosis.
- Mixed mass-forming/periductal-infiltrating type (20% of cases).

194. How do CAP protocols recommend assessing margins in intrahepatic cholangiocarcinoma?
- Document gross positive margins.
- Sample liver parenchyma nearest to the tumor and report the distance to the margin.
- Evaluate bile ducts at the margin for in situ carcinoma or dysplasia.

195. According to the AJCC, what does a T4 tumor classification for intrahepatic cholangiocarcinoma mean?
A tumor involving local extrahepatic structure by direct invasion.

196. What lymph nodes does CAP consider to be distant metastasis in intrahepatic cholangiocarcinoma?
Involvement of the celiac, periaortic, or pericaval lymph nodes are considered to be distant metastasis (pM1).

197. What is the most common risk factor for intrahepatic cholangiocarcinoma in North America?
Primary sclerosing cholangitis.

Note: in Asian countries, biliary parasites and recurrent pyogenic cholangitis are more common.

Perihilar Bile Duct Tumors

198. What is the current WHO classification of tumours arising in the biliary tree based on anatomic distribution?
- Tumors arising in the biliary tree are classified into 3 groups: intrahepatic, perihilar, and distal.
- Intrahepatic tumors are defined as those located within the liver parenchyma.
- Perihilar tumors are defined as those involving the hepatic duct bifurcation or the extrahepatic biliary tree proximal to the origin of the cystic duct.
- Distal tumors are defined as those arising between the junction of the cystic duct-bile duct and the ampulla of Vater.

199. What is Klatskin tumor?

Hilar carcinoma located at the confluence of left and right hepatic ducts.

200. How does the AJCC grade carcinomas of the perihilar bile ducts?

- GX: grade cannot be assessed.
- G1: well-differentiated.
- G2: moderately differentiated.
- G3: poorly differentiated.

201. What are the possible causes of local regional recurrence for perihilar bile duct tumor?

- Residual tumor at the resection margins.
- Tumors located along the dissected soft tissue margin in the portal area.
- Tumors that spread longitudinally along the duct wall.
- Perineural and lymphovascular invasion.

202. List some of the factors that influence the outcome of perihilar bile duct tumor.

- Completeness of surgical resection.
- Perineural and lymphatic invasion.
- Anatomic extent (stage) of disease at the time of resection.
- Lymph node metastases.

203. How common is it for a patient with bile duct carcinoma to have synchronous carcinomas of the gallbladder?

It occurs in approximately 5% of patients.

Extrahepatic Bile Duct Tumors

204. What are precursors for extrahepatic biliary duct carcinoma (EHBD)?

- Biliary intraepithelial neoplasia.
- Intraductal papillary neoplasm of the bile ducts.

205. What are the common mutations of EHBD carcinomas?

- *TP53*.
- *KRAS*.
- *MDM2* amplifications.

206. List the histologic features that can help differentiate bile duct adenocarcinoma from reactive changes.

- Perineural invasion.
- Haphazard arrangement of irregular glands instead of normal lobular arrangement.
- Loss of nuclear polarity and increased nuclear-cytoplasmic ratio.
- Cytoplasmic positivity for CEA by IHC.
- MUC1 and nuclear positivity for p53 by IHC

Note: CEA, MUC1, and MUC5AC are limited to the apical membrane in benign cells. MUC1 and MUC5AC are negative in intestinal type tumors.

207. How can frozen sections help in the surgical treatment of congenital extrahepatic biliary atresia?

- They can determine the caliber of the residual bile ducts in the portal hepatic scar.
- If > 100 μm, the Kasai procedure to restore bile flow has an 80–90% success rate.

208. What is the most important complication of choledochal cyst?

- Patients have a risk of carcinoma 20 times higher than the normal population.
- Carcinoma can develop in the cyst wall, gallbladder, or other parts of the biliary tree.

Distal Extrahepatic Bile Duct Tumors

209. What is the definition of distal tumors?

Common bile duct tumors arising between the junction of the cystic duct and the ampulla of Vater.

210. What are the histological types of tumors of the gallbladder and extrahepatic bile ducts according to the WHO classification?

- Benign epithelial tumors and precursors:
  - Adenoma.
  - Biliary intraepithelial neoplasia, low grade.
  - Biliary intraepithelial neoplasia, high grade.
- Intracystic papillary neoplasm with low grade intraepithelial neoplasia.
- Intracystic papillary neoplasm with high grade intraepithelial neoplasia.

(continued on next page)

- Intracystic papillary neoplasm associated with invasive carcinoma.
- Intraductal papillary neoplasm with low grade intraepithelial neoplasia.
- Intraductal papillary neoplasm with high grade intraepithelial neoplasia.
- Malignant epithelial tumors:
  · Adenocarcinoma, NOS.
  · Adenocarcinoma, intestinal type.
  · Clear cell adenocarcinoma, NOS.
  · Mucinous adenocarcinoma.
  · Poorly cohesive carcinoma.
  · Mucinous cystic neoplasm with associated invasive carcinoma.
  · Intraductal papillary neoplasm with associated invasive carcinoma.

· Intracystic papillary neoplasm with associated invasive carcinoma.
· Squamous cell carcinoma.
· Adenosquamous carcinoma.
· Undifferentiated carcinoma.
· Cholangiocarcinoma.
· Neuroendocrine tumor, NOS.
· Neuroendocrine tumor, grade 1.
· Neuroendocrine tumor, grade 2.
· Neuroendocrine tumor, grade 3.
· Neuroendocrine carcinoma.
· Large cell neuroendocrine carcinoma.
· Small cell neuroendocrine carcinoma.
· Mixed neuroendocrine-nonneuroendocrine neoplasm.

211. What is the AJCC T classification for distal extrahepatic bile duct tumors?

Tx: primary tumor cannot be assessed.

Tis: carcinoma in situ/high grade dysplasia.

T1: tumor invades the bile duct wall with a depth < 5 mm.

T2: tumor invades the bile duct wall with a depth of 5–12 mm.

T3: tumor invades the bile duct wall with a depth > 12 mm.

T4: tumor involves the celiac axis, the superior mesenteric artery, and/or hepatic artery.

212. Which histological type of carcinoma of the extrahepatic bile ducts has the best prognosis?

Papillary carcinoma.

213. Which histological types have a poorer prognosis?

- Signet-ring cell carcinoma.
- High grade neuroendocrine carcinoma.

- Undifferentiated carcinoma.

214. Which histological type is not graded?

Poorly differentiated neuroendocrine carcinoma.

215. What is the usual site of recurrence for tumors of the extrahepatic bile ducts?

- Most recurrences are locoregional and are usually at the surgical margins.

- They are usually residual tumors at the margins due to tumor spread along the wall or to perineural or lymphovascular invasion.

216. What feature of distal bile duct carcinomas makes them prone to have residual tumors at the margin?

They are often multifocal, and microscopic foci may be found away from the main mass.

217. What are the most important predictors of outcome in distal bile duct carcinomas?

- Stage of disease at presentation.

- Resectability: 5-year overall survival rate is 20–30% for resectable tumor, and 0% for unresectable cases.

218. Why should you pay special attention to the gallbladder in a resection specimen for a distal bile duct tumor?

Because 5% of patients also have carcinomas of the gallbladder.

219. Are perineural and lymphovascular invasion required elements or optional elements in reporting distal bile duct carcinomas?

They are required elements and should be specifically evaluated.

220. What should you keep in mind when evaluating perineural invasion in a patient with PSC?

Ducts affected by PSC can show perineural growth by benign hyperplastic intramural glands.

221. What are the features of distal bile ducts that can make classification as T2 or T3 difficult?

- The histology of the extrahepatic biliary tree varies along its length.
- The proximal ducts contain little smooth muscle compared to the distal bile ducts, which makes depth of invasion difficult to assess.

- Inflammatory changes and desmoplastic stromal responses to tumor may distort the duct.
- Periductal glands can be misinterpreted as invasive tumor glands.

222. How many lymph nodes does CAP recommend examining?
- A minimum number has not been determined, but the examination of at least 12 nodes is suggested.
- The regional lymph nodes are the same as those for carcinomas of the pancreas.

223. List 3 risk factors for biliary tract carcinomas.
- Primary sclerosing cholangitis.
- Biliary lithiasis and recurrent pyogenic cholangitis.
- Parasites (e.g., *Clonorchis sinensis*, *Opisthorchis viverrini*).

Mesenchymal Tumors of the Liver

224. What is the most common mesenchymal tumor of the liver?
Hemangioma.

225. What is the most common primary malignant mesenchymal neoplasm of the liver in adults?
Angiosarcoma.

226. What is the most common malignant hepatic mesenchymal neoplasm in children?
Embryonal sarcoma of the liver.

227. What is mesenchymal hamartoma (MH) of the liver?
A benign liver neoplasm composed of multicystic loose connective tissue and a ductal component with ductal plate malformation.

228. What is the difference between PEComa and angiolipoma? List important immunohistochemical markers.
- PEComa is a mesenchymal neoplasm composed of epithelioid-to-spindle cells showing variable expression of smooth muscle (desmins and/or SMA) and melanocytic markers (HMB045, Melan A, MITF, tyrosinase, PNL2).
  - The common locations for PEComas are the small and large bowels, pancreas, liver, and mesentery.
- Angiomyolipoma is a PEComa subtype composed of adipocytes and thick-walled, tortuous blood vessels.
  - Angyomyolipomas are nearly exclusively located in kidneys, pancreas, and liver.

229. What is the genetic syndrome associated with angiomyolipoma?
An associated syndrome is tuberous sclerosis.

Gallbladder
Cholelithiasis

230. Classify cholelithiasis and list 4 risk factors in each category.
- Cholesterol stones:
  - Advanced age.
  - Obesity and metabolic syndrome.
  - Hyperlipidemia syndromes.
  - Female sex hormones: pregnancy, oral contraceptives.
- Pigment stones:
  - Chronic hemolytic syndromes.
  - Biliary infection.
  - Ileal resection or bypass.
  - Ileal Crohn disease.

231. What are the 2 molecules involved in dissolving cholesterol into bile?
- Water soluble bile salts.
- Water insoluble lecithins.

232. Describe the conditions that facilitate the formation of cholesterol stones, and the conditions that facilitate the formation of pigment stones.
- Cholesterol gallstone formation (involves 4 simultaneous conditions):
  - Cholesterol supersaturation.
  - Hypomotility of the gallbladder.
  - Accelerated cholesterol nucleation in the bile.
  - Hypersecretion of mucus in the gallbladder.
- Black pigment stone:
  - Chronic extravascular hemolytic anemia (e.g., sickle cell anemia) increases the secretion of conjugated bilirubin into the bile.
  - Excess bilirubin in bile produces calcium bilirubinate.

(continued on next page)

- Brown pigment stone:
  - Bacterial contamination releases microbial β-glucuronidases.
- β-glucuronidases hydrolyze bilirubin glucuronides and result in an increase of unconjugated bilirubin in the biliary tree that exceeds its solubility.

233. List 5 common complications of cholelithiasis.

The spectrum of complications varies depending on where the stone is located in the biliary system: gallbladder, common bile duct, or intrahepatic ducts.

- Calculus cholecystitis, acute or chronic, hydrops/mucocele, empyema, perforation, fistulas.
- Obstructive cholestasis or pancreatitis.
- Cholangitis or hepatic abscess.
- Secondary biliary cirrhosis.
- Carcinoma of gallbladder.
- Gallstone ileus.

Note: in Bouveret syndrome, a large stone erodes into an adjacent loop of small bowel, causing intestinal obstruction. In Mirizzi syndrome, stones in the gallbladder neck or cystic duct compress the common bile duct extrinsically leading to jaundice.

Cholecystitis

234. List 5 complications of cholecystitis.
- Bacterial superinfection with cholangitis or sepsis.
- Gallbladder perforation and local abscess formation.
- Gallbladder perforation with diffuse peritonitis.
- Porcelain gallbladder with increased risk of cancer.
- Aggravation of preexisting medical illness.

235. List key risk factors for gallbladder carcinoma.
- Cholelithiasis.
- "Porcelain" gallbladder and hyalinizing cholecystitis.
- Choledochal cyst.
- Pancreatobiliary maljunction.
- Polyps.
- Primary sclerosing cholangitis.
- Aflatoxin B1.
- Salmonella typhi infection.
- Lynch syndrome (rare).
- Familial adenomatous polyposis (rare).

236. List 3 common causes of acalculous cholecystitis.
- Gallbladder ischemia due to severe volume depletion caused by:
  - Sepsis with hypotension.
  - Multisystem organ failure.
  - Major trauma and burns.
- Infections due to immunosuppression: CMV, HIV.
- Diabetes mellitus.

Gallbladder Polyps and Neoplasms

237. List at least 4 types of nonneoplastic and 2 types of neoplastic gallbladder polyps.
- Nonneoplastic:
  - Cholesterol polyp.
  - Hyperplastic/metaplastic polyp.
  - Fibro(myo)glandular polyp.
  - Adenomyoma.
  - Lymphoid polyp.
  - Inflammatory polyp.
- Neoplastic:
  - Pyloric gland adenoma.
  - Intracholecystic papillary neoplasm.

238. What types of metaplasia can be observed in the gallbladder?
- Pyloric gland metaplasia.
- Intestinal metaplasia.
- Gastric foveolar metaplasia.

239. What is the current WHO classification of preinvasive epithelial neoplasia of the gallbladder and extrahepatic bile ducts?
- Flat intraepithelial neoplasia:
  - Biliary intraepithelial neoplasia (BilIN), low grade.
  - Biliary intraepithelial neoplasia (BilIN), high grade.
- Mass-forming intraepithelial neoplasia:
  - Intracystic papillary neoplasm with low grade intraepithelial neoplasia.
  - Intracystic papillary neoplasm with high grade intraepithelial neoplasia.
  - Intraductal papillary neoplasm with low grade intraepithelial neoplasia.
  - Intraductal papillary neoplasm with high grade intraepithelial neoplasia.

240. Define intracystic papillary neoplasm (ICPN). What are the most common mutations? How is it staged?

- ICPN is a grossly visible, noninvasive mucosal-based neoplasm of the gallbladder.
- Histology: intraluminal growth of back-to-back glands, papillae, or tubulopapillary epithelial structures displaying low grade or high grade intraepithelial neoplasia.
- Morphological phenotypes:
  - Biliary.
  - Gastric.
  - Intestinal.
- Oncocytic.
- Most common mutations in ICPNs:
  - *KRAS.*
  - *GNAS.*
  - *TP53.*
- Staging: ICPNs with high grade dysplasia are staged as pTis.
  - The staging of ICPNs with associated invasive carcinoma follows that of gallbladder carcinoma.

241. Define intraductal papillary neoplasm (IPN) of the bile ducts and its common mutations.

- IPN is an intraductal, grossly visible, noninvasive biliary epithelial neoplasm with papillary or villous growth.
- The most common mutations are:
  - *KRAS.*
  - *TP53.*
  - Loss of *p16.*

242. What are the known risk factors for intraductal papillary neoplasm of the bile ducts?

- Primary sclerosing cholangitis.
- Hepatolithiasis.
- Liver fluke infections (clonorchiasis, opisthorchiasis).

243. What is the differential diagnosis of intraductal papillary neoplasm of the bile ducts?

- Micropapillary biliary intraepithelial neoplasia (BilIN).
- Intraductal tubulopapillary neoplasm.
- Intraductal polypoid metastasis from extrahepatic organs.

244. What are the common mutations of gallbladder carcinoma?

- *TP53.*
- *CDKNA* and *CDKN2B.*
- *ARID1A.*
- *PIK3CA.*
- *CTNNB1.*

245. What are the main histological patterns of adenocarcinoma of the gallbladder?

- Biliary-type adenocarcinoma.
- Intestinal-type adenocarcinoma.
- Mucinous adenocarcinoma.
- Clear cell carcinoma.
- Poorly cohesive carcinoma with or without signet ring cells.
- Adenosquamous carcinoma.
- Squamous cell carcinoma.

246. Define occult carcinoma in a cholecystectomy specimen.

Gallbladder carcinoma that is discovered during a pathologic evaluation of a resected specimen, but not recognized clinically or by imaging techniques.

247. What can a mucocele be mistaken for?

- A mucocele may be mistaken for a mucinous carcinoma.
- Muciphages may resemble signet ring cells, and sometimes they require immunohistochemical staining to differentiate.

248. What can be a pitfall for perineural invasion?

The ductal structures of adenomyomatous hyperplasia may present at the perineural spaces.

249. What are the benign entities in the differential diagnosis of adenocarcinoma of the gallbladder?

- Rokitansky-Aschoff sinuses.
- Adenomyomatous changes.
- Luschka ducts.

250. How do you distinguish in situ carcinoma in Rokitansky-Aschoff sinuses from invasive carcinoma?

- In situ carcinoma often shows:
  - Connection of epithelial invaginations to the luminal surface.
- Normal biliary epithelium admixed with neoplastic epithelium.
- Inspissated bile in long dilated spaces.
- Lack of invasion of smooth muscle bundles.

251. What lymph nodes are most frequently involved by gallbladder carcinoma?

The pericholedochal nodes.

252. What are the regional lymph nodes for gallbladder carcinoma and how is the nodal stage defined?

- The definition of regional lymph nodes has changed from location based-definitions to a number-based N category assessment:
  · N1: 1–3 positive lymph nodes.

- · N2: ≥ 4 positive lymph nodes.
- The recommendation is that at least 6 lymph nodes be harvested and evaluated.

Pancreas
Acute Pancreatitis

253. List 5 causes of acute pancreatitis.

- Metabolic — alcohol, hypercalcemia.
- Mechanical — cholelithiasis, trauma.
- Genetic — mutations in the cationic trypsinogen (*PRSS1*) and trypsin inhibitor (*SPINK1*) genes.

- Vascular — vasculitis, shock.
- Infection — e.g., mumps.

254. List 3 gross features of acute pancreatitis.

- Edema.
- Hemorrhage.

- Necrosis of pancreas parenchyma and peripancreatic fat.

255. List 3 mechanisms that can cause activation of pancreatic proenzymes.

- Obstruction of pancreatic duct by gallstones or alcohol induced thick duct secretions.
- Acinar injury from chemicals (e.g., alcohol, thiazides), infection (e.g., CMV, mumps), or mechanical processes (e.g., trauma, duodenal ulcer penetration).

- Metabolic activation of proenzymes (e.g., hypercalcemia, defective intracellular transport).

256. List the proenzymes and molecules activated by trypsin that contribute to tissue damage in pancreatitis.

- Phospholipase and lipase: cause fat necrosis.
- Elastase: damages vessel walls, causing hemorrhage.
- Proteinase: damages acinar structures.

See also Figure 15.1.

- Kallikrein: activates Hageman factor (factor XII) and the clotting cascade, and also activates the complement cascade, all of which results in small vessel thrombosis.

Pancreatic duct obstruction, or primary acinar injury, or defective intracellular transport

Activation of trypsin and other enzymes

- Phospholipase and lipase: cause fat necrosis
- Elastase: damages vessel walls, causing hemorrhage
- Proteinase: damages acinar structures
- Kallikrein: activates Hageman factor (factor XII) and the clotting cascade, and also activates the complement cascade, all of which results in small vessel thrombosis

FIGURE 15.1 Pathogenesis: autodigestion of the pancreatic substance by inappropriately activated pancreatic enzymes.

257. List 5 key complications of acute pancreatitis.

- Chronic pancreatitis.
- Medical emergency: disseminated intravascular coagulation (DIC), acute respiratory distress syndrome (ARDS), shock, acute tubular necrosis (ATN).

- Diffuse fat necrosis, hypocalcemia.
- Pancreas abscess, or pseudocyst.
- Long-term exocrine or endocrine insufficiency (fatty stool, diabetes).

Chronic Pancreatitis

258. List 3 key histologic findings of autoimmune pancreatitis (AIP).
- Duct centric lymphoplasmacytic infiltration and periductal fibrosis.
- Perivenulitis and obliterative thrombophlebitis.
- Increased numbers of IgG4 producing plasma cells.

Note: AIP can be divided into predominantly ductal and predominantly lobular subtypes.

259. List 3 key sequelae of chronic pancreatitis.
- Pancreatic insufficiency and diabetes mellitus.
- Severe chronic pain.
- Pancreatic pseudocysts.

260. List 3 main gross findings of chronic pancreatitis.
- Irregular scar.
- Dilated pancreatic duct containing secretions and calcifications.
- Pseudocysts and autodigestive fat necrosis in adjacent fat.

261. List 4 key histologic features of chronic pancreatitis.
- Acinar atrophy.
- Fibrosis.
- Irregular, distorted ducts.
- Pseudoincrease of islets of Langerhans.

262. What features differentiate chronic pancreatitis from pancreatic carcinoma?

FEATURE	CHRONIC PANCREATITIS	DUCTAL ADENOCARCINOMA*
Lesion distribution	• Diffuse, segmental, or focal.	• Head most common, often localized.
Gross features	• Irregular scar, dilated ducts with secretions and calcifications. • Pseudocysts. • Autodigestive fat necrosis in adjacent fat.	• Hard, solitary, poorly demarcated mass. • Dilated distal duct possible, but no pseudocysts. • No autodigestive fat necrosis in adjacent fat.
Histologic features	• Architecture: partial preservation of vaguely lobular architecture. • Ducts: ductal dilatation with protein plugs and intraductal calcifications. • Ductal epithelium with possible atrophy, metaplasia, and hyperplasia, but no dysplasia. • Acini: acinar atrophy with more prominent islets. • Stroma: patchy fibrosis and scarred area without glands; chronic inflammatory cells infiltration. • No vascular or perineural invasion.	• Architecture: tumor area without lobular architecture. • Ducts: neoplastic glands, irregular in shape, lined by atypical cells. • Nuclear variability and nuclear enlargement (> 4:1 rule). • Haphazard arrangement of the glands. • Glands with incomplete lumina. • Luminal necrosis. • Glands next to a muscular artery. • Naked glands in fat. • Acini: no acinar atrophy, no prominent islets. • Stroma: desmoplastic stroma surrounding tumor glands; fewer inflammatory cells. • Vascular or perineural invasion.

*Note: ductal adenocarcinoma can have features of obstructive pancreatitis distal to the tumor.

Pancreatic Adenocarcinoma and Related Entities

263. Define the anatomic subdivisions of head, body, and tail in the pancreas.
- Head: from the ampulla to the left border of the superior mesenteric vein.
- Body: from the left border of the superior mesenteric vein to the left border of the aorta.
- Tail: from the left border of the aorta to the splenic hilum.

264. Name the most common mutated oncogene and the most frequently inactivated tumor suppressor gene in pancreatic carcinoma.
- Most common mutated oncogene: *KRAS* gene (chromosome 12p).
- Most frequently inactivated tumor suppressor gene: *p16/CDKN2A* (chromosome 9p).

265. What other genes are implicated in pathogenesis of pancreatic ductal adenocarcinoma?
- *GNAS*.
- *RNF43*.
- *TP53*.
- *CDKN2A*.
- *SMAD4* (*DPC4*).

266. Which gene can be used in diagnostic molecular pathology for pancreatic adenocarcinoma?

SMAD4 (*DPC4*) mutations resulting in loss of SMAD4 (DPC4) protein.

267. What are the risk factors for pancreatic adenocarcinoma?
- Cigarette smoking.
- Obesity.
- Diet high in fat and low in vegetables and fruits.
- Low physical activity.
- Chemical exposure: benzene, dyes, petrochemicals.
- Hereditary pancreatitis.
- Chronic pancreatitis.
- Family history.
- Diabetes.

268. What are familial syndromes predisposing to pancreatic cancer and the implicated genes?

SYNDROME	GENES	PATHOLOGY
Lynch syndrome	• *MLH1*. • *MSH2*. • *MSH6*. • *PMS2*. • *EPCAM*.	• Medullary carcinoma. • Acinar cell carcinoma.
Hereditary breast and ovarian cancer syndrome	• *BRCA1*. • *BRCA2*. • *PALB2*.	• Ductal adenocarcinoma.
Familial atypical multiple mole melanoma syndrome	• *CDKN2a*.	• Ductal adenocarcinoma.
Hereditary pancreatitis	• *PRSS1*. • *SPINK1*. • *CPA1 or CPB1*.	• Ductal adenocarcinoma.
Peutz-Jeghers syndrome	• *STK11* (*LKB1*).	• Intraductal papillary mucinous neoplasm (IPMN).
Familial adenomatous polyposis	• *APC*.	• Ductal adenocarcinoma. • IPMN. • Pancreatoblastoma.

269. Classify the main histological types of tumors of the pancreas following the WHO classification.
- Benign epithelial tumors and precursors:
  · Serous cystadenoma, NOS.
  · Macrocystic (oligocystic) serous cystadenoma.
  · Solid serous adenoma.
  · Von Hippel-Lindau syndrome-associated serous cystic neoplasm.
  · Mixed serous-neuroendocrine neoplasm.
  · Glandular intraepithelial neoplasia, low grade.
  · Glandular intraepithelial neoplasia, high grade.
  · Intraductal papillary mucinous neoplasm with low grade dysplasia.
  · Intraductal papillary mucinous neoplasm with high grade dysplasia.
  · Intraductal oncocytic papillary neoplasm, NOS.
  · Intraductal tubulopapillary neoplasm.
  · Mucinous cystic neoplasm with low grade dysplasia.
  · Mucinous cystic neoplasm with high grade dysplasia.
- Malignant epithelial tumors:
  · Serous cystadenocarcinoma, NOS.
  · Intraductal papillary mucinous neoplasm with associated invasive carcinoma.
  · Intraductal oncocytic papillary neoplasm with associated invasive carcinoma.
  · Intraductal papillary neoplasm with associated invasive carcinoma.
  · Mucinous cystic neoplasm with associated invasive carcinoma.
  · Duct adenocarcinoma, NOS.
  · Colloid carcinoma.
  · Poorly cohesive carcinoma.
  · Signet-ring cell carcinoma.
  · Medullary carcinoma, NOS.
  · Adenosquamous carcinoma.
  · Hepatoid carcinoma.
  · Large cell carcinoma with rhabdoid phenotype.
  · Carcinoma, undifferentiated, NOS.
  · Undifferentiated carcinoma with osteoclast-like giant cells.

(continued on next page)

- Acinar cell carcinoma/cystadenocarcinoma.
- Mixed acinar-neuroendocrine carcinoma.
- Mixed acinar-endocrine-ductal carcinoma.
- Mixed acinar-ductal carcinoma.
- Pancreatoblastoma.
- Solid pseudopapillary neoplasm of the pancreas.
- Solid pseudopapillary neoplasm with high grade carcinoma.
  - Pancreatic neuroendocrine neoplasms:
    - Pancreatic neuroendocrine microadenoma.
    - Neuroendocrine tumor, NOS.

- Neuroendocrine tumor, grades 1–3.
- Nonfunctioning pancreatic neuroendocrine tumors (oncocytic, pleomorphic, clear cell, cystic).
- Functioning pancreatic neuroendocrine tumors (insulinoma, gastrinoma, VIPoma, glucagonoma, somatostatinoma).
- Neuroendocrine carcinoma, NOS.
  › Large cell neuroendocrine carcinoma.
  › Small cell neuroendocrine carcinoma.
- Mixed neuroendocrine-nonneuroendocrine neoplasm (MiNEN).

270. What are deceptive morphological patterns of pancreatic ductal adenocarcinoma one needs to be aware of at time of frozen sections or fine needle aspiration biopsies?
- Large duct pattern.
- Foamy gland pattern.
- Clear cell subtype.
- Cystic papillary pattern.

271. How does the AJCC grade pancreatic adenocarcinoma?
GX: grade cannot be assessed.
G1: well-differentiated.
G2: moderately differentiated.
G3: poorly differentiated.

Note: the tumor grade is assigned based on the highest grade seen, even if it is only a minor component (< 50% of the tumor).

272. What grade does CAP assign signet-ring cell carcinoma?
It is automatically assigned grade 3.

273. What is the criterion for diagnosing pancreatic colloid carcinoma? What is the immunoprofile and prognosis of this tumor?
- Diagnosis: ≥ 80% of the neoplastic epithelium is suspended in extracellular mucin pools.
- Immunohistochemistry: CDX2+/MUC2+ (intestinal differentiation).
- Prognosis: better prognosis than conventional ductal adenocarcinomas, with a 5-year survival rate > 55%.

274. What is the criterion diagnosing pancreatic micropapillary carcinoma? What is the prognosis?
- Diagnosis: ≥ 50% of the neoplasm is composed of small solid groups of cells suspended within stromal lacunae.
- Prognosis: poor.

275. What are the criteria for diagnosing pancreatic adenosquamous carcinoma?
Carcinoma demonstrating evidence of both adeno- and squamous differentiation with the squamous component of ≥ 30% of the neoplasm.

276. Which histological types of pancreatic adenocarcinoma are not graded in CAP protocols?
- Serous cystadenocarcinoma.
- Acinar cell carcinoma/acinar cell cystadenocarcinoma.
- Pancreatoblastoma.
- Solid pseudopapillary neoplasm.

277. Define the AJCC T staging of pancreatic carcinoma.
Tx: primary tumor cannot be assessed.
T0: no evidence of primary tumor.
Tis: carcinoma in situ, including:
   Pancreatic intraepithelial neoplasia, high grade.
   Intraductal papillary mucinous neoplasm with high grade dysplasia.
   Intraductal tubulopapillary neoplasm with high grade dysplasia.
   Intraductal oncocytic papillary neoplasm with high grade dysplasia.

   Mucinous cystic neoplasm with high grade dysplasia.
T1: tumor ≤ 2 cm in greatest dimension.
   T1a: tumor ≤ 0.5 cm in greatest dimension.
   T1b: tumor > 0.5 cm but < 1 cm in greatest dimension.
   T1c: tumor 1–2 cm in greatest dimension.
T2: tumor > 2 cm and ≤ 4 cm in greatest dimension.
T3: tumor > 4 cm in greatest dimension.
T4: tumor involving the celiac axis, superior mesenteric artery, and/or common hepatic artery, regardless of size.

278. How do you handle Whipple resection specimens?
- Identify and orient anatomical structures: stomach, duodenum, common bile duct (CBD), and pancreas. Ink the specimen. Leave the pancreas distal margin uninked for later orientation.
- Open the stomach along the greater curvature, across the anterior wall of the pylorus, and down the outer curvature of the duodenum. Record the dimensions of the stomach, duodenum, pancreatic head, CBD, and margins.
- Sample the margins: distal pancreas margin, uncinate margin, and the CBD, duodenum, and gastric margins.
- Using a probe, make a cut through the CBD, pancreatic duct, and ampulla of Vater.
- Identify and describe the lesion (size, color, consistency, cysts), its relation to different structures (duodenum, CBD, portal vein and/or mesenteric vessels), distance from margins (CBD, pancreas, duodenum, stomach, and retroperitoneal resection margin), and obstruction of ducts.
- Describe the nonneoplastic tissue (e.g., color, fibrosis, nodularity, fat necrosis, cysts, dilated ducts, calculi, anatomic variations).
- Fix the specimen overnight in 10% formalin.
- Prepare block samples:
  - Up to 6 blocks of tumor including relationship to pancreas, ducts, ampulla, duodenal mucosa, vascular groove, and surrounding soft tissue.
  - Margins if not sampled before.
  - Nonneoplastic pancreas: 1–2 including areas with normal and abnormal appearance.
  - Ampulla: 1 block.
  - Lymph nodes: submit as separate groups based on anatomical location.

279. What are the margins in a Whipple specimen?
- Proximal margin (stomach or duodenum).
- Distal margin (duodenum or jejunum).
- Common bile duct margin.
- Uncinate process margin (retroperitoneal).
- Pancreatic parenchymal resection margin.

280. Where in the pancreatic bed does local recurrence of pancreatic adenocarcinoma tend to occur?
In the area corresponding to the retroperitoneal (uncinate) margin and the deep retroperitoneal posterior surface of the pancreas, including the vascular groove of the portal and the superior mesenteric vein.

Note: the CAPP and AJCC recommend inking the posterior surface of the pancreas (including the vascular groove) and submitting sections of tumor at its closest location to this surface in addition to submitting the uncinate margin.

281. What are the critical margins for an intraductal tumor?
The critical margins are the common bile duct margin and the parenchymal resection margin.

282. Do pools of acellular mucin after chemoradiation represent residual tumor?
No.

283. Describe the histologic difference between pancreatic intraepithelial neoplasia (PanIN), low grade, and PanIN, high grade.
- Glandular intraepithelial neoplasia, low grade (formerly PanIN 1 and 2):
  - Architecture: flat or papillary mucinous epithelium.
  - Cytologic atypia: mild to moderate.
  - Mitoses: rare, nonatypical, and nonapical.
  - Absence of true cribriforming, luminal necrosis, or marked cytologic atypia.
- Glandular intraepithelial neoplasia, high grade (carcinoma in situ) (formerly PanIN 3):
  - Architecture: micropapillary or papillary, intraluminal noncohesive cell clusters; true cribriforming with intraluminal necrosis.
  - Cytologic atypia: severe with large nuclei and prominent nucleoli, significant nuclear pseudostratification, and loss of polarity.
  - Frequent mitoses, including atypical forms.

284. How does CAP subdivide regional lymph nodes (LN) surrounding the pancreas?
- The regional lymph nodes for pancreatic head and neck cancers include lymph nodes along common bile duct, common hepatic artery, portal vein, pyloric, anterior and posterior pancreaticoduodenal arcades, superior mesenteric vein, and right lateral wall of superior mesenteric artery.
- The regional lymph nodes for the pancreatic body and tail cancers include lymph nodes along common hepatic artery, celiac axis, splenic artery, and splenic hilum.
- Tumor involvement of other nodal groups is considered distant metastasis.
- Anatomic division of lymph nodes is not necessary, but separately submitted lymph nodes should be individually reported.

285. Define the AJCC N stages in pancreatic adenocarcinoma.

Nx: regional lymph nodes cannot be assessed.

N0: no regional lymph node metastases.

N1: metastasis in 1–3 regional lymph nodes.

N2: metastasis in ≥ 4 regional lymph nodes.

Note: a minimum of 12 lymph nodes has been suggested to achieve optimal staging.

286. How does CAP stage peritoneal seeding or ascitic peritoneal fluid containing cytologic evidence of malignancy?

As M1.

287. What are the precursor lesions of pancreatic ductal adenocarcinoma?
- Pancreatic intraepithelial neoplasia (PanIN).
- Intraductal papillary mucinous neoplasms (IPMN).
- Intraductal oncocytic papillary neoplasms (IOPN).
- Intraductal tubulopapillary neoplasms (ITPN).
- Mucinous cystic neoplasms (MCN).
- Acinar to ductal metaplasia.

Cystic Neoplasms of the Pancreas

288. List the pancreatic tumors that occur more commonly in female patients.
- MCN.
- Solid pseudopapillary neoplasm.
- Serous cystadenoma.

289. List key cystic neoplasms of the pancreas and their demographic characteristics.
- Serous cystadenoma: F:M 3:1, 60–70 years old.
- MCN: > 98% female, 40–50 years old.
- IPNM: M > F, 50–75 years old
- IOPN: F > M.
- ITPN: F > M.
- Solid pseudopapillary neoplasm: young females.

290. List the clinicopathological and molecular features that differentiate IPMN, MCN, and serous cystadenoma.

FEATURE	IPMN	MCN	SEROUS CYSTADENOMA
Age	• 50–75 years.	• 40–50 years.	• Middle-aged to elderly.
Gender	• M > F.	• > 98% F.	• F > M.
Clinical	• Bouts of pancreatitis.	• Nonspecific.	• Nonspecific.
Radiology	• Bulging papillae into duodenum lumen.	• Solitary multilocular cystic mass.	• CT honeycomb cyst.
Genes involved	• *GNAS*. • *KRAS*. • *TP53*. • *RNF43*.	• *KRAS*. • *TP53*. • *SMAD4*.	• *VHL* gene mutation.
Tumor location	• Head.	• Body or tail.	• Evenly distributed.
Involvement of large duct	• Duct epithelium involved.	• No connection with ducts.	• No connection with ducts.
Cyst configuration	• Multiple.	• Single, can be multilocular.	• Honeycomb cut surface.
Papilla formation	• Usually extensive.	• Usually minimal.	• No.
Lining epithelium	• Columnar mucin producing, or cuboidal eosinophilic with low or high grade dysplasia.	• Columnar mucin producing with low or high grade dysplasia.	• Cuboidal/flattened, clear cytoplasm rich in glycogen.
Ovarian stroma	• No.	• Present.	• No.
Adjacent pancreas	• Normal.	• Atrophy or scarring.	• Normal.
Immunohistochemistry	• Epithelium is positive for CK7, CK19, CA19-9, and CEA.	• Epithelium is positive for: CK7, CK8, CK18, CK19, EMA, CEA, and MUC5AC. • The ovarian-type stroma expresses SMA, MSA, desmin, ER, and PR. Luteinized cells stain for tyrosine hydroxylase, calretinin, and α-inhibin.	• Epithelium is positive for: PAS, inhibin, GLUT1, and MUC6. • Epithelium is negative for PAS-D.

291. How do you differentiate PanIN from IPMN?

FEATURE	PANIN	IPMN
Size	• < 0.5 mm.	• > 0.5–1 cm.
Mucin hypersecretion	• No.	• Yes.
Cystic dilation of duct	• Rare.	• Yes.
Tall papillae with stromal core	• No.	• Common.
MUC1 expression	• Yes for high grade PanIN.	• Yes for pancreatobiliary and oncocytic types.
MUC2 expression	• No.	• Yes for the intestinal type.
MUC5AC expression	• Yes.	• Yes.
Common mutations	• *KRAS*. • *CDKN2a* (*p16*).	• *KRAS*. • *GNAS*. • *RNF43*. • *TP53*.
DPC4 expression	• Retained (even in high grade).	• Usually retained.
Association with invasive colloid carcinoma	• No.	• Yes.

Note: the term *incipient IPMN* or *incipient intraductal oncocytic papillary neoplasm* can be applied to lesions 0.5–1.0 cm with papillary architecture, intestinal, or oncocytic differentiation, or a *GNAS* mutation.

292. What are histologic subtypes of intraductal pancreatic mucinous neoplasm (IPMNs)?
- Gastric type.
- Intestinal type.
- Pancreatobiliary type.

293. How are IPMNs classified based on degree of cytoarchitectural atypia?
- Low grade IPMNs.
- High grade IPMNs.

294. How are IPMNs classified based on anatomical distribution?
- Main-duct type: involves main pancreatic duct with segmental or diffuse dilatation. Most common location: head of the pancreas.
- Branch-duct type: involves smaller, secondary ducts without affecting the main pancreatic duct. Most common location: uncinate process.
- Mixed duct-type: combination of the other 2 types.

295. What types of invasive adenocarcinoma usually arise in association with IPMNs?
- Colloid carcinoma.
- Tubular (ductal) adenocarcinoma.

296. What is the main differential diagnosis of IPMN?
- PanIN.
- Simple mucinous cysts.
- MCN.
- Pancreatic IOPN.
- Pancreatic ITPN.

297. What is the molecular profile of pancreatic intraductal oncocytic papillary neoplasm (IOPN)?
- Mutations in *ARHGAP26*, *ASXL1*, *EPHA8*, and *ERBB4* genes.
- Lack of genetic alterations related to ductal adenocarcinoma and IPMNs (such as mutations in *KRAS*, *GNAS*, and *RNF43*).

298. What is the molecular profile of pancreatic ITPN?
- Panceatic ITPN has mutations in chromatin remodeling genes: *KMT2A, KMT2B, KMT2C,* and *BAP1*.
- It also has mutations in PI3K pathway genes (*PIK3CA, PTEN*).
- A subset of cases harbor *FGFR2* fusions.
- It lacks genetic alterations reported to be related to ductal adenocarcinoma and IPMNs (such as mutations in *KRAS*).

299. What is the differential diagnosis of ITPN? What is its immunoprofile?
- Differential diagnosis: pancreatobiliary-type IPMN.
- Immunoprofile of ITPN:
  · Positive: pancytokeratin, CK7/19, EMA (MUC1), MUC6.
- Negative: acinar markers (trypsin, etc.), neuroendocrine markers, MUC2, MUC5AC.

300. How do you differentiate ITPN from pancreatobiliary type IPMN?

ITPN: predominantly tubular architecture, diffuse high grade dysplasia, minimal intracellular mucin, and lack of MUC5AC expression.

301. List 2 key pancreatic cystic tumors that stain positively for the progesterone receptor.

- Solid pseudopapillary neoplasm: the neoplastic epithelial cells (but the cells are estrogen receptor-negative).
- Ovarian-type stroma of mucinous cystic neoplasm (the stromal cells can be estrogen receptor positive).

302. What are the main genes implicated in pathogenesis of serous cystadenoma?

- Somatic mutations in *VHL* (located on chromosome 3p25.3).
- Loss of heterozygosity of 3p.
- Allelic loss of chromosome 10q.

303. What are the 4 main macroscopic patterns of growth of serous cystadenomas?

- Microcystic serous cystadenomas.
- Macrocystic (oligocystic) subtypes.
- Solid serous cystadenomas.
- Diffuse serous cystadenomas (this particular subtype is closely associated with VHL syndrome).

304. What are positive special and immunohistochemical stains in serous cystadenoma?

- Special stains: PAS (+)/PAS-D (−) (highlights abundant glycogen).
- Immunohistohemical stains (epithelium): inhibin, GLUT1, and MUC6.

305. What is the single criterion of malignancy in pancreatic serous neoplasm (serous cystadenocarcinoma)?

Unequivocal distant metastasis beyond the pancreatic/peripancreatic bed.

Pancreatic Solid Pseudopapillary Neoplasm and Acinar Cell Carcinoma

306. What are the demographic characteristics and most common location of solid pseudopapillary neoplasm (SPN)?

- Affected population: adolescent girls and young women.
- Location (most common): tail of the pancreas; rarely in retropancreatic tissue, ovary, and testis.

307. What is the most common mutation in solid pseudopapillary neoplasm?

CTNNB1 exon 3 missense mutations/deletions (β-catenin) in 90–100% of cases.

308. What is the main differential diagnosis SPN?

- Pancreatic neuroendocrine tumors (grades 1–3) and neuroendocrine carcinoma.
- Acinar cell carcinoma.
- Pancreatoblastoma.
- Ductal adenocarcinoma.

309. Compare the clinical, morphological, and immunohistochemical characteristics of solid pseudopapillary neoplasm and other tumors that enter the differential diagnosis.

	NEUROENDOCRINE TUMORS (GRADES 1–3)	SOLID PSEUDOPAPILLARY NEOPLASM	ACINAR CELL CARCINOMA	PANCREATOBLASTOMA
Epidemiology	• No gender predilection. • 30–60 years old.	• Adolescent girls and young women (< 40 years old).	• Older patients (40–70 years old).	• Children and young adults (< 30 years old).
H&E	• Trabecular, nested, pseudoacinar architecture; "salt and pepper" stippled chromatin. • Usually well circumscribed, rarely cystic.	• Solid, pseudopapillary architecture. • Usually well circumscribed.	• Solid, trabecular, glandular, and acinar architecture. • Infiltrative growth pattern. • Granular cytoplasm; basal nuclear polarization.	• Solid and acinar patterns. • Lobulated growth. • Squamoid nests. • Cellular stroma.
CK7, CK19	• Variable.	• Negative.	• Variable.	• Positive.
CK8, CK18	• Positive.	• Occasionally positive.	• Positive.	• Positive.

(continued on next page)

(continued from previous page)

	NEUROENDOCRINE TUMORS (GRADES 1–3)	SOLID PSEUDOPAPILLARY NEOPLASM	ACINAR CELL CARCINOMA	PANCREATOBLASTOMA
EMA (MUC1)	• Negative	• Negative.	• Negative.	• Negative.
Chromogranin	• Positive.	• Negative.	• Focally positive.	• Focally positive.
Synaptophysin	• Strongly positive.	• Positive (focal, patchy).	• Focally positive.	• Focally positive.
Vimentin	• Negative.	• Strongly positive.	• Negative.	• Positive.
Progesteron receptor (PR)	• Negative.	• Strongly positive.	• Negative.	• Focally positive.
CD10	• Negative.	• Positive (perinuclear staining).	• Focally positive.	• Focally positive.
Nuclear β-catenin	• Negative.	• Positive (nuclear).	• Positive in 10%.	• Occasionally positive.
PAS-D	• Negative.	• Negative or scattered globules.	• Positive globules.	• Negative.
Trypsin, chymotrypsin, lipase	• Negative.	• Negative.	• Positive.	• Positive.
BCL-10	• Negative.	• Negative.	• Positive.	• Positive.

310. What is the prognosis of pancreatic acinar cell carcinoma?

Poor prognosis, with a median survival of about 19 months and a 5-year-survival rate of 25%.

311. What is characteristic of electron micrographs of acinar cell tumors?

Intracytoplasmic zymogen granules.

Pancreatoblastoma

312. What is the most common malignant pancreatic epithelial neoplasm of childhood? What are the associated genetic syndromes?

- Pancreatoblastoma is the most common pancreatic neoplasm of childhood.
- Associated genetic syndromes include:
- · Beckwith-Wiedemann syndrome.
- · Familial adenomatous polyposis.

313. What are the molecular abnormalities in pancreatoblastoma?

- Loss of heterozygosity of the short arm of chromosome 11p (in both sporadic cases and cases associated with Beckwith-Wiedemann syndrome).
- Alterations in APC/β-catenin pathways: *CTNNB1* mutations.

314. What are the histological features of pancreatoblastoma?

- Epithelial components:
  - · Acinar differentiation.
  - · Squamous nests — these are a defining component of pancreatoblastoma critical for establishing the diagnosis.
- · Neuroendocrine component.
- Stroma component: hypercellularity; rarely, heterologous differentiation (e.g., bone and cartilage).

Pancreatic Neuroendocrine Tumor

315. Classify pancreatic neuroendocrine neoplasms.

- Pancreatic neuroendocrine microadenoma: size < 5 mm and nonfunctional.
- Neuroendocrine tumors (PanNET), G1–G3 grades:
  - · Low grade (G1) (< 2 mitoses/2 mm^2 and/or Ki 67 proliferation index < 3%).
  - · Intermediate grade (G2) (2–20 mitoses/2 mm^2 and/or a Ki 67 proliferation index 3–20%).
- · High grade (G3) (> 20 mitoses/2 mm^2 and/or a Ki 67 proliferation index > 20%).
- Pancreatic neuroendocrine carcinoma (PanNEC):
  - · Small cell NEC.
  - · Large cell NEC.

316. List associated syndromes.
- Multiple endocrine neoplasia type 1 (*MEN1*).
- Von Hippel-Lindau disease.
- Neurofibromatosis type 1.
- Tuberous sclerosis.

317. What is the main differential diagnosis of PanNEC?
- Acinar cell carcinoma.
- Lymphoma.
- Melanoma.
- Metastatic carcinoma to pancreas.
- PanNETs, grade 3.

318. What are the molecular events in PanNETs and in PanNECs?
- Mutations in **PanNETs**:
  · *MEN1* gene (menin) — in 40% of PanNETs.
  · *DAXX* or *ATRX* (genes responsible for telomerase maintenance) — in 40%.
  · mTOR pathway genes (*TSC2* and *PTEN*) — in 15%.
  · *HIF1* genes.
  · *VHL* genes.
- Mutations in **PanNECs**:
  · *TP53*.
  · *RB1*.
  · *CDKN2a*.

319. What are the common growth patterns of PanNETs?
- Solid nesting pattern.
- Trabecular pattern.
- Gyriform pattern.
- Glandular pattern.
- Solid paraganglioma-like growth patterns.

320. What are the cytological subtypes of nonfunctioning PanNETs?
- Oncocytic subtype.
- Pleomorphic subtype.
- Clear cell subtype (reported often in association with VHL syndrome).

321. What is the main differential diagnosis of pancreatic neuroendocrine neoplasms?
- Pancreatic neuroendocrine carcinoma.
- Acinar cell carcinoma.
- Solid pseudopapillary neoplasm.
- Pancreatoblastoma.
- Ductal adenocarcinoma.
- Metastasis (from renal cell carcinoma, hepatocellular carcinoma, adrenal cortical carcinoma in particular).

322. What is the most common functioning PanNET?
Insulinoma.

323. What tumor of the pancreas is associated with Zollinger-Ellison syndrome (ZES)?
Gastrinoma.

324. What are the characteristic ultrastructural findings on electron microscopy of PanNETs?
Membrane-bound, electron-dense cytoplasmic neurosecretory granules.

325. How do you count Ki 67 and mitosis in pancreatic NETs?
- Ki 67: count at least 500 cells in the area of highest Ki 67 staining ("hot spot"); a notation is made if fewer cells are available.
- Mitosis: Count the number of mitoses per 2 mm^2, at least 10 mm^2 evaluated in the most mitotically active part of the tumor.

Note: if Ki 67 and mitosis are discordant, report the higher count as per the WHO guidelines.

326. What factors predict the prognosis of PanNETs?
- Proliferative rate (based on mitotic rate and Ki 67 proliferation) — this is the most important histological factor predictive of outcome.
- Tumor size (correlates with the tumor stage) — larger tumor size correlates with clinical aggressiveness and higher risk of metastasis.
- Extent of invasive growth (especially vascular invasion).
- Presence of necrosis.
- Status of regional lymph nodes.

327. What is the definition of pancreatic MiNEN according to the WHO classification of digestive tumours?

Neoplasms composed of morphologically recognizable neuroendocrine and nonneuroendocrine components, each constituting ≥ 30% of the tumor volume.

328. Define the TNM staging of pancreatic neuroendocrine tumors.

Primary tumor:

Tx: tumor cannot be assessed.

T1: tumor limited to pancreas, < 2 cm.

T2: tumor limited to pancreas, 2–4 cm.

T3: tumor limited to pancreas, > 4 cm; or tumor invades duodenum or bile duct.

T4: tumor invading adjacent organs (stomach, spleen, colon, adrenal gland) or the wall of large vessels (celiac axis or the superior mesenteric artery).

Regional lymph node:

Nx: regional lymph nodes cannot be assessed.

N0: no regional lymph node metastasis.

N1: regional lymph node metastasis.

Distant metastasis:

M0: no distant metastasis.

M1: distant metastasis.

M1a: metastasis confined to liver.

M1b: metastases in ≥ 1 extrahepatic site.

M1c: both hepatic and extrahepatic metastases.

329. Compare the immunohistochemical profile of intestinal type and pancreatobiliary type tumors.

IHC	INTESTINAL TYPE	PANCREATOBILIARY TYPE
MUC1	–	+
MUC2	+	–
MUC5AC	–	+
CK7	–	+
CK20	+	–
CDX2	+	–

330. How do you differentiate well-differentiated grade 3 pancreatic neuroendocrine tumor (WDNET G3) from poorly differentiated pancreatic large cell neuroendocrine carcinoma (PDNEC)?

	WDNET G3	PDNEC
Histomorphology	• Nested, organoid, or trabecular architecture, regular intratumoral vascular pattern, abundant granular cytoplasm, and stippled nuclei with inconspicuous nucleoli.	• Tumor necrosis, expansile and irregular nests with peripheral palisading, and rosettes/tubular structures within the large nests.
Co-existent with, or history of	• WDNET G1/G2.	• Adenocarcinoma, squamous cell carcinoma.
Mitosis	• < 20/10 high power fields.	• > 20/10 high power fields.
Ki67	• 20–55%.	• > 55%.
P53, RB or Smad4 mutation/loss	• No.	• Yes.
DAXX or ATRX loss	• Yes.	• No.

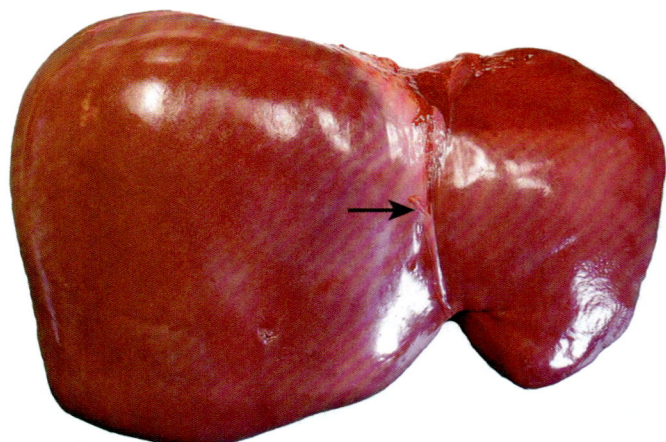

IMAGE 15.1 Normal liver, anterior view, right and left lobes; falciform ligament (arrow).

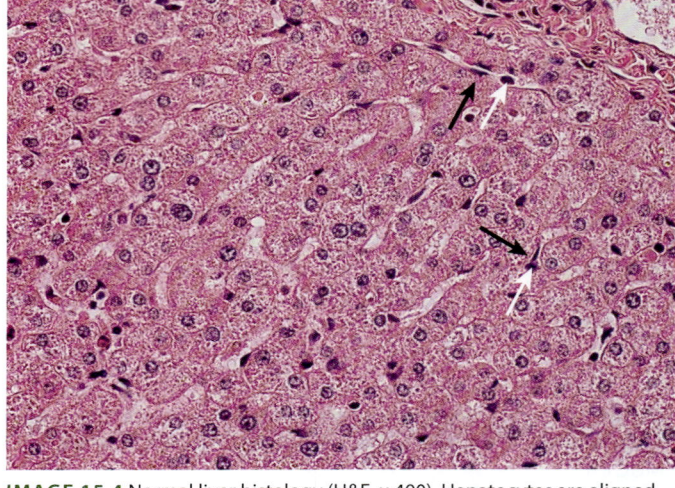

IMAGE 15.4 Normal liver histology (H&E, x 400). Hepatocytes are aligned into 1- to 2-cell thick plates and separated by sinusoidal spaces lined by sinusoidal endothelial cells (black arrow) containing Kupffer cells (white arrow).

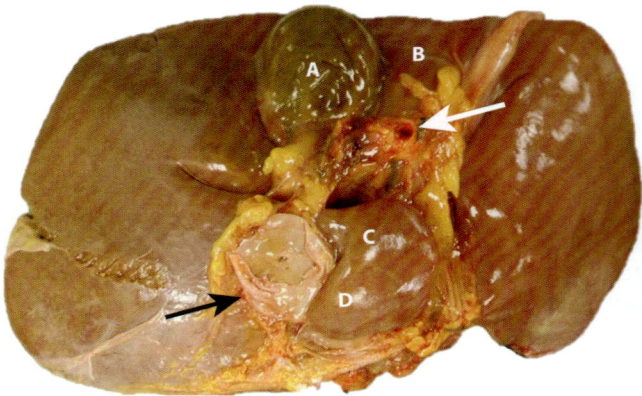

IMAGE 15.2 Normal liver, posterior view. Image A: gallbladder. Image B: quadrate lobe. Image C: caudate lobe. Image D: segment I. The white arrow indicates the porta hepatis, which contains the hepatic artery, portal vein, and common bile duct. The black arrow indicates the inferior vena.

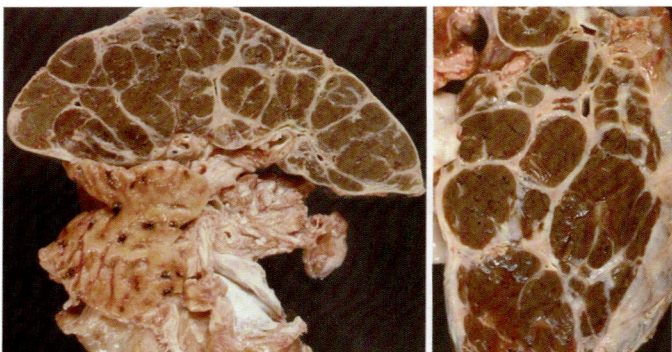

IMAGE 15.5 Cystic fibrosis with biliary cirrhosis. Variable sized regenerative nodules separated by fibrotic band forming a jigsaw pattern are present.

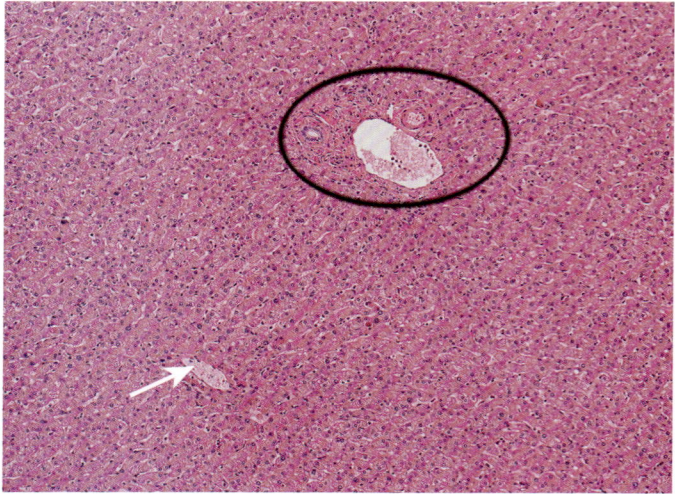

IMAGE 15.3 Normal liver histology: portal tract (circle) and central hepatic vein (arrow).

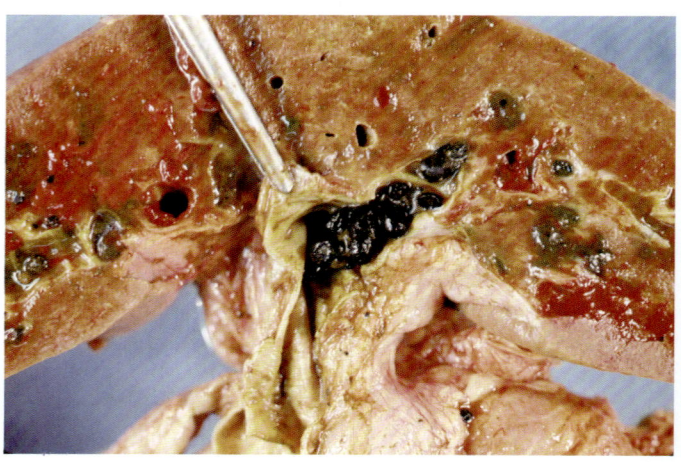

IMAGE 15.6 Hepatolithiasis. Pigmented calcium bilirubinate stones packed large hepatic bile duct are present. The liver parenchyma appears greenish due to cholestasis.

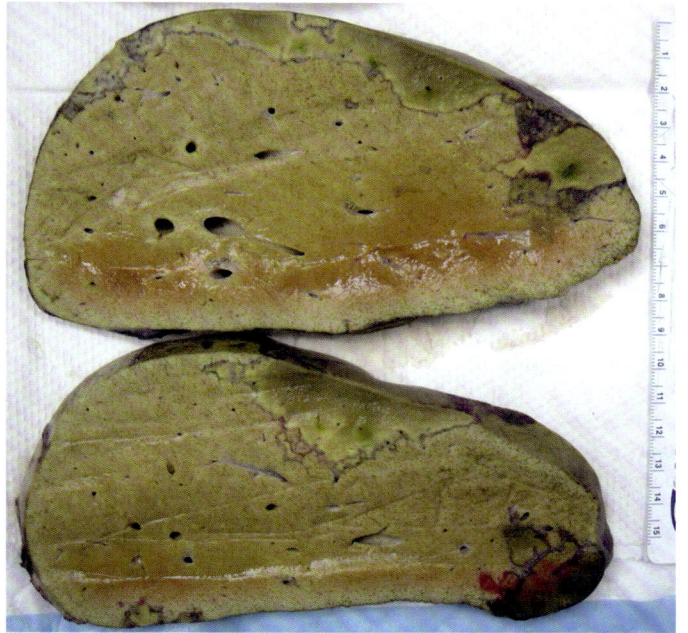

IMAGE 15.7 Liver infarct due to hepatic artery thrombosis. Note the wedge-shaped infarcts in the subcapsular area.

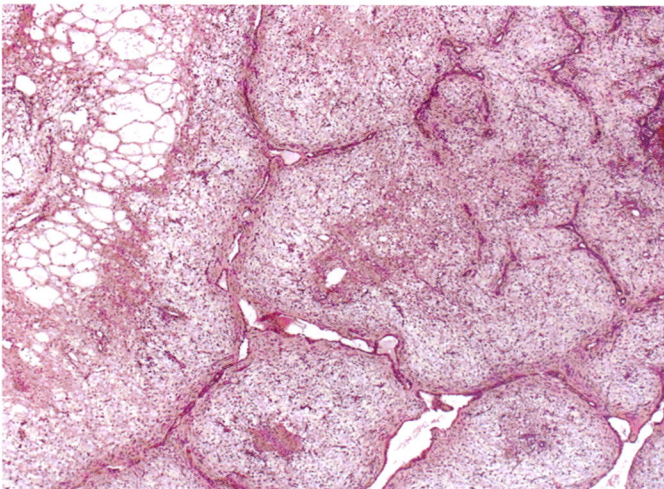

IMAGE 15.9 Liver mesenchymal hamartoma. Histologically this benign lesion is composed of haphazardly arranged bile ductules, myxoid stroma, liver cells islands and adipose tissue (H&E, x20).

Courtesy of Dr. Hanlin Wang.

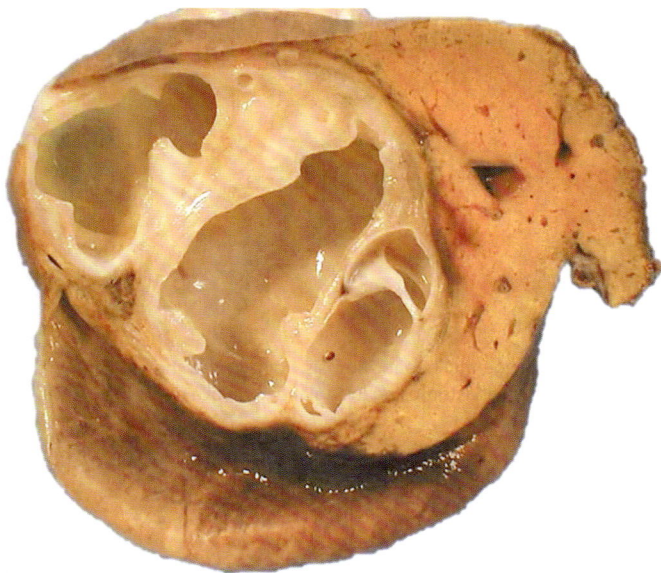

IMAGE 15.8 Liver mesenchymal hamartoma. The gross specimen shows a partially resected liver containing a well-circumscribed, cystic mass with myxoid stroma.

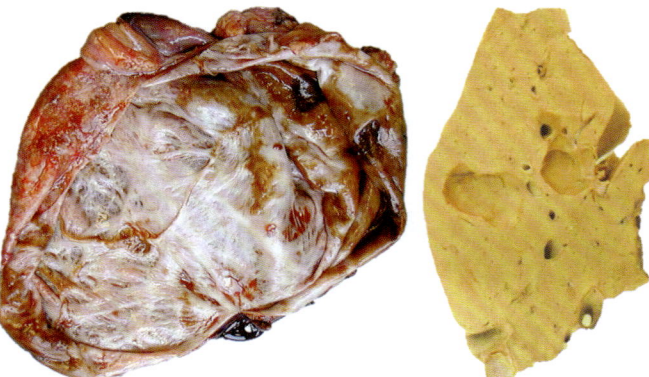

IMAGE 15.10 Simple cyst of the liver. Left: a single liver simple cyst measuring 11 cm in largest dimension. Right: multiple congenital simple cysts in the liver.

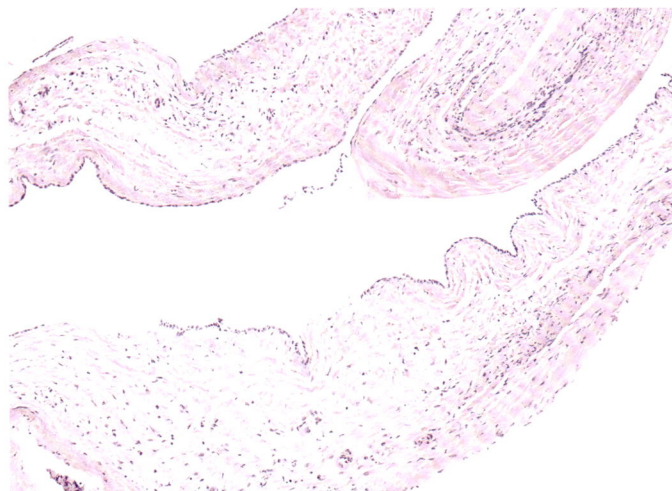

IMAGE 15.11 Simple benign liver cyst lined by a single layer of cuboidal epithelium (H&E, x40).

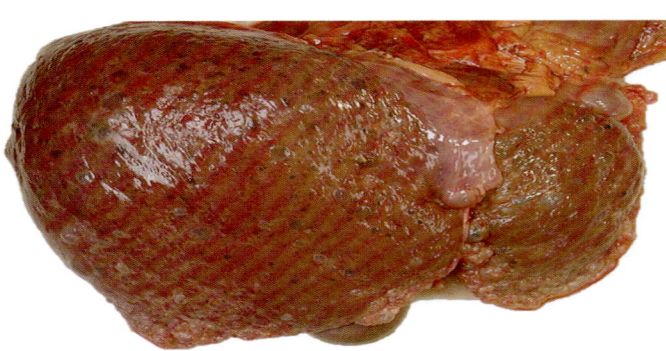

IMAGE 15.12 Adult polycystic liver disease. Numerous subcapsular cysts are seen.

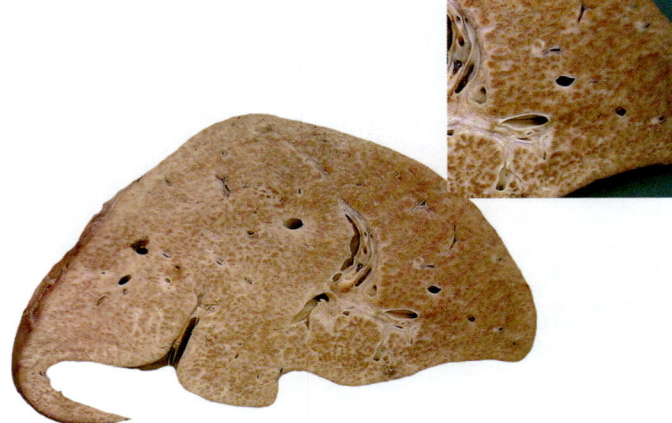

IMAGE 15.15 Congenital hepatic fibrosis. The images show prominent portal-to-portal bridging fibrosis.

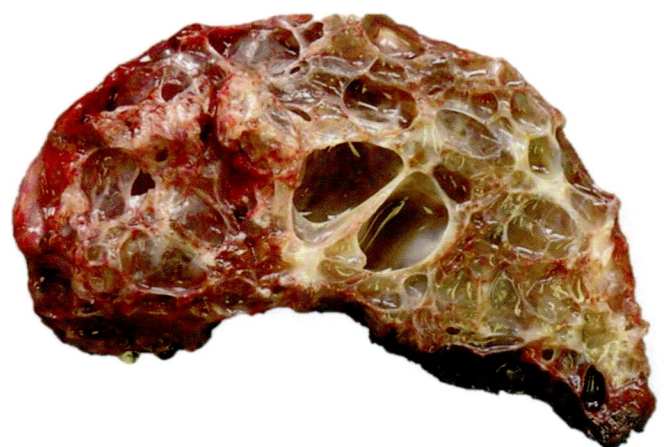

IMAGE 15.13 Adult polycystic liver disease. This cross-section of the liver shows variable sized cysts filled with clear or straw-colored fluid.

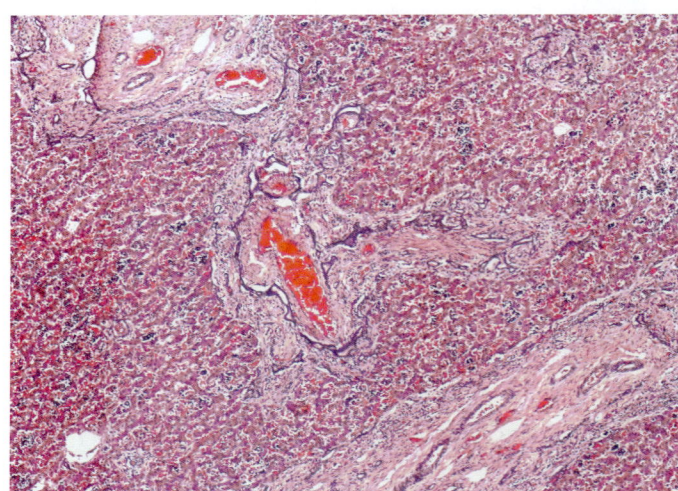

IMAGE 15.16 Congenital hepatic fibrosis. Portal tracts show extensive fibrosis and contain anastomosing irregular ectatic bile ducts (H&E, x40).

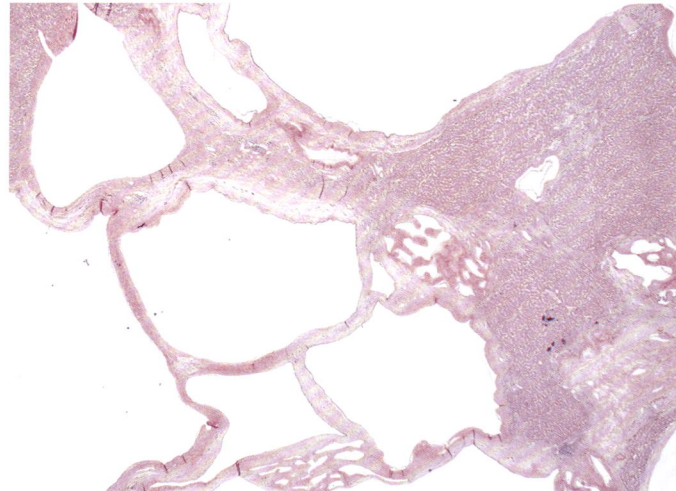

IMAGE 15.14 Polycystic liver disease. Note the normal liver tissue within the cyst septa (H&E, x10).

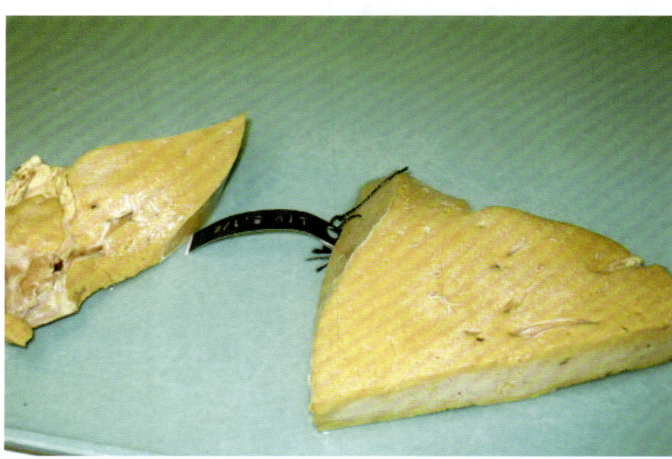

IMAGE 15.17 Fatty liver. Note the yellow color due to abundant lipid accumulation in hepatocytes.

Courtesy of Dr. Vincent Falk.

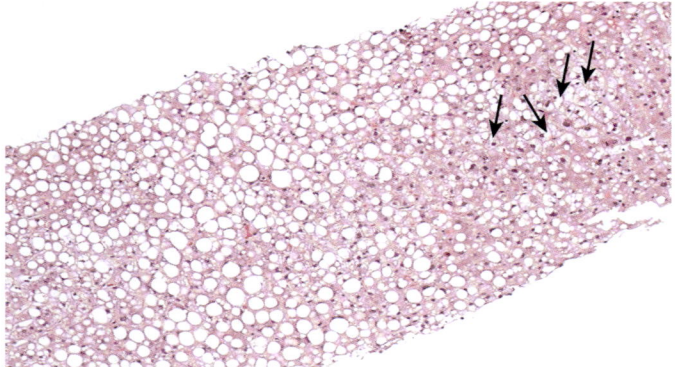

IMAGE 15.18 Nonalcoholic steatohepatitis (NASH). The image shows diffuse macrovesicular steatosis and numerous ballooned hepatocytes (black arrows) (H&E, x100).

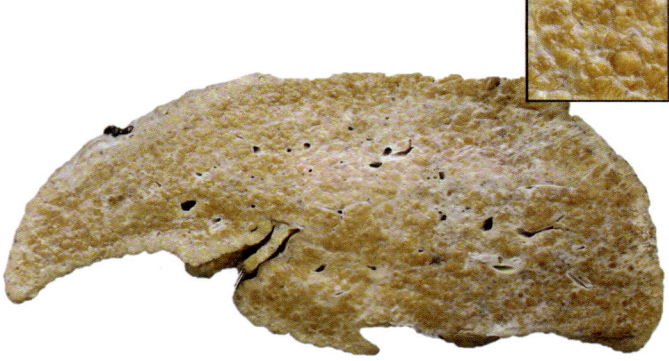

IMAGE 15.21 Micronodular cirrhosis (Laennec cirrhosis) due to end-stage alcoholic liver disease.

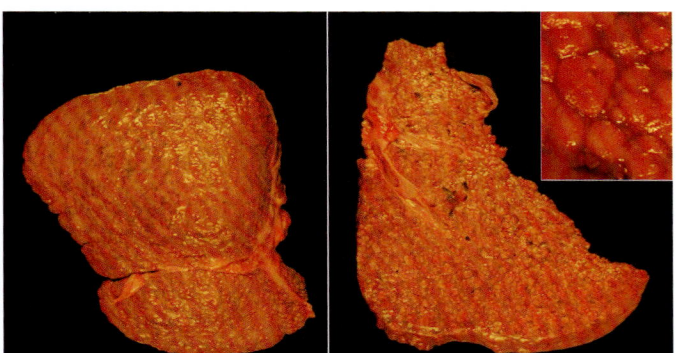

IMAGE 15.19 Liver cirrhosis. The images show diffuse replacement of liver parenchyma by fibrosis and regenerative nodules.

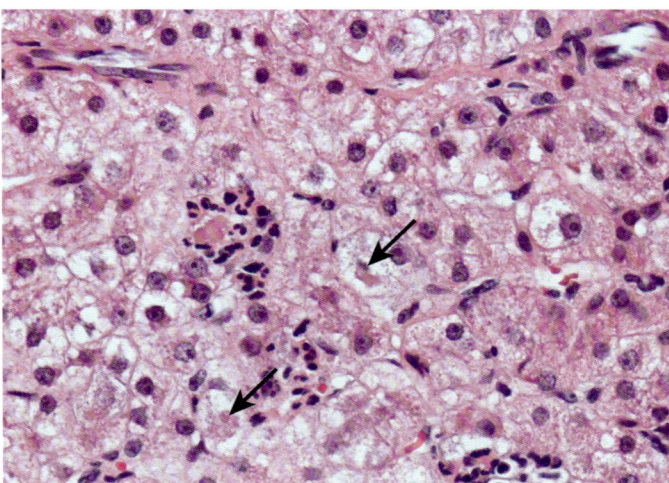

IMAGE 15.22 Alcoholic hepatitis. Hepatocytes show marked ballooning degeneration and intracytoplasmic Mallory bodies (black arrows). Mallory bodies can attract neutrophils (H&E, x400).

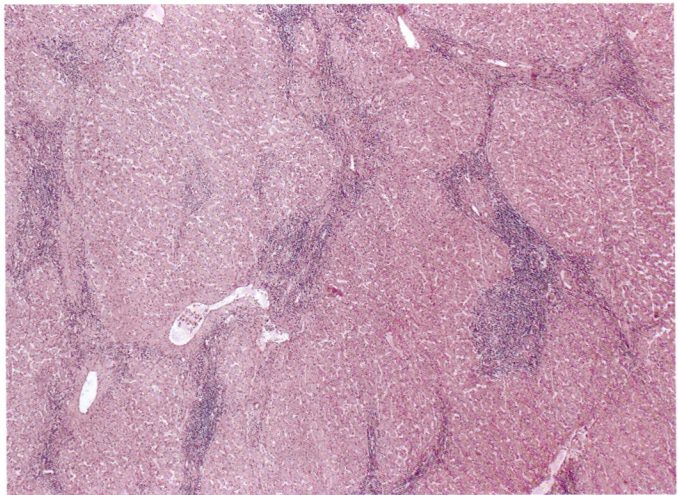

IMAGE 15.20 Liver with incomplete cirrhosis and ongoing inflammation (H&E, x40).

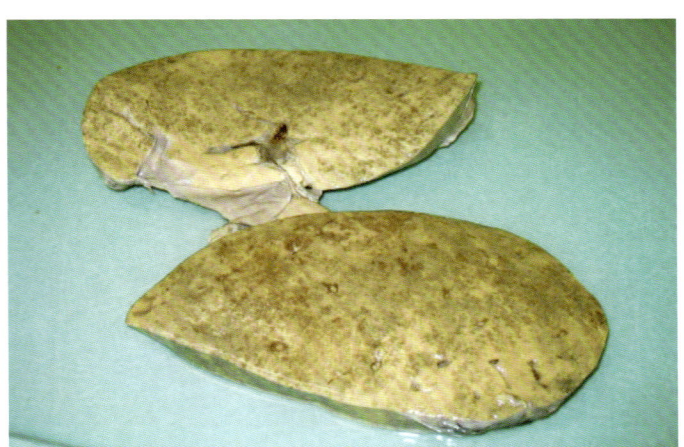

IMAGE 15.23 Liver with submassive necrosis. Note the pale yellow areas of necrosis scattered throughout the liver parenchyma.

Courtesy of Dr. Vincent Falck.

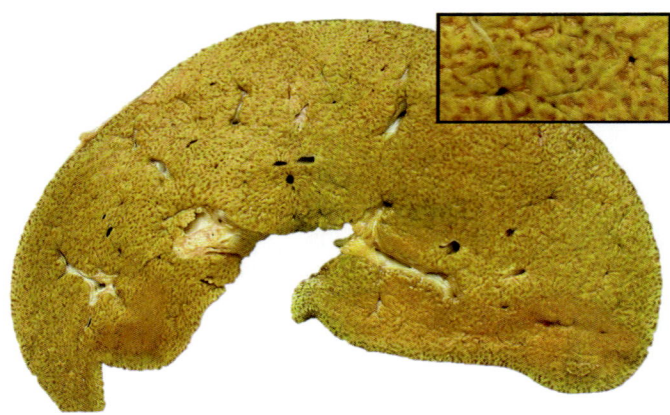

IMAGE 15.24 Fulminant liver failure due to acetaminophen overdose. The green-yellow color of the liver is caused by extensive steatosis, necrosis, and cholestasis. The brownish area in the inset highlights the remaining viable liver tissue.

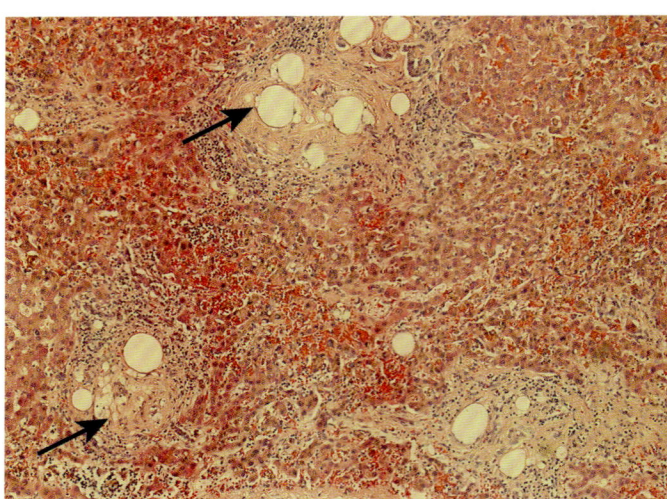

IMAGE 15.27 Mineral oil intake shows characteristic portal lipogranulomas (black arrows) (H&E, x100).

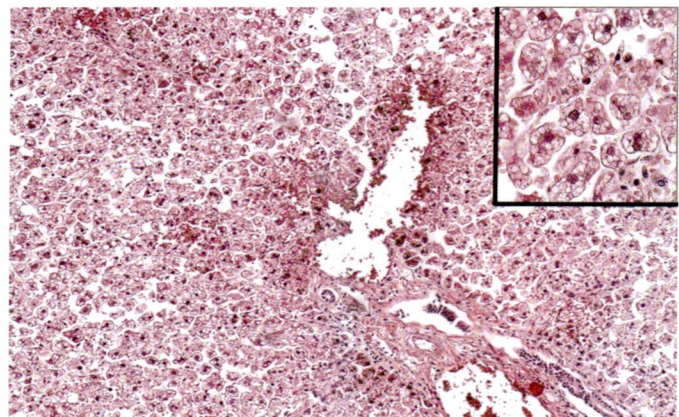

IMAGE 15.25 Acetaminophen toxicity. The image shows early coagulative necrosis characterized by disrupted hepatocellular plates, with individual hepatocytes showing typical features of microvesicular steatosis (main image: H&E, x100; inset: H&E, x400).

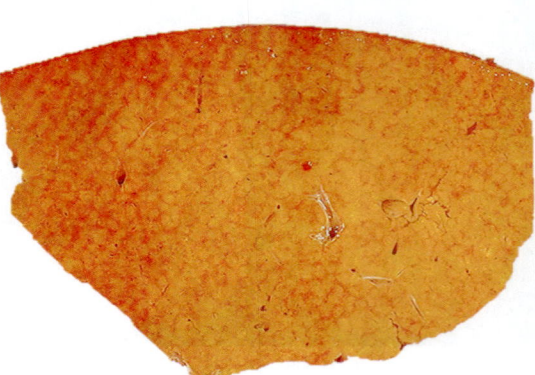

IMAGE 15.28 Amyloidosis. The liver weighed 3540 grams with a firm consistency. The cut surface is yellowish-brownish in color.

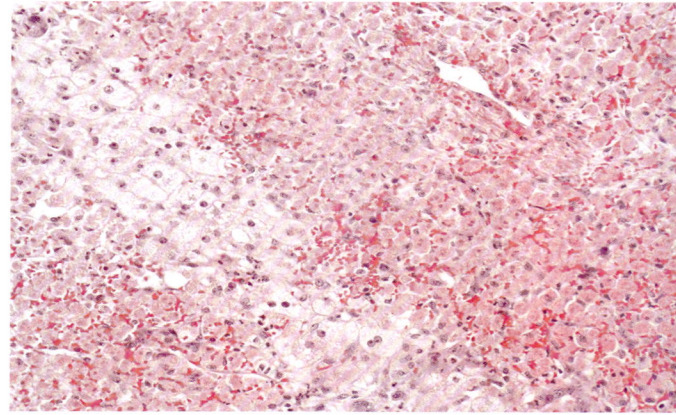

IMAGE 15.26 Acetaminophen toxicity. Massive early coagulative necrosis and individual hepatocytes showing microvesicular steatosis are present (H&E, x200).

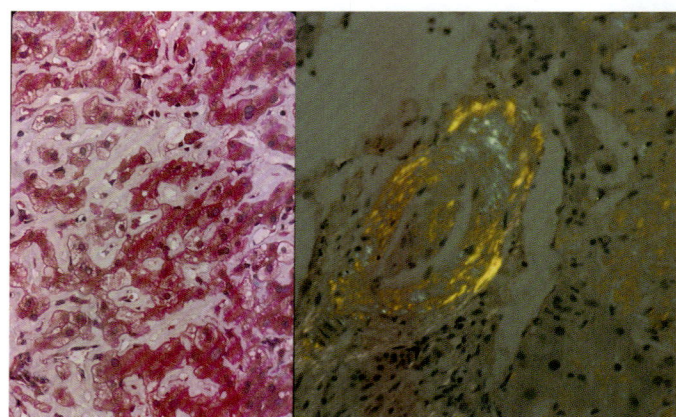

IMAGE 15.29 Amyloidosis. Left: amorphus material deposits within the sinusoidal spaces (H&E, x400). Right: polarized light shows green birefringence in the wall of a large artery (Congo red, x200).

Left: Courtesy of Dr. Vincent Falck. Right: Courtesy of Dr. Stefan Urbanski.

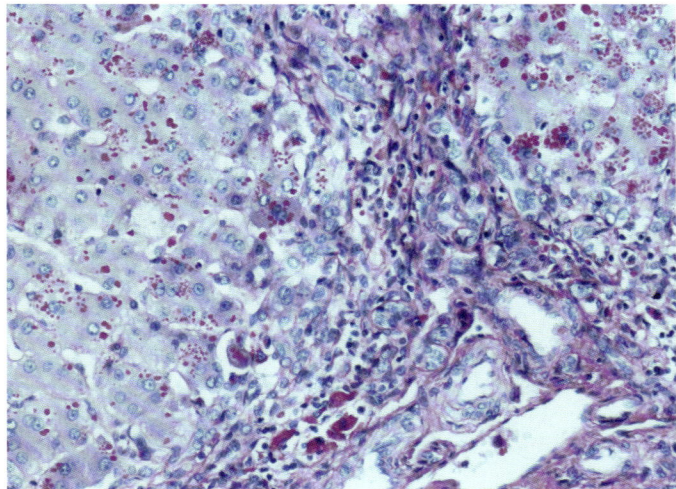

IMAGE 15.30 α₁-Antitrypsin deficiency. Distinct eosinophilic globules in the cytoplasm of periportal hepatocytes (PAS-D, x200).

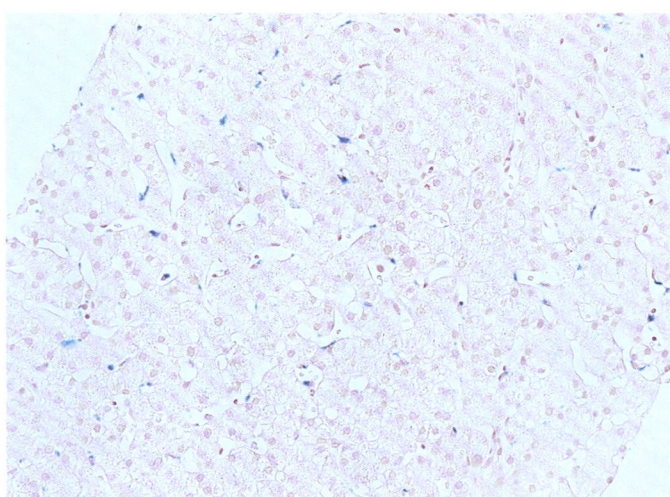

IMAGE 15.33 Hemosiderosis. Iron deposits in Kupffer cells are often caused by blood transfusion or hemolysis (Perl stain, x100).

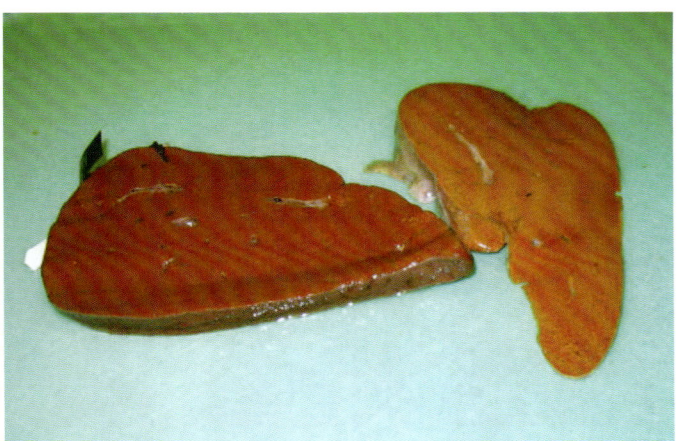

IMAGE 15.31 Hemochromatosis. Note the rusty brown color quite typical of iron overload in the liver.

Courtesy of Dr. Vincent Falck.

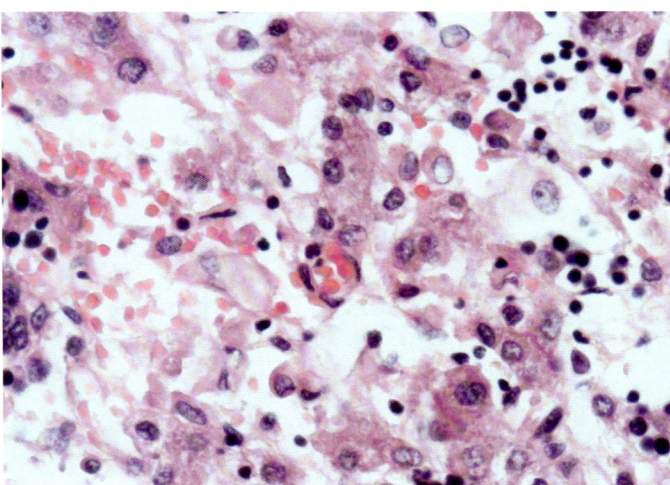

IMAGE 15.34 Gaucher disease. Pale staining Gaucher cells have a faintly striated cytoplasm (H&E, x400).

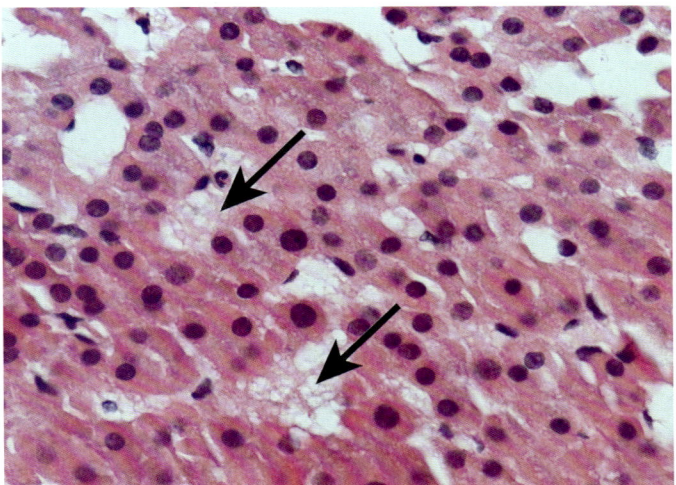

IMAGE 15.32 Hemochromatosis. Left: grade 1/4 (Perl stain, x100). Right: grade 4/4 (Perl stain, x40).

IMAGE 15.35 Amiodarone-induced phospholipidosis. The image shows a cluster of foam cells in lobular sinusoids (black arrows) (H&E, x400).

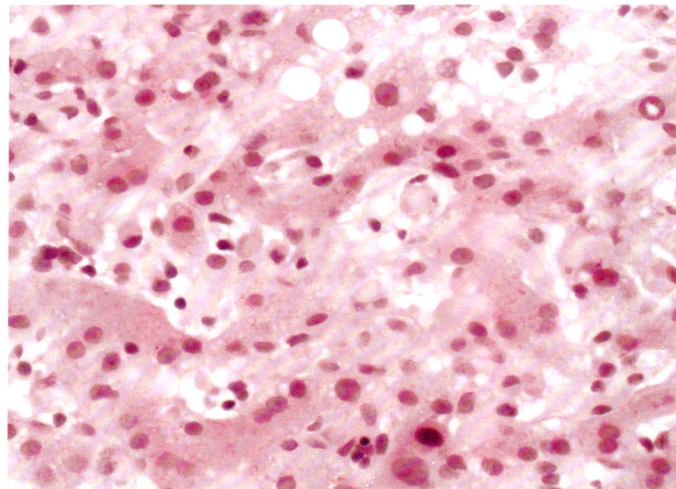

IMAGE 15.36 Hemophagocytic syndrome. Lymphocytes are engulfed by Kupffer cells (H&E, x400).

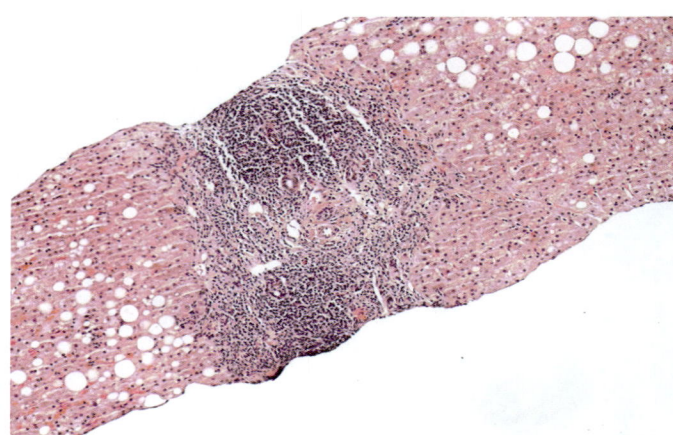

IMAGE 15.39 HCV (hepatitis C virus). The image shows dense lymphoid aggregate within the portal tract and patchy lobular fatty change (H&E, x100).

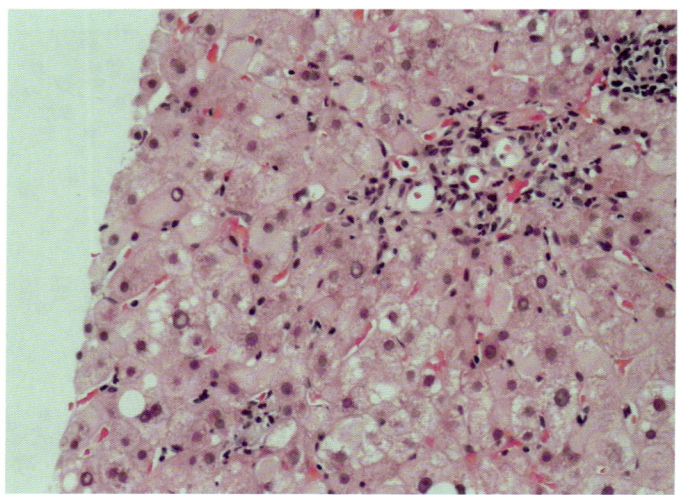

IMAGE 15.37 HBV (hepatitis B virus). The image shows ground-glass hepatocytes (H&E, x200).

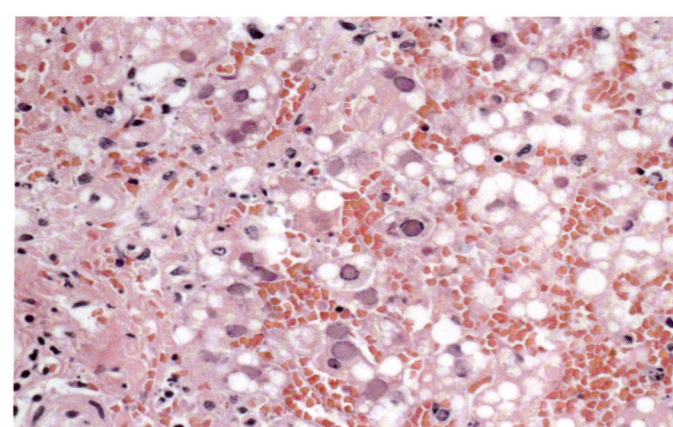

IMAGE 15.40 Herpes hepatitis. The image shows hepatocytes with Cowdry type A intranuclear viral inclusions present at the border between viable liver and an area of coagulative necrosis (H&E, x200).

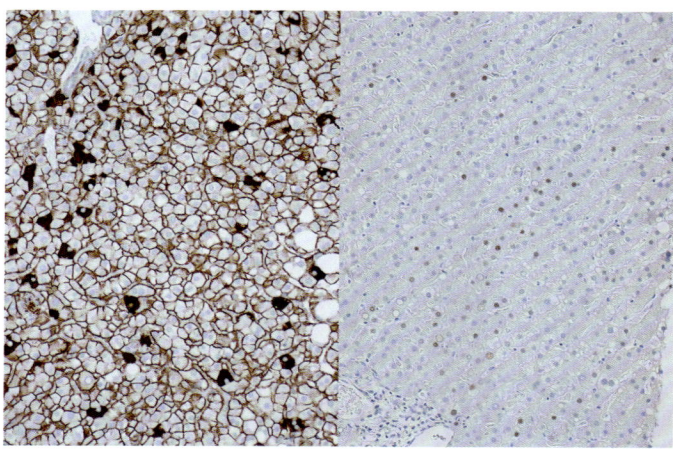

IMAGE 15.38 HBV. Left: HBSAg cytoplasmic staining. Right: HBcAg nuclear staining (imunoperoxidase, x200).

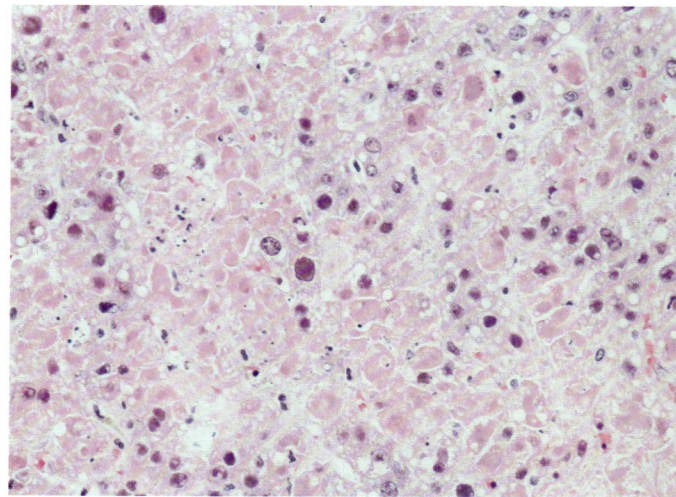

IMAGE 15.41 Adenovirus hepatitis. The image shows coagulative necrosis and intranuclear viral inclusions (H&E, x200).

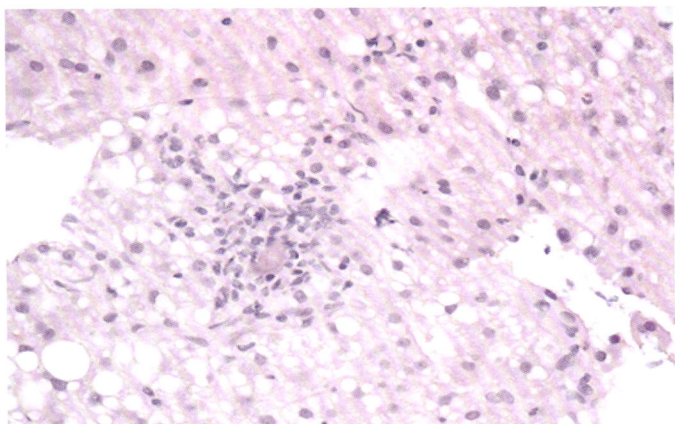

IMAGE 15.42 Cytomegalovirus (CMV) hepatitis. A microabscess with inflammatory cells surrounding a hepatocyte containing a large intranuclear viral inclusion (H&E, x200).

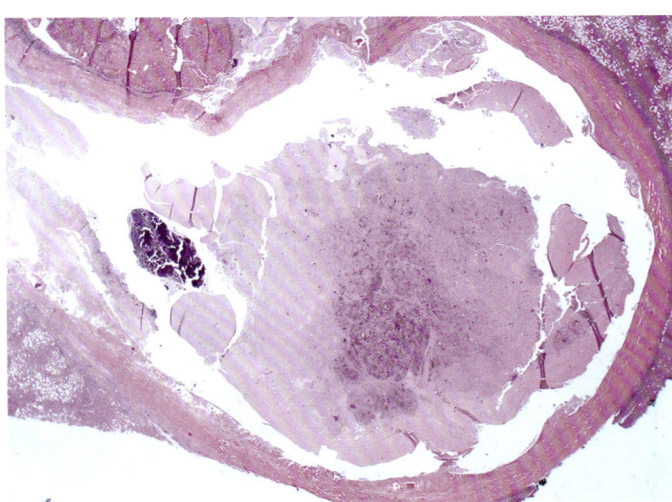

IMAGE 15.45 Histoplasmosis. The image shows a solitary, well-defined necrotic mass in the liver parenchyma, which is the usual presentation (H&E, x10).

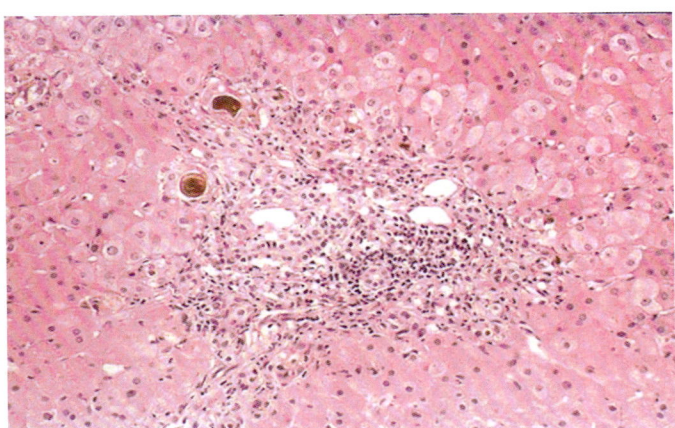

IMAGE 15.43 Sepsis. The image shows periportal mild bile ductular proliferation with intracanalicular cholestasis ("chloangitis lenta") (H&E, x100).

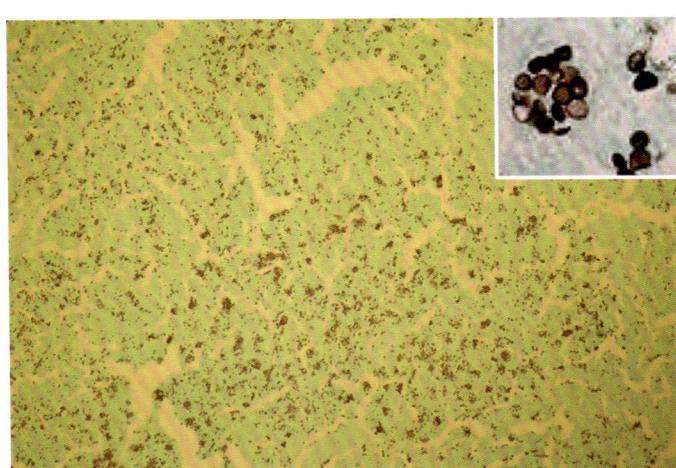

IMAGE 15.46 Histoplasmosis. On a necrotic background, numerous oval 2–4 μm yeasts with narrow based buds are shown. The cell wall is highlighted with methenamine silver stain (x10; inset: x400).

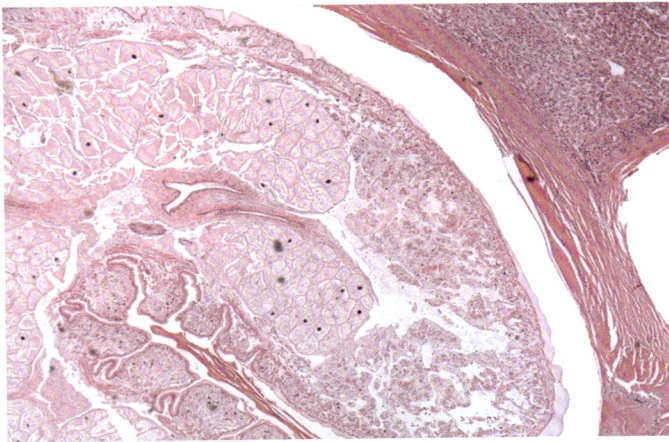

IMAGE 15.44 Liver tapeworm, microscopic (H&E, x40).

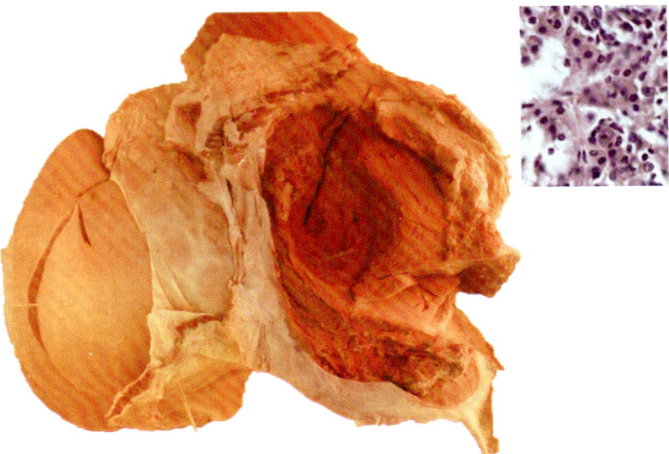

IMAGE 15.47 Liver amoeba abscess. An abscess cavity contains chocolate colored blood clots and necrotic tissue. The insert highlights the amoeba microorganisms (H&E, x400).

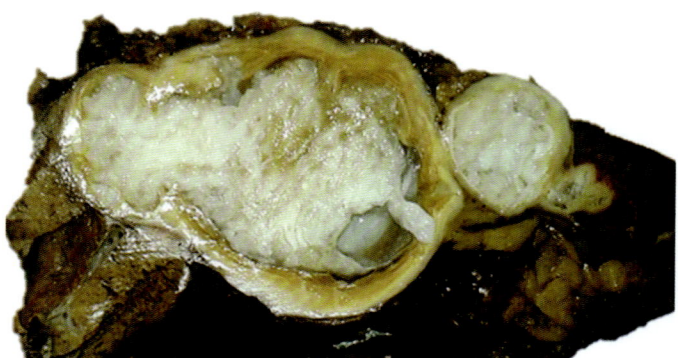

IMAGE 15.48 An echinococcus cyst showing many daughter cysts, some of which have a translucent cyst wall.

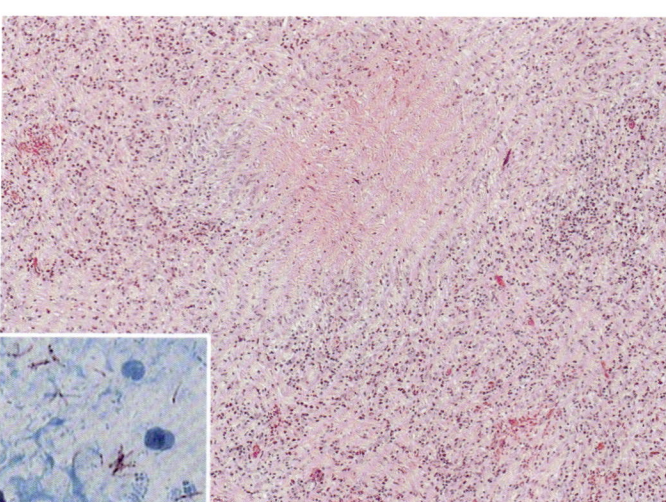

IMAGE 15.51 Necrotizing granuloma in a patient with tuberculosis (H&E, x40). Inset: *Mycobacterium tuberculosis* highlighted by Ziehl-Neelsen stain (x400).

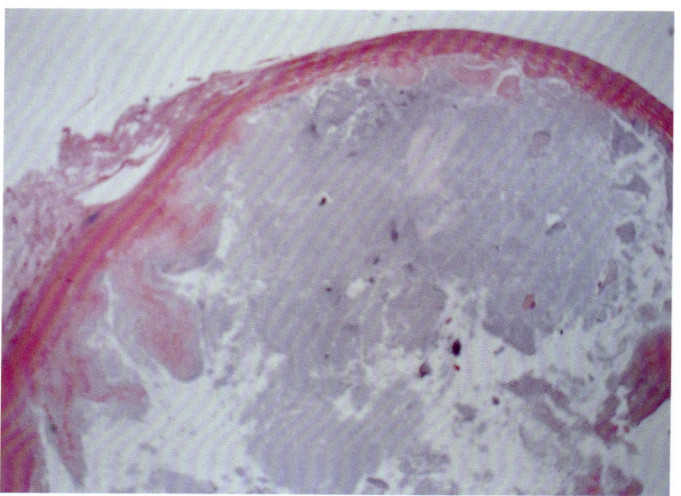

IMAGE 15.49 A hydatid cyst showing a laminated keratin-like cyst wall containing necrotic debris (H&E, x10).

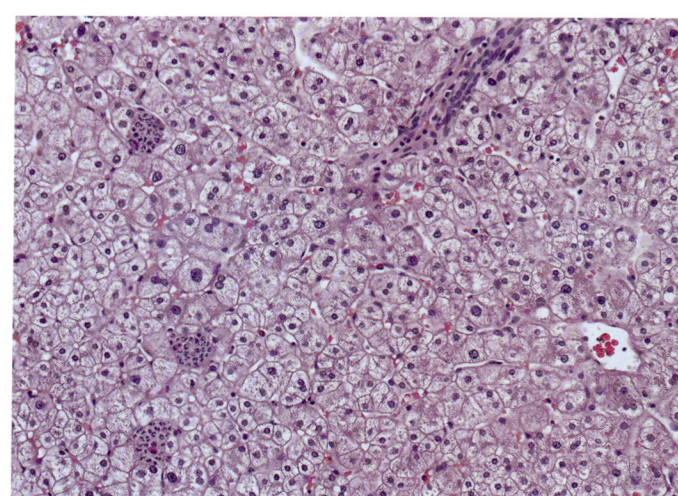

IMAGE 15.52 "Surgical hepatitis" showing multiple intralobular microabscesses and hepatocyte ballooning. There is no steatosis (H&E, x100).

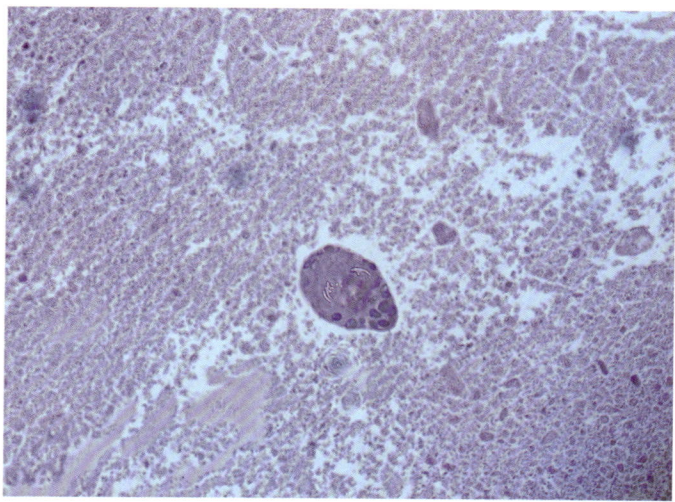

IMAGE 15.50 A hydatid cyst containing hooklets within the cyst fluid (H&E, x200).

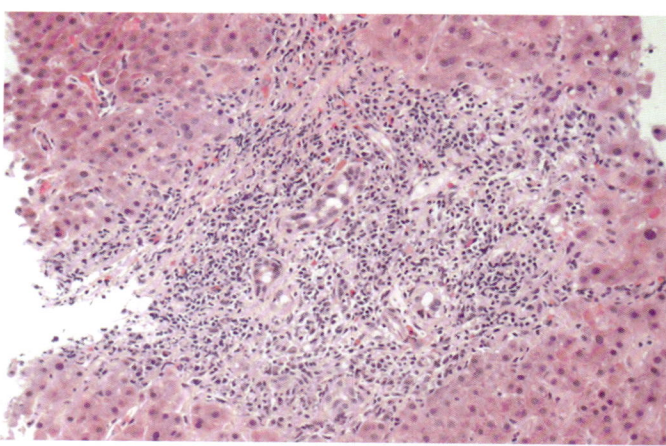

IMAGE 15.53 Autoimmune hepatitis. Interface hepatitis with numerous plasma cells (H&E, x200).

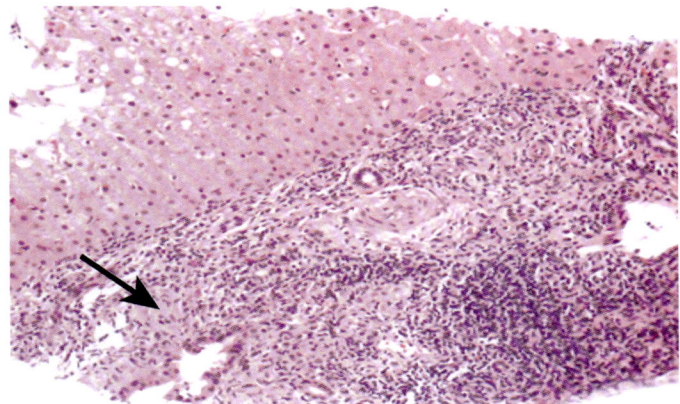

IMAGE 15.54 Primary biliary cirrhosis. The image shows a periductal granuloma (arrow) and portal dense lymphoid infiltrate (H&E, x200).

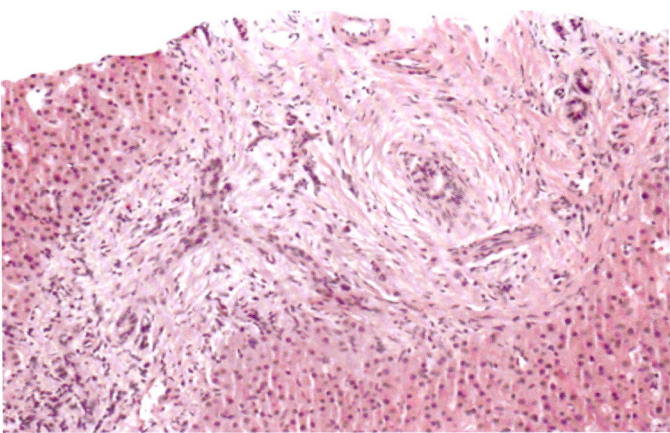

IMAGE 15.57 Extrahepatic biliary obstruction with portal edema and ductular proliferation (H&E, x200).

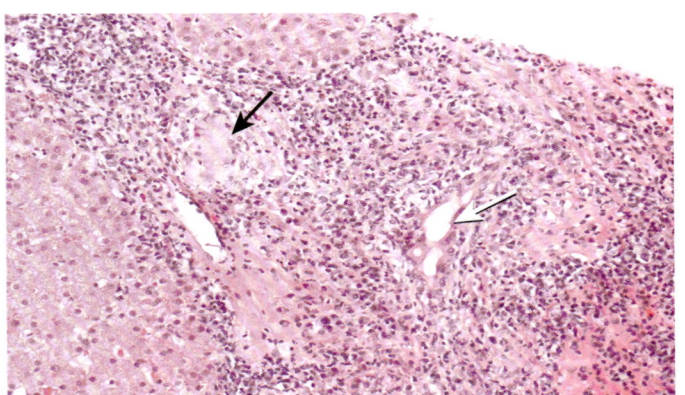

IMAGE 15.55 Overlap of autoimmune hepatitis and primary biliary cholangitis. The image shows periductal granuloma (black arrow), bile duct injury (white arrow), portal dense lymphoid infiltrate with interface hepatitis rich in plasma cells (H&E, x200).

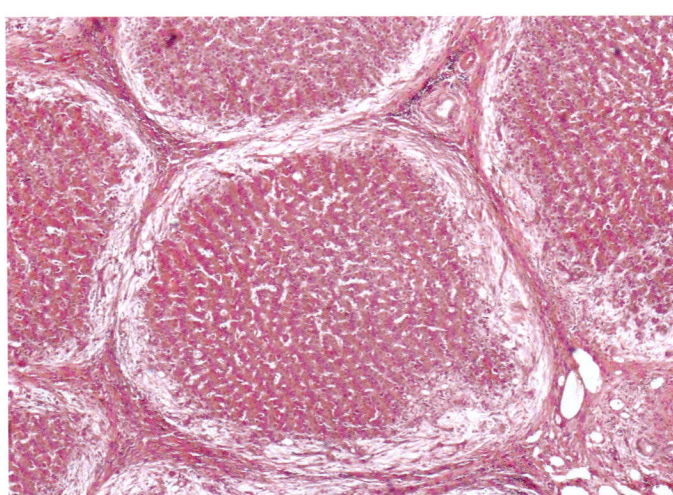

IMAGE 15.58 Biliary cirrhosis. The clear halo around the regenerative nodules (cholate stasis) is characteristic of biliary cirrhosis (H&E, x20).

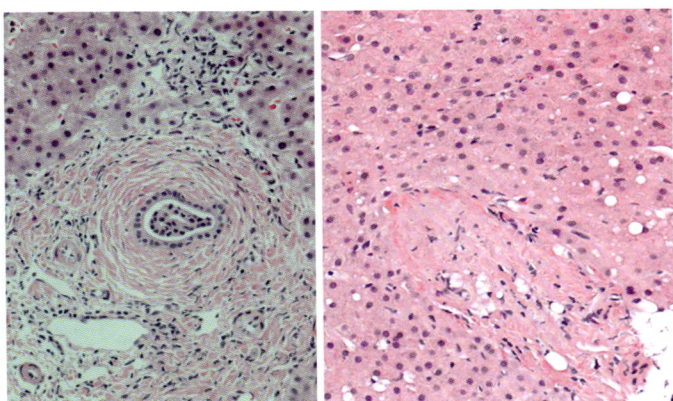

IMAGE 15.56 Primary sclerosing cholangitis. Left: periductal onionskin-type fibrosis (H&E, x200). Right: fibrous obliteration of a preexisting interlobular bile duct (H&E, x200).

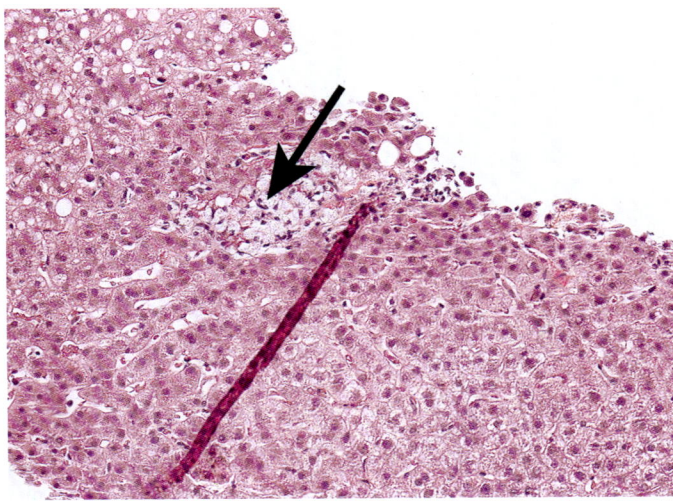

IMAGE 15.59 Pseudoxanthomatous change. In patients with cholestasis, clusters of foamy histiocytes (arrow) mimicking xanthomas are seen in the liver parenchyma (H&E, x200).

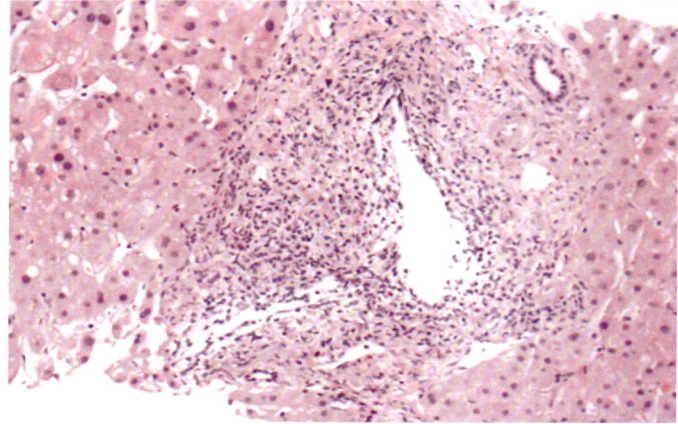

IMAGE 15.60 Liver allograft with acute cellular rejection. The image shows 3 features: mixed portal infiltrates with lymphoplasmacytes and eosinophils, vascular endothelialitis, and ductulitis (H&E, x200).

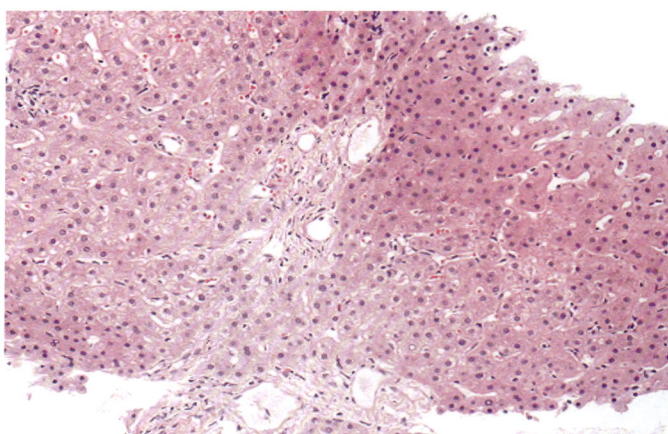

IMAGE 15.63 Ductopenia in a patient with late-stage chronic allograft rejection (H&E, x200).

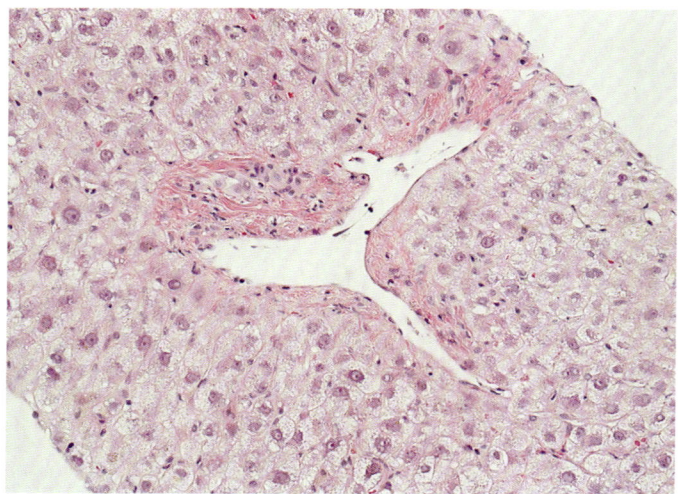

IMAGE 15.61 Early chronic rejection with partially destroyed duct. Notice the rarity of inflammatory cells in the portal tract (H&E, x200).

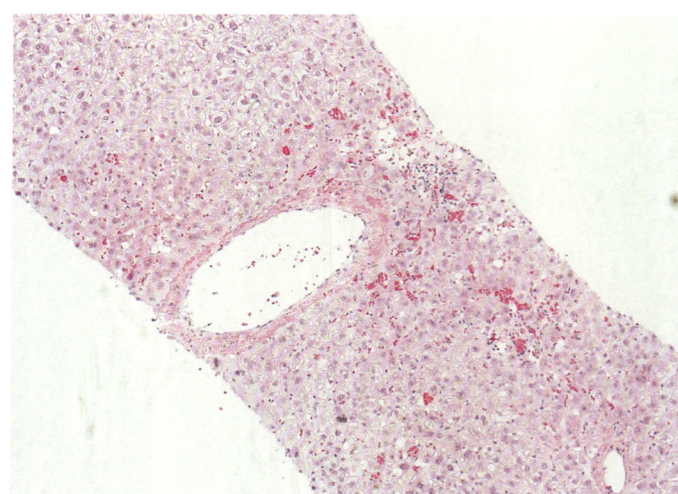

IMAGE 15.64 Chronic rejection with perivenular fibrosis and residual endothelialitis (H&E, x100).

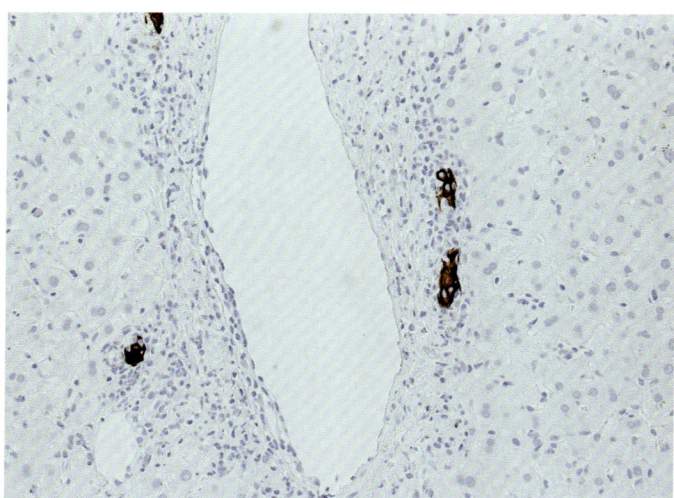

IMAGE 15.62 Ductal damage in early chronic rejection (CK19 stain, x200).

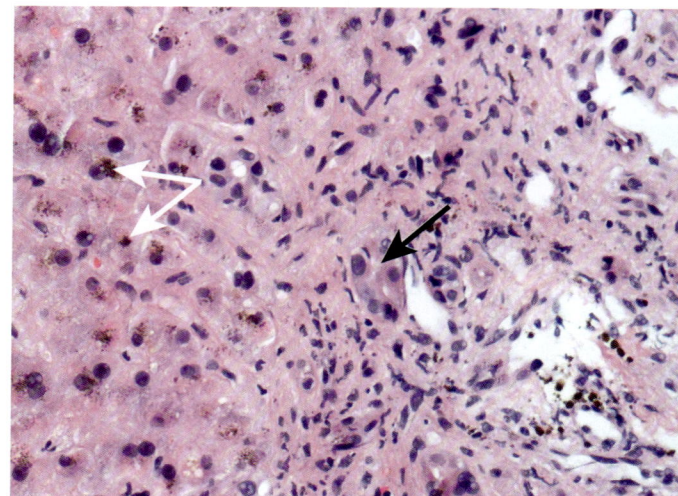

IMAGE 15.65 GVHD (graft versus host disease) with duct damage (characteristic "dysplastic ductal epithelium") (black arrow) and cholestasis (H&E, x400). Iron pigments white arrows) are also seen in the lobules due to repeated blood transfusion.

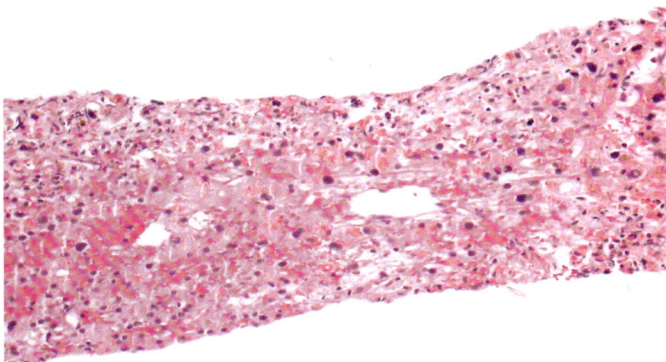

IMAGE 15.66 Sinusoidal obstruction syndrome. The image shows sinusoidal endothelial damage with red blood cell extravasation into the space of Disse (H&E, x200).

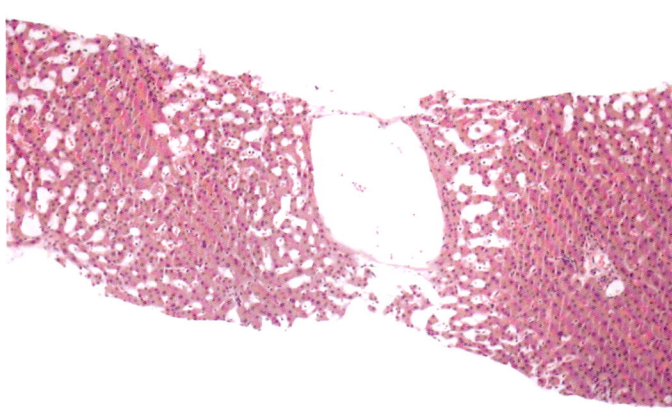

IMAGE 15.69 Congestive heart failure. Central vein and perivenular sinusoidal spaces show marked dilatation (H&E, x100).

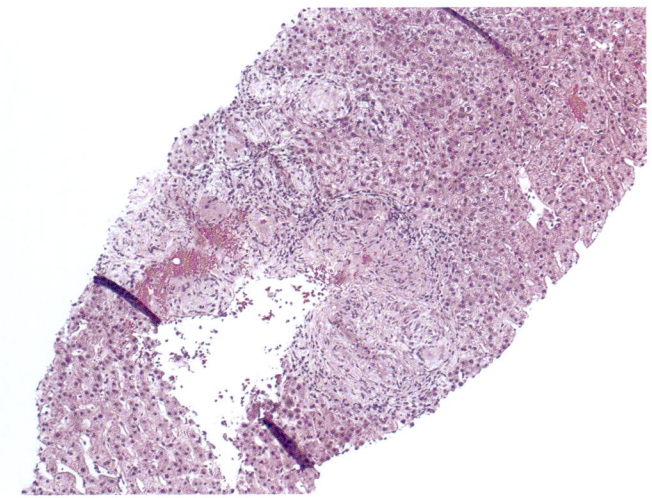

IMAGE 15.67 Sarcoidosis. Liver parenchyma contains multiple noncaseating sarcoid granulomas around periportal areas associated with scarce inflammation ("naked" granulomas) and fibrous bands that separate a large granuloma into several small granulomata (H&E, x100).

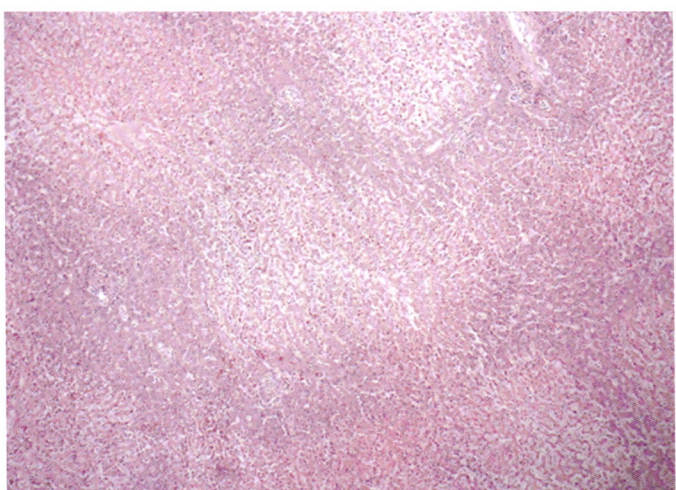

IMAGE 15.70 "Shock" liver. Perivenular hepatocyte necrosis extends to midzone without obvious inflammation (H&E, x100).

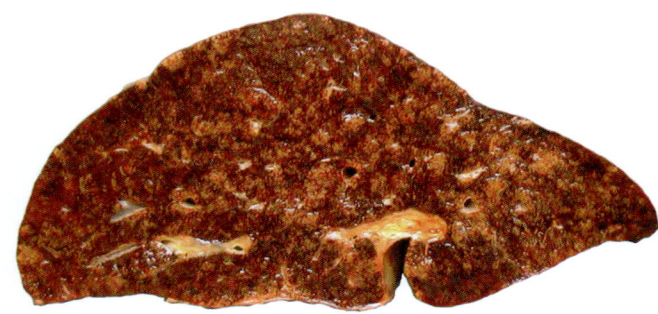

IMAGE 15.68 Congestive hepatopathy ("nutmeg liver"). The image shows prominent centrilobular congestion alternating with foci of more intact paler liver parenchyma.

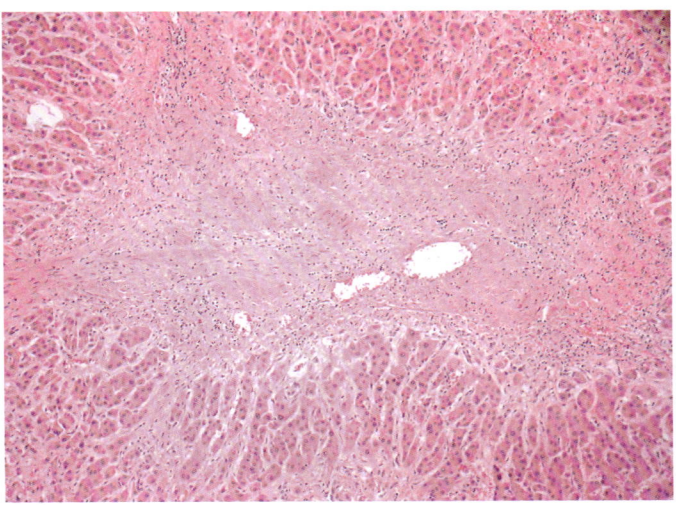

IMAGE 15.71 Bud-Chiari syndrome. The image shows a large hepatic vein with organized thrombosis and recanalization (H&E, x200).

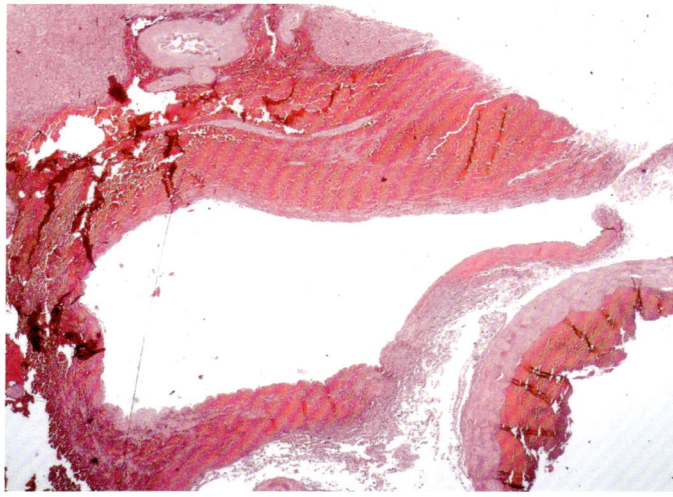

IMAGE 15.72 Arteriovenous malformation. The image shows a ruptured large, thick-walled vein and adjacent artery (H&E, x40).

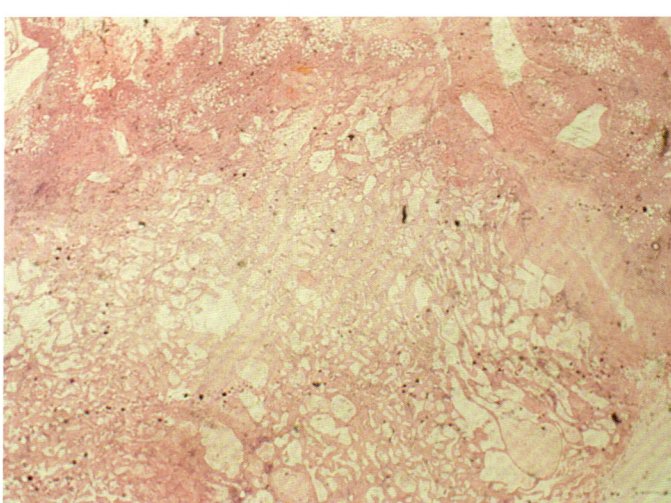

IMAGE 15.75 A cavernous hemangioma shows variable sized spaces lined by benign vascular endothelium and separated by fibrous septa (H&E, x20).

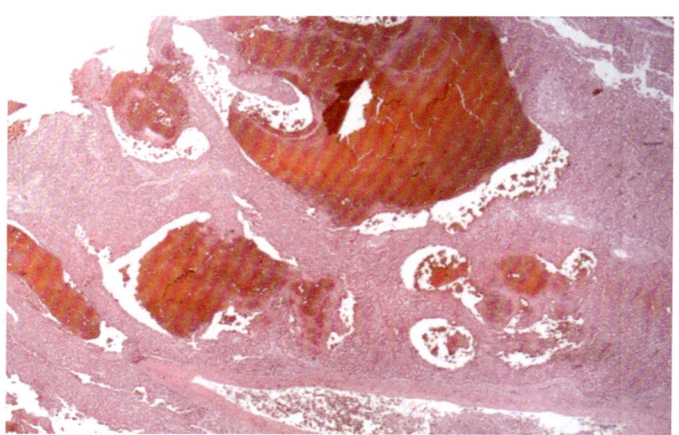

IMAGE 15.73 Peliosis hepatis. The image shows blood filled cystic areas with no distinct cellular lining (H&E, x20).

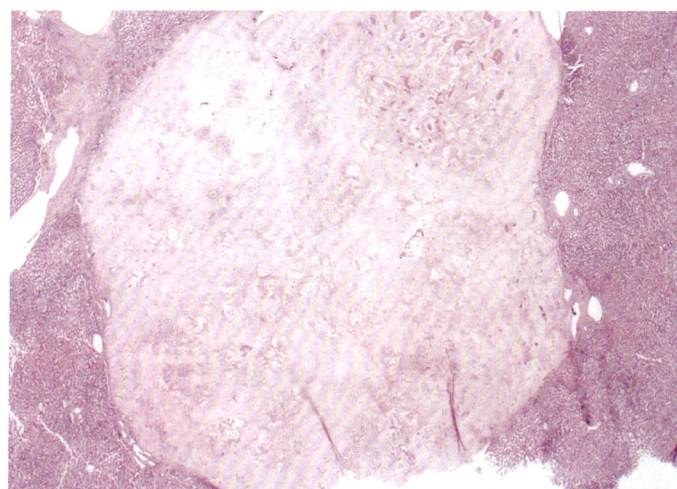

IMAGE 15.76 A sclerotic hemangioma shows a well-demarcated lesion with myxoid sclerotic stroma and shadows of vascular structures (H&E, x10).

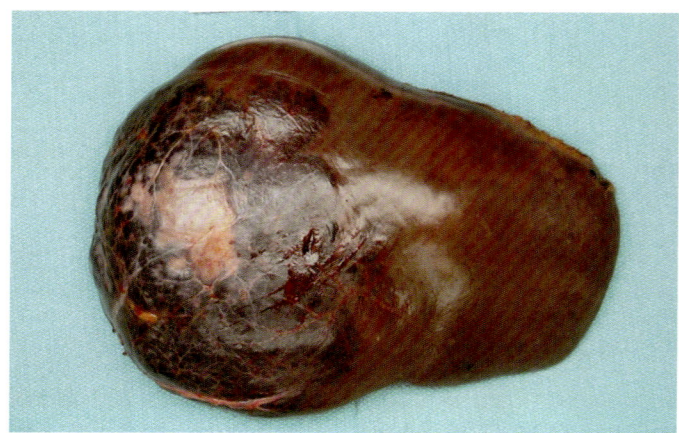

IMAGE 15.74 Liver hemangioma. This is a solitary, well-demarcated mass containing blood with a central area of fibrosis.

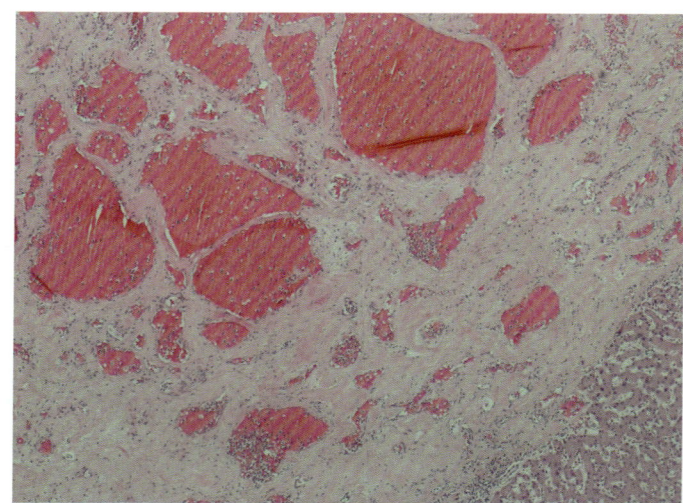

IMAGE 15.77 Sclerosing hemangioma. The tumor is partially sclerosed. A vascular silhouette can be seen in the sclerotic area (H&E, x10).

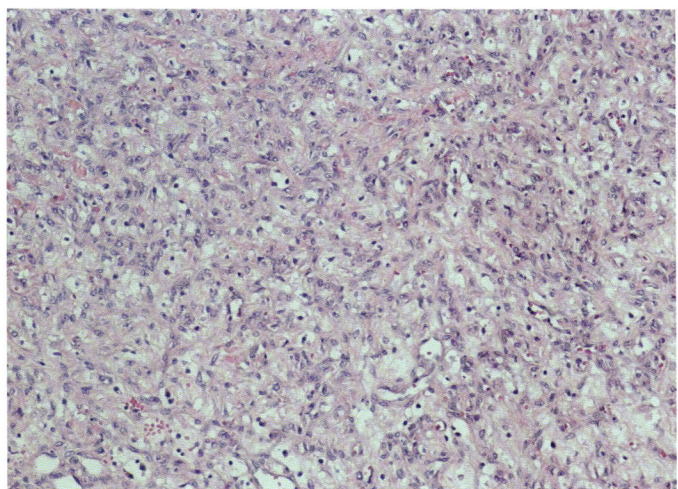

IMAGE 15.78 Infantile hemangioendothelioma. The image shows variable sized vascular channels and foci of extramedullary hematopoiesis (H&E, x200).

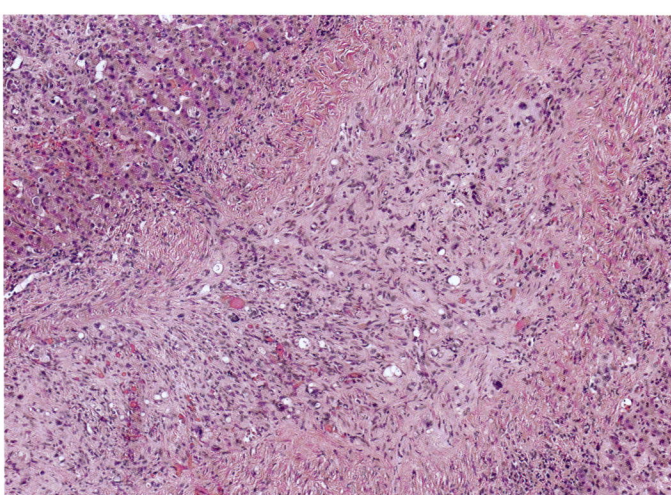

IMAGE 15.81 Epithelioid hemangioendothelioma. Atypical tumor cells grow within the lumen of a large hepatic vessel. Intracellular lumens are visible within the cytoplasm of some tumor cells (H&E, x100).

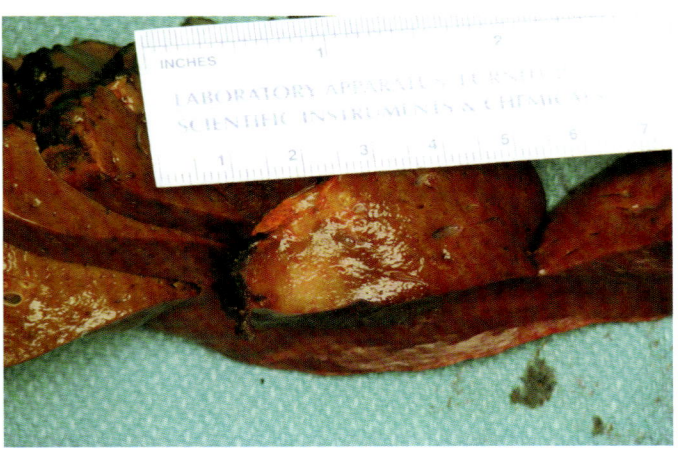

IMAGE 15.79 Epithelioid hemangioendothelioma. The white fleshy cut surface resembles a solid neoplasm rather than a vascular neoplasm.

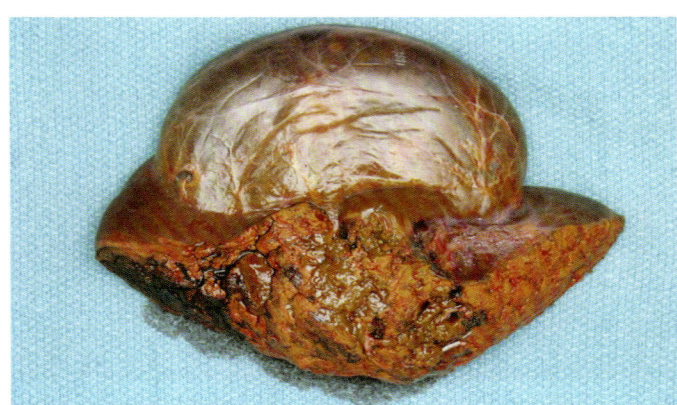

IMAGE 15.82 Liver angiosarcoma. The tumor shows extensive hemorrhage and necrosis. There is no clear demarcation from nonneoplastic parenchyma on cut section.

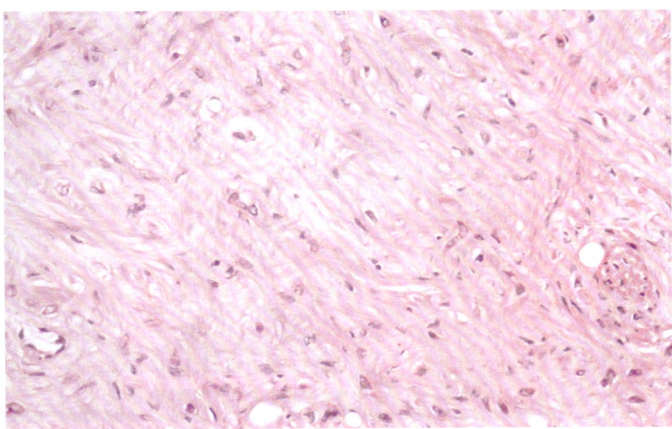

IMAGE 15.80 Epithelioid hemangioendothelioma. Within myxoid stroma, some tumor cells appear epithelioid and others form intracellular lumen (H&E, x200).

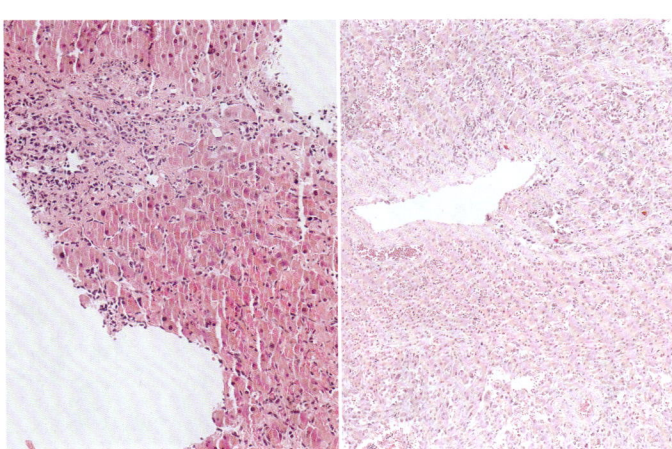

IMAGE 15.83 Angiosarcoma. Left: tumor cells invading into portal tracts and portal vein (H&E, x200). Right: tumor cells invading into the wall of a large hepatic vessel (H&E, x100).

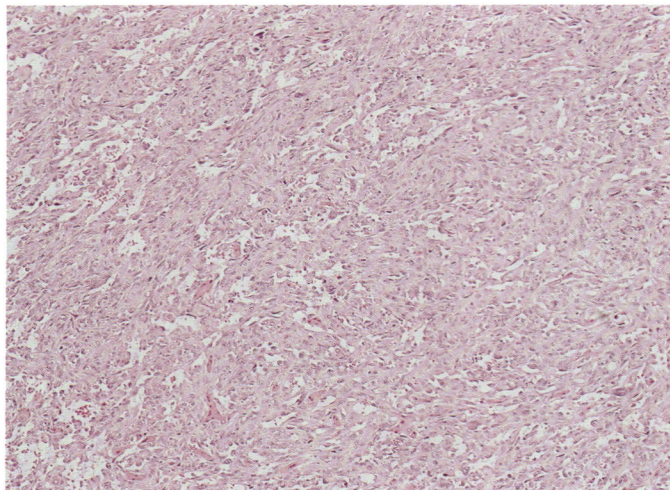

IMAGE 15.84 Angiosarcoma. The solid area shows atypical tumor cells and anastomosing vascular channels (H&E, x100).

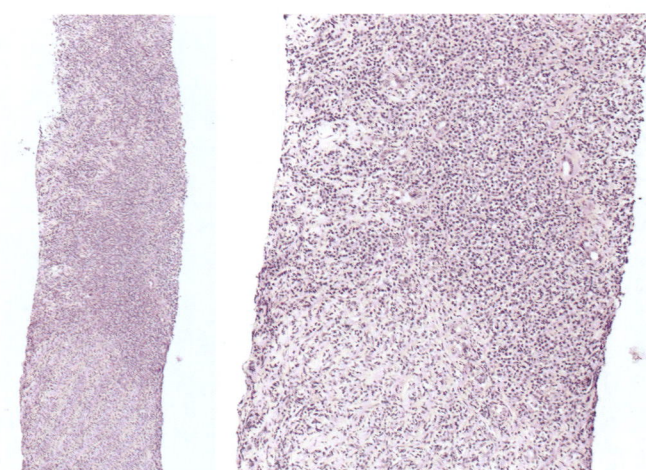

IMAGE 15.87 Inflammatory pseudotumor. This biopsy of a liver mass is composed entirely of inflammatory cells (H&E, left: x10; right: x40).

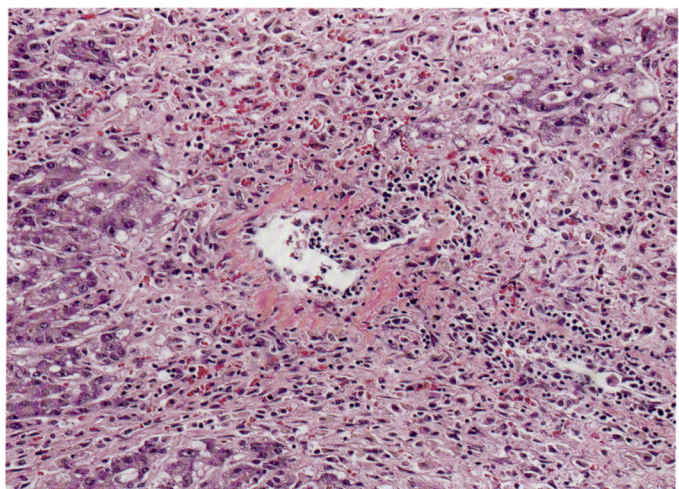

IMAGE 15.85 Drug (Tylenol)-induced vasculitis. The endothelium is lifted up by inflammatory cells. The vessel wall shows hyalinizing necrosis. There are also perivascular hepatocytes dropping out (H&E, x200).

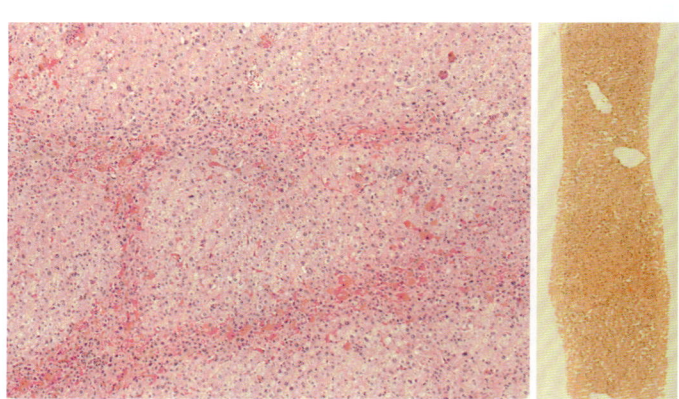

IMAGE 15.88 Nodular regenerative hyperplasia. Left: resection specimen shows nodularity, alternating thick and thin hepatocellular plates, and vascular congestion without fibrosis (H&E, x100). Right: biopsy specimen shows the contour of nodularity without fibrosis (H&E, x40).

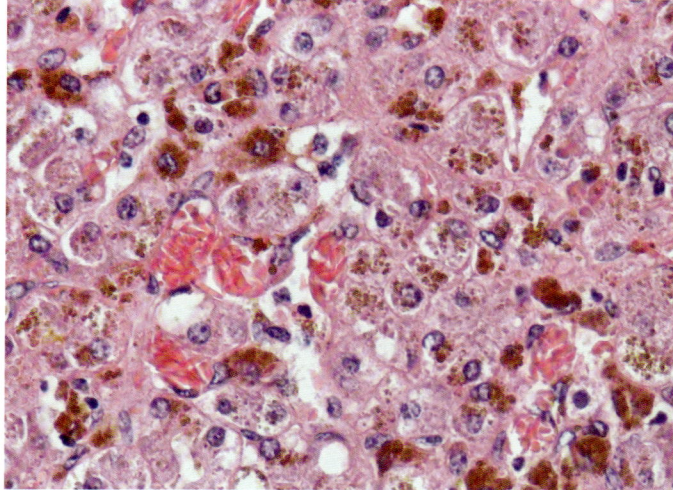

IMAGE 15.86 Sickle cell anemia. Sinusoids are dilated and contain sickled red blood cells. Hepatocytes show hemosiderin deposition (H&E, x400).

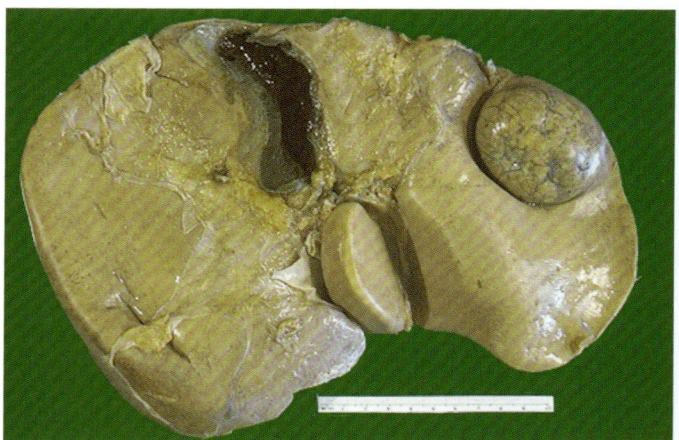

IMAGE 15.89 Hepatocellular adenoma. This is a subcapsular well-demarcated tumor bulging from under the surface of the left lobe.

Courtesy of Dr. Vincent Falck.

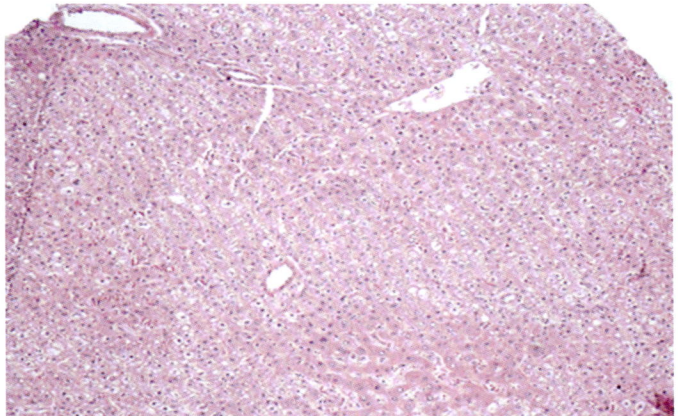

IMAGE 15.90 Hepatocellular adenoma. The lesion is composed of benign hepatocytes and aberrant vascular channels without an identifiable portal tract or central vein (H&E, x40).

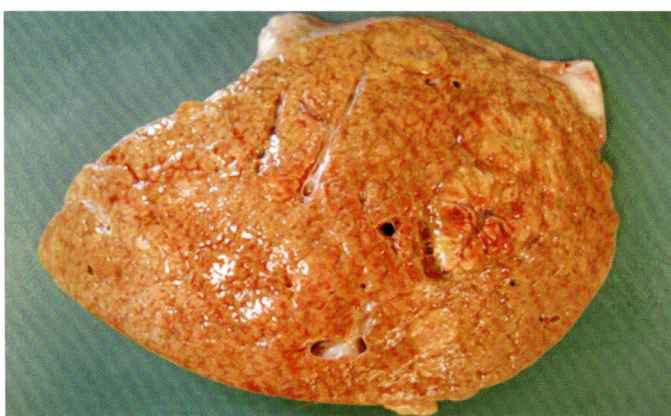

IMAGE 15.93 Focal nodular hyperplasia. On the right side of the image, there are 2 back-to-back nodular lesions with a central fibrous scar. The background liver is noncirrhotic.

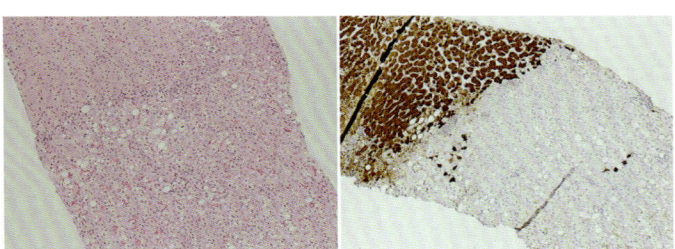

IMAGE 15.91 Hepatocellular adenoma, HNF-1α-inactivated subtype. Left: the image shows mild steatosis in the neoplastic tissue (below) and no steatosis in the normal liver (above) (H&E, 100x). Right: the image shows the absence of liver fatty acid binding protein (LFABP) immunostaining in neoplastic tissue (below) in contrast to the normal staining pattern in the normal liver parenchyma (above, immune peroxidase, x100).

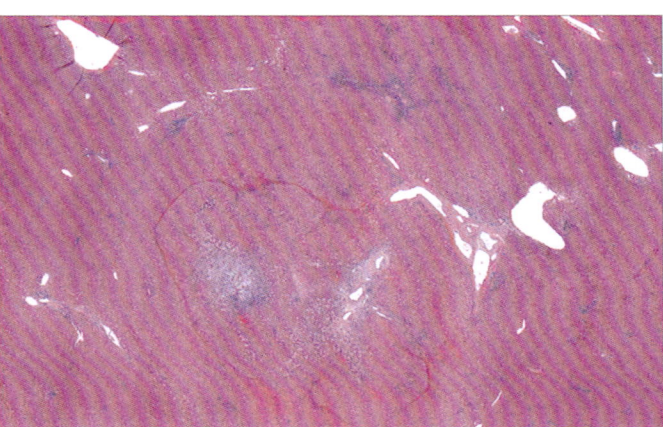

IMAGE 15.94 Focal nodular hyperplasia. This is a vague nodular lesion surrounded by normal liver parenchyma with a central scar, aberrant vessels, and proliferating ductules (H&E, x20).

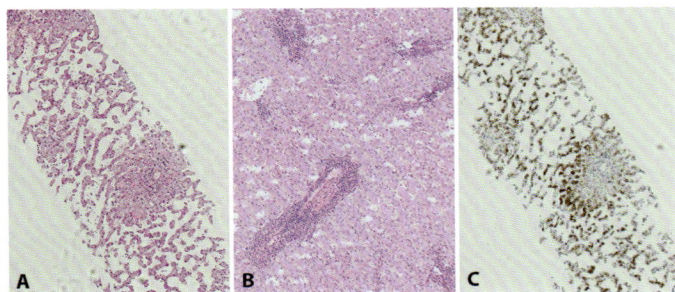

IMAGE 15.92 Hepatocellular adenoma, inflammatory subtype. Images A and B: sinusoidal dilatation, inflammatory cells, and thick-walled arteries are hallmarks of this tumor (H&E, x100). Image C: the neoplastic hepatocytes show strong intracytoplasmic serum amyloid protein A staining (immune peroxidase, x100).

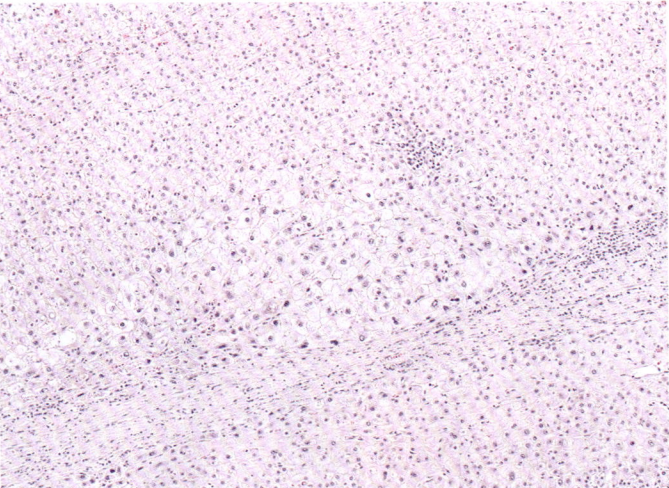

IMAGE 15.95 Small cell dysplasia (upper and lower part of the image) shows hepatocytes with small round nuclei, inconspicuous nucleoli, and scanty cytoplasm. Large cell dysplasia (middle part of the image) shows hepatocytes with large hyperchromatic nuclei (H&E, x100).

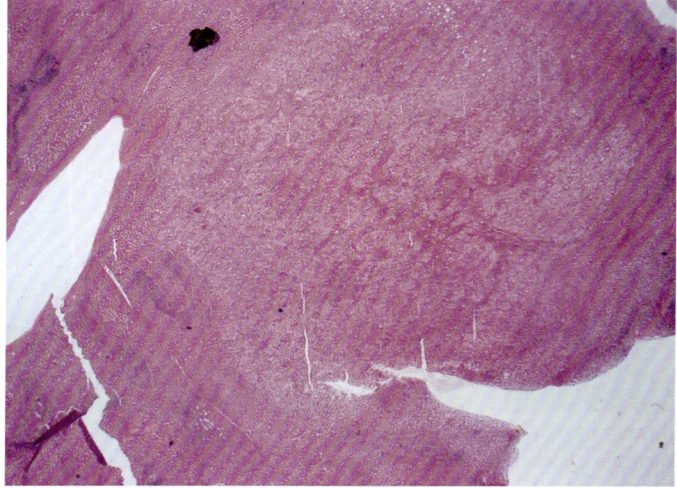

IMAGE 15.96 Early hepatocellular carcinoma. Grossly, this is a poorly defined lesion < 2 cm in diameter (H&E, x20).

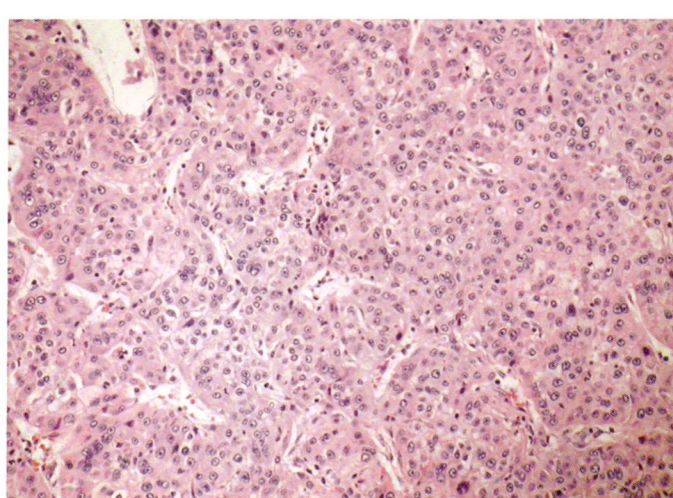

IMAGE 15.99 Hepatocellular carcinoma. Trabecular pattern (H&E, x200).

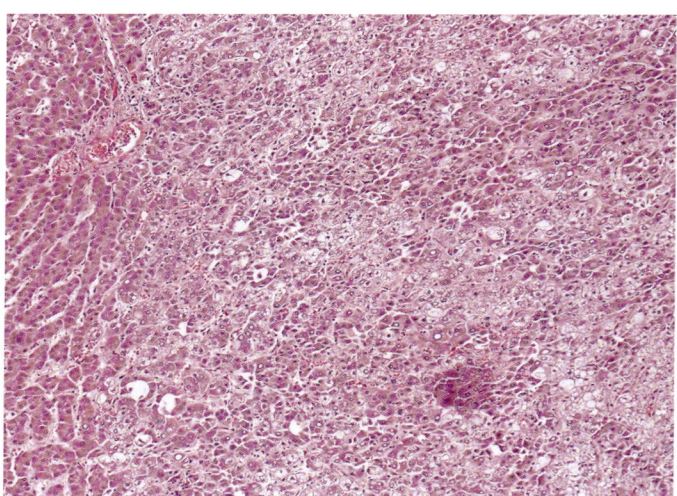

IMAGE 15.97 Early hepatocellular carcinoma. The image shows microscopic features of a well-differentiated hepatocellular carcinoma that merge imperceptibly with surrounding parenchyma (H&E, x100).

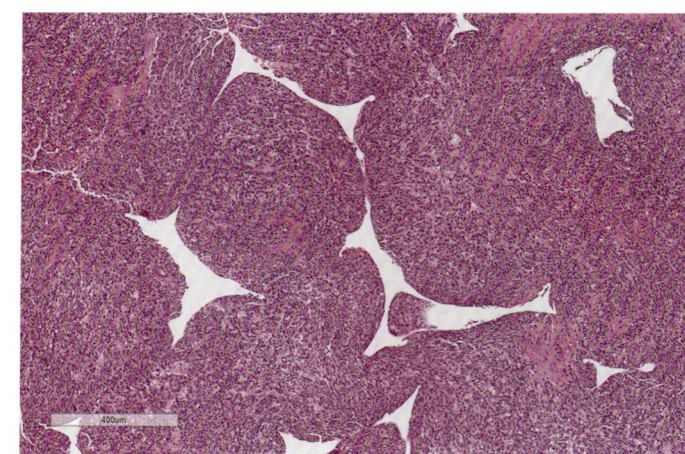

IMAGE 15.100 Hepatocellular carcinoma, macrotrabecular subtype. This subtype is associated with worse prognosis. (H&E, x400).

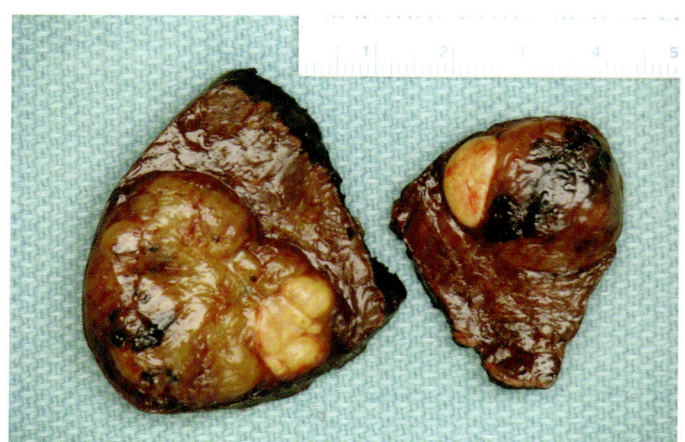

IMAGE 15.98 Hepatocellular carcinoma. This is a large heterogeneous tumor mass with areas of hemorrhage and necrosis.

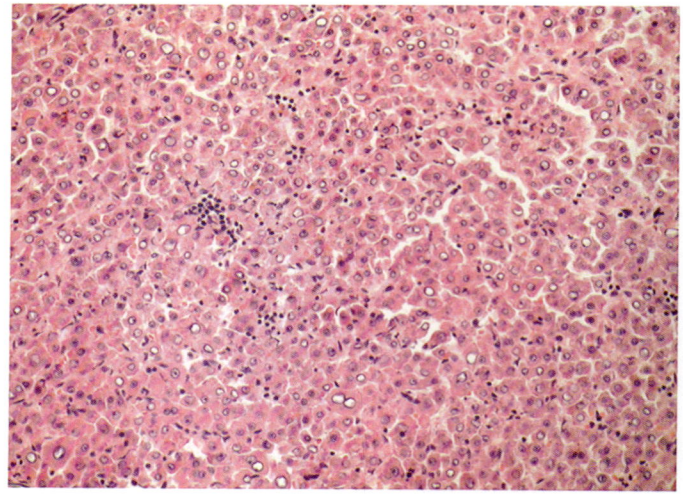

IMAGE 15.101 Hepatocellular carcinoma, solid pattern (H&E, x200).

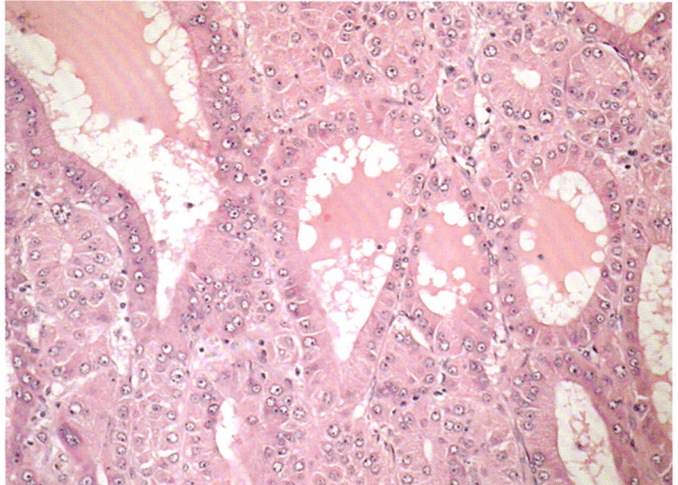

IMAGE 15.102 Hepatocellular carcinoma, pseudoglandular pattern (H&E, x400).

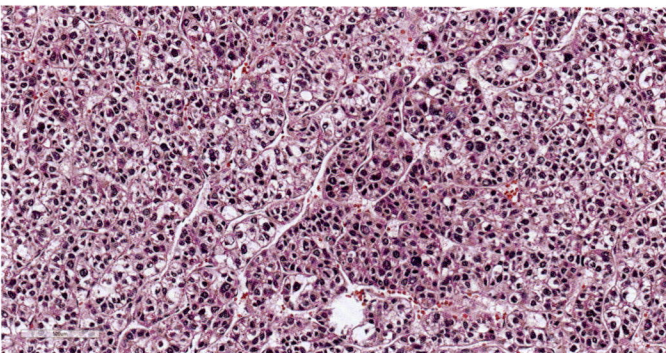

IMAGE 15.105 Hepatocellular carcinoma, chromophobe subtype. The tumor cells have clear cytoplasm and striking nuclear atypia (H&E, x200).

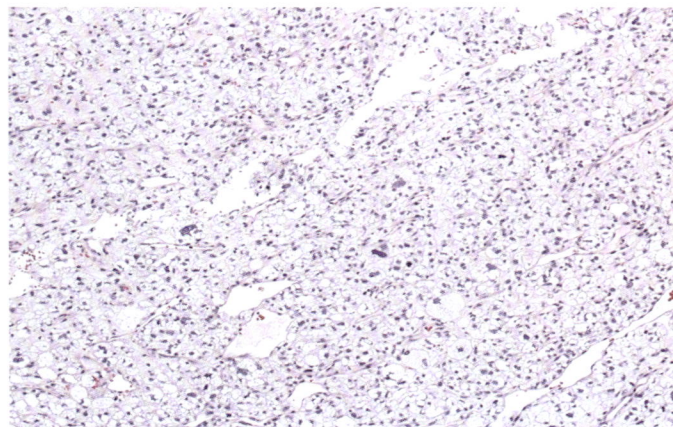

IMAGE 15.103 Hepatocellular carcinoma, clear cell subtype (H&E, x100).

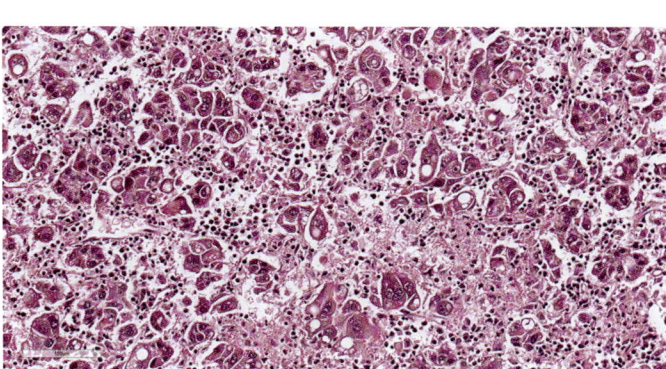

IMAGE 15.106 Hepatocellular carcinoma, lymphocyte-rich subtype (H&E, x200).

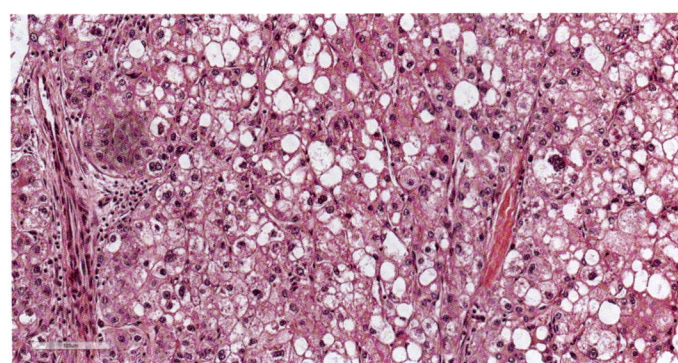

IMAGE 15.104 Hepatocellular carcinoma, steatohepatitic subtype (H&E, x200).

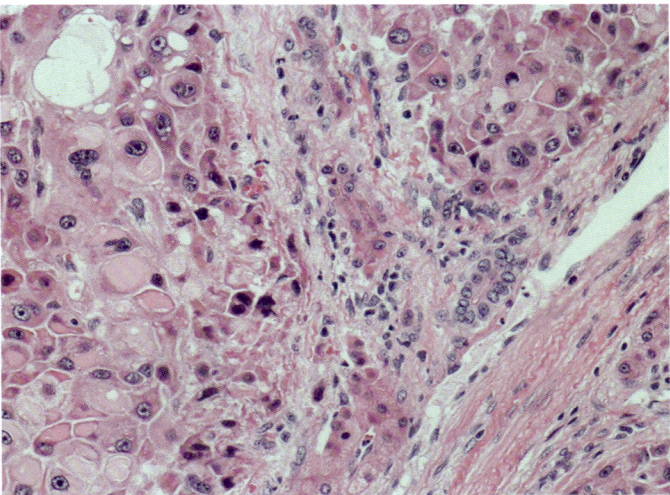

IMAGE 15.107 Fibrolamellar hepatocellular carcinoma. Tumor cells with abundant eosinophilic cytoplasm and occasional pale bodies are separated by fibrous stroma (H&E, x400).

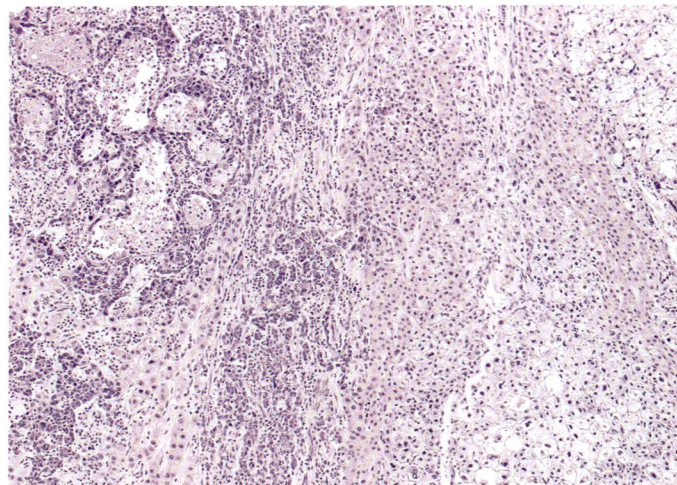

IMAGE 15.108 Mixed hepatocellular carcinoma (right side of image) and cholangiocarcinoma (left side of image) (H&E, x100).

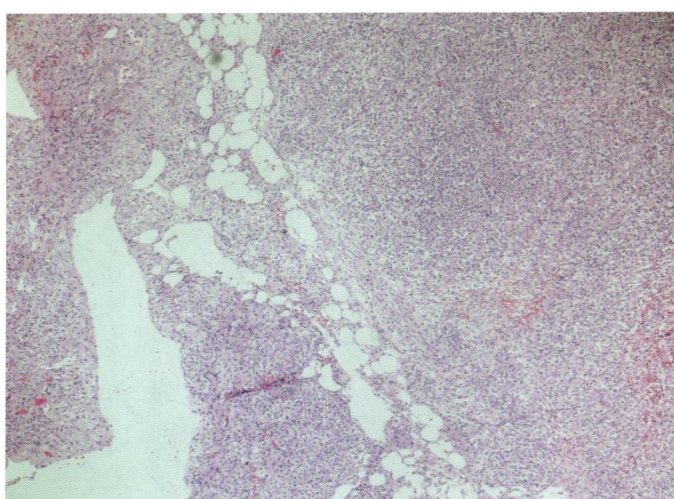

IMAGE 15.111 Liver angiomyolipoma. Liver parenchyma shows mixed vascular spaces, fat smooth muscle cells, and occasional hematopoietic elements (H&E, x40).

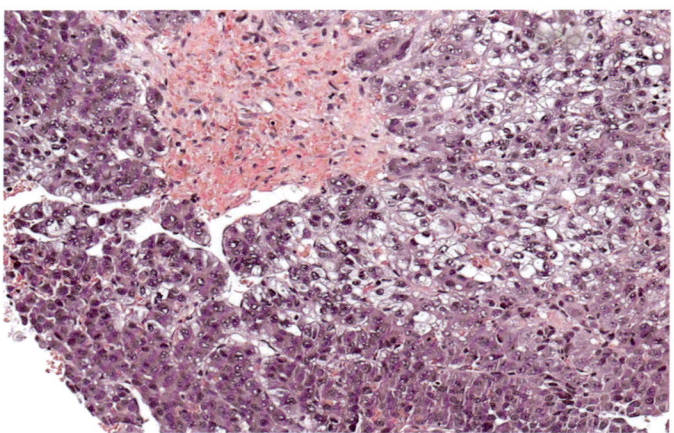

IMAGE 15.109 Hepatoblastoma with embryonal epithelium and focal mesenchymal component (H&E, x200).

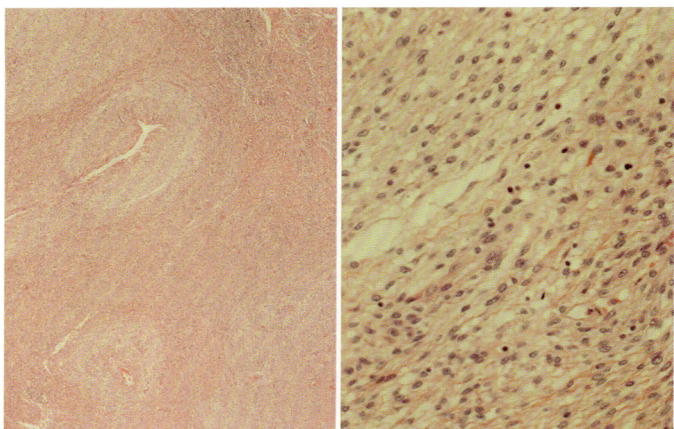

IMAGE 15.112 Follicular dendritic cell sarcoma. Left: the image shows a well- demarcated tumor with adjacent normal liver parenchyma and close relation of tumor cells with vessels (H&E, x40). Right: the image shows epithelioid spindle cells with oval nuclei and distinct nucleoli (H&E, x400). These tumor cells stain positive for CD21, CD23, and CD35.

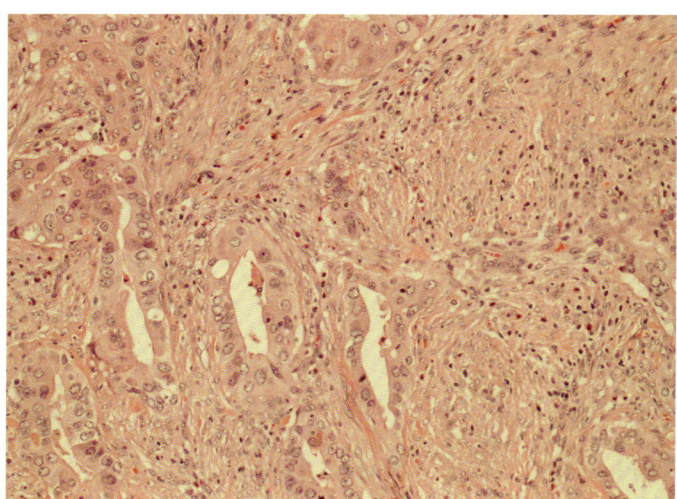

IMAGE 15.110 Liver carcinosarcoma. The image shows infiltrating malignant glands admixed with atypical spindle cells (H&E, x200).

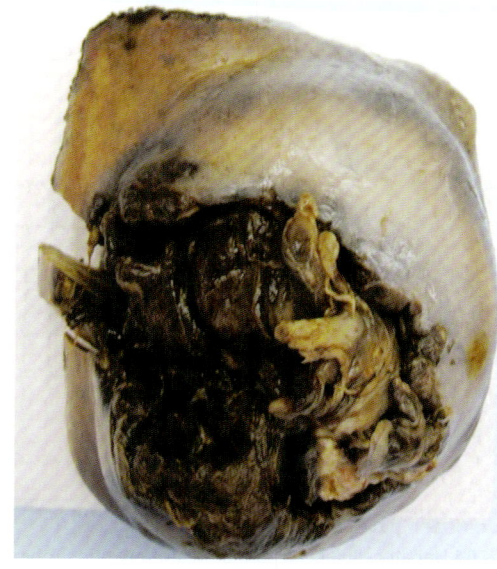

IMAGE 15.113 Liver embryonal sarcoma. The image shows a large hemorrhagic mass.

Courtesy of Dr. VH Nguyen.

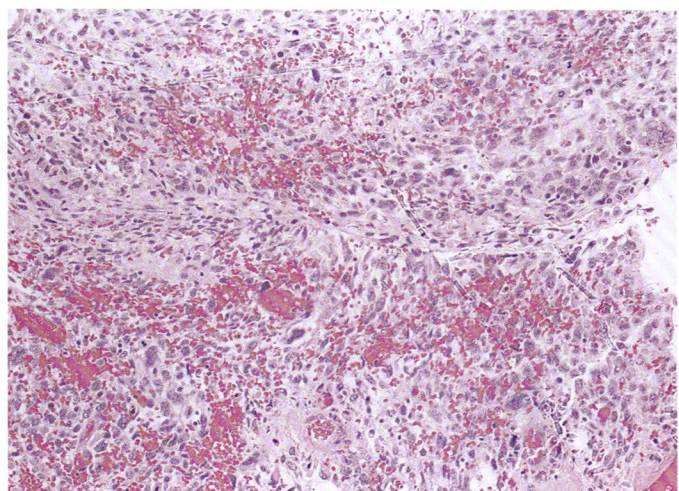

IMAGE 15.114 Liver embryonal sarcoma. The image shows hyperchromatic pleomorphic neoplastic cells with fresh hemorrhage (H&E, x200).

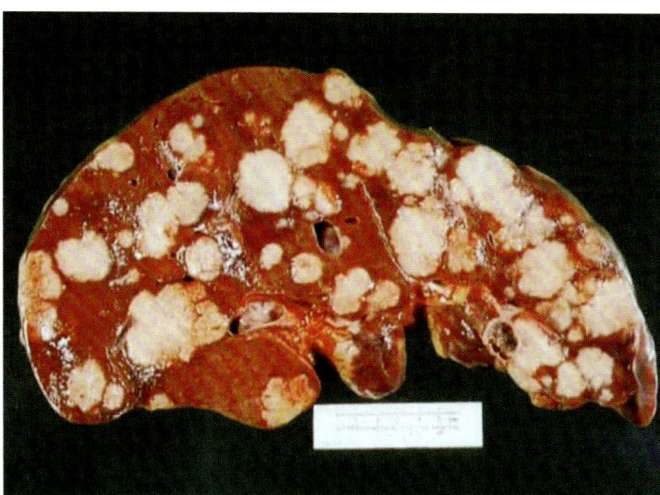

IMAGE 15.117 Liver with metastatic carcinoma. The image shows multiple tumor nodules randomly distributed throughout the liver.

Courtesy of Dr. Vincent Falck.

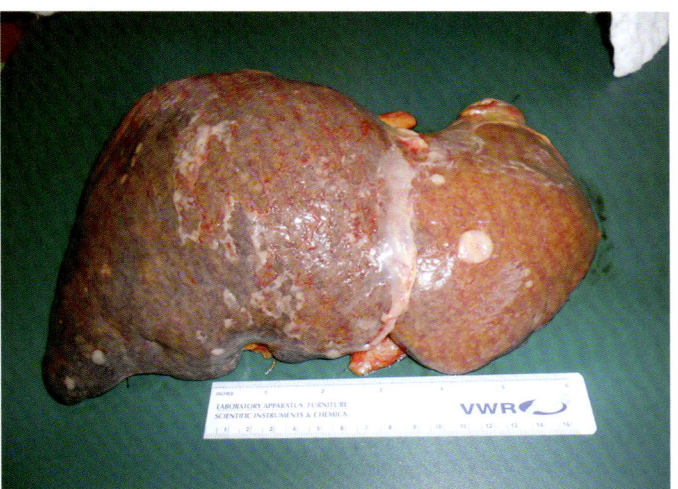

IMAGE 15.115 Liver involved by diffuse large B-cell lymphoma. The serosa of both lobes shows variable sized fleshy umbilicoid masses.

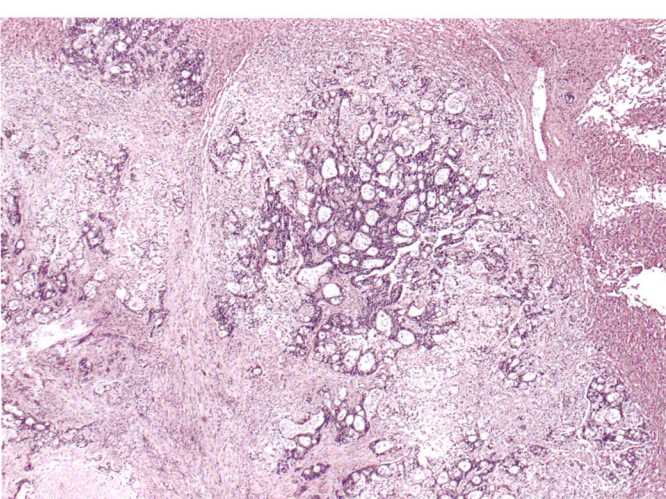

IMAGE 15.118 Metastatic colonic adenocarcinoma. The image shows tumor glands with characteristic intraluminal "dirty necrosis" (H&E, x40).

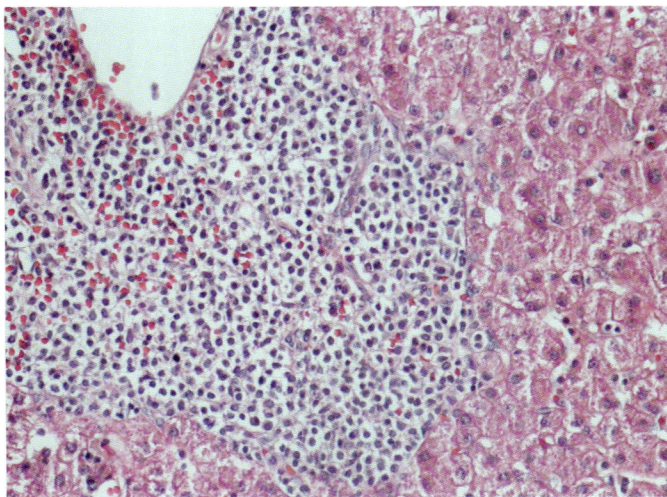

IMAGE 15.116 Hairy cell leukemia. The leukemia cells in the portal tract show characteristic clear cytoplasm (H&E, x400).

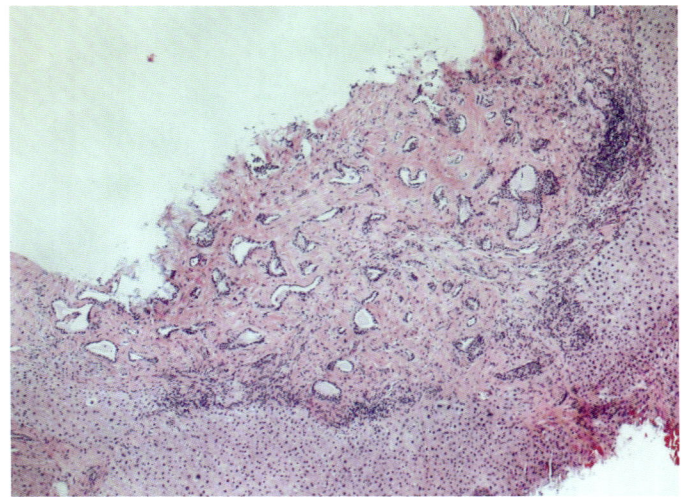

IMAGE 15.119 Bile duct hamartoma (Meyenburg complex). The image shows irregular branching glands with flat-cuboidal epithelial lining in fibrous stroma (H&E, x20).

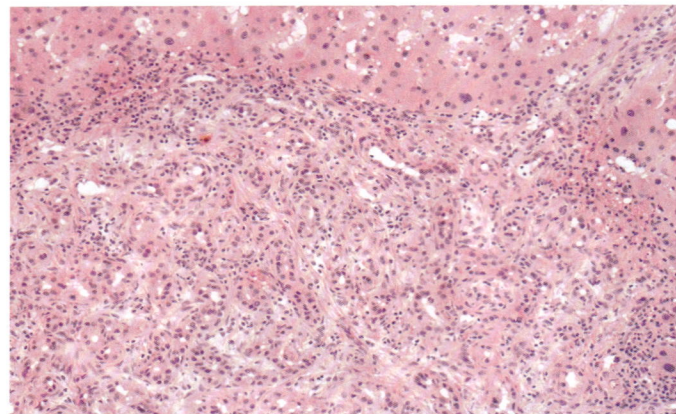

IMAGE 15.120 Bile duct adenoma. The image shows proliferation of benign tubules and glands within fibrous stroma. The lesion is sharply demarcated from the adjacent liver parenchyma (H&E, x100).

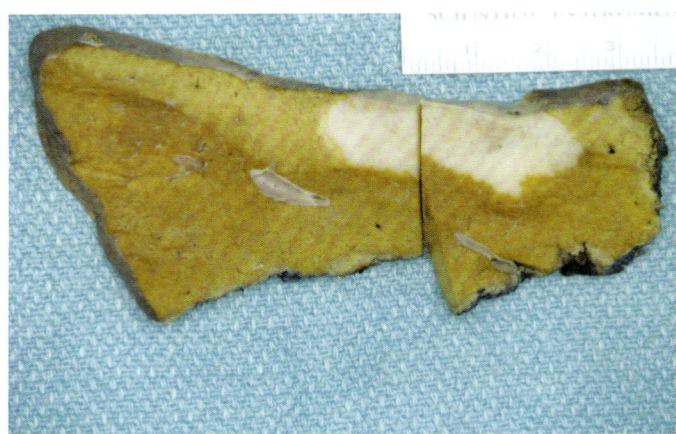

IMAGE 15.123 Cholangiocarcinoma. This is a solid tumor in the liver parenchyma with a whitish, fleshy cut surface.

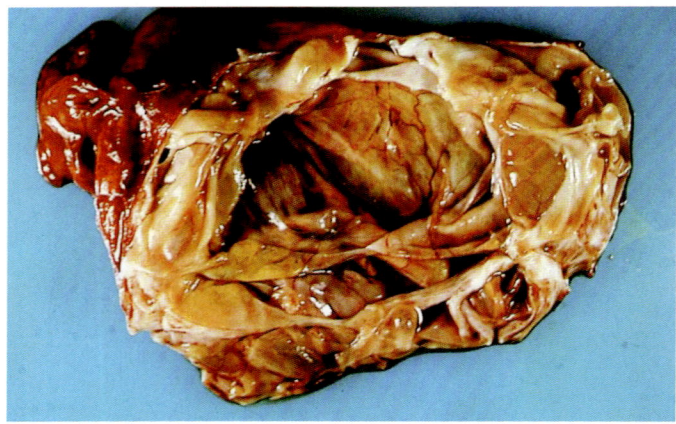

IMAGE 15.121 Mucinous cystic neoplasm of the liver. The cyst wall has been collapsed after opening and leaking of cystic contents.

Courtesy of Dr. Vincent Falck.

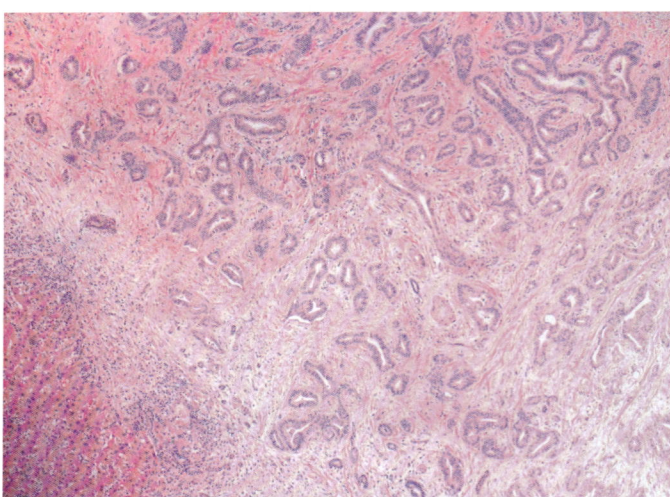

IMAGE 15.124 Intrahepatic cholangiocarcinoma. The image shows irregular malignant glands in desmoplastic stroma (H&E, x40).

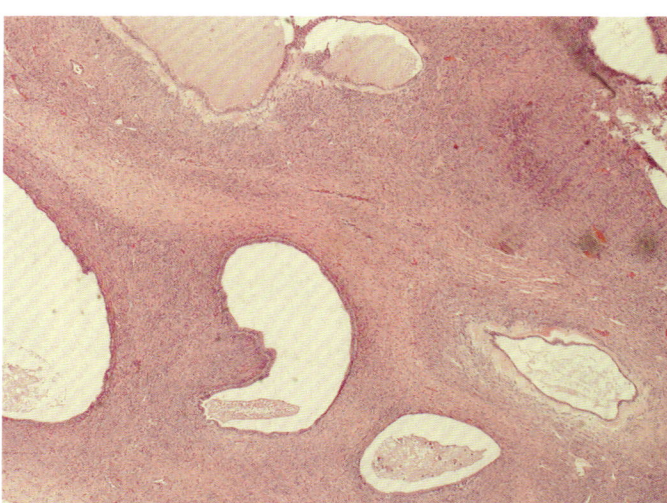

IMAGE 15.122 Mucinous cystic neoplasm of the liver with dense cellular ovarian-type stroma under the benign cyst epithelium (H&E, x40).

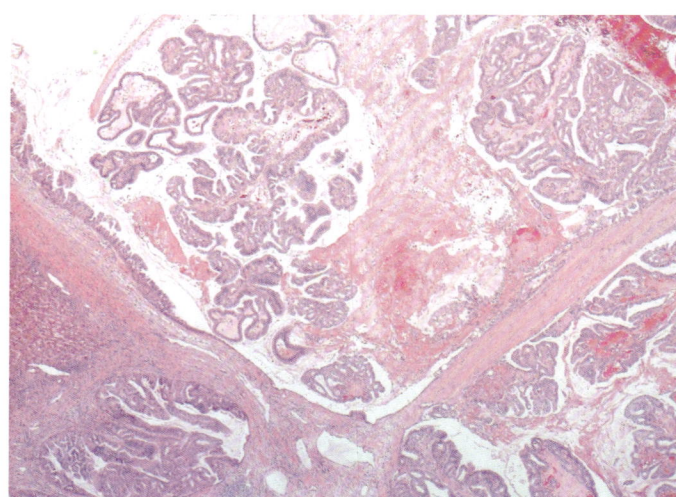

IMAGE 15.125 Mucinous cystic neoplasm of the liver with high grade intraepithelial neoplasia and associated invasive adenocarcinoma (H&E, x20).

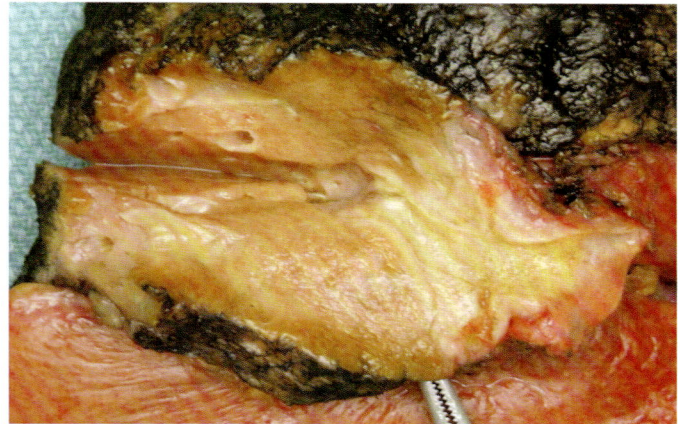

IMAGE 15.126 Hilar cholangiocarcinoma (Klatskin tumor) located at the confluence of the right and left hepatic bile ducts.

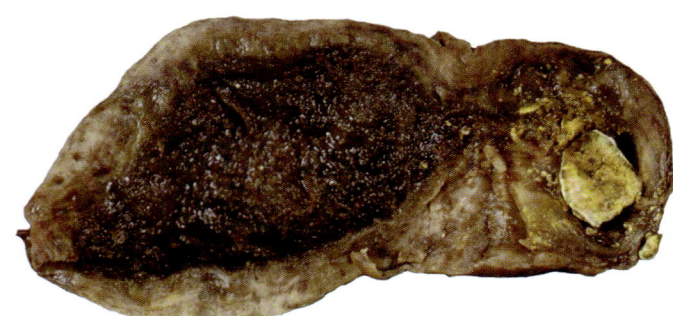

IMAGE 15.129 Acute calculous cholecystitis. Significantly thickened gallbladder wall with the gallstone obstructing the cystic duct is seen (at the right side of the image).

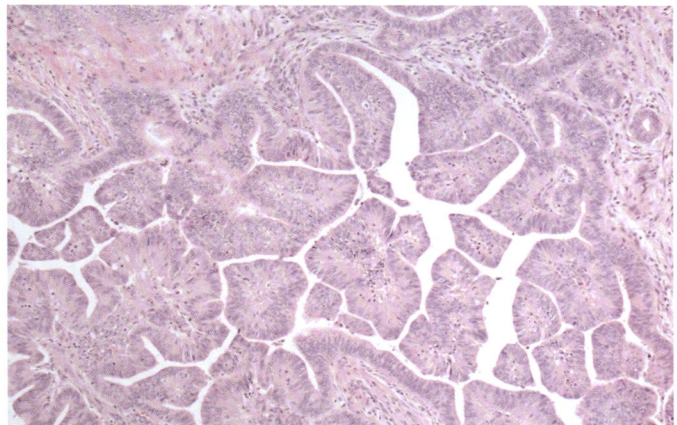

IMAGE 15.127 Common bile duct cholangiocarcinoma, papillary type (H&E, x100).

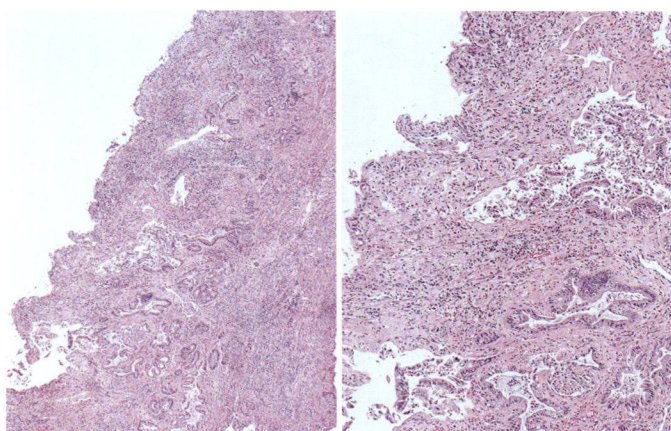

IMAGE 15.130 Acute cholecystitis. There is edema, surface erosion, and mixed neutrophilic and lymphoplasmacytic infiltration throughout the wall of the gallbladder (H&E; left: x40; right: x100).

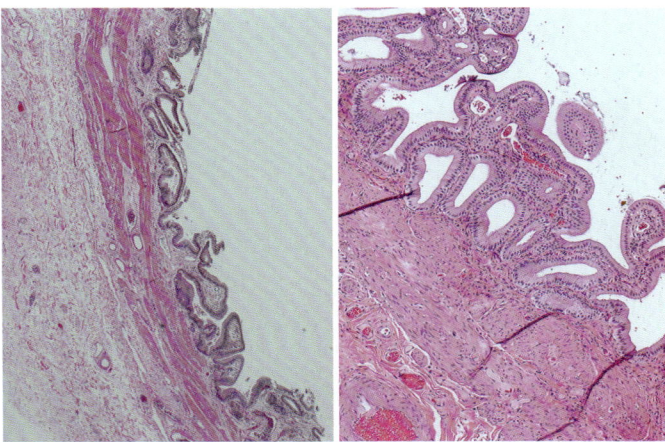

IMAGE 15.128 Normal gallbladder histology. The wall of the gallbladder consists of 3 layers: mucosa, muscularis propria, and serosa. Compared to the mucosa of the gastrointestinal tract, there is no muscularis mucosae and submucosa in the gallbladder (H&E; left: x20; right: x40).

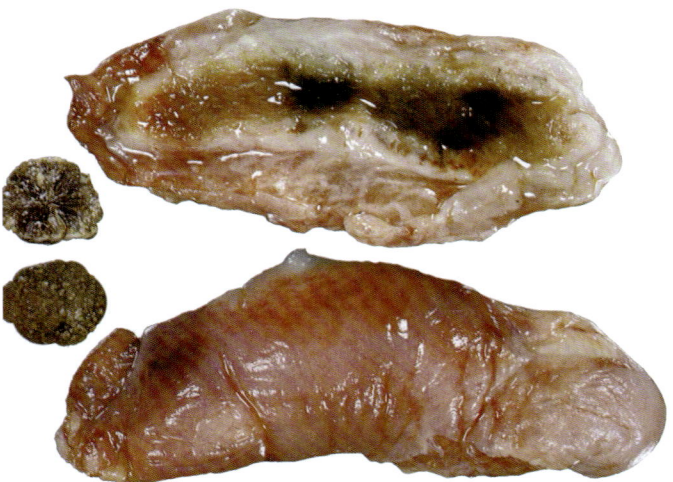

IMAGE 15.131 Chronic cholecystitis and cholelithiasis. Gallbladder shows significantly thickened wall.

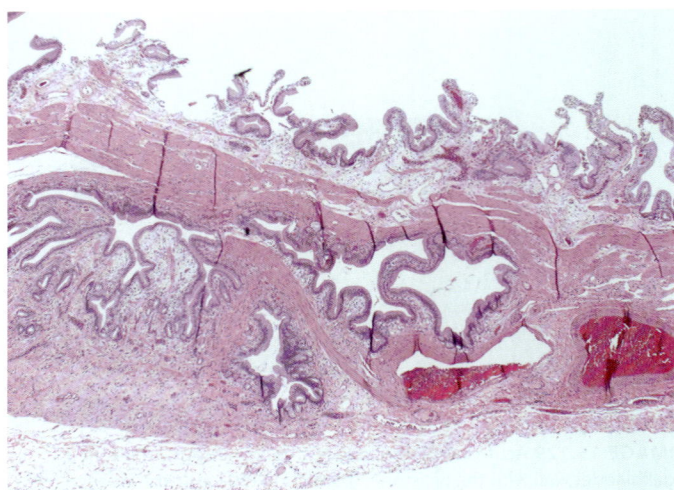

IMAGE 15.132 Chronic cholecystitis with Rokitansky-Aschoff sinuses (invaginations of mucosa through the muscularis propria into the muscularis propria and subserosa) (H&E, x100).

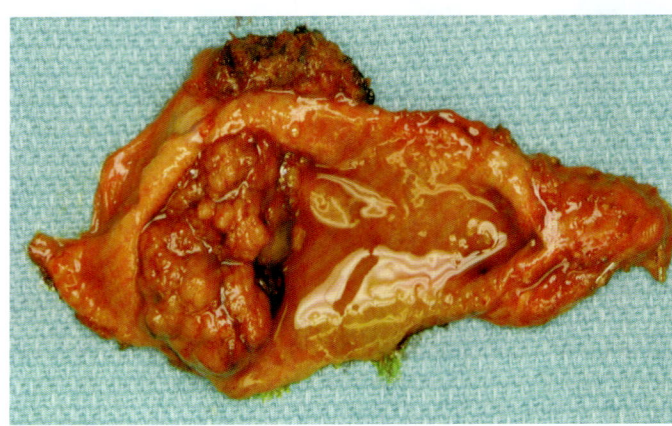

IMAGE 15.135 Gallbladder adenocarcinoma. The opened gallbladder contains a large exophytic tumor that partially fills the lumen.

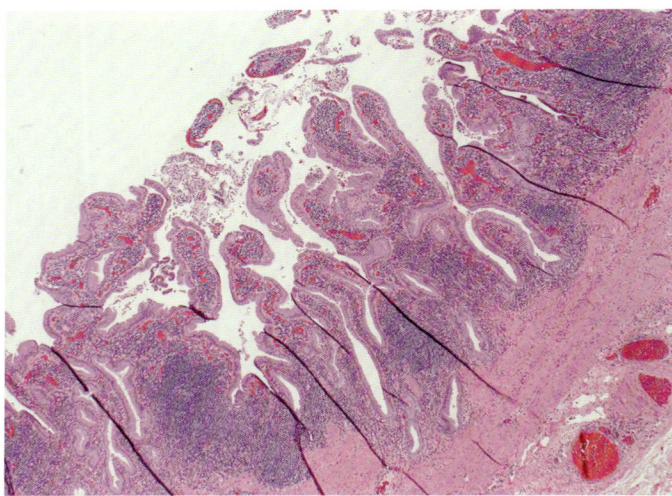

IMAGE 15.133 Follicular cholecystitis (H&E, x40). The image shows multiple lymphoid follicles distributed throughout the wall of the gallbladder.

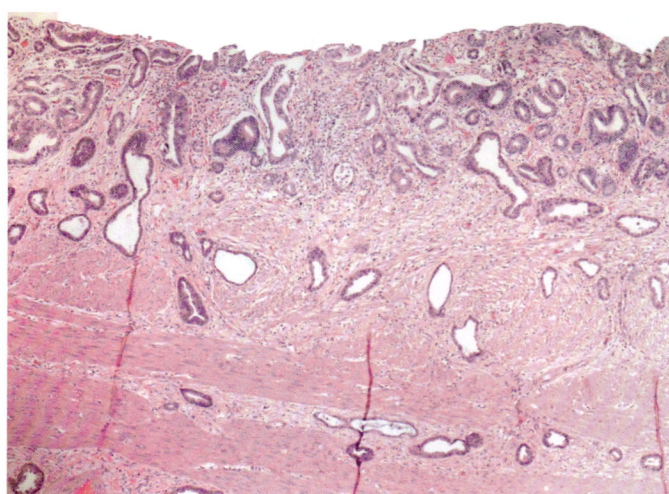

IMAGE 15.136 Gallbladder invasive adenocarcinoma (H&E, x40).

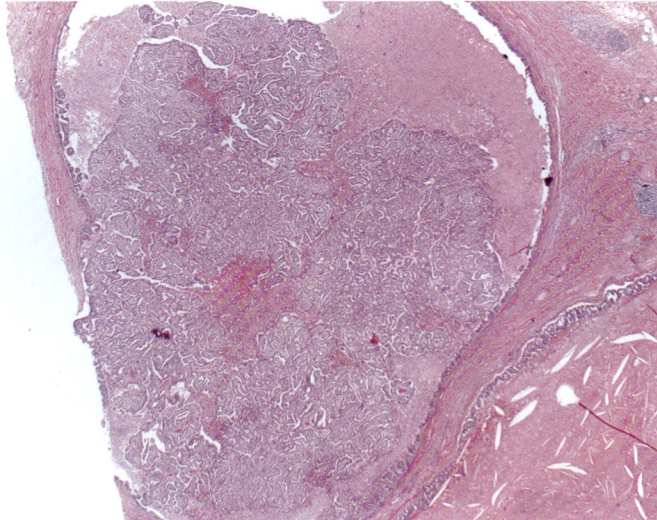

IMAGE 15.134 Intraductal tubulopapillary neoplasm (IPTN) of the common bile duct. It is characterized by predominantly tubular and focal solid growth patterns of biliary-type epithelium (H&E, x20).

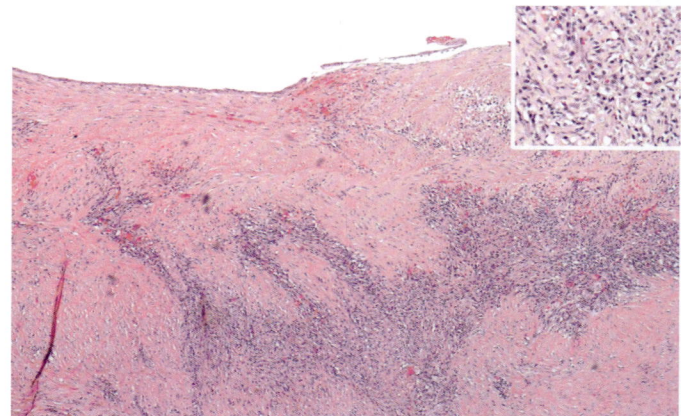

IMAGE 15.137 Xanthogranulomatous cholecystitis. The image shows a thickened fibrotic gallbladder wall infiltrated by mixed inflammatory cells with numerous foamy macrophages (main image: H&E, x40; inset: H&E, x200).

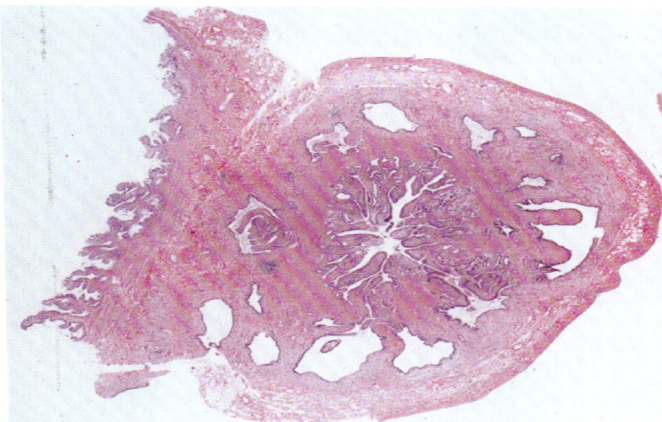

IMAGE 15.138 Adenomyoma of the gallbladder. A benign mass lesion at the fundus is formed by a cluster of herniated glands (Rokitansky-Aschoff sinuses) with muscle hypertrophy (H&E, x20).

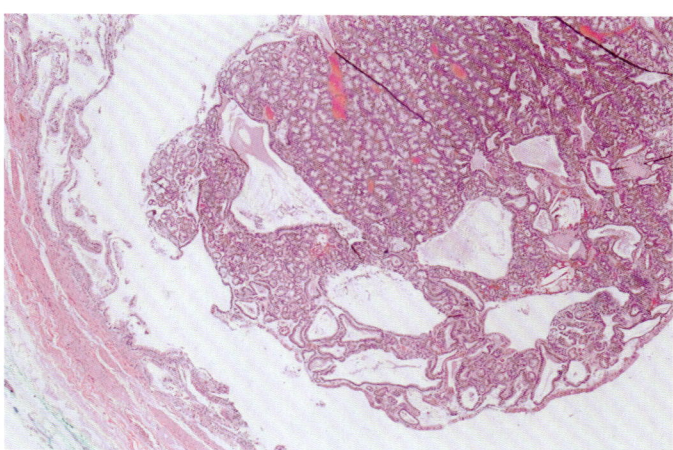

IMAGE 15.141 Gallbladder, intracholecystic papillary neoplasm (H&E, x20).

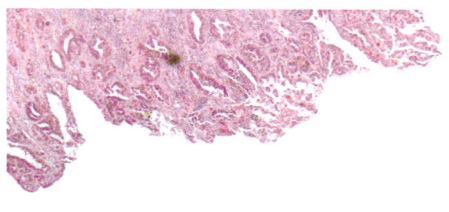

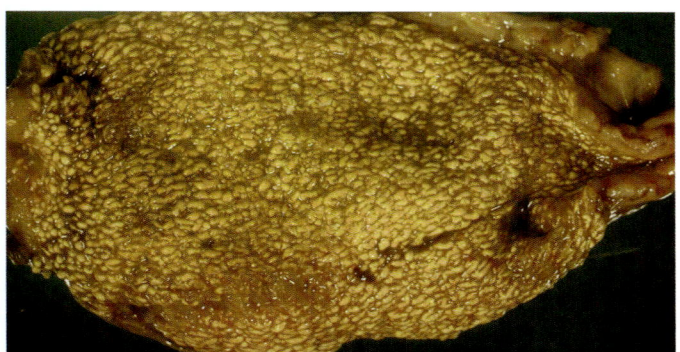

IMAGE 15.139 Cholesterolosis of the gallbladder (also known as "strawberry gallbladder").

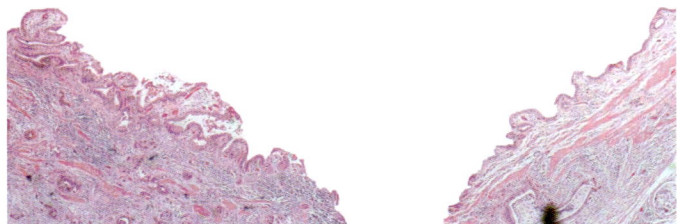

IMAGE 15.142 Cholangiocarcinoma. The tumor involves two-thirds of the common bile duct circumference (H&E, x40).

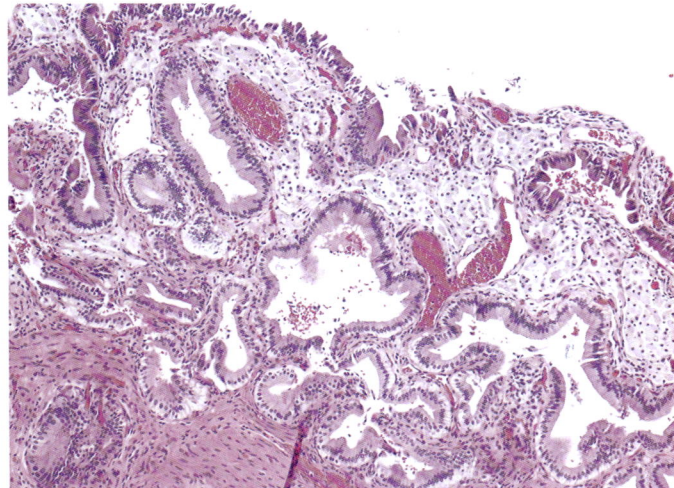

IMAGE 15.140 Cholesterolosis. The gallbladder mucosa contains many foamy macrophages in the lamina propria (H&E, x400).

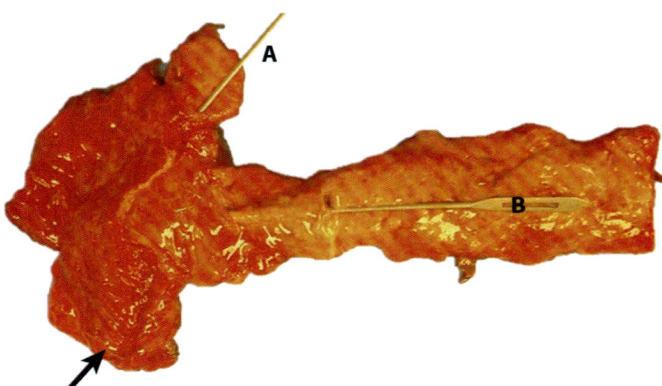

IMAGE 15.143 Normal pancreas with duodenum. The image shows the duodenum (arrow), common bile duct (probe A), and pancreatic duct (probe B).

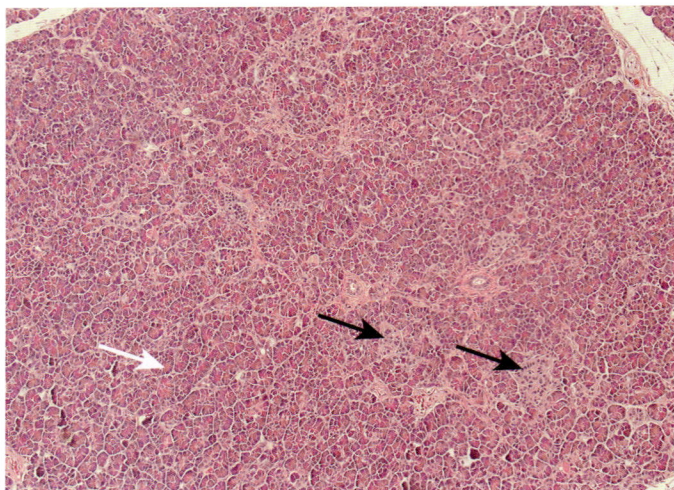

IMAGE 15.144 Normal pancreas histology. The exocrine pancreas consists of closely packed acini (white arrow). The endocrine pancreas (islets) (black arrow) is located within the exocrine lobules and secretes insulin, glucagon, somatostatin, and pancreatic polypeptide into the blood (H&E, x100).

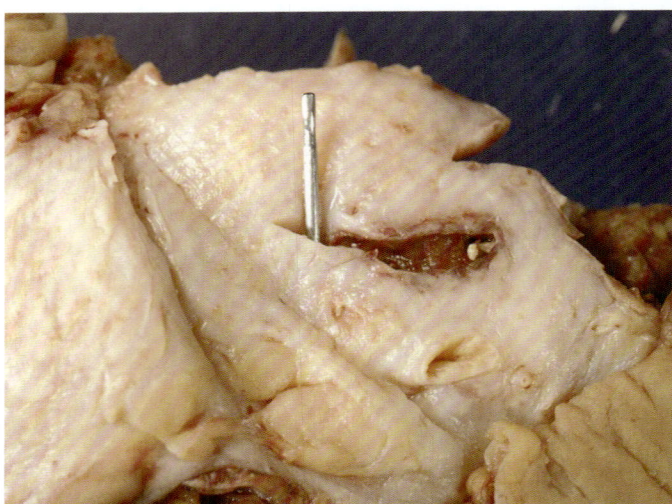

IMAGE 15.147 Chronic pancreatitis. The pancreas shows diffuse fibrosis of the pancreatic parenchyma and dilated pancreatic duct with concretions.

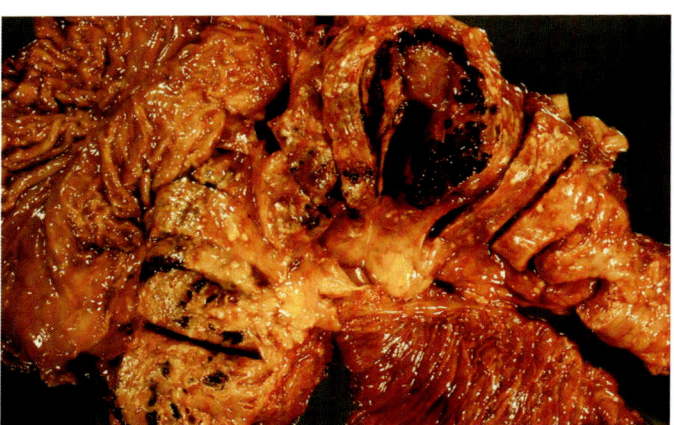

IMAGE 15.145 Acute hemorrhagic pancreatitis. The pancreas shows areas of hemorrhage and necrosis.

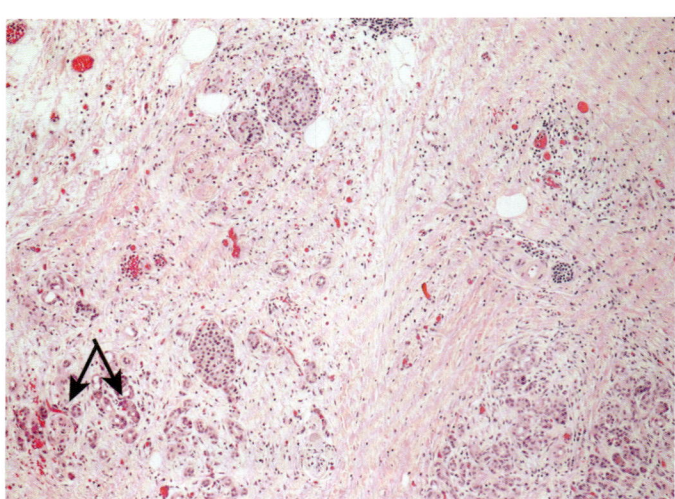

IMAGE 15.148 Chronic pancreatitis. The pancreas shows diffuse fibrosis of the pancreatic parenchyma, lobular arrangement of partially atrophic acini, acinar to ductal metaplasia (arrow), and pseudohyperplasia of islets of Langerhans (H&E, x100).

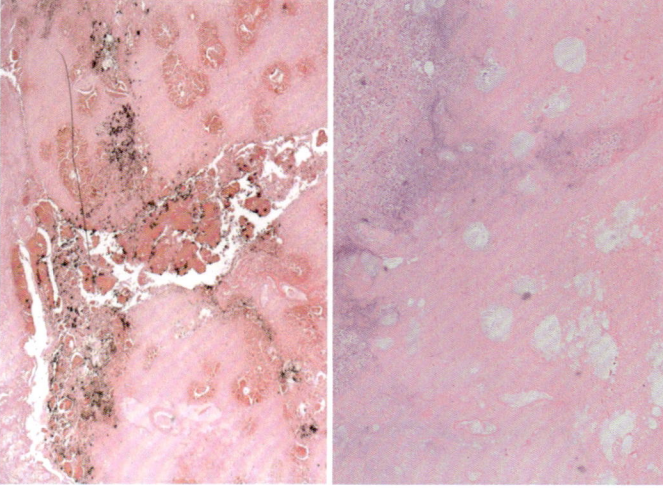

IMAGE 15.146 Acute hemorrhagic pancreatitis (two specimens). The pancreas shows diffuse hemorrhage and necrosis (H&E, x100).

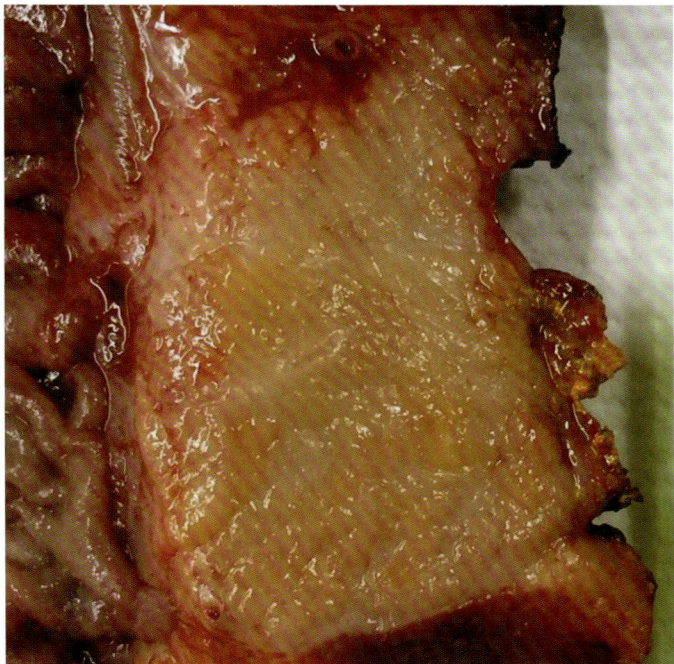

IMAGE 15.149 Chronic IgG4-related pancreatitis. The mass-forming lesion of IgG4-disease grossly mimics a neoplasm.

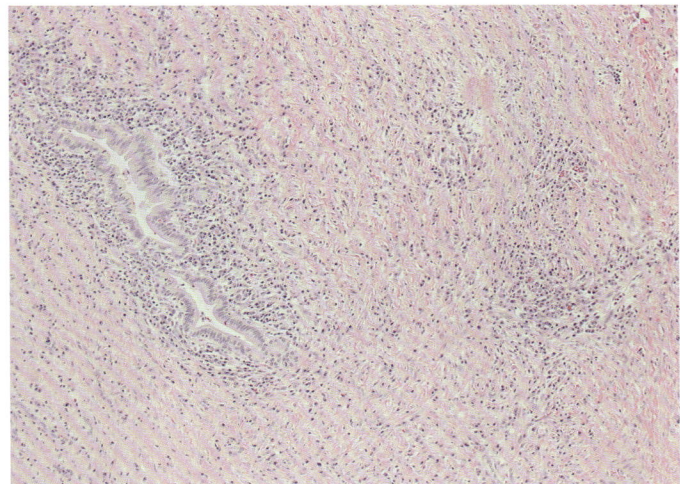

IMAGE 15.150 Chronic IgG4-related pancreatitis. The image shows duct-centric lymphoplasmacytic infiltration and periductal fibrosis (H&E, x100).

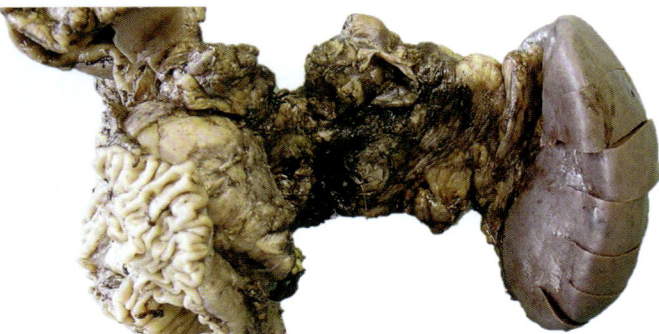

IMAGE 15.151 Pseudocyst arising in chronic active pancreatitis. Pancreatic pseudocysts are the result of autodigestion of the pancreas by pancreatic enzymes. It typically contains necrotic tissue, pancreatic enzymes, and degenerated blood, surrounded by granulation tissue and fibrosis.

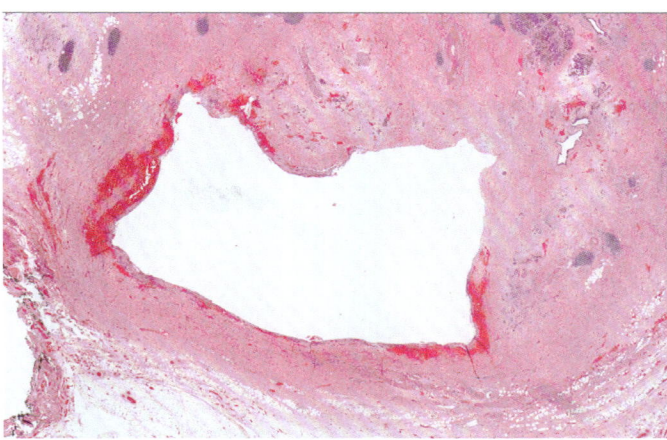

IMAGE 15.152 Pancreas pseudocyst. The cyst has no epithelial lining. Some inflammatory cells can be seen on the fibrous cyst wall (H&E, x10).

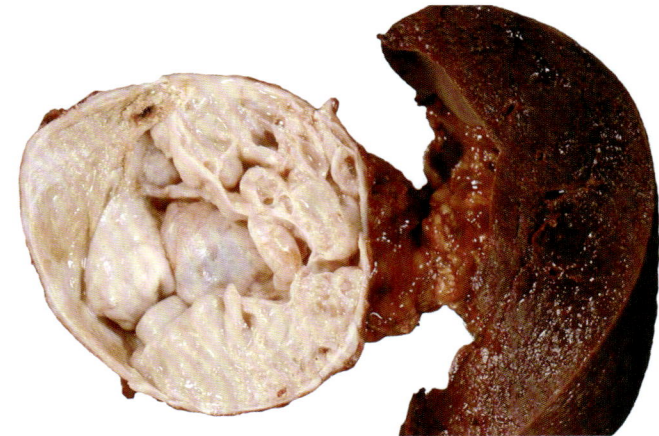

IMAGE 15.153 Pancreatic mucinous cystic neoplasm (cystadenoma). The tumor is usually 6–10 cm in size and formed by multiloculated cysts containing thick mucin.

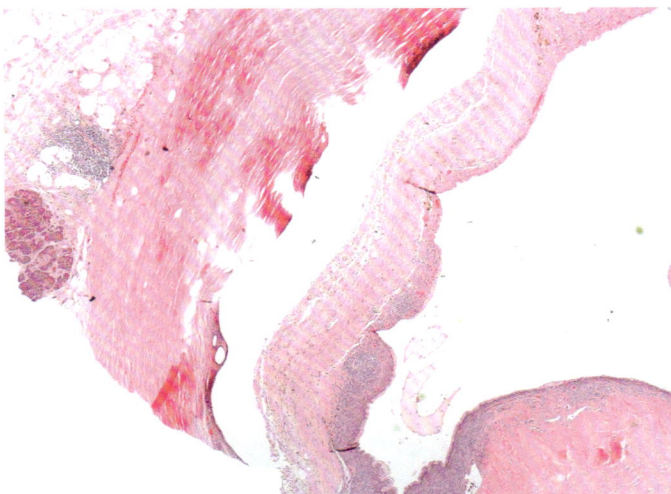

IMAGE 15.154 Pancreas mucinous cystic neoplasm with low grade dysplasia. The cyst is formed by a single layer of mucinous epithelium with a dense cellular ovarian-type stroma within its wall (H&E, x20).

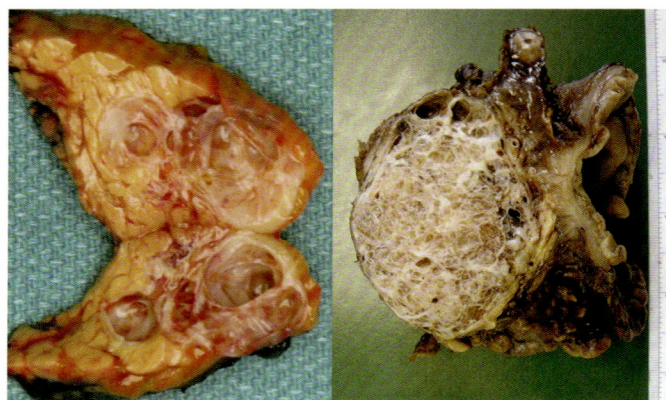

IMAGE 15.155 Pancreatic serous cystadenoma. The tumor typically shows a multilocular cystic neoplasm with a smooth, shiny internal surface, and it contains serous fluid. It is usually found in the tail of the pancreas.

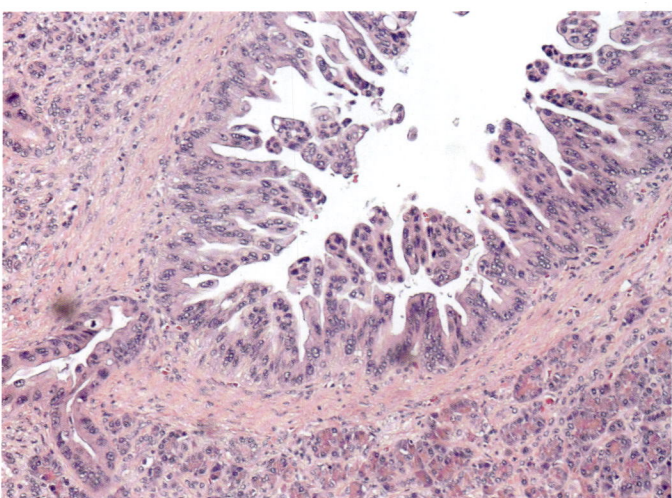

IMAGE 15.158 Pancreatic intraepithelial neoplasia, high grade (formerly PanIN-3). The image shows high grade nuclei with tufting (H&E, x200).

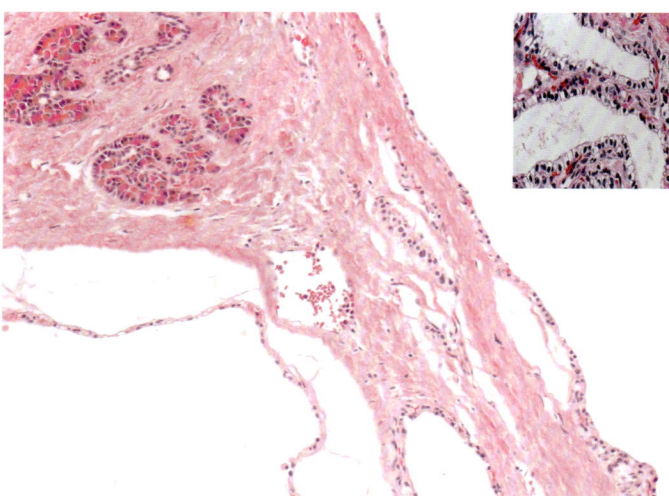

IMAGE 15.156 Serous cystadenoma pancreas (H&E, x40). Clear cytoplasm is highlighted in the inset from a different tumor (H&E, x200).

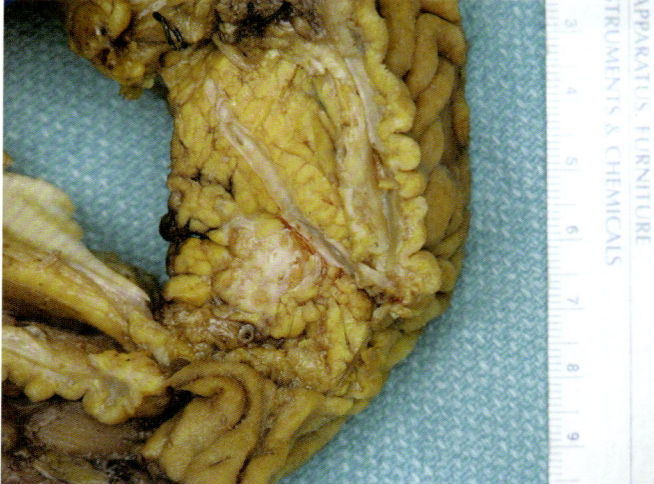

IMAGE 15.159 Pancreatic adenocarcinoma. The image shows a white fibrous mass at the head of pancreas. Its relation to pancreatic duct, common bile duct, and ampulla of Vater is illustrated.

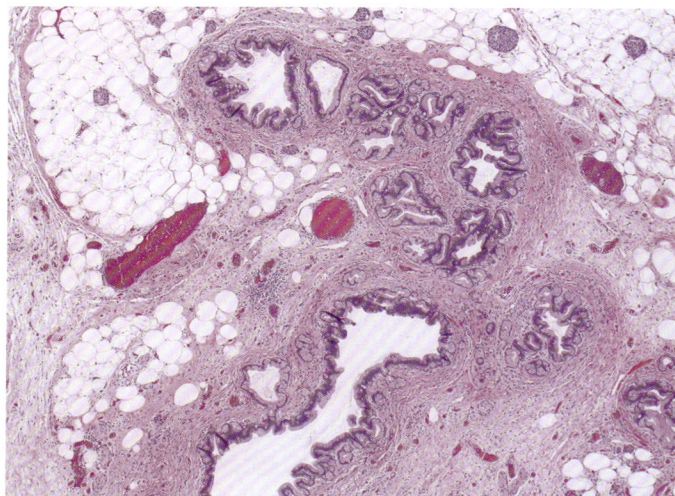

IMAGE 15.157 Pancreatic intraepithelial neoplasia, low grade (glandular intraepithelial neoplasia, low grade) (H&E, x40).

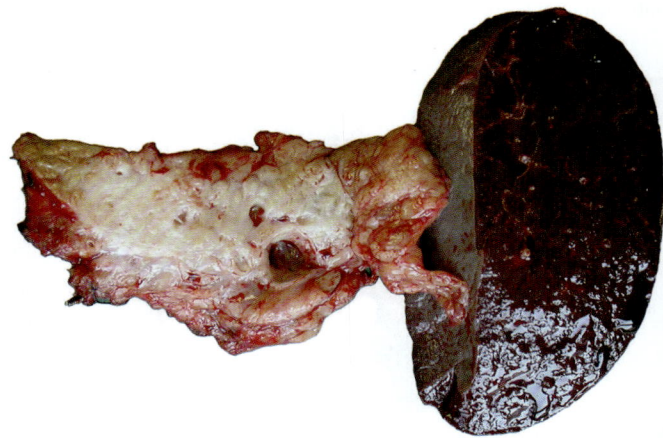

IMAGE 15.160 Invasive ductal adenocarcinoma of the distal pancreas. The tail of the pancreas shows a white tumor diffusely infiltrating the parenchyma but sparing the spleen.

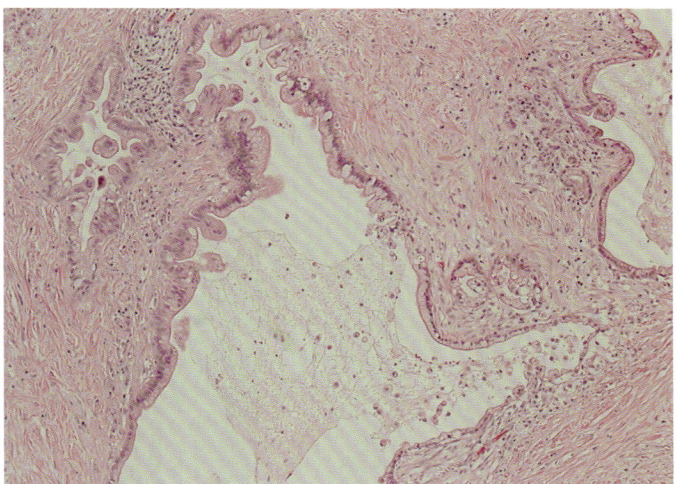

IMAGE 15.161 Well-differentiated pancreatic ductal adenocarcinoma (H&E, x100).

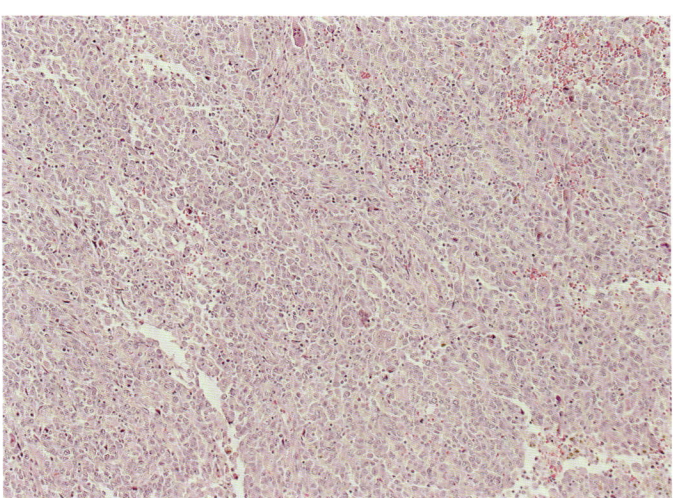

IMAGE 15.164 Undifferentiated invasive pancreatic ductal adenocarcinoma (H&E, x100).

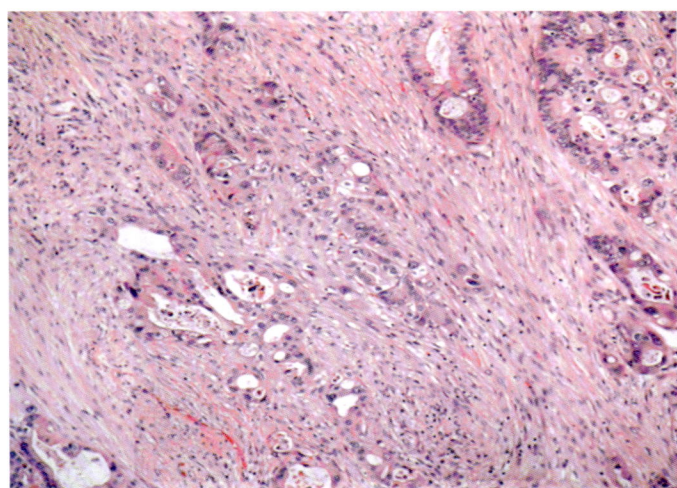

IMAGE 15.162 Pancreatic ductal adenocarcinoma, moderately differentiated (H&E, x200).

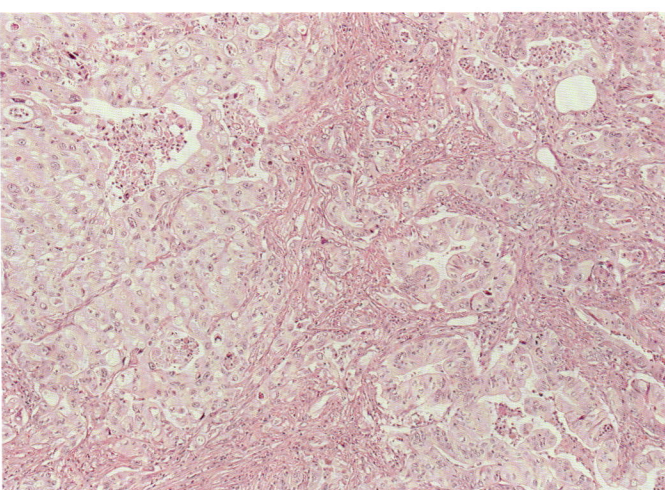

IMAGE 15.165 Adenosquamous carcinoma. Left: squamous cell carcinoma component. Right: invasive pancreatic ductal adenocarcinoma component (H&E, x100).

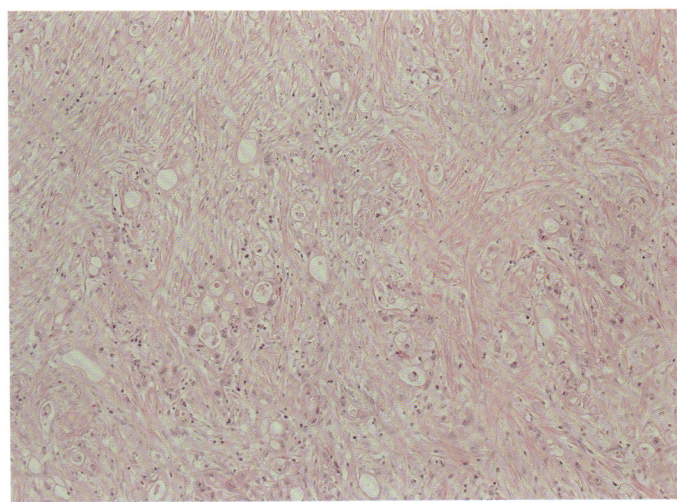

IMAGE 15.163 Poorly differentiated invasive pancreatic ductal adenocarcinoma (H&E, x100).

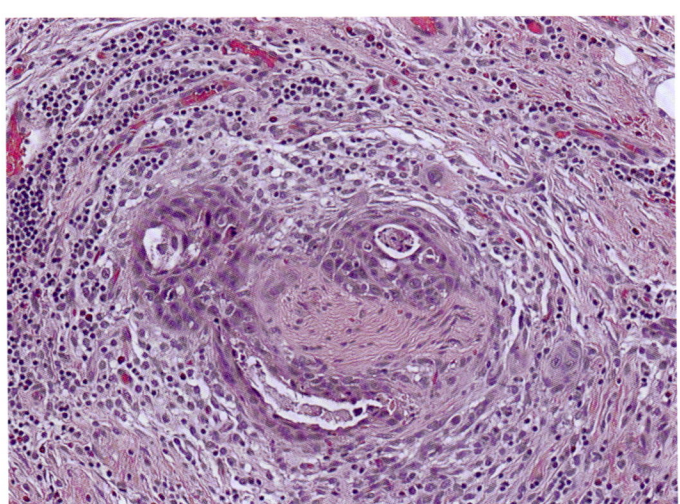

IMAGE 15.166 Pancreatic adenocarcinoma with perineural invasion (H&E, x100).

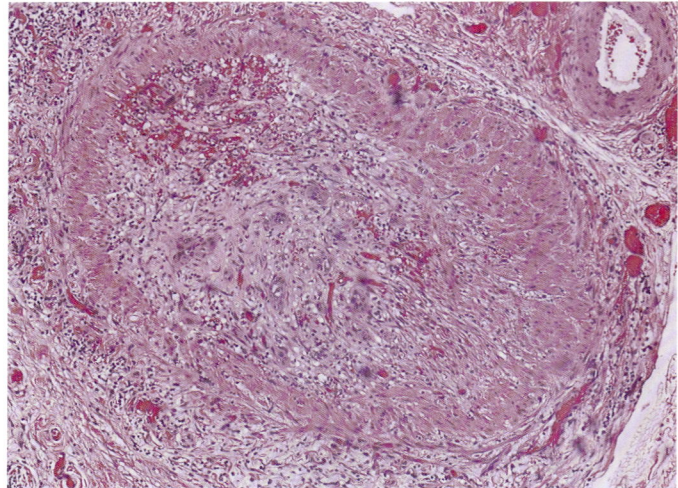

IMAGE 15.167 Pancreatic adenocarcinoma with large vessel invasion (H&E, x100).

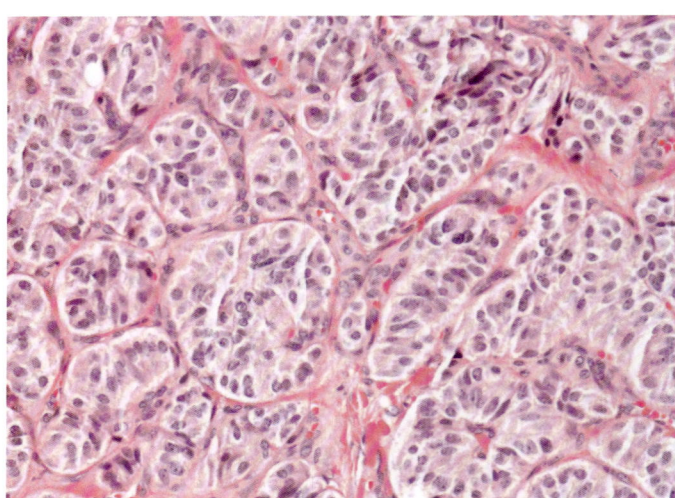

IMAGE 15.170 Pancreatic neuroendocrine tumor, grade 1. The image shows nests of tumor cells with characteristic "salt and pepper" nuclei in vascular stroma (H&E, x200).

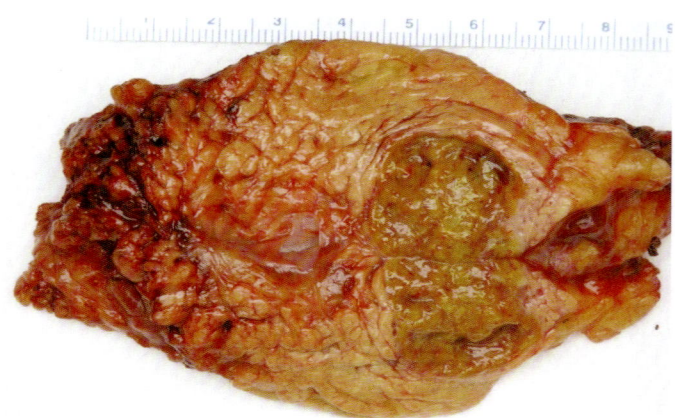

IMAGE 15.168 Pancreatic neuroendocrine tumor. This is a well-circumscribed neoplasm within the parenchyma of pancreas. The tumor has a characteristic yellowish homogenous cut surface.

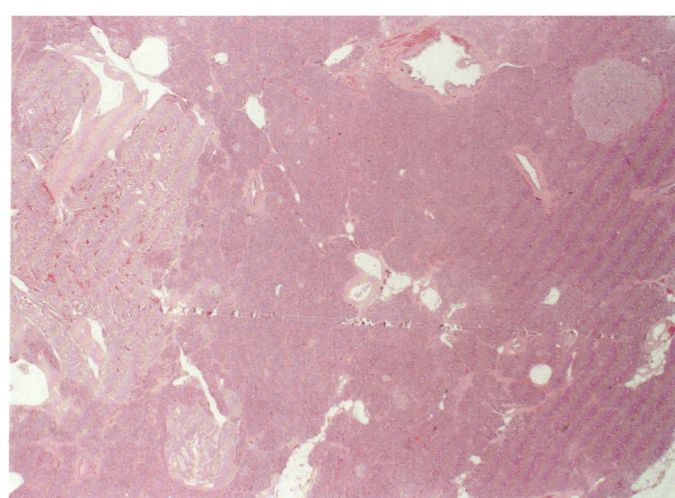

IMAGE 15.171 Multiple endocrine neoplasia type 1. The lower power image shows neuroendocrine hyperplasia (right upper) and neoplasia (left) (H&E, x20).

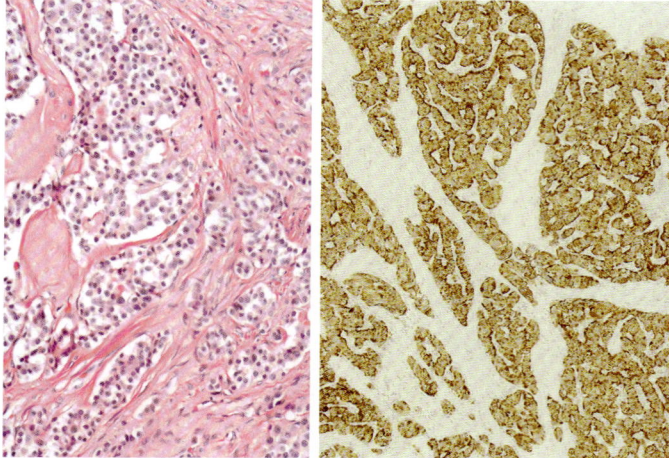

IMAGE 15.169 Insulinoma. Left: H&E, x100. Right: immunohistochemical staining with antibody against insulin immunoperoxidase, x100.

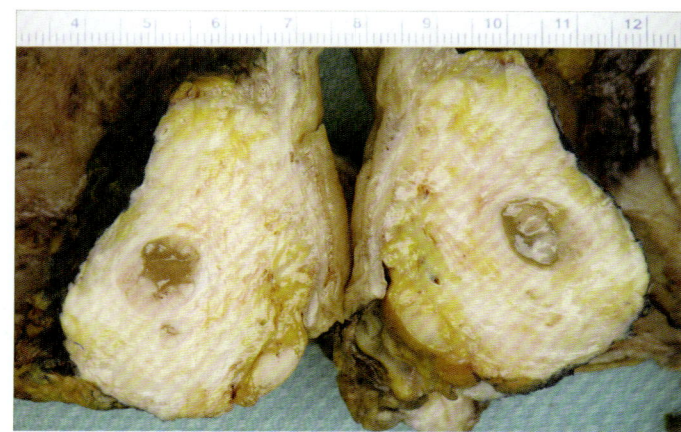

IMAGE 15.172 Intraductal papillary mucinous neoplasm (IPMN). This cross-section of pancreatic duct reveals a papillary lesion protruding into the dilated duct lumen with mucinous secretions.

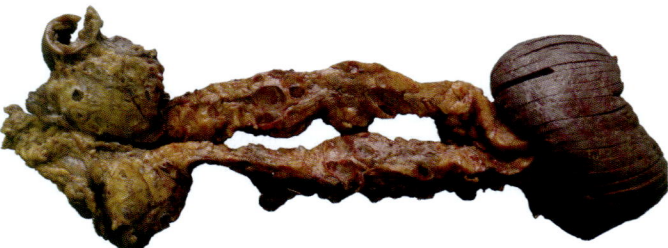

IMAGE 15.173 Intraductal papillary mucinous neoplasm involving both the main pancreatic duct and its branch ducts.

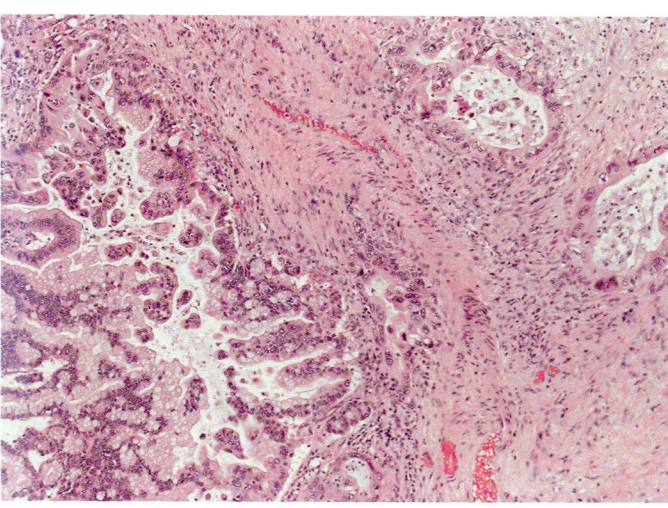

IMAGE 15.176 Intraductal papillary mucinous neoplasm, high grade, with associated invasive ductal carcinoma.

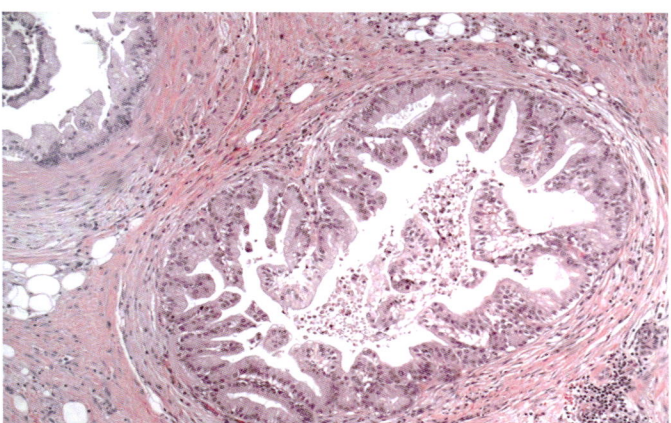

IMAGE 15.174 Intraductal papillary mucinous neoplasm with high grade dysplasia. Papillary proliferation of columnar mucinous cells project into the duct lumen with intraductal mucinous secretions (H&E, x100).

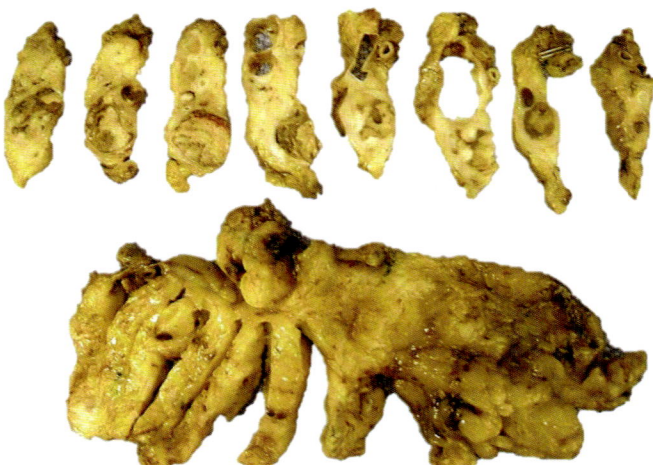

IMAGE 15.177 Intraductal tubulopapillary neoplasm. There is a solid tumor filling and expanding the dilated pancreatic duct lumen.

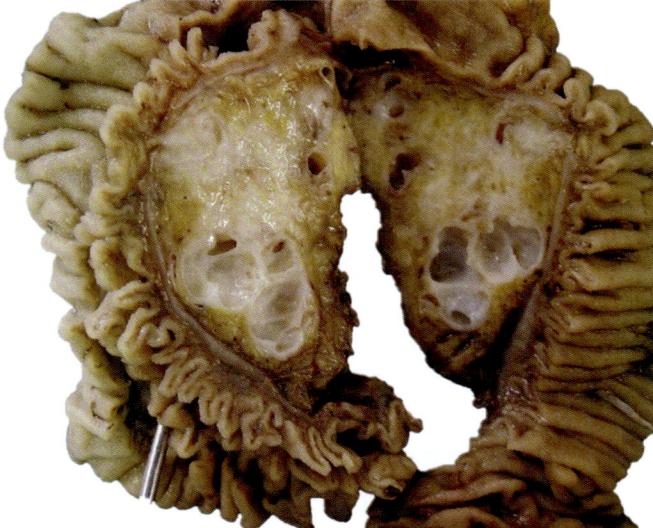

IMAGE 15.175 Invasive ductal adenocarcinoma arising from IPMN. This Whipple resection shows the head of the pancreas with a white tumor diffusely infiltrating the parenchyma surrounding the cystically dilated and tortuous duct of IPMN.

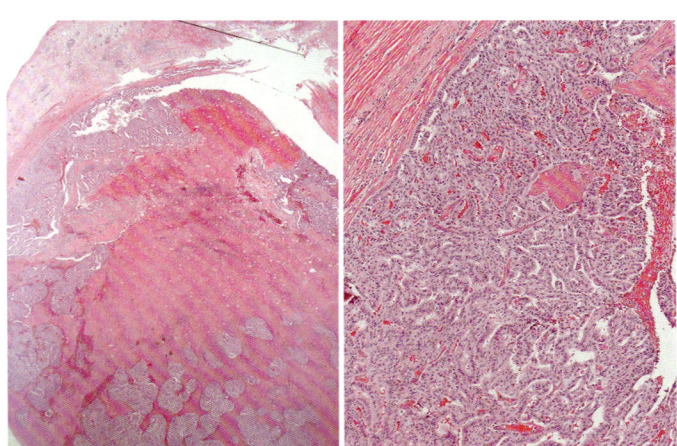

IMAGE 15.178 Intraductal tubulopapillary neoplasm. The dilated duct contains a neoplasm with tubulopapillary growth, uniform high grade cytological atypia, extensive necrosis, and absence of mucin (H&E: left, x10; right, x100).

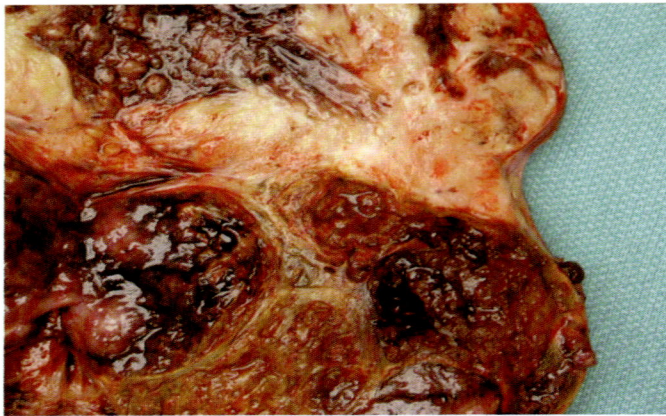

IMAGE 15.179 Solid pseudopapillary tumor. The tumor is well-demarcated from the remaining pancreas tissue without evidence of invasion, and it contains solid and cystic areas with focal hemorrhage and necrosis.

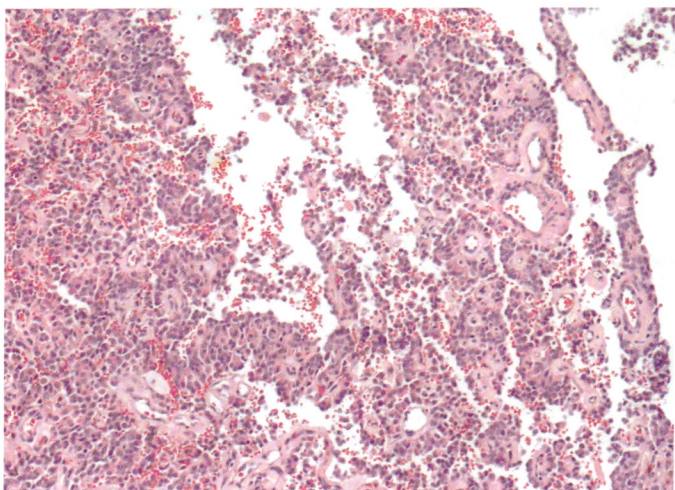

IMAGE 15.180 Pancreatic solid pseudopapillary tumor. Tumor cells between vessels are discohesive and degenerated, resulting in the formation of pseudopapillae (H&E, x100).

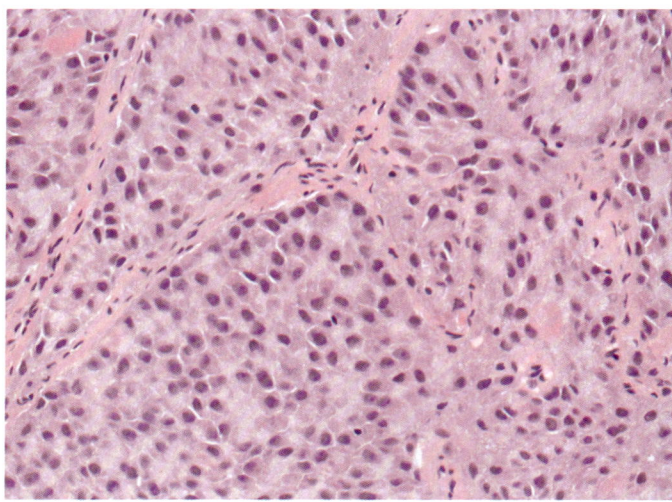

IMAGE 15.181 Pancreas acinar cell carcinoma. Tumor cells show abundant amorphous cytoplasm and form acinar architecture (H&E, x400).

References

1. Kleiner DE, Brunt EM, Van Natta M,et al. Design and validation of a histological scoring system for nonalcoholic fatty liver disease. Hepatology. 2005;41(6):1313-21. doi: 10.1002/hep.20701

2. WHO Classification of Tumours Editorial Board. WHO classification of tumours. 5th ed. Vol. 1, Digestive system tumours. Lyon (France): IARC; 2019.

Bibliography

Amin MB, Edge S, Greene F, et al, editors. AJCC cancer staging manual. 8th ed. New York: Springer; 2017.

Burgart LJ, Shi C, Adeyi OA, et al ; Cancer Committee, College of American Pathologists. Protocol for the examination of specimens from patients with carcinoma of the intrahepatic bile ducts (Version: IntrahepaticBileDuct 4.1.0.0) [Internet]. College of American Pathologists; 2020. Available from www.cap.org.

Burgart LJ, Shi C, Adsay NV, et al; Cancer Committee, College of American Pathologists. Protocol for the examination of specimens from patients with carcinoma of the gallbladder (Version: Gallbladder 4.1.0.0) [Internet]. College of American Pathologists; 2020. Available from www.cap.org.

Burgart LJ, Shi C, Adsay V, et al; Cancer Committee, College of American Pathologists. Protocol for the examination of specimens from patients with carcinoma of the exocrine pancreas (Version: PancreasExocrine 4.1.0.0) [Internet]. College of American Pathologists; 2020 Available from www.cap.org.

Burgart LJ, Shi C, Berlin J, et al; Cancer Committee, College of American Pathologists. Protocol for the examination of specimens from patients with carcinoma of the distal extrahepatic bile ducts (Version: Distal Extrahepatic Bile Duct 4.1.0.0) [Internet]. College of American Pathologists; 2020. Available from www.cap.org.

Burgart LJ, Shi C, Fitzgibbons PL, et al; Cancer Committee, College of American Pathologists. Protocol for the examination of specimens from patients with carcinoma of the perihilar bile ducts (Version: PerihilarBileDuct 4.1.0.0) [Internet]. College of American Pathologists; 2020. Available from www.cap.org.

Burgart LJ, Shi C, Fitzgibbons PL, et al; Cancer Committee, College of American Pathologists. Protocol for the examination of specimens from patients with hepatocellular carcinoma (Version: Hepatocellular 4.1.0.0) [Internet]. College of American Pathologists; 2020 Available from www.cap.org.

Burt AD, Ferrell LD, Hubscher SG. MacSween's pathology of the liver. 7th ed. Philadelphia (PA): Elsevier Ltd; 2022.

Centers for Disease Control and Prevention; Department of Health and Human Services, Division of Viral Hepatitis. Interpretation of hepatitis B serologic test results [Internet]. Center for Disease Control and Prevention; n.d. Available from www.cdc.gov/hepatitis.

Chen IY, Whitney-Miller CL, Liao X. Congenital hepatic fibrosis and its mimics: a clinicopathologic study of 19 cases at a single institution. Diagn Pathol. 2021;16(1):81. doi: 10.1186/s13000-021-01142-y

European Association for the Study of the Liver. EASL clinical practice guidelines: management of hepatocellular carcinoma. J Hepatol. 2018;69(1):182-236. PMID:29628281. doi: 10.1016/j.jhep.2018.03.019

Goldblum J, Lamps L, McKenny J, et al. Rosai and Ackerman's surgical pathology. 11th ed. Philadelphia (PA): Elsevier; 2017.

Graham RP, Jin L, Knutson DL, et al. DNAJB1-PRKACA is specific for fibrolamellar carcinoma. Mod Pathol. 2015;28(6):822-29. doi: 10.38/modpathol.2015.4

Honeyman JN, Simon EP, Robine N, et al. Detection of a recurrent DNAJB1-PRKACA chimeric transcript in fibrolamellar hepatocellular carcinoma. Science. 2014;343(6174):1010-14. doi: 10.1126/science.1249484

Kakar S, Burgart LJ, Batts KP, Garcia J, Jain D, Ferrell LD. Clinicopathologic features and survival in fibrolamellar carcinoma: comparison with conventional hepatocellular carcinoma with and without cirrhosis. Mod Pathol. 2005;18(11):1417-23. doi: 10.1038/modpathol.3800449

Kleiner DE, Brunt EM, Van Natta M, et al; Non-alcoholic Steatohepatitis Clinical Research Network. Design and validation of a histological scoring system for nonalcoholic fatty liver disease. Hepatology. 2005;41(6):1313-21. doi: 10.1002/hep.20701

Kleiner DE, Brunt EM, Van Natta M,et al. Design and validation of a histological scoring system for nonalcoholic fatty liver disease. Hepatology. 2005;41(6):1313-21. doi: 10.1002/hep.20701

Kumar V, Abbas AK, and Aster JC. Robbins and Cotran pathologic basis of disease. 10th edition. North York (ON): Elsevier Canada; 2020.

La Rosa S, Adsay V, Albarello L, et al. Clinicopathologic study of 62 acinar cell carcinomas of the pancreas: insights into the morphology and immunophenotype and search for prognostic markers. Am J Surg Pathol. 2012;36(12):1782-95. PMID:23026929. doi: 10.1097/PAS.0b013e318263209d

La Rosa S, Franzi F, Marchet S, et al. The monoclonal anti-BCL10 antibody (done 331.1) is a sensitive and specific marker of pancreatic acinar cell carcinoma and pancreatic metaplasia. Virchows Arch. 2009;454(2):133-42. PMID:19066953. doi: 10.1007/s00428-008-0710-x

Lalazar G, Simon SM. Fibrolamellar carcinoma: recent advances and unresolved questions on the molecular mechanisms. Semin Liver Dis. 2018;38(1):51-9. doi: 10.1055/s-0037-1621710

Lester SC. Manual of surgical pathology. 3rd ed. Philadelphia (PA): Elsevier Saunders; 2010.

Lokesh K, Prasad SR, Sunnapwar A, et al. Pancreatic neuroendocrine neoplasms: 2020 update on pathologic and imaging findings and classification. RadioGraphics. 2020;40(5);1240-62. doi: 10.1148/rg.2020200025

Longacre TA, editor. Mills and Sternberg's diagnostic surgical pathology. 7th ed. Philadelphia (PA): Wolters Kluwer; 2022.

Mayo SC, Mavros MN, Nathan H, et al. Treatment and prognosis of patients with fibrolamellar hepatocellular carcinoma: a national perspective. J Am Coll Surg. 2014;218(2):196-205. doi: 10.1016/jamcollsurg.2013.10.011

Nagtegaal ID, Odze RD, Klimstra D, et al. The 2019 WHO classification of tumours of the digestive system. Histopathology. 2020;76:182-88. doi: 10.1111/his.13975

Njei B, Konjeti VR, Ditah I. Prognosis of patients with fibrolamellar hepatocellular carcinoma versus conventional hepatocellular carcinoma: a systematic review and meta-analysis. Gastrointest Cancer Res. 2014;7(2):49-54. PMID: 24799971

Odze RD, Goldblum JR. Surgical pathology of the GI tract, liver, biliary tract, and pancreas. 4th ed. Philadelphia (PA): Elsevier; 2022.

Pandey CK, Karna ST, Pandey VK, Tandon M. Acute liver failure in pregnancy: challenges and management. Indian J Anaesth. 2015;59(3):144-49. doi: 10.4103/0019-5049.153035

Ranganathan S, Hicks J, Kim G, et al; Cancer Committee, College of American Pathologists. Protocol for the examination of specimens from pediatric patients with hepatoblastoma (Version: Hepatoblastoma 3.2.0.0) [Internet]. College of American Pathologists; 2016. Available from www.cap.org.

Shi C, Adsay V, Bergsland EK, et al; Cancer Committee, College of American Pathologists. Protocol for the examination of specimens from patients with tumors of the endocrine pancreas (Version: PancreasEndocrine 4.1.0.0) [Internet]. College of American Pathologists; 2020. Available from www.cap.org.

Sun Y, Zhou J, Wang L, et al. New classification of liver biopsy assessment for fibrosis in chronic hepatitis B patients before and after treatment. Hepatology. 2017;65(5):1438-50. doi: 10.1002/hep.29009

Tang LH, Basturk O, Sue JJ, et al. A practical approach to the classification of WHO grade 3 (G3) well-differentiated neuroendocrine tumor (WD-NET) and poorly differentiated neuroendocrine carcinoma (PD-NEC) of the pancreas. Am J Surg Pathol. 2016;40(9):1192-1202. doi: 10.1097/PAS.0000000000000662

Taskin OC, Clarke CN, Erkan M, et al. Pancreatic neuroendocrine neoplasms: current state and ongoing controversies on terminology, classification and prognostication. J Gastrointest Oncol. 2020;11(3):548-58. PMID: 32655934; PMCID: PMC7340800. doi: 10.21037/jgo.2020.03.07

Thompson ED, Wood LD. Pancreatic neoplasms with acinar differentiation: a review of pathologic and molecular features. Arch Pathol Lab Med. 2020; 144(7):808-15. doi: 10.5858/arpa.2019-0472-RA

WHO Classification of Tumours Editorial Board. WHO classification of tumours. 5th ed. Vol. 1, Digestive system tumours. Lyon (France): IARC; 2019.

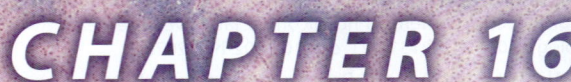

CHAPTER 16

Neuropathology

BASMA M. ALYAMANY,
HUDA T. ALGHEFARI,
JEFFREY T. JOSEPH,
JASON KARAMCHANDANI

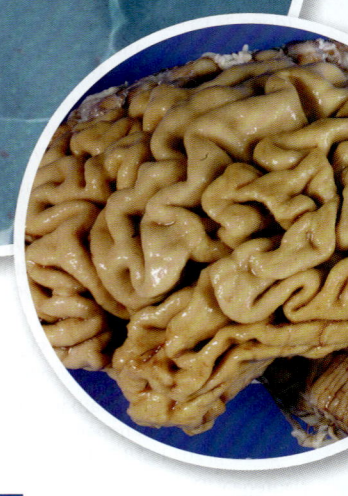

Neuropathology Exam Essentials

MUST KNOW

World Health Organization (WHO) classification

Neuropathology is a vast and complex field with many neoplastic and nonneoplastic lesions. Relatively speaking, primary tumors of the central nervous system (CNS) are infrequently examined in anatomic pathology and general pathology, hence we focus on lesions in the WHO classification that are common or high yield. Key CNS tumors that are part of syndromes are covered in the segment on genetic and systemic conditions.

- Before studying the WHO classification in depth, review the neuroanatomy and histology of major CNS components such as the cortex, white matter, and cerebellum.
- Key topics within primary CNS tumors include:
  · Astrocytoma.
  · Glioblastoma.
  · Oligodendroglioma.
  · Pilocytic astrocytoma.
  · Glial tumors as part of syndromes, such as subependymal giant cell astrocytoma (SEGA).
  · Meningiomas.
  · Pituitary and sellar tumors, including pituitary adenoma, craniopharyngioma,, and others.
  · Choroid plexus tumors.
  · Nonepithelial tumors, many of which cross over into other systems: solitary fibrous tumor (SFT),

lymphoma, sarcomas, germ cell tumors.
  · Peripheral nerve tumors: schwannoma, neurofibroma, perineurioma, malignant peripheral nerve sheath tumor (MPNST).
  · Neural-related tumors: chordoma, granular cell tumor, neurothekeoma.
  · The role of molecular pathology in the modern classification of CNS tumors.
  · Metastasis (don't forget about this).

AJCC and College of American Pathologists (CAP) protocols

AJCC and CAP have only 1 protocol for all tumors of the brain and spinal cord. Pertinent details include (although these are unlikely to be examined in great depth):

- Importance of radiologic correlation for CNS tumors.
- Importance of location.
- WHO grading (in-depth knowledge of CNS tumor grades is not expected).
- Biomarker studies (you likely only need superficial knowledge of some biomarkers for glial tumors).

Nonneoplastic diseases

This includes a variety of conditions, some of which overlap with areas such as forensic pathology and infectious disease. The exam is more likely to include classic lesions than esoteric lesions. High-yield topics include:

- Neurodegenerative diseases (focus on very common entities):
  - Alzheimer disease.
  - Parkinson disease, parkinsonism, and Lewy body dementia.
  - Demyelinating diseases, including multiple sclerosis.
  - Huntington disease and trinucleotide repeat diseases.
  - Amyotrophic lateral sclerosis (ALS).
  - Common stains used in neurodegenerative diseases (e.g., Luxol fast blue, [LFB], glial fibrillary acid protein [GFAP], Bielschowsky).
- Traumatic brain injuries (these are sometimes asked in relation to forensic pathology:
  - Skull fractures.
  - Basilar skull fracture.
  - Brain herniations, Duret hemorrhages.
  - Traumatic and nontraumatic causes of brain hemorrhages.
- Other:
  - Toxic and metabolic diseases, especially alcohol.
  - Meningitis and infections, including complications of HIV.
  - Prion disease.
  - Amyloid and amyloid angiopathy.
  - Hypoxic and ischemic changes, especially in relation to stroke.
  - Types of brain hemorrhages, including their location and relevant anatomic landmarks.
  - Aneurysms and vascular malformations.
  - Congenital malformations (e.g., anencephaly, holoprosencephaly, myelomeningocele, spina bifida).
  - Inflammatory myopathies.
  - Duchene and Becker muscular dystrophy.

Genetic and systemic conditions

- The CNS is a key area of manifestation for many syndromes and diseases. Study these syndromes not in isolation, but in conjunction with other organ systems in which they manifest. Key topics include:
  - Neurofibromatosis 1 and 2.
  - Von Hippel-Lindau disease.
  - Tuberous sclerosis.
  - Li-Fraumeni syndrome.
  - Cowden syndrome.
  - Turcot syndrome.
  - Gorlin syndrome.
  - SMARCB1 inactivation (rhabdoid tumor) syndrome.
- Many genetic diseases cause nonneoplastic lesions in the CNS. These are usually esoteric: don't spend too much time on them. Key topics include:
  - Trinucleotide repeat disorders.
  - Lysosomal storage disorders.
  - Leukodystrophies.
  - Mitochondrial and peroxisomal disorders.

- Systemic conditions with CNS changes (e.g., hemochromatosis, Wilson disease)

MUST SEE

Neuropathology is a field rich with entities that can show up as gross or microscopic images. The exam will likely focus on classic, typical diseases: hence, when providing answers, try not to be overly specific. For example, an infiltrating mass might be better described as high grade glioma, rather than as a specific type of glial cell and WHO grade.

- Key neoplastic images include:
  - Glioblastoma.
  - Pilocytic astrocytoma.
  - Oligodendroglioma.
  - Meningiomas.
  - Choroid plexus papilloma.
  - Pituitary and sellar tumors (e.g., pituitary adenoma, craniopharyngioma).
  - SFT, lymphoma, sarcomas, germ cell tumors.
  - Peripheral nerve tumors: schwannoma, neurofibroma, perineurioma, MPNST.
  - Granular cell tumor.
  - Chordoma.
  - Various metastasis, including ones that are hemorrhagic.
- Key nonneoplastic images include:
  - Alzheimer dementia.
  - Multiple sclerosis.
  - Parkinson disease.
  - ALS.
  - Huntington disease.
  - Neuronal changes in response to ischemia.
  - Recent and remote ischemic stroke.
  - Hemorrhagic stroke.
  - Ruptured berry aneurysm and arteriovenous malformation (AVM).
  - Bacterial and viral meningitis.
- Many findings overlap forensic pathology (see chapter 8), including:
  - Basilar skull fracture.
  - Duret hemorrhage.
  - Cerebral edema.
  - Various types of herniation: uncal, transtentorial, tonsillar, subfalcine, and others.
  - Coup contrecoup injury.
  - Cerebral cortex contusion.
  - Penetrating trauma and gunshot injuries, including skull fractures.
  - Epidural, subdural, and subarachnoid hemorrhage.
- Sometimes congenital and pediatric lesions can have specific appearances (see chapter 17), including:
  - Encephalocele.
  - Myelomeningocele.

- Spina bifida.
- Kernicterus.

- For each of the entities outlined in the Must See section, you should be comfortable generating a differential diagnosis and listing additional studies (e.g., histochemical or immunohistochemical stains).
- For entities that cross over into other chapters, the examinee should use them to complement this chapter.
- When studying in groups, practice:
  - Common forensic neuropathology findings, especially trauma related findings.
  - Classic neurodegenerative diseases, their gross and microscopic features.

- Thrombotic and ischemic diseases, especially stroke.
- Brain tumors (it is hard to predict which brain tumor might be examined; some possibilities include pituitary tumors, chordomas, and so on).
- You should be able to describe the grossing protocol for, and independently gross, the following specimens:
  - Brain biopsy.
  - Resection of brain mass.
  - Autopsy retrieval and cutting of brain.
  - Autopsy retrieval and examination of spinal cord.
- You should be able to describe and handle fresh specimens and frozen sections from brain biopsies, including making of smears.
- You should be able to describe and perform taking specimens for lymphoma workup.

MULTIPLE CHOICE QUESTIONS

1. The cell type that is **not** commonly found in the brain is:

  a. Neuron.
  b. Astrocyte.
  c. Lymphocyte.
  d. Microglia.
  e. Ependymal cell.

Answer: c

2. The pencil fibers of Wilson are a feature of which structure?

  a. Substantia nigra.
  b. Inferior olivary nucleus.
  c. Red nucleus.
  d. Putamen.
  e. Hippocampus.

Answer: d

3. Which of the following immunostains is a useful marker for neurons?

  a. Glial fibrillary acid protein (GFAP).
  b. Vimentin.
  c. Cytokeratin.
  d. APP.
  e. NeuN.

Answer: e

4. Which structure features neuromelanin pigmented neurons?

  a. Dentate nucleus.
  b. Substantia nigra.
  c. Caudate nucleus.
  d. Amygdala.
  e. Lateral geniculate body.

Answer: b

Neuromelanin is a nonenzymatically produced adduct of catecholamine byproducts. It accumulates in catecholaminergic neurons throughout the brainstem and is grossly visible in the substantia nigra and locus ceruleus.

5. Which of the following is **not** associated with fetal hypoxia or ischemic injury?

  a. Germinal matrix hemorrhage.
  b. Anencephaly.
  c. Periventricular leukomalacia.
  d. Schizencephaly-porencephaly.
  e. Subarachnoid hemorrhage.

Answer: b

Anencephaly results from a failure of neural tube closure, which occurs about the third to fourth week of gestation, long before fetal hypoxia or ischemic injuries develop. Periventricular leukomalacia is considered a border zone lesion that develops in the second and third trimesters. Germinal matrix hemorrhages are more common in the second trimester. Schizencephaly-porencephaly is thought to develop before or during early cortical gyration.

6. Which of the following is a likely associated finding or presentation of Chiari II malformation?

  a. Tuberous sclerosis.
  b. Germinal matrix hemorrhage.
  c. Periventricular leukomalacia.
  d. Ventricular enlargement.
  e. Heterotopia.

Answer: d

7. A 32-year-old man involved in a motorcycle accident has "raccoon eyes." Which is the most likely diagnosis?

  a. Subarachnoid hemorrhage.
  b. Basilar skull fracture.
  c. Diastatic fracture.
  d. Frontal depressed skull fracture.
  e. Tonsillar herniation.

Answer: b

8. Which vascular malformation is characterized by arterialized veins?

a. Arteriovenous malformation (AVM).
b. Venous angioma.
c. Cavernous angioma.
d. Capillary telangiectasia.
e. None of the above.

Answer: a

9. Which of the following statements concerning central pontine myelinolysis is **not** correct?

a. Rapid correction of hyponatremia is the cause.
b. It is usually located in the center of the pontine base.
c. It is associated with expanding mass lesions.
d. Similar lesions may occur outside the pons.
e. It has been associated with malnourished chronic alcoholics.

Answer: c

10. Which of the following would be the best stain to exclude amyloid angiopathy as a differential diagnostic consideration?

a. Periodic acid-Schiff (PAS).
b. Oil Red O.
c. Luxol fast blue (LFB).
d. Collagen IV.
e. Congo red.

Answer: e

11. Which characteristic antibody is the marker for Langerhans cell histiocytosis?

a. CD1a.
b. CD1b.
c. CD3.
d. CD8.
e. CD45.

Answer: a

12. Which of the following individuals are most likely to develop meningitis due to *Streptococcus pneumonia*?

a. A premature infant boy.
b. A 1-month-old baby girl.
c. An 18-year-old man.
d. A 60-year-old man.
e. None of the above.

Answer: d

13. Which is the most likely causative organism in rhombencephalitis?

a. Cytomegalovirus.
b. Rabies.
c. Herpes simplex virus, type 1 (HSV-1).
d. Human immunodeficiency virus (HIV).
e. West Nile virus.

Answer: c

14. A 42-year-old man with a history of renal transplant has developed multiple white matter lesions in both the brain and brain stem. The most likely diagnosis is:

a. Acute disseminated encephalomyelitis (ADEM).
b. Progressive multifocal leukoencephalopathy (PML).
c. Multiple sclerosis.
d. HIV leukoencephalopathy.
e. Subacute sclerosing panencephalitis (SSPE).

Answer: b

PML is caused by the JC virus, which infects predominantly astrocytes and oligodendrocytes. Infection of oligodendrocytes is lytic and causes the cell to die and its myelin to be lost. The multiple lesions are small or confluent foci of demyelination.

15. A 32-year-old man has multiple white matter lesions, many located periventricular. What is the most likely diagnosis?

a. Multiple sclerosis.
b. Cerebral autosomal dominant arteriopathy with subcortical infarcts and leukoencephalopathy (CADASIL).
c. Vasculitis.
d. Viral encephalitis.
e. Storage disease.

Answer: a

Multiple sclerosis is an inflammatory demyelinating disease that has a predilection for the periventricular region. Stretches of demyelination extending from the corpus callosum are called *Dawson's fingers*.

16. In the patient in question 15, a Luxol fast blue (LFB) stain shows large cells with staining of intracytoplasmic vacuoles in some of the periventricular white matter lesions. Which are the most likely cells?

a. Reactive astrocytes.
b. Macrophages.
c. Neutrophils.
d. Lymphocytes.
e. Eosinophils.

Answer: b

17. What is the most appropriate diagnosis for a 55-year-old man with rapidly progressive dementia and widespread spongiform cortical degeneration?

a. Creutzfeldt-Jakob disease.
b. Alzheimer disease.
c. Lewy body disease.
d. Gerstmann-Straussler-Scheinker disease.
e. New variant Creutzfeldt-Jakob disease.

Answer: a

18. The most likely diagnosis of a slowly growing tumor typically arising in the wall of the lateral ventricles in an 8-year-old girl with tuberous sclerosis is:

a. Cortical tuber.
b. Cortical dysplasia.
c. Subependymal giant cell astrocytoma.
d. Metastatic germ cell tumor.
e. Pilocytic astrocytoma.

Answer: c

19. The most likely location for a craniopharyngioma in a 12-year-old is:

a. Frontal lobe.
b. Fourth ventricle.
c. Cerebellum.
d. Suprasellar.
e. Pons.

Answer: d

20. Using the World Health Organization (WHO) schema for an ependymoma,* what is the most appropriate grade designation?

a. Grade 1.
b. Grade 2.
c. Grade 3.
d. Grade 4.
e. This tumor does not have a grade.

Answer: b

The pathologic grade of an ependymoma is significantly less relevant to the management of the patient than the extent of the surgical resection.

*This chapter uses the fifth edition of the WHO classification of tumors of the central nervous system.

21. How do you refer to the structures found in a pilocytic astrocytoma that contain multiple brightly eosinophilic inclusions?

a. Lewy bodies.
b. Corpora amylacea.
c. Marinesco bodies.
d. Granular bodies.
e. Rosenthal fibers.

Answer: d

22. Immunoreactivity with which antibody is most characteristic in glial neoplasms?

a. Glial fibrillary acid protein (GFAP).
b. S100 protein.
c. Vimentin.
d. Cytokeratin.
e. Epithelial membrane antigen (EMA).

Answer: a

23. The intermediate staining fibers on adenosine triphosphatase (ATPase) stained muscle section at pH 4.7 are:

a. Type 1.
b. Type 2A.
c. Type 2B.
d. Type 2C.
e. Type 3.

Answer: c

24. A 32-year-old woman has a heliotropic rash and proximal muscle weakness. Which is the most likely diagnosis if the muscle showed the presence of perifascicular atrophy on biopsy?

a. Dermatomyositis.
b. Neurogenic atrophy.
c. Muscular dystrophy.
d. Inclusion body myositis.
e. Gaucher disease.

Answer: a

25. The presence in a peripheral nerve of randomly oriented small bundles of axons surrounded by organized layers containing Schwann cells, fibroblasts, and perineurial cells is most likely to be encountered in the setting of:

a. Traumatic neuroma.
b. Amyloid neuropathy.
c. Vasculitic neuropathy.
d. Diabetic neuropathy.
e. Thiamine deficiency neuropathy.

Answer: a

26. Which of the following metazoan parasites is **not** associated with nervous system disease?

a. *Taenia solium*.
b. *Taenia saginata*.
c. *Schistosoma* species.
d. *Trichinella spiralis*.
e. *Echinococcus granulosus*.

Answer: b

27. Which of the following structures is most characteristic of embryonal tumor with abundant neuropil and true rosettes (ETANTR) and embryonal tumor with multilayered rosettes (ETMR)?

a. Homer-Wright rosette.
b. Ependymal rosette.
c. Ependymoblastoma rosette.
d. Flexner-Wintersteiner rosette.
e. Neurocytic rosette.

Answer: c

28. What feature does **not** distinguish a grade 2 from a grade 3 meningioma?

a. *TERT* promoter mutation.
b. Mitotic index ≥ 20/10 high power field (HPF).
c. Homozygous deletion of *CDKN2A* and/or *CDKN2B*.
d. Frank anaplasia.
e. Brain invasion.

Answer: e

29. Which of the following is **not** a typical feature of Parkinson disease?

a. Chorea-athetosis.
b. Stooped posture.
c. Masked facies or diminished facial expression.
d. Rigidity.
e. Tremor ("pill rolling").

Answer: a

Chorea-athetosis is a common feature in Huntington disease.

30. Which of the following is **not** typical of radiation effects?

a. Fibrinoid vascular necrosis.
b. Nuclear atypia.
c. Pseudopalisading necrosis.
d. Geographic necrosis.
e. Mineralization.

Answer: c

Pseudopalisading necrosis, with tumor cells aligned around small areas of necrosis, is characteristic of glioblastoma, including recurrent, actively proliferating glioblastoma that has occurred after radiation therapy.

Malformations and Developmental Diseases

31. Name at least 3 malformations resulting from neural tube defects.
- Anencephaly.
- Encephalocele.
- Spina bifida (spina dysraphism).
- Myelomeningocele.
- Chiari II malformation.

32. What are at least 2 developmental anomalies involving the cerebral cortex?
- Polymicrogyria.
- Pachygyria.
- Lissencephaly (classic) (agyria).
- Cobblestone lissencephaly.
- Periventricular nodular heterotopia.
- Laminar band heterotopia (double cortex).
- Holoprosencephaly.

33. Name 3 clinical settings in which microencephaly can appear.
- Fetal alcohol syndrome.
- Chromosome abnormalities.
- Infections acquired in utero (TORCH: toxoplasmosis, other infections, rubella, cytomegalovirus infection, herpes simplex).

34. List at least 3 features commonly associated with holoprosencephaly.
- Chromosome 13 trisomy.
- "Sonic hedgehog" deficit.
- Absence of the olfactory tracts.
- Absence of the gyrus rectus.
- Fusion of hemispheres.
- Ergot poisoning.

35. List the most common perinatal hemorrhages.
Acute, subdural, subarachnoid, subpial, intracerebral, white matter, subependymal, and choroid plexus.

36. Describe the mechanism of subdural hemorrhage in the perinatal period.
It is not related to asphyxia; it is related to perinatal distress during delivery involving compression and distortion of the head leading to disruption of the veins.

37. List the conditions associated with subependymal germinal plate/matrix hemorrhage.
- Coagulopathy.
- Congenital heart disease.
- Respiratory distress syndrome with hyaline membranes.
- Hypernatremia.

38. List the ultrasound grading of germinal matrix hemorrhage.
- Grade 1 — confined to germinal matrix.
- Grade 2 — germinal matrix and lateral ventricle, without ventricular dilatation.
- Grade 3 — germinal matrix and lateral ventricles, with acute dilatation by hematoma in ventricle.
- Grade 4 — grade 3 + hemorrhage into adjacent parenchyma.

39. List 6 key conditions associated with white matter necrosis/periventricular leukomalacia.
- Respiratory distress syndrome.
- Congenital heart disease.
- Septicemia.
- Shock.
- Intrauterine growth retardation (IUGR) with hypoglycemia.
- Meningoencephalitis.

40. Describe the clinical manifestation of white matter necrosis/periventricular leukomalacia (WMN/PVL).
It is initially nonspecific; later, patients develop spastic motor dysfunction.

41. Describe the pathogenesis of WMN/PVL.
- Perfusion at the boundary zone between ventriculopetal and ventriculofugal arteries, where metabolic requirements for myelination are high, is impaired.
- Developmental changes and selective vulnerability of oligodendrocyte precursor to free radicals and glutamate toxicity occur.
- Neonatal sepsis and endotoxemia increase anaerobic glycolysis and accumulation of lactic acid and free radical.
- Loss of cerebral autoregulation causes pressure-passive circulation.

42. List the 4 major features of Dandy-Walker syndrome and central nervous system (CNS) features associated with it.
- Features:
  - Vermal agenesis.
  - Cystically dilated fourth ventricle.
  - Enlarged posterior fossa.
  - Hydrocephalus.
- Associated CNS features:
  - Microcephaly.
  - Callosal agenesis.
  - Polymicrogyria and pachygyria.
- Aqueduct stenosis.
- Infundibular hamartoma.
- Occipital meningocele.
- Hindbrain abnormalities.
  - Cerebellar hypoplasia.
  - Cerebellar heterotopias.
  - Cerebellar cortical dysplasias.
  - Dentate dysplasia.
  - Olivary dysplasia and heterotopia.
  - Anomalies of the pyramidal tract decussation.

43. List 6 key systemic malformations associated with Dandy-Walker syndrome.
- Klippel-Feil syndrome.
- Cornelia de Lange syndrome.
- Cleft palate.
- Polycystic kidneys.
- Spina bifida.
- Polydactyly and syndactyly.

44. Define Chiari II syndrome.

Herniation of cerebellar vermis with malformation and downward displacement of brainstem.

45. Describe key anomalies associated with Chiari II syndrome.
- Brainstem:
  - Fusion of inferior colliculi; beak-like appearance to the quadrigeminal plate.
  - Indistinct pontomedullary junction; rod-shaped pons.
  - Looping of the lower medulla dorsally over the cervical cord.
- Dysplastic cranial nerves, olives, and pontine nuclei.
- Subependymal nodular heterotopias in lateral ventricles.
- Disordered cortical lamination.
- Abnormal upward course of the first 6 cervical spinal roots.
- Asymmetry or flattening of the cerebellar hemispheres.
- Lumbosacral myelomeningocele and hydrocephalus.

46. Describe the macroscopic appearance of the brain in alobar holoprosencephaly.
- Monoventricle.
- No interhemispheric fissure.
- Bizarre convolutional pattern.
- No gyri recti or olfactory structures.
- Dorsal surface of holosphere that continues as a delicate membrane, which is attached posteriorly to the tentorium.
- Fused basal ganglia and thalami.
- Hippocampus that makes continuous arch with the ventricle and attaches to the roof of the membrane.
- Absent corpus callosum and septum.
- Minimal white matter.

47. Name other systemic features in alobar holoprosencephaly.
- Craniofacial:
  - Cyclopia.
  - Fused ears.
  - Single nostril nose.
  - Microphthalmia.
  - Hypo/hypertelorism.
  - Agnathia.
  - Proboscis.
- Skeletal abnormalities:
  - Absent crista galli and lamina cribrosa.
  - Absent or shallow sella.
  - Absent falx and sagittal sinus.
  - Short narrow skull base.
- Circle of Willis:
  - The anterior cerebellar artery (ACA) and middle cerebellar artery (MCA) are replaced by forward directed branches of 1 or both internal carotids.
  - Dorsal cyst receives vascular supply from large choroidal arteries.

48. Describe the cerebral cortex in lobar holoprosencephaly.

It is continuous across the midline at the frontal pole, the orbital region, and above the callosum.

49. List key types of neuronal heterotopias.
- Diffuse.
- Nodular.
- Laminar.

50. What is the genetic mutation in fragile X syndrome?
- CGG premutation (55–200 repeat) expansion in the 5′ untranslated region of the *FMR1* gene.
- Cellular: RNA-mediated toxic gain of function.

51. What is a useful antibody for excluding polyglutamine repeat disorders?

1C2.

52. What is the pathognomonic histopathologic abnormality in fragile X syndrome?

Eosinophilic, ubiquitinated intranuclear inclusions in neurons and glial cells.

53. What is the mutation that causes Alexander disease?

GFAP gene.

54. What are the histologic locations of Rosenthal fibers in Alexander disease?

- Subpial.
- Perivascular.
- Subependymal.

55. List the pathologies in which Rosenthal fibers are found.

- Pilocytic astrocytoma.
- Hemangioblastoma.
- Benign brain tumors.
- Reactive conditions.
- Cortical dysplasia.
- Alzheimer disease.

56. What are the immunohistochemical stains used to stain Rosenthal fibers?

- Alpha B crystallin.
- GFAP.
- 27 kD heat shock protein.
- Ubiquitin.

57. What are the types of primary axial mesodermal defects?

- With herniation of the neural tissue: encephalocele and meningocele.
- Closed defects: split cord high.

58. What are the 3 tail bud defects?

- Spina bifida occulta.
- Split cord low.
- Hydromyelia.

59. Define kernicterus.

Selective yellow staining of deep grey matter and brainstem nuclei in bilirubin encephalopathy.

60. What is the pathogenesis of kernicterus?

- Bilirubin accumulates due to:
  · Excessive production.
  · Insufficient conjugation and excretion (unconjugated bilirubin is toxic).
- In the classic form of kernicterus, the bilirubin level is at least 30 mg/dL.
- Kernicterus follows hemolytic disease of newborns.
- Kernicterus is seen in small preterm infants with bilirubin as low as 10 mg/dL, who have suffered:
  · Asphyxia.
  · Acidosis.
  · Hypoglycemia.
  · Septicemia.
- Contributory factors include:
  · Damage to the blood-brain barrier.
  · Reduced binding of bilirubin to albumin during treatment with certain drugs or following hepatic necrosis.

61. What are the macroscopic and microscopic features of kernicterus?

- Macroscopy:
  · Characteristically affected areas.
  · Subthalamic nucleus.
  · Globus pallidus.
  · Lateral thalamus.
- Other affected areas:
  · Hippocampus (particularly the CA2 region).
  · Lateral geniculate nucleus.
  · Colliculi.
  · Substantia nigra.
  · Cranial nerve nuclei.
- Microcopy:
  · Accumulation of bilirubin causes neuronal necrosis and later gliosis and mineralization of affected neurons.

Reactions of the Central Nervous System to Injury

62. Name at least 4 reactions of astrocytes to injury.

- Gliosis.
- Cellular swelling.
- Rosenthal fibers.
- Corpora amylacea.
- Glial cytoplasmic inclusions.
- Alzheimer type II astrocyte.

63. List the histologic hallmarks of hypoxic-ischemic neurons.

- Eosinophilia of the neuronal cytoplasm.
- Loss of nuclear membrane integrity.
- Loss of Nissl substance.
- Pyknosis of the nucleus.
- Disappearance of the nucleolus.
- Karyorrhexis.

64. What are the major mechanisms and the major complication of cerebral edema?

- Major mechanisms (2):
  - Vasogenic caused by blood-brain barrier disruption and increased vascular permeability allowing fluid to shift from the intravascular compartment into the intercellular space.

- Cytotoxic caused by injury to the neuronal, glial, or endothelial cell membrane, and influx of fluid from the extracellular to intracellular space.
- Major complication:
  - Herniation and compression and occlusion of venous outflow.

65. List at least 3 types of herniations by anatomical site.

- Uncal/transtentorial downward through brainstem tentorial opening.
- Central (diencephalic) through tentorial opening.

- Transtentorial upward cerebellar.
- Subfalcine (cingulate gyrus) beneath falx cerebri.
- Cerebellar tonsillar through foramen magnum.

66. Name at least 3 lesions associated with severe "moving head" injury.

- Contusions.
- Diffuse axonal injury.

- Focal hemorrhagic lesions (corpus callosum and superior cerebellar peduncle lacerations).
- Vascular injury.

Intracranial Bleeding

67. List the major types of hemorrhages that affect the brain.

- Epidural hematoma.
- Subdural hematoma.
- Subarachnoid hematoma.

- Intraparenchymal hematoma.
- Intraventricular hematoma.

68. What is the most common pathogenesis of epidural hemorrhage?

Rupture of the middle meningeal artery due to trauma. Thin temporal bone skull fractures rupture the middle meningeal artery as it courses between the periosteum and pachymeninges (between layers of the cranial dura). The blood at arterial pressure dissects between the dural layers and causes an expansile lesion that has a lens shaped appearance. The expansion typically does not cross sutures or cross the midline.

69. What is the specific clinical feature of epidural hemorrhage?

Presence of a variable lucid interval between the moment of trauma and the development of neurological signs.

70. What is the cause of death in a case of epidural hematoma?

- Cerebral compression.

- Transtentorial herniation.

71. What are the pathogenesis and risk factors for subdural hemorrhages?

- Pathogenesis: rupture or tearing of the bridging veins at the point where they penetrate the dura.
- Risk factors:
  - Elderly patients with significant brain atrophy.

- Chronic alcoholics.
- Patients treated with anticoagulants.
- Repeated head injury (e.g., patients with seizure disorders).

72. What are the clinical features of subdural hemorrhage? What is the treatment?

- Clinical features:
  - It manifests in the first 48 hours after injury. Slowly progressive neurologic deterioration, including headache and confusion, is typical, but acute decompensation may occur. It is most common over the lateral aspects of the cerebral hemispheres and is bilateral in 10% of cases.

- There may be focal neurological signs due to the pressure exerted on the adjacent brain.
- Treatment:
  - Remove the blood and associated organizing tissue.

73. Name at least 3 common causes of subarachnoid hemorrhage.

- Rupture of saccular (berry) aneurysm.
- Superficial contusions and lacerations in brain trauma.

- Hemorrhagic superficial or extensive infarcts.
- Tumors.

74. What is the most common clinical feature of subarachnoid hemorrhage?

Headache, which the patient usually describes as "the worst headache of my life."

75. List at least 3 common causes of intraparenchymal hemorrhage.
- Congophilic angiopathy.
- Hypertension.
- Bleeding tumor.
- Infection.
- Vascular malformation.

76. What are the phases of the organization of subdural hematomas?
- Lysis of the clot (about 1 week).
- Growth of fibroblasts from the dural surface and capillaries into the hematoma (2 weeks).
- Vascular proliferation.
- Changes to membrane: becomes predominantly fibrous, often with calcifications (1–3 months).

77. Name 3 populations that are at increased risk for subdural hemorrhage compared to the general population.
- Elderly.
- Trauma patients.
- Patients with coagulopathies and bleeding diathesis.

78. List the features that distinguish intracerebral hemorrhage from a hemorrhagic cerebral infarct on pathological examination.
- Cerebral hemorrhage:
  - Solid clot.
  - Lines of Zahn.
- Hemorrhagic infarct:
  - Perivascular hemorrhage.
  - Lesion in specific vascular territory.

79. What is the location of Duret hemorrhages, what causes them, and what do they signify?
- Location: midline or parasagittal midbrain and rostral pons hemorrhages.
- Cause: avulsion of penetrating arteries arising from top of basilar artery.
- Significance: supratentorial brain herniation, either uncal herniation or diencephalic (also called "central," or "transtentorial") herniation, and coma from interruption of ascending reticular formation.

Trauma

80. List the types of skull fractures.
- Linear:
  - The inner and outer tables of skull are broken.
  - These fractures as associated with falls.
  - They may be extensive.
- Basilar:
  - These are linear skull fractures that run across the base of the skull.
  - They require considerable force and are usually associated with:
    › Road traffic accidents.
    › Fall from heights.
  - They have typical clinical signs related to blood in the sinuses, cerebrospinal fluid (CSF) leakage, and orbital and perimastoid bruising.
- Depressed:
  - Fractured bone moves downward.
  - Inner tables of the fracture surround the bone.
  - These are related to force applied to a small area.
- Comminuted:
  - This involves fragmentation of skull bones.
  - Depressed fractures are often comminuted.
- Compound:
  - This involves scalp laceration(s) that overlie skull fracture(s).
  - The cranial cavity becomes exposed.
  - Linear and depressed fractures can be compound.
- Ping-pong fractures:
  - These are seen in neonates and infants due to different biomechanical properties of developing skull bones.
- Diastatic:
  - These fractures extend along suture lines.
  - They are seen in neonates and infants.
- Development-associated:
  - These are seen in childhood.
  - They are due to dura and arachnoid extending between bone fragments, which prevents union and healing.

81. Describe lesions associated with rotational acceleration and deceleration of the brain.
- Diffuse axonal injury:
  - This is shearing of axons, which occurs in long white matter tracts:
    › Corpus callosum.
    › Internal capsule.
  - Findings at autopsy include:
    › Parasagittal gliding contusions.
    › Variably prominent punctate hemorrhages in the splenium of the corpus callosum and internal capsule, and in the dorsolateral areas of the rostral brainstem.

(continued on next page)

- Microscopy:
  › Axonal swellings if there is a period of survival after injury:
  › Visible on H&E after 12–18 hours.
  › Presence of amyloid precursor protein (APP) after 2–3 hours.

82. Define contusion and list the most common sites involved in the brain.
- Definition: a bruise on the surface of the brain (by definition, the overlying pia mater is intact in contusions but torn in lacerations).
- Common sites: the crests of gyri that come into contact with protuberances within the skull.
  - Frontal poles.
  - Orbital surface of the frontal lobes.
  - Temporal poles.
  - Lateral and inferior surfaces of the temporal lobes.
  - Cortex adjacent to the sylvian fissures.

83. List the types of brain herniation.
- Transcalvarial.
- Cingulate (subfalcine): brain herniates beneath falx cerebri.
- Uncal (transtentorial): brain herniates downward through the tentorial brainstem opening.
- Central (diencephalic): brain herniates through tentorial opening.
- Tonsillar (cerebellar): brain herniates through foramen magnum.

84. List the important consequences of uncal (transtentorial) brain herniation.
- Uncal brain herniation compresses and stretches the third and sixth cranial nerves.
- When the ipsilateral cerebral peduncle is compressed directly, a hemiparesis contralateral to the lesion may ensue.
- When the contralateral peduncle is displaced and compressed against the free edge of the tentorium (Kernohan notch), an ipsilateral hemiparesis may follow.
- If the adjacent posterior cerebral artery is compressed, there can be secondary infarction anywhere along its territory of distribution.

85. Define coup and contrecoup brain contusions.
- In coup contusions, the damaged brain tissue occurs beneath the point of impact.
- In contrecoup contusions, the identical structural damage to the surface of the brain occurs in a region diametrically opposite the point of external impact.

86. Name 2 key brainstem injuries that result from blunt force trauma.
- Pontomedullary rent (high-velocity lesions causing extreme hyperflexion- or hyperextension-type injuries).
- Hemorrhages within the brainstem:
  - Secondary to axial displacement causing large midline hemorrhages in the midbrain and pons (Duret hemorrhages).
  - Part of diffuse traumatic axonal injury with a dorsolateral localization.

87. List at least 5 common head and spinal injuries associated with nonaccidental injuries in children.
- Subdural hematomas, which are often bilateral and interhemispheric and may only be thin films.
- Scanty subarachnoid hemorrhage.
- Cerebral contusions.
- Retinal and optic nerve sheath hemorrhages.
- Traumatic axonal injury, particularly in the lower medulla or upper cervical cord.
- Diffuse brain swelling.

88. What is the mechanism of diffuse vascular injury?
- Diffuse vascular damage results from acute deformation, stretching, and tearing of small blood vessels.
- It mostly occurs in the frontal and temporal white matter, diencephalon, and brainstem.

89. What are the major mechanisms and the major complication of cerebral edema?
- Mechanisms:
  - Vasogenic edema can be seen in the setting of head injury, abscess, tumors, and hemorrhage; it results from injury to the blood-brain barrier, which leads to increased permeability of the microcirculation to macromolecules, particularly to proteins.
  - Cytotoxic edema results from excessive amounts of water entering 1 or more of the intracellular compartments of the CNS due to increased cellular concentration of osmotically active solutes; it is associated with systemic disturbances in fluid and electrolyte metabolism.
- Major complication:
  - Herniation and compression, and occlusion of venous outflow, can occur.

Cerebrovascular Disease

90. How much blood flows to the brain?
- Cerebral blood flow represents 15% of cardiac output and accounts for 20% of the total body oxygen consumption.
- Normal cerebral blood flow is approximately 50 ml per minute for each 100 g of tissue.

91. Define the concept of selective vulnerability and name a few neurons that are most sensitive to hypoxia-ischemia.
- Selective vulnerability: selective populations of cells are at increased risk during episodes of hypoxia-ischemia.
- Neurons are the most sensitive cells to ischemia, but their susceptibility varies greatly among different populations of neurons in different regions of the CNS.
- Most-sensitive neurons: large and located in the hippocampus (especially the Sommer sector/CA1 pyramidal neurons) and cerebellum with loss of pyramidal and Purkinje neurons.
- Neocortex can also be affected and a laminar neuronal loss is often encountered with loss especially from pyramidal neurons in the cerebral cortex layers III, V, and VI.
- Other areas: caudate and putamen, and the boundary zones between vascular distributions ("watershed" areas).

92. Name at least 5 factors that increase the risk of stroke.
- Increasing age.
- Male > female.
- Smoking.
- Hypertension.
- Atrial fibrillation.
- Carotid artery stenosis.
- Hyperlipidemia.
- Diabetes.
- Heart surgery.
- Heart vegetations.
- Antiphospholipid antibodies.
- Estrogen oral contraceptives.

93. List at least 3 early histopathological changes of an infarct (12–24 hours after the infarct).
- Astrocytic swelling.
- Interstitial edema.
- Nuclear pyknosis.
- Hypereosinophilia of neurons (red neurons).
- Microvacuolization of neurons and later karyorrhexis.

94. What are the subacute histopathological changes of an infarct?
- Infiltration by macrophages.
- Proliferation of vessels (neovascularization).
- Peripheral (reactive) gliosis.

95. List the 3 most common sites of primary thrombosis causing cerebral infarction.
- The carotid bifurcation.
- The origin of middle cerebral artery.
- The ends of the basilar artery.

96. Name at least 3 diseases associated with cerebral amyloid angiopathy (CAA).
- Alzheimer disease.
- Down syndrome.
- Hereditary cerebral hemorrhage with amyloidosis of Icelandic origin.
- Hereditary cerebral hemorrhage with amyloidosis of British origin.

97. Name at least 2 types of amyloid that produce CAA.
- β-Amyloid peptide, the most common amyloid subunit implicated in sporadic CAA and rarely in hereditary forms of CAA.
- The variant cystatin C in hereditary cerebral hemorrhage with amyloidosis of Icelandic type.
- The ABri and ADan subunits in familial British dementia and familial Danish dementia, respectively.
- Variant transthyretins in meningovascular amyloidosis.
- Disease associated prion protein (PrP^{sc}) in hereditary prion disease.
- Mutated gelsolin (AGel) in familial amyloidosis of Finnish type.
- Amyloid precursors protein mutations in hereditary cerebral hemorrhage with amyloidosis Dutch type.

98. What is the most common presentation of CAA?
Acute intracerebral, lobar hemorrhage with compression of the adjacent parenchyma.

99. Name the gene that is mutated in cerebral autosomal dominant arteriopathy with subcortical infarcts and leukoencephalopathy (CADASIL), and describe the histologic and electron microscopy findings in this disease.

- CADASIL is a rare hereditary form of stroke caused by mutations in the *NOTCH3* gene located on chromosome 19.
- Small arteries and arterioles in the deep white matter have thickened walls (media and adventitia) with granule deposition within the smooth muscle cells. These granules stain with PAS and appear as granular osmiophilic material ultrastructurally.

100. What are the most common sites of occurrence of saccular aneurysms?

- Middle cerebral artery trifurcation — 34%.
- Anterior communicating artery-anterior cerebral artery junction — 40%.
- Internal carotid artery-posterior communicating artery junction — 20%.
- Basilar posterior cerebral arteries.

101. What are the most common conditions associated with saccular aneurysms?

- Fibromuscular dysplasia.
- Autosomal dominant polycystic kidney disease.
- Ehlers-Danlos syndrome — types 4 and 6.
- Coarctation of aorta.
- Marfan syndrome.
- Neurofibromatosis type I.
- Pseudoxanthoma elasticum.

102. What are the hallmark histopathological findings of saccular aneurysms?

- The defective tunica media is gradually more attenuated as it approaches the neck of the aneurysm.
- The internal elastic lamina is absent within the aneurysm sac.
- Thickened hyalinized intima forms the sac.
- Adventitia covering the sac is continuous with that of the parent vessel.
- Hemosiderin deposition with phagocytosis may be present in the adjacent brain and meninges.

103. Name at least 3 vascular malformations and describe their histopathological features.

- Arteriovenous malformations — composed of an admixture of arteries, veins, and intermediate size vessels that are greatly enlarged and separated by gliotic neural parenchyma. The veins may show marked thickening or partial replacement of the media by hyalinized connective tissue (arterialized veins).
- Cavernous angioma — consists of large sinusoidal type vessels with thin collagenized walls, in apposition to each other and with little or no intervening neural tissue.
- Venous angioma — consists of veins of varying sizes separated by mostly normal parenchyma.
- Capillary telangiectasia — formed by capillary sized vessels separated by relatively normal brain parenchyma.
- Venous ectasia — dilated venous channel within brain parenchyma.

Infections of the Central Nervous System (CNS)

104. List at least 3 types of meningitis.

- Acute pyogenic (bacterial).
- Aseptic (typically viral).
- Chronic (tuberculosis; spirochetes (syphilis); certain fungi or yeast — e.g., *Cryptococcus meningitis*).
- Granulomatous (tuberculosis, most fungi and yeast, chemical or foreign material — e.g., ruptured epidermoid cyst).

105. What are the 3 most common microorganisms that can produce acute meningitis in a neonate?

- *Streptococcus agalactiae* (group B).
- *Escherichia coli*.
- *Listeria monocytogenes*.

106. What are the 3 most common microorganisms that can produce acute meningitis in children and adolescents?

- *Neisseria meningitides* — responsible for most epidemic outbreaks.
- *Hemophilus influenza*.
- *Streptococcus pneumonia*.

107. What are the clinical features of acute meningitis?

- Fever.
- Signs of meningeal irritation: headache, photophobia, nausea, vomiting, neck stiffness, irritability, altered mental status, and Kernig and Brudzinski signs.
- Focal neurologic signs and focal cranial nerve palsies, including gaze paresis caused by hydrocephalus.
- Seizures.
- Rarely coma.
- Petechial or purpuric rash in meningococcal meningitis.
- Ataxia and labyrinthitis in *Hemophilus influenzae* meningitis.

108. Describe the CSF findings in bacterial, viral, and fungal meningitis.

AGENT	OPENING PRESSURE (MM H₂O)	WBC COUNT (CELLS/ML)	GLUCOSE (MG/DL)	PROTEIN (MG/DL)	MICROBIOLOGY
Aseptic meningitis	• 90–200.	• 10–300. • Lymphocytes.	• Normal.	• Normal but may be slightly elevated.	• Negative findings on workup.
Bacterial meningitis	• 200–300.	• 100–5000. • > 80% PMNs.	• < 40.	• > 100.	• Specific pathogen demonstrated in 60% of Gram stains and 80% of cultures.
Cryptococcal meningitis	• 180–300.	• 10–200. • Lymphocytes.	• Reduced.	• 50–200.	• India ink. • Cryptococcal antigen. • Culture.
Tuberculous meningitis	• 180–300.	• 100–500. • Lymphocytes.	• Reduced, < 40.	• Elevated, > 100.	• Acid-fast bacillus stain. • Culture. • PCR.
Viral meningitis	• 90–200.	• 10–300. • Lymphocytes.	• Normal, but reduced in LCM and mumps.	• Normal but may be slightly elevated.	• Viral isolation, PCR assays.

Abbreviations: LCM = lymphocytic choriomeningitis; PCR = polymerase chain reaction; PMN = polymorphonuclear leukocyte; WBC = white blood cell.

109. List at least 3 gross features of acute meningitis.
- Cloudy or purulent leptomeninges.
- Engorged meningeal vessels, occasionally thrombosed.
- Sometimes ventriculitis in fulminant cases.
- Sometimes increased size of the ventricular system (hydrocephalus).
- Thrombosis of the superior sagittal sinus and/or transverse sinuses.

110. List at least 3 microscopic features of acute purulent meningitis.
- Numerous neutrophils and fibrin are present in the subarachnoid space.
- Treated cases have more lymphocytes, macrophages, and plasma cells present in the subarachnoid space.
- Gram stain can reveal the causative organism.
- Inflammatory infiltrate is extended along the Virchow Robin spaces into brain parenchyma.
- Vascular congestion is present.
- Thrombosis and vasculitis are present, which may lead to infarct, hemorrhage, and cerebral edema.
- It may extend to cause cerebritis, ependymitis, and ventriculitis.

111. Name at least 3 direct effects of HIV infection on the brain.
- HIV aseptic meningitis.
- HIV encephalitis.
- HIV leukoencephalopathy.
- HIV dementia complex.
- HIV vacuolar myelopathy.

112. List at least 3 microorganisms responsible for opportunistic infections of the brain in HIV infection.
- Toxoplasmosis encephalitis.
- Cytomegalovirus.
- Cryptococcal meningitis.
- Tuberculosis meningoencephalitis.
- JC virus (progressive multifocal leukoencephalopathy — PML).
- *Pneumocystis carinii* (very rare).

113. List at least 3 histopathological findings in HIV meningoencephalitis.
- Microglial nodules, which often contain the characteristic macrophage-derived multinucleate giant cells (positive staining for p24 antibody).
- Chronic inflammatory infiltrate.
- Microscopic foci of tissue necrosis and reactive gliosis.
- Perivascular multinucleated cells.

114. Name the causative agent and main histopathological findings in progressive multifocal leukoencephalopathy (PML).
- Causative agent: JC papovavirus, which is a DNA virus.
- Histopathology:
  · Multifocal, asymmetrical, isolated or merging demyelinated areas with macrophages and decreased number of axons, frequently located at the gray-white junction.
  · At the edge of these lesions: significantly enlarged oligodendrocyte nuclei with glassy inclusions, peripherally marginated chromatin, plus bizarre, atypical astrocytes.

115. List at least 3 major protozoa that can cause nervous system disease.
- *Plasmodium falciparum.*
- *Toxoplasma gondii.*
- *Trypanosoma brucei.*
- Amoeba (several different forms: *Acanthamoeba* species, *Nagleria fowleri, Balamuthia mandrillaris*).

116. Describe the pathogenesis of brain abscess.
- Direct spread:
  - Infection spreads from a septic focus in the paranasal sinus, middle ear, or dental root.
  - *Streptococcus milleri* is the most commonly implicated pathogen.
- Hematogenous spread:
  - In children, congenital heart disease with right-to-left shunting.
- In adults, septic emboli, usually from bronchiectasis, a lung abscess, or subacute endocarditis.
- Cranial trauma.
- Neurosurgery.
- Immunodeficiency, either disease-related (e.g., AIDS, leukemia) or iatrogenic (e.g., after organ or bone marrow transplantation).

117. List the 4 stages in the microscopic appearance of brain abscess.
- Focal suppurative encephalitis (days 1–2).
- Focal suppurative encephalitis with confluent central necrosis (days 2–7).
- Early encapsulation (days 5–14).
- Late encapsulation (from day 14).

Demyelinating Diseases

118. What are the pathological criteria to define a lesion as "demyelinating"?
- Loss of myelin: in active lesions, macrophages contain myelin debris, while chronic lesions are devoid of stainable myelin.
- Relative preservation of axons: in demyelination, axons are often damaged, swollen, or partially lost, but some remaining axons should be present.

Note: loss of both axons and myelin is not considered demyelination, since it frequently develops in ischemic injury. In Wallerian degeneration, some myelinated axons often remain in the affected tracts, in contrast to demyelinating lesions, in which all of the myelin is lost.

119. Define multiple sclerosis (MS).

Multiple sclerosis: inflammatory demyelinating disease characterized by episodes of focal neurologic deficits separated both in space (e.g., different anatomic locations) and time (occurring at different times; with relapsing and remitting episodes).

120. List at least 4 clinical features of MS.
- Unilateral visual impairment due to the involvement of the optic nerve — this is the classic initial manifestation, but it is not universally present.
- Spinal cord disease: limb weakness, spasticity, paresthesias, bladder dysfunction.
- Brainstem disease: nystagmus, internuclear ophthalmoplegia, other cranial nerve signs.
- Cerebellar disease: ataxia.
- Predominance in women (F:M = 2:1).
- Moderate pleocytosis (one-third of cases), elevated total protein level, and elevated IgG with oligoclonal IgG bands in CSF.

121. What are the gross findings in the brain and spinal cord of patients with MS?
- Variable number of gray, demyelinated, firm plaques in the white matter located especially in the periventricular region, optic nerve, and spinal cord.
- Atrophy and hydrocephalus ex vacuo with long-standing disease (also seen in Alzheimer disease).

122. What are the microscopic findings in the brain and spinal cord of patients with MS?
- Demyelinated plaques (defined as a loss of myelin with a relative preservation of axons) with sharp and/or diffuse borders.
- 2 categories of demyelinated plaques:
  - Active (with macrophages containing myelin).
    - › These are characterized by ongoing myelin breakdown, with abundant macrophages containing myelin debris (Luxol fast blue positive) and a relative preservation of axons.
    - › They become subacute plaques as they progress, which are characterized by loss of myelin and oligodendrocytes, presence of macrophages with PAS positive material, free neutral fat, astrocytosis, and perivascular lymphocyte inflammation (mostly T cells).
  - Inactive (macrophages absent).
    - › These have loss of myelin in the center accompanied by significant axonal loss and gliosis.

(continued on next page)

> Mature plaques have few oligodendrocytes and a mature gliotic background of astrocytes. Iron deposits may develop at the periphery (infrequent).
- Cortical demyelination:
  - Subpial demyelination (identified using myelin basic protein or proteolipid protein stains) with associated leptomeningeal chronic inflammation.
  - Intracortical plaques (identified using myelin basic protein or proteolipid protein stains).

123. What are shadow plaques?
- They are remyelinated lesions at the border between normal and affected white matter.
- Axons within them have abnormally thin myelin sheaths.

124. Discuss the pathogenesis of MS.
- While MS is likely to be a heterogeneous disease with differential involvement of inflammation throughout its progression, autoimmune T and B cell responses against CNS antigens remain a central component in the current view of MS pathogenesis.
- Myelin antigens are the prevalent targets, due to the often primarily demyelinating nature of inflammatory CNS lesions.
- Several lines of evidence indicate that B cells, plasma cells, and in particular, antibodies contribute to development and progression of MS.
- Among the putative antigens, more attention has been given to myelin oligodendrocyte glycoprotein (MOG).
- The disease is initiated by CD4+ TH1 T cells that react against self-myelin antigens and secrete cytokines such as interferon-gamma (IFN-γ) and tumor necrosis factor alpha (TNF-α).

125. What anatomic sites are involved in neuromyelitis optica (NMO) and what is the specific autoantibody involved in its pathogenesis?
- NMO is characterized by demyelination of the optic nerves and spinal cord. Microscopically, unlike multiple sclerosis, astrocytes are significantly diminished.
- The specific autoantibody is against aquaporin-4 (Aqp-4), which is a water channel protein that is expressed on astrocytes.

126. List some causes of demyelinating disease in the brain and spinal cord other than multiple sclerosis.
- Nutritional causes:
  - Chronic alcoholism — Marchiafava-Bignami disease with foci of demyelination in the corpus callosum.
  - Vitamin B$_{12}$ deficiency — subacute combined degeneration of the spinal cord.
  - Hyponatremia — central pontine and extrapontine myelinolysis.
- Toxin:
  - Inflammatory demyelination complication of treatment with 5-fluorouracil and its derivatives.
- Genetic causes:
  - Demyelination in adrenoleukodystrophy, adrenomyeloneuropathy, and other leukodystrophies.
  - Leber hereditary optic neuropathy.
- Infection:
  - Vacuolar myelopathy of AIDS.
- Other:
  - Acute disseminated encephalomyelitis — this differs from MS in the monophasic pattern of disease, and the close relationship of most lesions to small veins and venules.
  - Neuromyelitis optica.

Neurodegenerative Diseases

127. List at least 3 common early clinical features of Alzheimer disease.
- Short-term memory impairment.
- Lack of insight.
- Judgment and visuospatial impairment.
- Behavioral change (aggression, wandering, disinhibition).

128. What are the key gross features of Alzheimer disease?
- Generalized cortical atrophy, but usually sparing the primary cortices (primary motor, primary somatosensory, occipital lobes) and the cerebellum.
- Ventricular enlargement (hydrocephalus ex vacuo).
- Atrophy of the structures of the medial temporal lobe: hippocampus, entorhinal cortex, and amygdala.
- Loss of pigment in the locus ceruleus, but preservation of substantia nigra.

129. What are the most common histopathological changes of Alzheimer disease?
- Neuritic (senile) amyloid plaques.
- Neurofibrillary tangles.
- Neuropil threads.
- Hirano bodies.
- Granulovacuolar degeneration.
- Cerebral amyloid angiopathy.

130. What are the characteristic pathologic features that underlie Alzheimer disease?

- Extracellular accumulation of amyloid-β peptide (Aβ, mainly Aβ42), derived by proteolytic processing from amyloid precursor protein (APP), in the form of amyloid plaques.
- Intracellular linear accumulations of hyperphosphorylated tau protein in the form of neurofibrillary tangles and neuropil threads.
- Combination of Aβ42 and thickened neurites containing tau to form neuritic amyloid plaques.

- The "amyloid hypothesis": β-amyloid is derived through processing of amyloid precursor protein (APP). Once generated, the β-amyloid readily self-aggregates, first into small oligomers and eventually into large aggregates of fibrils (plaques). Small aggregates of β-amyloid are toxic to neurons (demonstrated in tissue culture) and can cause them to form hyperphosphorylated tau, which can then aggregate into neurofibrillary tangles.

131. Name at least 5 neurological diseases that have neurofibrillary tangles.

- Alzheimer disease.
- Progressive supranuclear palsy (PSP).
- Corticobasal degeneration (CBD).
- Pick disease.
- FTD-tau (frontotemporal dementia–tau).
- Postencephalic Parkinson disease (exceedingly rare today).

- Parkinsonian dementia complex of Guam (exceedingly rare today).
- Gerstmann-Straussler-Scheinker disease (inherited prion disease).
- Subacute sclerosing panencephalitis.
- Tuberous sclerosis.
- Niemann-Pick disease type C.
- Meningioangiomatosis.

132. Name 3 common nonmotor clinical findings in patients who have Lewy bodies.

- Attention deficits.
- Visual hallucinations, especially of small, animate objects or creatures.
- Postural hypotension.
- Bowel and bladder dysfunction.

- Masked or expressionless face.
- Adverse reaction to neuroleptics (e.g., haloperidol).
- Fluctuations in cognition, attention, and alertness.
- REM (rapid eye movement) sleep disorder.

133. Name at least 3 diseases that clinically exhibit parkinsonism.

- Parkinson disease, including rare inherited forms.
- Multiple system atrophy.
- Progressive supranuclear palsy.
- Corticobasal degeneration.

- Frontotemporal dementia with parkinsonism linked to chromosome 17.
- Postencephalic Parkinson disease (mostly historical).
- Parkinsonian dementia complex of Guam (very rare).

134. What are the microscopic features in Parkinson disease (PD)?

- Lewy bodies in the substantia nigra; also in many other sites, including nuclei of the major diffusely projecting systems (dorsal motor nucleus of the vagus, locus ceruleus, raphe nuclei, tuberomamillary hypothalamic nucleus, and basal nucleus of Meynert) and often in parts of the cortex.
- Lewy-related neurites (identified with ubiquitin or α-synuclein stains).

- Neuron loss, especially in the substantia nigra, but also in the nuclei of the major diffusely projecting systems (see above).
- Ballooned, eosinophilic neurons.
- Vacuolization of the entorhinal cortex.

135. Describe Lewy bodies.

- Single or multiple cytoplasmic, eosinophilic, round to elongated inclusions with a dense core surrounded by a pale halo.
- Composed of intermediate filaments (neurofilament), ubiquitin, and α-synuclein.

- Cortical Lewy bodies: intraneuronal, eosinophilic, rounded to oval inclusions in lower layers of cortex, usually without halos.

136. What is the immunohistochemical profile of Parkinson disease?

- α-Synuclein, ubiquitin, and neurofilament positivity in the Lewy bodies.

- α-Synuclein in Lewy related neurites.

137. Name at least 3 trinucleotide repeat expansion diseases.

- Huntington disease (CAG repeats).
- Friedreich ataxia (CAA repeats).
- Spinal and bulbar muscular atrophy (CAG repeats).
- Fragile X syndrome (CGG repeats).

- Myotonic dystrophy type 1 (CTG repeats).
- Spinocerebellar ataxia type I and III (CAG repeats).
- Dentatorubral-pallidoluysian atrophy (CAG repeats).

138. List at least 2 examples of triple repeat expansion diseases that occur in coding regions and at least 3 examples that occur in noncoding regions.

Expansions affecting noncoding regions				
DISEASE	**GENE**	**LOCUS**	**PROTEIN**	**REPEAT**
Fragile X syndrome	• *FMR1*.	• X.	• FMRP.	• CGG.
Friedreich ataxia	• *FXN*.	• 9.	• Frataxin.	• GAA.
Myotonic dystrophy	• *DMPK*.	• 19.	• Myotonic dystrophy protein kinase (DMPK).	• CTG.
Expansions affecting coding regions				
DISEASE	**GENE**	**LOCUS**	**PROTEIN**	**REPEAT**
Huntington disease	• *HTT*.	• 4.	• Huntington.	• CAG.
Spinocerebellar ataxia type 1	• *ATXN1*.	• 6.	• Ataxin-1.	• CAG.

139. What are the gross features of Huntington disease (HD)?
- Progressive atrophy of the caudate and putamen, and later the globus pallidus.
- Cortical atrophy in the frontal, temporal, and sometimes parietal lobes.
- Ventricular dilatation.

140. What is the name of the grading system used in Huntington disease?
Vonsattel grading.

141. What are the key microscopic features of HD?
Severe loss of neurons and astrocytosis in the caudate (especially the tail) and putamen, developing in a dorsomedial to ventrolateral and caudal to rostral pattern.

142. Name the gene involved in the pathogenesis of HD.
- HD is a progressive and invariably fatal autosomal dominant neurodegenerative disorder.
- It is caused by expansion of the CAG trinucleotide repeat in exon 1 within the huntingtin (*HTT*) gene on chromosome 4.
  - The *HTT* gene encodes the protein huntingtin, which is essential for normal neural development.
  - "Normal" *HTT* genes have fewer than 36 repeats.
- Abnormal (expanded) genes have 36 or more repeats.
- Genes with CAG repeat lengths between 36 and 39 show reduced penetrance, which means that only some people with these lengths will develop HD and the disease will manifest later in life.
- CAG repeats of 40 or more will always cause Huntington disease.

143. Name the characteristic gross and microscopic features of amyotrophic lateral sclerosis (ALS).
- Thin and dark anterior roots of the spinal cord.
- Atrophy of the precentral gyrus in cases of long duration.
- Reduction of the number of anterior horn lower motor neurons accompanied by reactive gliosis.
- Loss of myelinated axons in the anterior and lateral corticospinal tracts.
- Loss of neurons in the hypoglossal nucleus.
- Loss of Betz neurons in the primary motor cortex.
- Neurogenic atrophy of the skeletal muscles.

144. List at least 2 genes known to cause familial ALS.
- Copper/zinc superoxide dismutase 1 (*SOD1*) on chromosome 21 in ~20% of familial ALS cases and ~3% of sporadic cases.
- *TARDBP* gene on chromosome 1 encoding for the TAR DNA binding protein 43 (TDP-43).
- *FUS/TLS* gene (FUS: fused in sarcoma; TLS: translocation in liposarcoma).

145. List the major types of protein aggregates in neurodegenerative diseases.

AGGREGATE	DISEASE(S)	LOCATION(S)
Tau-immunoreactive neurofibrillary tangles	• AD. • PSP.	• AD: hippocampus, entorhinal cortex, cerebral cortex. • PSP: brainstem nuclei (substantia nigra and others).
Tau-immunoreactive neuronal inclusions	• FTD-tau.	• Cerebral cortex, especially frontal lobes.
Tau-immunoreactive astrocytic plaques or thorny astrocytes	• PSP. • CBD. • CTE.	• PSP & CBD: multiple locations, but especially basal ganglia. • CTE: cerebral cortex and underlying white matter.
Tau-immunoreactive, small cytoplasmic bodies (Pick bodies)	• Pick disease. • FTD-tau.	• Hippocampus (especially dentate gyrus), cerebral cortex.
Tau-immunoreactive ballooned neurons (Pick cells)	• CBD. • Pick disease.	• Involved cerebral cortex (often parietal lobes in CBD and frontal lobes in Pick disease).
Amyloid β	• AD.	• First in neocortex, followed by hippocampus, basal ganglia, and last in cerebellum.
α-Synuclein condensed, round cytoplasmic bodies (Lewy bodies)	• PD. • LBD.	• Diffusely projecting nuclei (substantia nigra, locus ceruleus, raphe nuclei, basal nucleus of Meynert, tuberomamillary nuclei), autonomic control centers, cerebral cortex.
α-Synuclein neuronal neurites (Lewy-related neurites)	• PD. • LBD.	• Hippocampus CA2.
α-Synuclein glial cytoplasmic inclusions	• MSA.	• Cerebellar white matter, pontine white matter, inferior olivary nucleus, basal ganglia.
TDP43-immunoreactive cytoplasmic deposits	• FTD-TDP. • ALS. • FTD-ALS.	• FTD: hippocampus dentate gyrus, superficial cerebral cortex. • ALS: low motor neurons in spinal cord and hypoglossal nucleus.
Polyglutamine aggregates	• HD. • SCA.	• Within neuronal nuclei (neuronal intranuclear inclusions).

Abbreviations: AD: Alzheimer disease; ALS: amyotrophic lateral sclerosis; CBD: corticobasal degeneration; CTE: chronic traumatic encephalopathy; FTD: frontotemporal dementia; HD: Huntington disease; LBD: Lewy body dementia; MSA: multiple system atrophy; PD: Parkinson disease; PSP: progressive supranuclear palsy. SCA: spinocerebellar atrophy.

146. What is the pathogenesis of prion disease of the CNS?
- The PrP is a normal 30 kDa cellular protein (PrP^C) present in neurons. It is encoded by the *PRNP* gene located on chromosome 20.
- In disease, the prion protein undergoes a conformational change from its normal α-helix-containing isoform (PrP^C) to an abnormal β-pleated sheet isoform (PrP^{sc} or PrP^{res}).
- The abnormal protein promotes further conversion to the abnormal prion protein material from the normal host protein.
- The neurons develop vacuoles within their cytoplasm and processes and die, although the exact mechanism is still not known.

147. Name at least 3 human prion diseases.
- Creutzfeldt-Jakob disease (CJD).
- New variant CJD.
- Gerstmann-Straussler-Scheinker disease.
- Kuru.
- Fatal familial insomnia.

148. List at least 2 characteristic histologic features of prion disease.
- Spongiform change.
- Neuron loss.
- Reactive gliosis.
- Kuru plaques — appear in 10% of cases and are extracellular deposits of aggregated abnormal protein (Congo red and PAS positive).

149. Name the main categories of genetic metabolic diseases affecting the CNS.
- Lysosomal storage diseases (neuronal storage diseases).
- Leukodystrophies.
- Mitochondrial disorders (mitochondrial encephalomyopathies).
- Peroxisomal diseases.

150. Describe the microscopic and ultrastructural changes that appear in Tay-Sachs disease.
- Ballooned neurons.
- Cytoplasmic neuronal vacuoles representing markedly distended lysosomes with gangliosides.

(continued on next page)

- Progressive destruction of neurons, proliferation of microglia, and accumulation of complex lipids in phagocytes.
- Cytoplasmic inclusions on electron microscopy, the most prominent being whorled configurations composed of "onionskin" layers of membrane within lysosomes.

- Ganglion cells in retina are swollen with gangliosides, particularly at the margins of the macula, giving the characteristic cherry red spot.

151. What are the gross features of the brain in infantile ceroidlipofuscinosis?
Severe atrophy, "walnut brain."

152. Name the underlying enzymatic defect in Farber disease.
Lysosomal ceramidase.

153. Describe the mode of transmission and the enzymatic defect in Fabry disease.
- Fabry disease is a rare, X-linked recessive disorder, due to a deficiency of the hydrolase enzyme α-galactosidase.
  · α-Galactosidase is coded on the long arm of the X chromosome (Xq21.33-q22).

- α-Galactosidase deficiency results in the accumulation of glycosphingolipids, particularly globotriaosylceramide especially within the vascular endothelial and smooth muscle cells.

154. What are the ultrastructural changes in Niemann-Pick disease?
The engorged lysosomes appear as vacuoles that often contain membranous cytoplasmic bodies resembling concentric lamellated myelin figures, called "zebra bodies."

155. Which is the most common lysosomal storage disease and what is its characteristic microscopic finding?
- Disease: Gaucher disease.

- Characteristic microscopic finding: Gaucher cells, which are large monocyte-macrophage cells with a fibrillary type of cytoplasm that have a "wrinkled tissue paper" appearance.

156. Name at least 2 mucopolysaccharidoses and describe their mode of inheritance.
- Type I, Hurler syndrome — autosomal recessive.
- Type II, Hunter syndrome — X-linked recessive.
- Type III, Sanfilippo syndrome (A, B, C, D) — autosomal recessive.
- Type IV, Morquio syndrome — autosomal recessive.
- Type VI, Maroteaux-Lamy syndrome — autosomal recessive.
- Type VII, Sly syndrome — autosomal recessive.

157. Name at least 2 glycogenoses that affect the skeletal muscle and name the underlying defect.
- Pompe disease (type II glycogenosis) due to deficit of acid maltase (α-1,4-glucosidase).
- Cori-Forbes disease (type III glycogenosis) due to deficit of amylo-1,6-glucosidase.
- McArdle disease (type V glycogenosis) due to deficit of phosphorylase.
- Tarui disease (type VII glycogenosis) due to deficit of phosphofructokinase.

158. Name at least 2 leukodystrophies.
- Metachromatic leukodystrophy.
- Adrenoleukodystrophy.
- Pelizaeus-Merzbacher disease.
- Canavan disease.
- Alexander disease.
- Vanishing white matter leukodystrophy.

159. What are the lysosomal enzyme defects causing leukodystrophy?
- Krabbe disease — galactocerebroside β-galactosidase deficiency.
- Metachromatic leukodystrophy — aryl sulfatase A deficiency.

160. Name the underlying enzymatic defect and the clinical features of Krabbe disease.
- Enzymatic defect:
  · Deficiency of galactocerebroside β-galactosidase.
- Clinical features:
  · Onset occurs in childhood.
- It is rapidly progressive.
- Patients experience:
  › Stiffness.
  › Weakness.
  › Gradually worsening difficulties in feeding.

161. Describe the microscopic changes in metachromatic leukodystrophy.
- Demyelination.
- Gliosis.
- Scattered macrophages with vacuolated cytoplasm in the white matter.
- The vacuoles show metachromasia with certain dyes such as toluidine blue because they contain complex crystalloid structures composed of sulfatides.

162. Name at least 3 mitochondrial encephalomyopathies.

- Mitochondrial encephalomyopathy, lactic acidosis, and stroke like episodes (MELAS).
- Myoclonic epilepsy and ragged red fibers (MERRF).
- Leigh syndrome (subacute necrotizing encephalopathy).
- Kearns-Sayre syndrome.
- Alpers disease.

163. Describe the clinical characteristics of Leigh syndrome.

- Onset in early childhood.
- Rapid progression.
- Arrest of psychomotor development.
- Feeding problems.
- Seizures.
- Extraocular palsies.
- Weakness with hypotonia.

164. What are peroxisomes, and what is their function?

- Tiny organelles in the cytoplasm of all nucleated cells.
- Function:
  · Processes integral to normal metabolism of the nervous system, adrenals, and liver:
    › Plasmalogen biosynthesis (important components in cell membranes and myelin).
    › Cholesterol biosynthesis.
    › Bile acid biosynthesis.
    › β-Oxidation of fatty acids (including very long chain fatty acids).
- Other functions:
  › Dolichol synthesis (through action of mevalonate kinase).
  › Glyoxalate transamination.
  › Peroxide-based respiration/peroxidatic oxidation.
  › Pipecolic acid oxidation.
  › Glutaric acid oxidation.
  › Phytanic acid α-oxidation.
  › Alcohol dehydrogenase (medium chain).

165. What are the 2 classifications of peroxisomal disorders? Give examples for each.

- Peroxisomes absent or severely reduced (defective peroxisomal membrane synthesis or import of matrix protein results in defective peroxisomal assembly and generalized enzyme defects).
  · Zellweger cerebrohepatorenal syndrome.
  · Neonatal adrenoleukodystrophy.
  · Infantile Refsum disease.
  · Zellweger-like syndrome.
  · Rhizomelic chondroplasia punctata (classic form).
  · Pseudoinfantile Refsum disease.
- Peroxisomes present, but possibly with structural abnormalities (single peroxisomal enzyme defect).
  · X-linked adrenoleukodystrophy.
- Pseudoneonatal adrenoleukodystrophy.
- Rhizomelic chondroplasia punctata.
- Bifunctional enzyme deficiency.
- Pseudo-Zellweger syndrome.
- Trihydroxycholestanoic acidemia.
- Pipecolic acidemia (isolated).
- Refsum disease.
- Atypical Refsum disease.
- Glutaric aciduria type 3.
- Primary hypoxaluria type 1.
- Acatalasemia.
- Mevalonic aciduria.
- Sjögren-Larsson syndrome.

166. What are the macroscopic features of Zellweger cerebrohepatorenal syndrome?

- Increased brain weight.
- Widespread gyral abnormalities:
- Pachygyria.
- Polymicrogyria.

Toxic and Acquired Metabolic Diseases

167. Describe the gross findings in the brains of alcoholics.

- Decreased brain weight.
- Frontal atrophy.
- Dilatation of the lateral ventricles.
- Atrophy of the vermis (occasionally).
- Hemorrhagic necrosis of mamillary bodies, with relative sparing of neurons.

168. List at least 4 clinical morphological findings in fetal alcohol syndrome.

- Intrauterine growth retardation.
- Short palpebral fissures.
- Epicanthal folds.
- Low nasal bridge.
- Short nose.
- Flat face.
- Indistinct philtrum.
- Thin upper lip.

169. Describe the pathophysiology of fetal alcohol syndrome.

- Alcohol crosses the placental blood barrier rapidly.
- The fetus depends on maternal hepatic detoxification:
  - The level of alcohol dehydrogenase in fetal liver is < 10%.
  - Amniotic fluid acts as a reservoir for alcohol, which leads to prolonged fetal exposure.
- Ethanol and its metabolite acetaldehyde alter fetal development by:
  - Disrupting cellular differentiation and growth.
  - Disrupting DNA and protein synthesis.
  - Inhibiting cell migration.

170. Describe the microscopic findings and main structures of Wernicke-Korsakoff syndrome.

- Acute phase:
  - Foci of hemorrhage and necrosis in the mammillary bodies, walls of the third ventricle and floor of the fourth ventricles, periaqueductal gray matter, and thalamus.
- Chronic phase:
  - Macrophage infiltration and deposition of hemosiderin and development of cystic spaces in involved structures.
- Mammillary body atrophy (occasionally).
- Lesions in the dorsomedial nucleus of the thalamus, which correlate well with the presence of memory disturbance and confabulation.
- Midline cerebellar degeneration (degeneration of the superior vermis) with Purkinje neurons loss, Bergmann gliosis, and depletion of the internal granular cell layer.

171. List the causes of intramyelinic edema.

- Toxins:
  - Hexachlorophane/hexachlorophene.
  - Triethyltin.
  - 5-Fluorouracil, tegofur, and carmofur.
  - Lithium.
- Nutritional deficiencies:
  - Subacute combined degeneration (vitamin B_{12} deficiency).
- Disorders of metabolism:
  - Mitochondrial encephalopathies.
  - Canavan disease (aspartoacylase deficiency).
  - Several other disorders of amino acid metabolism.
- Infections:
  - Vacuolar myelopathy in HIV infection.
  - Human T-lymphotropic virus type 1 associated myelopathy (HTLV-1 associated myelopathy [HAM]).

172. List the causes of distal degeneration of long axons in the CNS.

- Toxins:
  - Acrylamide:
    - Distal axonal swelling contains accumulation of neurofilament.
  - Carbon disulfide.
  - Cisplatinum:
    - This involves the posterior column only.
  - Clioquinol.
  - Hexacarbon solvents.
  - Organophosphorus:
    - In the early stages, distal axonal swellings contain accumulation of the smooth endoplasmic reticulum.
  - Thallium.
  - Neurolathyrism.
- System degenerations:
  - Motor neuron disease.
  - Hereditary spastic paraparesis.
  - Friedreich ataxia.
- Nutritional deficiencies:
  - Vitamin E deficiency.
  - Pellagra:
    - This results in chromatolysis, which affects:
      - Betz cells.
      - Neurons in the brainstem.
      - Spinal anterior horn cells.
  - Subacute combined degeneration is secondary to the myelinopathy.

173. List the causes of bilateral necrosis of basal ganglia.

- Toxic or hypoxic injury:
  - Carbon monoxide.
  - Cyanide.
  - Methanol.
  - Marchiafava-Bignami disease — associated with chronic alcoholism.
- Heroin and other causes of global cerebral hypoxia.
- Metabolic disorders:
  - Leigh disease.
  - Infantile holotopistic/bilateral striatal necrosis.
  - Wilson disease.

174. List the causes of multifocal necrotizing leukoencephalopathy (MNL).

- Amphotericin B.
- BCNU.
- Cisplatin.
- Cytosine arabinoside.
- Methotrexate.
- X-irradiation.
- AIDS.

Note: the white matter abnormalities in patients with previous carbon monoxide poisoning, global cerebral hypoxia, mitochondrial disorders can be confused with MNL but are usually less circumscribed and tend to contain prominent axonal swellings or to calcify.

175. List the causes of irreversible drug-induced parkinsonism.
- As a major manifestation of neurotoxicity:
  - Manganese.
    - › The substantia nigra is preserved.
    - › Gliosis and loss of neurons from the pallidum and subthalamic nucleus(and to a lesser extent from the caudate and putamen) occur.
  - MPTP.
    - › The pattern of neuronal loss closely resembles that of idiopathic Parkinson disease.
- As a rare manifestation of neurotoxicity:
  - Amphotericin B.
  - Cytosine arabinoside.
  - Carbon tetrachloride.
  - Cyclophosphamide.
  - Ethylene oxide.
  - Haloperidol.
  - Methotrexate.

176. Describe at least 2 distinct changes that develop following early fatal carbon monoxide exposure.
- Bilateral necrosis of the globus pallidus.
- Loss of neurons in the Sommer sector (CA1) of the hippocampus.
- Loss of Purkinje neurons.
- Loss of neurons of the layers III and V of the cerebral cortex.

177. What is psychic akinesia?
- This is an organic psychiatric syndrome.
- It is associated with exposure to low dose carbon monoxide.
- The presentation is characterized by:
  - Inactivity.
  - Lethargy.
  - Amotivational state.
- Imaging shows subtle abnormalities in the globus pallidus that do not represent pannecrosis.

178. Describe at least 3 microscopic changes in injuries produced by combined methotrexate and radiation.
- Focal areas of coagulative necrosis either scattered in the white matter, or located adjacent to the lateral ventricles or in the brainstem.
- Axonal spheroids in the surrounding axons.
- Dystrophic mineralization of the neurons.
- Adjacent gliosis.

179. What is the clinical triad of pellagra (vitamin B**3** deficiency)?
- Dermatitis.
- Diarrhea.
- Dementia.

180. What are the microscopic changes found in pellagra?
- Changes in the CNS occur predominantly in the later stages of pellagra.
- Betz cells and neurons in the pontine and cerebellar dentate nuclei show striking chromatolysis without associated microglial or astrocytic changes.
- Other neurons in the brain stem and the anterior horn cells of the spinal cord may also be affected.
- Symmetric degeneration of the dorsal columns (especially the gracile funiculi) and, to a lesser extent, the corticospinal tracts is present.

181. How can you distinguish between hypoxic ischemic injury and hypoglycemia on microscopy?
- In hypoglycemia:
  - Cerebellar Purkinje cells are spared.
  - Superficial distribution of neuronal necrosis is present.
  - The cortex, hippocampus, and caudate are the most common locations of neuronal loss.

182. What is the etiology of osmotic demyelination syndrome (ODS)?
- It is associated with hyponatremic conditions.
- It develops in patients with normal serum sodium concentrations.
- Incidence is high in liver transplant.
- Risk of developing ODS is related to the severity, duration, and speed of correction.
- It may occur after infusion of hypertonic saline into normonatremic patients.
- It is a complication of chronic malnutrition or debilitation.

183. List extrapontine areas that may be involved in ODS.
- Cerebellum.
- Lateral geniculate nucleus.
- External capsule.
- Extreme capsule.
- Subcortical cerebral white matter.
- Basal ganglia.
- Thalamus.
- Internal capsule.

184. What is the most common CNS complication of recreational drug use, and what is the etiology?

- The most common CNS complications of recreational drugs are cerebrovascular infarcts and hemorrhages, either parenchymal or subarachnoid.
- Causes include:
  - Emboli.
    › This is associated with cardiac arrhythmias, myocardial infarction, or endocarditis.
  - Vasospasm.
    › This involves the pharmacologic action of drugs such as:
      » Amphetamines.
      » Cocaine.
      » Phencyclidine.
      » Lysergic acid diethylamide (LSD).
      » Mescaline.
  - › It can be secondary to subarachnoid hemorrhage.
  - Vasculitis.
    › This is a complication of drugs including:
      » Amphetamines.
      » Phenylpropanolamine.
      » Heroin.
      » Methylphenidate.
      » Ephedrine.
      » Pseudoephedrine.
      » Pentazocine.
      » Tripelennamine.
      » Cocaine.
    › Angiography demonstrates segmental narrowing and dilatation of distal intracerebral arteries.

Nervous System Tumors

185. Name at least 3 common tumors that can develop in the cerebellar (infratentorial) region in children.

- Pilocytic astrocytoma.
- Medulloblastoma.
- Ependymoma.
- Choroid plexus papilloma.
- Atypical teratoid rhabdoid tumor (AT/RT).
- Diffuse pontine gliomas.

186. List the characteristic histologic features of the following tumors: pilocytic astrocytoma, glioblastoma, oligodendroglioma, ependymoma, and medulloblastoma.

- Pilocytic astrocytoma:
  - Low to moderate cellularity.
  - Biphasic pattern.
  - Bipolar cells with long hairlike processes.
  - Rosenthal fibers.
  - Microcysts.
  - Granular bodies/hyaline droplets.
  - Glomeruloid and hyalinized vessels (common).
- Glioblastoma:
  - Densely cellular with high nuclear pleomorphism.
  - Necrosis in a serpentine pattern with tumor cells along the edges of the necrotic regions (pseudopalisading).
  - Vascular or endothelial cell proliferation.
  - Mitotic figures.
  - Infiltrates as single cells.
- Oligodendroglioma:
  - Sheets of regular cells with round to oval nuclei containing finely granular chromatin surrounded by a clear halo of cytoplasm ("fried egg").
- Delicate network of anastomosing capillaries ("chicken wire").
- Calcifications in 90%.
- Secondary structures (perineuronal satellitosis, perivascular aggregation, subpial condensation) common.
- Mucin rich microcysts (common).
- Ependymoma:
  - Sharp demarcation from the adjacent CNS parenchyma.
  - Perivascular pseudorosettes typical.
  - True ependymal rosettes and canals in 5–10%.
  - Round to oval nuclei with small nucleoli and abundant granular chromatin.
- Medulloblastoma:
  - Small blue cells with high nuclear-cytoplasmic ratio.
  - Prominent mitotic activity.
  - Apoptosis (necrosis).
  - Homer Wright rosettes in about 30%.

187. Name at least 3 markers that the College of American Pathologists (CAP) identifies as the most relevant for molecular diagnostics of gliomas.

- 1p/19q deletion.
  - This codeletion is currently required for the diagnosis of oligodendroglioma.
  - Patients with tumors having this codeletion have a longer survival and show an enhanced response to chemotherapy and radiotherapy.
- *IDH1/IDH2* mutation.
  - This is a diagnostic marker for a subset of diffusely infiltrating gliomas.
  - It is present in all oligodendrogliomas, a majority of grade 2 and 3 astrocytomas, and a minority of glioblastomas.
  - *IDH1* mutations are more frequent than *IDH2* mutations; the R132H mutation is the most common and can be identified with an immunoperoxidase stain.

(continued on next page)

- It is associated with a hypermethylation phenotype (CpG island methylation G-CIMP).
- It is associated with a better prognosis.
- MGMT promoter methylation.
  - MGMT (O^6-methylguanine methyltransferase) is a DNA repair enzyme that repairs DNA strand breaks.
  - Methylation of the MGMT promoter diminishes the expression of the enzyme.
  - MGMT promoter methylation is present in about 40–50% of glioblastomas.
  - DNA alkylating agents cause DNA strand breaks, which would normally be repaired by MGMT; methylation diminishes MGMT expression and hence decreases the repair of these DNA breaks and allows the agents to be more effective.
  - MGMT methylation or "epigenetic silencing" is predictive for better response of glioblastoma to alkylating chemotherapy (e.g., temozolomide) combined with radiotherapy.
  - Methylation is associated with longer survival of glioblastoma patients, independent of other factors.
- *BRAF* point mutations, duplication/fusion.
  - This marker is helpful for the diagnosis of pleomorphic xanthoastrocytoma (V600E point mutation in about 66%), gangliogliomas (V600E mutations in about 20%), and pilocytic astrocytomas (V600E mutation in locations outside the cerebellum; fusion with KIAA1549 in about 80% of cerebellar cases).
  - *BRAF* mutations can rarely be found in glioblastomas, especially having large cells with epithelioid morphology.
  - Combination of *BRAF* genetic analysis and IDH mutation status is useful to distinguish pilocytic astrocytoma

and pleomorphic xanthoastrocytoma from diffusely infiltrating astrocytomas.
- *EGFR* amplification or mutations.
  - The epidermal growth factor receptor gene (*EGFR*) is located on chromosome 7p12.
  - EGFR is a receptor for both epidermal growth factor (EGF) and transforming growth factor alpha (TGF-α).
  - Increased EGFR signaling occurs either through gene amplification or through activating or constitutive mutations (e.g., vIII mutation).
  - *EGFR* gene amplification found in about 30–40% of "primary" or "de novo" glioblastomas (e.g., those that do not arise from lower grade astrocytomas) and 10% of anaplastic astrocytomas.
  - *EGFR* gene mutations are mutually exclusive with IDH mutations.
- Phosphatase and tensin homolog (*PTEN*) mutations.
  - *PTEN* is a tumor suppressor gene located on the long arm of chromosome 10 at 10q23.
  - Mutations are frequently found in high grade gliomas.
  - Mutations are practically absent in secondary glioblastomas.
  - LOH at 10q is:
    › Common in high grade astrocytoma and glioblastoma.
    › Less common in anaplastic oligodendrogliomas.
  - 10q LOH and *PTEN* mutations are poor prognostic markers for high grade astrocytomas and glioblastomas.
- *TP53* mutations.
  - This is a prognostic marker for shorter survival.
  - It is present in majority of diffuse astrocytomas (about 60%).
  - It is significantly more frequent in secondary than primary glioblastomas (65% versus 28%).

188. As described in CAP protocols, what is the effect of the mutated isocitrate dehydrogenase (IDH) protein in gliomas?
- Mutant forms encoded by either *IDH1* or *IDH2* lead to the production of the oncometabolite 2-hydroxyglutarate, which inhibits the function of numerous α-ketoglutarate-dependent enzymes.
- Inhibition of the family of histone demethylases and the TET family of 5-methylcytosine hydroxylases has a profound effect on the epigenetic status of mutated cells

and leads directly to a hypermethylator phenotype that has been referred to as the CpG island methylator phenotype (G-CIMP).
- Glial neoplasms having *IDH* gene mutations have a less malignant course, compared to histologically similar tumors without such mutations.

189. As described in CAP protocols, what is *ATRX*?
- *ATRX* is a gene that encodes a protein involved in chromatin remodeling.

- *IDH1* mutation and *TP53* mutation in infiltrating gliomas are strongly associated with inactivating mutations in the *ATRX* gene.

190. Describe the mechanism of telomere lengthening in *ATRX* mutations.
The mechanism is alternative lengthening of telomeres (ALT), in which telomerase-independent mechanisms directly add telomere DNA repeats onto the end of chromosomes (recombination-based mechanism).

191. Indicate the 3 major categories of adult diffuse gliomas and indicate their genetic signatures.
- Oligodendroglioma: codeletion of 1p and 19q; *IDH* mutation; also *CIC* and *FUBP1* mutations.
- Astrocytoma: *IDH* mutation; *ATRX* gene mutation or loss of ATRX expression (1p/19q not codeleted); also *TP53* mutations.

- Glioblastoma: *IDH* not mutated; *ATRX* not mutated; 1p/19q not codeleted; also *EGFR* amplified, *PTEN* mutated, loss of chromosome 10.

192. What are the WHO grades for diffuse infiltrating *IDH*-mutant astrocytomas and histologic criteria used in grading?

WHO GRADE AND DESIGNATION	HISTOLOGIC CRITERIA
Grade 2 astrocytoma	• Increased cellularity, nuclear atypia.
Grade 3 astrocytoma	• Nuclear atypia, increased cellular density, and mitotic figures (required).
Grade 4 astrocytoma	• Nuclear atypia, mitotic figures and endothelial proliferation, and/or necrosis (either of latter 2 required).

193. What is the immunohistochemical and molecular profile of oligodendrogliomas?
- *IDH1/2* mutation along with 1p19q codeletion.
- *TERT* promoter mutations.
- *ATRX* wild-type.
- No mutation of *TP53* — mutually exclusive with 1p/19q codeletion.

194. If you find atypia and endovascular proliferation in an oligodendroglioma, what is the WHO grade?

Grade 3 oligodendroglioma.

Note: grade 3 oligodendroglioma may histologically resemble glioblastoma, but as long as *IDH* is mutated and 1p/19q is codeleted, the tumor is still considered an anaplastic oligodendroglioma (WHO grade 3).

195. What is the most important prognostic factor for ependymomas?
- Extent of tumor resection.
- Microvascular proliferation, pseudopalisading necrosis, frequent mitoses, and a high cell density are important for grading, but less important than the extent of resection.

196. What are the 9 molecular subgroups of ependymoma?

LOCATION	GROUP	GENETICS	PATHOLOGY	PROGNOSIS
Supratentorial	• ST-EPN-RELA.	*RELA* fusion gene.	Classic/anaplastic.	• Poor.
	• ST-EPN-YAP1.	• *YAP1* fusion gene.	Classic/anaplastic.	• Good.
	• ST-SE.	• Balanced genome.	Subependymoma.	• Good.
Posterior fossa	• PF-EPN-A.	• Balanced genome.	Classic/anaplastic.	• Poor.
	• PF-EPN-B.	• Genome-wide polyploidy.	Classic/anaplastic.	• Good.
	• PF-SE.	• Balanced genome.	Subependymoma.	• Good.
Spinal	• SP-EPN.	• *NF2* mutation.	Classic/anaplastic.	• Good.
	• SP-MPE.	• Genome-wide polyploidy.	Myxopapillary.	• Good.
	• SP-SE.	• 6q deletion.	Subependymoma.	• Good.

197. What is the WHO grade assigned for ependymoma?

Grade 2 or 3.

198. What are the macroscopic and microscopic features of ependymoma?
- Macroscopy:
  - It is well circumscribed.
  - It may be cystic.
  - It has a hemorrhagic, cherry red appearance.
- Microscopy:
  - Classic features include:
    › Perivascular pseudorosettes.
    › True rosettes, lumina, canals.
    › Sheetlike growth pattern, hypercellular.
    › Highly fibrillar areas, sometimes with few nuclei.
    › Necrosis in posterior fossa (not an indicator of anaplasia).
  - Variants include:
    › Clear cell.
    › Papillary.
    › Tancyte.

199. What is the immunohistochemical profile of ependymoma?
- Positive for:
  - GFAP.
  - Epithelial membrane antigen (EMA).
    › Surfaces, especially true rosettes, canals, papilla.
    › Dot-like staining of microlumina.
  - CD56.
    › Throughout tumor and microlumina.
- Negative for:
  - Oligodendrocyte transcription factor 2 (OLIG2).

200. What are the ultrastructural features of ependymoma?
- Microlumina with microvilli.
- Cilia and ciliary apparatus.
- Runs of intermediate junctions, especially near microlumina.

201. What is the most common location for myxopapillary ependymoma and what is the cell of origin?
- Location: filum terminale.
- Cell of origin: radial glia.

202. What is the WHO grade assigned for myxopapillary ependymoma?
Grade 2.

203. What is the classic feature of myxopapillary ependymomas on imaging?
MRI shows a discrete, contrast-enhancing lesion.

204. What are the macroscopic and microscopic features of myxopapillary ependymoma?
- Macroscopy:
  - Well-circumscribed, encapsulated in some cases.
  - Spontaneous rupture with involvement of nerve roots or CSF dissemination possible.
  - Soft, myxoid with a translucent membrane.
- Microscopy:
  - Perivascular arrangement of epithelial cells around mucin.
  - Pseudopapillae, ribbons or strands of epithelial cells.
- Epithelial surfaces in some cases.
- Fibrillar tumor similar to tanycytic ependymoma, but often with perivascular myxoid substance.
- Microcysts.
- Dense sclerosis or infarction in some cases, absence of interspersed reticulin fibers, unlike schwannoma.
- Large, hyperchromatic pleomorphic nuclei without increased mitotic or Ki 67 rate (giant cell ependymoma) in occasional cases.

205. List the epigenetic modifications in glioblastoma.
- Hypermethylation of DNA:
  - Transcription of specific genes is shut down, resulting in the loss of protein product. This has impacts on genes and pathways that could potentially act as regulators. The result is:
    › Proliferation.
    › Apoptosis.
    › Migration.
    › Invasion.
  - *Rb*, *PTEN*, *TP53*, and *CDKN2/Ap16* are examples of tumor suppressor genes that are hypermethylated in some glioblastomas.
  - Hypermethylation of the MGMT promoter is associated with better survival.
  - A particular pattern of methylation called the glioma-CpG island methylator phenotype (G-CIMP) is strongly associated with:
    › Proneural gene expression phenotype.
    › *IDH1* mutation.
- Hypomethylation of DNA:
  - Global hypomethylation occurs in many primary glioblastomas (~80%).
  - The effect of hypomethylation may be inappropriate transcriptional activation of genes.
  - Marked global hypomethylation in glioblastoma has been associated with increased cellular proliferation, in part due to activation of oncogenes like *MAGEA1*.
- Hypomethylated repetitive sequences are also genetically unstable and are prone to copy-number aberrations.
- Aberrant histones:
  - Histones are protein components of chromatin that have functions in spooling DNA and regulating gene expression.
  - Anomalous histone H3K9 methylation and decreased H3K9 acetylation may predispose CpG islands to hypermethylation.
  - Mutations of histone deacetylase genes (*HDAC2, HDAC9*) and histone demethylases (*KDM3A, KDM3B*), and histone methyltransferases (*SETD7, MLL*) have been identified in glioblastoma.
- MicroRNA (miRNA):
  - Each of these short, noncoding RNAs (19–27 nucleotides) can potentially bind several different messenger RNA (mRNA) sequences, preventing translation or promoting degradation of the respective genes.
  - Different miRNAs are overexpressed or repressed in primary glioblastoma with various effects.
  - Increased levels of miRNA26a repress *PTEN* and *Rb* (upregulation of miRNA21 has an antiapoptotic effect).
  - In contrast, overexpression of miRNA-128 can block self-renewal capacity of stem cells in vitro.

206. What is the molecular profile of pediatric low grade gliomas?
- Duplications of portions of the *FGFR1* gene.
- Translocations involving *MYB*.

207. What is the diagnostic approach to diffuse high grade pediatric glioma?

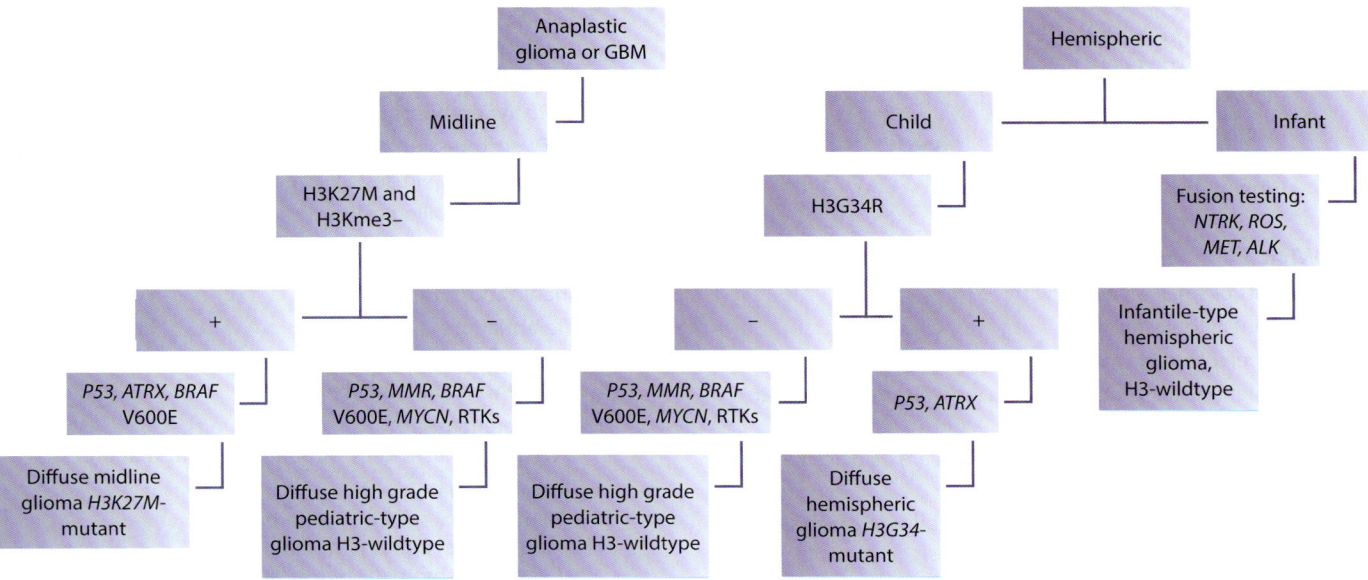

Abbreviations: GBM: glioblastoma; RTK: receptor tyrosine kinase.
Courtesy of Dr. Cynthia Hawkins.

208. List 3 types of choroid plexus tumors in the WHO classification.
- Papilloma, grade 1.
- Atypical papilloma, grade 2.
- Carcinoma, grade 3.

209. What are the microscopic features of choroid plexus papilloma and atypical papilloma?
- Papilloma:
  · More complex papillary architecture than normal plexus.
  · Surface of epithelium flat rather than normal cobblestone.
  · Transition to normal choroid plexus (common).
  · Foci with elongate, bipolar tumor cells (glial differentiation).
  · Acinar architecture (rare).
  · Prominent vascular hyalinization.
  · Calcification.
  › Focal oncocytic changes.
- Atypical papilloma:
  · ≥ 2 mitoses per 10 HPF.
  · Crowding.
  · Cytological atypia.
  · Pseudostratification.
  · Solid, nonpapillary areas.
  · Necrosis (possible).

210. What are the macroscopic and microscopic features of choroid plexus carcinoma?
- Macroscopy:
  · Fleshy.
  · Hemorrhage and necrosis — mainly in anaplastic types.
  · Invasive in some cases.
  · Intraoperative bleeding in some cases.
- Microscopy:
  · More cellular than papilloma.
  · Considerable inter- and intratumoral variation in degree of anaplasia.
  · Mitotically, no precise cutoff from atypical papilloma, but carcinoma generally ≥ 5–10 per 10 HPF; often ≥ 5 per 10 HPF in presence of solid areas.
  · Hypercellularity.
  · Necrosis.
  · Solid, nonpapillary areas (most cases).

211. What familial syndromes are associated with choroid plexus carcinoma?
- Li-Fraumeni cancer syndrome (germline *TP53* mutation).
- Aicardi cancer syndrome.

212. What is the most common intraocular tumor in children?
Retinoblastoma.

213. What crucial role does the retinoblastoma gene (*Rb*) play in the cell cycle?
- *Rb* encodes 110–114 kDa nuclear protein, which plays a crucial role in cell cycle progression by regulating cell cycle arrest.
  · Major checkpoint at G1.
  · Blocking S-phase entry and cell growth.
- *Rb* includes 3 "pocket proteins":
  · *Rb*/p105.
  · p107.
  · *Rb2*/p130.

(continued on next page)

- Forms of *Rb* include:
  - Active.
    - Hypophosphorylated.
    - Binds to E2F family of transcription factors which bind to DNA and inhibit transcription.
  - Inactive — leads to transcription.
    - Phosphorylated via cyclin D-CDK4/CDK6 complexes.
    - Inhibited by p16INK4a.
  - Caused by:
    - Loss of p16INK4a, leading to phosphorylation of *Rb* which inactivates the protein.
    - *Rb* mutations.
    - *Rb* hyperphosphorylation.
    - Overexpression of cyclin D.
    - DNA tumor viruses: SV40 T antigen, adenovirus.
    - Human papillomavirus.

214. What are the microscopic features of retinoblastoma?
- Sheets of small blue cells with:
  - Scant cytoplasm.
  - Hyperchromatic nuclei.
- Frequent necrosis of tumor cells (away from vessels and calcification).
- Flexner-Wintersteiner rosettes (nuclei are displaced away from lumen).
- Fluerettes (tumor cells arranged side by side which show differentiation toward photoreceptors).
- Azzopardi phenomena: basophilic deposits around blood vessels (also seen in small cell carcinoma).
- Frequent mitosis.

- Variable apoptosis.
- Differentiation:
  - Differentiated.
    - Presence of bipolar-like cells.
  - Undifferentiated.
    - Large anaplastic cells without rosette formation.
  - Retinocytoma.
    - Marked photoreceptor differentiation.
    - Abundant cytoplasm in cells.
    - Less hyperchromatic nuclei.
    - Presence of calcification, and absence of necrosis and mitotic activity.

215. Name 3 types of embryonal tumors and indicate the molecular signature.
- Medulloblastoma; several signatures or subtypes:
  - WNT-activated (nuclear β-catenin expression; filamin A and YAP1 expression); monsomy 6.
  - SHH (sonic hedgehog pathway — PTCH, SMO, SUFU mutations; GAB1, filamin A, and YAP1 expression); desmoplastic histology; 9q deletion.
  - Non-SHH/WNT (chromosome 17 abnormalities; no nuclear β-catenin; no GAB1 or YAP1 expression; MYC amplification).
- Pineoblastoma; complex; including mutation and loss of heterozygosity in *Rb1* (retinoblastoma) gene on chromosome 13.
- AT/RT (atypical teratoid/rhabdoid tumor); loss of INI1 (*SMARCB1*) expression; loss of heterozygosity at 22q11.2.
- ETANTR (embryonal tumor with abundant neuropil and true rosettes); high *LIN28A* expression; low *OLIG2* levels; amplification of miRNA cluster C19MC.
- Retinoblastoma; mutation and loss of heterozygosity in *Rb1* (retinoblastoma) gene on chromosome 13.

216. As described in CAP protocols, what is rhabdoid tumor predisposition syndrome (RTPS) and how is it diagnosed?
- RTPS is characterized by germline mutations of *SMARCB1/INI1* and manifested by a marked predisposition to the development of malignant rhabdoid tumors of infancy and early childhood.
- Up to one-third of atypical teratoid/rhabdoid tumors (AT/RTs) arise in the setting of RTPS, and the majority of these occur within the first year of life.
- Diagnosis:
  - Demonstration of a germline *SMARCB1* or *SMARCA4* mutation in a patient with MRT is sufficient for the diagnosis of RTPS1 or RTPS2, respectively.
  - Children with multiple MRTs or with affected siblings or other relatives are almost certain to be affected by RTPS themselves.
- Because of the risk associated with the RTPS, the germ line status of *SMARCB1*/INI1 is typically assessed for each new case of AT/RT.

217. What are the most common pediatric brain tumors between birth and 14 years of age?
- Pilocytic astrocytoma (PA) (19–23%).
- Malignant glioma (14%), especially pontine gliomas.
- Embryonal tumors such as medulloblastoma (13%).

218. Name at least 4 inherited syndromes associated with nervous system neoplasms and indicate their associated tumors.
- Cowden syndrome (*PTEN* gene) — dysplastic cerebellar gangliocytoma (Lhermitte-Duclos disease).
  - Mutations result in activation of the PI3K/AKT signaling pathway.
- Li-Fraumeni syndrome (*TP53* gene) — astrocytomas, glioblastomas, and medulloblastomas.
- Turcot syndrome (constitutional mismatch repair genes *MLH1*, *MSH2*, *MSH6*, and *PMS2*) — medulloblastoma or glioblastoma.

(continued on next page)

- Gorlin syndrome (*PTCH* or patched gene) — medulloblastoma.
  - Mutations cause an upregulation of sonic hedgehog signaling pathways.
- Tuberous sclerosis complex (*TSC1* and *TSC2* genes) — hamartomas within the CNS that take the form of cortical tubers and subependymal nodules; subependymal giant cell astrocytomas.
- Von Hippel-Lindau disease (*VHL* gene): hemangioblastomas of the CNS (cerebellum and retina) and cysts involving the pancreas, liver, and kidneys.

- Patients are at increased risk to develop renal cell carcinoma and pheochromocytoma.
- Neurofibromatosis, type 1 (*NF1* gene) — pigmented nodules of the iris (Lisch nodules), cutaneous hyperpigmented macules (café au lait spots), neurofibromas of peripheral nerves, optic nerve glioma, malignant peripheral nerve sheath tumors.
- Neurofibromatosis, type 2 (*NF2* gene) — often bilateral vestibular schwannomas, multiple meningiomas, spinal ependymoma.

219. What are the inactivating mutations in tuberous sclerosis and what are their associated proteins?
- *TSC1*:
  - Notes: is important for cell growth and turnover; affects chromosome 9.
  - Protein: hamartin.
- *TSC2*:
  - Notes: acts as tumor suppressor gene; affects chromosome 16; is the more common mutation in sporadic cases.
  - Protein: tuberin.

220. List the mode of inheritance and the gene involved in the following phakomatoses.

DISEASE	INHERITANCE	GENE/CHROMOSOME
Ataxia-telangiectasia	• Autosomal recessive.	• *ATM* chr 11.
Sturge-Weber syndrome (encephalofacial/ encephalotrigeminal angiomatosis)	• Sporadic.	• *GNAQ* chr 9.
Neurofibromatosis type 1	• Autosomal dominant.	• *NF1* chr 17.
Neurofibromatosis type 2	• Autosomal dominant.	• *NF2* chr 22.
Tuberous sclerosis	• Autosomal dominant/sporadic.	• *TSC1* chr /*TSC2* chr .
Von Hippel-Lindau disease	• Autosomal dominant.	• *VHL* chr 3.
Cowden syndrome	• Autosomal dominant.	• *PTEN* chr 10.
Gorlin-Goltz syndrome	• Autosomal dominant.	• *PTCH* chr 9 (encodes for SHH receptor).
Carney complex (melanotic schwannoma)	• Autosomal dominant.	• *PRKAR1A* chr 17.

221. What are 2 germline mutations in schwannomatosis?
- *SMARCB1* on 22q.
- *LZTR1* on 22q.

222. What is the characteristic clinical feature distinguishing schwannomatosis from neurofibromatosis type 2(NF2)?

Severe pain associated with the tumors is characteristic of schwannomatosis. This is a distinguishing feature from NF2, in which pain is rare and neurological deficits and polyneuropathy are common.

223. What is the function of the *SMARCB1* gene?
- *SMARCB1* encodes a protein which is a core subunit of mammalian SWI/SNF chromatin remodeling complexes.
  - It regulates the expression of many genes by using adenosine triphosphate (ATP) for sliding the nucleosomes along the DNA helix, facilitating or repressing transcription.
- SMARCB1 protein functions as a tumor suppressor via:
  - › Repression of *CCND1* gene expression.
  - › Induction of the *CDKN2A* gene.
  - › Hypophosphorylation of retinoblastoma protein, resulting in G0/G1 cell cycle arrest.

224. What are the sites of involvement in Li-Fraumeni cancer syndrome?
- Breast cancer.
- Soft tissue sarcomas.
- CNS tumors.
- Adrenal tumors.
- Bone tumors.

225. Cowden syndrome is an autosomal dominant disorder, caused by a germline mutation in *PTEN*. What is this syndrome characterized by?
- Patients have multiple hamartomas involving tissues derived from all 3 germ cell layers.
- They have a high risk of breast, epithelial thyroid, endometrial, renal, and colon cancers.

(continued on next page)

- Facial trichilemmomas are highly characteristic of Cowden syndrome.
- Adult-onset dysplastic cerebellar gangliocytoma (Lhermitte-Duclos disease) is also considered to be pathognomonic.

226. Name 3 types of tumors that involve the meninges or dura.
- Meningioma.
- Hemangiopericytoma.
- Melanocytoma or primary melanoma.
- B cell lymphoma of mucosa-associated lymphoid tissue (MALT).
- Leiomyosarcoma associated with Epstein-Barr virus (EBV) infection in immunosuppressed host.
- Metastases, especially prostate to dura.
- Hemangioblastoma.

227. What are the histologic criteria and grades for meningioma in the WHO classification?
- Grade 1: benign meningioma.
- Grade 2: atypical meningioma:
  · **Either:** 1) mitosis 4–19 in 10 consecutive HPF; or 2) unequivocal brain invasion (not only perivascular spread or indentation of brain without pial breach);
  · **Or** at least 3 of the following 5 histologic parameters:
    › Sheeting architecture (loss of whirling and/or fascicles).
    › Small cell formation.
    › Macronucleoli.
    › Hypercellularity.
    › "Spontaneous" necrosis.
- Grade 3: anaplastic (malignant) meningioma:
  · Any 1 of:
    › Mitosis ≥ 20/10 HPF.
    › Frank anaplasia (sarcoma, carcinoma, or melanoma-like histology).
    › Either of the following: *TERT* promoter mutation; or homozygous deletion of *CDKN2A* and/or *CDKN2B*.

228. List at least 3 gross features of meningioma.
- Rubbery or firm.
- Well-circumscribed and demarcated.
- Broad dural attachment.
- Invasion of underlying dura or of dural sinuses (common).
- Low grade tumors (typically): indentation, but no invasion, of brain.

229. Name common light microscopic features of meningioma.
- Formation of lobules, some partly demarcated by thin collagenous septae.
- Formation of whorls that recapitulate arachnoid granulations.
- Psammoma bodies, often in the center of whorls.
- Cells appearing to form a syncytium, in which individual cells seem to lack cell borders (ultrastructurally, the borders interdigitate).
- Bland, round-to-oval nuclei that occasionally contain pale cytoplasmic pseudoinclusions.

230. Name at least 3 histologic subtypes of grade 1 meningiomas.
- Meningothelial meningioma.
- Fibrous (fibroblastic) meningioma.
- Transitional (mixed) meningioma.
- Psammomatous meningioma.
- Angiomatous meningioma.
- Microcystic meningioma.
- Secretory meningioma.

231. List at least 3 features suggesting aggressive behavior of meningioma.
- Increased mitotic activity.
- Increased cellularity.
- Collections of small tumor cells with a high nuclear to cytoplasmic ratio.
- Macronucleoli or cells with prominent nucleoli.
- Patternless, sheetlike growth.
- Foci of "spontaneous" or "geographic" necrosis.
- Clear cell morphology.
- Chordoid morphology.
- Brain invasion.

232. What is the molecular signature of rhabdoid meningioma?
BAP1 inactivation.

233. List the immunohistochemical stains that are helpful in distinguishing meningioma from schwannoma.
- EMA — positive in meningioma and negative in schwannoma.
- S100 protein — strong and diffusely positive in schwannoma, but focal, patchy, or minimal staining in meningioma.

234. Name at least 3 common tumors that can develop in the sella turcica.
- Pituitary adenoma.
- Craniopharyngioma.
- Rathke cleft cyst.
- Meningioma.

235. List the subtypes of pituitary adenoma as defined by their transcription factors.
- PIT-1: thyrotroph, lactotroph, sommatotroph, mixed somatotroph-lactrotroph, mammosomatotroph, acidophil stem cell.
- TPit: corticotroph.
- SF1: gonadtotroph

236. List the aggressive pituitary adenomas.
- Sparsely granulated GH adenoma.
- Acidophil stem cell adenoma.
- Silent corticotroph adenoma.
- Crooke hyaline adenoma.
- Multihormonal adenoma; silent subtype.
- Lactotroph adenoma in men.

237. What are the 2 types of craniopharyngioma, and what are their molecular alterations?
- Admantinomatous craniopharyngioma: *CTNNB1*.
- Papillary craniopharyngioma: *BRAF* V600E.

238. Identify tumors that have the radiological appearance of a cyst with an enhancing nodule.
- Pilocytic astrocytoma.
- Pleomorphic xanthoastrocytoma.
- Ganglioglioma.
- Metastasis, especially metastatic adenocarcinoma.

239. Name at least 3 radiation effects that can be found in a treated tumor.
- Coagulative and fibrinoid parenchymal and vascular necrosis.
- Vascular hyalinization.
- Vascular telangiectasias.
- Rarefied hypocellular parenchyma.
- Dystrophic calcification.
- Radiation induced atypia (bizarre bubbly nuclei and abundant pink cytoplasm).
- Gliosis.
- p53 positive nuclei.

240. How do you stage nonembryonal CNS tumors?
CNS tumors are not staged.

241. How do you stage CNS embryonal tumors postoperatively?
- The staging system developed by Chang et al, including MRI examination of the CNS with a constrast agent and CSF cytology, has the following categories:
- M0: no evidence of subarachnoid or hematogenous metastasis.
- M1: microscopic tumour cells found in the cerebrospinal fluid.
- M2: gross nodular seeding demonstrated in the cerebellar/cerebral subarachnoid space or in the third or lateral ventricles.
- M3: gross nodular seeding the spinal subarachnoid space.
- M4: metastasis outside the cerebrospinal axis.

242. List the histopathological prognostic factors recommended for the clinical care of CNS tumors based on the eighth edition of the American Joint Committee on Cancer (AJCC) staging manual (2017).
- Accuracy of diagnosis.
- Grade of tumor (according to the 2016 WHO classification of CNS tumors).
- Presence and extent of mitosis, pleomorphism, necrosis, endothelial proliferation, oligodendroglial component, and gemistocytes.
- Proliferative fraction (Ki 67, MIB1).

243. List the molecular status required as clinical prognostic factors for CNS tumors.
- IDH mutation status required for gliomas for clinical care: level 1.
- 1p,19q deletions required for gliomas for clinical care: level 1.
- MGMT methylations status required for gliomas for clinical care: level 1.

244. List the clinical prognostic factors recommended for the care of CNS tumors based on the AJCC staging manual.
- Age of the patient: young favorable; > 65 years unfavorable.
- Location of the tumor: unilateral or multifocal.
- Eloquent or noneloquent brain area.
- Functional neutological status: Karnosfsky score, quality of life.
- Symptoms at presentation and duration before diagnosis: seizures and long duration of symptoms are favorable.
- Primary tumor or recurrent tumor.
- Extent of resection: biopsy, subtotal, radical, complete (gross).

Skeletal Muscle and Peripheral Nerve

245. Define the functional unit of the neuromuscular unit.

- Neuromuscular unit: the anterior horn neuron, its axon, and the muscle fibers it supplies, all of which are functionally dependent on each other.
  - The nerves innervating muscle fibers have their origin in lower motor neurons within the anterior horns of the spinal cord.
- The axons of these neurons branch to supply a variable number of muscle fibers, which in most muscles is several hundred.
- Each myofiber is innervated by only 1 lower motor neuron.
- Firing of a single lower motor neuron activates all of the myofibers it innervates.

246. List at least 3 major proteins in the composition of myelin in the peripheral nervous system (PNS).

- Myelin protein zero (MPZ).
  - A transmembrane protein, which functions in the compaction of the apposing lipid bilayers of myelin.
  - 50% of PNS myelin protein.
- Myelin basic protein (MBP).
  - Located on the internal surface of the bilayers at the major dense line of myelin.
- Peripheral myelin protein 22 (PMP22).
  - A 22 kDa transmembrane protein located in compacted myelin.
- Myelin-associated glycoprotein (MAG).
  - Glycoprotein in the immunoglobulin superfamily that stabilizes the connection between the Schwann cells and its underlying axon.

247. Describe the topology of the T-tubule system.

The T-tubule system is an invagination of the sarcolemmal membrane into the interior of the cell. It runs parallel to the Z bands and is accompanied on each side by sarcoplasmic reticulum, which store calcium to be released during contraction. The T-tubule system carries the action potential from the superficial neuromuscular junction to deep inside the myofiber.

248. What is the primary function of the T-tubule system?

- Involved in coupling excitation with contraction. T-tubules invaginations allow depolarization of the membrane to quickly penetrate to the interior of the cell.
  - During membrane depolarization, L-type calcium channels are activated.
- This activation leads to release of calcium from the sarcoplasmic reticulum.
- Release of calcium further depolarizes the cells and starts a cascade of events that leads to contraction.

249. What are the characteristics of the major muscle fiber types?

- 2 major fiber types: type 1 and type 2 defined on the basis of histochemistry and biology (see table below).

HISTOCHEMISTRY/BIOLOGY	TYPE 1	TYPE 2
Action	• Slow movements/sustained force.	• Rapid movements.
Fatigability	• Resistant.	• Sensitive.
Strength	• Weight bearing.	• Flight.
Mitochondrial content	• Many mitochondria.	• Fewer mitochondria.
Lipid content	• Abundant.	• Scant.
Glycogen content	• Scant.	• Abundant.

250. To evaluate mitochondrial disease, compare the following stains: Gomori one-step trichrome stain, cytochrome oxidase histochemistry, and succinate dehydrogenase immunoperoxidase.

- Gomori one-step trichrome stain: this binds to structural aspects of proteins. It stains mitochondria red and shows mitochondrial aggregation but does not assess mitochondrial function.
- Cytochrome oxidase histochemistry: this assays mitochondrial enzymatic activity. It represents the final step in oxidative phosphorylation and is lost in many electron transport disorders, but not all mitochondrial diseases. Key components of this enzyme are encoded in the mitochondrial genome.
- Succinate dehydrogenase (SDH) immunoperoxidase stains: an antibody to SDH would identify the mitochondria specific protein and hence show their distribution in the myofibers but would not assess whether the SDH was functional. This is in contrast to SDH histochemistry, which would assay both the distribution of mitochondria and their initial functioning in the Krebs cycle. SDH is encoded in the nucleus and can be intact even with the mitochondrial genome is defective.

251. What are the types of lipid metabolism disorders?
- Systemic (primary):
  - Carnitine deficiency.
  - Multiple acyl-CoA dehydrogenase deficiency.
  - Neutral lipid storage disease.
- Secondary:
  - Mitochondrial disease.
    - › Lipid storage secondary to oxidative phosphorylation.
  - Inflammation.
  - Drug-induced disorder.
  - Congenital myasthenic syndrome *DOK7* mutation.

252. What are conditions associated with myoglobinuria?
- Rhabdomyolysis.
- McArdle disease.
- Lipid storage myopathy:
  - Carnitine deficiency.
  - Lipin-1 (children) deficiency.
  - Carnitine palmitoyl transferase deficiency.
    - › CPT2.
  - Short chain acyl-CoA dehydrogenase deficiency.
  - Very long chain acyl-CoA dehydrogenase deficiency.
  - Trifunctional protein deficiency.
- Isolated myopathy.
- Progressive external ophthalmoplegia (PEO).
- Toxic myoglobinuria.
- Malignant hyperthermia .

253. Name conditions associated with polyglucosan bodies.
- Phosphofructokinase.
- *GBE1*-mutation-associated polyglucosan body myopathy.
- *GYG1*-mutation-associated polyglucosan body myopathy.
- Lafora disease.

254. What is the type of deficiency associated with type 2 glycogenosis (Pompe disease)?
Acid maltase.

255. What are the early histologic changes of Wallerian degeneration?
- It occurs in the first 24–36 hours after a nerve fiber is cut or crushed (CNS or PNS).
- It starts distal to the injury.
- It consists of the breakdown of axonal skeleton and the breaking apart of axonal membrane.
- The distal axon stump is initially still electrically excitable.

256. What are the later histologic changes of Wallerian degeneration?
- Later changes include degradation of the myelin sheath and infiltration by macrophages, which participate in the phagocytosis of axonal and myelin-derived debris.
- The nerve fiber's neurolemma remains a hollow tube.

257. How does a peripheral axon regenerate?
- Within 96 hours of the injury, the distal end of the portion of the nerve fiber proximal to the lesion sends out sprouts toward the hollow tubes.
- These sprouts are attracted by growth factors produced by Schwann cells in the tubes, eventually reinnervating the target tissue.

258. What are the most common reactions of muscle fibers to pathological processes?
- Internalized nuclei.
- Myofiber segmental necrosis.
- Myophagocytosis.
- Vacuolation.
- Increased endomysial connective tissue.
- Regeneration.
- Hypertrophy.
- Myofiber splitting.

259. Describe the main features that distinguish myopathic from neurogenic changes in the skeletal muscle.

MYOPATHIC	NEUROGENIC
• Single atrophic fibers.	• Group atrophy.
• Rounded fibers.	• Angular, atrophic fiber; nuclear bags.
• Internalized nuclei.	• No internalized nuclei.
• Checkerboard pattern intact.	• Fiber type grouping (on ATPase stains) — loss of checkerboard.
• Necrotic and basophilic (regenerating) fibers.	• No necrotic or basophilic fibers.
• Endomysial (within muscle bundle) fibrosis.	• No endomysial fibrosis.
• Inflammation.	• No inflammation.
• Normal NADH staining.	• Target and targetoid fibers.

260. Explain the phenomenon of fiber type grouping.

- This phenomenon appears in the setting of chronic denervation-reinnervation.
  - A single lower motor neuron innervates several to many hundreds of myofibers, which is termed the motor unit. This innervation determines whether a muscle fiber will be type 1 or type 2: all fibers of a motor unit are of the same type.
  - The myofibers of a single motor unit are scattered across the muscle, giving rise to a checkerboard pattern of alternating fiber types.
- When axonal degeneration occurs, the muscle fibers within the affected motor unit undergo denervation atrophy.
- The atrophic muscle fibers recover when reinnervation from a neighboring axon occurs. However, because the axon is from a different motor unit, the myofiber will assume the type of the neighboring axon.
- Thus, the number of myofibers belonging to that motor unit increases, and the "checkerboard" pattern becomes distorted by larger patches of myofibers of the same type — fiber type grouping.

261. Name at least 3 common causes of type 2 fiber atrophy.

- Disuse.
- Weight loss > 15%.
- Corticosteroid myopathy.
- Aging.
- Systemic diseases: paraneoplastic, collagen vascular.
- Spinal cord disease/pyramidal tract disease.

262. What is acute inflammatory demyelinating polyradiculopathy (Guillain-Barré syndrome) and what are the main histopathological changes?

- Description:
  - This is an acute onset immune mediated neuropathy, often preceded by an acute influenza-like illness (~60% cases).
  - Microorganisms shown to have a significant epidemiological association include *Campylobacter jejuni*, cytomegalovirus, Epstein-Barr virus, and *Mycoplasma pneumoniae*.
- Histopathological findings:
  - Main finding: presence of endoneurial and perivascular chronic inflammation (lymphocytes, plasma cells, and macrophages).
- The process mostly affects the nerve roots.
- The primary lesion is segmental demyelination affecting peripheral nerves.
- Electron microscopy can identify the early effects on myelin sheaths with cytoplasmic processes of macrophages penetrating the basement membrane of Schwann cells, particularly in the vicinity of nodes of Ranvier, and extending between the myelin lamellae, stripping away the myelin sheath from the axon.
- Remyelination follows demyelination.

263. Name at least 3 infectious diseases that can affect peripheral nerves.

- Leprosy (*Mycobacterium leprae*).
- Diphtheria.
- Varicella zoster (varicella-zoster virus).
- Lyme disease (*Borrelia burgdorferi*).
- HIV.

264. Name the mutations underlying hereditary motor sensory neuropathy type I (HMSN, or Charcot-Marie-Tooth disease, demyelinating type).

- Duplication of a large region on chromosome 17p11.2 (*PMP22* gene) in HMSN IA (70%).
- Point mutations in *MPZ* gene on chromosome 1q22–33 in HMSN IB (20%).
- Point mutations in *LITAF* gene on chromosome 16p12–13 in HMSN IC (< 10%).
- Point mutations in *EGR2* gene on chromosome 10q21–22 in HMSN ID (rare).

265. What are the main histopathological changes encountered in peripheral neuropathy associated with adult onset diabetes mellitus?

- Axonal degeneration — determines distal symmetric sensorimotor neuropathy.
- Segmental demyelination, and a relative loss of small myelinated and unmyelinated fibers.
- Loss of large myelinated fibers (sometimes).
- Thickening hyalinization of the endoneurial arterioles with intense PAS positivity in their walls and reduplication of their basement membrane by electron microscopy.

266. What are the types of vasculitis most commonly associated with nerve and muscle disease?

Polyarteritis nodosa (PAN) and hypersensitivity microvasculitis (a vasculitis associated with antineutrophil cytoplasmic antibodies [ANCA]).

267. List 4 types of myelin abnormalities and give an example of each.

- Macrophage stripping myelin.
  - Guillain-Barre syndrome.
- Hypomyelination.
  - Congenital hypomyelinating neuropathy (CHN):
    › Hypotonia and muscle weakness at birth resulting in slow development.
    › Pathology:
      » Marked reduction or even absence of myelin.

(continued on next page)

» Onion bulbs composed of basal lamina reduplication.
› Etiology:
  » Mutations of *PMP22, MPZ*, and *PRX*.
· Hypomyelination and congenital cataracts (HCC; also known as hypomyelinating leukodystrophy 5 [HLD5]).
  › *DRCTNNB1A* mutation.
• Uncompact myelin/wide spaced myelin.
· Widening of myelin lamellae (rarely seen in the absence of a dysclobulememia):
  › Waldenström macroglobulinemia.

› Monoclonal gammopathy of unknown significance (MGUS).
· Uncompacted myelin lamellae:
  › POEMS; also acute and chronic inflammatory demyelinating polyneuropathy (CIDP).
  › Hereditary neuropathy with pressure palsies, Charcot-Marie-Tooth disease type 1 (CMT-1), and inflammatory demyelinating polyradiculoneuritis.
• Hypermyelination:
· CIDP and in the spectrum of CMT.
· Tomaculous neuropathy (hereditary neuropathy with propensity to develop pressure palsies).

268. Name at least 3 causes of metabolic or nutritional peripheral neuropathies.
• Vitamin B$_1$ (thiamine) deficiency (beriberi).
• Vitamin B$_{12}$ deficiency.
• Vitamin B$_6$ deficiency.
• Vitamin E deficiency.
• Renal failure.
• Chronic ethanol consumption.

269. What are the 2 most common X-linked muscular dystrophies and what is the underlying genetic defect?
• 2 most common:
· Duchenne muscular dystrophy (DMD) — appears earlier in life and is the most severe and most common.
· Becker muscular dystrophy (BMD) — appears later in life.
• Genetic defect: mutations in *DMD* gene on Xp21 encoding dystrophin.
· Intragenic deletions of the *DMD* gene:
· Frameshift (65%).
· Duplications (10%).
· Frame shifting point mutations (presumed 25%).

270. Describe the major histopathological changes in DMD and BMD.
• Early stages:
· Variation in fiber size.
· Fiber splitting (which is a manifestation of fiber regeneration).
· Increased number of internalized nuclei (beyond the normal range; in adults, the normal range is considered 3–5%, while in children it is significantly less).
• Later stages:
· Degeneration (fiber necrosis) and regeneration (basophilic fibers) of muscle fibers.
· Hypercontracted fibers.
· Extensive endomysial fibrosis.
• Final stages:
· Muscle almost totally replaced by fat and connective tissue.

271. What are the 2 types of myotonic dystrophy and what are the mutations associated with them?
• Myotonic dystrophy type 1 (DM1):
· Expansion of CTG repeat in the 3′ untranslated region of a gene.
· Chromosome 19q.
  › Protein is a putative kinase (DMPK).
    » There are normally 4–40 CTG repeats.
    » In DM1, this increases to 50 or more.
    » There is a correlation between the size of repeat and clinically severity.
    » Genetic disorder anticipation is more common than in DM2.
• Myotonic dystrophy type 2 (DM2):
· Proximal myotonic myopathy.
· CCTG repeat expansion of the first intron of *ZNF9* gene.
  › There are normally 10–30 repeats.
  › In DM2, the number of repeats increases to many thousands.
  › Correlation between size of repeat and clinical severity is less clear than in DM1.
· Chromosome 3.
  › Zinc finger protein.
· No congenital forms.

272. What is the pathogenesis of myotonic dystrophy?
• Both disorders are a result of toxic RNA produced by expansion.
• Toxic RNA results in binding proteins:
· Muscleblind-like protein 1 abnormal alternative splicing and nuclear sequestration.

273. Give at least 2 histopathological features of myotonic dystrophy.
• Numerous internalized nuclei.
• Nuclear knots/nuclear bags.
• Excessive splitting of muscle spindles.
• Type 1 myofiber atrophy.
• Ring fibers — the myofibers have a subsarcolemmal band of cytoplasm that appears distinct from the center of the fiber.

274. What is the most common ion channel myopathy and what triggers the clinical symptoms?

- Most common: malignant hyperpyrexia (malignant hyperthermia).
  - Mutations in the *RYR1* and *CACNA1S* calcium channel genes, which increase the risk of developing malignant hyperthermia.
- Linkage with central core disease (produced by mutations of the *RYR1* gene). More than 50% of the type 1 fibers of patients with malignant hyperpyrexia show the presence of cores.
- Triggered by: anesthetics — most commonly halogenated inhalational agents and succinylcholine.

275. Name at least 2 congenital myopathies.

- Central core disease.
- Multicore disease.
- Nemaline myopathy.
- Myotubular (centronuclear) myopathy.
- Congenital fiber type disproportion.

276. What are the major histopathological and ultrastructural changes that appear in mitochondrial myopathies?

- "Ragged red fibers" (modified Gomori trichrome stain) — myofibers with an increased number of mitochondria located under the sarcolemma, which appear as irregular red aggregates.
- Cytochrome oxidase — negative fibers, which often overexpress succinate dehydrogenase.
- Increased number of mitochondria with irregular shapes on electron microscopy — some contain paracrystalline, "parking lot" inclusions, or alterations in the structure of cristae.

277. What are the major histopathological changes in dermatomyositis?

- Inflammation of the perimysial blood vessels and interfascicular septa is present (lymphocytes, plasma cells and rare eosinophils).
- Groups of atrophic fibers are present at the periphery of fascicles (perifascicular atrophy).
- Intramuscular capillaries show a marked reduction in number and the remaining capillary walls are thickened —
- changes that are believed to result from endothelial injury and fibrosis.
- Necrosis and phagocytosis of muscle fibers appear commonly in groups (microinfarcts).
- Capillary deposition of complement C5b-9 is present ("membrane attack complex").

278. Describe the clinical manifestations of inclusion body myositis.

- It occurs in older patients (> 50 years).
- It has an insidious onset.
- It begins with involvement of the distal muscles.
- Weakness can be asymmetric.
- Approximately half the patients have difficulty swallowing.

279. List 4 conditions associated with rimmed vacuoles.

- Inclusion body myositis (IBM).
- Myofibrillar myopathy.
- Hereditary inclusion body myopathy (HIBM):
  - *GNE*-mutation-associated HIBM.
- *VCP*-mutation-associated HIBM.
- Distal myopathies:
  - Welander distal myopathy.

280. Name at least 2 drugs that can induce myopathies.

- Chloroquine.
- Statins.
- Corticosteroids.
- Colchicines.
- Beta-blockers.
- D-penicillamine.

281. Name the most common findings in chloroquine-induced myopathy.

- Main finding: presence of vacuoles in ~50% of myocytes (vacuolar myopathy).
- 2 types of vacuoles:
- Autophagic membrane bound.
- Curvilinear bodies with short curved membranous structures with alternating light and dark zones.

282. Discuss the clinical presentation, clinical testing, pathological features, pathophysiology, and treatment of myasthenia gravis.

- Clinical presentation:
  - It presents as weakness, ptosis that worsens after use or throughout the day.
  - A myasthenic crisis is a rapidly progressive weakness that especially affects the respiratory muscles and hence is a medical emergency.
- Clinical test:
  - The "Tensilon test" involves administering Tensilon™ or edrophonium. Patients with myasthenia gravis typically improve for a short time after given edrophonium.
  - Edrophonium is a short acting acetylcholinesterase inhibitor that temporarily increases the concentration of acetylcholine at the neuromuscular junction.

(continued on next page)

- Pathological features:
  - These are only visible by electron microscopy.
  - The neuromuscular junction typically has reduced or very simplified junctional folds, and a diminished number and density of acetylcholine receptors.
- Pathophysiology:
  - Myasthenia gravis is thought to be an autoimmune disease in which the patient develops antibodies against their own acetylcholine receptors.
  - The disease is often associated with thymus pathology, including thymic hyperplasia, thymoma, and thymic atrophy or involution.
- Treatment includes:
  - Symptomatic treatment with acetylcholinesterase inhibitors, which act to increase the concentration of acetylcholine at the neuromuscular junction.
  - Plasmapheresis to remove the offending antibodies (short term solution).
  - Thymectomy (may be indicated when thymic pathology is present).

Laboratory Practices

283. Indicate the main components of a surgical pathology report on a brain tumor, as established by CAP.

- History (patient age, duration of symptoms), information about previous tumors or familial tumor syndromes, preoperative treatments, and relevant neuroimaging findings.
- Specimen type or procedure.
- Specimen handling (e.g., smear preparation, tissue held for electron microscopy).
- Specimen size.
- Laterality (side of tumor).
- Tumor site (location of tumor, especially what major layer or region is afflicted).
- Histologic type and grade, using the WHO classification and grading system.
- Margins (only for resections of malignant peripheral nerve sheath tumors).
- Ancillary studies.
- Additional pathologic findings.
- Comment(s).

284. What are common specimen handling procedures performed in neuropathology?

- Intraoperative cytologic preparations: smear, touch, and quash preparations.
- Intraoperative frozen sections.
- Routine, permanent formalin-fixed, paraffin embedded sections.
- Electron microscopy (retain a small portion in glutaraldehyde, or "embed and hold" for electron microscopy, as necessary).
- Frozen tissue, for possible molecular diagnostic studies (freeze fresh tissue as soon as possible and store).
- Snap-frozen muscle, for histochemical studies.
- Microbiology (for any suspected infectious disease).
- Flow cytometry (for suspected lymphomas or lymphoproliferative disorders).
- Air-dried smear preparations for select cytogenetics.

285. Compare and contrast smears and frozen sections for the evaluation of intraoperative biopsies, including their pros and cons.

	SMEAR	FROZEN SECTION
Speed of preparation	Fast.	Slow.
Speed of examination	Slower.	Faster.
Cytologic detail	Excellent.	Mediocre.
View entire cells	Yes.	No.
Examine architecture	Poor.	Good.
Sampling	Multiple sites.	Usually 1 site.
Evaluation of margins	Poor.	Good.
Conservation of tissue for other studies	Good.	Poor.
Evaluation of reticulin-rich tumors	Poor.	Good.

IMAGES: NEUROPATHOLOGY

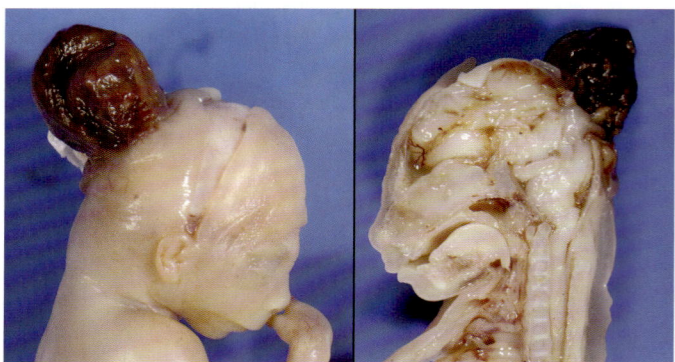

IMAGE 16.1 Parietal-occipital encephalocele. The skull is absent in the region and brain tissue has herniated through the defect. The area cerebrovasculosa is degenerated brain tissue in the encephalocele.

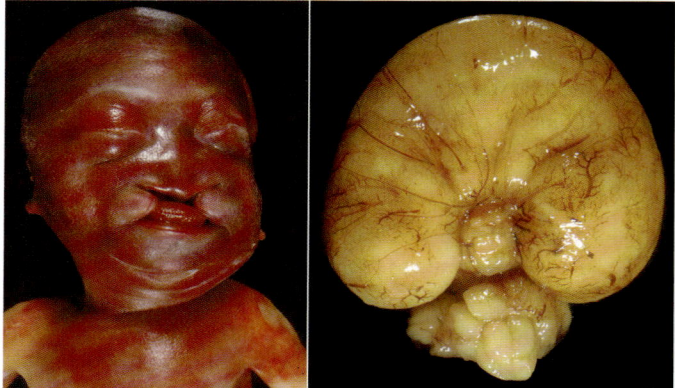

IMAGE 16.2 Holoprosencephaly. Left: the fetus has a central cleft lip, a flattened nose, and eyes that are too close together (hypotelorism). Right (ventral view): This infant had alobar holoprosencephaly; the cerebral hemispheres show no signs of an interhemispheric fissure.

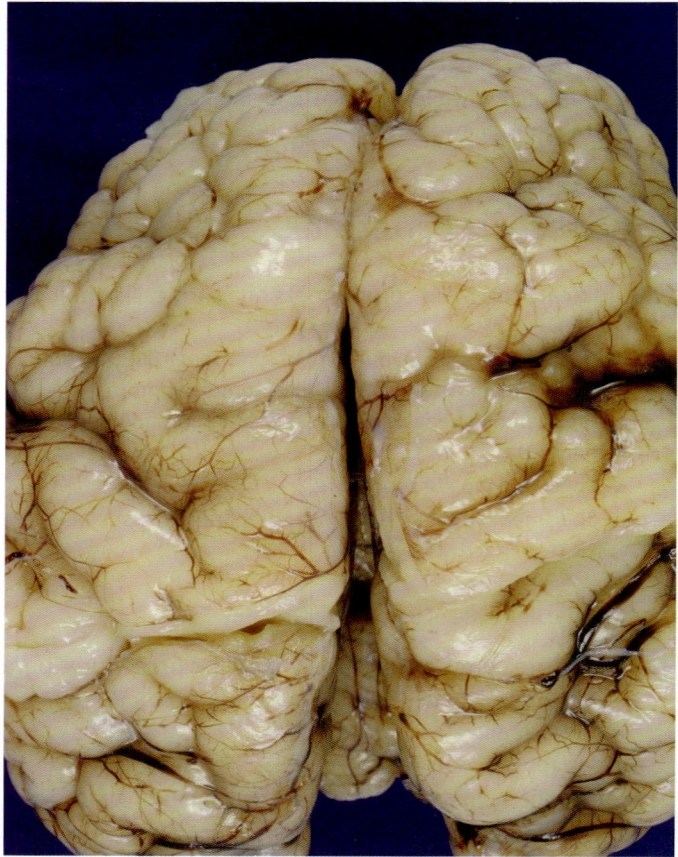

IMAGE 16.4 Pachygyria. In contrast to the smooth cortex of classic lissencephaly, this brain from an infant with Zellweger syndrome has widened but gnarly ("cobblestone") gyri on the superior surface. It lacks normal meningeal vessels, which are embedded in the brain tissue.

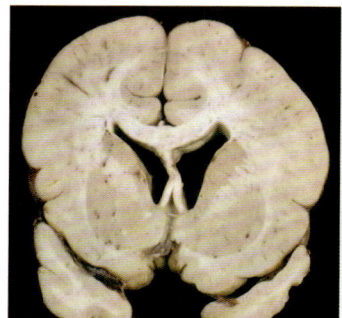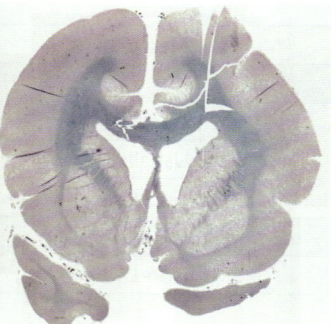

IMAGE 16.3 Lissencephaly. This child had classic or type 1 lissencephaly. The cerebral cortex displays few gyri and the cortex is vastly widened compared with the underlying white matter. Notice the better preservation of the temporal lobes and relatively normal structure of the basal ganglia.

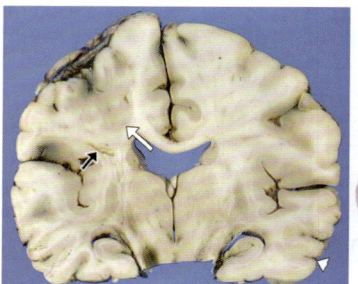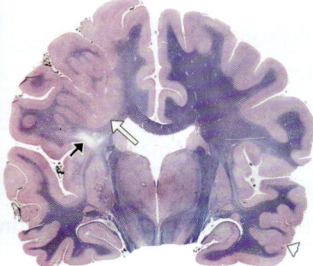

IMAGE 16.5 Polymicrogyria, gross and microscopic. The patient had a large schizencephalic lesion in the left frontal border zone, which was associated with a large region of polymicrogyria (white arrows). A smaller area of polymicrogyria was also present in the right temporal border zone region (white arrowheads). The patient had a much more recent infarct in near the insula (black arrows).

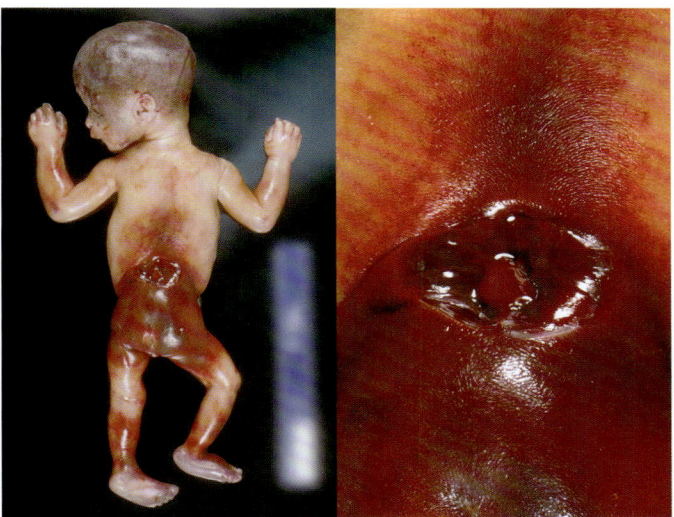

IMAGE 16.6 Myelomeningocele in a fetus with a Chiari II malformation.

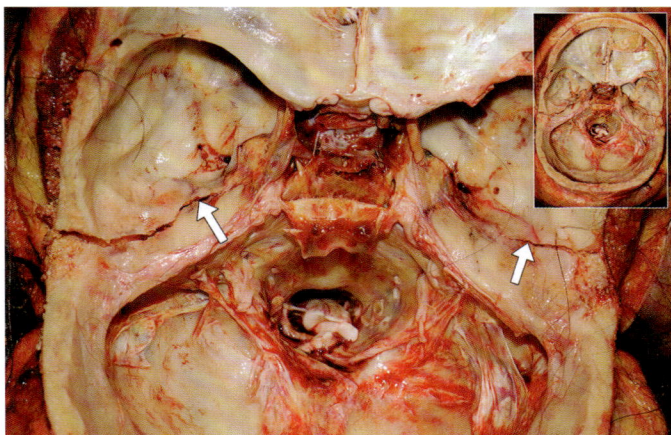

IMAGE 16.8 Basal skull fracture. The decedent was an alcoholic who had fallen the evening before her death. When the body was being transferred from the gurney to the autopsy table, it slipped and fell to the floor, and the head hit the occipital bone. The autopsy demonstrated a base of skull fracture across the front of the petrous ridges bilaterally (arrows). The bone lesion is typical of base of skull fractures, which often cross over both petrous ridges; however, it is atypical since it lacks hemorrhages into the bone. This fracture occurred postmortem.

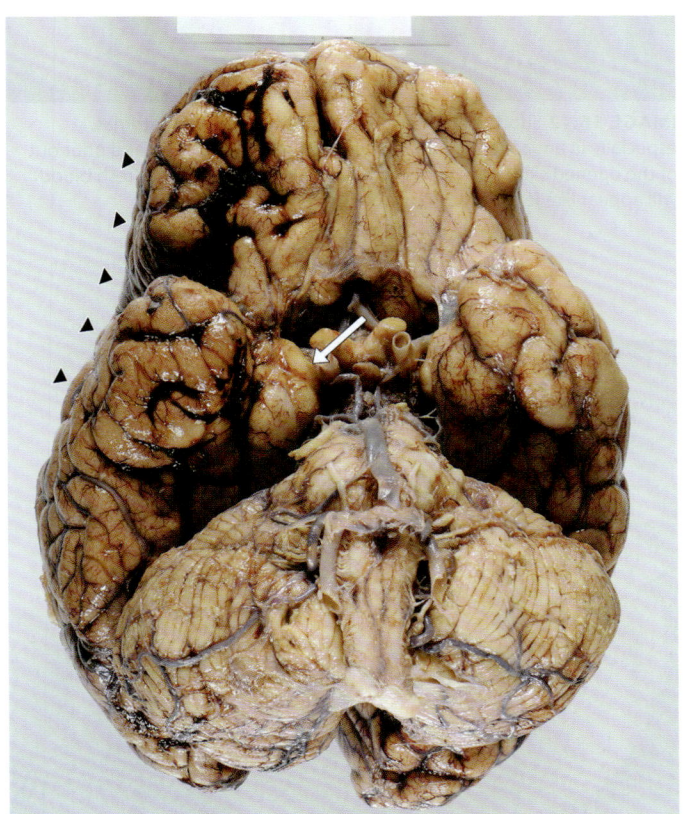

IMAGE 16.7 Uncal herniation. The patient developed a massive subdural hematoma over the right cerebral hemisphere that compressed the right brain inward (black arrowheads). This created a mass effect in the right hemisphere and caused terminal right uncal herniation (white arrow).

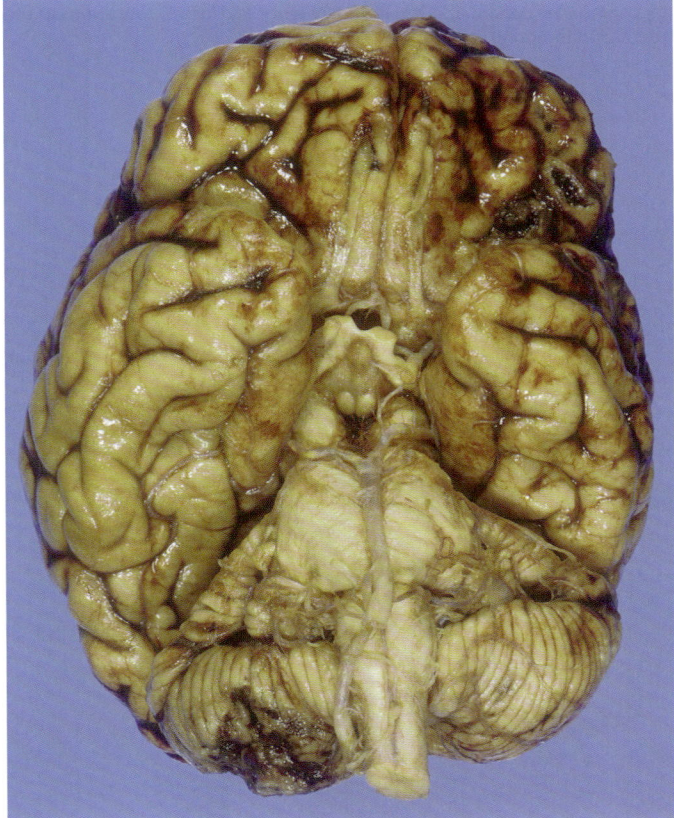

IMAGE 16.9 Acute coup-contrecoup contusions. The surface of the left orbitofrontal lobes is disrupted and hemorrhagic (contrecoup contusion); beneath the site of impact, the right posterior cerebellum has hemorrhagic changes (coup contusion). These contusions resulted from a fall on the occiput.

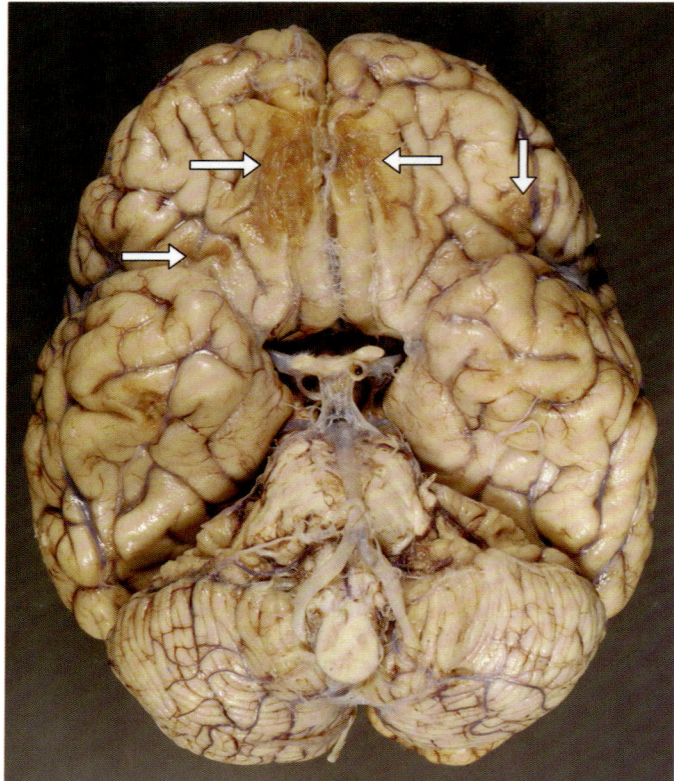

IMAGE 16.10 Remote contrecoup contusion. The patient had classic orbitofrontal chronic contrecoup contusions, as evidenced by superficial (gyral crest-to-crest but not deeper) tissue loss and extensive hemosiderin deposition. The patient also has more posterior and lateral contusions in the frontal and temporal lobes.

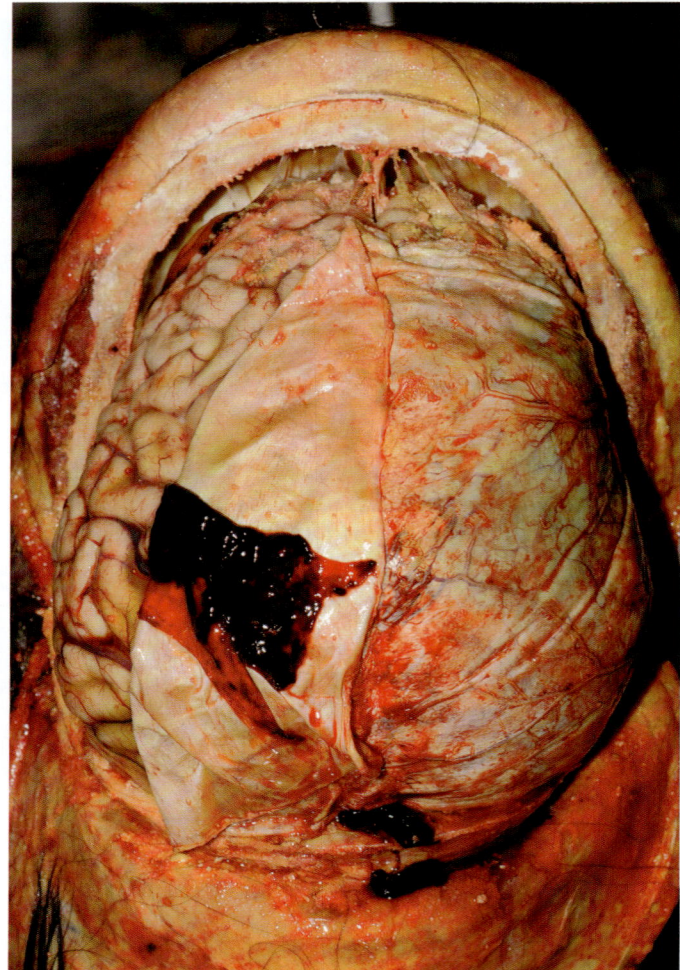

IMAGE 16.12 Subdural hemorrhage. Acute subdural hematomas, especially in anticoagulated patients, often have not clotted and pour out of the opened skull. In patients with normal coagulation, the fresh blood will appear like jelly.

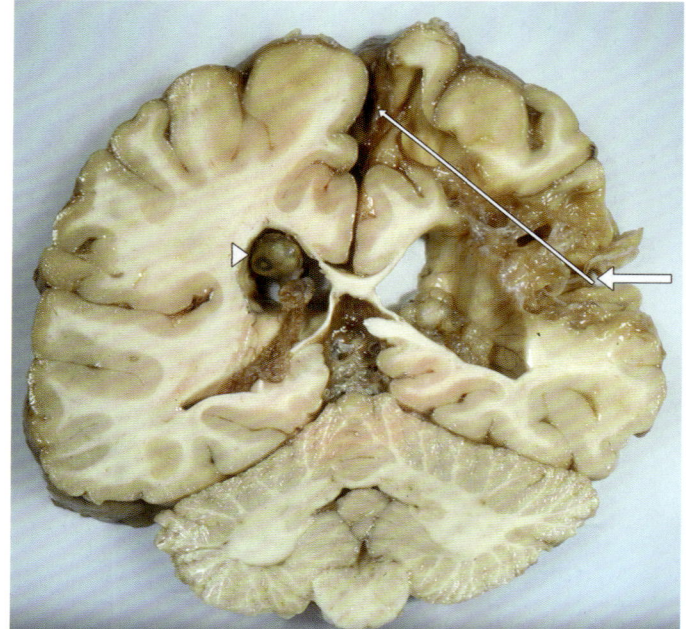

IMAGE 16.11 Remote gunshot wound. The bullet entered the skull on the right (large arrow) and dragged skin, scalp, and bone debris into the brain, which left a wide gap of destruction. The bullet then traveled through the brain to the top of the skull (narrow arrow), ricocheted off the skull bone, and then ended in the left lateral ventricle (arrowhead).

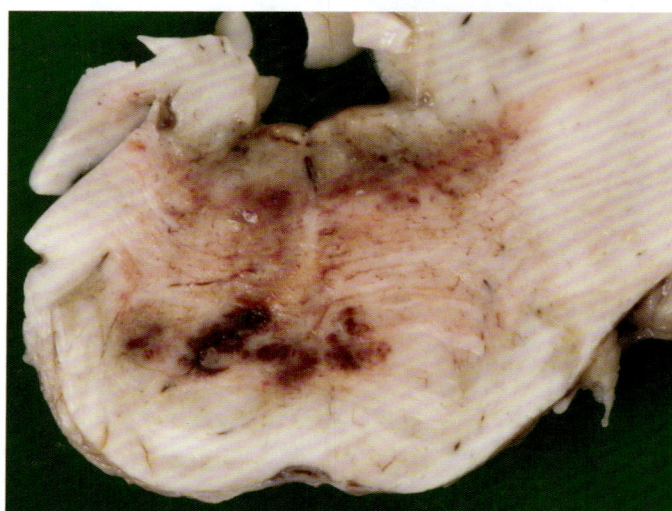

IMAGE 16.13 Duret hemorrhage. These typically develop in the midbrain and rostral pons.

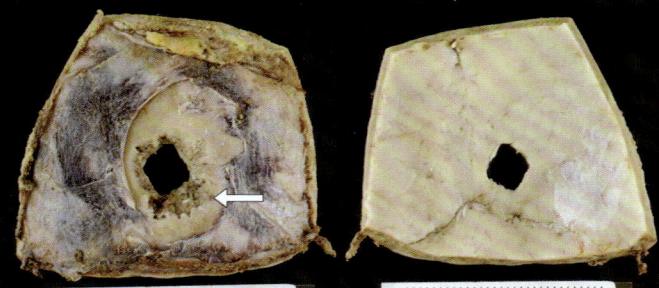

IMAGE 16.14 Exit wound. The decedent shot a handgun through his mouth. The bullet entered the skull at its base, traversed the pons, and then exited through the occipital bone. The bullet left a simple hole on the interior of the occipital bone, but fractured the outer skull table and caused the hole to be bevelled outward (exit wound).

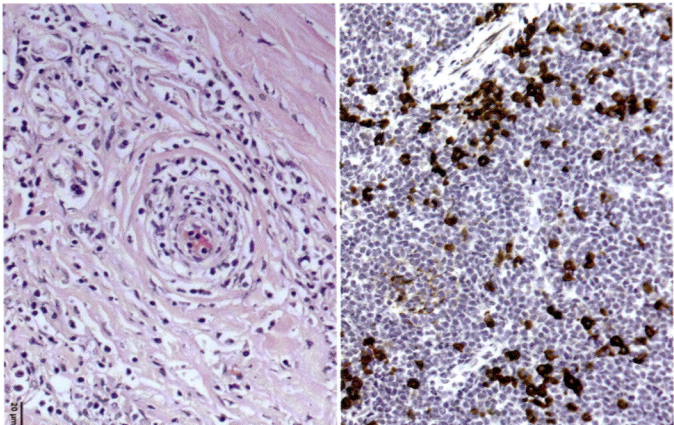

IMAGE 16.15 Central nervous system (CNS) IgG4 disease. IgG4 disease has been implicated in pachymeningitis (marked thickening of the dura) and hypophysitis. Left: H&E stained images show phlebitis, hyaline sclerosis, and abundant lymphoplasmacytic inflammation with admixed eosinophils. Right: immunohistochemistry directed against the IgG4 isoform shows increased numbers of IgG4-expressing plasma cells, both in absolute numbers, and as a percentage of IgG-expressing plasma cells (x40).

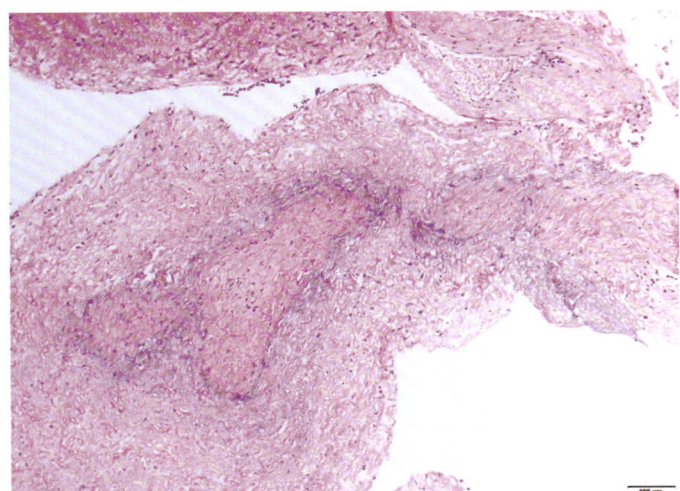

IMAGE 16.16 CNS rheumatoid arthritis. This H&E stained section shows the classic palisading necrobiosis of this immune-mediated inflammatory pathology. When this affects the CNS, the dura and leptomeninges are frequently involved.

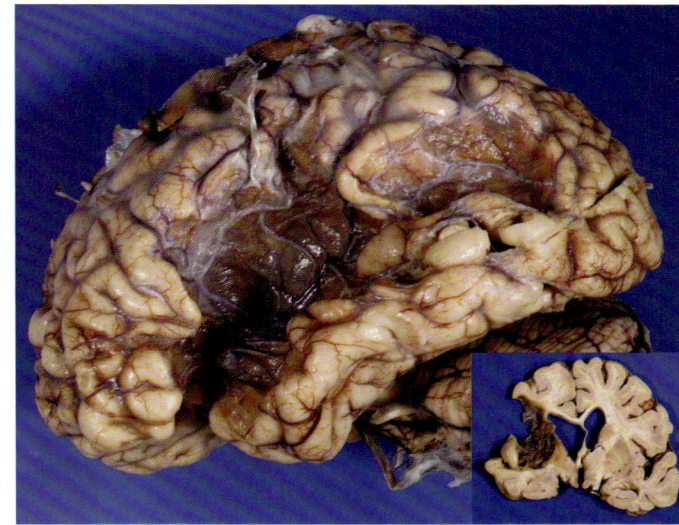

IMAGE 16.17 Left middle cerebral artery infarct. This infarct involved the major speech areas in the superior posterior temporal gyrus (Wernicke area) and the posterior frontal operculum (Broca area) and led to profound deficits in language.

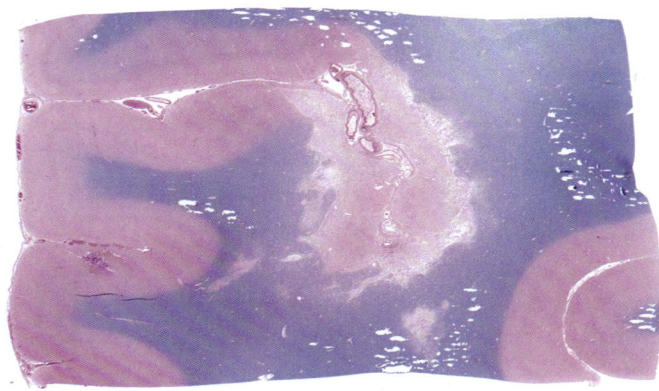

IMAGE 16.18 Recent infarct (H&E/LFB, x20). Embolic material is still present in the leptomeningeal artery. At this point, after a few weeks, the edema has subsided and the infarct is better circumscribed.

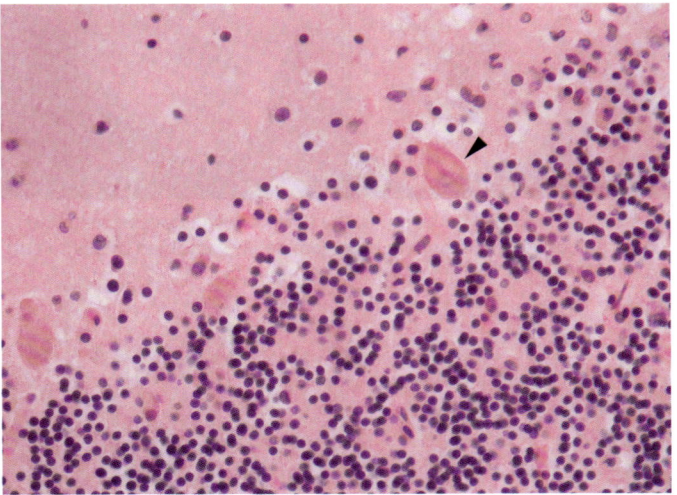

IMAGE 16.19 Red neuron (H&E, x400). The image shows eosinophilic cytoplasm, a disintegrating nucleus and nuclear membrane, and disappearance of the nucleolus.

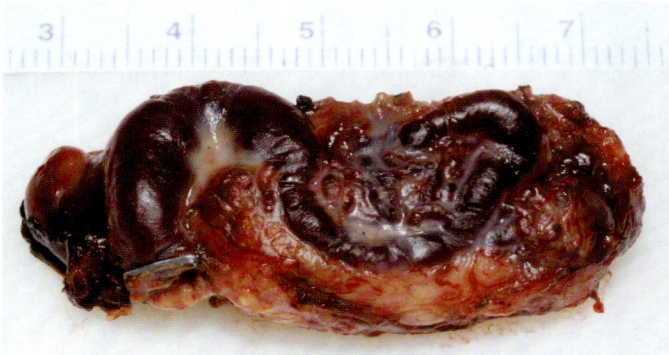

IMAGE 16.20 Arteriovenous malformation. This resection has the appearance of a "can of worms" within brain parenchyma.

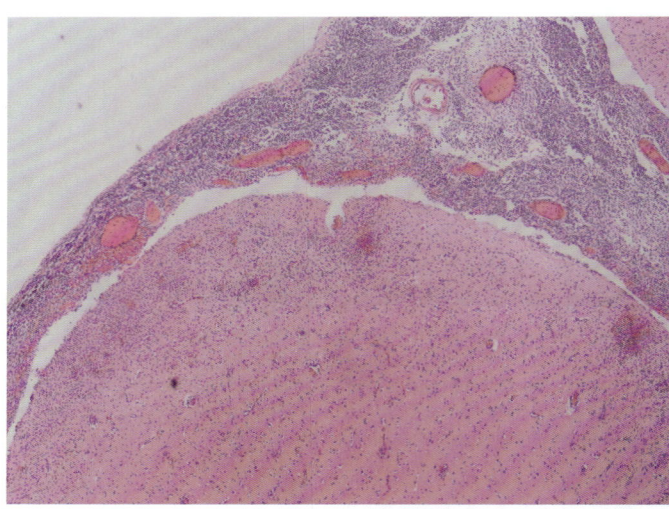

IMAGE 16.22 Acute bacterial meningitis (H&E, x40). The subarachnoid space is replete with neutrophils and the surface of the brain shows an acute cerebritis.

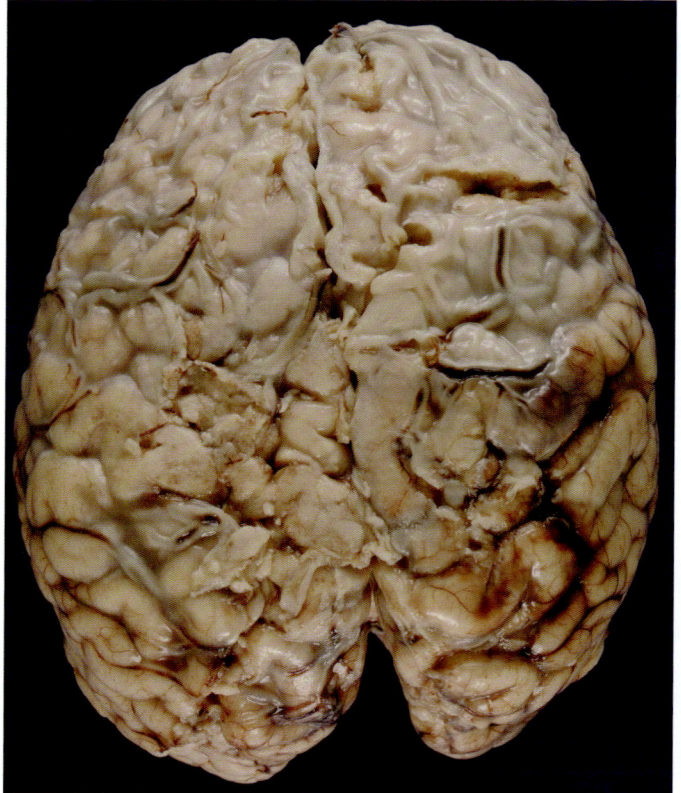

IMAGE 16.21 Purulent meningitis. The subarachnoid space beneath the leptomeninges of this infant has been completely subsumed by a purulent exudate.

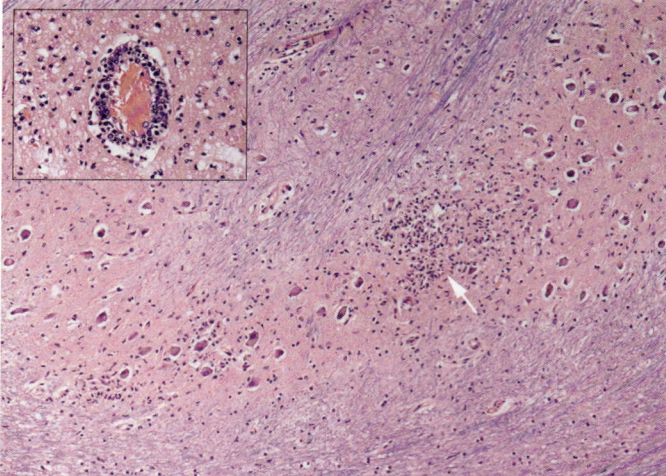

IMAGE 16.23 Acute viral encephalitis. Main image (H&E/LFB; x200): focal neuronal depletion, red neurons, and microglial nodules (arrow). Inset: perivascular inflammation (H&E, x400).

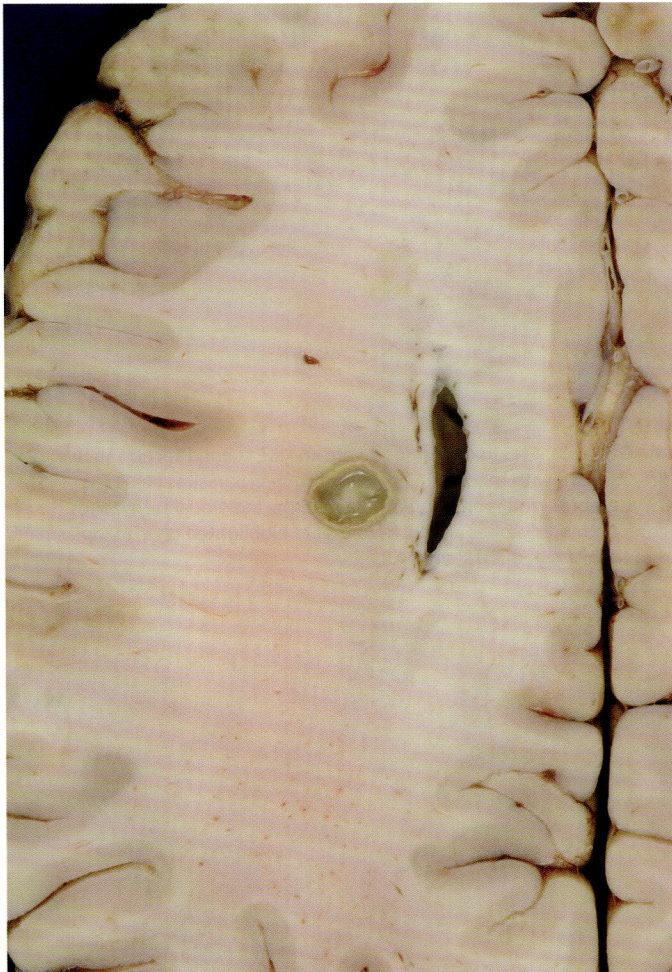

IMAGE 16.24 Cerebral abscess. This is a well-established abscess, at least several weeks old. This main area of purulent material has been "walled off" by a fibrous capsule.

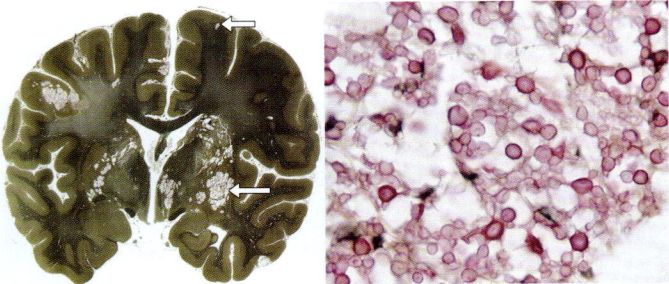

IMAGE 16.25 Cryptococcosis meningoencephalitis. Left: giant section displays multiple sites of "soap bubbles," which are vacuolated spaces around the long penetrating arteries in the base of the brain and in the cortical penetrating arteries (white arrows). Right (high magnification): *Cryptococcus neoformans* yeast polysaccharide cell walls stain pink with mucicarmine.

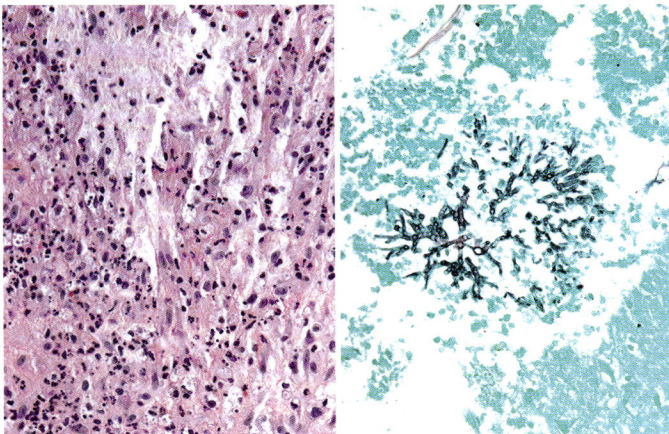

IMAGE 16.26 CNS aspergillosis. Left: this H&E stained section shows necrotic brain with acute inflammation. Right: this GMS stained section shows septate hyphal forms with acute angle branching (45°).

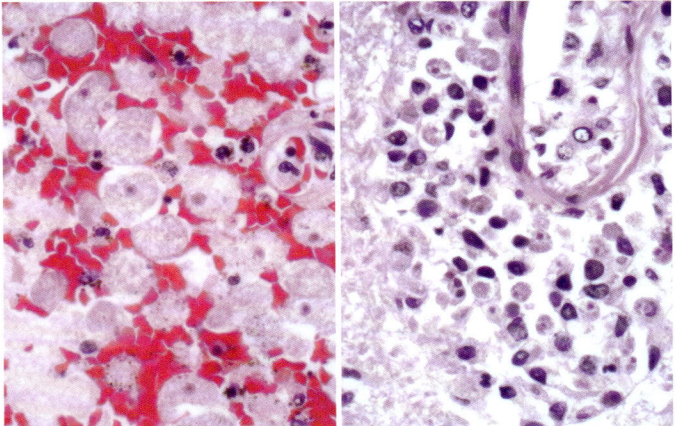

IMAGE 16.27 CNS amebiasis. These H&E (x60) stained sections show large foamy cells with small nuclei with prominent nucleoli. Left: the organism in this image is *Balamuthia*. Right: *Naegleria fowleri* shows a perivascular distribution. *Balamuthia* is larger than other amebic organisms, such as this.

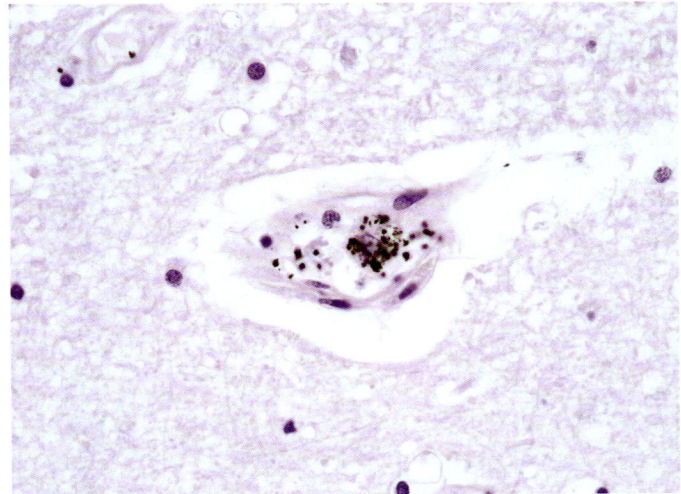

IMAGE 16.28 CNS malaria. H&E (x40) stained sections show dark, hyperchromatic protozoan organism inside red blood cells within CNS blood vessels. The organism in this image was *Plasmodium falciparum*.

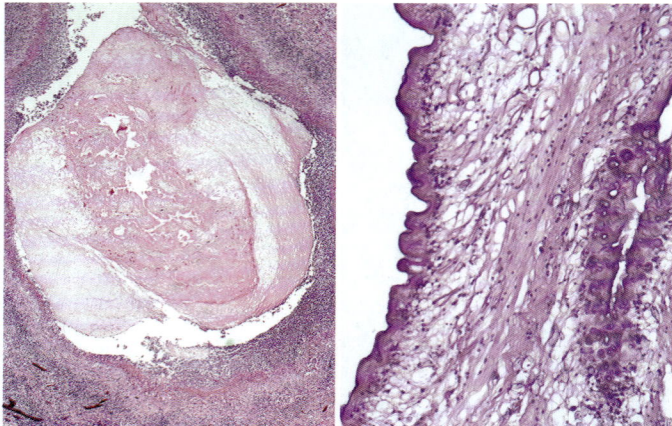

IMAGE 16.29 CNS neurocysticercosis. These H&E stained sections show a cavitating abscess with purulent debris surrounding a necrotic pork tapeworm (*Taenia solium*). Higher magnification images highlight the acellular cuticle. Left: x2. Right: x20.

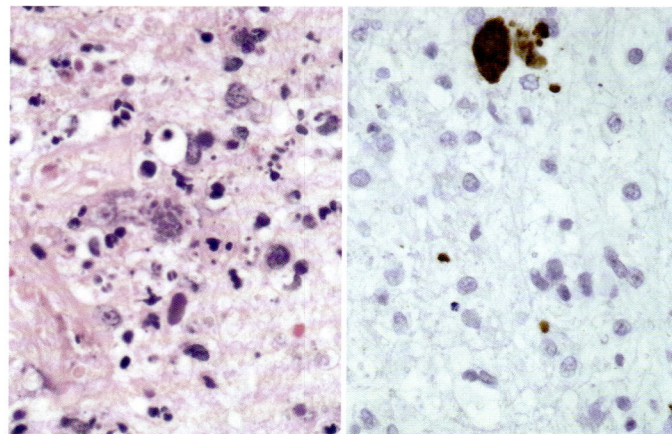

IMAGE 16.32 CNS toxoplasmosis. Left: an H&E stained section shows dirty necrosis with basophilic *Toxoplasma gondii* parasites (x40). The encysted bradyzoites are more stable than the individual tachyzoites. Right: both bradyzoites and tachyzoites are highlighted on a "toxoplasma" immunohistochemical stain (x40).

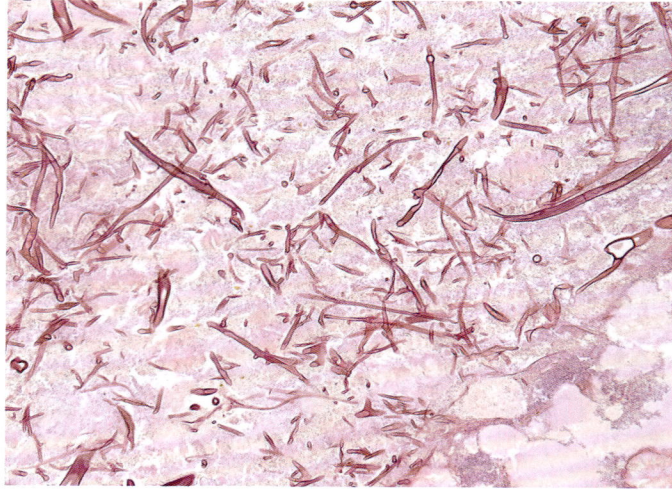

IMAGE 16.30 CNS mucormycosis. This H&E stained section shows the nonseptate ribbonlike hyphal structures. These hyphae can be darker on H&E and only stain weakly on GMS.

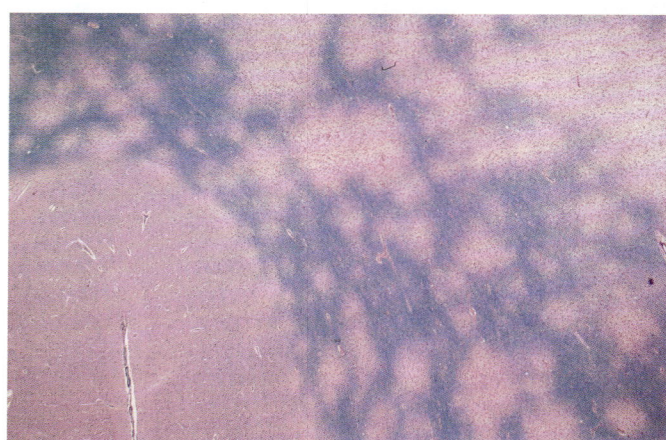

IMAGE 16.33 Progressive multifocal leukoencephalopathy (H&E/LFB, x12.5). Plaques of demyelination in the white matter and at the gray-white junction are devoid of LFB staining. This image is pathognomonic for PML.

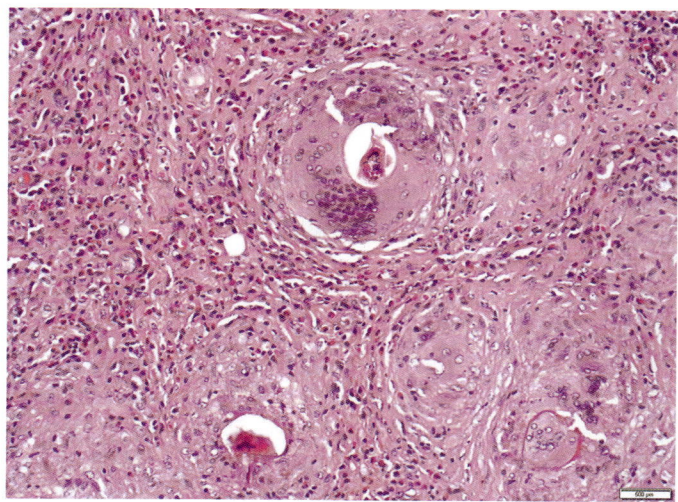

IMAGE 16.31 CNS schistosomiasis. This H&E stained section shows the intact parasitic flatworms eliciting a brisk immune response consisting of multinucleated giant cells and abundant eosinophils.

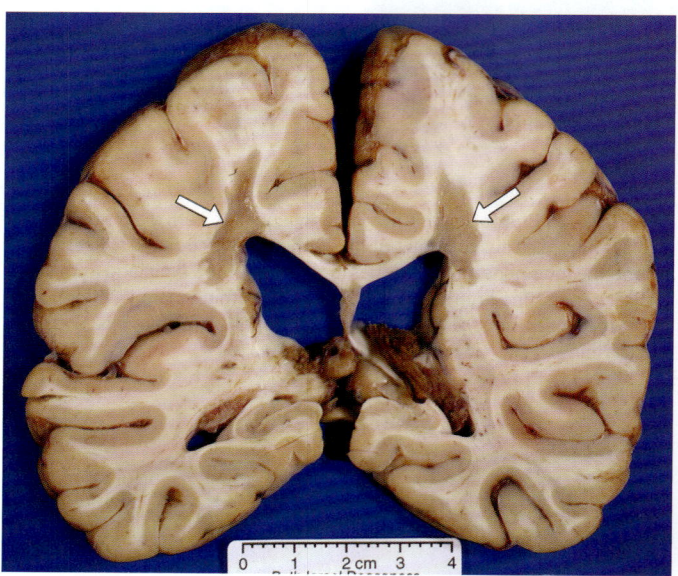

IMAGE 16.34 Multiple sclerosis. At the lateral corners of the lateral ventricles are irregular but bilateral demyelinated plaques (arrows).

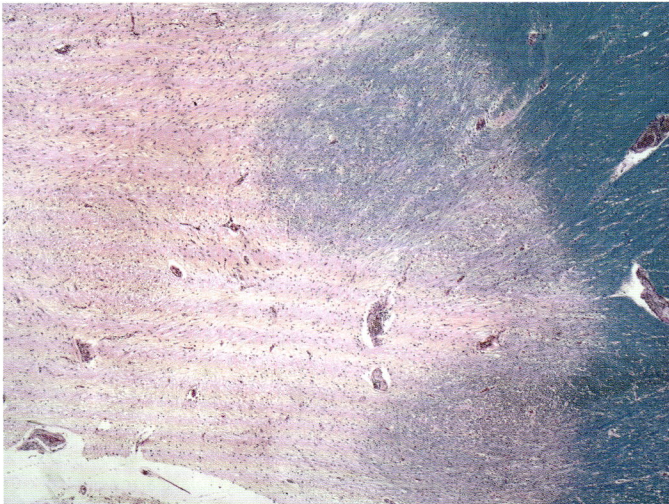

IMAGE 16.35 Chronic active multiple sclerosis plaque (H&E/LFB, x12.5). The left side is completely demyelinated, the right side is normal-appearing white matter, and the light blue areas are regions of remyelination ("shadow plaques").

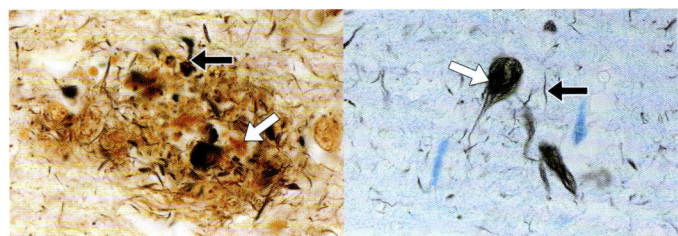

IMAGE 16.38 Alzheimer disease silver stains. Left: Bielschowsky stain of a neuritic amyloid plaque (x1000). The plaque has dense amyloid cores (white arrow) and dystrophic neurites (black arrow). Right: Gallyas stain (x1000), which shows a neurofibrillary tangle (white arrow) and a neuropil thread (black arrow) in fine detail.

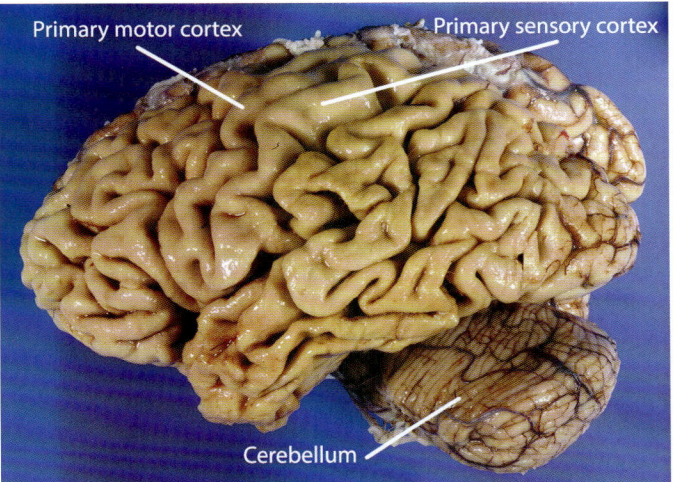

IMAGE 16.36 Alzheimer disease. The disease involves all lobes of the cortex, but spares by comparison the primary motor and sensory cortices. The cerebellum is uninvolved.

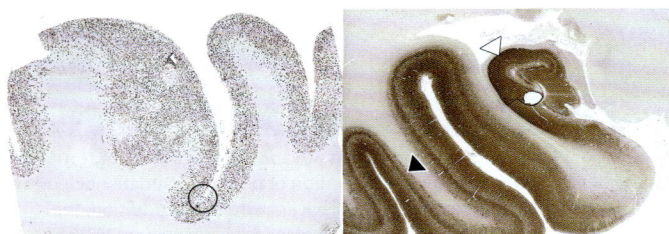

IMAGE 16.39 Alzheimer disease immunoperoxidase (entire slides). Left: amyloid-β (Aβ) immunostain shows the high density of amyloid plaques in Alzheimer disease, along with a few vessels having cerebral amyloid angiopathy (circled). Right: tau immunostain demonstrates the high level of tau deposition, containing both neurofibrillary tangles and neuropil threads in the CA1 region of the hippocampus (white arrowhead), as well as the layering of these features in neocortex (black arrowhead).

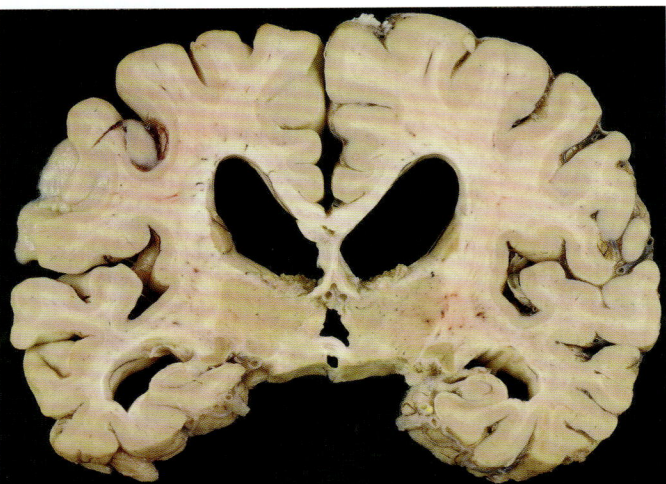

IMAGE 16.37 Alzheimer disease. The lateral ventricles, especially the temporal horns, are dilated and the hippocampi are shrunken.

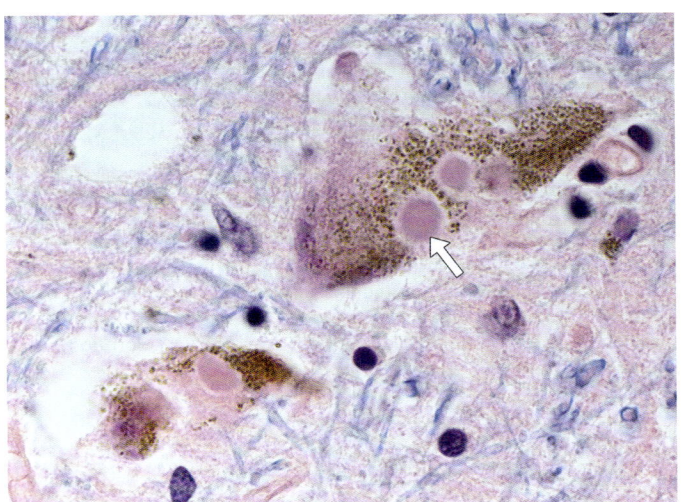

IMAGE 16.40 Lewy bodies (H&E/LFB, x1000). The image illustrates 2 pigmented neurons in the substantia nigra that have 2 or more classic or brainstem Lewy bodies (white arrow).

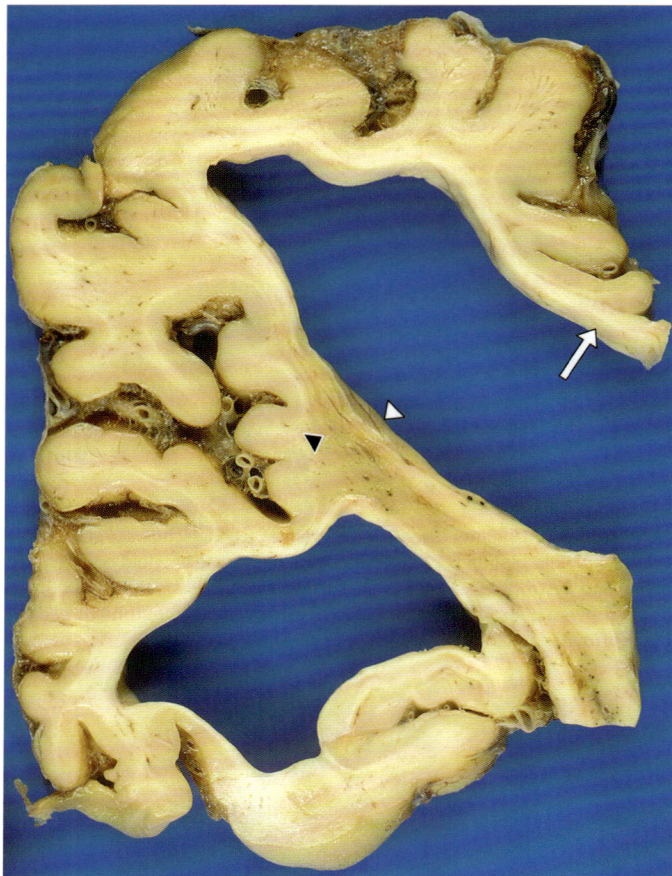

IMAGE 16.41 Huntington disease. This advanced case of Huntington disease demonstrates marked degeneration of both the caudate nucleus (white arrowhead) and the putamen (black arrowhead). In addition, the entire cerebral cortex is atrophic, which is also indirectly evident by the thinness of the corpus callosum (white arrow).

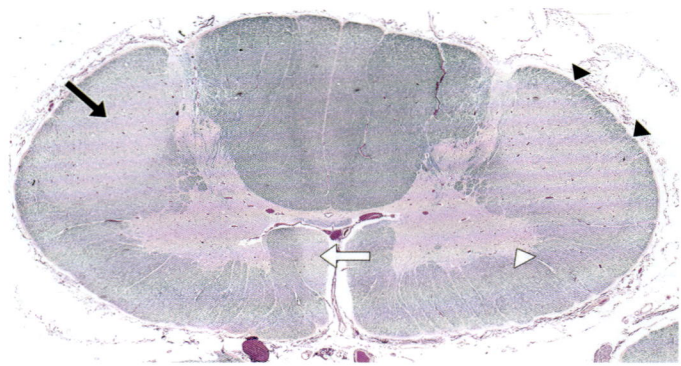

IMAGE 16.43 ALS (low magnification). Both the lateral (black arrow) and ventral (white arrow) corticospinal tracts in this cervical section have extensive loss of myelinated axons. Note the relative symmetry of the lateral loss but not the ventral tracts; this is a common anatomic variation in the ventral tracts. Adjacent dorsal spinocerebellar tracts (black arrowheads) are spared, which reflects the specificity of the loss. In addition, the ventral horns (white arrowhead) are shrunken and lack the usual clusters of the large lower motor neurons.

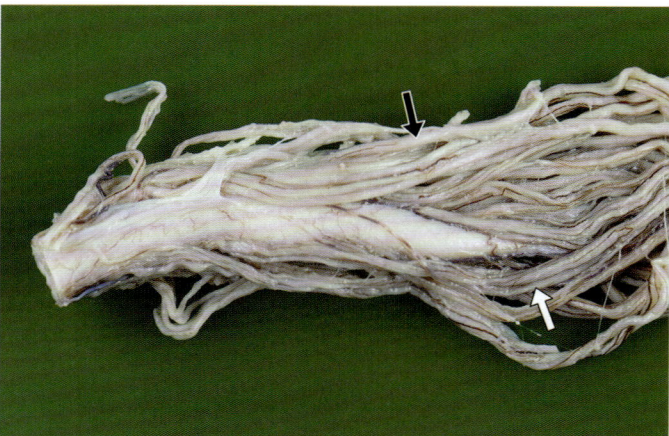

IMAGE 16.42 Amyotrophic lateral sclerosis (ALS). This view of the caudal end of the spinal cord illustrates the thicker, well-myelinated (whiter) dorsal roots (black arrow) and the thin ventral roots (white arrow) that have lost many of their large, myelinated lower motor axons (grayer color). Both roots should be the same white color.

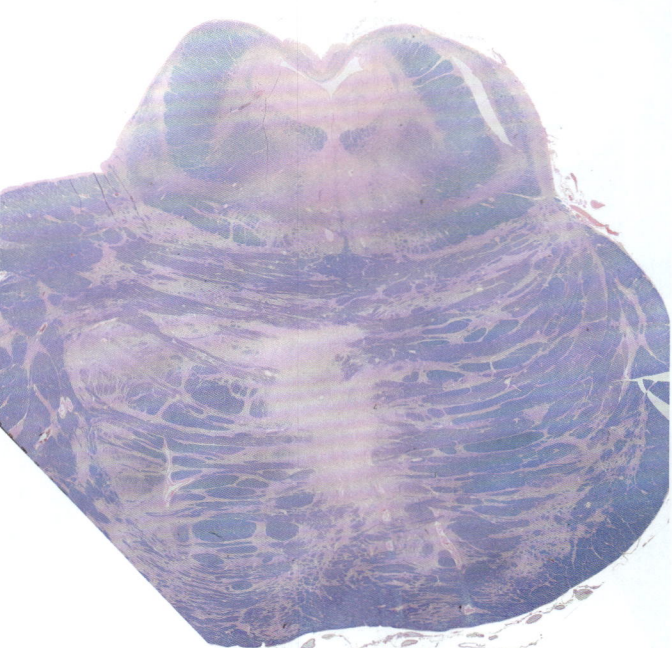

IMAGE 16.44 Central pontine myelinolysis (H&E/LFB, entire slide). Osmotic demyelination most often causes loss of myelinated axons but no neuron cell bodies within the center of the pontine base.

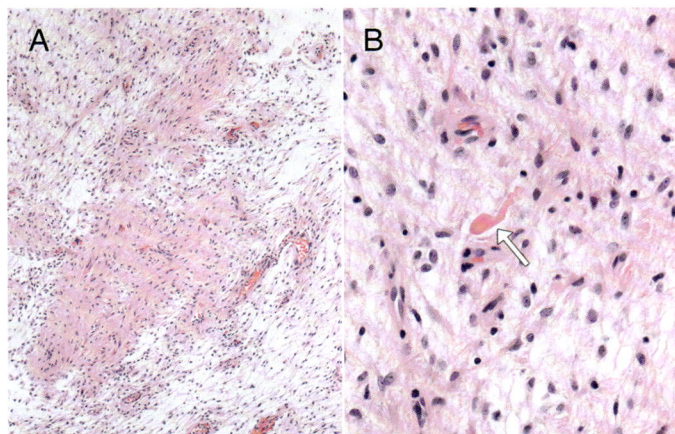

IMAGE 16.45 Pilocytic astrocytoma. Image A: an astrocytic tumor that has both loose and dense areas (x100). Both areas have fine processes. Image B (x400): high magnification reveals occasional Rosenthal fibers (arrow).

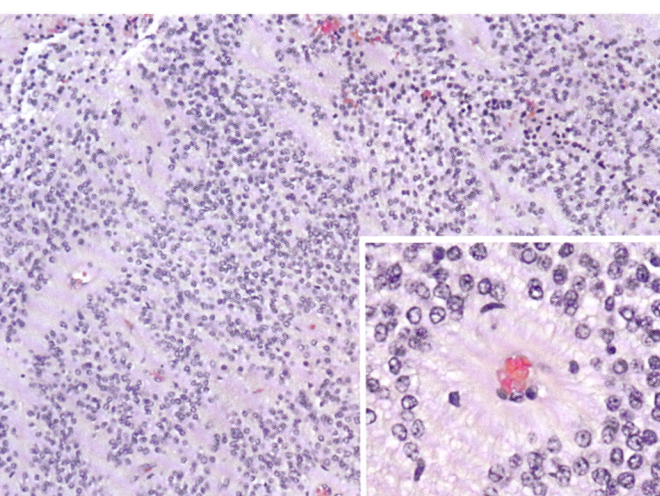

IMAGE 16.48 CNS ependymoma. These glial neoplasms feature conspicuous perivascular pseudorossettes, which are elaborate dense glial fibers that extend to the vessel wall comprising an anuclear zone.

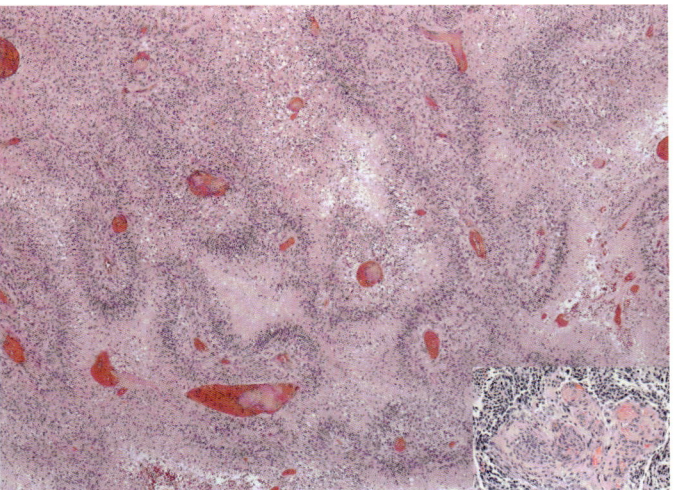

IMAGE 16.46 Glioblastoma. Main image: necrosis with pseudopalisading and vascular proliferation (H&E, x40). Inset: vascular proliferation (H&E, x200).

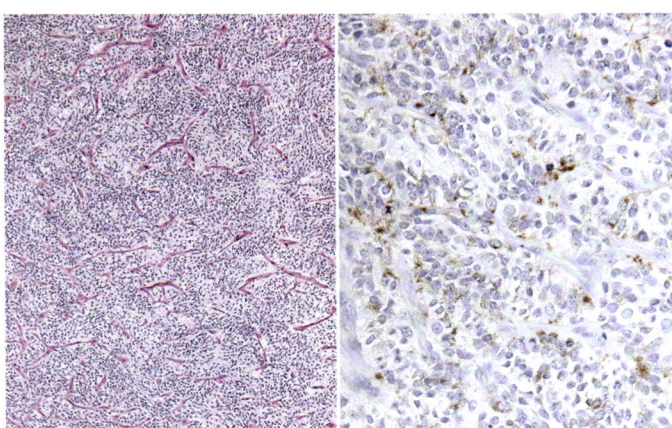

IMAGE 16.49 Clear cell ependymoma. This is a challenging morphological variant of ependymoma, in which the tumor cells have predominantly clear cytoplasm (seen in the left image). Immunohistochemistry for EMA shows perinuclear dot-like positivity.

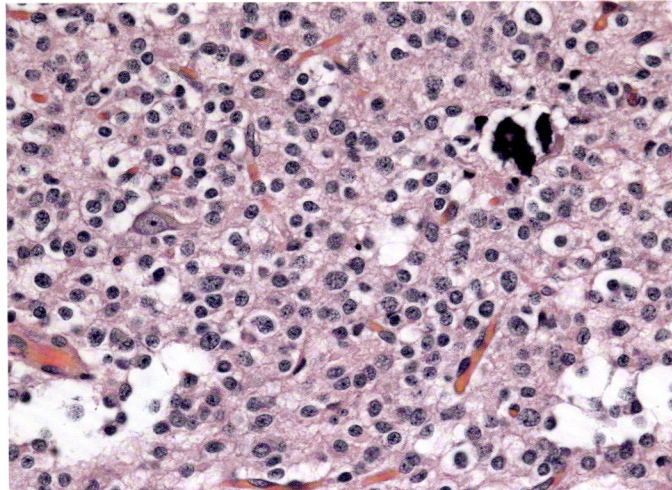

IMAGE 16.47 Oligodendroglioma (H&E, x200). Round nuclei, perinuclear halos ("fried eggs"), many thin capillaries ("chicken wire vasculature"), and microcalcifications are common features in oligodendroglioma.

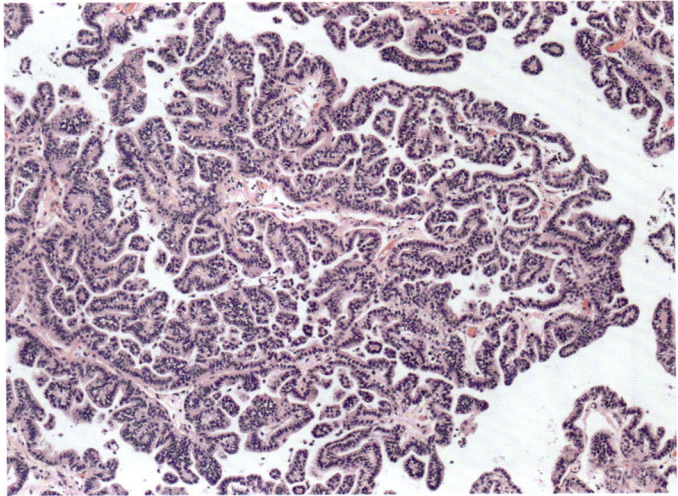

IMAGE 16.50 Choroid plexus papilloma (H&E, x200). This tumor is composed of neoplastic epithelial cells that line a fibrovascular core in papillary stalks.

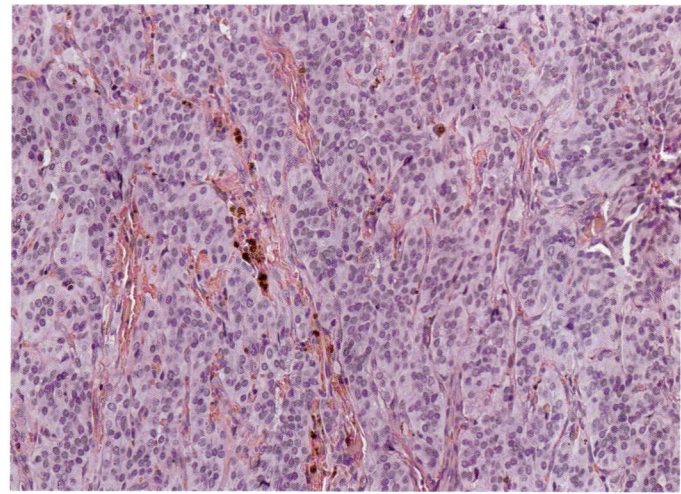

IMAGE 16.51 Paraganglioma (H&E, x200). Tumor cells form nests or balls of cells ("Zellballen").

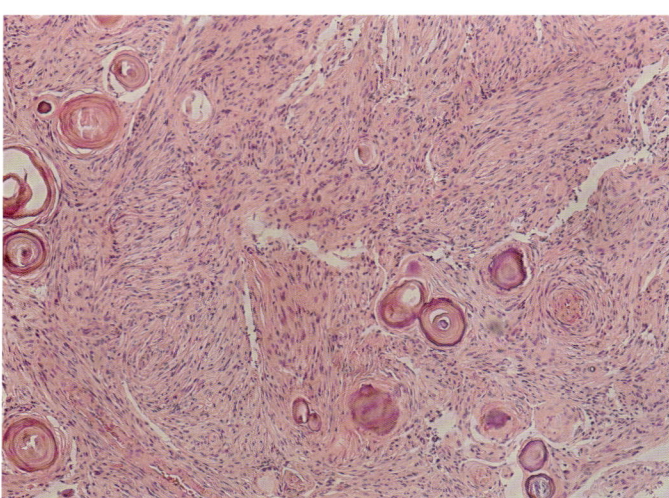

IMAGE 16.54 Meningioma. The image shows whorls and psammoma bodies (H&E, x100).

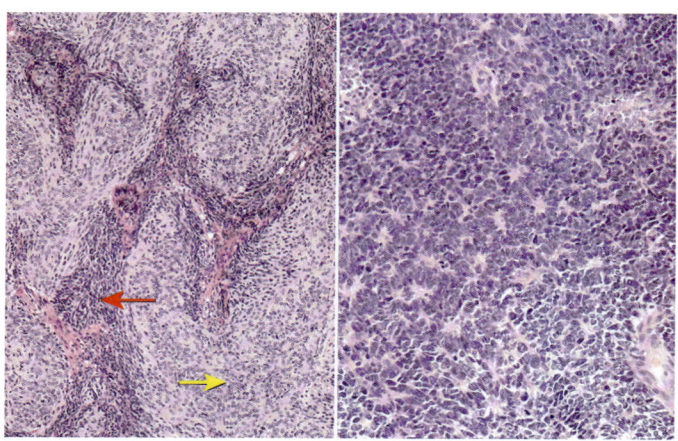

IMAGE 16.52 Medulloblastoma. Left (x100): a desmoplastic medulloblastoma, which has less-dense areas containing abundant neuropil that are separated by dense areas with primitive cells. Right: Homer-Wright rosettes. Medulloblastomas can show characteristic rosettes formed by the cytoplasm of these neoplastic embryonal cells with neuronal differentiation.

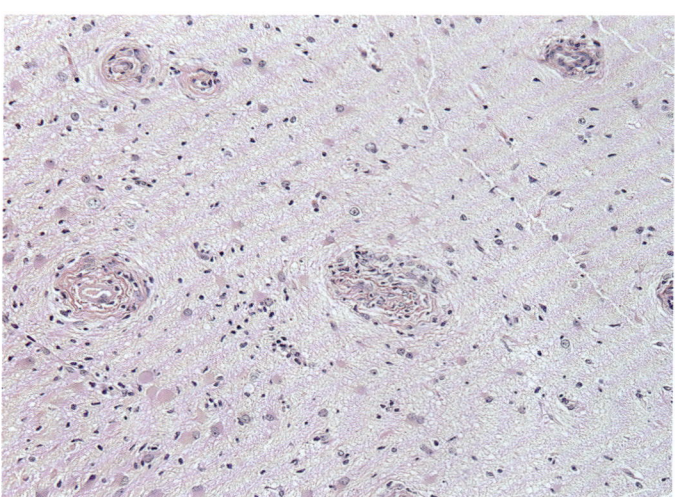

IMAGE 16.55 Meningioangiomatosis. This is a benign focal lesion of the leptomeninges and underlying cerebral cortex in which meningothelial cells are arranged around blood vessels, with no well-formed dural mass. This is associated with type 2 neurofibromatosis.

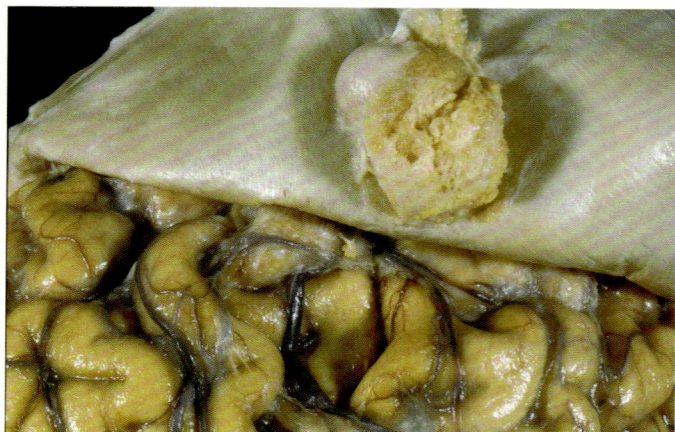

IMAGE 16.53 Meningioma. The tumor is well circumscribed, attached to the dura, and indents but does not adhere to or invade underlying brain.

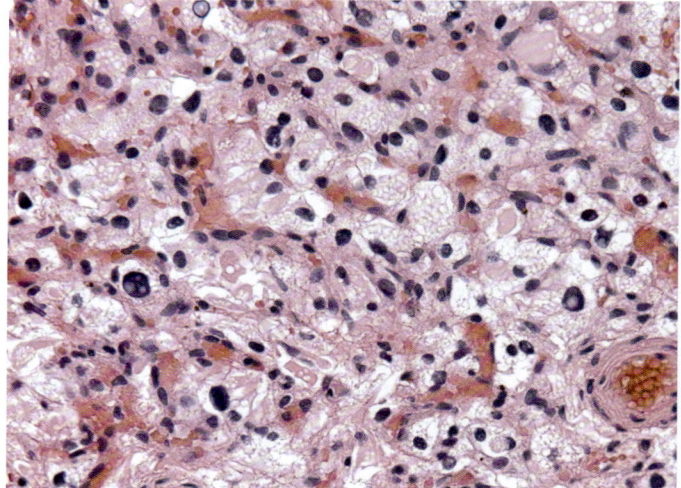

IMAGE 16.56 Hemangioblastoma. This highly vascular tumor contains many large, vacuolated stromal cells. Approximately a third of these tumors are associated with Von Hippel-Lindau syndrome, and close attention should be paid to exclude metastatic renal cell carcinoma.

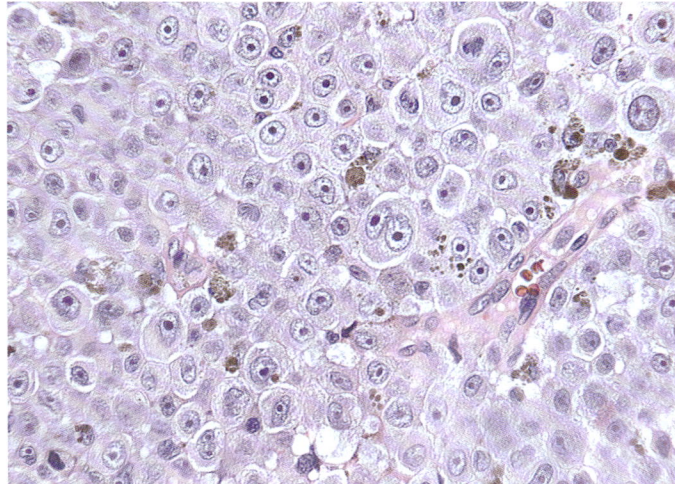

IMAGE 16.57 Primary CNS melanoma. The dura and falx can contain pigmented cells called "melanophores." These cells can give rise to primary melanocytic lesions which can be both benign and malignant. A primary malignant CNS melanoma is represented here. This tumor was seen in a pediatric patient with neurocutaneous melanosis.

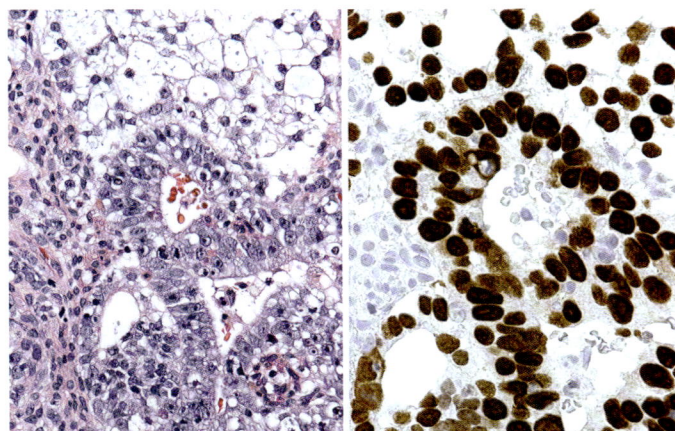

IMAGE 16.58 CNS yolk sac tumor. Primary germ cell neoplasms can occur in the CNS, typically in the midline in the pineal or suprasellar region. All forms and combinations of germ cell tumors are possible. Left: an H&E stained section of a primary CNS yolk sac tumor forming conspicuous Schiller-Duval bodies. Right: the tumor cell nuclei label with SALL4 by immunohistochemistry.

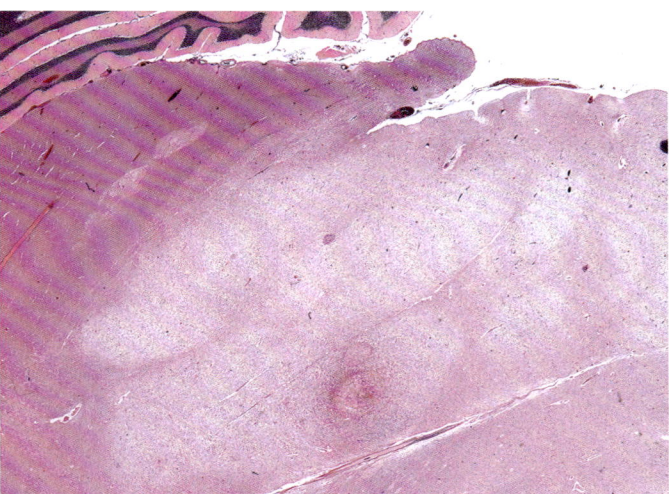

IMAGE 16.59 H3 K27-altered glioma. These tumors are frequently midline in younger patients, and are associated with an aggressive clinical course. This image shows tumor within the pons infiltrating into the cerebellum (also called "diffuse intrinsic pontine glioma").

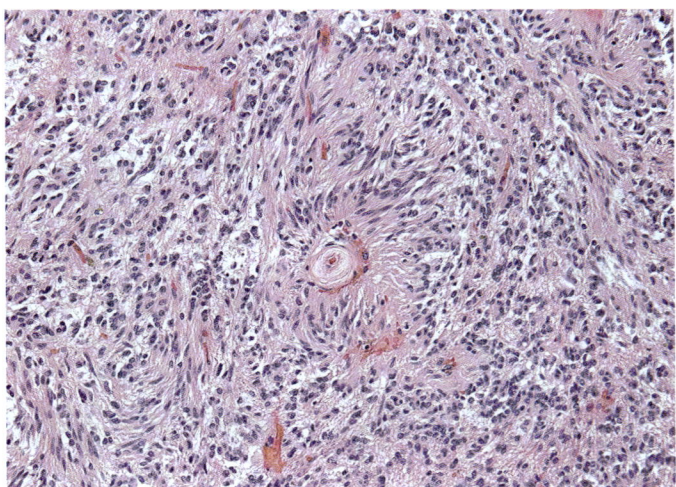

IMAGE 16.60 Angiocentric glioma. This H&E-stained section shows a cellular glial neoplasm where the spindled tumor cells are conspicuously arranged around blood vessels. These indolent tumors are associated with *MYB* fusion events.

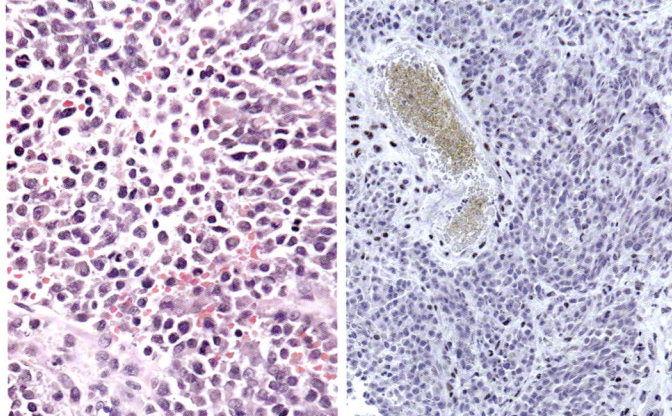

IMAGE 16.61 CNS atypical teratoid rhabdoid tumor. Left: this H&E-stained section shows a cellular embryonal neoplasm composed of atypical cells with manifold appearances. A subset of cells have abundant eosinophilic cytoplasm giving the cells a rhabdoid appearance. Right: these cells show no nuclear expression of INI1/*SMARCB1* by immunohistochemistry, with intact expression in the nonneoplastic endothelial cells.

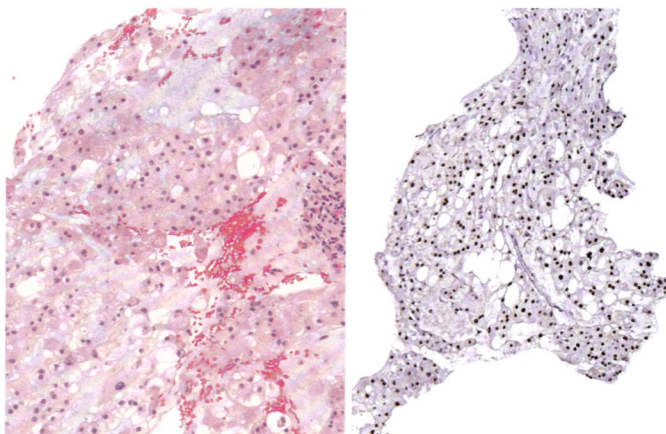

IMAGE 16.62 CNS chordoma. Left: an H&E stained section shows a neoplasm composed of epithelioid multivacuolated physaliferous ("bubble-bearing") cells arranged in cords separated by myxoid stroma. Right: the bubble-bearing cells show nuclear labelling with brachyury by immunohistochemistry.

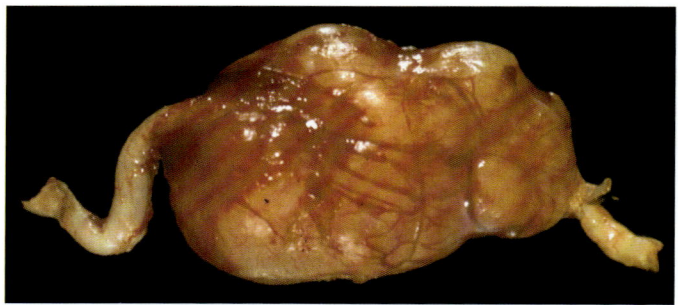

IMAGE 16.63 Schwannoma. These tumors push the peripheral nerve aside or splay it across the surface but do not cause nerve expansion beyond the tumor.

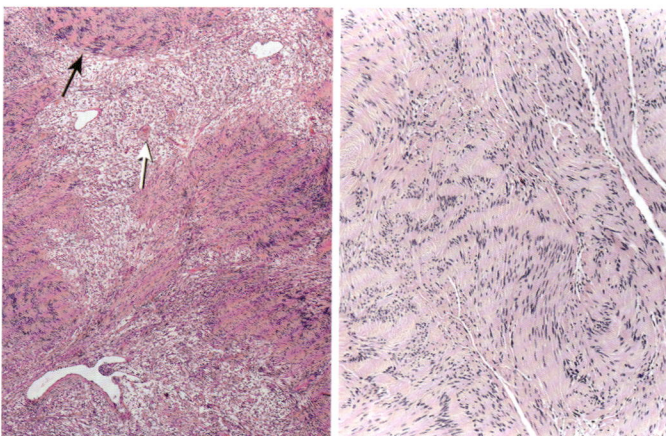

IMAGE 16.64 Schwannoma. (H&E, x100). Left: dense and loose areas, nuclear palisading (black arrow), and hyalinized vessels (white arrow). Right: Verocay bodies. Schwannomas are characterized by areas featuring prominent nuclear regimentation with central eosinophilic anuclear zone. These conspicuous palisades are called *Verocay bodies* after the pathologist who described this tumor, José Verocay.

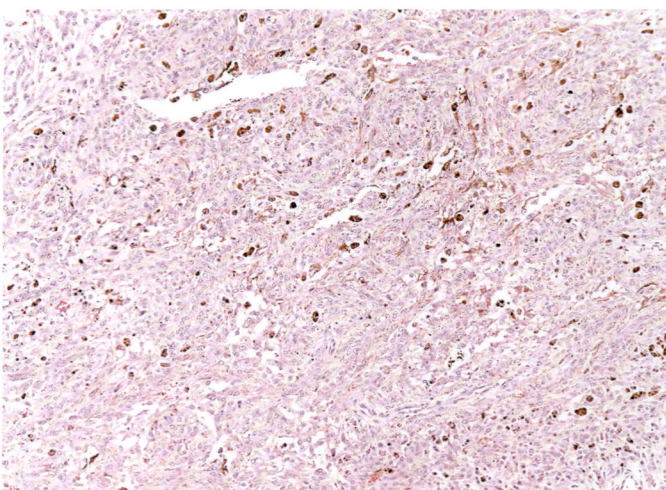

IMAGE 16.65 Malignant melanotic nerve sheath tumour. This is associated with Carney complex.

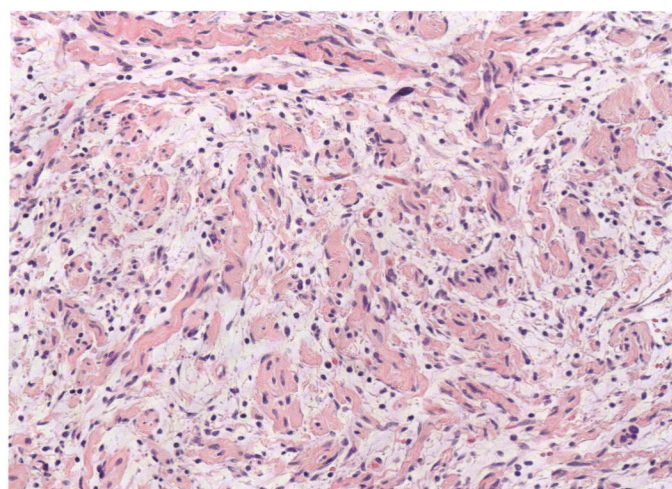

IMAGE 16.66 Neurofibroma (H&E, x200). In contrast to a Schwannoma, a neurofibroma expands the entire nerve. Residual axons, fibrous tissue, and Schwann cells form short, linear strands, which give the tumor the appearance of "shredded carrots."

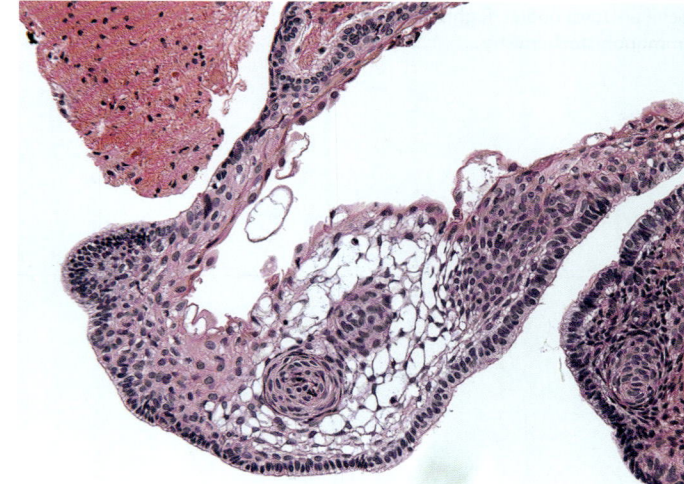

IMAGE 16.67 Craniopharyngiomas are epithelial neoplasms typically arising in the suprasellar region. The adamantinomatous variant, which features prominent stellate reticulum (right side of the image), is associated with WNT alterations.

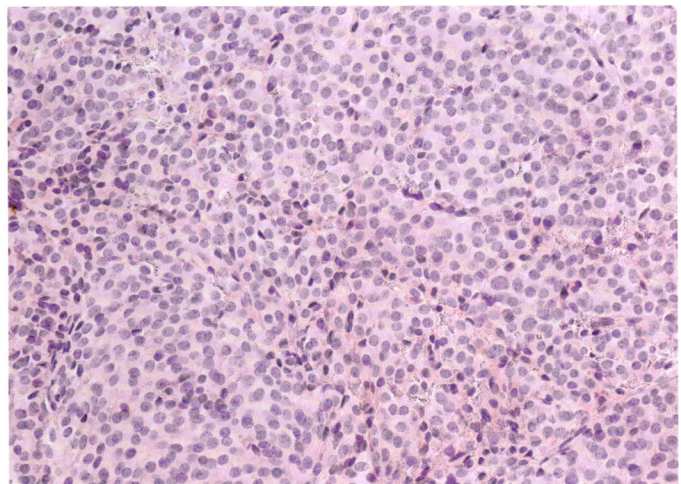

IMAGE 16.68 Pituitary adenoma (H&E, x200). These tumors have a notable monotomy, with uniform nuclei dispersed in reticulin-sparse, relatively uniform matrix.

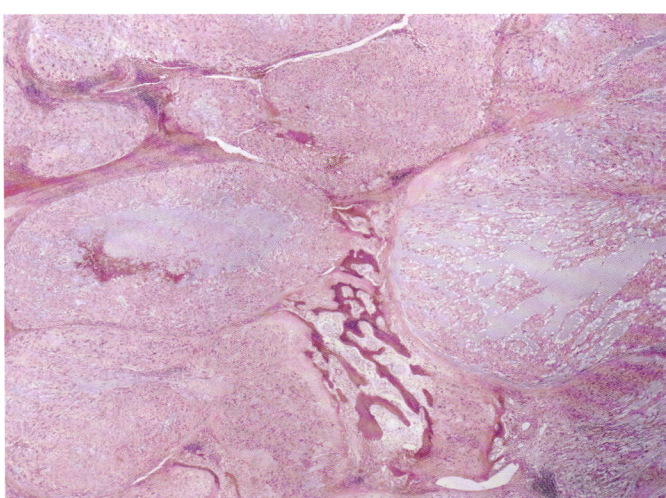

IMAGE 16.71 Chordoma (H&E, x20). Chordomas often display a nodular growth pattern, with cords of cells dispersed within a loose, myxoid matrix.

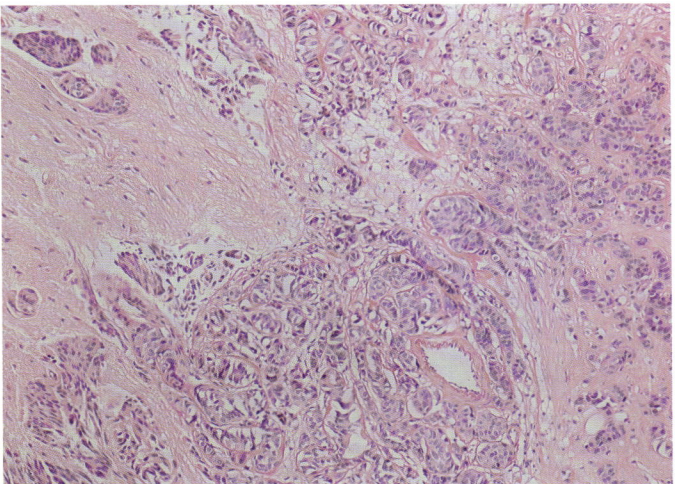

IMAGE 16.69 Metastatic breast carcinoma (H&E, x100).

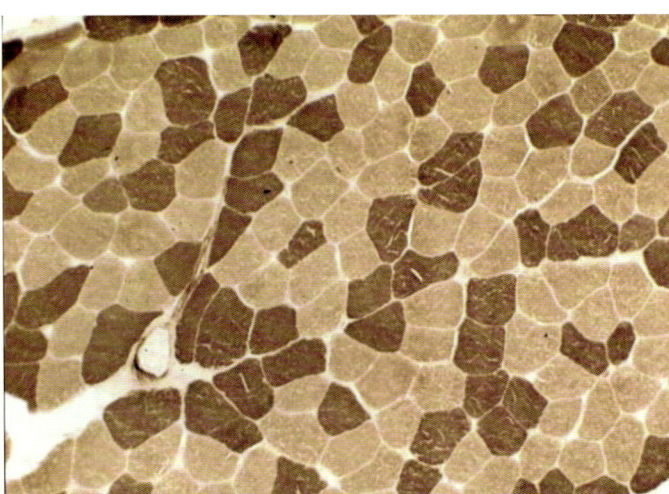

IMAGE 16.72 Normal skeletal muscle with ATPase reaction at pH 4.3 (x40). The image shows a mosaic pattern of different fiber types.

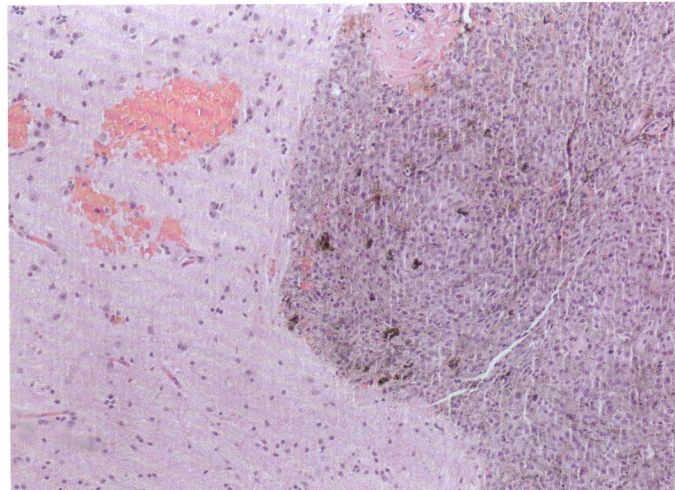

IMAGE 16.70 Metastatic melanoma (H&E, x100). Like many melanomas, this tumor has both melanin pigment and hemosiderin from hemorrhaging.

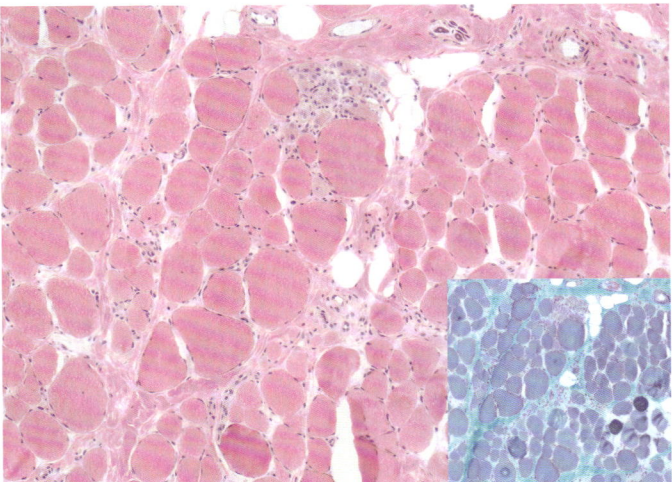

IMAGE 16.73 Duchenne muscular dystrophy. The images show myopathic changes, including fiber size variation, increased connective tissue between myofibers, degenerating myofibers, and some fatty replacement. Main image: H&E, x200. Inset: modified Gomori, x100.

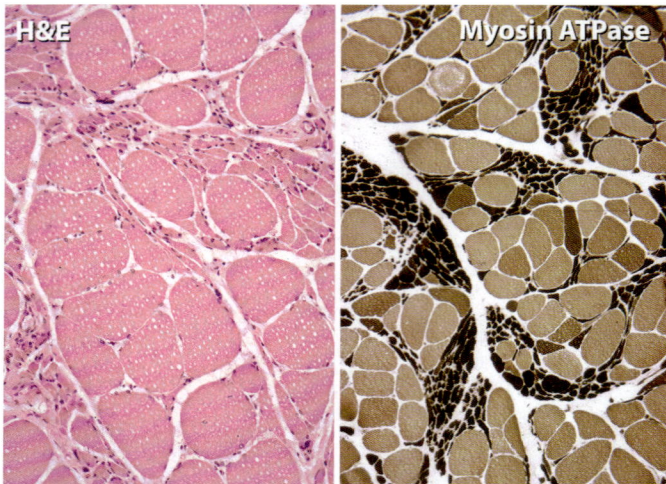

IMAGE 16.74 Chronic denervation. Left: small groups of atrophic myofibers (H&E, x400). Right: myofiber type grouping (ATPase at pH 4.3, x100).

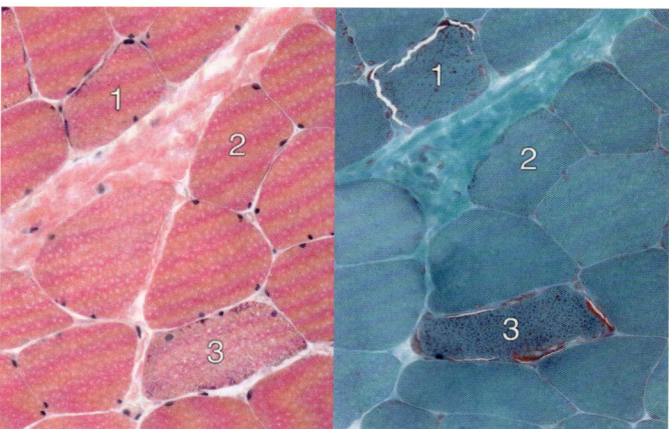

IMAGE 16.75 Ragged red fibers, routine stains. Left: the H&E stain on this frozen muscle shows subtle basophilia in fiber 3, minimal changes in fiber 1, and no changes in fiber 2. Right: in comparison, the Gomori trichrome of the identical fibers (at a different level) clearly shows increased red staining of fiber 3 and subtly increased red staining in fiber 1. It fails to show abnormal staining of fiber 2 (modified Gomori, x200).

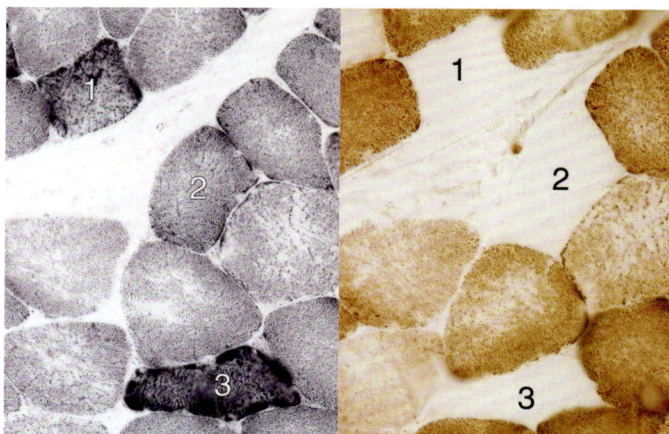

IMAGE 16.76 Ragged red fibers, histochemical stains (the same fibers as image 16.75). Left: succinate dehydrogenase, which reflects the overall density of mitochondria, shows abnormally increased staining in fibers 3 and 2, with a subtle increase in fiber 1 (succinate dehydrogenase, x200). Right: cytochrome oxidase demonstrates complete loss of this oxidative phosphorylation enzyme in all 3 fibers (cytochrome oxidase, x200).

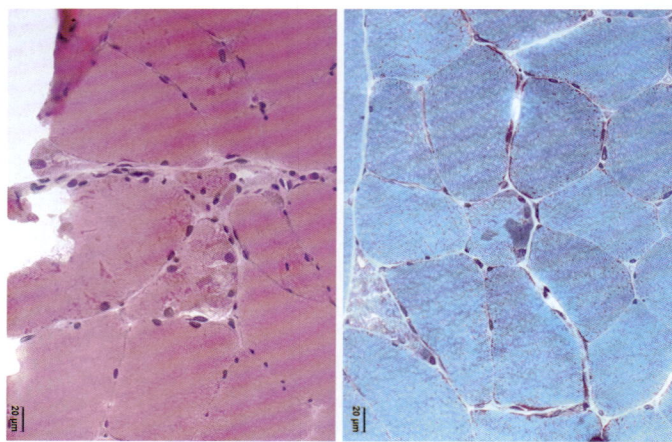

IMAGE 16.77 Myofibrillar myopathy. This group of myopathies results in intracellular aggregates of proteins. Left: the aggregates are amorphous with sharp but irregular borders, and frequently small and multiple. Right: these aggregates frequently have a blueish hue on a modified Gomori trichrome stain.

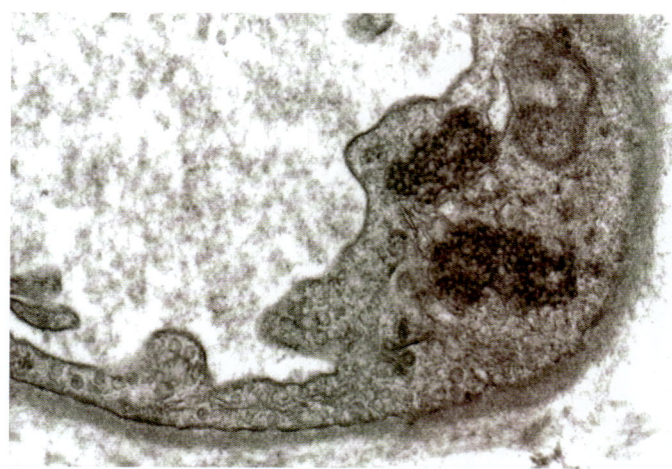

IMAGE 16.78 Tubuloreticular inclusions. These are ultrastructural findings seen within the cytoplasm in endothelial cells in pathologies linked to increased interferon production, including dermatomyositis (inflammatory myopathy with perifascicular pathology), HIV, and systemic lupus erythematosus (SLE).

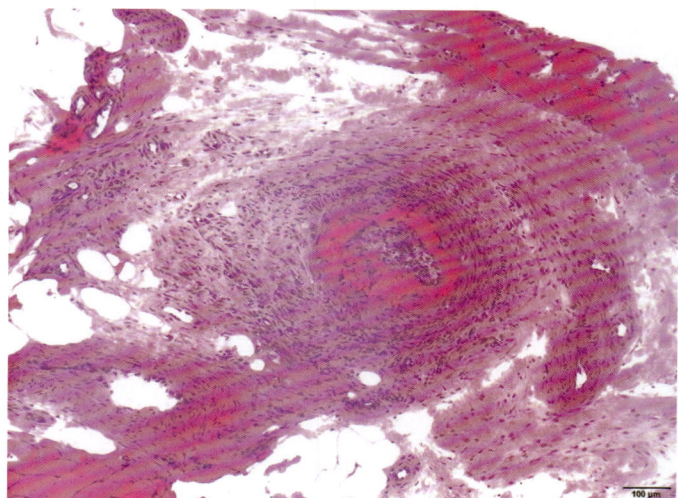

IMAGE 16.79 Acute vasculitis. This H&E-stained isopentane-frozen cryosection shows fibrinoid necrosis of the skeletal muscle artery, accompanied by transmural inflammation.

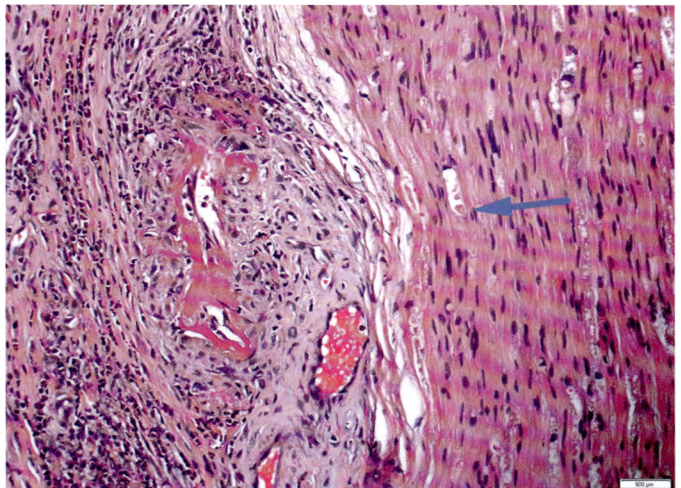

IMAGE 16.80 Acute vasculitis in peripheral nerve. This H&E stained section shows acute leukocytoclastic vasculitis with fibrinoid necrosis and transmural inflammation of the arterial wall. It is accompanied by acute Wallerian degeneration in the adjacent peripheral nerve.

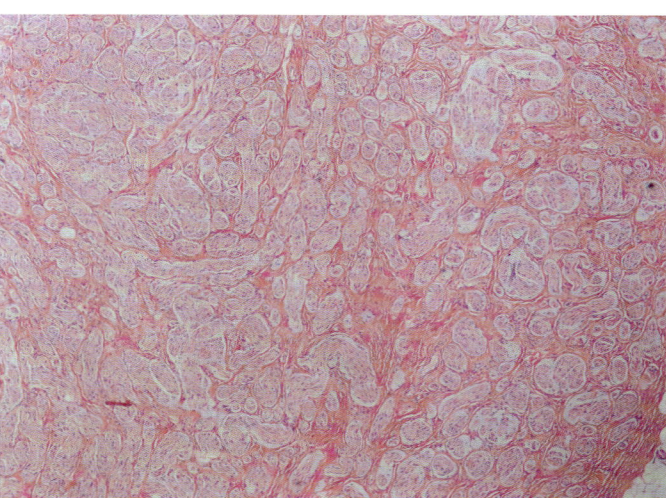

IMAGE 16.83 Traumatic neuroma (H&E, x40). This reactive process is a chaotic attempt of axons and their accompanying cells to regenerate. Instead of reforming the nerve fascicles, they form haphazard collections of small nerve endings.

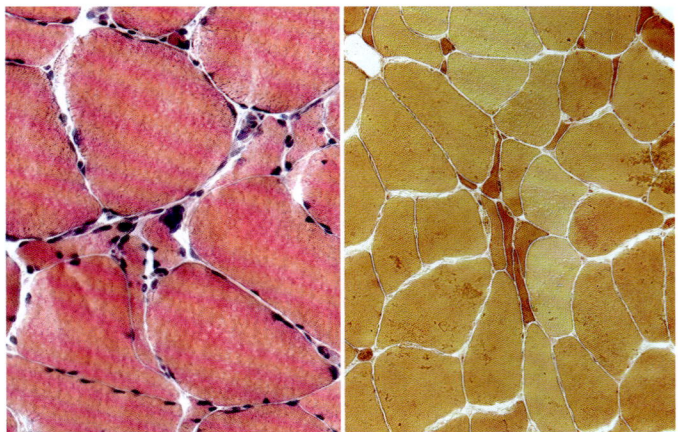

IMAGE 16.81 Denervation atrophy. Left: an H&E-stained section shows acutely angulated atrophic fibers and nuclear aggregates (nuclear bags). Right: the acutely angulated atrophic denervated fibers stain overly dark on an esterase enzyme histochemical preparation.

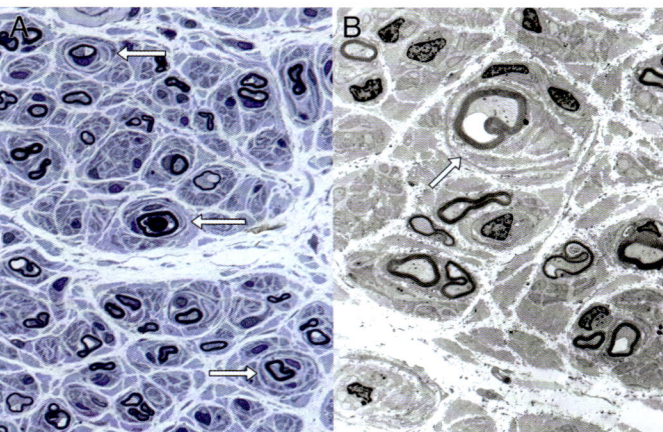

IMAGE 16.84 Chronic demyelination. Left: thick, toluidine blue stained section showing multiple "onion bulbs" (white arrows); significant loss of large, myelinated axons; and scattered, thinly myelinated axons. Right: electron micrograph showing multiple "onion bulbs" (white arrow).

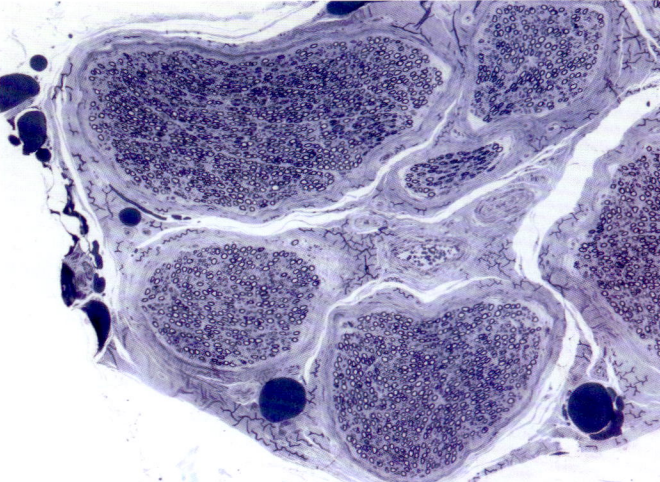

IMAGE 16.82 Normal nerve (toluidine blue, x20). This plastic, 1 micron section shows several nerve fascicles that have a perineurial sheath and connective tissue with vessels in their adventitia.

Bibliography

Agrawal S, Nadel S. Acute bacterial meningitis in infants and children: epidemiology and management. Paediatr Drugs. 2011;13(6):385-400. Medline:21999651. doi: 10.2165/11593340-000000000-00000

Amin MB, Edge S, Greene F, et al, editors. AJCC cancer staging manual. 8th ed. New York: Springer; 2017.

Boissé L, Gill MJ, Power C. HIV infection of the central nervous system: clinical features and neuropathogenesis. *Neurol Clin*. 2008;26(3):799-819. Medline:18657727. doi: 10.1016/j.ncl.2008.04.002

Brat DJ, Cagle P, Dillon D, et al; Cancer Biomarker Reporting Committee, College of American Pathologists. Template for reporting results of biomarker testing of specimens from patients with tumors of the central nervous system (Version: CNS Biomarkers 1.0.0.0) [Internet]. College of American Pathologists; 2014. Available from www.cap.org.

Castellani RJ, Rolston RK, Smith MA. Alzheimer disease. Dis Mon. 2010;56(9):484-546. Medline:20831921. doi 10.1016/j.disamonth.2010.06.001

Chabriat H, Joutel A, Dichgans M, et al. Cadasil. Lancet Neurol. 2009;8(7):643-53. Medline:19539236. doi 10.1016/S1474-4422(09)70127-9

Chang CH, Housepian EM, Herbert C Jr. An operative staging system and a megavoltage radiotherapeutic technic for cerebellar medulloblastomas. Radiology. 1969;93(6):1351-9. PMID: 4983156. doi: 10.1148/93.6.1351

Dubowitz V, Sewry C, Oldfors, editors. Muscle biopsy: a practical approach. 5th ed. North York (ON): Elsevier Canada; 2020.

Eberhart CG, Brat DJ, Cohen KJ, et al. Pediatric neuroblastic brain tumors containing abundant neuropil and true rosettes. Pediatr Dev Pathol. 2000;3(4):346-52. Medline:10890250. doi: 10.1007/s100249910049

Fenrich K, Gordon T. Canadian Association of Neuroscience review: axonal regeneration in the peripheral and central nervous systems—current issues and advances. Can J Neurol Sci. 2004;31(2):142-56. Medline:15198438. doi: 10.1017/S0317167100053798

Fischer MT, Wimmer I, Höftberger R, et al. Disease-specific molecular events in cortical multiple sclerosis lesions. Brain. 2013;136(Pt 6):1799-815. Medline:23687122. doi: org/10.1093/brain/awt110

Focosi D, Marco T, Kast RE, et al. Progressive multifocal leukoencephalopathy: what's new? Neuroscientist. 2010;16(3):308-23. Medline:20479473. doi: 10.1177/1073858409356594

Hattab EM, Bach SE, Cuevas-Ocampo AK, et al; Cancer Committee, College of American Pathologists. Protocol for the examination of specimens from patients with tumors of the brain/spinal cord. (Version: Brain/Spinal Cord 4.0.0.0) [Internet]. College of American Pathologists; 2018. Available from www.cap.org.

Jones DTW, Kocialkowski S, Liu L, et al. Tandem duplication producing a novel oncogenic BRAF fusion gene defines the majority of pilocytic astrocytomas. Cancer Res. 2008;68(21):8673-7. Medline:18974108. doi: 10.1158/0008-5472.CAN-08-2097

Kouri N, Whitwell JL, Josephs KA, et al. Corticobasal degeneration: a pathologically distinct 4R tauopathy. Nat Rev Neurol. 2011;7(5):263-72. Medline:21487420. doi: 10.1038/nrneurol.2011.43

Kumar V, Abbas AK, Aster J. Robbins and Cotran pathologic basis of disease. 10th ed. North York (ON): Elsevier Canada; 2020.

Kurschus FC, Wörtge S, Waisman A. Modeling a complex disease: multiple sclerosis. Adv Immunol. 2011;110:111-37. Medline:21762817. doi: 10.1016/B978-0-12-387663-8.00001-6

WHO Classification of Tumours Editorial Board. WHO classification of tumours. 5th ed. Vol. 6, Central nervous system tumours. Lyon (France): IARC, 2021.

Louis DN, Perry A, Burger P, et al; International Society of Neuropathology. International Society of Neuropathology — Haarlem consensus guidelines for nervous system tumor classification and grading. Brain Pathol. 2014;24(5):429-35. Medline:24990071. doi:10.1111/bpa.12171

Love S, Perry A, Ironside J, et al, editors. Greenfield's neuropathology. 9th ed. Boca Ranton (FL): CRC Press; 2015.

McKintosh E, Tabrizi SJ, Collinge J. Prion diseases. J Neurovirol. 2003;9(2):183-93. Medline:12707849. doi: 10.1080/13550280390194082

Norrby E. Prions and protein-folding diseases. J Intern Med. 2011;270(1):1-14. Medline:21481020. doi: 10.1111/j.1365-2796.2011.02387.x

Pfister SM, Korshunov A, Kool M, et al. Molecular diagnostics of CNS embryonal tumors. Acta Neuropathol. 2010;120(5):553-66. Medline:20882288. doi:10.1007/s00401-010-0751-5

Revesz T, Holton JL, Lashley T, et al. Genetics and molecular pathogenesis of sporadic and hereditary cerebral amyloid angiopathies. Acta Neuropathol. 2009;118(1):115-30. Medline:19225789. doi: 10.1007/s00401-009-0501-8

Riemenschneider MJ, Jeuken JWM, Wesseling P, et al. Molecular diagnostics of gliomas: state of the art. Acta Neuropathol. 2010;120(5):567-84. Medline:20714900. doi: 10.1007/s00401-010-0736-4

Shulman JM, De Jager PL, Feany MB. Parkinson's disease: genetics and pathogenesis. Annu Rev Pathol. 2011;6(1):193-222. Medline:21034221. doi: 10.1146/annurev-pathol-011110-130242

Von Deimling A, Korshunov A, Hartmann C. The next generation of glioma biomarkers: MGMT methylation, *BRAF* fusions and *IDH1* mutations. Brain Pathol. 2011;21(1):74-87. Medline:21129061. doi: 10.1111/j.1750-3639.2010.00454.x

Vonsattel JP, Myers RH, Stevens TJ, et al. Neuropathological classification of Huntington's disease. J Neuropathol Exp Neurol. 1985;44(6):559-77. Medline:2932539. doi:10.1097/00005072-198511000-00003

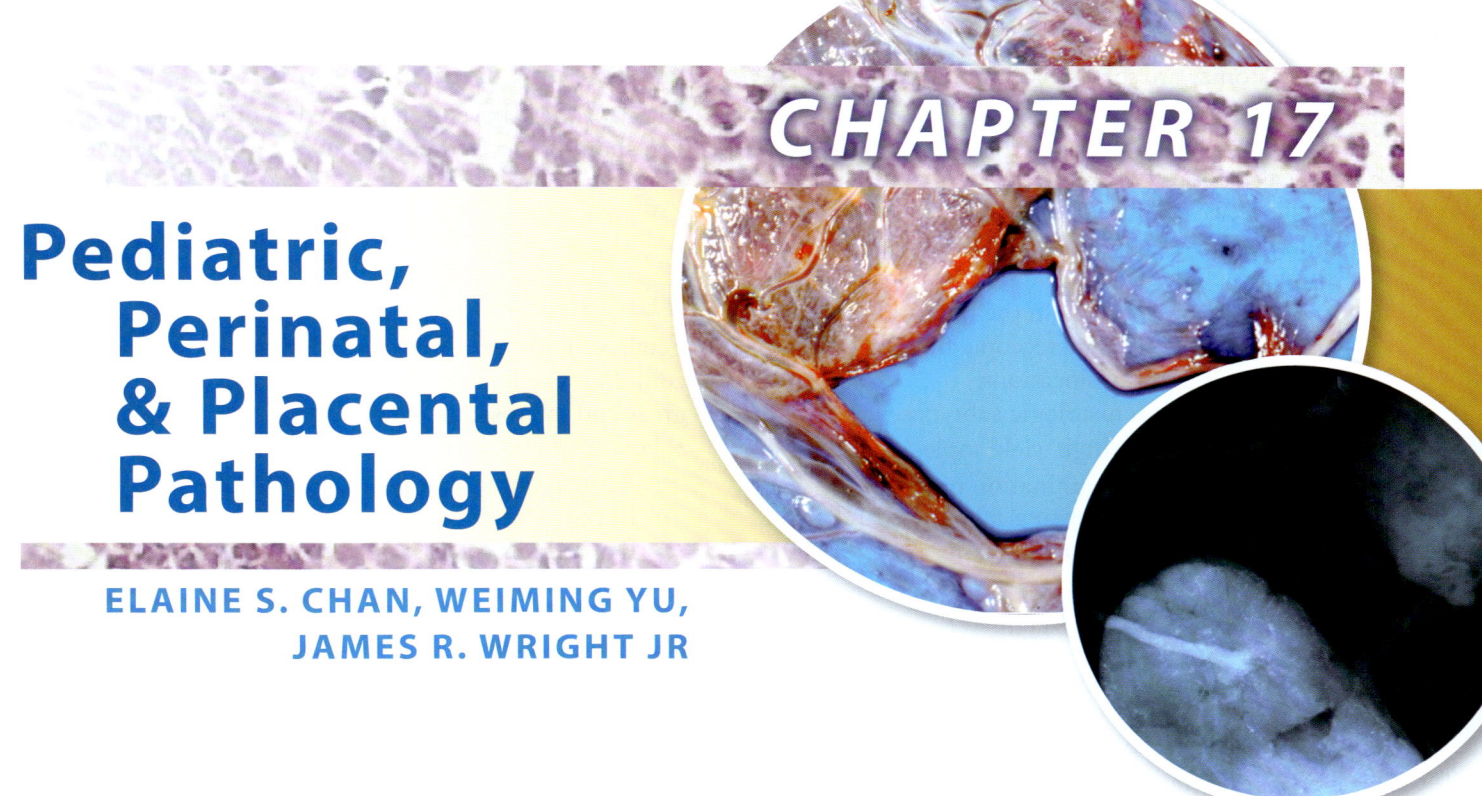

CHAPTER 17

Pediatric, Perinatal, & Placental Pathology

ELAINE S. CHAN, WEIMING YU, JAMES R. WRIGHT JR

Pediatric, Perinatal, and Placental Pathology Exam Essentials

MUST KNOW

General comments

- Pediatric tumors are present in numerous organs. For the purpose of studying, you should focus on organ-specific "blastomas," of which Wilms tumor (nephroblastoma) is the most high yield.
- The protocols of the AJCC and College of American Pathologists are helpful because they discuss the most common pediatric tumors; you could use them as a guide to high-yield entities.
- A topic not covered by CAP/AJCC protocols is Langerhan cell histiocytosis.
- Placental tumors are exceedingly rare: chorangioma is likely the only entity the exam might cover.
- Gestational trophoblastic tumors are covered in chapter 11 on gynecologic pathology.

AJCC and College of American Pathologists (CAP) protocols

- CAP/AJCC protocols include many pediatric, perinatal, and placental entities (including retinoblastoma). Although these entities are rarely encountered in clinical practice, they are reliable exam topics, especially the molecular changes in sarcomas (see chapter 2 on soft tissue tumors).
- Many pediatric tumors are covered in other chapters. Note that while leukemias are common in children, they are generally not high yield for the anatomic pathology exam.
- In general, ophthalmic pathology is an esoteric field. Nonetheless there are 2 classic features of retinoblastoma worth knowing:
  - Clinical presentation in children.
  - *Rb* gene, its role and relation to the two-hit hypothesis.
- Ewing sarcoma is among the most frequently examined entities in sarcoma. High-yield topics include:
  - Gross and radiologic bone findings.
  - Microscopic findings.
  - Treatment effect.
  - Cytogenetics and translocations.
  - Differential for small round blue cell tumors in children.
- In general, questions on germ cell tumors would be incorporated into the genitourinary or gynecologic sections. A few pertinent details related to pediatric germ cell tumors include:
  - Germ cell tumors outside of reproductive organs.
  - Prepubertal germ cell tumors in males.
  - Immature teratomas.
- Pediatric hepatoblastomas are rarely examined, but review subtypes of hepatoblastoma.

- Neuroblastomas are somewhat more frequently examined (see also chapter 16), including:
  - Histologic subtypes.
  - Clinical/laboratory testing.
  - Prognosis, especially as related to N-myc.
- Rhabdomyosarcoma is another high-yield sarcoma. Key topics include:
  - Gross findings, especially in the botryoid type.
  - Various subtypes and microscopic findings.
  - Cytogenetics and translocations.
  - Prognosis based on histologic subtypes.
- Wilms tumor is a very high-yield topic, including:
  - Gross handling and examination procedure, including weighing, assessing intactness, and so on.
  - Histology, and features of anaplasia.
  - Nephrogenic rests.
  - Margins.
  - Staging.
  - Syndromes related to Wilms tumor.

Nonneoplastic diseases

This area is important to placental and fetal pathology. You should note that a lot of placental pathology requires correlation with gross and microscopic findings. High-yield topics include:
- Fetus:
  - Fetal hydrops, causes, findings.
  - Causes of stillbirth, and ancillary studies.
  - Intrauterine growth retardation (IUGR), especially causes and complications.
  - Maternal factors that negatively affect the fetus or can cause congenital anomalies.
  - Cardiac malformations.
  - Omphalocele, gastroschisis.
  - Spina bifida and central nervous system (CNS) malformations (see chapter 16).
  - Twin-twin transfusion.
  - Oligo- and polyhydramnios.
  - Chromosomal anomalies (Down syndrome, other trisomies, Turner syndrome).
  - Fetal alcohol syndrome.
- Placenta:
  - Small- and large-sized placentas.
  - Multiple gestations.
  - Placental infarct.
  - Chorioamnionitis.
  - Villitis of unknown etiology.
  - Viral infections.
  - Membrane insertion anomalies.
  - Umbilical cord anomalies.
  - Preeclampsia, eclampsia and HELLP syndrome.
  - Fetal vascular malperfusion.
  - Maternal vascular malperfusion.
  - Complications of pregnancy by systemic diseases.

Genetic and syndromic conditions

Many of these have been covered in other chapters, so you should refer to them as well. Key topics include:
- Cystic fibrosis.
- Various chromosomal anomalies.

MUST SEE

Fetal/pediatric pathology and placental pathology contain many features that are grossly evident, so review gross and microscopic images.
- Fetal/pediatric entities include:
  - Acute lymphoblastic leukemia (ALL).
  - Burkitt lymphoma.
  - Langerhans cell histiocytosis.
  - Congenital pulmonary airway malformation (CPAM).
  - Retinoblastoma.
  - Ewing sarcoma.
  - Prepubertal teratoma.
  - Immature teratomas.
  - Teratomas outside of reproductive organs.
  - Yolk sac tumor.
  - Hepatoblastoma.
  - Neuroblastoma and ganglioneuromas.
  - Rhabdomyosarcoma.
  - Wilms tumor.
  - Rhabdoid tumor.
  - Fetal hydrops.
  - Hirschsprung disease.
  - IUGR.
  - Amniotic band syndrome.
  - Various heart malformations: tetralogy of Fallot, atrial septal defect (ASD)., atrioventricular septal defect (AVSD), ventricular septal defect (VSD), endocardial cushion defect, transposition of great arteries, patent ductus arteriosus (PDA).
  - Hydrops fetalis.
  - Omphalocele.
  - Gastroschisis.
  - Pyloric stenosis.
  - Spina bifida.
  - Diaphragmatic hernia.
  - Other CNS defects (see chapter 16).
  - Twin-twin transfusion.
  - Potter sequence.
  - Down syndrome.
  - Necrotizing enterocolitis.
  - Meckel diverticulum.
  - Situs inversus.
  - Autosomal recessive polycystic kidney disease.
  - Horseshoe kidney.
  - Multicystic renal dysplasia.
- Placental entities include:
  - Twin placenta.

- Placental infarct.
- Chorioamnionitis.
- Villitis.
- Cytomegalovirus (CMV).
- Herpes simplex virus (HSV).
- Circumvallate and circummarginate membranes.
- Velamentous cord insertion.
- Hypo- and hyper- coiled umbilical cord.
- True and false umbilical cord knots.
- Amnion nodosum.
- Fetus papyraceus.
- Chorangioma.

MUST DO

- For each of the entities outlined in the Must See section, you should be comfortable generating a differential diagnosis and listing additional studies (e.g., histochemical or immunohistochemical stains). For entities that overlap other chapters, use the other chapters to complement this chapter.
- When studying in groups, practice:
  - Pediatric small round blue cell tumors.
  - Common sarcomas and their molecular translocations.
- Wilms tumor, including grossing and associated syndromes.
- Using ancillary studies for pediatric lymphomas and sarcomas.
- Chromosomal anomalies, including trisomies 13, 18, 21, and Turner syndrome.
- Congenital conditions such as Hirschsprung disease, fetal hydrops, cystic fibrosis, and others.
- SIDS in the forensic context.
- Placental malformation and lesions that are diagnosed grossly.
- Preeclampsia.
- You should be able to describe the grossing protocol, and independently gross, the following specimens:
  - Soft tissue and bone resection for sarcoma.
  - Nephrectomy for Wilms tumor.
  - Products of conception.
  - Intact fetus of less than 20 weeks gestation.
  - Stillbirth at 20 or more weeks gestation, including those with genetic diseases.
  - Singleton placenta.
  - Twin and multiple-gestation placentas.
- You should be able to describe and perform lymphoma protocol for pediatric lymphoma and leukemia.

MULTIPLE CHOICE QUESTIONS

1. Which statement about prematurity is **false**?

a. Prematurity is defined as birth before 37 weeks gestation.

b. The incidence in the USA is ~10% but is higher among African-Americans.

c. Premature infants have higher morbidity and mortality rates.

d. Prematurity is the most common cause of neonatal mortality.

Answer: d

2. Which statement about respiratory distress syndrome (RDS) in newborns is **false**?

a. Has > 90% incidence in infants born at ≤ 28 weeks gestational age.

b. Has ~10% incidence in infants born at 34 weeks gestational age.

c. Has ~1% incidence in infants born at 37 weeks gestational age.

d. Never occurs in full term infants.

e. None of the above.

Answer: d

3. Identify the correct statement(s) about fetal growth restriction (FGR, or intrauterine growth retardation).

a. FGR can be divided into 3 main groups: fetal, placental, and maternal causes.

b. The most common fetal causes are chromosomal disorders, congenital malformations, and congenital TORCH group infections (TORCH: **t**oxoplasmosis, **o**ther infections, **r**ubella, **c**ytomegalovirus infection, **h**erpes simplex).

c. Uteroplacental insufficiency is an important cause.

d. Common maternal causes are preeclampsia, chronic hypertension, and behavioral causes (heavy smoking, alcohol consumption, drug use).

e. All of the above.

Answer: e

4. Which statement, from *a* to *d*, about FGR is **false**?

a. FGR can be divided into symmetric (proportionate) or asymmetric (i.e., relative sparing of the brain) types.

b. Placental causes tend to result in asymmetric FGR, as growth restriction generally occurs later in gestation due to limited nutrition or oxygenation.

c. Fetal causes usually result in symmetric FGR.

d. FGR is rarely associated with long-term morbidity, as postnatal growth can compensate.

e. None of the above.

Answer: d

5. Identify the correct statement(s) about the consequences of maternal smoking during pregnancy.

a. Associated with a higher incidence of spontaneous abortion.

b. Associated with a higher incidence of premature labor.

c. Associated with lower birth weight.

d. Associated with a higher incidence of sudden infant death syndrome (SIDS).

e. All of the above.

Answer: e

6. Which statement, from *a* to *d*, about the fetal consequences of maternal diabetes is **false**?

a. Fetal pancreas usually shows a marked increase in islet tissue and β cells.

b. Fetal macrosomia is common due to fetal hyperinsulinemia secondary to maternal hyperglycemia.

c. The placenta is almost always enlarged due to fetal hyperinsulinemia secondary to maternal hyperglycemia.

d. The incidence of major malformations is ~6–10%.

e. None of the above.

Answer: c

7. Which of the following is the least common cause of death in the first year of life?

a. SIDS.

b. Congenital anomalies.

c. Sequelae of prematurity and low birth weight.

d. Malignancies.

e. Maternal complications and injuries.

Answer: d

8. Identify the correct statement(s) about Chiari II (Arnold Chiari) malformation.

a. The cerebellar vermis is caudally displaced into the upper cervical spinal canal.

b. The fourth ventricle, midbrain, pons, and medulla are all elongated and caudally displaced.

c. Most (95%) are associated with a lumbosacral myelomeningocele.

d. The posterior fossa is not enlarged.

e. All of the above.

Answer: e

9. Which statement about cystic fibrosis (CF) or mucoviscidosis is **false**?

a. CF occurs due to abnormal function of a protein encoded by the *CFTR* gene on chromosome 7q31.2.

b. Symptoms can appear at anytime from birth until adolescence.

c. All patients with biallelic *CFTR* mutations eventually develop classic cystic fibrosis.

d. Heterozygous carriers have a higher rate of pulmonary and pancreatic diseases than the general population.

Answer: c

10. Which statement, from *a* to *d*, about CF is **false**?

a. It is the most common lethal genetic disease among Caucasians.

b. The carrier rate for Caucasians in the United States is ~1 in 20.

c. Its transmission is autosomal recessive but there is much phenotypic variation due to multiple mutations in the *CFTR* gene as well as effects of modifier genes.

d. Median life expectancy for patients with CF is approximately 50 years.

e. None of the above.

Answer: e

11. Which pathological finding is **not** highly characteristic of CF?

a. Nasal polyps containing large cystic glands with inspissated luminal secretions and a paucity of eosinophils.

b. Sweat gland morphologic abnormalities.

c. Azoospermia and infertility, often with congenital bilateral absence of the vas deferens.

d. Meconium ileus.

Answer: b

12. Pancreatic abnormalities characteristic of CF include which of the following?

a. Small pancreatic ducts plugged with mucus and dilatation of exocrine glands (early).

b. Near total atrophy and fibrosis of the exocrine pancreas (late).

c. Squamous metaplasia of the pancreatic duct epithelium due to malabsorption of vitamin A.

d. Pancreatic islets preserved within a fibrofatty stroma.

e. All of the above.

Answer: e

13. Which statement, from *a* to *d*, about gastrointestinal and hepatic findings in CF is **false**?

a. Meconium ileus is seen in 5–10% of patients at or near the time of birth.

b. Common hepatic findings in CF include bile ductular proliferation, containing amorphous pink concretions and portal inflammation.

c. Hepatic steatosis and focal biliary cirrhosis are rare.

d. Liver disease is now a common cause of death in adult CF patients.

e. None of the above.

Answer: c

14. The following statements concern the most common cause of death according to age. Which statements are correct?

a. Birth–1 year: congenital anomalies, prematurity and low birth weight, SIDS, and maternal complications and injuries.

b. 1–4 years: injuries resulting from accidents.

c. 5–9 years: injuries resulting from accidents.

d. 10–14 years: accidents, malignancies, suicide, homicide, and congenital malformations.

e. All of the above.

Answer: e

15. The following statements from *a* to *c* concern the most common cause of spontaneous abortion or stillbirth according to trimester. Which statement is **incorrect**?

a. First trimester: chromosomal anomalies.

b. Second trimester: infection.

c. Third trimester: placental insufficiency/cord accident.

d. None of the above.

Answer: d

16. Which birth defect has the highest prevalence?

a. Spina bifida.

b. Cleft palate.

c. Omphalocele.

d. Colonic atresia/stenosis.

e. Esophageal atresia/tracheoesophageal fistula.

Answer: b

17. Identify the correct statement(s) about Dandy-Walker malformations.

a. There is hydrocephalus.

b. There is cystic dilatation of the fourth ventricle.

c. The cerebellar vermis is hypoplastic or absent.

d. There is a large posterior fossa and elevation of the tentorium.

e. All of the above.

Answer: e

18. Which conditions support a diagnosis of diabetic embryopathy in the infant of a diabetic mother?

a. Single umbilical artery.

b. Sacral agenesis, caudal regression, sirenomelia, and neural tube defects.

c. Cardiac ventricular septal defects and transposition of the great vessels.

d. Meconium ileus.

e. All of the above.

Answer: e

19. Identify the correct statement(s) about omphalocele.

a. It is a type of abdominal wall defect allowing intestines, liver, and/or other organs to protrude.

b. Protrusion is through the base of the umbilical cord.

c. Protruding viscera are usually covered by a membrane.

d. It has an association with Beckwith-Wiedemann syndrome and chromosomal anomalies.

e. All of the above.

Answer: e

20. Which statement about gastroschisis is **false**?

a. It is a type of abdominal wall defect allowing intestines, liver, and/or other organs to protrude.

b. Protrusion is lateral to (usually to the right) and does not involve the umbilical cord; there is no membranous covering of viscera.

c. It has an association with Beckwith-Wiedemann syndrome.

d. It is often associated with specific histologic changes in the placenta.

e. None of the above.

Answer: c

21. Hazards of premature delivery include which of the following?

a. Hyaline membrane disease (neonatal respiratory distress syndrome).

b. Necrotizing enterocolitis.

c. Sepsis.

d. Germinal matrix hemorrhage and intraventricular hemorrhage.

e. All of the above.

Answer: e

22. Major risk factors for premature delivery include which of the following?

a. Preterm premature rupture of placental membranes.

b. Intrauterine infections.

c. Uterine abnormalities (fibroids, cervical incompetence).

d. Multiple gestation (e.g., twin pregnancy).

e. All of the above.

Answer: e

23. What is the best way to properly diagnose CF?

a. Measurement of nasal transepithelial potential difference in vivo.

b. Sweat test with persistently elevated chloride concentrations.

c. Sequencing the patient's *CFTR* gene.

d. Newborn screening by measuring immunoreactive trypsinogen blood levels.

e. A positive newborn screening test, meconium ileus at birth, and an appropriate family history.

Answer: c

24. Glycogenoses (glycogen storage diseases) include at least 10 inherited disorders, primarily characterized by glycogen accumulation in the liver, heart, and skeletal muscle. Almost all types are autosomal recessive. Which of the following statements are true about types of glycogenoses?

a. Type 1A (von Gierke disease) is due to glucose-6-phosphatase deficiency and characterized by hepatomegaly, hypoglycemia, and normal mental development, and is compatible with long life.

b. Type 2 (Pompe disease) is a lysosomal storage disease in which glycogen accumulates in most organs, and, usually, death via heart failure occurs before age 2.

c. Type 4 (Andersen disease) is very rare and due to the absence of a glycogen branching enzyme, which results in the accumulation of amylopectin-like polysaccharides in the liver; children usually die by age 2–4 from hepatic cirrhosis but can be cured by a liver transplant (transplantation, however, does not prevent nonhepatic complications of the disease).

d. Type 5 (McArdle disease) is characterized by the accumulation of glycogen in skeletal muscle due to muscle phosphorylase deficiency resulting in muscle spasms during exercise.

e. All of the above.

Answer: e

25. Identify the correct statement(s) small round blue cell tumor (SRBCT) of childhood.

a. SRBCT of childhood is a descriptive category of malignant pediatric neoplasm.

b. SRBCT is characterized by the presence of morphologically poorly differentiated cells with high nuclear–cytoplasmic ratios.

c. Correct identification of the specific tumor is important for therapy purposes.

d. Immunohistochemistry, cytogenetics, fluorescence in situ hybridization (FISH), molecular studies, and/or flow cytometry are needed for confirmation of diagnosis.

e. All of the above are true.

Answer: e

26. Which statement, from *a* to *d*, about Langerhans cell histiocytosis (LCH) is **false**?

a. LCH is a clonal proliferative disorder.

b. LCH can be focal with a self-limiting course.

c. LCH can be systemic with an aggressive course involving multiple organs.

d. Birbeck granules are found by electron microscopy in Langerhans cell.

e. None of the above.

Answer: e

27. Which statement about neuroblastoma is **false**?

a. Neuroblastoma is the most common extracranial solid tumor in childhood.

b. Most neuroblastoma occurs sporadically (1–2% are familial).

c. Germline mutations in the *ALK* gene are a major cause of familial predisposition to neuroblastoma.

d. The majority of neuroblastomas produce catecholamines, an important diagnostic feature.

e. Screening for neuroblastoma has improved overall mortality rates.

Answer: e

28. Which statement about anaplastic large cell lymphoma (ALCL) is **false**?

a. Most pediatric cases are null cell immunophenotype.

b. Most pediatric cases are *ALK* positive and have the translocation t(2;5).

c. CD30 is positive in both adult and pediatric ALCL.

d. Morphological variants include pleomorphic, sarcomatoid, histiocytic rich, neutrophilic rich, and small cell variant.

e. It affects patients of all ages.

Answer: a

29. Which statement about pediatric renal tumors is **false**?

a. The most common type of renal cell carcinoma in children is Xp11.2 translocation associated renal cell carcinoma.

b. Clear cell sarcoma of the kidney has a reciprocal translocation t(12;22)(q13;q12), resulting in the fusion of *EWSR1* and *ATF1* in > 90% of cases.

c. Congenital mesoblastic nephroma, the classic form, is histologically identical to infantile fibromatosis.

d. The cellular type of congenital mesoblastic nephroma is histologically and cytogenetically identical to infantile fibrosarcoma.

e. None of the above.

Answer: b

30. Which statement about Wilms tumor is **false**?

a. Some Wilms tumors (5–10%) involve both kidneys.

b. Most patients with Wilms tumor are associated with congenital malformation syndromes, including WAGR syndrome (WAGR: **W**ilms tumor, **a**niridia, **g**enitourinary anomalies, and mental **r**etardation), Denys-Drash syndrome, and Beckwith-Wiedemann syndrome.

c. The presence of anaplasia correlates with *TP53* mutations and emergence of resistance to chemotherapy.

d. Presence of histological anaplasia is a potent marker of adverse prognosis.

e. Gain-of-function mutations of the gene encoding β-catenin are found in 10% of sporadic Wilms tumors.

Answer: b

31. Which statement about pediatric spindle cell tumor (PSCT) is **false**?

a. Superficial PSCT is often excised while deep PSCT is assessed by incisional or core biopsies.

b. The main objectives for the pathologist are to establish the pathological diagnosis, assess margins, and harvest tissue for biological investigations (pathologic-genetic-prognostic information).

c. PSCT is categorized as benign, intermediate (locally recurrent, rarely metastasizing), and malignant.

d. Fibrous hamartoma of infancy is considered a borderline malignancy.

e. Nodular fasciitis can have rearrangements of *USP6*.

Answer: d

32. Which statement about inflammatory myofibroblastic tumor (IMT) is **false**?

a. It is a neoplasm composed of spindle cells accompanied by a lymphoplasmacytic infiltration.

b. Approximately 50% of cases have clonal rearrangement of *ALK* gene at 2p23.

c. Immunohistochemistry reveals reactivity with smooth muscle actin and desmin.

d. IMT is considered a benign tumor.

e. Some patients have fever, night sweats, weight loss, and malaise, probably related to the secretion of cytokines (interleukin 6).

Answer: d

33. Which statement about infantile fibrosarcoma is **false**?

a. It affects children ≤ 2 years of age.

b. It has the t(12;15) (p13;q25) *ETV6-NTRK3* gene fusion.

c. The histological and cytogenetic features are similar to cellular congenital mesoblastic nephroma.

d. It is always present at birth.

e. The principal sites of involvement are the extremities.

Answer: d

34. Which of the following statements about congenital pulmonary airway malformation (CPAM) is **false**?

a. CPAM is a hamartomatous lesion of the lung that can be separated into 5 major types: type 0 to 4.

b. CPAM type 1 (larger cysts) accounts for 65% of cases.

c. CPAM type 2 (medium cysts)

d. CPAM type 3 (small cysts) accounts for 5% of cases.

e. CPAM is also called "congenital cystic adenomatoid malformation" (CCAM).

can be associated with other congenital anomalies.

Answer: e

35. Which statement about extrachorial placentation is **false**?

a. It exists when the villous tissue extends outward beyond the chorionic vascular plate.

b. It takes 2 forms: circummargination and circumvallation.

c. When running your finger over the transition point where circumvallate membranes disconnect

d. from the extrachorial placenta, there is a ridge of debris, fibrin and old hemorrhage.

d. Neither type of extrachorial placentation has known clinical consequences.

e. Both types of extrachorial placentation can be partial or complete.

Answer: d

36. Identify the correct statement(s) about amnion nodosum.

a. It represents small nodules of baby hair and squames pressed onto the fetal surface of the placental membranes.

b. It is most likely seen in the third trimester.

c. It is associated with oligohydramnios.

d. Only answers a and c are true.

e. Answers a, b, and c are true.

Answer: e

37. Identify the correct statement(s) about placental avascular villi.

a. Placental villi deprived of fetal circulation become avascular.

b. Placentas of stillborn fetuses with long-term intrauterine retention become diffusely avascular.

c. Placentas with fetal vascular malperfusion (fetal thrombotic vasculopathy) develop multifocal avascular villi.

d. Only answers a and c are true.

e. Answers a, b, and c are true.

Answer: e

38. Identify the correct statement(s) about chorangiomas.

a. They are placental hemangiomas.

b. They are likely hamartomatous rather than neoplastic lesions.

c. If large, they can cause polyhydramnios.

d. Only answers a and c are true.

e. Answers a, b, and c are true.

Answer: e

39. Which statement about monozygotic twins is **false**?

a. Fertilization involves a single egg and sperm with subsequent splitting.

b. The timing of the splitting can result in either diamniotic monochorionic (DiMo) or monoamniotic monochorionic (MoMo) placentation.

c. All monochorionic twin placentas support monozygotic twins.

d. All monozygotic twins have monochorionic placentas.

e. Conjoined twins are always monozygotic.

Answer: d

40. Which statement about dizygotic twins is **false**?

a. Fertilization involves 2 eggs and 2 sperms.

b. All dichorionic twin placentas support dizygotic twins.

c. All dizygotic twins have dichorionic placentas.

d. Dizygotic twins may have separate placentas or a fused placenta.

e. Dizygotic twins have separate placental circulations even if they have a fused placenta.

Answer: b

41. Which type of twin placenta is associated with the highest mortality rate?

a. Diamniotic dichorionic (DiDi).

b. Diamniotic monochorionic (DiMo).

c. Monoamniotic monochorionic (MoMo).

d. All have the same mortality rate.

Answer: c

42. Which of the following **cannot** account for dizygotic twin A being larger than the dizygotic twin B?

a. Differences in placental size or vascular territories (A > B).

b. Velamentous cord insertions in the twin B portion of the placenta.

c. Twin-twin transfusion syndrome (TTTS).

d. Single umbilical artery in the twin B portion of the placenta.

e. All of the above could account for dizygotic twin A being larger than B.

Answer: c

Congenital Anomalies (Morphologic Defects Present at Birth)

43. Define each of the following 3 terms, which clarify the nature of congenital anomalies, and list at least 1 common example of each.

- Malformations:
  · Definition: primary errors of morphogenesis in which there is an intrinsically abnormal developmental process.
  · Examples: syndactyly, polydactyly, cleft lip, cleft palate, congenital heart diseases.
- Disruptions:
  · Definition: secondary destruction of an organ or body region that was previously normal (i.e., an extrinsic disturbance in morphogenesis). Disruptions are not heritable, hence they are not associated with increased risk of recurrence in subsequent pregnancies.
  · Example: amniotic bands.
- Deformations:
  · Definition: an extrinsic disturbance of development rather than an intrinsic error or morphogenesis (i.e., structural anomalies secondary to abnormal mechanical forces, usually uterine constraint).
  · Example: clubfoot due to bicornuate uterus, leiomyomas, oligohydramnios.

44. Define each of the following 2 terms, which clarify the nature of multiple congenital anomalies, and list a common example of each.

- Sequence:
  · Definition: a cascade of anomalies initiated by a single aberration.
  · Example: oligohydramnios (Potter) sequence.
- Malformation syndrome:
  · Definition: a group of congenital anomalies that may be pathologically related, but that do not result from a single aberration.
  · Example: Down syndrome.

45. Describe the Potter sequence.

- Chronic oligohydramnios (often caused by amniotic fluid leakage, renal agenesis, bladder outlet obstruction, or severe toxemia of pregnancy) causes fetal compression with a classic phenotype including many of these features:
  · Flattened facies with compressed nose and low set, posteriorly rotated ears.
  · Small chest circumference due to pulmonary hypoplasia caused by absence of adequate intrauterine inhalation of amniotic fluid. (Note: pulmonary hypoplasia is often the cause of death.)
  · Talipes equinovarus (clubfeet).
  · Hip dislocation due to compression.
  · Note: amnion nodosum is a characteristic placental finding.

46. Define the following organ-specific terms.

- Agenesis: absence of the organ primordium.
- Aplasia: failure of the organ primordium to develop beyond its primitive form.
- Atresia: abnormal absence or closure of an organ orifice or passage.
- Hypoplasia: under or incomplete development or decreased size of an organ due to decreased numbers of cells.
- Hyperplasia: increased size of an organ due to increased number of cells.
- Hypertrophy: increased size of an organ due to increased size of individual cells.
- Hypotrophy: decreased size of an organ due to decreased size of individual cells.

Placenta

47. List 5 reasons for examining a placenta.

- Obtain information useful in the management of the mother, the neonate, and/or future pregnancies.
- Identify pathological processes.
- Assess neonate's risk for short-term or long-term sequelae.
- Exclude retained placenta.
- Explain adverse outcomes — can help if litigation is possible.

Note: most institutions have formal guidelines indicating which placentas should be examined by a pathologist. The need for examination can be categorized as maternal, fetal, or placental.

48. How can you differentiate between an artery and a vein on the chorionic plate when grossing a placenta?

Arteries cross over veins.

49. List the common causes of a large placenta.
- Twin pregnancy.
- Placental edema.
- Maternal diabetes mellitus.
- Chronic intrauterine infections.
- Severe fetal anemia.
- Rh incompatibility.
- Fetal α-thalassemia major.
- Placental chorangiomas.
- Metabolic storage disease.

50. List the common causes of a small placenta.
- Intrauterine growth retardation.
- Chromosomal anomalies.
- Intrauterine infection.
- Maternal vascular malperfusion.

51. List the gross and histologic findings in a placental infarct.
- The placenta shows coagulative necrosis of a group of localized villi secondary to maternal vascular malperfusion.
- Size can vary markedly: smaller infarcts are generally wedge shaped but the villi immediately beneath the chorionic plate are often spared.
- Color depends on age of the infarct (with increasing age: dark red, brown, yellow, white).
- Intervillous spaces are patent early but later filled by fibrin and obliterated.
- Adjacent villi have increased syncytial knots.

Ascending Fetal Infection

52. What broad categories of organisms are usually transmitted to fetuses by the cervicovaginal (ascending) route? In what 2 ways can this occur? What pathological findings are often seen in the placenta?
- Organisms: mostly bacterial and a few viral infections such as herpes simplex virus type 2 (HSV-2).
- Mechanism: inhaling infected amniotic fluid in utero or passing through an infected birth canal during delivery.
- Pathological findings: chorionitis and chorioamnionitis (maternal response in severe cases; fetal inflammatory response in some cases (funisitis or chorionic vasculitis).

53. List the usual chronological sequence of placental histologic findings associated with an "ascending" infection.
- Acute subchorionitis (neutrophilic infiltration of subchorionic layer of the placental disc).
- Acute chorionitis (neutrophilic infiltration of chorion layer of the placental disc and/or membranes).
- Acute chorioamnionitis (neutrophilic infiltration of chorion and amnion layers of the placental disc and/or membranes).
- Acute chorioamnionitis with acute chorionic vasculitis, umbilical cord vasculitis, and funisitis.

54. What broad categories of maternal blood-borne infections can be transmitted to the fetus via the placenta? What is the main placental histologic feature?
- Infections:
  - Most parasitic (e.g., toxoplasmosis, malaria) and viral infections are transmitted via the placenta.
  - A few bacterial infections also are transmitted in this manner (e.g., syphilis, listeriosis).
- Histology:
  - The histologic findings are characterized by chronic villitis: multifocal involvement of chorionic villi by mononuclear cell inflammation, often patchy.
- Presence of plasma cells suggests cytomegalovirus (CMV) or syphilis.
- Listeriosis has multifocal acute villitis with microabscesses.
- Note: most cases of chronic villitis are not associated with maternal infections and are known as villitis of unknown etiology.

Twin Placentation

55. List the types of twin placentation.
- Dichorionic diamniotic twin placentas (2 discs).
- Dichorionic diamniotic twin placenta (fused, 1 disc).
- Monochorionic diamniotic twin placenta.
- Monochorionic monoamniotic twin placenta.

56. Describe the gross findings of twin placentation.

- It can have 1 or 2 disc(s).
- Most have a dividing membrane, which is either thick and opaque (dichorionic) or thin and translucent (monochorionic). The exception is monochorionic and monoamniotic (MoMo) twins.
- If monochorionic (and especially if twins have discordant weights), look for evidence of twin-twin transfusion. This is characterized by an arteriovenous vascular anastomosis (i.e., on the fetal surface, an artery and a vein will both dive into a shared cotyledon; injecting colored fluid into the artery will fill the vasculature within the cotyledon and drain out the vein). There may also be a dark-pale line of demarcation on the maternal surface.

57. Describe the histologic differences in the dividing membrane of a monochorionic versus a dichorionic placenta.

The presence or absence of chorion between 2 layers of amnion in the dividing membrane (DM) determines whether a twin placentation is monochorionic (has no chorion tissue in DM) or dichorionic (has chorionic tissue in DM). This requires either a section of a dividing membrane roll or a T-section.

58. Describe zygosity determination.

- Twins are of different sex: twins are dizygotic.
- Placenta is monochorionic: twins are monozygotic.
- Placenta is dichorionic: most twins (~80%) are dizygotic, but can be monozygotic.

Placental Disorders

59. What are the features of chronic histiocytic intervillositis (CHI)?

- It is defined as an infiltrate of histiocytic-predominant mononuclear cells in the intervillous space.
- It is thought to represent an abnormal cell-mediated immune response at the maternal-fetal interface.
- It is associated with adverse fetal outcome, including first and second trimester miscarriage and impaired growth.
- It has a 25% recurrence rate.
- Sometimes occurs with massive perivillous (intervillous) fibrin deposition.

60. Compare and contrast massive perivillous (intervillous) fibrin deposition and maternal floor infarction.

- These lesions are believed to be closely related.
- Massive perivillous (intervillous) fibrin deposition is characterized by diffuse intervillous fibrin deposition involving > 50% of the placenta; the placenta tends to be thick, firm, and pale.
- Maternal floor infarction presents as a layer of fibrin deposition surrounding the basal villi, with the other villi spared.
- Both are associated with second trimester fetal loss or growth retardation.
- Both tend to recur in subsequent pregnancies and can be associated with chronic histiocytic intervillositis.

61. Describe the gross features, microscopic features, and clinical significance of choriangiomas.

- Gross features:
  - Small: appear as well-demarcated, firm round nodules on cut surfaces of placental slices. They are often dark red, but their color can be variable.
  - Large: may appear as bulging protuberances on fetal surface, or may be pedunculated, which may undergo torsion and infarction.
  - Multiple lesions in the same placenta: called "choriangiomatosis."
- Microscopic features:
  - They usually have capillary-sized vessels and scanty stroma. Occasionally stroma predominates.
  - Foci of infarction may be present.
- Clinical significance:
  - Small lesions are insignificant.
  - Large lesions can cause polyhydramnios due to transudation or antepartum bleeding due to rupture.
  - Very large lesions can cause obstruction or can avulse during vaginal delivery, or can cause fetal cardiomegaly or anemia.

62. Describe the gross features, microscopic features, and clinical significance of velamentous cord insertion.

- Gross features:
  - Umbilical cord inserts into, and traverses, free membranes.
- Microscopic features:
  - Chorionic vessels can sometimes be seen in the membrane roll.
- Clinical significance:
  - Chorionic vessels are very susceptible to tearing during labor and delivery.
  - It is associated with small-for-gestational-age babies.

63. Describe the gross features, microscopic features, and clinical significance of circumvallate placenta.

- Gross features:
  - Placental membranes fold onto themselves, forming a lip at the junction of extraplacental membranes and fetal surface of the placental disc.
  - Circumvallate membranes are rolled back on themselves, forming a raised white ring at the point of transition of the fetal surface of the placenta to the gestational sac.
  - Categories include "complete" (circumferential) or "partial" circumvallate placenta.
- Note: circumvallate placenta is 1 of 2 types of extrachorial placenta. The other type is circummarginate, which has a flat transition and no known clinical consequences.
- Microscopic features:
  - Fibrin and infarcted chorionic villi are folded over surface with double membranes.
- Clinical significance:
  - Complete circumvallate placenta has an increased frequency of low birth weight, perinatal mortality, antepartum bleeding, premature labor, and fetal hypoxia.

Preeclampsia

64. What are the clinical manifestations of preeclampsia?

- Pregnancy induced hypertension and proteinuria develop after 20 gestational weeks.
- Subcutaneous edema is usually present.
- Epigastric pain/liver tenderness is common in preeclamptic patients with HELLP syndrome.
- Note: if preeclampsia is not successfully treated, it may progress to eclampsia (i.e., addition of tonic-clonic seizures).

65. What are the placental gross and histologic findings of preeclampsia?

- Small placental size.
- Multiple infarcts due to maternal vascular malperfusion.
- Decidual vasculopathy: lack of physiologic conversion (smooth muscle persists), thrombosis, and acute atherosis (fibrinoid necrosis plus macrophages).
- Villous "hypermaturity" or accelerated villous maturation.

Cytogenetic Analysis of Abortus Tissue

66. Why is cytogenetic analysis of abortus tissue done?

- About 50% of early pregnancy losses have chromosomal anomalies.
- The analysis may provide insight for parents as to the probability of recurrences.
- It is usually only medically indicated when parents have 3 or more pregnancy losses.

67. What are the limitations of cytogenetic analysis for abortus tissue?

- Fetal tissue may be contaminated by maternal cells.
- For karyotyping, fetal cells must be grown in tissue culture to obtain metaphases. Lack of viable fetal tissue prevents karyotyping. This can often be circumvented by using placental tissue, which tends to be more viable.

Lately, karyotyping is often replaced by molecular testing. Rapid aneuploidy detection (RAD) using quantitative-fluorescence PCR is a faster and often less labor intensive way to detect common aneuploidies involving chromosomes 13, 18, 21, X, and Y.

68. What is the pathologist's role in cytogenetic analysis of abortus tissue?

- A pathologist should examine tissue from an abortus to select appropriate fetal tissue.
- If the suitability of the selected tissue is uncertain, the pathologist submits identical tissue for overnight histology processing and then examines it to confirm viability and fetal origin.

Autopsies on Macerated Stillborn Fetuses

69. What is the value of performing autopsies on macerated stillborn fetuses?

- Demonstrate the presence or absence of malformations — combinations of findings may suggest a syndrome or a heritable condition.
- Demonstrate the presence or absence of various types of infections.
- Demonstrate the presence or absence of intrauterine stress — via grading of thymic involution, meconium aspiration, and/or pseudofollicular changes in the adrenal cortex.

(*continued on next page*)

- Determine approximate gestational age of the fetus (e.g., by measuring foot lengths, counting glomerular generations in developing kidney).
- Determine the presence or absence of intrauterine growth retardation.
- Obtain tissue for cytogenetics.
- Determine status of the fetus when the mother became infected: in mothers with ascending infections (chorioamnionitis), histologic findings in the placenta such as chorionic vasculitis or funisitis or demonstration of inhaled neutrophils in the fetal lung can confirm that the fetus was alive when the mother became infected.
- Predict outcomes of future pregnancies: completely negative findings in an autopsy can help assure parents that the probability of a poor outcome in the next pregnancy is relatively low.

70. How do you estimate the duration of fetal death before delivery?
- Degree of maceration allows very crude estimates:
  - Mild: red skin with skin slippage and peeling indicates 0–1 day.
  - Moderate: extensive peeling and red serous fluid in chest and abdomen, calvarial slippage indicates 2–7 days.
  - Severe: yellow-brown liver +/− mummification indicates > 14 days.
- Presence of diffuse avascular villi and obliteration of vessels in stem villi in the placenta can help further estimate the timing of fetal demise: > 2 weeks.

Chromosomal Anomalies

71. List the main common autopsy findings in an intrauterine/neonatal death with the following chromosomal anomalies: trisomy 13, trisomy 18, trisomy 21, and monosomy X.
- Trisomy 13 (Patau syndrome, incidence is 1:5000 births):
  - Central nervous system (CNS) and eyes: absence of olfactory bulbs; holoprosencephaly; incomplete development of forebrain; microopthalmia; coloboma of iris.
  - Craniofacial: microcephaly; abnormal ears; cleft lip and/or palate; parietooccipital scalp defect; occasionally midface anomalies such as cyclopia and proboscis.
  - Hands/feet: polydactyly.
  - Heart: ventricular septal defect (VSD), patent ductus arteriosus (PDA), or atrial septal defect (ASD).
  - Other: small for gestational age (SGA), inguinal or umbilical hernia, pancreatic-splenic fusion, single umbilical artery.
- Trisomy 18 (Edward syndrome, incidence is 1:3000 births):
  - CNS and eyes: no major characteristic finding.
  - Craniofacial: small mouth, micrognathia, low set abnormal ears.
  - Hands/feet: index finger overlaps third finger, fifth finger overlaps fourth finger, short dorsiflexed toe.
  - Heart: valvular abnormalities, VSD, ASD, PDA.
  - Other: SGA, short sternum.
- Trisomy 21 (Down syndrome, incidence is 1:700 births):
  - CNS and eyes: open operculum in brain.
  - Craniofacial: flat facies, oblique palpebral fissures, epicanthal folds.
  - Hands/feet: simian creases, other abnormal dermatoglyphics, short metacarpals and phalanges, sandal deformity of feet.
  - Heart: atrioventricular septal defect (canal), VSD.
  - Other: SGA.
- Monosomy X (Turner syndrome, incidence is 1:2500 births, most are "early lethal"):
  - CNS and eyes: no major characteristic finding.
  - Craniofacial: edema associated with massive nuchal cystic hygroma.
  - Hands/feet: marked edema of dorsal surfaces.
  - Heart: coarctation of aorta.
  - Other: SGA in females; generalized hydrops; often relatively normal ovaries at birth (note: "streak ovaries" develop later); horseshoe kidneys; duplication of renal pelvis.

Note: none of the above findings is always present, even in full trisomies or monosomies; findings in mosaics may be absent or less severe.

Turner Syndrome in Adolescent and Young Women

72. What genetic abnormalities cause Turner syndrome?
- Approximately 50% of cases: complete monosomy X (45, XO).
- Approximately 50% of cases: partial monosomy X (i.e., complete or partial deletion of small arm of chromosome X) or mosaics.

73. What are the manifestations of Turner syndrome in adolescent girls and young women?

- Phenotypic female:
  - Short stature.
  - Hypogonadism.
  - "Streak ovaries" (fibrous stroma but absence of ova and follicles).
- Failure in development of secondary sex characteristics (genitalia remain infantile, little pubic hair).
- Short webbed neck.
- Broad chest with widely spaced nipples.
- Congenital heart disease (25–50% of cases).
- Melanocytic nevi.

Down Syndrome

74. What genetic abnormalities cause Down syndrome?

- Most (95%) have trisomy 21 (usually due to meiotic nondisjunction).
- Some (3%) are due to translocations.
- Some (2%) are mosaics.
- Note: it is among the most common chromosomal disorders.
  - Incidence is 1:700 births.
  - Maternal age has strong influence: > 45 years, incidence is 1:25 births.

75. What are the manifestations of Down syndrome?

- Mental retardation.
- Flat facial profile.
- Oblique palpebral fissures.
- Epicanthal folds.
- Congenital heart disease (50% of cases).
- Increased incidence of acute leukemia (usually lymphoblastic).
- Alzheimer changes in brain in 40s.
- Diminished life expectancy (approximately 60 years is the current life expectancy).

Intrauterine Infections

76. List the main autopsy findings in an intrauterine/neonatal death from the following intrauterine infections: congenital herpes, congenital CMV, and congenital toxoplasmosis.

- Congenital herpes:
  - Microcephaly, hydrocephaly, microphthalmia.
- Congenital CMV:
  - Microcephaly, hydrocephaly, microphthalmia.
  - Necrotizing meningoencephalitis.
  - Arterial and periventricular calcification.
  - Giant cell hepatitis, cholangitis.
- Viral inclusions in lungs and kidneys.
- Congenital toxoplasmosis:
  - Most: asymptomatic.
  - Severe disease: hydrocephaly or microcephaly, intracranial calcifications, hepatosplenomegaly, jaundice, chorioretinitis, cerebrospinal fluid pleocytosis.
  - Visible organisms in multiple organs and tissues.

Teratogen

77. How does the timing of exposure to teratogens during pregnancy affect the severity of fetal anomalies produced?

- 0–3 weeks gestation:
  - Severe insult will result in abortion.
  - Less severe insult has little apparent affect.
- 3–9 weeks gestation:
  - Embryo is undergoing organogenesis and is very susceptible to malformations.
- Organs and structures differ in susceptibility from week to week during this time frame, depending on when they are formed.
- 9 weeks until birth:
  - Organogenesis is mostly complete, and organs are growing and maturing.
  - Already formed fetal organs are susceptible to growth retardation and organ damage.

78. List at least 5 well-documented teratogens.

- Thalidomide.
- Folate antagonists.
- Ethanol.
- Androgenic hormones.
- Warfarin.
- Retinoic acid.
- Valproic acid.

79. Provide 2 examples of dysmorphogenic features caused by environmental teratogens that can be recapitulated by genetic defects in pathways targeted by the teratogens.

- Consumption of cyclopamine, a plant teratogen, by a pregnant sheep results in lambs with cyclopia and holoprosencephaly. This teratogen is an inhibitor of hedgehog signaling in embryos. Some patients with holoprosencephaly possess Hedgehog gene mutations.

- Valproic acid, an antiepileptic drug, is a teratogen that disrupts expression of homeobox (HOX) protein transcription factors that are critical for limb, vertebrae, and craniofacial development.

Fetal Alcohol Syndrome

80. What are the classic findings of fetal alcohol syndrome? How is fetal alcohol syndrome different from fetal alcohol spectrum disorders (FASD)?

- Classic findings:
  - Growth retardation (prenatal and postnatal).
  - Microcephaly.
  - Atrial septal defect.
  - Short palpebral fissures.
  - Maxillary hypoplasia.
- Difference compared to FASD:
  - FASD is characterized by subtle cognitive or behavioral defects.

Retinoic Acid

81. During embryogenesis, what phenotypes are associated with excessive exposure to retinoic acid? What phenotypes are associated with retinoic acid deficiency?

- Excess (e.g., treatment for severe acne): retinoic acid embryopathy (craniofacial defects including cleft lip and palate; CNS defects; cardiac defects). Cleft palate is thought to be due to deregulation of the transforming growth factor-β (TGF-β) signaling pathway.
- Deficiency: ocular, genitourinary, cardiovascular, pulmonary, and diaphragmatic malformations.

Congenital Rubella Syndrome

82. What findings are characteristic of congenital rubella syndrome? What is the at-risk period for maternal infection?

- Characteristic tetrad:
  - Cataracts.
  - Congenital heart defects (persistent ductus arteriosus, pulmonary artery stenosis, ventricular septal defect, and tetralogy of Fallot).
  - Deafness.
  - Mental retardation.
- At-risk period:
  - Shortly before conception until the sixteenth week of gestation.
  - Highest risk: first 8 weeks of pregnancy, when the organs are forming.

Herpes Simplex Virus

83. List the main autopsy findings in a neonatal death following intrapartum (acute perinatal) infection with herpes simplex virus.

- Hepatoadrenal necrosis.
- Vesicular skin rash.
- Vesicular/ulcerated stomatitis, esophagitis.
- Necrotizing pneumonitis.
- Chorioretinitis.

Parvovirus B19

84. What are the usual consequences of infection with parvovirus B19 during pregnancy versus during childhood?

- Pregnancy:
  - Most women infected during pregnancy deliver a normal baby.
  - Rarely, the infection precipitates congenital anemia, hydrops fetalis, and spontaneous abortion, often during the second trimester. In these instances, characteristic intranuclear viral inclusions can often be identified in fetal nucleated red blood cells.
- Childhood:
  - Infection in childhood results in erythema infectiosum (fifth disease of childhood).

Fetal Hydrops

85. Fetal hydrops refers to the excessive accumulation of fluid in the fetus during intrauterine life. What is the most severe form and what are 3 key less severe, localized forms?

- Most severe: hydrops fetalis (a progressive, generalized edema that is usually lethal).
- Less severe: pleural effusion, peritoneal effusion (ascites), cystic hygroma (postnuchal edema).

86. List the 3 major causes of nonimmune hydrops (very broad categories) and give at least 1 specific example of each.

- Structural or functional cardiovascular defects: malformations, tachyarrhythmia, high output failure.
- Chromosomal: Turner syndrome, trisomy 21, trisomy 18.
- Fetal anemia: homozygous α-thalassemia, parvovirus B19.

87. List 4 other less common causes of nonimmune hydrops.

- Infections other than parvovirus — CMV, syphilis, toxoplasmosis.
- Malformations — especially thoracic (e.g., congenital pulmonary airway malformation, diaphragmatic hernia) or urinary tract.
- Twin-twin transfusion.
- Metabolic disorders.

88. Define immune hydrops.

Immune hydrops: hemolytic disorder caused by blood group antigen incompatibility between mother and fetus.

89. What is the etiology and pathogenesis of immune hydrops?

- It occurs when a fetus inherits red blood cell (RBC) antigens (usually Rh) from the father that are foreign to the mother.
- Rh+ RBCs cross into the mother's circulation from the fetus via the placenta and stimulate an Rh- mother to produce antibodies against Rh (D antigen).
- Maternal IgG antibodies can cross back into the fetal circulation via the placenta and bind to fetal Rh+ RBCs.
- Fetal RBCs are lysed, resulting in anemia, increased unconjugated bilirubin, hydrops fetalis, and often kernicterus.

90. Why is Rh disease uncommon in the first pregnancy?

Maternal exposure to fetal RBCs occurs in the last trimester when placental villi cytotrophoblasts are absent, or during delivery. Exposure initially invokes an IgM antibody response and IgM, unlike IgG, does not cross the placental barrier.

91. Describe prophylaxis for immune hydrops.

Rh negative mothers receive Rhesus immune globulin containing anti-D antibodies at 28 weeks gestation and within 72 hours of delivery, as well as after abortions.

92. How does fetal hemolysis caused by maternal-fetal ABO incompatibility differ from that caused by Rh incompatibility? Why?

- ABO incompatibility, occurring in approximately 20% to 25% of pregnancies, usually has no adverse effect. Only 1 in 200 cases causes clinically apparent hemolytic disease and even these are less severe than Rh-induced hemolysis. Also, it is not unusual for firstborns to be affected.
- Reasons include:
  - Most anti-A and anti-B antibodies are IgM and don't cross the placenta.
  - Neonatal RBCs express A and B blood group antigens poorly.
  - Fetal cells other than RBCs express them and can absorb transferred antibodies.

93. Under what circumstances is ABO hemolytic disease of the newborn most likely to occur?

It occurs almost exclusively in blood group A or B infants born to group O mothers who possess preformed IgG antibodies directed at group A and/or B antigens. This explains how this can occur in first pregnancies.

94. Describe changes in incidence of immune hydrops.

Immune hydrops was formerly the most common case of fetal hydrops, but because of the success of prophylaxis, nonimmune hydrops has surpassed it.

95. What are the 2 common signs and symptoms of excessive destruction of red blood cells in neonates?

- Anemia.
- Jaundice.

Sudden Infant Death Syndrome (SIDS)

96. Define SIDS.

SIDS (sudden infant death syndrome) is the death of an infant < 1 year that cannot be explained by clinical history, examination of the death scene, or autopsy.

97. What is the distinction between SIDS and SUID?

- SUID stands for sudden unexpected infant death — a subset of these are true SIDS cases.
- The incidence of SIDS has decreased precipitously since the early 1990s partly because of behavioral changes (e.g., having babies sleep on their backs rather than prone or on their sides).
- Careful complete autopsies with histology, microbiology, biochemical, and molecular testing have determined causes for many deaths formerly diagnosed as SIDS (e.g., viral myocarditis, congenital heart diseases, unexpected infections, genetic or metabolic disorders).
- Since SIDS is a diagnosis of exclusion, discovery of a cause precludes a SIDS diagnosis and results in a SUID diagnosis.

98. What is the "triple risk" model of SIDS? List at least 8 parental, infant, or environmental risk factors for SIDS.

- The triple-risk model identifies SIDS as a multifactorial condition that occurs when 3 overlapping factors intersect: (1) a vulnerable infant, (2) a critical developmental period in homeostatic control, and (3) an exogenous stressor.
- Risk factors include:
  · Young maternal age (< 20 years).
  · Maternal smoking during pregnancy.
  · Drug abuse in either parent.
  · Short intergestational intervals.
  · Late or no prenatal care.
  · Poverty.
  · Brainstem abnormalities with associated defective arousal and cardiorespiratory control.
  · Prematurity and/or low birth weight.
  · Male sex.
  · Product of a multiple birth.
  · SIDS in a prior sibling.
  · Germline polymorphisms in autonomic nervous system genes.
  · Antecedent respiratory infections.
  · Prone or side sleeping position.
  · Sleeping on a soft surface.
  · Cosleeping in first 3 months of life.
  · Hyperthermia.

Respiratory Distress Syndrome (RDS) in Newborns

99. List causes of neonatal respiratory distress.

- Neonatal respiratory distress syndrome (hyaline membrane disease).
- Excessive sedation of the mother.
- Fetal head injury, or aspiration of blood or amniotic fluid, at delivery.
- Cord accident causing intrauterine hypoxic insult.

100. What is the pathogenesis of RDS in newborns?

- RDS is caused by surfactant deficiency (normally, type 2 pneumocytes generate dipalmitoyl phosphatidylcholine [lecithin]; this combined with smaller amounts of phosphatidylglycerol and surfactant-associated proteins becomes surfactant).
- Surfactant reduces the surface tension required to keep alveoli open. Normally, the first breath requires a large inspiratory pressure and subsequent breaths require less work, as normal lungs retain 40% residual air.
- When surfactant is deficient, each breath requires the same work as the first.
- Administration of exogenous surfactant to extremely premature infants provides some protection.
- Prenatal administration of steroids can reduce the severity of RDS in premature neonates.

101. What are the gross features of RDS in newborns?
- Lungs are normal size, but solid and not aerated.
- Lungs are poorly aerated and do not float in water.
- Lungs have a reddish purple color like normal liver.

102. What are the microscopic features of RDS in newborns?
- Pink hyaline membranes (composed of fibrin and cell debris derived chiefly from necrotic type 2 pneumocytes) are present in respiratory bronchioles, alveolar ducts, and alveoli.
- Alveoli are poorly developed, and those present are collapsed.
- There is a paucity of neutrophilic inflammation.
- If survival > 48 hours, the lung will show reparative changes: alveolar epithelial proliferation, and sloughing of hyaline membranes and phagocytosis by macrophages.

103. Infants who recover from RDS are at increased risk for what conditions?
- Patent ductus arteriosus.
- Intraventricular hemorrhage.
- Necrotizing enterocolitis.
- Retinopathy of prematurity (retrolental fibroplasia).
- Bronchopulmonary dysplasia.

104. List at least 3 risk factors for neonatal hyaline membrane disease.
- Preterm delivery (but weight appropriate for gestational age).*
- Caesarean delivery.
- Male infant.
- Diabetic mother.

*Note: administration of corticosteroids decreases risk by enhancing lung maturity; lecithin/sphingomyelin ratio > 2:1 is protective.

105. List 2 serious complications of oxygen therapy.
- Retrolental fibroplasia (retinopathy of prematurity).
- Bronchopulmonary dysplasia.

106. Describe the 2-stage pathogenesis of retrolental fibroplasias.
- Phase 1: during the hyperoxic phase, vascular endothelial growth factor (VEGF) expression is markedly decreased, resulting in endothelial cell apoptosis.
- Phase 2: after returning to room air oxygen levels, the VEGF level increases, resulting in retinal vessel neovascularization fundamental to the lesion.

Necrotizing Enterocolitis

107. What are the clinical, gross, and histologic characteristics of necrotizing enterocolitis (NEC)? What is the etiology/pathogenesis?
- Clinical:
  - Clinical signs include bloody stools, abdominal distension, and circulatory collapse. Radiographs often show gas in intestinal wall.
  - Infants are often premature (incidence is 1:10 in very low birth weight infants).
  - If detected early, medical management may be possible, but often the involved bowel must be resected.
  - Necrotizing enterocolitis has high perinatal mortality; survivors often develop fibrotic strictures.
  - Probiotic therapies are being studied.
- Gross:
  - Distended, friable, and congested bowel (typically involving the terminal ileum, cecum, and ascending colon), which may progress to gangrene and perforation.
- Histologic:
  - Mucosal or transmural coagulative necrosis, ulceration, bacterial colonization, and often submucosal gas bubbles (pneumatosis intestinalis) are present.
  - Reparative changes (i.e., granulation tissue and fibrosis) are present.
- Etiology/pathogenesis:
  - The cause is unknown and probably multifactorial.
  - Alteration of the microbiome associated with enteral feeding seems likely.
  - Infectious agents (none uniformly cultured) may also contribute.
  - Increased mucosal permeability due to elevated inflammatory mediators such as platelet activating factor (PAF) permits migration of gut bacteria.

Gaucher Disease

108. Describe the genetics of Gaucher disease.
- It is an autosomal recessive disorder resulting from mutations in the gene encoding glucocerebrosidase, causing glucocerebrosidase deficiency, and leading to glucocerebrosides (generated from catabolism of glycolipids derived from cell membranes of dying red blood cells and white blood cells) to accumulate in cells.
- Three patterns are due to different allelic mutations in the structural gene for the enzyme.

109. List the subtypes and clinical consequences of Gaucher disease.
- Type I (classical or chronic nonneuronopathic): adult, noncerebral form (99% of all cases).
  - Reduced but detectable enzyme levels.
  - Storage limited to macrophages throughout organs and bone marrow without involving the brain. Massive splenomegaly and complications of hypersplenism (anemia and thrombocytopenia) are characteristic findings.
  - Symptoms: arise in adults, predominantly in people of European Jewish (Ashkenazi) descent.
  - Survival: compatible with long life.
- Type II (acute neuronopathic): infantile acute cerebral pattern.
  - Undetectable enzyme levels.
  - Progressive CNS involvement.
  - Hepatosplenomegaly (often), but not the primary problem.
  - No predilection for people of Jewish decent.
  - Early death.
- Type III (subacute neuronopathic): intermediate pattern.
  - Systemic involvement, like type I.
  - CNS involvement in second or third decade.

Niemann-Pick Disease

110. Describe the genetics of Niemann-Pick disease.

It is an autosomal recessive disorder characterized by lysosomal accumulation sphingomyelin due to deficiency of sphingomyelinase (usually) — causes sphingomyelin and cholesterol to accumulate in reticuloendothelial system and parenchymal cells.

111. List the major subtypes and clinical consequences of Niemann-Pick disease.
- Type A (severe infantile form — most common type):
  - Sphingomyelinase deficient.
  - Extensive neurologic involvement.
  - Progressive wasting.
  - Early death (< 3 years).
- Type B:
  - Sphingomyelinase deficient.
  - Development of symptoms from infancy to adulthood.
  - Milder symptoms than Type A.
  - Organomegaly, but no CNS involvement.
- Other types: very rare.

Phenylketonuria

112. Describe the genetics of phenylketonuria.

It is an autosomal recessive disorder, resulting in deficiency of phenylalanine hydroxylase (PAH) — affected infants can't convert phenylalanine into tyrosine, and have high levels of phenylalanine in blood (hyperphenylalaninemia). Not all *PAH* gene mutations cause a severe deficiency and neurologic damage (so-called benign hyperphenylalaninemia).

113. What are the pathological consequences of phenylketonuria?
- Affected infants are normal at birth, but if untreated, hyperphenylalaninemia leads to severe mental retardation in < 6 months. Treatment is dietary control of phenylalanine levels during CNS development.
- Pathologic examination shows decreased brain weight, defective myelination, and gliosis.
- Patients have:
  - Seizures and other neurologic abnormalities.
  - Decreased pigmentation of hair and skin (due to a deficiency of tyrosine, a precursor of melanin).
  - A musty odor.
  - Eczema.

114. How is phenylketonuria usually diagnosed in the newborn baby and how does the workup normally proceed?
- Phenylketonuria is usually found by neonatal screening of a blood spot.
- Primary diagnosis is biochemical (i.e., highly elevated serum phenylalanine levels), not molecular, as > 500 mutant alleles have been identified.

(continued on next page)

- Once diagnosed, the specific mutation can be established to allow testing for family members for carrier status.
- Some (2%) cases are not due to *PAH* mutations but rather to abnormalities with an enzyme cofactor tetrahydrobiopterin BH$_4$. This variant can't be treated by dietary restriction.

115. What is maternal phenylketonuria (PKU)? How can it be prevented?
- Women of childbearing age, if born with PKU and treated with dietary restriction at birth, are clinically normal and sometimes discontinue dietary treatment.
- These women have hyperphenylalaninemia. If they become pregnant without reestablishing dietary control, phenylalanine or its metabolites cross the placenta causing microcephaly, mental retardation, and sometimes congenital heart disease in the infant, even though the infant is a heterozygote.
- Prevention: maternal phenylalanine dietary restrictions should be reinstituted before pregnancy.

Galactosemia

116. Describe the genetics of galactosemia.
- It is an autosomal recessive disorder of galactose metabolism resulting from the accumulation of galactose-1-phosphate in tissues. Its 2 variants are caused by a deficiency of galactokinase or a deficiency of galactose-1-phosphate uridyl transferase (GALT).
  - Galactokinase deficiency causes a mild form of galactosemia that is not associated with intellectual disability.
  - GALT deficiency causes a severe form of galactosemia.
- Mechanism: the major carbohydrate in milk, lactose, is broken down by the intestinal microvilli into glucose and galactose by lactase in the intestinal microvilli. Galactose is converted to glucose via 4 linked chemical reactions. The first reaction utilizes the enzyme galactokinase and the second uses GALT.

117. What are the pathological consequences of galactosemia?
- GALT deficiency results:
  - Galactose-1-phosphate accumulates in the liver, eyes (lens), brain, and other organs.
  - Infants fail to thrive from birth, and develop diarrhea and vomiting as soon as they are started on milk.
  - Jaundice and hepatomegaly (initially fatty change, later cirrhosis), cataracts, and mental retardation develop within months (neuronal dropout, gliosis, edema in dentate nuclei of cerebellum and olivary nuclei of medulla).
  - Aminoaciduria develops due to impaired kidney function.
  - *E. coli* septicemia may develop due to impaired neutrophil bactericidal activity.
  - Newborns may also develop hemolysis and coagulopathy.
  - Dietary restriction during first 2 years of life permits almost normal development (however, these patients may still develop a speech disorder, gonadal failure, and ataxia when they get older).
- Galactokinase deficiency produces only a mild form of the disease without mental retardation.

Branchial Cleft Cysts

118. Describe the locations of first, second, and third branchial cleft cysts.
- First branchial cleft cysts are adjacent to the external auditory canal, the pinnae, or the parotid gland, extending to the level of the mandible angle.
- Second branchial cleft cysts result from persistence of cervical sinus; many types are possible.
- Third branchial cleft cysts are rare and occur in the lateral neck.

Thyroglossal Duct

119. What is the embryogenesis of thyroglossal duct and what are the gross and histologic findings in thyroglossal ducts remnants?
- The thyroglossal duct is a vestigial remnant of the tubular development of the thyroid gland.
- Location of remnants: midline neck anterior to trachea.
- Diameter: usually 2–3 cm.
- Parts of duct may be obliterated and other parts may form a cystic swelling filled with mucinous secretions.
- Cyst lining is variable (squamous high in neck; respiratory columnar epithelium low in neck).
- Thyroid follicles may or may not be present.

Cystic Fibrosis (CF)

120. Describe the characteristic pulmonary histology of CF.
- Bronchioles distended with thick mucous.
- Marked hyperplasia and hypertrophy of mucous secreting cells lining the respiratory tract.
- Chronic bronchitis, bronchiectasis, and abscesses.

121. List the 3 most common infectious organisms for CF patients and a fourth group of highly problematic organisms.
- *Staphylococcus aureus*.
- *Hemophilus influenzae*.
- *Pseudomonas aeruginosa* (particularly alginate producing forms) — 80% of patients with classic CF who are > 18 years old harbor this organism.
- *Burkholderia cepacia* complex (includes 9 or more different species), a group of pseudomonads that can lead to "cepacia syndrome" — this is a highly problematic organism and 3.5% of patients with classic CF who are > 18 years harbor this organism.

122. What are the most common causes of CF death in North America?
- Chronic lung infections, obstructive pulmonary disease, and cor pulmonale (80% of deaths).
- Complications post lung transplantation.
- Liver disease (adults).

123. Name and locate the gene that causes CF, describe the major features of its normal gene product, and explain the protein's normal function.
- Name: cystic fibrosis transmembrane conductance regulator (*CFTR*) gene.
- Location: chromosome 7q31.2.
- Features: CFTR protein is 1480 amino acids and consists of 2 transmembrane domains (each with 6 α-helices), 2 cytoplasmic nucleotide-binding domains (NBDs), and a regulatory domain (R) containing protein kinase A and C phosphorylation sites.
- Mechanism: the 2 transmembrane domains form a channel through which chloride passes; agonist binding increases cyclic adenosine monophosphate (cAMP) and activates protein kinase A, which causes phosphorylation of R and, in conjunction with adenosine triphosphate (ATP) binding NBD, opens the chloride channel.
- *CTFR* also regulates other ion channels including outwardly rectifying chloride channels, inwardly rectifying potassium channels (Kirb.I), gap junction channels, and the epithelial sodium channel (ENaC).

124. More than 2000 CF associated gene mutations have been described. How are these classified and how do they figure in the heterogeneity of the manifestations of cystic fibrosis?
- Only 5 of 2000 disease causing mutations have a frequency in CF patients > 1%.
- There are 6 broad classes of mutations:
  - Class I — defective protein synthesis (null mutations).
  - Class II — abnormal protein folding, processing, and trafficking (processing mutations).
  - Class III — defective regulation (gathering mutations).
  - Class IV — decreased conductance (conduction mutations).
  - Class V — reduced abundance (production mutations).
- Class VI — decreased membrane CFTR stability (instability mutations).
- Class I, II, and III mutations are "severe"; any combination of these from the mother and the father result in essentially zero CFTR protein function and the classic full CF phenotype (pancreatic insufficiency, sinopulmonary infections, and gastrointestinal symptoms).
- Classes IV to VI are "mild"; 1 of these mutations on either allele results in some CFTR protein function and a milder CF phenotype that does not usually include pancreatic insufficiency. Such patients may present with few features of CF and are classified as "nonclassic" or atypical CF.

125. Explain the role of genetic and environmental modifiers in the pulmonary manifestations of CF.
- Genetic: genes other than *CFTR* can modify the severity of manifestations in various organs. Mutations in genes that affect neutrophil function can exacerbate pulmonary infections.
- Environmental: bacteria capable of producing alginate are able to use this gel to protect themselves from cellular or humoral immune response.

126. How does bicarbonate ion transport figure in the manifestations of CF?

CFTR regulates ion channels other than chloride. In some mutations, bicarbonate transport is adversely affected. In these instances, pancreatic insufficiency occurs as epithelial secretions are too acidic, resulting in mucin plugging of pancreatic ducts and precipitating atrophy of the exocrine pancreas.

Hirschsprung Disease

127. What is the pathogenesis of Hirschsprung disease?
- Submucosal (Meissner) plexus and myenteric (Auerbach) plexus ganglion cells develop from neural crest cells that migrate to and populate the bowel wall during development.
- Aganglionic megacolon occurs when this does not happen normally, resulting in a distal (rectal) aganglionic segment that may extend proximally to the sigmoid or beyond.
- Functional obstruction occurs, resulting in dilatation, sometimes massive, proximal to the aganglionic segment.

128. What genetic abnormality causes Hirschsprung disease and what is its incidence?
- Most cases (especially short segment) are sporadic.
- Heterozygous loss-of-function mutations in the receptor tyrosine kinase RET account for most of familial and ~15% of sporadic Hirschsprung disease cases.
- Incidence: ~1 in 5000 live births, but is increased in children with Down syndrome, which accounts for ~10% of all cases.

129. What are the 2 major histologic features in colonic resections with Hirschsprung disease?
- Ganglion cells are absent in submucosal (Meissner) plexus and myenteric (Auerbach) plexus.
- Hypertrophic nerve fibers in submucosa are usually present.

130. Name an immunohistochemical stain that can help diagnose Hirschsprung disease.
- Calretinin immunostain helps diagnose Hirschsprung disease because:
  - Immunoreactivity of small nerve fibers in the lamina propria and muscularis mucosa is present in normal bowels.
- The absence of such immunoreactivity supports a diagnosis of Hirschsprung disease.

Heterotopia and Hamartoma

131. Define heterotopia. Provide at least 2 examples and describe the clinical significance of heterotopias.
- Heterotopia is microscopically normal cells or tissues present in abnormal locations (*choristoma* is a synonym).
- Examples of heterotopia include:
  - Pancreatic tissue in the wall of the small intestine.
  - Pancreatic or gastric tissue in a Meckel diverticulum.
- Adrenal cortical rests in a variety of sites, such as adjacent to a gonad.
- Thymic rest adjacent to the thyroid.
- Heterotopia is usually an incidental finding and has no clinical significance; rarely, can give rise to a primary neoplasm in an unexpected site.

132. Define hamartoma.
- Hamartoma is a focal overgrowth of normal, mature cells or tissues native to an organ, but not reproducing the normal architecture of the surrounding normal tissue.
- The distinction between hamartoma and benign neoplasm is sometimes not clear.

Benign Tumors

133. List 3 common broad categories of benign tumors with unique features in infancy and childhood, and then list what makes them unique.
- Hemangioma.
  - This is the most common tumor of infancy. It is usually cutaneous (face or scalp).
  - Capillary hemangiomas tend to be more cellular than in adults.
  - Hemangiomas can be a manifestation of an underlying hereditary disorder.
  - Infantile hemangioma often regress spontaneously.
- Lymphangioma/lymphangiectasis.
  - Lymphangioma is a localized benign tumor/hamartoma composed of cystic lymph channels. It often occurs in soft tissues of neck, axilla, where it tends to increase in size and may encroach on vital structures.
  - Lymphangiectasis is similar but less localized, often involving an extremity. Lymphangiectasis is not progressive.
- Fibromatosis/congenital-infantile fibrosarcoma.
  - This is generally associated with an excellent prognosis, unless it affects vital structures.

(continued on next page)

- Characteristic chromosomal translocation is t(12;15) (p13;q25) generating an ETV6 (transcription factor)-NTRK3 (a tyrosine kinase) fusion protein (also called ETV6-TRKC), which is constitutively active with signaling through the PI3K/AKT pathways. This fusion transcript is unique to infantile fibrosarcoma.

Teratoma

134. Describe sacrococcygeal teratomas.
- Teratomas are tumors composed of elements derived from 3 germ layers.
- They often produce massive congenital lesions.
- They usually occur in females.
- Other congenital anomalies are present in ~10% of sacrococcygeal teratomas (often hindgut or cloacal region).
- Their behavior has the following features:
  · About 75% are mature and ~13% immature.
  · Some (~12%) contain additional germ cell tumor(s) (mixed with yolk sac tumor or rarely embryonal carcinoma).

135. Describe mature ovarian teratomas.
- They represent 70% of all ovarian tumors in girls < 15 years.
- Mature cystic teratomas are most common (sebaceous material, hair, teeth).
- The vast majority are benign.
- Some (1–2%) undergo degeneration, usually to squamous cell carcinoma (invasive or in situ).
- Patients have an excellent prognosis, unless cancer has penetrated the capsule.

Malignancies by Age Range

136. Match age range predilections (0–4, 5–9, and 10–14 years) to the following childhood malignancies.
- Leukemia (usually acute lymphoblastic): 0–4 and 5–9.
- Retinoblastoma: 0–4.
- Neuroblastoma: 0–4 and 5–9.
- Wilms tumor: 0–4.
- Hepatoblastoma: 0–4.
- Hepatocellular carcinoma: 5–9 and 10–14.
- Soft tissue sarcoma/rhabdomyosarcoma: all age categories.
- Teratoma: 0–4.
- CNS tumors (usually posterior fossa: medulloblastoma, ependymoma, pilocytic astrocytoma): 0–4 and 5–9.
- Ewing sarcoma: 5–9 and 10–14.
- Osteogenic sarcoma: 10–14.
- Thyroid carcinoma: 10–14.
- Lymphoma: 5–9 and 10–14.
- Hodgkin disease: 10–14.

137. List the differential diagnoses of malignant small round blue cell tumors, based on site, in children.
- Head: medulloblastoma; atypical teratoid/rhabdoid tumors (AT/RT), neuroblastoma; retinoblastoma; olfactory neuroblastoma (esthesioneuroblastoma); rhabdomyosarcoma.
- Thorax: Askin tumor (malignant small cell tumor of thoracopulmonary origin, Ewing family of tumors), rhabdomyosarcoma, lymphoma, pleuropulmonary blastoma.
- Abdomen: neuroblastoma, rhabdomyosarcoma, lymphoma, Wilms tumor, Ewing sarcoma, desmoplastic small round cell tumor.

138. Describe the handling of tissue in diagnosis of small round blue cell and spindle cell tumors in pediatrics.
- Fresh tissue (cytogenetics, flow cytometry).
- Frozen tissue (biological studies).
- Touch imprints (cytology of the tumor).
- Formalin fixed tissue (routine histology, immunohistochemistry, molecular studies).
- Electron microscopy.
- Note: specific report guidelines are available for pediatric sarcomas in general and for specific tumors (Ewing sarcoma, neuroblastoma, rhabdomyosarcoma).

139. List the types of small round blue cell tumors with distinct molecular abnormalities that can aid diagnosis and prognosis.
- Neuroblastoma:
  · MYCN amplification, 1p deletion, 11q deletion, and/or 17q gain; DNA index.
- Burkitt lymphoma:
  · c-MYC gene (chromosome 8) translocations t(2;8), t(8;14), or t(8;22).

(continued on next page)

- Alveolar rhabdomyosarcoma:
  - Fusion of the *FOXO1* gene (13q14) to either the *PAX3* or *PAX7* gene.
    - *PAX3/FOXO1* fusion gene, t(2;13) — these patients have a 4-year overall survival rate of 64%.
    - *PAX7/FOXO1* fusion gene, t(1;13) — these patients have a 4-year overall survival rate of 86%.
- Ewing sarcoma:
  - EWS (*EWSR1*) gene on chromosome 22 and *FLI1* (ETS family of transcription factors) on chromosome 11.
  - *FLI1/EWSR1* fusion, t(11;22)(q24;q12) — 90–95% of cases.
  - *ERG/EWSR1* fusion, t(21;22)(q22;q12).

- Some of the less common ES translocations substitute *FUS* (ch16) for *EWSR1*, or involve other ETS partners including *ETV1*, *ETV4*, or *FEV*.
- Wilms tumor:
  - No single cytogenetic or molecular abnormality has been consistently abnormal in Wilms tumor or its host, but constitutional deletions of the *WT-1* tumor suppressor gene at 11p13 often predispose the patient to development of Wilms tumors.
- Desmoplastic small round cell tumor.
  - *EWS/WT1* fusion, t(11;22)(p13;q12).

Neuroblastoma

140. List 3 histologic features of neuroblastoma.
- Nesting pattern: usually ill-defined organoid nests with thin fibrovascular septa.
- Neuroblasts — various differentiation:
  - Nucleus: from small blue round to progressively enlarged, vesicular.
- Cytoplasm: from scanty to abundant.
- Neurofibrillary processes (neuropil).
- Differentiation toward ganglion cells.
- Homer-Wright pseudorosettes.
- Schwannian stroma: < 50% of the tumor.

141. List 5 differential diagnoses of neuroblastoma.
- Lymphoma.
- Ewing sarcoma.
- Rhabdomyosarcoma.
- Desmoplastic small round cell tumor.
- Wilms tumor.

142. How does the International Neuroblastoma Pathology Classification (INPC) classify neuroblastoma?
- The INPC distinguishes between 2 prognostic groups of untreated neuoblastoma:
  - Favorable histology (FH).
  - Unfavorable histology (UH).
- Classification is according to the amount of Schwannian stroma, ganglionic differentiation, the mitotic and karyorrhectic index (MKI), and the age of the patient.
- Neuroblastoma Schwannian stroma poor (3 subtypes based on the degree of neuroblastic differentiation: undifferentiated, poorly differentiated, differentiating).
- Ganglioneuroblastoma, nodular (composite, Schwannian stroma-rich/stroma-dominant and stroma-poor).
- Ganglioneuroblastoma, intermixed (Schwannian stroma-rich).
- Ganglioneuroma (Schwannian stroma-dominant).

143. List key prognostic parameters of neuroblastoma.
- Tumor stage (International Neuroblastoma Risk Group Staging System [INRGSS]), which relies only on pretreatment imaging, patient age, and clinical extent of disease):
  - Stage L1— localized tumor not involving vital structures as defined by the list of image-defined risk factors and confined to 1 body compartment.
  - Stage L2 — locoregional tumor with presence of ≥ 1 image-defined risk factors.
  - Stage M — distant metastatic disease (except stage MS).
  - Stage MS — metastatic disease in children < 18 months with metastases confined to skin, liver, and/or bone marrow with minimal marrow involvement.
- Prognostic parameters of low-risk or intermediate-risk neuroblastoma:
  - It has favorable prognosis, with survival rates > 95%.
  - It usually occurs in patients < 18 months of age.
  - Patients commonly have gains of whole chromosomes and are hyperdiploid.
- Prognostic parameters of high-risk neuroblastoma:
  - It has a long-term survival rate of < 50%.
  - It typically occurs in children > 18 months.
  - It is often metastatic to bone.
  - Segmental chromosome abnormalities (gains or losses) and/or *MYCN* gene amplification are common.
  - Patients are near diploid or near tetraploid by flow cytometry; rarely, they harbor exonic mutations.

144. What are the key genomic characteristics of neuroblastic tumors?

- *MYCN* amplification: this is the most prognostically relevant genetic alteration in neuroblastoma; *MYCN* gene amplification is associated with high-risk neuroblastic tumors and poor patient prognosis.
- *ALK* mutation and amplification: this is seen in a subset of neuroblastic tumors and in the germ line of patients with a familial predisposition to neuroblastic tumors; *ALK* aberrations are associated with higher risk and worse prognosis.
- *ATRX* mutation: this is found in 2–3% of all neuroblastic tumors; majority of high-stage tumors in older children and adolescents have *ATRX* mutations (*ATRX* mutations very rarely seen in congenital and infantile tumors).
- DNA index: near diploid/tetraploid is unfavorable, while hyperdiploid (near triploid) tumors have a better prognosis, though the prognostic effects of DNA index appear to be limited to patients diagnosed < 1 year of age.
- Hemizygous deletion of the distal short arm of chromosome 1.
- Segmental chromosomal aberrations (e.g., 1p deletion, 11q deletion, and/or 17q gain): there are associated with high-risk tumors.
- Alterations in the numbers of whole chromosomes: these are associated with lower-risk tumors.

145. List some immunohistochemical stains useful in diagnosing the following small round blue cell tumors: rhabdomyosarcoma, neuroblastoma, and Ewing sarcoma.

- Rhabdomyosarcoma:
  · Desmin, muscle specific actin, myoD1, myogenin.
- Neuroblastoma:
  · PGP9.5, NB84, synaptophysin, and neuron-specific enolase.
- Ewing sarcoma:
  · CD99 (CD99 is positive in many small round blue cell tumors; therefore, additional immunohistochemical stains are used to rule out other entities).

146. List 2 biochemical markers for neuroblastoma.

- These include vanillylmandelic acid (VMA) and homovanillic acid (HVA) in urine or blood.
- Catecholamines may not be increased in undifferentiated neuroblastomas.

Wilms Tumor

147. Name and briefly describe 3 key syndromes associated with an increased risk of developing Wilms tumors.

- WAGR syndrome:
  · Patients have a lifetime risk of ~33% of developing Wilms tumor.
  · Syndrome characteristics include **W**ilms, **a**niridia, **g**enitourinary anomalies, and intellectual disability (formerly referred to as mental **r**etardation).
  · Patients have a germline deletion of 11p13, which includes *WT1* (*Wilms tumor 1* gene) and *PAX6*, an adjacent autosomal dominant gene for aniridia.
  · Germline deletion of *WT1* represents the "first hit" (i.e., of the "2 hit theory" of tumor suppressor genes).
  · Tumor development occurs after a mutation in the second *WT1* allele ("second hit").
- Denys-Drash syndrome:
  · Patients have a lifetime risk of ~90% of developing Wilms tumor.
  · Syndrome characteristics include Wilms tumor, gonadal dysgenesis (male pseudohermaphroditism), and early-onset nephropathy (diffuse mesangial sclerosis).
  · Patients carry a germline dominant–negative missense mutation in the zinc-finger region of *WT1*, which interferes with the function of the other normal allele.
  · Wilms tumor is generally associated with biallelic inactivation of *WT1*.
  · Patients have high risk for gonadoblastoma.
- Beckwith-Wiedemann syndrome (BWS):
  · Syndrome characteristics include macrosomia, organomegaly, macroglossia, hemihypertrophy, omphalocele, and adrenal cytomegaly.
  · Chromosomal band 11p15.5 (also known as WT2 locus) distal to *WT1* is a region with multiple genes normally expressed from only 1 of 2 parental alleles, with the other transcriptionally silenced (i.e., imprinting) via methylation of the promoter region.
  · *IGF-2* resides in this region and is normally expressed only by the paternal allele.
  · In some Wilms tumors, reexpression of the maternal allele (loss of imprinting) leads to overexpression of the IGF-2 protein. Overexpression of this growth factor may contribute to macrosomia, organomegaly, and increased risk of Wilms tumor.
  · In other instances, there is duplication of the transcriptionally active paternal allele leading to overexpression of *IGF-2* (uniparental paternal disomy).

148. Describe common histologic features in Wilms tumor and how histologic appearance affects prognosis.

- Classic triphasic appearance:
  - Tumor has blastemal (sheets of small blue cells), stromal (fibroblastic, myxoid, occasionally skeletal muscle), and epithelial (abortive tubules and glomeruli) components.
  - The percentage of each component is highly variable.
  - Rarely, heterologous elements may be present (squamous epithelium, mucinous epithelium, smooth muscle, fat, cartilage, osteoid, neurogenic tissue).
- Prognosis:

- Overall cure rate for Wilms tumors is currently ~90%.
- Some patients who are likely to do poorly can be identified on H&E slide.
- Presence of anaplasia (large, hyperchromatic nuclei and abnormal mitoses), seen in ~5% of tumors, correlates with presence of *p53* mutations and chemotherapy resistance.
- Even when anaplasia is restricted to the kidney (i.e., no extrarenal spread), the prognosis is adversely affected.

Nephrogenic Rests

149. Define nephrogenic rests.

Nephrogenic rests are abnormally persistent clusters of embryonal kidney cells, putative precursor lesions of Wilms tumors, seen adjacent to 25%–40% of unilateral tumors and almost 100% of bilateral tumors. Some histologically resemble Wilms tumor while others are sclerotic.

150. What is the significance of nephrogenic rests?

The presence of nephrogenic rests in resected specimens must be documented, as patients have an increased risk of developing Wilms tumor in the contralateral kidney and must be closely monitored.

Ewing Sarcoma

151. What are sites of predilection for Ewing sarcoma?

- Long bones.
- Pelvis.

- Note: arises in medullary cavities.

152. What are the radiologic findings of Ewing sarcoma?

- Destructive lytic tumor extending into soft tissue.
- Elevation of periosteum.

- "Onionskin" layering.

153. What are the histologic findings of Ewing sarcoma?

- Sheets of uniform small round blue cells.
- Homer-Wright rosettes.
- Sparse intercellular stroma.

- Few or no mitoses.
- Intracytoplasmic glycogen (clear cytoplasm).
- CD99+ and vimentin+.

154. What are the cytogenetics of Ewing sarcoma?

- Most cases (95%) involve t(11;22)(q24;q12) translocation (fuses the *EWSR1* gene in chromosome 22 to the *FLI1* gene on chromosome 11).
- Some cases involve t(21;22) (*EWSR1-ERG*).

- Various other translocations fuse the *EWS* to other members of the ETS transcription factor family.
- The exact fusion site varies among tumors.

155. List at least 4 tumors with involvement of the *EWSR1* gene.

- Ewing sarcoma family of tumors.
- Desmoplastic small round cell tumor.
- Angiomatoid fibrous histiocytoma.
- Clear cell sarcoma of soft parts.

- Extraskeletal myxoid chondrosarcoma.
- Extraskeletal chondrosarcoma.
- Myoepithelioma.

156. List 4 immunostains useful in the diagnosis of pediatric small round blue cell tumors and 4 immunostains for spindle cell tumors.

- Small round cell tumors: CD99, WT1, CD45, CD56, synaptophysin, desmin, myogenin, INI1, TdT.

- Spindle cell tumors: actin, desmin, S100, pancytokerain, EMA, CD34, CD117, β-catenin, myogenin, BCL-2.

Aneurysmal Bone Cyst (ABC)

157. What is the clinical presentation of and treatment for ABC?
- It occurs in the first 2 decades of life.
- It has rapid onset of pain and swelling.
- The most common treatment is curettage and bone grafting; other treatments are also available.

158. Where does ABC most commonly arise?
- Long bones (metaphysis) — 50–60%.
- Vertebrae and sacrum — 20–30%.

159. What are the radiologic findings of ABC?
- X-ray: sharply defined, expansile osteolytic lesion with thin sclerotic borders.
- CT: fluid-fluid levels.

160. What are the gross and histologic findings of ABC?
- Honeycombing and cystic spaces.
- Septi of solid and hemorrhagic tissue.
- Cystic spaces filled with blood and separated by septa containing fibroblasts, osteoclast-like giant cells, and woven bone.
- Numerous hemosiderin-laden macrophages.
- Reactive bone formation.

161. What is the differential diagnosis of ABC?
- Telangiectatic osteosarcoma.
- Giant cell tumor.

162. What is the pathogenesis of ABC?
- Rearrangements of chromosome 17p13 lead to *USP6* overexpression.
- Secondary ABC (not a neoplasm) do not have *USP6* rearrangements.

Epstein-Barr Virus (EBV) Infection

163. What type of virus is EBV and what is the pathogenesis of EBV infection?
- Type of virus:
  - Herpes-type virus.
- Pathogenesis:
  - Infects B lymphocytes — interaction between the viral glycoprotein gp350 and the complement receptor CR2 (CD21), which is expressed on B lymphocytes.
  - Establishes a latent infection in most B cells that persists throughout life.
  - Also infects epithelial cells.

164. List at least 2 EBV gene products expressed in EBV infected B cells.
- EBV nuclear antigens (EBNA-1, EBNA-2, EBNA-3).
- Latent membrane proteins (LMP1, LMP2) localized in the plasma membrane of infected B cells.
- Nonpolyadenylated nuclear RNAs, EBER1 and EBER2 (which are often used to detect the presence of EBV within a cell).

165. List at least 5 diseases associated with EBV infection.
- Infectious mononucleosis (100%).
- Burkitt lymphoma (endemic > 90%, nonendemic 15%–20%).
- Nasopharyngeal carcinoma (100%).
- Chronic active EBV infection (100%).
- Hodgkin lymphoma (mixed cellularity 70%, lymphocyte-rich 40%, nodular sclerosis usually EBV negative).
- Primary CNS lymphoma (> 90%).
- Posttransplant lymphoproliferative disorder.
- Oral hairy leukoplakia (100%).
- EBV-associated smooth muscle tumor (100%).
- Extranodal NK/T cell lymphoma, nasal type.
- Angioimmunoblastic T cell lymphoma.
- EBV-associated gastric carcinoma.

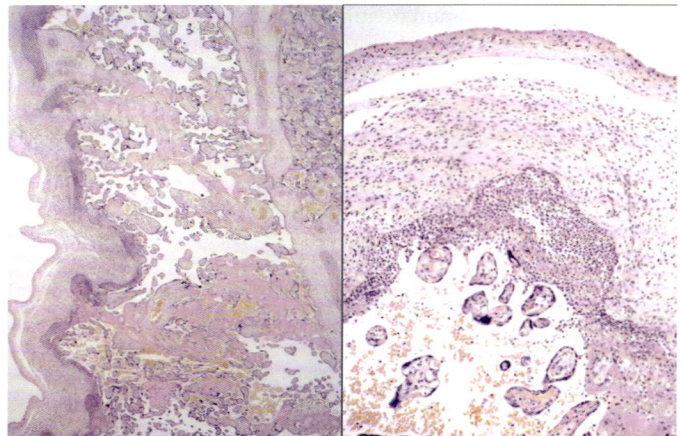

IMAGE 17.1 Chorioamnionitis: acute inflammatory cell infiltrate in the layers of chorion and amnion (lower magnification on the left, higher magnification on the right).

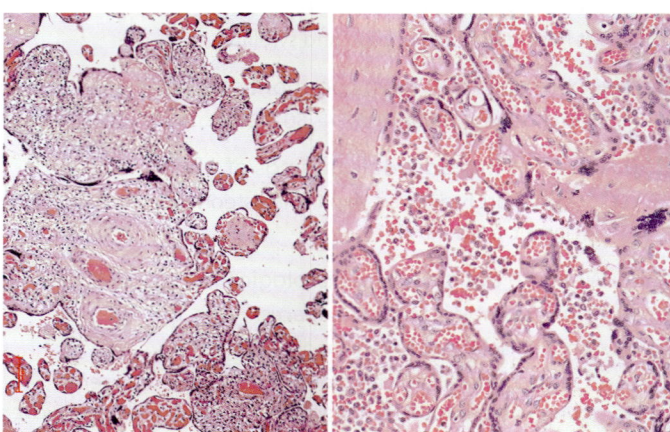

IMAGE 17.4 Left: villitis of unknown etiology (VUE). Lymphohistiocytic inflammation involving the chorionic villi is present. Right: chronic histiocytic intervillositis. Chronic inflammatory cells, mostly histiocytes, within the intervillous space are present.

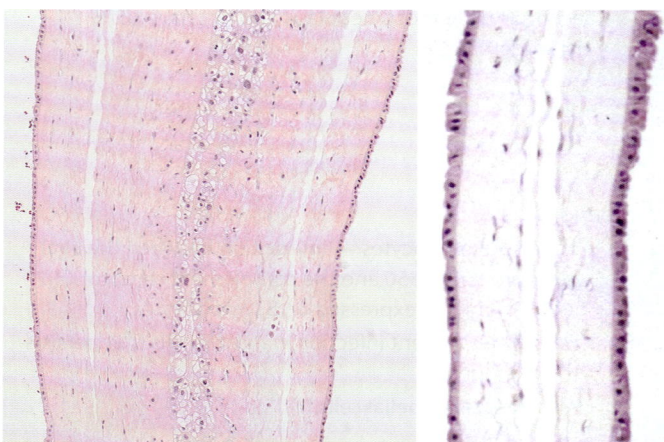

IMAGE 17.2 Left: dichorionic diamnionic dividing membrane. Right: monochorionic diamnionic dividing membrane.

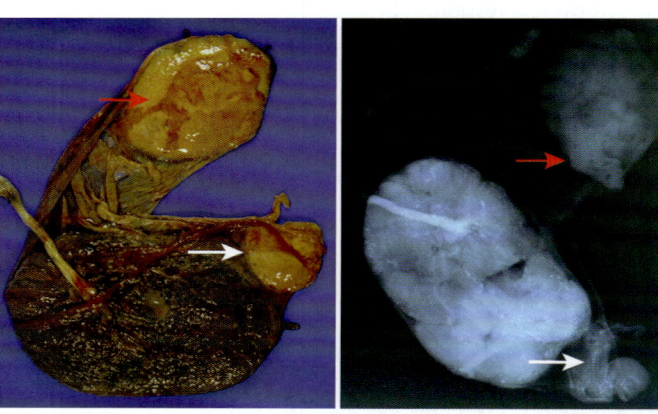

IMAGE 17.5 Fetus papyraceous. Left: the image shows the demise of 1 cotwin in a twin pregnancy with atrophic and fibrotic placenta (red arrow) and mummified fetus (white arrow). Right: X-ray reveals remnant of fetal skeletal structure.

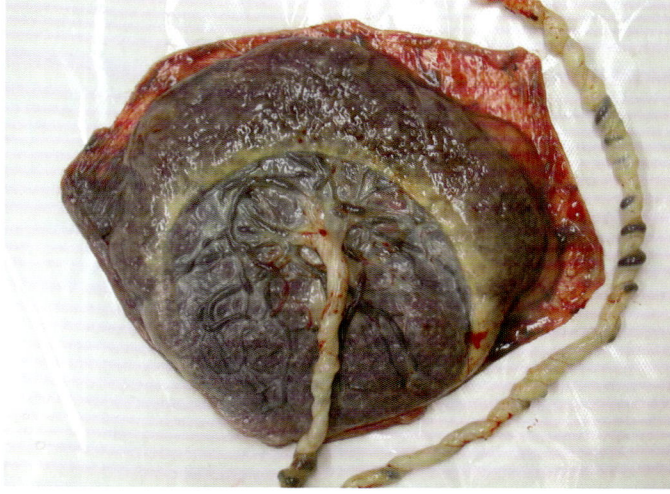

IMAGE 17.3 Placenta circumvallate. Fetal membranes insert in the disc away from the peripheral margin with a concentric ridge.

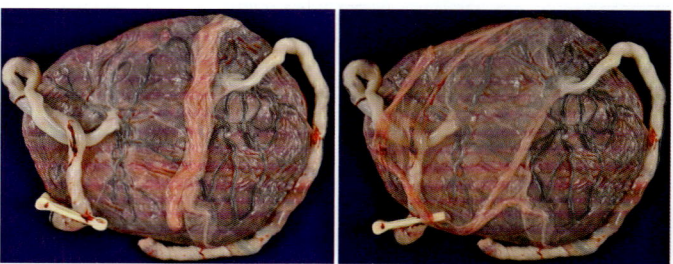

IMAGE 17.6 Left: dichorionic diamnionic twin placenta. Note the thick and opaque dividing membrane. Right: monochorionic diamnionic twin placenta. Note the thin and transparent dividing membrane.

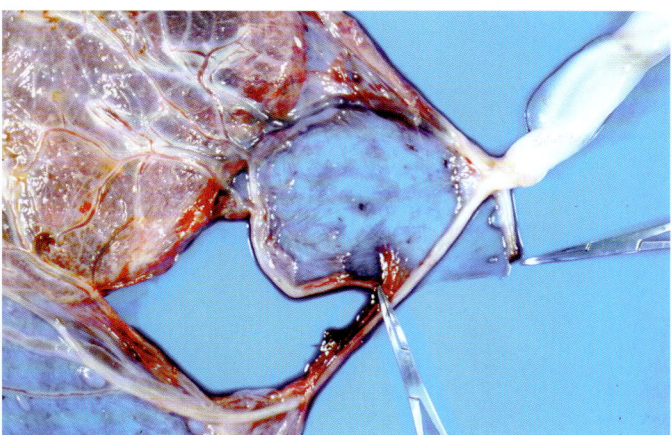

IMAGE 17.7 Velamentous insertion of umbilical cord with vasa previa rupture.

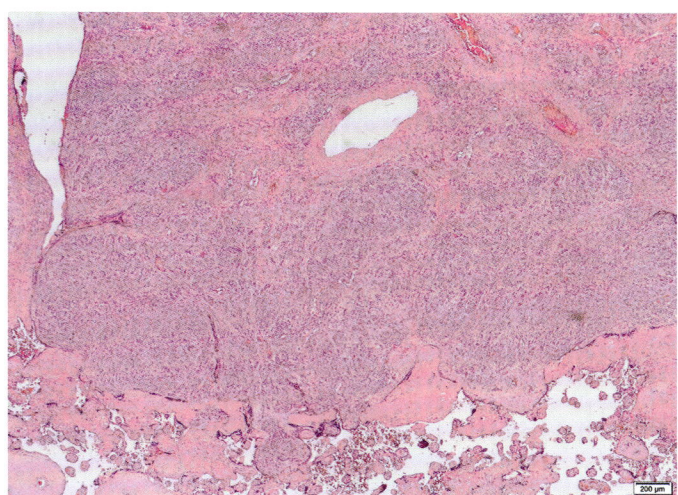

IMAGE 17.10 Chorangiomatosis. The image shows abnormally vascularized stem villi with small anastomosing capillaries at periphery surrounding stem vessels. Pericytes and stromal collagenization are present.

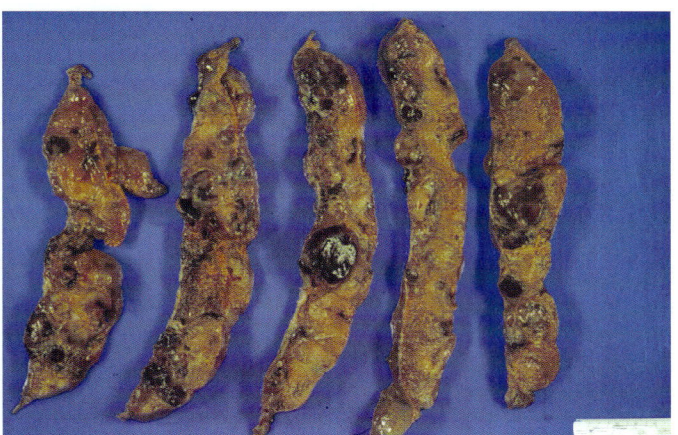

IMAGE 17.8 Chorangiomatosis. The image shows multiple dark red nodular lesions in the placental disc parenchyma.

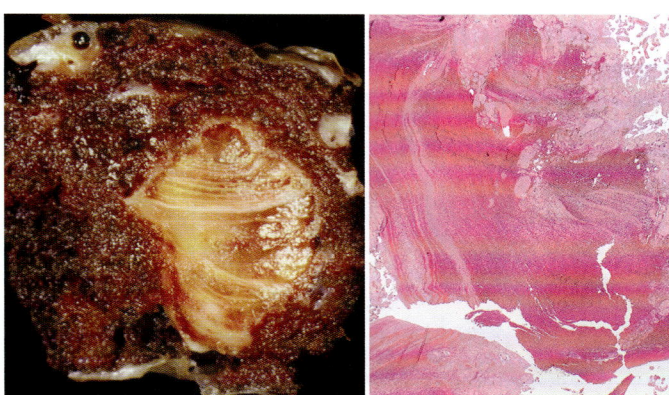

IMAGE 17.11 Intervillous thrombus. Left: the image shows a localized, circumscribed blood clot in the maternal intervillous space with lines of Zahn. Right: this is a microscopic image of intervillous thrombus. Note the laminated appearance.

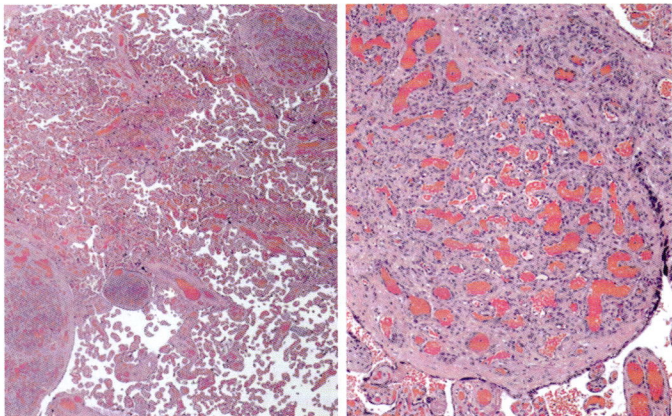

IMAGE 17.9 Multiple chorangiomas. Left: multifocal angiomatous nodules of varying sizes. Right: higher power view; small capillaries surrounded by pericytes, merging imperceptivity into surrounding villous stroma.

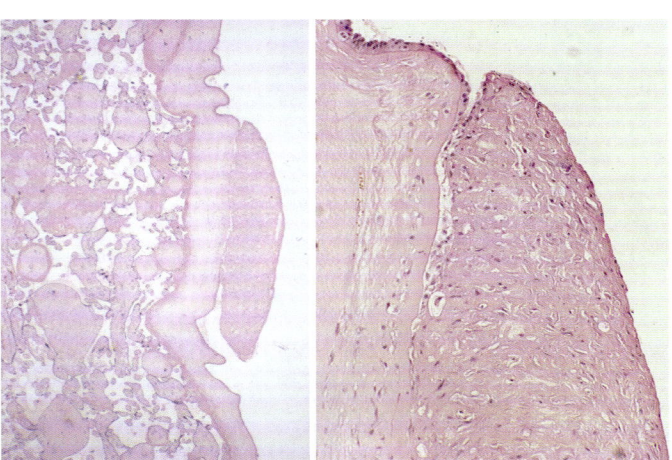

IMAGE 17.12 Amnion nodosum: a nodular aggregate of heterogeneous granular, eosinophilic materials containing scattered squames and cell debris (lower magnification on the left, higher magnification on the right).

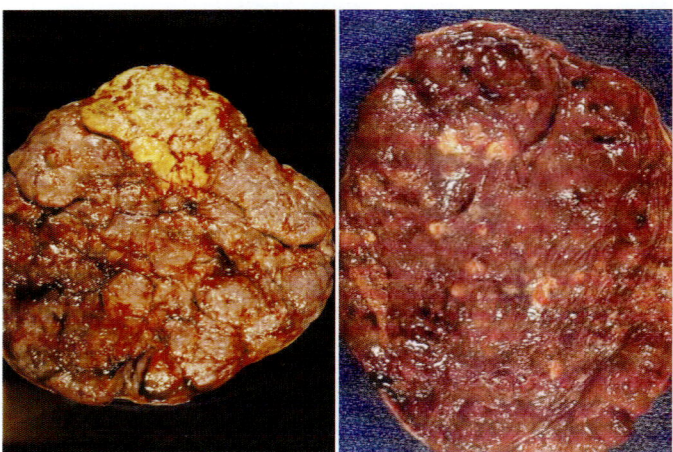

IMAGE 17.13 Placental infarct. Left: a gray-white firm area of old infarct. Right: multifocal small infarcts.

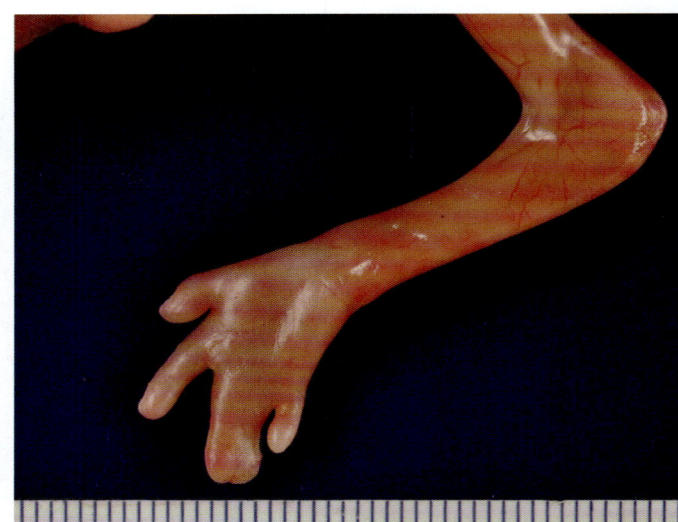

IMAGE 17.16 Classic third and fourth fingers syndactyly in triploidy syndrome.

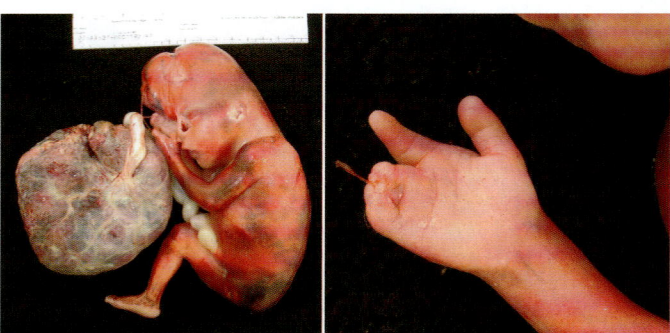

IMAGE 17.14 Amnion bands. Left: amnion adheres to the head with irregular distortion of craniofacial structure. Right: multiple amputations of the fingers.

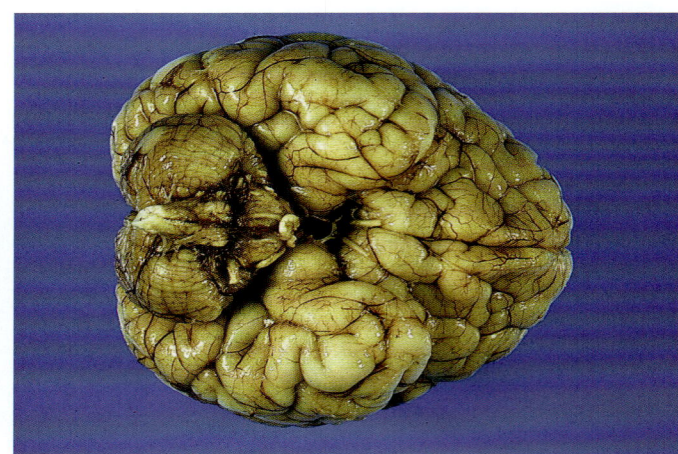

IMAGE 17.17 Arhinencephaly. The image shows absence of olfactory bulb and tracts.

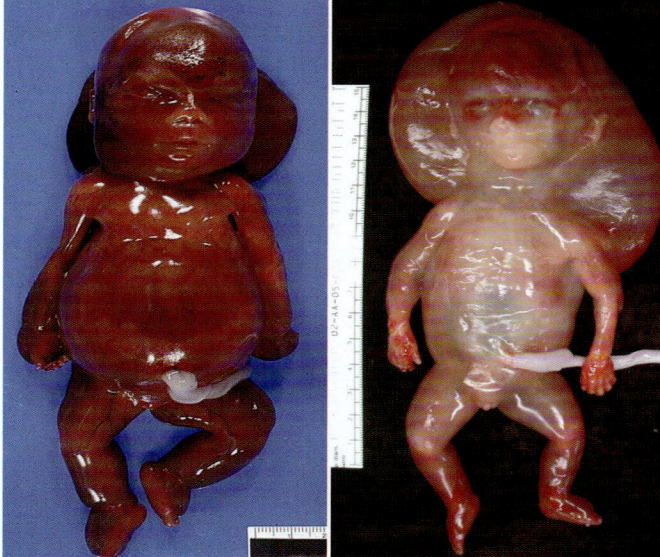

IMAGE 17.15 Left: Hydrops fetalis with generalized edema. Right: cystic hygroma.

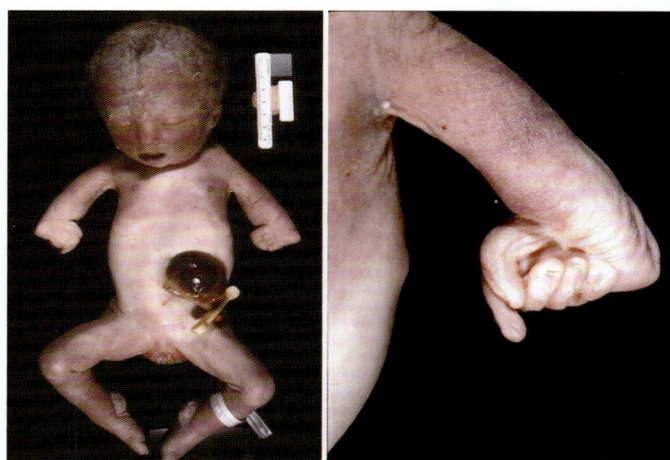

IMAGE 17.18 Bilateral radial aplasia, bilateral absence of thumbs, omphalocele, diastasis recti abdominis, hypoplasia of labia majora, short bifid sternum.

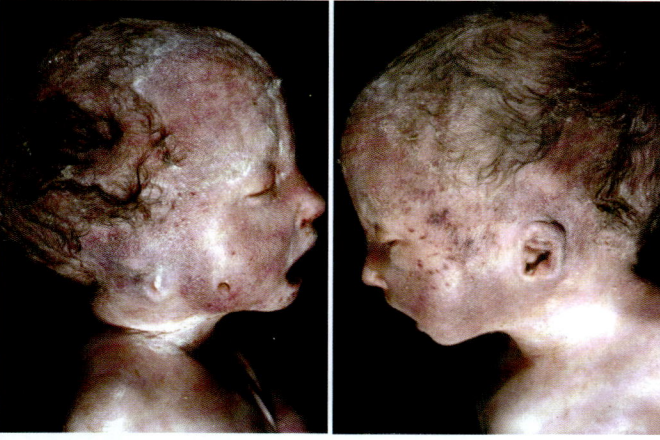

IMAGE 17.19 Trisomy 18. The image shows prominent occiput; rudimentary right ear with atresia of external auditory canal and skin tag on cheek; low-set small left ear.

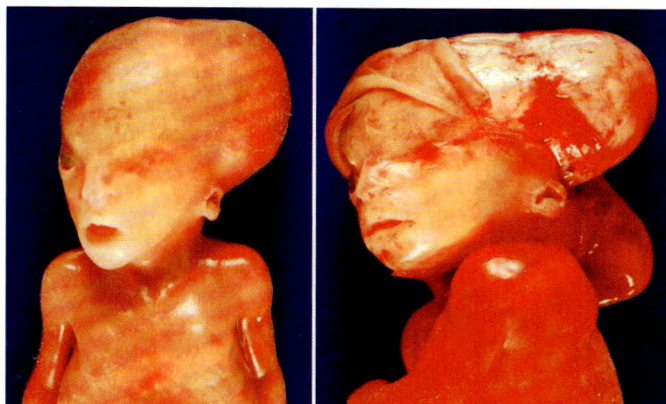

IMAGE 17.22 Encephalocele. The image shows a large fluctuant and bulging mass of the posterior cranium.

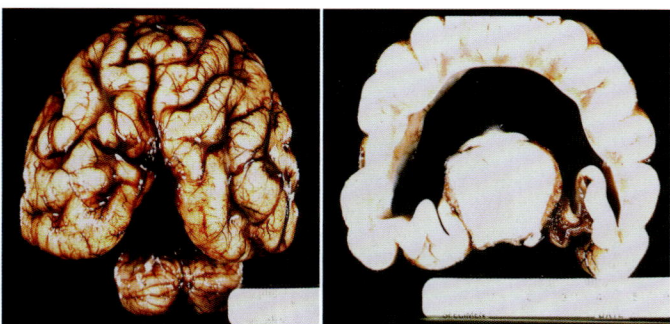

IMAGE 17.20 Alobar holoprosencephaly. Left: undivided holosphere with macrogyric convolutions. Right: single ventricle representing lateral and third ventricles.

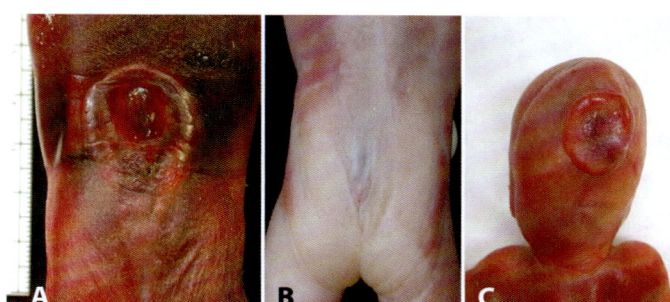

IMAGE 17.23 Lumbosacral myelomeningocele. Image A: an open lesion with vascular connective tissue and disorganized neural tissue. Image B: a closed cystic mass covered by skin. Image C: meningocele at the back of the head.

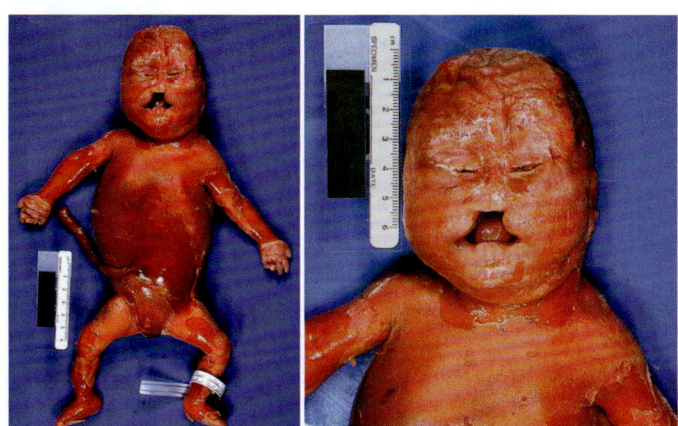

IMAGE 17.21 Stillborn male fetus at 30 weeks. The image shows microcephaly, absent external nose, bilateral cleft lip, total cleft palate, intrauterine growth retardation.

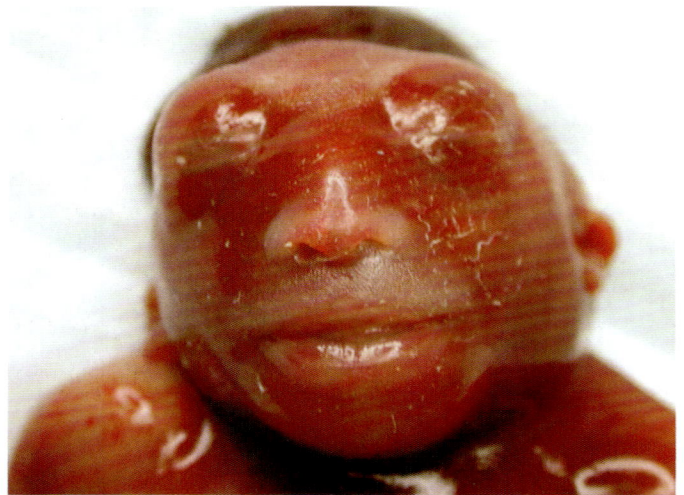

IMAGE 17.24 Anencephaly. Note the absence of skull vault, bulging of eyes, short neck, and cerebrovasculosa.

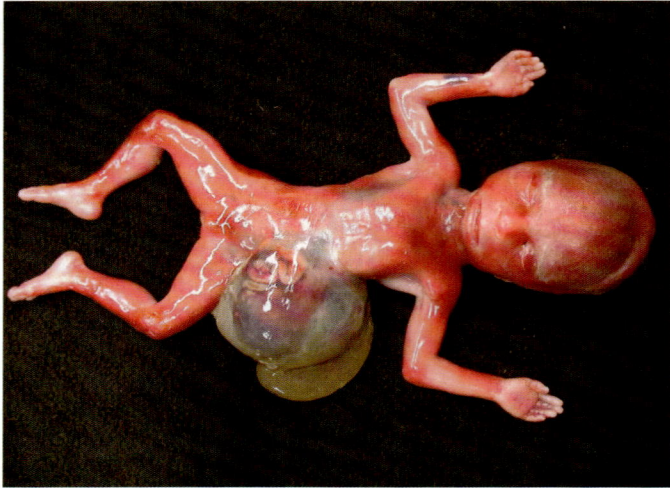

IMAGE 17.25 Omphalocele. The abdominal visceral organs are covered by amnion and peritoneum.

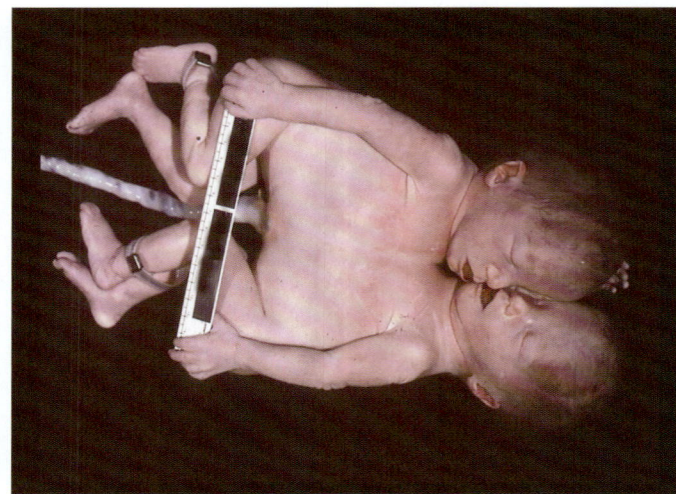

IMAGE 17.28 Thoracopagus-type conjoined twins.

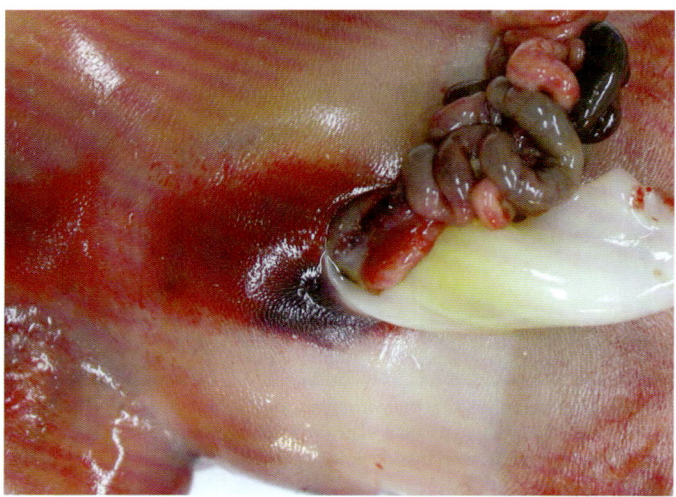

IMAGE 17.26 Gastroschisis. The image shows an abdominal wall defect located lateral to the umbilical ring. The protruding abdominal visceral organs are not covered by a sac.

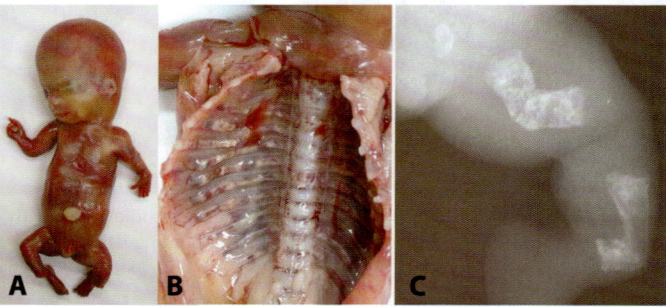

IMAGE 17.29 Osteogenesis imperfecta type II. Image A: infant with short limbs, multiple bone fractures. Image B: continuously beaded ribs due to multiple fractures. Image C: multiple fractures of femur and tibia.

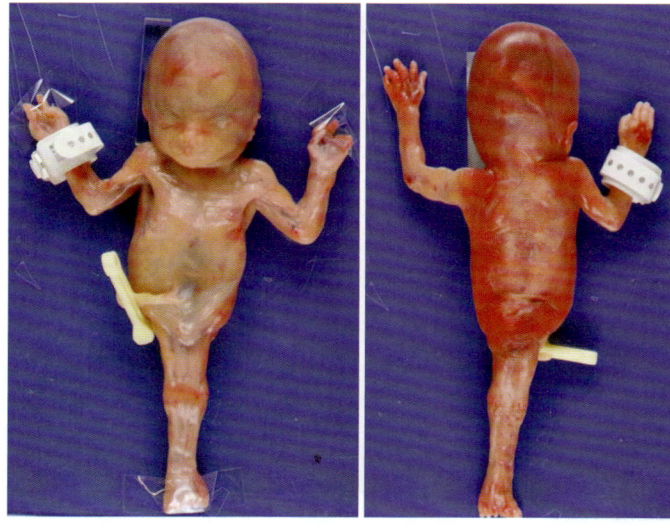

IMAGE 17.27 Sirenomelia.

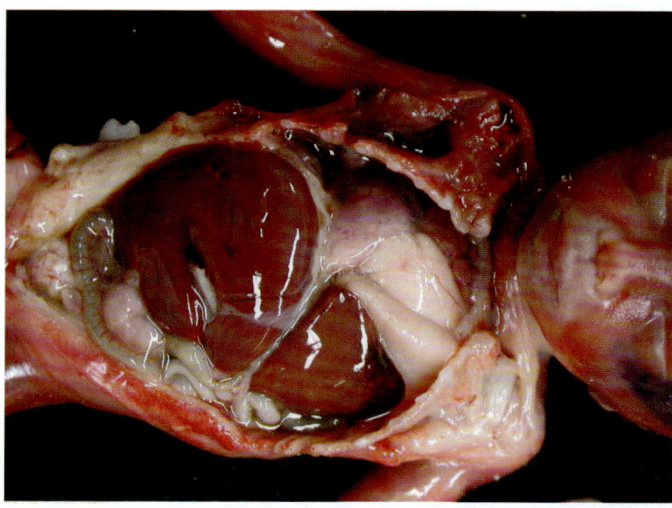

IMAGE 17.30 Diaphragmatic hernia. The stomach, spleen, and part of the intestine are herniated into the left side of the chest cavity.

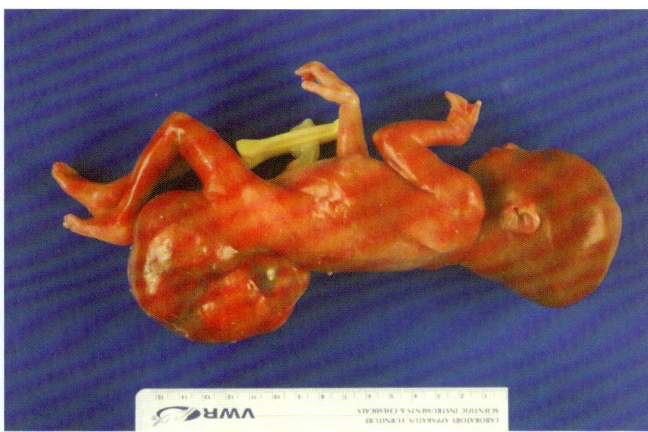

IMAGE 17.31 Sacrococcygeal teratoma in a newborn baby.

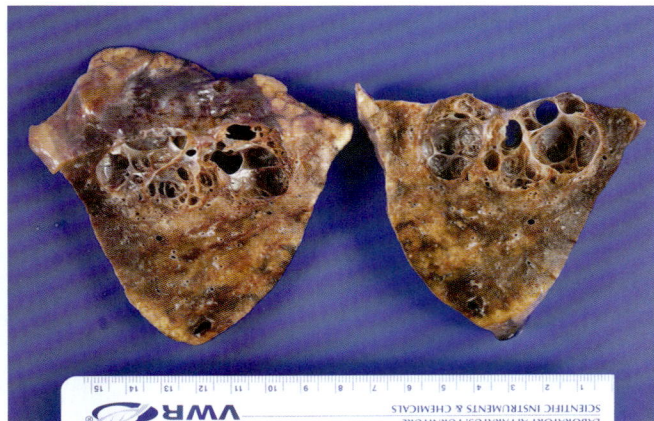

IMAGE 17.32 Congenital pulmonary airway malformation (CPAM) type 1 (large cyst type).

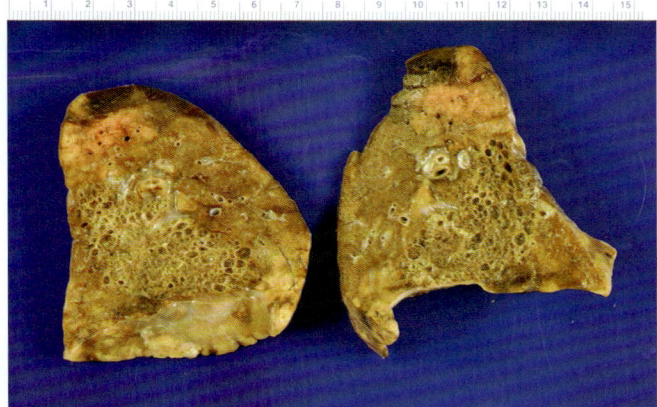

IMAGE 17.33 Congenital pulmonary airway malformation (CPAM) type 2 (small cyst type).

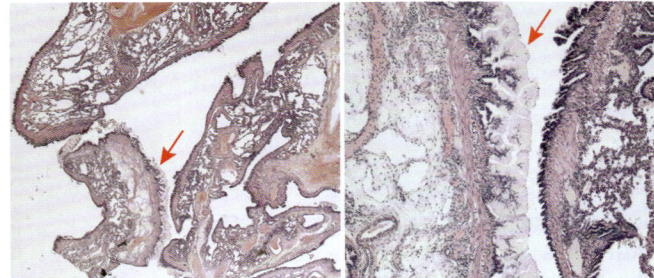

IMAGE 17.34 Congenital pulmonary airway malformation (CPAM) type 1 (large cyst type). The right image is a detail of the left image. Multiple large and small cysts, and ciliated pseudostratified columnar epithelial lining are present. Note the mucus cells (arrows).

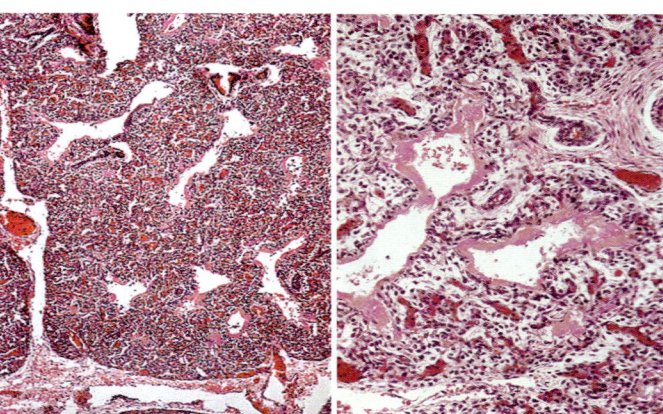

IMAGE 17.35 Hyaline membrane disease. Left: atelectasis, widespread collapse of distal air spaces, dilated terminal bronchioles. Right: anuclear eosinophilic hyaline membrane, composed of both necrotic epithelial cells and fibrin and other proteins.

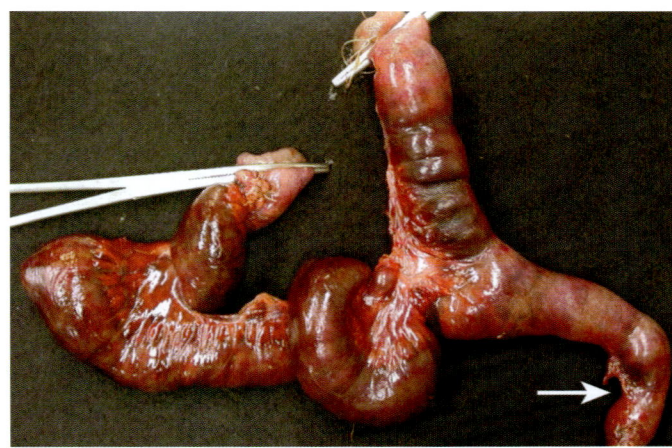

IMAGE 17.36 Meckel diverticulum. The diverticulum is located 100 cm proximal to the ileocecal valve, resulting from a failure of the omphalomesenteric duct to resorb by the eighth week.

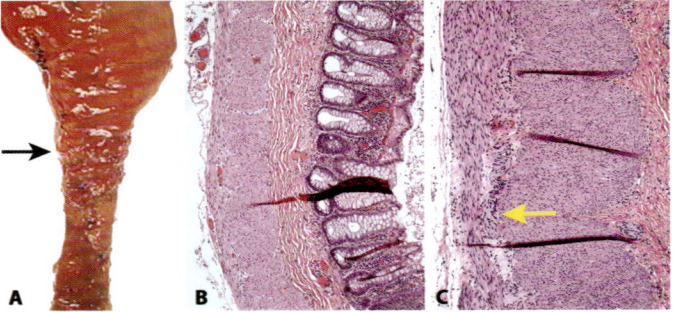

IMAGE 17.37 Hirchsprung disease. Image A: gross specimen showing transition between dilated proximal rectum and narrowed distal rectum (black arrow). Image B: absence of ganglion cells in the submucosal and myenteric plexuses of the colonic wall. Image C: hypertrophic nerve fibers in the colon wall (yellow arrow).

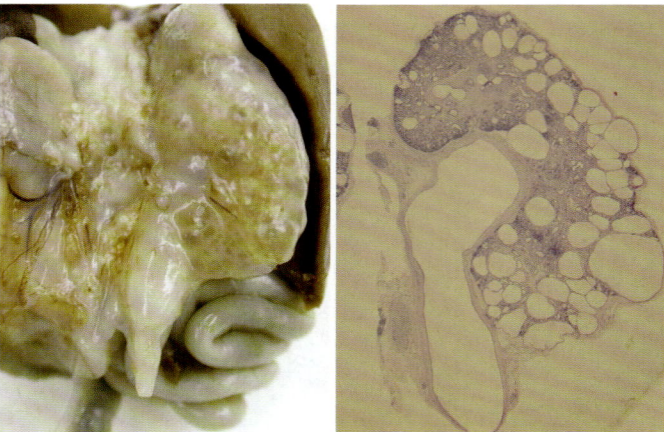

IMAGE 17.38 Renal multicystic dysplasia, gross and microscopic.

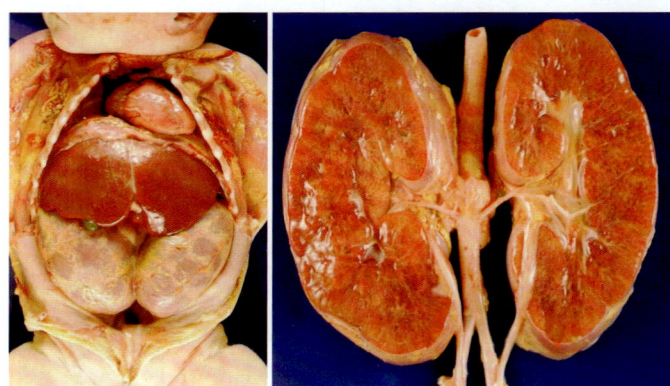

IMAGE 17.41 Autosomal recessive polycystic kidney disease. Left: enlargement of both kidneys with displacement of abdominal organs. Right: radially oriented fusiform cysts with a "spongy" appearance replacing the entire cortex.

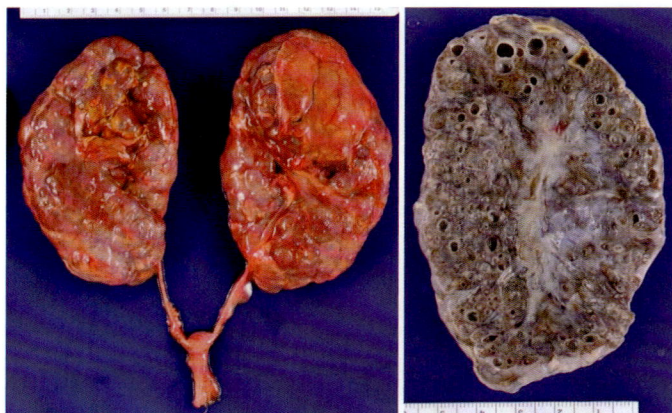

IMAGE 17.39 Diffuse cystic renal dysplasia, syndromal in ciliopathy. Both kidneys are reniform with patent hypoplastic ureters and bladder. Small round cysts through the renal parenchyma are present. (Left: before fixation in formalin. Right: after fixation and sectioning.)

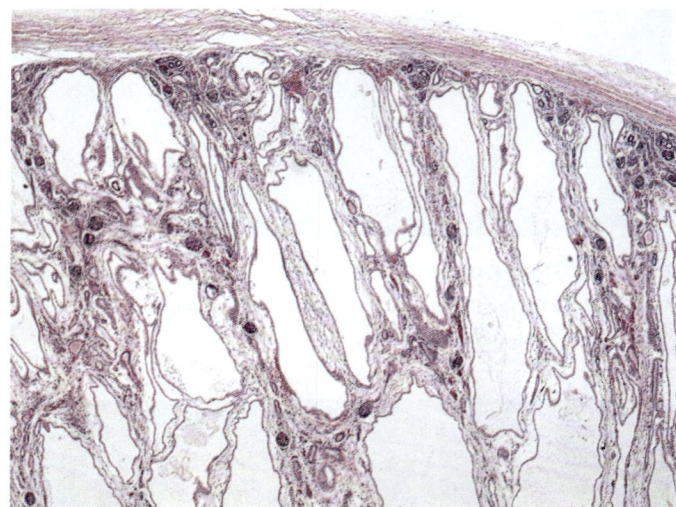

IMAGE 17.42 Autosomal recessive polycystic kidney disease. Cysts derived from dilated collecting ducts in a radiating arrangement are interspaced with normal glomeruli and tubules. There are no glomerular cysts, no fibrosis, and no inflammation.

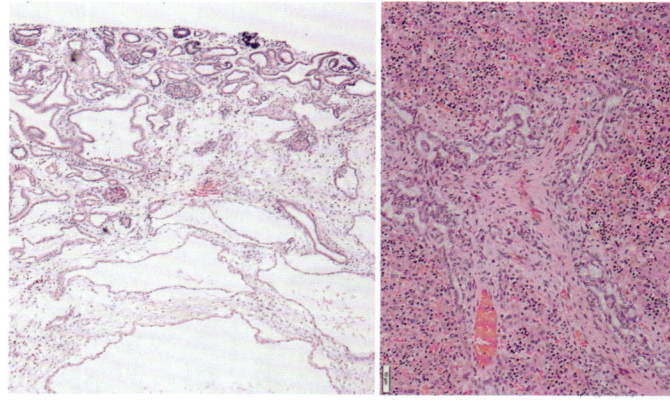

IMAGE 17.40 Diffuse cystic dysplasia in Meckel Gruber syndrome, 20 weeks gestation, ciliopathy. Left: deficient nephrogenesis, disproportionately large number of dilated and dysplastic collecting ducts. Right: hepatic ductal plate malformation, congenital hepatic fibrosis.

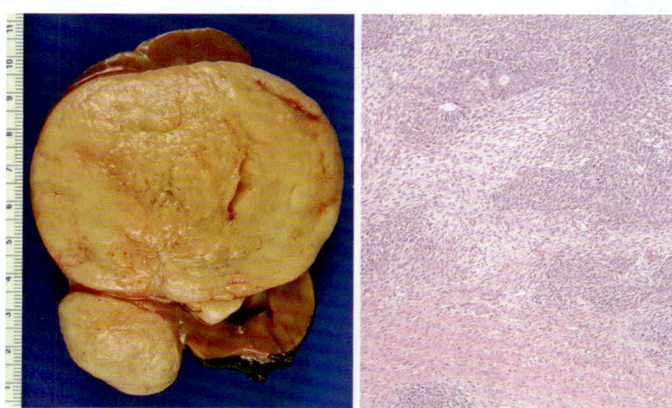

IMAGE 17.43 Wilms tumor. Left: large, well-circumscribed renal mass. Right: characteristic triphasic components of the tumor tissue.

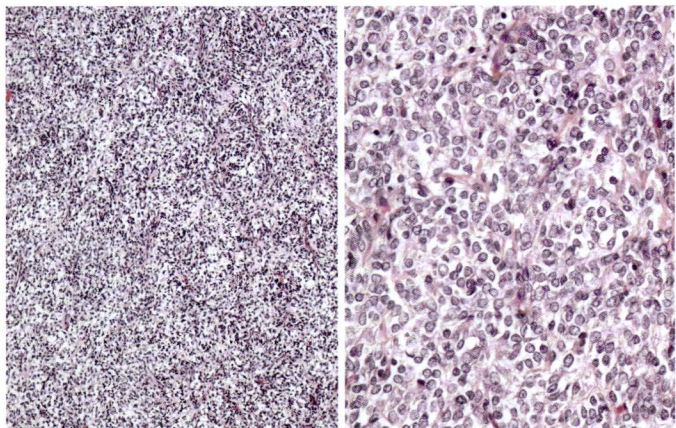

IMAGE 17.44 Clear cell sarcoma of the kidney (H&E, left: x20, right: x100). The image shows classic "chicken wire" pattern with fibrovascular septa subdividing the tumor into cords 6–10 cells in width, composed of polygonal cells with pale nuclei. The extracellular matrix is clear.

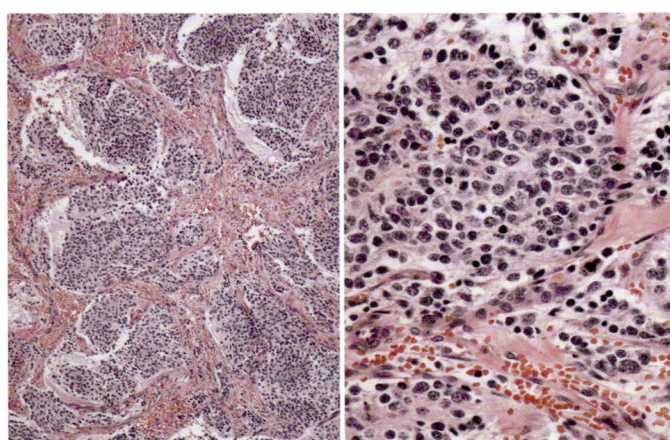

IMAGE 17.47 Neuroblastoma. Left: small blue round cells arranged in a nesting pattern. Right: high magnification shows cytoplasmic neuropil differentiation.

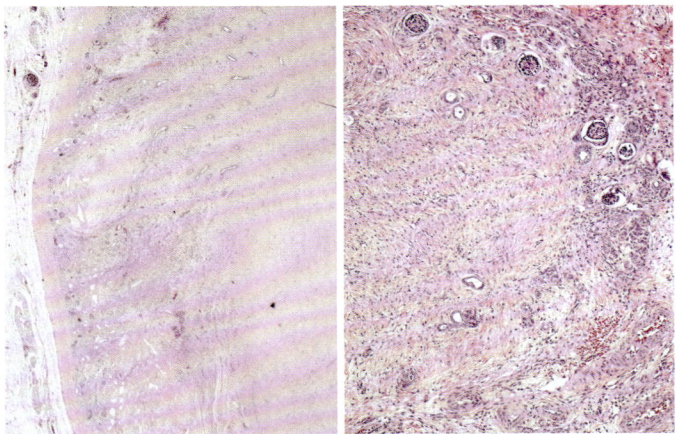

IMAGE 17.45 Mesoblastic nephroma, classic type: ill-defined infiltrate composed of elongated fibroblastic spindle cells in the kidney, entrapping glomeruli and renal tubules (lower magnification on the left, higher magnification on the right).

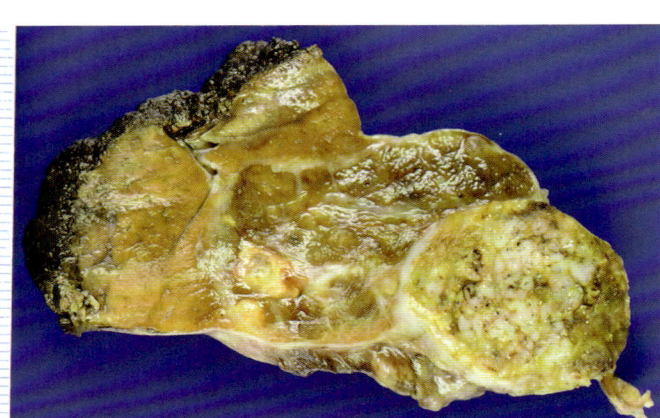

IMAGE 17.48 Hepatoblastoma. Nonneoplastic liver (arrow) and tumor (asterisk).

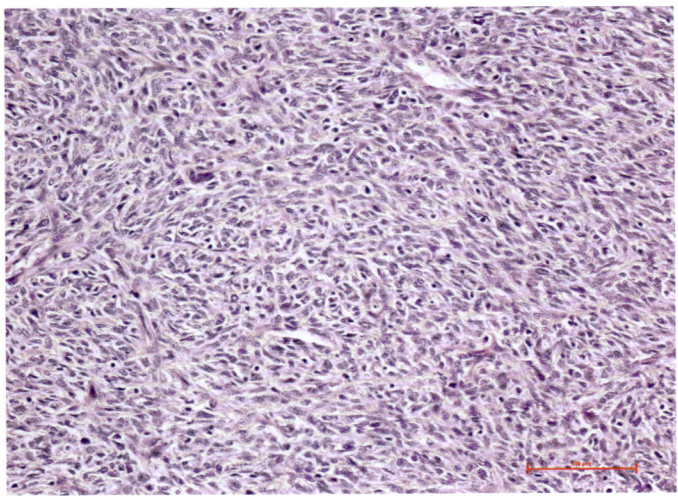

IMAGE 17.46 Mesoblastic nephroma, cellular type.

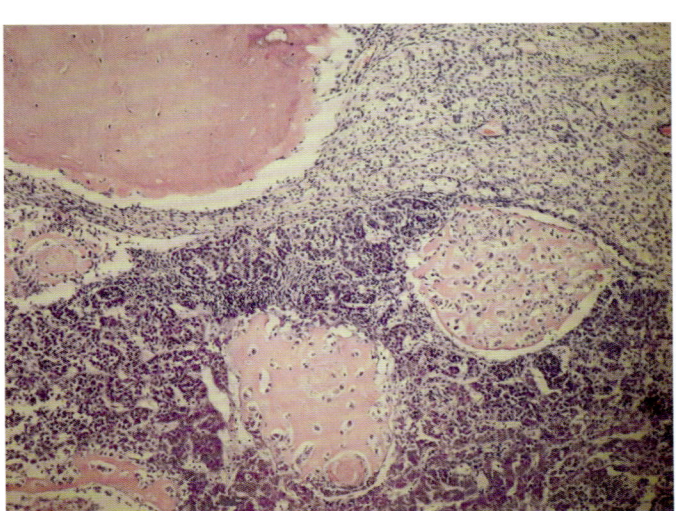

IMAGE 17.49 Hepatoblastoma with mixed epithelial and mesenchymal components.

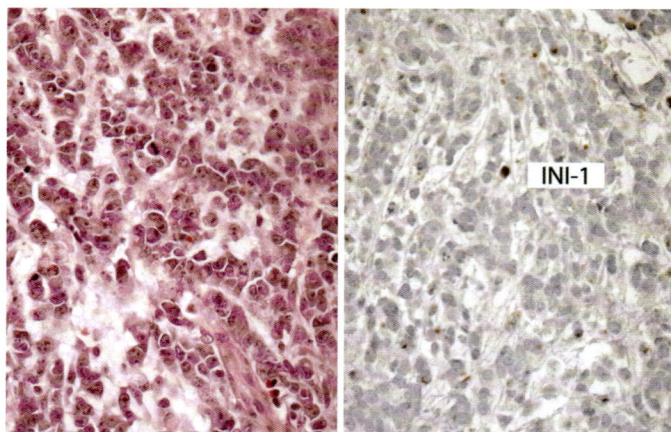

IMAGE 17.50 Rhabdoid tumor. Left: tumor cells have vesicular nuclei, prominent nucleoli, and cytoplasmic eosinophilic bodies. Right: loss of nuclear INI1 expression in tumor cells. Note that the background lymphocytes are appropriately positive for INI1.

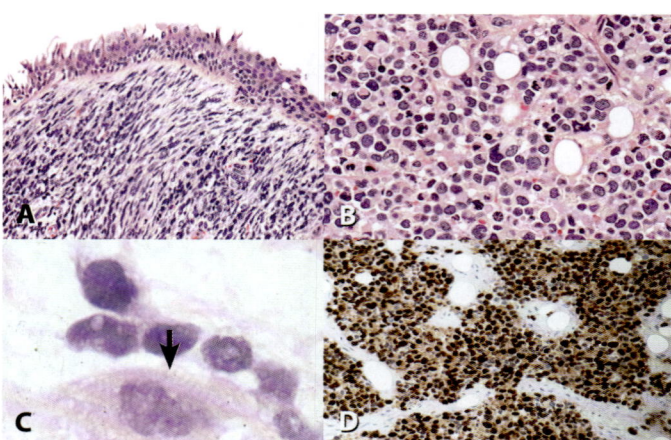

IMAGE 17.53 Rhabdomyosarcoma. Image A: botryoid type. Image B: solid variant (alveolar type). Image C: rhabdomyoblastic differentiation (arrow: cross striations). Image D: myogenin stain.

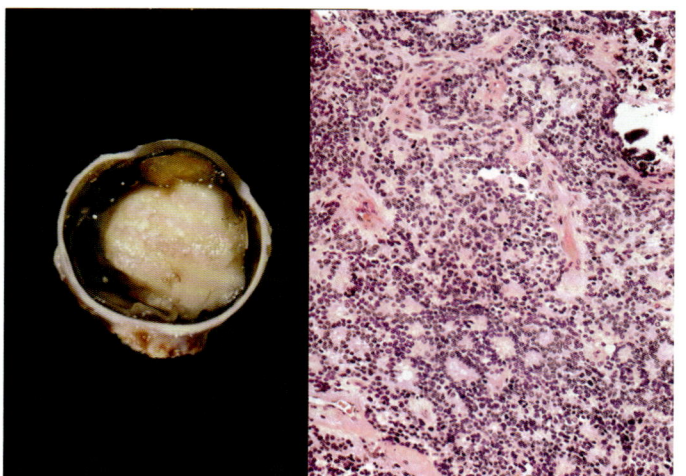

IMAGE 17.51 Retinoblastoma. Left: endophytic growth of eye tumor . Right: small blue round tumor cells with Flexner-Wintersteiner and Homer-Wright rosettes.

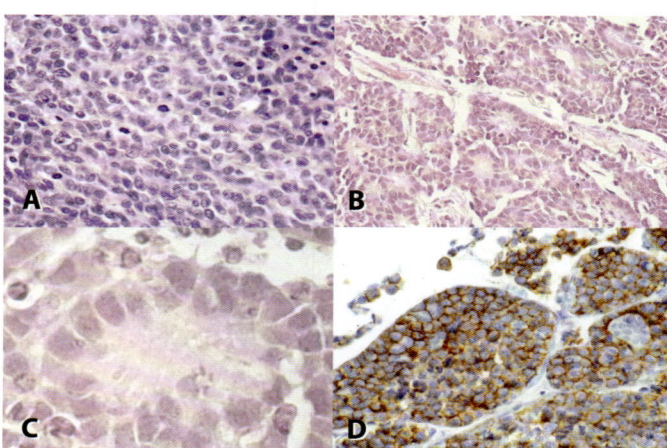

IMAGE 17.54 Small round cell tumor. Image A: undifferentiated pattern. Image B: prominent rosette pattern. Image C: Homer-Wright rosette. Image D: CD99 membranous immunostain.

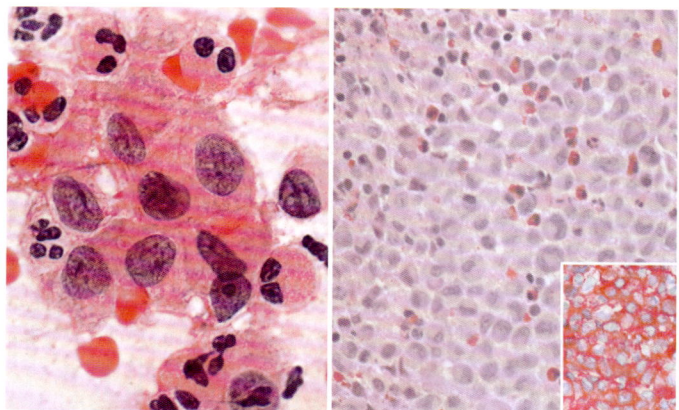

IMAGE 17.52 Langerhans cell histiocytosis. Left: Imprints, Langerhans cell phenotype (grooved nuclei and ample cytoplasm). Right: H&E stain. Inset: CD1a stain.

Bibliography

Cohen M, Scheimberg I, editors. Essentials of surgical pediatric pathology. Cambridge (UK): Cambridge University Press; 2014. doi: 10.1017/CBO9781139237000

Goldblum JR, Folpe AL, Weiss SW. Enzinger and Weiss soft tissue tumors. 7th ed. Philadelphia (PA): Elsevier; 2020.

Husain AN, Stocker JT, Dehner LP. Stocker and Dehner's pediatric pathology. 5th ed. Philadelphia (PA): Wolters Kluwar; 2021.

Kaplan CG. Color atlas of gross placental pathology. 2nd ed. New York: Springer, 2016.

Kumar V, Abbas AK, Aster J. Robbins and Cotran pathologic basis of disease. 10th ed. North York (ON): Elsevier Canada; 2020.

Mackinnon AC, editor. Pediatric neoplasia: advances in molecular pathology and translational medicine. NY: Humana Press; 2012.

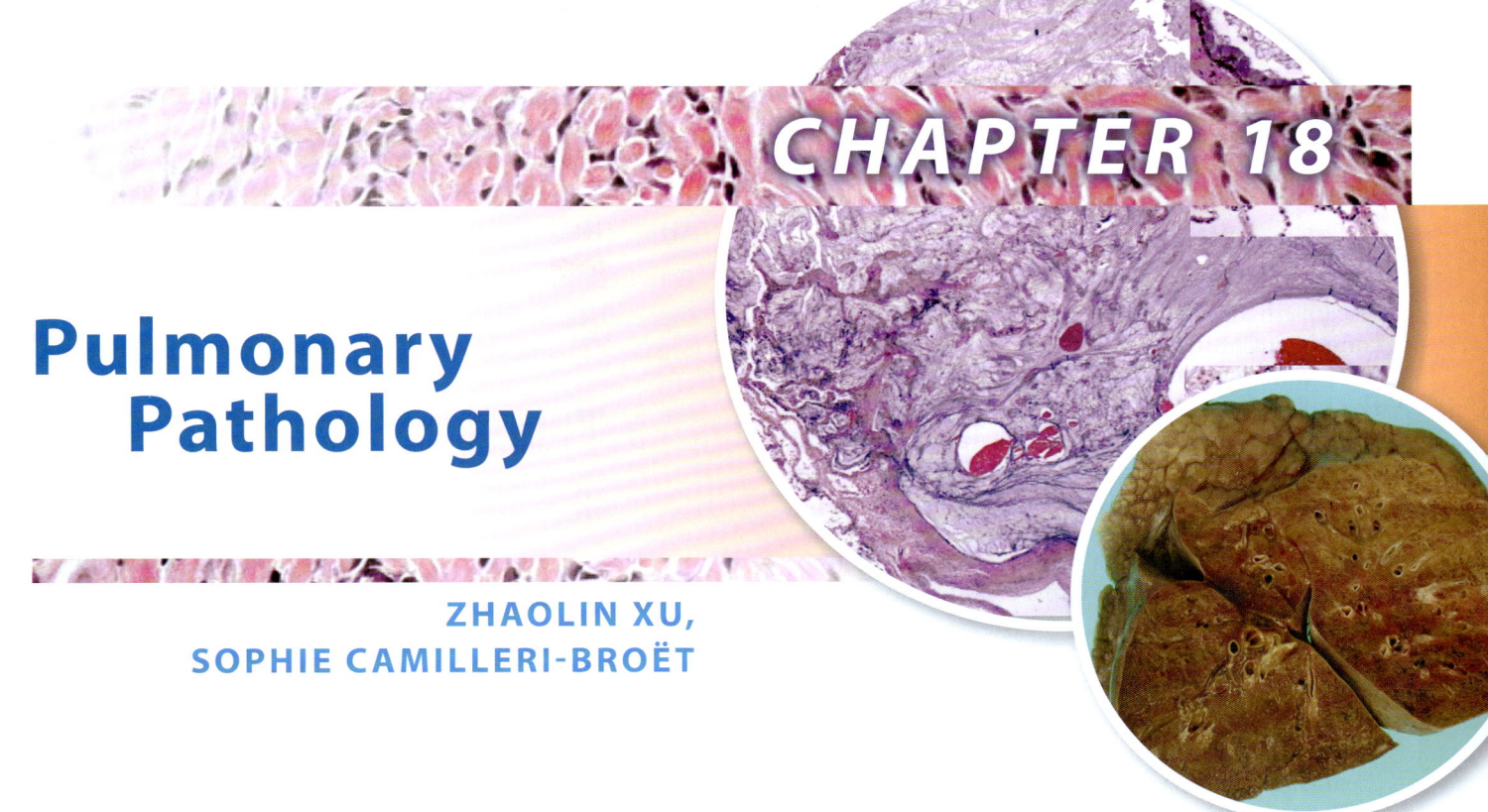

CHAPTER 18

Pulmonary Pathology

ZHAOLIN XU, SOPHIE CAMILLERI-BROËT

Pulmonary Pathology Exam Essentials

MUST KNOW

World Health Organization (WHO) classification

This chapter covers tumors of the lung, pleura, and thymus.

- Although the WHO classification of lung tumors appears extensive, these tumors can be organized into a few most-frequent tumors and related entities:
  · Adenocarcinoma, their variants and biomarkers.
  · Squamous cell carcinoma and variants.
  · Early lesions (e.g., in situ carcinomas).
  · Neuroendocrine tumors.
  · Mesenchymal tumors.
  · Hematolymphoid tumors.
  · Metastases.
- Tumors of the pleura are less diverse, but the differential diagnosis between mesothelial malignancies and reactive changes may be challenging. They include:
  · Malignant mesothelioma and variants.
  · Hematolymphoid tumors.
  · Mesenchymal tumors such as solitary fibrous tumor.
- Tumors of the thymus are rare and are mainly represented by:
  · Thymomas.
  · Thymic carcinomas.

College of American Pathologists (CAP) protocol and AJCC staging

- Overall, the lung sampling and reporting protocol is relatively straightforward. However, the area of lung cancer biomarker testing has become a major topic in the last few years. Key topics include:
  · Grossing and sampling of lung tumors.
  · Tumor staging factors (pT staging factors), including tumor size and pleural invasion.
  · How to classify tumors with multiple histologic subtypes.
  · Multifocal tumors.
  · Spread through air spaces (STAS) phenomenon.
  · Margins on a lobectomy specimen, segmentectomy, or wedge.
  · Biomarker testing: selection, methods, main biomarkers tested.
  · Sensitizing and resistant mutations in *EGFR*, *ALK*, and *ROS1* rearrangements.
  · Cytologic approaches.
- Generally, a very few topics regarding malignant mesothelioma may be examined. These include:
  · Histological subtypes.
  · General considerations in pT staging.
  · Additional findings in cases of chronic asbestos exposure.

- How to differentiate malignant mesothelioma from reactive changes.
- How to differentiate lung adenocarcinoma from malignant mesothelioma (very important).

Nonneoplastic diseases

- The lung has a number of inflammatory and infectious diseases that make excellent topics for the oral component of the exam. You should devote as much study time to nonneoplastic diseases as to tumors.
- For inflammatory lung disease, study a "histologic pattern" first (as with dermatoses). From the histologic pattern, you can narrow down the differential diagnosis with history, radiology findings, ancillary testing, and so on. Often a particular pattern may have many causes, and the oral exam may not require you to clarify a single diagnosis. Use a classification that suits the pattern best:
  - Acute hyaline changes: think causes of diffuse alveolar damage (DAD) or acute interstitial pneumonia.
  - Infectious pneumonia: think viral, bacterial, fungal, parasitic, mycobacterial, etc.
  - Changes with chronic obstructive pulmonary disease (COPD): think emphysema and chronic bronchitis.
  - Chronic fibrosis: think usual interstitial pneumonia (UIP), nonspecific interstitial pneumonia (NSIP), drug reaction, collagen vascular disease, asbestosis, etc.
  - Interstitial cellular infiltrate: think hypersensitivity pneumonitis, lymphocytic interstitial pneumonia (LIP), cellular NSIP, etc.
  - Alveolar filling: think bronchopneumonia, eosinophilic pneumonia, desquamative interstitial pneumonia (DIP), respiratory bronchiolitis interstitial lung disease (RBILD), pulmonary alveolar proteinosis, pulmonary edema, pneumocystis pneumonia, etc.
  - Nodules and mass like lesions: think silicosis, hyalinizing granuloma, sarcoidosis, pneumoconiosis, granulomatosis with polyangiitis and other granulomatous inflammation, etc.
  - Cystic changes: think emphysema, bullae formation, lymphangioleiomyomatosis (LAM), bronchiectasis, cystic fibrosis, Birt-Hogg-Dubé syndrome, pulmonary Langerhans cell histiocytosis, honeycombing, infection related, etc.
  - Granulomata: think infection-related (mycobacterial, fungal, etc.) and noninfection-related entities (hypersensitivity pneumonitis, sarcoidosis, collagen vascular disease, drug reaction, granulomatous vasculitis, foreign body reaction, amyloidosis, etc.).
  - Vascular changes: think congestive heart failure (CHF), pulmonary edema, embolism/infarct, pulmonary hypertension, etc.
  - Bronchiectasis: think cystic fibrosis, obstructing mass, foreign body, chronic airway inflammation/ infection, genetic cause, etc.
  - Pulmonary hemorrhage: think autoimmune disorders (Goodpasture syndrome, etc.), vasculitis, infection, toxic exposure, drug reaction, cardiac disorder, coagulation disorder, trauma, idiopathic entity, etc.

Genetic and syndromic conditions

Generally, this is a minor topic. The lung can be an organ of manifestation for genetic diseases that primarily affect other organs. Key topics include:
- Syndromes with increased risk of lung cancer (e.g., Peutz-Jeghers syndrome, DICER syndrome).
- Genetic diseases with lung symptoms (e.g., cystic fibrosis, Birt-Hogg-Dubé syndrome).

MUST SEE

Tumors and nonneoplastic lesions are both are high-yield topics. For nonneoplastic lesions, it may be helpful to correlate gross findings with radiologic findings, some of which may be pathognomonic (e.g., honeycombing).

- The main tumors are:
  - Adenocarcinoma in situ and minimally invasive adenocarcinoma.
  - Adenocarcinoma and histological variants.
  - Contrast metastatic adenocarcinoma to lung primary adenocarcinoma.
  - Squamous cell carcinoma and variants.
  - Typical and atypical neuroendocrine tumor (NET), large cell neuroendocrine carcinoma, and small cell carcinoma.
  - NUT carcinoma.
  - Sclerosing pneumocytoma.
  - Pulmonary hamartoma.
  - PEComatous tumors.
  - Inflammatory myofibroblastic tumor.
  - Synovial sarcoma.
  - MALT lymphoma.
  - Langerhans cell histiocytosis.
  - Metastatic carcinoma, sarcoma, and melanoma (don't forget about these).
  - Malignant mesothelioma.
  - Solitary fibrous tumor.
  - Thymoma and thymic carcinoma (see chapter 13).
- The main nonneoplastic lesions are:
  - Pulmonary infections including bacterial-, viral-, fungal-, and mycobacterial-related changes.
  - Asthma.
  - Emphysema.
  - Chronic bronchitis.
  - Pulmonary edema.
  - Pulmonary alveolar proteinosis.
  - Pulmonary hemorrhage.
  - Bronchiectasis.
  - DAD.

- UIP.
- NSIP.
- RBILD.
- DIP.
- Cryptogenic organizing pneumonia.
- LIP.
- LAM.
- Fat emboli and foreign body emboli in the autopsy setting.
- Amyloidosis.
- Pulmonary hypertension.
- Pulmonary eosinophilic pneumonia.
- Asbestosis, pneumoconiosis.
- Sarcoidosis.
- Hypersensitivity pneumonitis.
- Granulomatous inflammation.

MUST DO

- For each of the entities outlined in the Must See section, you should be comfortable generating a differential diagnosis and listing additional studies (e.g., histochemical or immunohistochemical stains).

For entities that overlap other chapters, use the other chapters to complement this chapter.
- When studying in groups, practice:
  - Granulomatous diseases, including occupational safety aspects for frozen section and autopsy when it comes to infectious causes.
  - Metastatic tumors to the lung.
  - Interstitial pneumonia, and how to use clinical history and radiologic findings to aid in your diagnosis.
  - Recent advances in lung biomarker testing.
  - Adenocarcinoma versus pleural mesothelioma.
- You should be able to describe the grossing protocol, and independently gross, the following specimens:
  - Core biopsy of lung.
  - Surgical resections: wedge resection, segmentectomy, lobectomy, pneumonectomy.
  - Pleural biopsy.
- You should be able to describe and handle a frozen section of a lung nodule with possible infectious etiology.
- You should be able to describe and perform taking a lung tumor specimen for ancillary and molecular studies.

MULTIPLE CHOICE QUESTIONS

1. Which statement about desmoplastic small round cell tumors is true?

a. They are a variant of small cell carcinoma.

b. They most often present as solitary nodules or masses arising from the lung parenchyma.

c. They are indolent neoplasms with a relatively

good prognosis for patients.

d. The tumor cells are positive for cytokeratin (AE1/AE3) and desmin.

e. The tumor cells are positive for S100 and/or neuroendocrine markers.

Answer: d

2. Which statement is true about diffuse idiopathic pulmonary neuroendocrine cell hyperplasia?

a. It is regarded as a preinvasive lesion.

b. It mainly involves the alveolar wall.

c. It is a congenital disorder.

d. It is mainly seen in individuals with a history of smoking.

e. It is positive for S100.

Answer: a

3. Which statement about respiratory papilloma is **incorrect**?

a. It is a papillary lesion covered by squamous or mixed squamous and columnar epithelium.

b. Dysplasia can occur but only in the squamous epithelium.

c. It is associated with human papillomavirus.

d. It often arises from the alveolar wall.

e. It presents as an endobronchial lesion.

Answer: d

4. Which statement about pulmonary hamartoma is **incorrect**?

a. Pulmonary hamartoma is a benign neoplasm.

b. Pulmonary hamartoma is composed of at least 2 mesenchymal elements (chondroid, fat, connective tissue, etc.) with

entrapped respiratory epithelium.

c. Cellular atypia is usually present.

d. Surgical resection is the treatment of choice.

e. Grossly, it is a firm well-circumscribed nodule.

Answer: c

5. All the following *EGFR* mutations are sensitive to first generation tyrosine kinase inhibitors (TKIs) for lung adenocarcinomas **except**:

a. Exon 18 mutation.
b. Exon 19 mutation.
c. Exon 21 L858R mutation.
d. Exon 20 T790M mutation.
e. Exon 21 L861Q mutation.

Answer: d

6. Which statement about molecular abnormalities in lung cancer is **incorrect**?

a. *ALK* translocations are associated with nonsmoking.
b. *KRAS* and *EGFR* mutations are usually mutually exclusive.
c. *KRAS* mutations are found more often in smokers.
d. *ROS1* and *ALK* translocations are associated with an increased expression of their protein.
e. Molecular analysis is performed only in nonsmoker patients.

Answer: e

7. Which statement about neuroendocrine tumors is correct?

a. Carcinoid tumors are strongly associated with smoking.
b. Typical carcinoid tumors show no necrosis and < 2 mitoses per 2 mm².
c. The presence of necrosis is always associated with a high grade tumor (large cell neuroendocrine tumor [LCNEC] or small cell lung carcinoma [SCLC]).
d. Ki 67 staining is key for the differential diagnostic between atypical carcinoid and LCNEC.
e. Small cell carcinomas are p40 positive.

Answer: b

8. Which of these statements about diagnostic features of minimally invasive adenocarcinoma is **incorrect**?

a. It is a small tumor, measuring < 3 cm.
b. Lepidic architecture is predominant.
c. Invasive component measures 5 mm in greatest dimension.
d. Any histologic subtype other than a lepidic pattern (such as acinar, papillary, micropapillary, solid, colloid) is considered invasive.
e. Spreading through air spaces is not considered an invasive pattern.

Answer: e

9. Which statement about lymphangioleiomyomatosis is **incorrect**?

a. Stain for estrogen receptor (ER) is often positive.
b. Almost all patients are female.
c. Characteristic radiologic changes are multiple small nodular lesions in the lung.
d. The lesional cells are usually HMB-45 positive.
e. It could be associated with tuberous sclerosis.

Answer: c

10. All of the following statements about pulmonary Langerhans cell histiocytosis are correct **except**:

a. Almost all patients have a history of cigarette smoking.
b. It is considered a malignant disorder.
c. The lesional cells have nuclear grooves and slightly eosinophilic cytoplasm.
d. Positive CD1a is characteristic.
e. Lesions are bronchiolocentric.

Answer: b

11. All of the following statements about minute meningothelioid nodules are correct **except**:

a. They are usually an incidental finding.
b. They have no clinical significance.
c. They are usually located around venues at the peripheral zones of the lung.
d. They used to be known as chemodectoma.
e. The lesional cells are usually positive for neuroendocrine markers.

Answer: e

12. Which statement about asthma is **incorrect**?

a. The immediate response of an asthmatic attack is mediated by IgA.
b. Both intrinsic and extrinsic types exist.
c. The mechanism of the disorder is mainly type 1 hypersensitivity reaction.
d. The precipitating factors include allergens, chemical agents, fungal organisms, and drugs.
e. Asthma is a chronic relapsing inflammatory disorder.

Answer: a

13. Which statement about the pulmonary immune response is correct?

a. Soluble antigens elicit a significant increase in the number of phagocytic cells.

b. Particulate antigens cause rapid increase in antigen presenting cell activities especially by dendritic cells.

c. Particulate antigens are associated with immune responses

characterized by antigen elimination and immune diversion.

d. Soluble antigens trigger antigen presenting cell activities only at a high volume of soluble antigens.

e. Soluble antigens are rapidly ingested by alveolar macrophages.

Answer: c

14. Which statement is true for hypersensitivity pneumonitis?

a. It is a type I hypersensitivity reaction.

b. Presence of poorly formed granuloma is a feature.

c. Presence of numerous eosinophils is a feature.

d. It is mainly seen in pediatric patients.

e. It is an acute disease process.

Answer: b

15. Which statement about the immunopathology of asthma is correct?

a. The immediate immune response is mediated by IgG.

b. Atopy is the strongest risk factor for the development of asthma.

c. Chronic lymphocytic inflammation is part of the disease process

and is predominantly Th1 subset cells.

d. Only type I hypersensitivity reaction is involved in an asthmatic attack.

e. IL-2 is the key cytokine involved in IgE synthesis.

Answer: b

16. Which statement about asthma is correct?

a. Asthma occurs in atopic and non-atopic forms.

b. It is mainly a type II hypersensitivity reaction.

c. Macrophages are the main antigen presenting cells.

d. Formation of Charcot-Leyden crystals is mainly related to alveolar macrophages.

e. The mediators and cytokines causing asthma attacks are mainly released from eosinophils.

Answer: a

17. All of the following statements about eosinophilic granulomatosis with polyangiitis (Churg-Strauss syndrome) are correct **except**:

a. Asthma is a common clinical presentation.

b. It presents with necrotizing granulomatous vasculitis.

c. It presents with peripheral eosinophilia with eosinophils making up > 10% of the white

blood cell differential count.

d. It is usually c-ANCA positive (ANCA: antineutrophil cytoplasmic antibody).

e. Bronchoalveolar lavage shows a high percentage of eosinophils (often > 30%).

Answer: d

18. Common pulmonary involvement in Behcet syndrome includes all of the following **except**:

a. Atelectasis.

b. Aneurysm.

c. Arteriobronchial fistulas.

d. Pulmonary infarcts.

e. Lymphocytic and necrotizing vasculitis.

Answer: a

19. Diffuse panbronchiolitis has all of the following features **except**:

a. Chronic sinusitis in the majority of patients.

b. Marked elevation of serum cold agglutinins.

c. Interstitial foamy macrophages.

d. Japanese heritage in the majority of patients.

e. Usually, elevated immunoglobulin levels.

Answer: e

20. All of the following statements about pulmonary botryomycosis are correct **except**:

a. It is an infection caused by nonfilamentous bacteria.

b. Most cases occur in immunocompromised individuals.

c. Sulfur granules are present.

d. It is diagnosed based on the presence of

granules that consist of gram-positive cocci or gram-negative bacilli.

e. It can take the form of endobronchial infections, tumor-like lesions, and diffuse pneumonia.

Answer: b

21. All the following pathologic lesions/disorders are related to silica dust exposure **except**:

a. Pulmonary alveolar proteinosis.

b. Caplan syndrome.

c. Lung cancer or mesothelioma.

d. Mixed dust pneumoconiosis.

e. Progressive massive fibrosis.

Answer: c

22. Which statement about rounded atelectasis is **incorrect**?

a. It is caused by localized obstruction of a small airway.

b. It is a pleural based lesion.

c. It is related to asbestos exposure.

d. It is accompanied by marked pleural and septal fibrosis.

e. Most patients are asymptomatic.

Answer: a

23. Which statement about acute interstitial pneumonia is correct?

a. It is an acute stage of viral pneumonia.

b. Antibiotic treatment is usually effective.

c. High fever is usually a common symptom.

d. Mechanical ventilation is most likely required.

e. Significant increase of lymphocytes in the blood is characteristic.

Answer: d

24. Which of following statements about pulmonary alveolar proteinosis is correct?

a. It is a disorder of protein metabolism.

b. The main etiology is related to viral infection.

c. It may be a presentation of acute silicosis.

d. The characteristic finding in electromicroscopic examination is Birbeck granules.

e. The most common clinical presentation is respiratory failure.

Answer: c

25. Which of the following is not a shared feature of diffuse alveolar damage and left heart failure?

a. Difficult breathing.

b. Pulmonary arterial wedge pressure > 18 mmHg.

c. Diffuse and bilateral ground-glass opacities on radiologic images.

d. Absence of leg edema (usually).

e. Pulmonary edema (possible).

Answer: b

26. The following statements describe Birt-Hogg-Dubé syndrome **except**:

a. It is an autosomal dominant disorder.

b. There is pulmonary cyst formation.

c. Benign tumors occur in the head and neck.

d. Pneumonthorax is a complication.

e. If a renal cell carcinoma has developed, the most common type is clear cell renal cell carcinoma.

Answer: e

27. The following statements about the pulmonary lymphatic system are correct **except**:

a. The lymphatic distribution is around bronchial vascular bundles, and along the septa and the pleura.

b. The lymphatics are very rich in the alveolar septa.

c. Chylothorax is mainly caused by damage of the thoracic duct.

d. The lymphoid tissue shows decreasing levels of complexity toward the alveolus.

e. Some people have intraparenchymal or subpleural lymph nodes.

Answer: b

28. What is the most common pulmonary histologic change in cystic fibrosis patients?

a. Dilatation of the small airways with inflammation.

b. Centriacinar emphysema.

c. Pleural effusion.

d. Lung cancer.

e. Eosinophilic pneumonia.

Answer: a

29. The most common pulmonary histologic change in chronic rejection after lung transplant is:

a. Significant peribronchial lymphocytic infiltrate.

b. Significant perivascular lymphocytic infiltrate.

c. Organizing pneumonia.

d. Constrictive bronchiolitis.

e. Diffuse pulmonary interstitial fibrosis.

Answer: d

SHORT ANSWER QUESTIONS
Tumors of the Lung
ADENOCARCINOMA

30. List the 5 main architectural patterns of lung adenocarcinomas.
- Lepidic adenocarcinoma.
- Acinar adenocarcinoma.
- Papillary adenocarcinoma.
- Micropapillary adenocarcinoma.
- Solid adenocarcinoma.

31. What are the diagnostic criteria and clinical significance for micropapillary adenocarcinoma?
- As the major component, tumor cells grow in papillary tufts that lack fibrovascular cores, floating within the alveolar space.
- This component must be distinguished from spread through air spaces (STAS).
- The micropapillary subtype is a poor prognosis factor for overall survival and for recurrence in patients with limited resections.

32. List 3 immunohistochemical stains usually positive for primary lung adenocarcinoma.
- Thyroid transcription factor-1 (TTF-1) (about 70–75%).
- Napsin-A (about 80%).
- Cytokeratin 7 (CK7).

33. What is the significance of TTF-1 staining in lung cancer?
- Poorly differentiated carcinoma: TTF-1 nuclear staining favors lung adenocarcinoma (around 75% positive); it is typically negative in squamous cell carcinoma.
- Adenocarcinoma: TTF-1 nuclear staining favors primary lung origin; it is usually negative in lung metastases (except for thyroid origin).
- Neuroendocrine tumor: TTF-1 nuclear staining favors high grade neuroendocrine carcinoma such as small cell carcinoma (~90%) or large cell neuroendocrine carcinomas (~50%); it is usually negative in carcinoids.

34. What is the definition and clinical significance of lung adenocarcinoma spread through air spaces (STAS)?
- Definition: STAS consists of free-floating tumor cell clusters or single tumor cells that are present in air spaces, in the surrounding lung parenchyma, beyond the edge of the tumor.
- Clinical significance: STAS represents tumor aerogenous spread and is considered as a pattern of invasion. It is associated with increased rate of locoregional recurrence for patients with early stage adenocarcinomas who undergo sublobar lung resection (wedge, segmentectomy).

35. List the 2 architectural patterns of lung adenocarcinoma associated with poorer prognosis.
- Solid adenocarcinoma.
- Micropapillary adenocarcinoma.

SQUAMOUS CELL CARCINOMA

36. List the 3 main subtypes of squamous cell carcinoma.
- Keratinizing squamous cell carcinoma.
- Nonkeratinizing squamous cell carcinoma.
- Basaloid squamous cell carcinoma.

37. List 3 immunohistochemical stains usually positive for squamous cell carcinoma (in contrast to adenocarcinoma).
- High molecular weight keratin, such as cytokeratin 5/6 (CK5/6).
- P63.
- P40.

38. What are the main entities in the differential diagnosis for lung squamous cell carcinoma?
- Metastatic squamous cell carcinoma from the upper gastrointestinal tract or the head and neck — there is no specific immunohistochemical marker for a lung primary.
- Metastatic urothelial carcinoma, more often GATA3+ and CK20+.
- Thymic squamous cell carcinoma when there is involvement of the anterior mediastinum.
- Squamous metaplasia in peripheral lung parenchyma following diffuse alveolar damage.

39. What are the main histological features of basaloid squamous cell carcinoma?

- Architecture: solid of trabecular growth, peripheral palisading, possible rosettes.
- Abrupt keratinization (without progressive squamous differentiation).
- Small monomorphic cells, hyperchromatic nuclei, absent/small nucleoli.

- High mitotic rate.
- Comedo-type necrosis.
- Immunostains: p40+, p63+, CK5/6+; no expression of TTF-1 or neuroendocrine markers.

Note: tumors showing > 50% of basaloid component are classified as basaloid squamous cell carcinoma.

40. What are the main entities in the differential diagnosis for basaloid squamous cell carcinoma?

- Neuroendocrine carcinomas (small cell, large cell).
- Poorly differentiated squamous cell carcinoma or adenocarcinoma.

- Adenoid cystic carcinoma.
- NUT carcinoma.

PREINVASIVE LESIONS AND EARLY ADENOCARCINOMA OF THE LUNG

41. Compare the diagnostic criteria and prognosis of adenocarcinoma in situ (AIS) and minimally invasive adenocarcinoma (MIA).

AIS	MIA
• Solitary tumor with a pure lepidic growth. • Size ≤ 3 cm. • No invasion: stromal, vascular, pleural invasion or invasive pattern (i.e., acinar, papillary, micropapillary, solid, etc.) or STAS (spread through air spaces). • Prognosis: 100% disease-free survival if the lesion is completely resected.	• Solitary tumor with a predominant lepidic growth. • Size ≤ 3 cm. • Invasive component ≤ 0.5 cm (includes stromal invasion and invasive architectural patterns). • Exclusion criteria: · Invasion of vessels, air spaces or pleura. · Tumor necrosis. · STAS (spreads through air spaces). • Prognosis: 100% disease-free survival if the lesion is completely resected.

42. What are the diagnostic criteria for squamous cell carcinoma in situ?

- It involves the full thickness of the epithelium, without maturation.
- Large cells with marked anisokaryosis and pleomorphism are present.

- Increased nuclear-cytoplasmic ratio, coarse chromatin, and nuclear angulations and folding are present.
- Mitotic figures are present through the full thickness.

43. List the diagnostic criterion and describe the clinical significance of diffuse idiopathic pulmonary neuroendocrine cell hyperplasia (DIPNECH).

- Diagnostic criterion: generalized proliferation of pulmonary neuroendocrine cells is present in the mucosa of airways.
- Clinical significance:
  · These lesions may be incidental findings or associated with chronic respiratory symptoms (asthma-like).

- · DIPNECH is a chronic slowly progressive disease. Neuroendocrine cells may invade locally to form tumorlets (frequent) or develop into carcinoid tumors (usually typical).

PULMONARY NEUROENDOCRINE TUMORS

44. List and describe the diagnostic criteria of the 4 main categories of neuroendocrine tumors.

- Typical carcinoid: neuroendocrine epithelial malignancy with < 2 mitoses per 2 mm^2 and lacking necrosis.
- Atypical carcinoid: carcinoid tumors with 2–10 mitoses per 2 mm^2 and/or foci of necrosis.
- Large cell neuroendocrine carcinoma: nonsmall-cell lung cancer (NSCLC) that shows neuroendocrine morphology and expresses immunohistochemical neuroendocrine markers (at least 1 positive marker with clear cut staining in > 10% of tumor cells is mandatory).

- Small cell carcinoma: malignant epithelial malignancy that consists of small cells with scant cytoplasm, poorly defined cell borders, fine chromatin nuclear molding, and absent or inconspicuous nuclei. Most of them show crushed artifacts, extensive necrosis, high mitotic rate, and expression of neuroendocrine markers.

45. What is a combined small cell carcinoma?

- It is the admixture of small cell carcinoma with components of any type of nonsmall-cell carcinoma (e.g., adenocarcinoma, squamous cell carcinoma).
- For combined small cell and large cell carcinoma, large cells should make up at least 10% of the cells present.

46. What is the difference between a large cell neuroendocrine carcinoma, an NSCLC with neuroendocrine differentiation, and a large cell carcinoma with neuroendocrine morphology?

- Large cell neuroendocrine carcinoma is an NSCLC that shows neuroendocrine morphology **and** expresses immunohistochemical neuroendocrine markers.
- NSCLC with neuroendocrine differentiation is an NSCLC (adenocarcinoma, squamous cell carcinoma or large cell carcinoma) without neuroendocrine morphology but that demonstrates neuroendocrine differentiation by immunohistochemistry (IHC) or on electron microscopy.
- Large cell carcinoma with neuroendocrine morphology has neuroendocrine morphology and negative neuroendocrine markers.

47. What are the main diagnostic criteria for neuroendocrine cell hyperplasia, tumorlet, and carcinoid?

- Neuroendocrine cell hyperplasia: proliferation of neuroendocrine cells confined to the epithelium of the airways without penetration through the basement membrane.
- Tumorlet: proliferation of neuroendocrine cells in the bronchioles, extending into surrounding tissue and measuring ≤ 0.5 cm in size.
- Carcinoid: proliferation of neuroendocrine cells that forms a nodular lesion measuring > 0.5 cm in size.

48. List the 3 commonly used neuroendocrine immunomarkers, and comment on subcellular location and usefulness.

- Chromogranin: this provides cytoplasmic staining (secretory vesicles); it is specific but not sensitive for neuroendocrine cells; it is more sensitive in carcinoid tumors than high grade neuroendocrine tumors; it is focal or weak when positive in small cell carcinomas.
- Synaptophysin: this provides cytoplasmic staining; it has good specificity for neuroendocrine tumors.
- CD56: this provides mostly membrane staining; it is the most sensitive and the least specific; it should be interpreted only with the appropriate morphological context.

OTHER EPITHELIAL TUMORS

49. What is large cell carcinoma?

- It is undifferentiated nonsmall-cell carcinoma.
- It is a diagnosis of exclusion: large cell carcinoma lacks the architectural, cytological, and immunohistochemical features of small cell carcinoma, adenocarcinoma, and squamous cell carcinoma.
- Diagnosis requires resected tumors.

Note: for a small sample (biopsy/cytology), the appropriate terminology would be *nonsmall-cell carcinoma, not otherwise specified*.

50. What are the diagnostic criteria of adenosquamous carcinoma?

- It is an admixture of adeno and squamous cell carcinoma components.
- Each component is > 10% of the tumor.
- It may be suggested on small specimen, but definite diagnosis requires a resection specimen.

51. How is pleomorphic carcinoma distinguished from carcinosarcoma?

- Pleomorphic carcinoma is a poorly differentiated carcinoma composed of any type of non–small cell carcinoma (adenocarcinoma, squamous cell carcinoma) that contains ≥ 10% spindle and/or giant cells, or a carcinoma consisting only of spindle and giant cells. Expression of epithelial markers (such as keratin, TTF-1, p40) in the pleomorphic elements help the diagnosis. These tumors are aggressive, often high stage and are associated with a poor prognosis.
- Carcinosarcoma consists of a mixture of nonsmall-cell carcinoma (more often squamous cell carcinoma) and sarcoma-containing heterologous elements, such as rhabdomyosarcoma, chondrosarcoma, and osteosarcoma. The prognosis is usually poor.

52. What are classic histologic features of pulmonary blastoma?

- It has a biphasic pattern.
- The primitive epithelial component presents as a malignant gland growing in tubules that resemble fetal bronchioles.
- The tubules/glands are lined by pseudostratified, nonciliated columnar cells and often have subnuclear or supranuclear vacuoles giving an endometrioid appearance.
- The primitive epithelial component is embedded in a sarcomatous mesenchyme with an embryonic appearance, composed of small oval and spindle cells in a myxoid stroma. Foci of rhabdomyosarcoma, chondrosarcoma or osteosarcoma may be present.

53. What are the histological features of lymphoepithelioma-like carcinoma? What is its clinical significance?

- This is a poorly differentiated carcinoma with a syncytial pattern of growth, large tumor cells with prominent nucleoli, marked lymphocytic infiltrate, and pushing borders.
- IHC shows a squamous lineage (p40, p63, CK5/6).
- The presence of EBV in the epithelial tumor cells is detected by EBER1 in situ hybridization.
- Lymphoepithelioma-like carcinoma is a rare tumor (< 1%). The overall survival is better than other carcinomas.

54. Define NUT carcinoma and describe its main clinical, histological, and genetic features.

- Definition: this is an aggressive, poorly differentiated carcinoma associated with a rearrangement in the *NUT* gene.
- Clinical features: it manifests as a large mass extending into hilar structures (referred to as "NUT midline carcinoma").
  · It often presents at advanced stages that are not eligible for surgery. The prognosis is usually poor.
- Histopathology: it features sheets and nests of intermediate monomorphic cells with prominent nucleoli. Focally abrupt foci of keratinization may be seen. Infiltrating neutrophils are often prominent.
- IHC: variable results are obtained with epithelial markers. Squamous markers (i.e., p40) are more often expressed than TTF-1 or neuroendocrine markers. Diffuse nuclear staining is present with NUT antibody.
- Genetic features: it involves a chromosomal translocation between the *NUT* gene (*NUTM1*) on chromosome 15q14 and different partners (i.e., *BRD4*, *BRD3*).

55. List and define the 4 salivary gland-type tumors occurring in the lung.

- Mucoepidermoid carcinoma: it consists of mucin-secreting cells, squamous/squamoid cells, and intermediate-type cells.
- Adenoid cystic carcinoma: it consists of epithelial and myoepithelial cells. Architecture may be cribriform, tubular, and solid.
- Epithelial-myoepithelial carcinoma: this is a low grade malignant tumor consisting of an inner layer of duct-like structures of epithelial cells and a surrounding layer of myoepithelial cells with spindle, clear cell, or plasmacytoid features.
- Pleomorphic adenoma: this is a benign tumor consisting of epithelial cells and modified myoepithelial cells intermingled with myxoid or chondroid stroma.

56. List and define the 3 types of papillomas of the lung.

- Squamous cell papilloma: papillary tumor with arborizing fibrovascular cores covered by stratified squamous epithelium.
- Glandular papilloma: papillary tumor lined by stratified/pseudostratified columnar epithelium (interspersed ciliated and mucinous cells may be present).
- Mixed squamous cell and glandular papilloma: papillary tumor with a mixed squamous and glandular epithelium (≥ 1/3).

Note: all 3 lesions are benign and endobronchial. Complete excision should be curative.

57. Describe the 2 neoplastic cells types present in sclerosing pneumocytoma.

- Cuboidal surface cells: these are similar to type II pneumocytes (they may have intranulclear inclusions and vacuolated cytoplasm). They are positive for pancytokeratin, epithelial membrane antigen, TTF-1, and napsin-A.
- Round stromal cells: these are bland cells with well-defined borders and often eosinophilic cytoplasm. They are positive for TTF-1 and epithelial membrane antigen, and usually negative for pancytokeratin.

58. List the 4 growth patterns of a sclerosing pneumocytoma.

- Most tumors have at least 3 of 4 primary growth patterns:
  · Solid.
  · Papillary.
  · Sclerosing.
  · Hemorrhagic.

MESENCHYMAL TUMORS

59. What is pulmonary hamartoma?

- It is the most common benign neoplasm.
- It most often manifests as peripheral, solitary, usually asymptomatic lesions, and approximately 10% present endobronchially.
- They are composed of varying amounts of at least 2 mesenchymal elements (chondroid or chondromyxoid tissue, fat, myxoid fibrous connective tissue, etc.) combined with entrapped respiratory epithelium.
- IHC is not usually necessary for diagnosis.

60. Define the 3 main forms of PEComatous tumors. What is the cell of origin and associated IHC of these cells?

- Cell of origin: perivascular epithelioid cells (PECs).
- IHC: PECs typically stain for melanocytic markers (HMB-45, Melan A, Mitf) and myogenic markers (actin, myosin). They may also be estrogen receptor (ER) and progesterone receptor (PR) positive.
- The 3 forms are:
  - Lymphangioleiomyomatosis (LAM): this is the most frequent form with a diffuse multicystic proliferation, now considered a low grade neoplasm (clonal nature, mutations in the *TSC2* gene with an invasive and metastatic potential). It occurs most commonly in women with pneumothorax, either sporadically or in association

with tuberous sclerosis. Histologically, it consists of thin-walled cysts with proliferation of plump spindle-shaped "myoid" cells.
  - PEComa (or clear cell tumor): this is a well-circumscribed, peripheral, localized, solitary lesion. Histologically, it consists of rounded/oval cells with clear or eosinophilic cytoplasm (glycogen-rich, PAS+), forming solid sheets around sinusoidal blood vessels. PEComas of the lung are usually cured by excision.
  - Diffuse proliferation with overlapping features between lymphangioleiomyomatosis and clear cell tumor (exceptional).

61. Describe the histopathological features of inflammatory myofibroblastic tumor.

- Monomorphic spindle cells, arranged in a fascicular pattern, with pale eosinophilic cytoplasm and ovoid vesicular nuclei, with myofibroblastic differentiation (positive for SMA and desmin).
- Chronic inflammatory infiltrate with numerous plasma cells.
- ALK1 positivity and *ALK* gene rearrangement in ~50% of cases.

Note: these tumors are usually cured by resection.

LYMPHOHISTIOCYTIC TUMORS

Note: most lymphohistiocytic tumors of the lung are morphologically similar to those in other sites (see chapter 13 on hematological pathology). Specificity of lung lymphomas is emphasized.

62. Describe the main histopathological features of a pulmonary extranodal marginal zone lymphoma of mucosa-associated lymphoid tissue (MALT lymphoma).

- Diffuse infiltration of small B cells (with possible plasmacytoid differentiation) with the following immunoprofile: CD20+, CD79a+, BCL-2+, often CD43+, CD10–, CD23– and Bcl-6–.
- Reactive follicles, which are best seen when highlighted by IHC (CD21).
- Lymphoepithelial lesions, which are frequently observed but are not pathognomonic (may be seen in benign lesions).

63. Describe the main clinical and histopathological features of lymphomatoid granulomatosis.

- This is a rare disorder occurring in immunocompromised patients.
- It is considered an EBV-associated B-cell lymphoproliferative disorder, with a prominent background T-cell reaction.
- It consists of bilateral, multiple, poorly defined pulmonary nodules/masses.
- A polymorphous lymphoid infiltrate is present with 2 key features:
  - Angiocentric location, with transmural involvement.
  - Large EBV-positive B cells (on EBER in situ hybridization), with immunoblastic-like or Reed-Sternberg-like features.

64. Describe the main clinical, histopathological, and genetic features of the pulmonary Langerhans cell histiocytosis (PLCH).

- PLCH presents as an interstitial lung disease or with spontaneous pneumothorax. It is highly associated with smoking.
- It consists of cellular proliferations of Langerhans cells along small airways (bronchiolocentric) with rounded or stellate nodules.
- Langerhans cells are positive for S100 and CD1a.
- In healed cases (one-fourth are asymptomatic), the diagnosis may be raised based on the presence of stellate centrilobular stellate scars.
- V600E mutations in the *BRAF* gene have been described in some cases.

65. Describe the main histopathological features of Erdheim-Chester disease.

- It consists of lipid-laden foamy histiocytes (CD68+, CD1a-) and giant cells infiltration along the distribution of the pulmonary lymphatics: visceral pleura, bronchovascular bundles, and interlobular septa.
- It is associated with fibrosis and chronic inflammation.
- *BRAF* V600E mutations have been detected in half of the patients.

METASTATIC CANCER IN THE LUNG

66. How do you differentiate primary from secondary metastatic adenocarcinoma?

FEATURE	PRIMARY	METASTATIC
Clinical history	• Smoking status.	• History of another primary tumor.
CT and gross analyses	• Spiculated edge. • Often single.	• Demarked/smooth edge. • More often multiple.
Micro	• Often mixed patterns. • Possible presence of in situ component (i.e., lepidic pattern).	• Morphology reminding a nonlung primary (i.e.,enteric, endometrioid). • Comparison with the primary tumor.
IHC	• TTF-1+. • CK7+/CK20 +/–. • Napsin-A+.	• CK7–/CK20+/CDX2+: colorectal cancer. • TTF-1+/thyroglobulin+/PAX8+: thyroid cancer. • ER+/PR+/GATA3+/mammaglobin+: breast cancer. • PSA+/PAP+/NKX3.1+: prostate cancer. • PLAP+/AFP+/SALL4+: germ cell tumor. • AFP+/HepPar1+/arginase1+/glypican3+: hepatocellular carcinoma.

Abbreviations: AFP: α1-fetoprotein; CT: computed tomography; PAP: prostatic acid phosphatase; PLAP: placental alkaline phosphatase; PSA: prostate specific antigen.

GROSSING AND SAMPLING OF LUNG CANCER

67. List the main parameters for describing a lung resection specimen for a primary lung cancer.

- Type of resection: pneumonectomy, lobectomy, segmentectomy, wedge.
- Pleural puckering.
- Presence of additional tissue: parietal pleura, chest wall, mediastinal pleura, azygos vein, etc.
- Unique/multiple lesions.
- Tumor location: central/peripheral, segment involved.
- Tumor size, necrosis, appearance.
  - If multiple lesions are present, all lesions should be described separately, with the distance between the lesions.
- Tumor relationship with the visceral pleura.
- Tumor relationship with airways.
- Distance of tumor to margins.
  - Lobectomy/pneumonectomy: bronchial, vascular.
  - Segmentectomy or extended lobectomy (lobectomy + wedge): bronchial, vascular, parenchymal.
  - Wedge resection: parenchymal.
- Nontumoral parenchyma (obstructive pneumonitis, fibrosis, emphysema, etc.).
- Lymph nodes: on the specimen (mainly N1), on separate containers for N2 stations.

68. List the main sampling required for a lung resection specimen for a primary lung cancer.

- Margins: submit the bronchial and vascular margins, and the parenchymal margin (depending on the type of resection).
- Tumor:
  - One full slide is preferred for: 1) small tumors with possible lepidic component (allowing estimating the size of the invasive component), and 2) postneoadjuvant treatment (estimation of the percentage of viable tumor).
  - Sample tumor involvement with the pleura (peripheral tumors), surrounding parenchyma (STAS, LVI), and/or airways (central tumor).
- If multiple lesions are present, all separate lesions should be submitted, with nontumoral parenchyma between separate lesions.
- Additional tissue present; submit this to assess possible invasion (parietal pleura, chest wall, mediastinal pleura, azygos vein, etc.).
- Nontumoral parenchyma.
- Lymph nodes:
  - Sample lymph nodes on the specimen (mainly N1).
  - Submit lymph nodes in separate containers for interlobar, hilar, and N2 stations. The specimens are usually fragmented and difficult to count. All stations should be submitted separately.

69. Describe the lymph node map of the International Association for the Study of Lung Cancer (IASLC).

- N3 lymph nodes:
  - Supraclavicular zone:
    - › Station 1: low cervical, supraclavicular, and sternal notch nodes.
- N2 lymph nodes:
  - Upper zone:
    - › Station 2: upper paratracheal nodes.
    - › Station 3: prevascular and retrotracheal nodes.
    - › Station 4: lower paratracheal lymph nodes.
  - Aortopulmonary zone:
    - › Station 5: subaortic nodes.
    - › Station 6: para-aortic (ascending aorta or phrenic) nodes.
- Subcarinal zone:
  - › Station 7: subcarinal nodes.
- Lower zone:
  - › Station 8: paraesophageal (below carina) nodes.
  - › Station 9: pulmonary ligament nodes.
- N1 lymph nodes:
  - Hilar/interlobar zone:
    - › Station 10: hilar nodes.
    - › Station 11: interlobar nodes.
  - Peripheral zone:
    - › Station 12: lobar nodes.
    - › Station 13: segmental nodes.
    - › Station 14: subsegmental nodes.

PATHOLOGY REPORTS FOR LUNG CANCER, STAGING, AND FROZEN SECTIONS

70. What is the rationale for frozen sections for a lung nodule?

- To establish a cancer diagnosis on a wedge resection before doing further surgery (e.g., lobectomy).
- To evaluate resection margins: parenchymal (wedge resection, bronchial or vascular).
- To confirm or rule out metastatic lesions before doing further surgery.

71. List the main parameters for reporting lung cancer.

- Specimen: type, procedure, integrity, laterality.
- Tumor: site, focality.
- Tumor size (for nonmucinous adenocarcinomas with a lepidic component, the size of the invasive component is used for staging).
- Histologic type, according to the most recent World Health Organization (WHO) classification (including subtype and for adenocarcinoma semiquantitative recording of architectural patterns in 5% increments).
- Histologic grade (optional).
- Lymphatic and vascular invasion.
- STAS.
- Extension of tumor: visceral pleura invasion, other tissue attached (parietal pleura, chest wall, etc.).
- Resection margins (e.g., bronchial, vascular, parenchymal, other tissues).
- Lymph node status (each submitted stations should be reported separately including N1 and N2).
- Pathologic stage, according to the most recent staging system (IASLC/AJCC).
- Other tumor related findings such as multiple tumor lesions (location and nature), evidence of atelectasis (lobar or 1 side of lung), obstructive pneumonia, etc.
- Additional pathologic findings (nontumoral lung parenchyma).
- Ancillary studies.

72. What is the American Joint Committee on Cancer (AJCC) T staging for lung cancer?*

CATEGORY	INDICATOR
TX	• Primary tumor cannot be assessed. – **or** – • Tumor proven by presence of malignant cells in sputum or bronchial washings, but not visualized by imaging or bronchoscopy.
T0	• No evidence of primary tumor.
Tis	• Carcinoma in situ. · Squamous cell carcinoma in situ. · Adenocarcinoma in situ: a pure lepidic pattern ≤ 3 cm in greatest dimension.
T1	• Tumor ≤ 3 cm in greatest dimension surrounded by lung visceral pleura, without bronchoscopic evidence of invasion more proximal than the lobar bronchus (i.e., not in the main bronchus).
T1mi	• Minimally invasive adenocarcinoma: tumor ≤ 3 cm in greatest dimension with a predominantly lepidic pattern and ≤ 0.5 cm invasion in greatest dimension.
T1a	• Tumor ≤ 1 cm in greatest dimension. – **or** – • A superficial spreading tumor of any size whose invasive component is limited to the bronchial wall and may extend proximal to the main bronchus.
T1b	• Tumor > 1 cm but ≤ 2 cm in greatest dimension.
T1c	• Tumor > 2 cm but ≤ 3 cm in greatest dimension.
T2	• Tumor > 3 cm but ≤ 5 cm in greatest dimension. – **or** – • Tumor involves main bronchus, but without involvement of carina. – **or** – • Tumor invades visceral pleura. – **or** – • Associated with atelectasis or obstructive pneumonitis that extends to the hilar region, involving part or all of the lung. · T2a Above features if tumor ≤ 4 cm. · T2b Above features if tumor > 4 cm but ≤ 5 cm.
T2a	• Tumor > 3 cm but ≤ 4 cm in greatest dimension.
T2b	• Tumor > 4 cm but ≤ 5 cm in greatest dimension.
T3	• Tumor > 5 cm but ≤ 7 cm in greatest dimension. – **or** – • Tumor directly invades any of the following: parietal pleura, chest wall (including superior sulcus tumors), phrenic nerve, parietal pericardium. – **or** – • Separate tumor nodule(s) in same lobe as the primary.
T4	• Tumor > 7 cm in greatest dimension. – **or** – • Tumor of any size that invades any of the following: diaphragm, mediastinum, heart, great vessels, trachea, recurrent laryngeal nerve, esophagus, vertebral body, or carina. – **or** – • Separate tumor nodule(s) in an ipsilateral lobe different from that of the primary.

*This chapter uses the eighth edition of the AJCC classification.

73. What is the AJCC N staging for lung cancer?

CATEGORY	INDICATOR
Nx	• Regional lymph nodes cannot be assessed.
N0	• No regional lymph node metastasis.
N1	• Metastasis in ipsilateral peribronchial and/or ipsilateral hilar lymph nodes and intrapulmonary nodes, including involvement by direct extension.
N2	• Metastasis in ipsilateral mediastinal and/or subcarinal lymph node(s).
N3	• Metastasis in contralateral mediastinal, contralateral hilar, ipsilateral or contralateral scalene, or supraclavicular lymph node(s).

74. What is the AJCC M staging for lung cancer?

CATEGORY	INDICATOR
M0	• No distant metastasis.
M1a	• Separate tumor nodule(s) in contralateral lung. – or – • Tumor with pleural or pericardial nodules. – or – • Malignant pleural or pericardial effusion.
M1b	• Single extrathoracic metastasis in a single organ (including involvement of a single nonregional node).
M1c	• Multiple extrathoracic metastases in a single organ or in multiple organs.

75. List 3 situations of pleural extension with their respective staging.
- Direct invasion of the visceral pleura and < 4 cm: stage pT2a.
- Direct invasion of the parietal pleura and < 7 cm: stage pT3.
- Visceral or pericardial nodule(s), separate for the primary lung tumor: stage M1a.

76. How do you stage multiple lung carcinomas?
- Multiple primary lung carcinomas should be staged separately.
- Intrapulmonary metastases are staged according to the location of the metastatic nodule(s):
  - Separate tumor nodule(s) in same lobe as the primary: stage pT3.
  - Separate tumor nodule(s) in an ipsilateral lobe different from that of the primary: stage pT4.
  - Separate tumor nodule(s) in contralateral lung: stage M1a.

77. Define visceral pleural invasion, and describe PL1 and PL2 invasion, including their staging.
- Visceral pleural invasion is present when the tumor cells invade the visceral pleura **beyond** the external elastic layer.
- PL1 visceral pleural invasion does not extend to the visceral pleural surface.
- PL2 visceral pleural invasion does extend to the visceral pleural surface.
- PL1 and PL2 are staged pT2a.

78. What are the TNM stage groupings?

STAGE	T	N	M
Occult carcinoma	TX	N0	M0
0	Tis	N0	M0
IA1	T1mi	N0	M0
1A2	T1a	N0	M0
1A3	T1b	N0	M0
	T1c	N0	M0
IB	T2a	N0	M0
IIA	T2b	N0	M0
IIB	T1a	N1	M0
	T1b	N1	M0
	T1c	N1	M0
	T2a	N1	M0
	T2b	N1	M0
	T3	N0	M0
IIIA	T1a	N2	M0
	T1b	N2	M0
	T1c	N2	M0
	T2a	N2	M0
	T2b	N2	M0
	T3	N1	M0
	T4	N0 or N1	M0
IIIB	T1a	N3.	M0
	T1b	N3.	M0
	T1c	N3.	M0
	T2a	N3.	M0
	T2b	N3.	M0
	T3	N2.	M0
	T4	N2.	M0
IIIC	T3	N3.	M0
	T4	N3.	M0
IVA	Any T	Any N.	M1a or M1b
IVB	Any T	Any N	M1c

CLASSIFICATION IN SMALL BIOPSIES AND CYTOLOGY

79. Why is subtyping important in small biopsies and cytology specimens?

- Most lung cancers are inoperable and should be treated on the results of small biopsies and cytology specimens.
- It has been reported life-threatening hemorrhage for squamous cell carcinomas treated by bevacizumab (mAB targeting VEGF).
- Molecular studies should be initiated on small samples in case of adenocarcinoma.

80. List and define the 4 main categories of small biopsies and cytology specimens for adenocarcinoma and squamous cell carcinoma.

- Adenocarcinoma, __* pattern present: when the morphological adenocarcinoma pattern is clearly recognized. (*Note: describe the identifiable architectural pattern — i.e., acinar, papillary, etc.)
- Nonsmall-cell carcinoma, favor adenocarcinoma: when no differentiation is clearly recognized, but supported by IHC (e.g., TTF-1 positive/p40 negative).
- Squamous cell carcinoma: when morphological squamous cell patterns are clearly recognized (e.g., intercellular bridges, keratinization).
- Nonsmall-cell carcinoma, favor squamous cell carcinoma: when no differentiation is clearly recognized, but supported by IHC (e.g., p40 positive/TTF-1 negative).

Note: the term *nonsmall-cell carcinoma, not otherwise specified* should be used as little as possible, only when more specific diagnosis is not possible. In situ carcinoma and minimally invasive carcinomas cannot be diagnosed on a small biopsy.

81. When classifying a poorly differentiated carcinoma, a simple immunohistochemical panel using 2 antibodies is sufficient in most cases. What is included this panel?

- The panel includes TTF-1 for glandular differentiation and p40 for squamous differentiation.

- In small specimens, the tissue sample should be managed for diagnosis (H&E, IHC), biomarkers, and molecular testing (see note).

Note: when more than 1 fragment is present, it is useful to submit the material in 2 blocks: 1 block will be used for IHC and the other block will be spared for molecular analysis. Also, serial sections are not recommended for cancer diagnosis.

BIOMARKERS IN NONSMALL-CELL CARCINOMA OF THE LUNG

82. Describe the 3 main genetic alterations in lung adenocarcinoma, including analysis techniques and clinical significance.

	EGFR	ALK	ROS1
Alteration	• Activation mutation.	• Gene rearrangement.	• Gene rearrangement.
Most frequent alterations	• Exon 19 deletion. • Exon 21 Leu858Arg. • Exon 20 insertion or Thr790Met.	Most frequent fusion partners: • *EML4*. • *KIF5B*. • *TFG*.	Most frequent fusion partners: • *CD74*. • *EZR*. • *SDC4*. • *TPM3*.

Main analysis techniques	• PCR.
	• Sequencing.
	• Next-generation sequencing (NGS).
		• IHC: negative/positive/equivocal.
		• All equivocal cases should be confirmed by a molecular technique:
		  · FISH (break apart).
		– or –
		  · NGS (RNA).
			• IHC: negative/positive/equivocal.
			• All equivocal and positive case should be confirmed by a molecular technique:
			  · FISH (break apart).
			– or –
			  · NGS (RNA).

Clinical significance	• Exon 19 and 21: response to EGFR TKI. • Exon 20: resistance to EGFR TKI.	• Response to therapy with a targeted inhibitor, such as crizotinib and ceritinib.	• Response to therapy with a targeted inhibitor, such as crizotinib.

Note: other genes such as *KRAS*, *BRAF*, *NRAS*, *RET*, *MET*, *ERRB2* mutations, as well as other fusions such as *NTRK*, may be tested by NGS.

83. What are the recommended items to report for molecular biomarkers?

- Specimen adequacy and quality test (DNA quantity and quality).
- Tumor cell content (TCC): the percentage in either in the whole section or in the selected area when microdissection for tumor cell enrichment is needed.
- Specimen type (e.g., lung adenocarcinoma).
- Results of mutational analysis or rearrangement.
- Method used.
- Genes and exons or partners that have been assessed.

84. What are the most common *EGFR* mutations?

- Exon 19 deletion.
- Exon 21 Leu858Arg (L858R).
- Exon 20 insertion and Thr790Met.

85. What is the incidence of *KRAS* and *EGFR* mutations? Describe their clinical characteristics.

- *KRAS* mutations are the most common oncogenic alteration in lung adenocarcinoma in Western countries (North America and western Europe), occurring in about 20–30% of cases. The frequency is lower in East Asia (about 10% of cases). *KRAS* mutation is associated with smoking history.
- The frequency of *EGFR* mutations is about 10% in Western countries and up to 40–50% in East Asia. They are associated with nonsmokers and are more frequent in women.
- Mutations of *KRAS* and *EGFR* are typically mutually exclusive.

86. List the codons where the most common *KRAS* mutations occur.

- Codon 12.
- Codon 13.
- Codon 61.

87. What results in suboptimal specimens?
- Improper fixation, which could lead to failure of molecular techniques (under- or overfixation, improper fixative other than formalin, decalcification, etc.).
- Low tumor cell content — the cutoff for acceptable tumor content depends on the method used by the laboratory (usually around 10%).

Note: formalin-fixed, paraffin-embedded (FFPE) specimens or fresh, frozen, or alcohol-fixed specimens are appropriate for molecular testing. For cytology, cell blocks are preferred over smear preparations.

88. What are the 3 "must-test genes"? What are the main indications for testing?
- The must-test genes are *EGFR*, *ALK*, and *ROS1*.
- The main indications are advanced stage adenocarcinomas, large cell carcinomas, and carcinomas of mixed histology with an adenocarcinoma component, regardless of smoking status.
- Note also:
  · In early stages, no clear recommendations have been issued (reflex testing in early stages may be performed when available).
- Primary tumor or metastatic lesions are equally suitable for testing.
- In multiple primary lung adenocarcinomas, each tumor may be tested.
- Other histologies (squamous cell carcinoma, small cell tumors) may be tested when occurring in an unusual clinical context (young age, nonsmoker).

89. Describe the main indications, techniques, results, and clinical consequences of PD-L1 testing in NSCLC.
- Immunotherapy that targets PD-1 or PD-L1 by monoclonal antibodies is beneficial in highly immunogenic tumors, such as NSCLC expressing the PD-L1 protein.
- PD-L1 testing is indicated for all nonsmall-cell lung cancers (including squamous histology).
- The testing technique is IHC for PD-L1 expression, as a predictive biomarker for both PD-1 and PD-L1 inhibitors. Several companion diagnostic assays are available.
- Tumor Proportion Score (TPS) is reported with 1% increment.
- Patients whose tumors show a TPS ≥ 50% or TPS ≥ 1% are eligible for PD-1 inhibitor pembrolizumab in either first-line (in a metastatic setting) or second-line therapy, respectively.

90. What is the recommended turnaround time for molecular testing?
Molecular testing results should be available within 2 weeks (10 working days) of receiving the specimen in the testing laboratory.

91. What is the role of *KRAS* analysis in selecting patients for targeted therapy with EGFR TKIs?
- *KRAS* mutation testing is not recommended as a sole determinant of EGFR TKI therapy.
- Note also that, considering that *KRAS*, *EGFR* and *ALK* mutations are mutually exclusive, a *KRAS* mutated case will not be eligible to anti-*EGFR* or anti-*ALK* targeted therapy.

92. Which *EGFR* mutation is tested in the setting of an acquired EGFR TKI resistance?
Secondary *EGFR* T790M mutation.

93. What methods are used for *ALK* testing?
- ALK IHC: this is considered a screening method, with proper positive/negative controls. Results are given as: positive, negative, equivocal. All equivocal cases should be tested by a second technique (FISH or molecular).
- *ALK* FISH assay using dual-labeled break-apart probes.
- NGS: this may detect *ALK* gene rearrangement and its fusion partner.

Tumors of the Pleura

94. List 3 subtypes of malignant mesothelioma.
- Epithelioid.
- Sarcomatoid, including desmoplastic.
- Biphasic.

95. Describe key cytology features of malignant mesothelioma.
- The cytology specimen is usually cellular.
- Cells are arranged in sheets, clusters, morulae, and papillae in 3-dimensional configurations and sometimes with psammoma bodies.
- Features of mesothelial lineage are apparent (e.g., doublets and triplets of cells, apposing cell borders, cells clasping each other, dense biphasic cytoplasm with peripheral fading, clusters of cells with knobby or smooth contours).

(continued on next page)

- Cytologic appearance ranges from pleomorphic to bland, and often lacks the significant atypia seen in carcinoma.
- Differentiation of mesothelioma from benign mesothelial hyperplasia with reactive atypia may be very difficult or impossible in cytologic specimens.

96. How can IHC help differentiate malignant epithelioid mesothelioma from bronchogenic adenocarcinoma?

- On IHC, malignant epithelioid mesothelioma has:
  - Positive mesothelial markers: calretinin, CK5/6, WT1, D2-40.
  - Negative adenocarcinoma makers (see below).
  - Loss of expression of BAP1.
- On IHC, lung adenocarcinoma has:
  - Positive adenocarcinoma markers: TTF-1, napsin-A, BerEP4, MOC31, carcinoembryonic antigen (CEA) monoclonal, other tissue-specific markers (e.g., mammaglobin, PAX8).
  - Negative mesothelial markers.

97. What is the definition of localized malignant mesotheliomas?

- Its histological features are indistinguishable from diffuse malignant mesothelioma.
- It is a localized nodular lesion with no evidence of diffuse pleural spread.

Note: rare lesions with better prognosis than diffuse mesotheliomas may be cured by surgical excision.

98. How do you differentiate an epithelioid mesothelioma from atypical mesothelial hyperplasia?

	EPITHELIOID MESOTHELIOMA	ATYPICAL MESOTHELIAL HYPERPLASIA
Invasion (main, robust criterion)	• Invasion of deep tissue (fat, lung parenchyma, etc.).	• No invasion of the deep tissue.
General architecture (highlighted by pankeratin immunostain)	• Expansile nodules. • Complex/disorganized pattern. • More cellular in deep areas.	• Surface growth. • More cellular on surface. • Less cellular in deep areas.
Mesothelial cells	• Complex papillae. • Bland tumor cells. • Few mitoses.	• Simple papillae. • Cell atypia confined on surface. • Possible numerous mitoses.
Vessels	• Irregular organization.	• Perpendicular to the surface.
Necrosis	• Usually sign of malignancy.	• Absent.
BAP1 immunostain	• Loss of expression.	• No loss of expression.

99. How can IHC help differentiate sarcomatoid malignant mesothelioma from sarcomatoid carcinoma?

- Sarcomatoid malignant mesothelioma has no expression of adenocarcinoma markers; low expression of mesothelial markers calretinin, CK5/6, WT1, and D2-40; and loss of BAP1.
- Sarcomatoid carcinoma has no expression of mesothelial markers; and possible positivity for adenocarcinoma markers, including TTF-1, napsin-A, BerEP4, MOC31, CEA monoclonal, and other tissue-specific markers (e.g., mammaglobin, PAX8).
- Note that both tumors are pankeratin positive.

100. Describe key cytology features of desmoplastic mesothelioma.

- It has atypical spindle cells in a dense, hyalinized, fibrous patternless stroma constituting at least 50% of the tumor.
- Invasion of deep tissue is the most reliable criterion to distinguish desmoplastic mesothelioma from organizing pleuritis.
- Other criteria include bland necrosis, and cellular/sarcomatoid nodules.
- This diagnosis is very difficult, especially in small biopsies.

101. To diagnose a mesothelioma as biphasic, how much of the tumor should the epithelioid and sarcomatoid components represent?

Each component should represent ≥ 10% of the tumor.

102. What is a well-differentiated papillary mesothelioma?

- It is a rare tumor of mesothelial origin.
- It has papillary architecture (fibrous core) with a single-cell layer of bland mesothelial cells.
- It exhibits superficial growth, without invasion.
- It is an indolent tumor and a separate entity from diffuse epithelioid malignant mesothelioma.

103. What additional features should be looked for in the resection specimen?

- Asbestos bodies.
- Pleural plaques.
- Pulmonary interstitial fibrosis (asbestosis).
- Inflammation.

104. What is the pT classification of malignant pleural mesothelioma?

pTx: primary tumor cannot be assessed.

pT0: no evidence of primary tumor.

pT1: tumor limited to the ipsilateral parietal pleura with or without involvement of visceral, mediastinal or diaphragmatic pleura.

pT2: tumor involving each of the ipsilateral pleural surfaces (parietal, mediastinal, diaphragmatic, and visceral pleura) with at least 1 of the following:

   Involvement of the diaphragmatic muscle.

   Extension of tumor from the visceral pleura into the underlying pulmonary parenchyma.

pT3: locally advanced but potentially resectable tumor that involves all of the ipsilateral pleural surfaces (parietal, mediastinal, diaphragmatic, and visceral pleura) with at least 1 of the following:

   Involvement of the endothoracic fascia.

   Extension into mediastinal fat.

   Solitary completely resectable focus of tumor extending into the soft tissues of the chest wall.

   Nontransmural involvement of the pericardium.

pT4: locally advanced, technically unresectable tumor; tumor involving all of the ipsilateral pleural surfaces (parietal, mediastinal, diaphragmatic, and visceral pleura) with at least 1 of the following:

   Diffuse extension or multifocal masses of tumor in the chest wall, with or without associated rib destruction.

   Direct diaphragmatic extension of the tumor to the peritoneum.

   Direct extension of the tumor to the contralateral pleura.

   Direct extension of the tumor to a mediastinal organ.

   Direct extension of the tumor into the spine.

   Tumor extending through to the internal surface of the pericardium with or without a pericardial effusion, or tumor involving the myocardium.

Note: most malignant mesotheliomas show a nonresectable advanced stage and have poor prognosis.

105. What is the pN classification of malignant pleural mesothelioma?

pNx: regional lymph nodes cannot be assessed.

pN0: no regional lymph node metastases.

pN1: metastases in the ipsilateral bronchopulmonary, hilar, or mediastinal lymph nodes.

pN2: metastases in the contralateral mediastinal, ipsilateral, or contralateral supraclavicular lymph nodes.

106. What is the AJCC TNM staging of malignant pleural mesothelioma?

	PRIMARY TUMOR	LYMPH NODE METASTASIS	DISTANT METASTASIS
Stage I			
• Stage IA	T1	N0	N0
• Stage IB	T2 or T3	N0	N0
Stage II	T1 or T2	N1	M0
Stage III			
• Stage IIIA	T3	N1	M0
• Stage IIIB	T1–3	N2	M0
	T4	N0–2	M0
Stage IV	T0–4	N0–2	M1

107. What is a primary effusion lymphoma?

- It consists of a proliferation of large, HHV-8-positive, atypical B cells with immunoblastic appearance and plasma cell-like phenotype (CD20–, CD138+).
- It presents as an effusion in serous body cavities.
- It occurs in immunocompromised patients.

Note: EBV may be detected by in situ hybridization but LMP1 is indetectable (type I latency).

108. What is a diffuse large B-cell lymphoma associated with chronic inflammation (DLBCL-CI)?

- It is an EBV-associated B-cell neoplasm (type III latency with positivity for LMP1 and EBNA2).
- It occurs in body cavities in a context of long-standing chronic inflammation (e.g., chronic tuberculosis).

109. What are the main clinical and histopathological characteristics of a solitary fibrous tumor?

- It is a slow-growing neoplasm, arising from the visceral pleura.
- It has uniform fibroblastic spindle cells, hyalinization, and branching hemangiopericytoma-like vessels. Rare mitoses may be seen.
- On IHC, it is CD34+ (not specific) and STAS6 positive (the most sensitive and specific marker). Pankeratin is usually negative.

Note: local recurrence and metastasis may occur (10% of the cases). A high mitotic rate (> 4 mitoses per 2 mm²) is the most reliable indicator of aggressive behavior.

Tumors of the Thymus

110. List and define the 5 main thymoma subtypes in the WHO classification.*

- Type A thymoma: thymic epithelial neoplasm composed of bland spindle tumor cells, with few/no immature lymphocytes.
- Type AB thymoma: thymic epithelial neoplasm composed of an admixture of type A component and type B–like component (rich in immature T cells). A sharp separation of type A and type B–like areas is often present.
- Type B1 thymoma: thymic epithelial neoplasm that resembles the normal thymus with few dispersed epithelial cells (without clusters) in a dense background of immature T cells (cortex-like).
- Type B2 thymoma: thymic epithelial neoplasm with a minority of epithelial cells organized in small clusters in a dense background of immature T cells.
- Type B3 thymoma: thymic epithelial neoplasm composed of numerous epithelial cells (solid growth pattern) with a minority of immature T cells.

*This chapter uses the fifth edition of the WHO classification of thoracic tumors.

111. What are the main clinical and histological features of thymic squamous cell carcinoma?

- This is a malignant neoplasm; it is the most common subtype of thymic carcinoma (around 70% of cases).
- It is often poorly defined, with invasion of mediastinal structures.
- It has the morphological features of squamous cell carcinoma (with intercellular bridges and keratinization in well differentiated cases); it lacks normal thymic cytoarchitecture.
- The 5-year survival is around 60%, and significantly associated with completeness of resection and stage.

112. How do you differentiate a thymic carcinoma and a type B3 thymoma by histology?

	TYPE B3 THYMOMA	THYMIC SQUAMOUS CELL CARCINOMA
Growth	• Lobular.	• Sheets, islands and cords.
Invasion of adjacent structures	• Pushing type.	• Infiltrative.
Stroma reaction	• No desmoplasia.	• Desmoplasia.
Differentiation	• No squamous differentiation.	• Intercellular bridges keratinization.
IHC	• CD5–. • CD117–. • Presence of immature T cells.	• CD5+ (80%). • CD117+ (80%). • Absence of immature T cells.

113. List common anterior mediastinal tumors.

- Thymic epithelial tumor: thymoma, thymic carcinoma, neuroendocrine tumor.
- Lymphoma: Hodgkin/non-Hodgkin lymphoma.
- Germ cell tumor (e.g., seminoma)/teratoma.
- Thyroid tumor/substernal goiter.
- Carcinoma (i.e., metastasis).

114. What is a primary mediastinal large B-cell lymphoma?

- It is an aggressive large B-cell lymphoma (positive for B-cell lineage antigens such as CD20 and CD79a) arising in the anterior mediastinum (putative thymic B-cell origin).
- No widespread extrathoracic lymph node or bone marrow involvement is present.

115. What does the College of American Pathologists (CAP) require as the main data to report for thymoma?*

- Histological type.
- Transcapular invasion: encapsulated, microscopic invasion, macroscopic invasion.
- Tumor extension: confined to thymus, invasion of mediastinal fat and/or adjacent structures.
- Margins.
- Treatment effect.
- Lymphovascular invasion.
- Regional lymph nodes.
- Pleural or pericardial dissemination (implants).
- Stage (pTNM, AJCC 8th Edition, +/– Masaoka-Koga system).

*This chapter uses the 4.1.0.0 version of the CAP protocol.

Case Scenario

A 60-year-old man has a chest wall mass. Microscopy shows poorly formed neoplastic glands infiltrating desmoplastic stroma.

116. What is your differential diagnosis?

- Metastatic adenocarcinoma.
- Malignant epithelioid mesothelioma.
- Primary lung adenocarcinoma extending to the chest wall.

117. How do you work up adenocarcinoma from an unknown site?

- Check clinical presentation, past medical history, and family cancer history.
- Review radiologic images searching for possible primary tumor elsewhere.
- Review slides from previous biopsy specimens of cancer if available.
- Perform IHC — e.g., TTF-1, napsin-A for lung adenocarcinoma; GATA3/ER/PR for breast cancer, ER/PR/PAX8 for gynecologic cancer; PSA/PAP/NKX3.1 for prostate cancer; CK7/CK20/CDX2 to confirm colorectal cancer; thyroglobulin/PAX8/TTF-1 for thyroid cancer.

118. How is mesothelioma differentiated from lung adenocarcinoma?

FEATURE	MESOTHELIOMA	ADENOCARCINOMA
GROSS		
Location	• Pleural based.	• Lung based.
Pattern	• Diffuse.	• Single nodule/mass.
Pleural effusion	• Present.	• Usually absent.
MICROSCOPIC		
Biphasic	• Possibly present.	• Absent.
Sarcomatoid	• Possibly present.	• Absent.
Cytology	• Possibly low grade.	• Usually high grade.
IMMUNOSTAINS		
Calretinin	+	–
CK5/6	+	–
WT1	+	–
D2-40	+	–
CEA monoclonal	–	+/–
LeuM1 (CD15)	–	+/–
BerEP4	–	+/–
MOC31	–	+/–
TTF-1	–	+/–
Napsin-A	–	+/–
Other adenocarcinoma markers from other origin (breast, thyroid, etc.)	-	+/–
HISTOCHEMICAL STAINS		
Periodic acid-Shiff/diastase	–	+/–

A pleural biopsy specimen from a 66-year-old man most likely shows metastatic melanoma on microscopy.

119. What is your differential diagnosis?

- Metastatic carcinoma.
- Metastatic or primary sarcoma.
- Malignant lymphoma.
- Malignant mesothelioma.
- Desmoplastic small round cell tumor.
- Others (e.g., small blue cell tumor, germ cell tumor).

120. List 4 IHC stains you would prefer for making the diagnosis.

- S100.
- Cytokeratin (AE1/AE3).
- Leukocyte common antigen (LCA).
- Vimentin.

121. What other information about this patient would be relevant?

- History of melanoma and other neoplastic disorders.
- Cancer type, location, extent and stage, and treatment if there is a history of cancer.
- Family history of cancer.
- Occupational history, such as a history of asbestos exposure.
- Smoking history.
- Radiologic images (e.g., CT scan, positron emission tomography scan).
- Previous biopsy or cytology results.
- Any systemic disorders, and immune status.

122. List stains for melanoma.

- S100.
- HMB-45.
- Melan-A.
- SOX10.

Hypersensitivity Pneumonitis (Extrinsic Allergic Alveolitis)

123. What is the pathogenesis of hypersensitivity pneumonitis?

- It is triggered by an immunologic reaction to inhaled organic antigens or simple chemicals.
- It is a combination of immune complex (type III) and T cell mediated (type IV) hypersensitivity reactions.

124. List 5 pathogens that cause hypersensitivity pneumonitis.

- *Saccharopolyspora rectivirgula* in moldy hay, seen in "farmer's lung."
- *Thermoactinomyces sacchari,* seen in sugarcane workers.
- *Cryptostroma corticale* (fungus), seen in maple bark workers.
- Proteins from birds, seen in bird keepers.
- Fungi growing in stagnant water in air conditioners, swimming pools, and central heating units.

125. Describe the clinical presentation of hypersensitivity pneumonitis at different stages.

- Acute:
  · Patients are usually previously sensitized individuals.
  · Symptoms have an abrupt onset (within hours) and include fever, chills, cough, chest tightness, dyspnea.
  · Symptoms subside over hours or days.
- Subacute:
  · Symptoms develop insidiously over days or weeks.
  · Cough and dyspnea are the main symptoms.
  · Other features include:
    › Diffuse crackles on auscultation.
    › A restrictive pattern and mild hypoxemia on pulmonary function tests.
- Chronic:
  · Symptoms develop insidiously and include dyspnea with a dry cough, fatigue, and malaise.
  · Patients may not experience or remember any acute episodes of the disease.
  · It presents disabling and often irreversible respiratory findings such as pulmonary fibrosis.
  · Pulmonary function tests show a restrictive pattern and hypoxia.
  · Symptoms and signs could also be related to airway obstruction.
  · The inciting antigen is often difficult to detect or never identified.

126. Describe the pathologic changes of hypersensitivity pneumonitis at different stages.

- Acute:
  · A neutrophilic infiltrate in the alveoli and respiratory bronchioles (acute alveolitis and bronchiolitis).
  · Diffuse alveolar damage (possible).
- Subacute:
  · Lymphocytic interstitial infiltrate (alveolitis).
  · Poorly formed granulomas.

(continued on next page)

- Focal organizing pneumonia (fibroblastic polyps/plugs).
- Eosinophils and neutrophils usually not prominent.
- Chronic:
  - Cellular chronic bronchiolitis with peribronchiolar interstitial mononuclear cell infiltrate (alveolitis).

- Poorly formed nonnecrotizing granulomas.
- Focal organizing pneumonia (fibroblastic polyps/plugs).
- Eosinophils: scant or absent.
- Interstitial fibrosis (possible).

127. List the 3 most consistent and diagnostic histologic features (triad) of hypersensitivity pneumonitis.

- A temporally uniform chronic interstitial pneumonia with peribronchiolar accentuation (alvrolitis).
- Nonnecrotizing granulomas (often poorly formed).

- Foci of organizing changes (fibroblastic polyps/plugs)/ organizing pneumonia.

128. List 3 findings in bronchoalveolar lavage specimens from patients with hypersensitivity pneumonitis.

- A marked lymphocytosis (often > 50%) with the phenotype of CD3+/CD8+/CD56+/CD57+/CD10–.

- A decreased CD4:CD8 ratio (< 1:0).
- Increased numbers of mast cells (> 1%).

Chronic Bronchitis

129. What is the clinical definition of chronic bronchitis?

Persistent cough with sputum production for at least 3 months in at least 2 consecutive years, in the absence of any other identifiable causes.

130. Describe the pathogenesis of chronic bronchitis.

- Long-standing irritation by inhaled substances such as tobacco smoke and environmental dust results in hypersecretion of mucus in the large airways and hypertrophy of the submucosal glands.
- Proteases released from neutrophils and matrix metalloproteinases stimulate mucus hypersecretion.

- As chronic bronchitis persists, there is also a marked increase in goblet cells of small airways leading to excessive mucus production that causes airway obstruction.
- Cigarette smoke interferes with ciliary action of the respiratory epithelium, and may cause direct damage to airway epithelium. It inhibits the ability of leukocytes to clear bacteria and predisposes affected individuals to infection.

131. List 4 important pathogenetic factors of chronic bronchitis.

- Cigarette smoking.
- Environmental causes.

- Chronic irritation/inflammation.
- Infections.

132. List 4 microscopic features of chronic bronchitis.

- Chronic inflammation of the airways — predominantly lymphocytes.
- Mucous gland hyperplasia of the trachea and bronchi.
- Reid index > 0.4 — assessed by the ratio of the thickness of the mucous gland layer to the thickness of the wall

between the basement membrane of the bronchial epithelium and the perichondrium of the bronchial cartilage.
- Marked narrowing of bronchioles — caused by mucus plugging, inflammation, and fibrosis.

Emphysema

133. Define emphysema.

An abnormal permanent enlargement of the airspaces distal to the terminal bronchiole, accompanied by the destruction of alveolar walls without obvious fibrosis.

134. Describe the pathogenesis of emphysema.

- An imbalance of proteases and their inhibitors leads to the destruction of lung tissue.
- Inflammatory cells, mediators, and oxidative stress also play important pathogenetic roles.

- Cigarette smoking plays a major role in the pathogenesis of centriacinar emphysema.
- α1-Antitrypsin deficiency is associated with the development of panacinar emphysema.

135. List 4 common types of emphysema and define each type.

- Centriacinar (centrilobular): distention and destruction involving proximal portion of the acinus, mainly the respiratory bronchioles.
- Panacinar (panlobular): distention and destruction involving the entire acinus, causing diffuse and bilateral lung involvement.
- Paraseptal (distal): distention and destruction involving the distal portion of the acinus, such as alveolar ducts and alveoli, often in the subpleural and paraseptal regions.
- Irregular: irregular airspace enlargement and tissue destruction associated with a scar.

136. List at least 4 causes of emphysema.

- Cigarette smoking — the most common cause of centriacinar emphysema.
- Chronic inflammation.
- α1-Antitrypsin deficiency — the most common cause of panacinar emphysema.
- Scarring — the most common cause of irregular emphysema.
- Others: intravenous drug abuse, genetic disorders such as Marfan syndrome.

Granulomatous Lesions of the Lung

137. Define granuloma.

- A granuloma is a focus of chronic inflammation consisting of a microscopic aggregation of macrophages/histiocytes surrounded by mononuclear leukocytes.
  - The macrophages are often transformed into "epithelioid" appearance.
- The "epithelioid" cells often fuse to form multinucleate giant cells, with nuclei arranged 1 of 2 ways:
  › Peripherally (Langerhans-type giant cell).
  › Haphazardly (foreign body–type giant cell).

138. List 5 examples of nonnecrotizing granulomas.

- Sarcoidosis.
- Berylliosis.
- Sarcoid reaction.
- Hypersensitivity pneumonitis (extrinsic allergic alveolitis).
- Foreign body granuloma.

139. List 5 examples of necrotizing granulomas.

- Tuberculosis and atypical mycobacteriosis.
- Mycoses:
  · Histoplasmosis.
  · Cryptococcosis.
  · Blastomycosis.
  · Coccidioidomycosis.
- Rare bacterial diseases:
  · *Treponema pallidum* — syphilitic gumma.
- Necrotizing sarcoid granulomatosis.
- Rheumatoid nodule.

140. List 3 examples of granulomas accompanied by necrotizing bronchiolitis.

- Tuberculosis and atypical mycobacteriosis.
- Mycoses.
- Bronchocentric granulomatosis.

141. List 5 examples of granulomatous vasculitis.

- Granulomatosis with polyangiitis.
- Eosinophilic granulomatosis with polyangiitis.
- Sarcoidosis.
- Giant cell arteritis.
- Takayasu arteritis.

Pulmonary Langerhans Cell Histiocytosis (Pulmonary Eosinophilic Granuloma)

142. What are the 2 synonyms for pulmonary Langerhans cell histiocytosis?

- Pulmonary eosinophilic granuloma.
- Histiocytosis X.

143. Describe the clinical features of pulmonary Langerhans cell histiocytosis (pulmonary eosinophilic granuloma).

- Almost all adult patients have a history of smoking.
- Clinical presentation is variable from asymptomatic to a rapidly progressive condition.
- Common symptoms and signs include dyspnea, nonproductive cough, chest pain, fatigue; and pneumothorax (25% of cases).

(continued on next page)

- Extrapulmonary involvement (e.g., bone, lymph nodes) occurs in about 10–15% of cases.
- Langerhans cell histiocytosis can occur in children either as an isolated lung disease or as a multisystem disorder.

- Routine lab tests are nonspecific.
- Pulmonary function tests may show a reduced diffusing capacity of the lungs for carbon monoxide (DCLO).

144. List 2 classic radiological changes of pulmonary Langerhans cell histiocytosis (pulmonary eosinophilic granuloma).

- A symmetric, bilateral nodular or reticulonodular pattern more prominent in the centrilobular (peribronchiolar) regions of the upper and middle zones of the lung.

- Often, small cystic changes with bizarre shapes of various sizes.

145. List 4 microscopic features of pulmonary Langerhans cell histiocytosis (pulmonary eosinophilic granuloma).

- Multiple nodular lesions centered on bronchioles with a stellate border.
- Lesions composed of Langerhans cells with moderate eosinophilic cytoplasm, indistinct cell borders, bean shaped nuclei, and prominently grooved nuclear membranes.

- Variable numbers of eosinophils.
- A spectrum of the disease process from cellular infiltrate to stellate fibrotic tissue.

146. List 4 positive IHC stains for pulmonary Langerhans cell histiocytosis (pulmonary eosinophilic granuloma).

- S100.
- CD1a.

- Vimentin.
- CD68.

147. List 2 common extrapulmonary organs involved in Langerhans cell histiocytosis.

- Bone.
- Lymph node.

148. What is the characteristic ultrastructural feature of Langerhans cells?
Birbeck granules.

Cystic Fibrosis (CF)

149. Describe the etiology and pathogenesis of CF.

- CF gene located on chromosome 7 (7q3) encodes a 1480 amino acid protein known as cystic fibrosis transmembrane regulator (CFTR).
- CFTR expressed in epithelial cells in the lung, gastrointestinal tract, and other organs.
- Mutations in CFTR result in:

  · An inability of airway epithelial cells to secrete salt (and secondarily water).
  · Excessive reabsorption of salt and water with consequent desiccation of luminal secretions.
- Mucous plugging and decreased clearance predispose affected individuals to bacterial growth, resulting in recurrent infection.

150. Describe the clinical features of CF in the respiratory and gastrointestinal tract.

- Respiratory tract:
  · Wheezing.
  · Persistent cough with production of thick mucus (sputum).
  · Recurrent lung infection.
  · Inflamed nasal passages or a stuffy nose.
  · Nasal polyps.
  · Recurrent sinusitis.
- Gastrointestinal tract:
  · Intestinal blockage, particularly in newborns (meconium ileus).
  · Foul-smelling, greasy stools (steatorrhea).

  · Malabsorption.
  · Chronic or severe constipation.
  · Rectal prolapse.
- Other features:
  · Exercise intolerance.
  · Salty taste when kissed.
  · Hypoproteinemia.
  · Vitamin deficiency.
  · Unexplained hypochloremic alkalosis.
  · Absence of sperm in semen.
  · Failure to thrive.

151. List pulmonary pathological findings of CF.

- Acute and chronic bronchitis, bronchiolitis, and pneumonia.
- Purulent mucous plugging.
- Bronchiectasis and bronchostenosis.
- Constrictive bronchiolitis and peribronchiolar scarring.

- Abscess formation.
- Atelectasis.
- Emphysema/air trapping.
- Interstitial inflammatory cell infiltrate and fibrosis.

152. List 3 gross findings of CF in the lungs.
- Bronchiectasis and purulent airway mucus.
- Atelectasis and pneumonic consolidation.
- Emphysematous changes with bullae formation.

153. List 5 extrapulmonary lesions of CF.
- Sinusitis.
- Nasal polyps.
- Pancreatitis.
- Biliary cirrhosis.
- Acrodermatitis.

154. What 2 microorganisms frequently cause lung infections in patients with CF?
- *Staphylococcus aureus.*
- *Hemophilus influenzae.*

Diffuse Alveolar damage

155. Define diffuse alveolar damage.
- Diffuse alveolar damage is a histologic pattern of acute lung injury that occurs in a variety of clinical settings.
- Clinically, it often presents as acute respiratory distress syndrome (ARDS).
- Histologically, hyaline membrane formation and/or interstitial organizing changes are present.

156. List at least 10 causes of diffuse alveolar damage.
- Infection.
- Shock.
- Trauma — lung contusion, fat embolism, head injury.
- Inhalation injury — smoke, oxygen, corrosive chemical.
- Aspiration of gastric contents.
- Drugs.
- Metabolic disorders — pancreatitis, uremia.
- Radiation.
- Hematologic disorders — disseminated intravascular coagulation (DIC), transfusion associated.
- Idiopathic (also known as acute interstitial pneumonia).
- Others (e.g., burns, high altitude, near drowning, venous air embolism, intravenous contrast material).

157. What is the radiologic appearance of diffuse alveolar damage?
- Within 12–24 hours from the clinical onset: decreased lung volume, otherwise unremarkable.
- After 12–24 hours: patchy airspace consolidation initially, then confluent and diffuse involvement quickly.
- With improvement clinically, gradual replacement of consolidation by ground-glass appearance and, later, reticular opacities.

158. List the main histologic features of diffuse alveolar damage.
- Acute phase (exudative phase; usually occurs within a week of clinical onset):
  · Pulmonary congestion, interstitial and intraalveolar edema, fibrin deposition.
  · Damage to the alveolar walls.
  · Hyaline membrane formation.
- Organizing phase (proliferative phase):
  · Type 2 pneumocyte proliferation.
  · Interstitial fibroblast proliferation with edematous change of the stroma.
  · Fibrotic thickening of the alveolar septa.
- Fibrotic phase (chronic phase):
  · Interstitial fibrosis.
  · "Honeycomb" changes.

159. Describe the pathogenesis of diffuse alveolar damage.
- Lung injury is caused by an imbalance of proinflammatory and antiinflammatory mediators, in favor of a proinflammatory state.
- Activated neutrophils release a variety of mediators (e.g., oxidants, proteases, platelet activating factor, and leukotrienes).
- Above mechanisms result in:
  · First, damage to the alveolar capillary endothelial cells and epithelial cells.
  · Then, increased vascular permeability, loss of diffusion capacity, and widespread surfactant abnormalities.
  · Finally, ischemic injury (because endothelial injury also triggers the formation of microthrombi).
- Hyaline membranes result from inspissation of protein rich edema fluid and debris of dead alveolar epithelial cells.
- The balance between the destructive and protective factors determines the degree of tissue injury and clinical severity.

Lymphangioleiomyomatosis

160. What is lymphangioleiomyomatosis (LAM)?
- LAM is now considered a low grade destructive metastasizing neoplasm.
- It is a PEComatous tumor.
- The lesional cells usually have growth promoting biallelic mutations in the tuberous sclerosis gene *TSC2* and also show evidence of clonal origin with invasive and metastatic potential.

161. Describe the clinical presentation of LAM.
- It most often occurs as a sporadic disease, but is also seen in tuberous sclerosis complex.
- It mostly occurs in young women of childbearing age, 20–40 years old at the onset (> 70% of cases).
- It occurs much more commonly in Caucasians than other racial groups.
- Main symptoms include dyspnea, cough, and chest pain.
- Complications include spontaneous pneumothorax, hemoptysis, chylothorax, chyloperitoneum, chyluria, and chylopericardium.

162. List 2 radiological features of LAM.
- Cystic spaces randomly distributed in both lungs.
- A diffuse and bilateral reticular pattern with hyperinflation.

163. List 4 disorders possibly associated with LAM.
- Tuberous sclerosis.
- Micronodular pneumocyte hyperplasia.
- Angiomyolipoma.
- Clear cell tumor (PEComa).

164. List 2 main histologic features of LAM.
- Variable sized cystic spaces lined by plaque-like or nodular aggregates of smooth muscle-like spindle cells.
- Spindle cells possibly admixed with more rounded epithelioid cells (representing perivascular epithelioid cells or epithelioid smooth muscle cells).

165. List positive IHC stains useful for the diagnosis of LAM.
- HMB-45.
- Melan A.
- Microphthalmia transcription factor, also known as melanocyte inducing transcription factor (MITF).
- Alpha-actin (smooth muscle actin).
- ER/PR.

Idiopathic Interstitial Pneumonia

166. What are the types of idiopathic interstitial pneumonias?
- Usual interstitial pneumonia (idiopathic pulmonary fibrosis).
- Nonspecific interstitial pneumonia.
- Desquamative interstitial pneumonia.
- Acute interstitial pneumonia (diffuse alveolar damage).
- Cryptogenic organizing pneumonia.
- Respiratory bronchiolitis interstitial lung disease.
- Unclassifiable idiopathic interstitial pneumonias.
- Other rare types:
  · Idiopathic lymphoid interstitial pneumonia.
  · Idiopathic pleuroparenchymal fibroelastosis.

167. What is idiopathic pleuroparenchymal fibroelastosis?
- It is an interstitial fibroelastotic change in the pleural/subpleural region, predominantly in the upper lobes, with unknown etiology.
- A median age of 57 years with no sex predilection.
- Approximately half of patients have a history of recurrent pulmonary infections, and pneumothorax is common.
- A minority has familial interstitial lung disease and nonspecific autoantibodies.
- Histologically, there is pleural/subpleural and intraalveolar fibroelastosis. In some cases, it may mimic a UIP pattern.
- Disease progression occurs in about 60% of patients with the disease, and death in about 40% of cases.

168. What is acute fibrinous and organizing pneumonia?
- It is a histologic pattern that can occur in the clinical spectrum of diffuse alveolar damage and organizing pneumonia.
- It may be idiopathic or associated with collagen vascular disease, hypersensitivity pneumonitis, or a drug reaction.
- The main CT findings are bilateral basal opacities and areas of consolidation.
- The histologic appearance is intraalveolar fibrin deposition with organizing pneumonia. Typical hyaline membranes of DAD are absent.

169. What is familial interstitial pneumonia (FIP)?

- Idiopathic interstitial pneumonias (IIP) have been reported in closely related family members in 2–20% of cases. Despite the genetic predisposition, FIP is still classified as IIP.
- In about 20% of FIP there are heterozygous mutations such as SFTPC (1%), SFTPA2 (1%), TERT (15%), and TERC (1%).
- Most FIP families (80%) have evidence of vertical transmission, suggesting single autosomal dominant mechanisms, but most responsible genes have not yet been identified.
- A common variant in the promoter of the MUCB gene is likely associated with the development of both familial and sporadic idiopathic pulmonary fibrosis.
- FIP can be indistinguishable from nonfamilial cases on CT and lung biopsy; therefore, all patients with suspected IIP should be questioned about relevant family history as this may guide gene mutation search.

Usual Interstitial Pneumonia (UIP)

170. What is UIP?

- UIP is a specific form of chronic fibrosing interstitial lung disease.
- UIP also refers to an idiopathic clinicopathologic entity synonymous with idiopathic pulmonary fibrosis (IPF).
- As a histologic pattern, it is also seen in a variety of clinical settings, including collagen vascular disease and drug reaction.

171. Describe the clinical features of UIP.

- Patients are usually between 50 and 70 years of age, M > F.
- Patients experience an insidious onset of dyspnea and nonproductive cough; most patients have clubbing (40–75%).
- Constitutional symptoms are uncommon.
- The typical pulmonary function tests show a restrictive pattern and impairment of gas exchange.
- The clinical course has a slow progression and patients have a poor prognosis (overall, a downhill clinical course) with the mean survival varying from 3 to 5 years.

172. List at least 3 common causes of a usual interstitial pneumonia pattern.

- Idiopathic.
- Collagen vascular disease.
- Drug reaction.
- Others — e.g., pneumoconiosis (asbestosis), radiation pneumonitis.

173. What are the main histologic features of UIP?

- Patchy lung involvement with peripheral/paraseptal predominance and intervening preserved normal alveolar architecture.
- Temporally variegated appearance with dense collagen fibrosis, fibroblastic foci, and "honeycomb" change.
- Others (e.g., interstitial inflammation, focal smooth muscle proliferation, focal alveolar macrophage accumulation, lymphoid aggregates).

Nonspecific Interstitial Pneumonia (NSIP)

174. List the main clinical features of NSIP.

- Idiopathic.
- Chronic disease process.
- Average age: mid-40s to mid-50s, slightly more common in women.
- Shortness of breath and dry cough.
- Restrictive pattern on pulmonary function test.
- Distinct disease entity.

175. List the main pathologic features of NSIP.

- Diffuse and temporal uniform disease process.
- Dense or loose interstitial fibrosis with various degrees of interstitial chronic inflammatory cell infiltrate and type 2 pneumocyte hyperplasia.
- Preserved alveolar architecture (usually).
- 2 possible patterns:
  - Cellular pattern (associated with significantly better prognosis).
  - Fibrotic pattern.
- No granulomatous inflammation (usually); inconspicuous or absent fibroblastic foci; no significant eosinophils or prominent alveolar macrophages.

Desquamative Interstitial Pneumonia (DIP)

176. List the main clinical features of DIP.
- It is idiopathic.
- Most patients present in their fourth to fifth decade of life.
- It is almost exclusively seen in patients with a cigarette smoking history.
- Most patients present with a subacute illness (weeks to months).
- Shortness of breath and cough are present.
- Pulmonary function tests demonstrate a restrictive pattern.

177. List the main pathologic features of DIP.
- Diffuse and temporal uniform disease process.
- Mild to moderate alveolar septal thickening with interstitial fibrosis and mild chronic inflammatory cell infiltrate.
- Prominent accumulation of alveolar macrophages.
- Lack of lung architecture remodeling or honeycomb fibrosis.
- Absent or inconspicuous fibroblastic foci or organizing pneumonia.

Respiratory Bronchiolitis Interstitial Lung Disease (RBILD)

178. List the main clinical features of RBILD.
- It is idiopathic.
- The mean age of onset is about mid-30s with no sex predilection.
- Almost all patients have a cigarette smoking history.
- Patients have mild shortness of breath and cough or no obvious symptoms.
- Pulmonary function tests demonstrate no significant change or a mild restrictive pattern.

179. List the main pathologic features of RBILD.
- Focal and patchy disease process near small airways.
- Accumulation of brown dusty alveolar macrophages within the respiratory bronchioles and adjacent alveolar spaces.
- Possible interstitial fibrosis involving the walls of the respiratory bronchioles and surrounding alveolar septa.
- No granulomatous formation or organizing changes.

Organizing Pneumonia

180. List the causes of organizing pneumonia.
- Idiopathic (cryptogenic organizing pneumonia, which was known as bronchiolitis obliterans organizing pneumonia).
- Collagen vascular disease.
- Drug reaction.
- Infection.
- Nonspecific reaction adjacent to other lesions (e.g., abscess, neoplasm, infarct).
- Others (e.g., viral infection, radiation, hemorrhage).

181. Describe the clinical features of cryptogenic organizing pneumonia.
- Acute/subacute onset, usually in patients 40–60 years old.
- Most common symptoms: nonproductive cough, shortness of breath.
- Flu-like illness with fever, malaise, fatigue, and weight loss.
- Restrictive defect on pulmonary function testing; possible obstructive defect in a small percentage of patients.

182. List the microscopic features of organizing pneumonia.
- Intraluminal organizing fibrosis with fibroblastic polyps/plugs in distal airspaces including bronchioles, alveolar ducts, and alveoli.
- Uniform temporal appearance and a patchy distribution.
- Mild interstitial chronic inflammation.
- Preservation of lung architecture.

183. List the conditions associated with the organizing pneumonia pattern.
- Cryptogenic organizing pneumonia.
- Collagen vascular diseases.
- Drug reaction.
- Hypersensitivity pneumonitis.
- Infection — e.g., viral, bacteria, HIV, pneumocystis pneumonia (PCP).
- Radiation.
- Hemorrhage.
- Nonspecific reaction adjacent to other lesions — tumor, abscess, infarct, obstruction.

Acute Interstitial Pneumonia

184. What is the etiology of acute interstitial pneumonia?
Idiopathic.

185. What is common in the clinical presentation of acute interstitial pneumonia?
- It typically presents with a prodromal illness resembling an upper respiratory tract viral infection.
- The disease process is rapidly progressive with acute respiratory failure follows.
- Cough and dyspnea are commonly seen.
- Profound hypoxemia is almost always present.

186. What are the histologic findings of acute interstitial pneumonia?
- These are identical to the histologic changes seen in diffuse alveolar damage:
  - Exudative phase:
    › Hyaline membranes.
    › Pulmonary edema.
    › Alveolar wall damage.
    › Variable inflammatory cells.
- Organizing phase:
  › Significant alveolar septal thickening with interstitial fibroblast proliferation.
  › Type 2 pneumocyte proliferation.
  › Variable inflammatory cells.
- Fibrotic phase.

Asbestos Related Disease

187. List 6 disorders associated with asbestos exposure.
- Asbestosis.
- Benign asbestos effusion.
- Hyaline pleural plaques.
- Rounded atelectasis.
- Lung carcinoma.
- Malignant mesothelioma.

188. List the methods for identifying or quantifying asbestos fibers in the lungs.
- Quantifying asbestos bodies in tissue sections with H&E stain and/or Prussian blue stain.
- Counting asbestos bodies in lung-tissue digest preparations with a light microscope.
- Counting uncoated asbestos fibers in lung-tissue digest preparations with a phase microscope.
- Counting uncoated asbestos fibers with an appropriately equipped electron microscope.

189. What are the histologic criteria for the diagnosis of asbestosis?
- The presence of both of the following are sufficient for the pathologic diagnosis of asbestosis:
- Pulmonary interstitial fibrosis resembling usual interstitial pneumonia or nonspecific interstitial pneumonia pattern with or without associated pleural fibrosis.
- Asbestos bodies.

Note: a finding of no asbestos bodies in tissue sections does not necessarily exclude a diagnosis of asbestosis.

Pulmonary Hypertension

190. What is the WHO classification of pulmonary hypertension?
- Group 1: pulmonary arterial hypertension (PAH).
- Group 2: pulmonary hypertension due to left-sided heart disease.
- Group 3: pulmonary hypertension due to lung diseases and/or hypoxia.
- Group 4: chronic thromboembolic pulmonary hypertension (CTEPH).
- Group 5: pulmonary hypertension with unclear or multifactorial etiologies:
  - Hematologic disorders (e.g., myeloproliferative disorders).
  - Systemic disorders (e.g., sarcoidosis, pulmonary Langerhans cell histiocytosis, lymphangioleiomyomatosis, neurofibromatosis, vasculitis).
  - Metabolic disorders (e.g., glycogen storage disease, Gaucher disease, thyroid disorders).
  - Miscellaneous conditions (e.g., tumor obstruction, mediastinal fibrosis, chronic renal failure on dialysis).

191. What is the etiology of pulmonary arterial hypertension?
- Subgroup 1: idiopathic PAH (IPAH).
- Subgroup 2: heritable PAH, including those with *BMPR2* and *ALK2* gene mutations.
- Subgroup 3: drug- and toxin-induced PAH:
  · Aminorex.
  · Fenfluramine derivatives.
  · Toxic rapeseed oil.
  · Other drugs as possible risk factors for PAH (amphetamine and amphetamine derivatives, cocaine, L-tryptophan, phenylpropanolamine, St. John's wort, leflunomide, phentermine, mazindol, dasatinib, and interferon.).
- Subgroup 4: conditions with known localization of lesions in the small pulmonary arterioles:
  · Collagen-vascular disease (scleroderma/CREST syndrome).
  · Congenital left-to-right shunts.
  · Portopulmonary hypertension.
  · HIV-associated pulmonary hypertension.
  · Schistosomiasis.

192. List 5 histologic changes of primary pulmonary arterial hypertension.
- Medial hypertrophy and muscularization of arterioles.
- Cellular proliferation of intima and concentric intimal fibrosis.
- Angiomatoid lesions.
- Plexiform lesions.
- Fibrinoid necrosis.

193. What is the Heath and Edwards grading system?
- It was designed for assessing the severity of pulmonary hypertension secondary to congenital heart disease, especially in the presence of a left-to-right shunt.
- It is not reliable for assessing the severity of noncongenital heart disease–related primary pulmonary arterial hypertension.
- There are 6 grades:
  · Grade 1: hypertrophy of the media of muscular pulmonary arteries, extension of muscle into the wall of pulmonary arterioles.
  · Grade 2: hypertrophy of the media of muscular pulmonary arteries, proliferation of intimal cells in arterioles and small muscular arteries.
  · Grade 3: hypertrophy of the media of muscular pulmonary arteries, subendothelial fibrosis, concentric masses of fibrous tissue, and reduplicated internal elastic lamina occlude the vascular lumen of arterioles and small muscular arteries.
  · Grade 4: progressive generalized arterial dilatation with intimal fibrous occlusion and plexiform lesions.
  · Grade 5: prominent plexiform lesions and angiomatoid lesions with intraalveolar hemosiderin-filled macrophages.
  · Grade 6: necrotizing arteritis with thrombosis and fibrinoid necrosis of the arterial wall.

194. What are the histologic changes in pulmonary venoocclusive disease?
- Pulmonary veins and venules.
  · Obstructive intimal fibrosis, initially of a loose texture.
  · Recanalization and septa formation.
  · Scarcity of recent thrombi.
  · Medial hypertrophy and arterialization.
- Pulmonary arteries.
  · Sometimes intimal fibrosis, often with recent thrombi.
  · Sometimes medial hypertrophy.
- Lung tissue.
  · Prominent hemosiderosis, focal congestion, and interstitial fibrosis.

Pulmonary Aspergillosis

195. What are 3 types of pulmonary aspergillosis?
- Colonization of *Aspergillus* to form fungus ball (mycetoma).
- Hypersensitivity reaction (allergic bronchopulmonary aspergillosis).
- Invasive aspergillosis (*Aspergillus* pneumonia).

196. List 5 examples of hypersensitivity reaction related to aspergillosis.
- Allergic bronchopulmonary aspergillosis.
- Bronchocentric granulomatosis.
- Mucoid impaction.
- Hypersensitivity pneumonitis.
- Eosinophilic pneumonia.

197. List 5 clinical manifestations related to invasive aspergillosis.
- Acute invasive aspergillosis.
- Chronic necrotizing aspergillosis.
- Necrotizing pseudomembranous tracheobronchitis.
- Empyema.
- Bronchopleural fistula.

Silicosis

198. What is the pathogenesis of silicosis?
- Silica particles are inhaled and deposited in lung tissue.
- The particles damage the lung tissue via direct cytotoxicity, or by the production of oxidants and other mediators to cause fibrosis.

199. List 5 disorders or pathologic changes associated with silica exposure.
- Acute silicoproteinosis.
- Nodular silicosis.
- Silicotuberculosis.
- Rheumatoid pneumoconiosis (Caplan syndrome).
- Mixed dust fibrosis, diffuse interstitial fibrosis, and pleural fibrosis.

200. What is the characteristic histology of nodular silicosis?
- In early/cellular silicosis, there is aggregation of dust laden macrophages producing centriacinar dust macules.
- Silicotic nodules are composed of discrete nodular dense collagen fibrosis, which may become calcified or hyalinized, or develop central degenerative changes.
- Polarized light reveals weakly birefringent silica particles and more strongly birefringent silicate particles within the nodules and in the surrounding dust filled macrophages.
- It may accompanied by progressive massive fibrosis, and diffuse interstitial fibrosis may occur.

Note: silicotic fibrosis in lymph nodes alone does not meet the diagnostic criteria for silicosis.

Sarcoidosis

201. What is sarcoidosis?
- A multiorgan disease of nonnecrotizing granulomatous inflammation with unknown etiology.
- Age group: young adults often 20–40 years old.
- Gender: a slight female predominance.
- Race: Swedes, Danes, and African Americans seem to have the highest prevalence rates in the world.

202. List 4 histologic findings of sarcoidosis in the lungs.
- Well-formed nonnecrotizing granulomas, which may become confluent and hyalinized.
- Distribution of granulomas along lymphatic routes — i.e., around bronchovascular bundles, along the pleura and septa.
- It may accompanied by vasculitis.
- It may contain some inclusion bodies — e.g., Schaumann bodies, asteroid bodies, crystalline inclusions (birefringent calcium carbonate or calcium oxalate crystals).

203. List 5 differential diagnoses of sarcoidosis.
- Fungal infection.
- Mycobacterium and atypical mycobacterium infection.
- Hypersensitivity pneumonitis.
- Berylliosis and other inhaled substances such as talc, aluminum.
- Sarcoidal reaction (e.g., as seen in malignancies, collagen vascular disease, vasculitis syndromes).

204. List the 5 extrapulmonary sites often involved in sarcoidosis.
- Lymph nodes.
- Liver.
- Eyes.
- Spleen.
- Skin.

Pulmonary Edema

205. List the causes of pulmonary edema.
- Increased hydrostatic pressure (increased pulmonary venous pressure).
  - Left sided heart failure (common).
  - Volume overload.
  - Pulmonary vein obstruction.
- Decreased oncotic pressure (less common).
  - Hypoalbuminemia.
  - Nephrotic syndrome.
- Liver disease.
- Infections: pneumonia, septicemia.
- Inhaled gases: oxygen, smoke.
- Liquid aspiration: gastric contents, near drowning.
- Drugs and chemicals.
- Shock, trauma.
- Radiation.

206. List the histologic changes of pulmonary edema.
- Alveolar capillaries are engorged.
- Alveolar spaces are filled with homogeneous or very fine granular pink material.
- Hemosiderin laden macrophages ("heart failure" cells) may be present.
- In long-standing cases of pulmonary congestion, fibrosis and thickening of the alveolar walls may occur.

Asthma

207. List the types of asthma.
- Extrinsic (atopic).
- Intrinsic.
- Occupational.
- Others — e.g., drug related (aspirin induced), obstructed, persistent.

208. List 5 histologic findings of asthma.
- Thickening of bronchial/bronchiolar basement membranes and subbasement membrane fibrosis.
- Increase in the size of submucosal glands.
- Goblet cell hyperplasia.
- Hypertrophy and/or hyperplasia of the bronchial wall smooth muscle.
- Mucus plugs with many eosinophils.

209. What are Charcot-Leyden crystals and Curschmann spirals?
- Charcot-Leyden crystals: slender, rhomboid shaped orangeophilic structures derived from the breakdown products of eosinophil granules.
- Curschmann spirals: coiled or corkscrew shaped casts of bronchioles formed by inspissated mucus.

Cor Pulmonale

210. What are the 4 main groups of disorders that predispose patients to cor pulmonale? (List 2 disorders in each group).
- Pulmonary parenchymal disorders.
  - Chronic obstructive pulmonary disease.
  - Diffuse pulmonary interstitial fibrosis.
- Pulmonary vascular disorders.
  - Primary pulmonary hypertension.
  - Recurrent pulmonary thromboembolism.
- Disorders affecting chest wall movement.
  - Marked obesity (sleep apnea).
  - Neuromuscular disorders.
- Disorders inducing pulmonary arterial constriction.
  - Hypoxemia.
  - Chronic altitude sickness.

211. List 2 acute causes of cor pulmonale.
- Massive pulmonary embolism.
- Exacerbation of chronic cor pulmonale.

212. List 2 gross pathological changes of the heart in cor pulmonale patients.
- Dilatation of the right ventricle.
- Right ventricular hypertrophy.

Kartagener Syndrome

213. What are 2 synonyms for Kartagener syndrome?
- Immotile cilia syndrome.
- Primary ciliary dyskinesia.

214. What is the ultrastructure of normal cilia?
- Normal cilia are 3–6 μm in length, with the main body formed by an axoneme, which consists of a central pair and 9 peripheral doubles of microtubules.
- Each doublet has a complete tubule (A subfiber) and attached 3-quarter circles of B subfiber.
- Two rows of dynein arms from the A subfiber protrude toward the B subfiber of the adjacent doublet, and 1 radial spoke extends toward the central pair.

215. List 4 common clinical presentations of Kartagener syndrome.
- Bronchiectasis and respiratory tract infection.
- Sinusitis.
- Situs inversus.
- Infertility in male patients.

216. List key ultrastructural features of Kartagener syndrome.
- Absent or shortened dynein arms.
- Absence of radial spokes.
- Absence, transposition, or disarrangement of microtubules.
- Presence of compound cilia and ciliary disorientation.

Birt-Hogg-Dubé Syndrome

217. What is Birt-Hogg-Dubé syndrome?
- It is a rare, complex, genetic disorder.
- It has 3 main clinical findings: noncancerous (benign) skin tumors; lung cysts and/or a history of pneumothorax; and various types of renal tumors.

218. What is the most common skin tumor in Birt-Hogg-Dubé syndrome?
- Fibrofolliculoma.
- It typically occurs on the face, neck, and upper torso.

219. What are the 2 common renal tumors in Birt-Hogg-Dubé syndrome?
- Chromophobe subtype of renal cell carcinoma.
- Oncocytoma.

220. What is the genetic alteration in Birt-Hogg-Dubé syndrome?
- It is caused by mutations in the *FLCN* gene.
- It is autosomal dominant disorder.

Pulmonary Alveolar Proteinosis (PAP)

221. What are the clinical features of PAP?
- The age of presentation is usually 30–50 years, and the male-to-female ratio is 2:1.
- Etiology is both idiopathic and "secondary."
- The mechanisms involve overproduction of surfactant by type 2 pneumocytes or impairment of its clearance by macrophages.
- Signs and symptoms include insidious onset, dry cough, shortness of breath with exertion, fatigue, and low grade fever.
- Physical examination is usually normal.
- Patients have markedly elevated serum levels of lung surfactant proteins A and D.
- Pulmonary function tests demonstrate a restrictive pattern.
- CT of the chest reveals bilateral ground-glass opacities with interlobular septal thickening, giving a "crazy paving" appearance.

222. What are the histologic features of PAP?
- It consists of an accumulation of eosinophilic proteinaceous granular material within the alveolar spaces.
- Small and dense globular clumps of eosinophilic material is present.
- These proteinaceous material may stain with the PSA stain and antibody to surfactant apoprotein.
- Electron microscopy reveals concentrically laminated myelin figures and lamellar bodies.

223. What conditions are associated with PAP?
- PAP can be idiopathic or associated with:
  - Infection such as bacteria (*Nocardia*), mycobacteria, fungi, virus.
  - Inorganic dust exposure such as silicosis, aluminum.
  - Immunodeficiency.
  - Lymphoma/leukemia.
  - Others such as Fanconi anemia, lysinuric protein intolerance, etc.

Bronchocentric Granulomatosis

224. What is bronchocentric granulomatosis?
- Bronchocentric granulomatosis is a destructive, granulomatous lesion of the bronchi and bronchioles.
- It is generally believed to represent a nonspecific response to a variety of types of airway injury.

225. What are its causes and associated disorders?
- Allergic reaction:
  - Allergic bronchopulmonary fungal disease.
  - Allergic aspergillosis with mucoid impaction.
- Infectious:
  - Mycobacterial.
  - Fungal.
  - Parasitic (pulmonary echinococcosis).
  - Influenza A virus.

(continued on next page)

- Noninfectious:
  - Granulomatosis with polyangiitis.
  - Rheumatoid arthritis.
  - Ankylosing spondylitis.

- Chronic granulomatous disease.
- Diabetes insipidus.
- Idiopathic.

226. What histologic changes does it involve?
- The airways are infiltrated by neutrophils, eosinophils, and necrotic debris surrounded by foreign body giant cells.
- Necrotizing granulomatous inflammation, involving and destroying the bronchial and/or bronchiolar wells with a palisading histiocytic reaction, is present.

- Fragmented elastic tissue (with elastic stain).
- The distal lung parenchyma may show obstructive pneumonia and scattered granulomas.
- No fibrinoid necrosis of the vessels is present.

Case Scenario

Microscopy of a lung wedge resection from a 55-year-old male shows granulomatous inflammation.

227. What is your differential diagnosis?
- Infection (e.g., fungi, TB, atypical mycobacterium).
- Sarcoidosis.
- Hypersensitivity pneumonitis.
- Reactions to inhaled substances (e.g., talc, aluminum).

- Berylliosis.
- Necrotizing sarcoid granulomatosis.
- Sarcoid-like reaction (e.g., due to malignancies, collagen vascular disease, vasculitis syndromes).

228. Describe an appropriate approach to the case.
- Obtain a clinical history: symptoms and signs, family history, medical history, drug history, radiologic appearance, other relevant details.
- Determine the type of granulomas:
  - Necrotizing granuloma.
    › Fungal infection.
    › Tuberculosis.
    › Atypical mycobacterial infection.
    › Rheumatoid nodule.
  - Nonnecrotizing granuloma:
    › Sarcoidosis.
    › Berylliosis.
    › Hypersensitivity pneumonitis.
    › Sarcoid reaction.
- Determine the distribution of the granulomas:

  - In sarcoidosis and berylliosis, the granulomas are arranged in a lymphatic distribution (i.e., around bronchial vascular bundles, along the septa, and along the pleura.
  - In tuberculosis, the granulomatous inflammation often occurs in the apex and/or superior segment of the lower lobe.
  - In hypersensitivity pneumonitis, the lesions are usually near small airways.
  - Other causes are either near small airways or randomly distributed.
- Perform special stains and other molecular procedures if necessary, to rule out infectious etiology, especially fungal infection and TB.
- If acid-fast bacilli are identified, the public health office, the lab supervisor, and exposed individuals should be notified.

229. What clinical information would you like to obtain?
- Medical history: such as multiorgan involvement of granulomatous inflammation, drug history, vasculitis and ANCA status, collagen vascular disease, immune status.
- History of close contact individuals with TB or other infectious granulomatous disorders.

- History of recent travel to places with a high incidence of granulomatous disease.
- Living conditions: birds in the home, hot tub in the home, or home that is isolated, damp, and old.
- Details of the onset of the disease and its duration, symptoms, and signs, and any medical treatment to date.

230. What ancillary studies would you order?
- PAS/diastase and Gomori methenamine-silver (GMS) stains for fungi.
- Ziehl-Neelsen stain and/or other methods if necessary for acid fast bacilli (e.g., auramine-rhodamine fluorescent

stain, Fite stain, polymerase chain reaction, BACTEC radio respiratory detection system).
- Gram stain for bacteria.

231. What do you do if TB is suspected on frozen section?
- Take universal precaution measures.
- Use an N95 mask.
- Inform the surgeon/operating room staff immediately.
- Request the surgeon to take a tissue culture if possible.

- Take a sample for tissue culture from frozen section lab if necessary.
- Decontaminate the equipment, surface of the workstation, and the cryostat in the frozen section lab.

(continued on next page)

- After frozen section, keep the specimen in formalin for a couple of days before grossing to make sure the specimen is fully fixed.

- Report to the lab supervisor.
- Inform the occupational office and public health office if TB is confirmed.

Case Scenario

A 30-year-old man presented with diffuse lung infiltrate and bilateral areas of ground-glass attenuation on a chest CT. Microscopy shows diffuse foamy exudates within alveolar spaces.

232. What is the most possible diagnosis?
- The patient is most likely immune suppressed or deficient, especially if HIV positive.
- In such a setting, pneumocystis pneumonia (PCP) is the most common lung infection.

233. How do you tell different fungi apart by morphology?

FUNGI	MORPHOLOGY
Candida	• Oval yeast-like cells. · Diameter: 2–6 μm. · Accompanied by mycelial forms with pseudohyphae. · Pseudohyphae: elongated yeast-like cells, 3–5 μm in width that line up in chains. · Note: true hyphae are occasionally present.
Aspergillus	• Septate hyphae. · Width: 3–6 μm. · Generally uniform. · Growth pattern: parallel, with septa at regular intervals. · Branching: dichotomous at acute angles, often at 45°.
Zygomycetes (including *Mucor*)	• Broad hyphae. · Width: 5–25 μm. · Often twisted or folded due to the thin wall. · Branching: irregular, but sometimes with angles of 90°.
Histoplasma	• Yeast-like forms. · Diameter: 2–4 μm. · Structure: single budding with a narrow base. · Note: occasionally darkly stained foci are present, similar to those seen in *Pneumocystis jirovecii*.
Cryptococcus	• Yeast-like forms. · Diameter: 4–6 μm (may range 2–20 μm). · Structure: single budding with a narrow base. · Capsule: presents as a halo that is positive for mucin stains such as mucicarmine, PAS/diastase, and Alcian blue.
Blastomyces	• Yeast-like forms. · Diameter: 8–15 μm. · Structure: single budding with a broad base, a thick and refractile wall, and multiple nuclei.
Coccidioides	• Mature spherules. · Diameter: 30–200 μm. · Refractile wall: 1–2 μm thick. · Spherule contents: uninucleate endospores 2–5 μm in diameter. · Note: immature spherules also present, of various sizes and lacking endospores.
Pneumocystis jiroveci	• Round to oval cysts. · Diameter: 5–7 μm. • Structure: prominent grooves or folds. · Darkly stained foci: represent discoid thickenings of the cyst capsule, a tiny central dot often present. · Tissue section: an intraalveolar foamy exudate is present in which the organisms appear as small "bubbles."

234. What special stains confirm fungal infection?

- PAS positive and diastase resistant.
- GMS positive.

Note: *Candida* is also positive on Gram stain.

235. What other information about this patient would be relevant?

- Travel history.
- Immune status.
- History of cancer.
- History of chemotherapy or radiation therapy.
- History of organ/bone marrow transplantation.

236. How do you handle a wedge lung biopsy for nonneoplastic lung tissue?

- Request fresh tissue in saline to be sent immediately to the lab from the operating room (OR).
- Apply universal precautions during the procedure.
- Take a small piece of the tissue for culture in a sterilized condition, if this was not done in the OR.
- Measure the specimen.
- Inject formalin gently into the tissue using a 16–18 gauge needle with a syringe.
- Submerge the tissue in formalin for approximately 1 hour.
- Slice the tissue perpendicular or parallel to the surface to obtain a sufficient plane.
- Place the tissue into cassettes and resubmerge in formalin for further fixation.
- Follow the routine procedure for tissue processing.

Case Scenario

A 38-year-old man presents with geographic necrosis, granulomatous inflammation, and vasculitis in his lungs.

237. What is your differential diagnosis?

- Granulomatosis with polyangiitis (previously referred to as Wegener granulomatosis).
- Infection.
- Necrotizing sarcoid granulomatosis.
- Eosinophilic granulomatosis with polyangiitis (also known as Churg-Strauss syndrome).
- Bronchocentric granulomatosis such as allergic bronchopulmonary aspergillosis.
- Rheumatoid arthritis.

238. What is your favored diagnosis?

Granulomatosis with polyangiitis.

239. Define ANCAs and describe how to detect them.

- ANCAs: antineutrophil cytoplasmic antibodies, a heterogeneous group of autoantibodies directed against enzymes of neutrophil primary granules, monocyte lysosomes, and endothelial cells.
- Detection:
  · Indirect immunofluorescence assays. There are 2 major immunofluorescence patterns according to their intracellular distribution when using ethanol fixation:
    › c-ANCA: proteinase 3 located in primary granules in the cytoplasm, yielding a cytoplasmic staining pattern.
    › p-ANCA: myeloperoxidase (MPO) dissolved from the primary granules attaches to the cell nucleus, yielding a perinuclear staining pattern.
  · Antigen detection using enzyme-linked immunosorbent assay (ELISA) based on the target antigens:
    › Antiproteinase-3 (c-ANCA).
    › Antimyeloperoxidase (p-ANCA).

240. What is the significance of positive ANCA tests?

- Although not entirely specific, antiproteinase-3 (c-ANCA) is typical of granulomatosis with polyangiitis, and antimyeloperoxidase (p-ANCA) is more likely seen in patients with microscopic polyangiitis and eosinophilic granulomatosis with polyangiitis (Churg-Strauss syndrome).
- ANCAs are useful diagnostic markers for ANCA associated vasculitides, and their titers may reflect the degree of inflammatory activity. ANCA titers also rise with recurrent disease and are therefore useful in clinical management.
- Although the precise mechanisms are unknown, ANCA can directly activate neutrophils and may thereby stimulate neutrophils to release reactive oxygen species and proteolytic enzymes.

241. What additional information is helpful if granulomatosis with polyangiitis is suspected?

- Check the patient's clinical history and presentation, especially symptoms and signs in head and neck regions, upper and lower respiratory tract, kidney, and other organ systems.
- Check renal functions.
- ANCA status.
- Radiologic findings.
- Keep the differential diagnosis in mind as listed above.

242. What organs does granulomatosis with polyangiitis involve?
- It is a systemic granulomatous inflammatory process.
- It predominantly affects the head and neck, the upper and lower respiratory tract, and the kidneys.
- It may also involve other organ systems (e.g., eyes, joints, skin, pericardium, central and peripheral nervous system).

Case Scenario

A lung biopsy specimen shows features of Cytomegalovirus (CMV) pneumonia.

243. What is CMV?
- It is a herpesvirus with a double stranded DNA that contains the genetic information to approximately 33 structural proteins.
- It measures 120–200 nm and has an envelope derived from the nuclear membrane.
- It replicates in the host cell nucleus.

244. What are the pathologic patterns of CMV pneumonia?
- A CMV associated with minimal inflammation or lung injury pattern.
- A miliary pattern.
- A diffuse interstitial pneumonitis pattern.
- A hemorrhagic pneumonia pattern.

245. How do you diagnosis CMV pneumonia?
- Diagnosis requires:
  · Histologic evaluation +/– IHC for CMV.
  · Culture.
- Serologic signs of CMV infection are inadequate for a diagnosis of CMV pneumonia.
- Findings of CMV in urine, blood, or respiratory secretions indicate the presence of CMV organisms, but not necessarily that the organisms are pulmonary pathogens.

246. What other types of infection can be caused by CMV?
- Congenital and perinatal infections.
- Infectious mononucleosis.
- Hepatitis.
- Opportunistic infections in transplant patients, AIDS patients, and other individuals with immunodeficiency.
- Posttransfusion infections.
- Infection in those receiving immunosuppressive therapy.

247. Describe how to handle an infectious fresh wedge lung biopsy specimen.
- Apply universal precautions.
- Use an N95 mask (recommended).
- Handle the specimen at a workstation with a ventilated hood.
- Take a piece of tissue for culture in a sterilized condition, if this was not done in the OR.
- Fix the tissue well in formalin before grossing.
- Decontaminate the equipment and surfaces of the workstation.

Case Scenario

The lung wedge biopsy specimen from a 37-year-old man shows mostly organizing changes.

248. What is your differential diagnosis?
- Cryptogenic organizing pneumonia — previously known as bronchiolitis obliterans organizing pneumonia (BOOP).
- Infection induced changes.
- Acute interstitial pneumonia/diffuse alveolar damage.
- Drug reaction.
- Hypersensitivity pneumonitis.
- Others (e.g., collagen vascular disease, nonspecific reaction, etc.).

249. What are the primary and secondary causes of organizing pneumonia?
- Primary:
  · Cryptogenic organizing pneumonia.
- Secondary:
  · Infection.
  · Collagen vascular disease.
  · Drug reaction.
  · Nonspecific reaction adjacent to other lesions (e.g., abscess, neoplasm, infarct).
  · Others (e.g., aspiration, radiation, hemorrhage, granulomatosis with polyangiitis, hypersensitivity pneumonitis, cocaine abuse, myelodysplastic syndrome).

250. How do you distinguish organizing pneumonia from usual interstitial pneumonia (UIP)?

FEATURE	ORGANIZING PNEUMONIA	UIP
CLINICAL		
Mean age	• 56.	• 64.
Duration of symptoms	• 1–6 months.	• 1–3 years.
Response to steroids	• Good.	• Poor.
Prognosis	• Good.	• Poor.
PATHOLOGIC		
Distribution	• Patchy, centered near airways.	• Patchy, subpleural and paraseptal predominant.
Temporal appearance	• Uniform.	• Heterogenous.
Fibroblastic foci	• Absent.	• Characteristic.
Fibroblastic polyps/plugs	• Characteristic.	• Focal and minimal.
Dense fibrosis	• Absent.	• Characteristic.
Honeycomb	• Absent.	• Often present.

251. What is the clinical behavior of cryptogenic organizing pneumonia?

- Clinical presentation mimics community acquired pneumonia.
- Onset is usually in the fifth or sixth decade of life.
- It has an acute/subacute clinical course.
- Main symptoms include nonproductive cough and dyspnea.
- Routine lab tests are nonspecific.
- Pulmonary function tests usually show a restrictive defect.
- It has a good response to steroids.

IMAGES: PULMONARY PATHOLOGY

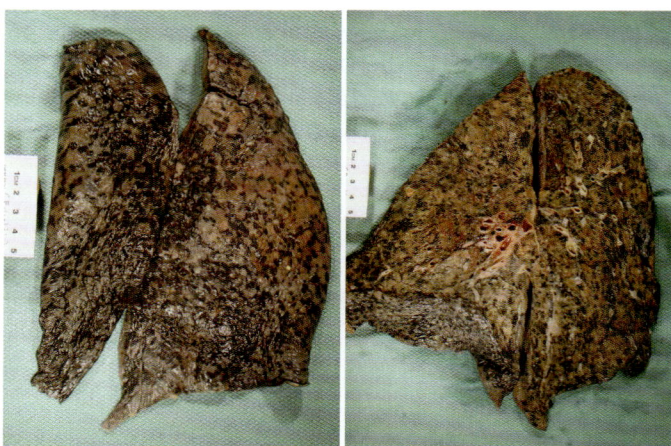

IMAGE 18.1 Simple coal worker's pneumoconiosis. There are numerous coal dust macules and small black nodules.

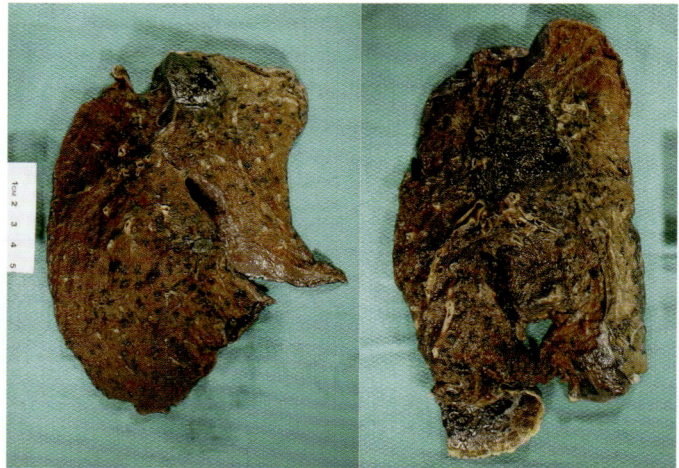

IMAGE 18.2 Complicated coal worker's pneumoconiosis. In addition to numerous coal dust macules and small pigmented nodules, there are bilateral large black masses.

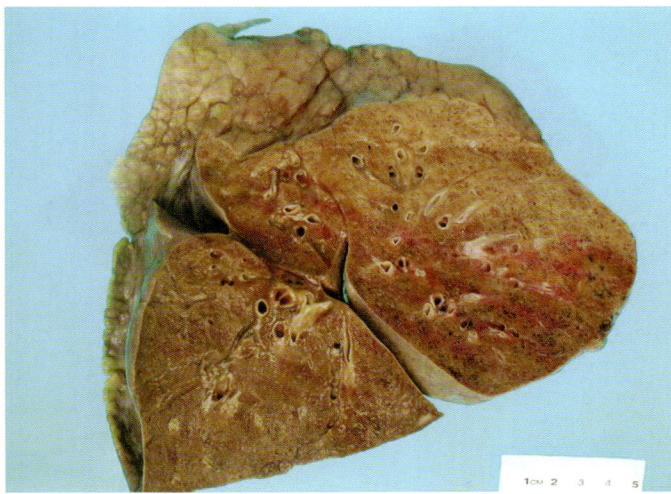

IMAGE 18.3 Diffuse alveolar damage. There is congestion and consolidation, especially in the lower lobe.

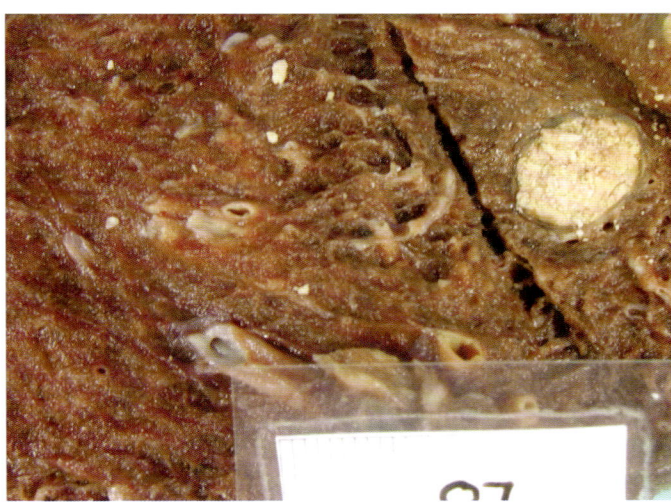

IMAGE 18.6 Coccidioidomycosis. The image shows a well-demarcated nodular lesion with necrosis.

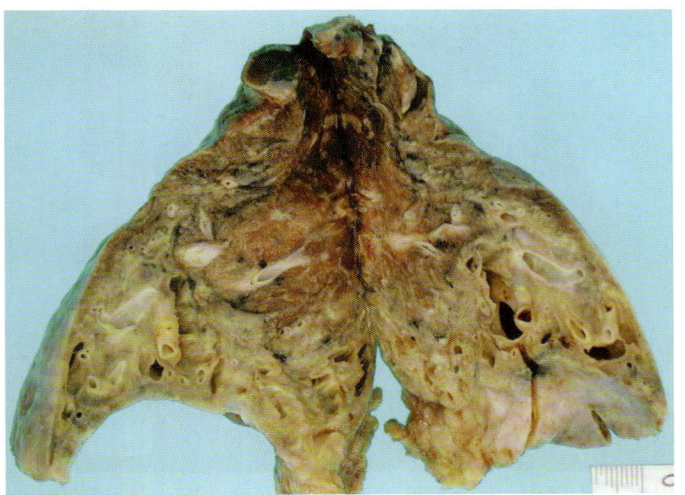

IMAGE 18.4 Intralobar sequestration. There is an ill-defined area of consolidation with prominent and dilated vessels.

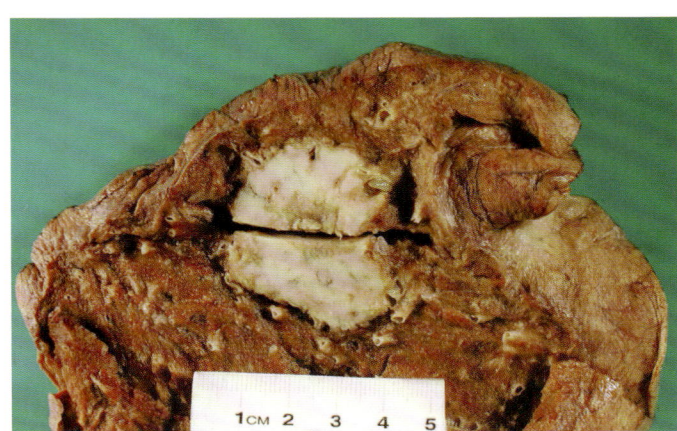

IMAGE 18.7 Pulmonary hyalinizing granuloma grossly resembling lung cancer.

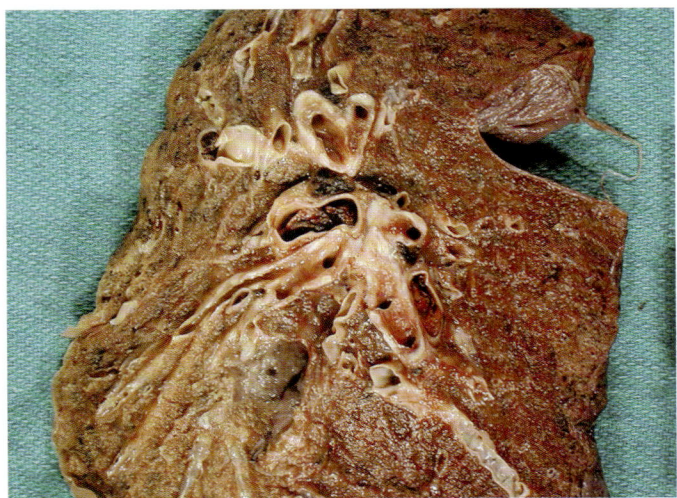

IMAGE 18.5 Pulmonary emboli. Organized emboli are present within large pulmonary arteries.

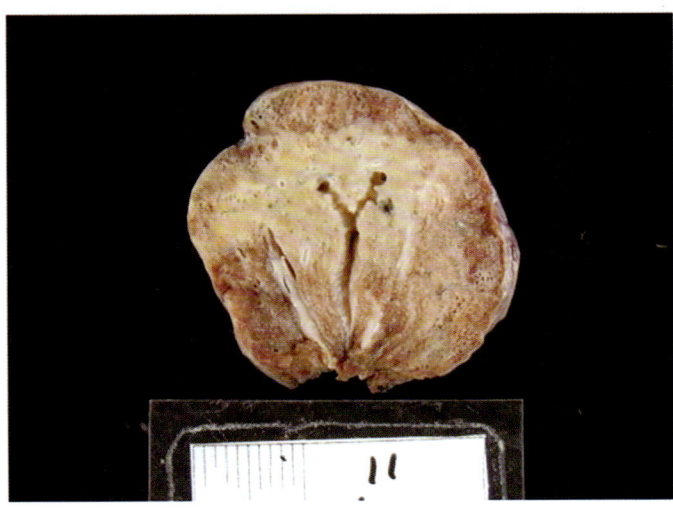

IMAGE 18.8 Localized interstitial fibrosis with mass-like appearance resembling a neoplastic process.

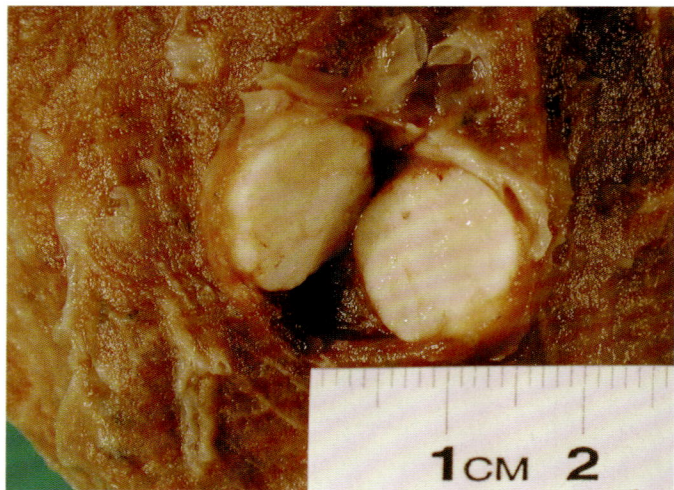

IMAGE 18.9 Pulmonary chondroid hamartoma.

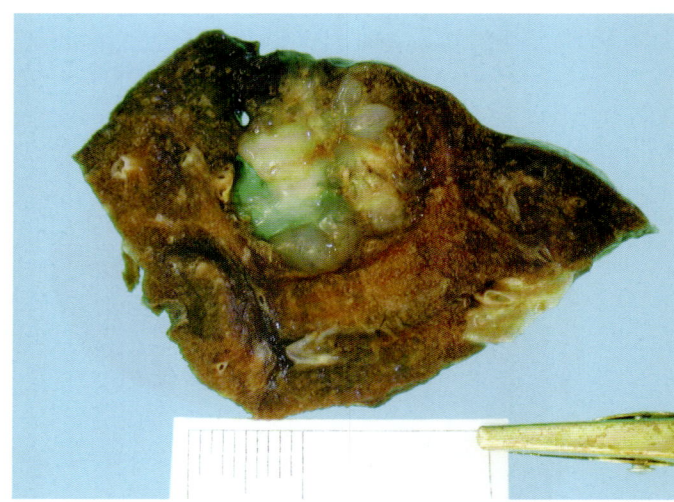

IMAGE 18.12 Adenocarcinoma with prominent mucin accumulation.

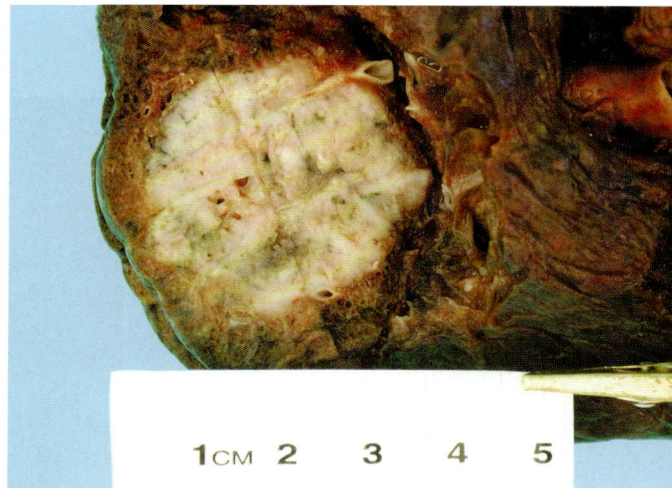

IMAGE 18.10 Bronchogenic adenocarcinoma in a peripheral location of lung.

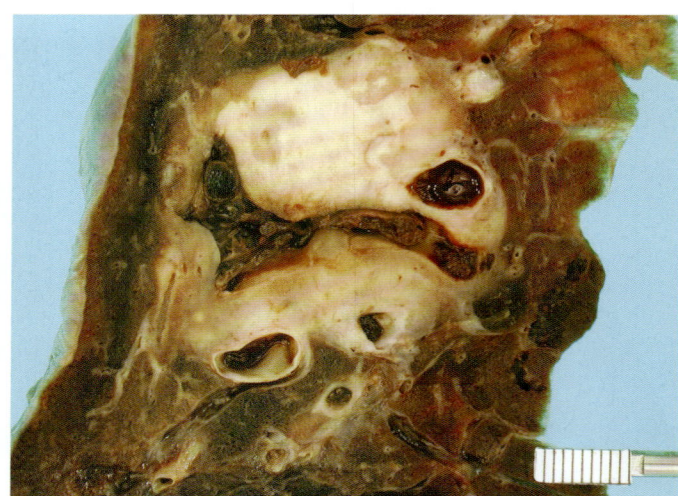

IMAGE 18.13 Lymphomatoid granulomatosis shows its close proximity to large vessels with thrombi and focal hemorrhage.

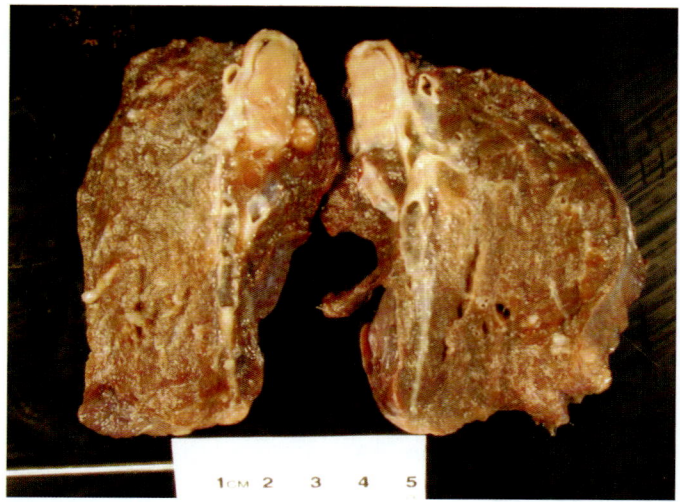

IMAGE 18.11 Carcinoid tumor that protrudes into the bronchial lumen causing obstruction. Note the yellow-tan color on the cut surface.

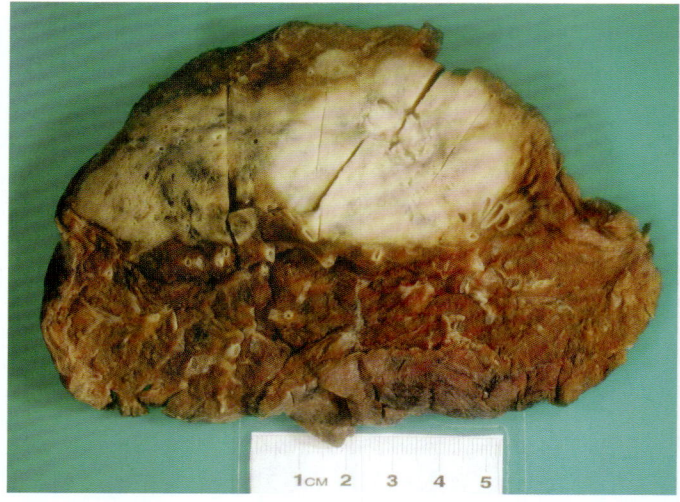

IMAGE 18.14 Adenosquamous carcinoma. The solid mass on the right is squamous cell carcinoma while the lesion on the left side is well-differentiated adenocarcinoma with prominent lepidic pattern on microscopic examination.

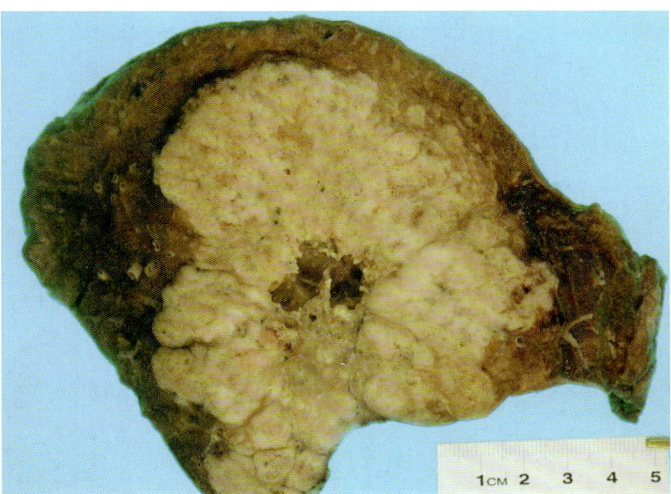

IMAGE 18.15 Squamous cell carcinoma with central necrosis and cavitation.

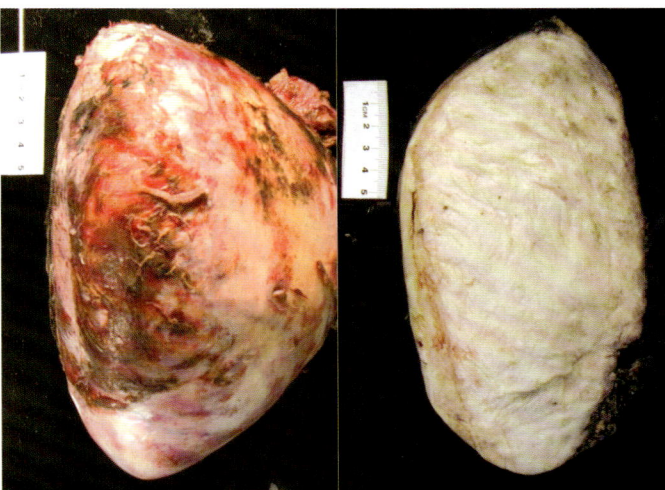

IMAGE 18.18 Chest wall desmoid fibromatosis. This is a large thoracic mass about 22 × 13 × 10 cm arising from the chest wall and growing toward the thoracic cavity.

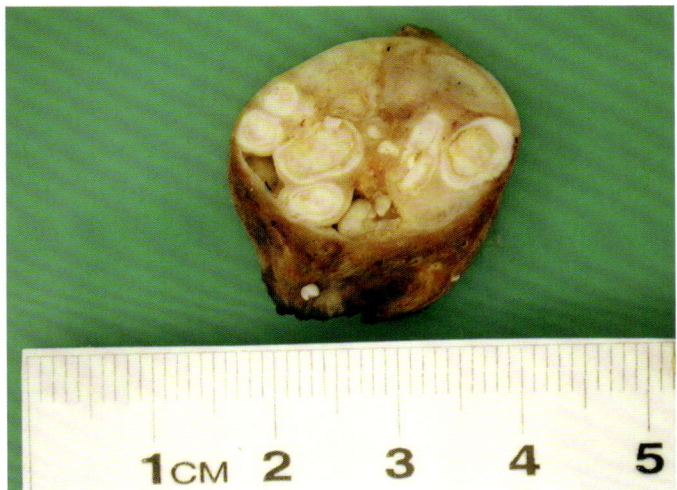

IMAGE 18.16 Metastatic teratoma. This patient had a testicular mixed germ cell tumor including teratoma components, which had been treated with surgery and chemotherapy.

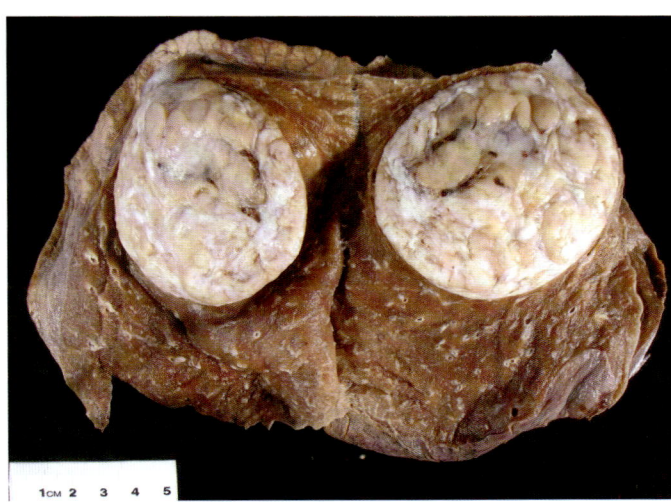

IMAGE 18.19 Solitary fibrous tumor. The image shows a well-demarcated pleura based mass.

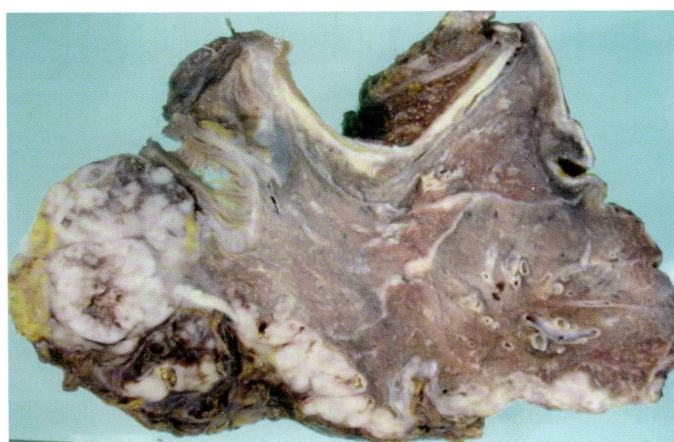

IMAGE 18.17 Malignant mesothelioma. The image shows pleural based nodular lesions and fibrous pleural thickening.

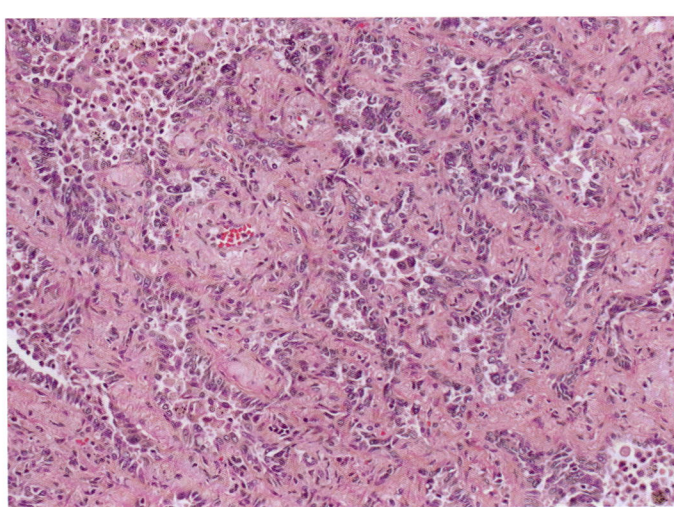

IMAGE 18.20 Adenocarcinoma, acinar pattern. Tumor cells form glandular structures with various sizes and irregular shapes (H&E, x200).

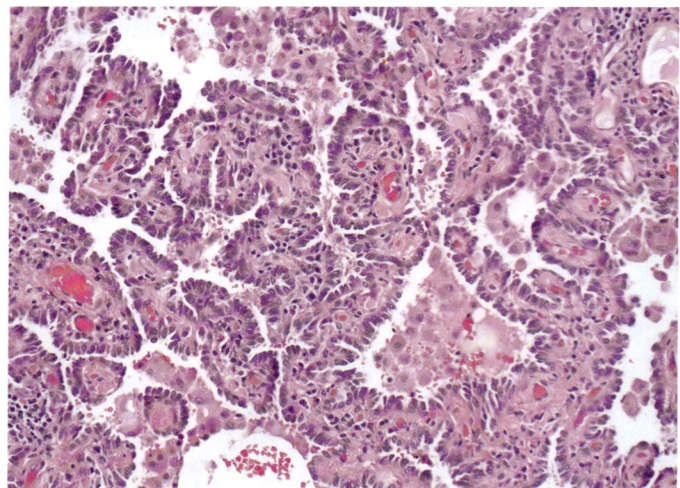

IMAGE 18.21 Adenocarcinoma, papillary pattern. Tumor cells form papillary configuration with fibrovascular cores (H&E, x200).

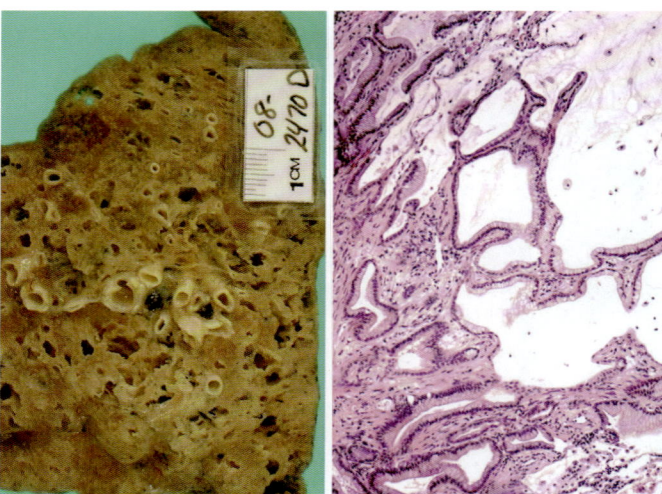

IMAGE 18.24 Invasive mucinous adenocarcinoma. Left: this gross image shows that the tumor occupies almost the entire lobe and has a glistening gelatinous appearance. Right: the tumor cells have bland and basally located nuclei (H&E, x100).

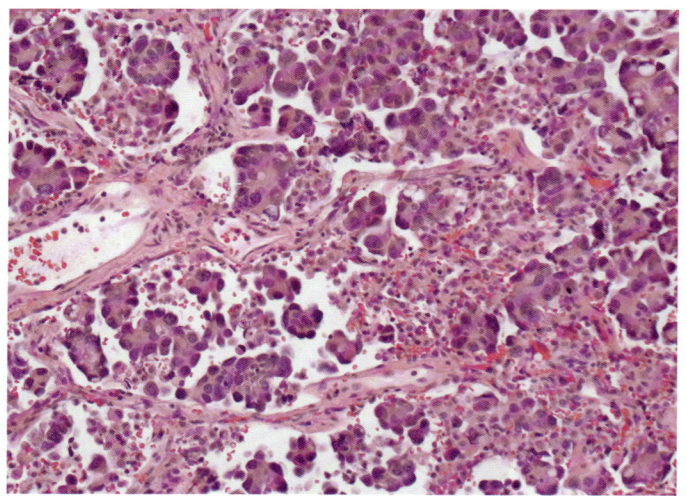

IMAGE 18.22 Adenocarcinoma, micropapillary pattern. Tumor cells form micropapillary clusters without fibrovascular cores floating within the air spaces (H&E, x200).

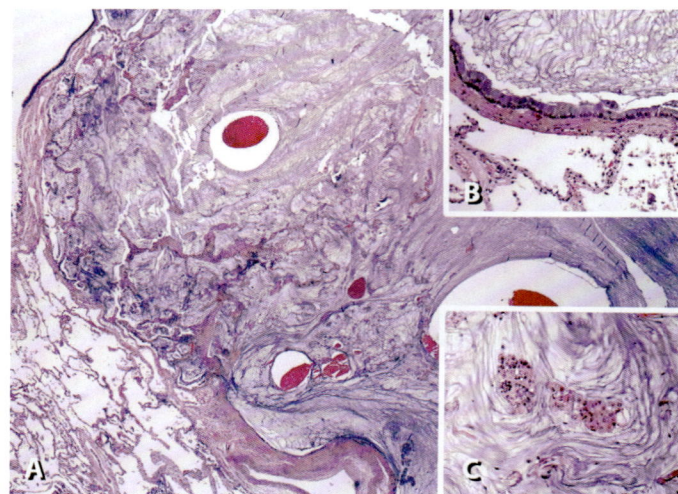

IMAGE 18.25 Colloid adenocarcinoma. Image A: H&E, x20. Image B: a large pool of mucin partially lined by bland mucinous epithelium. Image C: a small cluster of bland tumor cells floating within the mucin pool.

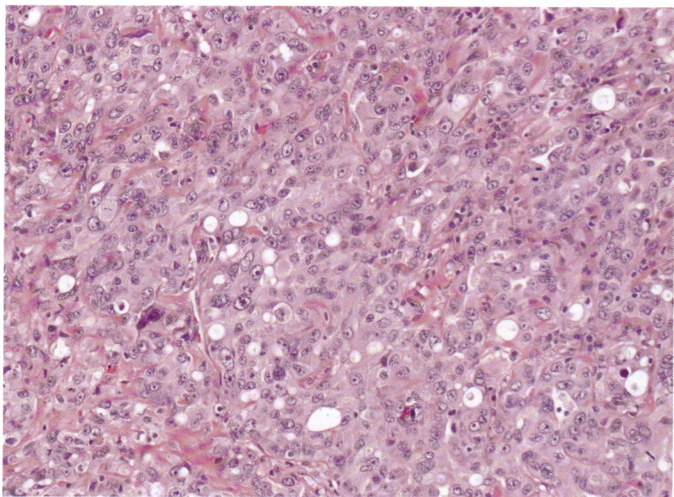

IMAGE 18.23 Adenocarcinoma, solid pattern. Tumor cells form solid sheets or nests with scattered vacuolar changes but no obvious tubular or glandular structures (H&E, x200).

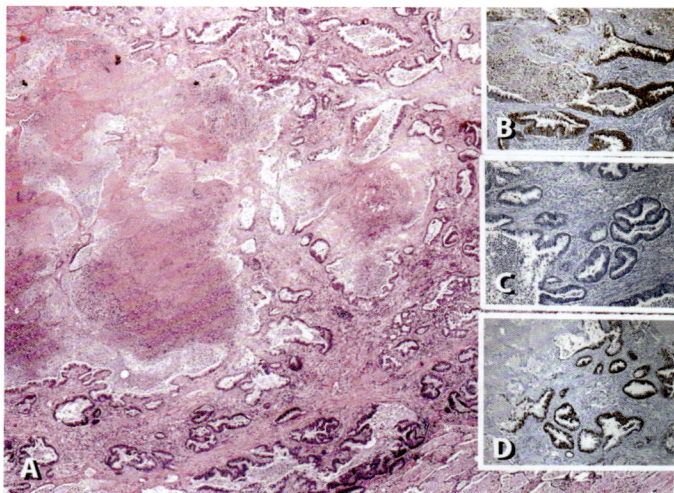

IMAGE 18.26 Adenocarcinoma, enteric type. Image A: morphologically, this tumor is difficult to differentiate from metastatic colonic adenocarcinoma (H&E, x40). The inset images show immunostains (image B: CK7; image C: CK20; image D: TTF-1).

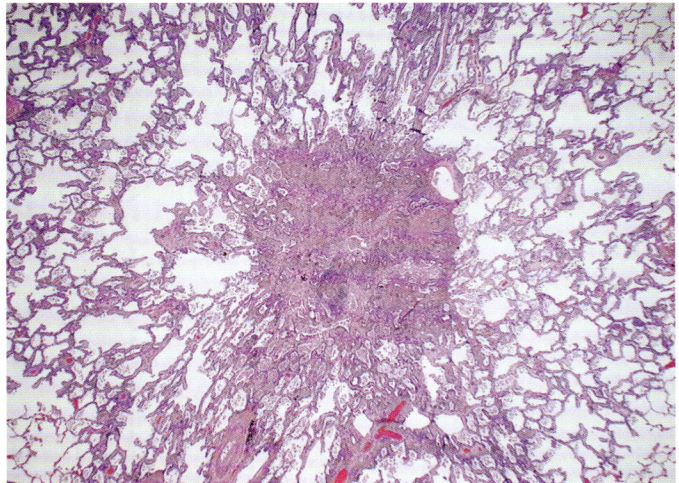

IMAGE 18.27 Minimally invasive adenocarcinoma showing a lepidic growth pattern with a focal invasive component that is < 0.5 cm in size (H&E, x20).

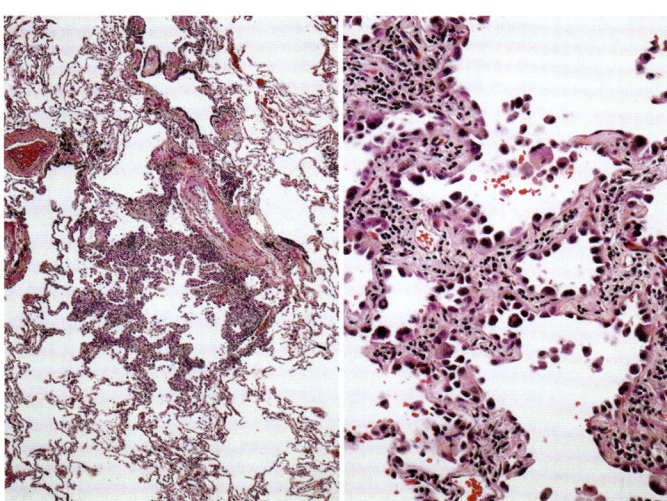

IMAGE 18.30 Atypical adenomatous hyperplasia. The lesion is usually < 5 mm in size. There is a focal proliferation of slightly atypical cuboidal to low columnar epithelial cells along the alveolar wall, and slight thickening of the alveolar septa that resembles but falls short of criteria for nonmucinous AIS. Left: H&E, x20. Right: H&E, x100.

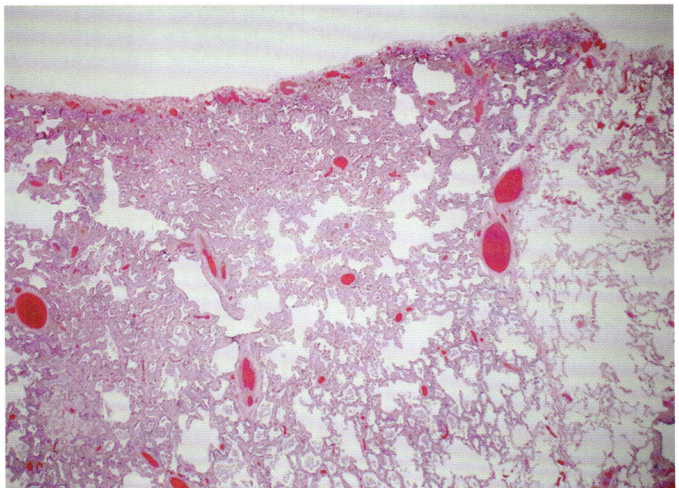

IMAGE 18.28 Adenocarcinoma in situ (nonmucinous type) shows a pure lepidic pattern without evidence of stromal invasion (H&E, x20).

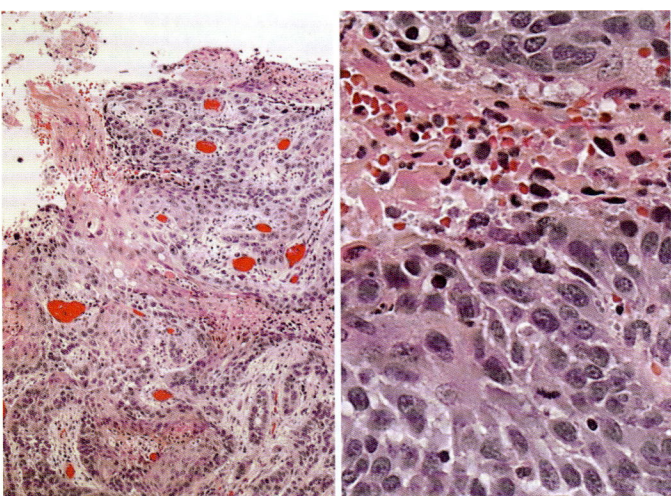

IMAGE 18.31 Squamous cell carcinoma showing keratin formation and intercellular bridges Left: H&E, x100. Right, H&E, x400.

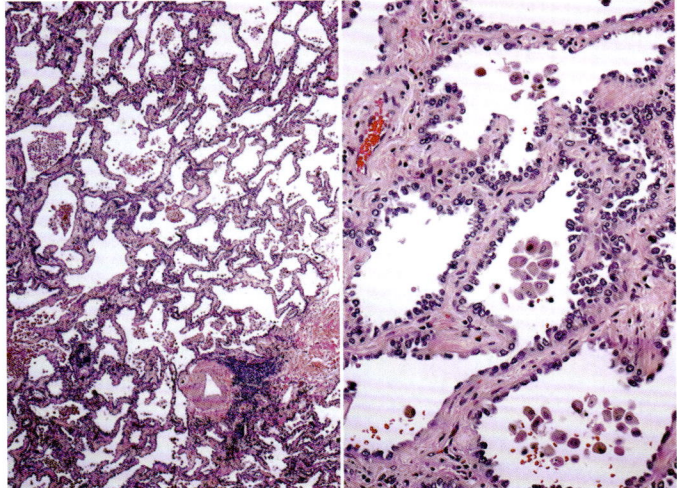

IMAGE 18.29 Adenocarcinoma, lepidic pattern. Left: H&E, x40. Right: H&E, x100.

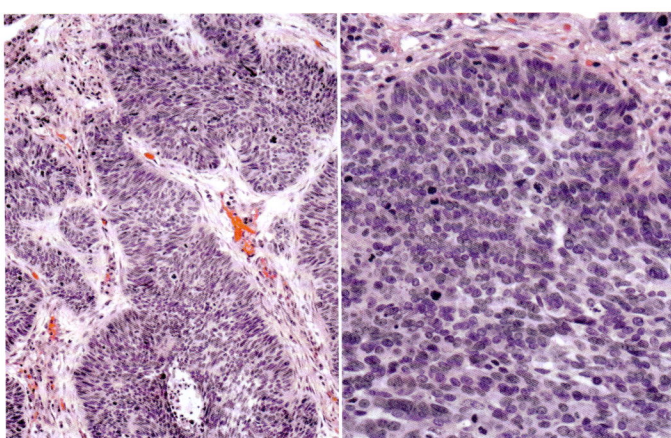

IMAGE 18.32 Basaloid squamous cell carcinoma. The tumor cells are relatively small with a basaloid appearance and peripheral palisading. Neuroendocrine markers are all negative. Left: H&E, x40. Right: H&E, x200.

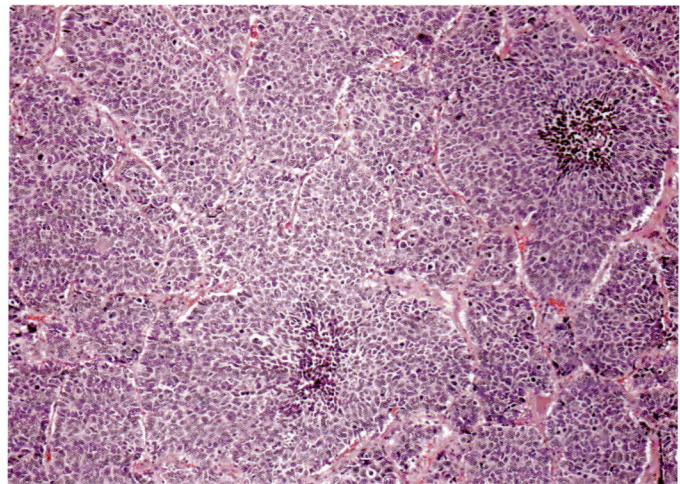

IMAGE 18.33 Large cell carcinoma. It is an undifferentiated carcinoma of nonsmall cell type (H&E, x100). Neuroendocrine markers are negative in this case.

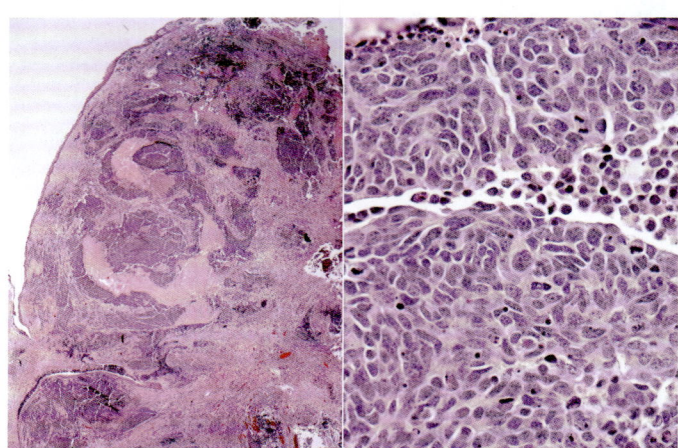

IMAGE 18.36 Large cell neuroendocrine carcinoma. Left: the tumor has prominent necrosis (H&E, x20). Right: the tumor cells are intermediate to large in size with "salt and pepper" chromatin and frequent mitoses (H&E, x400).

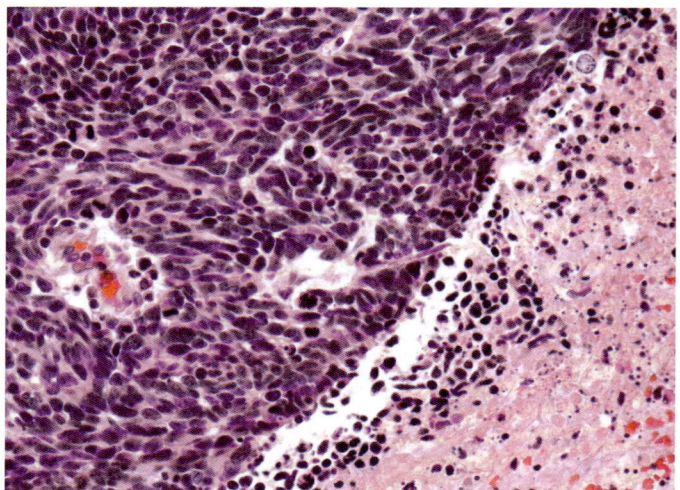

IMAGE 18.34 Small cell carcinoma. Tumor cells are small (usually < 3x resting lymphocytes) with hyperchromatic nuclei, nuclear molding, inconspicuous nucleoli, frequent mitoses, and prominent tumor cell necrosis (H&E, x200).

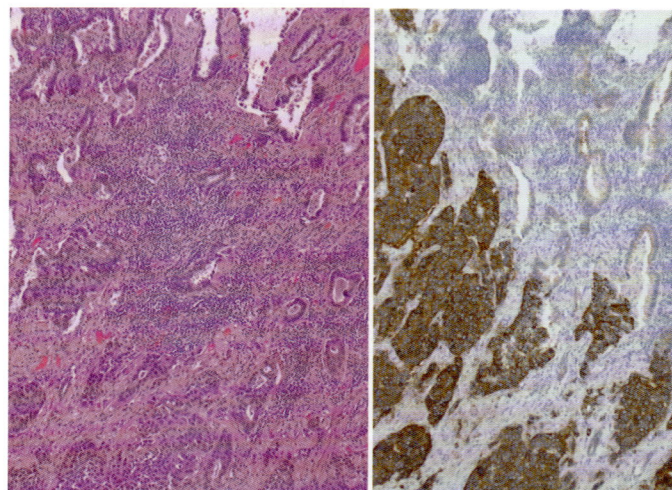

IMAGE 18.37 Combined large cell neuroendocrine carcinoma with adenocarcinoma component. Left: H&E x100. Right: synaptophysin stain, x100.

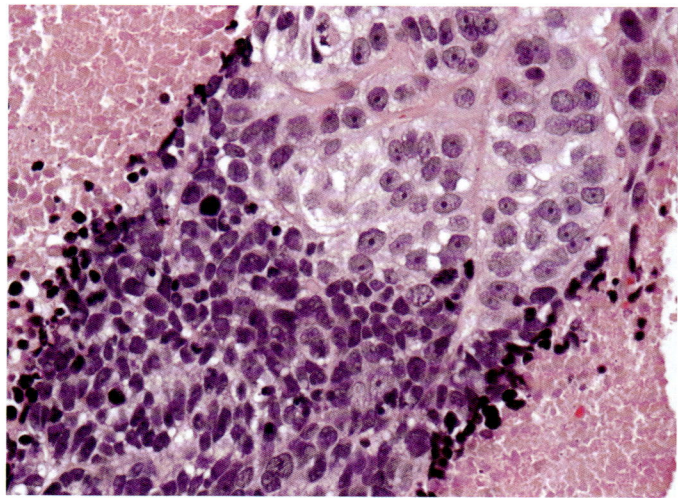

IMAGE 18.35 Combined small cell carcinoma with squamous cell carcinoma component in the upper right corner (H&E, x400).

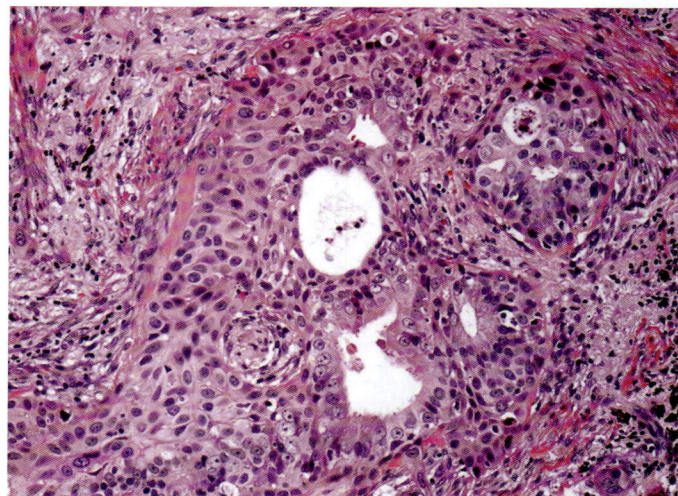

IMAGE 18.38 Adenosquamous carcinoma. The tumor shows neoplastic glandular structures and squamous differentiation (H&E, x200).

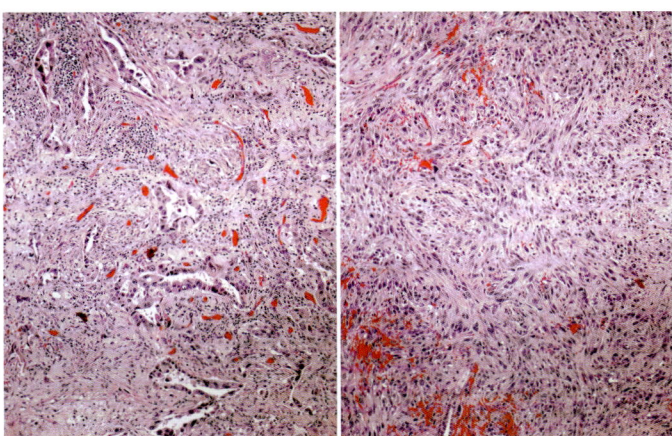

IMAGE 18.39 Pleomorphic carcinoma. There is a mixture of malignant glands and sarcomatoid spindle cells. Left and right: H&E, x100.

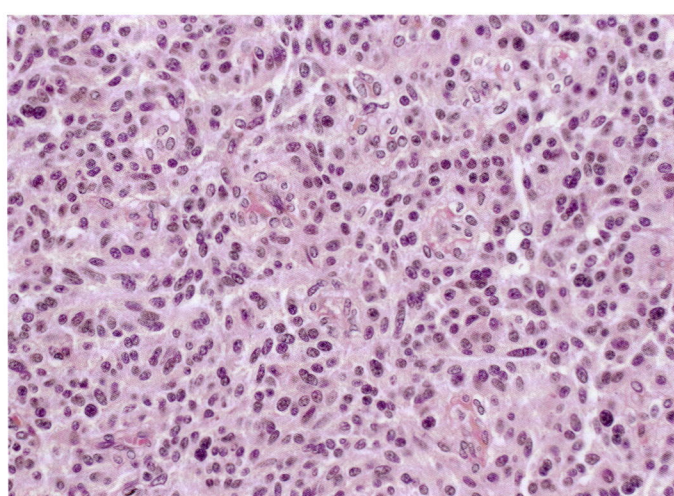

IMAGE 18.42 Typical carcinoid. Tumor cells have a monotonous appearance with slightly eosinophilic and granular cytoplasm (H&E, x400).

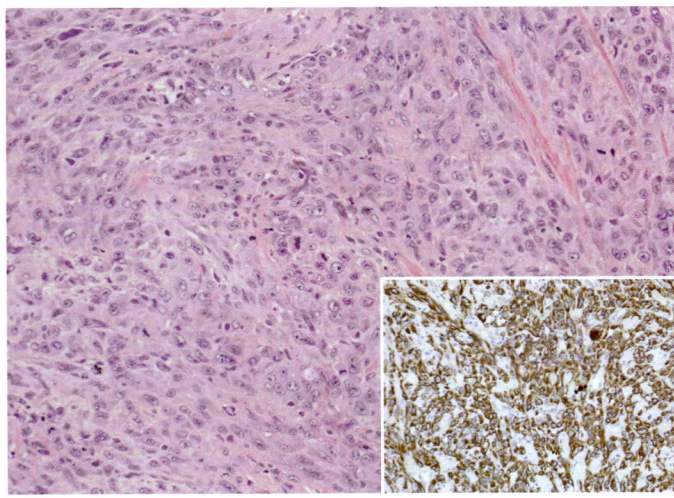

IMAGE 18.40 Pleomorphic carcinoma. The tumor shows malignant epithelioid cells and spindle cells (H&E, x200). AE1/AE3 stain is positive in both components (inset image).

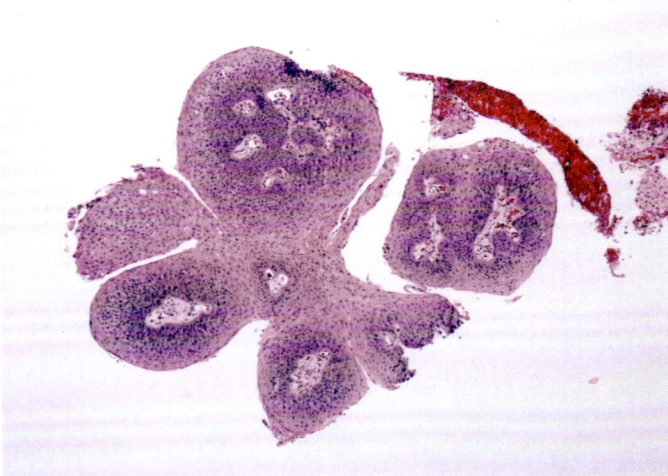

IMAGE 18.43 Squamous papilloma. This is an endobronchial lesion composed of benign squamous epithelium with a papillary configuration (H&E, x40).

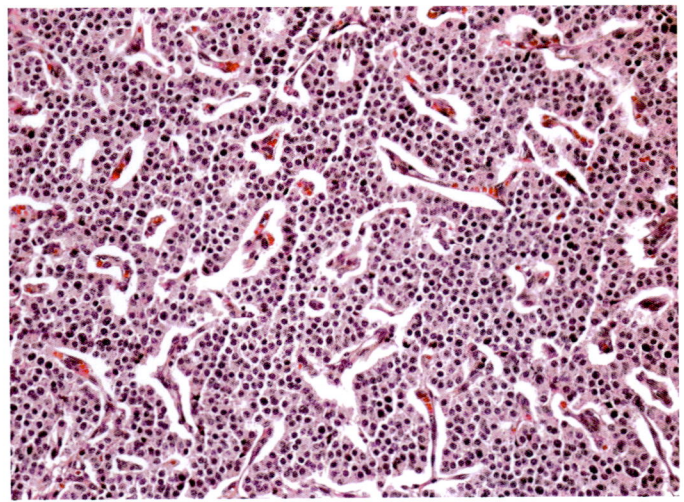

IMAGE 18.41 Typical carcinoid. Tumor cell nests are surrounded by delicate vasculature with no tumor cell necrosis and mitosis (H&E, x100).

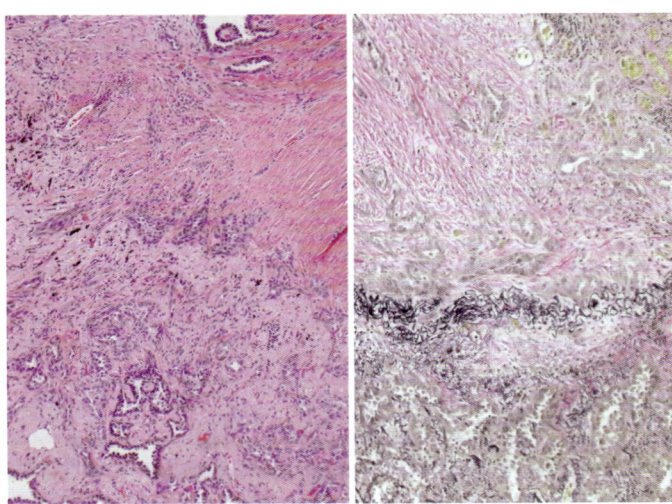

IMAGE 18.44 Adenocarcinoma invading though visceral pleura. Left: H&E, x100. Right: elastic stain, x100.

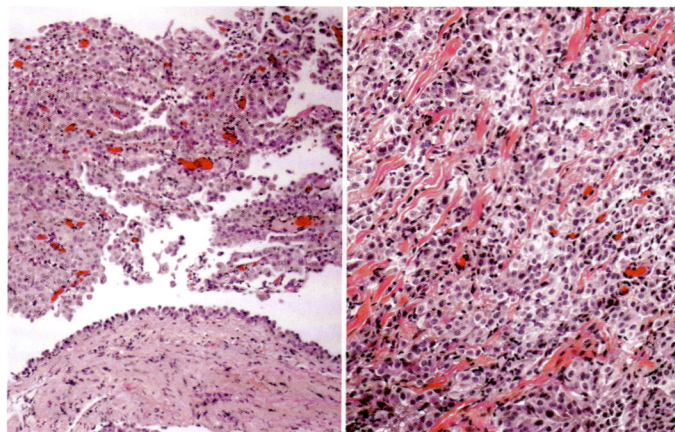

IMAGE 18.45 Epithelioid malignant mesothelioma. Left: focal tubular and papillary architecture (H&E, x40). Right: stromal invasion (H&E, x100).

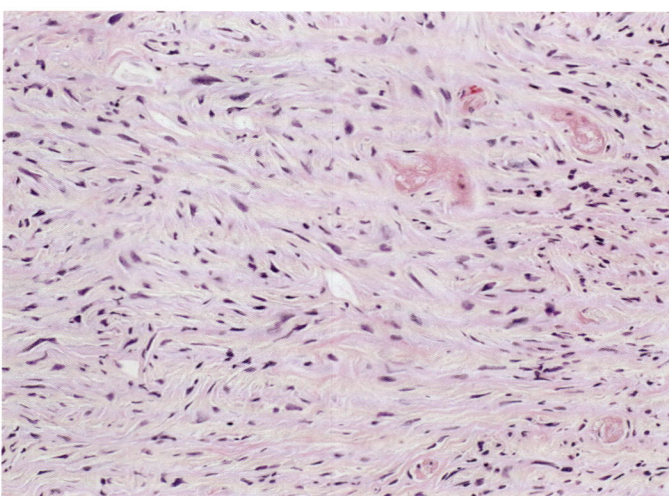

IMAGE 18.48 Desmoplastic malignant mesothelioma shows atypical spindle tumor cells interspersed with prominent fibrous stroma (H&E, x200).

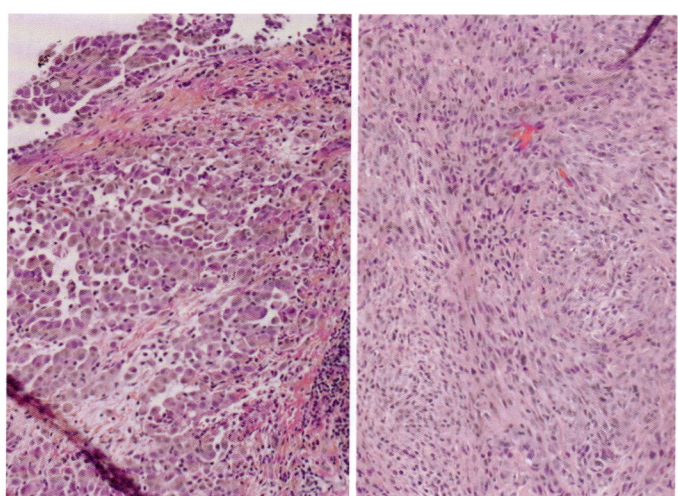

IMAGE 18.46 Biphasic malignant mesothelioma. Left: a tumor with epithelioid component (H&E, x200). Right: a tumor with sarcomatoid component (H&E, x200).

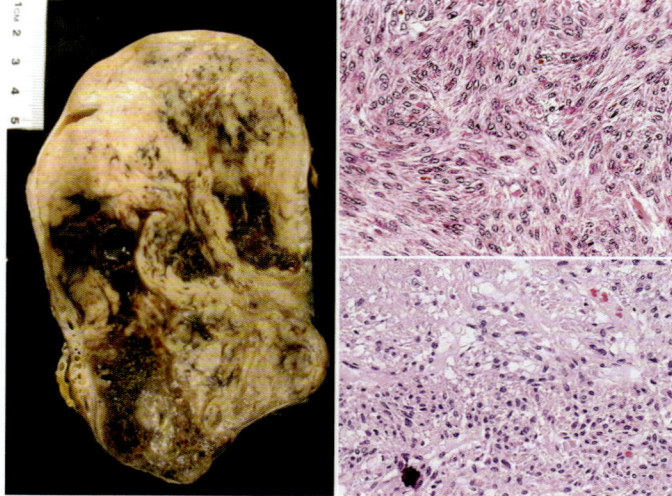

IMAGE 18.49 Mediastinal low grade leiomyosarcoma. Left: the tumor is a solid mass with areas of hemorrhage and small cystic degeneration. Right upper: tumor cells with bland nuclear features (H&E, x200). Right lower: focal calcification and a focal area of necrosis (H&E, x100). Tumor cells stain positive for smooth muscle markers (not shown).

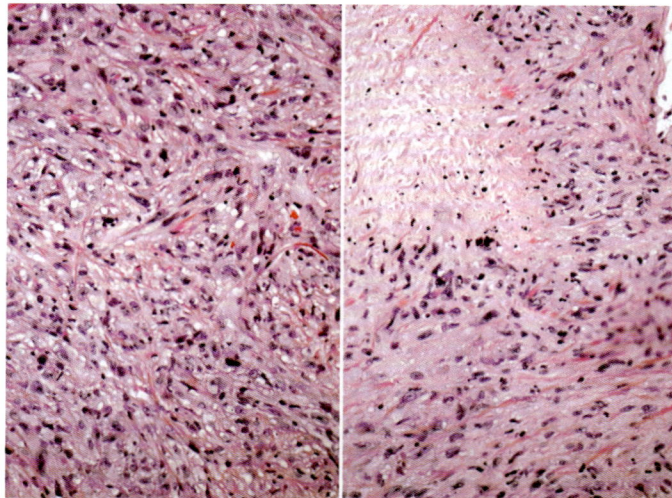

IMAGE 18.47 Sarcomatoid malignant mesothelioma. Left: spindle shaped tumor cells in a haphazard arrangement (H&E, x200). Right: focal tumor cell necrosis (H&E, x200).

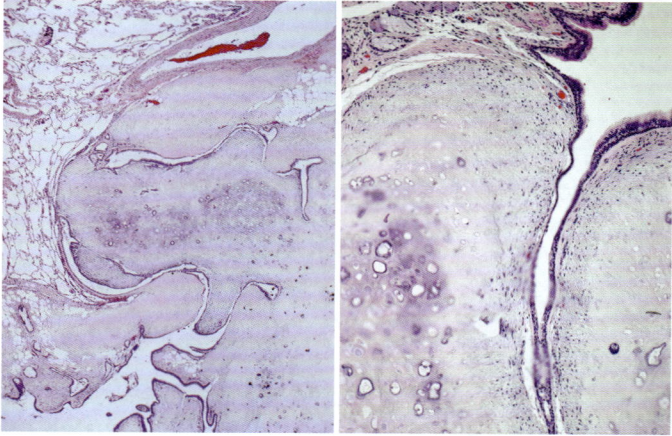

IMAGE 18.50 Pulmonary hamartoma. Left: the tumor is composed of cartilage and some benign adipose tissue with the surface covered by respiratory epithelium (H&E, x20). Right: at the periphery of the cartilage, there are myxoid stroma with some stromal cells (H&E, x100).

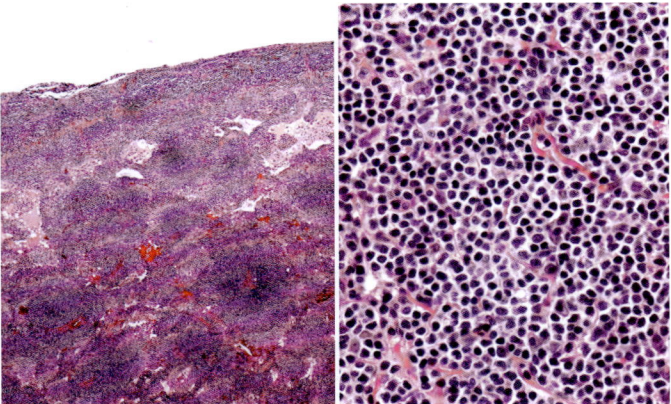

IMAGE 18.51 MALT lymphoma. The image shows a nodular lesion composed of centrocyte-like cells within the lung parenchyma and extending to the visceral pleura. Left: H&E, x20. Right: H&E, x100. The tumor cells are strongly and diffusely positive for CD20 (not shown).

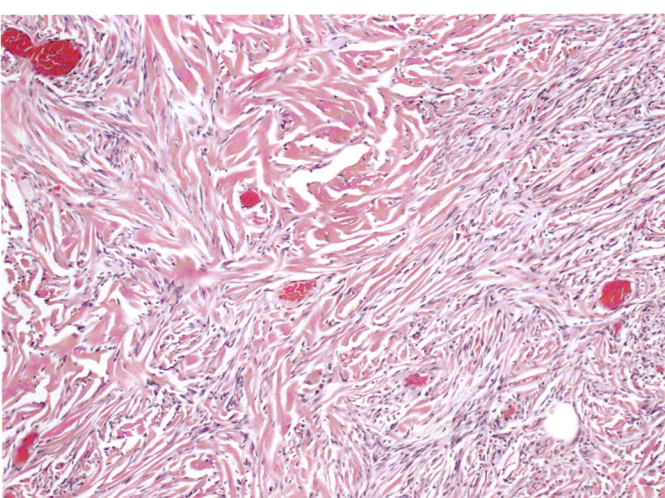

IMAGE 18.54 Solitary fibrous tumor. The tumor shows a low cellularity and prominent fibrotic stroma (H&E, x100).

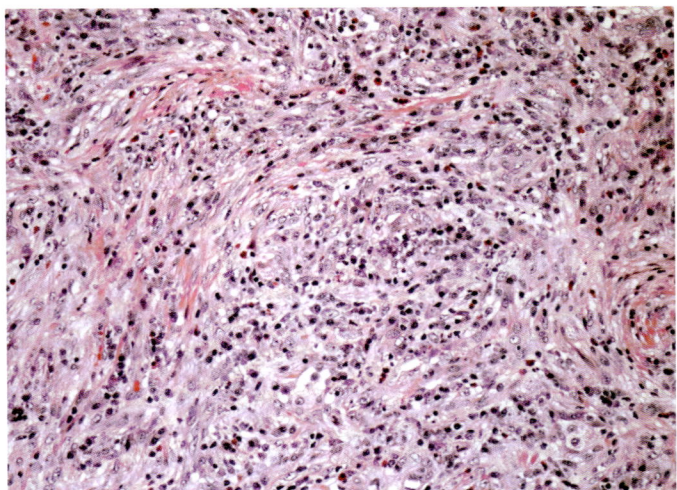

IMAGE 18.52 Inflammatory pseudotumor. The tumor is composed of bland spindle mesenchymal cells accompanied by plasmacyte rich mixed inflammatory infiltrates (H&E, x100).

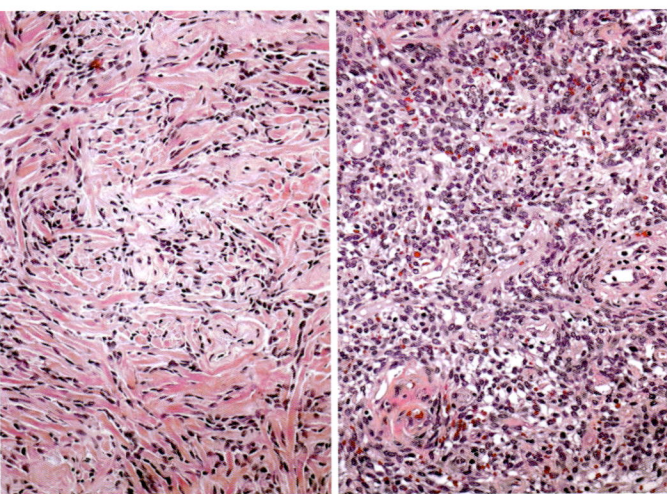

IMAGE 18.55 Solitary fibrous tumor. The tumor demonstrates a "patternless pattern" and variable cellularity. Left: H&E, x100. Right: H&E, x100.

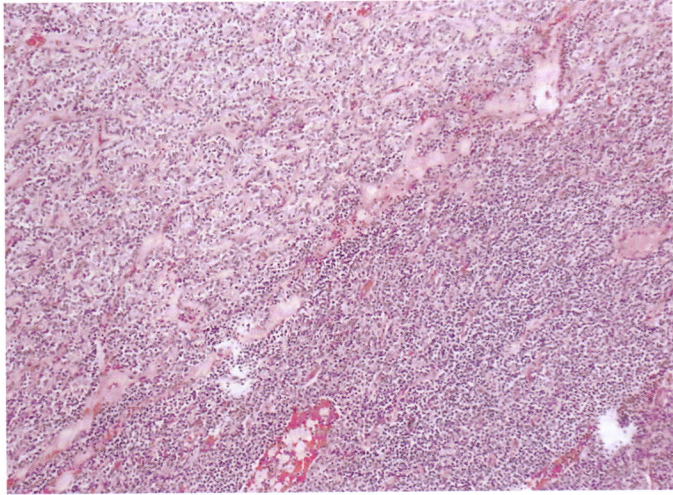

IMAGE 18.53 Thymoma type AB showing both type A component (left upper corner) and type B component (right lower corner) (H&E, x100).

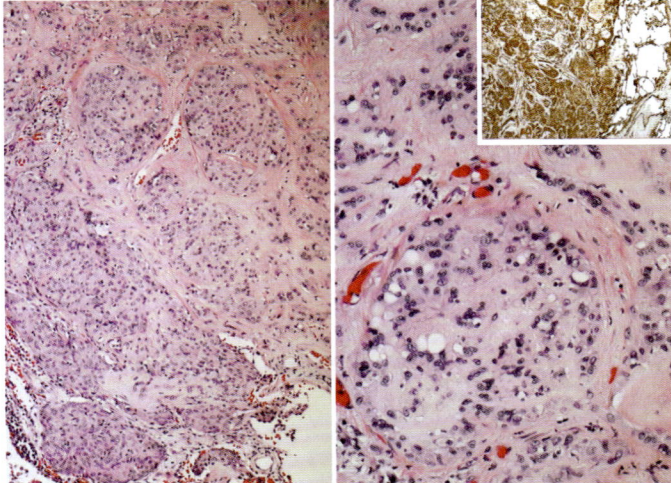

IMAGE 18.56 Epithelioid hemangioendothelioma. Left: the tumor has a lobular appearance with a myxohyaline stroma (H&E, x40). Right: there are small vacuoles in the tumor cells with a signet ring appearance (H&E, x200). Inset image shows tumor cells positive for the vascular marker CD31.

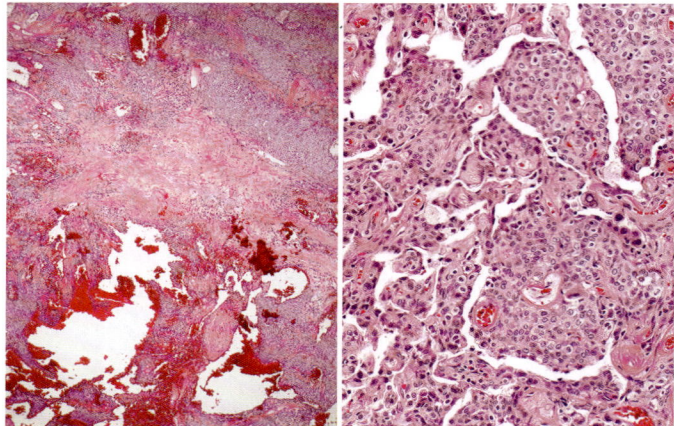

IMAGE 18.57 Sclerosing pneumocytoma. Left: a combination of solid tumor cells, sclerotic area, and hemorrhagic areas (H&E, x40). Right: papillary groups with a surface layer of cuboidal cells and also rounded tumor cells in the stroma (H&E, x200).

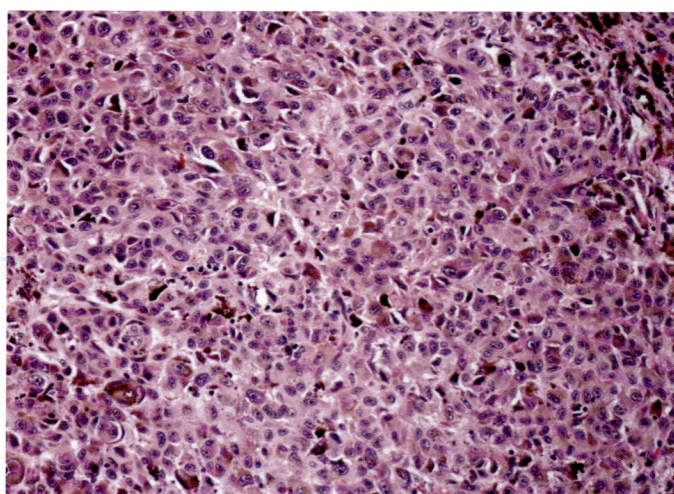

IMAGE 18.60 Metastatic melanoma. The patient had a history of skin melanoma and presented with multiple lung nodules. The tumor consists of large pleomorphic cells with intracellular melanin pigment (H&E, x200).

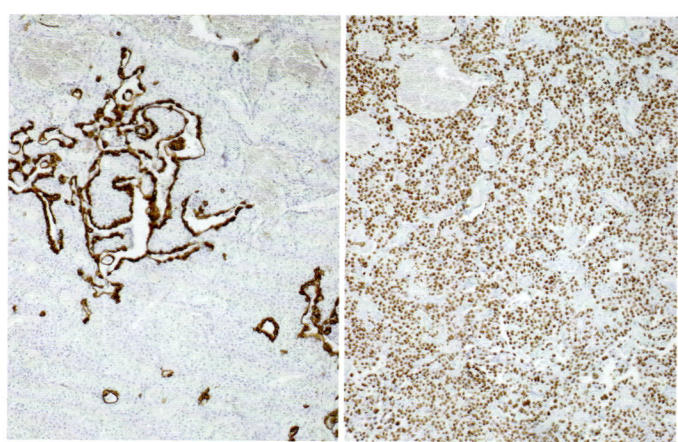

IMAGE 18.58 Sclerosing pneumocytoma. Left: the surface tumor cells are positive for keratin stain (AE1/AE3), but the tumor cells in the stroma are negative for the stain. Right: the tumor cells are positive for TTF-1 stain.

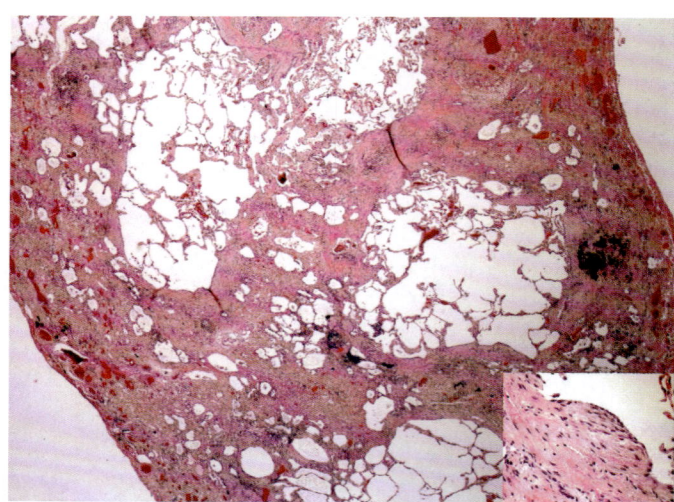

IMAGE 18.61 Usual interstitial pneumonia (UIP). The image shows patchy interstitial fibrosis with peripheral predominance and intervening preserved alveolar architecture (H&E, x20). Inset image: a fibroblastic focus adjacent to dense fibrosis.

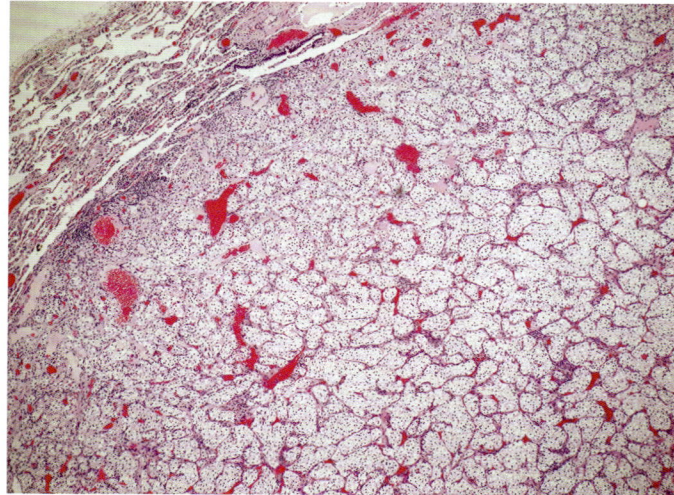

IMAGE 18.59 Metastatic clear cell renal cell carcinoma. The tumor cells have clear cytoplasm with a rich vascular network surrounding the tumor nests. (H&E, x40).

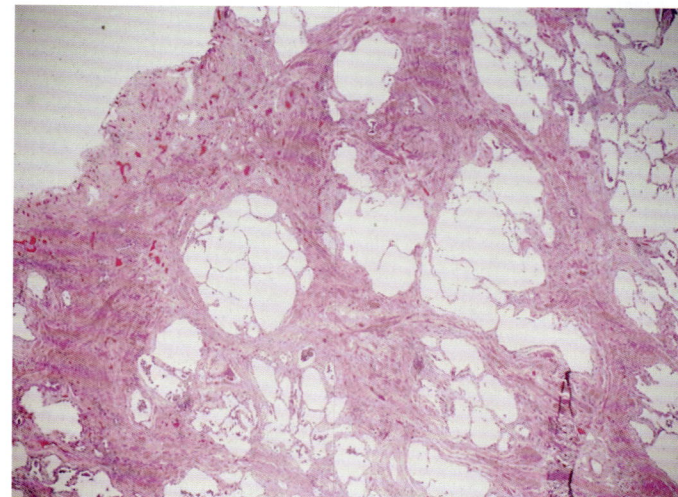

IMAGE 18.62 UIP. There is focal interstitial collagen fibrosis with intervening preserved alveolar architecture (H&E, x40).

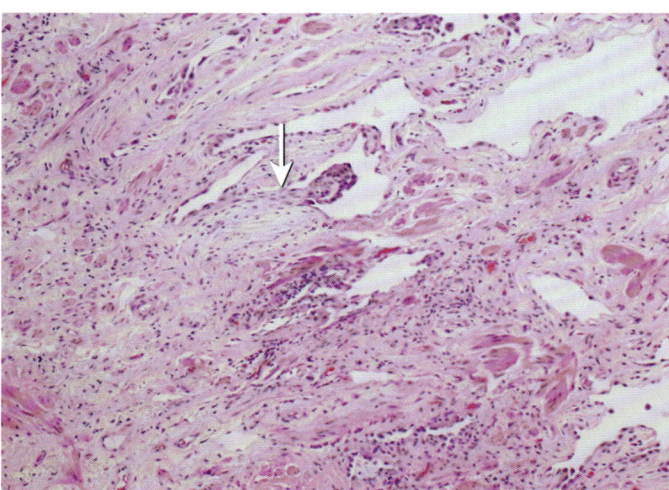

IMAGE 18.63 UIP. The image shows collagen fibrosis with a fibroblastic focus (arrow) (H&E, x100).

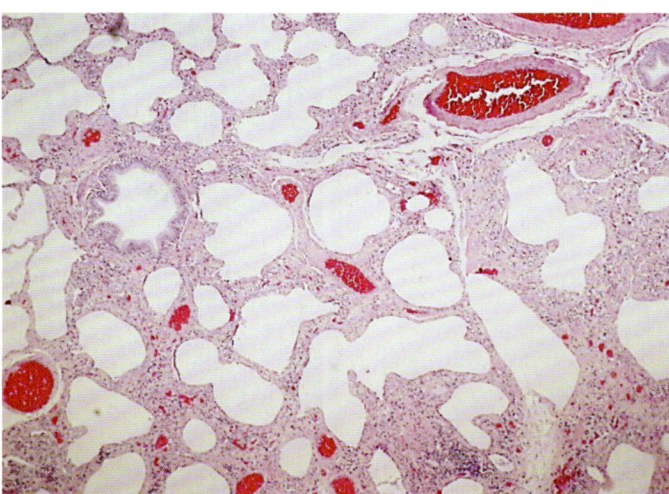

IMAGE 18.66 NSIP, fibrotic phase. It has a temporally uniform appearance with fibrotic thicken of the alveolar wall (H&E, x40).

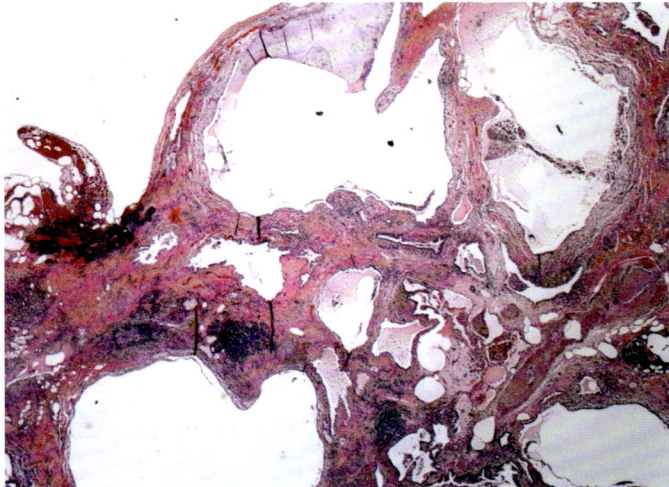

IMAGE 18.64 "Honeycomb" lung shows remodeling of lung architecture with cystic spaces surrounded by fibrosis (H&E, x20). It is often seen in usual interstitial pneumonia.

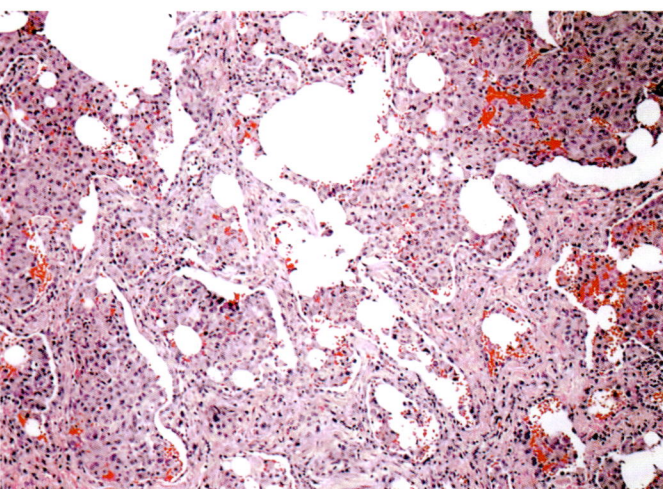

IMAGE 18.67 Desquamative interstitial pneumonia. It shows intraalveolar accumulation of macrophages accompanied by thick alveolar septa with mild interstitial fibrosis. The pulmonary changes are diffuse and temporally uniform (H&E, x100).

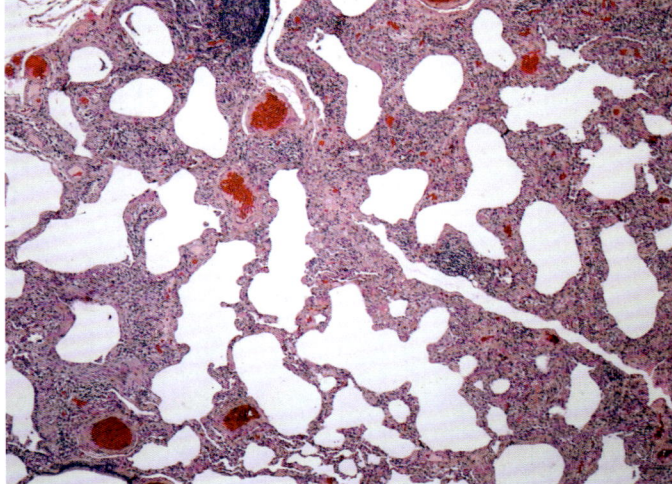

IMAGE 18.65 Nonspecific interstitial pneumonia (NSIP), cellular phase. It is characterized by diffuse fibrotic thickening of the alveolar wall with an interstitial mononuclear cell infiltrate. It has a temporally uniform appearance (H&E, x40).

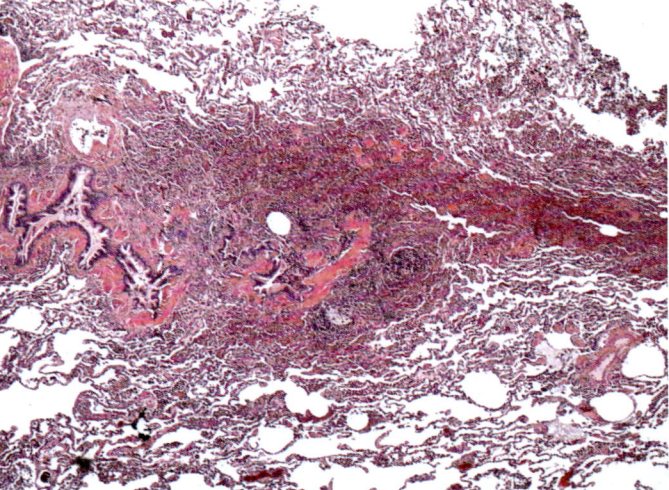

IMAGE 18.68 Respiratory bronchiolitis interstitial lung disease. Lung parenchyma adjacent to terminal bronchioles/respiratory bronchioles shows accumulations of brown dusty macrophages and subtle interstitial fibrosis (H&E, x20).

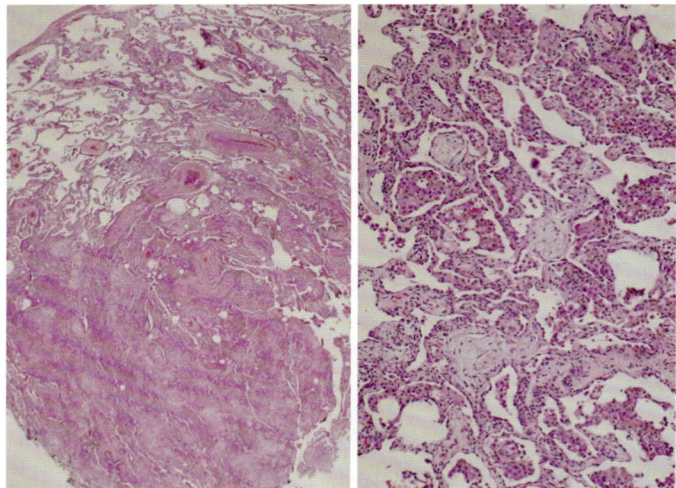

IMAGE 18.69 Organizing pneumonia. There are fibroblastic polyps/plugs protruding into alveolar spaces accompanied by scattered inflammatory cells. It is temporally uniform and is often centered around airways. Left: H&E, x20. Right: H&E, x100.

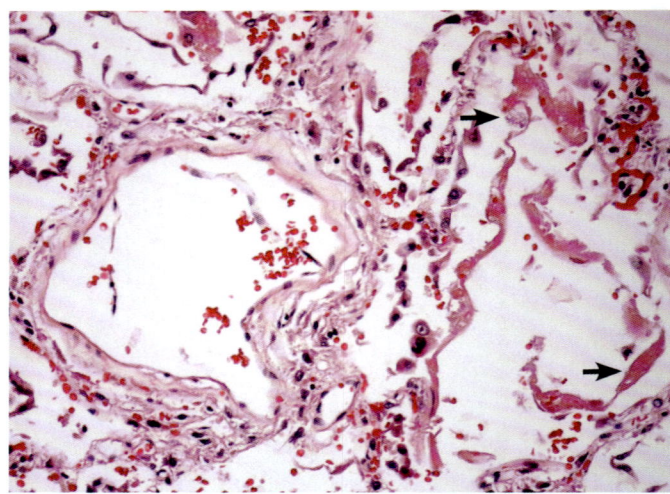

IMAGE 18.72 Diffuse alveolar damage, exudative phase. It is characterized by damage of the alveolar wall with hyaline membrane formation (H&E, x200).

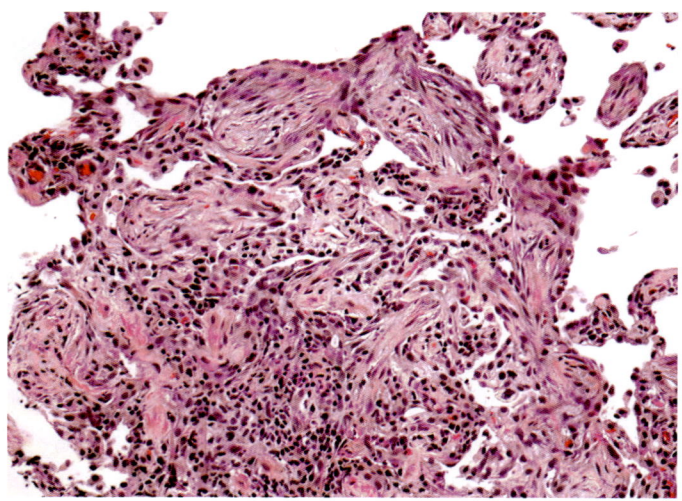

IMAGE 18.70 Organizing pneumonia. There are fibroblastic polyps/plugs to form a nodular lesion (H&E, x100).

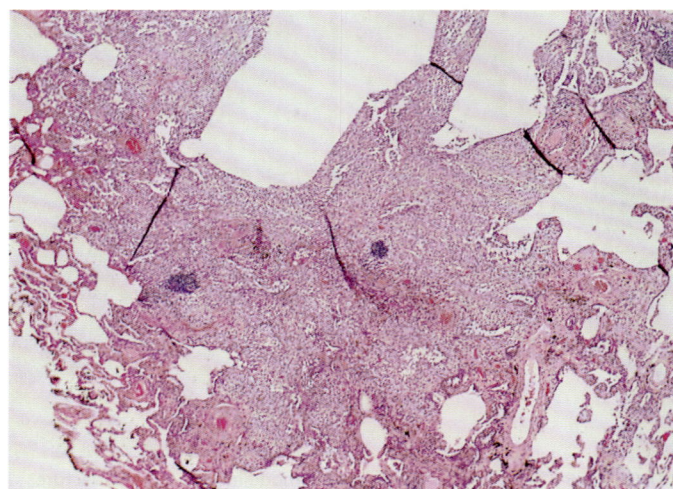

IMAGE 18.73 Pulmonary Langerhans cell histiocytosis (also called "pulmonary eosinophilic granuloma"). This presented as a small and stellate shaped lesion (H&E, x40).

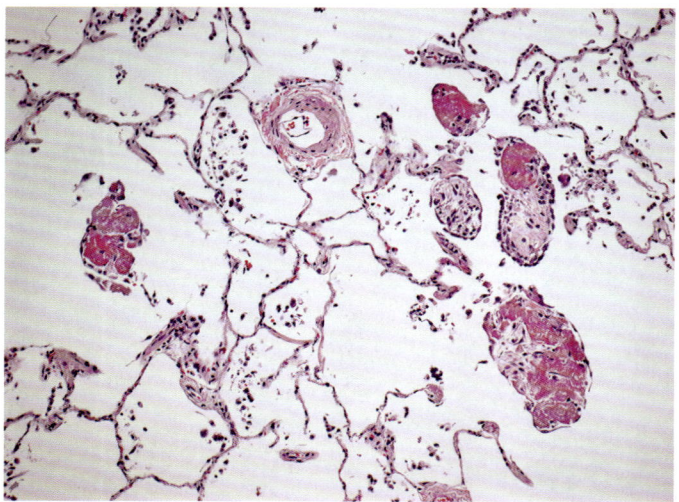

IMAGE 18.71 Fibrinous organizing pneumonia. There are fibrinous exudates within the alveolar spaces which are partially organized by fibroblastic change (H&E, x100).

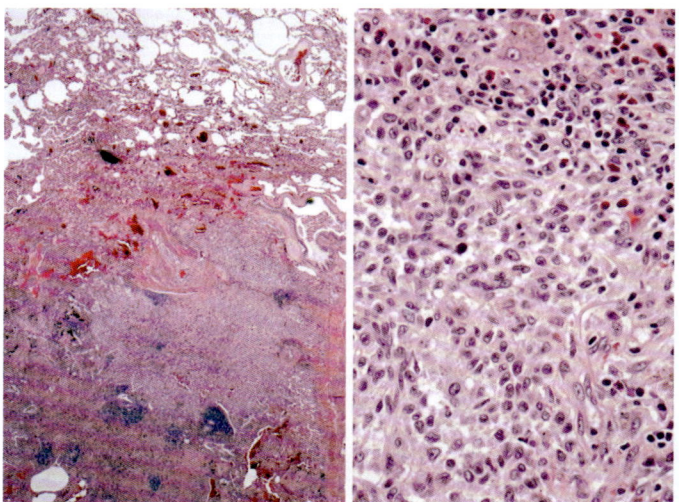

IMAGE 18.74 Pulmonary Langerhans cell histiocytosis. Left: the image shows a low power view (H&E, x40). Right: the Langerhans cell has a characteristic coffee-bean-shaped nucleus with a prominent nuclear groove, eosinophilic cytoplasm, and an indistinct cell border, as well as variable numbers of eosinophils within the lesion (H&E, x200).

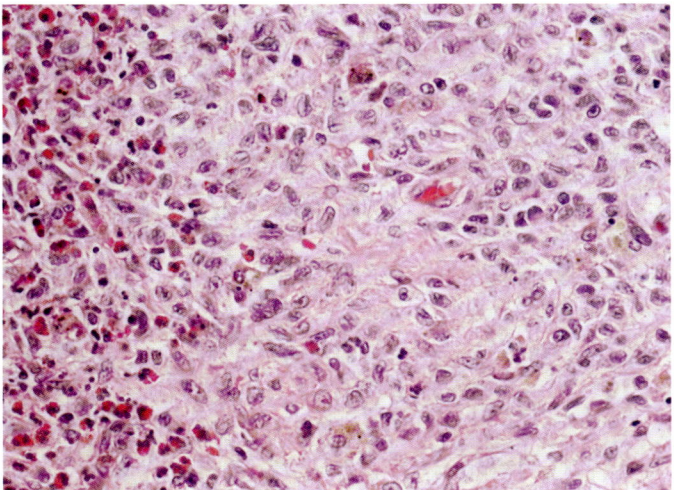

IMAGE 18.75 Pulmonary Langerhans cell histiocytosis shows the Langerhans cells with nuclear grooves (H&E, x400).

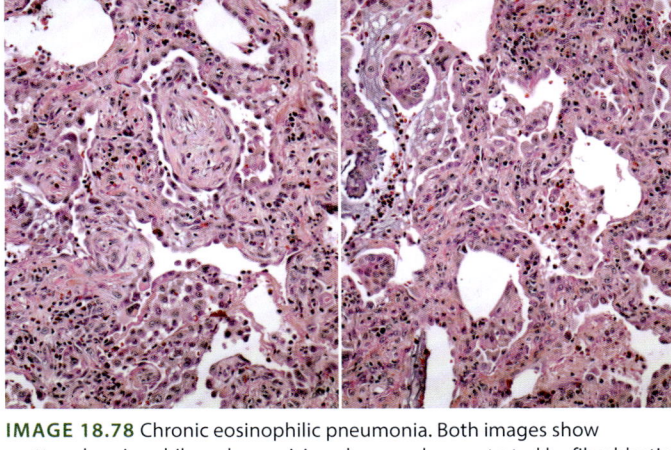

IMAGE 18.78 Chronic eosinophilic pneumonia. Both images show scattered eosinophils and organizing changes demonstrated by fibroblastic polyps/plugs (H&E, x100).

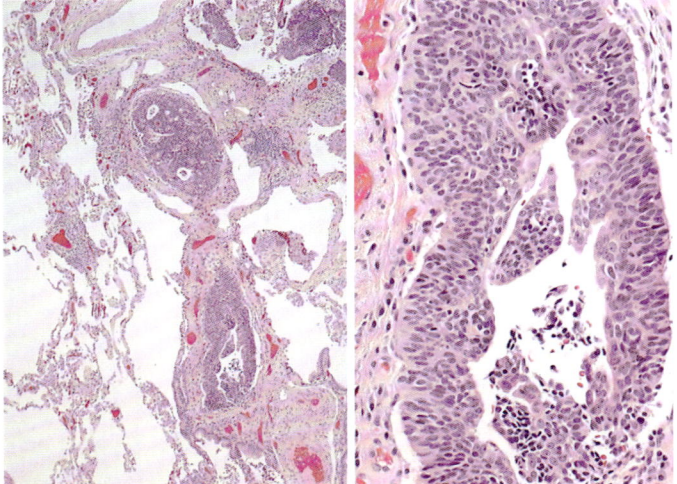

IMAGE 18.76 Diffuse idiopathic pulmonary neuroendocrine cell hyperplasia. There is a focal proliferation of neuroendocrine cells in the bronchial epithelium involving many areas. Left: H&E, x40. Right: H&E, x200.

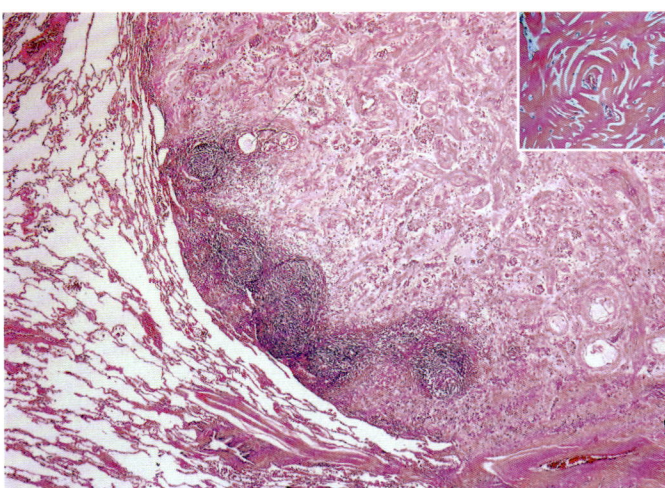

IMAGE 18.79 Pulmonary hyalinizing granuloma. The image shows a well-demarcated nodule composed of dense collagen with lymphoid aggregates at the periphery (H&E, x40). Inset image: lamellar hyaline collagen around small blood vessels.

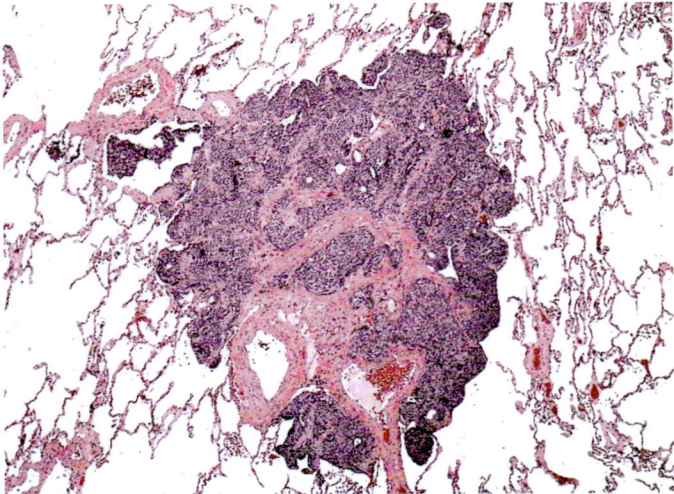

IMAGE 18.77 Tumorlet. Neuroendocrine cell proliferation forms a small nodular lesion < 0.5 cm (H&E, x40).

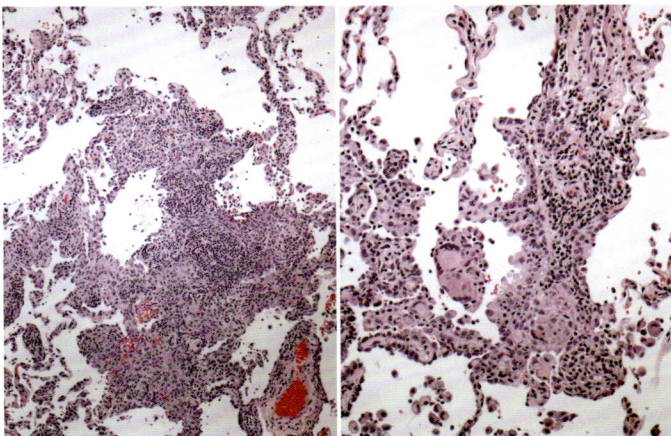

IMAGE 18.80 Hypersensitivity pneumonitis. There is alveolitis with mononuclear cell infiltrate in the alveolar septa, often centered in peribronchial regions accompanied by scattered poorly formed granulomas. Left: H&E, x20. Right: H&E, x40.

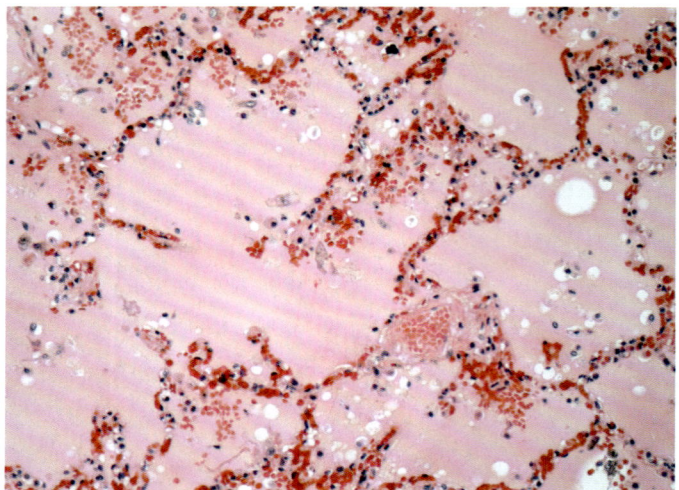

IMAGE 18.81 Pulmonary edema. The image shows homogeneous pink material with some red blood cells inside the alveolar spaces accompanied by congestion of alveolar capillaries (H&E, x100).

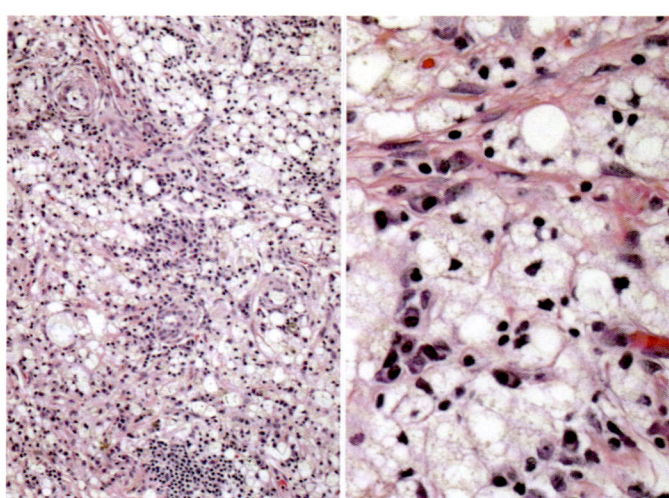

IMAGE 18.84 Lipoid pneumonia. There are numerous foamy macrophages and fat droplets indicative of exogenous lipoid pneumonia. Left: H&E, x40. Right: H&E, x200.

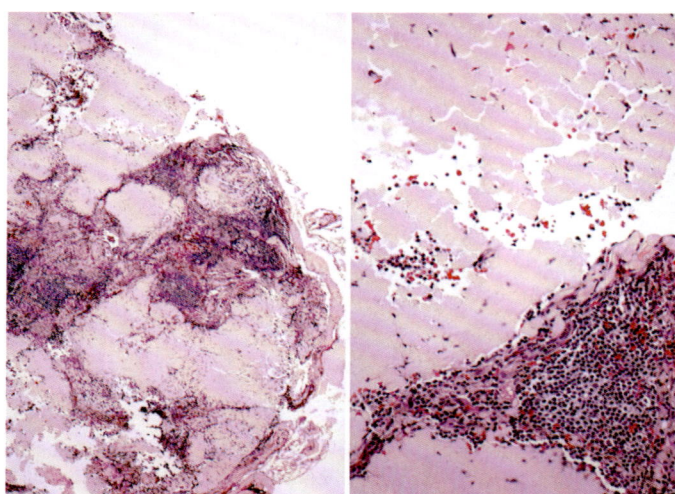

IMAGE 18.82 Amyloidosis. It involves a mediastinal lymph node that is partially replaced by amorphous pink material. Left: H&E, x20. Right: H&E, x100).

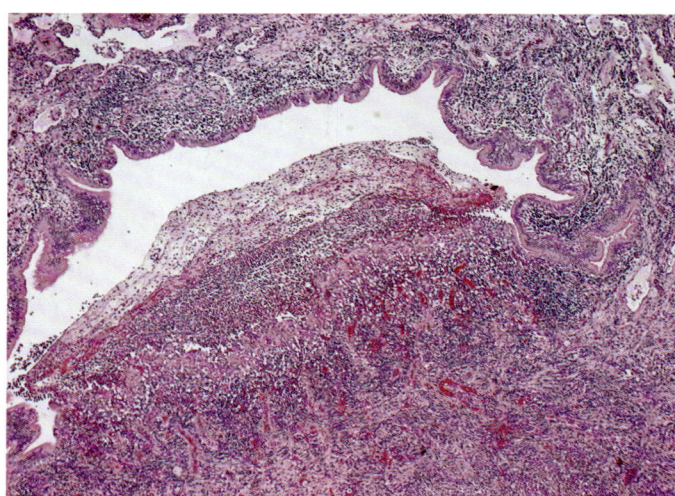

IMAGE 18.85 Bronchocentric granulomatosis. The bronchial epithelium is partially replaced by histiocytes and an infiltrate with a high proportion of inflammatory cells (H&E, x40).

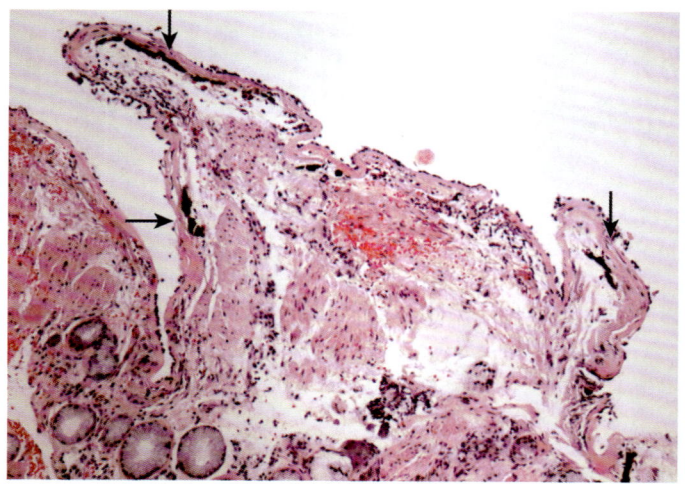

IMAGE 18.83 Metastatic calcification. There is focal calcium deposition (arrows) along the basement membrane of the bronchial epithelium (H&E, x40). It is often seen in patients with chronic renal failure.

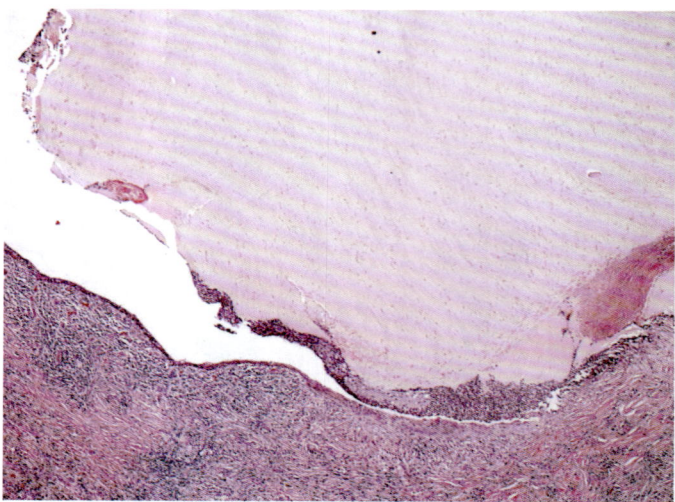

IMAGE 18.86 Bronchocentric granulomatosis. There is an inflammatory cell infiltrate and focal damage of the bronchial epithelium as well as accumulation of mucus (H&E, x40).

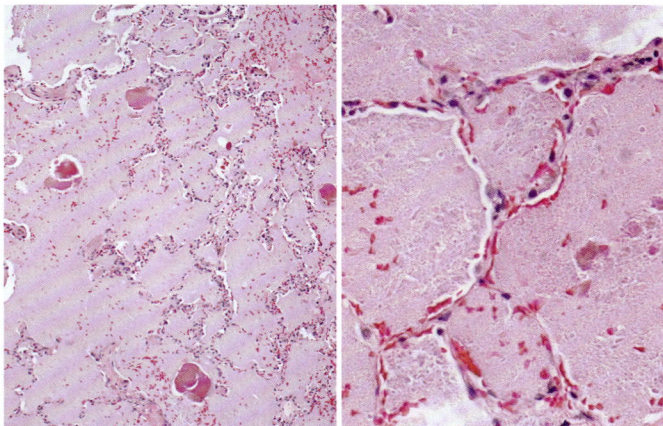

IMAGE 18.87 Pulmonary alveolar proteinosis. The alveolar spaces are filled with granular proteinaceous material, including a few dense eosinophilic substances. Left: H&E, x100. Right: H&E, x400.

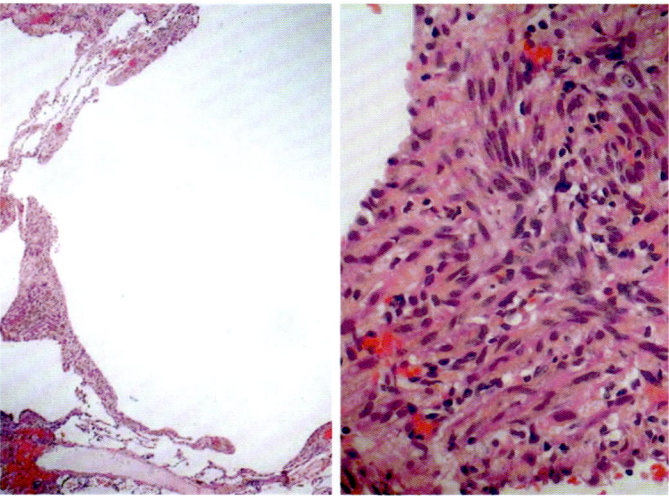

IMAGE 18.90 Lymphangioleiomyomatosis. The image shows a cystic structure with focal spindle cell proliferation in the cyst wall. Left: H&E, x20. Right: H&E, x200. The spindle cells are positive for HMB-45, alpha-actin, ER, and PR (not shown).

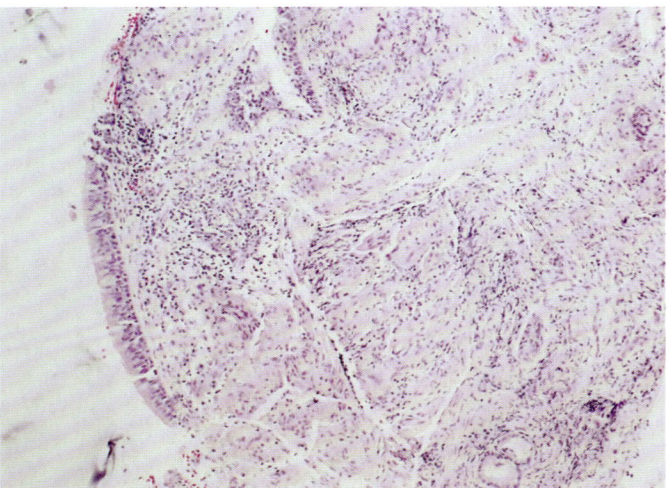

IMAGE 18.88 Sarcoidosis. There are nonnecrotizing granulomas involving the bronchial wall (H&E, x100).

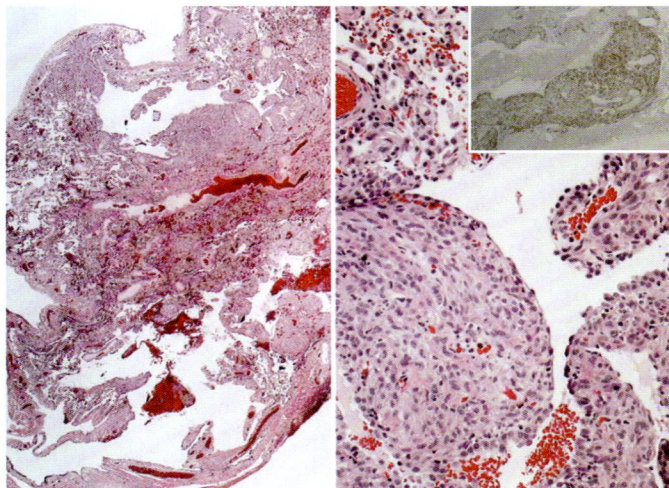

IMAGE 18.91 Lymphangioleiomyomatosis. There are irregular cystic spaces with a proliferation of spindle shaped cells in the wall. Left: H&E, x20. Right: H&E, x100. Inset image: HMB45.

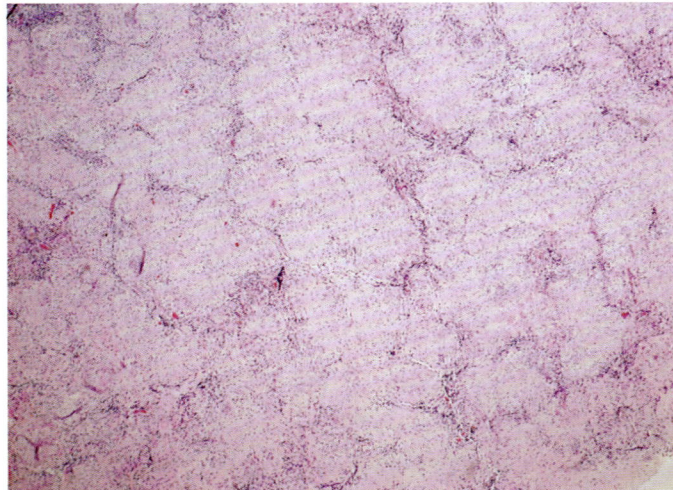

IMAGE 18.89 Sarcoidosis. A mediastinal lymph node shows numerous nonnecrotizing granulomas, which replace the entire nodal tissue (H&E, x40).

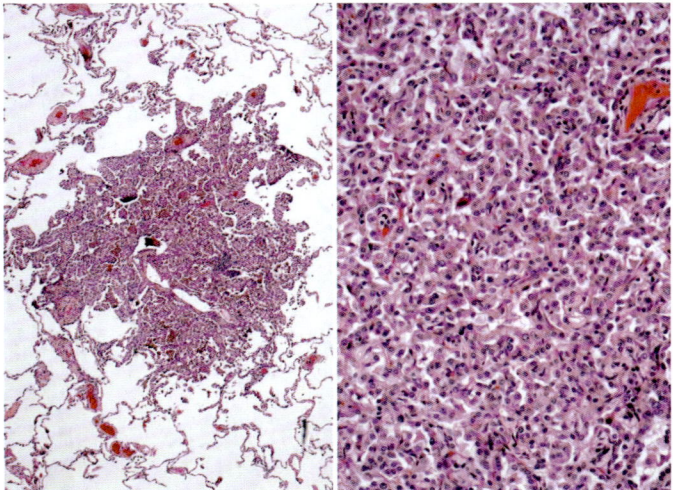

IMAGE 18.92 Micronodular pneumocyte hyperplasia. The image shows an ill-defined nodular lesion composed of hyperplastic cuboidal type 2 pneumocytes. It is often seen in patients with tuberous sclerosis and may coexist with lymphangioleiomyomatosis. Left: H&E, x40. Right: H&E, x200.

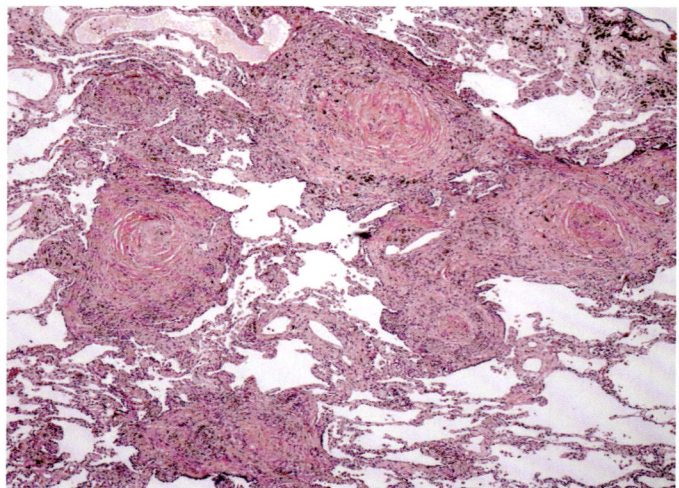

IMAGE 18.93 Silicosis, early stage. There are multiple small nodular lesions with dense acellular collagen in the center surrounded by prominent dust laden macrophages (H&E, x40).

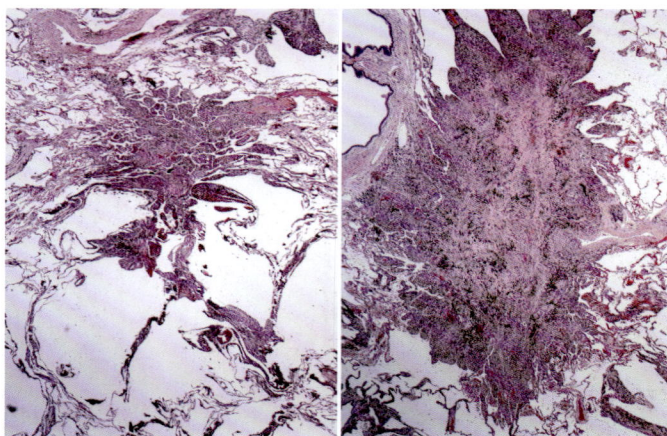

IMAGE 18.96 Simple coal worker's pneumoconiosis. Left: a coal dust macule with prominent dust laden macrophages and emphysematous change (H&E, x20). Right: a coal dust nodule < 1.0 cm in size composed of prominent dust laden macrophages and deposition of coal dust pigments with central collagen fibrosis (H&E, x20).

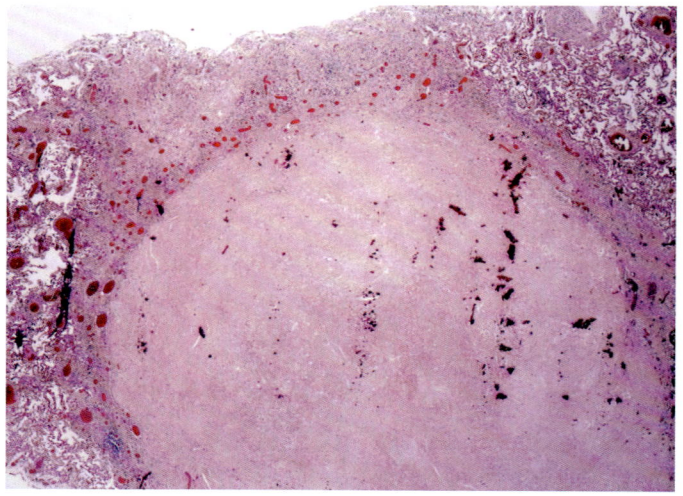

IMAGE 18.94 Silicosis. The image shows a demarcated silicotic nodule composed of dense collagen fibrosis without cellular component (H&E, x20).

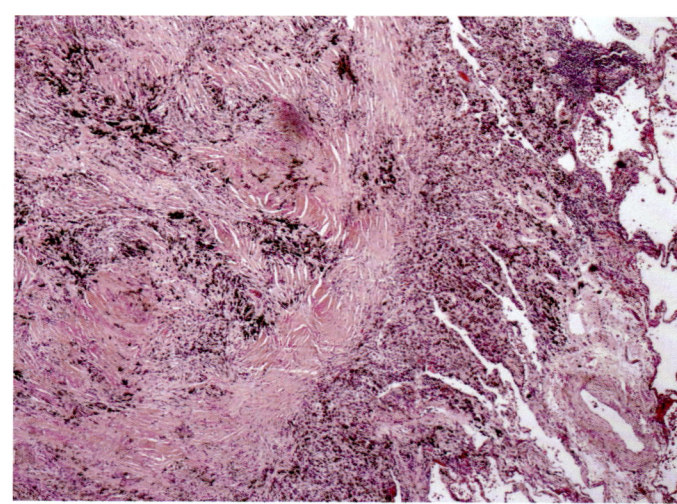

IMAGE 18.97 Complicated coal worker's pneumoconiosis. There is a large fibrotic mass with prominent dust laden macrophages and deposition of coal dust pigments (H&E, x20).

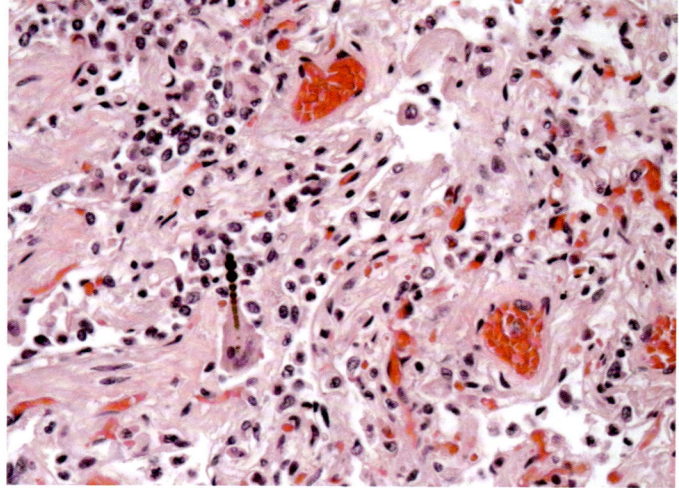

IMAGE 18.95 Asbestos body. The image shows a thin and lucent central core coated with beaded brown hemosiderin particles (H&E, x400).

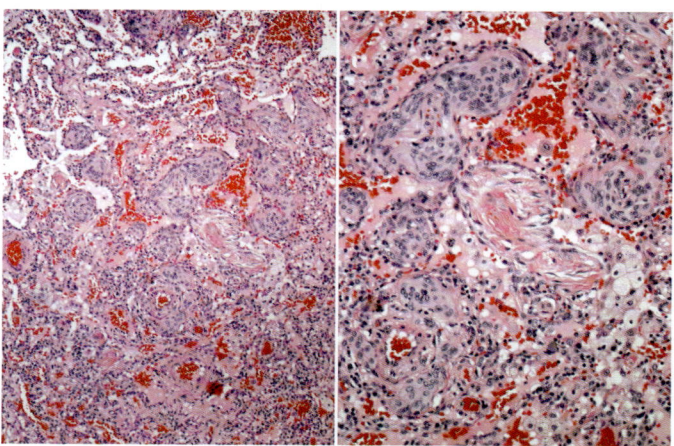

IMAGE 18.98 Minute meningothelioid nodule. There are aggregates of bland small round-to-oval cells associated with small blood vessels. Left: H&E, x40. Right: H&E, x100.

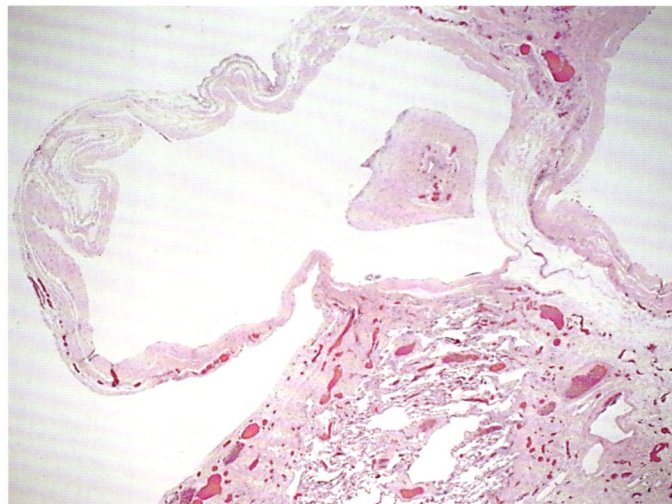

IMAGE 18.99 Bleb. It presents a small subpleural thin-walled air-containing space which is usually < 1–2 cm (H&E, x20).

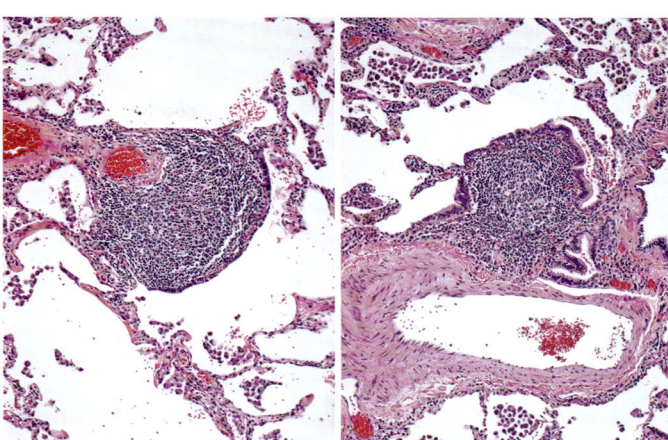

IMAGE 18.102 Follicular bronchiolitis. The image shows lymphoid follicles with germinal centers adjacent to small airways. Left and right: H&E, x100.

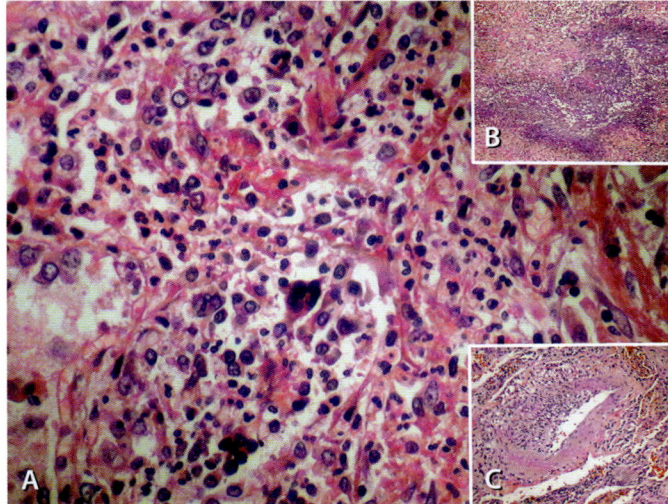

IMAGE 18.100 Granulomatosis with polyangiitis, previously known as Wegener granulomatosis. Image A: an inflammatory background with multinucleated giant cells (H&E, x400). Image B: zones of basophilic necrosis. Image C: granulomatous vasculitis.

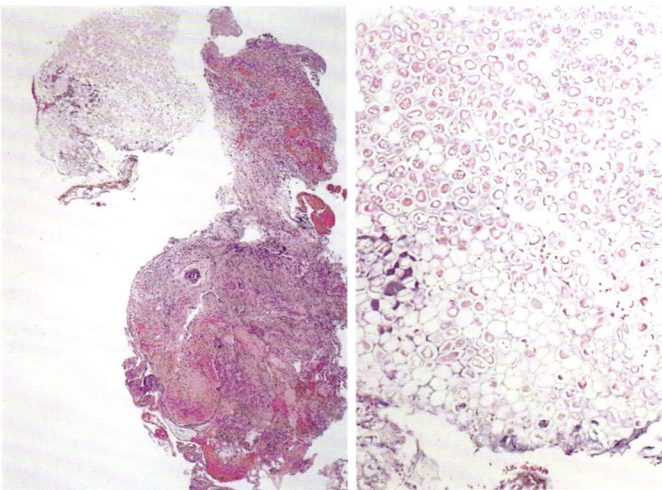

IMAGE 18.103 Aspiration. Heavily inflamed bronchial mucosa with a fragment of foreign tissue. Left: H&E, x20. Right: H&E, x100.

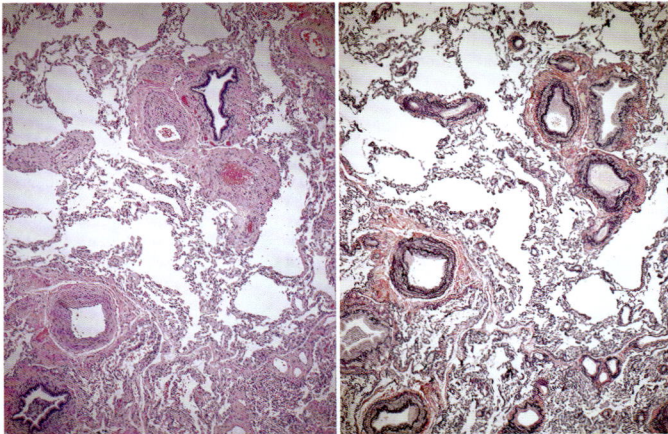

IMAGE 18.101 Early pulmonary hypertension. Left: there is focal and mild intima thickening in small pulmonary arteries with mild narrowing of the vascular lumen (H&E, x40). Right: the elastic stain highlights the vascular changes.

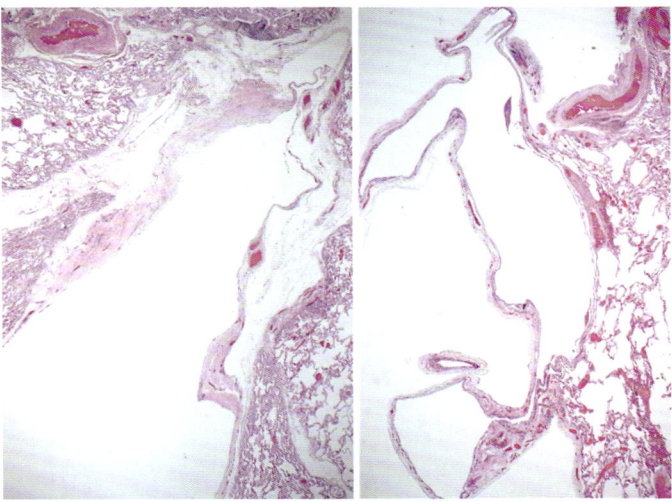

IMAGE 18.104 Birt-Hogg-Dubé syndrome. There are multiple thin-walled cystic structures in the lung. Left: H&E, x20. Right: H&E, x20.

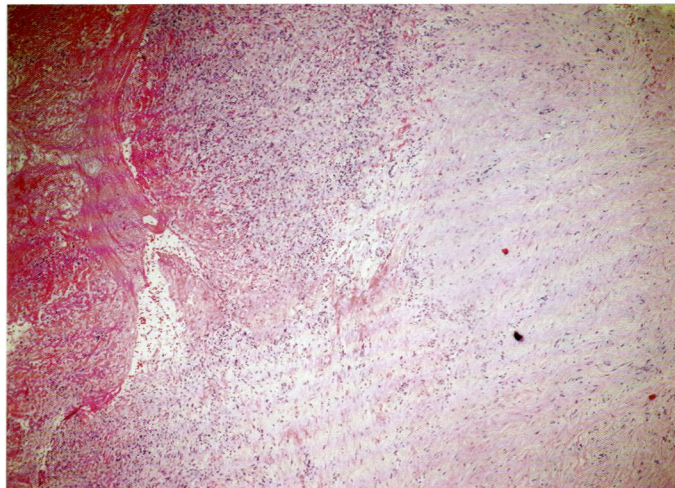

IMAGE 18.105 Fibrinous pleuritis with fibrosis. It demonstrates zonation with high cellularity near the surface (left) and low cellularity at the bottom (right) (H&E, x40).

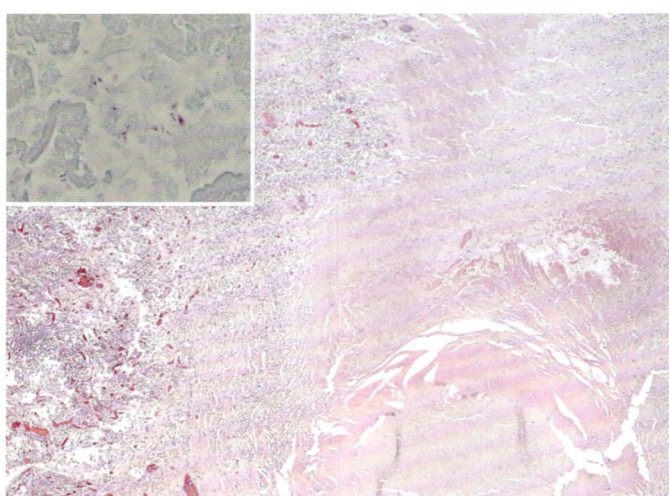

IMAGE 18.108 Atypical mycobacterial infection. There is a necrotizing granuloma (H&E, x40). Inset image: acid-fast bacilli are demonstrated by Ziehl-Neelsen stain.

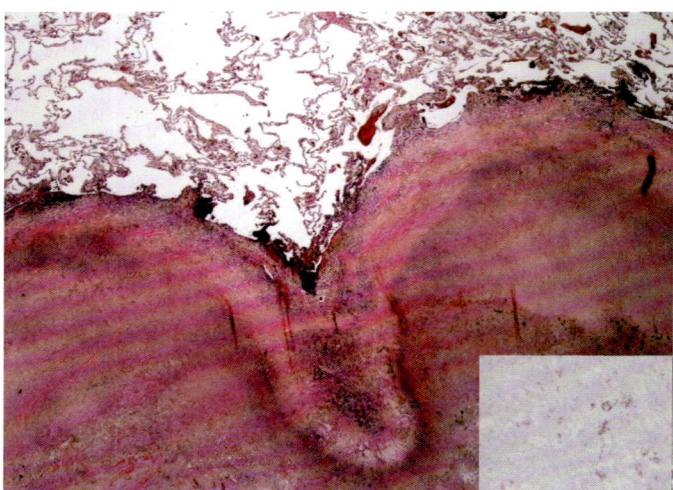

IMAGE 18.106 Pulmonary tuberculosis. The image shows a large confluent necrotizing granulomatous lesion (H&E, x20). Inset image: mycobacteria are demonstrated by Ziehl-Neelsen stain.

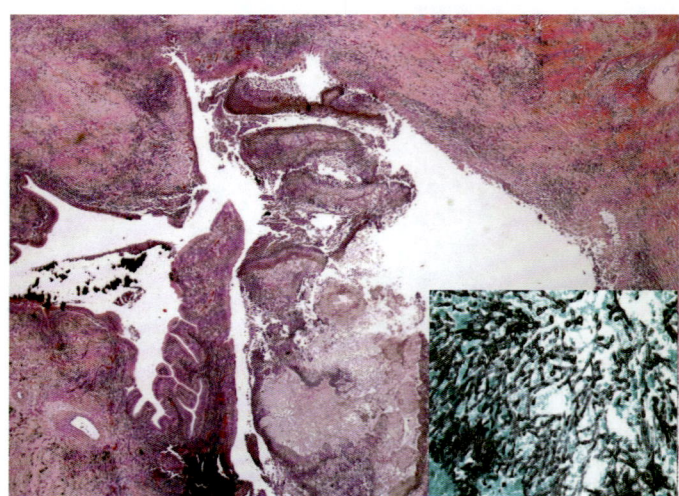

IMAGE 18.109 Chronic necrotizing aspergillosis. The bronchial epithelium in this cystically dilated airway is largely denuded and replaced by granulation tissue. The central lower area shows a cluster of fungal organisms (Main image: H&E, x20. Inset image: GMS stain, x40).

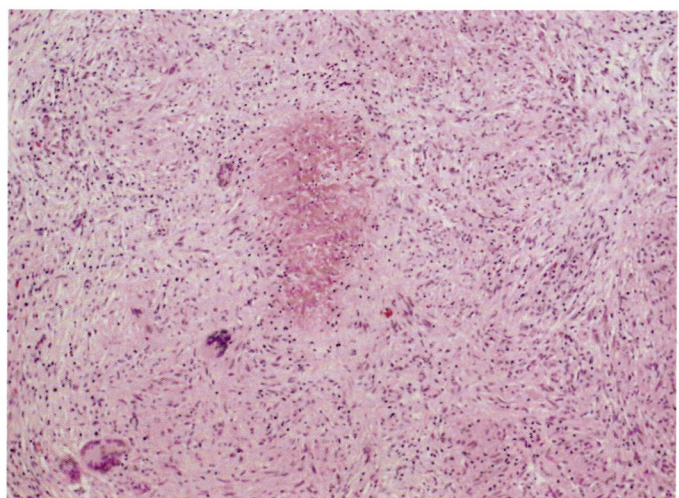

IMAGE 18.107 Pulmonary tuberculosis. It demonstrates necrotizing granulomatous inflammation with multinucleated giant cells (H&E, x100).

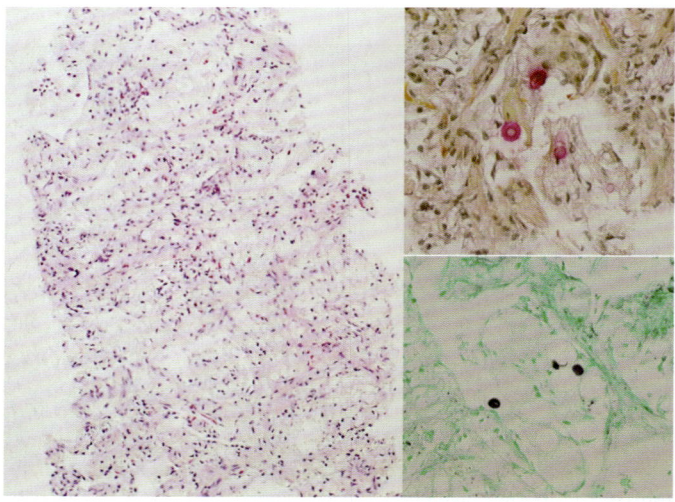

IMAGE 18.110 Cryptococcosis. Left: H&E x100. Right upper: mucicarmine stain highlighting a mucinous wall (x200). Right lower: GMS stain (x200).

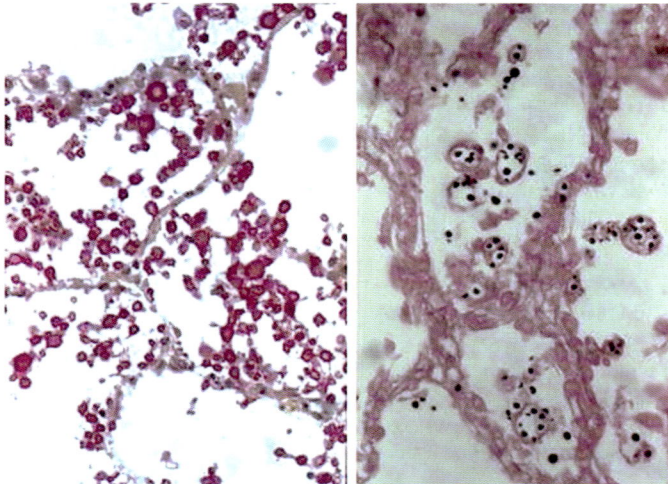

IMAGE 18.111 Cryptococcosis. Left: cryptococcus has a mucinous capsule highlighted by PAS with diastase stain (x200). Right: the mucinous capsule becomes a halo on GMS stain (x200).

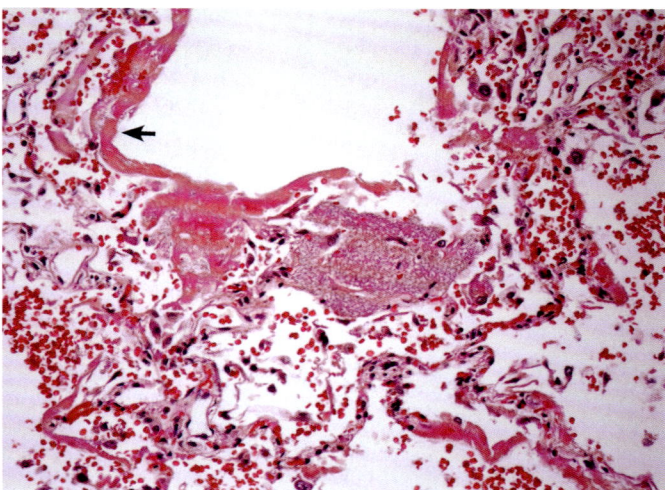

IMAGE 18.114 *Pneumocystis jiroveci* pneumonia with diffuse alveolar damage. There is characteristic foamy exudate within the alveolar spaces. The surrounding lung tissue shows features of diffuse alveolar damage with hyaline membrane formation (H&E, x100).

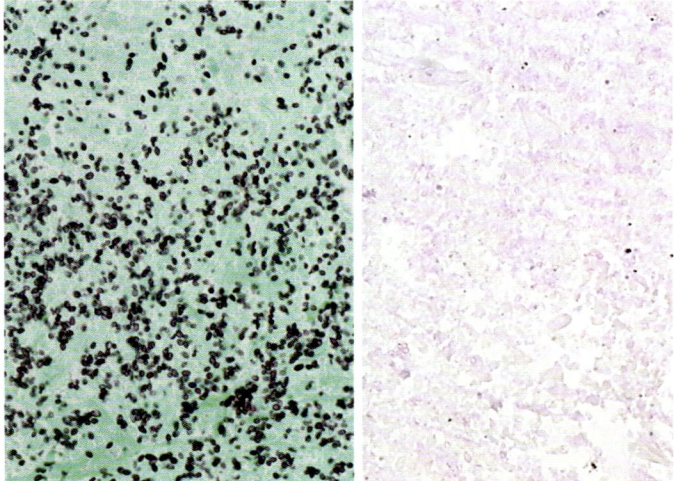

IMAGE 18.112 Histoplasmosis. Left: the organisms are well demonstrated by GMS stain (x400). Right: the organisms are difficult to see on a PAS/diastase slide (x400).

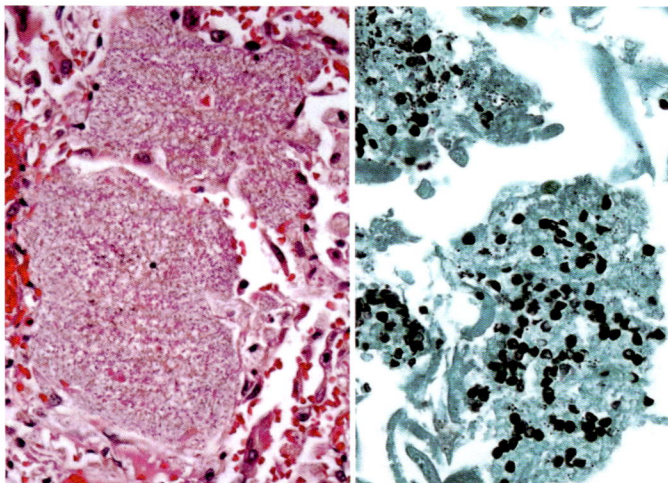

IMAGE 18.115 *Pneumocystis jirovecii* pneumonia. Left: foamy exudates within the alveolar spaces with tiny dots in the center of many bubbles (H&E, x400). Right: round, oval, or cup-shaped microorganisms measuring 5–7 μm in diameter (GMS stain, x400).

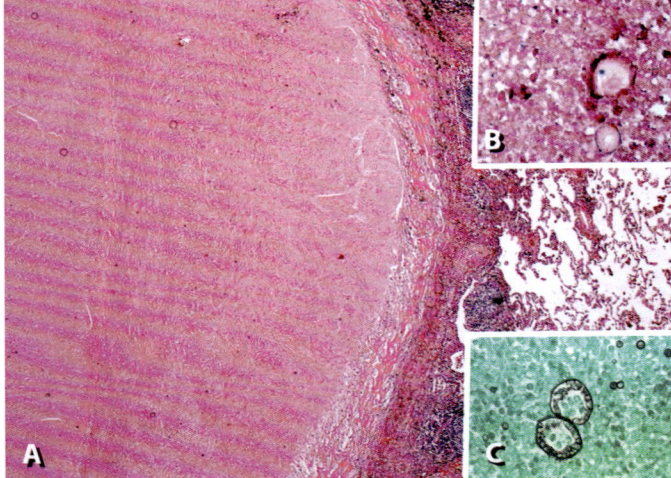

IMAGE 18.113 Coccidioidomycosis. Image A: a necrotizing granuloma (H&E, x20). Image B: immature and mature spherules within the granuloma (H&E, x200). Image C: the mature spherules contain multiple endospores (GMS stain, x200).

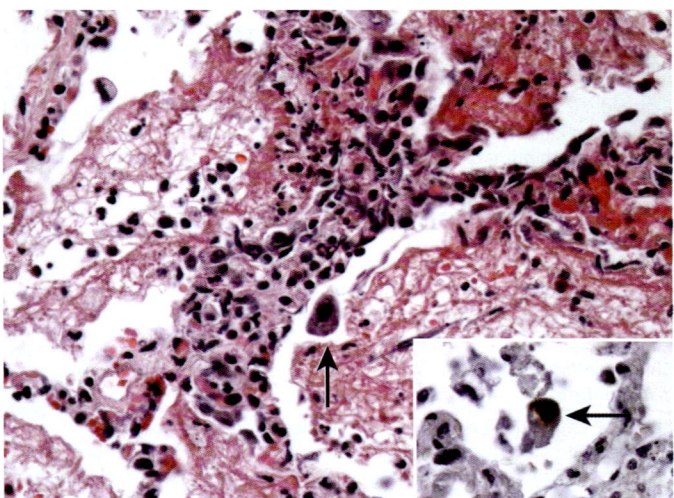

IMAGE 18.116 CMV infection with acute lung injury/diffuse alveolar damage. A CMV inclusion (arrow) is shown in the center of the field (H&E, x200). Inset image: the inclusion (arrow) is highlighted by a CMV stain.

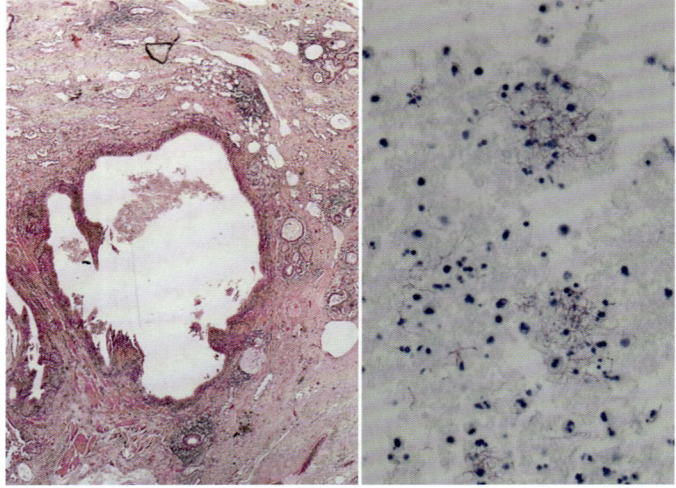

IMAGE 18.117 Nocardiosis. A dilated bronchiole with amorphous material is surrounded by fibrotic stroma and scattered inflammatory cells. Left: H&E x40. Right: modified acid-fast stain, x400.

Bibliography

Amin MB, Edge SB, Greene FL, et al, editors. AJCC cancer staging manual. 8th ed. New York: Springer; 2017.

Galiè N, Humbert M, Vachiery JL, et al. 2015 ESC/ERS guidelines for the diagnosis and treatment of pulmonary hypertension. Eur Respir J. 2015;46(4):903-75. Medline:26318161. doi: 10.1183/13993003.01032-2015

Goldblum JR, Lamps LW, McKenny J, et al. Rosai and Ackerman's surgical pathology. 11th ed., vol. 2. Philadelphia (PA): Elsevier; 2017.

Kumar V, Abbas AK, Aster J. Robbins and Cotran pathologic basis of disease. 10th ed. North York (ON): Elsevier Canada; 2020.

Lindeman NI, Cagle PT, Beasley MB, et al. Molecular testing guideline for selection of lung cancer patients for EGFR and ALK tyrosine kinase inhibitors: guideline from the College of American Pathologists, International Association for the Study of Lung Cancer, and Association for Molecular Pathology. Arch Pathol Lab Med. 2013;137(6):828-60. doi: 10.1097/JTO.0b013e318290868f

Longacre TA, editor. Mills and Sternberg's diagnostic surgical pathology. 7th ed. Philadelphia (PA): Wolters Kluwar; 2022.

Marx A, Chan JKC, Coindre JM, et al. The 2015 World Health Organization classification of tumors of the thymus: continuity and changes. J Thorac Oncol. 2015;10(10):1383-95. Medline:26295375. doi: 10.1097/JTO.0000000000000654

Rusch VW, Asamura H, Watanabe H, et al; IASLC Staging Committee. The IASLC lung cancer staging project: a proposal for a new international lymph node map in the forthcoming seventh edition of the TNM classification for lung cancer. J Thoracic Oncology. 2009;4(5):568-77.

Schneider F, Butnor KJ, Beasley MB, et al; Cancer Committee, College of American Pathologists. Protocol for the examination of specimens from patients with primary non-small cell carcinoma, small cell carcinoma, or carcinoid tumors of the lung (Version: Lung 4.1.0.0) [Internet]. College of American Pathologists; 2019. Available from www.cap.org.

Schneider F, Roden A, Dacic S, et al; Cancer Committee, College of American Pathologists. Protocol for the examination of specimens from patients with malignant pleural mesothelioma (Version: PleuralPericard 4.1.0.0) [Internet]. College of American Pathologists; 2021. Available from www.cap.org.

Shimosato Y, Mukai K, Matsuno Y, editors. Tumors of the mediastinum. Washington, DC: ARP and AFIP; 2010.

Sholl LM, Cagle PT, Lindeman NI, et al; Cancer Biomarker Reporting Committee, College of American Pathologists. Template for reporting results of biomarker testing of specimens from patients with non-small cell carcinoma of the lung (Version: Lungbiomarker 1.3.0.2) [Internet]. College of American Pathologists; 2016. Available from www.cap.org.

Travis WD, Brambilla E, Nicholson AG, et al; the WHO Editorial Panel. The 2015 World Health Organization classification of lung tumors: impact of genetic, clinical and radiologic advances since the 2004 classification. J Thorac Oncol. 2015;10(9):1243-60. Medline:26291008. doi: 10.1097/JTO.0000000000000630

Travis WD, Colby TV, Koss MN, et al, editors. Non-neoplastic disorders of the lower respiratory tract. Washington, DC: ARP and AFIP; 2002.

Travis WD, Costabel U, Hansell DM, et al; ATS/ERS Committee on Idiopathic Interstitial Pneumonias. An official American Thoracic Society/European Respiratory Society statement: update of the international multidisciplinary classification of the idiopathic interstitial pneumonias. Am J Respir Crit Care Med. 2013;188(6):733-48. Medline:24032382. doi: 10.1164/rccm.201308-1483ST

WHO Classification of Tumours Editorial Board. WHO classification of tumours. 5th ed. Vol. 5, Thoracic tumours. Lyon (France): IARC; 2021.

WHO Classification of Tumours Editorial Board. WHO classification of tumours. 4th ed. Vol. 7, WHO classification of tumours of the lung, pleura, thymus, and heart. Lyon (France): IARC; 2015.

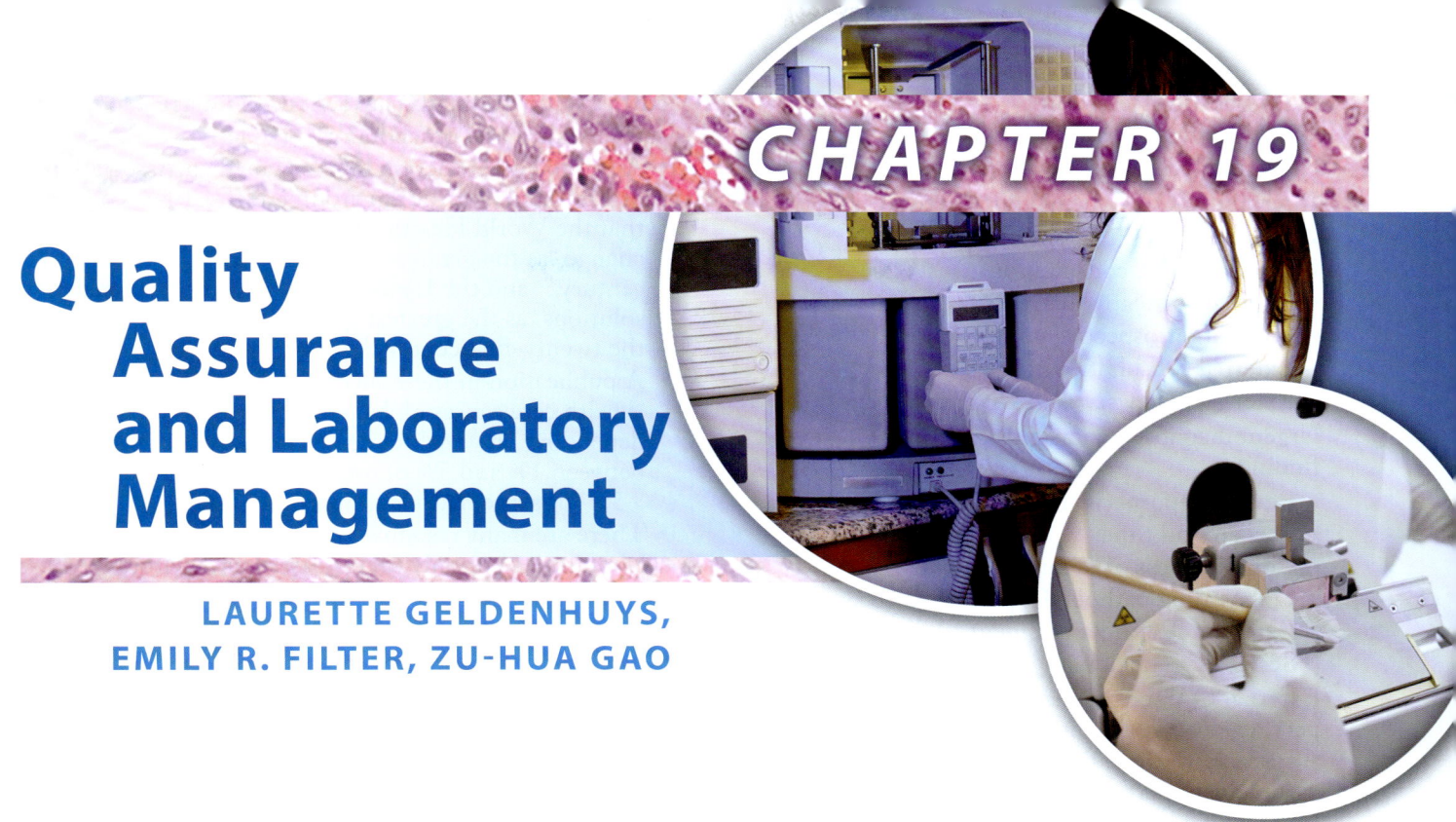

CHAPTER 19

Quality Assurance and Laboratory Management

LAURETTE GELDENHUYS, EMILY R. FILTER, ZU-HUA GAO

Quality Assurance (QA) and Laboratory Management Exam Essentials

In recent years, an ever-growing emphasis on nonmedical expert CanMEDS roles has made QA a common topic in the written and practical components of the exam. QA and laboratory management are vast topics. A way to approach them is to use your own institutional experience to identify common scenarios encountered in the pathology laboratory, and to get involved in QA exercises at your institution for hands-on experience.

MUST KNOW
- You should be comfortable answering questions about the following key topics:
  - Basic concepts in QA.
  - Surgical pathology QA.
  - Intraoperative consultation QA.
  - Autopsy pathology QA.
  - Cytopathology QA.
  - Laboratory management.
  - Risk management.
- In addition, you should be familiar with:
  - The Pan-Canadian quality assurance recommendations for interpretive pathology.
  - Emerging topics in laboratory management.

Pan-Canadian quality assurance recommendations for interpretive pathology[1]
- These recommendations were developed through a collaboration between the Canadian Association of Pathologists/Association cannadienne des pathologistes (CAP-ACP) and the Canadian Partnership Against Cancer, engaging a network of interpretative pathology experts across Canada.
- They aim to "enhance patient safety through promoting more consistent and high quality pathology quality assurance across the country" by providing a "framework of quality recommendations for interpretive pathology that could be implemented into existing and developing provincial quality assurance programs across Canada."
- Key topics include:
  - Foundational elements:
    › Governance and QA programs.
    › Accreditation.
    › Human resource plan, workload measurement and sufficient staffing.
    › Appropriate training, licensure, credentialing, and continuing professional development.
    › Privacy, confidentiality, disclosure, and duty to report.
    › Informatics and quality documentation systems.
    › Appropriate pathologist workspace and related tools.
  - Interpretive pathology testing cycle:
    › Preinterpretive protocols.

- › Diagnostic assessment.
- › Prospective peer review.
- › Postinterpretive protocols (pathology report).
- · Interpretive QA policies and procedures (QAPPs):
  - › Intradepartmental consultation.
  - › Intraoperative consultation.
  - › Internal correlative activities.
  - › Internal retrospective reviews/audits.
  - › External consultation.
  - › External reviews.
- · Urgent diagnoses, and significant and unexpected findings.
  - › Revised reports (with addenda, amendments).
  - › Turnaround time.
  - › Completeness of reporting.
  - › Onboarding pathologist performance assessment.
  - › External QA and assessment.
  - › Service satisfaction.
- · External QA and assessment, including pathologist peer review assessment.
- · Approach to expression of concern regarding a pathologist's performance.
- · Patient safety checklists for surgical pathology.

Emerging topics in laboratory management

In the last few years, laboratory professional wellness and sustainability have emerged as topics of increasing importance in laboratory management. It is beyond the scope of this chapter to delve into these important topics. However, pathologists, particularly those aspiring to leadership, should make every opportunity to learn more about these fields, and incorporate these principles into their practice.

Laboratory professional wellness

Several health-care institutions and professional bodies offer resources to support medical professional wellness, and medical schools are creating administrative positions to support faculty wellness. Examples include:
- The Canadian Medical Association: Physician Health and Wellness.[2]
- The Royal College of Physician and Surgeons of Canada: Wellness Resources for Health Professionals.[3]

Sustainability

As health advocates, all physicians, including pathologists, and in particular pathologist leaders, must advocate for urgent climate action, and make a focus on sustainability part of laboratory practice.
- A call to climate action by the Canadian Association of Physicians for the Environment (CAPE)[4] states that the World Health Organization sees climate change "as the greatest health threat of the twenty-first century,"[5] and the Lancet Commission sees climate solutions "as the greatest global health opportunity of the twenty-first century."[6]
- A publication in the Lancet in July 2020 states that "health care causes global environmental impacts that, depending on which indicator is considered, range between 1% and 5% of total global impacts, and are > 5% for some national impacts."[7]
- There are many resources available to assist laboratories not only to decrease their environmental impacts, but also significantly reduce health-care spending in the process. An excellent resource that may serve as an introduction to understanding the climate crisis from the perspective of the health-care industry is the CAPE Climate Change Toolkit.[8]

MUST SEE

You should review the following documents from your institution:
- Organizational chart.
- Hiring guidelines.
- Laboratory budget.
- Contracts and leases with vendors.
- Standard operating procedures, such as for grossing and specimen processing.
- Guidelines on handling of errors.
- QA committee meeting minutes.

MUST DO

Consider improving your understanding of QA and laboratory management by:
- Serving on a QA committee.
- Participating in a QA project.
- On encountering a QA issue, following it up and seeing how it was resolved.
- Talking to technical mangers and staff about issues they encounter in the laboratory.

Basic Concepts in QA[9-16]

1. **What is quality?**

   The Canadian Council on Health Services Accreditation defines quality as the "degree of excellence; in the context of health care, it is the extent to which an organization meets client/patient/resident needs and exceeds their expectations."

2. **What is quality assurance (QA)?**

   A system for reviewing procedures used by those who regularly perform a service or produce a product with the goal of ensuring that standards have been met.

3. **Why do we need QA in a pathology laboratory?**

   - To provide documentation that the laboratory functions to an acceptable standard.
   - To identify the source of an error or areas that need to be improved.
   - To promote processes for reducing error and improving patient care.

4. **What is proficiency testing?**

   A process for evaluating unknown specimens, carried out by pathologists or laboratories, in which the results are retained and evaluated against a reference standard and compared with the results from other participating laboratories.

5. **What is quality control?**

   A system of routine techniques and activities performed to control the quality of the product being produced or the service being provided.

6. **List 3 examples of quality control.**

   - On slide positive and negative controls in immunohistochemistry (IHC).
   - Daily assessment of hematoxylin and eosin (H&E) stain quality.
   - Daily checking of the temperature and pH value of a staining solution.

7. **What is a quality manual?**

   The International Organization for Standardization (ISO) describes a quality manual as "a document specifying the quality management system of an organization." It contains all of the laboratory's policies.

8. **What is a medical error?**

   The failure of a planned action to be completed as intended, or the use of an incorrect plan to achieve an aim.

9. **What is a pathology error?**

   The failure of a diagnostic or surgical procedure to be followed by a timely, accurate, and complete pathology report that describes the disease and the findings in a manner that is concise and readily understandable.

10. **What is a near miss?**

    An incident that has no impact due to timely intervention or chance.

11. **What is a critical incident?**

    An incident that significantly alters treatment or results in death or disability. This type of incident must be reported to the Provincial Minister of Health.

12. **What is a nonconformity report?**

    A report on tests that have not been performed to the appropriate standard (i.e. a laboratory error).

13. **What is an adverse event?**

    The Health Insurance Reciprocal of Canada defines an adverse event as "an unexpected event in health-care delivery that results in harm to a patient and that is related to the care and/or services provided to the patient rather than to the patient's underlying medical condition. This includes an incident, in the course of health-care treatment, that results in a recognized risk of a nontrivial adverse outcome or consequence at some future time."

14. **What are examples of activities in pathology of the physician competencies defined by the CanMEDS framework?**

    - *Communicator*: quality reports, critical values, rounds.
    - *Collaborator*: interaction with pathology peers and clinicians.
    - *Medical expert*: diagnostic expertise.

(continued on next page)

- *Leader (Manager)*: quality management, resources management, workload assessment, client satisfaction.
- *Health advocate*: infection control, critical values, education.
- *Scholar*: teaching, research, conferences, continuing professional development.
- *Professional*: respecting the call schedule, punctuality, appropriate behavior.

15. What is the difference between guidelines and standards?
- Guidelines are a recommended strategy or range of strategies of laboratory practice. Variation due to patient-specific or laboratory-specific factors is a reasonable expectation.
- Standards are accepted principles of laboratory practice in which variation is not expected.

16. How is QA achieved?
- QA is achieved by measuring a set of performance indicators to determine whether performance conforms to accepted standards, and by seeking to improve performance when accepted standards are not met.
- It is done on a continuing basis.
- Reports should be generated at least annually and discussed with laboratory personnel.

Surgical Pathology QA

17. What does quality mean in surgical pathology?
- Quality indicates that a pathology report is:
  - Timely.
  - Accurate.
  - Complete, clearly communicating all necessary information.

18. What QA procedures apply to surgical pathology?

QUALITY ASSURANCE PHASE	QUALITY ASSURANCE PROCEDURES
Preanalytical phase	**Monitoring** • Specimen delivery timeliness and specimen condition. • Adequacy of clinical history, including completeness and relevance. • Specimen identification errors. • Lost specimens. • Errors in accessioning, fixation, grossing, embedding, cutting and staining.
Analytical phase	**Prospective procedures** • Intradepartmental consultations. • Consensus conferences. **Retrospective procedures*** • Intraoperative consultation-permanent section correlation. • Cytology-histology correlation. • Targeted case reviews. • Intra- and interdepartmental case conferences. • Interinstitutional consultations. *Note that random case reviews are no longer recommended.
Postanalytical phase	• Monitoring turnaround time. • Reviewing report quality, such as use of synoptic reporting and standard terminology. • Reviewing amended reports. • Reviewing record-keeping and storage systems.

19. List 5 types of peer review.
- Intraoperative consultation-permanent section correlation.
- Cytology-histology correlation.
- Intradepartmental consultation.
- Interinstitutional consultations.
- Audits.

20. List 5 types of pathology audit.
- Random review.
- Targeted review.
- Retrospective review.
- Prospective review.
- Accountability review.

21. List 5 quality assurance processes that might reveal diagnostic discrepancies.
- Peer review.
- Reviews of previous cases in light of follow-up.
- Interdisciplinary conferences or tumor boards.
- Clinician requested reviews.
- Amended report rate.

22. What is a critical diagnosis in anatomical pathology?

Any anatomical pathology result that has the potential to negatively impact patient care if not communicated in an urgent and timely fashion.

23. List examples of critical diagnoses in anatomical pathology.
- Crescents in > 50% of glomeruli in a kidney biopsy specimen.
- Transplant rejection.
- Leukocytoclastic vasculitis.
- Fat in a colonic endoscopic polypectomy specimen.
- Uterine contents without villi or trophoblasts.
- Fat in an endometrial curettage specimen.
- Mesothelial cells in an endocardial biopsy specimen.
- Malignancy in superior vena cava syndrome.
- Neoplasms causing paralysis.
- Unexpected or discrepant findings:
  · Unexpected malignancy.
  · Significant disagreement between intraoperative consultation and final diagnoses.
  · Significant disagreement between immediate interpretation and final diagnosis by fine needle aspiration biopsy (FNAB).
  · Significant disagreement and/or change between diagnoses of primary pathologist and external pathologist consulted.
- Infections:
  · Any invasive organism in specimens from immunocompromised patients.
  · Acid-fast bacilli in immunocompromised and immunocompetent patients.
  · Bacteria in heart valve or bone marrow.
  · Herpes simplex viral changes in gynecologic samples of near-term pregnant patients.
  · Bacteria or fungi in cerebrospinal or orbital fluid cytology.
  · Pneumocystis organisms, fungi, or viral cytopathic changes in bronchoalveolar lavage, bronchial washing, brushing cytology specimens, or FNAB specimens.

24. How should critical diagnoses be reported?
- Urgent (same day) verbal notification of the submitting clinician is required in cases of unexpected malignancy or identification of organisms in an immunocompromised patient.
- Timely notification should otherwise be initiated based on the findings and professional judgment.
- The notification date, time, and method (e.g., telephone call, email, fax, etc.) should be documented in the report.

25. List the components of a complete surgical pathology report.
- Patient identification: name, date of birth, health card number, hospital number.
- Physician identification.
- Dates when specimens were collected, received, processed, reported.
- Diagnosis.
- Gross description:
  · Labeling.
  · Container in which received.
  · Medium in which received, whether fresh, in saline, in formalin, or other.
  · Whether opened.
  · Orientation.
  · Dimensions, weight if relevant, other features.
  · Sampling, whether in toto or representative.
  · Block description.
- Microscopic description.
- If relevant:
  · Special stains.
  · IHC.
  · Biomarkers and molecular testing.
  · Immunofluorescence.
  · Electron microscopy.
  · Adequacy statements.
  · References.
  · Additional comments.
  · Intraoperative consultation diagnosis.
  · Cancer synoptic report.
  · Communication with physician.
  · Details if corrected report.
  · Details if amended report.
  · Addendum.
- Diagnostic SNOMED coding.
- Optional quality-type coding.

26. What are the College of American Pathologists (CAP) standards for acceptable turnaround times for reporting intraoperative consultations, surgical pathology specimens, and autopsies?
- Intraoperative consultations: 90% of cases reported within 20 minutes per block.
- Surgical pathology specimens: 80% of routine cases reported within 2 working days.
- Different benchmarks outside of the United States have acceptable turnaround times in the range of 2–7 days.
- Autopsy, preliminary report: 3 working days.
- Autopsy, final report: 30 working days for routine cases, 3 months for complex cases.

27. Compare the guidelines of the Canadian Association of Pathologists (CAP-ACP) and the College of American Pathologists (CAP) for the retention of pathology material and records.

RETENTION GUIDELINES	MINIMUM PERIOD	
	CAP-ACP[17]	CAP[18]
SURGICAL PATHOLOGY		
Wet tissue	4 weeks after final report.	2 weeks after final report.
Frozen tissue	Up to 20 years.	
Paraffin blocks	20 years.	10 years.
Slides	20 years.	10 years.
Consultation	Indefinitely.	
Paper requisition	2 years.	
Reports		10 years.
PEDIATRIC PATHOLOGY		
Wet tissue	4 weeks after final report.	
Paraffin blocks*	20 years.	
Slides	20 years.	
Consultation	Indefinitely.	
Paper requisition	2 years.	
CYTOPATHOLOGY (GYNECOLOGIC AND NONGYNECOLOGIC)		
Cell blocks	20 years.	
Slides, negative and unsatisfactory	5 years.	Gynecologic cytology glass slides: 5 years.
Slides, suspicious and positive	20 years.	
Slides, fine needle aspiration	20 years.	Nongynecologic cytology glass slides (including FNAB): 10 years.
Slides, male fertility	1 year.	
Consultation	Indefinitely.	
Paper requisition	2 years.	
Reports	Indefintely.	10 years.
AUTOPSY PATHOLOGY		
Wet tissue	3 months after final report.	3 months after final report.
Paraffin blocks*	10 years.	10 years.
Slides	10 years.	10 years.
Report and consent		10 years.
Hospital autopsy records	Indefinitely.	
Coroner/medical examiner	As per general autopsy, or at discretion of the coroner's/medical office/forensic pathologist.	Detailed guidelines, see reference.
ELECTRON MICROSCOPY		
Blocks, slides, grids, prints, digital images	20 years.	10 years.
MEDICAL RENAL BIOPSIES[19]		
Light microscopy		
Slides	20 years or more.	
Blocks	20 years or more.	
Immunofluorescence		
Slides	1 month after case verification in refrigerator.	
Frozen tissue	20 years or more at −70 degrees C.	
Images	Indefinitely.	
Electron microscopy		
Blocks, slides, grids	20 years or more.	
Images	Indefinitely.	

*For special pediatric cases, such as in children's hospitals, 50 years is the recommended minimum retention period for paraffin blocks.

Intraoperative Consultation QA

28. What are the QA indicators for intraoperative consultation?
- Turnaround time.
- Intraoperative consultation-permanent section discordant rate.

29. List 4 causes of intraoperative consultation-permanent section discordance.
- Technical issue: 10%.
- Interpretative error: 40%.
- Sampling error: 40%.
- Incorrect or incomplete clinical history: 10%.

30. Categorize intraoperative consultation-permanent section correlation results, and the thresholds for acceptable deferral and discordance rates, as recommended by the Association of Directors of Anatomic and Surgical Pathology (ADASP).
- Agreement.
- Deferral, appropriate.
- Deferral, inappropriate, 10% threshold.
- Disagreement, minor.
- Disagreement, major 3% threshold.

Note: the denominator must be consistent (blocks, specimens, or cases).

31. Categorize the clinical impact of intraoperative consultation-permanent section discordance.
- No clinical significance.
- Minor or questionable significance.
- Major or potentially major significance.

Note: discrepancies must be reconciled in the final report.

AUTOPSY PATHOLOGY QA

32. What are some of the QA elements in autopsy pathology?
- Was the preautopsy process timely and complete?
- Were permissions appropriate and the paperwork complete?
- Were the clinical questions and medicolegal issues addressed?
- Was clinicopathological correlation provided in the report?
- Were safety regulations adhered to during the autopsy?
- Was consultation sought, when required, for subspecialty expertise?
- Were findings documented via digital photographs?
- Were tissue blocking and slide preparation timely and of good quality?
- Were ancillary studies used appropriately?
- Were preliminary and final reports within the accepted timeframe?
- Were cases reviewed at morbidity and mortality rounds?
- Was a peer review process followed?

34. List the components of a complete autopsy report.
- Consent.
- Clinical information and any questions to be answered by the autopsy.
  · This is the clinician's responsibility to provide.
- Gross findings.
- Microscopic findings.
- Primary diagnosis and comments.
- Cause of death.

Cytopathology QA[20–23]

35. What are elements in a cytology quality assurance manual?
- Laboratory personnel.
- Physical facilities and equipment.
- Requisition forms, specimen collection, and accessioning.
- Preparation and staining techniques.
- Pathologist's responsibilities.
- Cytotechnologist's responsibilities.
- Screening practices.
- Diagnostic practices.
- Reporting.
- Records.
- Gynecologic cytology utilization registry.
- QA practices.
- Performance evaluation.
- Continuing education practices.

36. What are the standard staining techniques used for cytopathologic specimens?
- For gynecologic specimens: Papanicolaou staining.
- For fixed nongynecologic specimens: Papanicolaou staining.
- For air-dried nongynecologic specimens: Romanowsky-type staining.
- For cell-block preparations: hematoxylin-based stains.

37. How should stain quality be monitored in the laboratory?
- Staining quality should be monitored daily with appropriate correction of suboptimal results.
- Stains should be filtered or replaced regularly to maintain potency and freedom from contamination.

38. What qualifications does a director of cytopathology require?
The director must be a legally qualified physician with qualifications in anatomical pathology and cytopathology. It is recommended that the director have extra training and/or experience in cytopathology and laboratory management to oversee the quality of the laboratory.

39. What responsibilities for QA does a director of cytopathology have?
- Update laboratory manuals (at least annually).
- Generate laboratory QA reports (at least annually).
- Conduct regular meetings (at least quarterly) with all laboratory personnel to discuss laboratory performance and measures for quality improvement as necessary.
- Facilitate laboratory-based continuing education opportunities for all laboratory personnel.
- Identify deficiencies in knowledge, attitude, and skill of laboratory personnel.
- Facilitate remedial training for laboratory personnel as needed.

40. How should cytology specimens be screened?
- All nongynecological and all gynecologic specimens must be screened by a cytotechnologist.
- Hierarchical screening by a senior cytotechnologist or second mandatory screening by another cytotechnologist may be carried out in some labs for some gynecologic and nongynecologic specimens.
- Automated screening by approved commercial devices may be used in some labs following protocols recommended by the manufacturer and regulatory bodies.

41. What are the responsibilities and expectations of associate cytopathologists in a department?
- They should:
  · Have malpractice insurance.
  · Consult, as needed, with cytotechnologists, laboratory and clinical colleagues, and other allied health-care providers.
  · Keep up-to-date by reviewing current literature and participating in continuing education practices relating to cytopathology.
  · Maintain diagnostic competence: report a sufficient variety of gynecologic and nongynecologic material each year.
  · Obtain pertinent clinical information.
  · Report all cytology cases referred to them by cytotechnologists.
  · Provide appropriate feedback on case material to cytotechnologists.

42. What is the recommended reporting terminology?
- The most current edition of the Bethesda System for Reporting Cervical Cytology should be used for reporting gynecologic cytology. Specimens from the lower anogenital tract (vagina, anus) may also be reported using this terminology.
- For nongynecologic cytology, it is recommended that reports use clear interpretive terminology and follow published classification systems.

43. List the rescreening methods for gynecologic cytology specimens. Why are rescreening procedures carried out?
- Methods include:
  · Prospective rescreening: targeted, random, rapid, or prescreening.
  · Retrospective rescreening.
- A cytotechnologist with established competence carries out all manual rescreening.
- The aim of rescreening procedures is to identify false negative results.

44. What is the target rate of prospective rescreening for gynecologic cytology specimens?
A total of 10% of all negative gynecologic cytology specimens should be prospectively rescreened. These slides will be selected through a combination of random and targeted rescreening methods.

45. What is a prospective targeted rescreen?
- This involves rescreening a slide if the patient belongs to a high risk group.
- High risk patients include those with:
  · Clinical history of vaginal bleeding or spotting.
  · History of cervical/vaginal/vulvar carcinoma.
  · Previous cytology reported as ≥ atypical squamous or glandular cells within the last 2 years.
  · Abnormal cervix on speculum examination.
  · History of DES exposure.

46. What is a prospective random rescreen?
- This involves rescreening 10% of randomly selected negative gynecologic cytology slides.
- It is of questionable value in detecting false negatives.

47. What is a prospective rapid rescreen?
- This involves rescreening all negative gynecologic cytology slides for a specified time period (< 1 minute) after a routine screen. The use of this method precludes the 10% random rescreen.
- There is increased detection of false negatives with this technique.

48. What is a prospective rapid prescreen?
- This involves reviewing all gynecologic cytology slides for abnormal cells (< 2 minutes) prior to the full routine screen (≥ 6 minutes). The use of this method precludes the 10% rescreen.
- There is increased detection of false negatives with this technique.

49. What is involved in retrospective rescreening of gynecologic cytology specimens?
- If a current sample shows an abnormality of high grade squamous intraepithelial lesion (HSIL), adenocarcinoma in situ (AIS), or malignancy, the screening cytotechnologist retrieves and rescreens the patient's negative gynecologic cytology slides obtained within the previous 5 years. All slides are then referred to the pathologist for review.
- A corrected report is issued only when findings on rescreening change the patient's current management.
- The findings are used for educational feedback.

50. What are the indications for cytology-histology correlation?
- Nongynecologic cytology: malignant cases should be correlated with corresponding or subsequent tissue biopsy and/or autopsy material when feasible. Correlation of FNAB results with concurrent surgical pathology samples is also recommended.
- Gynecologic cytology: comparison with concurrent colposcopic histology samples should be carried out to monitor noncorrelation rates. Diagnoses of invasive carcinoma, HSIL, and AIS should be compared with follow-up biopsy results taken within 6 months following cytologic diagnosis.

51. What is the purpose of a follow-up program in cytology?
- A follow-up program involves correlating cytological diagnoses with biopsy, resection, or autopsy diagnoses.
  - It can help resolve apparent cytologic-histologic discrepancies.
- It can streamline and standardize laboratory diagnostic criteria.
- It can provide valuable continuing education material for laboratory staff and trainees.

52. What are 4 potential applications of high risk human papillomavirus (hrHPV) testing in gynecologic cytology?
- Primary HPV screening.
- An up-front cotesting approach in which both a hrHPV test and cervical cytology specimen are obtained at the time of patient screening.
- Triage of an abnormal cytology result using a hrHPV test— this improves the sensitivity and specificity for disease detection and targeted colposcopic referral.
- HPV genotyping — this allows for selective reporting of specific HPV types (e.g., HPV 16 and 18) associated with an increased risk of precancerous lesions to facilitate colposcopic referral.

53. What is the hrHPV positivity rate in gynecologic cases with a cytologic diagnosis of atypical squamous cells of undetermined significance (ASC-US)? What is the underlying risk of HSIL in ASC-US cases?
- High risk HPV is identified in 40–50% of ASC-US cases.
- Among women with ASC-US, 10-20% have an underlying HSIL (CIN2 or CIN3).

54. What are the recommended laboratory target rates for the ASC:SIL ratio, and for use of the ASC-H and atypical glandular cell (AGC) diagnostic categories, according to the Bethesda System for Reporting Cervical Cytology?
- ASC:SIL ratio:
  - This should not exceed 3:1. A higher ratio suggests overuse of ASC diagnostic categories.
- ASC-H:
  - This is expected to represent < 10% of all ASC interpretations.
- Of these, 30–40% will have underlying HSIL.
- AGC:
  - This is expected to represent < 1% (0.1- 0.8%) of cases.
  - On follow-up, high grade lesions are identified in 10–40% of cases and are more often squamous (HSIL) than glandular.

55. How should performance indicators be documented by the cytology laboratory?

- Performance indicators should be documented at least annually, and include:
  - Productivity rates for each cytotechnologist and cytopathologist.
  - Individual performance indicators (delivered confidentially).
- Overall laboratory performance, which should be shared with all personnel.
- Specimen adequacy, which may be communicated to individual health-care providers.

Note: no national standard exists: laboratories should aim for equivalency with comparable laboratories and published data.

56. List at least 5 gynecologic cytology performance indicators.

- The total number and rates of unsatisfactory specimens for the laboratory, each cytotechnologist, cytopathologist, and health-care provider.
- The total number and rates of each major diagnostic category for the laboratory, each cytotechnologist, and each pathologist.
- The false negative/positive rate on 10% rescreening.
- The hrHPV positivity rate in ASC cases, if available.
- The ASC:SIL ratio for the laboratory overall and for each cytopathologist. The ASC includes ASC-US and ASC-H, while the SIL includes LSIL and HSIL diagnostic categories.
- The cytohistological correlation rates for HSIL, ASC-H, AIS, and malignancy.
- The false negative/positive rate in cytology–histology correlation.
- Screening misses of ASC-H or AGC or other abnormality that changes management.
- The laboratory turnaround time (from receiving specimen to finalized report).

57. List at least 5 nongynecologic cytology performance indicators.

- The total number of cases categorized by anatomic site and specimen type.
- The total number and rates of unsatisfactory cases for the laboratory, and each cytotechnologist and cytopathologist.
- The major diagnostic category rates (e.g., unsatisfactory, negative, atypical, suspicious, malignant) for the laboratory overall and for major nongynecological specimen types.
- Correlation of results of FNAB specimens with their corresponding surgical material — at a minimum, the malignant diagnoses should be correlated.
- Major and minor discrepancy rates between cytotechnologist and cytopathologist diagnoses.
- The laboratory turnaround time (from receiving specimen to finalized report).

58. List 3 postanalytical performance indicators that can be monitored by the cytopathology laboratory.

- The number of corrected and supplemental cytology reports issued by the laboratory and/or by individual cytopathologists.
- The number of internal and external cytology consultations.
- The number of external review requests, the reasons for external consultation, and any diagnostic discrepancies.

59. What performance indicator should be carried out in specimens obtained via rapid on-site evaluation (ROSE)?

A comparison of the initial specimen adequacy assessment/preliminary diagnosis versus the final diagnosis.

60. What are 3 aspirator outcome performance indicators?

- FNAB unsatisfactory rates.
- FNAB complication rates/outcomes.
- FNAB service satisfaction (e.g., clinician feedback survey).

61. List 4 continuing education practices in cytopathology.

- Keeping up to date through review of current cytology journals.
- Consulting appropriate, current cytology textbooks.
- Attending scientific meetings, review courses, or specialty conferences.
- Attending lectures or symposia.

62. What is the workload limit for cytotechnologists in the United States and Canada?

- US workload limit:
  - The primary screening maximum is 100 slides/24 hours; at least 8 hours screening time is needed for 100 slides (i.e., the maximum rate is 12.5 slides/hour). Secondary review is not regulated.
- Canadian workload limit:
  - If cytotechnologists are exclusively screening without other duties, the maximum is 60–80 slides in an average 8-hour working day.
- If other duties are required in addition to screening, there should be a proportionally reduced workload (e.g., 4 hours of screening time means 30–40 slides total).
- Laboratories using automated screening technologies (field of view [FOV] method) should adjust the number of slides screened by cytotechnologists. Slides with FOV-only review are considered equivalent to 0.5 slides (or half a slide). Slides that require both FOV and full manual review are considered equivalent to 1.5 slides.

63. Under what conditions is a cytology case referred from a cytotechnologist to a cytopathologist?

- The following cases in gynecologic cytology must be referred:
  - All cases of NILM with reparative changes.
  - All cases of ASC or AGC, for reporting.
- All nongynecologic cytology must be signed out by a cytopathologist.
- The report must document the names of the screening cytotechnologist and the cytopathologist.

64. Compare the United States and Canada regarding the guidelines for retaining blocks, slides, and paper records.

See the answer to question 27.

65. List at least 3 sources of external proficiency testing.

- College of American Pathologists (CAP) (PAP, nongynecologic).
- American Society of Clinical Pathologists (ASCP) (CheckPath program).
- Laboratory Services of Ontario, which administers the Quality Management Program (now compulsory for laboratories in Ontario and Quebec) and uses the CheckPath program of the ASCP and the PAP program of CAP.

66. List examples of critical diagnoses in cytopathology.

See the answer to question 23.

67. How should critical cytologic diagnoses be reported?

See the answer to question 24.

68. List 3 scenarios in which obtaining a prospective second opinion may be prudent in cytopathology.

- A sample obtained from an unusual anatomic location.
- Cytologic diagnoses that may result in "high stakes" treatment decisions (e.g., positive ureteric brushings with subsequent nephroureterectomy).
- A major discordance between a cytotechnologist and cytopathologist diagnostic interpretation.

Laboratory Management

69. How would you develop a QA program in anatomical pathology?

- Establish a QA committee that includes a medical leader, a technical manager, and a QA coordinator.
- Develop a QA plan based on CAP standards and anatomical pathology workflow.
  - Preanalytical: from specimen collection, through delivery to the laboratory and processing in the laboratory, to when the slide is ready for the pathologist to review.
  - Analytical: from when the pathologist receives the slide to report verification.
- Postanalytical: from report verification to when the clinician acts on it.
- Draw up a quality manual, a document that specifies the quality management system of the laboratory.
- Convene regular committee meetings to review, monitor, and evaluate various aspects of the laboratory service to ensure that standards of quality are being met.
- Identify quality improvement opportunities and manage unexpected events.

70. What are the steps in a quality improvement initiative?

- Identify a process that needs to be improved by establishing realistic goals or responding to deficiencies.
- Measure the current level of performance for that process.
- Determine the target or desirable level of performance.
- Design and implement an intervention to achieve the desired level of performance.
- Monitor performance.
- Assess and document the improvement.

Note: these steps may need to be repeated.

71. List 4 important types of quality management documents.

- Policy: statement of intent, what is to be done, and why.
- Process: the interrelated steps involved in an activity, which often involves a number of individuals and which may be illustrated with a flow chart.
- Standard operating procedures: specific details of how an individual performs an activity.
- Forms: documentation of what was done.

72. What are universal precautions in laboratories?

- Universal precautions apply to handling of human tissue; blood; and body fluids such as semen, and pleural, peritoneal, pericardial, synovial, cerebrospinal and amniotic fluid.
- All specimens of blood and body fluids should be placed in a well-constructed container with a secure lid to prevent leakage during transport.
- Workers should routinely use appropriate barriers — including gloves, aprons, masks, and protective eyewear or face shields — to prevent skin and mucous membrane exposure when they expect to come into contact with blood or other body fluids.
- Workers should wear gloves when processing blood or other body fluids, such as when removing tops from vacuum tubes.
- Workers should use biological safety cabinets for procedures that have a high potential to generate droplets, such as blending, sonicating, and vigorous mixing.

- Workers should not use their mouths for pipette procedures.
- Workers should wash their hands and other skin surfaces immediately and thoroughly if contaminated with blood or other body fluids.
- Workers should decontaminate after spills, and should decontaminate equipment after use.
- Workers should wash their hands after completing a laboratory task, and should remove protective clothing before leaving the laboratory.
- Workers should take precautions to prevent injuries caused by needles, scalpels, and other sharp instruments or devices during procedures. After sharp instruments are used, they should be placed in puncture resistant containers for disposal. The puncture resistant containers should be located as close as practical to the area where they are used.

Note: the American Centers for Disease Control and Prevention, the Canadian Centre for Occupational Health and Safety, and provincial colleges of physicians and surgeons publish recommendations for preventing the transmission of HIV and other blood-borne pathogens.

73. What information is required on a requisition form?

- Patient name.
- Date of birth.
- Provincial health card number.
- Hospital identification number.
- Address.

- Name of requesting health-care provider.
- Anatomic site and laterality of specimen.
- Appropriate clinical history.
- Date and time of specimen collection.

74. What information is required on a specimen-container label?

- Patient name.
- Date of birth.

- Identifying number.
- Anatomic site and laterality of the specimen.

75. What are some standard practices in specimen accessioning?

- Specimens should only be accessioned if ordered by an appropriate health-care provider.
- A clear rejection policy should be developed and communicated to all users of the laboratory.

- Specimens should be accessioned with a unique number.
- Time and date of specimen receipt should be recorded.
- The accessioning number should be recorded on each slide.

76. How should slides be labeled?

- Each slide should have 2 unique identifiers; it should also have a barcode if the laboratory uses a barcoding and tracking system.

- One identifier should include the patient's last name and initials.

77. What advantages does computerization have in laboratories?

- Computerization facilitates:
  · Accessioning.
  · Reporting.

  · Archiving records.
  · Accessing data for QA practices.

78. If you were employed in a small hospital and wished to establish an IHC service with limited resources, which 4 stains would you initially choose?

- Pancytokeratin to identify carcinoma.
- CD45 to identify lymphoma.

- S100 to identify melanoma.
- A neuroendocrine marker such as synaptophysin, CD56 or chromogranin.

Note: vimentin can be positive in sarcomas and also many carcinomas, and hence is not particularly useful.

Risk Management

79. What are the processes involved in handling an adverse event?
- Incident review and root cause analysis.
- Performance review and performance management.
- Disclosure.
- Identifying and managing medicolegal consequences.
- Managing media relations.

80. What is root cause analysis?
- Root cause analysis is a method of problem solving that identifies root causes. Removing a root cause from a problem-fault sequence prevents the recurrence of a problem.
- QA data collection alone does not result in change to behaviors or processes. It helps locate the problem, but change requires understanding the reason the problem exists.
- Monitoring of and response to events should take place as close as possible to the time of sign-out to minimize the impact of an error.

81. What is the purpose of root cause analysis?

The purpose is to identify the causes, factors, or sources of variation that led to a specific event, result, or defect in a product or process.

82. How is root cause analysis done?
- A variety of techniques can be used to uncover root causes, such as cause mapping, change analysis, using the Ishikawa fishbone diagram, and the "5 whys."
- At its most basic, the process poses 3 questions:
  - · What was the problem?
  - · What were the causes of the problem?
  - · What actions should be taken to prevent the problem from recurring?

83. What should you do if you notice that one of your colleagues has made a diagnostic error that could impact the care of the patient?
- Discuss the case with your colleague.
- If your colleague agrees with the change in diagnosis, they should inform the clinician and issue an amended report.
- If your colleague disagrees with the change in diagnosis, a third opinion should be sought, either internally or externally.
- Notify the clinician so that no irreversible clinical management takes place before the disagreement is resolved.
- If your colleague refuses to seek a third opinion, notify the Laboratory Medical Director.

84. A surgeon approaches you because he or she strongly disagrees with a diagnosis your colleague has made. What do you do?
- Obtain clinical information from the surgeon as to the nature of the disagreement and the surgeon's reasons for not approaching your colleague directly.
- Review the case.
- Discuss the situation with your colleague.
- If there is any new information, collaborate with your colleague to issue an addendum, or corrected or amended report.

85. If the surgeon asks you to review all the cases your colleague signs out, what do you do?
- Clarify the reason for the surgeon's request.
- Contact the Laboratory Medical Director to manage the issue.

86. A review reveals that your colleague makes many errors. What do you do?
- Contact the Laboratory Medical Director to manage the issue.
- Document all details.
- The Laboratory Medical Director may temporarily suspend the pathologist from signing out the specific types of case on which the pathologist tends to make errors, and arrange for remedial training so the pathologist can reestablish their competency.
- If the pathologist refuses to undergo remedial training, the Laboratory Medical Director must seek advice from the institution's Vice President, Medical, or the Provincial College of Physicians and Surgeons.

87. What should you do if you are subject to an accountability review?

Contact the Canadian Medical Protective Association (CMPA).

Note: audits performed as part of a routine QA process are afforded protection. However, accountability reviews which concern the performance of individual pathologists, are not afforded protection and are not confidential.

Interpretive Pathology

This section quotes from the Pan-Canadian quality assurance recommendations for interpretive pathology[1] with permission from the Canadian Partnership Against Cancer.

FOUNDATIONAL ELEMENTS

88. What are the foundational elements for interpretive pathology QA?

- Appropriate governance, and oversight at jurisdictional and institutional level; and linkage to existing QA programs.
- Accreditation.
- A human resource plan, workload measurement and sufficient staffing.
- Appropriate training, licensure, credentialing and continuing professional development.
- Privacy, confidentiality, disclosure and duty to report.
- Informatics and quality documentation systems.
- Appropriate pathologist workspace and related tools.

89. What QA oversight should be in place in a laboratory?

- A laboratory medical director.
- A single QA committee, or 2 committees.
- A technical/administrative QA committee, with authority from the health authority, to provide oversight for technical laboratory services, by implementing a quality management system, including policies and procedures for achieving optimal results, and ongoing quality improvement.
- A professional/interpretive QA committee, chaired by an appropriate pathologist, reporting to an institutional-level senior QA committee that is responsible for implementing and monitoring of QA within the laboratory specialty.

Laboratory medical directors implement and monitor the practice guidelines and/or standards by:
- Developing a QA plan and implementing QAPPs.
- Regularly reviewing QA metrics and monitoring of compliance.
- Reporting on the performance of the quality management system and areas for improvement.
- Providing of a forum for peer discussion and resolution of quality issues.
- Identifying of acceptable QA targets/metrics.

90. What should a human resource plan for medical, scientific, technical and support staff address?

- Laboratory services, including administrative and academic responsibilities.
- QA activities in the laboratory.
- Anticipating and responding to changes in staffing, including staff turnover and retirement.

91. What should an effective workload measurement system include?

- A transparent system that is based on the specimen volume and complexity; ancillary investigations such as immunohistochemistry, molecular testing, immunofluorescence and electron microscopy; reporting requirements; and clinical information.
- Activities related to QA and patient care.
- Other professional activities, including administrative and academic.
- Evaluation of laboratory and individual pathologist workload levels to ensure adequate staffing.

92. List some workload measurement systems widely implemented nationally or internationally.

- The guidelines on staffing and workload for histopathology and cytopathology departments.[24]
- The Canadian Association of Pathologists workload model.[25]
- Work2Quality: guidelines for workload measurement in pathology professional practices.[26]

93. Which support staff are required for maximum pathologist efficiency?

- Pathologists require adequate numbers of competent technical staff, secretarial staff, and qualified and skilled pathologists' assistants (PAs).
- At the local and organizational level, it is possible to develop new ways of working that will free pathologists
- from tasks that can be done by other providers such as histotechnologists and PAs.
- This will allow pathologists to focus on interpretation and diagnosis.

94. What should be done when for a period appropriate expertise is not available?

Cases should be referred out.

95. What must the informatics systems in a laboratory support?

- A laboratory information system (LIS) for pathology case management.
- Synoptic reporting:
  - Generation of synoptic reports in a standardized format.
  - Integration of electronic synoptic pathology data into existing provincial and national e-Health infrastructure,
- such as provincial electronic health records and provincial cancer registries.
- QA activities:
  - Generation of indicators to measure completeness and compliance with necessary clinical indicators.

Note: access to documentation of QA activities should be restricted to appropriate individuals as per institutional/jurisdictional policies.

933

- Workload capture.

- New technology:
  - Digital pathology and telepathology.

96. What elements constitute an appropriate pathologist workspace and related tools?

- Pathologists require a quiet office, with adequate space, efficient design, sufficient illumination and appropriate ventilation.
- Workspace and equipment should be designed or positioned to reduce the risks of ergonomic distress disorders and accidents.
- Pathologists should not work in isolation. Their offices should ideally be located in close proximity to other colleagues or linked through technologies that facilitate sharing of cases and interprofessional communication.
- Microscopes and equipment used in the laboratory should be of high quality, and be cleaned and maintained on a

regular basis. All equipment should be replaced/updated on a regular basis, as appropriate.
- Pathologists should be provided with an appropriate communication system commensurate with the industry standard.
- Pathologists should have access to the most current decision support tools to remain up to date on the most recent evidence and advances in the field, to make an informed and accurate diagnosis.
- There should be proper processes and adequate resources to perform ancillary testing and/or to seek second medical opinions, internally or externally.

INTERPRETIVE PATHOLOGY TESTING CYCLE

97. What are the elements of the interpretive pathology testing cycle from the perspective of the pathologist as medical practitioner?

- Preinterpretive phase:
  - The pathologist assesses elements such as specimen identification, presence of clinical information, the quality and completeness of the gross description, and the quality of slides prepared.
- Interpretive phase:
  - This involves the actual analysis of the case material and covers the following key activities: correlation of the morphology with the clinical and imaging information; correlation with prior or concurrent pathology results; sharing the case with colleagues (peer review); taking

additional blocks from the specimen; and utilization of ancillary techniques such as immunohistochemistry or molecular diagnostics to further work up the case. The product of the interpretive phase is the pathology report.
- Postinterpretive phase:
  - This involves ensuring that the pathology report maintains proper patient identification, and is timely, accurate and complete. This phase also deals with delivering the report to a referring physician(s). This may be done electronically, in hard copy and/or verbally, where appropriate.

PREINTERPRETIVE PHASE

98. Which material should be submitted to the laboratory, and examined microscopically?

There should be evidence-based policies and procedures to define material from the operating room exempt from submission to the laboratory, and those specimens that do not require a microscopic assessment.

99. Which measures should be in place to minimize the risk of case mix-ups?

- Multidepartmental (clinical departments in addition to anatomical pathology) policies that reduce the risk of case mix-ups.

- A comprehensive bar-coding system, or similar positive patient identification system, to track specimens from time of collection, through the pathologist's office, to report release and electronic delivery.

100. Who can perform gross examination?

Gross examination must be performed by a pathologist, a pathology resident, or other qualified personnel, such as a PA or grossing technologist, who are under the supervision of a pathologist.

101. What should occur prior to the pathologist's assessment of a case?

- Patient demographics, specimen identification and integrity, should be reviewed and verified.
- Clinical information included on the requisition should be reviewed; if any or all of this information is missing, its absence should be documented.
- In cases where additional clinical information is deemed necessary, the pathologist should review the electronic medical records where available, and/or results of

diagnostic imaging and/or laboratory studies, or contact the referring physician or other appropriate personnel.
- Discrepancies should be managed in line with the relevant QAPP.
- The quality of technical preparation should be monitored, and any concerns, errors or deficiencies should be documented, and appropriate corrective actions put in place.

102. Who can perform microscopic examination?

A pathologist must perform all microscopic examinations, with the exception of cervical cytology and peripheral blood smears. The cervical cytology and blood smears that must be reviewed by a pathologist should be determined based on guidelines from the Canadian Society of Cytopathology, the Canadian Hematology Society, and other organizations.

103. Which elements do the pathologists synthesize to create the final report, including diagnosis?

- Gross features.
- Microscopic features.
- Relevant clinical information.
- Relevant previous and concurrent pathology results/ findings, including intraoperative consultations.
- Relevant additional studies, such as:
  · Additional blocks.
- Additional block levels.
- Special stains.
- Immunohistochemistry.
- Biomarker and molecular tests.
- Immunofluorescence.
- Electron microscopy.
- Internal and/or external expert opinion/consultation.

PEER REVIEW

104. List the types of peer review.

- Prospective — prior to case verification.
- Retrospective — after case verification.
  · Multidisciplinary case rounds.
  · Case lookbacks during the process of evaluating current cases.

– and –
- Intrainstitutional.
- Extrainstitutional.

Note: the CAP-ACP developed guidelines for pathology review in the research context.[27]

105. What are the purposes of peer review?

- Elimination of significant errors before they affect patient care decisions or patient outcomes.
- Identification of system flaws and individual pathologist's knowledge deficits, allowing corrective action to be taken.

106. What are the requirements for case review?

- Timeliness.
- Incorporation into normal laboratory work flow.
- Professionalism.
- Independent analysis.
- Formal documentation.
- Targeted review of difficult, or significant and unexpected diagnoses.
- Protection from civil legal action.

POSTINTERPRETIVE PHASE: PATHOLOGY REPORT

107. Which final actions should the pathologist take prior to report verification?

- Reconfirm positive patient/specimen identification.
- Check the report for accuracy, completeness and appropriate formatting/usability.
- Ensure the report is in a standardized format, and contains standard terminology, scoring, grading and staging systems, and clear language.
- Reconcile discrepancies between elements of the report.

108. Which factors are relevant to the timeliness of the report?

- Clinical urgency.
- Specimen type.
- Whether additional investigations and consultations are required.

109. Which procedures should be followed related to report delivery?

- Patient confidentiality should be maintained.
- There should be protocols for electronic and hard copy (where appropriate) delivery of reports to ordering physicians.
- Significant and unexpected diagnoses and changes to the report that may impact patient management should be
personally communicated to the treating physician as soon as possible.
- There should be audits of receipt and integrity of electronic and hard copy reports.
- Transcription, verification and delivery errors should be monitored and managed through a nonconforming event management system.

110. Which QAPPs are required to support a robust internal and external interpretive QA program in the pathology laboratory?

- Intradepartmental consultation.
- Intraoperative consultation.
- Internal correlative activities.
- Internal retrospective reviews/audits.
- External consultation.
- External reviews.
- Urgent diagnoses, and significant and unexpected findings.
- Revised (addended, amended) reports.
- Turnaround time.
- Completeness of reporting.
- Onboarding pathologist performance assessment.
- External QA/assessment.
- Service satisfaction.

111. What is required, in addition to having QAPPs guiding these activities?

- There should be a system to document these activities.
- All discrepancies should be resolved and documented.
- The results should be reported by the Professional/Interpretive QA Committee on a regular basis.
- These data should be used to inform continuous quality improvement activities.

112. Which diagnoses require timely communication to licensed caregivers?

- Urgent diagnoses for medical conditions which require treatment as soon as possible.
- Significant, unexpected diagnoses or findings which are clinically unusual or unforeseen and should be addressed at some point in the patient's course.
- These should be communicated to the licensed caregiver in a timely manner to ensure that they are aware of these unexpected results, and to ensure proper treatment.

113. How should these be documented?

- This communication should be documented in the report.
- There should be a process to ensure that the message is received correctly.

114. What are the definitions of addended, amended and corrected reports, as recommended by the Pan-Canadian Guidelines?

- Addended or supplementary report:
  - Adds information to a previously completed pathology report.
  - This information does not change the diagnosis or any data elements related to the diagnosis.
  - For clear communication these may appear at the top of the report.
  - It may be used for example to add ancillary test results.
- Amended or corrected report:
  - Changes information in the finalized report.
  - The reason for the amendment must be included in the report. Reasons for amendments fall into two categories.
    - › Correction of information not related to the diagnosis, such as errors in transcription, patient identification, specimen site, and report defects — corrected report, in some jurisdictions.
    - › Correction of diagnosis and/or other data related to the diagnosis — amended report in some jurisdictions.
  - Amendments that may lead to a change in treatment must be communicated to the responsible physician, and this must be documented in the report.
  - For clear communication these may replace the original report.
  - Amended reports that significantly alter synoptic report data fields should automatically overwrite those data fields within the synoptic report database.

115. List some reasons for addended and amended reports.

- Retrospective reviews.
- Acquisition of new information related to ancillary testing.
- Receipt of additional clinical information.

116. How are microscopic discrepancies classified?

- A diagnosis which one is surprised to see from any pathologist, such as an obvious cancer reported as benign. This type of error should be investigated.
- A diagnosis which is fairly clearly incorrect, but which one is not surprised to see a small percentage of pathologists
- such as a moderately difficult diagnosis, or missing a small clump of malignant cells in an otherwise benign biopsy.
- A diagnosis where inter-observer variation is known to be large, such as disagreements between 2 adjacent tumor grades, or any very difficult diagnosis.

117. When in particular, and how should the performance of pathologists be audited?

- An audit, preferably targeted, should be performed on a proportion of cases reported by all recently hired pathologists or a pathologist returning to practice after an extended absence.
- The results of the audit should be monitored by the Professional/Interpretive QA Committee on a regular basis.
- If the performance of the pathologist is in question, the Laboratory Medical Director or designate requires access to all of the data.
- Pathologists should be aware of the auditing process and results.

118. How should service satisfaction be monitored?

At appropriate intervals, feedback from consulting clinicians should be solicited with an aim to improve product quality. Such feedback may potentially uncover problems that have not been identified by other QA activities. Feedback can be solicited through surveys, as well as by monitoring complaints and compliments. Monitoring client satisfaction is particularly helpful before, during and after implementing changes or new services.

EXTERNAL QA AND ASSESSMENT (EQA)

119. What is EQA?

EQA, which is sometimes called external proficiency testing (EPT), is an interlaboratory peer program that allows assessment of technical and diagnostic performance compared to other laboratories using the same methods, instrumentation, and analysis.

121. What is the purpose of EQA?

EQA can provide laboratories and pathologists with the necessary information to help them:

- Maintain and improve technical and diagnostic quality.
- Improve inter-laboratory and inter-pathologist agreement, and raise standards.
- Detect equipment faults, identify reagent problems, and identify diagnostic discordance.
- Compare performance across different technical methods.

122. Which pathologists should participate?

All pathologists should participate in EQA programs, where available and appropriate, which have been designed to reflect the specific functions of the laboratory, and the scope of practice of the pathologist.

123. What are Class II IHC tests and how should the results of these be monitored?

- Class II IHC tests are prognostic and/or predictive tests that trigger specific treatment decisions independent of morphologic findings and classification.
- All laboratories performing Class II marker IHC should participate in EPT.
- EPT programs for IHC should utilize validated test materials, be statistically and temporally relevant, have established parameters for acceptable performance, and should have comparative results viewable by all participants.
- Laboratories should report EPT performance results to the Departmental QA Committee and to the appropriate regulatory/accreditation agency, if required.
- All laboratories performing class II IHC testing should monitor biomarker positivity rates for comparison with nationally recognized standards, and report these rates to the Departmental QA Committee and to the appropriate regulatory/accreditation agency, if required.

PATHOLOGIST PEER REVIEW ASSESSMENT

124. What are the requirements for pathologists related to peer review assessment?

Pathologists should participate in existing peer review assessments that are part of their licensing and regulatory body.

APPROACH TO EXPRESSION OF CONCERN REGARDING A PATHOLOGIST'S PERFORMANCE

125. How should an expression of concern regarding a pathologist's performance be managed?

A policy that outlines how expressions of concern regarding a pathologist's performance are handled should be available at all institutions delivering interpretive pathology services. The CAP-ACP developed guidelines that could be adopted for local use.[28]

PATIENT SAFETY CHECKLISTS IN SURGICAL PATHOLOGY

126. What tools can be used to enhance patient safety in surgical pathology?

The CAP-ACP guidelines include patient safety checklists that could be adapted for local use.

References

1. Canadian Partnership Against Cancer. Pan-Canadian quality assurance recommendations for interpretive pathology [Internet]. Canadian Partnership Against Cancer; 2016 November. Available from https://www.partnershipagainstcancer.ca/topics/quality-interpretive-pathology-report/.

2. Canadian Medical Association: physician health and wellness [Internet]. Ottawa (ON): Canadian Medical Association; [updated 2022; cited 2022 August 11]. Available from https://www.cma.ca/physician-health-and-wellness.

3. Royal College of Physicians and Surgeons of Canada: wellness resources for health professionals [Internet]. Ottawa (ON): Royal College of Physicians and Surgeons of Canada; [updated 2022; cited 2022 August 11.]. Available from https://www.royalcollege.ca/rcsite/documents/about/covid-19-wellness-resources-hp-e.

4. Perrotta K, Howard C; Canadian Medical Association; Canadian Nurses Association; Urban Public Health Network; Canadian Public Health Association. Call to action on climate change and health [Internet]. Toronto (ON): Canadian Association of Physicians for the Environment; c2019. Available from https://www.cfpc.ca/CFPC/media/PDF/Call-to-Action-Full-logos-updated-EN-June-25-2019.pdf

5. World Health Organization. WHO Director-General addresses Human Rights Council on climate change [Internet]. Geneva: World Health Organization; 2016. Available from https://www.who.int/director-general/speeches/detail/who-director-general-addresses-human-rights-council-on-climate-change.

6. Watts N, Adger WN, Agnolucci P, et al. Healthy and climate change policy responses to protect public health. Lancet. 2015;386(10006). doi: 10.1016/S0140-6736(15)60854-6

7. Lenzen M, Malik A, Li M, et al. The environmental footprint of health care: a global assessment. Lancet Planet Health. 2020;4(7):e271–e279. doi: 10.1016/S2542-5196(20)30121-2. PMID: 32681898.

8. Perrotta K, editor. Climate change toolkit for health professionals [Internet]. Toronto (ON): Canadian Association of Physicians for the Environment; 2019 April 29. Available from https://cape.ca/category/climate-health-and-policy/climate-change-toolkit/.

9. College of American Pathologists: accreditation checklists [Internet]. Northfield (IL): College of American Pathologists; [updated 2022; cited 2022 August 11]. Available from https://www.cap.org/laboratory-improvement/accreditation/accreditation-checklists.

10. Dahl J. Quality, assurance, diagnosis, treatment, and patient care. Patient Safety & Quality Healthcare [Internet]. 2006 March/April [cited 2022 August 11]. Available from: http://www.psqh.com/marapr06/pathologist.html.

11. Nakhleh R, Coffin C, Cooper K; Association of Directors of Anatomic and Surgical Pathology. Recommendations for quality assurance and improvement in surgical and autopsy pathology. Am J Clin Pathol. 2006;126(3):337-40. Medline:16880147. doi: 10.1309/2TVBY2D8131FAMAX

12. Nakhleh RE. Core components of a comprehensive quality assurance program in anatomic pathology. Adv Anat Pathol. 2009;16(6):418-23. Medline:19851132. doi: 10.1097/PAP.0b013e3181bb6bf7

13. Nakhleh RE, Fitzgibbons PL. Quality management in anatomic pathology: promoting patient safety through systems improvement and error reduction. Northfield (IL): College of American Pathologists; 2005.

14. Renshaw AA. Measuring and reporting errors in surgical pathology: lessons from gynecologic cytology. Am J Clin Pathol. 2001;115(3):338-41. Medline:11242788. doi: 10.1309/M2XP-3YJA-V6E2-QD9P

15. Torlakovic EE, Riddell R, Banerjee D, et al; Canadian Association of Pathologists — Association canadienne des pathologistes National Standards Committee. Canadian Association of Pathologists — Association canadienne des pathologistes National Standards Committee/Immunohistochemistry: best practice recommendations for standardization of immunohistochemistry tests. Am J Clin Pathol. 2010;133(3):354–65. Medline:20154273. doi: 10.1309/AJCPDYZ1XMF4HJWK

16. Troxel DB. Error in surgical pathology. Am J Surg Pathol. 2004;28(8):1092–5. Medline:15252317. doi: 10.1097/01.pas.0000126772.42945.5c

17. Canadian Association of Pathologists — Association canadienne des pathologistes. The retention and use of human biologic material [Internet]. Ottawa (ON): Canadian Association of Pathologists; 2005. Available from https://www.cap-acp.org/guide_retention-human-biologic-material.php.

18. College of American Pathologists. Minimum period of retention of laboratory records and materials [Internet]. Northfield (IL): College of American Pathologists; 2020 September [cited 2022 August 11]. Available from https://elss.cap.org.

19. Nephropathology Special Interest Group. Retention guidelines for medical renal biopsies [Internet]. Kingston (ON): Nephropathology Special Interest Group; 2015 July 17 [cited 2022 August 11]. Available from https://www.cap-acp.org/Nephro.php.

20. Nayar R, Wilbur D, editors. The Bethesda system for reporting cervical cytology. 3rd ed. New York: Springer; 2015.

21. Institute for Quality Management in Healthcare. Consensus practice recommendation - gynecologic and non-gynecologic cytology [Internet]. Toronto (ON): IQMH; 2015 [revised 2015 February 10; cited 2022 August 10]. Available from https://qview.ca/qview/FileView.aspx?resourceid=716661.

22. College of American Pathologists. Minimum period of retention of laboratory records and materials [Internet]. Northfield (IL): College of American Pathologists; 2020 September [cited 2022 August 11]. Available from https://elss.cap.org.

23. Canadian Society of Cytopathology. Canadian Society of Cytopathology guidelines for practice & quality assurance in cytopathology [Internet]. Kingston (ON): Canadian Society of Cytopathology; [revised 2019; cited 2022 August 11]. Available from http://cytopathology.ca/wp-content/uploads/2019/04/CSC-cyto_guidelines-final-2019.-docx.pdf.

24. Royal College of Pathologists. Guidelines on staffing and workload for histopathology and cytopathology departments [Internet]. 4th ed. London (UK): Royal College of Pathologists; 2015 September. Available from https://www.rcpath.org/uploads/assets/aaae5525-894f-472c-ae2dfa281829e3d1/g107_guidelinesstaffingworkload_sep15.pdf.

25. Canadian Association of Pathologists — Association canadienne des pathologistes. The Canadian Association of Pathologists workload model [Internet]. Kingston (ON): Canadian Association of Pathologists; 2018 [updated 2020 July 15; cited 2022 August 11]. Available from https://www.cap-acp.org/cmsUploads/CAP/File/CAP-ACP%20Workload%20AP%20HP%20Model%20%2020200801.pdf.

26. Path2Quality. Work2Quality: guidelines for workload measurement in pathology professional practices [Internet]. Version 1.2. Path2Quality; 2012 September 6. Available from https://www.cap-acp.org.

27. Duggan MA, Goswami R, Magliocco AM, et al; Canadian Association of Pathologists — (Association canadienne des pathologistes) Working Group. Guidelines for the review of pathology in the research context. Surgery. 2013;154(1):111–15. PMID: 23499018. doi: 10.1016/j.surg.2013.02.009

28. Canadian Association of Pathologists — Association canadienne des pathologistes. Canadian Association of Pathologists' (CAP-ACP) guidelines for the investigation of alleged irregularities in surgical pathology practice [Internet]. Kingston (ON): Canadian Association of Pathologists: 2011 January 12 [cited 2022 August 11]. Available from https://cap-acp.org/cmsUploads/CAP/File/Investigation%20of%20Lab%20Med%20Irregularities%20Final%20-%20Revised20141030.pdf.

Contributors to the Third Edition

Huda Alghefari MD, FRCPC
Department of Pathology and Laboratory Medicine
Western University
London, Ontario, Canada

Basma M. AlYamany, MBBS
Neuropathology Fellow
University of Western Ontario
London, Ontario, Canada

Sylvia L. Asa, MD, PhD, FRCPC, FCAP, FRCPath (Hon)
Professor of Pathology
Case Western Reserve University
University Hospitals Cleveland Medical Center
Cleveland, Ohio, USA

Manon Auger, MDCM (McG), FRCP(C)
Professor
Department of Pathology
McGill University
Montreal, Quebec, Canada

Penny J. Barnes, MD, FRCP(C)
Professor
Department of Pathology
Dalhousie University
Halifax, Nova Scotia, Canada

Martin Bullock, MD, FRCPC
Professor
Departments of Pathology and Surgery
Dalhousie University
Head and Neck Pathologist
Queen Elizabeth II Health Sciences Centre
Halifax, Nova Scotia, Canada

Sophie Camilleri-Broët, MD, PhD (Paris)
Associate Professor
Department of Pathology
McGill University
Montreal, Quebec, Canada

Elaine S. Chan
Clinical Assistant Professor
Department of Pathology and Laboratory Medicine
Alberta Children's Hospital
University of Calgary
Calgary, Alberta, Canada

Ivan Chebib, MD, FRCPC
Director of Cytopathology, Massachusetts General Hospital
Assistant Professor of Pathology, Harvard Medical School
Boston, Massachusetts, USA

Elizaveta Chernetsova, MD, FRCPC
Staff Pathologist (gastrointestinal and liver pathology)
Ottawa Hospital
Ottawa, Ontario, Canada

Gertruda Evaristo, MD
Resident Physician
Department of Pathology
McGill University
Montreal, Quebec, Canada

Emily R. Filter, BScN, MD, FRCPC, DRCPSC
Assistant Professor
Department of Pathology
Dalhousie University, QEII Health Sciences Centre
Halifax, Nova Scotia, Canada

Yuan Gao, MD, FRCPC
Assistant Clinical Professor
Department of Pathology and Laboratory Medicine
University of Alberta
Edmonton, Alberta, Canada

Zu-hua Gao, MD, PhD, FRCPC, FCAHS
Professor and Head
Department of Pathology and Laboratory Medicine
University of British Columbia
Vancouver, British Columbia, Canada

Laurette Geldenhuys, MBBCH, FFPATH, MMED, FRCPC, MAEd, FCAP
Professor
Department of Pathology and Medicine
Dalhousie University
Halifax, Nova Scotia, Canada

Guangming Han, MD, FRCPC
Clinical Associate Professor
Department of Pathology and Laboratory Medicine
University of British Columbia
Vancouver, British Columbia, Canada

Jeffrey T. Joseph, MD, PhD
Professor
Departments of Pathology and Laboratory Medicine, and Clinical Neurosciences
Foothills Medical Centre
Calgary, Alberta, Canada

Yonca Kanber, MD (Turkey), FRCPC
Associate Professor
Department of Pathology
McGill University
Montreal, Quebec, Canada

Jason Karamchandani, MD (Stanford)
Associate Professor
Department of Pathology
McGill University
Montreal, Quebec, Canada

Moosa Khalil, MBBCh, FRCPC, FCAP
Clinical Associate Professor
Department of Pathology and Laboratory Medicine, University of Calgary
Alberta Precision Laboratories
Calgary, Alberta, Canada

Lik Hang Lee, MD, FRCPC
Clinical Assistant Professor
St. Paul's Hospital
Department of Pathology and Laboratory Medicine
University of British Columbia
Vancouver, British Columbia, Canada

Thai Yen Ly, MD, FRCPC
Assistant Professor
Department of Pathology
Dalhousie University
Halifax, Nova Scotia, Canada

Jennifer Merrimen, MD, FRCPC
Associate Professor
Departments of Pathology and Urology
Dalhousie University
Halifax, Nova Scotia, Canada

Ann Marie Nelson, MD
Pathologist
InPaLa Consulting
Washington, DC, USA

Tuyet Nhung Ton Nu, MSc, MD, FRCPC
Assistant Professor
Department of Pathology
McGill University
Montreal, Quebec, Canada

Sylvia Pasternak, MD, FRCPC
Associate Professor
Department of Pathology
Division of Clinical Dermatology and Cutaneous Science
Dalhousie University
Halifax, Nova Scotia, Canada

Bibianna Purgina, MD, FRCPC
Pathologist and Associate Professor
Department of Pathology and Laboratory Medicine
University of Ottawa
Ottawa, Ontario, Canada

Simon F. Roy, MD
Clinical Fellow
Department of Dermatology
Yale School of Medicine
New Haven, Connecticut, USA

Meer-Taher Shabani-Rad, MD, FRCPC
Clinical Associate Professor
Department of Pathology and Laboratory Medicine
University of Calgary
Calgary, Alberta, Canada

Thomas Shi, MD, FRCPC, DABP
Pathologist
Dr. Everett Chalmers Hospital
Horizon Health NB
Fredericton, New Brunswick, Canada

Vincent Quoc-Huy Trinh, MD, MSc, FRCPC
Clinical Fellow and Research Instructor
Clinical Assistant Professor
Department of Pathology and Cellular Biology
Université de Montréal
Montreal, Quebec, Canada

John P. Veinot, MD, FRCPC
Professor
Department of Pathology and Laboratory Medicine
University of Ottawa
Ottawa, Ontario, Canada

Jennifer Vuong, MD, MSc, FRCPC
Clinical Assistant Professor
Department of Pathology and Laboratory Medicine
University of Calgary
Calgary, Alberta, Canada

Alfredo E. Walker, MB.BS, FRCPath, DMJ (Path), MFFLM, MCSFS
Assistant Professor, Vice Chair, and Director of Education, Department of Pathology and Laboratory Medicine, Faculty of Medicine, University of Ottawa
Forensic Pathologist/Coroner, Eastern Ontario Regional Forensic Pathology Unit, Ottawa Hospital General Campus
Ottawa, Ontario, Canada

Noreen M. Walsh, MD, FRCPC, FRCPath (UK)
Professor
Department of Pathology, Division of Clinical Dermatology and Cutaneous Science
Dalhousie University
Halifax, Nova Scotia, Canada

Cheng Wang, MD, FRCPC
Associate Professor
Department of Pathology and Urology
Dalhousie University
Halifax, Nova Scotia, Canada

Yinong Wang, MD, FACP
Clinical Associate Professor, Department of Pathology and Laboratory Medicine, University of Calgary
Alberta Precision Laboratories
Calgary, Alberta, Canada

James R. Wright, Jr, MD, PhD
Professor
Department of Pathology & Laboratory Medicine
Alberta Children's Hospital
University of Calgary
Calgary, Alberta, Canada

Zhaolin Xu, MD, FRCPC, FCAP
Professor
Department of Pathology
Queen Elizabeth II Health Sciences Centre
Dalhousie University
Halifax, Nova Scotia, Canada

Hua Yang, MD, FRCPC
Clinical Associate Professor
Department of Pathology and Laboratory Medicine
University of Calgary
Calgary, Alberta, Canada

Weiming Yu, MD, FRCPC
Clinical Associate Professor
Department of Pathology and Laboratory Medicine
Alberta Children's Hospital
University of Calgary
Calgary, Alberta, Canada

Image Index

parenchyma, 909
respiratory syncytial virus infection, 682
tuberculosis, 684
lung adenocarcinoma, 900–903, 905
lung FNA specimens, 231–234
lymphadenitis, 637, 638, 639
lymphangioleiomyomatosis, 913
lymph node
histiocytic necrotizing lymphadenitis, 639
histiocytic proliferation, 651
HIV, 641, 682
Kaposi sarcoma, 641
metastases, 148
mixed hyperplasia, 637
pathology, 627–653
radioactive seed-labeled (axillary), 149
lymph node (axillary) FNA specimens, 241
lymph node (mediastinal) FNA specimen, diffuse
large B-cell lymphoma, 242
lymph node (neck) FNA specimens, 241
lymphomatoid papulosis, 648
lymphomatoid polyposis, 642
lymphophagocytosis (emperipolesis), 651
lymphoplasmacytic lymphoma, 643

M

macrocytic red cells, 627
malaria infections, 689, 811
malignant melanotic nerve sheath tumor, 818
malignant peripheral nerve sheath tumor
(MPNST), 106
mammary analog secretory carcinoma (now
called secretory carcinoma), 578
mantle cell lymphoma (MCL), 641, 642
manual strangulation, 346, 364
Marfan syndrome, 193
marginal zone lymphoma, 298, 425, 642, 643,
646
Masson tumor (intravascular papillary
endothelial hyperplasia), 195
mastitis, 153, 154
mastoid ecchymosis (battle sign), 362
mechanical heart valve prosthesis with
thrombosis, 178, 179, 199
Meckel diverticulum, 425, 855
medullary carcinoma, 482
thyroid, 239, 240, 310, 328
medulloblastoma, 816
megakaryocytic proliferation with giant variants,
631
melanoma
malignant, 289, 290
metastatic, 241, 819, 908
nasal, 581
primary CNS, 817
in situ, 289
vulvar, 548
melanosis coli, 426
Ménétrier disease, 419
meningioangiomatosis, 816
meningioma, 816
meningitis, 683, 810
Merkel cell carcinoma, 296, 297
mesenteric artery ostia, 189
mesenteric gliomatosis, 436
mesoblastic nephroma, 857
mesothelioma

arising from the tunica vaginalis, 495
epithelioid, 236
malignant, 495, 548, 901, 906
normal mesothelial cells, 235
metabolic acidosis, 341
metanephric adenoma, 476
metaplasia, 484, 497
metaplastic carcinoma, 146, 147
metastatic
appendiceal mucinous carcinoma, 155
breast carcinoma, 154, 819
calcification, 912
carcinoma, 184, 755
choriocarcinoma, 155
colonic adenocarcinoma, 298, 755
melanoma, 241, 819, 908
paraganglioma in cervical lymph node, 329
renal cell carcinoma to the palate, 592
signet-ring cell carcinoma to the ovary, 540
teratoma, 901
Meyenburg complex (bile duct hamartoma), 755
microcephaly, 853
microcystic adnexal carcinoma, 295
microcytic red cells, 627, 628
microglandular adenosis (MGA), 141
micronodular pneumocyte hyperplasia, 913
minute meningothelioid nodule, 914
mitral annular calcification, 178
mitral valve
in acute bacterial endocarditis, 180
with acute bacterial endocarditis, 180
with fungal infective endocarditis, 196
infective endocarditis perforated aneurysm,
199
myxomatous, 178
with nonbacterial thrombotic endocarditis
(marantic), 179
prolapse, 180
ruptured papillary muscle and, 181, 182, 183
mixed epithelial and stromal tumor, 476
mixed germ cell tumor of testis, 493, 494
mixed germ cell tumor with embryonal
carcinoma and teratoma, 494
mixed hyperplastic-adenomatous polyp, 431
molluscum contagiosum, 299, 548, 683
Monckeberg medial calcinosis, 196
Mongolian spot, 367
monochorionic diamnionic, 850
monocytoid hyperplasia, 641
morphea, 153, 280, 281
mucinous micropapillary carcinoma, 146
mucoepidermoid carcinoma, 240, 576
Mucor infection, 686
mucormycosis, 232, 473, 812
mucosa associated lymphoid tissue (MALT)
lymphoepithelial lesion in, 418
lymphoma, 154, 421, 907
mucosa associated T-cell lymphoma, 425
mucosa ulcer with raised edges, 432
mucosal erosion-stress ulcer, 417
mucous membrane pemphigoid, 591
multiple endocrine neoplasia type 1, 764
multiple sclerosis, 812, 813
mummification and skeletonization, 357
muscular artery with intima, media, and
adventitia, 192
mycobacterial infection, 423, 916

Mycobacterium avium-intracellulare complex
(MAI) infection, 684
Mycobacterium tuberculosis, in liver, 684, 744
mycosis fungoides, 297
mycotic bacterial aneurysm, 194
myelodysplastic syndrome (MDS), 632
myelomeningocele, 807, 853
myocardial contraction bands, 186
myocardial infarction, 159, 181–183
acute, 338
of the posterior wall of the left ventricle, 349
ruptured myocardial free wall, 358
myocarditis, 183, 187
myocardium with atheroembolic debris, 187
myofibrillar myopathy, 820
myofibroblastoma, 152
myofibroma, 103
myopericytoma, 103
myxofibrosarcoma, 109
myxoma, 107, 153, 185, 198
myxomatous mitral valve, 178

N

Naegleria fowleri, 811
nasal type hemangiopericytoma, 583
nasopharyngeal angiofibroma, 583
nasopharyngeal carcinoma, undifferentiated
type, 587
neck and head pathology, 572–593
necrobiosis lipoidica, 281
necrosis
acute tubular, 475
adenoid cystic carcinoma, solid pattern with
comedo-like necrosis, 577
avascular, 110
caseous pericardial, 184
coagulative, 740
fat, 97
gangrenous, 192
kidney papillary, 474
liver with submassive necrosis, 739
myocardial infarct with transmural necrosis
and free wall rupture, 182
perivenular hepatocyte necrosis, 747
segmental necrotizing arteritis with fibrinoid
necrosis, 194
squamous cell carcinoma with central
necrosis and cavitation, 901
necrotizing arteritis, segmental, 194
Neisseria gonorrhea salpingitis, 683
nematodes *Capillaria philippinensis,* 422
neoplasia
germ cell neoplasia in situ, 491
intraepithelial, 498, 542, 548, 762
multiple endocrine neoplasia type 1, 764
neuroendocrine, 764
nephrogenic metaplasia, 484
neuroblastoma, 857
adrenal, 318
olfactory, 579
neurocysticercosis, 812
neuroendocrine hyperplasia and neoplasia, 764
neuroendocrine tumor
appendiceal well-differentiated, 435
gastric, 421
ileal, 331
pancreatic, 243, 764
primary, 147
rectal well-differentiated, 433